プロメテウス
解剖学コア アトラス
PROMETHEUS
Atlas of Anatomy

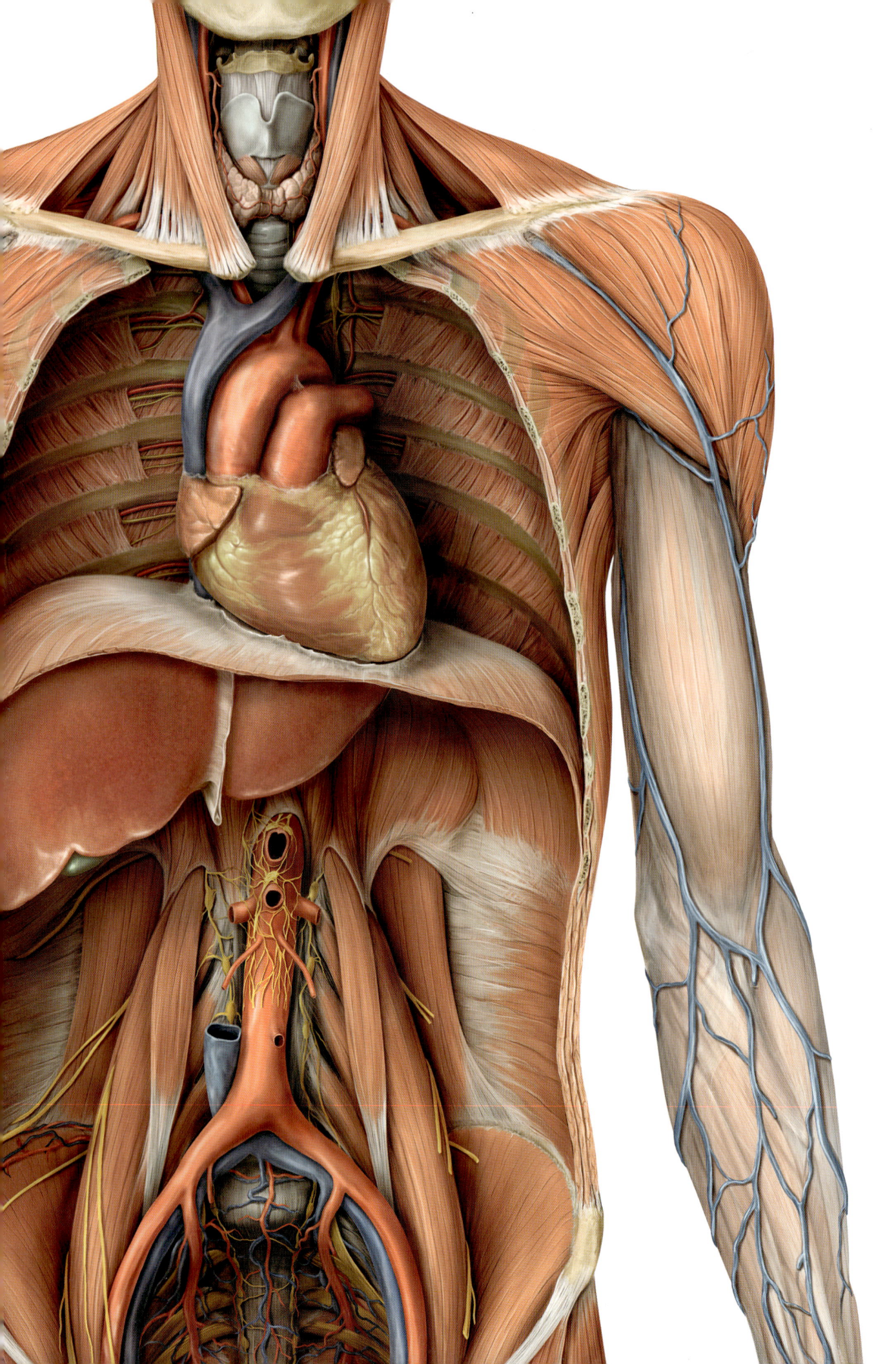

PROMETHEUS
Atlas of Anatomy

Edited by
Anne M. Gilroy
Brian R. MacPherson
Lawrence M. Ross

Based on the work of
Michael Schünke
Erik Schulte
Udo Schumacher

Illustrations by
Markus Voll
Karl Wesker

Thieme
Stuttgart・New York

プロメテウス
解剖学コア アトラス

監訳
坂井 建雄　　順天堂大学医学部　教授

訳
市村 浩一郎　順天堂大学医学部
澤井 直　　　順天堂大学医学部

医学書院

著者

Anne M.Gilroy
University of Massachusetts, Worcester, MA

Brian R.MacPherson
University of Kentucky Medical School, Lexington, KY

Lawrence M.Ross
University of Texas Medical School at Houston

執筆協力

Michael Schünke
Erik Schulte
Udo Schumacher

イラスト

Markus Voll
Karl Wesker

注意

医学は常に発展途上にあって進歩し続けている科学分野です．人類の医学知識はたゆまぬ研究と臨床経験によって現在も成長を続けており，とくに治療や薬物療法に関しては，その質・量ともに日々高まっています．本書で採用した用量や投薬方法の記述に関しては，著者および発行者ともに，制作時点での水準に照らして最新の内容となるように最大限の配慮を施しています．

しかしながら，本書における各種薬剤の用量や投薬方法に関する記載は，臨床上の投薬や用量に対して保証や責任を負うものではありません．服用あるいは投薬する際には，薬剤に添付されている使用上の注意を読んで注意深く検討する必要があります．また，服用量や服用スケジュールに関する本書と添付文書との相違に関しては，必要に応じて医師や専門家にお問い合わせください．このような対応は，使用頻度の少ない薬剤や新規に導入された医薬品でとくに大切で，服用量や服用スケジュールについては，使用者が自己責任のもとに設定しなければなりません．

Authorized translation of the First original English language edition
"Atlas of Anatomy", by Anne M. Gilroy/Brian R. MacPherson/Lawrence M. Ross,
based on the work of Michael Schünke, Erik Schulte, and Udo Schumacher,
illustrations by Markus Voll and Karl Wesker

Copyright © of the original English language edition 2008 by
Thieme Medical Publishers, Inc., New York, USA.
© First Japanese edition 2010 by Igaku-Shoin Ltd., Tokyo
Printed and bound in Japan.

プロメテウス解剖学コア アトラス

発　行　2010年6月1日　第1版第1刷
　　　　2012年8月1日　第1版第2刷
監訳者　坂井建雄（さかい たつお）
発行者　株式会社　医学書院
　　　　代表取締役　金原　優
　　　　〒113-8719　東京都文京区本郷1-28-23
　　　　電話 03-3817-5600（社内案内）
印刷・製本　三美印刷

本書の複製権・翻訳権・上映権・譲渡権・公衆送信権（送信可能化権を含む）は㈱医学書院が保有します．

ISBN978-4-260-00746-7

本書を無断で複製する行為（複写，スキャン，デジタルデータ化など）は，「私的使用のための複製」など著作権法上の限られた例外を除き禁じられています．大学，病院，診療所，企業などにおいて，業務上使用する目的（診療，研究活動を含む）で上記の行為を行うことは，その使用範囲が内部的であっても，私的使用には該当せず，違法です．また私的使用に該当する場合であっても，代行業者等の第三者に依頼して上記の行為を行うことは違法となります．

JCOPY〈㈳出版者著作権管理機構　委託出版物〉

本書の無断複写は著作権法上での例外を除き禁じられています．複写される場合は，そのつど事前に，㈳出版者著作権管理機構（電話03-3513-6969，FAX 03-3513-6979，info@jcopy.or.jp）の許諾を得てください．

訳者序

　21世紀に入って，人間の健康と生命をまもる医療に対する社会からの期待と要求が高まっている．多くの若者が医師とそれに関連する職種をめざして，医学の専門的な知識と技術を学んでいる．人体の構造と機能について知る解剖学は，医学を学ぶための最重要の基礎であり，その教材に対するニーズもますます高まっている．人体の構造そのものが大きく変化するわけではないが，コンピューターによる画像処理や情報技術の発展，さらに画像診断技術の普及を背景に，解剖学の教材も大きく進化し，印象的で理解しやすいものが数多く登場している．その中でも，2005年にドイツで出版された『プロメテウス解剖学アトラス』全3冊は，高品質の解剖図と洗練された編集により，圧倒的な迫力と内容をもつ新しい時代の解剖学教材として世界的に高い評価を得てきた．その日本語訳も好評を博し，数多くの読者に迎えられた．

　本書『プロメテウス解剖学コア アトラス』は，このプロメテウスのドイツ語版をもとに，アメリカで新たに編集された1冊本の解剖学アトラスの日本語訳である．3冊本のプロメテウスに掲載された高品質の解剖図を生かしながら，人体解剖実習での使いやすさを重視して全体の構成を部位別に改め，頁の構成を見開きの形にまとめてある．さらに，理解を助けるための概念的な模式図や，要約の表を多数付け加えて，コンパクトでわかりやすいまったく新たな解剖学教材を実現したものである．アトラスと銘打ってはいるが，解剖図だけを配した従来の解剖アトラスの域をはるかに超えて，これ一冊で解剖学の学習を可能にする統合的な教材となっている．

　翻訳にあたっては，若手の優秀な解剖学者である市村と澤井が日本語訳の作業を行い，坂井が全体に目を通して監訳を担当した．とくに3冊本の『プロメテウス解剖学アトラス』および解剖学用語との内容および用語の整合性に配慮した．日本語訳にあたっては瑕疵がないように細心の注意をしたつもりではあるが，至らぬところは監訳者の責である．

　本書『プロメテウス解剖学コア アトラス』が，多くの学生たちに行き渡り，よりよい医療者となるべくその基礎となる解剖学の学習に役立てていただけることを願うものである．

坂井建雄

2009年12月1日
八王子の寓居にて

まえがき

　本書の著者らはそれぞれ，Michael Schünke, Erik Schulte, Udo Schumacher による『プロメテウス解剖学アトラス』のために創られた解剖図の傑出した詳細さ精確さ美麗さに，驚嘆し感銘を受けた．これらの図は，過去50年間において解剖学教育に付け加えられた最も意義あるものと感じ，好奇心と情熱のある健康科学の学生向けに簡潔な1冊の解剖学アトラスを創ろうと取り組む際の礎として，これらの卓抜なイラストを使おうと決めた．

　われわれが最初に取り組んだのは，この膨大な図版の集成から，現在の解剖実習において最も教育的で実例となるものを選び出すことであった．しかしながら，1冊の解剖アトラスを創り上げることは，単に図を選び出す以上のことであると，われわれは理解するようになった．すなわち，それぞれの図は大量の細部まで伝える一方，強調と指示文字は清潔で落ち着いたものでなければならない．そのため数百の解剖図を新たに描いたり修正したりして，この新しい解剖アトラスに相応しいものにした．さらに，必要に応じて重要な模式図や単純化して要約した表を付け加えた．また数十の関連する医用画像と関連する重要な臨床事項を，適切な場所に加えた．また体表解剖図には質問を付して，診察において最重要の解剖学的事項に学生の注意を向けるようにした．これらの主要事項の要点は部位ごとに配置して，解剖実習において使いやすいようにした．それぞれの部位の中で，さまざまな要素を系統的に吟味し，それに続いて部位の中で局所的な画像を器官系と結びつけるようにした．このすべてにおいて，解剖学的構造について臨床的な視点をとった．この本の特色である見開き構成によって，読者の目は探求する領域・話題に引きつけられる．

　これらの努力は，明晰で情熱ある学生たちに解剖学という学問を教える百年近い歳月の成果であり，ここから包括的で使いやすい教材かつ参考書が生み出されることを願うものである．

　われわれはThieme社の人たちによる専門的な支援に感謝したい．Cathrin E. Schulz, M. D.（編集主幹，教育編集部）は丁重に締切を想い出させてくれ，問題の解決にいつでもつきあってくれた．このことに感謝しすぎることはない．さらに重要なのは，彼女がわれわれを励まし，支援し，敬意を表してくれたことである．

　とくに感謝したい人として，Bridget Queenan（企画編集者）は，情報の可視化と直感的な流れに飛び抜けた才能をもち，原稿を編集し発展させてくれた．彼女が，この間に多くの細部を受け取り，図版と指示文字の変更の要求にいつも我慢強く対応してくれたことにとくに感謝する．

　最大の感謝を捧げる人として，Elsie Starbecker（上席制作編集者）は，2,200を超える図版をもつこのアトラスを，細心の注意をもって迅速に制作してくれた．最後に，校正の段階でチームに加わってくれた，Rebecca McTavish（企画編集者）にも感謝したい．かれらの勤勉な仕事が，この解剖学アトラスを実現したのである．

Anne M. Gilroy
Brian R. MacPherson
Lawrence M. Ross

2008年3月
Worcester, MA, Lexington, KY, Houston, TX

献辞

　父のFrancis Gilroyは医学に献身し，そのことは父が思っていた以上に私を励ましてくれた．私の学生たちは，人体解剖に対する私の情熱を優しく受け容れ，ときにはその情熱を分かち合ってくれた．そして誰よりも私の息子達であるColinとBryanの愛情と援助を何よりも大切に覚えている．

　私の友人であり指導者のDr. Ken McFadden（アルベルタ大学解剖学部門）は，私が成功するために必要な人体解剖教育の修練を受けることを保証してくれた．過去30年間に私が教えた何千人もの専門課程の学生たちに対してこの技術を磨いた．学問において私が享受した成功は，妻のCynthia Longの絶えざる援助，関与，励ましなしにはあり得なかった．

　私の妻のIreneに，子どもたちのChip，Jennifer，JocelynとBarryに，Tricia，Scott，KatieとSnapperに，Treyに，また私に教えてくれた学生たちにも本書を捧げる．

謝辞

　ドイツにおいて権威ある賞に輝いた解剖学シリーズの原著者であるMichael Schünke，Erik Schulte，Udo Schumacher各氏の長年にわたる仕事に感謝する．

　アドヴァイザリー委員会の人たちの寄与に心から感謝する．

- Bruce M. Carlson, MD, PhD
  University of Michigan, Ann Arbor, Michigan
- Derek Bryant（Class of 2011）
  University of Toronto Medical School, Burlington, Ontario
- Peter Cole, MD
  Glamorum Healing Centre, Orangeville, Ontario
- Michael Droller, MD
  The Mount Sinai Medical Center, New York, New York
- Anthony Firth, PhD
  Imperial College London, London
- Mark H. Hankin, PhD
  University of Toledo, College of Medicine, Toledo, Ohio
- Katharine Hudson（Class of 2010）
  McGill Medical School, Montreal, Quebec
- Christopher Lee（Class of 2010）
  Harvard Medical School, Cambridge, Massachusetts
- Francis Liuzzi, PhD
  Lake Erie College of Osteopathic Medicine, Bradenton, Florida
- Graham Louw, PhD
  University of Cape Town Medical School, University of Cape Town
- Estomih Mtui, MD
  Weill Cornell Medical College, New York, New York
- Srinivas Murthy, MD
  Harvard Medical School, Boston, Massachusetts
- Jeff Rihn, MD
  The Rothman Institute, Philadelphia, Pennsylvania
- Lawrence Rizzolo, PhD
  Yale University, New Haven, Connecticut
- Mikel Snow, PhD
  University of Southern California, Los Angeles, California
- Kelly Wright（Class of 2010）
  Wayne State University School of Medicine, Detroit, Michigan

序 言

　この解剖学アトラスは，これまで作られた1巻本の人体解剖図譜の中で最も素晴らしいものであると私は思う．これには2つの要素がある．図とその構成の方法である．

　画家のMarkus VollとKarl Weskerは，解剖図の洗練の新しい標準を作り上げた．洗練された半透明の使用と，光と陰の繊細な表現により，読者はあらゆる構造を精確に3次元的に理解することができる．

　著者らは，図の配置を工夫して，学生が人体のイメージを明確に頭の中に作り上げるのに必要な情報の流れを与えている．見開きのそれぞれの頁には，必要な教材が揃っており，経験深く思慮深い教師の手腕をさりげなく見せている．私自身，学生の頃にこの本を使いたかったものだ．それができる今の学生たちをうらやましく思う．

Robert B. Acland

2008年3月
Louisville, KY

目 次

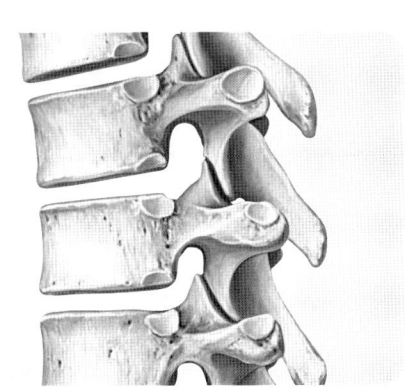

背 部

1．骨，靱帯，関節

- 脊柱：概観 … 2
- 脊柱：構成要素 … 4
- 頸椎 … 6
- 胸椎と腰椎 … 8
- 仙骨と尾骨 … 10
- 椎間円板 … 12
- 脊柱の関節：概観 … 14
- 脊柱の関節：頭蓋との連結 … 16
- 脊柱の靱帯：概観，頸部脊柱 … 18
- 脊柱の靱帯：胸腰部脊柱 … 20

2．筋

- 背部の筋：概観 … 22
- 頸部脊柱の固有筋 … 24
- 固有背筋 … 26
- 個々の筋(1) … 28
- 個々の筋(2) … 30
- 個々の筋(3) … 32

3．神経，血管

- 背部の動脈と静脈 … 34
- 背部の神経 … 36
- 背部の神経と血管(局所解剖) … 38

4．体表解剖

- 体表解剖 … 40

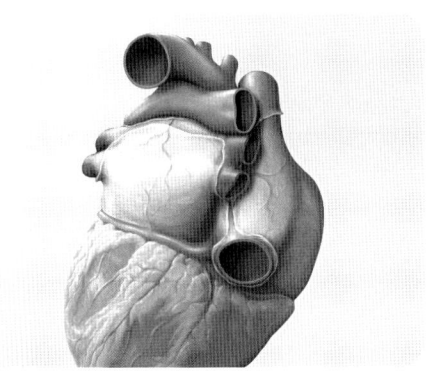

胸 部

5．胸壁

- 胸部の骨格 … 44
- 胸骨と肋骨 … 46
- 胸郭の関節 … 48
- 胸壁の筋 … 50
- 横隔膜 … 52
- 横隔膜の神経と血管 … 54
- 胸壁の動脈と静脈 … 56
- 胸壁の神経 … 58
- 胸壁の神経と血管の位置 … 60
- 女性の乳房 … 62
- 女性乳房のリンパ管 … 64

6．胸腔

- 胸腔の区分 … 66
- 胸腔の動脈 … 68
- 胸腔の静脈 … 70
- 胸腔のリンパ管 … 72
- 胸腔の神経 … 74

7．縦隔

- 縦隔：概観 … 76
- 縦隔の構造 … 78
- 胸腺と心膜 … 80
- 原位置の心臓 … 82
- 心臓：表面と部屋 … 84
- 心臓：弁 … 86
- 心臓の動脈と静脈 … 88
- 心臓の刺激伝導と神経支配 … 90
- 心臓：X線像 … 92
- 出生前・後の循環 … 94
- 食道 … 96
- 食道の神経と血管 … 98
- 縦隔のリンパ管 … 100

8. 胸膜腔
- 胸膜腔……102
- 原位置の肺……104
- 肺：X線像……106
- 肺の気管支肺区域……108
- 気管と気管支樹……110
- 呼吸機構……112
- 肺動脈と肺静脈……114
- 気管気管支樹の神経と血管……116
- 胸膜腔のリンパ管……118

9. 体表解剖
- 体表解剖……120

腹部・骨盤

10. 骨，靱帯，関節
- 下肢帯……124
- 男性骨盤と女性骨盤……126
- 骨盤の靱帯……128

11. 腹壁
- 腹壁の筋……130
- 鼠径部と鼠径管……132
- 腹壁と鼠径ヘルニア……134
- 会陰部……136
- 腹壁の筋……138
- 骨盤底の筋……140

12. 腹腔
- 腹腔・骨盤腔の区分……142
- 腹膜腔……144
- 網嚢……146
- 腸間膜と後壁……148
- 骨盤の内容……150
- 腹膜の位置関係……152
- 骨盤と会陰……154
- 水平断……156

13. 内臓
- 胃……158
- 十二指腸……160
- 空腸と回腸……162
- 盲腸，虫垂，結腸……164
- 直腸と肛門管……166
- 肝臓：概観……168
- 肝臓：肝区域と肝葉……170
- 胆嚢と胆管……172
- 膵臓と脾臓……174
- 腎臓と副腎：概観……176
- 腎臓と副腎：詳説……178
- 尿管……180
- 膀胱……182
- 膀胱と尿道……184

14. 生殖器
- 生殖器の概観……186
- 子宮と卵巣……188
- 腟……190
- 女性の外生殖器……192
- 女性生殖器の神経と血管……194
- 陰茎，陰嚢，精索……196
- 精巣と精巣上体……198
- 男性の付属生殖腺……200
- 男性生殖器の神経と血管……202
- 生殖器の発生……204

15. 動脈と静脈
- 腹部の動脈……206
- 腹大動脈と腎動脈……208
- 腹腔動脈……210
- 上腸間膜動脈と下腸間膜動脈……212
- 腹部の静脈……214
- 下大静脈と腎静脈……216
- 門脈……218
- 上腸間膜静脈と下腸間膜静脈……220
- 骨盤の動脈と静脈……222
- 直腸と生殖器の動脈と静脈……224

16. リンパ系
- 腹部と骨盤部のリンパ節……226
- 後腹壁のリンパ節……228
- 前腹部内臓のリンパ節……230
- 腸のリンパ節……232
- 生殖器のリンパ節……234

17. 神経系
- 自律神経叢……236
- 腹部内臓の神経支配……238
- 腸の神経支配……240
- 骨盤の神経支配……242
- 自律神経支配：概観……244
- 自律神経支配：泌尿器と生殖器……246

18. 体表解剖
- 体表解剖……248

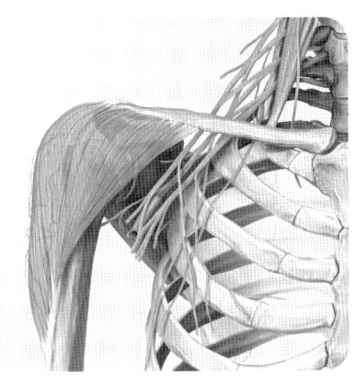

上肢

19．肩と上腕
上肢の骨 ···················· 252
鎖骨と肩甲骨 ···················· 254
上腕骨 ···················· 256
肩の関節 ···················· 258
肩の関節：肩関節（肩甲上腕関節） ···················· 260
肩峰下腔と肩峰下包 ···················· 262
肩と上腕の前面にある筋(1) ···················· 264
肩と上腕の前面にある筋(2) ···················· 266
肩と上腕の後面にある筋(1) ···················· 268
肩と上腕の後面にある筋(2) ···················· 270
個々の筋(1) ···················· 272
個々の筋(2) ···················· 274
個々の筋(3) ···················· 276
個々の筋(4) ···················· 278

20．肘と前腕
橈骨と尺骨 ···················· 280
肘関節 ···················· 282
肘関節の靱帯 ···················· 284
橈尺関節 ···················· 286
前腕の筋(1) ···················· 288
前腕の筋(2) ···················· 290
個々の筋(1) ···················· 292
個々の筋(2) ···················· 294
個々の筋(3) ···················· 296

21．手首と手
手首と手の骨 ···················· 298
手首と手の関節 ···················· 300
手首と手の靱帯 ···················· 302
指の靱帯 ···················· 304
手の筋：浅層と中間層 ···················· 306
手の筋：中間層と深層 ···················· 308
手背 ···················· 310
個々の筋(1) ···················· 312
個々の筋(2) ···················· 314

22．神経と脈管
上肢の動脈 ···················· 316
上肢の静脈とリンパ管 ···················· 318
腕神経叢とその枝 ···················· 320

腕神経叢の鎖骨上部からの枝，後神経束 ···················· 322
後神経束：橈骨神経と腋窩神経 ···················· 324
内側・外側神経束 ···················· 326
正中神経，尺骨神経 ···················· 328
上肢の皮静脈，皮神経 ···················· 330
肩と腋窩の後部 ···················· 332
肩の前面 ···················· 334
腋窩の局所解剖 ···················· 336
上腕と肘の局所解剖 ···················· 338
前腕の局所解剖 ···················· 340
手根の局所解剖 ···················· 342
手掌の局所解剖 ···················· 344
手背の局所解剖 ···················· 346
断面解剖 ···················· 348

23．体表解剖
体表解剖(1) ···················· 350
体表解剖(2) ···················· 352

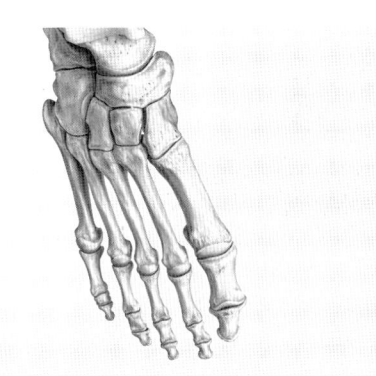

下肢

24．骨盤と大腿
下肢の骨 ···················· 356
下肢帯と寛骨 ···················· 358
大腿骨 ···················· 360
股関節：概観 ···················· 362
股関節：靱帯と関節包 ···················· 364
骨盤部と大腿の前面にある筋(1) ···················· 366
骨盤部と大腿の前面にある筋(2) ···················· 368
骨盤部と大腿の後面にある筋(1) ···················· 370
骨盤部と大腿の後面にある筋(2) ···················· 372
個々の筋(1) ···················· 374
個々の筋(2) ···················· 376
個々の筋(3) ···················· 378

25．膝と下腿
脛骨と腓骨 ···················· 380
膝関節：概観 ···················· 382
膝関節：靱帯，関節包，滑液包 ···················· 384
膝関節：靱帯と半月 ···················· 386
十字靱帯 ···················· 388
膝関節腔 ···················· 390
下腿の前面と外側面にある筋 ···················· 392

XIII

下腿の後面にある筋	394
個々の筋(1)	396
個々の筋(2)	398

26．足首と足

足の骨	400
足の関節(1)	402
足の関節(2)	404
足の関節(3)	406
足首と足の靱帯	408
土踏まずと足底弓	410
足底の筋	412
足の筋と腱鞘	414
個々の筋(1)	416
個々の筋(2)	418

27．神経と脈管

下肢の動脈	420
下肢の静脈とリンパ管	422
腰仙骨神経叢	424
腰神経叢の枝	426
腰神経叢の枝：閉鎖神経と大腿神経	428
仙骨神経叢の枝	430
仙骨神経叢の枝：坐骨神経	432
下肢の皮神経と皮静脈	434
鼠径部の局所解剖	436
殿部の局所解剖	438
大腿の前面と後面の局所解剖	440
下腿の後面と内側面の局所解剖	442
下腿の外側面と前面の局所解剖	444
足底の局所解剖	446
大腿と下腿の断面解剖	448

28．体表解剖

体表解剖	450

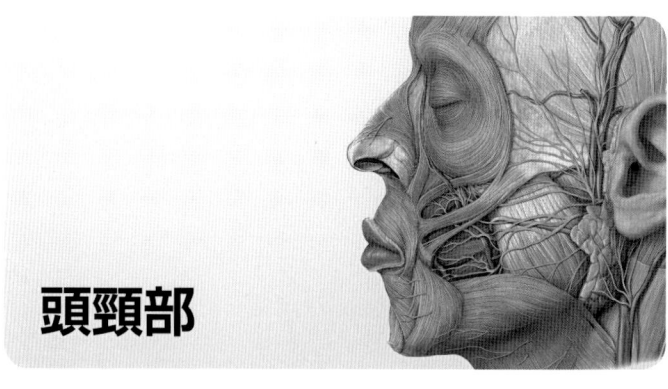

頭頸部

29．頭部の骨

頭蓋：側面と前面	454
頭蓋：後面と頭蓋冠	456
頭蓋底	458
篩骨と蝶形骨	460

30．頭部・顔面の筋

表情筋と咀嚼筋	462
頭部の筋，起始と停止	464
頭部の筋(1)	466
頭部の筋(2)	468

31．脳神経

脳神経の概観	470
脳神経：嗅神経(CN I)と視神経(CN II)	472
脳神経：動眼神経(CN III)，滑車神経(CN IV)，外転神経(CN VI)	474
脳神経：三叉神経(CN V)	476
脳神経：顔面神経(CN VII)	478
脳神経：内耳神経(CN VIII)	480
脳神経：舌咽神経(CN IX)	482
脳神経：迷走神経(CN X)	484
脳神経：副神経(CN XI)と舌下神経(CN XII)	486

32．頭部・顔面の神経と血管

顔面の神経支配	488
頭頸部の動脈	490
外頸動脈：前枝，内側枝，後枝	492
外頸動脈：終枝	494
頭頸部の静脈	496
顔面浅層の局所解剖	498
耳下腺咬筋部と側頭窩の局所解剖	500
側頭下窩の局所解剖	502
翼口蓋窩の局所解剖	504

33．眼窩と眼

眼窩の骨	506
眼窩の筋	508
眼窩の神経と血管	510

眼窩の局所解剖……………………………………………512
　眼窩と眼瞼…………………………………………………514
　眼球…………………………………………………………516
　角膜，虹彩，水晶体………………………………………518

34．鼻腔と鼻
　鼻腔の骨……………………………………………………520
　副鼻腔………………………………………………………522
　鼻腔の神経と血管…………………………………………524

35．側頭骨と耳
　側頭骨………………………………………………………526
　外耳と外耳道………………………………………………528
　中耳：鼓室…………………………………………………530
　中耳：耳小骨連鎖と鼓膜…………………………………532
　中耳：中耳の動脈…………………………………………534
　内耳…………………………………………………………536

36．口腔・咽頭
　口腔の骨……………………………………………………538
　顎関節………………………………………………………540
　歯……………………………………………………………542
　口腔の筋……………………………………………………544
　口腔の神経支配……………………………………………546
　舌……………………………………………………………548
　口腔と唾液腺の局所解剖…………………………………550
　扁桃と咽頭…………………………………………………552
　咽頭筋………………………………………………………554
　咽頭の神経と血管…………………………………………556

37．頸部
　頸部の骨と靱帯……………………………………………558
　頸部の筋肉（1）……………………………………………560
　頸部の筋肉（2）……………………………………………562
　頸部の筋肉（3）……………………………………………564
　頸部の動脈と静脈…………………………………………566
　頸部の神経支配……………………………………………568
　喉頭：軟骨と構造…………………………………………570
　喉頭：筋と区分……………………………………………572
　喉頭の神経と血管，甲状腺と副甲状腺（上皮小体）……574
　頸部の局所解剖：部位と筋膜……………………………576
　前頸部の局所解剖…………………………………………578
　前頸部と外側頸三角部の局所解剖………………………580
　外側頸三角部の局所解剖…………………………………582
　後頸部の局所解剖…………………………………………584
　頸部のリンパ管……………………………………………586

38．体表解剖
　体表解剖……………………………………………………588

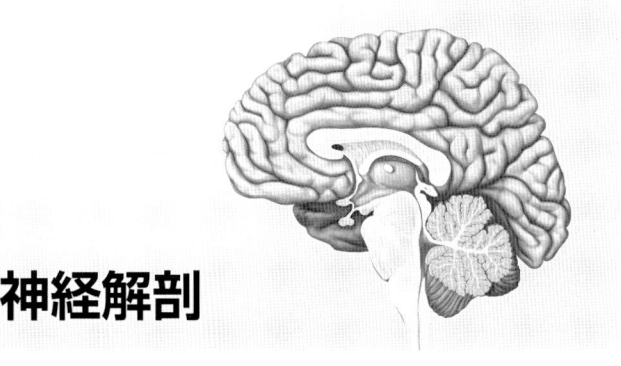

神経解剖

39．脳と脊髄
　神経系：概観………………………………………………592
　大脳…………………………………………………………594
　大脳と間脳…………………………………………………596
　間脳，脳幹，小脳…………………………………………598
　脊髄…………………………………………………………600
　髄膜…………………………………………………………602
　脳室と脳脊髄液の空間……………………………………604

40．脳と脊髄の血管
　硬膜静脈洞と脳の静脈……………………………………606
　脳の動脈……………………………………………………608
　脊髄の動脈と静脈…………………………………………610

41．機能系
　神経回路：概観……………………………………………612
　一般感覚と運動の伝導路…………………………………614
　特殊感覚の伝導路（1）……………………………………616
　特殊感覚の伝導路（2）……………………………………618
　特殊感覚の伝導路（3）……………………………………620

42．自律神経系
　自律神経系…………………………………………………622

付録

　体表解剖に関する問題の解答……………………………626
　英文索引……………………………………………………628
　和文索引……………………………………………………659

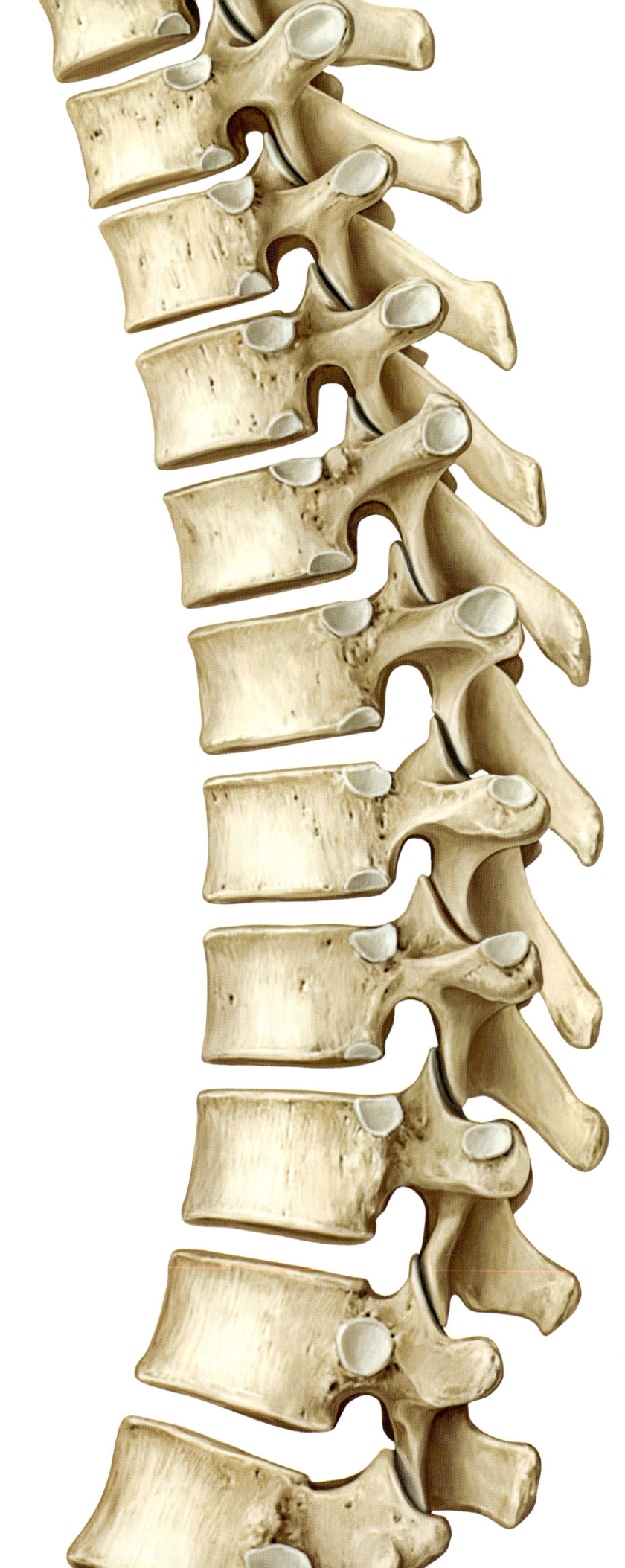

背部
Back

1. 骨，靱帯，関節
脊柱：概観 …………………………………………… 2
脊柱：構成要素 ……………………………………… 4
頸椎 …………………………………………………… 6
胸椎と腰椎 …………………………………………… 8
仙骨と尾骨 …………………………………………… 10
椎間円板 ……………………………………………… 12
脊柱の関節：概観 …………………………………… 14
脊柱の関節：頭蓋との連結 ………………………… 16
脊柱の靱帯：概観，頸部脊柱 ……………………… 18
脊柱の靱帯：胸腰部脊柱 …………………………… 20

2. 筋
背部の筋：概観 ……………………………………… 22
頸部脊柱の固有筋 …………………………………… 24
固有背筋 ……………………………………………… 26
個々の筋（1） ………………………………………… 28
個々の筋（2） ………………………………………… 30
個々の筋（3） ………………………………………… 32

3. 神経，血管
背部の動脈と静脈 …………………………………… 34
背部の神経 …………………………………………… 36
背部の神経と血管（局所解剖） ……………………… 38

4. 体表解剖
体表解剖 ……………………………………………… 40

脊柱：概観
Vertebral Column: Overview

脊柱は4つの領域（頸部，胸部，腰部，仙骨部）に区分される．脊柱の頸部と腰部は前方に弯曲し（前弯），胸部と仙骨部は後方に弯曲する（後弯）．

図1.1 脊柱
左外側方から見たところ．

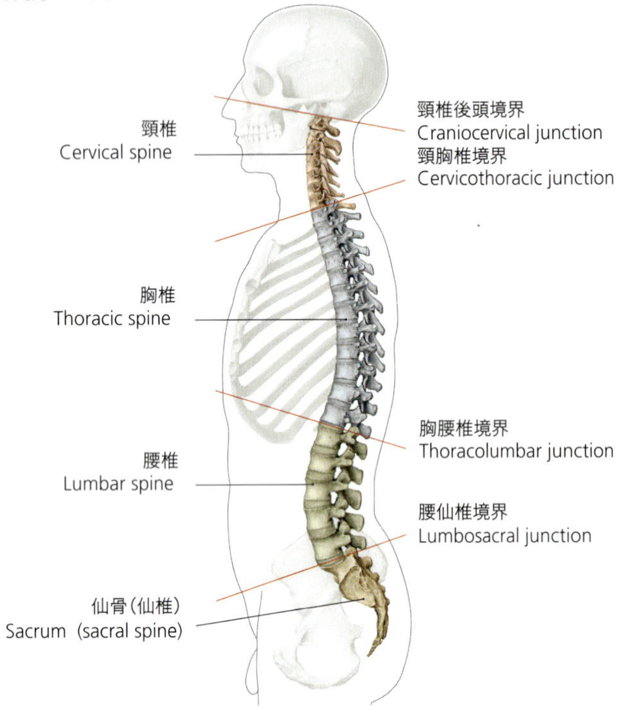

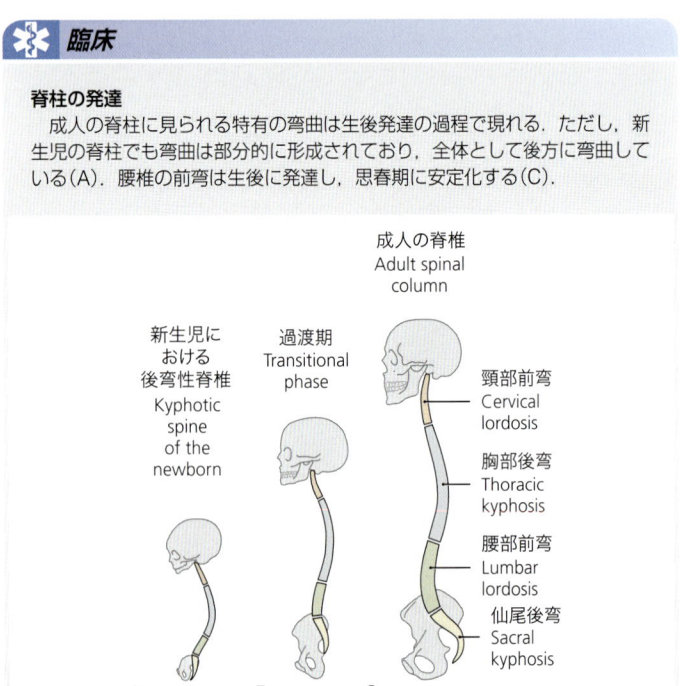

A 脊柱の4領域．

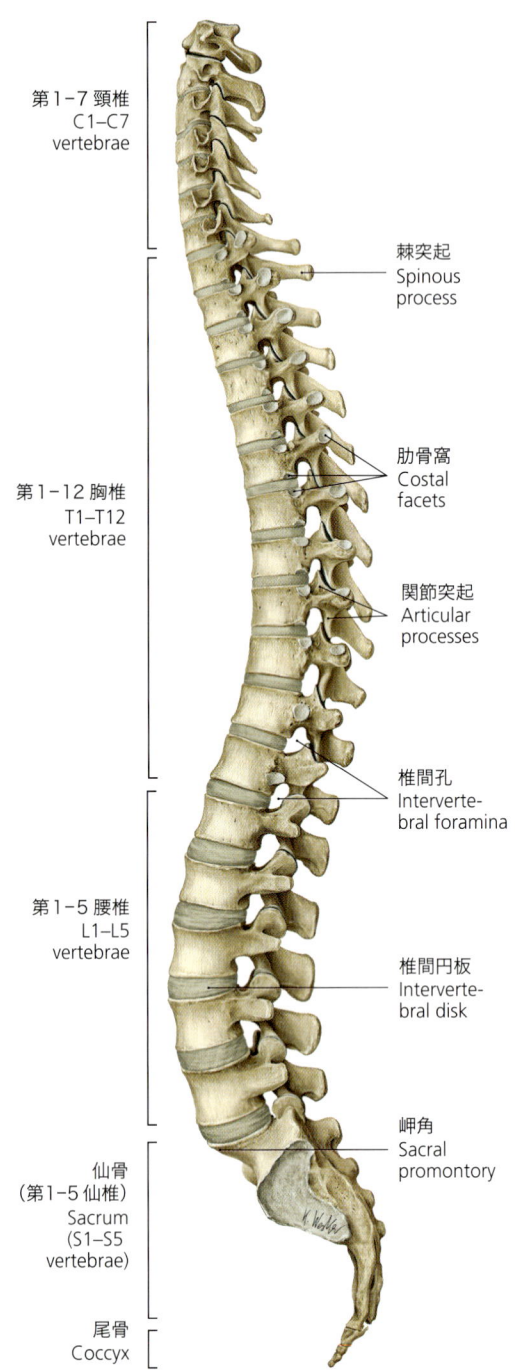

B 骨性脊柱（脊柱の骨・軟骨部分）．

臨床

脊柱の発達

成人の脊柱に見られる特有の弯曲は生後発達の過程で現れる．ただし，新生児の脊柱でも弯曲は部分的に形成されており，全体として後方に弯曲している（A）．腰椎の前弯は生後に発達し，思春期に安定化する（C）．

図1.2　脊柱の解剖学的正位置
左外側方から見たところ.

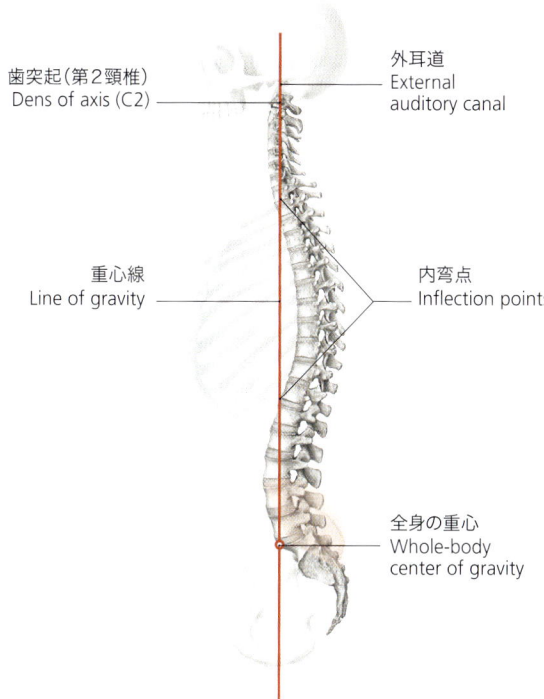

A 重心線．重心線は脊柱における特定の場所を通る．頸部と胸部，胸部と腰部の境界は脊柱の変曲点であり，重心線はこの2つの点を通る．重心線はさらに下方へ続き，重心（仙骨の岬角の前方）を通り，股関節，膝，踵へと連なる．

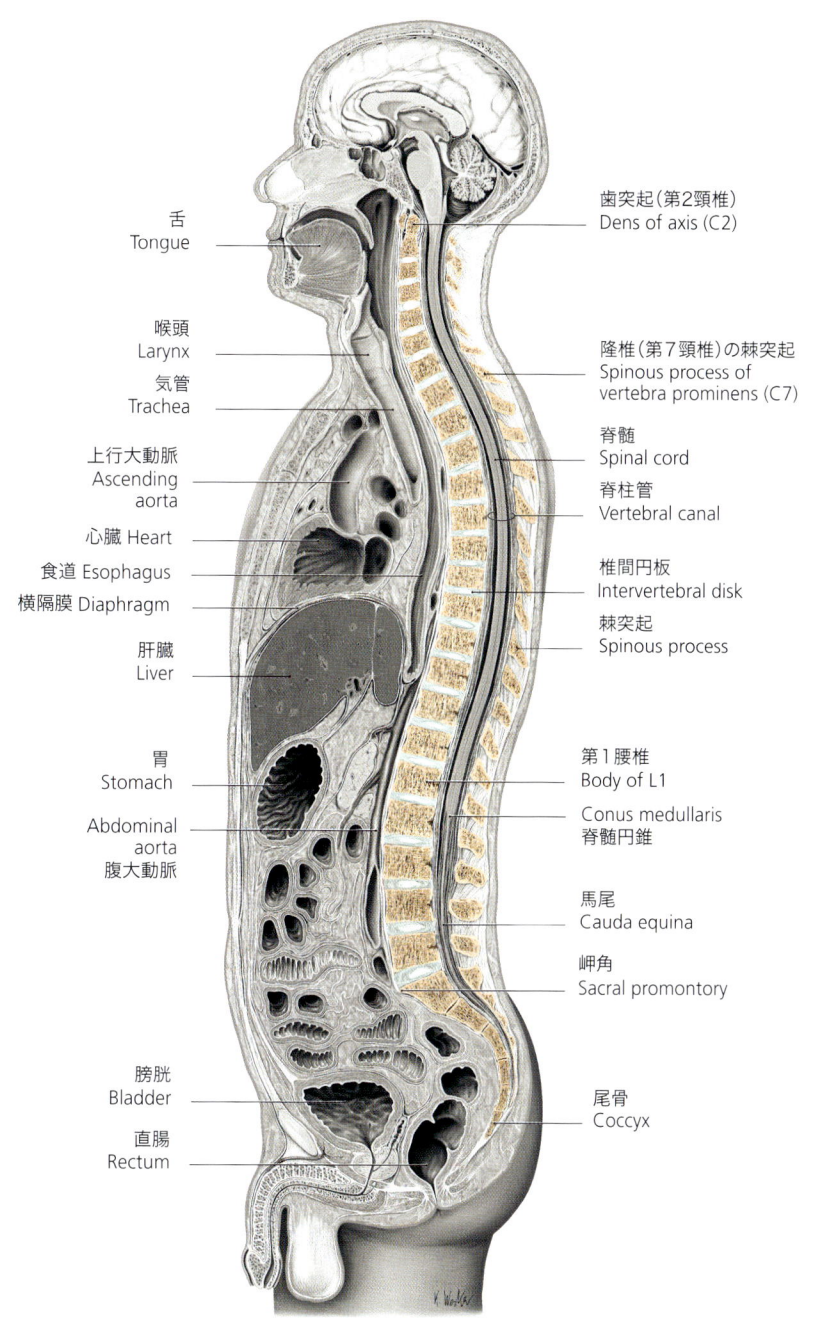

B 成人男性の正中矢状断面.

脊柱：構成要素
Vertebral Column: Elements

図1.3 脊柱を構成する骨

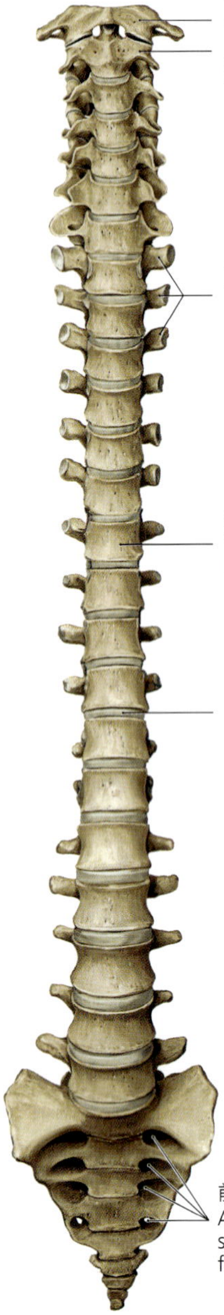

- 第1-7頸椎 C1—C7 vertebrae
  - 環椎（第1頸椎）Atlas (C1)
  - 軸椎（第2頸椎）Axis (C2)
- 第1-12胸椎 T1—T12 vertebrae
  - 横突起 Transverse process
  - 椎体 Vertebral body
  - 椎間円板 Intervertebral disk
- 第1-5腰椎 L1—L5 vertebrae
- 仙骨（癒合した第1-5仙椎）Sacrum (fused S1—S5 vertebrae)
  - 前仙骨孔 Anterior sacral foramina
- 尾骨 Coccyx

A 前方から見たところ．

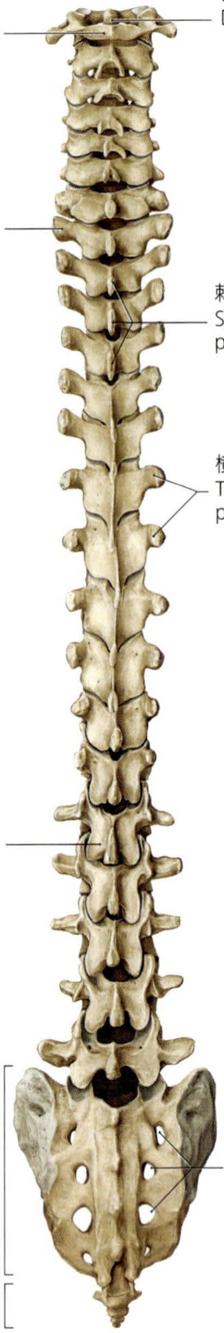

- 環椎（第1頸椎）Atlas (C1)
- 歯突起（第2頸椎）Dens of axis (C2)
- 隆椎（第7頸椎）Vertebra prominens (C7)
- 棘突起 Spinous processes
- 横突起 Transverse processes
- 第1腰椎 L1
- 仙骨 Sacrum
  - 後仙骨孔 Posterior sacral foramina
- 尾骨 Coccyx

B 後方から見たところ．

図1.4 目印として役立つ棘突起

後方から見たところ．これらの触知しやすい棘突起は理学的診察を行ううえで重要な目印となる．

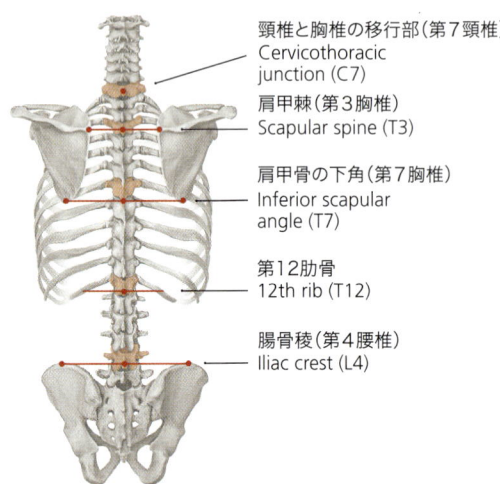

- 頸椎と胸椎の移行部（第7頸椎）Cervicothoracic junction (C7)
- 肩甲棘（第3胸椎）Scapular spine (T3)
- 肩甲骨の下角（第7胸椎）Inferior scapular angle (T7)
- 第12肋骨 12th rib (T12)
- 腸骨稜（第4腰椎）Iliac crest (L4)

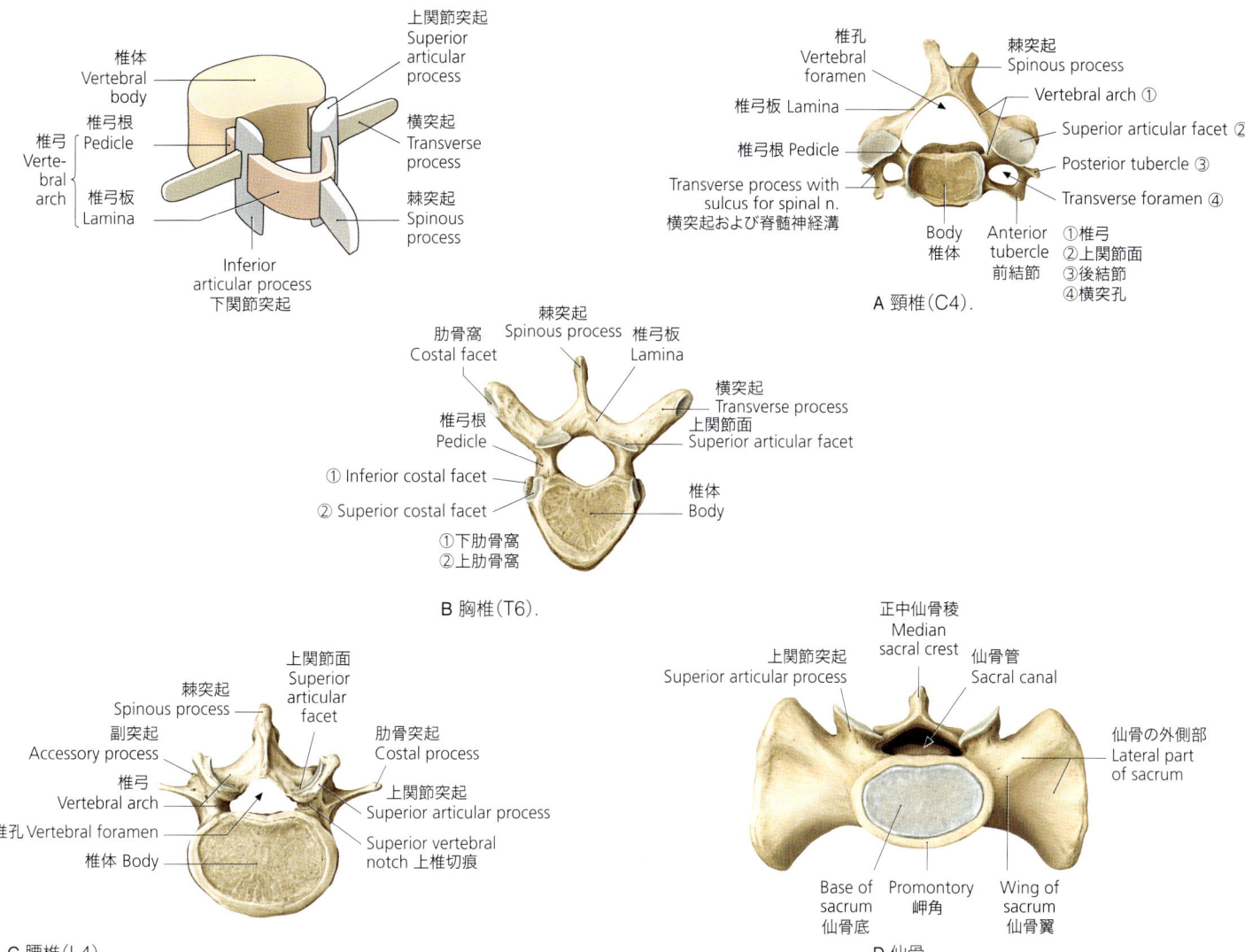

図1.5 椎骨の構成要素
左後上方から見たところ．例外（環椎C1と軸椎C2）を除いた全ての椎骨は同じ構成要素によって形成されている．

図1.6 典型的な椎骨
上方から見たところ．

A 頸椎（C4）．
①椎弓
②上関節面
③後結節
④横突孔

B 胸椎（T6）．

C 腰椎（L4）．

D 仙骨．

椎骨	椎体	椎孔	横突起	関節突起	棘突起
頸椎* C3-C7	小さい（腎臓型）	大きい（三角形）	小さい（C7では消失していることもある），前結節と後結節が横突孔を囲む	上後方もしくは下前方を向く，関節面は水平面から約45°傾いている	短い（C3-C5），二分する（C3-C6），長い（C7）
胸椎 T1-T12	中間（ハート型），肋骨窩（肋骨頭との関節面）が見られる	小さい（円形）	強大，下方のものほど短い，T1-T10では横突肋骨窩（肋骨との関節面）が見られる	後方（やや外側）もしくは前方（やや内側）を向く，関節面は前額面内にある	長い，後下方に向かって伸び，突起の先端は直ぐ下にある椎体の高さにまで達する
腰椎 L1-L5	大きい（腎臓型）	中間（三角形）	肋骨原基は椎弓根に融合して肋骨突起となり，"横突起"状の形態をとる．本来の横突起は乳頭突起・副突起に変化する	後内側（内側）もしくは前外側（外側）を向く，関節面は矢状面内にある．上関節突起の後面に乳頭突起が見られる	短い，幅が広い
仙椎（仙骨） S1-S5（癒合）	底から尖にかけて小さくなる	連なって仙骨管を形成する	発生期にできる肋骨と融合している（肋骨についてはpp.44-47参照）	仙骨の上関節突起は上後方を向く，関節面は前額面内にある	連なって正中仙骨稜を形成する

*C1（環椎）とC2（軸椎）は非典型的な椎骨であり，詳しくはp.6-7を参照．

頸椎
Cervical Vertebrae

 頸部脊柱を構成する7つの椎骨（頸椎）は一般的な椎骨の形態からかけ離れている．頸椎は頭部の重量を支えつつ，首をあらゆる方向に動かすことを可能にしている．C1とC2はそれぞれ環椎，軸椎という別名で知られている．また，C7は触知しやすい長い棘突起を持つため，隆椎とも呼ばれる．

図 1.7　頸部脊柱
左外側方から見たところ．

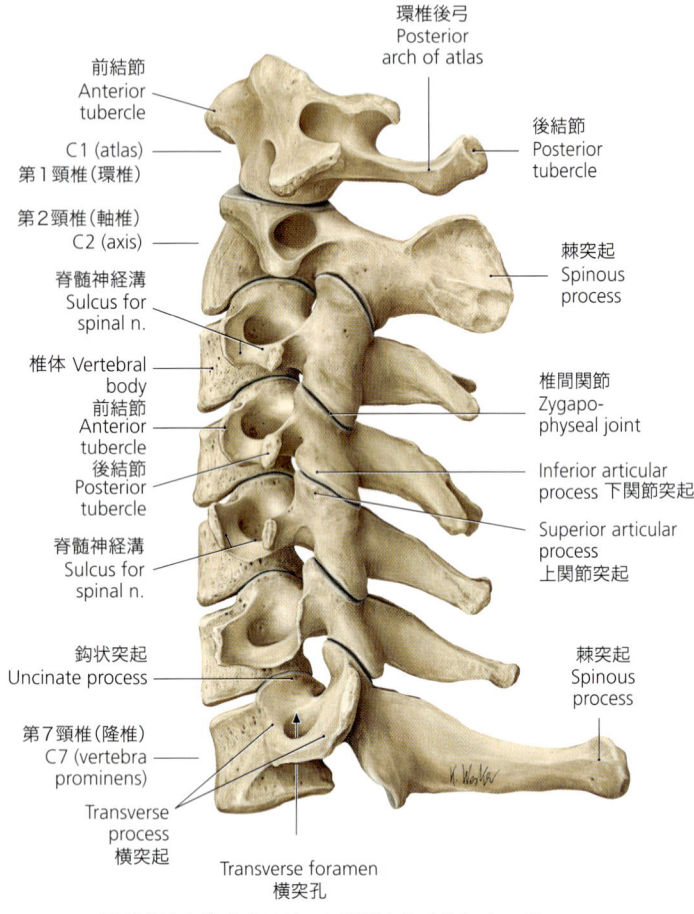

A　頸部脊柱を構成する骨，左外側方から見たところ．

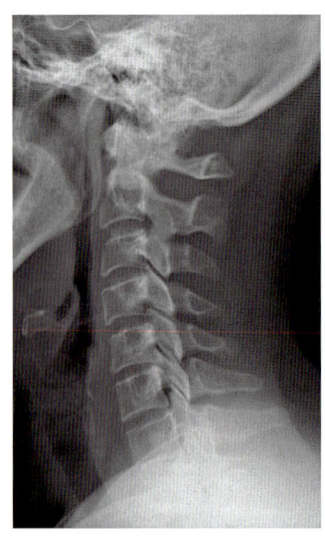

B　頸部脊柱のX線写真，左側面像．

図 1.8　環椎（第1頸椎，C1）

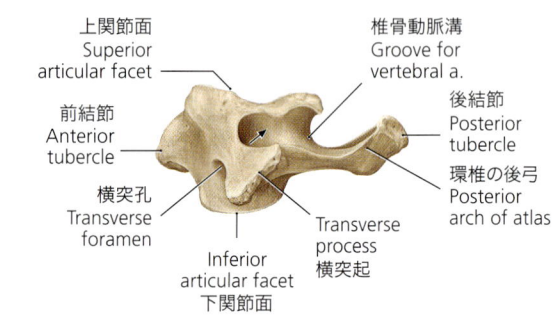

A　左外側方から見たところ．

図 1.9　軸椎（第2頸椎，C2）

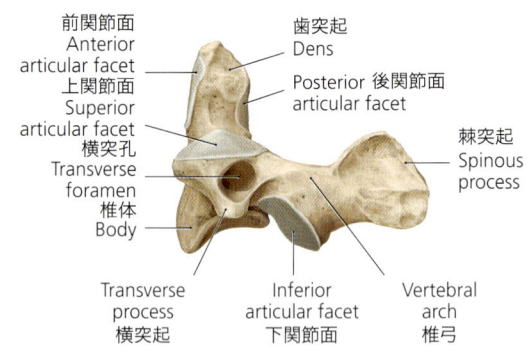

A　左外側方から見たところ．

図 1.10　典型的な頸椎（第4頸椎，C4）

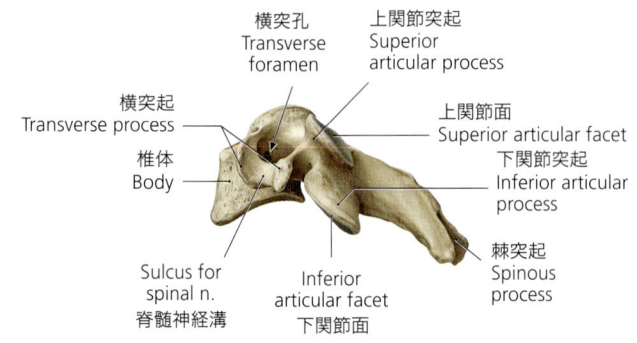

A　左外側方から見たところ．

臨床

頸部脊柱の外傷

頸部脊柱は過伸展に起因する外傷（例えば，むち打ち症）を受けやすい部位である．これは頭部が通常の可動域をはるかに超えて後方に引っ張られた場合に生じる．頸部脊柱に最も多い外傷は，軸椎歯突起の骨折，外傷性頸椎すべり症（椎体の前方へのずれ），環椎骨折である．患者の予後は，損傷された脊髄の高さによって大きく異なる（p.600参照）．

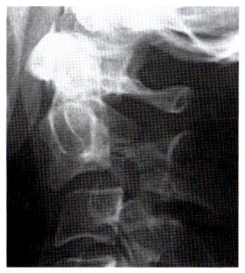

左のX線写真は，シートベルトを着用しなかったがために，ダッシュボードに打ち付けられた患者のものである．頸部の過伸展により，C2（軸椎）の椎弓が骨折し，さらにC2とC3をつなぐ靱帯が裂け，外傷性頸椎すべり症を発症している．このタイプの骨折はしばしば「ハングマン骨折」と呼ばれる．

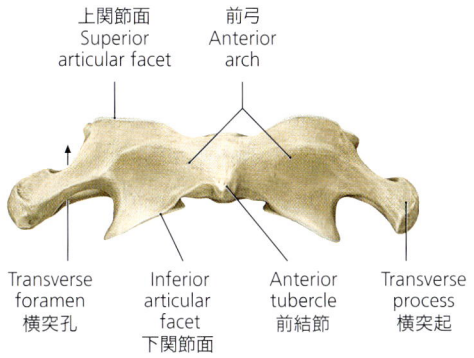

B 前方から見たところ．

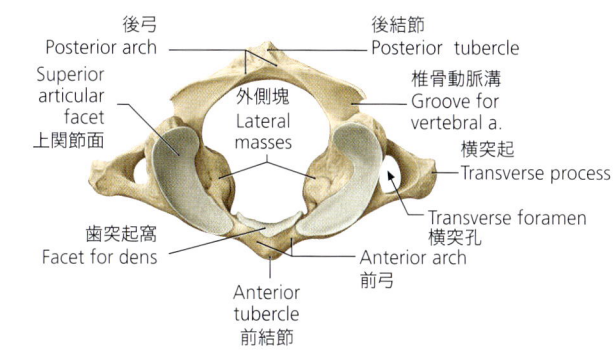

C 上方から見たところ．

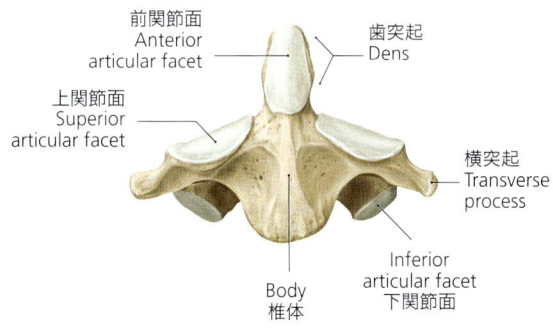

B 前方から見たところ．

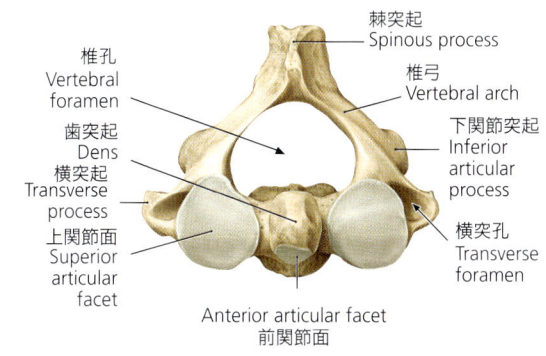

C 上方から見たところ．

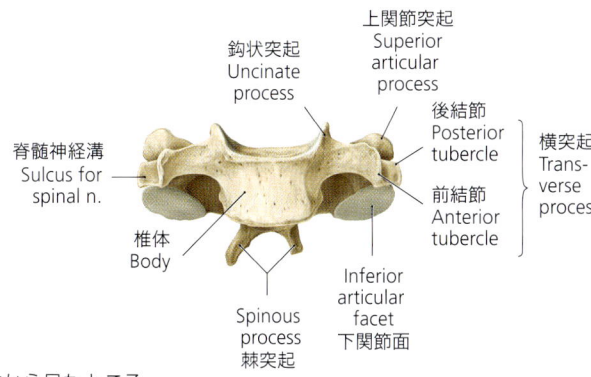

B 前方から見たところ．

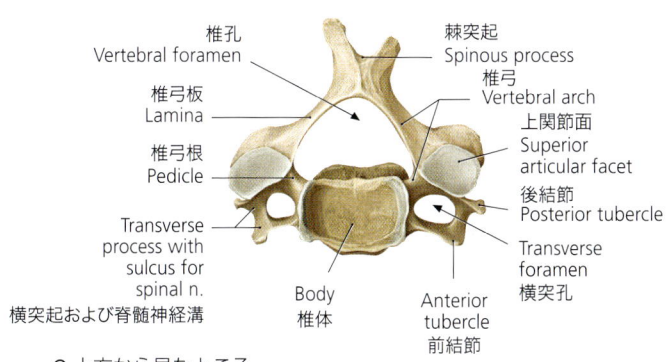

C 上方から見たところ．

胸椎と腰椎
Thoracic & Lumbar Vertebrae

図 1.11 胸部脊柱
左外側方から見たところ．

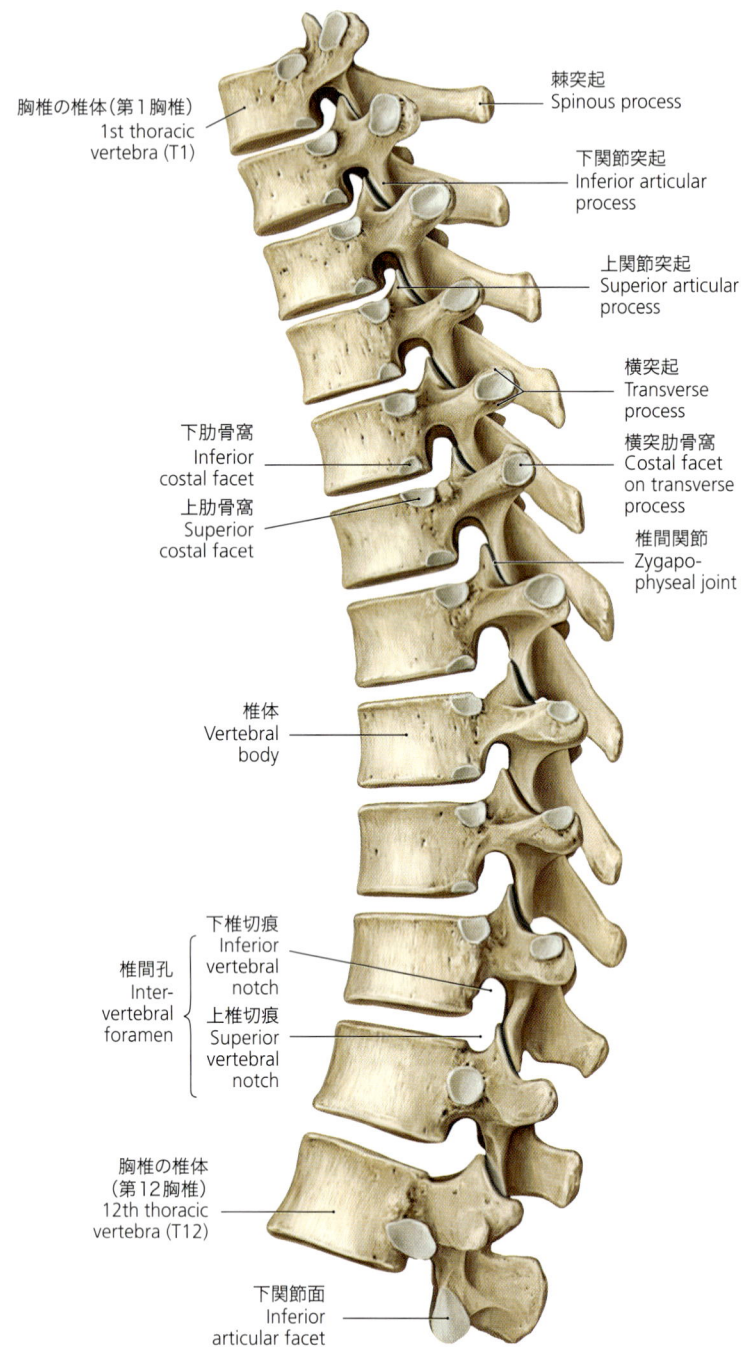

図 1.12 典型的な胸椎（第 6 胸椎，T6）

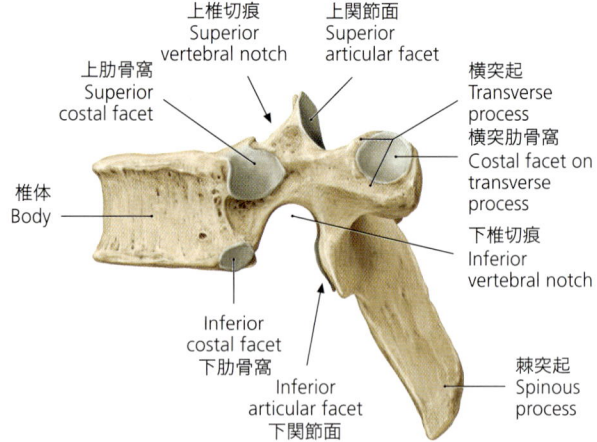

A 左外側方から見たところ．

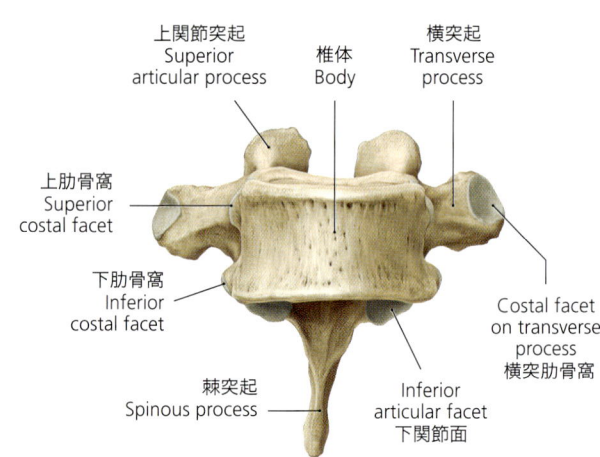

B 前方から見たところ．

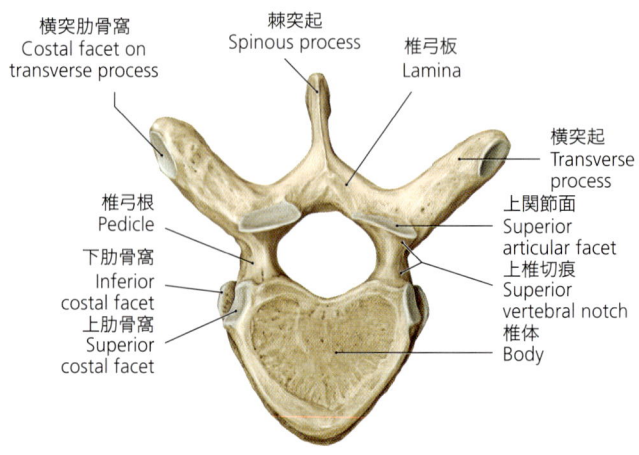

C 上方から見たところ．

図 1.13　腰部脊柱
左外側方から見たところ.

図 1.14　典型的な腰椎（第 4 腰椎，L4）

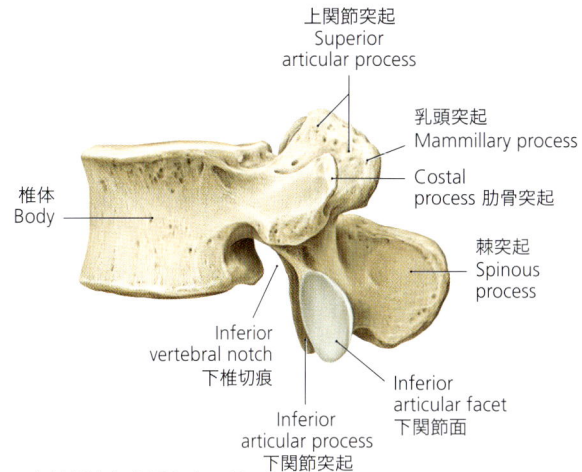

A　左外側方から見たところ.

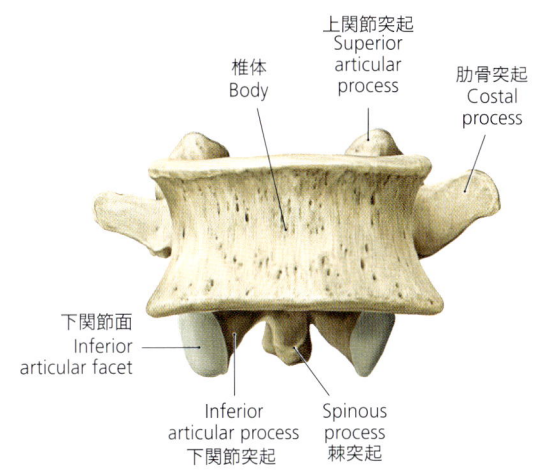

B　前方から見たところ.

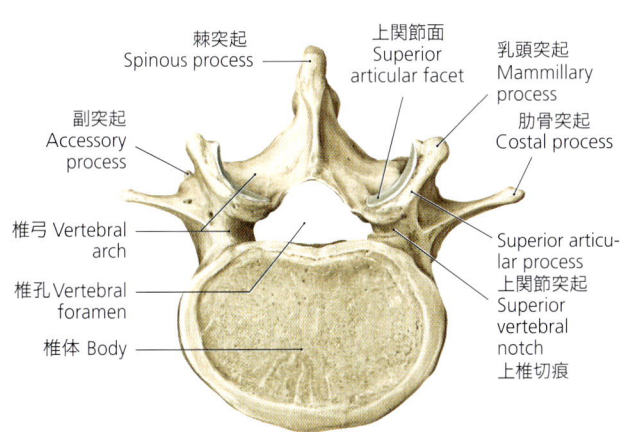

C　上方から見たところ.

臨床

骨粗鬆症

脊柱は骨格の退行性疾患（変形性関節症や骨粗鬆症）に最も侵されやすい部位である．骨粗鬆症では，骨成分の吸収（溶出）量が沈着量を上回るため，骨量が減少する．この疾患では，腰椎の圧迫骨折とそれにともなう背部痛が見られる場合がある．

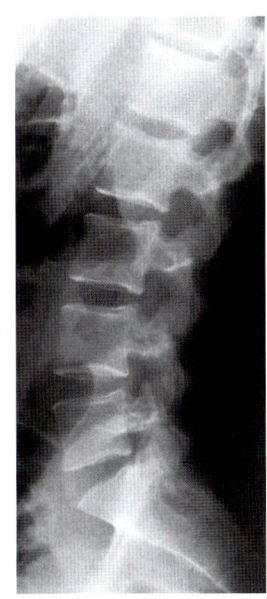

A　正常な腰部脊柱の X 線写真．左側面像．

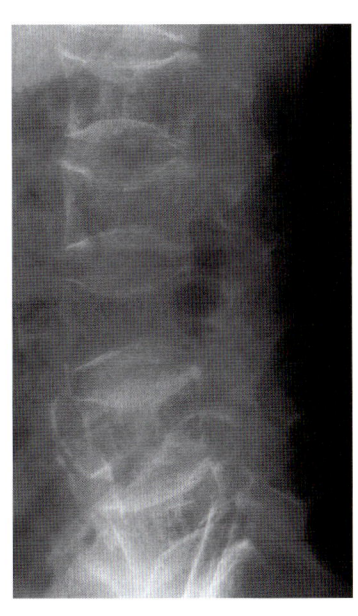

B　骨粗鬆症患者の X 線写真．椎体の骨密度が減少し，骨梁が疎になっている．圧迫骨折も認められる．

仙骨と尾骨
Sacrum & Coccyx

 仙骨は生後に癒合した5つの仙椎からなる．仙骨底は第5腰椎と，仙骨尖は尾骨とそれぞれ連結する．尾骨は3〜4個の痕跡的な椎骨（尾椎）が連なったものである．

図1.15 仙骨と尾骨

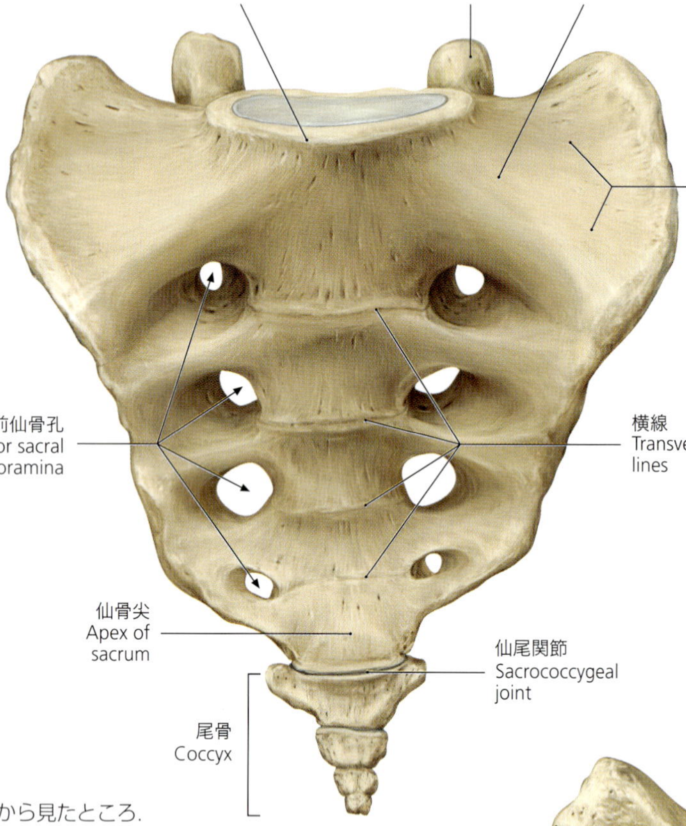

A 前方から見たところ．

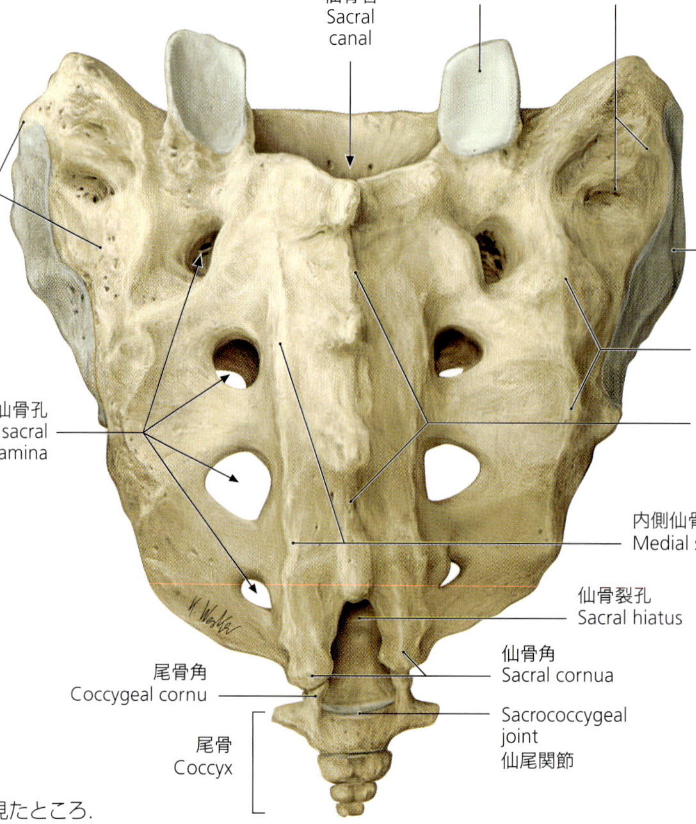

B 後方から見たところ．

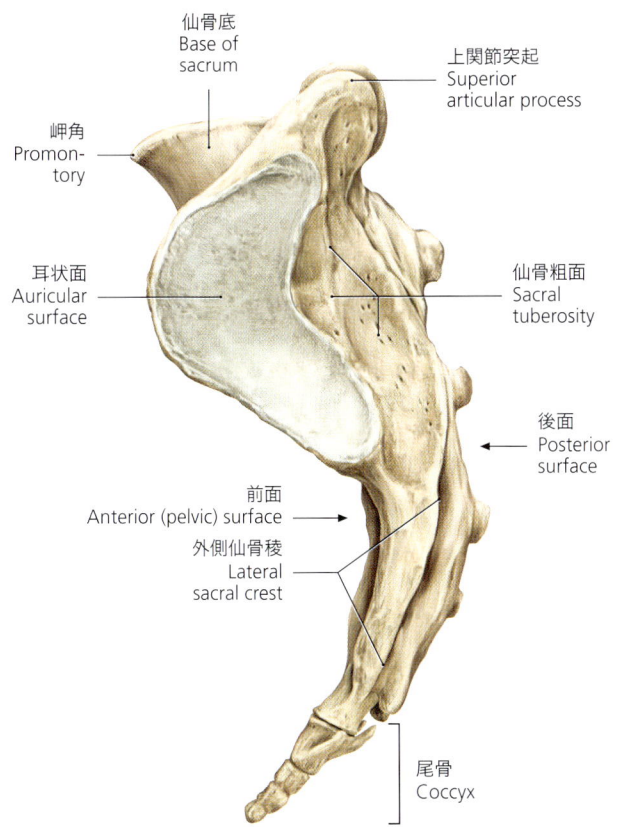

C 左外側方から見たところ．

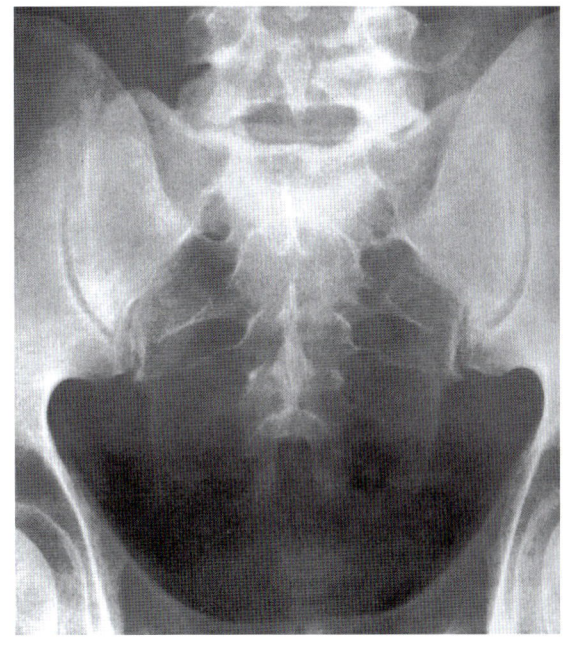

D 仙骨のX線写真，前後像．

図 1.16 仙骨

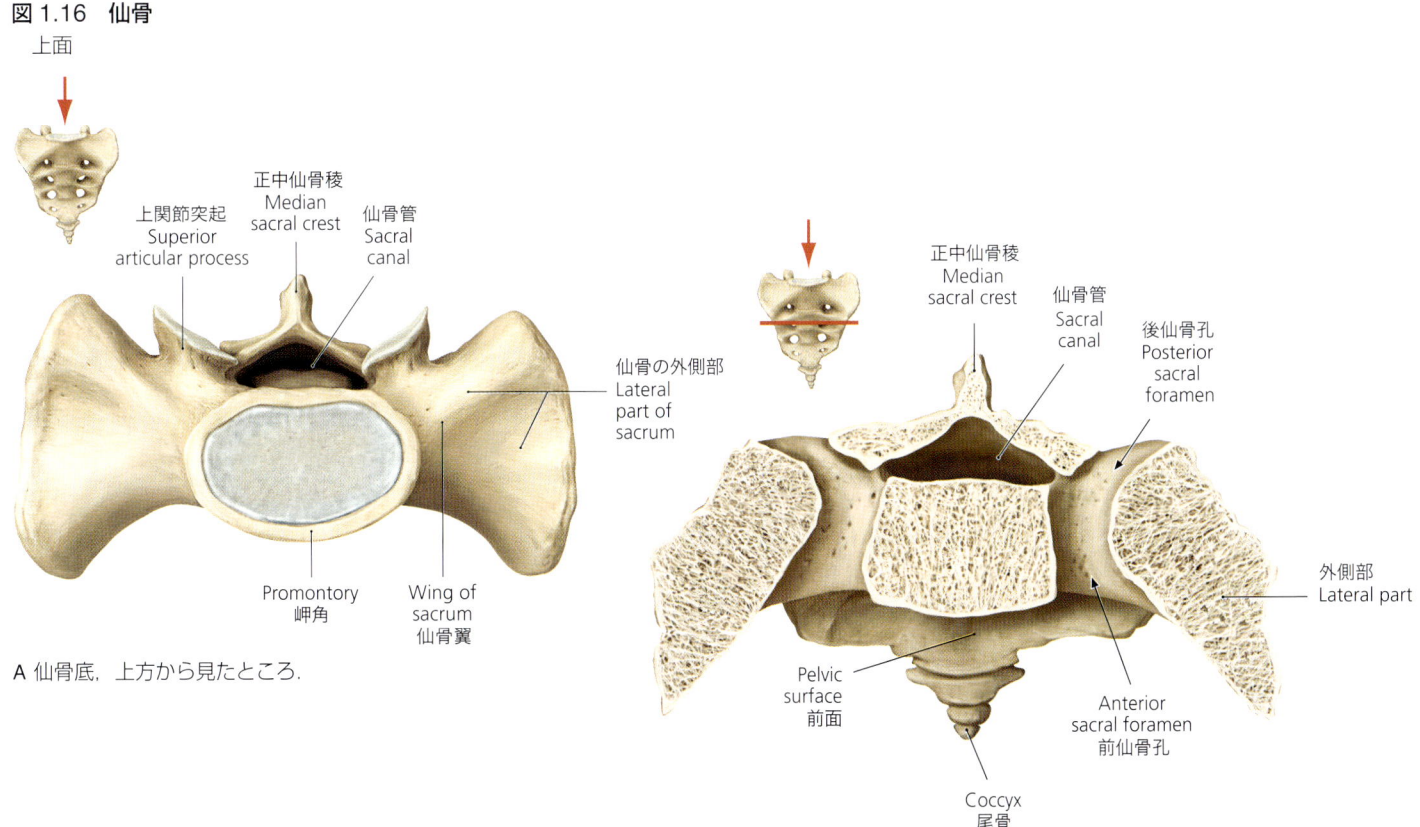

A 仙骨底，上方から見たところ．

B 第2仙椎を通る横断面．前仙骨孔と後仙骨孔を示している．上方から見たところ．

椎間円板
Intervertebral Disks

図 1.17 脊柱内での椎間円板の位置
第11-12胸椎の矢状断面（右半分）．左外側方から見たところ．椎間円板は椎体と椎体の間にできる空間を占めている（椎間関節についてはp.14参照）．

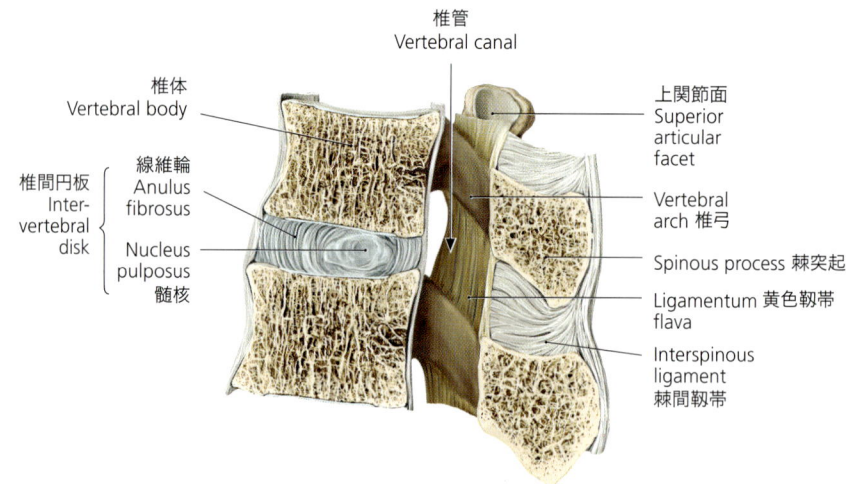

図 1.18 椎間円板の構造
前上方から見たところ．椎間円板の前半分と硝子軟骨板の右前4分の1が除去されている．椎間円板は外側にある線維輪と内側にあるゼラチン質の核（髄核）からなる．

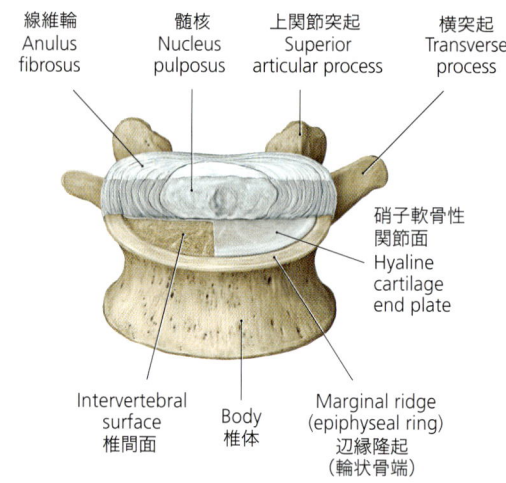

図 1.19 椎間円板と椎孔の関係
第4腰椎，上方から見たところ．

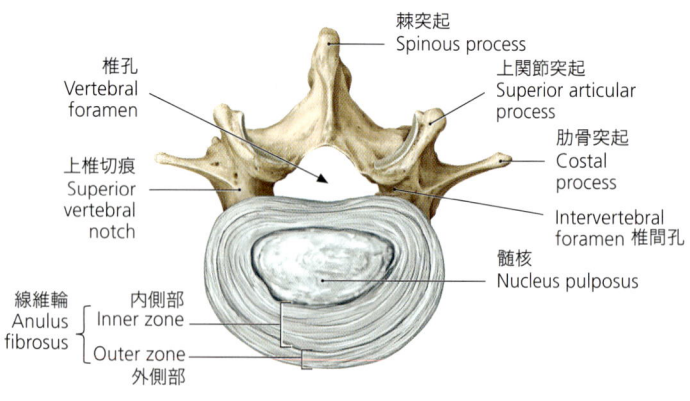

図 1.20 線維輪の外層
第3-4腰椎とその間の椎間円板，前方から見たところ．

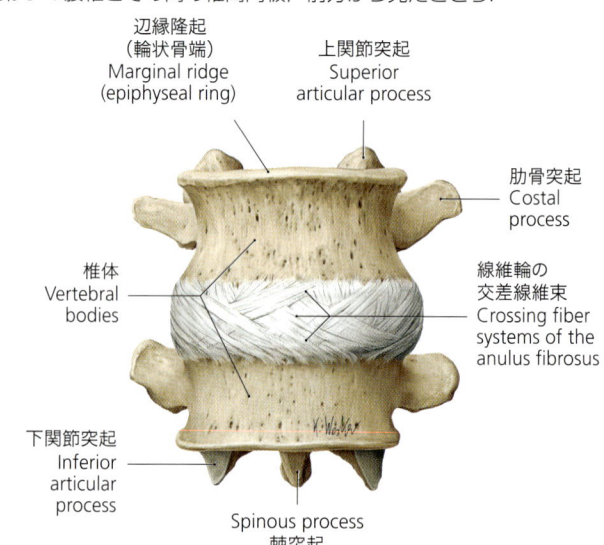

臨床

腰部脊柱の椎間板ヘルニア

加齢にともない，線維輪は外力に対する抵抗性が弱くなり，負荷がかかった状態では髄核が線維輪の脆弱な部分から突出することがある．さらに，もし線維輪が破断してしまった場合には，髄核が逸脱し椎間孔の内容物（神経根と血管）を圧迫することもある．このような患者はしばしば激しい背部痛に襲われる．痛みは圧迫された神経根に対応するデルマトーム（皮膚分節，p.600 参照）でも感じられる．神経根の運動神経の部分が傷害された場合には，その神経が支配する筋の筋力低下や萎縮が見られる．特定の神経根が分布する筋やデルマトームを検査することは，ヘルニアの生じた高さを診断するうえで重要となる．例：第1仙骨神経は腓腹筋とヒラメ筋を支配しているので，この神経根が圧迫されると，爪先立ちや爪先歩きが困難になる（p.398 参照）．

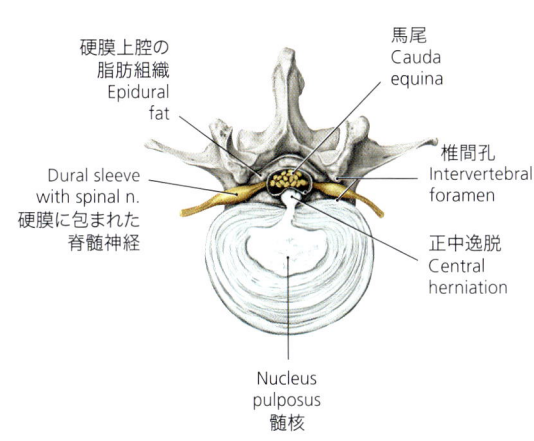

A 上方から見たところ．

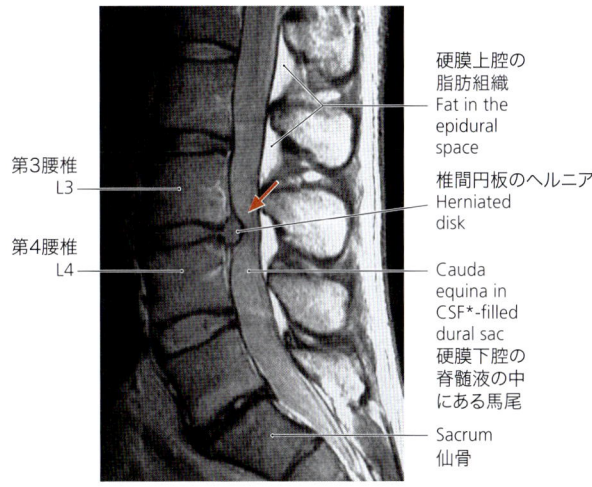

B MR像（正中矢状断 T2 強調像）．

＊CSF（cerebrospinal fluid）脳脊髄液

後方ヘルニア（A, B） MR像において，椎間円板（L3 と L4 の間）が後方に向かって著しく突出しているのがわかる（経靱帯性のヘルニア）．硬膜嚢はヘルニアの部位で深く陥没している．

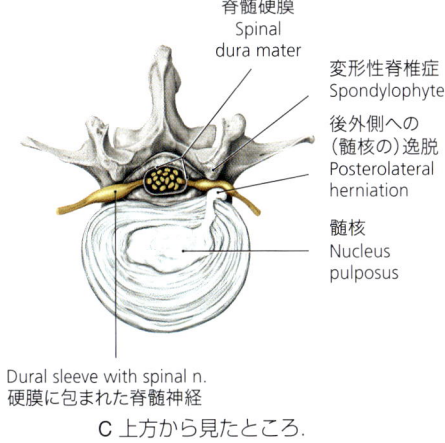

C 上方から見たところ．

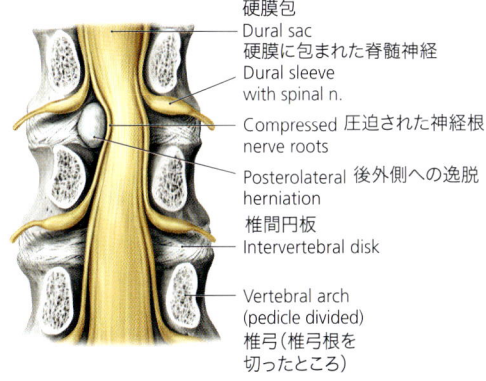

D 後方から見たところ．椎弓移動．

後外方ヘルニア（C, D） 逸脱した髄核が椎間孔に入り込み，神経根を圧迫する場合がある．もし，逸脱した髄核がより内側に位置する場合は，その高さの椎間孔から出る神経根は圧迫されず，下位の椎間孔から出る神経根が圧迫される．

脊柱の関節：概観
Joints of the Vertebral Column: Overview

表 1.2　脊柱の関節

頭蓋と脊柱の連結		
①	環椎後頭関節	後頭骨-C1
②	環軸関節	C1-C2
椎体の関節		
③	鉤椎関節	C3-C7
④	椎体間関節	C1-S1
椎弓の関節		
⑤	椎間関節	C1-S1

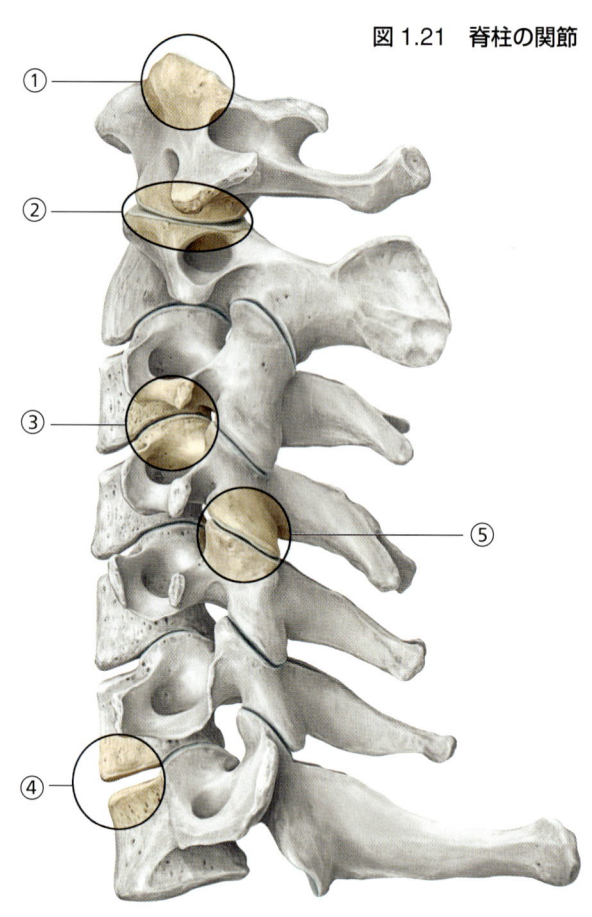

図 1.21　脊柱の関節

図 1.22　椎間関節
椎間関節の配列は脊柱の各部位で異なり，運動の大きさや方向を決めている．

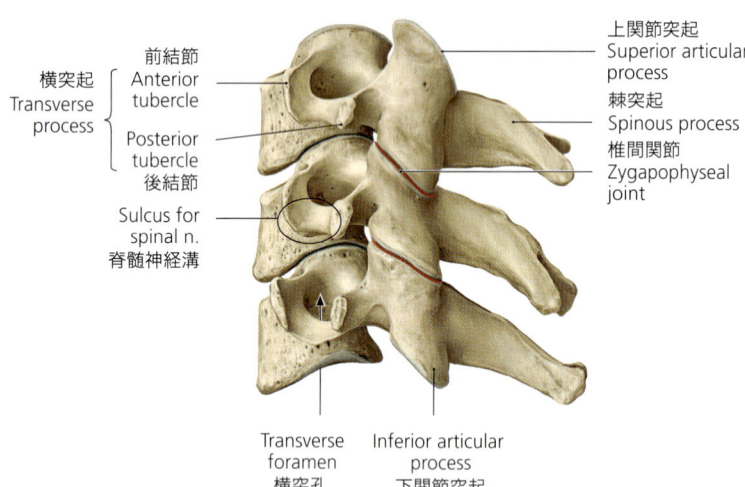

A 頸部脊柱，左外側方から見たところ．椎間関節の関節面は水平面より45°傾いた面にある．

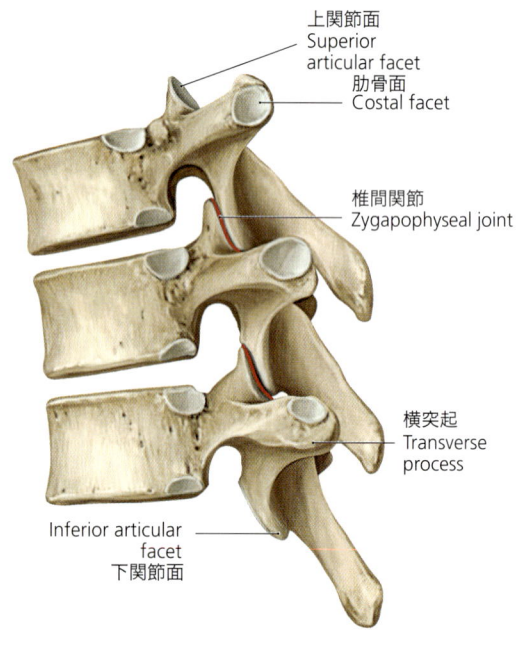

B 胸部脊柱，左外側方から見たところ．椎間関節の関節面は前額面にある．

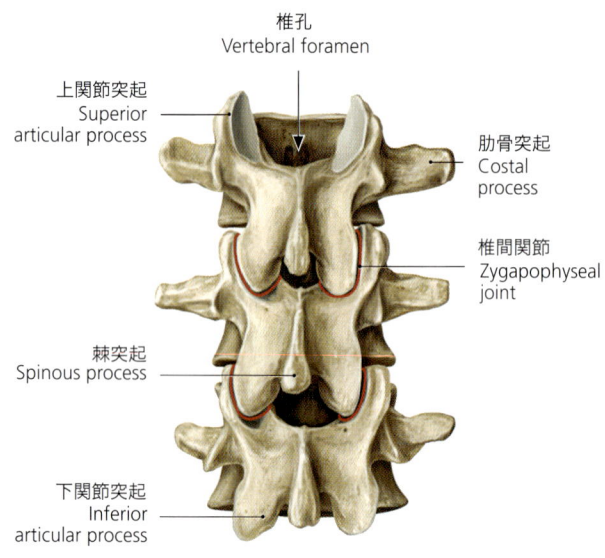

C 腰部脊柱，左外側方から見たところ．椎間関節の関節面は矢状面にある．

図 1.23　鉤椎関節

前方から見たところ．鉤椎関節は小児期に形成され，C3-C6 の鉤状突起とひとつ上位の椎体との間にできる．この関節は椎間円板（軟骨）の中に裂隙が生じて形成される．この裂隙が大きく広がると，椎間円板ヘルニアに罹患する危険性が増す（p.13 参照）．

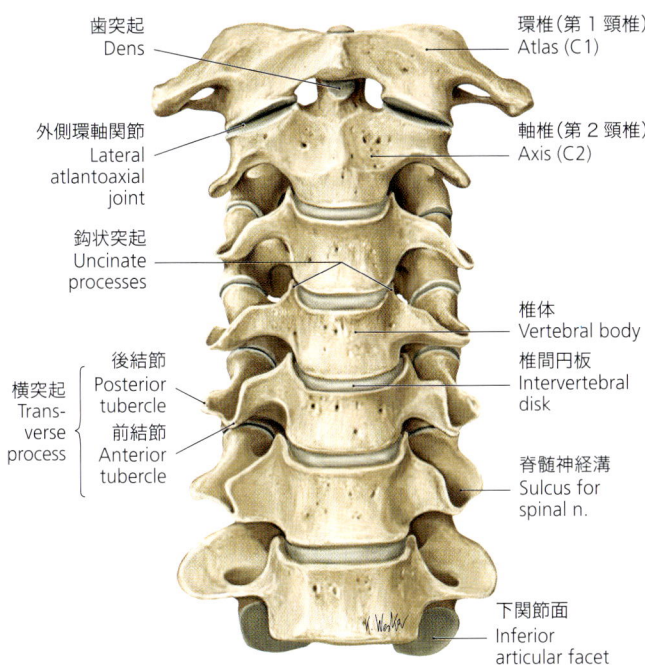

A　18 歳男性の頸部脊柱における鉤椎関節，前方から見たところ．

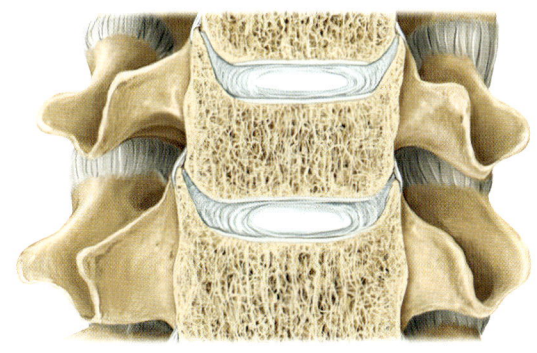

B　鉤椎関節（拡大図），全額断面，前方から見たところ．

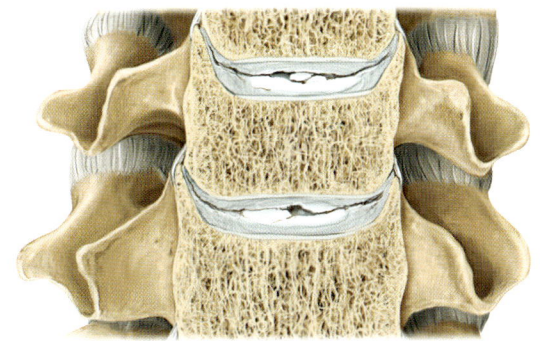

C　椎間円板内に形成された裂隙，全額断面，前方から見たところ．

臨床

脊髄神経と椎骨動脈は鉤状突起に近接している

脊髄神経と椎骨動脈はそれぞれ椎間孔と横突孔を通る．鉤椎関節の変形性関節症によって骨棘（骨組織が外方へ増生したもの）が形成され，この骨棘が脊髄神経と椎骨動脈の両者を圧迫することがある．また，骨棘によって慢性的な頸部痛が生じる場合もある．

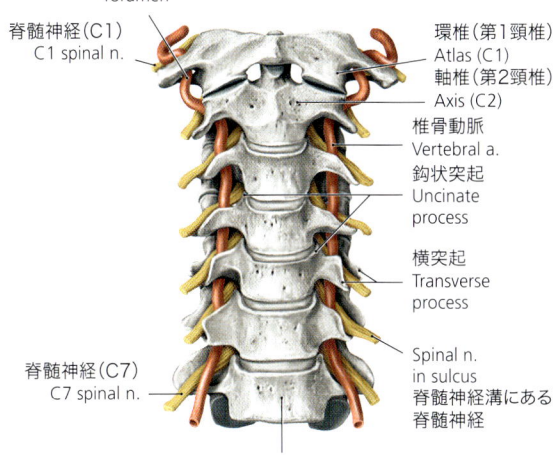

A　頸椎，前方から見たところ．

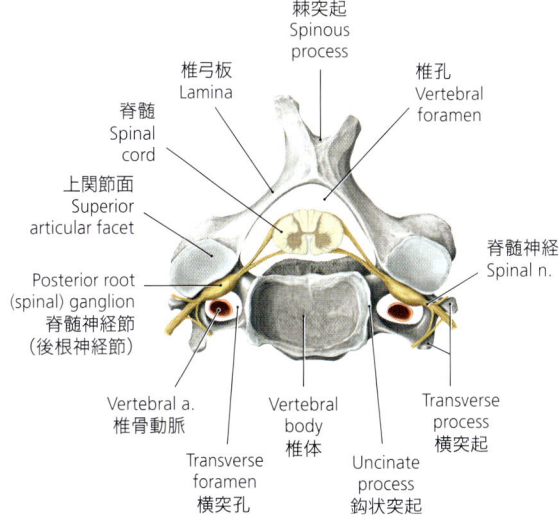

B　第 4 頸椎，上方から見たところ．

脊柱の関節：頭蓋との連結
Joints of the Vertebral Column: Craniovertebral Region

図 1.24　頭蓋と脊柱の連結

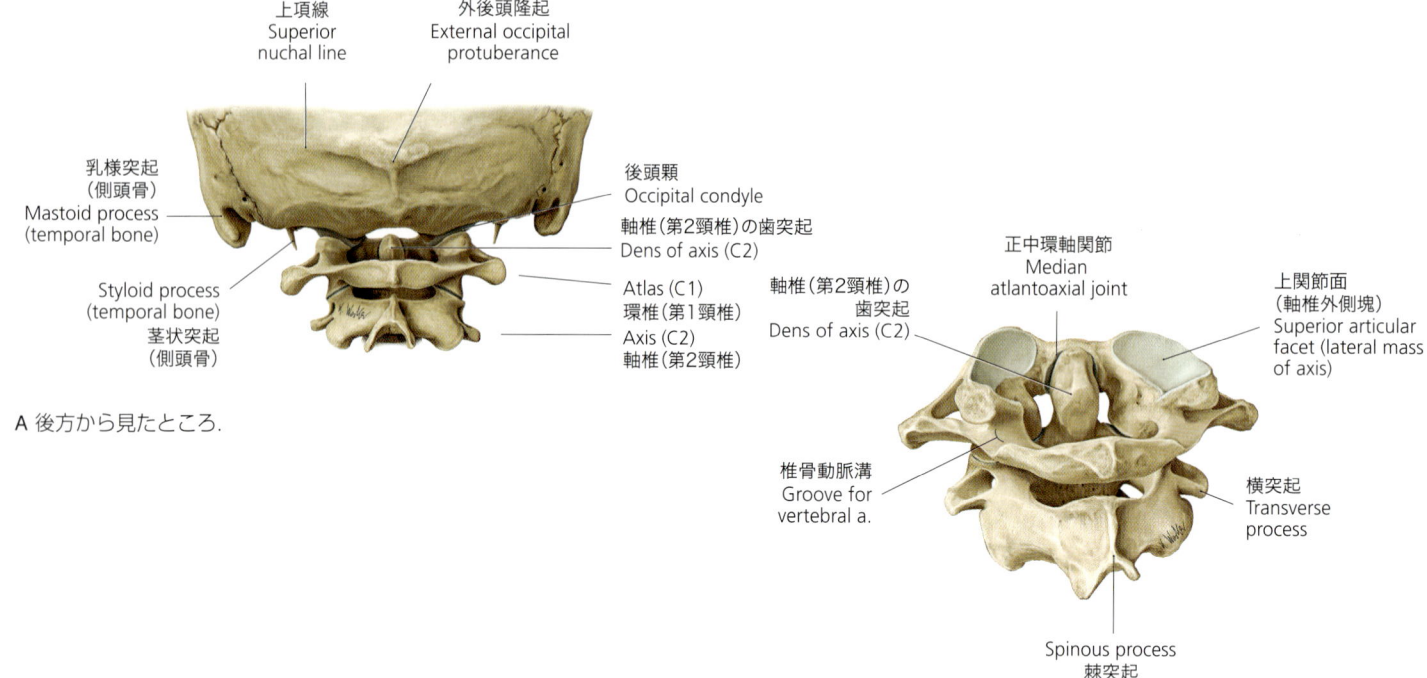

A 後方から見たところ．

B 環椎と軸椎，後上方から見たところ．

図 1.25　頭蓋と脊柱を連結する靱帯の剖出
後方から見たところ．

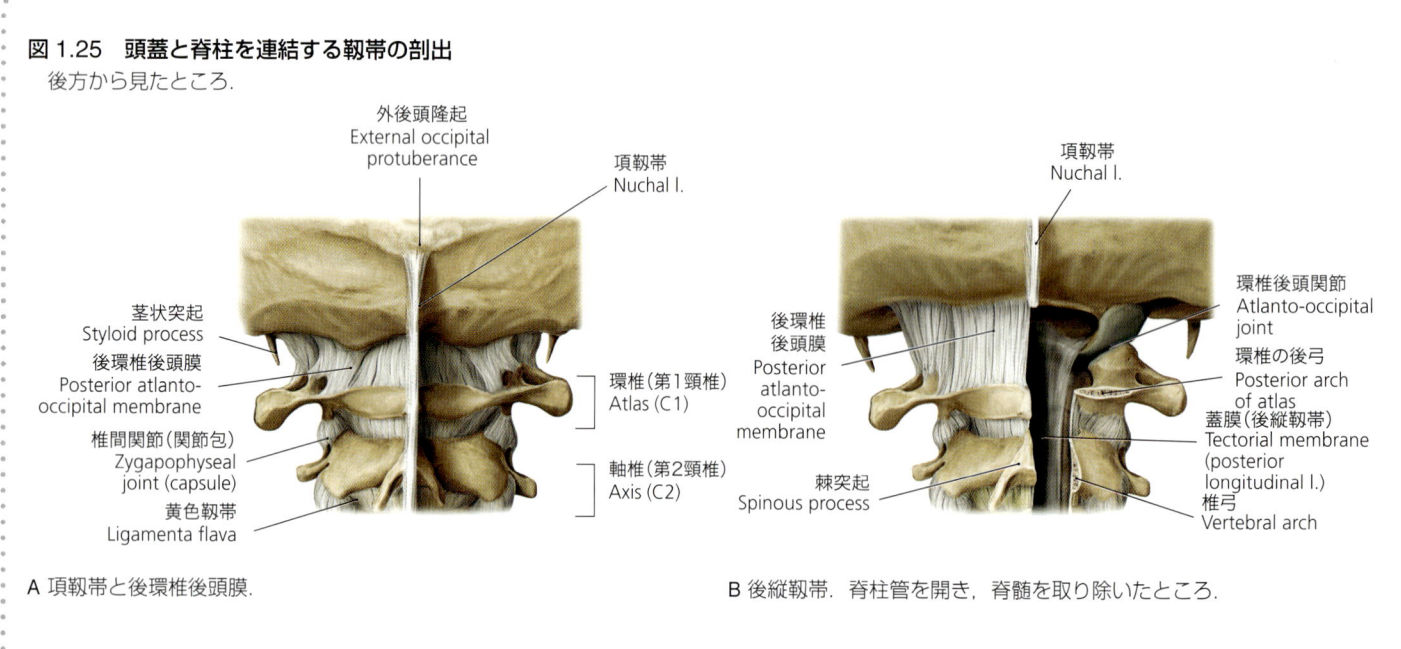

A 項靱帯と後環椎後頭膜．

B 後縦靱帯．脊柱管を開き，脊髄を取り除いたところ．

環椎後頭関節は，後頭骨にある突出した後頭顆と環椎（C1）にある窪んだ上関節面の間に形成される1対の関節である．環軸関節は環椎（C1）と軸椎（C2）の間に形成され，外側にある1対と正中にある1つの関節からなる．

図1.26 頭蓋と脊柱を連結する靱帯

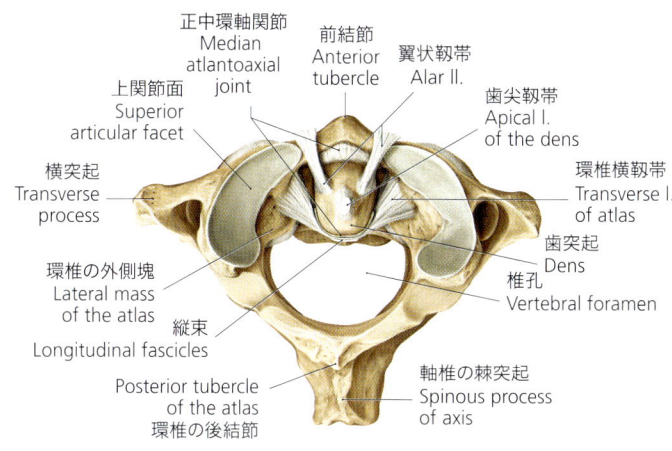
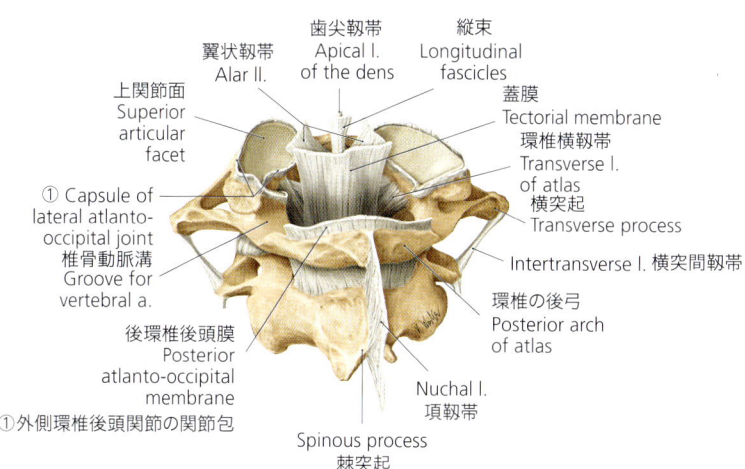

A 正中環軸関節の靱帯，上方から見たところ．環椎の歯突起窩は関節包によって隠れている．

B 頭蓋と脊柱を連結する靱帯，左後上方から見たところ．軸椎の歯突起は蓋膜によって隠れている．

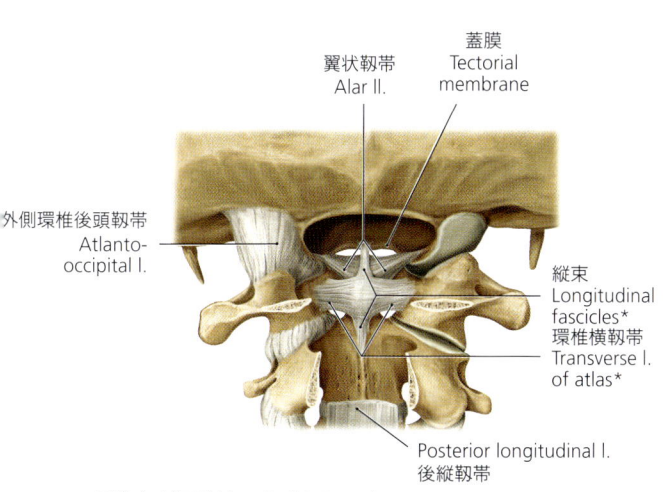
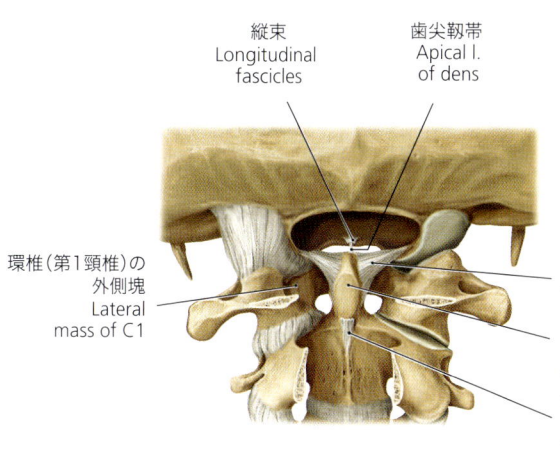

C 環椎十字靱帯（*）．蓋膜を取り除いたところ．

D 翼状靱帯と歯尖靱帯．環椎横靱帯と縦束（上3分の2）を取り除いたところ．

脊柱の靱帯：概観，頸部脊柱
Vertebral Ligaments: Overview & Cervical Spine

 脊柱の靱帯は椎骨を連結し，脊髄を大きな荷重やせん断ストレスから保護する．またこれらの靱帯によって脊柱の可動域は制限される．

靱帯は椎体の靱帯と椎弓の靱帯に分けられる．

図 1.27　脊柱の靱帯
左後上方から見たところ．

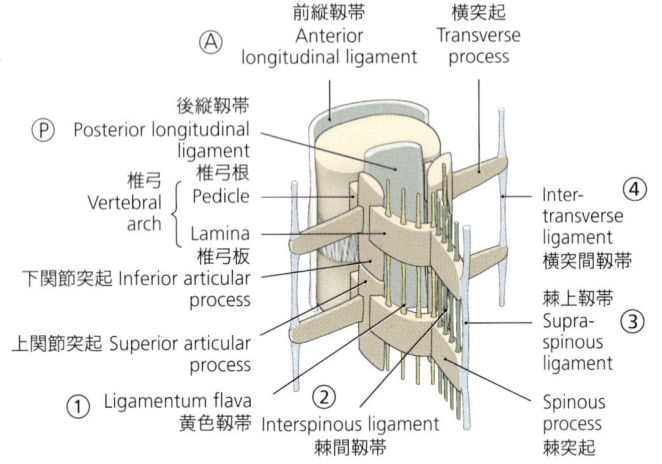

表 1.3　脊柱の靱帯

靱帯	位置
椎体の靱帯	
Ⓐ　前縦靱帯	椎体の前面に沿っている
Ⓟ　後縦靱帯	椎体の後面に沿っている
椎弓の靱帯	
①　黄色靱帯	椎弓板の間
②　棘間靱帯	棘突起の間
③　棘上靱帯	棘突起の後縁に沿っている
④　横突間靱帯	横突起の間
項靱帯*	外後頭隆起とC7の棘突起の間

*棘上靱帯が後方（矢状方向）に広がったもの．

図 1.28　前縦靱帯
前方から見たところ．頭蓋底を取り除いてある．

①環椎後頭関節（外側環椎後頭靱帯）
②外側環軸関節（関節包）

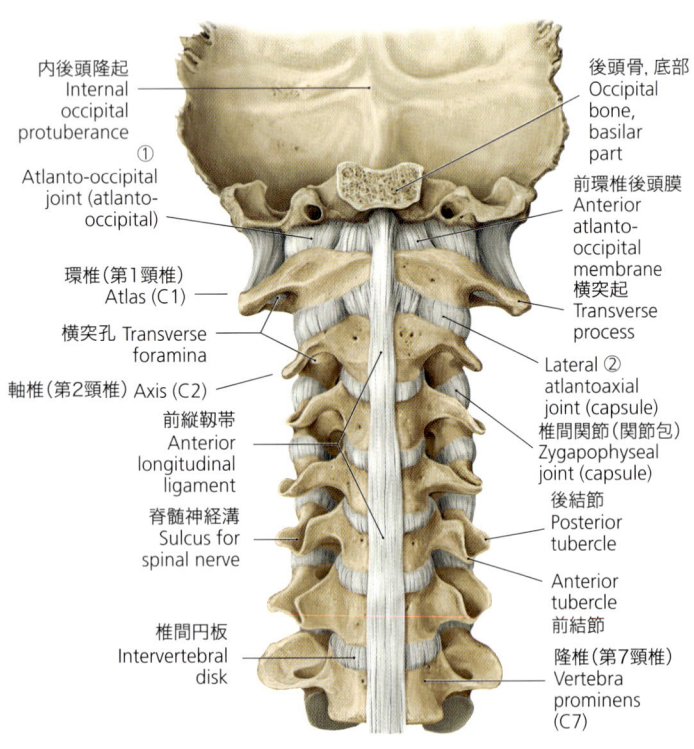

図 1.29　後縦靱帯
後方から見たところ．脊柱管を開き，脊髄を取り除いてある．蓋膜は後縦靱帯が上方へ広がったものである．

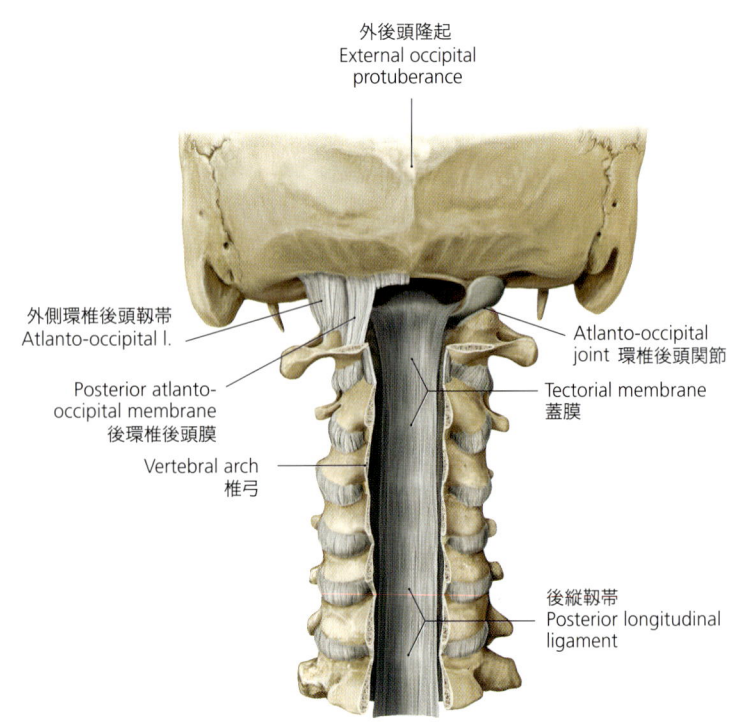

図 1.30 頸部脊柱の靱帯

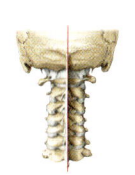

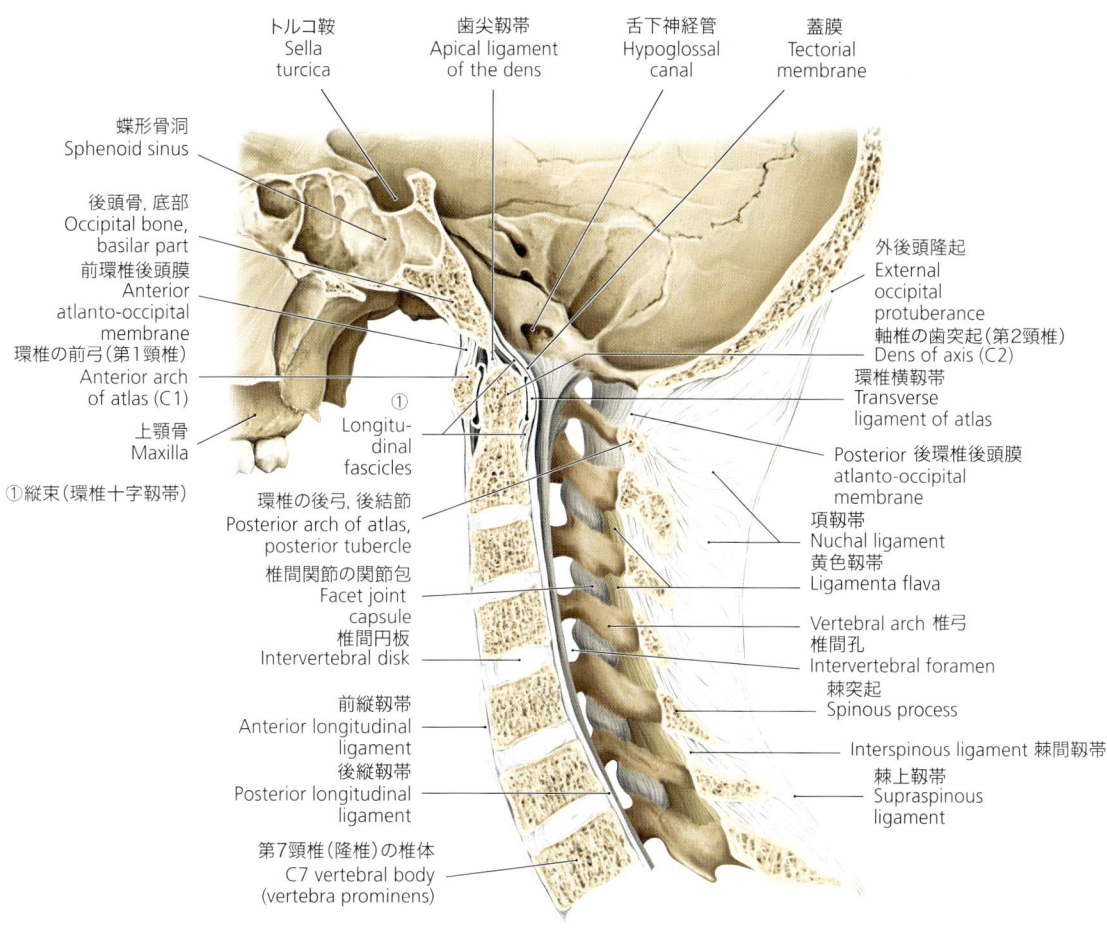

主な標示（上図）:
- トルコ鞍 Sella turcica
- 歯尖靱帯 Apical ligament of the dens
- 舌下神経管 Hypoglossal canal
- 蓋膜 Tectorial membrane
- 蝶形骨洞 Sphenoid sinus
- 後頭骨, 底部 Occipital bone, basilar part
- 前環椎後頭膜 Anterior atlanto-occipital membrane
- 環椎の前弓（第1頸椎）Anterior arch of atlas (C1)
- 上顎骨 Maxilla
- ①縦束（環椎十字靱帯）① Longitudinal fascicles
- 環椎の後弓, 後結節 Posterior arch of atlas, posterior tubercle
- 椎間関節の関節包 Facet joint capsule
- 椎間円板 Intervertebral disk
- 前縦靱帯 Anterior longitudinal ligament
- 後縦靱帯 Posterior longitudinal ligament
- 第7頸椎（隆椎）の椎体 C7 vertebral body (vertebra prominens)
- 外後頭隆起 External occipital protuberance
- 軸椎の歯突起（第2頸椎）Dens of axis (C2)
- 環椎横靱帯 Transverse ligament of atlas
- 後環椎後頭膜 Posterior atlanto-occipital membrane
- 項靱帯 Nuchal ligament
- 黄色靱帯 Ligamenta flava
- 椎弓 Vertebral arch
- 椎間孔 Intervertebral foramen
- 棘突起 Spinous process
- 棘間靱帯 Interspinous ligament
- 棘上靱帯 Supraspinous ligament

A 正中矢状断, 左側方から見たところ. 項靱帯は棘上靱帯が後方（矢状方向）に広がったもので, 隆椎（C7）から後頭骨の外後頭隆起に至る.

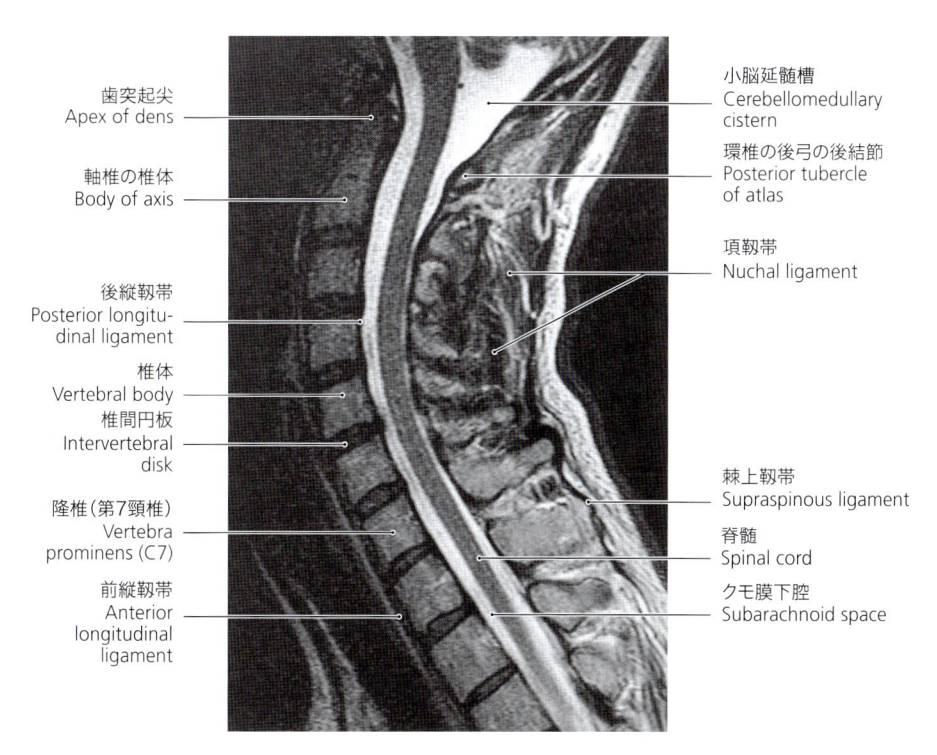

主な標示（下図 MR像）:
- 歯突起尖 Apex of dens
- 軸椎の椎体 Body of axis
- 後縦靱帯 Posterior longitudinal ligament
- 椎体 Vertebral body
- 椎間円板 Intervertebral disk
- 隆椎（第7頸椎）Vertebra prominens (C7)
- 前縦靱帯 Anterior longitudinal ligament
- 小脳延髄槽 Cerebellomedullary cistern
- 環椎の後弓の後結節 Posterior tubercle of atlas
- 項靱帯 Nuchal ligament
- 棘上靱帯 Supraspinous ligament
- 脊髄 Spinal cord
- クモ膜下腔 Subarachnoid space

B MR像（正中矢状断 T2強調像）, 左側像.

1 骨、靱帯、関節

脊柱の靭帯：胸腰部脊柱
Vertebral Ligaments: Thoracolumbar Spine

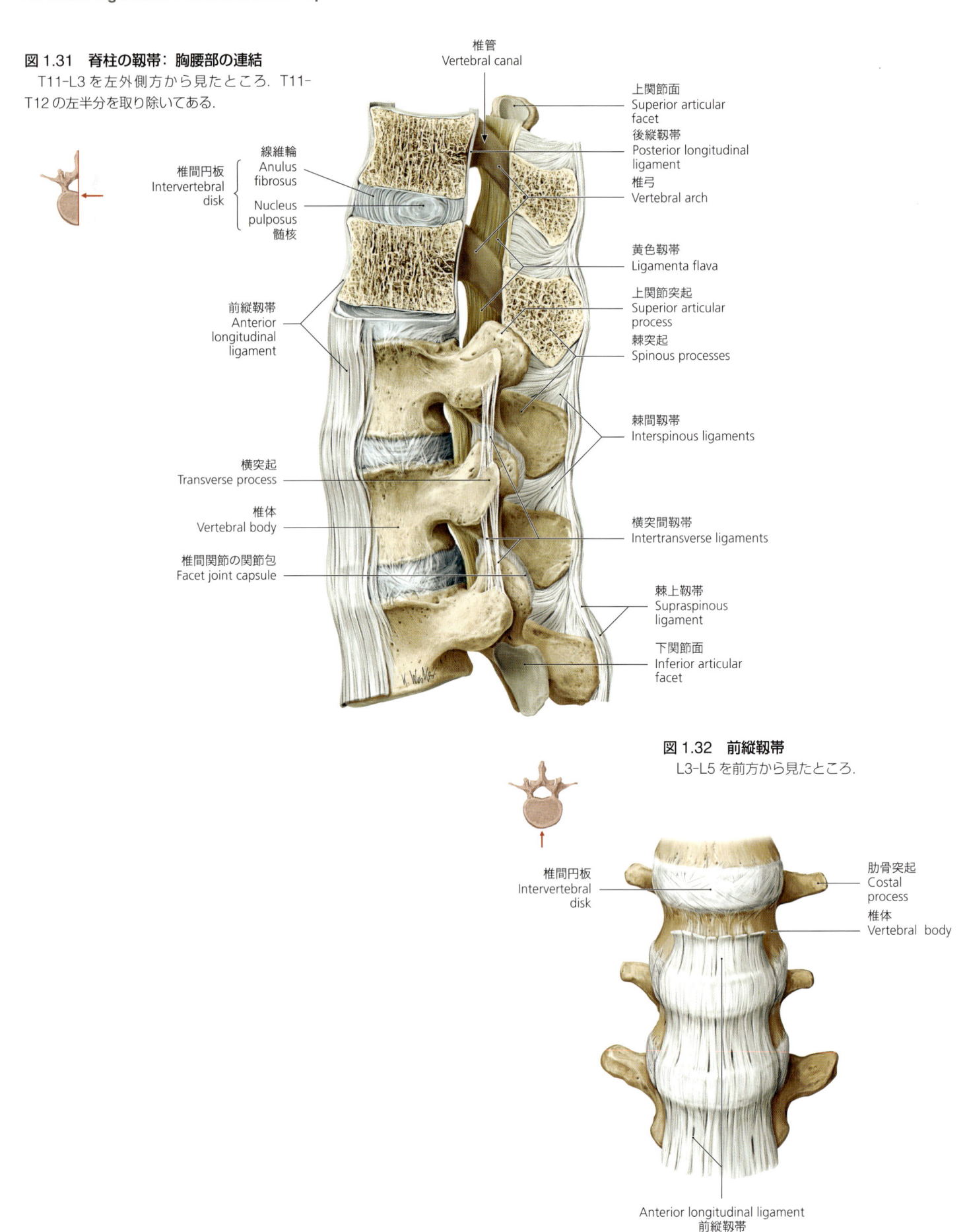

図 1.31 脊柱の靭帯：胸腰部の連結
T11-L3 を左外側方から見たところ．T11-T12 の左半分を取り除いてある．

- 椎間円板 Intervertebral disk
  - 線維輪 Anulus fibrosus
  - 髄核 Nucleus pulposus
- 前縦靭帯 Anterior longitudinal ligament
- 横突起 Transverse process
- 椎体 Vertebral body
- 椎間関節の関節包 Facet joint capsule
- 椎管 Vertebral canal
- 上関節面 Superior articular facet
- 後縦靭帯 Posterior longitudinal ligament
- 椎弓 Vertebral arch
- 黄色靭帯 Ligamenta flava
- 上関節突起 Superior articular process
- 棘突起 Spinous processes
- 棘間靭帯 Interspinous ligaments
- 横突間靭帯 Intertransverse ligaments
- 棘上靭帯 Supraspinous ligament
- 下関節面 Inferior articular facet

図 1.32 前縦靭帯
L3-L5 を前方から見たところ．

- 椎間円板 Intervertebral disk
- 肋骨突起 Costal process
- 椎体 Vertebral body
- Anterior longitudinal ligament 前縦靭帯

図 1.33 黄色靱帯と横突間靱帯

L2–L5 を前方から見たところ．L2–L4 の椎体を取り除き，脊柱管を開いてある．

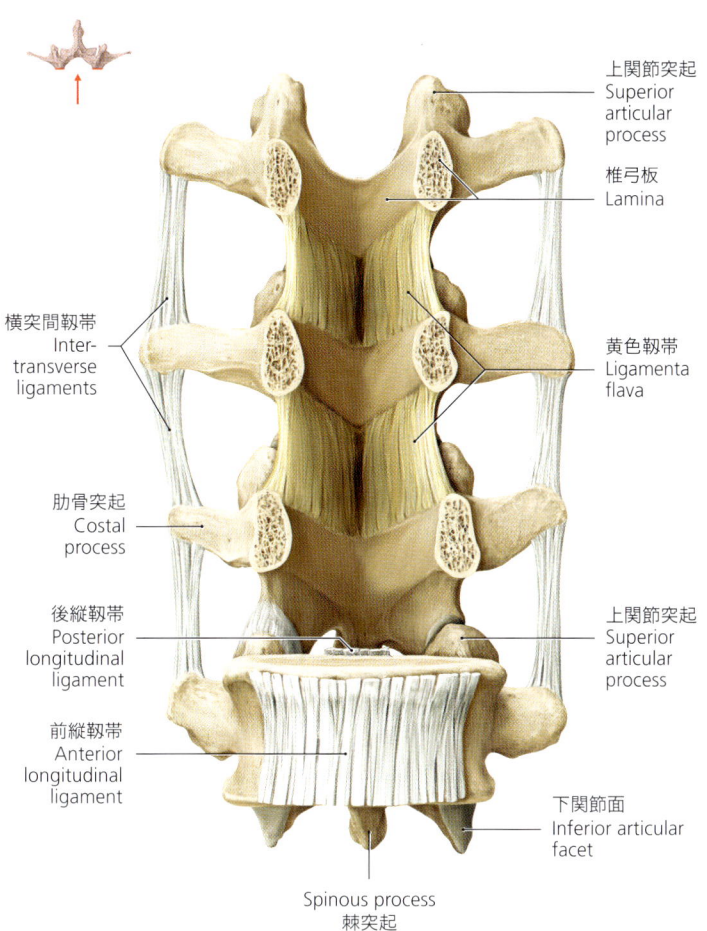

- 上関節突起 Superior articular process
- 椎弓板 Lamina
- 横突間靱帯 Inter-transverse ligaments
- 黄色靱帯 Ligamenta flava
- 肋骨突起 Costal process
- 後縦靱帯 Posterior longitudinal ligament
- 上関節突起 Superior articular process
- 前縦靱帯 Anterior longitudinal ligament
- 下関節面 Inferior articular facet
- Spinous process 棘突起

図 1.34 後縦靱帯

L2–L5 を後方から見たところ．L2–L4 の椎弓を椎弓根の部分で切り取り，脊柱管を開いてある．

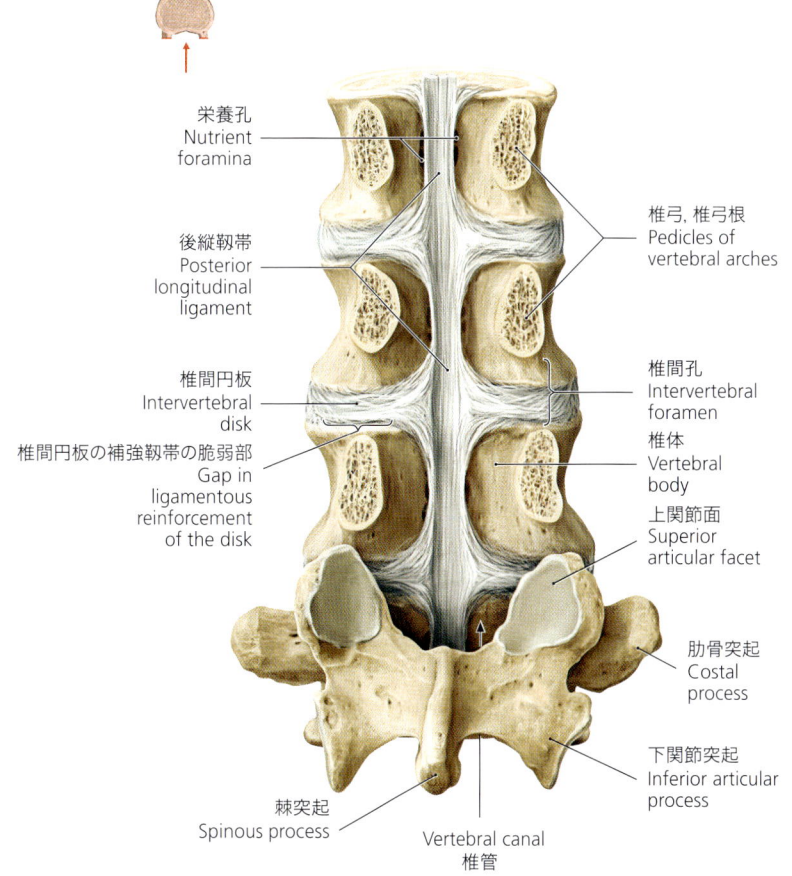

- 栄養孔 Nutrient foramina
- 後縦靱帯 Posterior longitudinal ligament
- 椎間円板 Intervertebral disk
- 椎間円板の補強靱帯の脆弱部 Gap in ligamentous reinforcement of the disk
- 椎弓, 椎弓根 Pedicles of vertebral arches
- 椎間孔 Intervertebral foramen
- 椎体 Vertebral body
- 上関節面 Superior articular facet
- 肋骨突起 Costal process
- 下関節突起 Inferior articular process
- 棘突起 Spinous process
- Vertebral canal 椎管

背部の筋：概観
Muscles of the Back: Overview

背部の筋は2つのグループ（外来背筋と固有背筋）に区分され，両者は胸腰筋膜の浅葉によって分けられる．表層にある外来背筋は，上肢の筋が背部に入り込んだものと考えられている．外来背筋については第4部で扱う．

図2.1　表層にある外来背筋
後方から見たところ．右側では僧帽筋と広背筋が取り除かれ，胸腰筋膜が見えている．*Note*：胸腰筋膜の浅葉が広背筋の腱膜起始部によって補強されている．

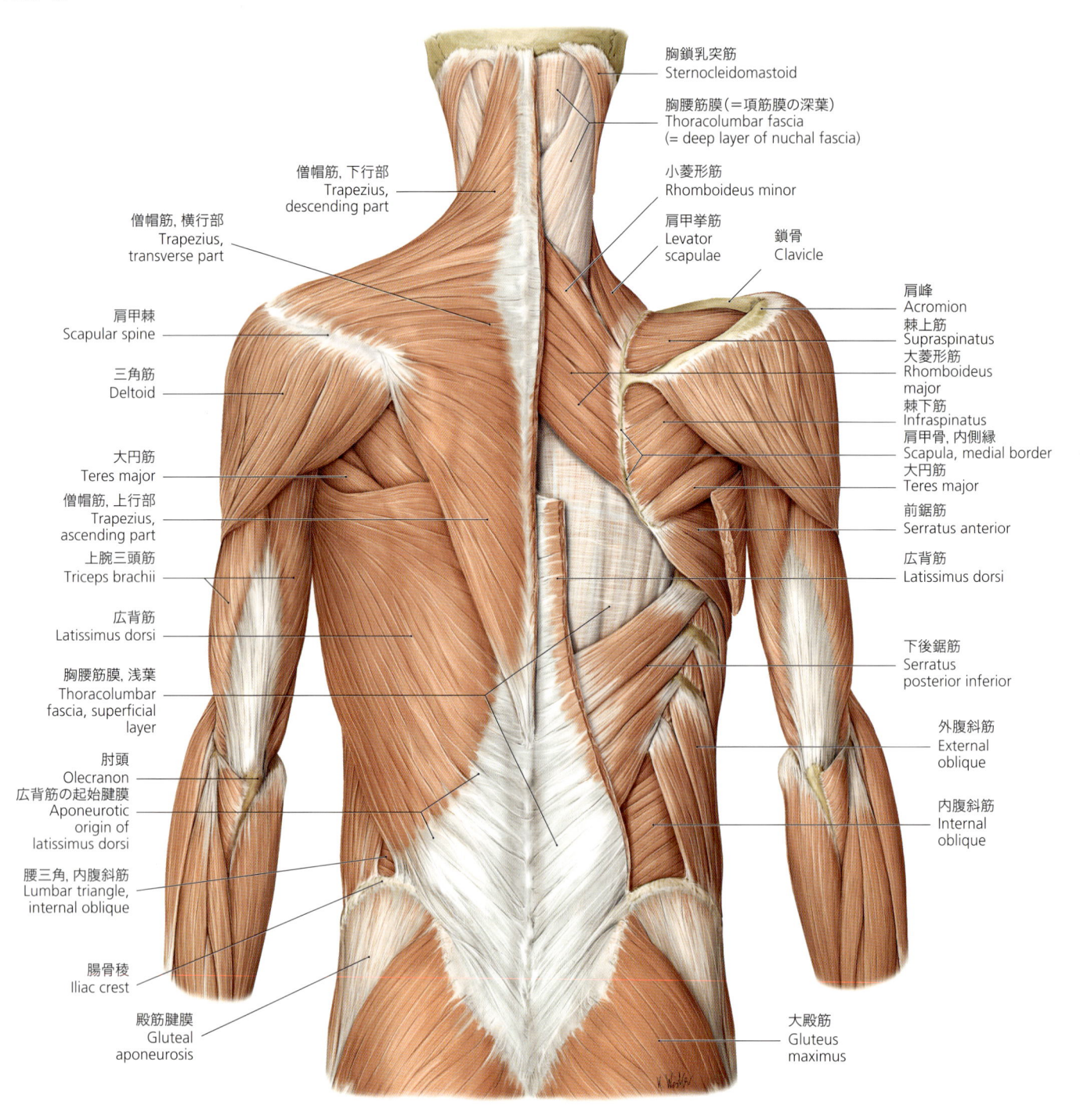

図2.2 胸腰筋膜

横断面を上方から見たところ．固有背筋は骨と線維で形成された管の中に隔離されている．この管を作るのは，胸腰筋膜，椎弓，棘突起，横突起である．胸腰筋膜は浅葉と深葉からなり，両者は固有背筋の外側縁で合わさっている．胸腰筋膜の浅葉は，頸部において項筋膜の深葉に連なる．深葉はさらに頸筋膜の椎前葉に連なる．

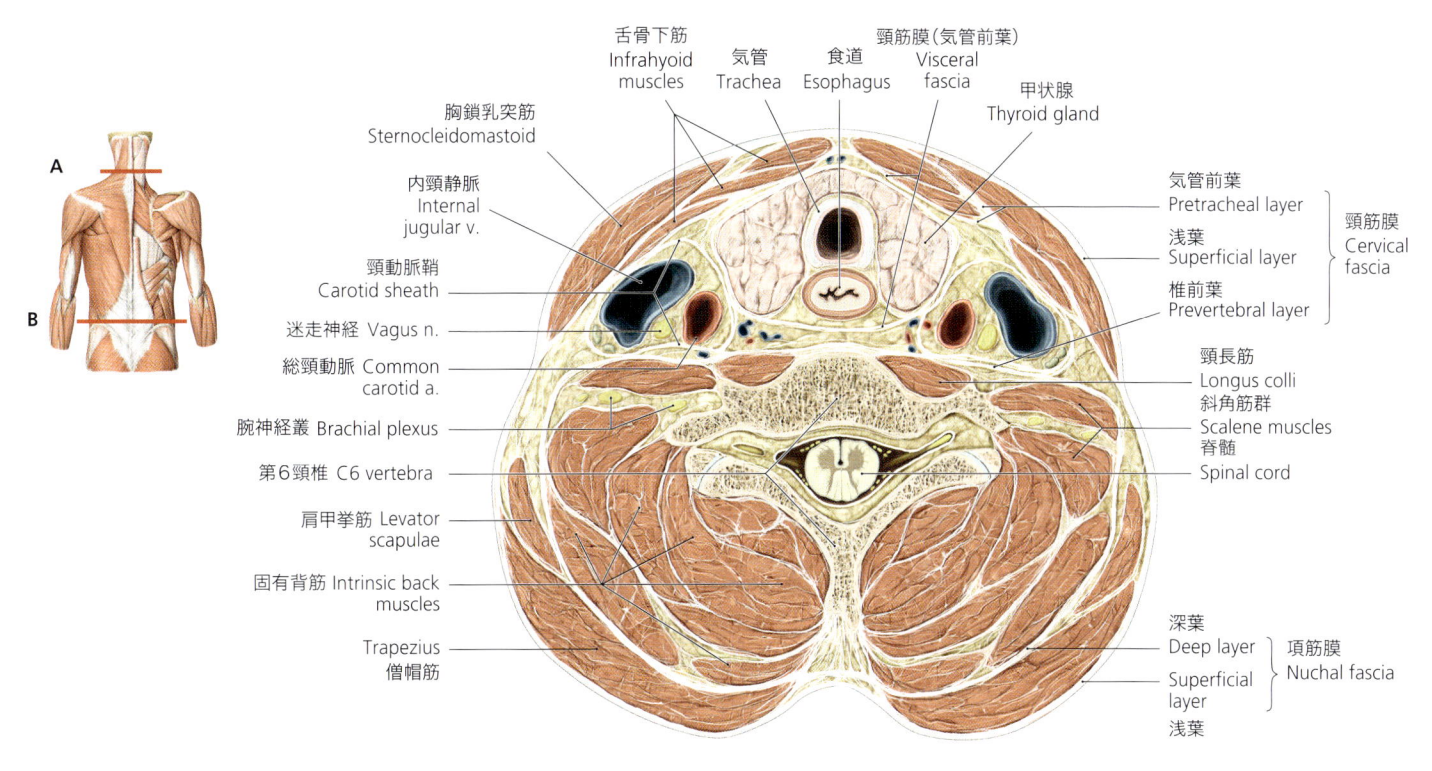

A C6の高さでの横断面．上方から見たところ．

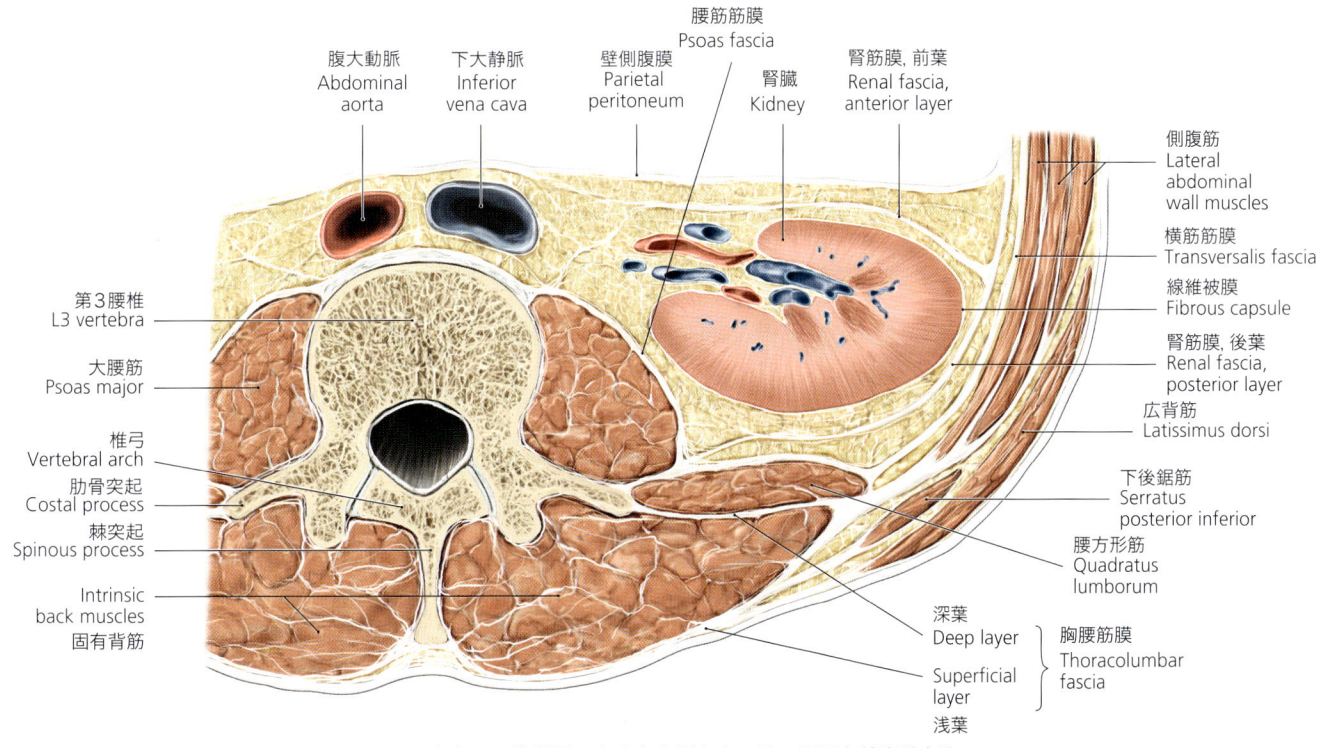

B L3の高さでの横断面．上方から見たところ．馬尾と前腹壁を取り除いてある．

頸部脊柱の固有筋
Intrinsic Muscles of the Cervical Spine

図 2.3　項部の筋
　後方から見たところ．右側では僧帽筋，胸鎖乳突筋，板状筋，半棘筋が取り除かれ，後頭下筋群が見えている．

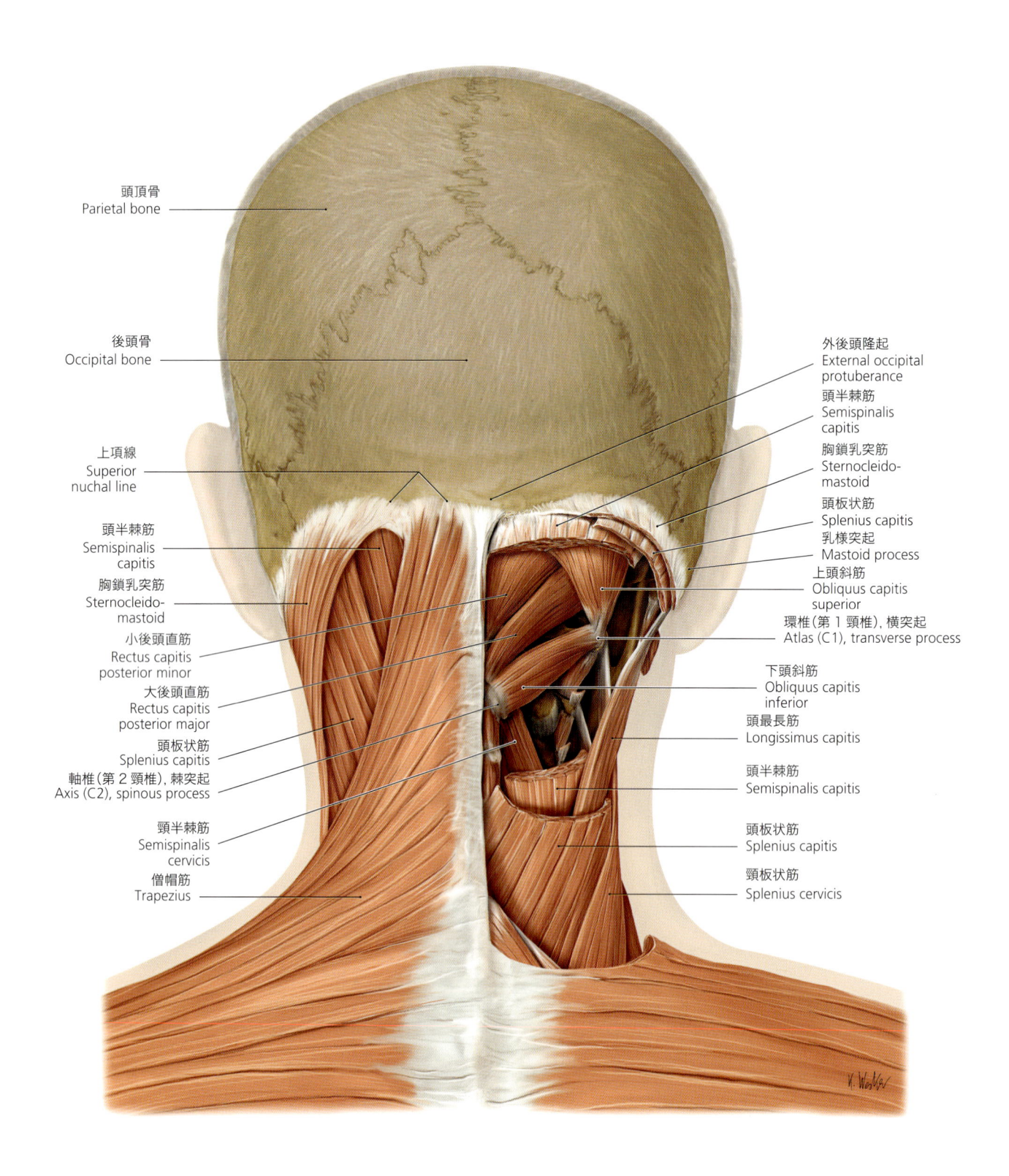

図2.4 短い項筋（後頭下筋群）

後方から見たところ．図2.6を参照．

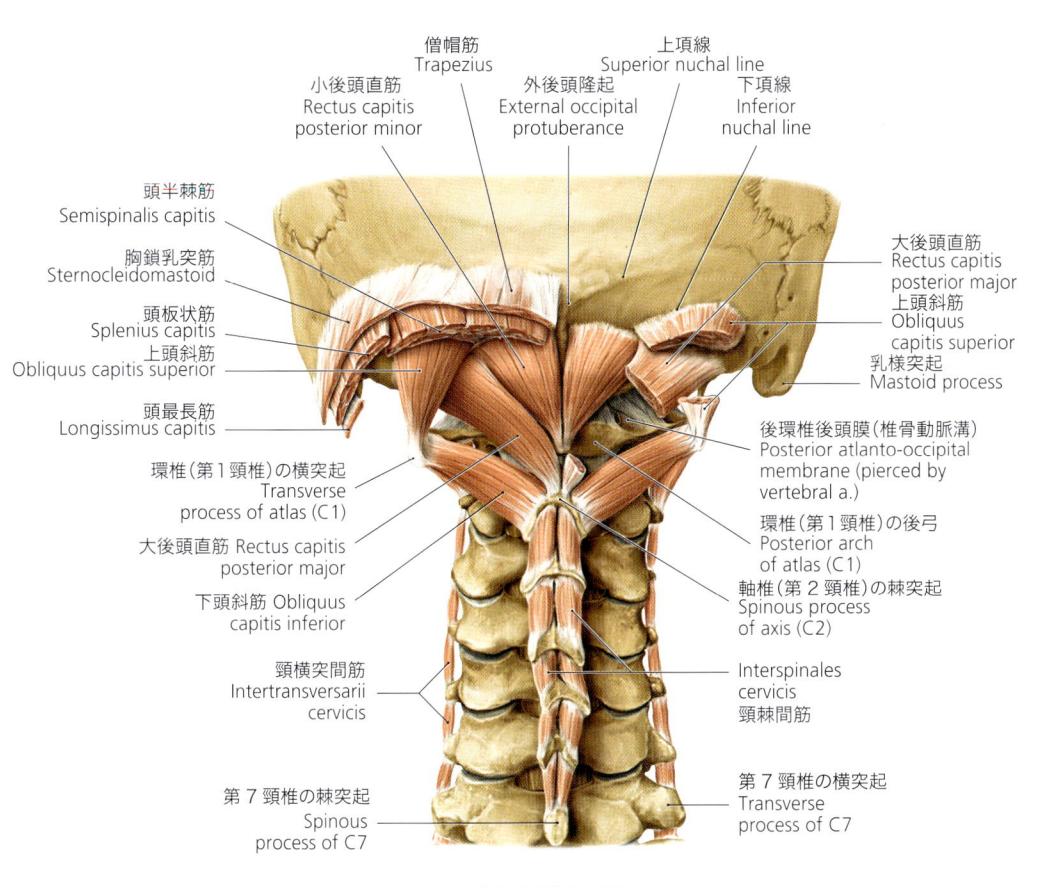

A 短い項筋の走行．

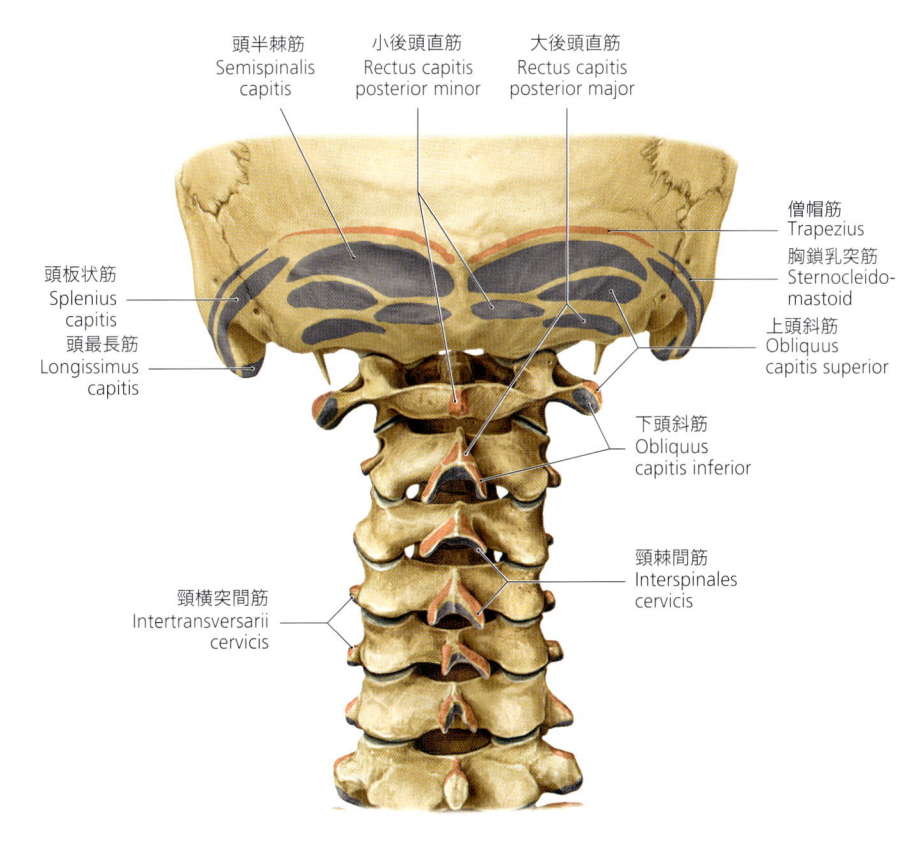

B 後頭下領域における筋の起始（赤）と停止（青）．

固有背筋
Intrinsic Muscles of the Back

> 外来背筋（僧帽筋，広背筋，肩甲挙筋，菱形筋）は第4部で扱う．後鋸筋は外来背筋の中間部と考えられているが，ここでは固有背筋の浅部に含める．

図 2.5　固有背筋
後方から見たところ．胸腰筋膜，固有背筋（浅部，中間部，深部）を順に剖出したところ．

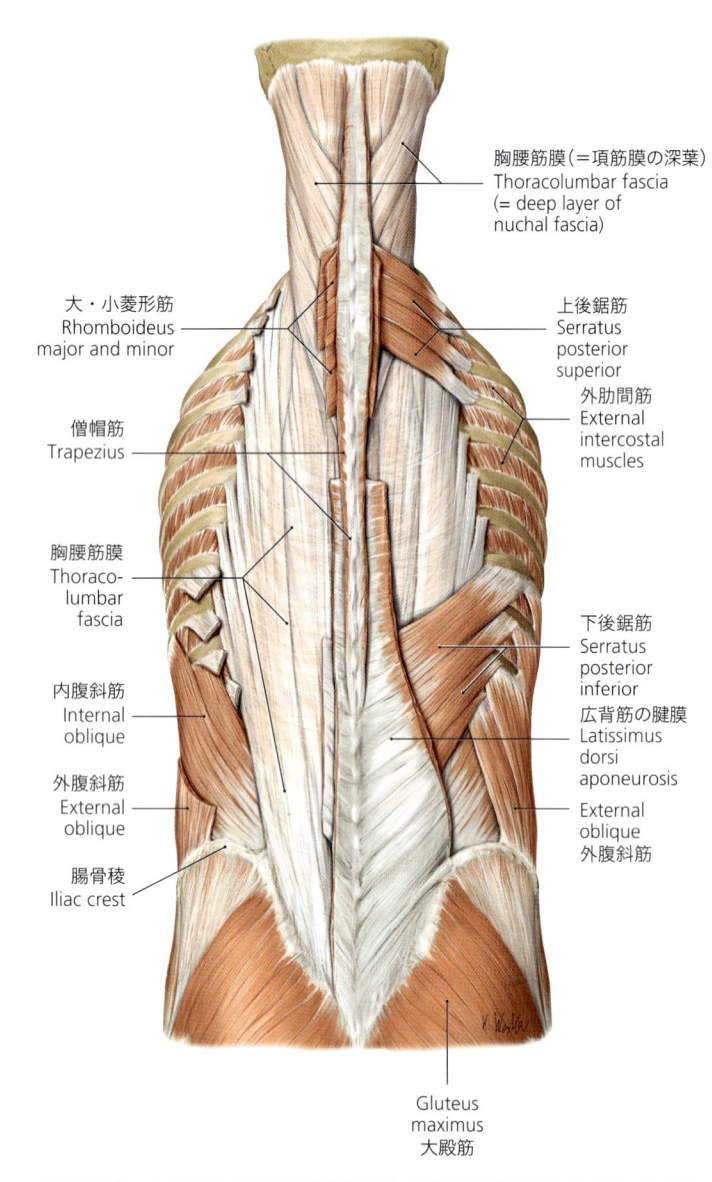

左図ラベル：
- 胸腰筋膜（＝項筋膜の深葉）Thoracolumbar fascia (= deep layer of nuchal fascia)
- 大・小菱形筋 Rhomboideus major and minor
- 上後鋸筋 Serratus posterior superior
- 僧帽筋 Trapezius
- 外肋間筋 External intercostal muscles
- 胸腰筋膜 Thoracolumbar fascia
- 下後鋸筋 Serratus posterior inferior
- 広背筋の腱膜 Latissimus dorsi aponeurosis
- 内腹斜筋 Internal oblique
- 外腹斜筋 External oblique
- 外腹斜筋 External oblique
- 腸骨稜 Iliac crest
- 大殿筋 Gluteus maximus

A 胸腰筋膜．上肢帯と外来背筋（後鋸筋と広背筋の腱膜起始部を除く）が取り除かれ，胸腰筋膜の浅葉が見えている．

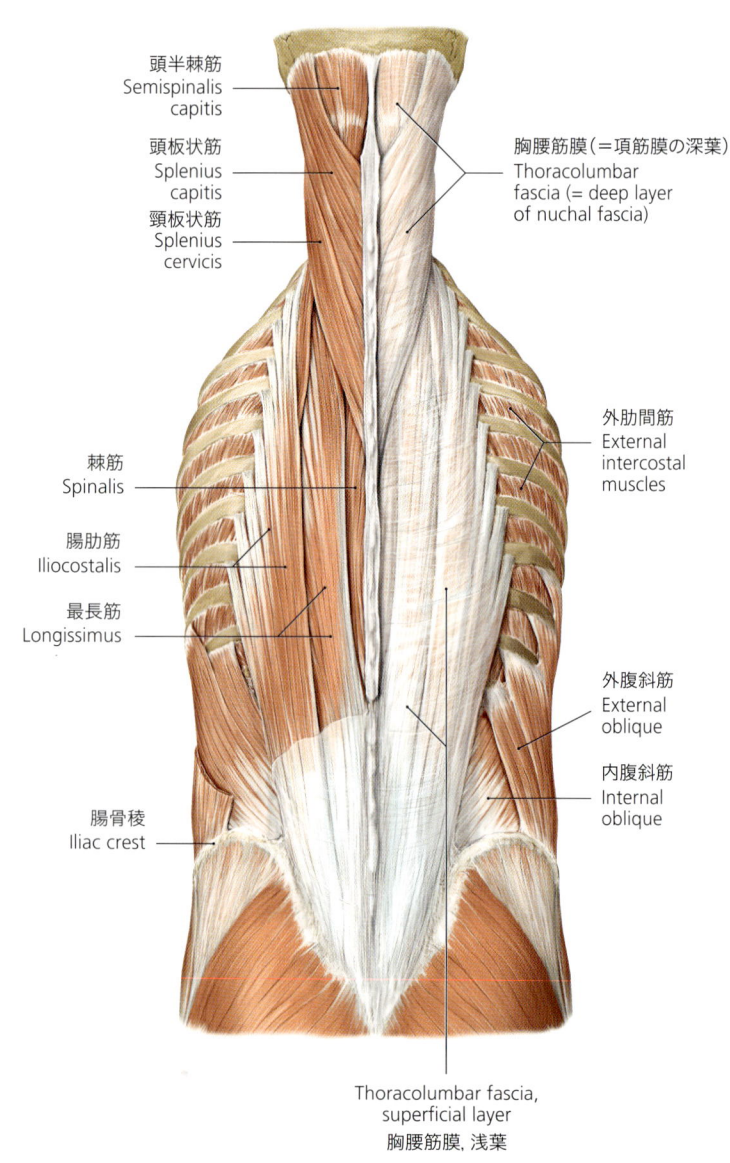

右図ラベル：
- 頭半棘筋 Semispinalis capitis
- 頭板状筋 Splenius capitis
- 頸板状筋 Splenius cervicis
- 胸腰筋膜（＝項筋膜の深葉）Thoracolumbar fascia (= deep layer of nuchal fascia)
- 棘筋 Spinalis
- 腸肋筋 Iliocostalis
- 最長筋 Longissimus
- 外肋間筋 External intercostal muscles
- 外腹斜筋 External oblique
- 内腹斜筋 Internal oblique
- 腸骨稜 Iliac crest
- 胸腰筋膜，浅葉 Thoracolumbar fascia, superficial layer

B 固有背筋の浅部と中間部．左側では胸腰筋膜が取り除かれ，脊柱起立筋と板状筋が見えている．

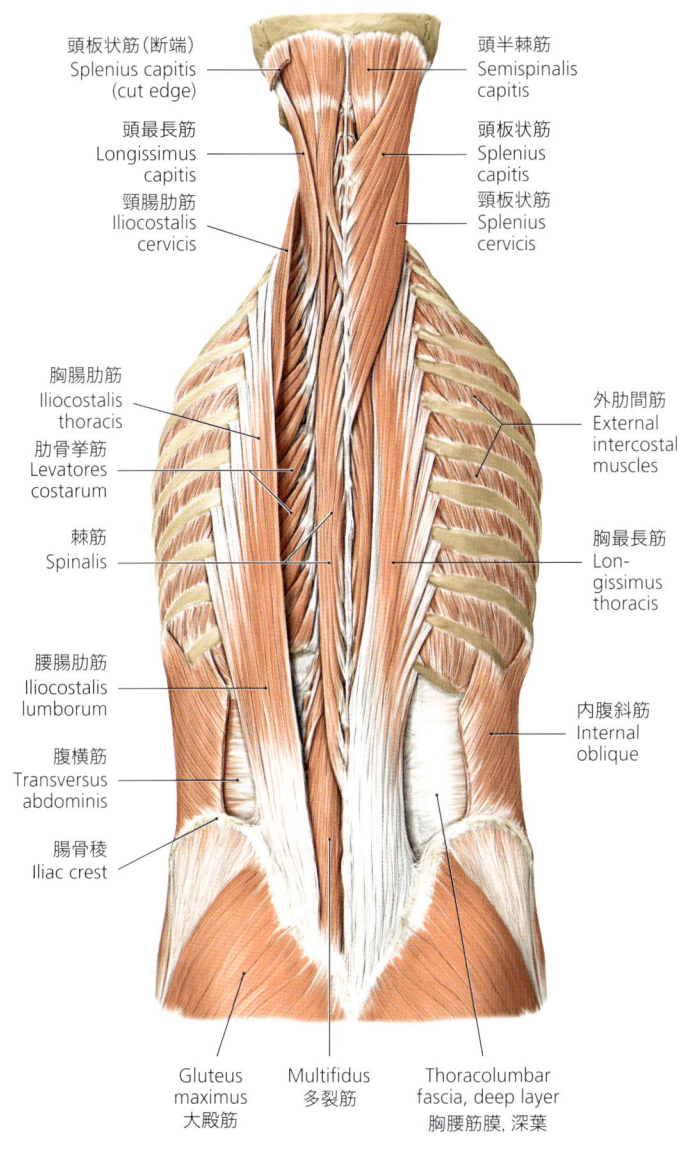

C 固有背筋の中間部と深部．左側では板状筋，頸最長筋，胸最長筋が取り除かれ，固有背筋の深部が見えている．また右側では腸肋筋が取り除かれている．*Note*：胸腰筋膜の深葉が内腹斜筋と腹横筋の起始となる．

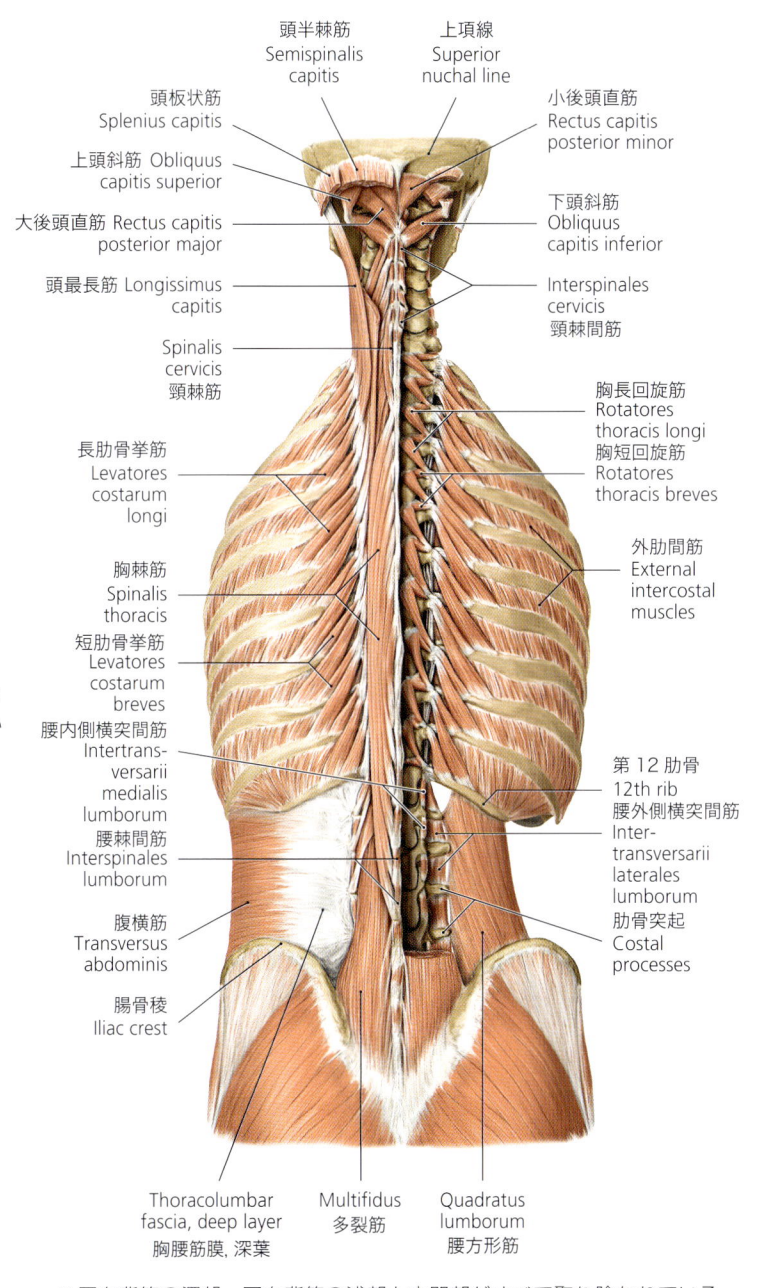

D 固有背筋の深部．固有背筋の浅部と中間部がすべて取り除かれている．また右側では，胸腰筋膜の深葉，棘筋，半棘筋，多裂筋が取り除かれ，回旋筋，横突間筋，腰方形筋が見えている．

個々の筋（1）
Muscle Facts (I)

図2.6　短い項筋（後頭下筋）

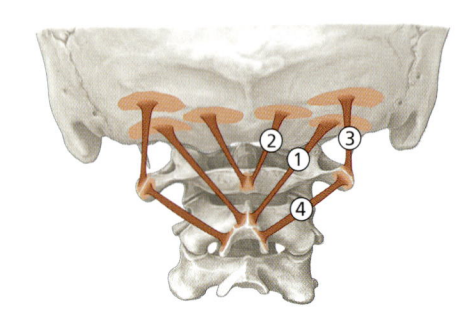

A 後方から見たところ．

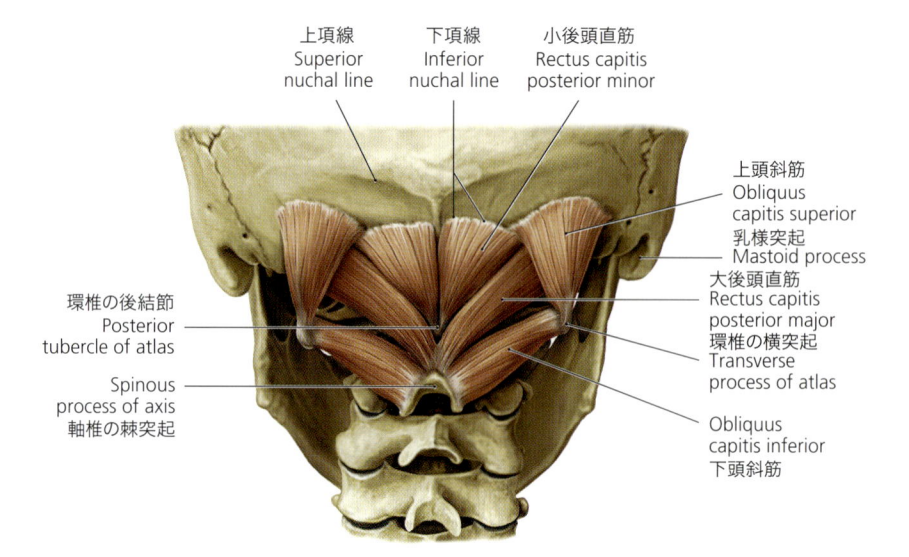

B 短い項筋，後方から見たところ．

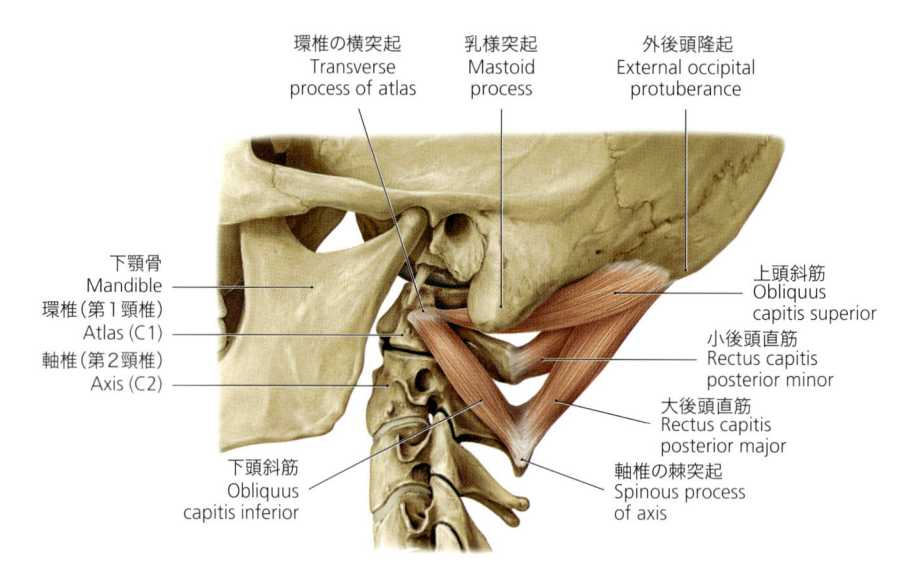

C 短い項筋，左側方から見たところ．

表2.1　短い項筋（後頭下筋）

筋		起始	停止	神経支配	作用
後頭直筋	①大後頭直筋	C2（棘突起）	後頭骨（下項線の中央3分の1）	C1の後枝（後頭下神経）	両側：頭を後屈させる，片側：頭を同側に回旋させる
	②小後頭直筋	C1（後結節）	後頭骨（下項線の内側3分の1）		
頭斜筋	③上頭斜筋	C1（横突起）	後頭骨（下項線の中央3分の1，大後頭直筋の停止の上方）		両側：頭を後屈させる 片側：頭を同側に傾けるとともに反対側に回旋させる
	④下頭斜筋	C2（棘突起）	C1（横突起）		両側：頭を後屈させる，片側：頭を同側に回旋させる

図2.7 椎前筋

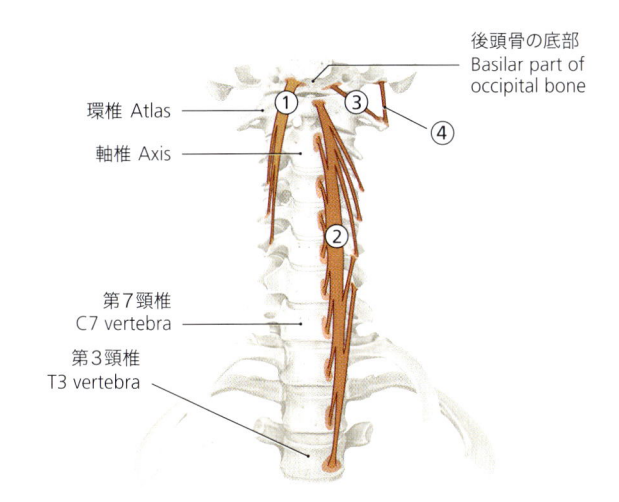

環椎 Atlas
軸椎 Axis
後頭骨の底部 Basilar part of occipital bone
第7頸椎 C7 vertebra
第3頸椎 T3 vertebra

A 前方から見たところ.

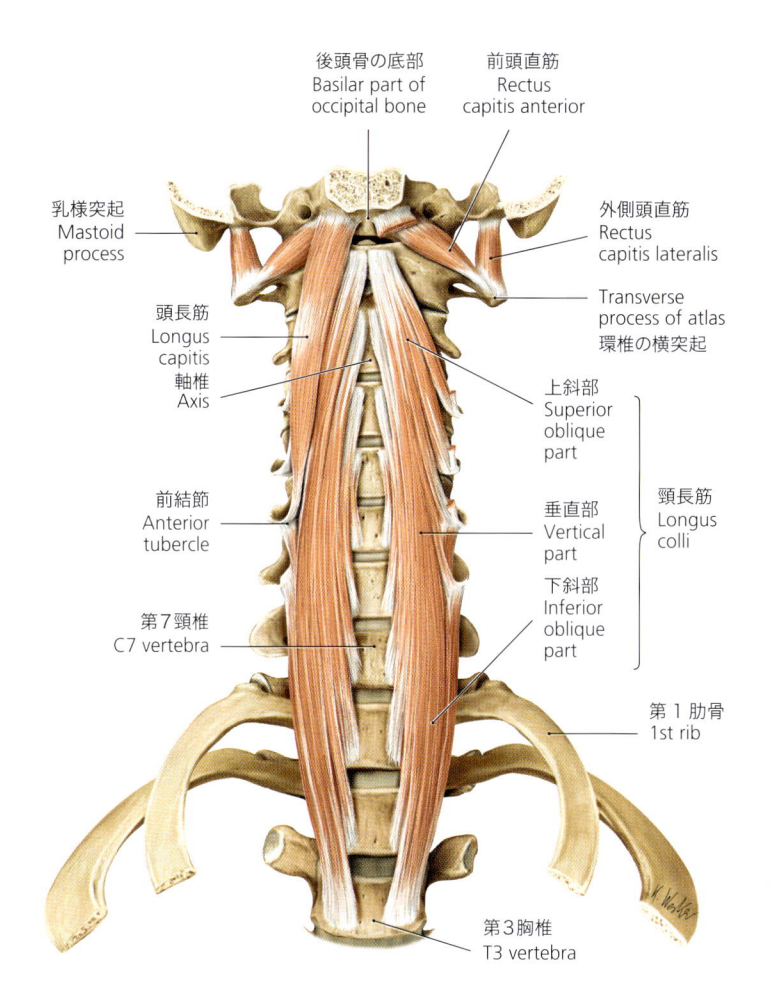

後頭骨の底部 Basilar part of occipital bone
前頭直筋 Rectus capitis anterior
乳様突起 Mastoid process
外側頭直筋 Rectus capitis lateralis
Transverse process of atlas 環椎の横突起
頭長筋 Longus capitis
軸椎 Axis
上斜部 Superior oblique part
前結節 Anterior tubercle
垂直部 Vertical part
下斜部 Inferior oblique part
頭長筋 Longus colli
第7頸椎 C7 vertebra
第1肋骨 1st rib
第3胸椎 T3 vertebra

B 椎前筋, 前方から見たところ. 頸部内臓と左の頭長筋が取り除かれている.

表2.2　椎前筋

筋		起始	停止	神経支配	作用
①頭長筋		C3-C6（横突起, 前結節）	後頭骨（底部）	頸神経叢からの枝（C1-C3）	両側: 頭を前屈させる 片側: 頭を同側に傾け, やや回旋させる
②頸長筋	垂直（内側）部	C5-T3（椎体の前面）	C2-C4（椎体の前面）	頸神経叢からの枝（C2-C6）	両側: 頸部脊柱を前屈させる 片側: 頸部脊柱を同側に側屈・回旋させる
	上斜部	C3-C5（横突起, 前結節）	C1（横突起, 前結節）		
	下斜部	T1-T3（椎体の前面）	C5-C6（横突起, 前結節）		
頭直筋	③前頭直筋	C1（外側塊）	後頭骨（底部）	C1（前枝）	両側: 環椎後頭関節で前屈させる 片側: 環椎後頭関節で側屈させる
	④外側頭直筋	C1（横突起）	後頭骨（底部, 後頭顆よりも外側）		

個々の筋(2)
Muscle Facts (II)

固有背筋は3層(浅層, 中間層, 深層)に分けられ, それぞれ脊髄神経の後枝によって支配される. 後鋸筋は脊髄神経の前枝(肋間神経)によって支配され, 本来は外来背筋に分類される. しかし, 後鋸筋は固有背筋を解剖する際に現れるので, 本項に含めてある.

表2.3 固有背筋の浅層

筋		起始	停止	神経支配	作用
後鋸筋	①上後鋸筋	項靱帯, C7-T3(棘突起)	第2-4肋骨(上縁)	第2-5肋間神経	肋骨を引き上げる
	②下後鋸筋	T11-L2(棘突起)	第8-12肋骨(肋骨角付近の下縁)	第9-12胸神経(前枝)	肋骨を引き下げる
板状筋	③頭板状筋	項靱帯, C3-T3(棘突起)	後頭骨(上項線の外側部, 乳様突起)	第1-6頸神経(後枝の外側枝)	両側:頭と頸部脊柱を後屈させる 片側:頭を同側に側屈・回旋させる
	④頸板状筋	T3-T6(棘突起)	C1-C2(横突起)		

図2.8 固有背筋の浅層(模式図)
右側, 後方から見たところ.

図2.9 固有背筋の中間層(模式図)
右側, 後方から見たところ. これらの筋は総称して脊柱起立筋と呼ばれる.

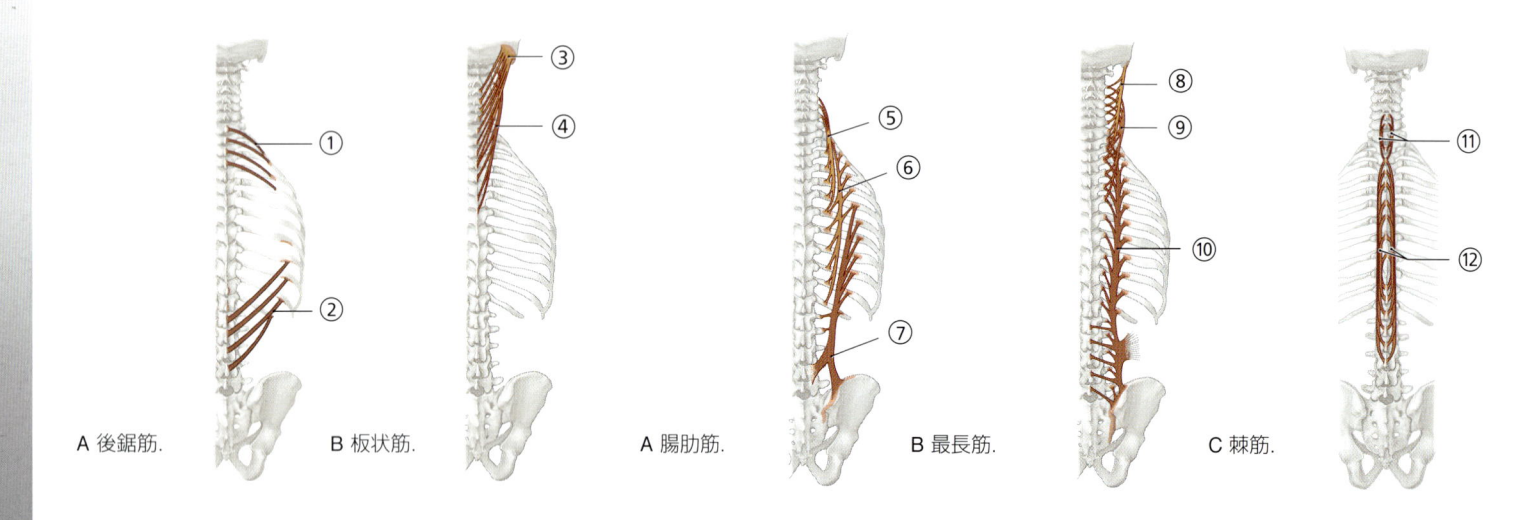

A 後鋸筋. B 板状筋. A 腸肋筋. B 最長筋. C 棘筋.

表2.4 固有背筋の中間層

筋		起始	停止	神経支配	作用
腸肋筋	⑤頸腸肋筋	第3-7肋骨	C4-C6(横突起)	第8頸神経-第1腰神経(後枝の外側枝)	両側:脊柱を伸展させる 片側:脊柱を同側に側屈させる
	⑥胸腸肋筋	第3-12肋骨	第1-6肋骨		
	⑦腰腸肋筋	仙骨, 腸骨稜, 胸腰筋膜	第6-12肋骨, 胸腰筋膜(深葉), 上位腰椎(肋骨突起)		
最長筋	⑧頭最長筋	C4-C7(横突起, 前結節), T1-T3(横突起)	側頭骨(乳様突起)	第1頸神経-第5腰神経(後枝の外側枝)	両側:頭部を後屈させる 片側:頭部を同側に側屈・回旋させる
	⑨頸最長筋	T1-T6(横突起)	C2-C5(横突起)		両側:脊柱を伸展させる 片側:脊柱を同側に側屈させる
	⑩胸最長筋	仙骨, 腸骨稜, 腰椎(棘突起), 下位胸椎(横突起)	第2-12肋骨, 腰椎(肋骨突起), 胸椎(横突起)		
棘筋	⑪頸棘筋	C5-T2(棘突起)	C2-C5(棘突起)	脊髄神経の後枝	両側:頸胸部の脊柱を伸展させる 片側:頸胸部の脊柱を同側に側屈させる
	⑫胸棘筋	T10-L3(棘突起の外側面)	T2-T8(棘突起の外側面)		

図 2.10 固有背筋の浅層と中間層
後方から見たところ.

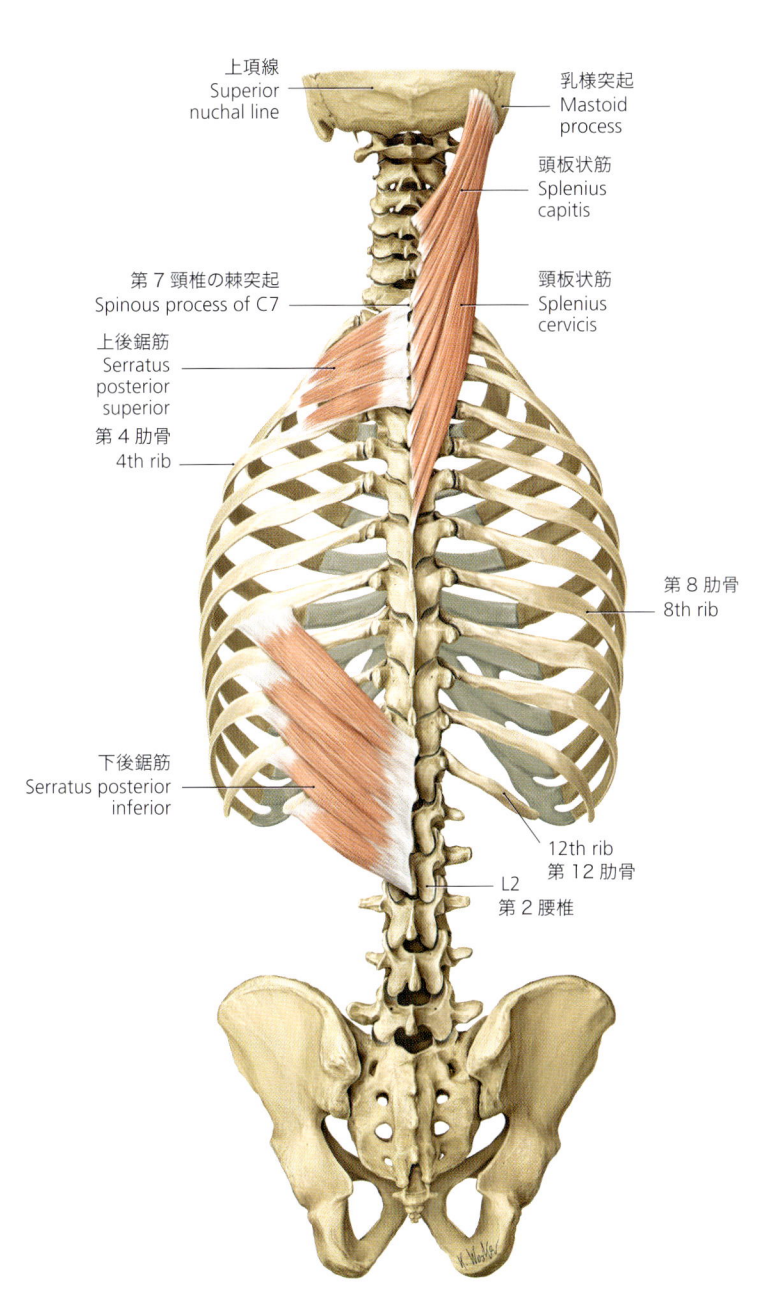

A 板状筋と後鋸筋.

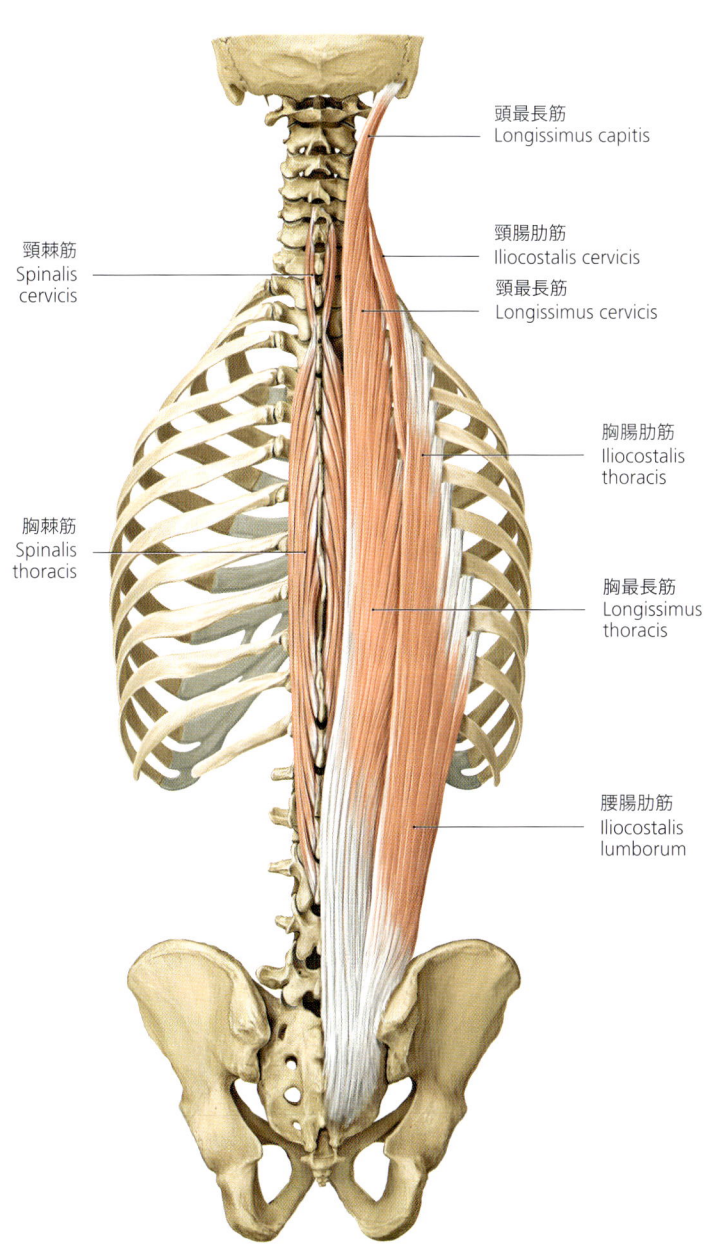

- 上項線 Superior nuchal line
- 乳様突起 Mastoid process
- 頭板状筋 Splenius capitis
- 第 7 頸椎の棘突起 Spinous process of C7
- 頸板状筋 Splenius cervicis
- 上後鋸筋 Serratus posterior superior
- 第 4 肋骨 4th rib
- 第 8 肋骨 8th rib
- 下後鋸筋 Serratus posterior inferior
- 12th rib 第 12 肋骨
- L2 第 2 腰椎

B 脊柱起立筋：腸肋筋，最長筋，棘筋.

- 頭最長筋 Longissimus capitis
- 頸棘筋 Spinalis cervicis
- 頸腸肋筋 Iliocostalis cervicis
- 頸最長筋 Longissimus cervicis
- 胸腸肋筋 Iliocostalis thoracis
- 胸棘筋 Spinalis thoracis
- 胸最長筋 Longissimus thoracis
- 腰腸肋筋 Iliocostalis lumborum

個々の筋(3)
Muscle Facts (III)

> 固有背筋の深層はさらに2つのグループ（横突棘筋と深分節筋）に分けられる．横突棘筋は椎骨の横突起と棘突起の間を走る．

表2.5　横突棘筋

筋		起始	停止	神経支配	作用
回旋筋	①短回旋筋	T1-T12（胸椎の横突起と1つ上位の椎骨の棘突起を結ぶ）		脊髄神経の後枝	両側：頸部の脊柱を伸展させる， 片側：脊柱を反対側に回旋させる
	②長回旋筋	T1-T12（胸椎の横突起と2つ上位の椎骨の棘突起を結ぶ）			
	③多裂筋	C2-仙骨（横突起と3～5つ上位の椎骨の棘突起を結ぶ）			両側：頸部の脊柱を伸展させる， 片側：脊柱を同側に側屈させ，反対側に回旋させる
半棘筋	④頭半棘筋	C4-T7（横突起，関節突起）	後頭骨（上項線と下項線の間）		両側：頸胸部の脊柱を伸展させる，また頭部を後屈させる（頭椎関節を安定化させる） 片側：頭部と頸胸部の脊柱を同側に側屈させ，反対側に回旋させる
	⑤頸半棘筋	T1-T6（横突起）	C2-C5（棘突起）		
	⑥胸半棘筋	T6-T12（横突起）	C6-T4（棘突起）		

図2.11　横突棘筋（模式図）
後方から見たところ．

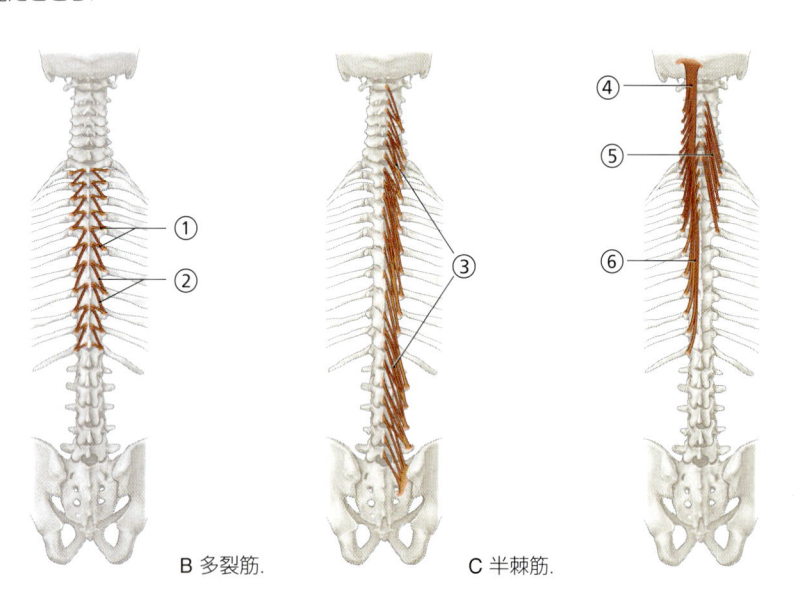

A 回旋筋．　B 多裂筋．　C 半棘筋．

図2.12　深分節筋（模式図）
後方から見たところ．

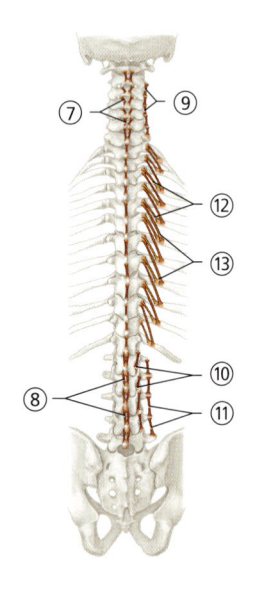

表2.6　深分節筋

筋		起始	停止	神経支配	作用
棘間筋*	⑦頸棘間筋	C1-C7（隣接する頸椎の棘突起を結ぶ）		脊髄神経の後枝	頸部と腰部の脊柱を伸展させる
	⑧腰棘間筋	L1-L5（隣接する腰椎の棘突起を結ぶ）			
横突間筋*	頸前横突間筋	C2-C7（隣接する頸椎の前結節を結ぶ）		脊髄神経の前枝	両側：頸部と腰部の脊柱を伸展，安定化させる 片側：頸部と腰部の脊柱を同側に側屈させる
	⑨頸後横突間筋	C2-C7（隣接する頸椎の後結節を結ぶ）			
	⑩腰内側横突間筋	L1-L5（隣接する腰椎の乳頭突起を結ぶ）		脊髄神経の後枝	
	⑪腰外側横突間筋	L1-L5（隣接する腰椎の肋骨突起を結ぶ）			
肋骨挙筋	⑫短肋骨挙筋	C7-T11（横突起）	1つ下位の肋骨の肋骨角		両側：胸部脊柱を伸展させる 片側：胸部脊柱を同側に側屈させ，反対側に回旋させる
	⑬長肋骨挙筋		2つ下位の肋骨の肋骨角		

*棘間筋と横突間筋の両者は脊柱の全体にわたって存在する．

図 2.13 固有背筋の深層
後方から見たところ．

労働者用ラベル：
- 上項線 Superior nuchal line
- 下項線 Inferior nuchal line
- 頭半棘筋 Semispinalis capitis
- 頸半棘筋 Semispinalis cervicis
- 第7頸椎の棘突起 Spinous process of C7
- 胸半棘筋 Semispinalis thoracis
- 横突起 Transverse process
- 棘突起 Spinous process
- Rotatores longi 長回旋筋
- 短回旋筋 Rotatores breves
- 肋骨突起 Costal processes
- 多裂筋 Multifidus
- 仙骨 Sacrum

A 横突棘筋：回旋筋，多裂筋，半棘筋．

- 頸棘間筋 Interspinalis cervicis
- 頸後横突間筋 Intertransversarii posteriores cervicis
- 長肋骨挙筋 Levatores costarum longi
- 短肋骨挙筋 Levatores costarum breves
- Intertransversarii mediales lumborum 腰内側横突間筋
- Interspinalis lumborum 腰棘間筋
- Intertransversarii lateralis lumborum 腰外側横突間筋

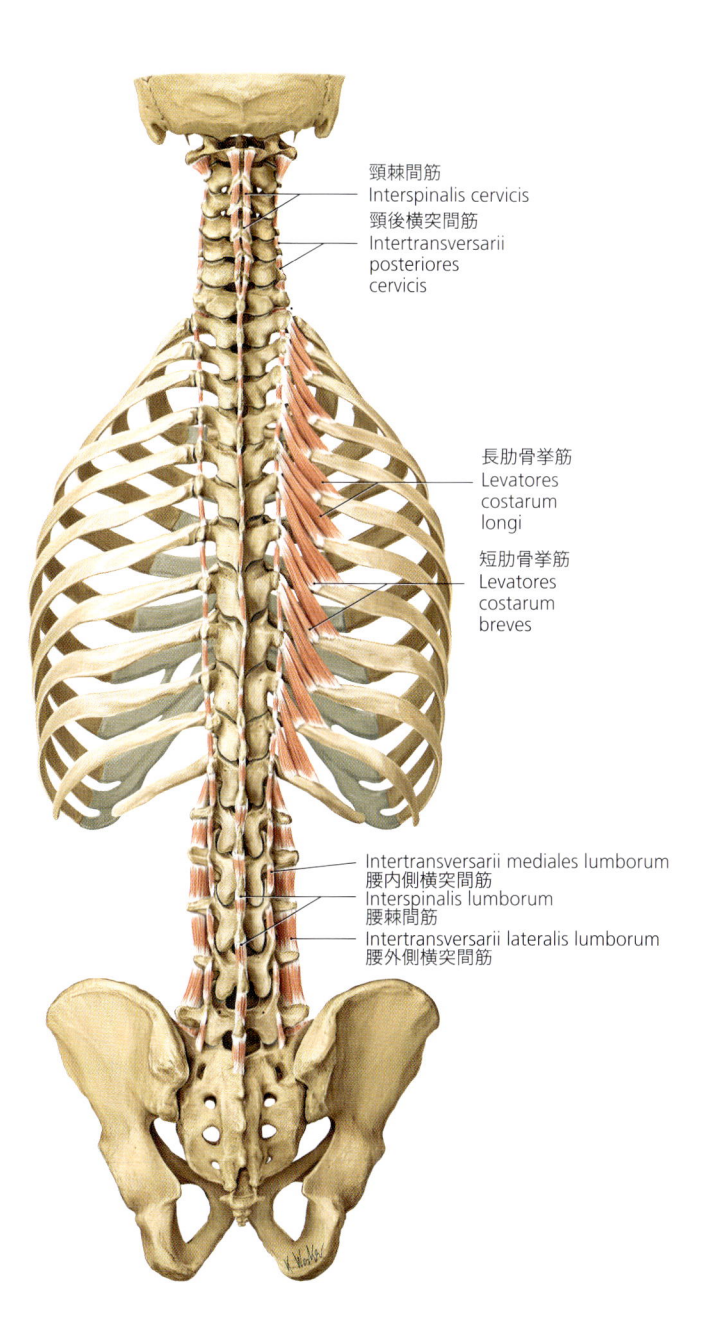

B 深分節筋：棘間筋，横突間筋，肋骨挙筋．

背部の動脈と静脈
Arteries & Veins of the Back

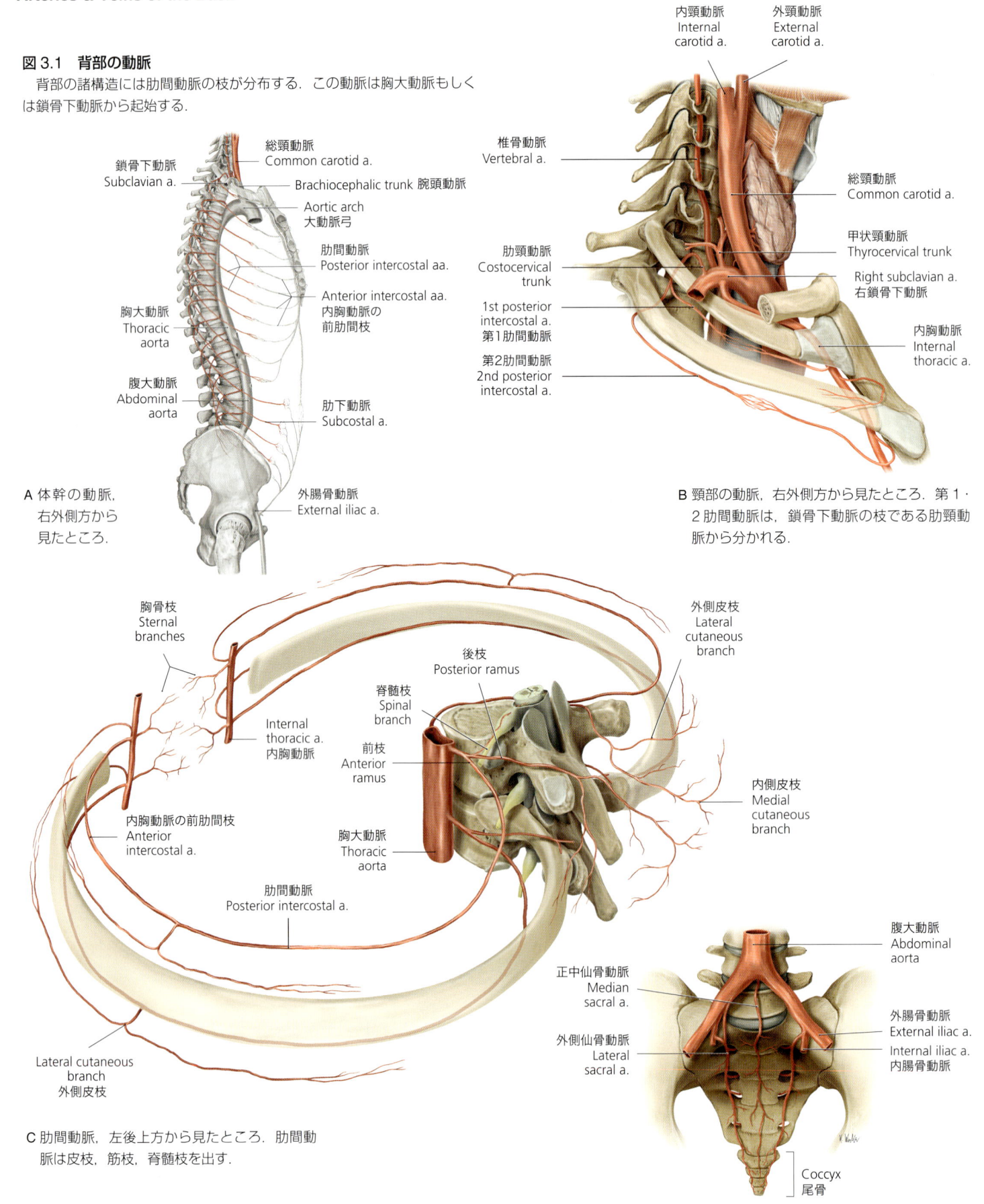

図3.1 背部の動脈
背部の諸構造には肋間動脈の枝が分布する．この動脈は胸大動脈もしくは鎖骨下動脈から起始する．

A 体幹の動脈，右外側方から見たところ．

- 鎖骨下動脈 Subclavian a.
- 総頸動脈 Common carotid a.
- Brachiocephalic trunk 腕頭動脈
- Aortic arch 大動脈弓
- 肋間動脈 Posterior intercostal aa.
- Anterior intercostal aa. 内胸動脈の前肋間枝
- 胸大動脈 Thoracic aorta
- 腹大動脈 Abdominal aorta
- 肋下動脈 Subcostal a.
- 外腸骨動脈 External iliac a.

B 頸部の動脈，右外側方から見たところ．第1・2肋間動脈は，鎖骨下動脈の枝である肋頸動脈から分かれる．

- 内頸動脈 Internal carotid a.
- 外頸動脈 External carotid a.
- 椎骨動脈 Vertebral a.
- 総頸動脈 Common carotid a.
- 甲状頸動脈 Thyrocervical trunk
- 肋頸動脈 Costocervical trunk
- Right subclavian a. 右鎖骨下動脈
- 第1肋間動脈 1st posterior intercostal a.
- 第2肋間動脈 2nd posterior intercostal a.
- 内胸動脈 Internal thoracic a.

C 肋間動脈，左後上方から見たところ．肋間動脈は皮枝，筋枝，脊髄枝を出す．

- 胸骨枝 Sternal branches
- 内胸動脈 Internal thoracic a.
- 内胸動脈の前肋間枝 Anterior intercostal a.
- 後枝 Posterior ramus
- 脊髄枝 Spinal branch
- 前枝 Anterior ramus
- 胸大動脈 Thoracic aorta
- 外側皮枝 Lateral cutaneous branch
- 内側皮枝 Medial cutaneous branch
- 肋間動脈 Posterior intercostal a.
- 外側皮枝 Lateral cutaneous branch

D 仙骨の動脈，前方から見たところ．

- 腹大動脈 Abdominal aorta
- 正中仙骨動脈 Median sacral a.
- 外側仙骨動脈 Lateral sacral a.
- 外腸骨動脈 External iliac a.
- 内腸骨動脈 Internal iliac a.
- Coccyx 尾骨

図 3.2 背部の静脈

背部の静脈は，上肋間静脈，半奇静脈，上行腰静脈などを介して，奇静脈へ連なる．脊柱内部の静脈血は椎骨静脈叢に流れ込む．この静脈叢は脊柱に沿って連なっている．

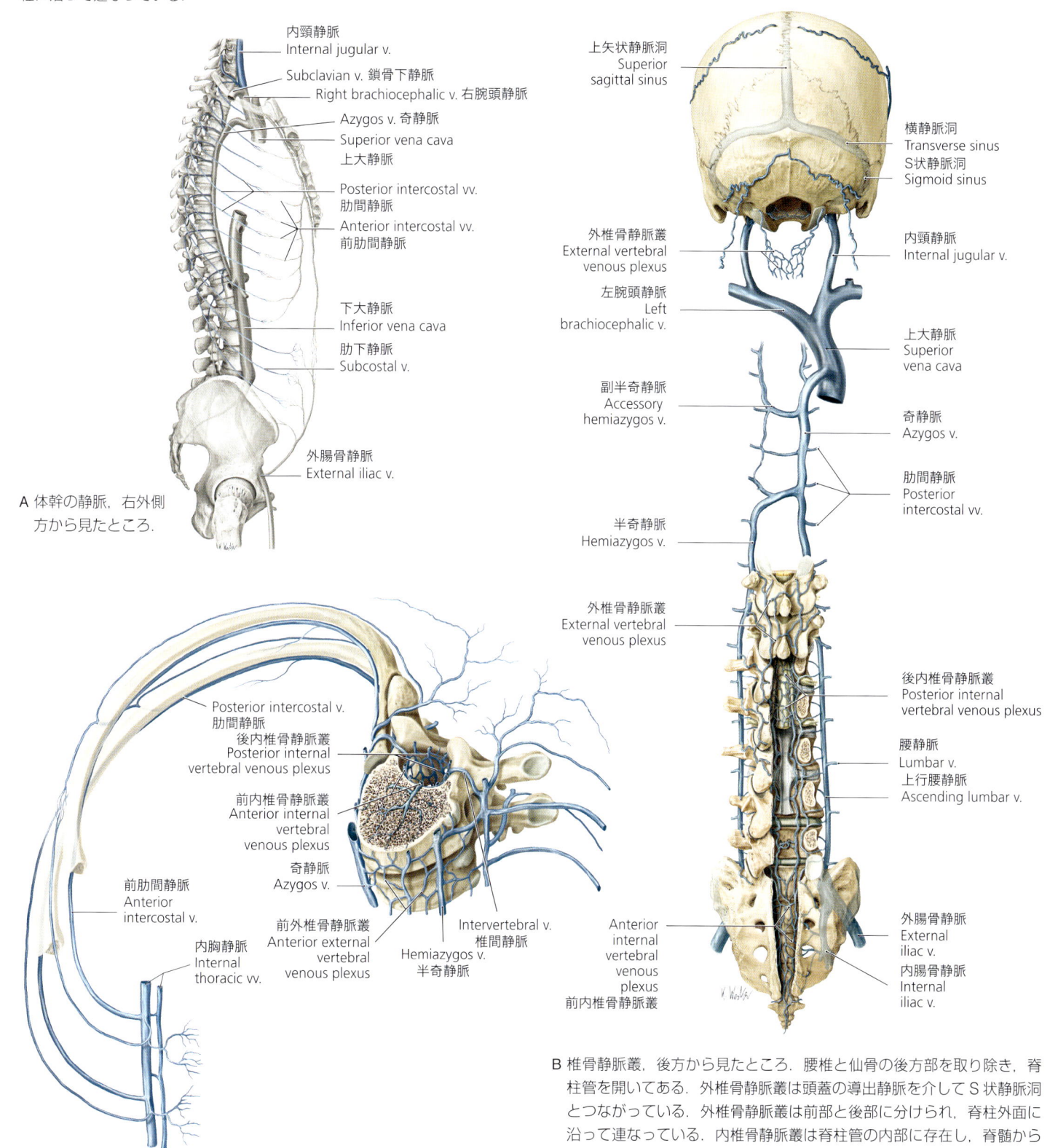

A 体幹の静脈，右外側方から見たところ．

C 肋間静脈と椎骨静脈叢，左前上方から見たところ．肋間静脈は肋間動脈・神経と同じように走行する（pp.34，36 参照）．*Note*：前外椎骨静脈叢が奇静脈とつながっている．

B 椎骨静脈叢，後方から見たところ．腰椎と仙骨の後方部を取り除き，脊柱管を開いてある．外椎骨静脈叢は頭蓋の導出静脈を介してS状静脈洞とつながっている．外椎骨静脈叢は前部と後部に分けられ，脊柱外面に沿って連なっている．内椎骨静脈叢は脊柱管の内部に存在し，脊髄からの静脈血が流れ込む．内椎骨静脈叢も前部と後部に分けられる．

3 神経、血管

背部の神経
Nerves of the Back

> 背部の諸構造には脊髄神経の枝が分布する．脊髄神経の後枝は固有背筋を支配し，前枝は外来背筋を支配する．

図3.3 背部の神経

脊髄神経(T1–T11)の前枝は肋間神経となる．この神経は肋骨に沿って走り，外側皮枝と前皮枝を分枝する．

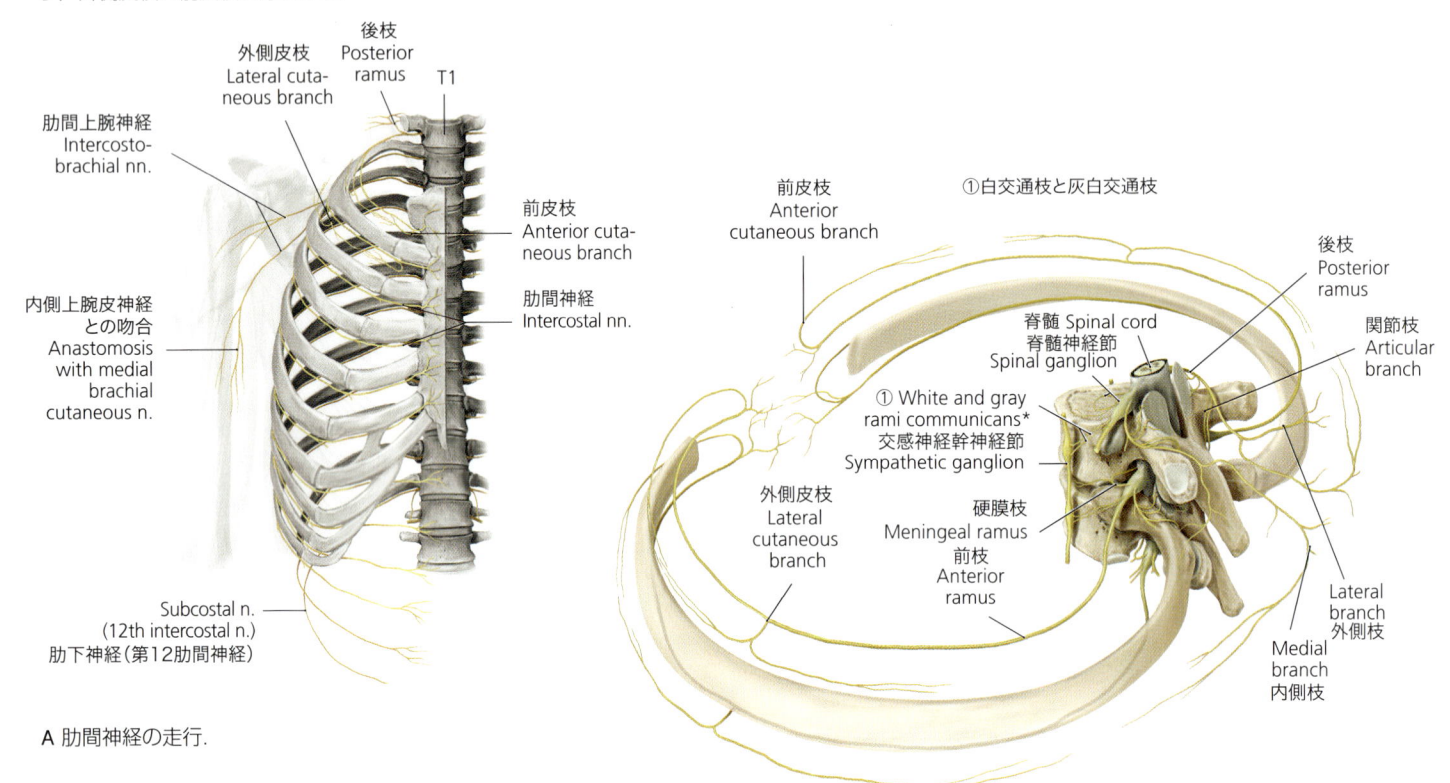

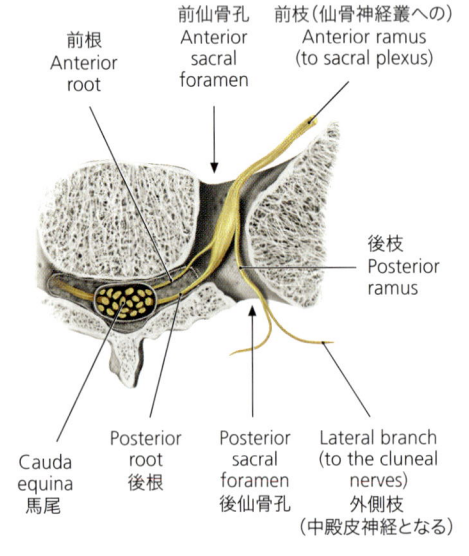

A 肋間神経の走行．

主な標識：
- 後枝 Posterior ramus
- 外側皮枝 Lateral cutaneous branch
- 肋間上腕神経 Intercostobrachial nn.
- 内側上腕皮神経との吻合 Anastomosis with medial brachial cutaneous n.
- 前皮枝 Anterior cutaneous branch
- 肋間神経 Intercostal nn.
- 肋下神経（第12肋間神経）Subcostal n. (12th intercostal n.)

B 脊髄神経の枝，左後上方から見たところ．脊髄神経の後枝は，椎間関節に枝を出し，筋枝と皮枝に分かれる．脊髄神経(T1–T11)の前枝は肋間神経となる(T12の前枝は肋下神経となる)．

主な標識：
- 前皮枝 Anterior cutaneous branch
- ①白交通枝と灰白交通枝
- 脊髄 Spinal cord
- 脊髄神経節 Spinal ganglion
- 後枝 Posterior ramus
- 関節枝 Articular branch
- ① White and gray rami communicans*
- 交感神経幹神経節 Sympathetic ganglion
- 外側皮枝 Lateral cutaneous branch
- 硬膜枝 Meningeal ramus
- 前枝 Anterior ramus
- 外側枝 Lateral branch
- 内側枝 Medial branch

C 仙骨孔における仙骨神経の枝．左の仙骨孔を通る横断面，上方から見たところ．

主な標識：
- 前根 Anterior root
- 前仙骨孔 Anterior sacral foramen
- 前枝（仙骨神経叢への）Anterior ramus (to sacral plexus)
- 後枝 Posterior ramus
- 馬尾 Cauda equina
- 後根 Posterior root
- 後仙骨孔 Posterior sacral foramen
- 外側枝（中殿皮神経となる）Lateral branch (to the cluneal nerves)

表3.1 脊髄神経の枝

枝			分布
硬膜枝			脊髄硬膜，脊柱の靱帯
後枝	内側枝	関節枝	椎間関節
		筋枝	固有背筋
		皮枝	後頭部，後頸部，背部，殿部の皮膚
	外側枝	皮枝	
		筋枝	固有背筋
前枝	外側皮枝		胸郭側壁の皮膚
	前皮枝		胸郭前壁の皮膚

*白交通枝と灰白交通枝は交感神経幹と脊髄神経とを結び，それぞれ節前線維と節後線維を含む(p. 622参照)．

図 3.4 項部の神経

右側，後方から見たところ．背部と同様に，項部の諸構造にも脊髄神経の後枝に由来する運動神経と感覚神経が分布する．C1-C3 の後枝は別名が付いており，後頭下神経（C1），大後頭神経（C2），第 3 後頭神経（C3）と呼ばれる．小後頭神経と大耳介神経は C2-C4 の前枝に由来し，頭部と頸部の前外側部の皮膚に分布する．また，C1-C4 の前枝は頸神経ワナを形成する．このワナから出る枝は舌骨下筋を支配する（p.562 参照）．

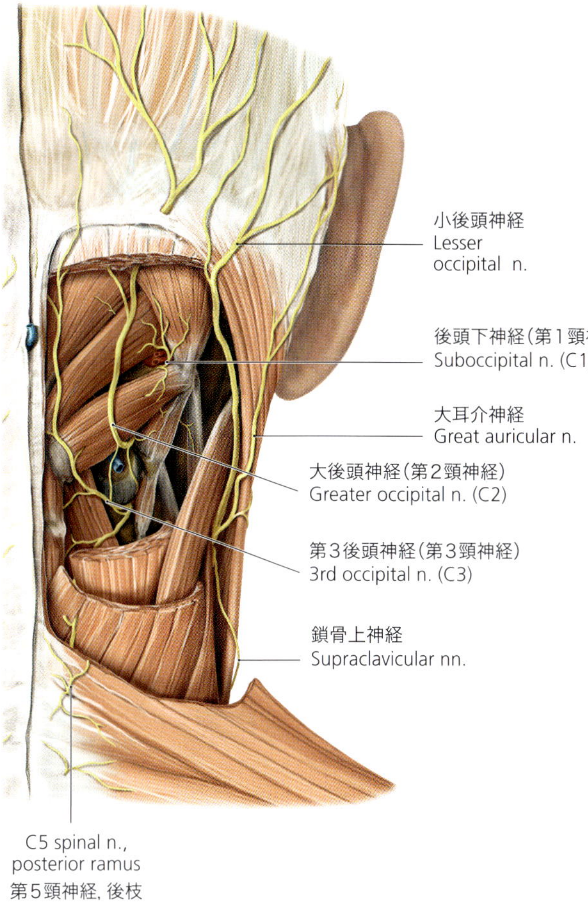

- 小後頭神経 Lesser occipital n.
- 後頭下神経（第1頸神経）Suboccipital n. (C1)
- 大耳介神経 Great auricular n.
- 大後頭神経（第2頸神経）Greater occipital n. (C2)
- 第3後頭神経（第3頸神経）3rd occipital n. (C3)
- 鎖骨上神経 Supraclavicular nn.
- C5 spinal n., posterior ramus 第5頸神経，後枝

図 3.5 背部皮膚の神経分布

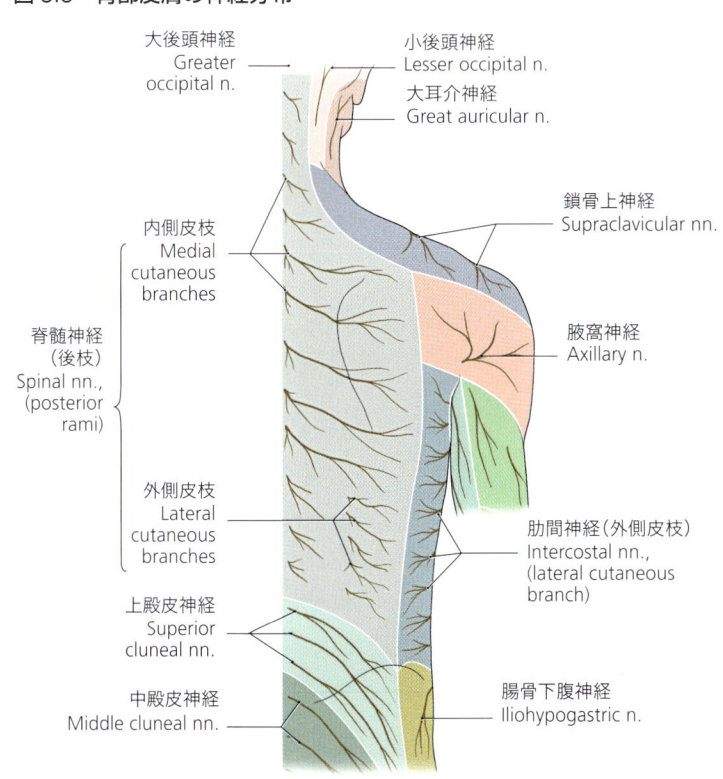

- 大後頭神経 Greater occipital n.
- 小後頭神経 Lesser occipital n.
- 大耳介神経 Great auricular n.
- 鎖骨上神経 Supraclavicular nn.
- 内側皮枝 Medial cutaneous branches
- 腋窩神経 Axillary n.
- 脊髄神経（後枝）Spinal nn., (posterior rami)
- 外側皮枝 Lateral cutaneous branches
- 肋間神経（外側皮枝）Intercostal nn., (lateral cutaneous branch)
- 上殿皮神経 Superior cluneal nn.
- 中殿皮神経 Middle cluneal nn.
- 腸骨下腹神経 Iliohypogastric n.

A 背部の皮神経とその分布．

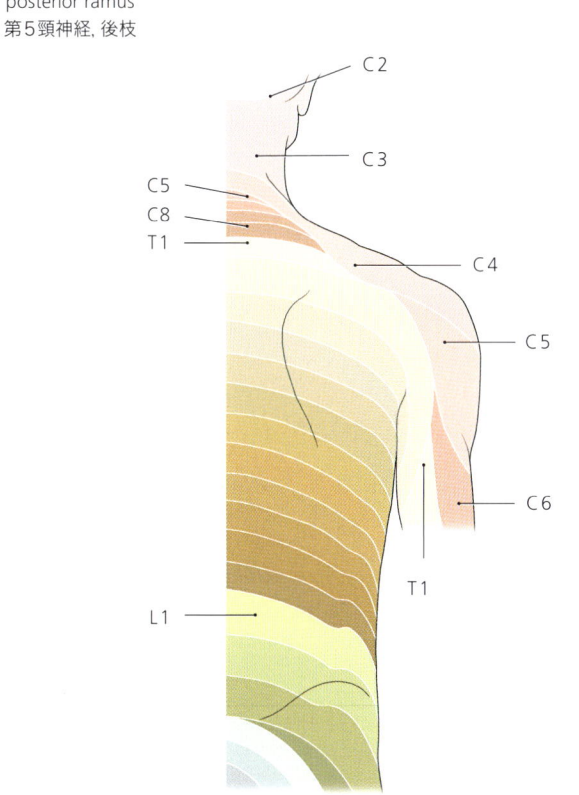

B デルマトーム：背部の皮膚における脊髄神経の分節状分布．*Note*：C1 は純運動神経であり，したがって C1 のデルマトームは存在しない．

背部の神経と血管（局所解剖）
Neurovascular Topography of the Back

図3.6 項部の神経と動脈
後方から見たところ．僧帽筋，胸鎖乳突筋，頭板状筋，頭半棘筋を取り除き，後頭下領域が剖出されている．

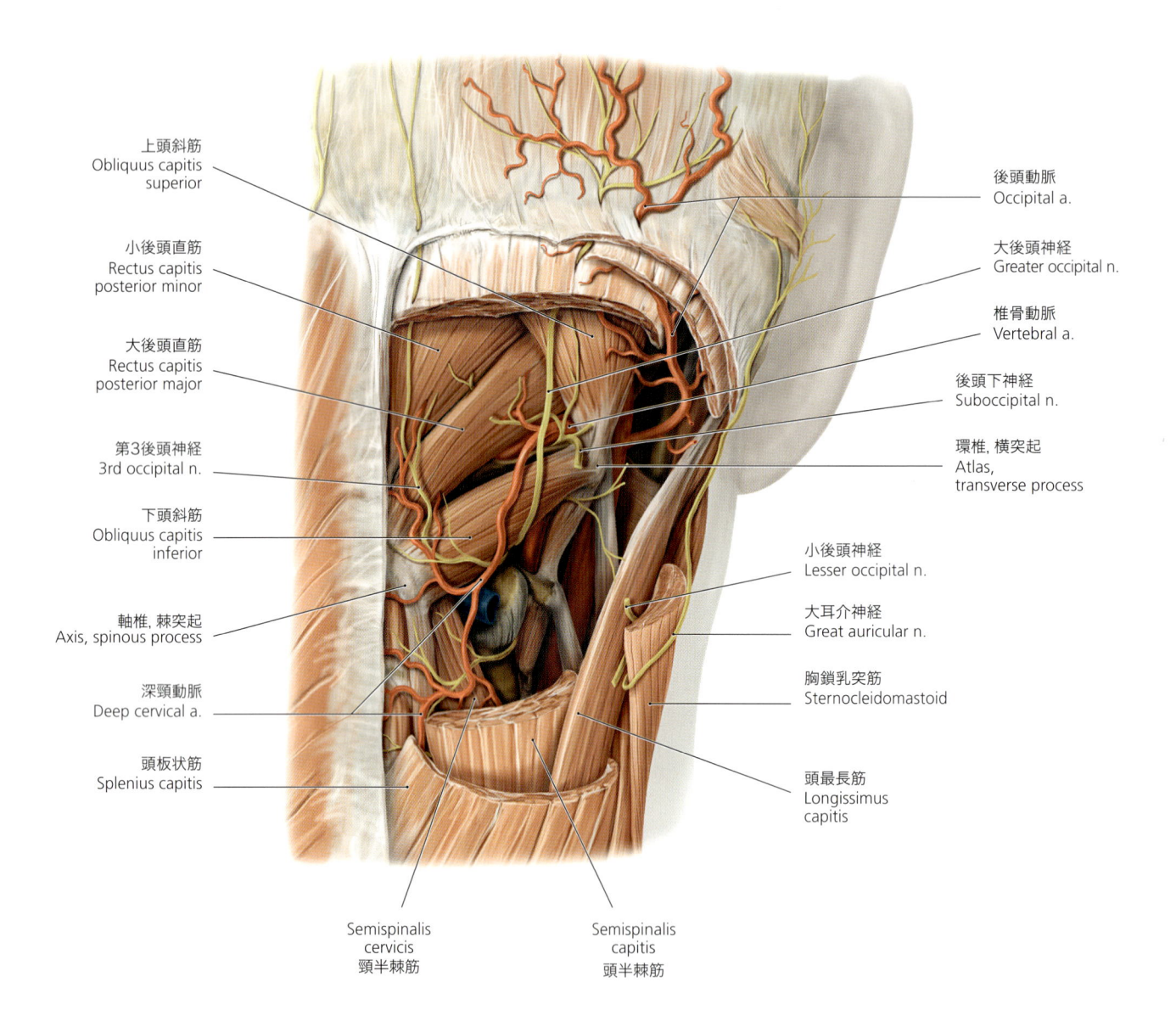

- 上頭斜筋 Obliquus capitis superior
- 小後頭直筋 Rectus capitis posterior minor
- 大後頭直筋 Rectus capitis posterior major
- 第3後頭神経 3rd occipital n.
- 下頭斜筋 Obliquus capitis inferior
- 軸椎，棘突起 Axis, spinous process
- 深頸動脈 Deep cervical a.
- 頭板状筋 Splenius capitis
- Semispinalis cervicis 頸半棘筋
- Semispinalis capitis 頭半棘筋
- 後頭動脈 Occipital a.
- 大後頭神経 Greater occipital n.
- 椎骨動脈 Vertebral a.
- 後頭下神経 Suboccipital n.
- 環椎，横突起 Atlas, transverse process
- 小後頭神経 Lesser occipital n.
- 大耳介神経 Great auricular n.
- 胸鎖乳突筋 Sternocleidomastoid
- 頭最長筋 Longissimus capitis

図 3.7 背部の神経と動静脈

後方から見たところ．筋の筋膜（胸腰筋膜の浅葉を除く）と右の広背筋が取り除かれ，右の僧帽筋が反転されている．頸横動脈は僧帽筋の深層を肩甲骨の内側縁に沿って走る．

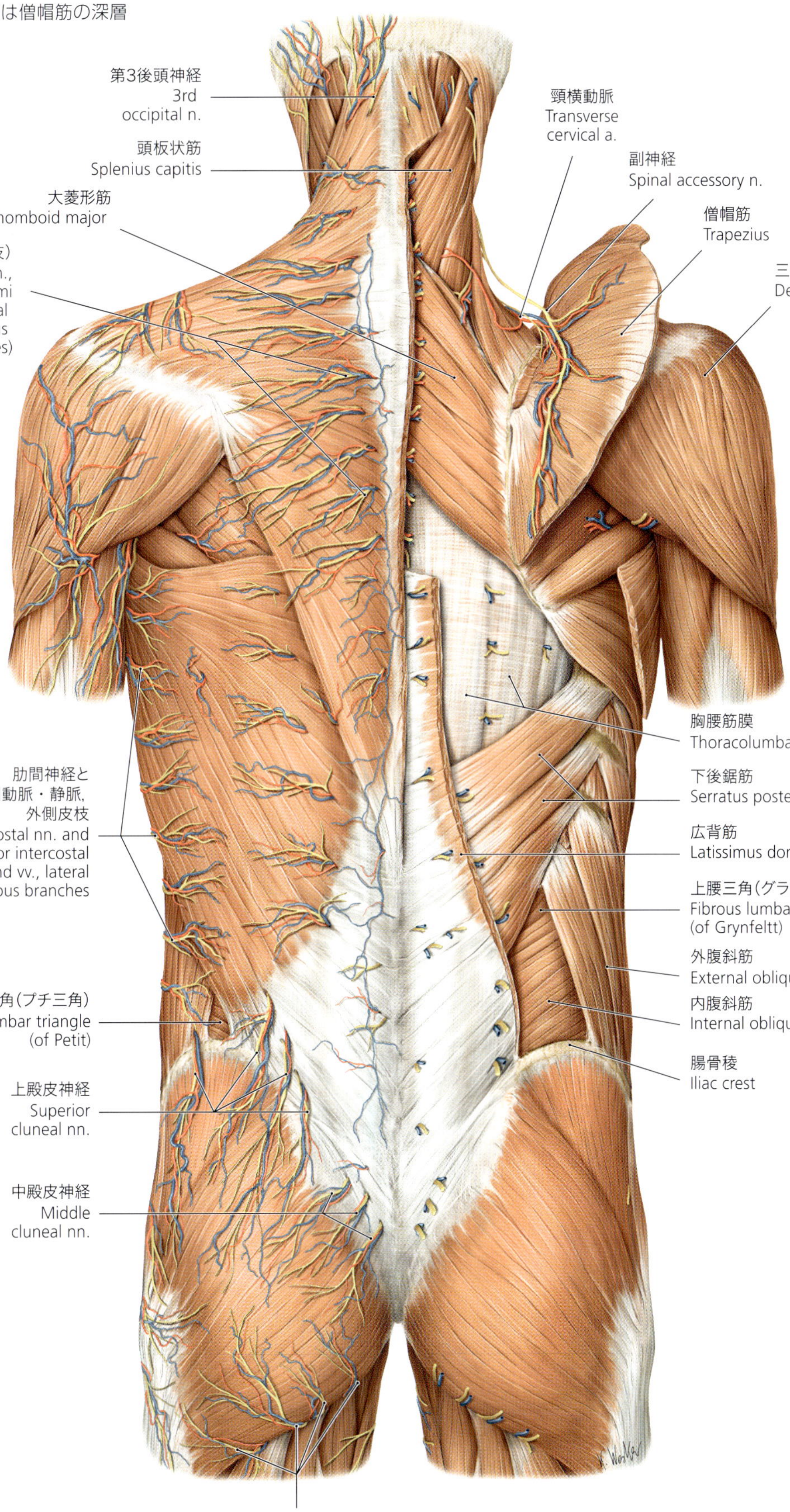

- 第3後頭神経 3rd occipital n.
- 頭板状筋 Splenius capitis
- 大菱形筋 Rhomboid major
- 脊髄神経, 後枝（内側皮枝）Spinal nn., posterior rami (medial cutaneous branches)
- 頸横動脈 Transverse cervical a.
- 副神経 Spinal accessory n.
- 僧帽筋 Trapezius
- 三角筋 Deltoid
- 胸腰筋膜 Thoracolumbar fascia
- 下後鋸筋 Serratus posterior inferior
- 広背筋 Latissimus dorsi
- 上腰三角（グランフェルト三角）Fibrous lumbar triangle (of Grynfeltt)
- 外腹斜筋 External oblique
- 内腹斜筋 Internal oblique
- 腸骨稜 Iliac crest
- 肋間神経と肋間動脈・静脈, 外側皮枝 Intercostal nn. and posterior intercostal aa. and vv., lateral cutaneous branches
- 下腰三角（プチ三角）Iliolumbar triangle (of Petit)
- 上殿皮神経 Superior cluneal nn.
- 中殿皮神経 Middle cluneal nn.
- Inferior cluneal nn. 下殿皮神経

体表解剖
Surface Anatomy

図 4.1 体表から触知できる構造
後方から見たところ．

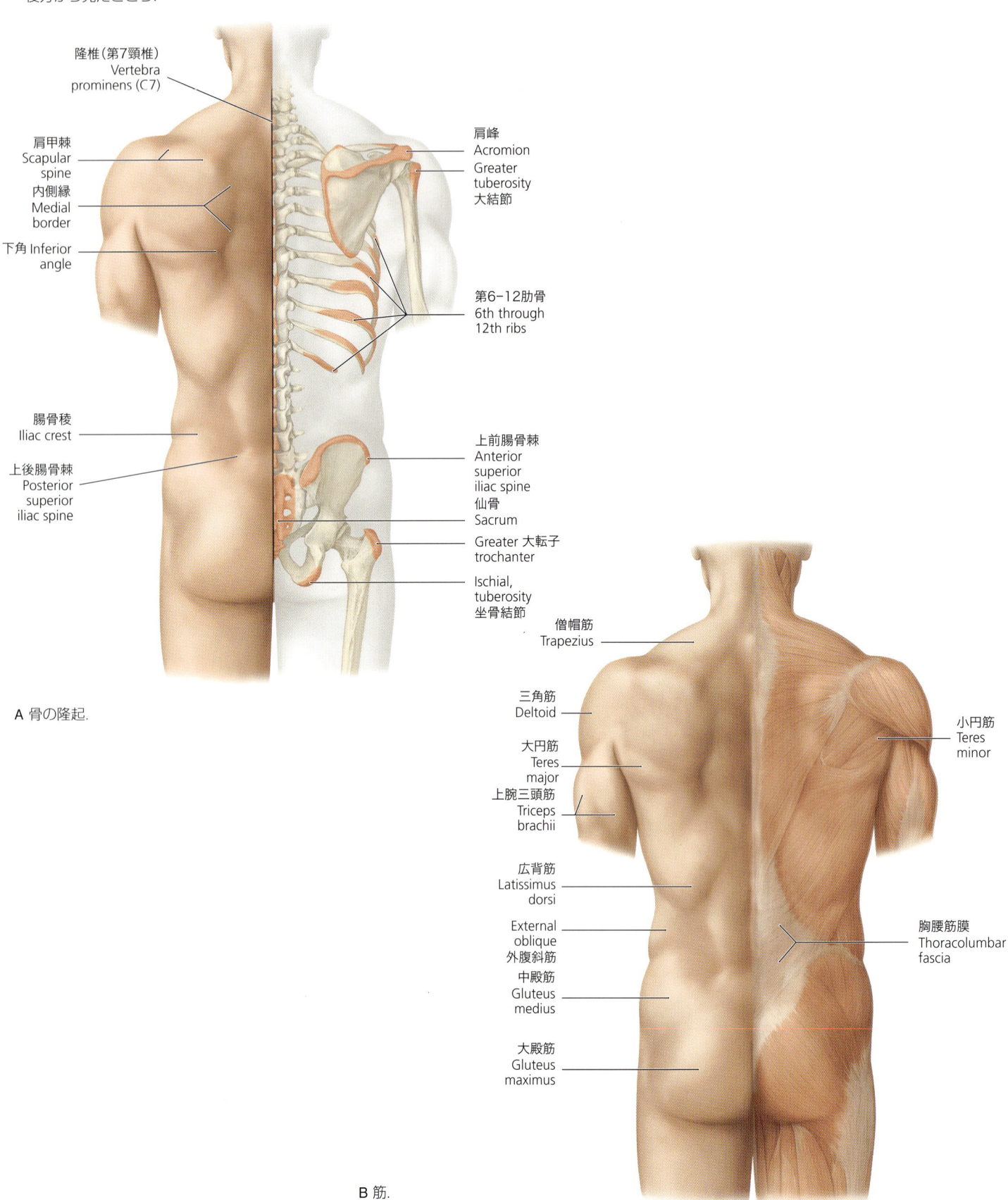

A 骨の隆起．

- 隆椎（第7頸椎）Vertebra prominens (C7)
- 肩甲棘 Scapular spine
- 内側縁 Medial border
- 下角 Inferior angle
- 腸骨稜 Iliac crest
- 上後腸骨棘 Posterior superior iliac spine
- 肩峰 Acromion
- 大結節 Greater tuberosity
- 第6-12肋骨 6th through 12th ribs
- 上前腸骨棘 Anterior superior iliac spine
- 仙骨 Sacrum
- 大転子 Greater trochanter
- 坐骨結節 Ischial tuberosity

B 筋．

- 僧帽筋 Trapezius
- 三角筋 Deltoid
- 大円筋 Teres major
- 上腕三頭筋 Triceps brachii
- 広背筋 Latissimus dorsi
- 外腹斜筋 External oblique
- 中殿筋 Gluteus medius
- 大殿筋 Gluteus maximus
- 小円筋 Teres minor
- 胸腰筋膜 Thoracolumbar fascia

図4.2 背部の体表解剖
後方から見たところ．

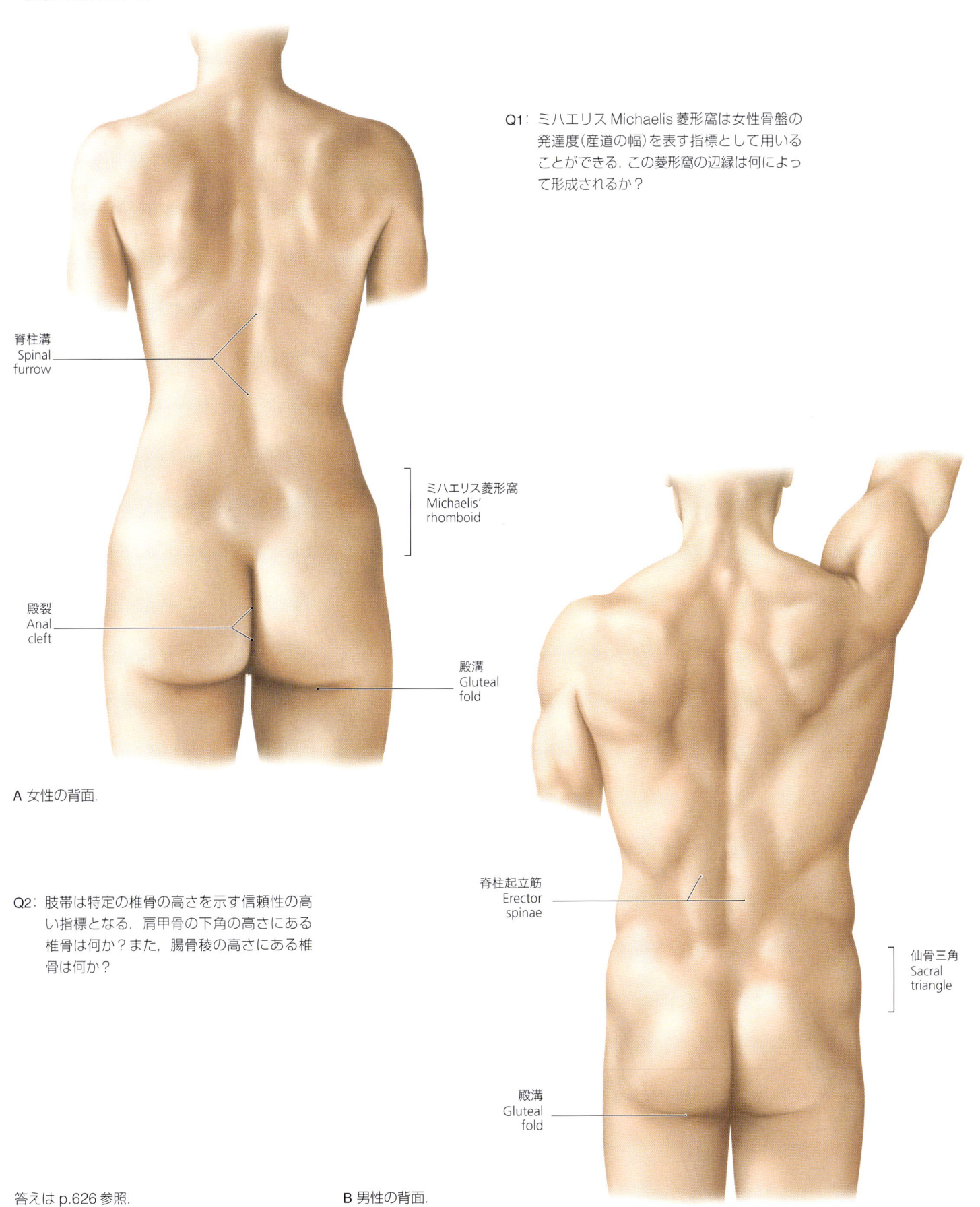

Q1: ミハエリス Michaelis 菱形窩は女性骨盤の発達度（産道の幅）を表す指標として用いることができる．この菱形窩の辺縁は何によって形成されるか？

脊柱溝
Spinal furrow

ミハエリス菱形窩
Michaelis' rhomboid

殿裂
Anal cleft

殿溝
Gluteal fold

A 女性の背面．

Q2: 肢帯は特定の椎骨の高さを示す信頼性の高い指標となる．肩甲骨の下角の高さにある椎骨は何か？また，腸骨稜の高さにある椎骨は何か？

脊柱起立筋
Erector spinae

仙骨三角
Sacral triangle

殿溝
Gluteal fold

答えは p.626 参照．

B 男性の背面．

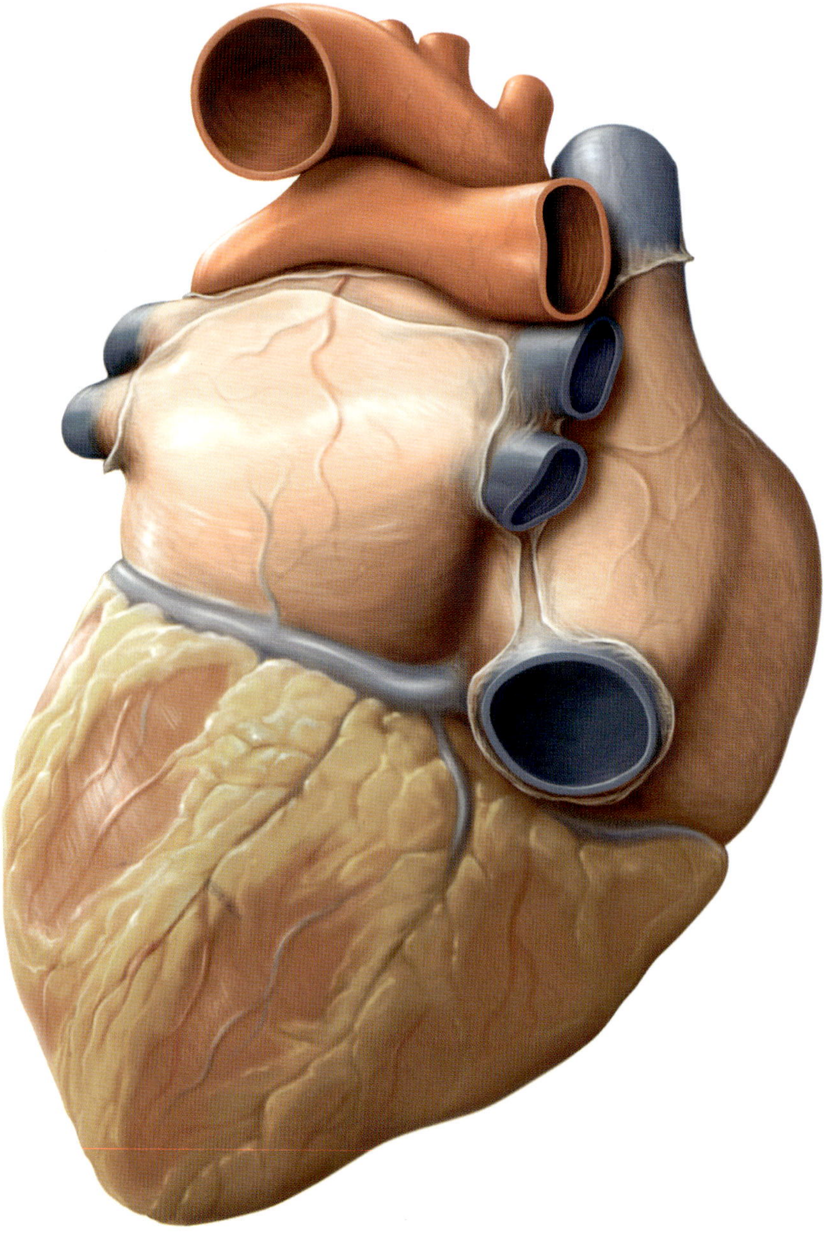

胸 部
Thorax

5. 胸壁
- 胸部の骨格……………………………………44
- 胸骨と肋骨……………………………………46
- 胸郭の関節……………………………………48
- 胸壁の筋………………………………………50
- 横隔膜…………………………………………52
- 横隔膜の神経と血管…………………………54
- 胸壁の動脈と静脈……………………………56
- 胸壁の神経……………………………………58
- 胸壁の神経と血管の位置……………………60
- 女性の乳房……………………………………62
- 女性乳房のリンパ管…………………………64

6. 胸腔
- 胸腔の区分……………………………………66
- 胸腔の動脈……………………………………68
- 胸腔の静脈……………………………………70
- 胸腔のリンパ管………………………………72
- 胸腔の神経……………………………………74

7. 縦隔
- 縦隔：概観……………………………………76
- 縦隔の構造……………………………………78
- 胸腺と心膜……………………………………80
- 原位置の心臓…………………………………82
- 心臓：表面と部屋……………………………84
- 心臓：弁………………………………………86
- 心臓の動脈と静脈……………………………88
- 心臓の刺激伝導と神経支配…………………90
- 心臓：X線像…………………………………92
- 出生前・後の循環……………………………94
- 食道……………………………………………96
- 食道の神経と血管……………………………98
- 縦隔のリンパ管………………………………100

8. 胸膜腔
- 胸膜腔…………………………………………102
- 原位置の肺……………………………………104
- 肺：X線像……………………………………106
- 肺の気管支肺区域……………………………108
- 気管と気管支樹………………………………110
- 呼吸機構………………………………………112
- 肺動脈と肺静脈………………………………114
- 気管気管支樹の神経と血管…………………116
- 胸膜腔のリンパ管……………………………118

9. 体表解剖
- 体表解剖………………………………………120

胸部の骨格
Thoracic Skeleton

胸部の骨格は，12個の脊柱(p.8)，12対の肋骨および肋軟骨，胸骨からなる．呼吸に関与するほかに，生命維持に必要な臓器を適度に保護している．一般に，女性の胸郭は男性よりも狭く短い．

図 5.1 胸部の骨格

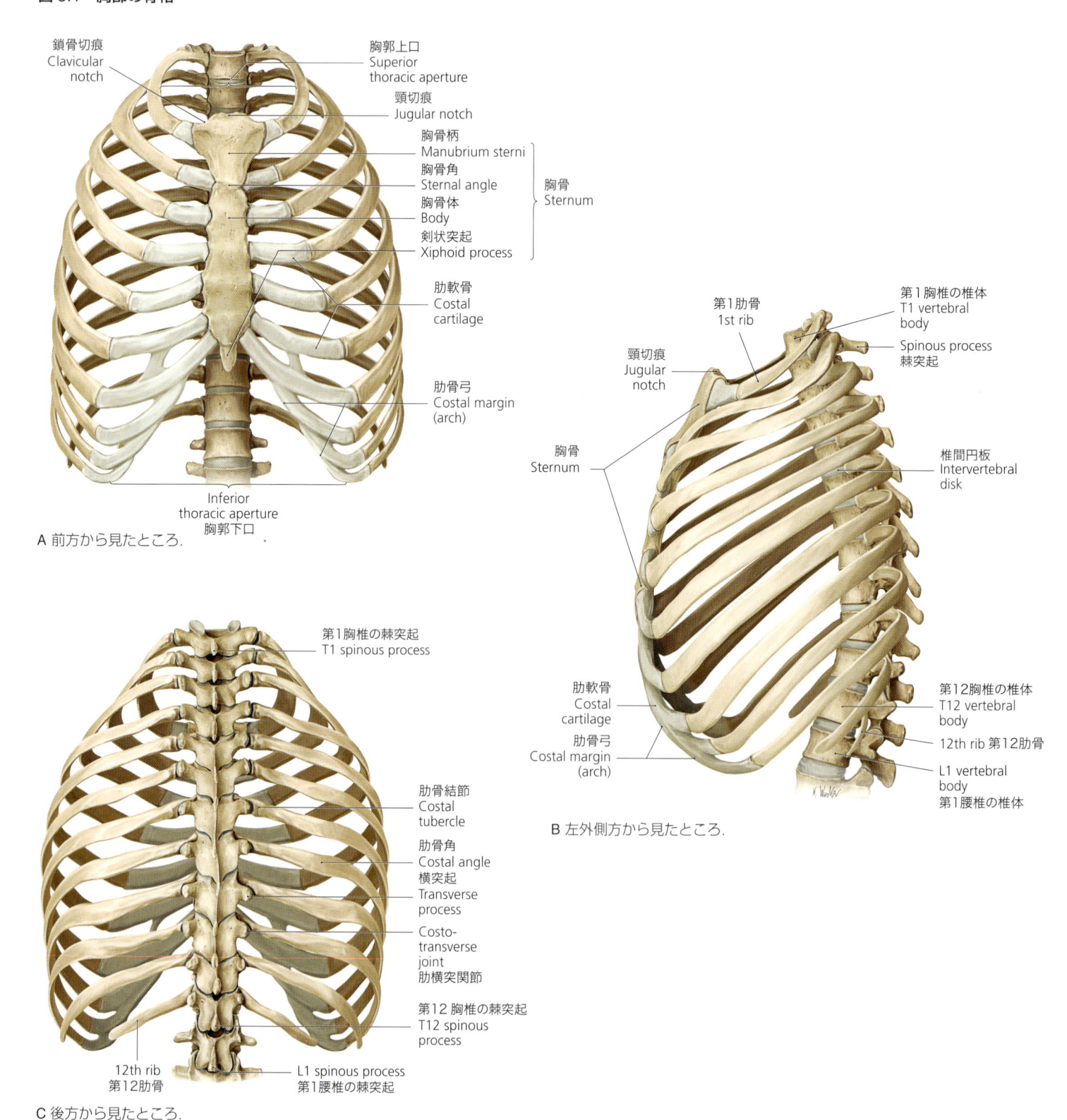

鎖骨切痕 Clavicular notch
胸郭上口 Superior thoracic aperture
頸切痕 Jugular notch
胸骨柄 Manubrium sterni
胸骨角 Sternal angle
胸骨体 Body
剣状突起 Xiphoid process
胸骨 Sternum
肋軟骨 Costal cartilage
肋骨弓 Costal margin (arch)
Inferior thoracic aperture 胸郭下口

A 前方から見たところ．

第1肋骨 1st rib
第1胸椎の椎体 T1 vertebral body
Spinous process 棘突起
頸切痕 Jugular notch
胸骨 Sternum
椎間円板 Intervertebral disk
肋軟骨 Costal cartilage
肋骨弓 Costal margin (arch)
第12胸椎の椎体 T12 vertebral body
12th rib 第12肋骨
L1 vertebral body 第1腰椎の椎体

B 左外側方から見たところ．

第1胸椎の棘突起 T1 spinous process
肋骨結節 Costal tubercle
肋骨角 Costal angle
横突起 Transverse process
Costo-transverse joint 肋横突関節
第12胸椎の棘突起 T12 spinous process
12th rib 第12肋骨
L1 spinous process 第1腰椎の棘突起

C 後方から見たところ．

図 5.2 胸部の構造
第 6 肋骨を上方から見たところ．

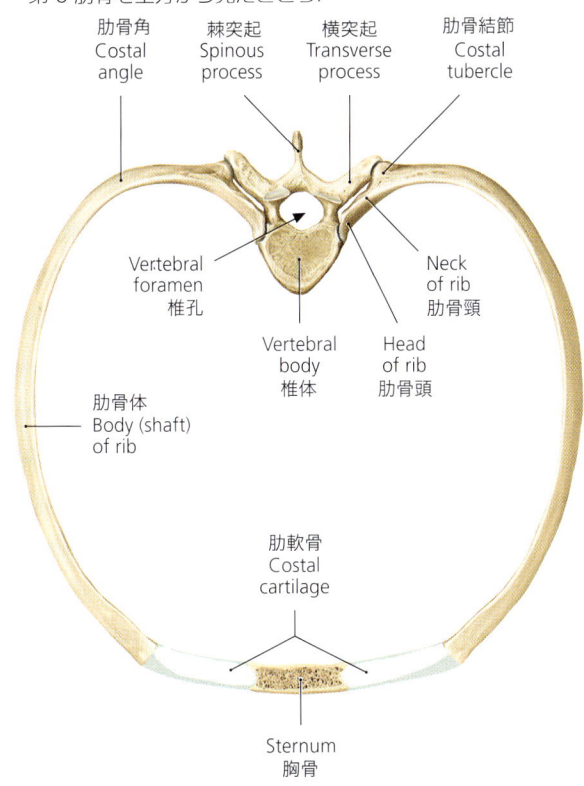

- 肋骨角 Costal angle
- 棘突起 Spinous process
- 横突起 Transverse process
- 肋骨結節 Costal tubercle
- 椎孔 Vertebral foramen
- 肋骨頸 Neck of rib
- 椎体 Vertebral body
- 肋骨頭 Head of rib
- 肋骨体 Body (shaft) of rib
- 肋軟骨 Costal cartilage
- 胸骨 Sternum

表 5.1 胸部の要素

椎骨		
肋骨	骨性部（肋骨）	肋骨頭
		肋骨頸
		肋骨結節
		肋骨体（肋骨角を含む）
	軟骨部（肋軟骨）	
胸骨（真肋の肋軟骨とのみ関節する．図 5.3 を参照）		

図 5.3 肋骨の分類
左外側方から見たところ．

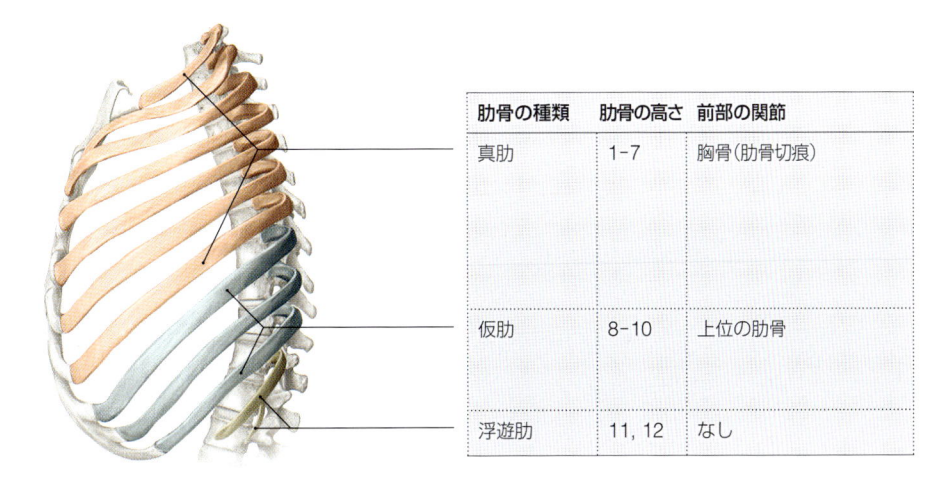

肋骨の種類	肋骨の高さ	前部の関節
真肋	1-7	胸骨（肋骨切痕）
仮肋	8-10	上位の肋骨
浮遊肋	11, 12	なし

胸骨と肋骨
Sternum & Ribs

図 5.4　胸骨
　胸骨は刀状の骨で，胸骨柄，胸骨体，剣状突起からなる．胸骨体と胸骨柄との結合部（胸骨角）は盛り上がっているのが特徴で，第 2 肋骨の関節の目印となる．胸骨角は内部構造の重要な指標である．

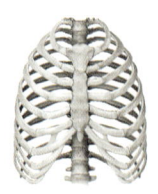

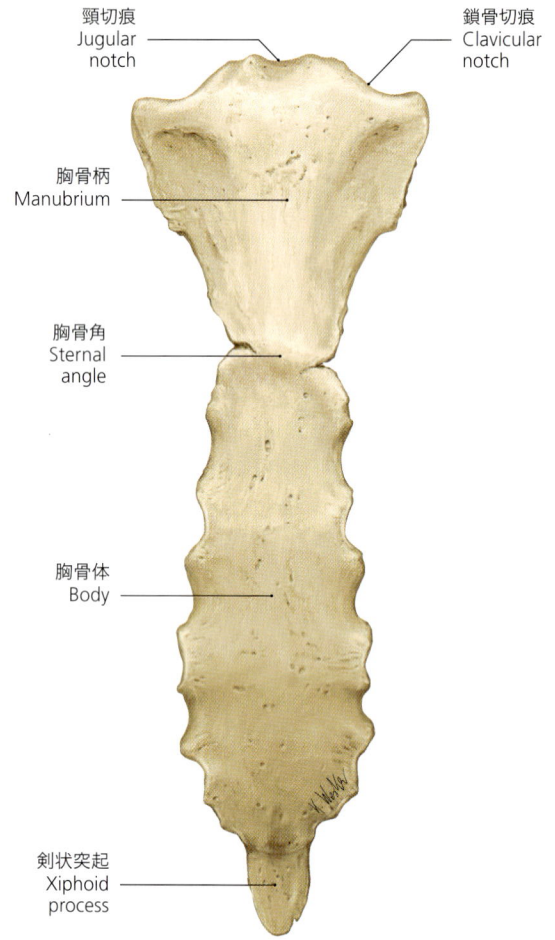

- 頸切痕　Jugular notch
- 鎖骨切痕　Clavicular notch
- 胸骨柄　Manubrium
- 胸骨角　Sternal angle
- 胸骨体　Body
- 剣状突起　Xiphoid process
- 第1肋骨切痕　1st costal notch
- 第2-7肋骨切痕　2nd through 7th costal notches

A 前方から見たところ．

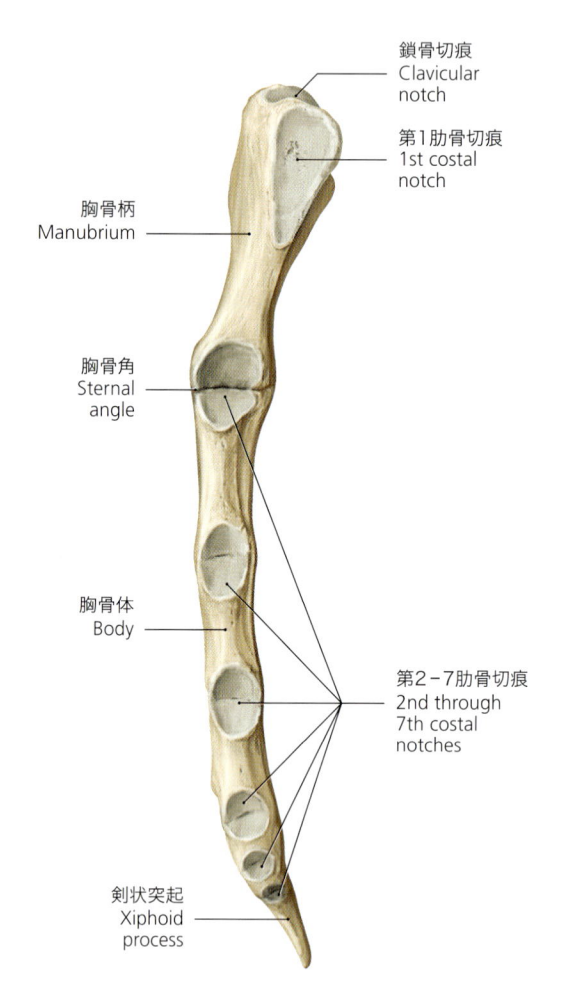

B 左外側方から見たところ．肋骨切痕は真肋の肋軟骨と関節をなす場所である（図 5.3 参照）．

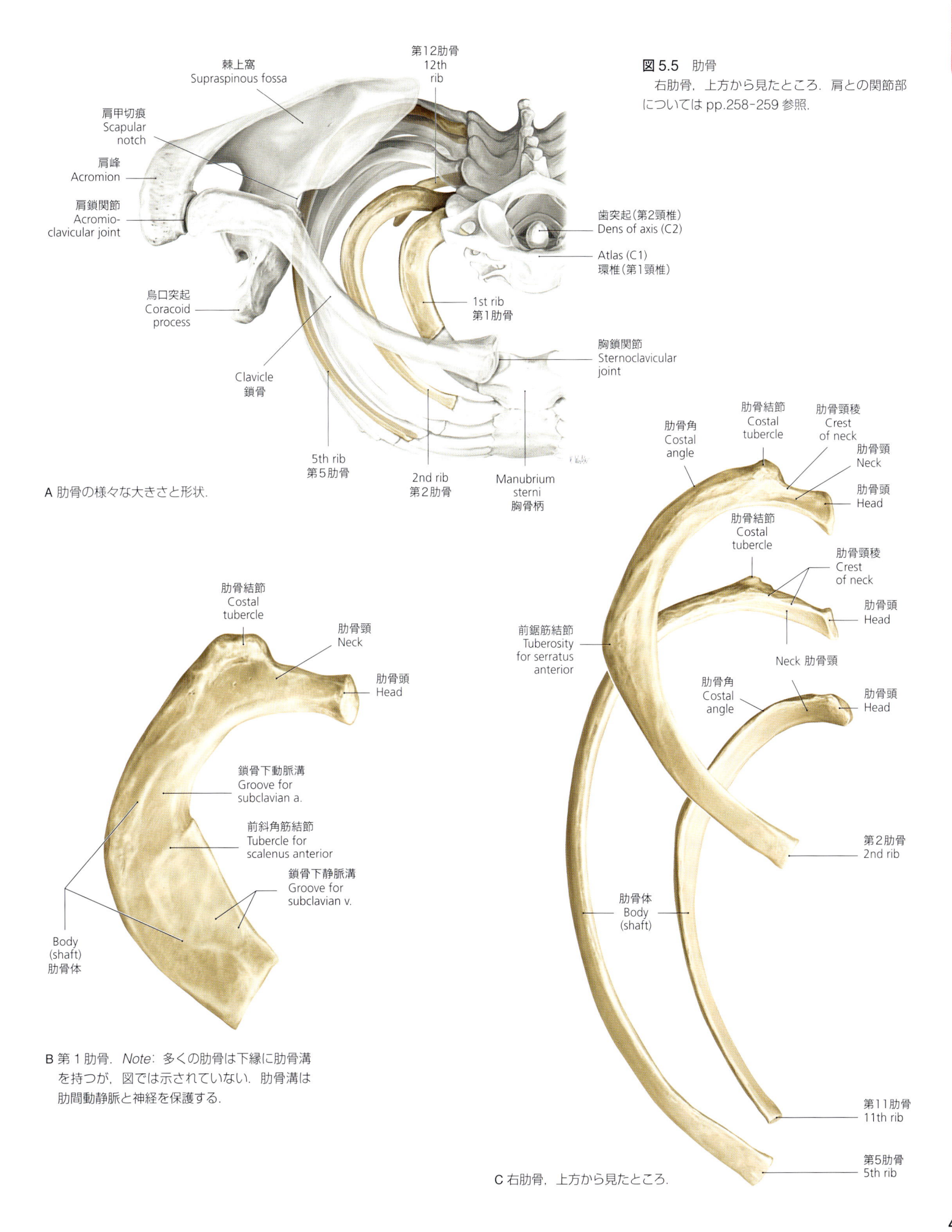

図5.5 肋骨
右肋骨，上方から見たところ．肩との関節部については pp.258-259 参照．

A 肋骨の様々な大きさと形状．

- 棘上窩 Supraspinous fossa
- 肩甲切痕 Scapular notch
- 肩峰 Acromion
- 肩鎖関節 Acromio-clavicular joint
- 烏口突起 Coracoid process
- Clavicle 鎖骨
- 5th rib 第5肋骨
- 2nd rib 第2肋骨
- Manubrium sterni 胸骨柄
- 第12肋骨 12th rib
- 1st rib 第1肋骨
- 歯突起（第2頸椎）Dens of axis (C2)
- Atlas (C1) 環椎（第1頸椎）
- 胸鎖関節 Sternoclavicular joint

B 第1肋骨．*Note*：多くの肋骨は下縁に肋骨溝を持つが，図では示されていない．肋骨溝は肋間動静脈と神経を保護する．

- 肋骨結節 Costal tubercle
- 肋骨頸 Neck
- 肋骨頭 Head
- 鎖骨下動脈溝 Groove for subclavian a.
- 前斜角筋結節 Tubercle for scalenus anterior
- 鎖骨下静脈溝 Groove for subclavian v.
- Body (shaft) 肋骨体

C 右肋骨，上方から見たところ．

- 肋骨角 Costal angle
- 肋骨結節 Costal tubercle
- 肋骨頸稜 Crest of neck
- 肋骨頸 Neck
- 肋骨頭 Head
- 前鋸筋結節 Tuberosity for serratus anterior
- 肋骨体 Body (shaft)
- 第2肋骨 2nd rib
- 第11肋骨 11th rib
- 第5肋骨 5th rib

胸郭の関節
Joints of the Thoracic Cage

横隔膜は安静時の呼吸の主要筋である(p.52 参照). 胸壁の筋肉 (p.50 参照)は努力呼吸を助ける.

図 5.6 胸郭の運動

深吸息時(赤); 深呼息時(青). 深吸息時には胸骨の横径, 矢状径および胸骨下角が大きくなる. 横隔膜の下降によってさらに胸腔容量が増加する.

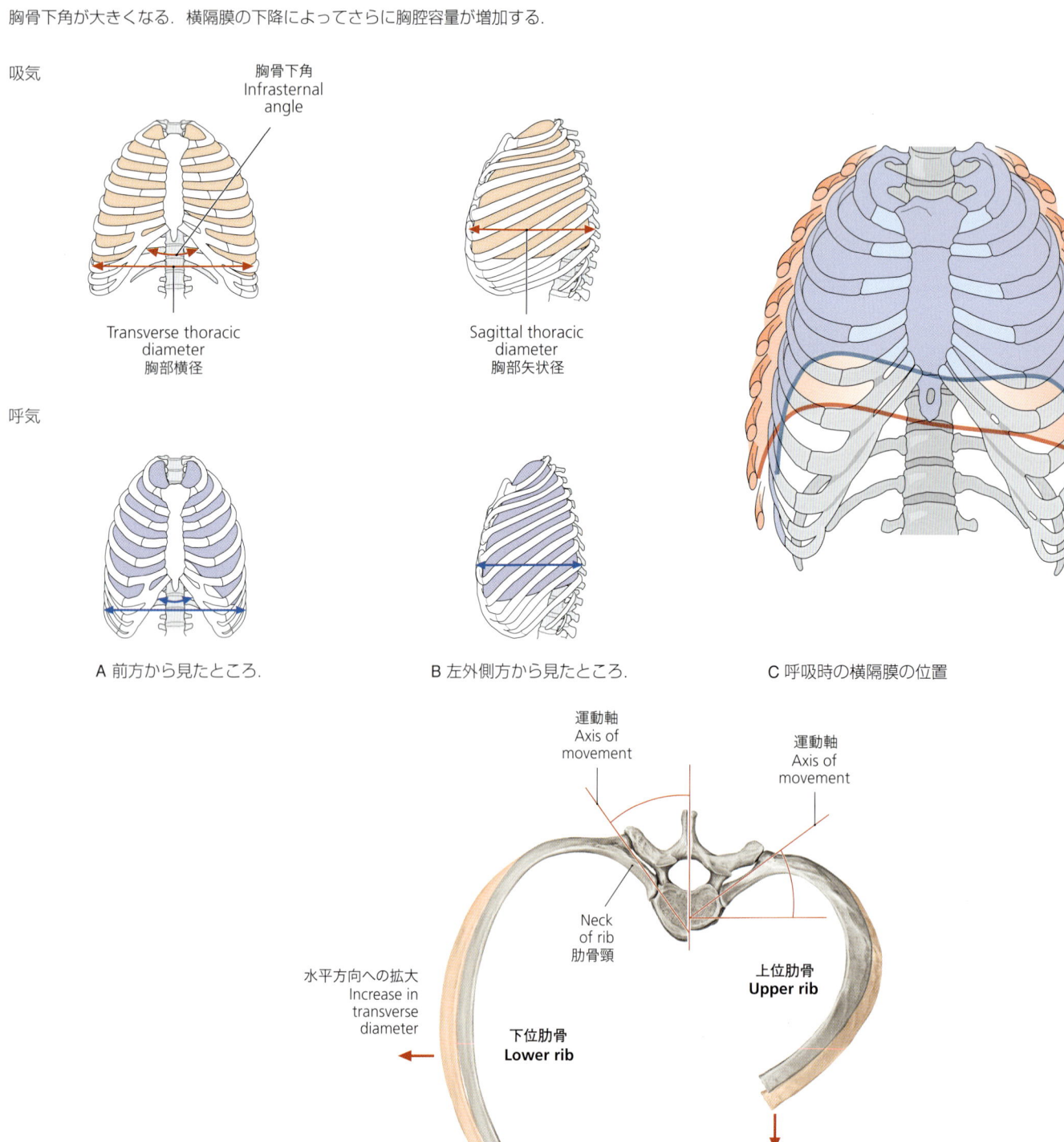

吸気

胸骨下角
Infrasternal angle

Transverse thoracic diameter
胸部横径

Sagittal thoracic diameter
胸部矢状径

呼気

A 前方から見たところ.

B 左外側方から見たところ.

C 呼吸時の横隔膜の位置

運動軸
Axis of movement

運動軸
Axis of movement

Neck of rib
肋骨頸

上位肋骨
Upper rib

水平方向への拡大
Increase in transverse diameter

下位肋骨
Lower rib

Increase in sagittal diameter
矢状方向への拡大

D 肋骨の運動軸, 上方から見たところ.

図 5.7 胸肋関節

前方から見たところ，胸骨は右半で前頭断されている．真の関節は第 2–5 肋骨にのみ見られ，第 1，6，7 肋骨は軟骨結合によって胸骨に付着する．

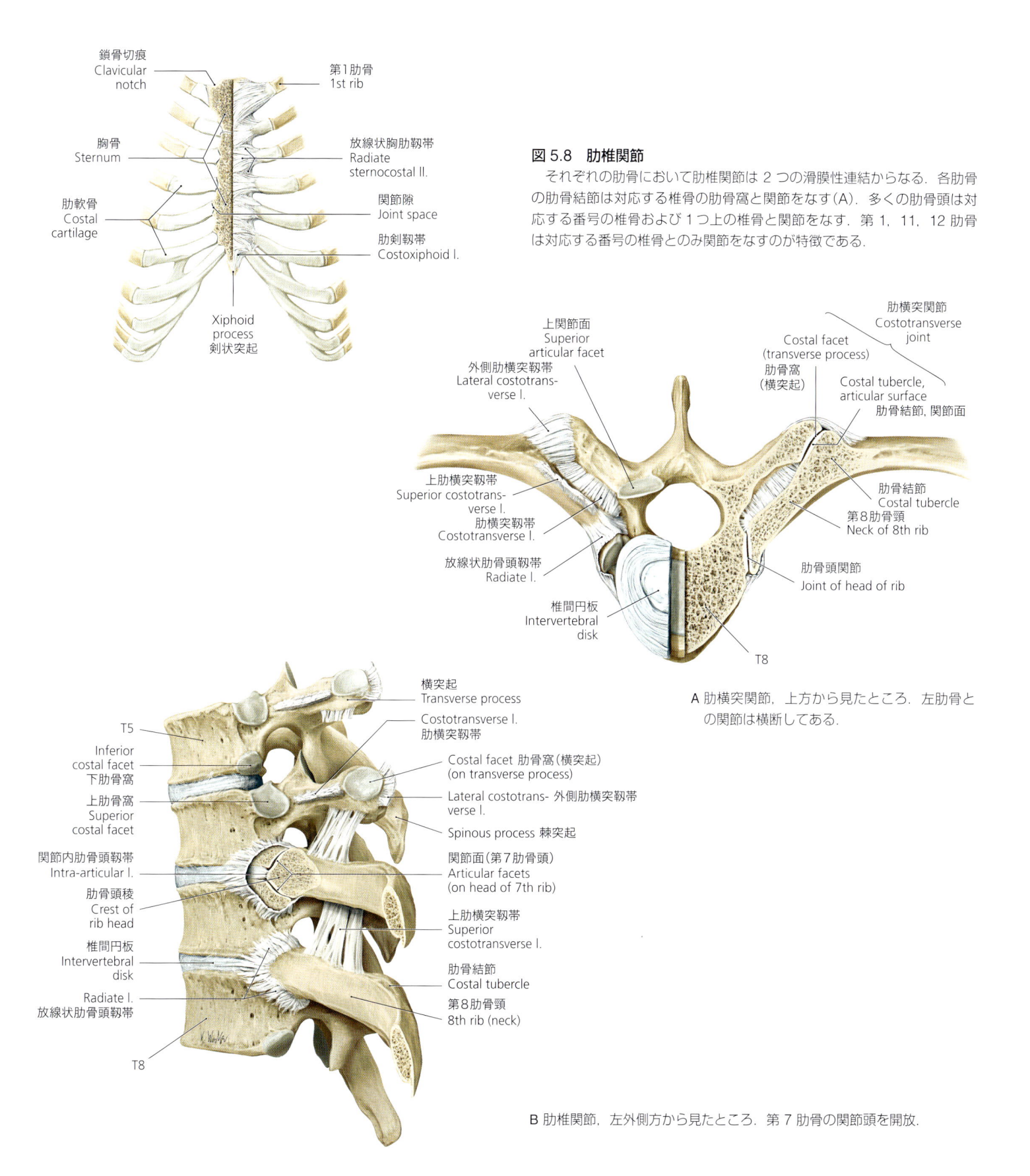

鎖骨切痕 Clavicular notch
第1肋骨 1st rib
胸骨 Sternum
放線状胸肋靱帯 Radiate sternocostal l.
肋軟骨 Costal cartilage
関節隙 Joint space
肋剣靱帯 Costoxiphoid l.
Xiphoid process 剣状突起

図 5.8 肋椎関節

それぞれの肋骨において肋椎関節は 2 つの滑膜性連結からなる．各肋骨の肋骨結節は対応する椎骨の肋骨窩と関節をなす（A）．多くの肋骨頭は対応する番号の椎骨および 1 つ上の椎骨と関節をなす．第 1，11，12 肋骨は対応する番号の椎骨とのみ関節をなすのが特徴である．

上関節面 Superior articular facet
外側肋横突靱帯 Lateral costotransverse l.
肋横突関節 Costotransverse joint
Costal facet (transverse process)
肋骨窩（横突起）
Costal tubercle, articular surface
肋骨結節, 関節面
上肋横突靱帯 Superior costotransverse l.
肋横突靱帯 Costotransverse l.
放線状肋骨頭靱帯 Radiate l.
椎間円板 Intervertebral disk
肋骨結節 Costal tubercle
第8肋骨頸 Neck of 8th rib
肋骨頭関節 Joint of head of rib
T8

A 肋横突関節，上方から見たところ．左肋骨との関節は横断してある．

T5
Inferior costal facet 下肋骨窩
上肋骨窩 Superior costal facet
関節内肋骨頭靱帯 Intra-articular l.
肋骨頭稜 Crest of rib head
椎間円板 Intervertebral disk
Radiate l. 放線状肋骨頭靱帯
T8
横突起 Transverse process
Costotransverse l. 肋横突靱帯
Costal facet 肋骨窩（横突起）(on transverse process)
Lateral costotransverse l. 外側肋横突靱帯
Spinous process 棘突起
関節面（第7肋骨頭）Articular facets (on head of 7th rib)
上肋横突靱帯 Superior costotransverse l.
肋骨結節 Costal tubercle
第8肋骨頭 8th rib (neck)

B 肋椎関節，左外側方から見たところ．第 7 肋骨の関節頭を開放．

胸壁の筋
Thoracic Wall Muscle Facts

> 胸壁の筋肉は胸式呼吸の主要筋であり，努力呼吸時には他の筋肉も働く．大胸筋と前鋸筋は肩とともに扱い（pp.264-267 参照），後鋸筋は背中とともに扱う（p.30 参照）．

図 5.9　胸壁の筋肉

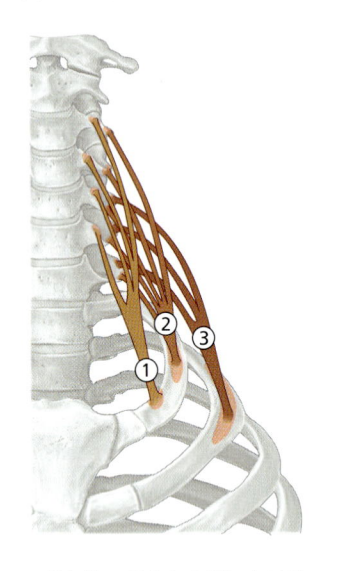

A 斜角筋，前方から見たところ．　　B 肋間筋，前方から見たところ．　　C 胸横筋，後方から見たところ．

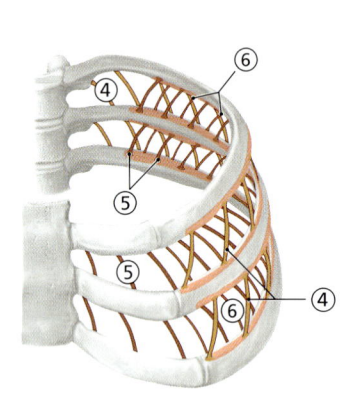

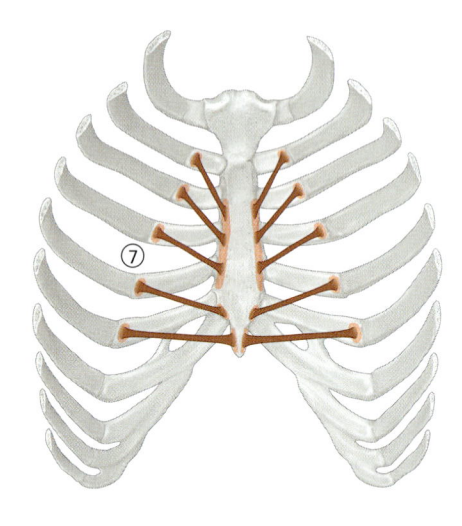

表 5.2　胸壁の筋肉

筋		起始	停止	神経支配	作用
斜角筋	①前斜角筋	第 3-6 頸椎の横突起の前結節	第 1 肋骨の前斜角筋結節	頸・腕神経叢（C3-C6）の枝	・肋骨可動時は，上位の肋骨を挙上する（吸気時） ・肋骨の動きを固定すると，（片側の収縮は）同側に頸椎を屈曲し，（両側の収縮）頸を屈曲する
	②中斜角筋	第 4-6 頸椎の横突起の後結節	第 1 肋骨の鎖骨下動脈溝の後ろ側		
	③後斜角筋		第 2 肋骨の外側面		
肋間筋	④外肋間筋	肋骨の下縁から起こり，隣接する下位の肋骨の上縁に付着する（肋骨結節から骨軟骨性接合部まで斜め前下方に走行する）		肋間神経（T1-T11）	肋骨を挙上する（吸気時），肋間隙を支持し，胸郭を安定する
	⑤内肋間筋	肋骨の上縁から起こり，隣接する上位の肋骨の下縁に付着する（肋骨角から胸骨まで斜め前上方に走行する）			肋骨を引き下げる（呼気時）
	⑥最内肋間筋				
肋下筋		下位肋骨の下縁から 2，3 個下の肋骨の内側面		下位の肋間神経	肋骨を挙上する（吸気時）
⑦胸横筋		胸骨体と剣状突起（内側面）	第 2-6 肋骨（肋軟骨の内側面）	肋間神経（T2-T7）	肋骨を引き下げる（呼気時）

図 5.10　胸壁の筋肉

前方から見たところ．外肋間筋は前方では外肋間膜になっている．内肋間筋は後方では内肋間膜となっている（図 5.11 では取り除いている）．

図 5.11　胸横筋

前方から見たところ．胸郭を開き，前壁の後面を見せる．

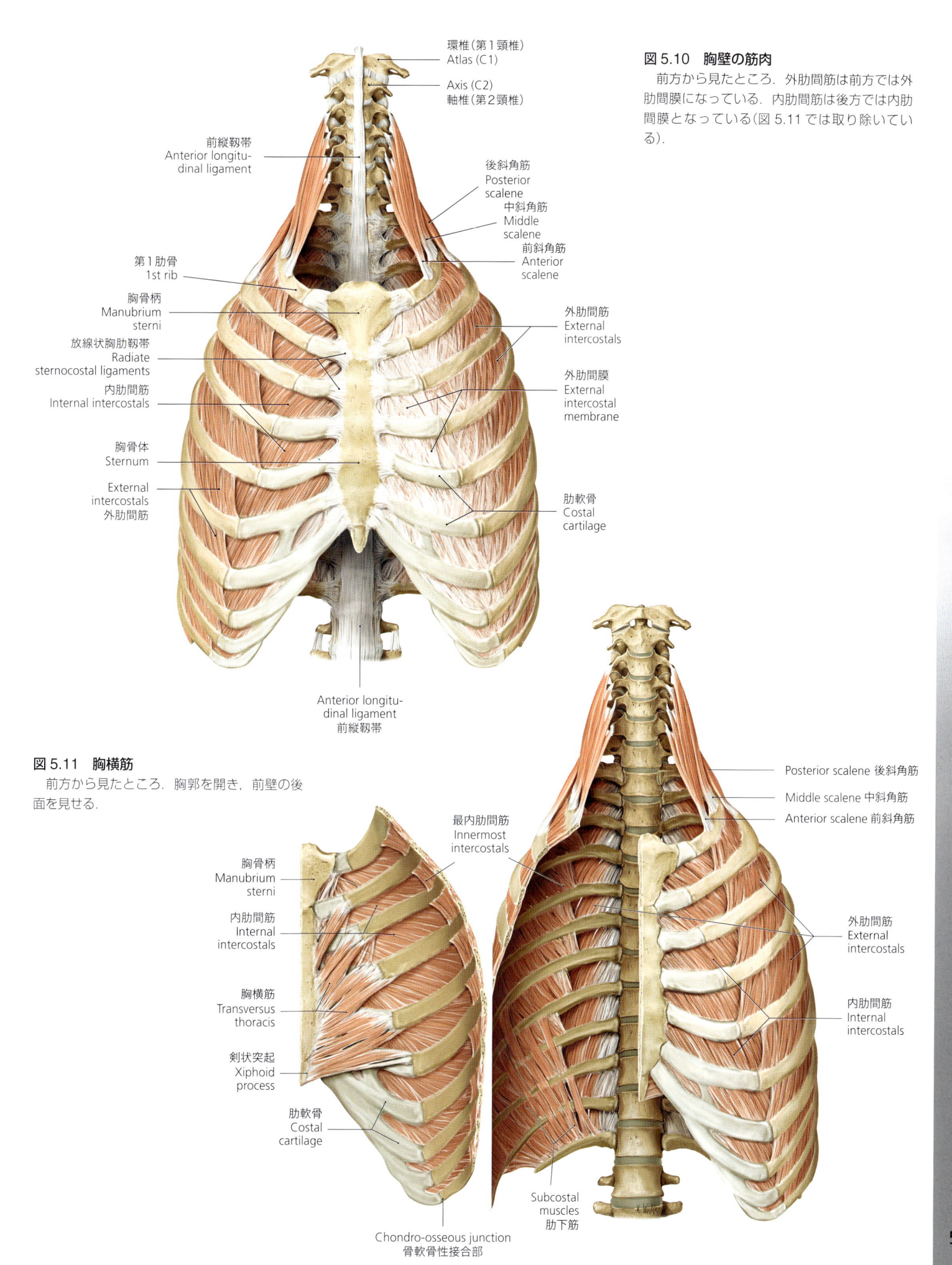

横隔膜
Diaphragm

図 5.12 横隔膜
胸部と腹部を隔てる横隔膜は非対称の2つの頂部と3つの開口部（大動脈，大静脈，食道のための．図5.13B参照）を持つ．

図中ラベル（B 後方から見たところ）:
- 鎖骨 Clavicle
- 肩甲骨 Scapula
- 静脈孔 Caval aperture
- 第12肋骨 12th rib
- 第1腰椎, 横突起 L1, tranverse process
- 腰肋三角 Lumbocostal triangle

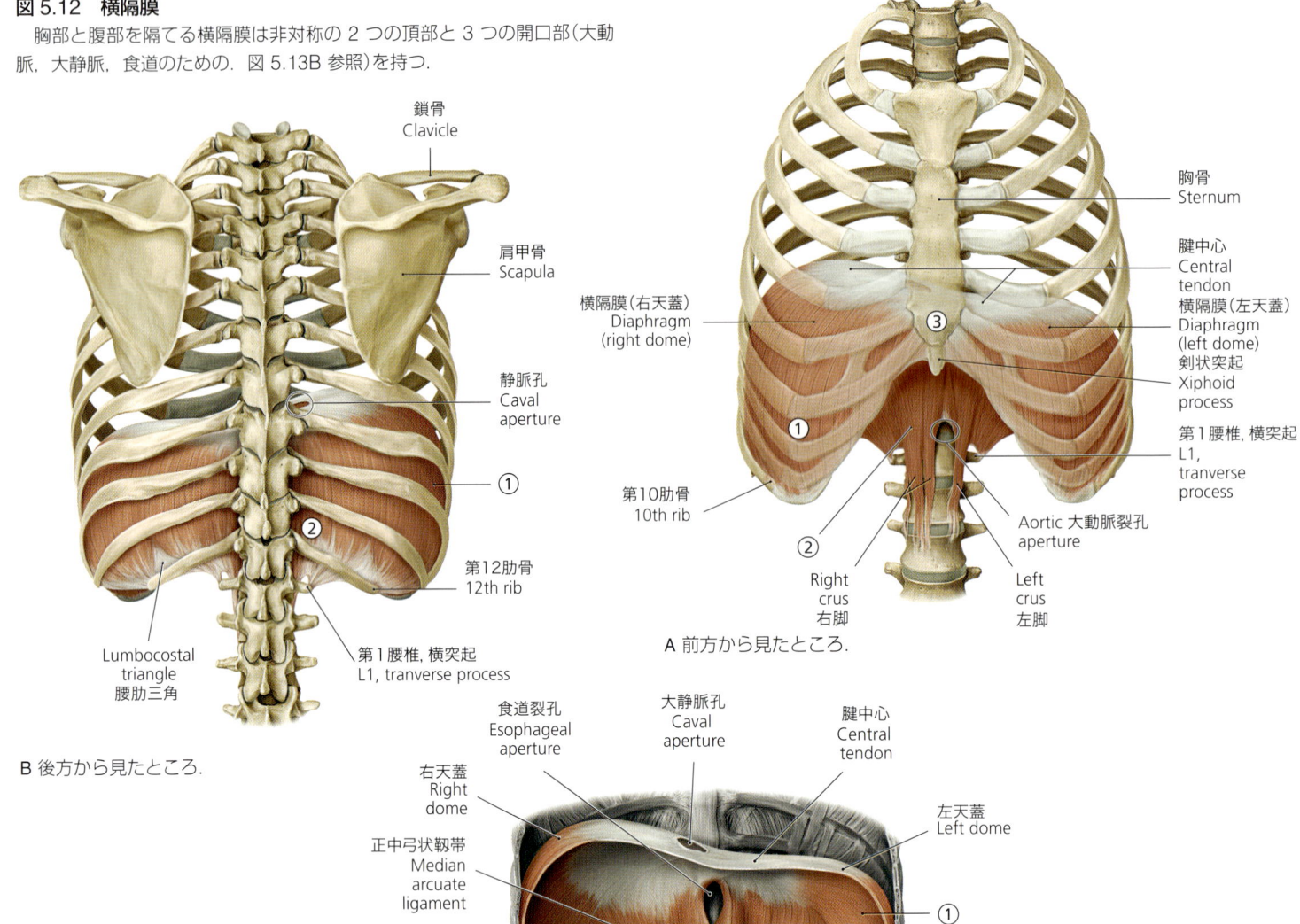

図中ラベル（A 前方から見たところ）:
- 胸骨 Sternum
- 腱中心 Central tendon
- 横隔膜（右天蓋）Diaphragm (right dome)
- 横隔膜（左天蓋）Diaphragm (left dome)
- 剣状突起 Xiphoid process
- 第1腰椎, 横突起 L1, tranverse process
- 第10肋骨 10th rib
- 大動脈裂孔 Aortic aperture
- 右脚 Right crus
- 左脚 Left crus

図中ラベル（C 中間位の横隔膜の冠状断）:
- 食道裂孔 Esophageal aperture
- 大静脈孔 Caval aperture
- 腱中心 Central tendon
- 右天蓋 Right dome
- 左天蓋 Left dome
- 正中弓状靭帯 Median arcuate ligament
- Right crus
- 外側弓状靭帯 Lateral arcuate ligament
- 腰方形筋 Quadratus lumborum
- 大腰筋 Psoas major
- 小腰筋 Psoas minor
- 大動脈裂孔 Aortic aperture
- 内側弓状靭帯 Medial arcuate ligament
- 腹横筋 Transversus abdominis

表 5.3　横隔膜

筋		起始	停止	神経支配	作用
横隔膜	①肋骨部	第7-12肋骨（肋骨弓の下縁）	腱中心	頸神経叢の横隔神経（C3-C5）	呼吸（横隔膜・胸郭呼吸運動）の最も重要な筋である．また，腹腔内臓への加圧を助ける（腹圧負荷）
	②腰椎部	内側部：第1-3腰椎椎体，椎間円板，（右脚・左脚として）前縦靭帯 外側部：内側・外側弓状靭帯			
	③胸骨部	剣状突起の後面			

図5.13 原位置の横隔膜

A 上方から見たところ．

- 胸骨 Sternum
- 横隔膜（胸骨部）Diaphragm (sternal part)
- 腱中心 Central tendon
- 大静脈孔 Caval aperture
- 肋間筋 Intercostal muscles
- 食道裂孔 Esophageal aperture
- T8
- 肋骨 Rib
- 胸内筋膜 Endothoracic fascia
- 固有背筋 Intrinsic back muscles
- 大動脈裂孔 Aortic aperture
- 横隔膜（肋骨部）Diaphragm (costal part)

B 下面．

- 大静脈孔 Caval aperture
- 胸肋三角 Sternocostal triangle
- 胸骨 Sternum
- 横隔膜（胸骨部）Diaphragm (sternal part)
- 腹直筋 Rectus abdominis
- 腱中心 Central tendon
- 横隔膜（肋骨部）Diaphragm (costal part)
- 食道裂孔 Esophageal aperture
- 左脚 Left crus
- 腰肋三角（ボクダレク三角）Lumbocostal triangle (Bochdalek's triangle)
- 広背筋 Latissimus dorsi
- 外側弓状靱帯 Lateral arcuate ligament
- 内側弓状靱帯 Medial arcuate ligament
- 脊柱起立筋 Erector spinae
- 椎体 Vertebral body
- 大腰筋 Psoas major
- 腰方形筋 Quadratus lumborum
- 腹横筋 Transversus abdominis
- 内腹斜筋 Internal oblique
- 右脚 Right crus
- 外腹斜筋 External oblique
- 大動脈裂孔 Aortic aperture
- 正中弓状靱帯 Median arcuate ligament

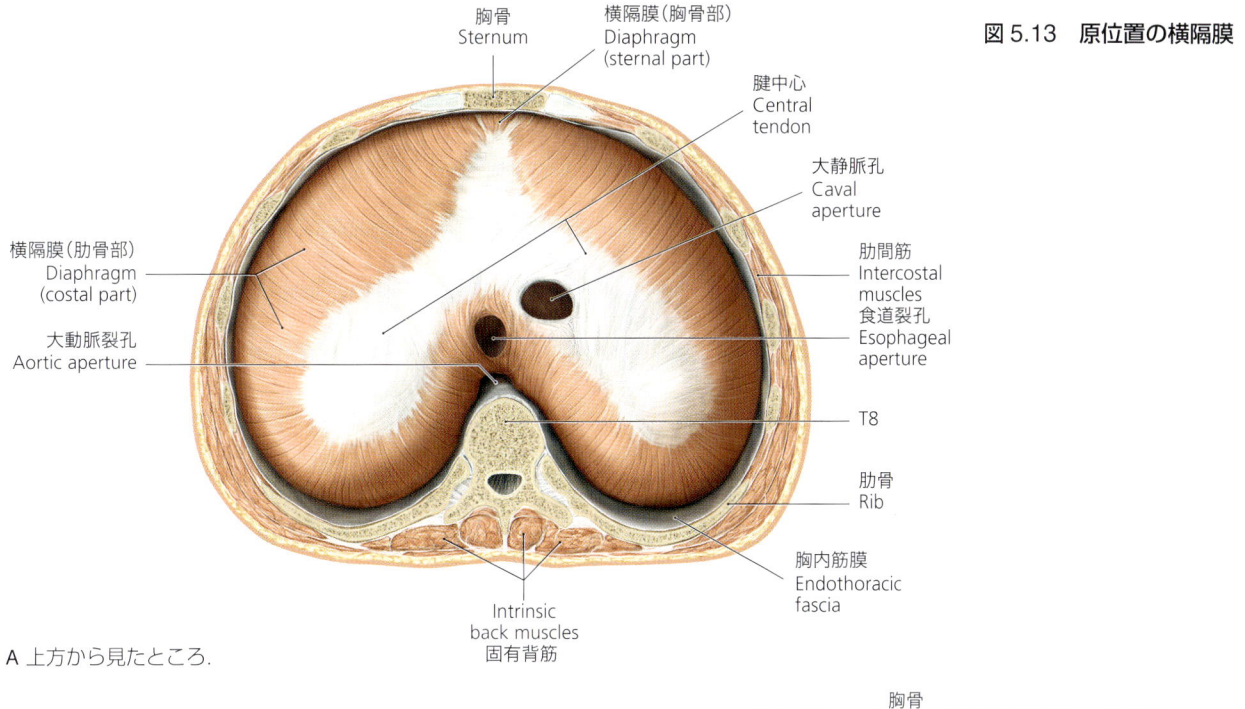

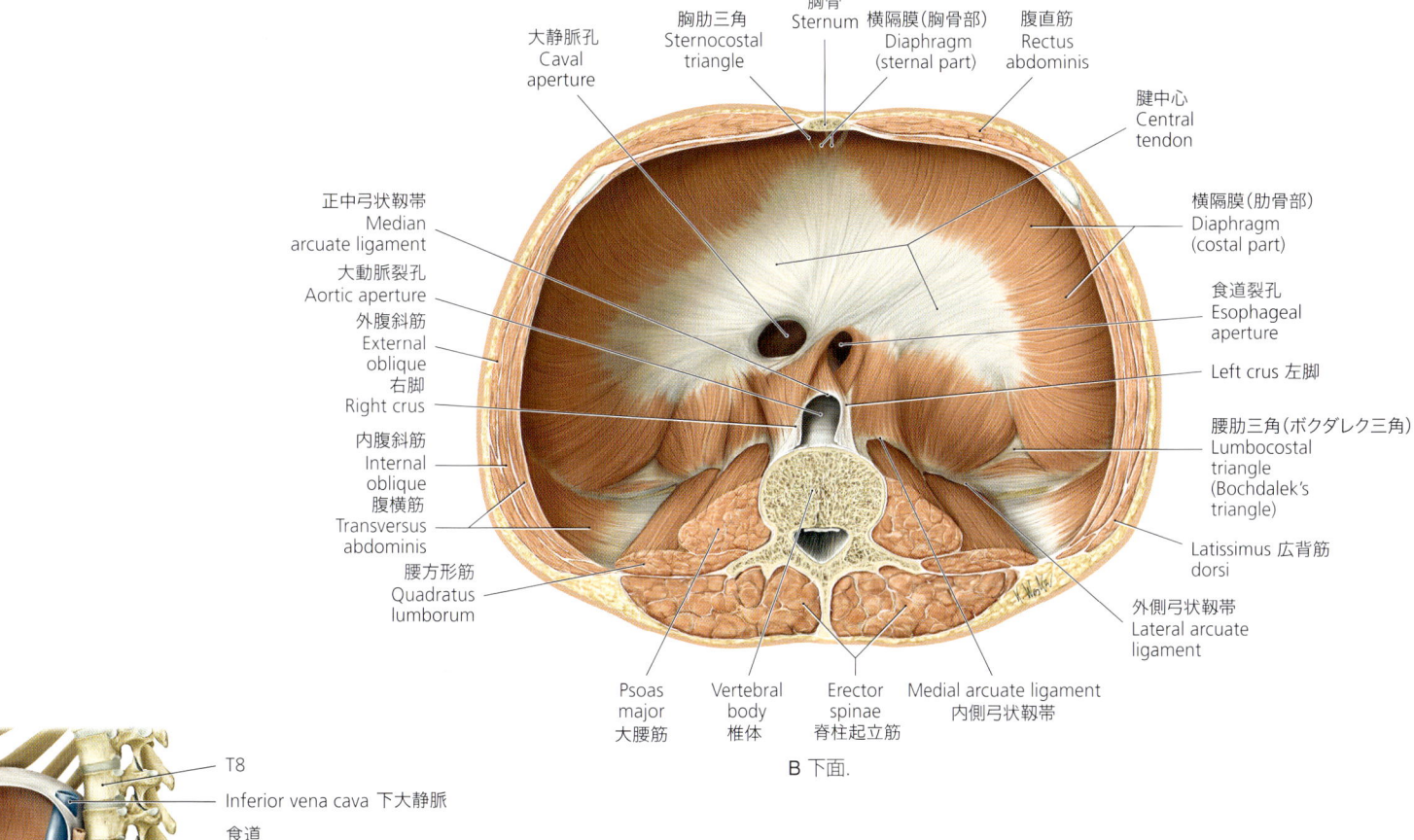

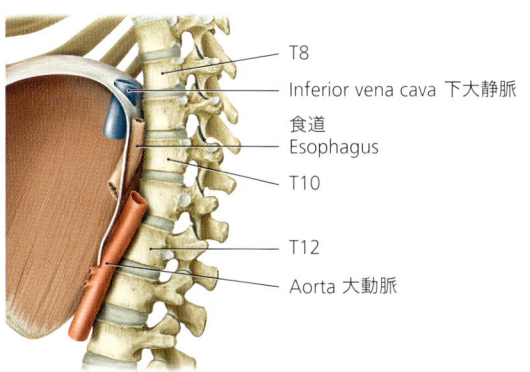

C 横隔膜の開口部，左外側方から見たところ．

- T8
- 下大静脈 Inferior vena cava
- 食道 Esophagus
- T10
- T12
- 大動脈 Aorta

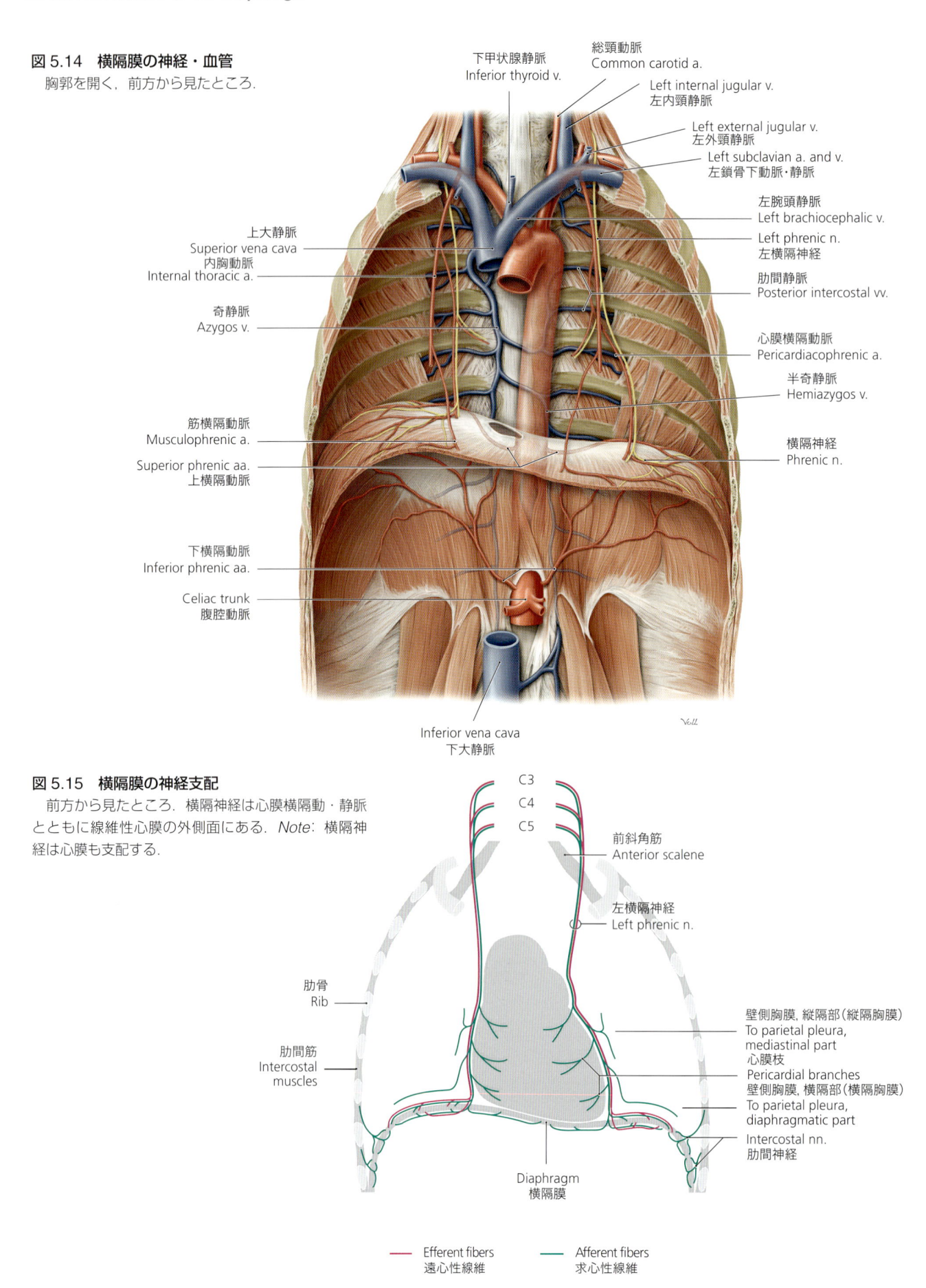

横隔膜の神経と血管
Neurovasculature of the Diaphragm

図 5.14 横隔膜の神経・血管
胸郭を開く，前方から見たところ．

主要な構造：
- 下甲状腺静脈 Inferior thyroid v.
- 総頸動脈 Common carotid a.
- Left internal jugular v. 左内頸静脈
- Left external jugular v. 左外頸静脈
- Left subclavian a. and v. 左鎖骨下動脈・静脈
- 左腕頭静脈 Left brachiocephalic v.
- Left phrenic n. 左横隔神経
- 上大静脈 Superior vena cava
- 内胸動脈 Internal thoracic a.
- 肋間静脈 Posterior intercostal vv.
- 奇静脈 Azygos v.
- 心膜横隔動脈 Pericardiacophrenic a.
- 半奇静脈 Hemiazygos v.
- 筋横隔動脈 Musculophrenic a.
- 上横隔動脈 Superior phrenic aa.
- 横隔神経 Phrenic n.
- 下横隔動脈 Inferior phrenic aa.
- Celiac trunk 腹腔動脈
- Inferior vena cava 下大静脈

図 5.15 横隔膜の神経支配
前方から見たところ．横隔神経は心膜横隔動・静脈とともに線維性心膜の外側面にある．*Note*：横隔神経は心膜も支配する．

- C3, C4, C5
- 前斜角筋 Anterior scalene
- 左横隔神経 Left phrenic n.
- 肋骨 Rib
- 肋間筋 Intercostal muscles
- 壁側胸膜，縦隔部（縦隔胸膜）To parietal pleura, mediastinal part
- 心膜枝 Pericardial branches
- 壁側胸膜，横隔部（横隔胸膜）To parietal pleura, diaphragmatic part
- 肋間神経 Intercostal nn.
- Diaphragm 横隔膜

— Efferent fibers 遠心性線維
— Afferent fibers 求心性線維

表 5.4	横隔膜の血管			
動脈	起始		静脈	流域
下横隔動脈（主要な供給源）	腹大動脈，時には腹腔動脈から起始		肋間静脈	
上横隔動脈	胸大動脈		上横隔静脈	右側：奇静脈へ，左側：半奇静脈へ
心膜横隔動脈	内胸動脈		右上肋間静脈	
筋横隔動脈				

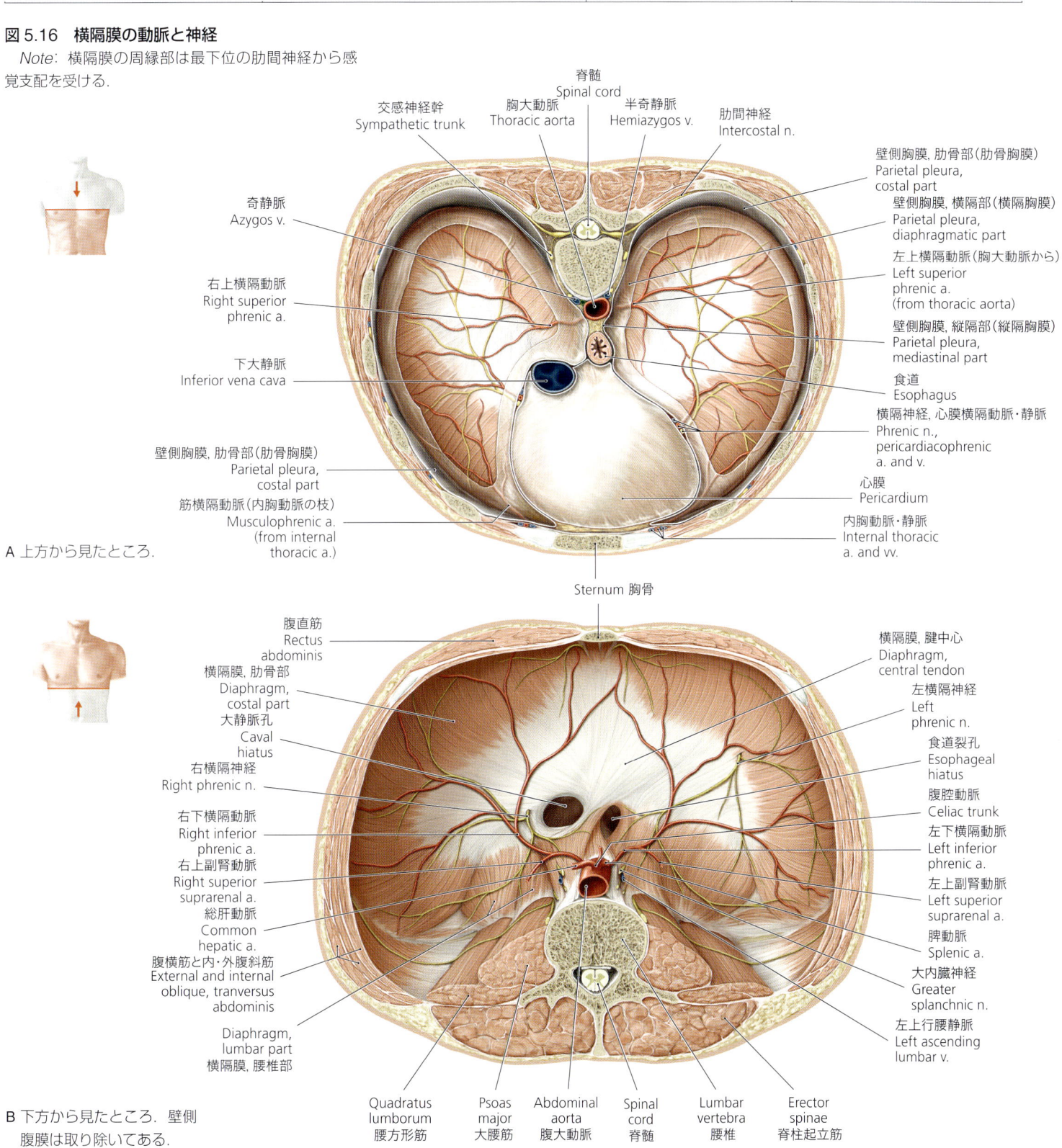

図 5.16　横隔膜の動脈と神経

Note：横隔膜の周縁部は最下位の肋間神経から感覚支配を受ける．

A　上方から見たところ．

B　下方から見たところ．壁側腹膜は取り除いてある．

胸壁の動脈と静脈
Arteries & Veins of the Thoracic Wall

> 肋間動脈は内胸動脈の前肋間枝と吻合し，胸壁の構造を栄養する．肋間動脈は胸大動脈から分岐するが，第1および第2肋間動脈は肋頸動脈の枝の最上肋間動脈から起こる．

図5.17 胸壁の動脈
前方から見たところ．

表5.5　胸壁の動脈

起始	枝
鎖骨下動脈	最上胸動脈
	外側胸動脈
	胸肩峰動脈
	第1-2肋間動脈（p.34 参照）
胸大動脈	肋間動脈（第3-12）
内胸動脈	前肋間枝
	筋横隔動脈
	上腹壁動脈

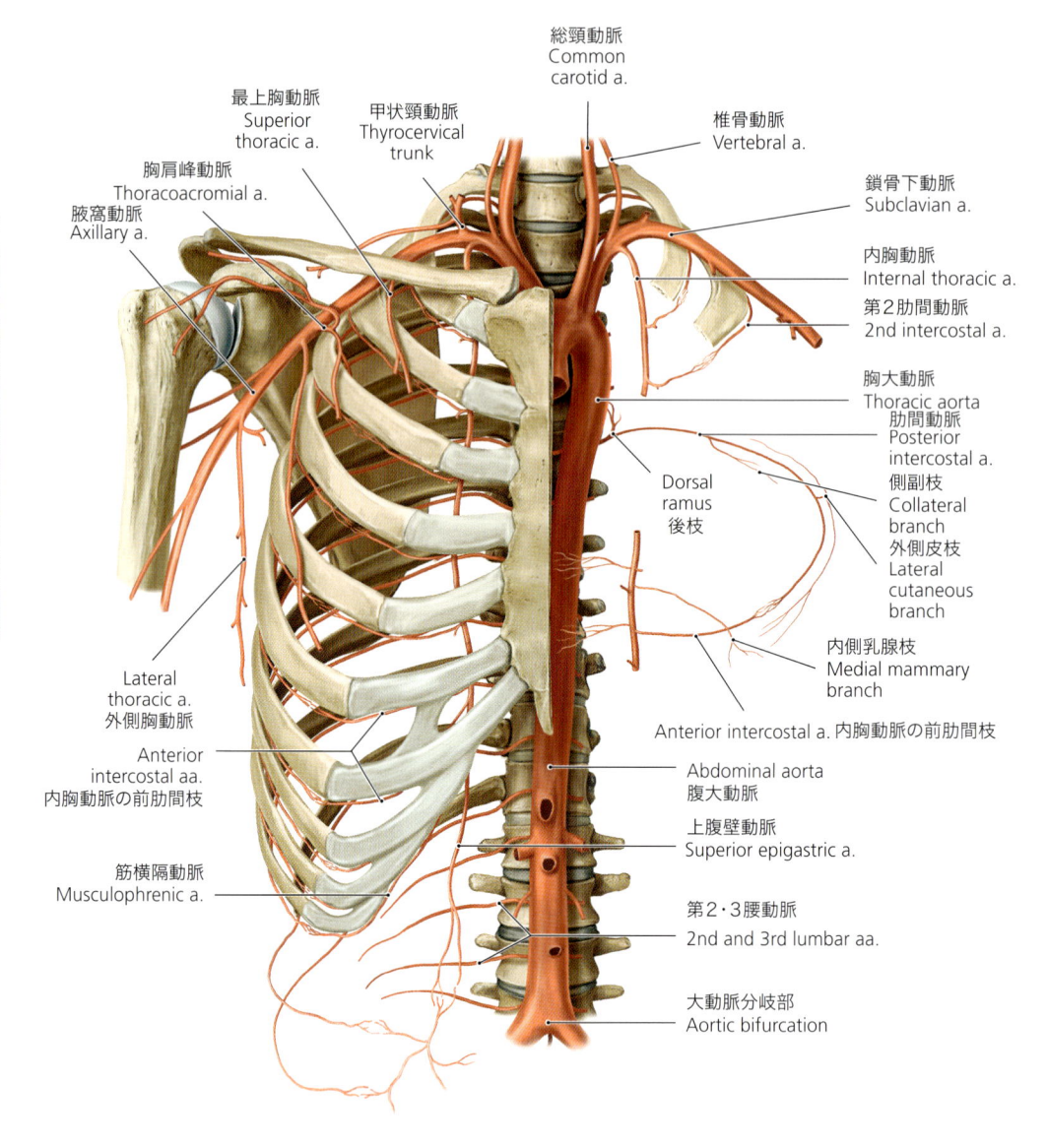

図5.18 肋間動脈の枝
上方から見たところ．

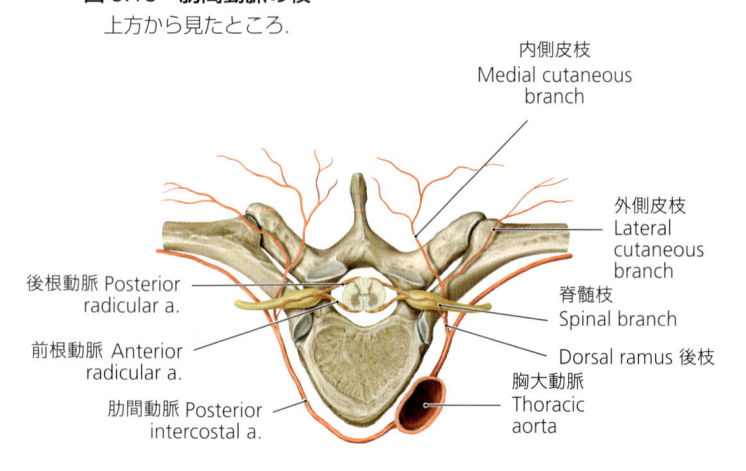

表5.6　肋間動脈の枝

動脈	枝		支配
肋間動脈	後枝	脊髄枝	脊髄
		外側皮枝	後胸壁
		内側皮枝	
	側副枝		外胸壁
内胸動脈の前肋間枝	外側皮枝*		前胸壁

*外側皮枝の外側乳腺枝は内胸動脈の内側乳腺枝とともに乳房を支配する．

肋間静脈は主に奇静脈系へと連絡するが，内胸静脈にも注ぐ．血液は最終的には上大静脈を介して心臓に戻る．肋間静脈は肋間動脈と同様の位置に分布するが，脊柱の静脈は脊椎を全長にわたって横切る椎骨静脈叢を作る（p.35 参照）．

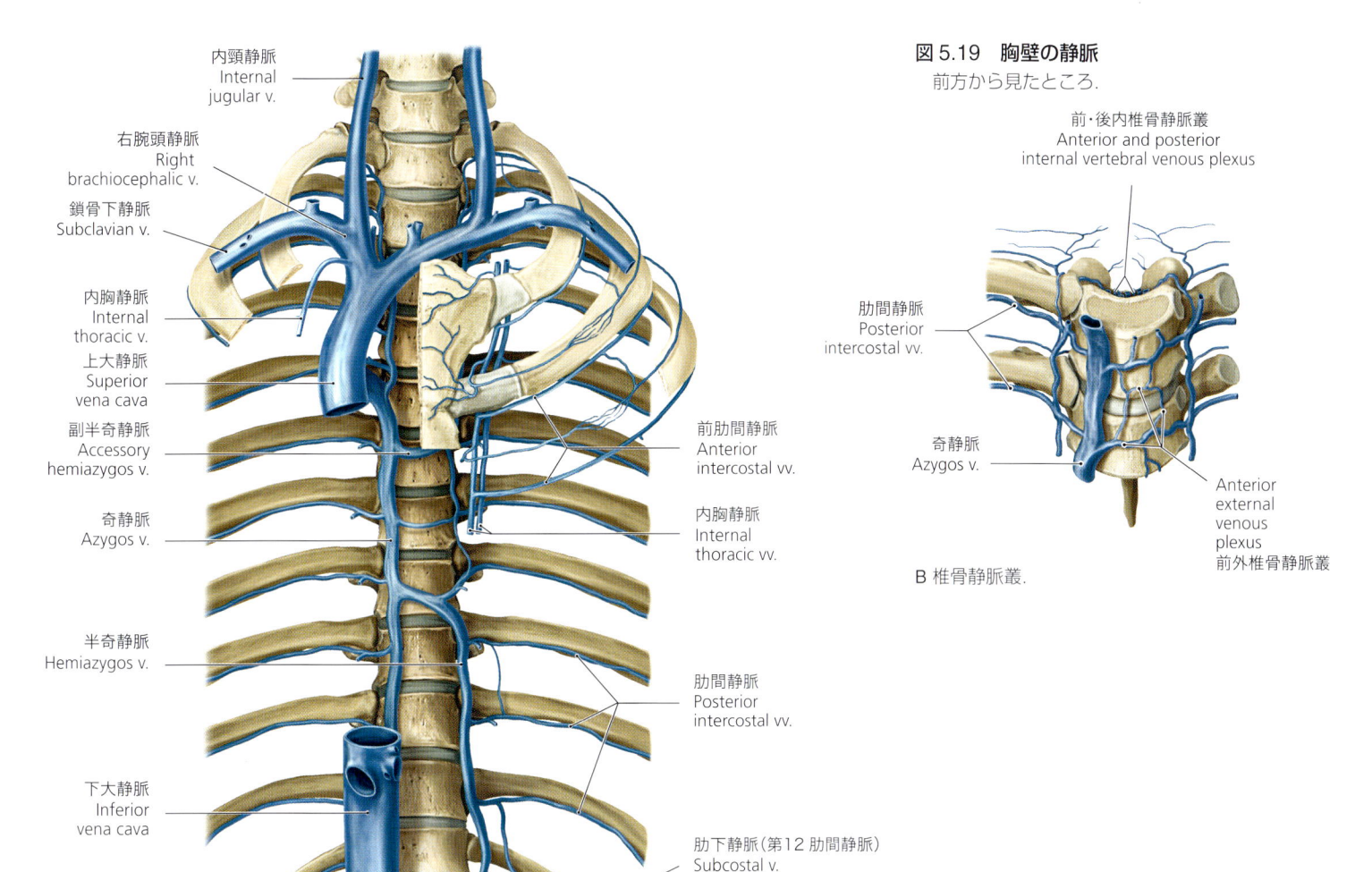

図 5.19　胸壁の静脈
前方から見たところ．

- 内頸静脈 Internal jugular v.
- 右腕頭静脈 Right brachiocephalic v.
- 鎖骨下静脈 Subclavian v.
- 内胸静脈 Internal thoracic v.
- 上大静脈 Superior vena cava
- 副半奇静脈 Accessory hemiazygos v.
- 奇静脈 Azygos v.
- 半奇静脈 Hemiazygos v.
- 下大静脈 Inferior vena cava
- 前肋間静脈 Anterior intercostal vv.
- 内胸静脈 Internal thoracic vv.
- 肋間静脈 Posterior intercostal vv.
- 肋下静脈（第12 肋間静脈）Subcostal v. (12th intercostal v.)
- 第1腰静脈 1st lumbar v.

A 前方から見たところ．胸郭を開く．

- 前・後内椎骨静脈叢 Anterior and posterior internal vertebral venous plexus
- 肋間静脈 Posterior intercostal vv.
- 奇静脈 Azygos v.
- 前外椎骨静脈叢 Anterior external venous plexus

B 椎骨静脈叢．

図 5.20　皮静脈
前方から見たところ．胸腹壁静脈は上大静脈・下大静脈閉塞時の潜在的な浅層の側副路である．

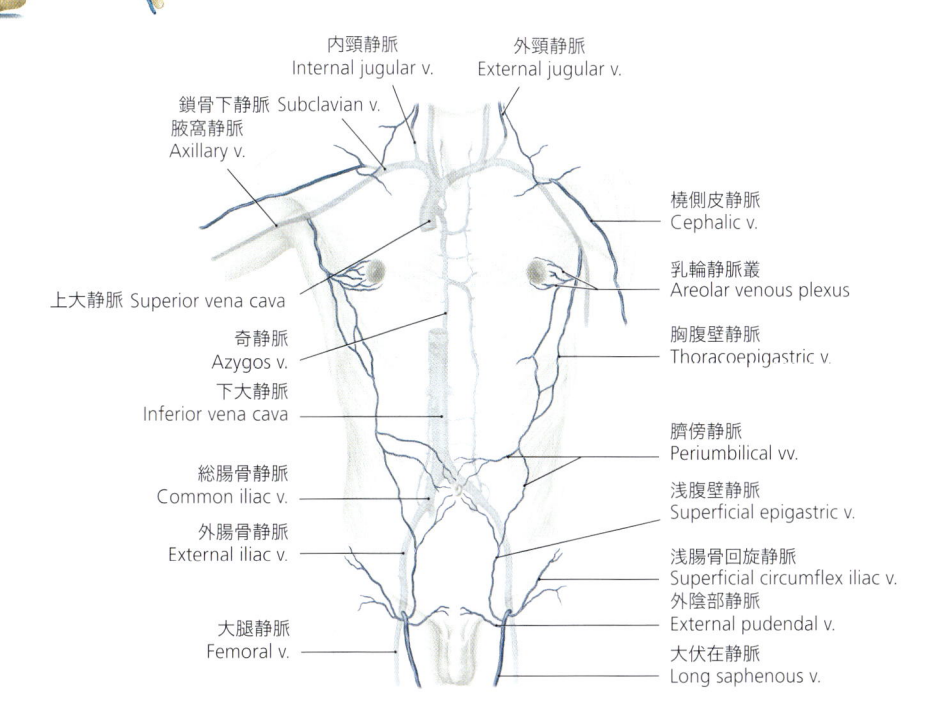

- 内頸静脈 Internal jugular v.
- 外頸静脈 External jugular v.
- 鎖骨下静脈 Subclavian v.
- 腋窩静脈 Axillary v.
- 上大静脈 Superior vena cava
- 奇静脈 Azygos v.
- 下大静脈 Inferior vena cava
- 総腸骨静脈 Common iliac v.
- 外腸骨静脈 External iliac v.
- 大腿静脈 Femoral v.
- 橈側皮静脈 Cephalic v.
- 乳輪静脈叢 Areolar venous plexus
- 胸腹壁静脈 Thoracoepigastric v.
- 臍傍静脈 Periumbilical vv.
- 浅腹壁静脈 Superficial epigastric v.
- 浅腸骨回旋静脈 Superficial circumflex iliac v.
- 外陰部静脈 External pudendal v.
- 大伏在静脈 Long saphenous v.

胸壁の神経
Nerves of the Thoracic Wall

図 5.21　肋間神経
前方から見たところ．第 1 肋骨が取り除かれ，第 1，2 肋間神経が見えている．

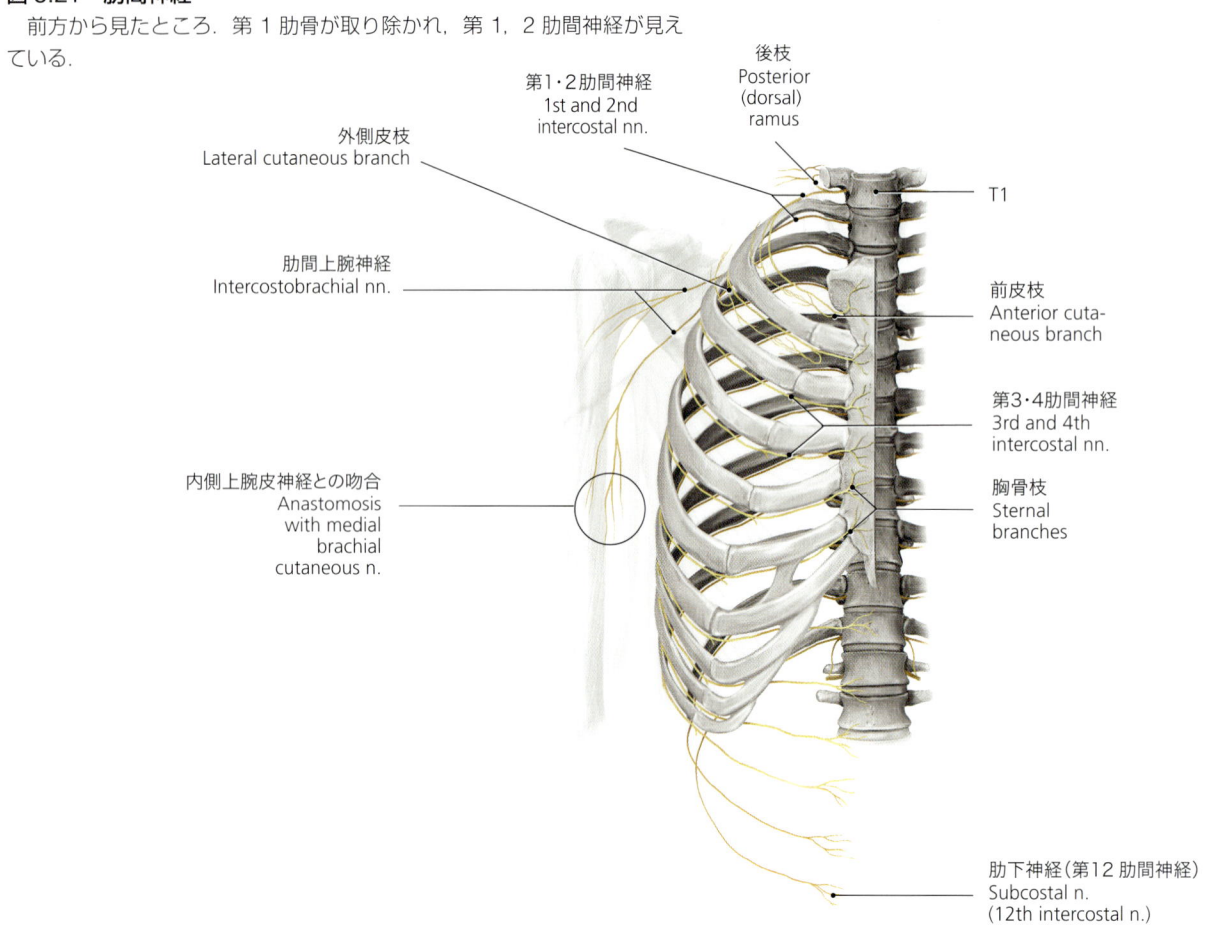

- 外側皮枝　Lateral cutaneous branch
- 第1・2肋間神経　1st and 2nd intercostal nn.
- 後枝　Posterior (dorsal) ramus
- T1
- 肋間上腕神経　Intercostobrachial nn.
- 前皮枝　Anterior cutaneous branch
- 第3・4肋間神経　3rd and 4th intercostal nn.
- 内側上腕皮神経との吻合　Anastomosis with medial brachial cutaneous n.
- 胸骨枝　Sternal branches
- 肋下神経（第12肋間神経）　Subcostal n. (12th intercostal n.)

図 5.22　胸壁．末梢感覚皮神経

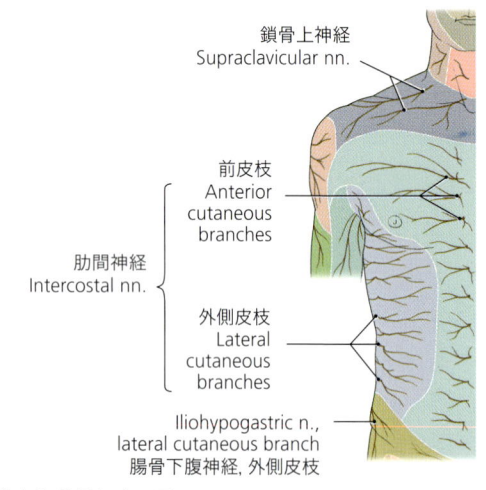

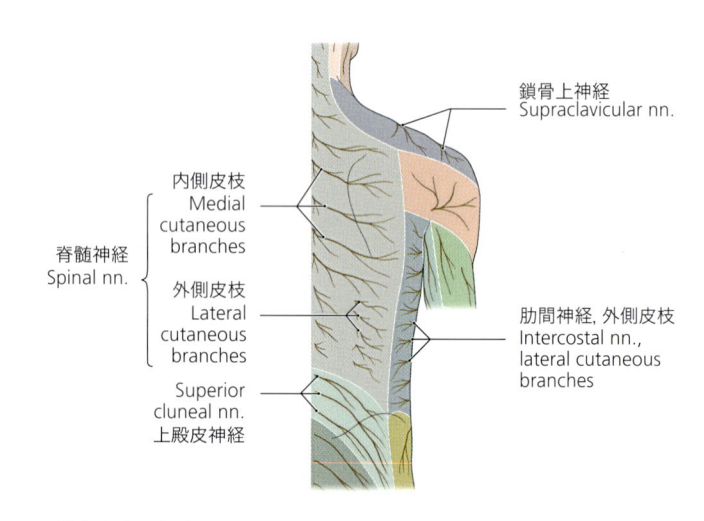

- 鎖骨上神経　Supraclavicular nn.
- 前皮枝　Anterior cutaneous branches
- 肋間神経　Intercostal nn.
- 外側皮枝　Lateral cutaneous branches
- Iliohypogastric n., lateral cutaneous branch　腸骨下腹神経，外側皮枝
- 鎖骨上神経　Supraclavicular nn.
- 内側皮枝　Medial cutaneous branches
- 脊髄神経　Spinal nn.
- 外側皮枝　Lateral cutaneous branches
- 肋間神経，外側皮枝　Intercostal nn., lateral cutaneous branches
- Superior cluneal nn.　上殿皮神経

A 前方から見たところ．　　B 後方から見たところ．

図 5.23 脊髄神経の枝

上方から見たところ．後根と前根が結合して作られる，約 1 cm の脊髄神経が椎間孔を通過し，脊柱管の外に出る．その後枝は背部の皮膚と固有背筋を支配し，前枝は肋間神経をなす．さらに詳細については p.36 参照．

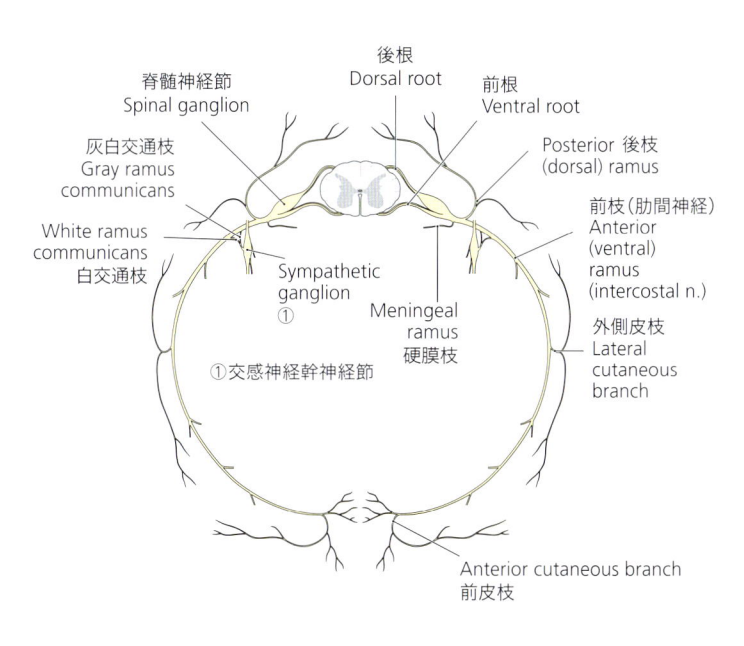

- 脊髄神経節 Spinal ganglion
- 灰白交通枝 Gray ramus communicans
- White ramus communicans 白交通枝
- 後根 Dorsal root
- 前根 Ventral root
- Posterior (dorsal) ramus 後枝
- 前枝（肋間神経）Anterior (ventral) ramus (intercostal n.)
- Sympathetic ganglion ①
- ①交感神経幹神経節
- Meningeal ramus 硬膜枝
- 外側皮枝 Lateral cutaneous branch
- Anterior cutaneous branch 前皮枝

図 5.24 肋間神経の経路

冠状断，前方から見たところ．

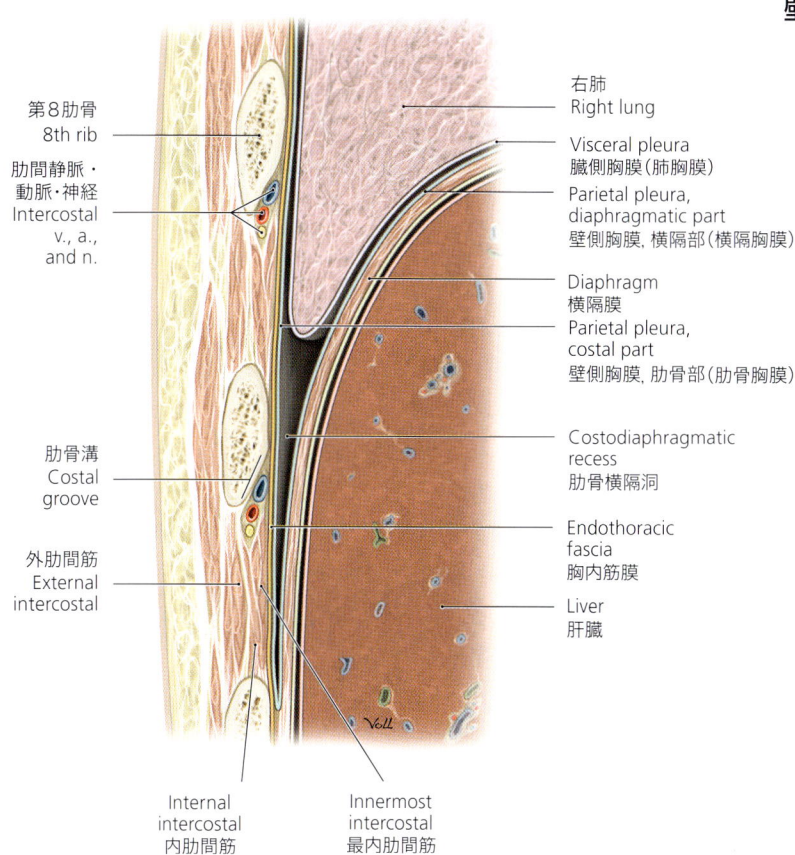

- 第8肋骨 8th rib
- 肋間静脈・動脈・神経 Intercostal v., a., and n.
- 肋骨溝 Costal groove
- 外肋間筋 External intercostal
- Internal intercostal 内肋間筋
- Innermost intercostal 最内肋間筋
- 右肺 Right lung
- Visceral pleura 臓側胸膜（肺胸膜）
- Parietal pleura, diaphragmatic part 壁側胸膜，横隔部（横隔胸膜）
- Diaphragm 横隔膜
- Parietal pleura, costal part 壁側胸膜，肋骨部（肋骨胸膜）
- Costodiaphragmatic recess 肋骨横隔洞
- Endothoracic fascia 胸内筋膜
- Liver 肝臓

図 5.25 胸壁のデルマトーム

Landmarks：第 4 胸神経は一般に乳頭を含み第 6 胸神経は剣状突起より上の皮膚を支配する．

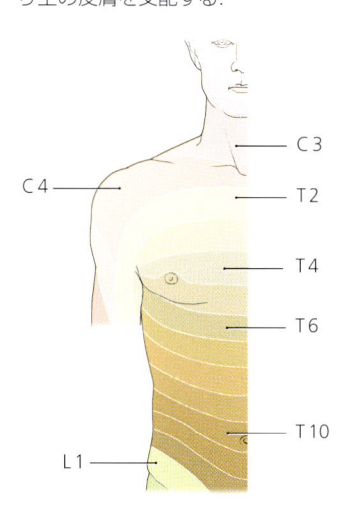

A 前方から見たところ．

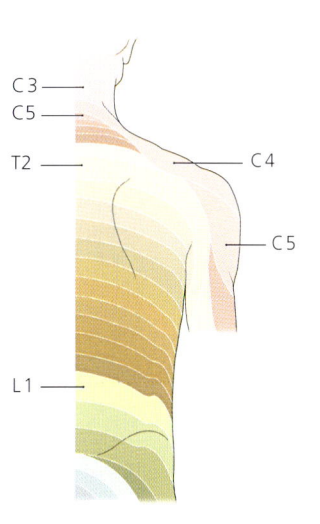

B 後方から見たところ．

胸壁

胸壁の神経と血管の位置
Neurovascular Topography of the Thoracic Wall

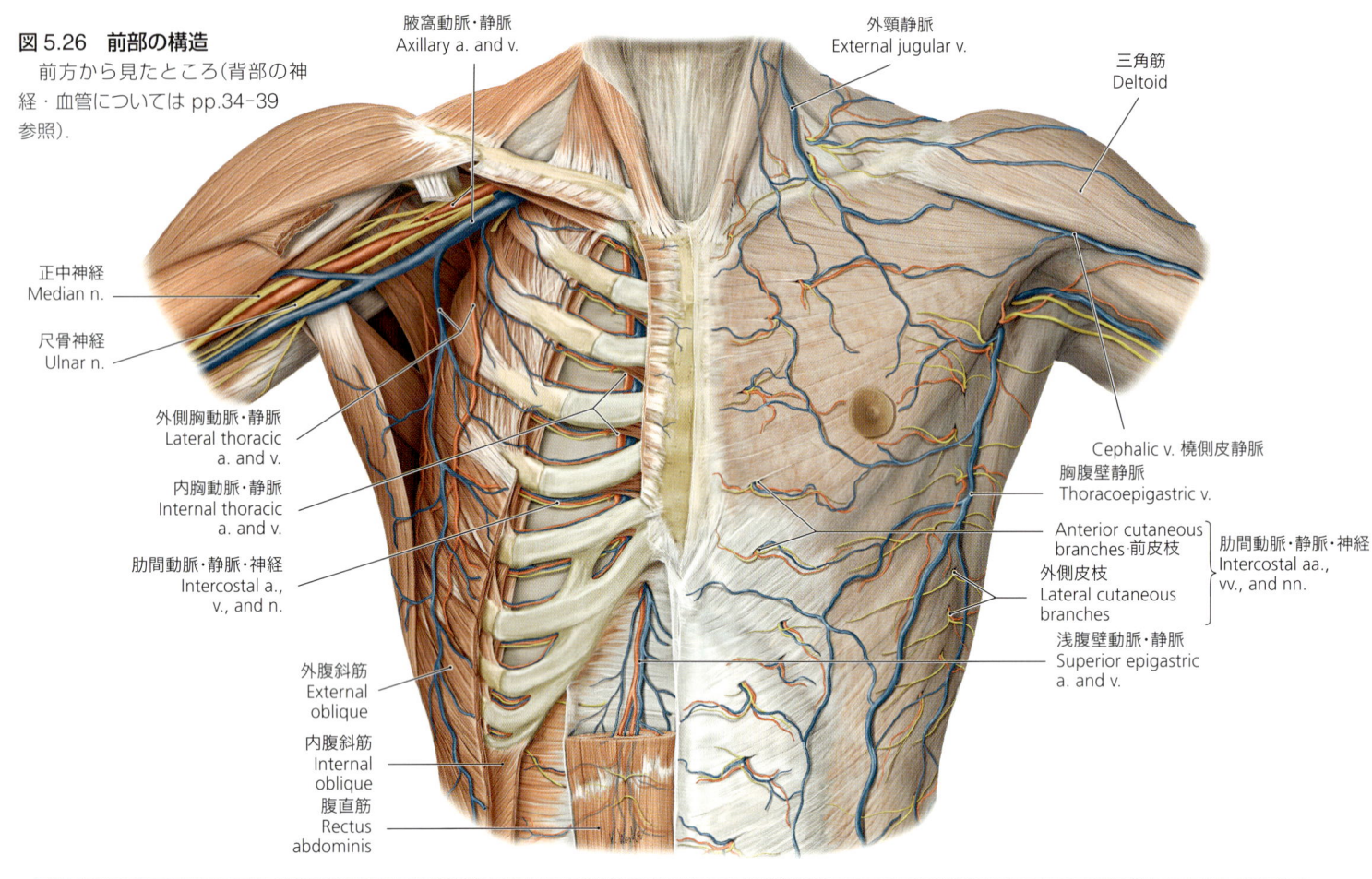

図 5.26　前部の構造
前方から見たところ（背部の神経・血管については pp.34-39 参照）．

Labels:
- 腋窩動脈・静脈 Axillary a. and v.
- 外頸静脈 External jugular v.
- 三角筋 Deltoid
- 正中神経 Median n.
- 尺骨神経 Ulnar n.
- 外側胸動脈・静脈 Lateral thoracic a. and v.
- 内胸動脈・静脈 Internal thoracic a. and v.
- 肋間動脈・静脈・神経 Intercostal a., v., and n.
- 外腹斜筋 External oblique
- 内腹斜筋 Internal oblique
- 腹直筋 Rectus abdominis
- Cephalic v. 橈側皮静脈
- 胸腹壁静脈 Thoracoepigastric v.
- 前皮枝 Anterior cutaneous branches
- 外側皮枝 Lateral cutaneous branches
- 肋間動脈・静脈・神経 Intercostal aa., vv., and nn.
- 浅腹壁動脈・静脈 Superior epigastric a. and v.

臨床

胸腔チューブの挿入

気管支癌に起因する胸水のような，胸膜腔に貯留する異常な滲出液には胸腔チューブが必要である．一般に，座位で最も有効な穿刺部位は後腋窩線沿いの第 7-8 肋間とされている．チューブは肋骨上縁で挿入される．これは肋間動脈・静脈・神経を傷つけないためである．虚脱した肺についての詳細は p.113 参照．

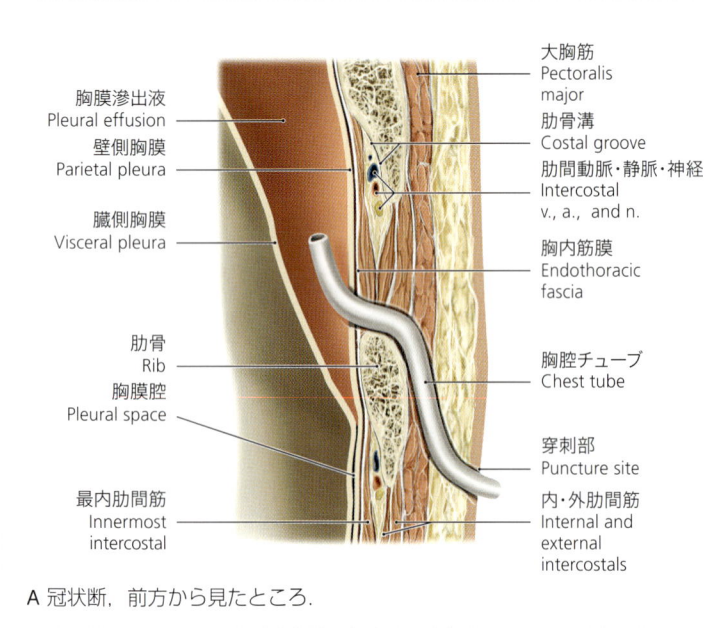

Labels (cross-section):
- 胸膜滲出液 Pleural effusion
- 壁側胸膜 Parietal pleura
- 臓側胸膜 Visceral pleura
- 肋骨 Rib
- 胸膜腔 Pleural space
- 最内肋間筋 Innermost intercostal
- 大胸筋 Pectoralis major
- 肋骨溝 Costal groove
- 肋間動脈・静脈・神経 Intercostal v., a., and n.
- 胸内筋膜 Endothoracic fascia
- 胸腔チューブ Chest tube
- 穿刺部 Puncture site
- 内・外肋間筋 Internal and external intercostals

A　冠状断，前方から見たところ．

B　胸腔チューブは胸壁に垂直に挿入していく．

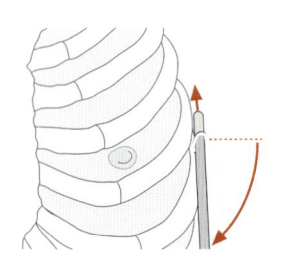

C　肋骨にあてた後，チューブの向きを変え，胸壁に平行に皮下のチューブを進めていく．

D　肋骨上縁でチューブは肋間筋を貫き，胸腔に進める．

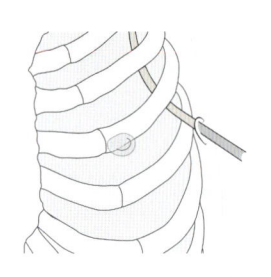

図 5.27 断面における肋間の構造

横断，前上方から見たところ．

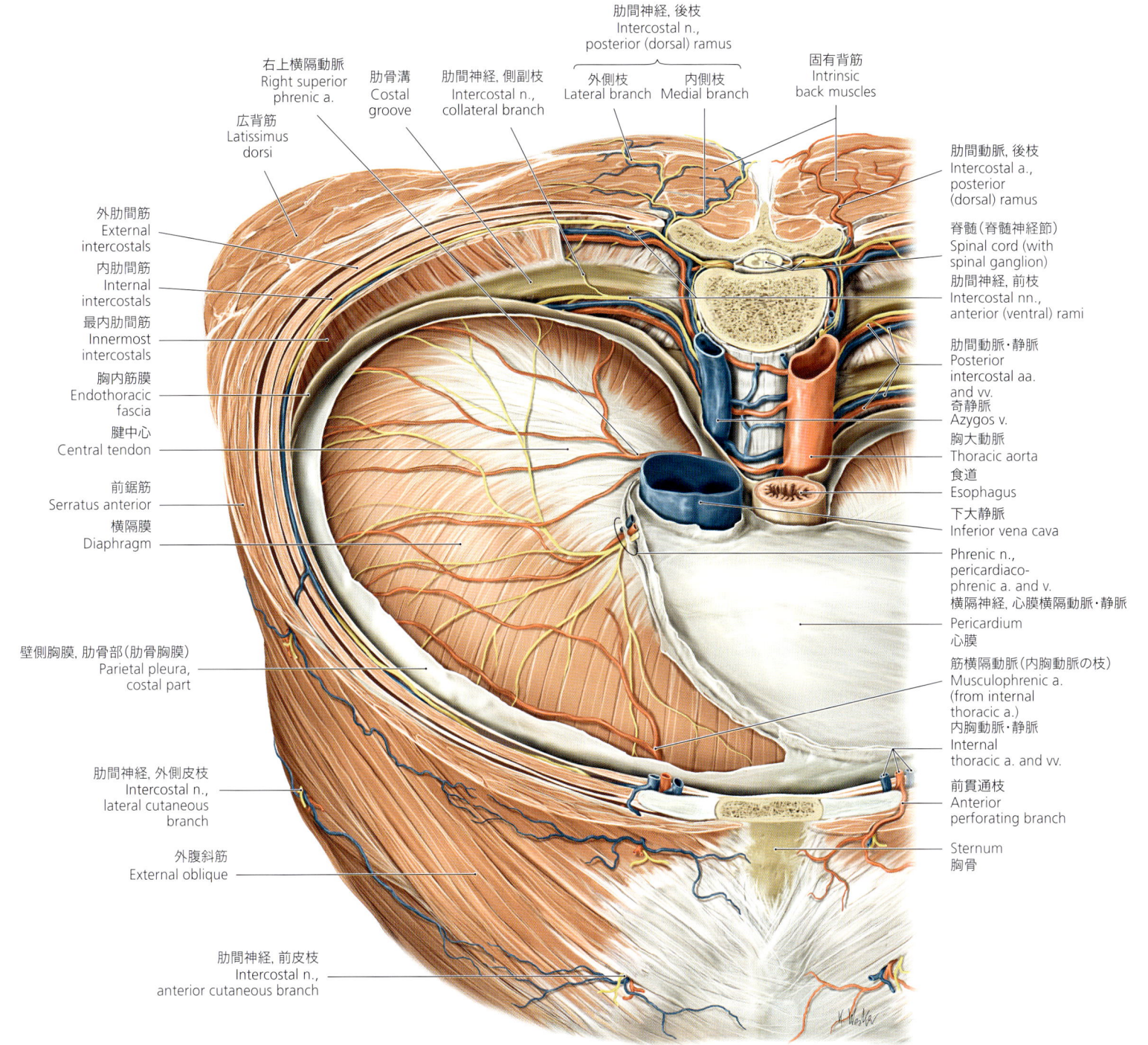

女性の乳房
Female Breast

女性の乳房は皮下組織層内の汗腺が変形したもので，腺組織，線維性の間質，脂肪からなる．乳房は第 2-6 肋骨に広がり，胸筋膜，腋窩筋膜，浅腹筋膜と結合組織によって緩く結合している．このほか乳房提靱帯によっても支えられる．乳房組織が腋窩まで伸び出した腋窩尾も多く見られる．

図 5.28 女性の乳房
右乳房，前方から見たところ．

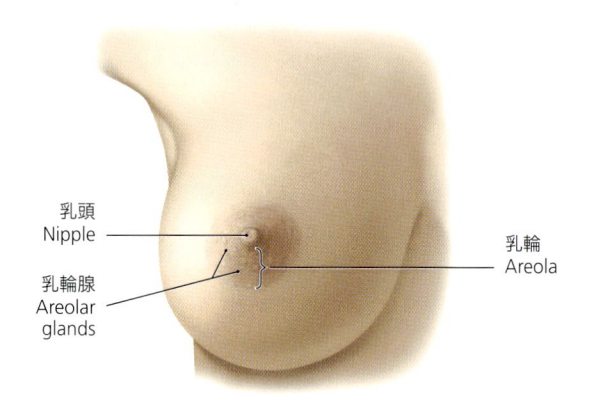

- 乳頭 Nipple
- 乳輪腺 Areolar glands
- 乳輪 Areola

図 5.29 乳腺堤
乳腺の痕跡は両性で乳腺堤を作る．通常は胸部の対のみが残るが，時にはヒトでも副乳として残る．

図 5.30 胸への栄養血液

- 腋窩動脈・静脈 Axillary a. and v.
- 外側胸動脈・静脈 Lateral thoracic a. and v.
- 内側乳腺枝 Medial mammary branches
- 外側乳腺枝 Lateral mammary branches
- 鎖骨下動脈・静脈 Subclavian a. and v.
- 内胸動脈・静脈 Internal thoracic a. and v.
- 貫通枝 Perforating branches
- 乳腺枝 Mammary branches

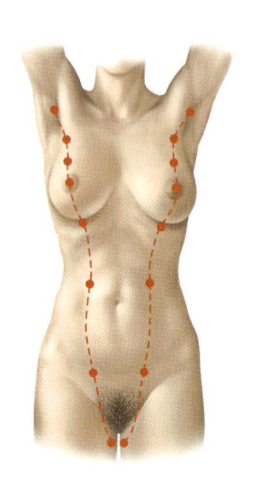

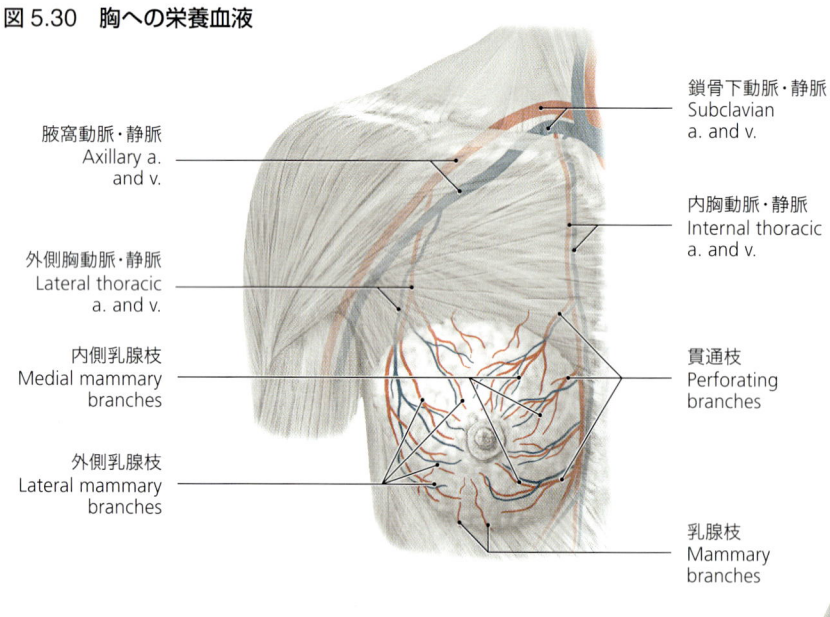

図 5.31 乳房の感覚神経支配

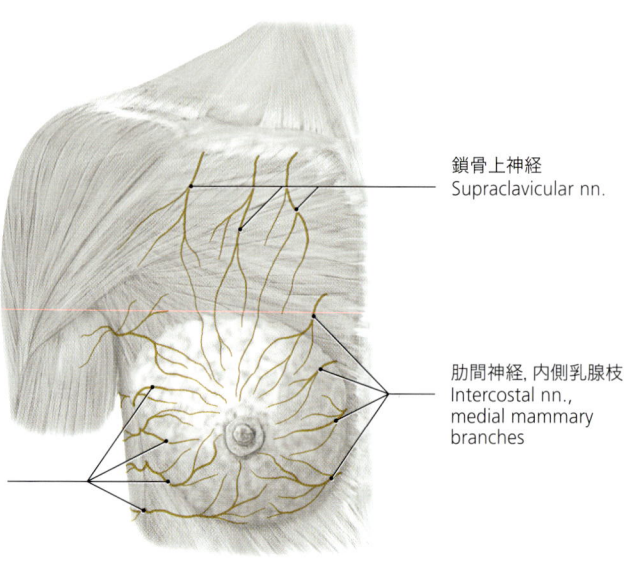

- 鎖骨上神経 Supraclavicular nn.
- 肋間神経, 内側乳腺枝 Intercostal nn., medial mammary branches
- 肋間神経, 外側乳腺枝 Intercostal nn., lateral mammary branches

腺組織は 10〜20 個の乳腺葉からなり，それぞれに乳管がある．乳管は色素沈着の強い乳輪の中心にある盛り上がった乳頭に開口する．乳管開口部周辺には乳管洞と呼ばれる拡張した領域がある．乳輪の高まりには乳輪腺の開口部（脂腺）がある．腺と乳管は血流の豊富な固い線維性組織で囲まれている．

図 5.32　乳房の構造

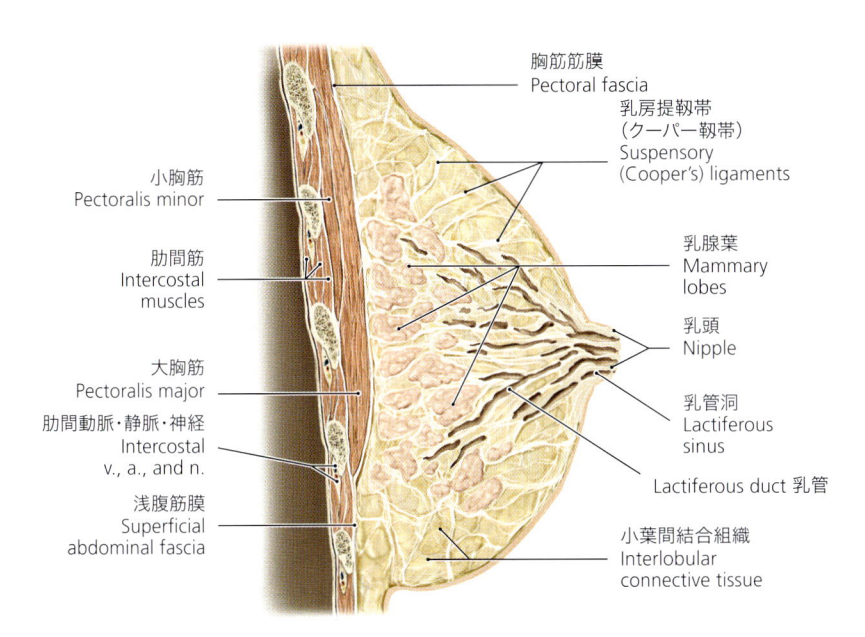

胸筋筋膜 Pectoral fascia
乳房提靱帯（クーパー靱帯） Suspensory (Cooper's) ligaments
小胸筋 Pectoralis minor
肋間筋 Intercostal muscles
大胸筋 Pectoralis major
肋間動脈・静脈・神経 Intercostal v., a., and n.
浅腹筋膜 Superficial abdominal fascia
乳腺葉 Mammary lobes
乳頭 Nipple
乳管洞 Lactiferous sinus
Lactiferous duct 乳管
小葉間結合組織 Interlobular connective tissue

A 鎖骨中線での矢状断．

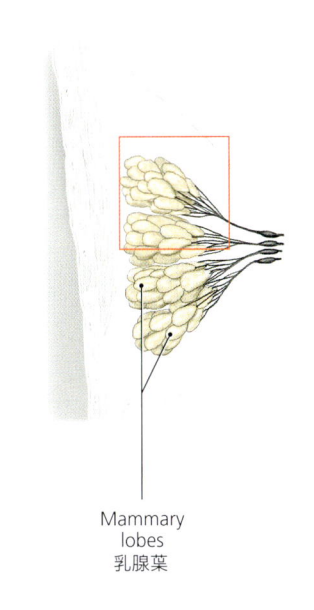

Mammary lobes 乳腺葉

B 導管系と葉．矢状断．ここで示した非授乳乳腺では，小葉に痕跡的な腺房の束が含まれる．

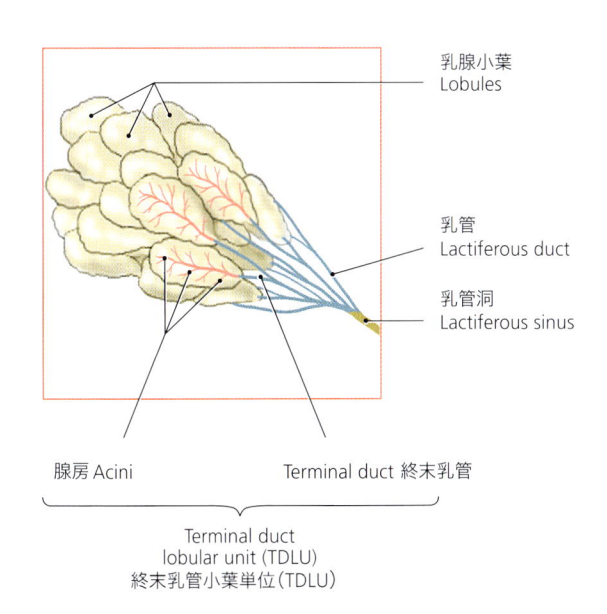

乳腺小葉 Lobules
乳管 Lactiferous duct
乳管洞 Lactiferous sinus
腺房 Acini　　**Terminal duct 終末乳管**
Terminal duct lobular unit (TDLU)
終末乳管小葉単位（TDLU）

C 終末乳管小葉単位（TDLU）．小葉を作る腺房の束は終末乳管によって空になる．これらの構造はまとめて TDLU として知られる．

女性乳房のリンパ管
Lymphatics of the Female Breast

乳房のリンパ管（ここでは示されていない）は浅，皮下，深の3リンパ管系に分けられる．これらは主に腋窩リンパ節に集まるが，小胸筋との関係で分類される（表 5.7）．乳房の内側部は内胸動脈に沿って分布する胸骨傍リンパ節によって灌流される．

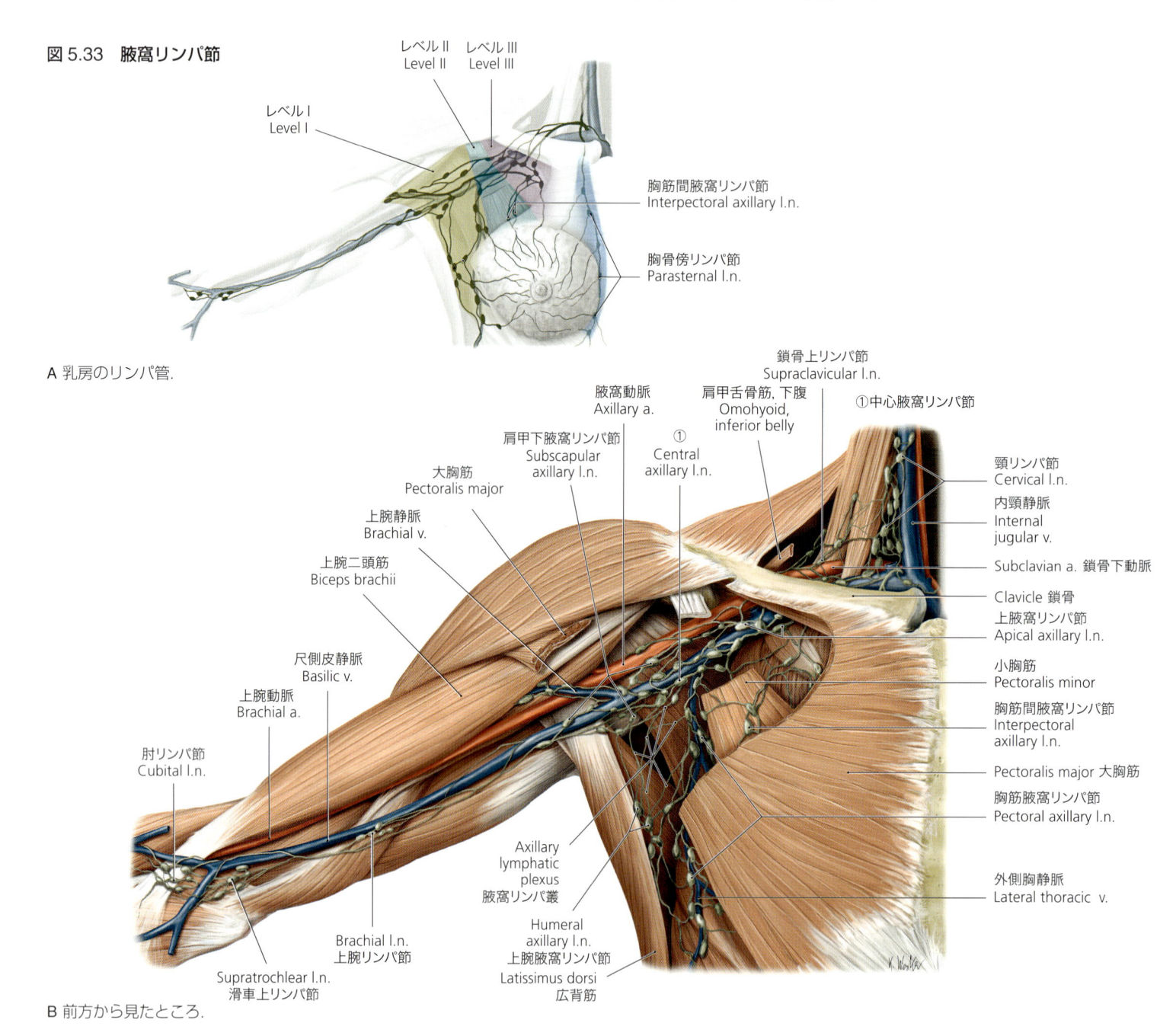

図 5.33 腋窩リンパ節

A 乳房のリンパ管．

B 前方から見たところ．

表 5.7 腋窩リンパ節のレベル

レベル	位置		リンパ節
I	下腋窩グループ	小胸筋の外側	胸筋腋窩リンパ節
			肩甲下腋窩リンパ節
			上腕腋窩リンパ節
			中心腋窩リンパ節
II	中腋窩グループ	小胸筋の浅層	胸筋間腋窩リンパ節
III	上腋窩グループ	小胸筋の内側	上腋窩リンパ節

臨床

乳癌

小葉内結合組織の幹細胞は乳管の増殖と腺房の分化に必要な細胞の著しい増殖に働く．これが悪性乳癌の頻発部位である終末乳管小葉単位（TDLU）を構成する．

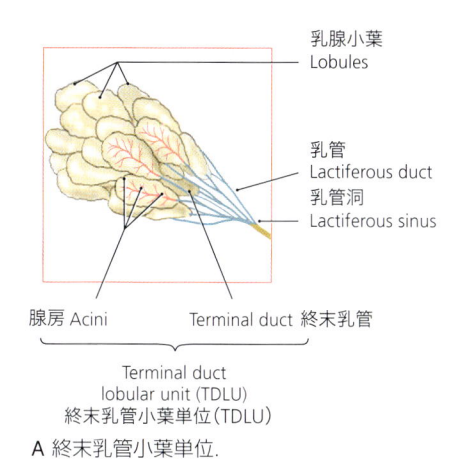

A 終末乳管小葉単位．

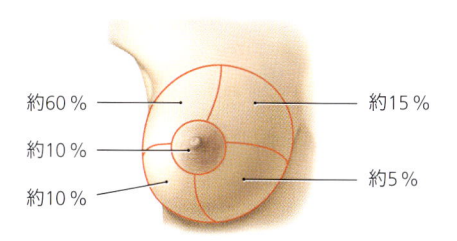

B 悪性腫瘍の部位別発生比率．

乳房腫瘍はリンパ管を通して広がる．胸骨傍リンパ節を経て正中線を越えて反対側に広がることもあるが，深リンパ管系（レベルIII）が特に重要である．乳癌の生存率は腋窩リンパ節の各レベルに属するリンパ節への転移の広さに強く左右される．転移の波及度合いは放射標識コロイド（テクネチウム99m標識硫黄マイクロコロイド）によるシンチグラフ法で測定される．腫瘍から最初にリンパを受け入れる見張りリンパ節は放射標識によって初めに標識される．認識された後は，見張りリンパ節除去を行い，組織学的に癌組織の検査が行われる．この方法は腋窩リンパ節転移のレベルを98％の精度で予測する．

転移	5年生存率
レベルI	65%
レベルII	31%
レベルIII	～0%

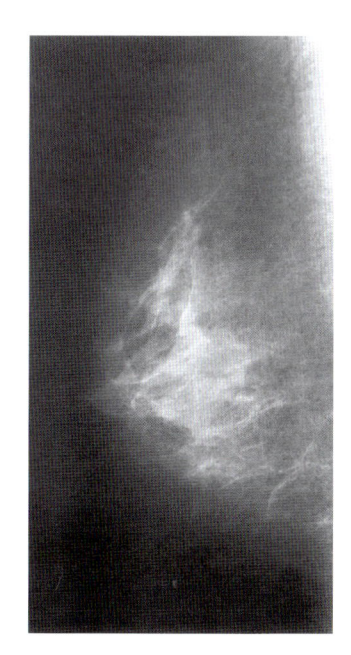

C 正常マンモグラフィ．

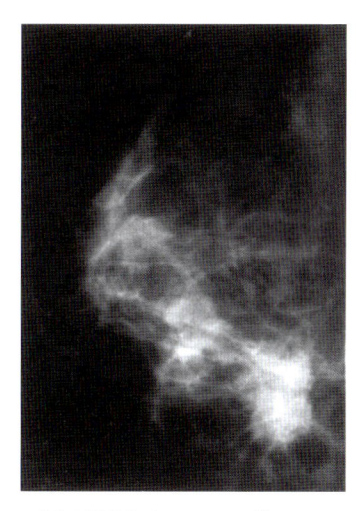

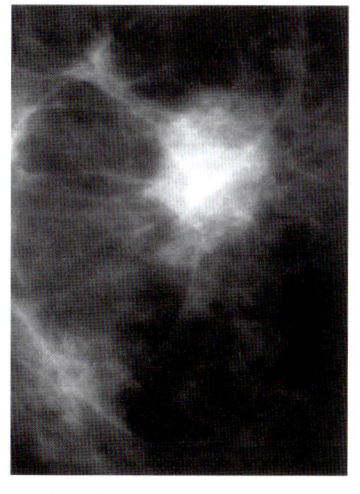

D 浸潤性乳管癌のマンモグラフィ．大きな病変が乳房組織の周辺構造を変化させている．

胸腔の区分
Divisions of the Thoracic Cavity

胸腔は大きく縦隔(p.76)と2つの胸膜腔(p.102)の3つの領域に分けられる.

図6.1 胸腔
冠状断，前方から見たところ．

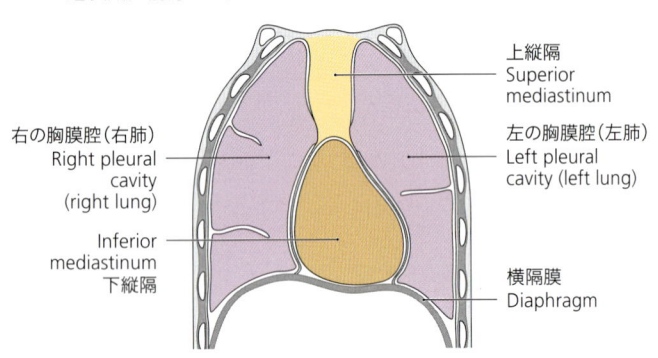

A 胸腔の区分．

表6.1 胸腔の主要構造

縦隔	上縦隔		胸腺，大血管，気管，食道，胸管
	下縦隔	前縦隔	胸腺
		中縦隔	心臓，心膜，大血管の根部
		後縦隔	胸大動脈，胸管，食道，奇静脈系
胸膜腔	右胸膜腔		右肺
	左胸膜腔		左肺

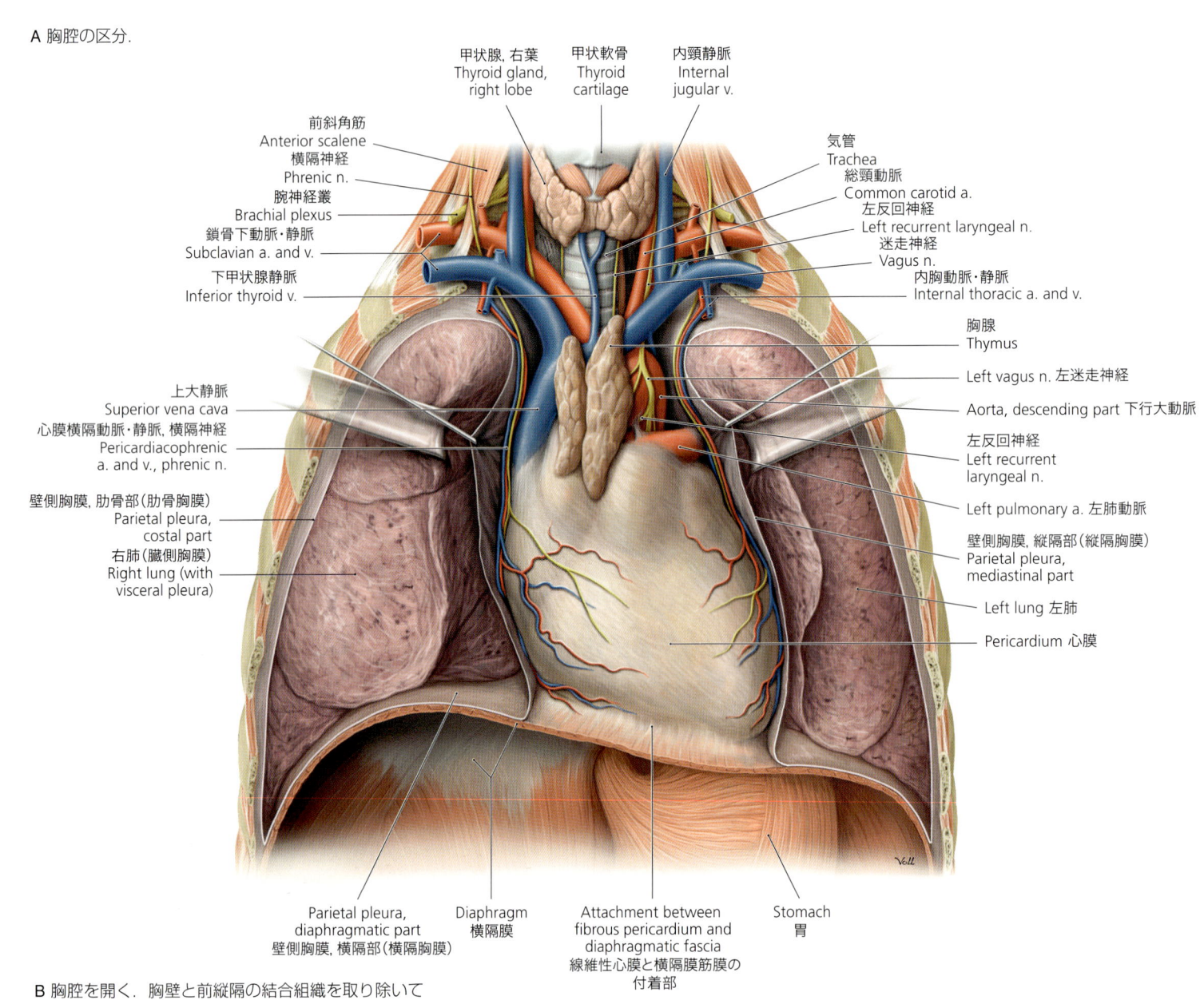

B 胸腔を開く．胸壁と前縦隔の結合組織を取り除いている．

図6.2 縦隔の区分

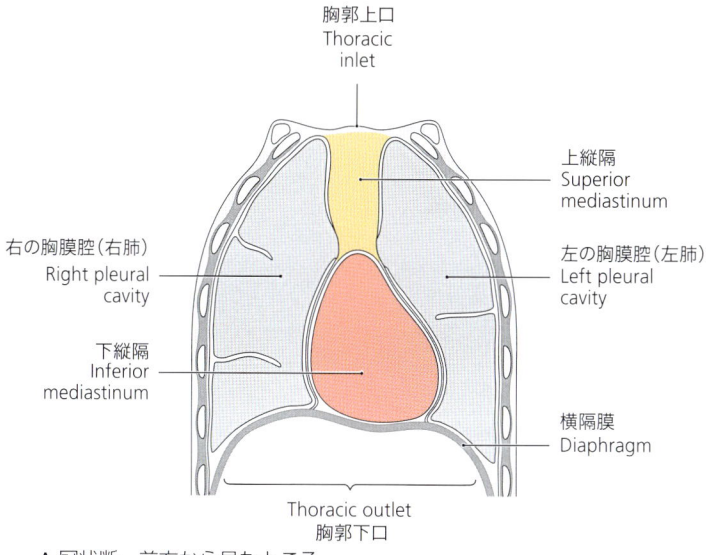

A 冠状断，前方から見たところ．

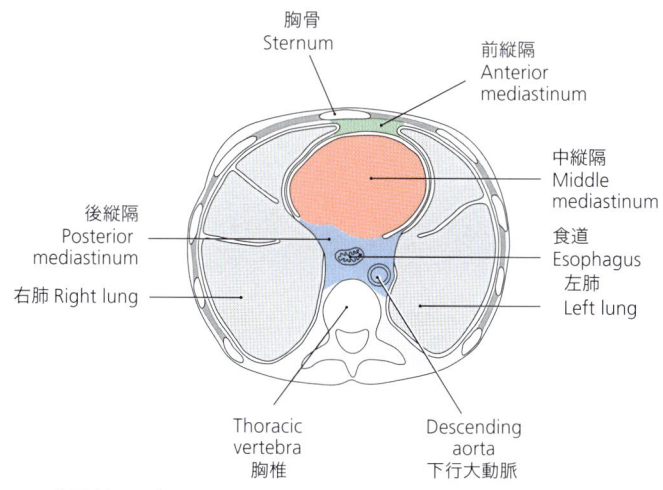

- 胸郭上口 Thoracic inlet
- 上縦隔 Superior mediastinum
- 右の胸膜腔(右肺) Right pleural cavity
- 左の胸膜腔(左肺) Left pleural cavity
- 下縦隔 Inferior mediastinum
- 横隔膜 Diaphragm
- 胸郭下口 Thoracic outlet

C 水平断，下方から見たところ．

- 胸骨 Sternum
- 前縦隔 Anterior mediastinum
- 中縦隔 Middle mediastinum
- 後縦隔 Posterior mediastinum
- 食道 Esophagus
- 右肺 Right lung
- 左肺 Left lung
- 胸椎 Thoracic vertebra
- 下行大動脈 Descending aorta

B 正中矢状断，外側方から見たところ．

- 食道，頸部 Esophagus, cervical part
- 胸郭上口 Thoracic inlet
- 食道，胸部 Esophagus, thoracic part
- 後縦隔 Posterior mediastinum
- 気管 Trachea（頸部 Cervical part／胸郭部 Thoracic part）
- 上縦隔 Superior mediastinum
- 胸骨(体) Sternum (body)
- 前縦隔 Anterior mediastinum
- 中縦隔 Middle mediastinum
- 横隔膜 Diaphragm

図6.3 胸部の水平断

胸部のCTスキャン，下方から見たところ．

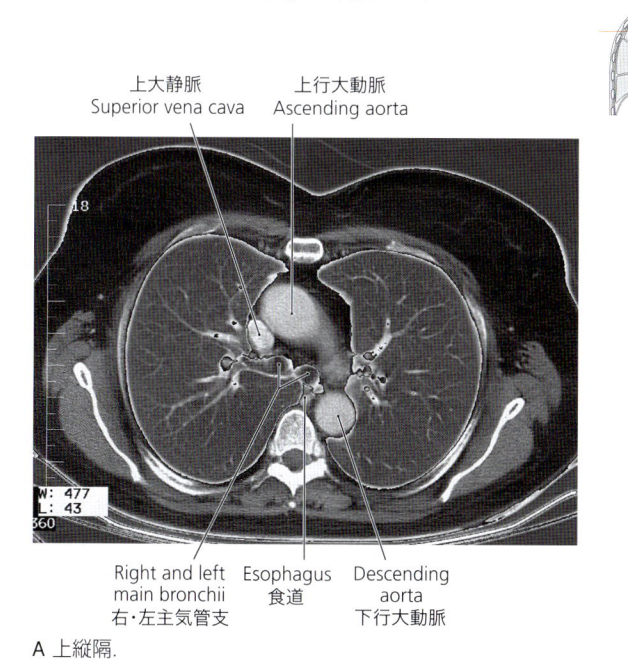

A 上縦隔．
- 上大静脈 Superior vena cava
- 上行大動脈 Ascending aorta
- 右・左主気管支 Right and left main bronchii
- 食道 Esophagus
- 下行大動脈 Descending aorta

B 下縦隔．
- 下大静脈 Inferior vena cava
- 食道 Esophagus
- 奇静脈 Azygos v.
- 下行大動脈 Descending aorta

胸腔の動脈
Arteries of the Thoracic Cavity

大動脈弓からは腕頭動脈，左総頸動脈，左鎖骨下動脈の3つの大きな枝が分かれる．大動脈弓を経て大動脈は下行し，胸骨角の高さで胸大動脈となり，横隔膜の大動脈裂孔を通過後に腹大動脈となる．

図6.4 胸大動脈

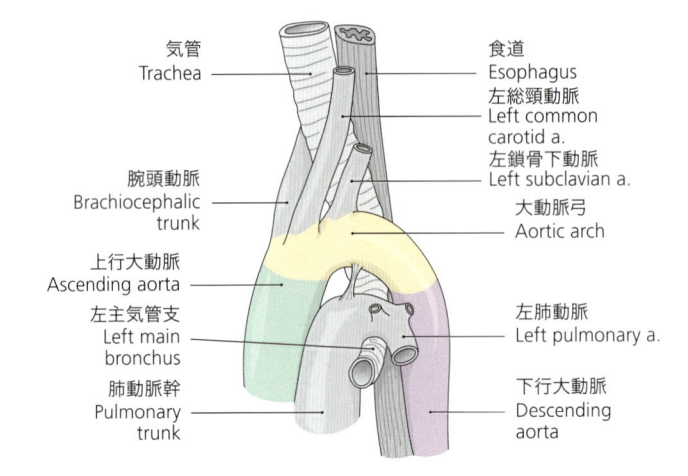

- 気管 Trachea
- 食道 Esophagus
- 左総頸動脈 Left common carotid a.
- 左鎖骨下動脈 Left subclavian a.
- 腕頭動脈 Brachiocephalic trunk
- 大動脈弓 Aortic arch
- 上行大動脈 Ascending aorta
- 左主気管支 Left main bronchus
- 左肺動脈 Left pulmonary a.
- 肺動脈幹 Pulmonary trunk
- 下行大動脈 Descending aorta

A 大動脈の部分，外側方から見たところ．
Note：大動脈弓の始まりと終わりは胸骨角（p.46参照）の高さである．

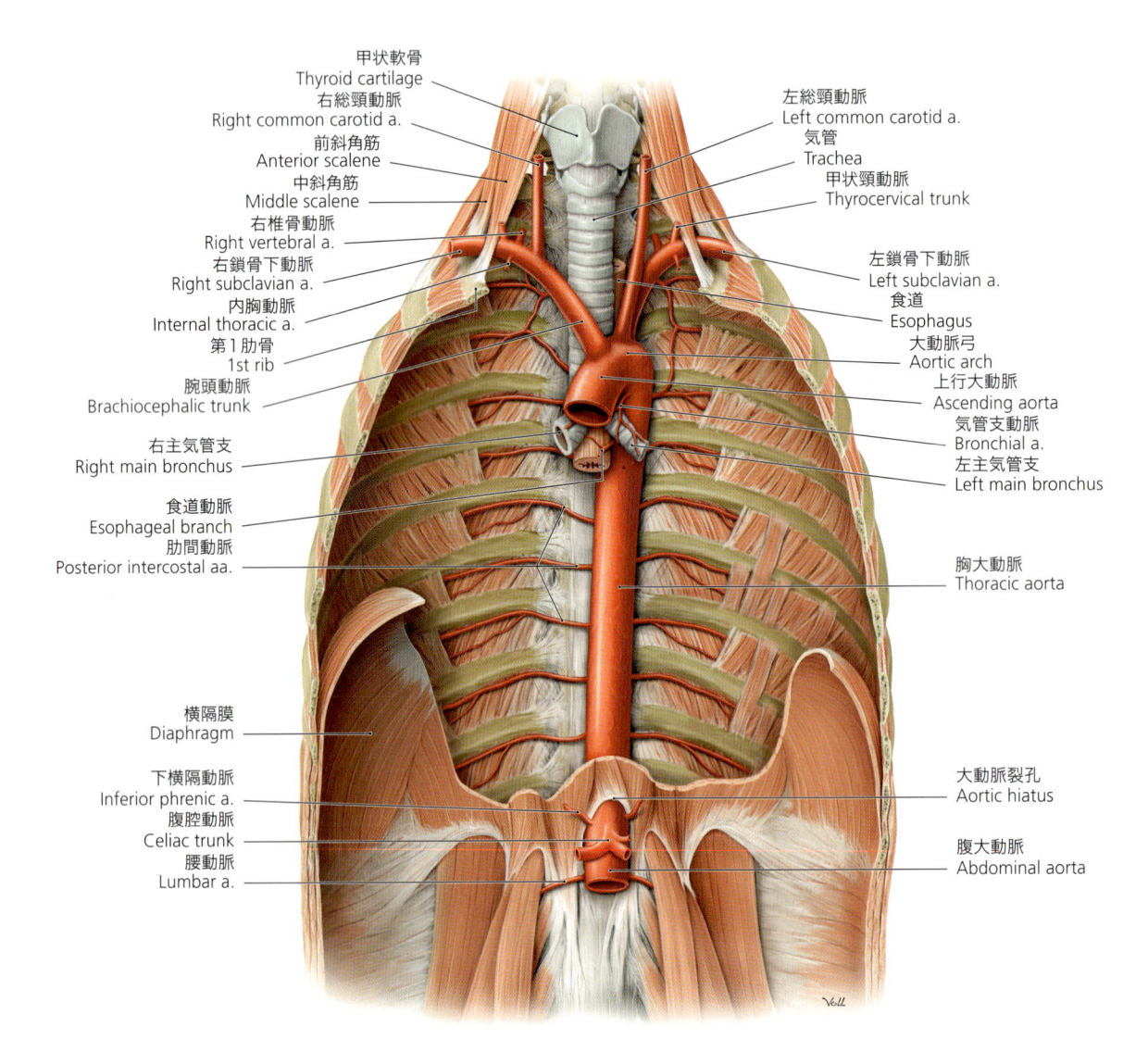

- 甲状軟骨 Thyroid cartilage
- 右総頸動脈 Right common carotid a.
- 前斜角筋 Anterior scalene
- 中斜角筋 Middle scalene
- 右椎骨動脈 Right vertebral a.
- 右鎖骨下動脈 Right subclavian a.
- 内胸動脈 Internal thoracic a.
- 第1肋骨 1st rib
- 腕頭動脈 Brachiocephalic trunk
- 右主気管支 Right main bronchus
- 食道動脈 Esophageal branch
- 肋間動脈 Posterior intercostal aa.
- 左総頸動脈 Left common carotid a.
- 気管 Trachea
- 甲状頸動脈 Thyrocervical trunk
- 左鎖骨下動脈 Left subclavian a.
- 食道 Esophagus
- 大動脈弓 Aortic arch
- 上行大動脈 Ascending aorta
- 気管支動脈 Bronchial a.
- 左主気管支 Left main bronchus
- 胸大動脈 Thoracic aorta
- 横隔膜 Diaphragm
- 下横隔動脈 Inferior phrenic a.
- 腹腔動脈 Celiac trunk
- 腰動脈 Lumbar a.
- 大動脈裂孔 Aortic hiatus
- 腹大動脈 Abdominal aorta

B 原位置の胸大動脈，前方から見たところ．心臓，肺，横隔膜の一部を切り取っている．

表6.2　胸大動脈の枝

胸部内臓は胸大動脈からの直接枝と鎖骨下動脈からの間接枝によって栄養される．

枝			栄養される領域
腕頭動脈	右鎖骨下動脈		左鎖骨下動脈を参照
	右総頸動脈		
左総頸動脈			頭部と頸部
左鎖骨下動脈	椎骨動脈		
	内胸動脈	前肋間枝	前胸壁
		胸腺枝	胸腺
		縦隔枝	後縦隔
		心膜横隔動脈	心膜，横隔膜
	甲状頸動脈	下甲状腺動脈	食道，気管，甲状腺
	肋頸動脈	最上肋間動脈	胸壁
下行大動脈	臓側枝		心臓，心膜，気管支，気管，食道
	壁側枝	肋間動脈	後胸壁
		左・右上横隔動脈	横隔膜

臨床

動脈解離

大動脈の内膜裂傷によって大動脈壁のレベルで血流が分離し，偽腔が作られ，潜在的に生死に関わる大動脈破裂につながる．症状としては呼吸困難と血流不足が見られ，突然激しい痛みを感じる．急性動脈解離は上行大動脈によく起こり，一般的に外科手術が必要である．これより遠位の動脈解離は，合併症（灌流を回復するためにステントの挿入を必要とするような臓器への血流障害など）がない場合には，保存的に治療される．

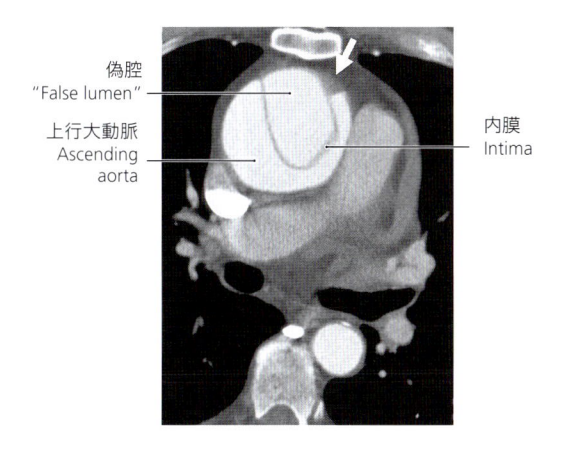

A　動脈解離．内膜の一部はまだ大動脈壁の結合組織と結合している（矢印）．

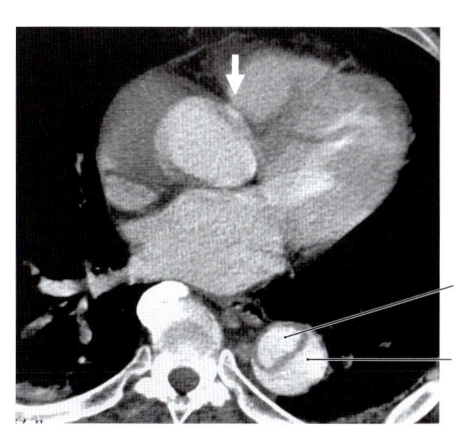

B　冠状動脈への血流は障害されていない（矢印）．

胸腔の静脈
Veins of the Thoracic Cavity

上大静脈は両腕頭静脈が第 2-3 胸椎間の高さで合流してでき，奇静脈系からの血流が流入する（下大静脈は胸部に枝を持たない）．

図 6.5　上大静脈と奇静脈系

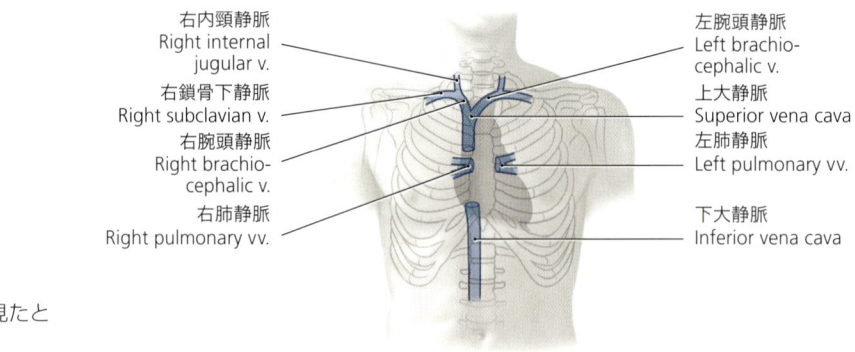

右内頸静脈 Right internal jugular v.
右鎖骨下静脈 Right subclavian v.
右腕頭静脈 Right brachio-cephalic v.
右肺静脈 Right pulmonary vv.
左腕頭静脈 Left brachio-cephalic v.
上大静脈 Superior vena cava
左肺静脈 Left pulmonary vv.
下大静脈 Inferior vena cava

A 胸への大静脈の投影．前方から見たところ．

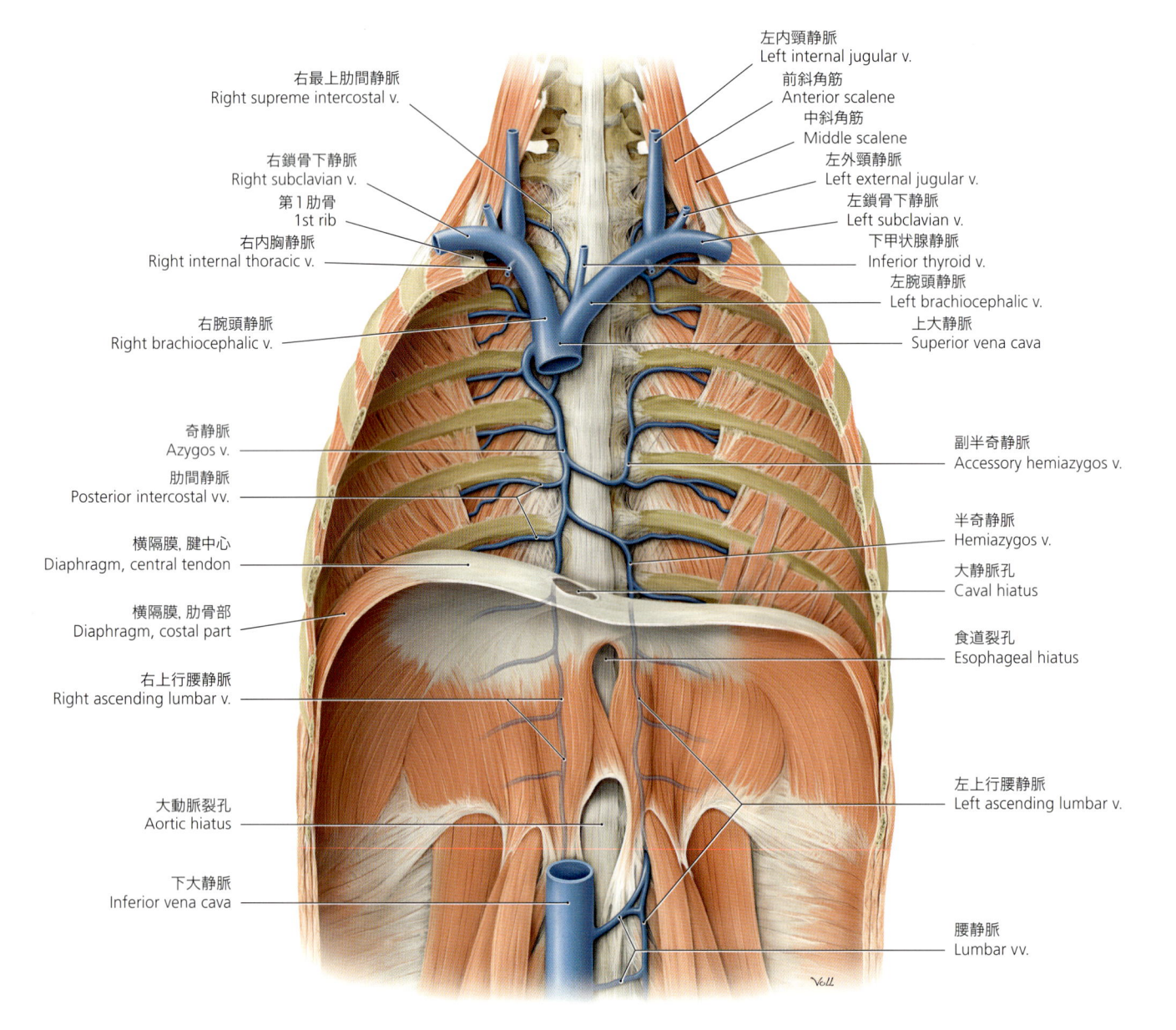

右最上肋間静脈 Right supreme intercostal v.
右鎖骨下静脈 Right subclavian v.
第1肋骨 1st rib
右内胸静脈 Right internal thoracic v.
右腕頭静脈 Right brachiocephalic v.
奇静脈 Azygos v.
肋間静脈 Posterior intercostal vv.
横隔膜, 腱中心 Diaphragm, central tendon
横隔膜, 肋骨部 Diaphragm, costal part
右上行腰静脈 Right ascending lumbar v.
大動脈裂孔 Aortic hiatus
下大静脈 Inferior vena cava

左内頸静脈 Left internal jugular v.
前斜角筋 Anterior scalene
中斜角筋 Middle scalene
左外頸静脈 Left external jugular v.
左鎖骨下静脈 Left subclavian v.
下甲状腺静脈 Inferior thyroid v.
左腕頭静脈 Left brachiocephalic v.
上大静脈 Superior vena cava
副半奇静脈 Accessory hemiazygos v.
半奇静脈 Hemiazygos v.
大静脈孔 Caval hiatus
食道裂孔 Esophageal hiatus
左上行腰静脈 Left ascending lumbar v.
腰静脈 Lumbar vv.

B 胸腔の静脈．胸郭を開く．前方から見たところ．

表6.3　上大静脈の胸部支脈

本幹	支脈		流域
左・右腕頭静脈	下甲状腺静脈		食道，気管，甲状腺
	左・右内頸静脈		頭部，頸部，上腕
	左・右外頸静脈		
	左・右鎖骨下静脈		
	最上肋間静脈		
	心膜静脈		
	左上肋間静脈		
奇静脈系（左側：副半奇静脈，右側：奇静脈）	臓側枝		気管，気管支，食道
	壁側枝	肋間静脈	内胸壁，横隔膜
		左・右上横隔静脈	
		右上肋間静脈	
内胸静脈	胸腺静脈		胸腺
	縦隔枝		後縦隔
	前肋間静脈		前胸壁
	心膜横隔静脈		心膜
	筋横隔静脈		横隔膜

注意：上縦隔の構造からの静脈は，気管静脈・食道静脈・縦隔静脈を経由して腕頭静脈に直接注ぐこともある．

図6.6　奇静脈系
前方から見たところ．

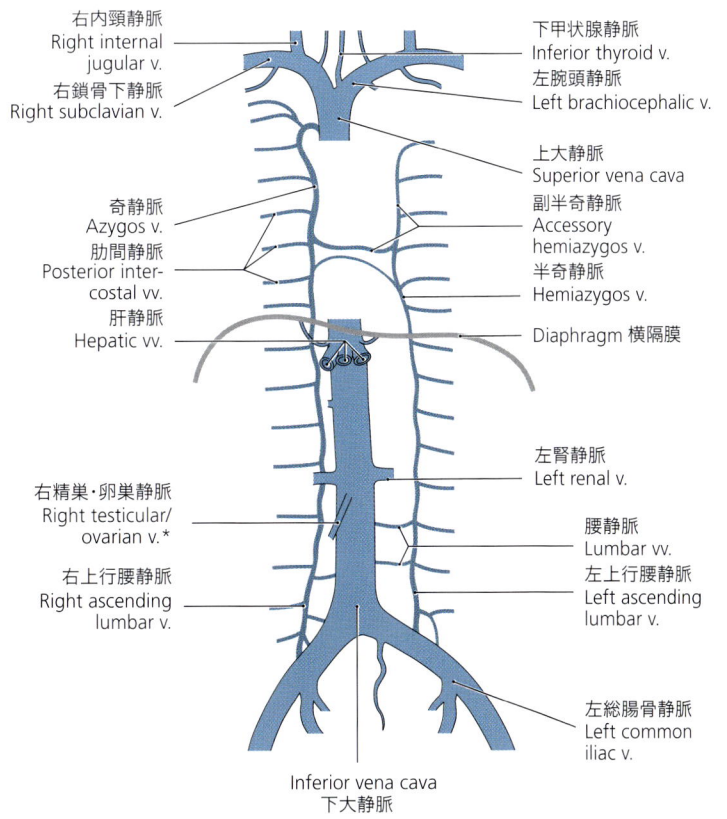

*左精巣・卵巣静脈は左腎静脈から起こる．

胸腔のリンパ管
Lymphatics of the Thoracic Cavity

人体の主要なリンパ管は胸管である．胸管は，腹部の第1腰椎の高さの乳ビ槽から始まり，左内頸静脈と鎖骨下静脈の合流部に注ぐ．

右リンパ本幹は右内頸静脈と鎖骨下静脈の合流部に注ぐ．

図 6.7 胸部のリンパ本幹
前方から見たところ．胸郭を開く．

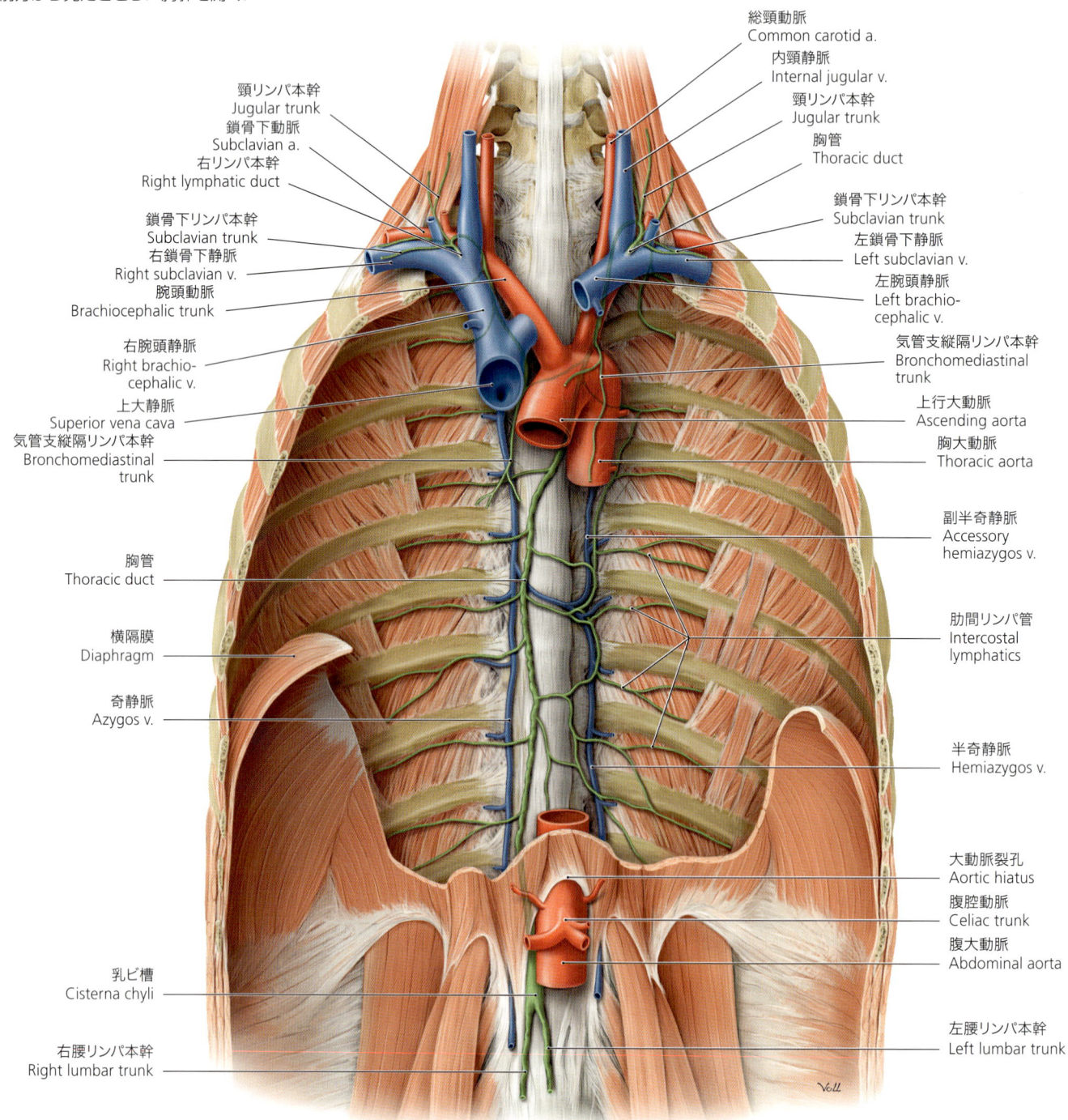

図 6.8 胸部のリンパ管の経路

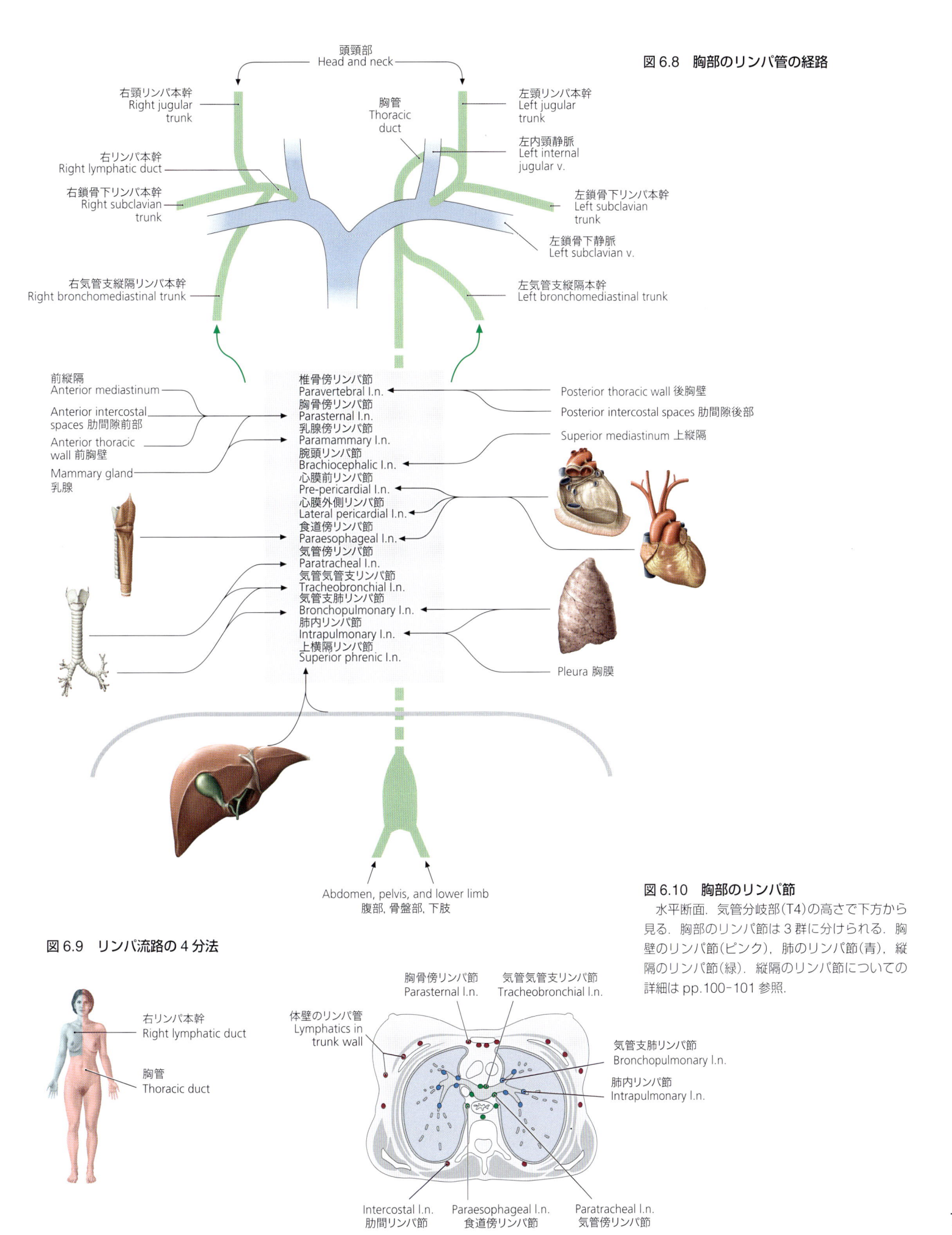

- 頭頸部 Head and neck
- 右頸リンパ本幹 Right jugular trunk
- 左頸リンパ本幹 Left jugular trunk
- 胸管 Thoracic duct
- 左内頸静脈 Left internal jugular v.
- 右リンパ本幹 Right lymphatic duct
- 右鎖骨下リンパ本幹 Right subclavian trunk
- 左鎖骨下リンパ本幹 Left subclavian trunk
- 左鎖骨下静脈 Left subclavian v.
- 右気管支縦隔リンパ本幹 Right bronchomediastinal trunk
- 左気管支縦隔本幹 Left bronchomediastinal trunk

- 前縦隔 Anterior mediastinum
- 肋間隙前部 Anterior intercostal spaces
- 前胸壁 Anterior thoracic wall
- 乳腺 Mammary gland
- 椎骨傍リンパ節 Paravertebral l.n.
- 胸骨傍リンパ節 Parasternal l.n.
- 乳腺傍リンパ節 Paramammary l.n.
- 腕頭リンパ節 Brachiocephalic l.n.
- 心膜前リンパ節 Pre-pericardial l.n.
- 心膜外側リンパ節 Lateral pericardial l.n.
- 食道傍リンパ節 Paraesophageal l.n.
- 気管傍リンパ節 Paratracheal l.n.
- 気管気管支リンパ節 Tracheobronchial l.n.
- 気管支肺リンパ節 Bronchopulmonary l.n.
- 肺内リンパ節 Intrapulmonary l.n.
- 上横隔リンパ節 Superior phrenic l.n.

- Posterior thoracic wall 後胸壁
- Posterior intercostal spaces 肋間隙後部
- Superior mediastinum 上縦隔
- Pleura 胸膜

- Abdomen, pelvis, and lower limb 腹部，骨盤部，下肢

図 6.9 リンパ流路の 4 分法

- 右リンパ本幹 Right lymphatic duct
- 胸管 Thoracic duct

図 6.10 胸部のリンパ節

水平断面．気管分岐部(T4)の高さで下方から見る．胸部のリンパ節は 3 群に分けられる．胸壁のリンパ節（ピンク），肺のリンパ節（青），縦隔のリンパ節（緑）．縦隔のリンパ節についての詳細は pp.100-101 参照．

- 胸骨傍リンパ節 Parasternal l.n.
- 気管気管支リンパ節 Tracheobronchial l.n.
- 体壁のリンパ管 Lymphatics in trunk wall
- 気管支肺リンパ節 Bronchopulmonary l.n.
- 肺内リンパ節 Intrapulmonary l.n.
- Intercostal l.n. 肋間リンパ節
- Paraesophageal l.n. 食道傍リンパ節
- Paratracheal l.n. 気管傍リンパ節

胸腔の神経
Nerves of the Thoracic Cavity

胸部の神経支配はほとんどが自律神経で，交感神経幹または副交感神経性の迷走神経に由来する．例外は，心膜と横隔膜を支配する横隔神経（p.54）と胸壁を支配する肋間神経（p.58）の2つである．

図6.11 胸部にある神経
前方から見たところ．胸部を開く．

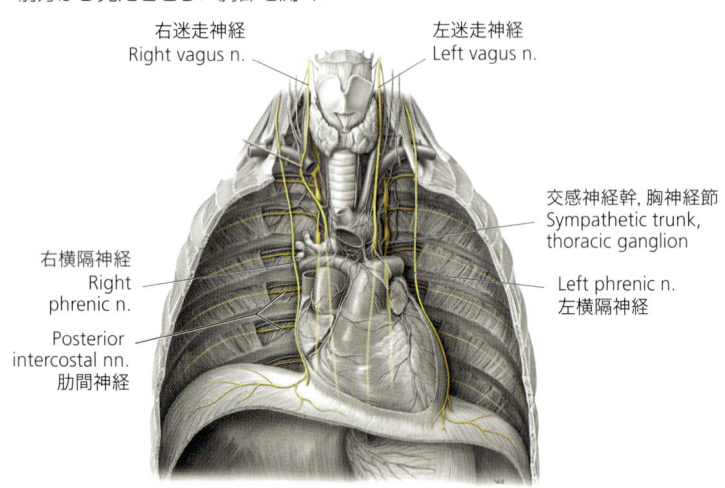

A 胸部の神経支配．

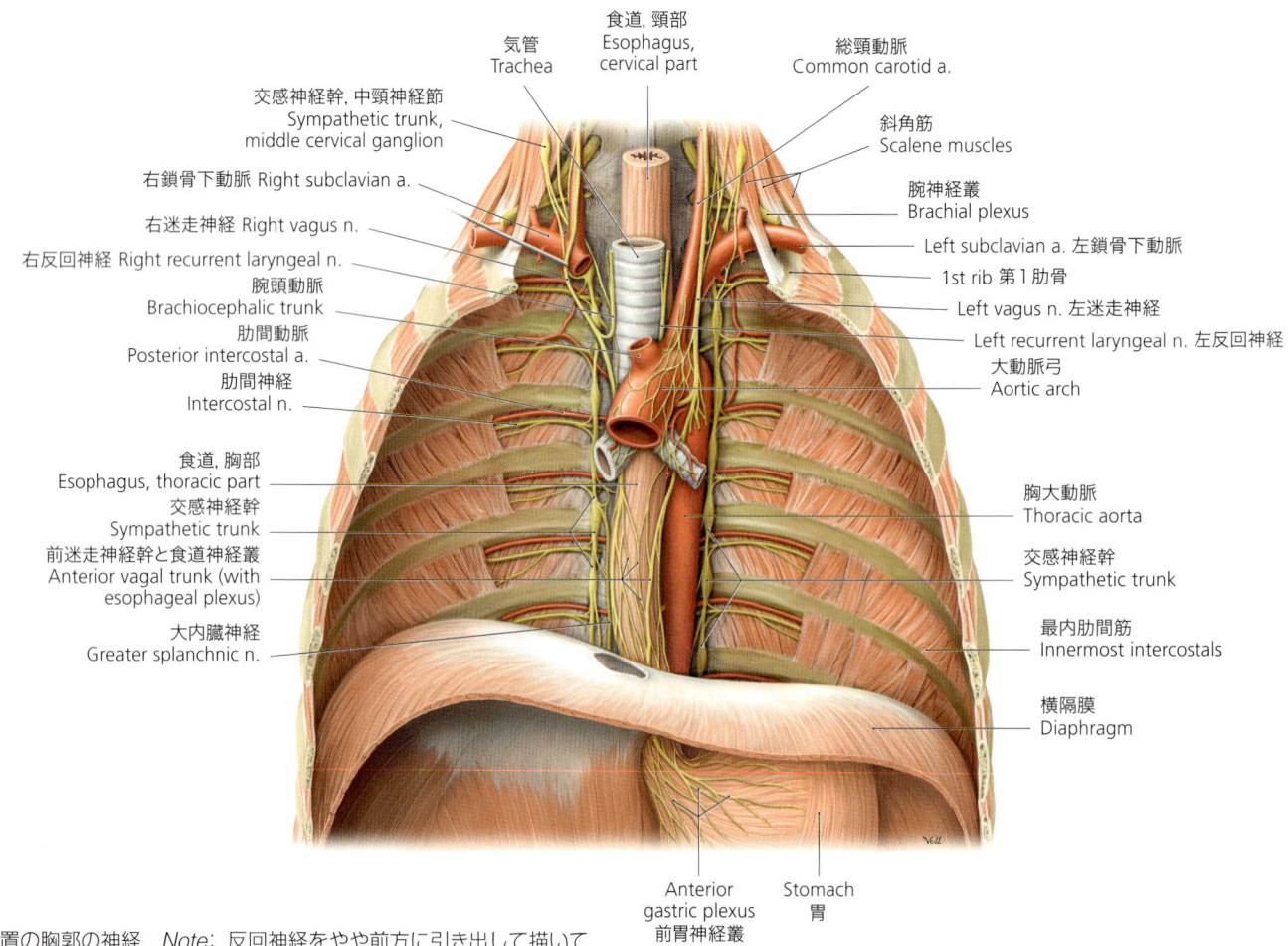

B 原位置の胸郭の神経．*Note*：反回神経をやや前方に引き出して描いている．通常は反回神経は気管と食道の間の溝に入り込んでいるために，甲状腺の手術の際に傷つきやすい．

自律神経系は平滑筋，心筋，腺を支配する．自律神経系は交感神経系（赤）と副交感神経系（青）に分けられ，どちらも血流，分泌，内臓機能を調節する．

図 6.12 胸部の交感神経系と副交感神経系

交感神経系 Sympathetic nervous system

- 上頸神経節 Superior cervical ganglion
- 中頸神経節 Middle cervical ganglion
- 星状神経節 Stellate ganglion
- 頸心臓神経 Cervical cardiac nn.
- 外頸動脈神経叢 External carotid plexus
- 内頸動脈神経叢 Internal carotid plexus
- 総頸動脈神経叢 Common carotid plexus
- 椎骨動脈神経叢 Vertebral plexus
- 鎖骨下動脈神経叢 Subclavian plexus
- 胸大動脈神経叢 Thoracic aortic plexus
- 肺神経叢 Pulmonary plexus
- 心臓神経叢 Cardiac plexus
- Sympathetic trunk 交感神経幹
- Greater and lesser splanchnic nn. 大・小内臓神経

C8, T1–T12, L1, L2

副交感神経系 Parasympathetic nervous system

- 迷走神経 Vagus n. (CN X)
- 上喉頭神経 Superior laryngeal n.
- 喉頭 Larynx
- Recurrent laryngeal n. 反回神経
- Pharyngeal plexus ① ①咽頭神経叢
- Esophageal plexus ② ②食道神経叢
- Pulmonary plexus ③ ③肺神経叢
- 心臓枝 Cardiac branches
- 迷走神経幹 Vagal trunks

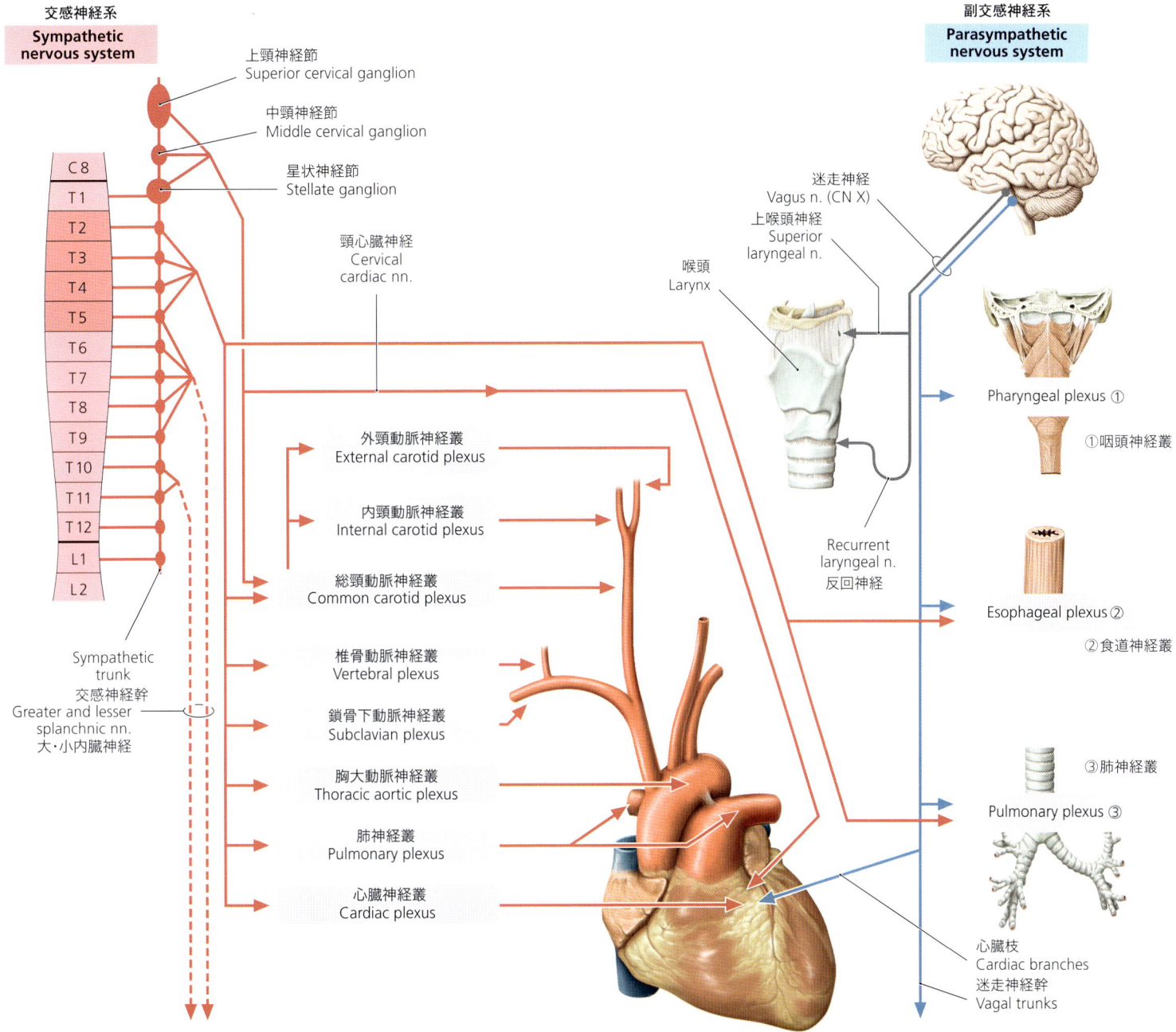

表6.4　末梢の交感神経系

節前線維の起始*	神経節細胞	節後線維の経路	標的
脊髄	交感神経幹	肋間神経に伴行	胸壁の血管と腺
		胸郭内の動脈に伴行	標的器管
		大・小内臓神経に集まる	腹部

*節前ニューロンの軸索は前根を経由して脊髄を離れ，交感神経節で節後ニューロンとシナプスを作る．

表6.5　末梢の副交感神経系

節前線維の起始	運動性節前線維の経路*		標的
脳幹	迷走神経 (CN X)	心臓枝	心臓神経叢
		食道枝	食道神経叢
		気管枝	気管
		気管支枝	肺神経叢（気管支，肺の血管）

*副交感神経系の神経節細胞は支配器官内に散在していて顕微鏡レベルでしか確認できない．迷走神経は運動性の節前線維をこれらの標的まで運ぶ．
CN = cranial nerve（脳神経）

縦隔：概観
Mediastinum: Overview

胸部

縦隔は左右の肺を包む胸膜の間にある空間であり，上部・下部の2つの領域に分けられる．下縦隔はさらに前縦隔，中縦隔，後縦隔に分けられる．

図7.1 縦隔の区分

A 模式図．

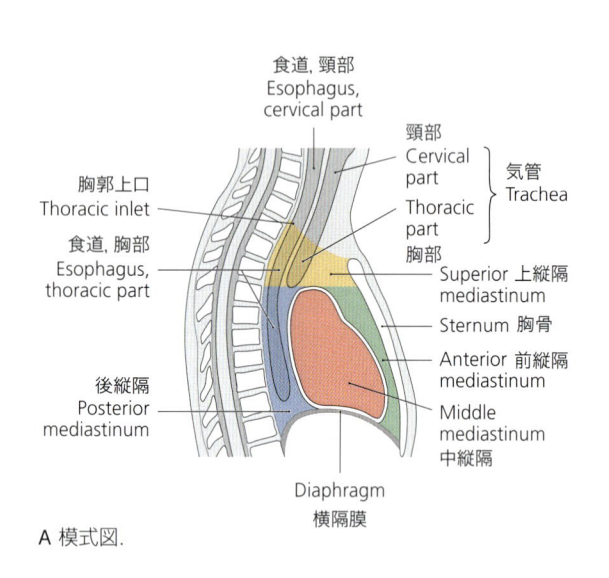

表7.1 縦隔の構成要素

	上縦隔	下縦隔		
		前縦隔	中縦隔	後縦隔
器官	・胸腺 ・気管 ・食道 ・胸管	・胸腺（小児においては，図7.5参照）	・心臓 ・心膜	・食道
動脈	・胸大動脈 ・腕頭動脈 ・左総頸動脈 ・左鎖骨下動脈	・小さい血管	・上行大動脈 ・肺動脈幹とその枝 ・心膜横隔動脈	・胸大動脈
静脈と リンパ管	・上大静脈 ・腕頭静脈 ・胸管	・小さな血管， リンパ管， リンパ節	・上大静脈 ・奇静脈 ・肺静脈 ・心膜横隔静脈	・奇静脈 ・半奇静脈 ・胸管
神経	・迷走神経 ・左反回神経 ・心臓神経 ・横隔神経	・なし	・横隔神経	・迷走神経

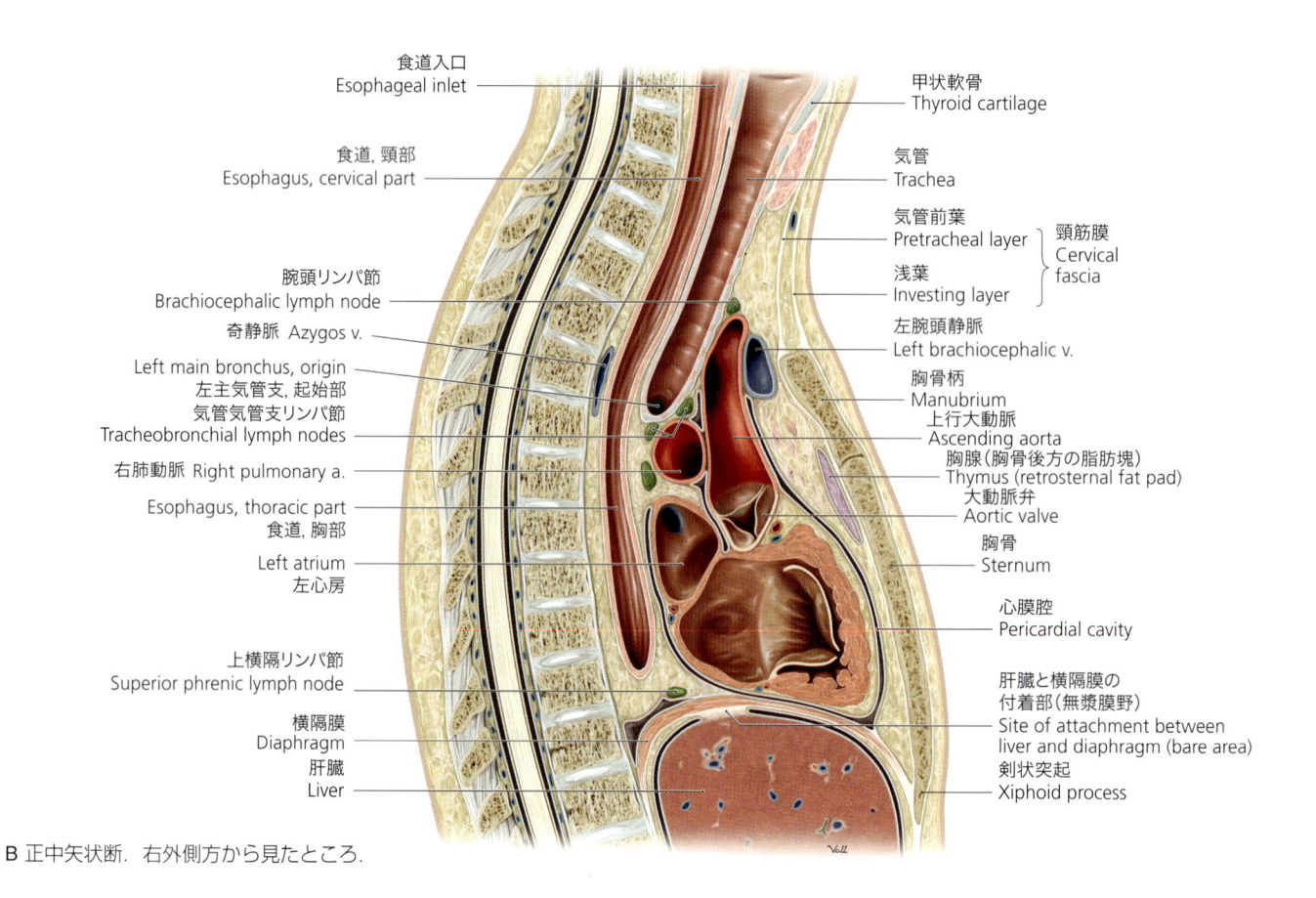

B 正中矢状断．右外側方から見たところ．

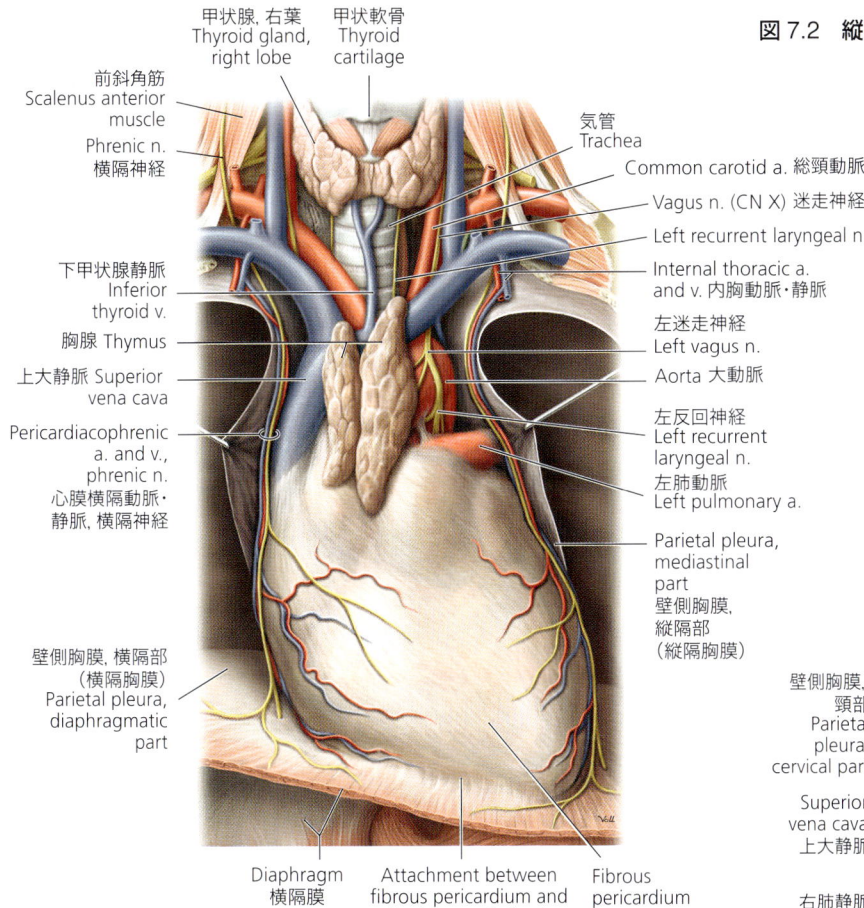

図 7.2 縦隔の内容

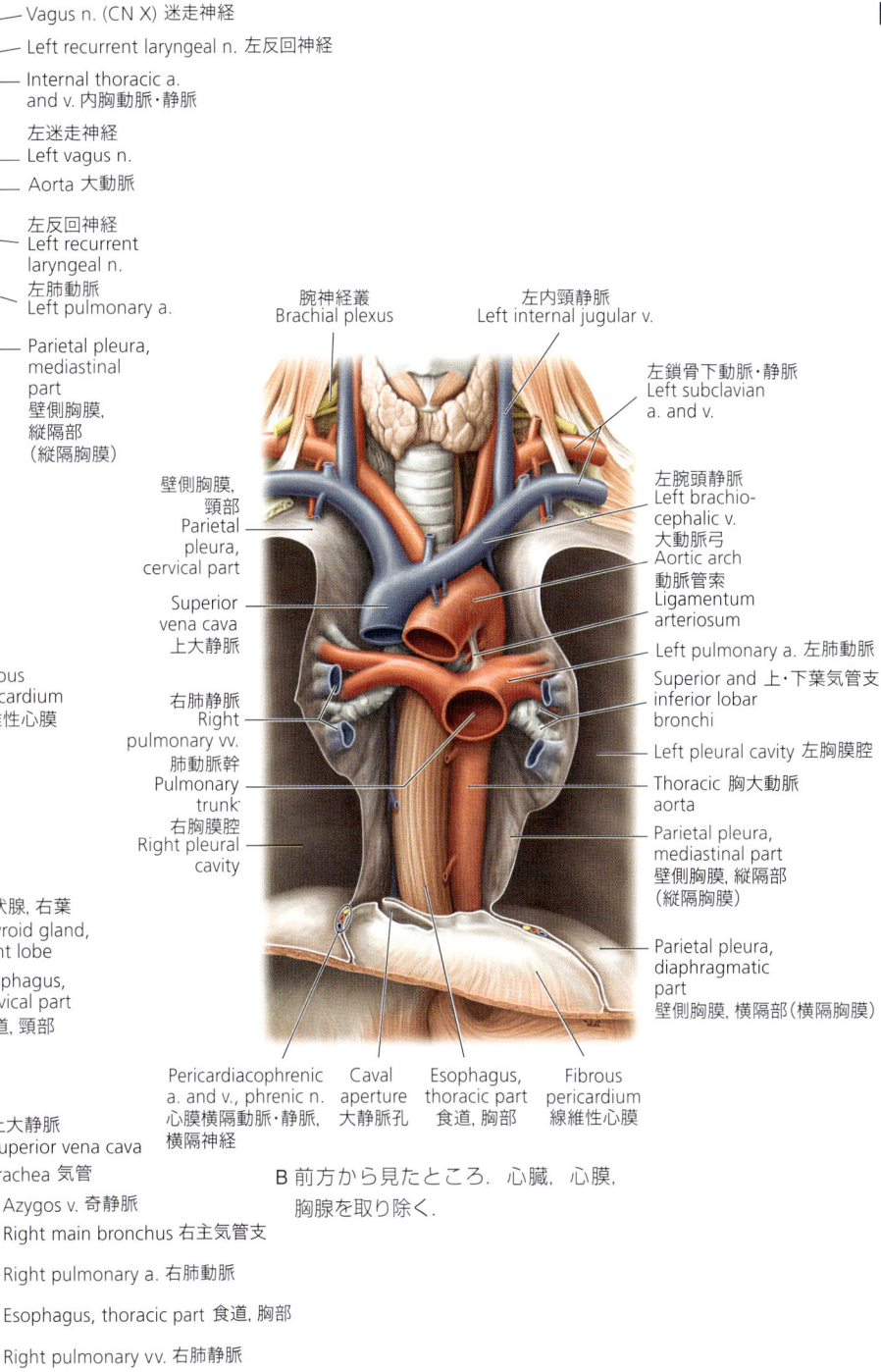

A 縦隔を前方から見たところ.

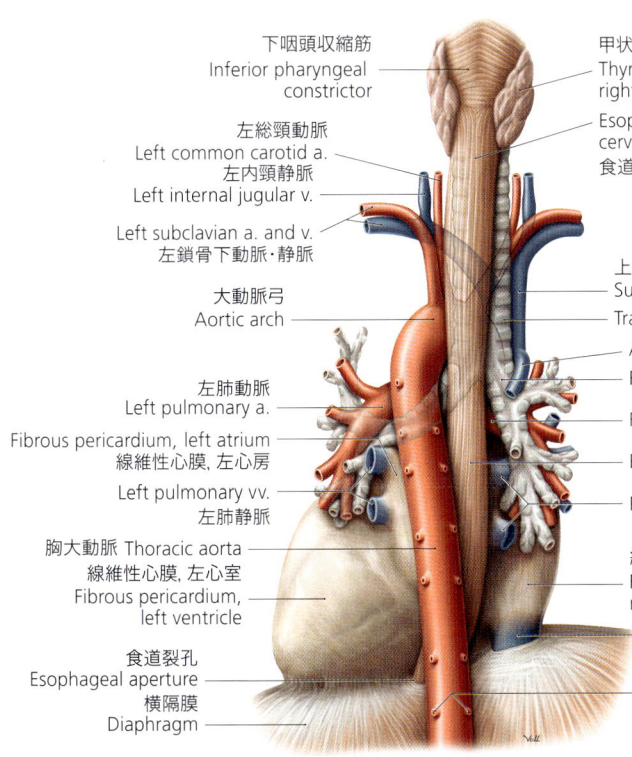

B 前方から見たところ. 心臓, 心膜, 胸膜を取り除く.

C 後方から見たところ.

縦隔の構造
Mediastinum: Structures

図 7.3　縦隔

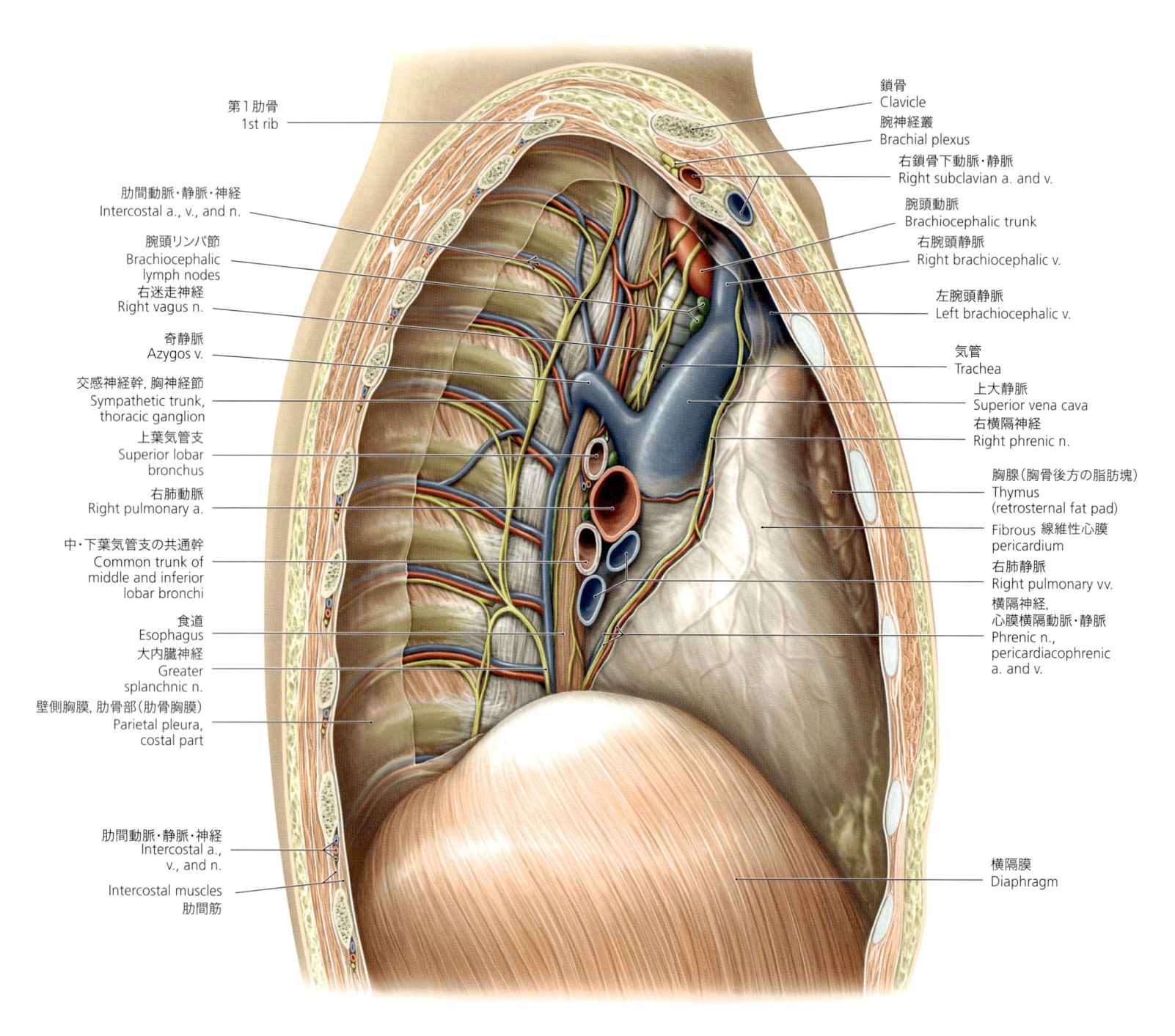

- 第1肋骨 / 1st rib
- 肋間動脈・静脈・神経 / Intercostal a., v., and n.
- 腕頭リンパ節 / Brachiocephalic lymph nodes
- 右迷走神経 / Right vagus n.
- 奇静脈 / Azygos v.
- 交感神経幹, 胸神経節 / Sympathetic trunk, thoracic ganglion
- 上葉気管支 / Superior lobar bronchus
- 右肺動脈 / Right pulmonary a.
- 中・下葉気管支の共通幹 / Common trunk of middle and inferior lobar bronchi
- 食道 / Esophagus
- 大内臓神経 / Greater splanchnic n.
- 壁側胸膜, 肋骨部（肋骨胸膜）/ Parietal pleura, costal part
- 肋間動脈・静脈・神経 / Intercostal a., v., and n.
- 肋間筋 / Intercostal muscles

- 鎖骨 / Clavicle
- 腕神経叢 / Brachial plexus
- 右鎖骨下動脈・静脈 / Right subclavian a. and v.
- 腕頭動脈 / Brachiocephalic trunk
- 右腕頭静脈 / Right brachiocephalic v.
- 左腕頭静脈 / Left brachiocephalic v.
- 気管 / Trachea
- 上大静脈 / Superior vena cava
- 右横隔神経 / Right phrenic n.
- 胸腺（胸骨後方の脂肪塊）/ Thymus (retrosternal fat pad)
- 線維性心膜 / Fibrous pericardium
- 右肺静脈 / Right pulmonary vv.
- 横隔神経, 心膜横隔動脈・静脈 / Phrenic n., pericardiacophrenic a. and v.
- 横隔膜 / Diaphragm

A　傍矢状断，右側方から見たところ．上縦隔と下縦隔（中縦隔と後縦隔）の間に多くの構造があることに注意．

鎖骨	Clavicle
腕神経叢	Brachial plexus
左鎖骨下動脈・静脈	Left subclavian a. and v.
食道	Esophagus
左上肋間静脈	Left superior intercostal v.
左迷走神経	Left vagus n.
動脈管索	Ligamentum arteriosum
左横隔神経	Left phrenic n.
左肺動脈	Left pulmonary a.
左肺静脈	Left pulmonary vv.
線維性心膜	Fibrous pericardium
心膜外側リンパ節	Lateral pericardial lymph node
左迷走神経, 横隔神経, 心膜横隔動脈・静脈	Left vagus n., Phrenic n., pericardiacophrenic a. and v.
上横隔リンパ節	Superior phrenic lymph node
横隔膜	Diaphragm
第1肋骨	1st rib
肋間動脈・静脈・神経	Intercostal a., v., and n.
胸管	Thoracic duct
大動脈弓	Aortic arch
左反回神経	Left recurrent laryngeal n.
交感神経幹	Sympathetic trunk
副半奇静脈	Accessory hemiazygos v.
左主気管支	Left main bronchus
胸大動脈(下行大動脈)	Thoracic aorta (descending aorta)
壁側胸膜, 肋骨部(肋骨胸膜)	Parietal pleura, costal part
半奇静脈	Hemiazygos v.
肋間筋	Intercostal muscles
肋間動脈・静脈・神経	Intercostal a., v., and n.

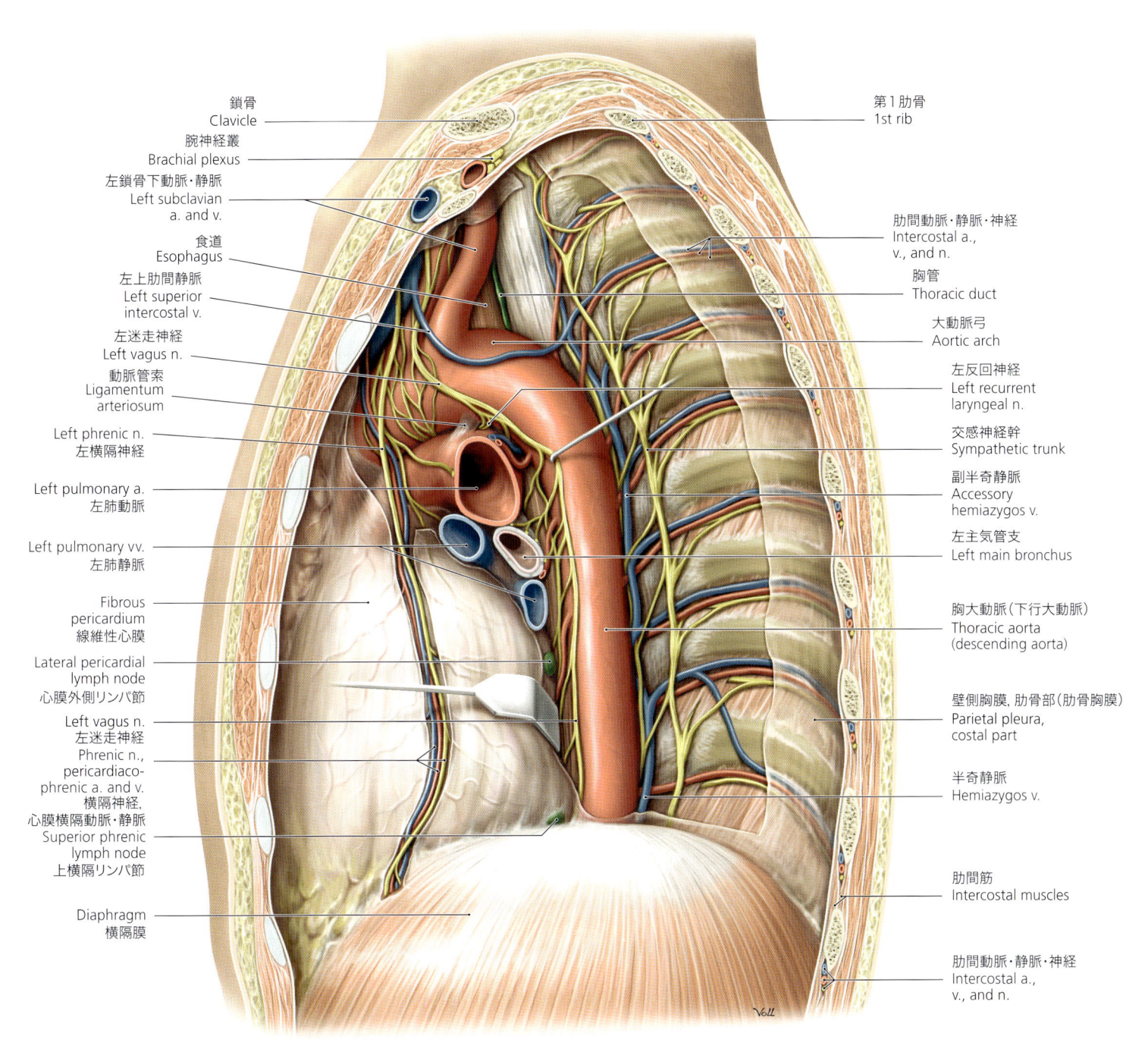

B 傍矢状断，左外側方から見たところ．左肺と壁側胸膜を取り除く．後縦隔の構造が見える．

胸腺と心膜
Thymus & Pericardium

図 7.4　原位置の胸腺と心膜
冠状断を前方から見たところ．胸腺は上縦隔にある．

図 7.5　胸腺
前方から見たところ．2歳の小児の縦隔を開く．胸腺はこの年頃ではよく発達し，下方では前縦隔に達する（図 7.4 と比較せよ）．胸腺は幼児期の間は発達し，思春期には性ホルモンの循環量が多くなり，胸腺が退縮する．

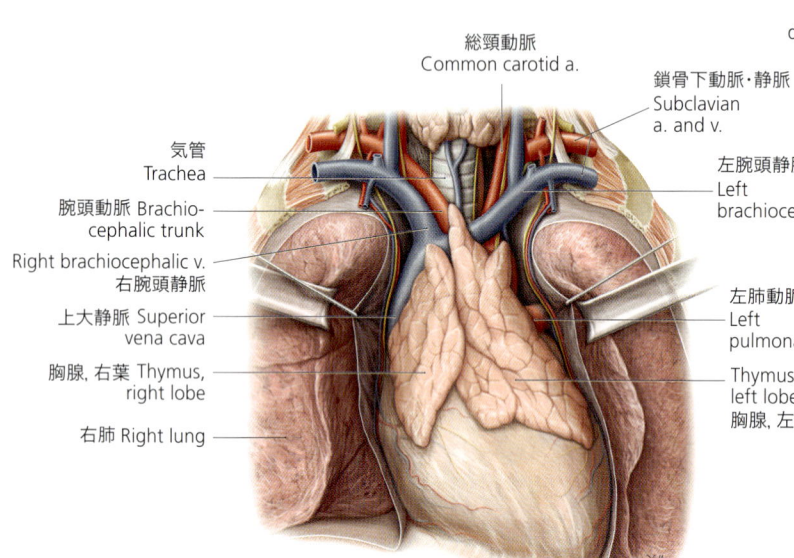

図 7.6　心膜
前方から見たところ．胸郭を開き，線維性心膜を翻転する．

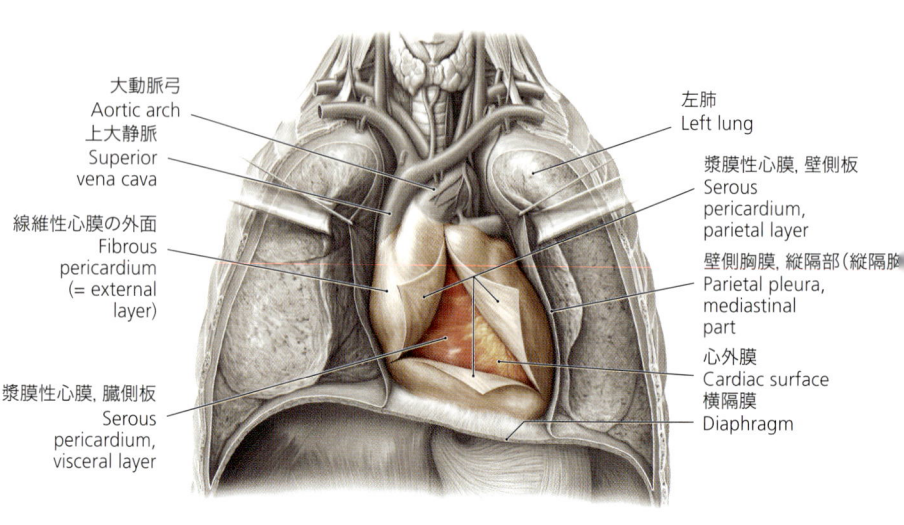

図 7.7 漿膜性心膜の折れ返り

前方から見たところ．漿膜性心膜の壁側板と臓側板は心臓の大血管の近位部で連続している．動脈付近の折れ返り部と静脈付近の折れ返り部分の間にある空洞が心膜横洞である（B を参照）．

A 縦隔の矢状断．漿膜性心膜の壁側板と臓側板の連続に注意．

B 心膜．心臓は取り除く．前方から見たところ．

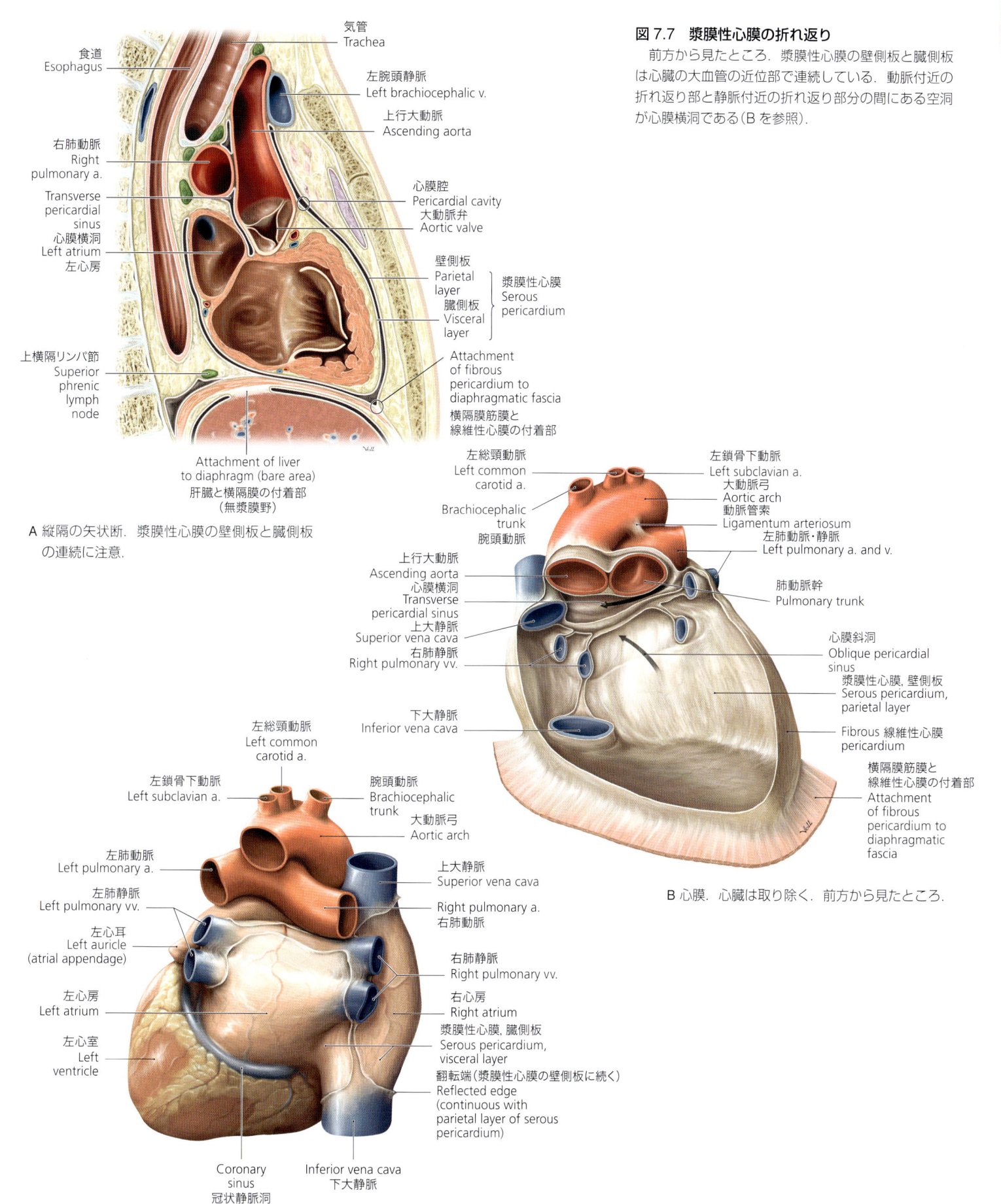

C 後方から見たところ．心臓は線維性心膜から取り除く．漿膜性心膜の壁側板の折れ返りの切れ端に注意．

原位置の心臓
Heart in Situ

心臓は胸骨後方で，下縦隔の中縦隔に位置する．心臓は胸腔左側に投影される．

図 7.8 心臓の位置関係

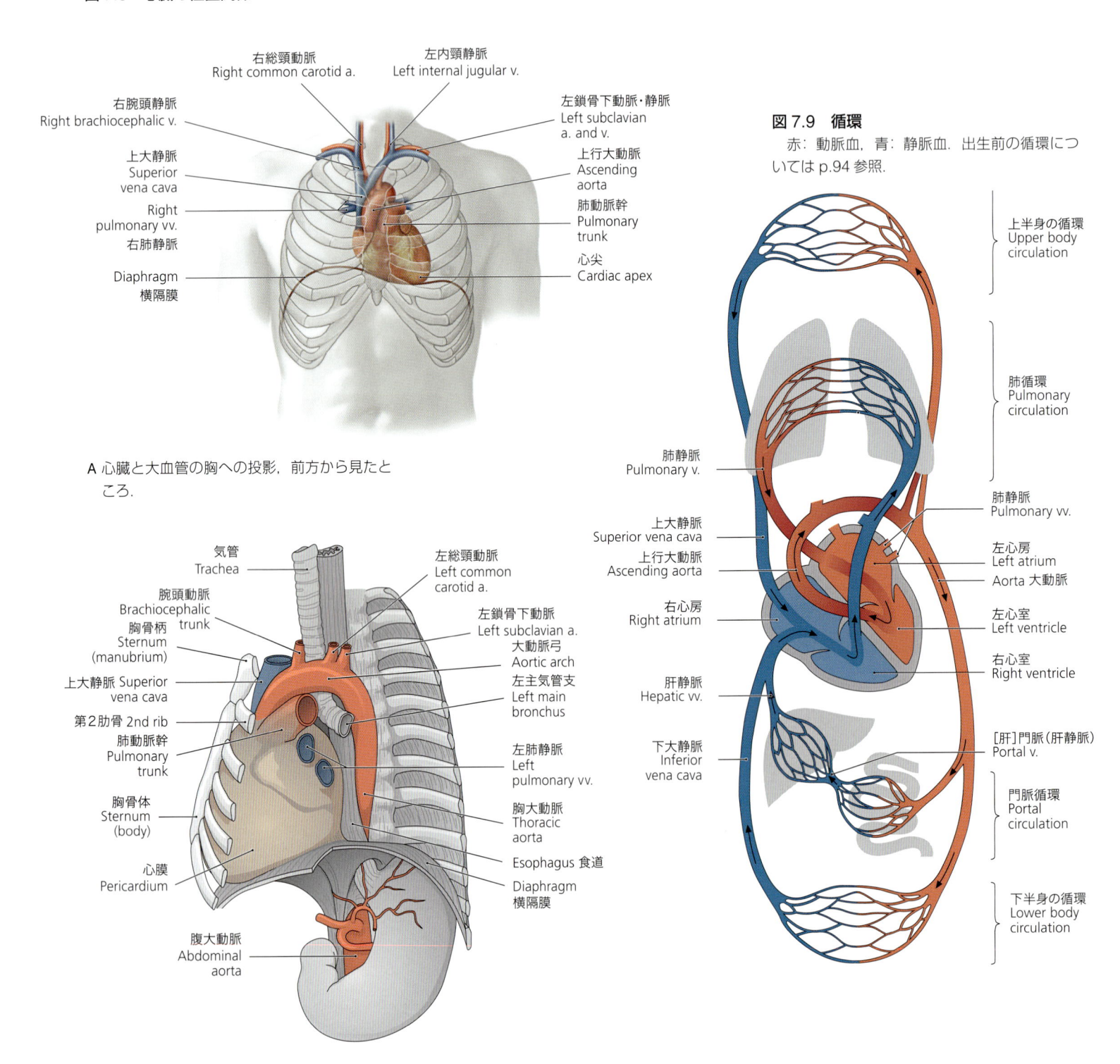

- 右総頸動脈 Right common carotid a.
- 左内頸静脈 Left internal jugular v.
- 右腕頭静脈 Right brachiocephalic v.
- 左鎖骨下動脈・静脈 Left subclavian a. and v.
- 上大静脈 Superior vena cava
- 上行大動脈 Ascending aorta
- 右肺静脈 Right pulmonary vv.
- 肺動脈幹 Pulmonary trunk
- 心尖 Cardiac apex
- 横隔膜 Diaphragm

A 心臓と大血管の胸への投影，前方から見たところ．

- 気管 Trachea
- 左総頸動脈 Left common carotid a.
- 腕頭動脈 Brachiocephalic trunk
- 胸骨柄 Sternum (manubrium)
- 左鎖骨下動脈 Left subclavian a.
- 大動脈弓 Aortic arch
- 上大静脈 Superior vena cava
- 左主気管支 Left main bronchus
- 第2肋骨 2nd rib
- 肺動脈幹 Pulmonary trunk
- 左肺静脈 Left pulmonary vv.
- 胸骨体 Sternum (body)
- 胸大動脈 Thoracic aorta
- 心膜 Pericardium
- 食道 Esophagus
- 横隔膜 Diaphragm
- 腹大動脈 Abdominal aorta

B 左外側方から見たところ．

図 7.9 循環

赤：動脈血，青：静脈血．出生前の循環については p.94 参照．

- 上半身の循環 Upper body circulation
- 肺循環 Pulmonary circulation
- 肺静脈 Pulmonary v.
- 上大静脈 Superior vena cava
- 上行大動脈 Ascending aorta
- 右心房 Right atrium
- 肝静脈 Hepatic vv.
- 下大静脈 Inferior vena cava
- 肺静脈 Pulmonary vv.
- 左心房 Left atrium
- 大動脈 Aorta
- 左心室 Left ventricle
- 右心室 Right ventricle
- [肝]門脈（肝静脈）Portal v.
- 門脈循環 Portal circulation
- 下半身の循環 Lower body circulation

図 7.10　原位置の心臓
前方から見たところ．

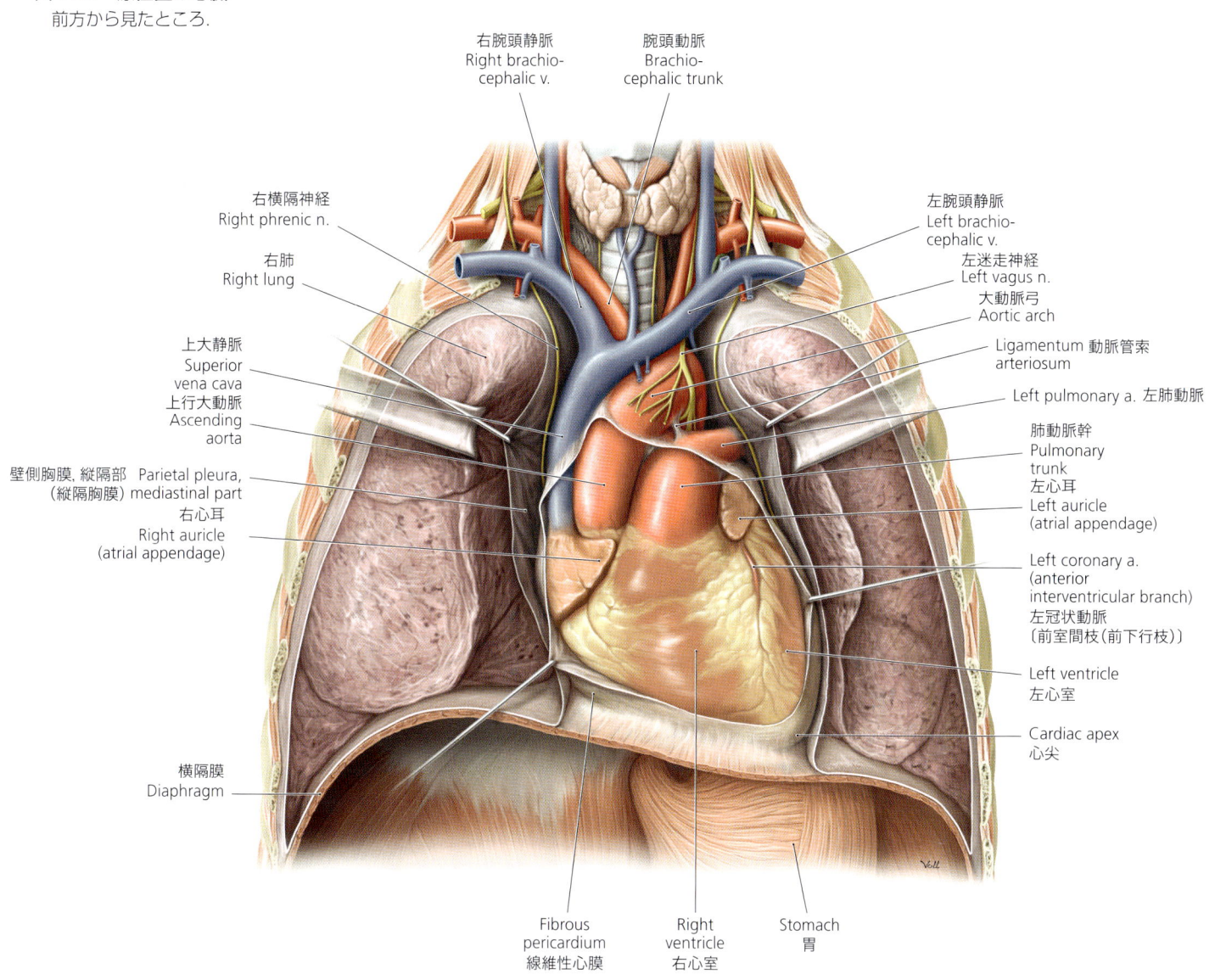

心臓：表面と部屋
Heart: Surfaces & Chambers

> 漿膜性心膜臓側板が折り返って漿膜性心膜壁側板になることに注意．

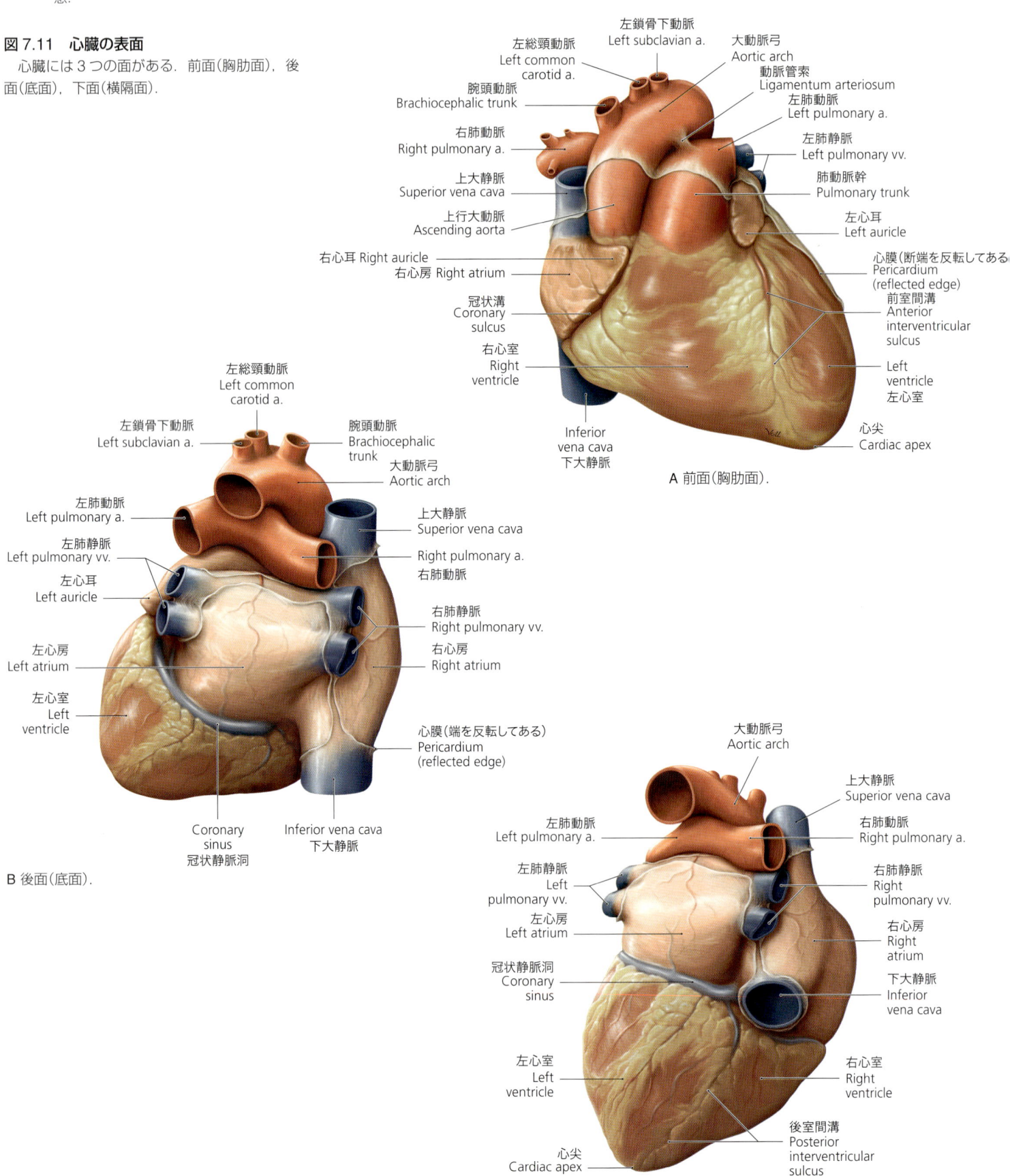

図 7.11 心臓の表面
心臓には3つの面がある．前面（胸肋面），後面（底面），下面（横隔面）．

A 前面（胸肋面）．

B 後面（底面）．

C 下面（横隔面）．

図 7.12 心臓の室

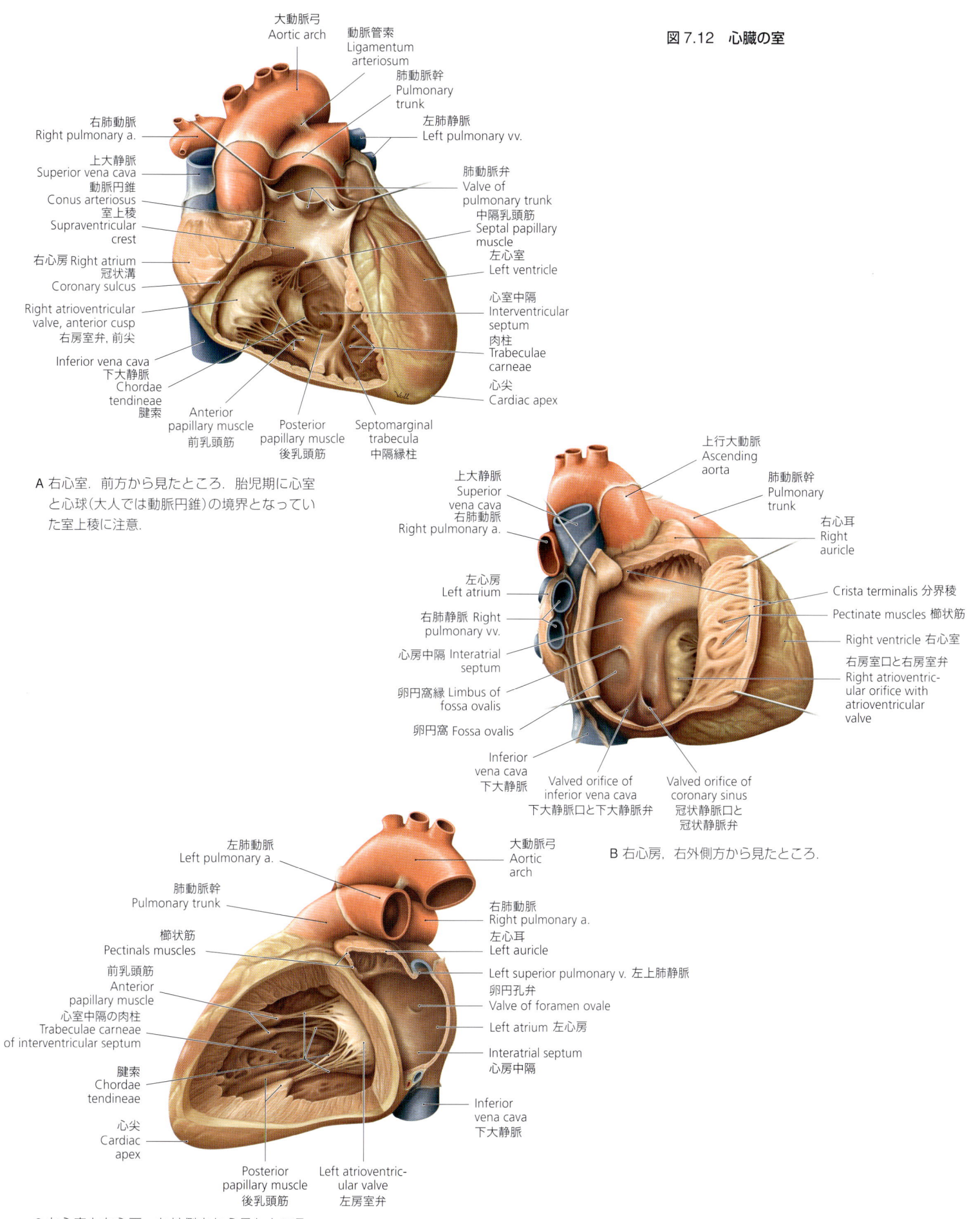

A 右心室．前方から見たところ．胎児期に心室と心球（大人では動脈円錐）の境界となっていた室上稜に注意．

B 右心房，右外側方から見たところ．

C 左心室と左心房，左外側方から見たところ．心室壁に特徴的な不規則な肉柱に注意．

心臓：弁
Heart: Valves

心臓弁は半月弁と房室弁の2つに分類される．2つの半月弁（大動脈弁と肺動脈弁）は心臓の2本の大血管基部にあり，心室から大動脈と肺動脈への血流を調節している．2つの房室弁（左房室弁と右房室弁）は心房と心室の境界にある．

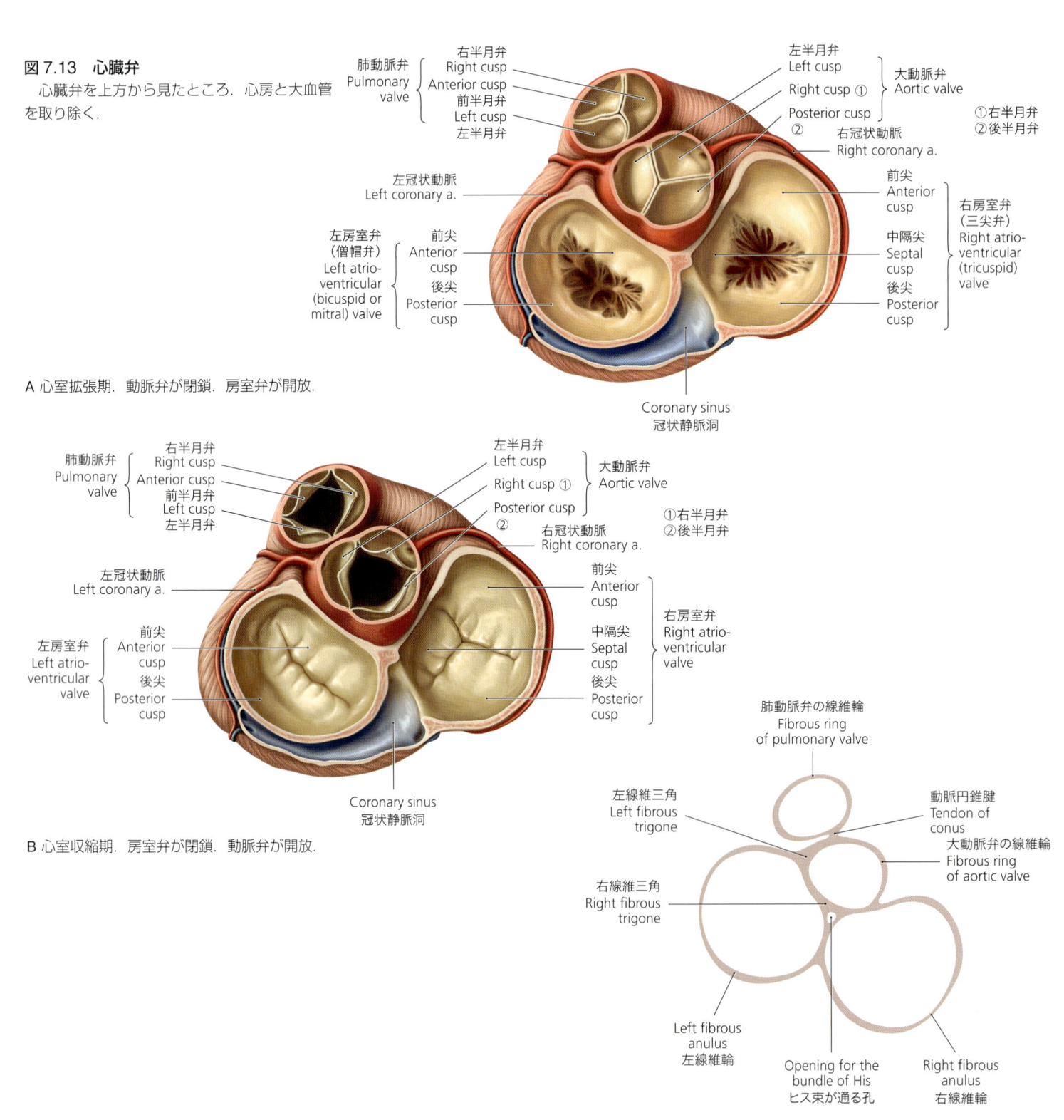

図 7.13 心臓弁
心臓弁を上方から見たところ．心房と大血管を取り除く．

肺動脈弁 Pulmonary valve
- 右半月弁 Right cusp／前半月弁 Anterior cusp
- 左半月弁 Left cusp／左半月弁

大動脈弁 Aortic valve
- 左半月弁 Left cusp
- 右半月弁 Right cusp ①
- 後半月弁 Posterior cusp ②
- ①右半月弁 ②後半月弁

右冠状動脈 Right coronary a.
左冠状動脈 Left coronary a.

左房室弁（僧帽弁）Left atrio-ventricular (bicuspid or mitral) valve
- 前尖 Anterior cusp
- 後尖 Posterior cusp

右房室弁（三尖弁）Right atrio-ventricular (tricuspid) valve
- 前尖 Anterior cusp
- 中隔尖 Septal cusp
- 後尖 Posterior cusp

冠状静脈洞 Coronary sinus

A 心室拡張期．動脈弁が閉鎖．房室弁が開放．

B 心室収縮期．房室弁が閉鎖．動脈弁が開放．

肺動脈弁の線維輪 Fibrous ring of pulmonary valve
動脈円錐腱 Tendon of conus
大動脈弁の線維輪 Fibrous ring of aortic valve
左線維三角 Left fibrous trigone
右線維三角 Right fibrous trigone
左線維輪 Left fibrous anulus
右線維輪 Right fibrous anulus
ヒス束が通る孔 Opening for the bundle of His

C 心臓の骨格．心臓の骨格は密な線維結合組織から作られる．線維輪と線維三角は心房と心室を隔てており，機械的に堅固にし，電気的絶縁体になり（刺激伝導系についてはp.90参照），心筋と弁尖の付着部にもなっている．

図 7.14 動脈弁
弁を縦方向に切って開く．

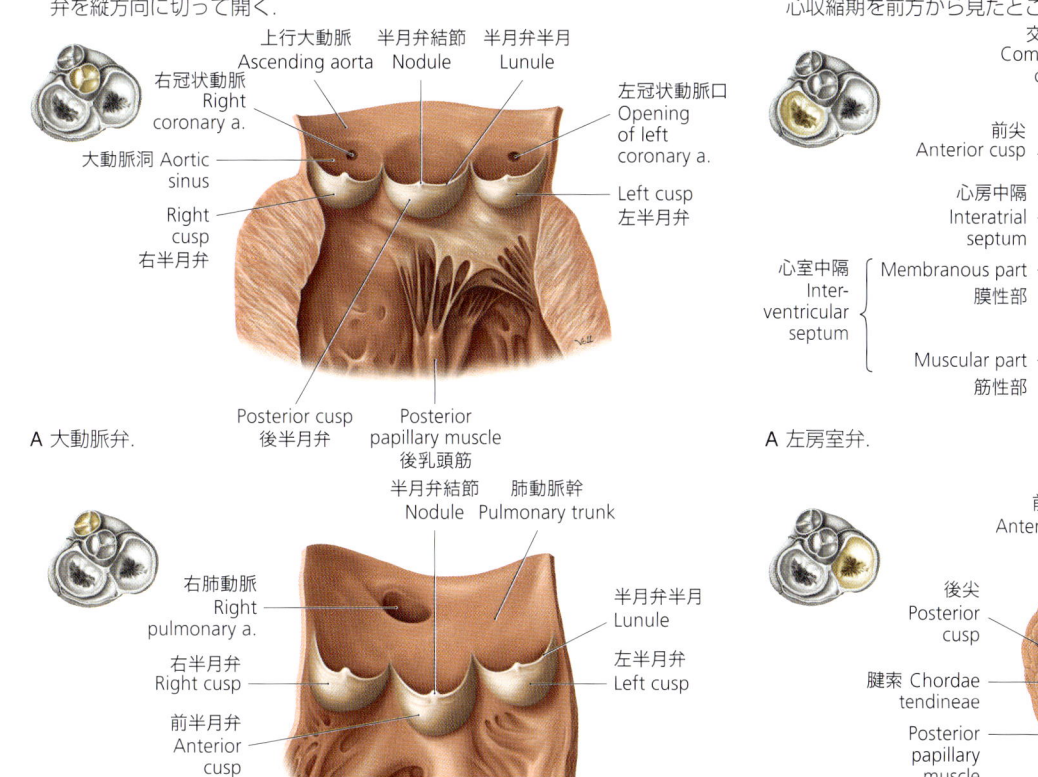

A 大動脈弁．
- 上行大動脈 Ascending aorta
- 半月弁結節 Nodule
- 半月弁半月 Lunule
- 右冠状動脈 Right coronary a.
- 左冠状動脈口 Opening of left coronary a.
- 大動脈洞 Aortic sinus
- Right cusp 右半月弁
- Left cusp 左半月弁
- Posterior cusp 後半月弁
- Posterior papillary muscle 後乳頭筋

B 肺動脈弁．
- 半月弁結節 Nodule
- 肺動脈幹 Pulmonary trunk
- 右肺動脈 Right pulmonary a.
- 半月弁半月 Lunule
- 右半月弁 Right cusp
- 左半月弁 Left cusp
- 前半月弁 Anterior cusp

図 7.15 房室弁
心収縮期を前方から見たところ．

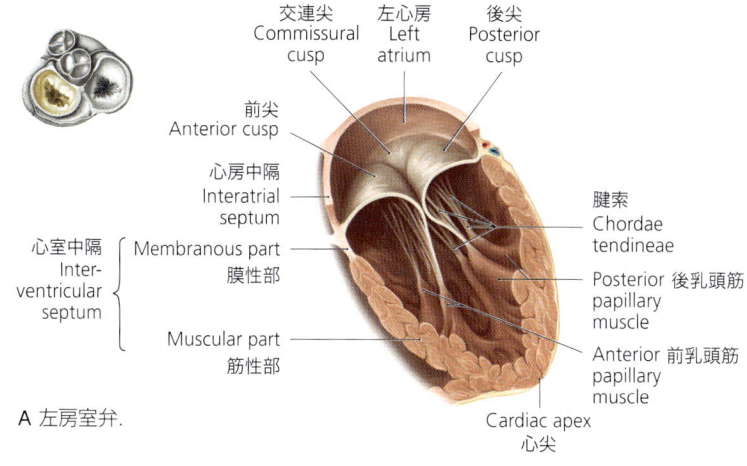

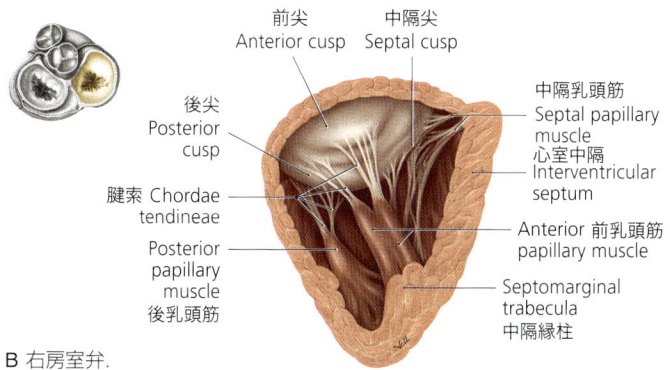

A 左房室弁．
- 交連尖 Commissural cusp
- 左心房 Left atrium
- 後尖 Posterior cusp
- 前尖 Anterior cusp
- 心房中隔 Interatrial septum
- 腱索 Chordae tendineae
- 心室中隔 Interventricular septum
  - 膜性部 Membranous part
  - 筋性部 Muscular part
- 後乳頭筋 Posterior papillary muscle
- 前乳頭筋 Anterior papillary muscle
- 心尖 Cardiac apex

B 右房室弁．
- 前尖 Anterior cusp
- 中隔尖 Septal cusp
- 後尖 Posterior cusp
- 中隔乳頭筋 Septal papillary muscle
- 心室中隔 Interventricular septum
- 腱索 Chordae tendineae
- 前乳頭筋 Anterior papillary muscle
- 後乳頭筋 Posterior papillary muscle
- 中隔縁柱 Septomarginal trabecula

臨床

心臓弁の聴診

半月弁と房室弁の閉鎖で生じる心音は，弁を通過する血流を介して伝導される．心臓弁の疾患では弁を通過するときに乱流が起こり，色をつけて示した領域に雑音が生じる．そのため，この心音は血流の下流で聞こえる．その聴診部位を濃色の円で示す．

- 大動脈弁 Aortic valve
- 肺動脈弁 Pulmonary valve
- 右房室弁 Right atrioventricular valve
- 左房室弁 Left atrioventricular valve

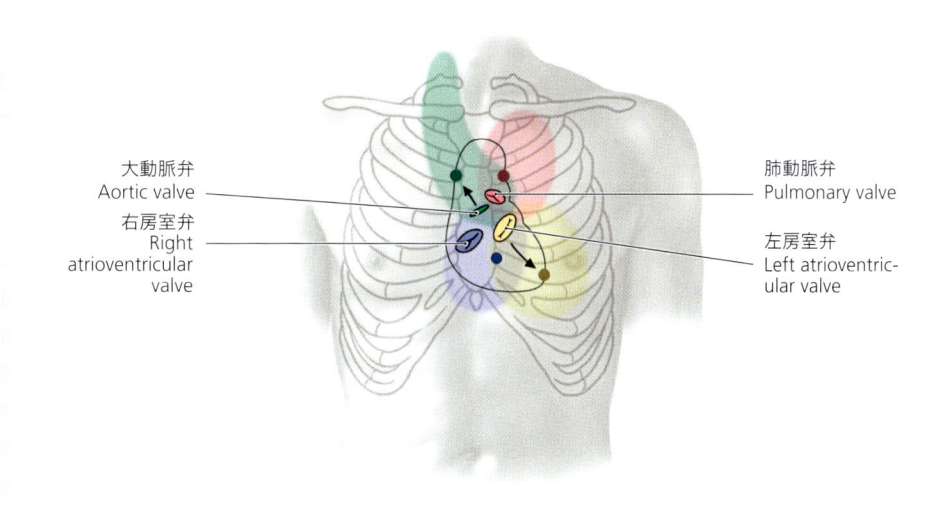

表7.2 心臓弁の位置と聴診部位

弁	解剖学的投影位置	聴診部位
大動脈弁	第3肋骨の高さの胸骨左縁	胸骨周辺の右第2肋間
肺動脈弁	第3肋軟骨の高さの胸骨左縁	胸骨周辺の左第2肋間
左房室弁	左側第4・5肋軟骨間	鎖骨中線上の左第5肋間あるいは心尖部
右房室弁	第5肋軟骨の高さの胸骨	胸骨周辺の左第5肋間

心臓の動脈と静脈
Arteries & Veins of the Heart

図 7.16　冠状動脈と心臓静脈

A　前方から見たところ．

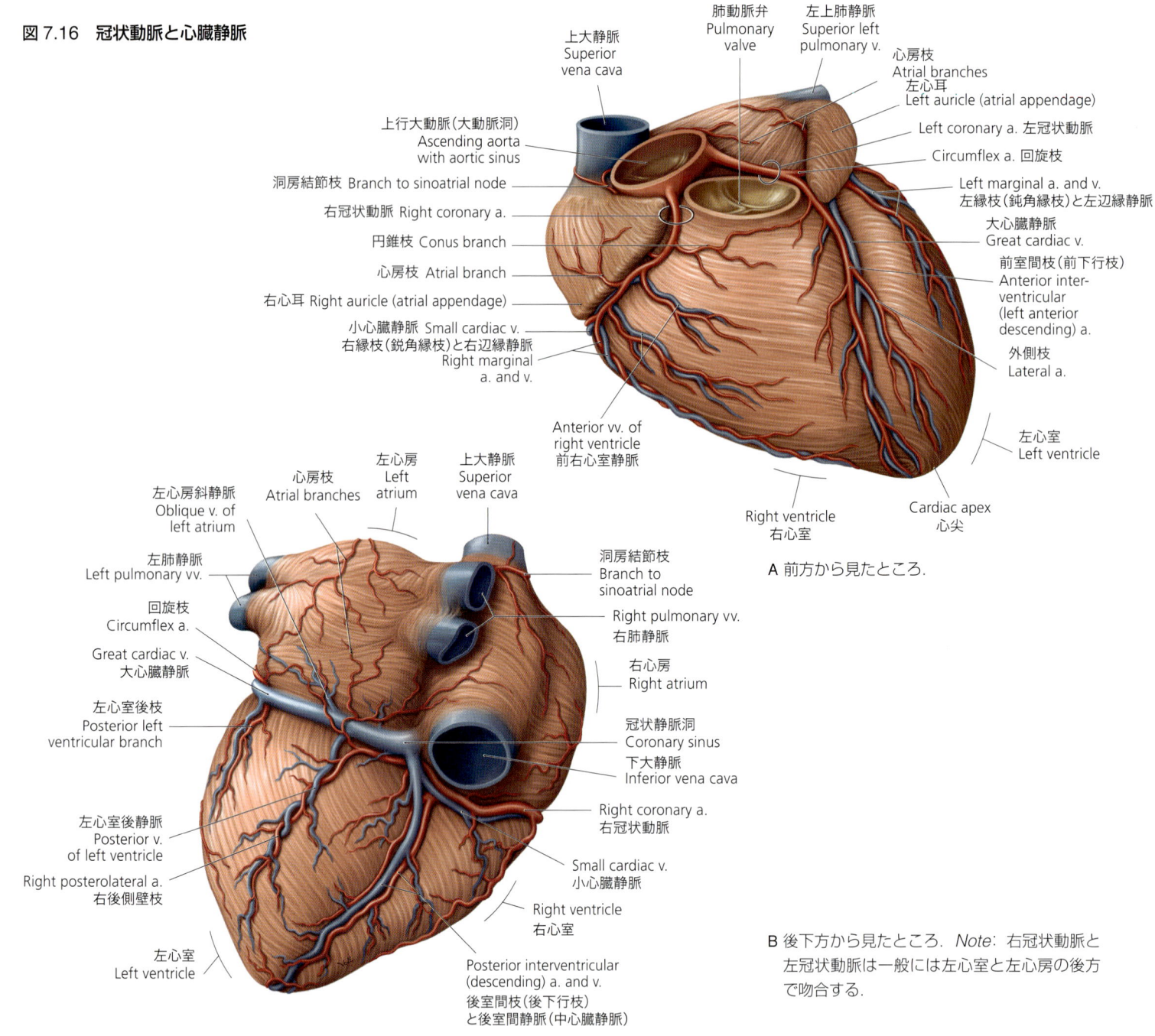

B　後下方から見たところ．Note：右冠状動脈と左冠状動脈は一般には左心室と左心房の後方で吻合する．

表 7.3	冠状動脈の枝
左冠状動脈	右冠状動脈
回旋枝 ・心房枝 ・左縁枝（鈍角縁枝） ・左心室後枝	洞房結節枝
	円錐枝
	心房枝
	右縁枝（鋭角縁枝）
前室間枝（前下行枝） ・円錐枝 ・外側枝 ・心室中隔枝	後室間枝（後下行枝） ・心室中隔枝
	房室結節枝
	右後側壁枝

表 7.4	心臓静脈の分布	
静脈	枝	流入
前心臓静脈（図には示していない）		右心耳
大心臓静脈	前室間静脈	冠状静脈洞
	左辺縁静脈	
	左心房斜静脈	
左心室後静脈		
後室間静脈（中心臓静脈）		
小心臓静脈	前右心室静脈	
	右辺縁静脈	

図 7.17 冠状動脈の分布

心臓を前方と後方から見たところ．心室の水平断の上面．冠状動脈の分布は人によって異なる．右冠状動脈とその枝（緑）；左冠状動脈とその枝（赤）

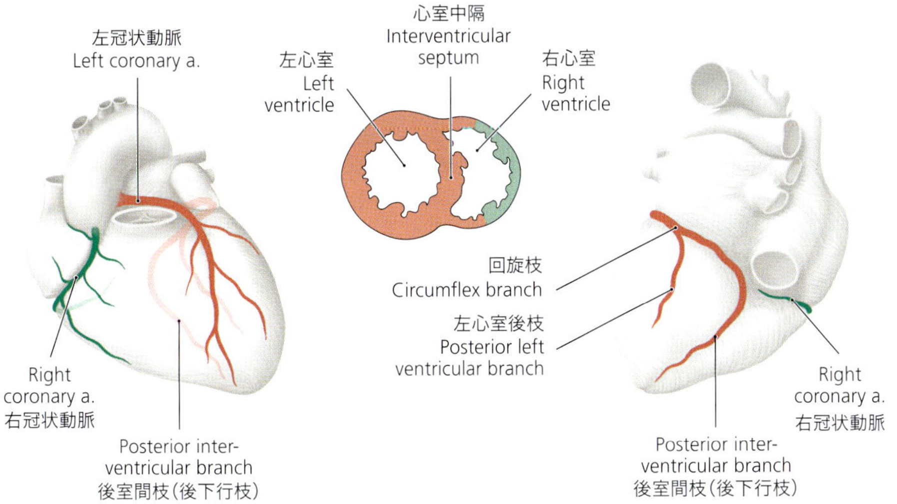

- 左冠状動脈 Left coronary a.
- 心室中隔 Interventricular septum
- 左心室 Left ventricle
- 右心室 Right ventricle
- Right coronary a. 右冠状動脈
- 回旋枝 Circumflex branch
- 左心室後枝 Posterior left ventricular branch
- Right coronary a. 右冠状動脈
- Posterior interventricular branch 後室間枝（後下行枝）
- Posterior interventricular branch 後室間枝（後下行枝）

A 左冠状動脈優位型（約 15％）．

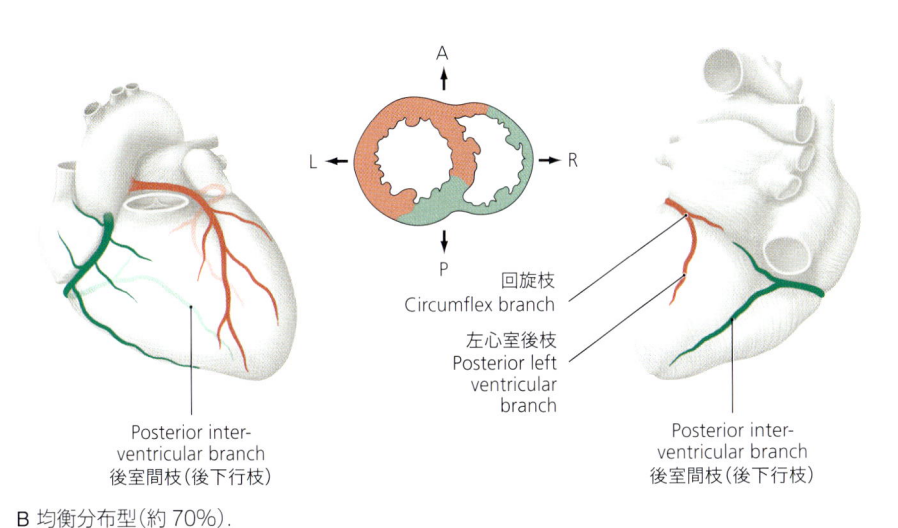

B 均衡分布型（約 70％）．

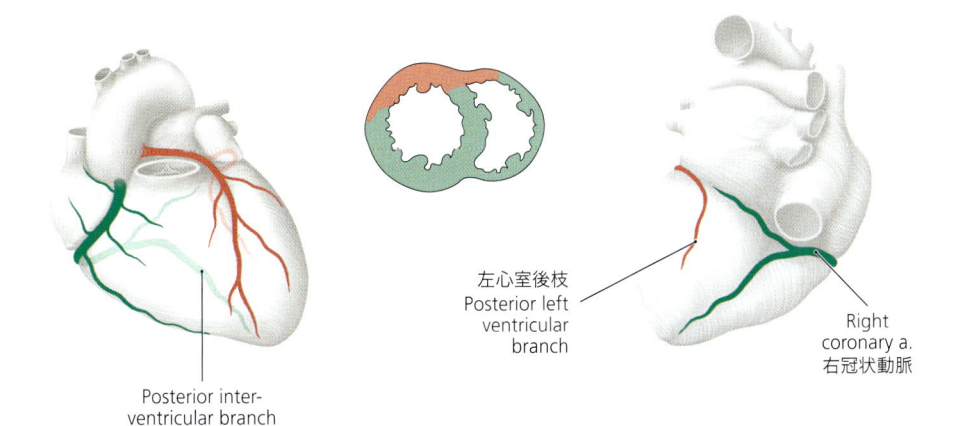

C 右冠状動脈優位型（約 15％）．

臨床

冠血流の障害

冠状動脈は吻合によって互いに連絡しているが，機能の面では終動脈である．血流不足の原因として最も多いのはアテローム性動脈硬化症であり，血管壁に斑点が沈着して血管腔が狭くなる．血管狭窄が亢進した場合には，冠血流が阻害され，胸痛（狭心症）が起こる．この胸痛はまずは労作時に起こるが，安静時にも続くようになり，典型的な部位（左腕，頭頸部の左側）に放散する．心筋梗塞は血流不足によって心筋細胞が壊死して起こる．梗塞の部位と広がりは障害された血管によって決まる．

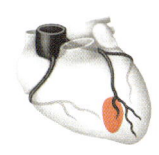

A 心尖上部前壁梗塞．

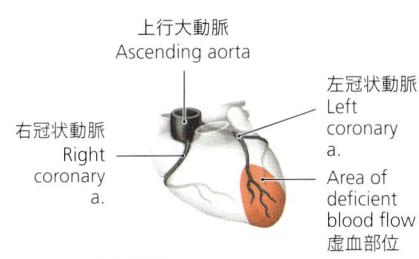

- 上行大動脈 Ascending aorta
- 右冠状動脈 Right coronary a.
- 左冠状動脈 Left coronary a.
- Area of deficient blood flow 虚血部位

B 心尖前壁梗塞．

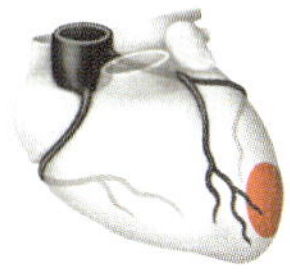

C 前外側壁梗塞．

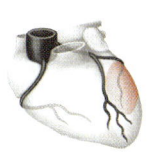

D 後外側壁梗塞．

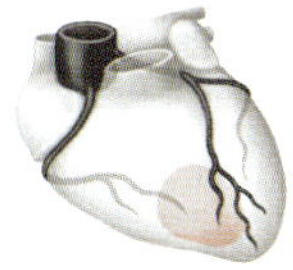

E 後壁梗塞．

心臓の刺激伝導と神経支配
Conduction & Innervation of the Heart

心筋の収縮は刺激伝導系によって調節される．特殊心筋細胞からなる刺激伝導系は心臓の興奮を発生させ伝導させる．刺激伝導系には心房に位置する2つの結節，ペースメーカーと呼ばれる洞房結節（SA）と房室結節（AV）がある．

図7.18 心臓刺激伝導系

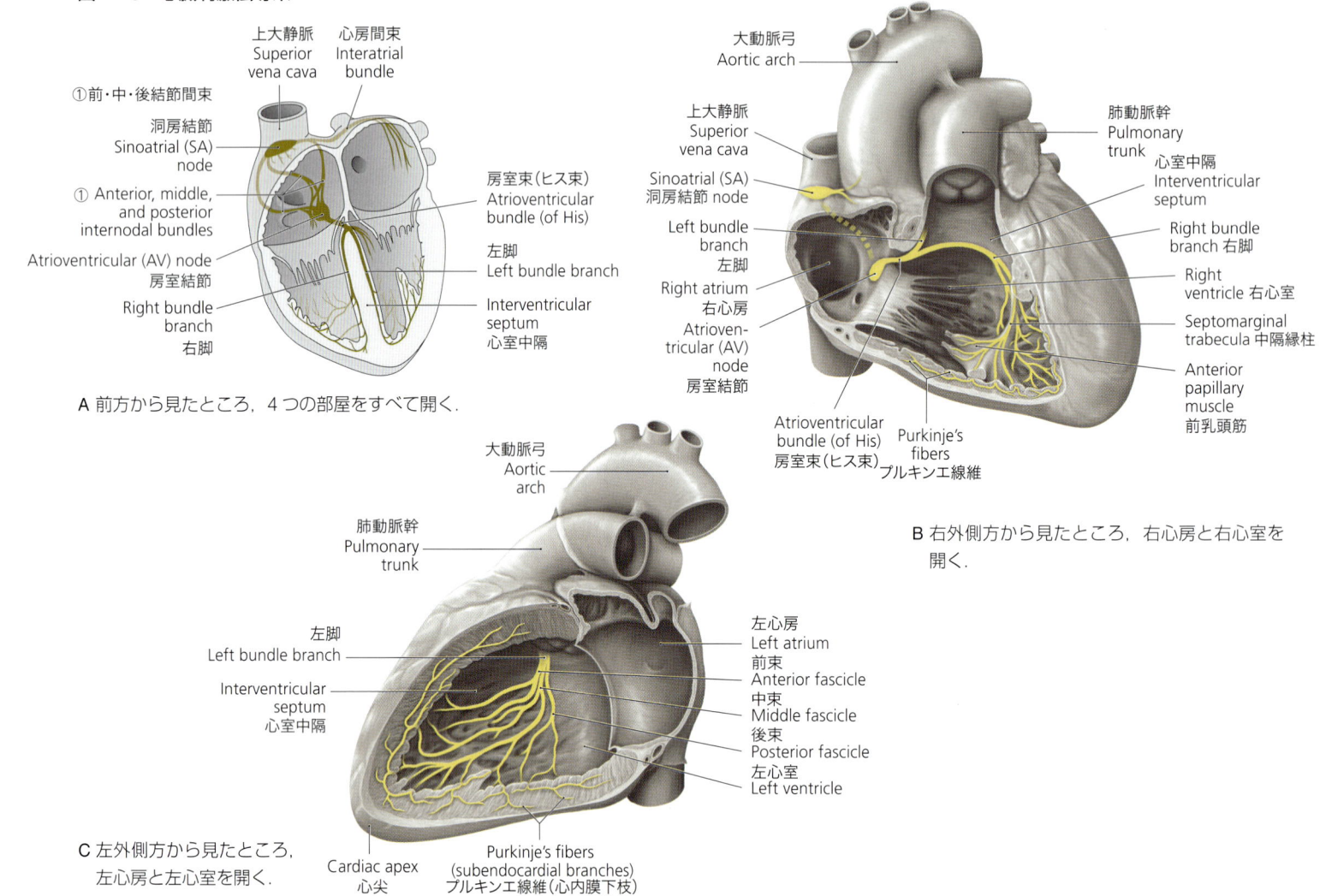

A 前方から見たところ，4つの部屋をすべて開く．

B 右外側方から見たところ，右心房と右心室を開く．

C 左外側方から見たところ，左心房と左心室を開く．

臨床

心電図

心臓の刺激は心臓を巡り，電極で検知される．3極軸あるいはベクトル（アイントーフェンの四肢誘導）に沿って別々に心臓の電気活動を記録することで，心電図が作られる．心電図は心周期（心拍）を記録し，1つの周期は一連の波，分節，間隔からなる．その波形は心臓の刺激の電動が正常か異常（例えば心筋梗塞や心拡張）かを決定するのに役立つ．*Note*: 3つの電極が必要とされるが，標準的な心電図検査ではそのほか少なくとも2つの電極が追加される（Goldberger, Wilson 誘導）

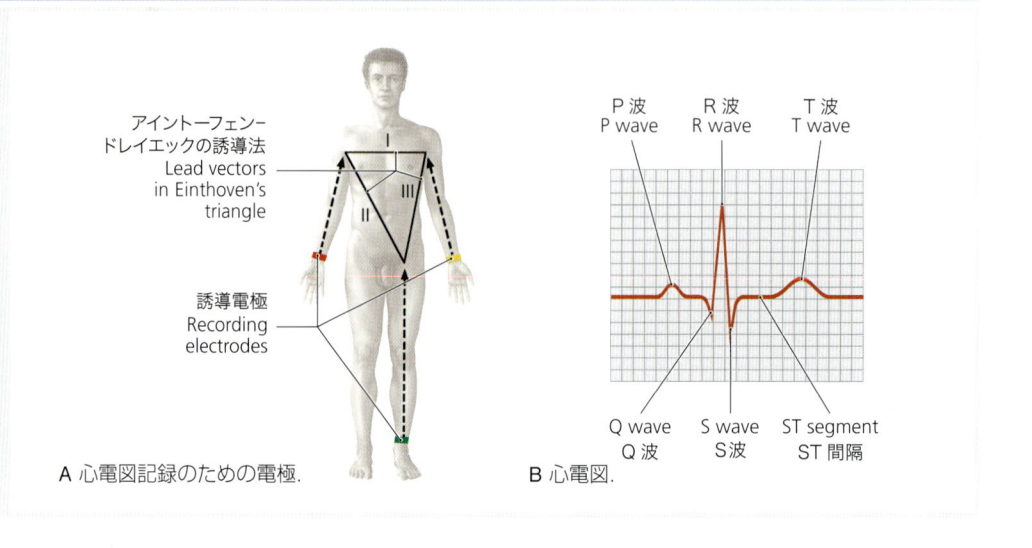

A 心電図記録のための電極．

B 心電図．

交感神経支配：第1-6胸髄節からの節前線維が頸部と胸部上部の交感神経節でシナプスを作る線維を送る．3本の頸心臓神経と胸心臓枝は心臓神経叢を作る．

副交感神経支配：節前線維とその枝は，一部は頸神経節に由来する心臓枝を介して心臓に至る．洞房結節付近や冠状動脈に沿ってシナプスを形成する．

図7.19 心臓の自律神経支配

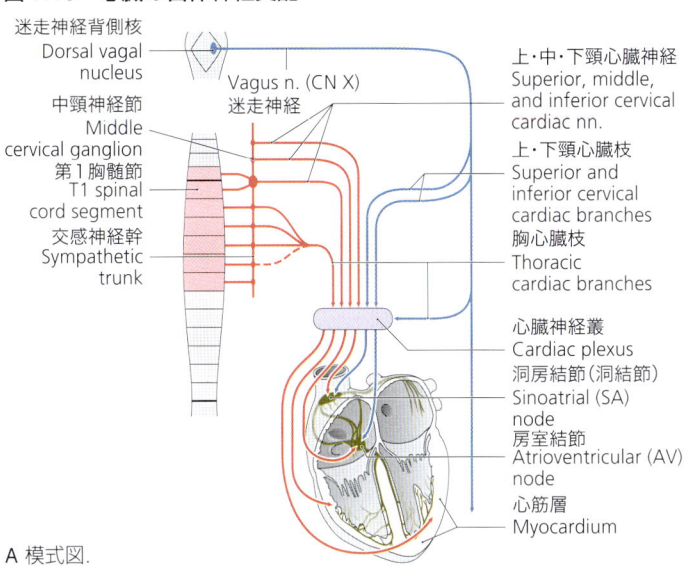

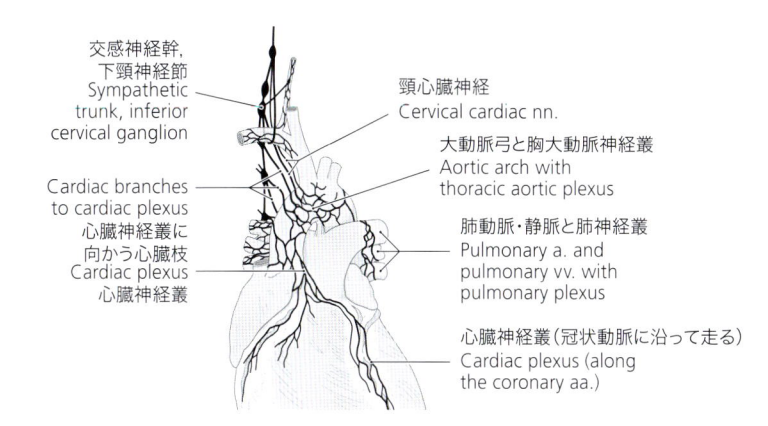

A 模式図．

B 心臓の自律神経叢．右外側方から見たところ．心臓神経叢，胸大動脈神経叢，肺神経叢の間の連絡に注意．

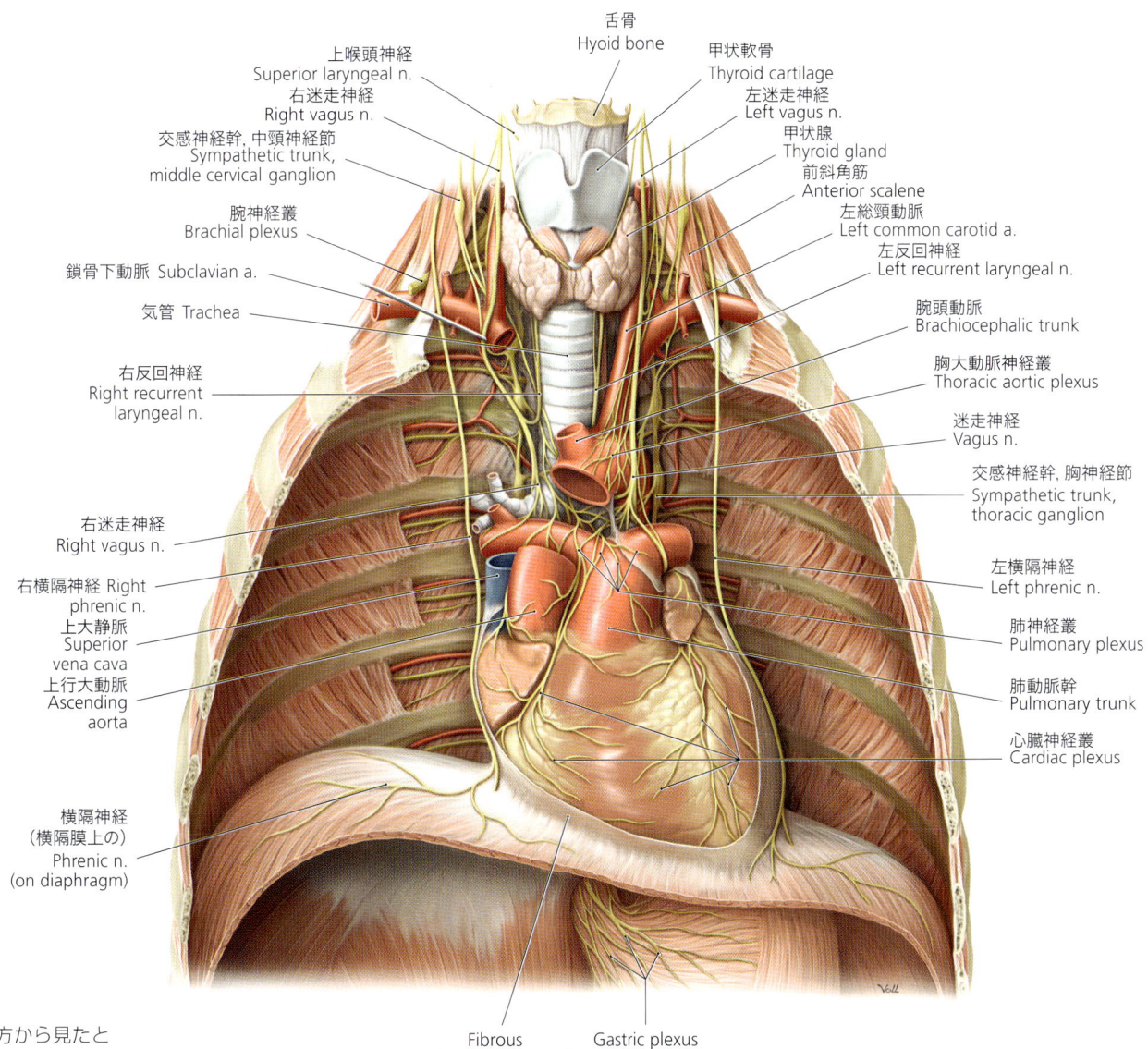

C 心臓の自律神経．前方から見たところ．胸郭を開く．

心臓：X線像
Heart: Radiology

表 7.5　心臓の辺縁

辺縁	規定構造
右心縁	右心房
	上大静脈
尖部	左心室
左心縁	大動脈弓（大動脈隆起）
	肺動脈幹
	左心房
	左心室
下縁	左心室
	右心室

図 7.20　心臓の境界と配置

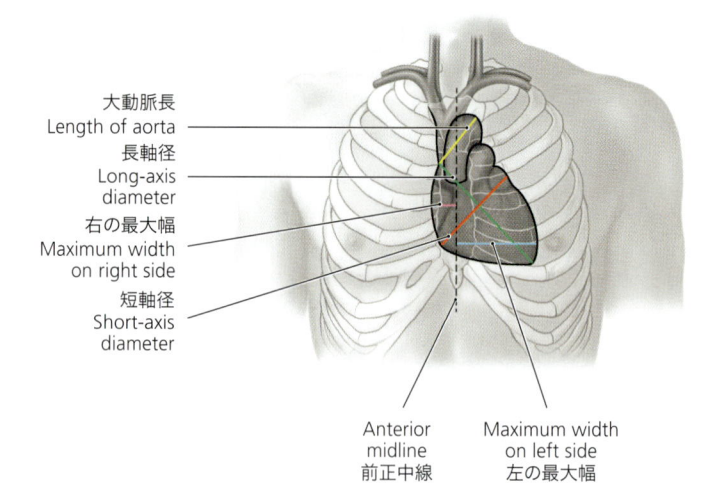

- 大動脈長　Length of aorta
- 長軸径　Long-axis diameter
- 右の最大幅　Maximum width on right side
- 短軸径　Short-axis diameter
- Anterior midline　前正中線
- Maximum width on left side　左の最大幅

図 7.21　心臓のX線像

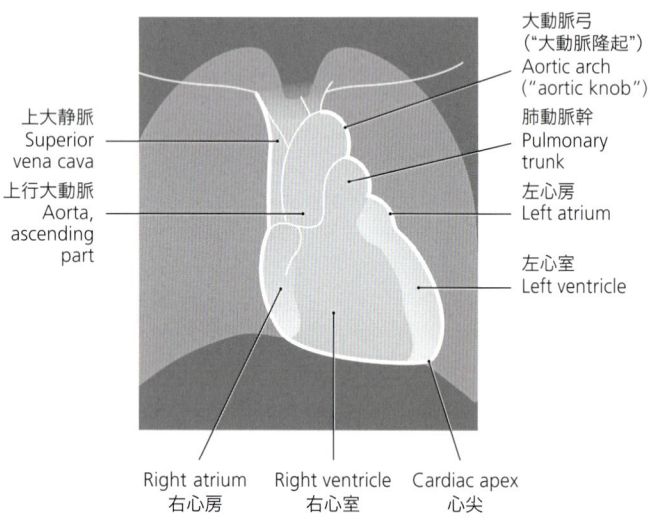

A　前方から見たところ．

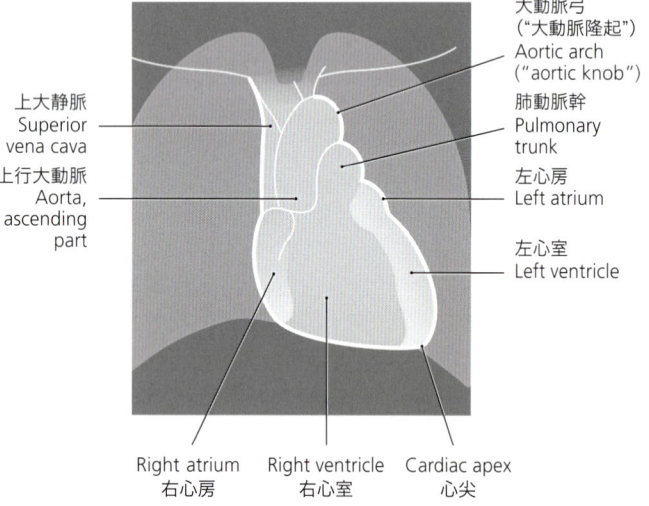

- 上大静脈　Superior vena cava
- 上行大動脈　Aorta, ascending part
- 大動脈弓（"大動脈隆起"）　Aortic arch ("aortic knob")
- 肺動脈幹　Pulmonary trunk
- 左心房　Left atrium
- 左心室　Left ventricle
- 右心房　Right atrium
- 右心室　Right ventricle
- 心尖　Cardiac apex

B　胸部X線前後像．

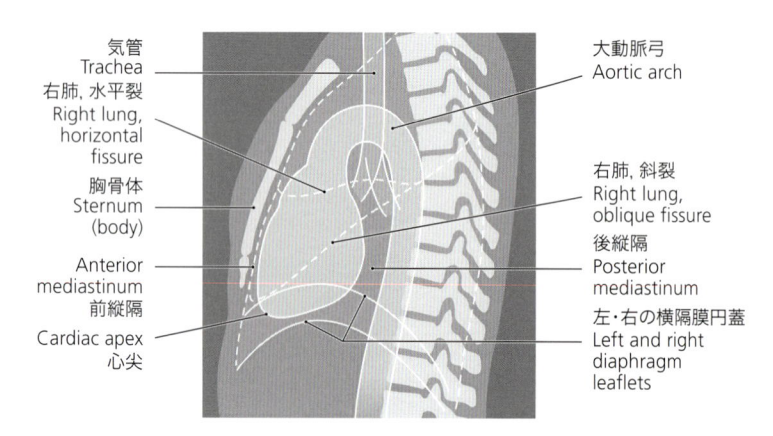

C　外側方から見たところ．横隔膜の円蓋と肺が見える．動脈弓は左主気管支の上に架かっている．後縦隔と比較して前縦隔が狭いことに注意．

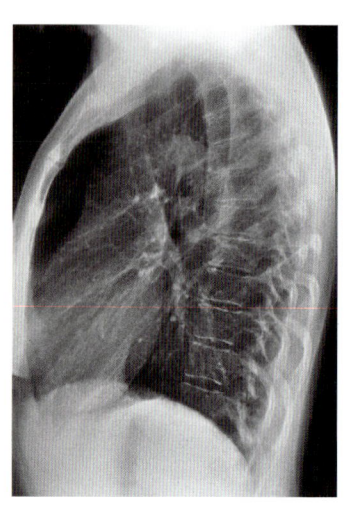

- 気管　Trachea
- 右肺，水平裂　Right lung, horizontal fissure
- 胸骨体　Sternum (body)
- Anterior mediastinum　前縦隔
- Cardiac apex　心尖
- 大動脈弓　Aortic arch
- 右肺，斜裂　Right lung, oblique fissure
- 後縦隔　Posterior mediastinum
- 左・右の横隔膜円蓋　Left and right diaphragm leaflets

D　胸部X線左側面像．

図 7.22 水平断面での心臓

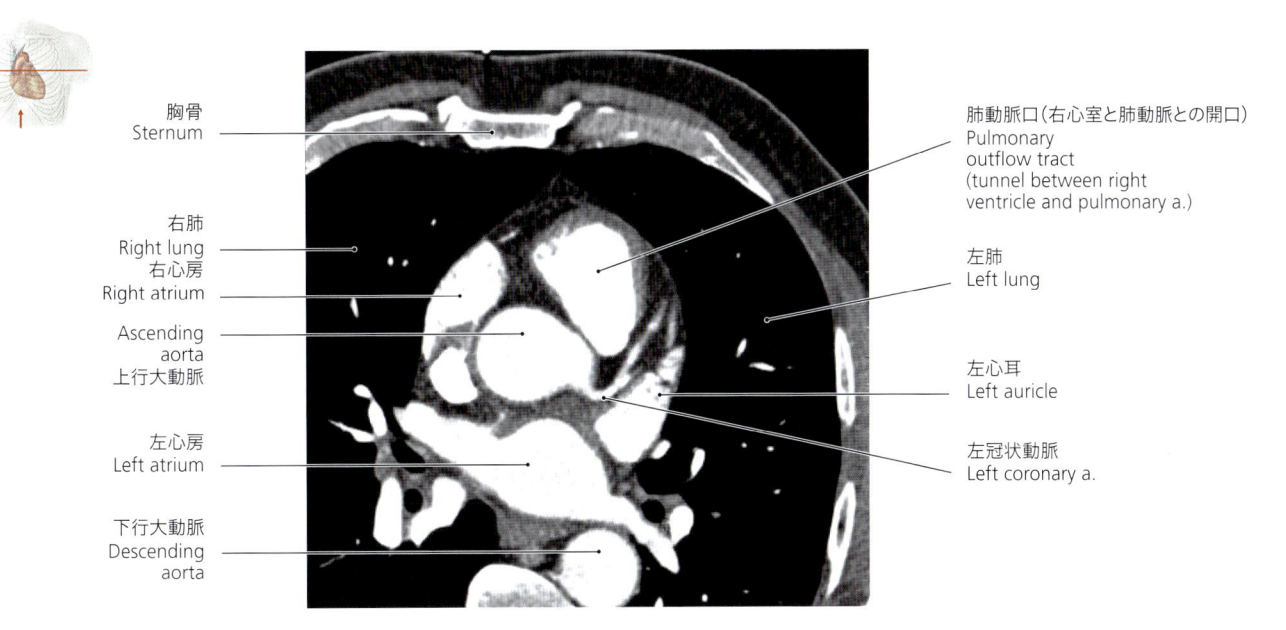

A 正常な胸郭の MR 像．心臓の各室は信号強度が高いために明瞭に描出されるが，肺は描出されない．

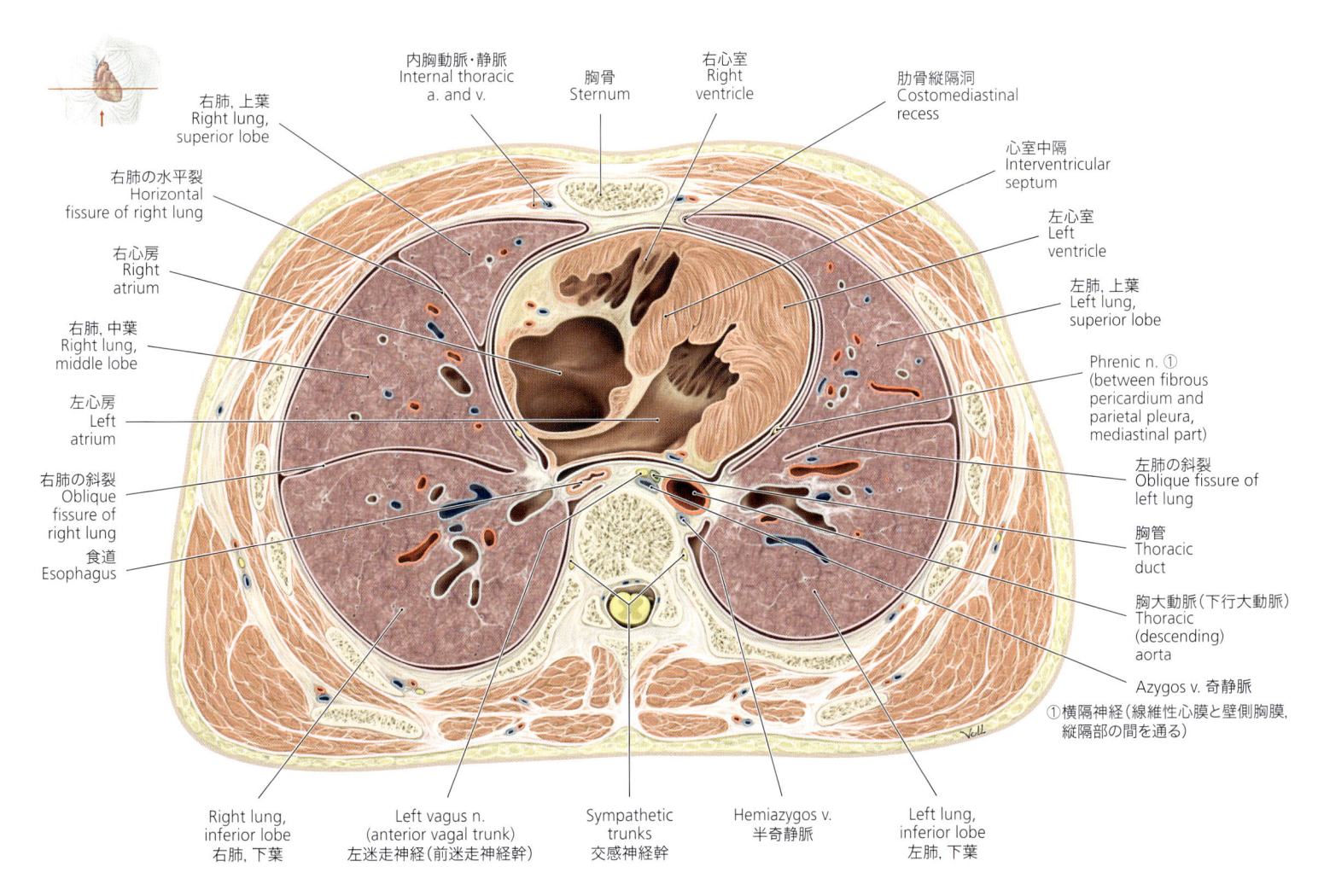

ラベル（図A）：
- 胸骨 / Sternum
- 右肺 Right lung
- 右心房 Right atrium
- Ascending aorta 上行大動脈
- 左心房 Left atrium
- 下行大動脈 Descending aorta
- 肺動脈口（右心室と肺動脈との開口）Pulmonary outflow tract (tunnel between right ventricle and pulmonary a.)
- 左肺 Left lung
- 左心耳 Left auricle
- 左冠状動脈 Left coronary a.

B 第8胸椎の高さにおける水平断，上方から見たところ．

ラベル（図B）：
- 右肺，上葉 Right lung, superior lobe
- 右肺の水平裂 Horizontal fissure of right lung
- 右心房 Right atrium
- 右肺，中葉 Right lung, middle lobe
- 左心房 Left atrium
- 右肺の斜裂 Oblique fissure of right lung
- 食道 Esophagus
- 内胸動脈・静脈 Internal thoracic a. and v.
- 胸骨 Sternum
- 右心室 Right ventricle
- 肋骨縦隔洞 Costomediastinal recess
- 心室中隔 Interventricular septum
- 左心室 Left ventricle
- 左肺，上葉 Left lung, superior lobe
- Phrenic n. ① (between fibrous pericardium and parietal pleura, mediastinal part)
- 左肺の斜裂 Oblique fissure of left lung
- 胸管 Thoracic duct
- 胸大動脈（下行大動脈）Thoracic (descending) aorta
- Azygos v. 奇静脈
- ①横隔神経（線維性心膜と壁側胸膜，縦隔部の間を通る）
- Right lung, inferior lobe 右肺，下葉
- Left vagus n. (anterior vagal trunk) 左迷走神経（前迷走神経幹）
- Sympathetic trunks 交感神経幹
- Hemiazygos v. 半奇静脈
- Left lung, inferior lobe 左肺，下葉

出生前・後の循環
Pre- & Postnatal Circulation

図 7.23 出生前の循環
Fritsch and Kühnel による.

① 胎盤からの酸素と栄養に富んだ胎児血が臍静脈を通って胎児に運ばれる.
② この血液のほぼ半分は肝臓を迂回し(静脈管を通って),下大静脈に入る. 残りは門脈に入り肝臓に栄養と酸素を与える.
③ 下大静脈から右心房に入った血液は(肺はまだ機能していないので)右心室を迂回して右-左シャントである卵円孔を通って左心房に入る.
④ 上大静脈から右心房に入った血液は右心室に入り,肺動脈幹に向かう. この血液のほとんどは右-左シャントである動脈管を通って大動脈に入る.
⑤ 大動脈の動脈血の一部は内腸骨動脈から起こる1対の臍動脈を通って胎盤に戻る.

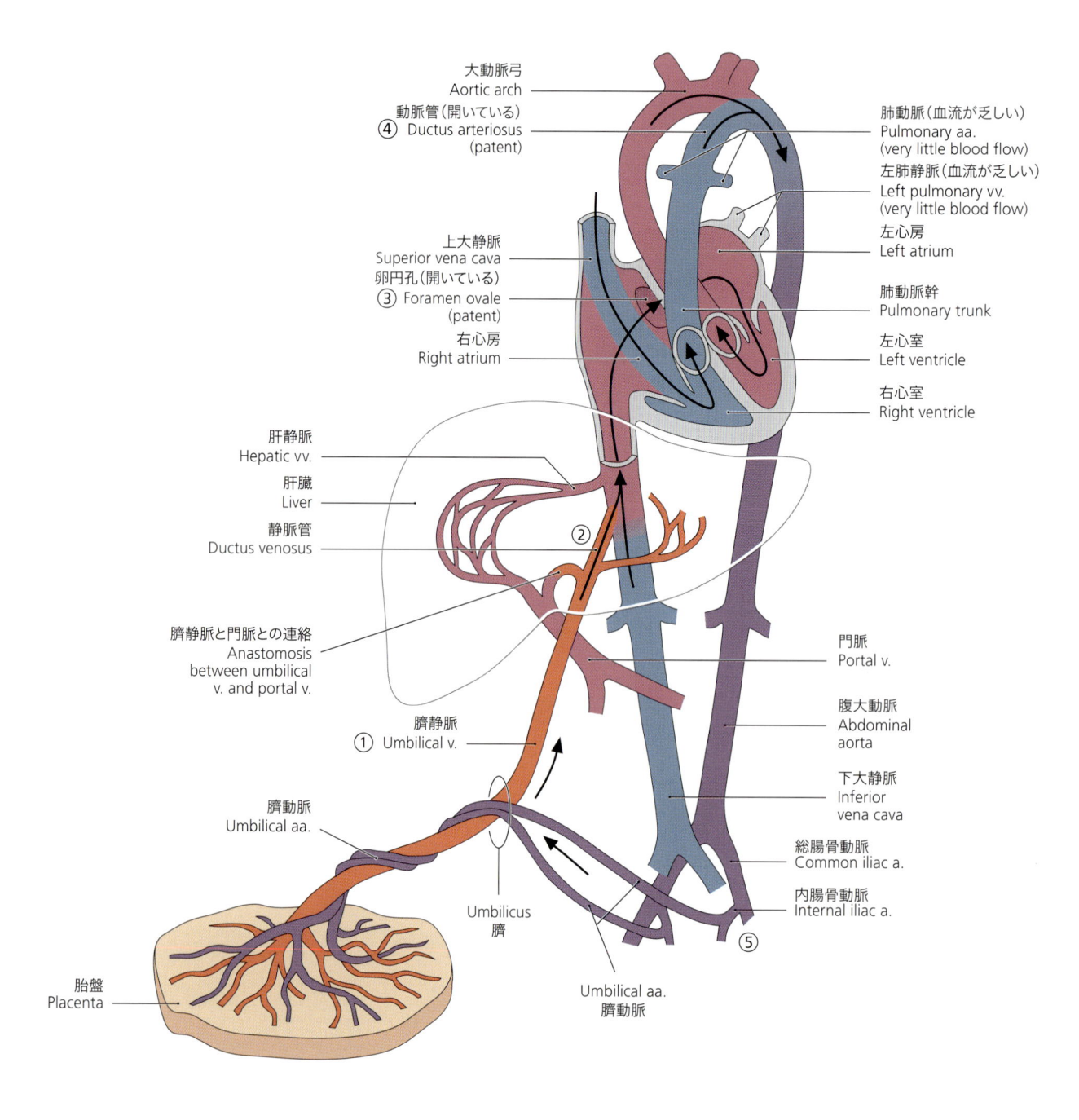

大動脈弓 Aortic arch
動脈管(開いている) Ductus arteriosus (patent) ④
肺動脈(血流が乏しい) Pulmonary aa. (very little blood flow)
左肺静脈(血流が乏しい) Left pulmonary vv. (very little blood flow)
上大静脈 Superior vena cava
左心房 Left atrium
卵円孔(開いている) Foramen ovale (patent) ③
肺動脈幹 Pulmonary trunk
右心房 Right atrium
左心室 Left ventricle
右心室 Right ventricle
肝静脈 Hepatic vv.
肝臓 Liver
静脈管 Ductus venosus
臍静脈と門脈との連絡 Anastomosis between umbilical v. and portal v.
門脈 Portal v.
臍静脈 Umbilical v. ①
腹大動脈 Abdominal aorta
下大静脈 Inferior vena cava
総腸骨動脈 Common iliac a.
臍動脈 Umbilical aa.
内腸骨動脈 Internal iliac a. ⑤
Umbilicus 臍
Umbilical aa. 臍動脈
胎盤 Placenta

①出生時に肺呼吸が始まると，肺の血管抵抗が低下し，右肺動脈幹からの血液が肺静脈に入る．
②卵円孔と動脈管が閉ざされて，胎児の右-左シャントがなくなる．このときに心臓において肺循環と体循環が分離される．
③新生児が胎盤から離されると，臍静脈と静脈管と同様に臍動脈は（近位部をのぞいて）閉塞する．
④代謝を必要とする血液が肝臓を通過するようになる．

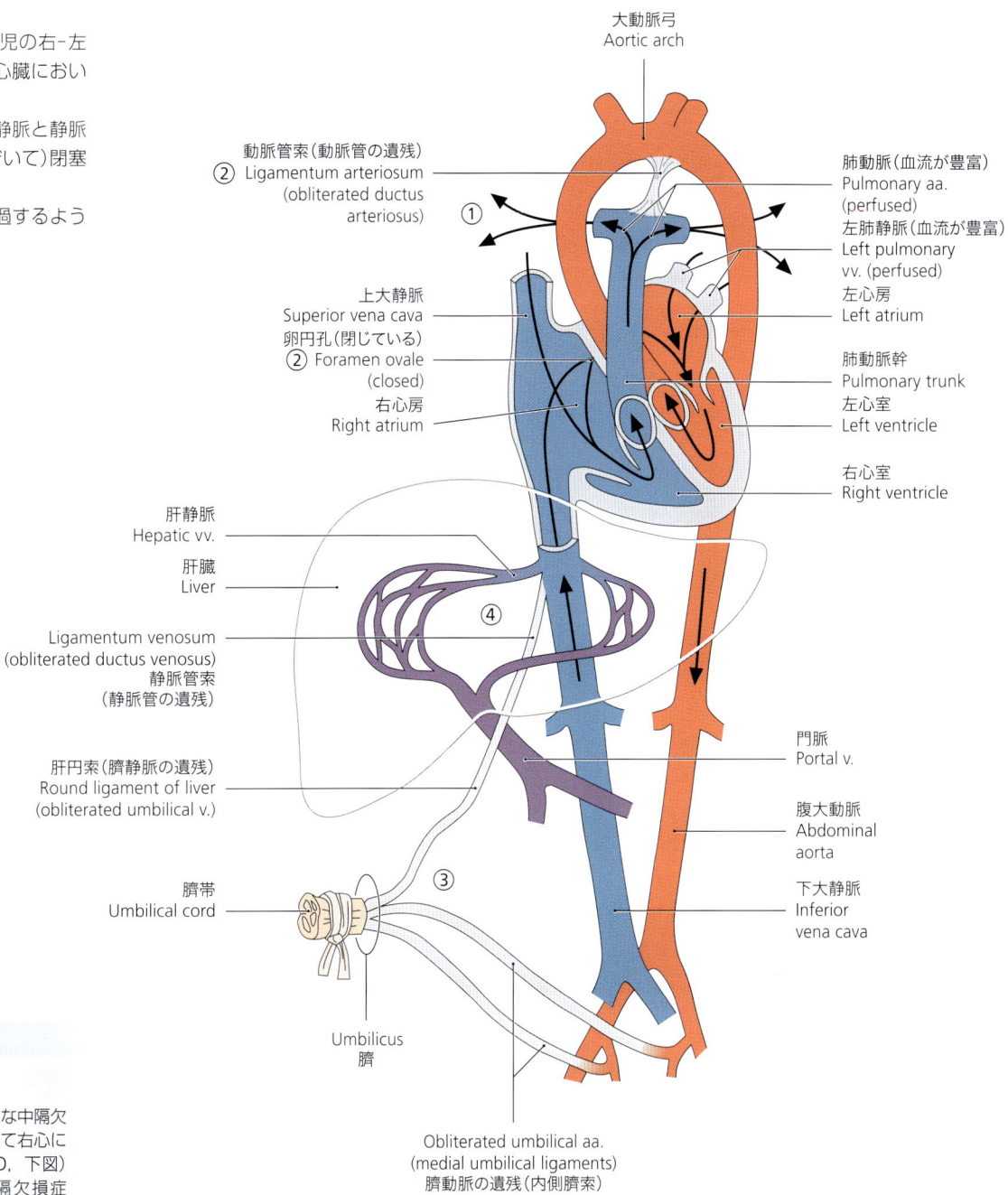

図7.24 出生後の循環
Fritsch and Kühnel による．

大動脈弓 Aortic arch
動脈管索（動脈管の遺残）② Ligamentum arteriosum (obliterated ductus arteriosus)
肺動脈（血流が豊富）Pulmonary aa. (perfused)
左肺静脈（血流が豊富）Left pulmonary vv. (perfused)
上大静脈 Superior vena cava
卵円孔（閉じている）② Foramen ovale (closed)
左心房 Left atrium
右心房 Right atrium
肺動脈幹 Pulmonary trunk
左心室 Left ventricle
右心室 Right ventricle
肝静脈 Hepatic vv.
肝臓 Liver
Ligamentum venosum (obliterated ductus venosus)
静脈管索（静脈管の遺残）
肝円索（臍静脈の遺残）Round ligament of liver (obliterated umbilical v.)
門脈 Portal v.
腹大動脈 Abdominal aorta
下大静脈 Inferior vena cava
臍帯 Umbilical cord
Umbilicus 臍
Obliterated umbilical aa. (medial umbilical ligaments)
臍動脈の遺残（内側臍索）

臨床

中隔欠損症

先天的な心臓疾患の中で最も一般的な中隔欠損症では，収縮期に左心の血液が誤って右心に入ってしまう．心室中隔欠損症（VSD，下図）は最も一般的な型である．心房中隔欠損症（ASD）の最も一般的な型では，卵円孔が開いたままであり，胎児のシャントが不十分にしか閉じなかったことで生じる．

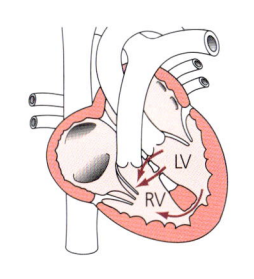

表7.6	胎児の循環器系構造からの派生物
胎児の構造	成人の遺残物
動脈管	動脈管索
卵円孔	卵円窩
静脈管	静脈管索
臍静脈	肝円索
臍動脈	内側臍索

食道
Esophagus

食道は頸部（第6頸椎-第1胸椎），胸部（第1胸椎-横隔膜食道裂孔），腹部（横隔膜-胃）の3つの部分に分けられる．食道は胸大動脈のや や右側を下行し，胸骨剣状突起の下で横隔膜をやや左側で貫通する．

図 7.25 食道：位置と狭窄部位

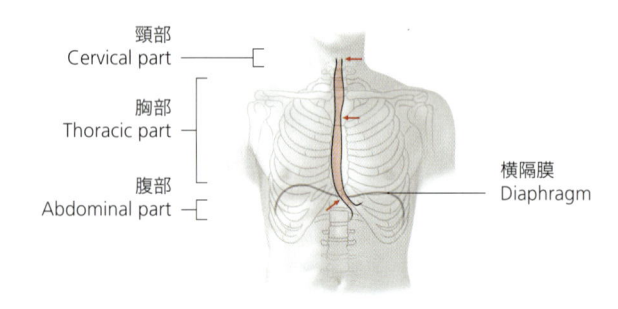

- 頸部 Cervical part
- 胸部 Thoracic part
- 腹部 Abdominal part
- 横隔膜 Diaphragm

A 胸壁への食道の投影．食道の狭窄部位は矢印で示してある．

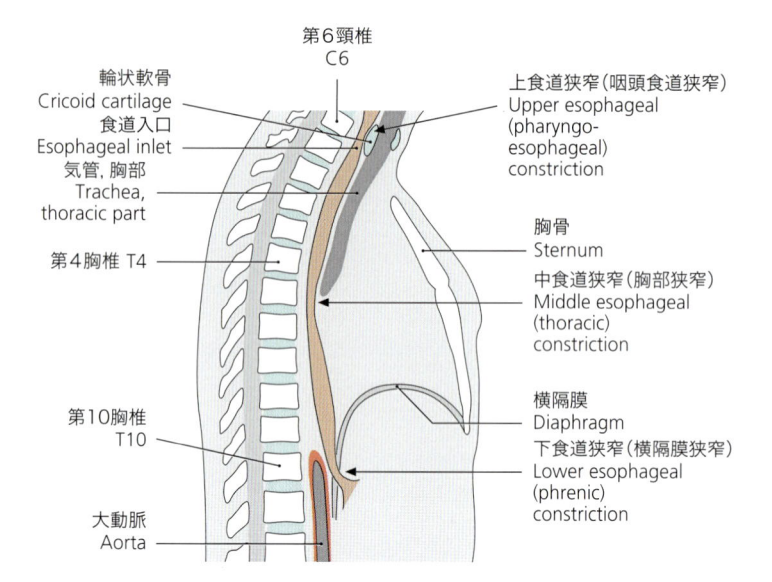

- 第6頸椎 C6
- 輪状軟骨 Cricoid cartilage
- 食道入口 Esophageal inlet
- 気管, 胸部 Trachea, thoracic part
- 第4胸椎 T4
- 第10胸椎 T10
- 大動脈 Aorta
- 上食道狭窄（咽頭食道狭窄） Upper esophageal (pharyngo-esophageal) constriction
- 胸骨 Sternum
- 中食道狭窄（胸部狭窄） Middle esophageal (thoracic) constriction
- 横隔膜 Diaphragm
- 下食道狭窄（横隔膜狭窄） Lower esophageal (phrenic) constriction

B 食道の狭窄部位, 右外側方から見たところ．

図 7.26 原位置の食道
前方から見たところ．

- 気管, 頸部 Trachea, cervical part
- 食道, 頸部 Esophagus, cervical part
- 腕神経叢 Brachial plexus
- 左内頸静脈 Left internal jugular v.
- 腕頭動脈 Brachiocephalic trunk
- 左鎖骨下動脈・静脈 Left subclavian a. and v.
- 右腕頭静脈 Right brachiocephalic v.
- 左腕頭静脈 Left brachiocephalic v.
- 壁側胸膜, 頸部 Parietal pleura, cervical part
- 大動脈弓 Aortic arch
- 動脈管索 Ligamentum arteriosum
- 上大静脈 Superior vena cava
- 左肺動脈 Left pulmonary a.
- 右肺動脈 Right pulmonary a.
- 上・下葉気管支 Superior and inferior lobar bronchi
- 右肺静脈 Right pulmonary vv.
- 胸大動脈 Thoracic aorta
- 肺動脈幹 Pulmonary trunk
- 壁側胸膜, 縦隔部（縦隔胸膜） Parietal pleura, mediastinal part
- 壁側胸膜, 横隔部（横隔胸膜） Parietal pleura, diaphragmatic part
- 食道, 胸部 Esophagus, thoracic part
- 線維性心膜 Fibrous pericardium
- 胃 Stomach

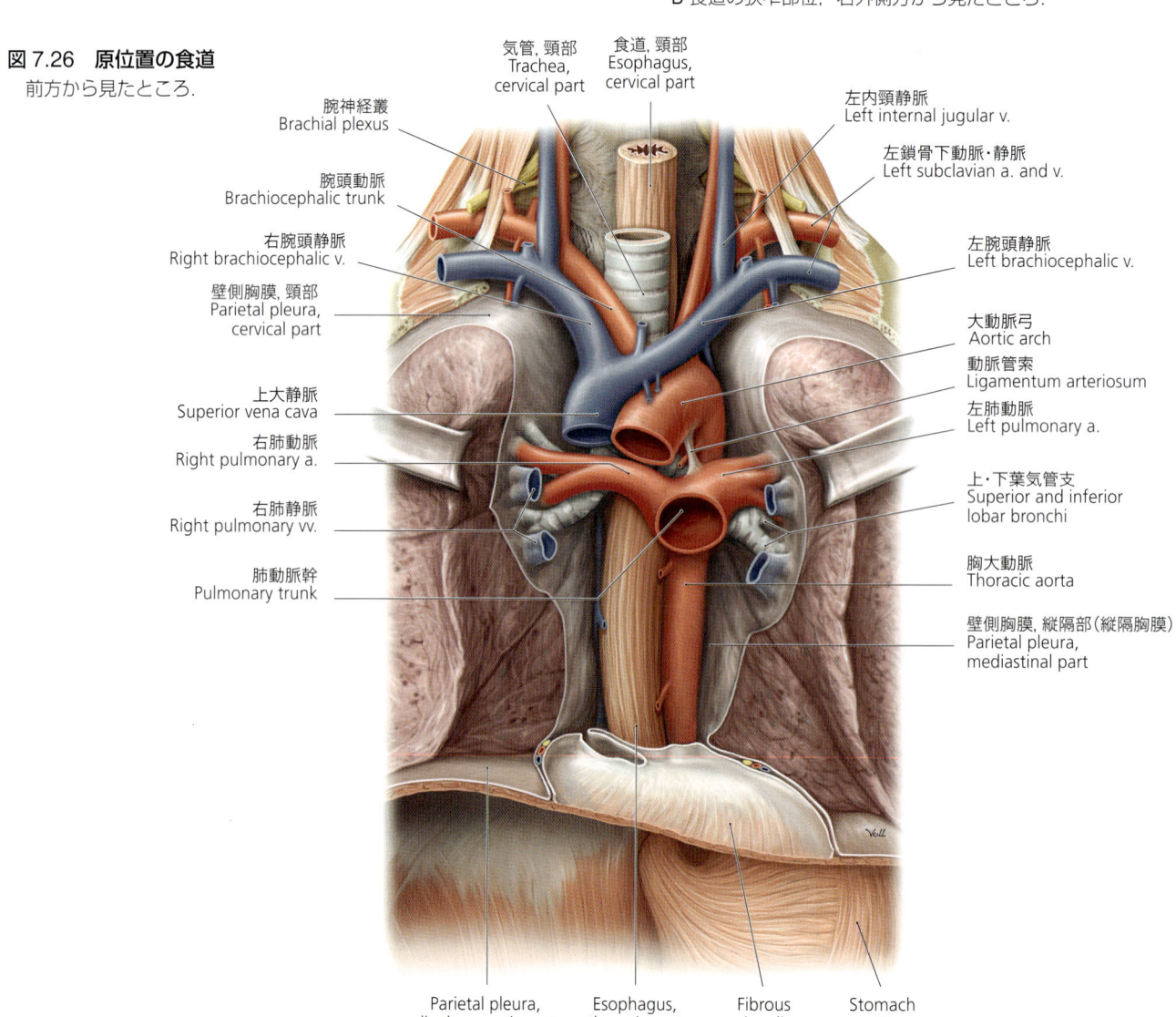

図 7.27　食道の構造

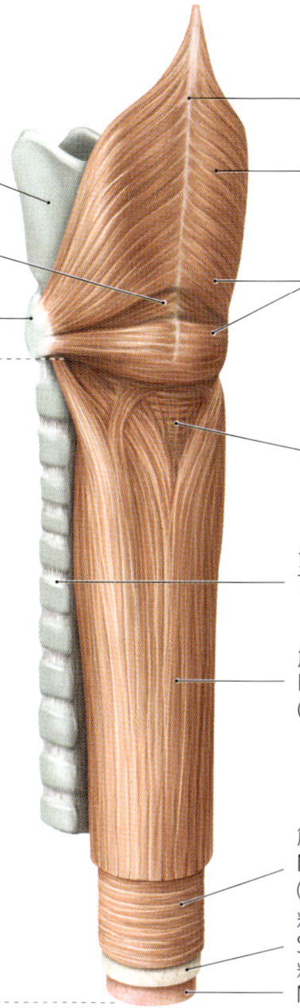

- 甲状軟骨 Thyroid cartilage
- キリアン三角 Killian's triangle
- 輪状軟骨 Cricoid cartilage
- 食道 Esophagus
- ①下咽頭収縮筋, 甲状咽頭部
- ②下咽頭収縮筋, 輪状咽頭部
- 咽頭縫線 Pharyngeal raphe
- Inferior pharyngeal ① constrictor, thyro-pharyngeal part
- Inferior pharyngeal ② constrictor, crico-pharyngeal part
- 筋層（輪筋層）Muscular coat (circular layer)
- 気管 Trachea
- 筋層（縦筋層）Muscular coat (longitudinal layer)
- 筋層（輪筋層）Muscular coat (circular layer)
- 粘膜下組織 Submucosa
- 粘膜 Mucosa

A 食道の壁．左後方から見たところ．喉頭(p.552)，気管(p.110)．

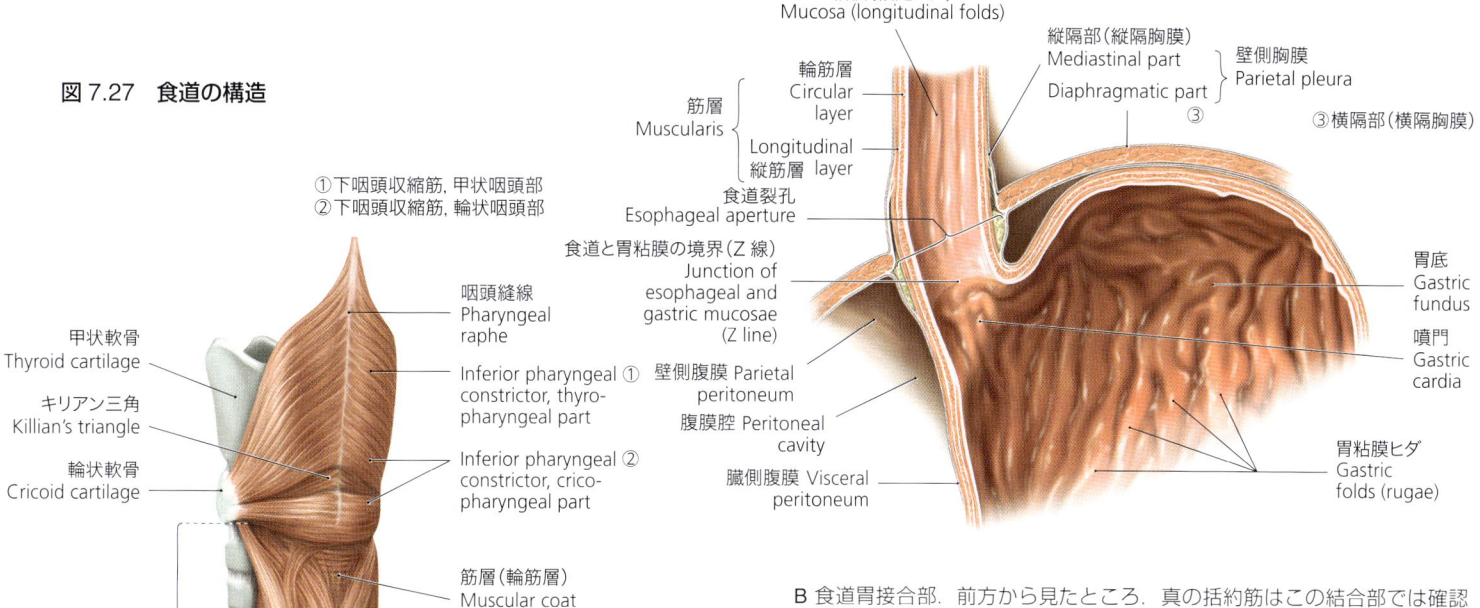

- 粘膜（縦走ヒダ）Mucosa (longitudinal folds)
- 輪筋層 Circular layer ｝筋層 Muscularis
- 縦筋層 Longitudinal layer
- 食道裂孔 Esophageal aperture
- 食道と胃粘膜の境界(Z線) Junction of esophageal and gastric mucosae (Z line)
- 壁側腹膜 Parietal peritoneum
- 腹膜腔 Peritoneal cavity
- 臓側腹膜 Visceral peritoneum
- 縦隔部（縦隔胸膜）Mediastinal part
- 横隔部 Diaphragmatic part
- ③ 壁側胸膜 Parietal pleura
- ③横隔部（横隔胸膜）
- 胃底 Gastric fundus
- 噴門 Gastric cardia
- 胃粘膜ヒダ Gastric folds (rugae)

B 食道胃接合部．前方から見たところ．真の括約筋はこの結合部では確認できない．その代わりに横隔膜食道裂孔の筋肉が括約筋として機能しており，ジグザグ状であるのでZ線と呼ばれることが多い．

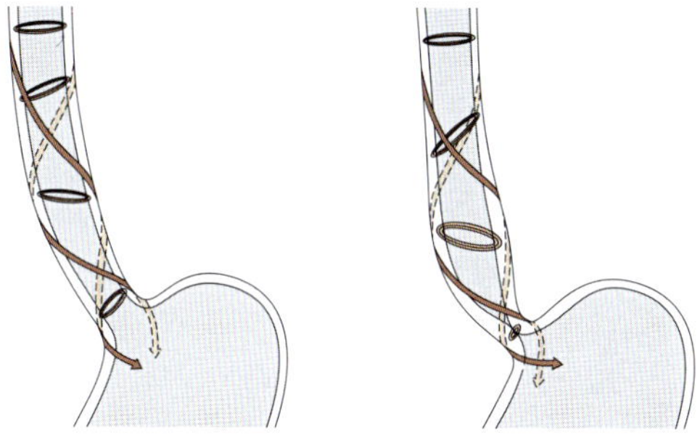

C 食道の筋の機能的構造．

臨床

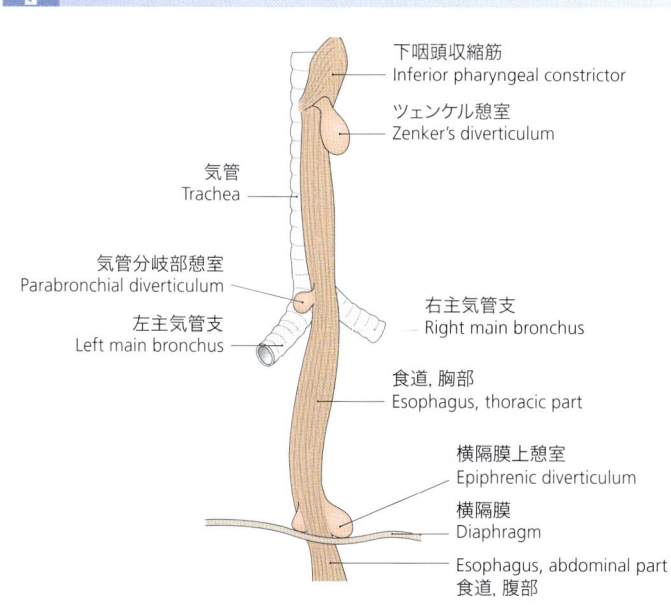

食道憩室

憩室（異常外嚢あるいは嚢）は，一般的に食道壁の脆弱な部位に発生する．食道憩室には主に3つのタイプがある．

- 下咽頭憩室：喉頭と咽頭の接合部に起こる外嚢．ツェンケル憩室(Zenker diverticulum)も含まれる(70%)．
- "真性"牽引性憩室：典型的な脆弱な部分では起こらず，全層の突出によって起こる．これらは一般的にリンパ管炎のような炎症によって起こり，食道が気管支や気管支リンパ節に近づく部分で発生する（胸部憩室あるいは気管支分岐部憩室）．
- "偽性"内圧性憩室：（例えば正常な嚥下中に）食道圧の上昇によって筋層の脆弱な部分を突き抜けて，粘膜および粘膜下組織が脱出したもの．横隔膜の食道裂孔上で起こる傍裂孔憩室および横隔膜上憩室を含む(10%)．

- 下咽頭収縮筋 Inferior pharyngeal constrictor
- ツェンケル憩室 Zenker's diverticulum
- 気管 Trachea
- 気管分岐部憩室 Parabronchial diverticulum
- 左主気管支 Left main bronchus
- 右主気管支 Right main bronchus
- 食道, 胸部 Esophagus, thoracic part
- 横隔膜上憩室 Epiphrenic diverticulum
- 横隔膜 Diaphragm
- 食道, 腹部 Esophagus, abdominal part

食道の神経と血管
Neurovasculature of the Esophagus

交感神経支配：節前線維は第2-6胸髄節に由来する．節後線維は交感神経鎖から起こり，食道神経叢に入る．
副交感神経支配：節前線維は迷走神経背側核から起こり，迷走神経を経由してよく発達した食道神経叢を作る．
Note：節後線維は食道壁にある．食道の頸部への線維は反回神経を経由する．

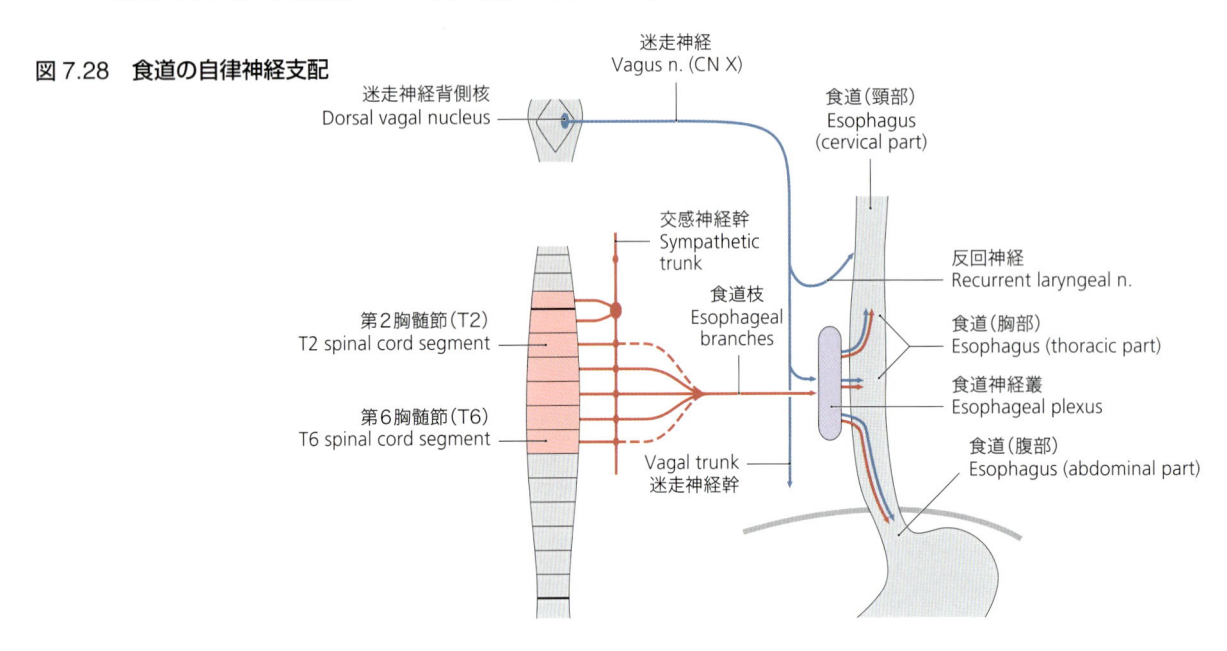

図7.28 食道の自律神経支配

図7.29 食道神経叢
左・右迷走神経は最初は食道の左側・右側を下行する．食道神経叢に枝を出し始めると左迷走神経は前面，右迷走神経は後面に移動する．迷走神経が腹部に入るときに，前・後迷走神経幹と名前を変える．

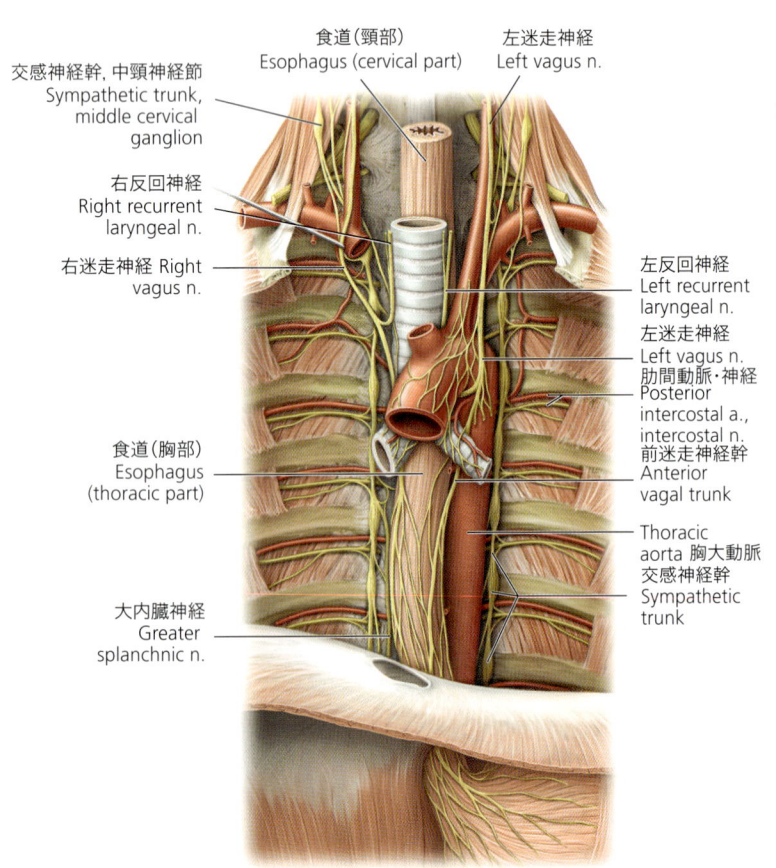

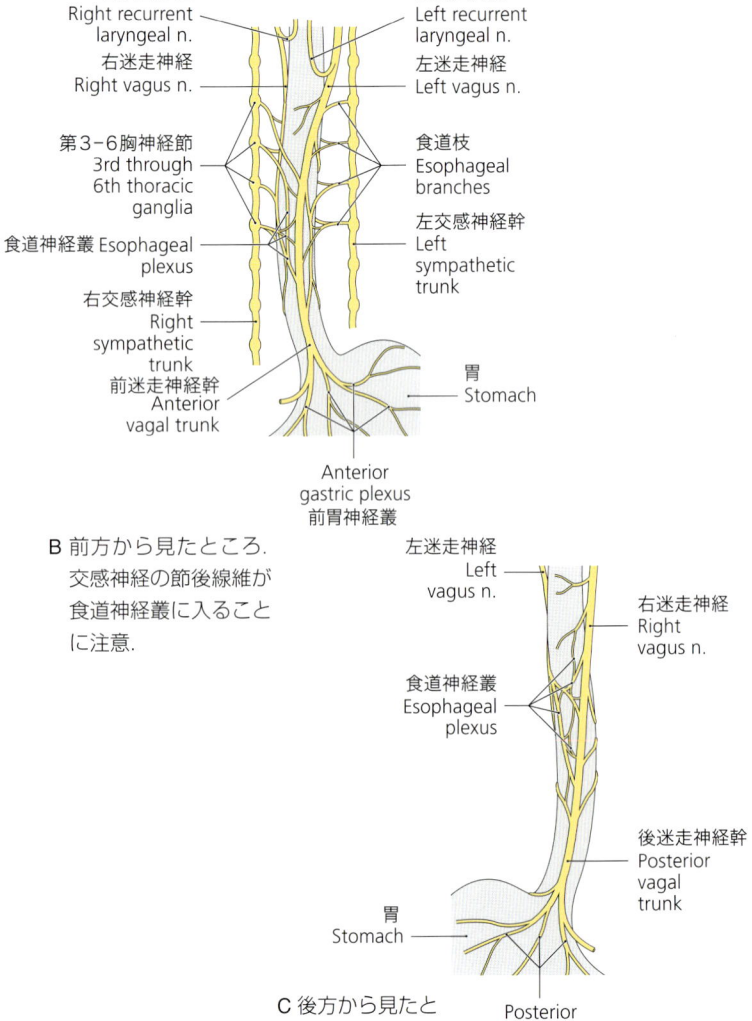

A 原位置の食道神経叢，前方から見たところ．

B 前方から見たところ．交感神経の節後線維が食道神経叢に入ることに注意．

C 後方から見たところ．

図 7.30 　食道の動脈
前方から見たところ.

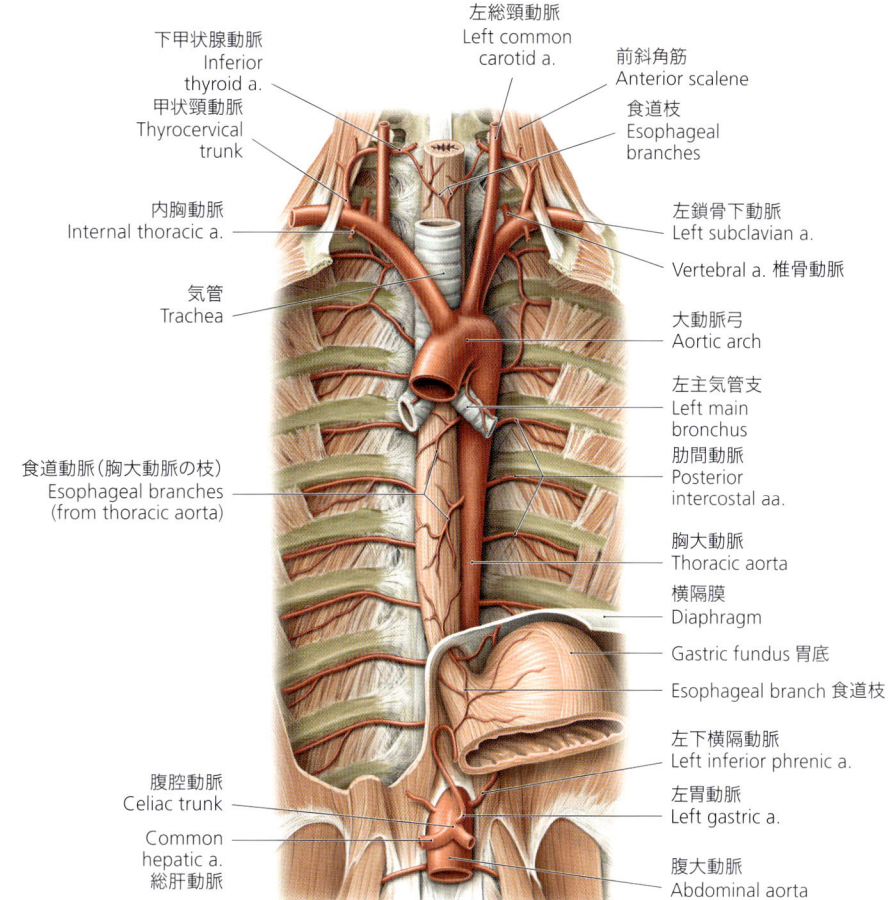

図 7.31 　食道の静脈
前方から見たところ.

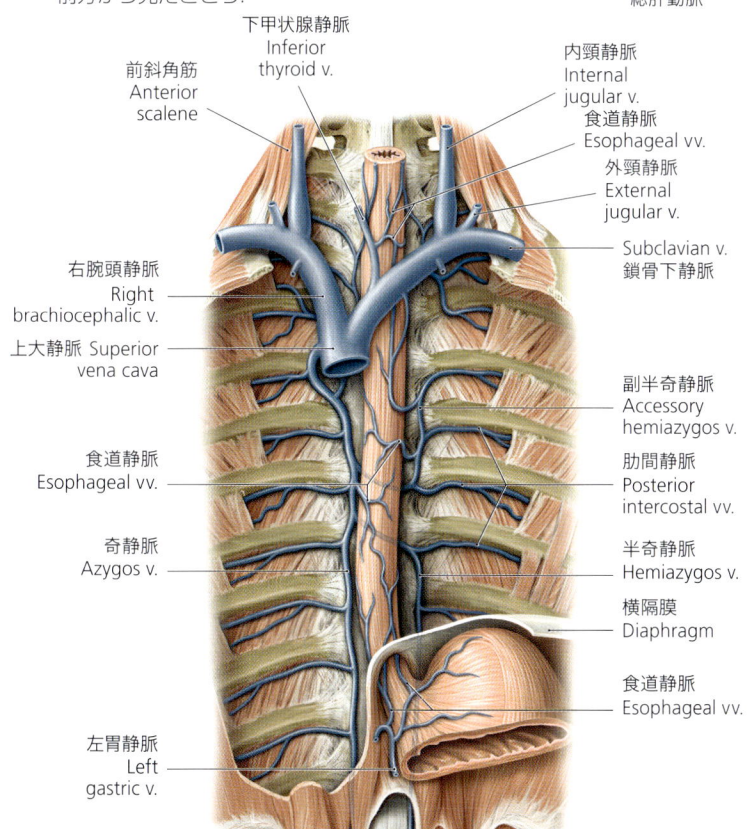

表 7.7	食道の血管	
区分	食道の動脈の起始	食道の静脈の分布
頸部	下甲状腺動脈	下甲状腺静脈
	稀に，総頸動脈の甲状頸動脈からの直接の枝	左腕頭静脈
胸部	大動脈（4，5本の食道動脈）	左上部：副半奇静脈あるいは左腕頭静脈
		左下部：半奇静脈
		右部：奇静脈
腹部	左胃動脈	左胃静脈

縦隔

縦隔のリンパ管
Lymphatics of the Mediastinum

上横隔リンパ節は横隔膜，心膜，食道下部，肺，肝臓からリンパを集め，気管支縦隔リンパ本幹に注ぐ．腹部にある下横隔リンパ節は横隔膜，肺の下葉からのリンパを集め，腰リンパ本幹に注ぐ．
Note: 心膜からのリンパもまた上方に向かって腕頭リンパ節に注ぐ．

図 7.32　縦隔と胸腔のリンパ節
左前方から見たところ．

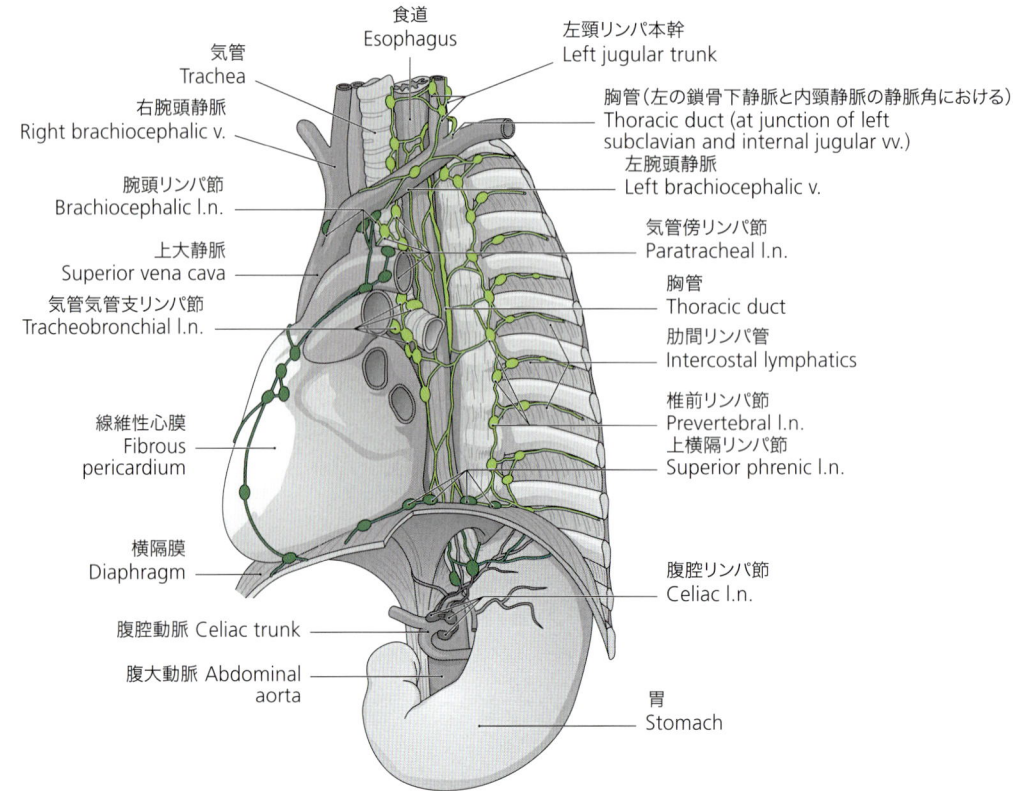

図 7.33　心臓のリンパ流路
心臓では特徴的な"交差した"リンパ流路がある．左心房と左心室からのリンパは右静脈角に流れ，右心房と右心室からのリンパは左静脈角に流れる．

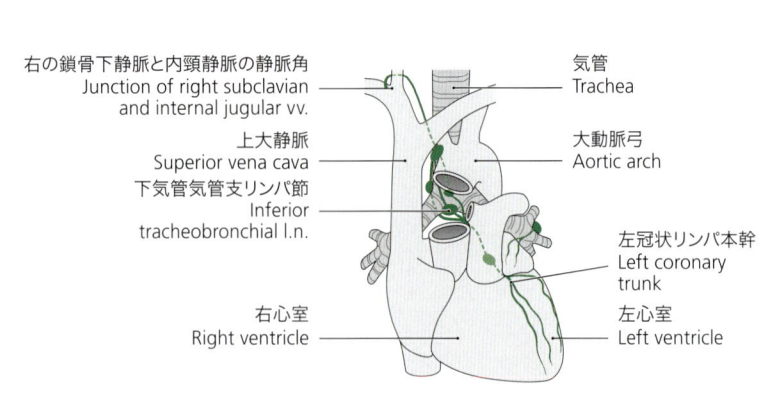

A 左心のリンパ流路，前方から見たところ．

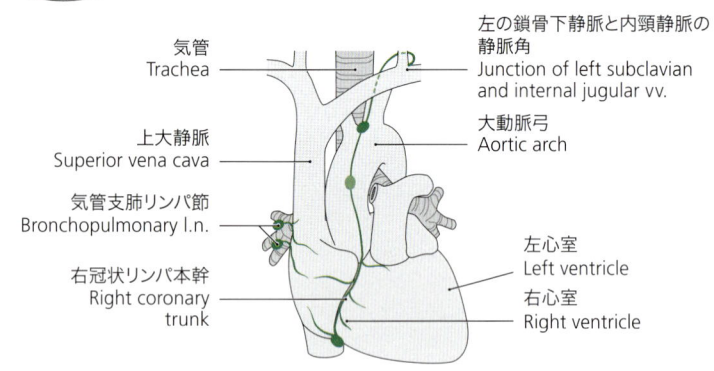

B 右心のリンパ流路，前方から見たところ．

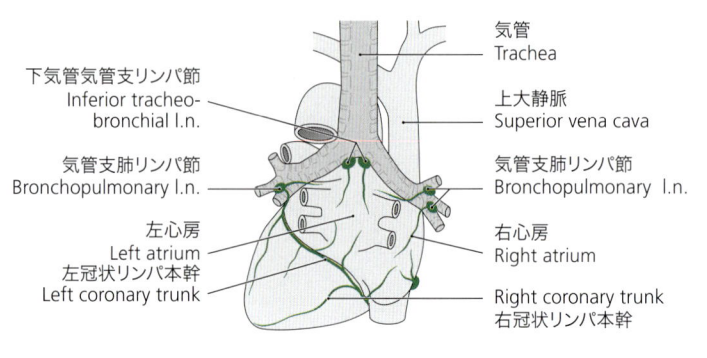

C 後方から見たところ．

食道傍リンパ節は食道からのリンパを運ぶ．食道の頸部では上方に向かい，主に深頸リンパ節に排導し，そして頸リンパ本幹へ流入する．食道の胸部では気管支縦隔リンパ節に排導し，2方向に分かれ，上半分は上方に向かい，下半分は上横隔リンパ本幹を経由して下方に向かう．気管支肺リンパ節と気管傍リンパ節は肺，気管支，気管からリンパを集め，気管支縦隔リンパ本幹に注ぐ（p.118参照）．

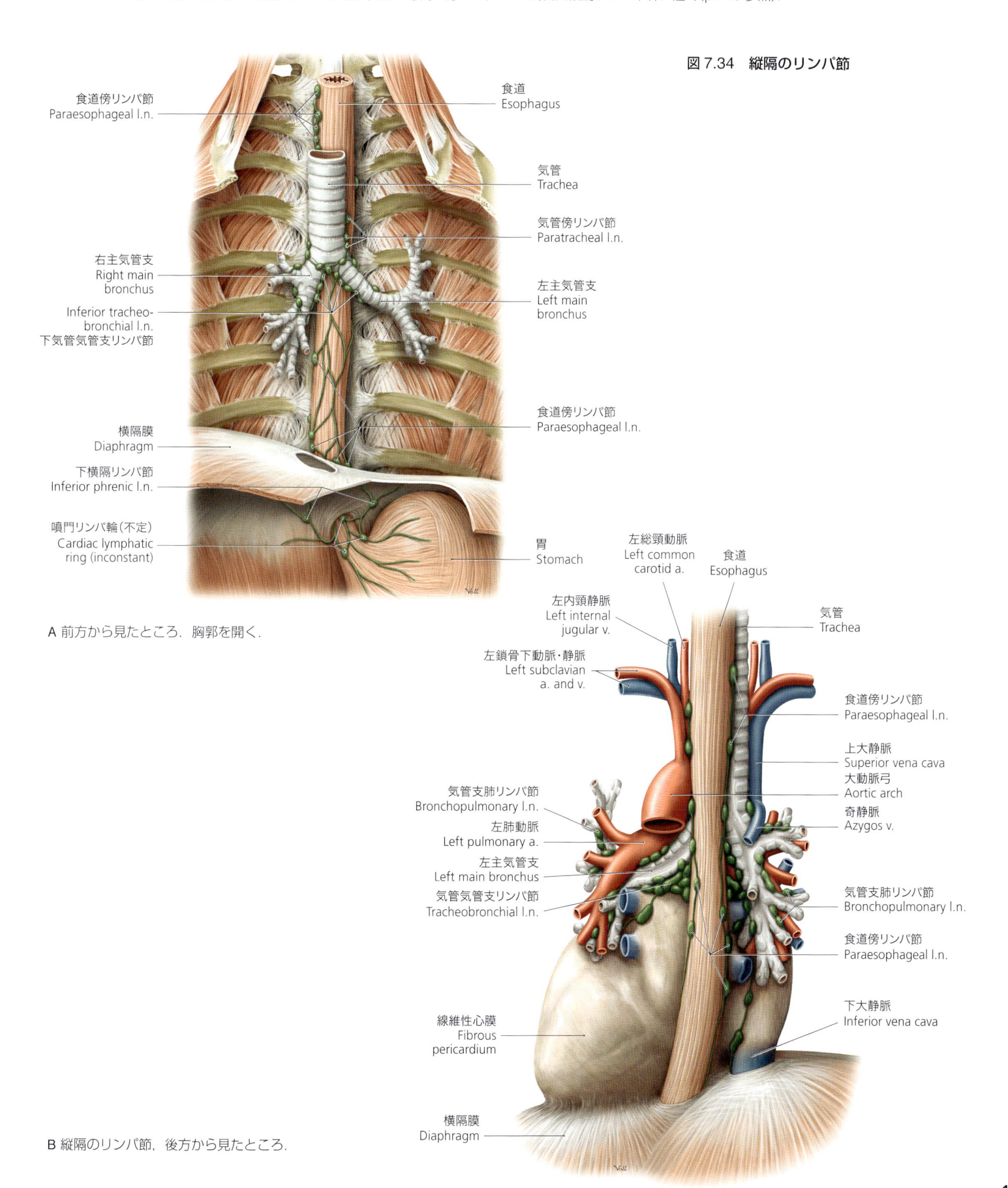

図7.34　縦隔のリンパ節

A　前方から見たところ．胸郭を開く．

B　縦隔のリンパ節，後方から見たところ．

胸膜腔
Pleural Cavity

> 左右の胸膜腔には左右の肺が含まれる．両肺は縦隔によって互いに隔てられ，陰圧となっている（pp.112-113 の呼吸のメカニズムを参照）．

図 8.1　胸膜腔
胸膜腔と肺が胸郭の骨格に投影される．

右腕頭静脈 Right brachiocephalic v.
上大静脈 Superior vena cava
右肺静脈 Right pulmonary vv.
右肺 Right lung
横隔膜 Diaphragm
肝臓, 右葉 Liver, right lobe
Stomach 胃
左腕頭静脈 Left brachiocephalic v.
大動脈弓 Aortic arch
Left lung 左肺
Pulmonary trunk 肺動脈幹
Heart 心臓
肝臓, 左葉 Liver, left lobe
Left pleural cavity 左胸膜腔
Transverse colon 横行結腸

A 前方から見たところ．

第 1 胸椎 T1 vertebra
左肺 Left lung
横隔膜 Diaphragm
脾臓 Spleen
左の副腎 Left suprarenal gland
T12 vertebra 第 12 胸椎
Transverse colon 横行結腸
右肺 Right lung
Parietal pleura 壁側胸膜
肝臓 Liver
右の腎臓 Right kidney
Ascending colon 上行結腸

B 後方から見たところ．

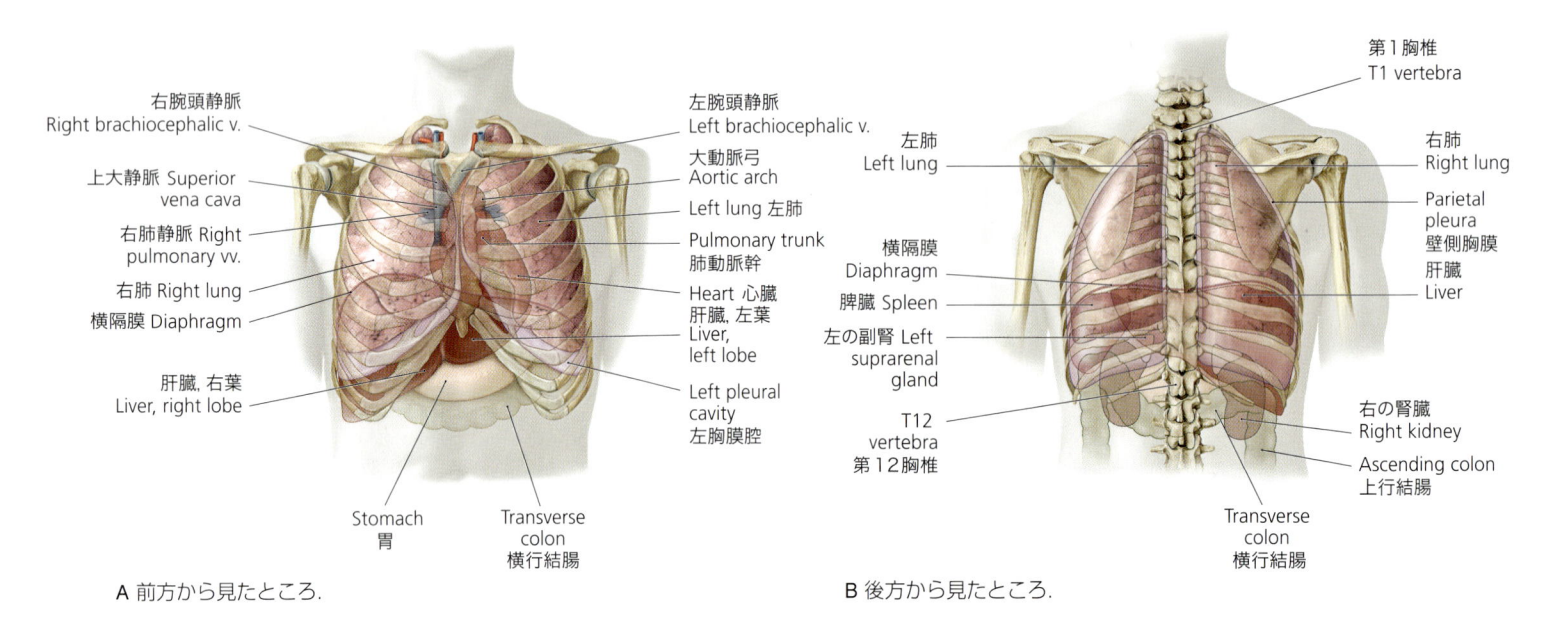

図 8.2　胸膜腔と肺の境界

MC 鎖骨中線　St 胸骨線

A 前方から見たところ．

中腋窩線 MA

B 右外側方から見たところ．

PV 椎骨傍線　MC 鎖骨中線

C 後方から見たところ．

中腋窩線 MA

D 左外側方から見たところ．

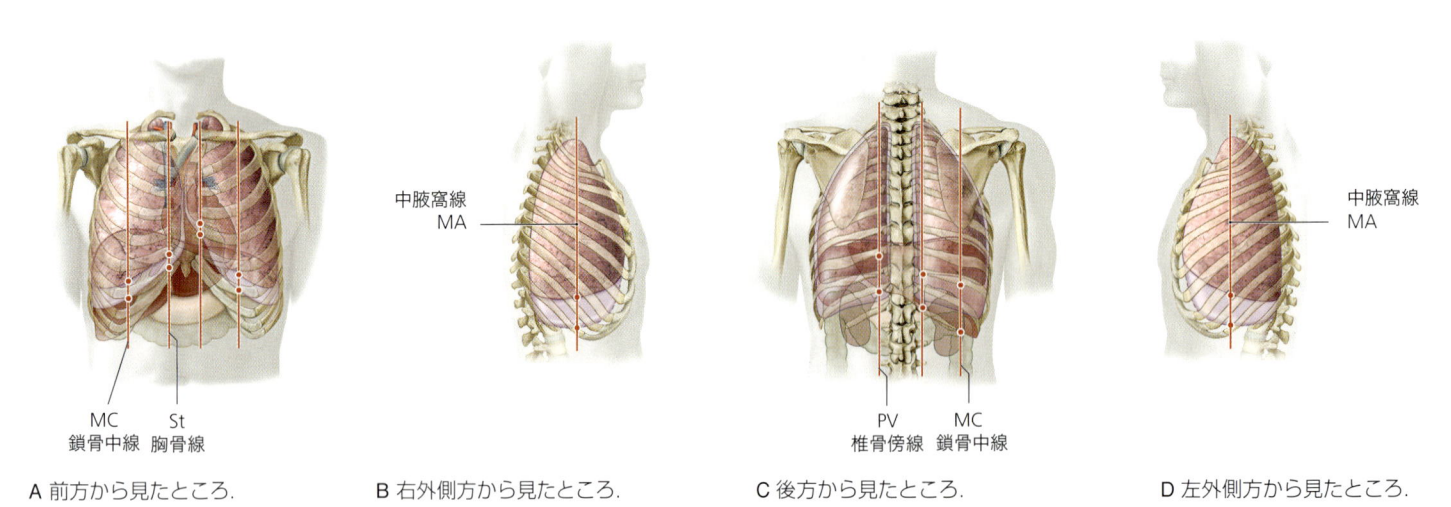

表 8.1　胸膜腔境界部と基準点

基準線	右の壁側胸膜	右肺	左肺	左の壁側胸膜
胸骨線（ST）	第 7 肋骨	第 6 肋骨	第 4 肋骨	第 4 肋骨
鎖骨中線（MC）	第 8 肋軟骨	第 6 肋骨	第 6 肋骨	第 8 肋骨
中腋窩線（MA）	第 10 肋骨	第 8 肋骨	第 8 肋骨	第 10 肋骨
椎骨傍線（PV）	第 12 胸椎	第 10 肋骨	第 10 肋骨	第 12 胸椎

図 8.3 壁側胸膜

胸膜腔は 2 つの漿膜で囲まれる．臓側胸膜（肺胸膜）は肺を包み，壁側胸膜は胸腔の内面を覆う．壁側胸膜の 4 つの部分である肋骨胸膜・横隔胸膜・縦隔胸膜・胸膜頂は連続している．

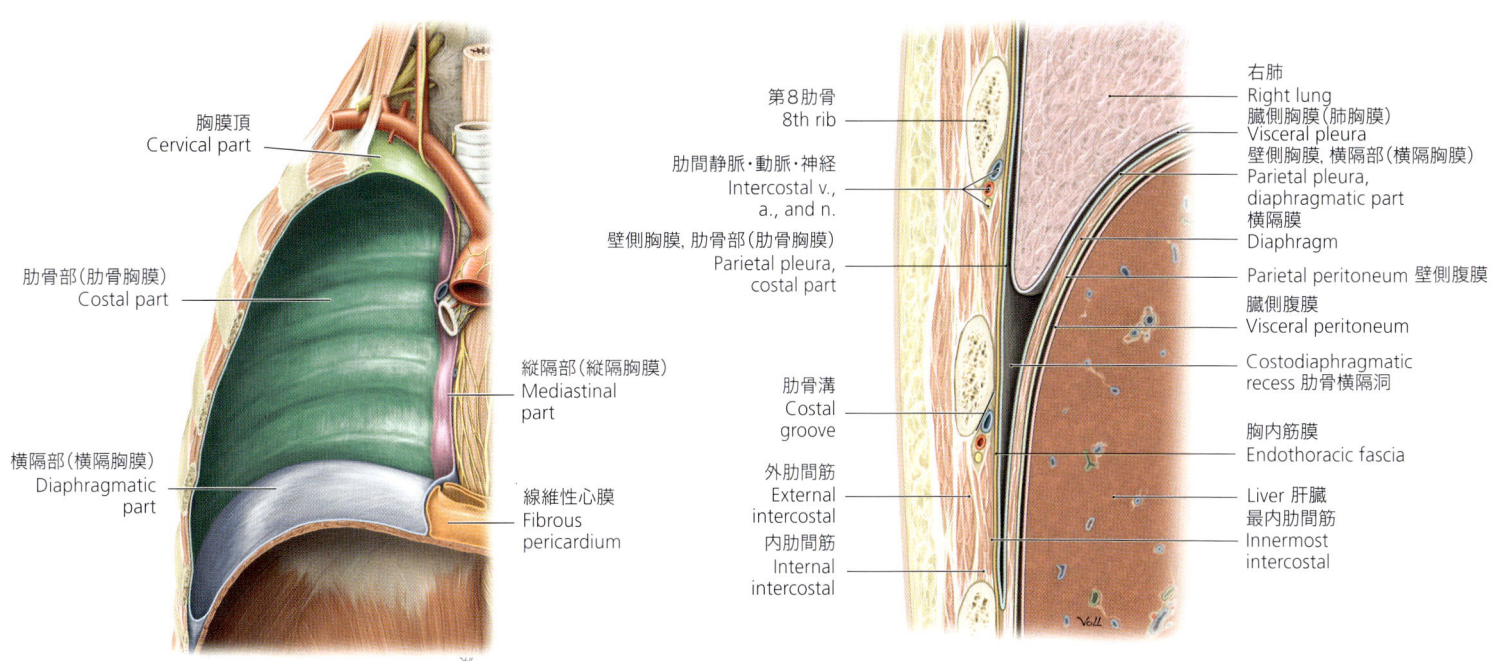

A 壁側胸膜の部分．右胸膜腔を開く．前方から見たところ．

B 肋骨横隔洞．冠状断，前面．横隔胸膜の胸郭内面への折り返り（肋骨胸膜に移行）が肋骨横隔洞を作る．

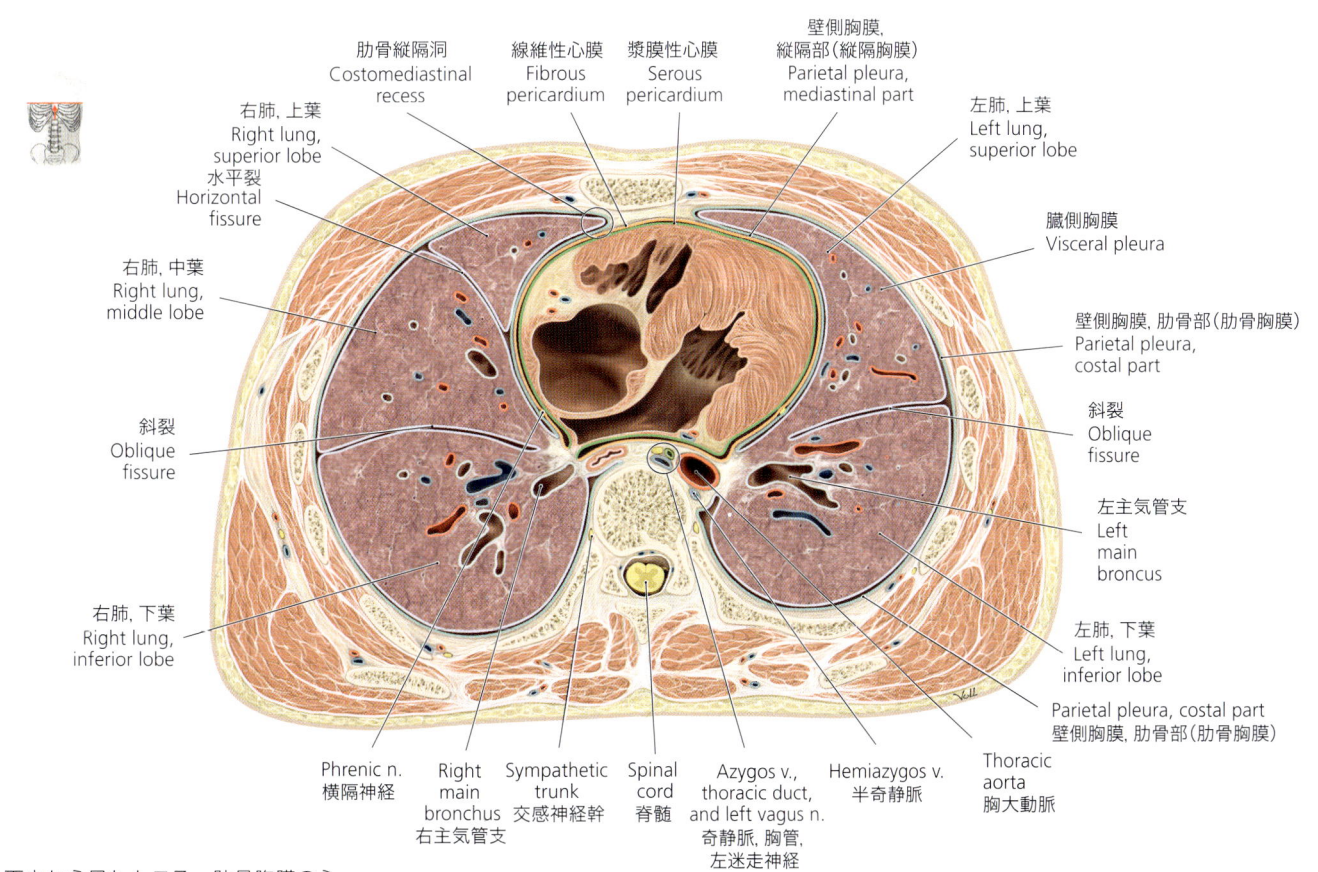

C 水平断，下方から見たところ．肋骨胸膜の心膜への折り返りが肋骨縦隔洞を作る．

原位置の肺
Lungs in Situ

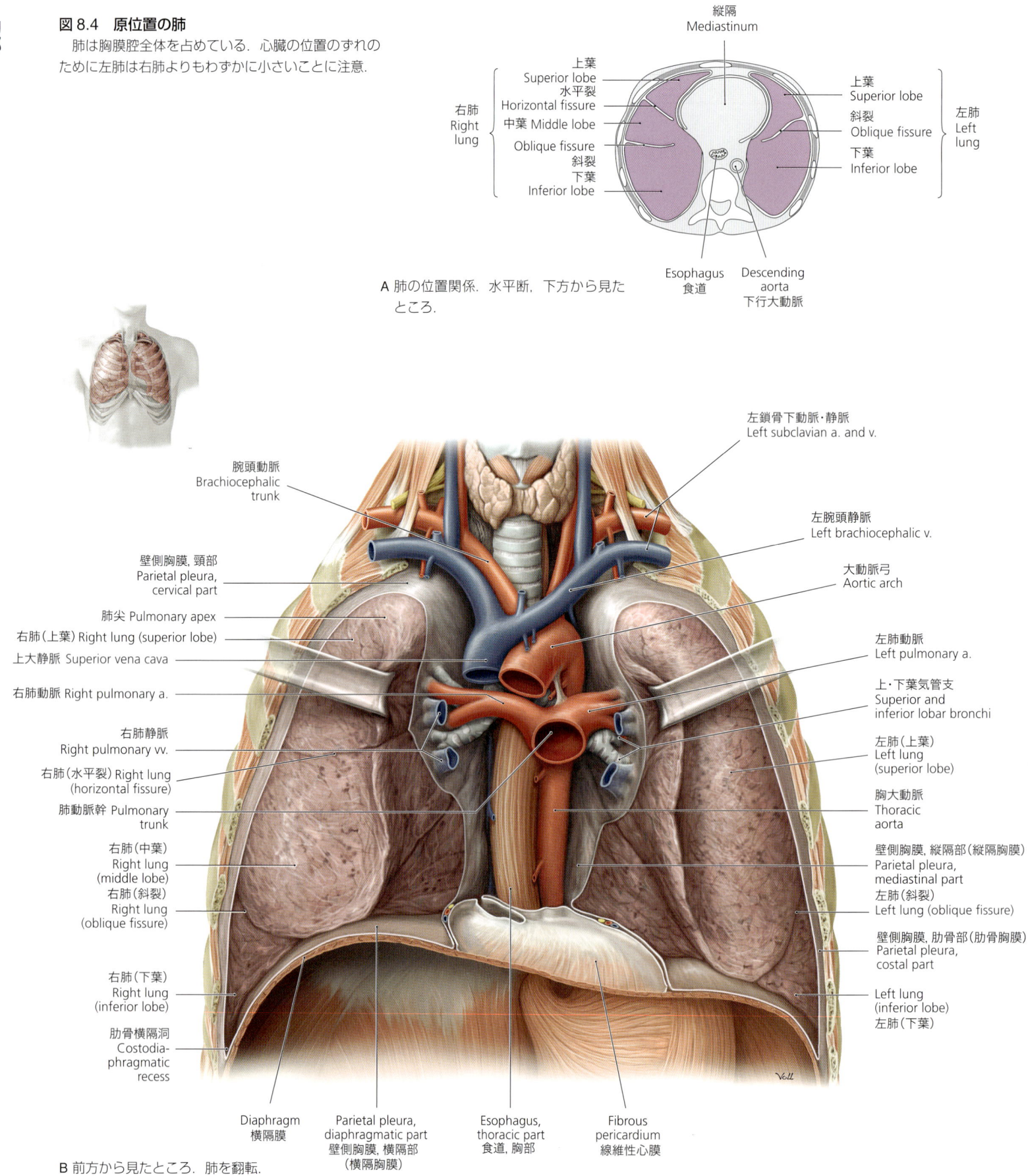

図 8.4 原位置の肺
肺は胸膜腔全体を占めている．心臓の位置のずれのために左肺は右肺よりもわずかに小さいことに注意．

A 肺の位置関係．水平断，下方から見たところ．

- 縦隔 Mediastinum
- 上葉 Superior lobe
- 水平裂 Horizontal fissure
- 中葉 Middle lobe
- 斜裂 Oblique fissure
- 下葉 Inferior lobe
- 右肺 Right lung
- 上葉 Superior lobe
- 斜裂 Oblique fissure
- 下葉 Inferior lobe
- 左肺 Left lung
- 食道 Esophagus
- 下行大動脈 Descending aorta

B 前方から見たところ．肺を翻転．

- 腕頭動脈 Brachiocephalic trunk
- 壁側胸膜，頸部 Parietal pleura, cervical part
- 肺尖 Pulmonary apex
- 右肺（上葉）Right lung (superior lobe)
- 上大静脈 Superior vena cava
- 右肺動脈 Right pulmonary a.
- 右肺静脈 Right pulmonary vv.
- 右肺（水平裂）Right lung (horizontal fissure)
- 肺動脈幹 Pulmonary trunk
- 右肺（中葉）Right lung (middle lobe)
- 右肺（斜裂）Right lung (oblique fissure)
- 右肺（下葉）Right lung (inferior lobe)
- 肋骨横隔洞 Costodiaphragmatic recess
- 左鎖骨下動脈・静脈 Left subclavian a. and v.
- 左腕頭静脈 Left brachiocephalic v.
- 大動脈弓 Aortic arch
- 左肺動脈 Left pulmonary a.
- 上・下葉気管支 Superior and inferior lobar bronchi
- 左肺（上葉）Left lung (superior lobe)
- 胸大動脈 Thoracic aorta
- 壁側胸膜，縦隔部（縦隔胸膜）Parietal pleura, mediastinal part
- 左肺（斜裂）Left lung (oblique fissure)
- 壁側胸膜，肋骨部（肋骨胸膜）Parietal pleura, costal part
- 左肺（下葉）Left lung (inferior lobe)
- 横隔膜 Diaphragm
- 壁側胸膜，横隔部（横隔胸膜）Parietal pleura, diaphragmatic part
- 食道，胸部 Esophagus, thoracic part
- 線維性心膜 Fibrous pericardium

右肺は斜裂と水平裂によって上葉，中葉，下葉の3葉に分けられる．左肺は斜裂によって上葉と下葉の2葉に分けられる．両肺の肺尖は頸の基部に入り込んでいる．肺門は気管支や神経・脈管が肺に出入りする部位．

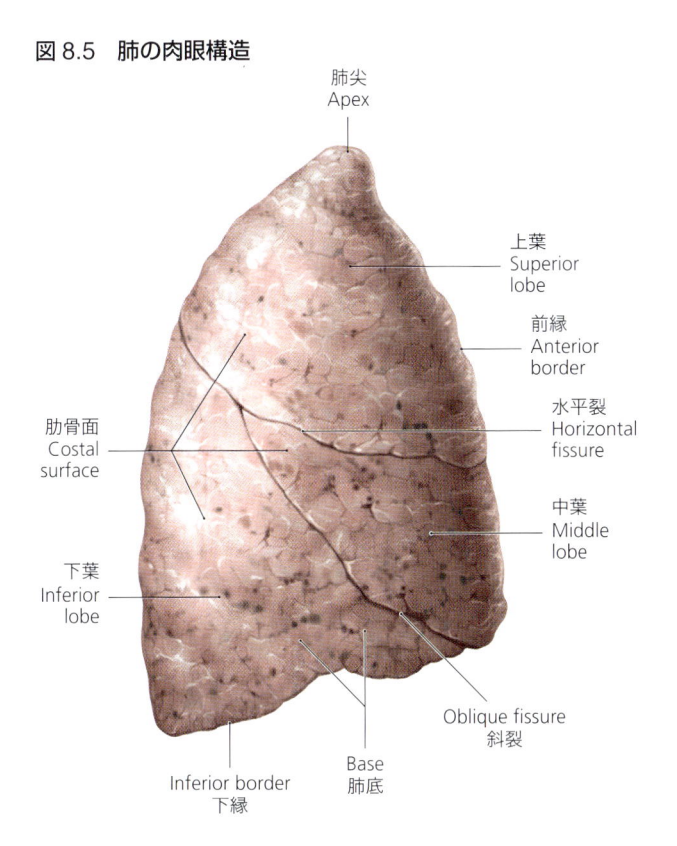

図 8.5 肺の肉眼構造

A 右肺，外側方から見たところ．

B 左肺，外側方から見たところ．

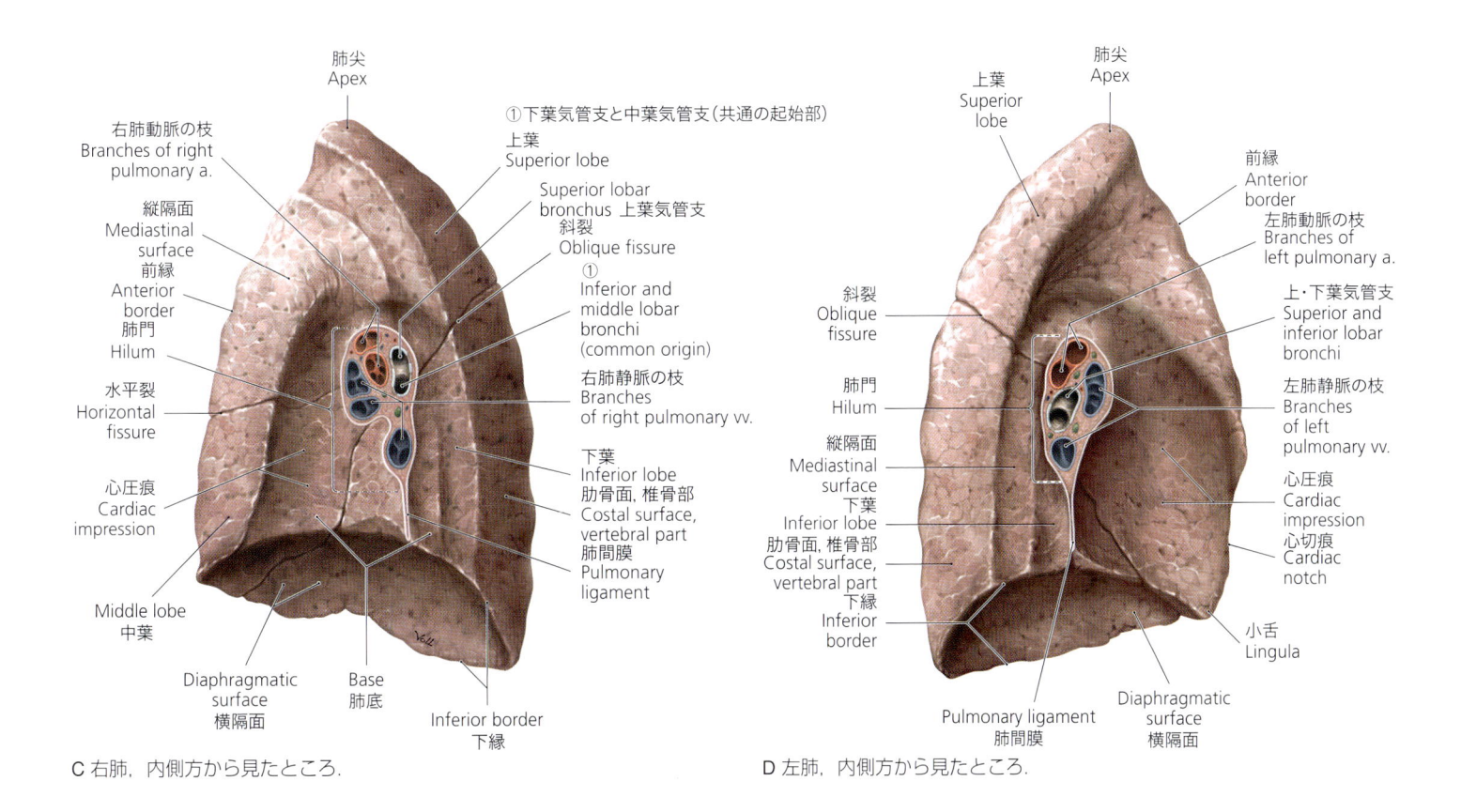

C 右肺，内側方から見たところ．

D 左肺，内側方から見たところ．

肺：X線像
Lung: Radiology

胸部X線像において，肺は部位によって異なる透過性を示す．肺門の近傍部（肺に主気管支と血管が出入りする部分）は，径の小さい血管と区域気管支を含む肺の周縁よりX線透過性が低い．さらに，肺門の近傍部は心臓に覆われる．これらの"影"は，X線像で白く明るい領域となる（X線像は陰画であり，光を透過しない領域が明るくなる）．

図 8.6　肺のX線像

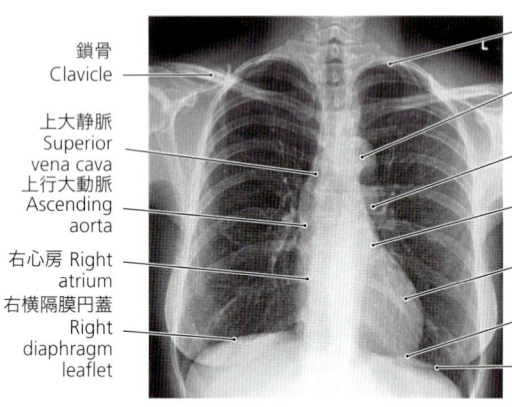

A 正常肺のX線前後像．

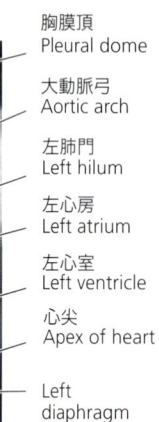

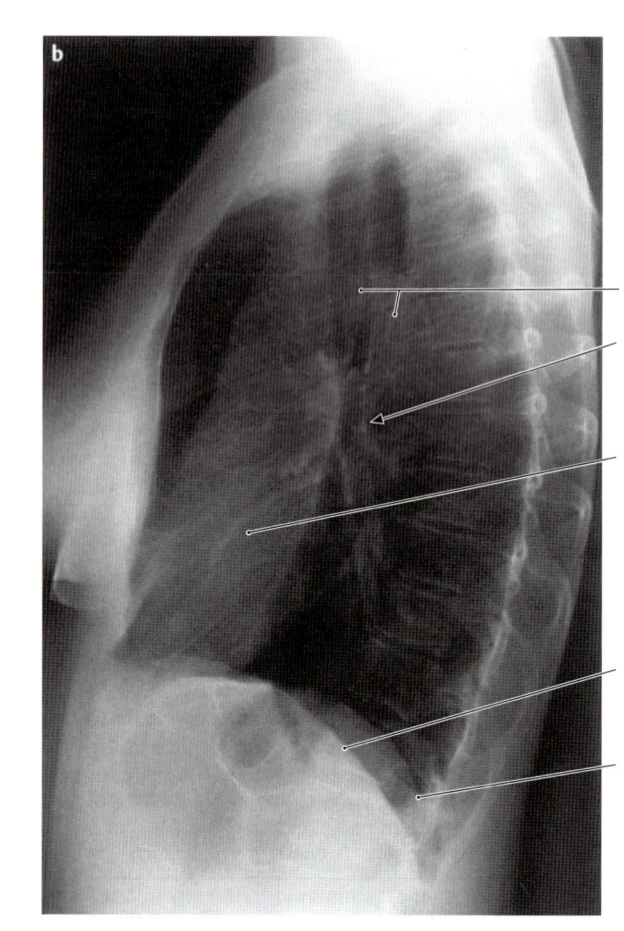

ラベル：鎖骨 Clavicle／上大静脈 Superior vena cava／上行大動脈 Ascending aorta／右心房 Right atrium／右横隔膜円蓋 Right diaphragm leaflet／胸膜頂 Pleural dome／大動脈弓 Aortic arch／左肺門 Left hilum／左心房 Left atrium／左心室 Left ventricle／心尖 Apex of heart／左横隔膜円蓋 Left diaphragm leaflet

B 正常肺のX線側面像．

ラベル：大動脈弓 Aortic arch／中食道狭窄（胸部狭窄）Middle esophageal (thoracic) constriction／左心室 Left ventricle／右横隔膜円蓋 Right diaphragm leaflet／左横隔膜円蓋 Left diaphragm leaflet

図 8.7　肺の非透過性

右肺を外側方と前方から見たところ．非透過性（X線透過性の低下）は肺領域の疾患で見られる．液体浸潤（炎症）や組織増殖（腫瘍）によって非透過性がさらに強くなる．この非透過性は，もともとはX線透過性が高い肺の周縁部において検出しやすい．*Note*：肺区域縁に認められる非透過性は，ほぼ常に肺炎による．

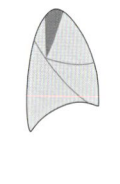

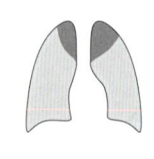

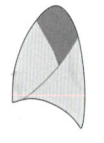

A 肺尖区における非透過性．

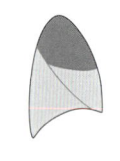

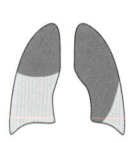

B 上葉の非透過性．

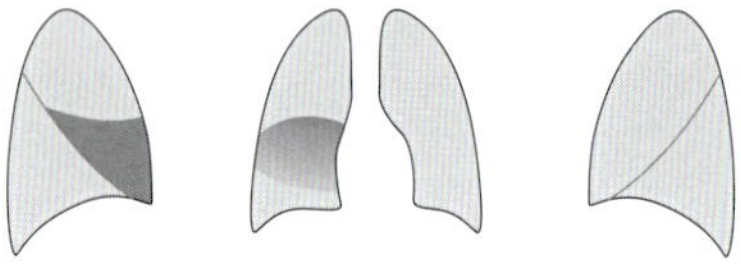

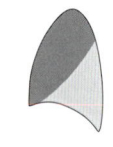

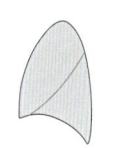

C 中葉の非透過性．*Note*：左肺には中葉はない．

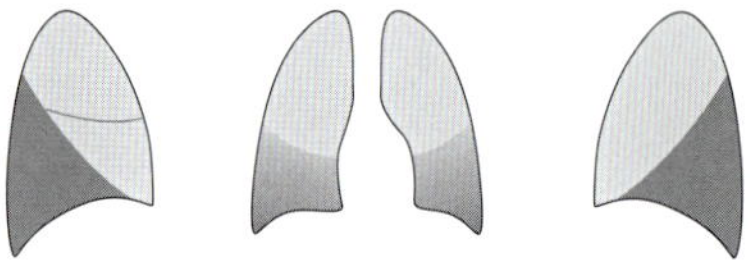

D 下葉の非透過性．

臨床

肺の疾患

肺の非透過性の増大は区域縁とは必ずしも対応しない．肺の液体浸潤は肺X線像に特徴的な"影"を作る．

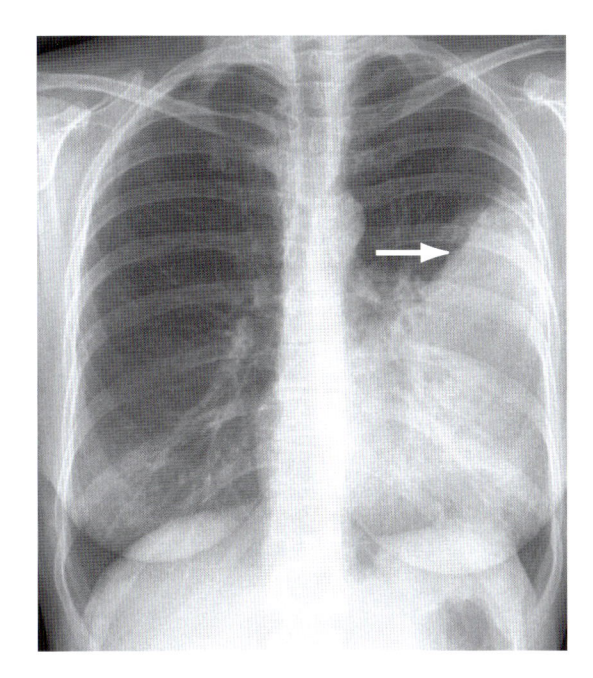

A 小舌肺炎．水平裂が見える（矢印）．*Note*：第IVと第V区域の非透過性が増大しているために，ここでは心臓を見るのが難しくなっている．

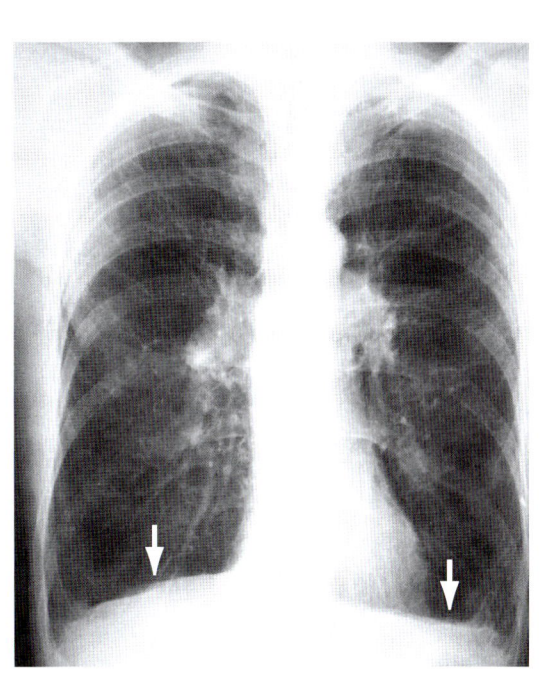

B 肺気腫．胸部X線像により横隔膜の低下（横隔膜頂の平坦化）が顕著になり，これと対応して心陰影の方向が変化する．心臓は横隔膜が低位にあることで鉛直方向に伸びる（X線側面像では胸骨後腔が広がっていることが明らかになる）．肺動脈は中枢側では拡張するが，区域レベルでは劇的に細くなる．

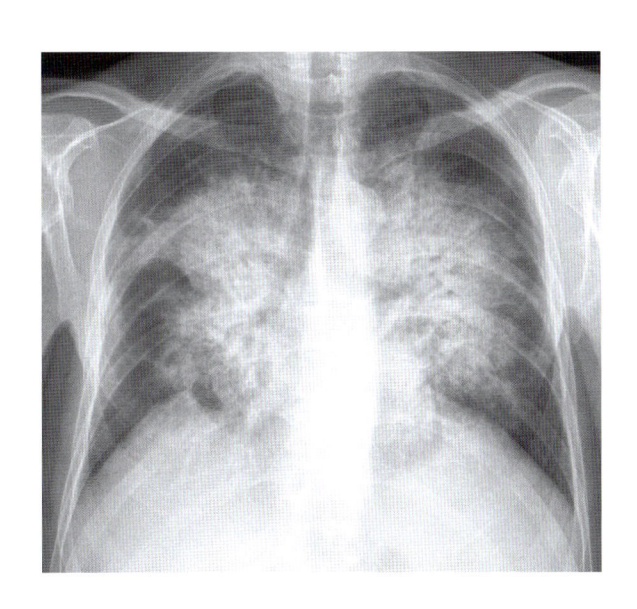

C 急性の心筋梗塞から併発した肺水腫．血管が拡張し，可視の管腔構造の数が増加している．この像は肺水腫と両側性の胸水による蝶形陰影を示している．

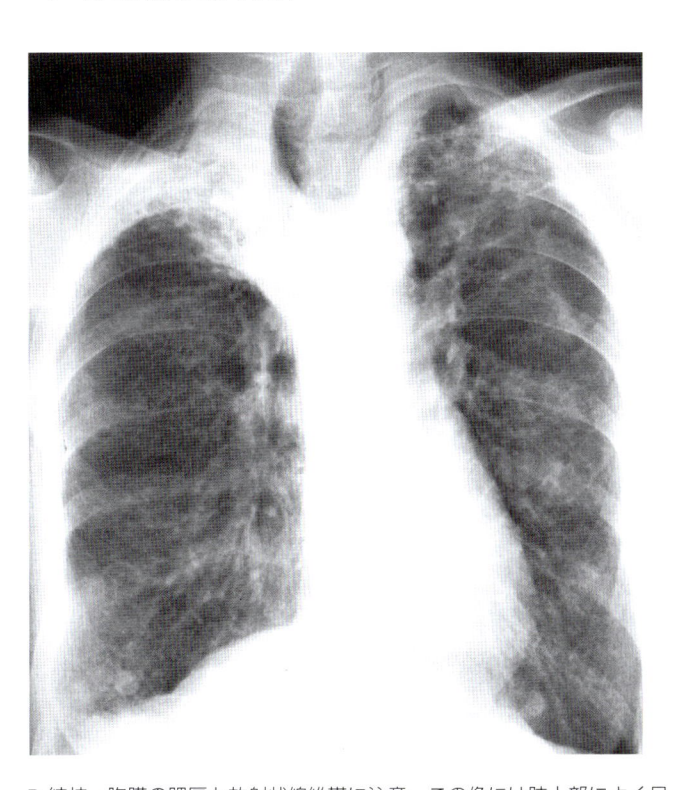

D 結核．胸膜の肥厚と放射状線維帯に注意．この像には肺上部によく見られる結核腫がない．

肺の気管支肺区域
Bronchopulmonary Segments of the Lungs

> 肺の各葉はさらに気管支肺区域へと分けられ，それぞれに区域気管支が通る．*Note*：肺区域は肺表面では識別されず，その根本となる気管支によって識別される．

図 8.8 肺区域
前方から見たところ．気管と気管支樹の詳細については pp.110-111 参照．

右肺 Right lung　　　気管と気管支樹 Trachea and bronchial tree　　　左肺 Left lung

水平裂 Horizontal fissure
斜裂 Oblique fissure
斜裂 Oblique fissure

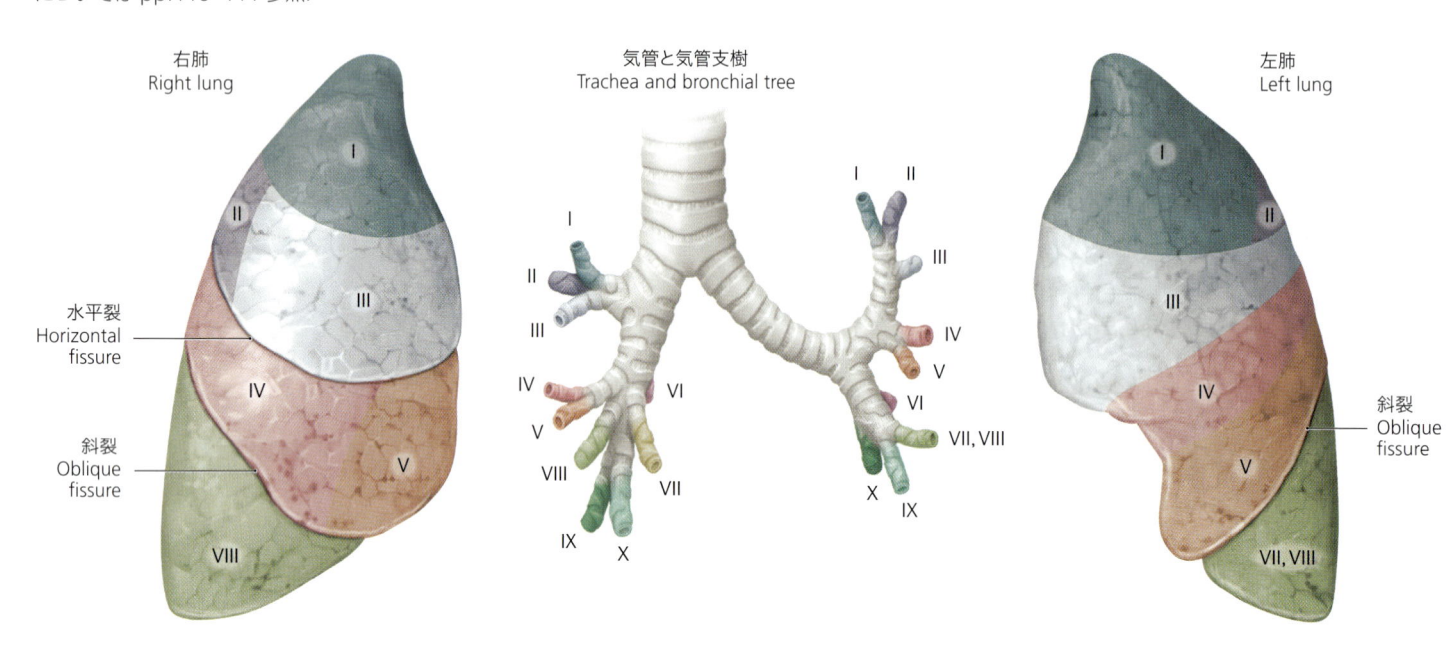

図 8.9 前後方向の気管支造影図
右肺を前方から見たところ．

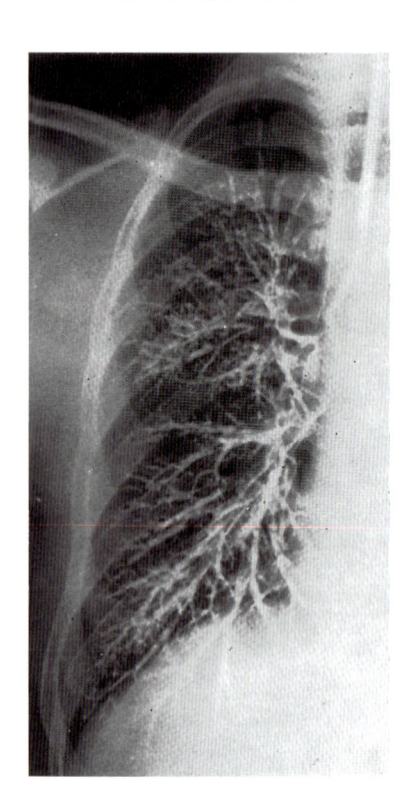

表 8.2　肺の区域構造

各区域には同名の区域気管支が分布する（例：肺尖区には肺尖枝が分布）．気管と気管支樹の詳細については pp.110-111 参照．

右肺			左肺
上葉			
I	肺尖区	肺尖後区	I
II	後上葉区		II
III		前上葉区	III
中葉			小舌
IV	外側中葉区	上舌区	IV
V	内側中葉区	下舌区	V
下葉			
VI	上-下葉区		VI
VII	内側肺底区		VII
VIII	前肺底区		VIII
IX	外側肺底区		IX
X	後肺底区		X

図 8.10　右肺：気管支肺区域

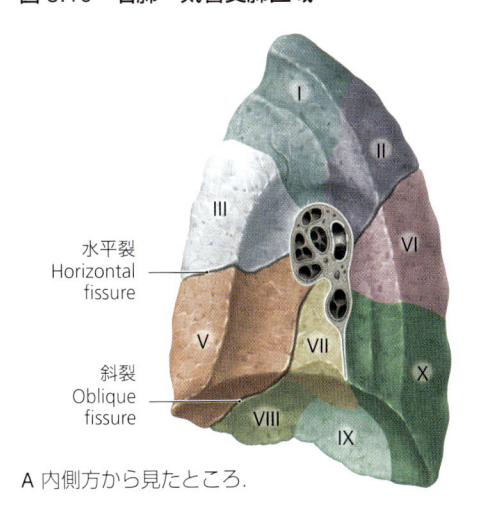

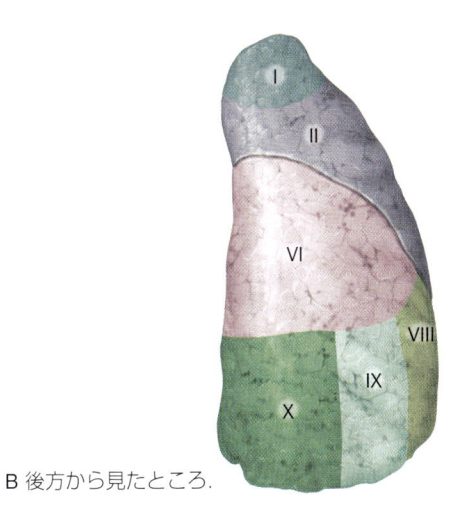

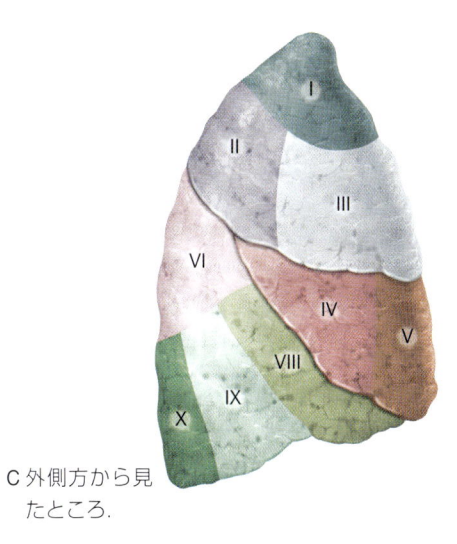

A 内側方から見たところ．　　B 後方から見たところ．　　C 外側方から見たところ．

水平裂　Horizontal fissure
斜裂　Oblique fissure

図 8.11　左肺：気管支肺区域

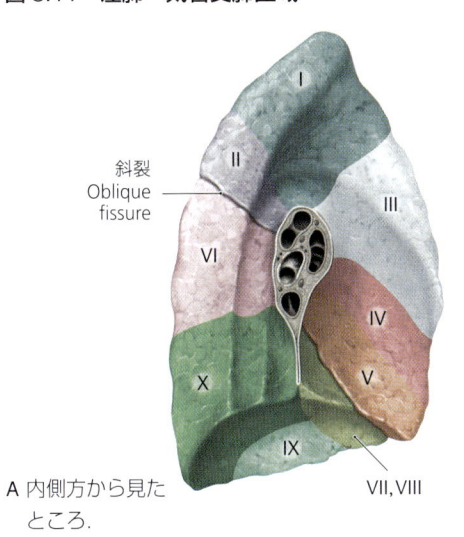

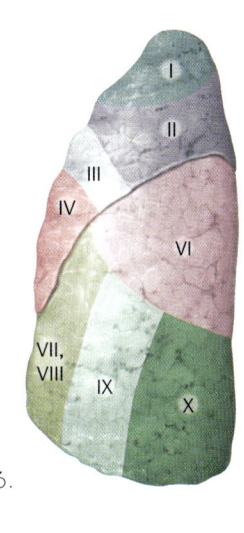

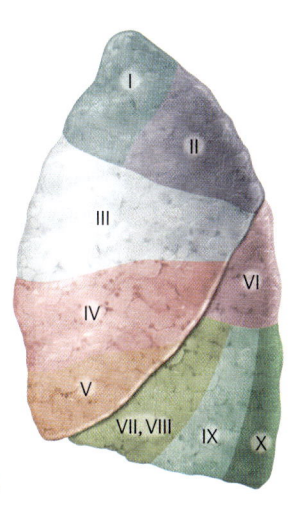

A 内側方から見たところ．　　B 後方から見たところ．　　C 外側方から見たところ．

斜裂　Oblique fissure

臨床

肺の部分切除

肺癌，肺気腫，肺結核においては肺の障害部位を外科的に取り除く必要がある．外科医は損傷した組織を切除する際には，葉・区域の解剖学的区分を利用する．

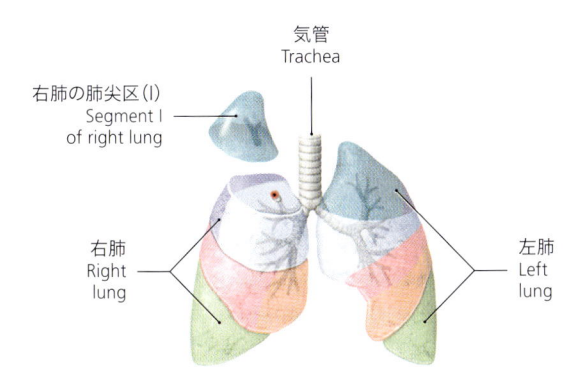

気管　Trachea
右肺の肺尖区（I）　Segment I of right lung
右肺　Right lung
左肺　Left lung
右肺の上葉　Superior lobe of right lung

A 区域切除術（楔状切除）：1つかそれ以上の区域の切除．　　B 肺葉切除術：葉の切除．　　C 肺切除術：肺全体の切除．

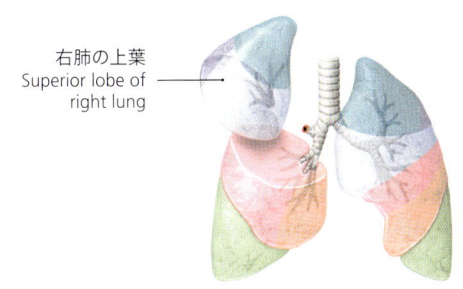

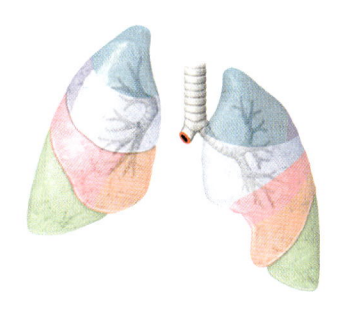

気管と気管支樹
Trachea & Bronchial Tree

胸骨角の高さ近辺で，最下にある気管軟骨は前後方向に伸び，気管竜骨となる．気管は気管竜骨で二分され，右主気管支と左主気管支となる．どちらの主気管支も対応する肺へ葉気管支を送る．

図8.12 気管
甲状腺の構造についてはp.574参照．

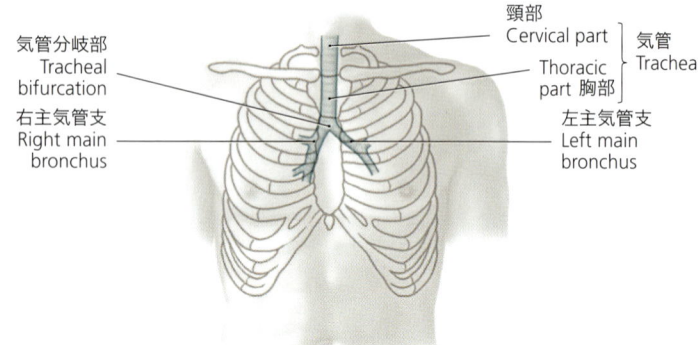

- 気管分岐部 Tracheal bifurcation
- 頸部 Cervical part
- 胸部 Thoracic part
- 気管 Trachea
- 右主気管支 Right main bronchus
- 左主気管支 Left main bronchus

A 気管の胸への投影．

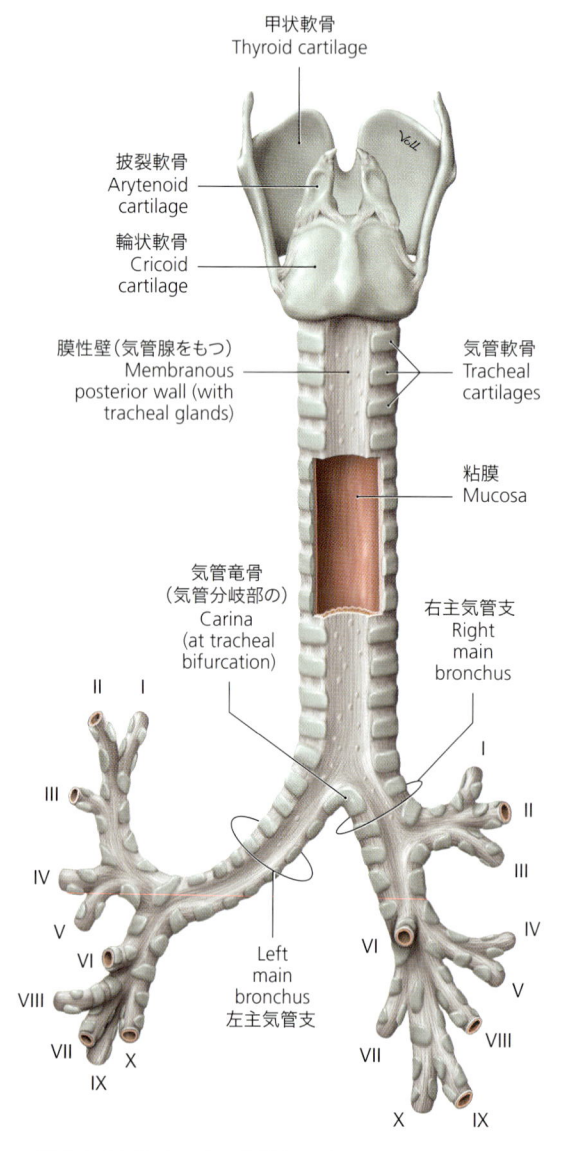

- 甲状軟骨 Thyroid cartilage
- 披裂軟骨 Arytenoid cartilage
- 輪状軟骨 Cricoid cartilage
- 膜性壁（気管腺をもつ）Membranous posterior wall (with tracheal glands)
- 気管軟骨 Tracheal cartilages
- 粘膜 Mucosa
- 気管竜骨（気管分岐部の）Carina (at tracheal bifurcation)
- 右主気管支 Right main bronchus
- 左主気管支 Left main bronchus

C 後方から見たところ．後壁を開く．

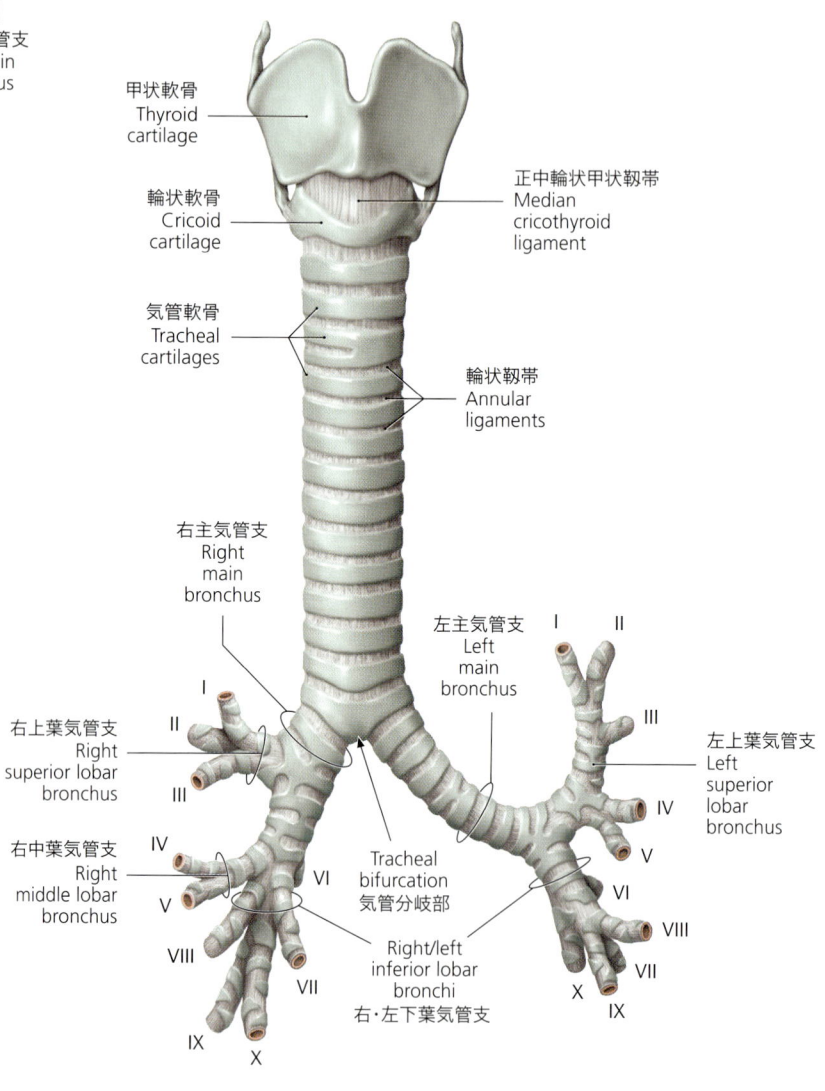

- 甲状軟骨 Thyroid cartilage
- 輪状軟骨 Cricoid cartilage
- 正中輪状甲状靱帯 Median cricothyroid ligament
- 気管軟骨 Tracheal cartilages
- 輪状靱帯 Annular ligaments
- 右主気管支 Right main bronchus
- 左主気管支 Left main bronchus
- 右上葉気管支 Right superior lobar bronchus
- 左上葉気管支 Left superior lobar bronchus
- 右中葉気管支 Right middle lobar bronchus
- 気管分岐部 Tracheal bifurcation
- Right/left inferior lobar bronchi 右・左下葉気管支

B 前方から見たところ．

臨床

異物吸引
幼児は潜在的に異物を吸引する危険性が高い．一般的に，異物は左より右主気管支に入りやすい．気管分岐部で左主気管支は急角度で曲がっているが，右主気管支は比較的垂直に近いからである．

気管支樹の伝導部は気管分岐部から終末細気管支に及び，その間にある気管支の各分岐も含む．呼吸部は呼吸細気管支，肺胞管，肺胞嚢，肺胞を含む．

図8.13 気管支樹

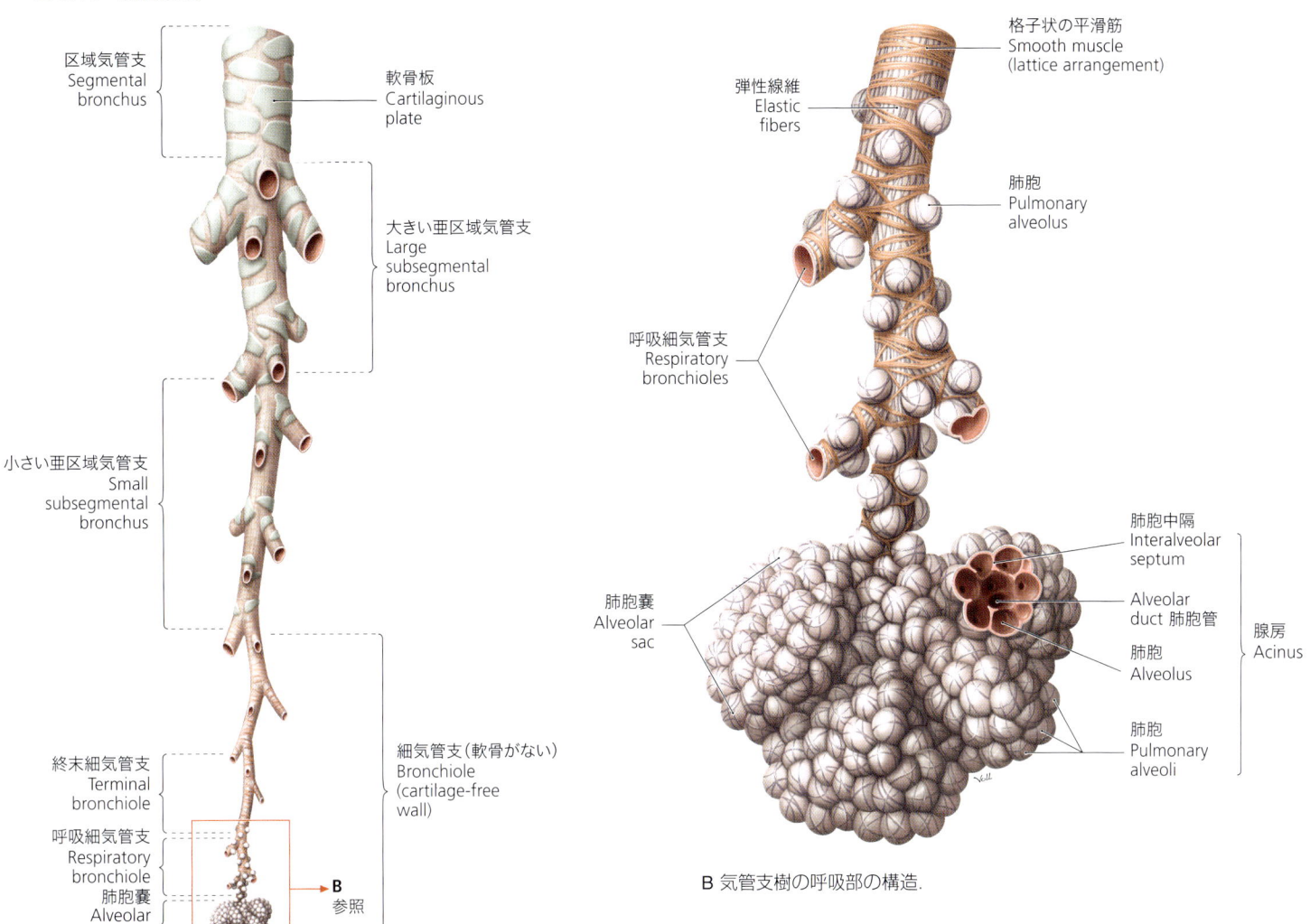

A 気管支樹の区分．

区域気管支 Segmental bronchus
軟骨板 Cartilaginous plate
大きい亜区域気管支 Large subsegmental bronchus
小さい亜区域気管支 Small subsegmental bronchus
終末細気管支 Terminal bronchiole
細気管支（軟骨がない）Bronchiole (cartilage-free wall)
呼吸細気管支 Respiratory bronchiole
肺胞嚢 Alveolar sacs

B 気管支樹の呼吸部の構造．

格子状の平滑筋 Smooth muscle (lattice arrangement)
弾性線維 Elastic fibers
肺胞 Pulmonary alveolus
呼吸細気管支 Respiratory bronchioles
肺胞嚢 Alveolar sac
肺胞中隔 Interalveolar septum
肺胞管 Alveolar duct
肺胞 Alveolus
肺胞 Pulmonary alveoli
腺房 Acinus

C 肺胞内面を覆う上皮．

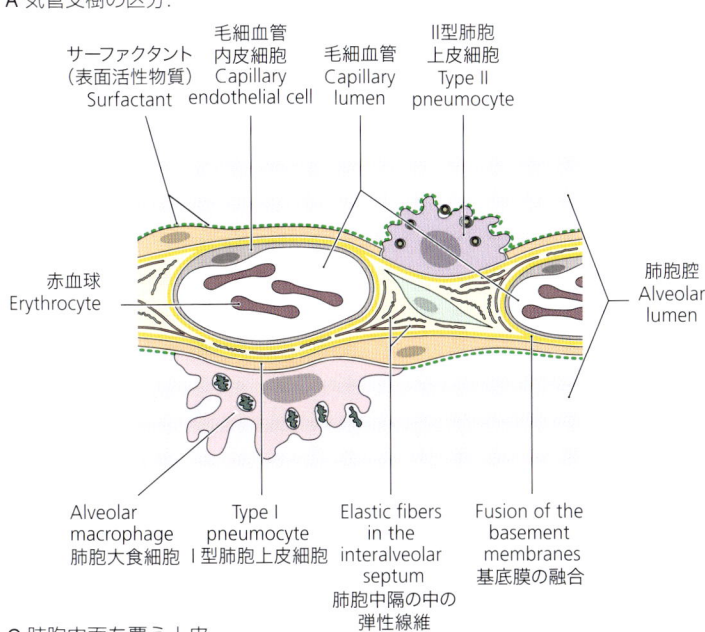

サーファクタント（表面活性物質）Surfactant
毛細血管内皮細胞 Capillary endothelial cell
毛細血管 Capillary lumen
II型肺胞上皮細胞 Type II pneumocyte
赤血球 Erythrocyte
肺胞腔 Alveolar lumen
肺胞大食細胞 Alveolar macrophage
I型肺胞上皮細胞 Type I pneumocyte
肺胞中隔の中の弾性線維 Elastic fibers in the interalveolar septum
基底膜の融合 Fusion of the basement membranes

臨床

呼吸不全
気管支レベルでの呼吸不全の最も一般的な原因は喘息である．肺胞レベルでの呼吸不全は拡散距離の増大，低換気（肺気腫），液体浸潤（肺炎など）から起こる．

拡散距離
ガス交換は肺胞で肺胞腔と血管腔の間で行われる（図8.13C参照）．毛細血管内皮細胞の基底膜はI型肺胞上皮細胞の基底膜と融合することで，交換が行われる距離が0.5μmとなっている．この拡散距離を増大させる疾患（浮腫液貯留あるいは炎症）では呼吸不全となる．

肺胞の状態
慢性閉塞性肺疾患において起こる肺気腫のような疾患では，肺胞の破壊や損傷が起こる．これによってガス交換に必要な肺胞表面積が減少する．

サーファクタントの産生
サーファクタントは肺胞の表面張力を減少させ，肺をふくらみやすくするリン脂質蛋白である．低出生体重児の未熟な肺は，しばしば十分なサーファクタントを産出できず，呼吸障害を起こす．サーファクタントは肺胞上皮細胞で産出され吸収される．I型肺胞上皮細胞はサーファクタントを再吸収し，II型肺胞上皮細胞はサーファクタントを産出し，分配する．

呼吸機構
Respiratory Mechanics

呼吸の機構は，肺の拡張と収縮を伴う胸腔容積量のリズミカルな増減に基づく．吸息（赤）：横隔膜の各部が収縮すると横隔膜が吸息位に下がり，胸膜腔容積が鉛直方向に増大する．胸郭の筋肉（外肋間筋と他に斜角筋，軟骨間の筋，後鋸筋）の収縮によって肋骨が持ち上げられ，胸膜腔容積が矢状方向と横方向に増大する（図 8.15 A, B）．胸膜腔の表面張力によって臓側胸膜と壁側胸膜が密着し，胸郭容積の変化から肺の容量の変化が起こる．これは特に胸膜洞において明らかである．機能的残気量（吸息と呼息の間の休止時の位置）では，肺は胸膜洞の内腔に進入しない．胸膜腔が拡張して，胸膜腔内圧が陰圧になる．大気圧との差から空気の流入が起こる（吸息）．呼息（青）：受動呼息時に，胸郭の筋肉は弛緩し，横隔膜が呼息位に戻る．肺の収縮は肺圧を高め，肺から空気を外に押し出す．強制呼息では，内肋間筋が（胸横筋膜と肋骨下粘膜とともに）受動的な弾性反動の場合よりも大きく素早く，能動的に胸郭を押し下げることができる．

図 8.14　呼吸による胸腔容積の変化
吸息時（赤），呼息時（青）．

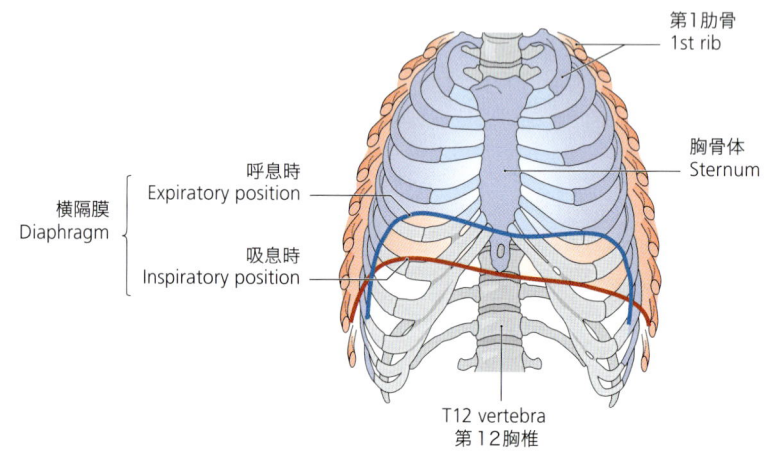

図 8.15　吸息：胸膜腔の拡張
A 前方から見たところ．
B 左外側方から見たところ．
C 前外側方から見たところ

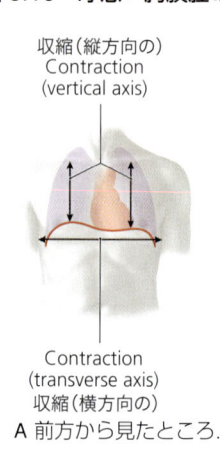

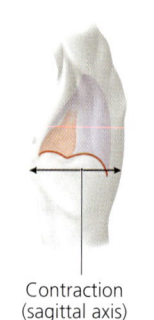

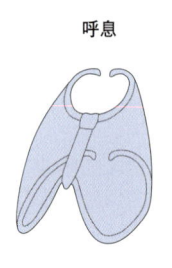

図 8.16　呼息：胸膜腔の縮小
A 前方から見たところ．
B 左外側方から見たところ．
C 前外側方から見たところ．

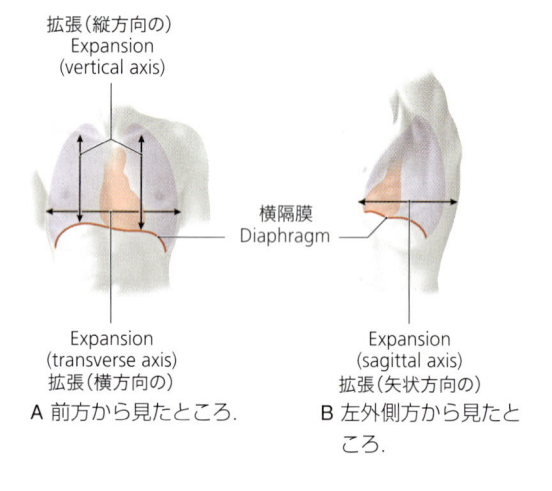

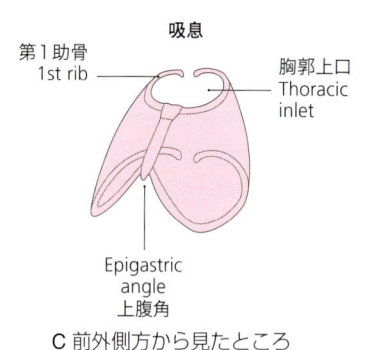

図 8.17　呼吸による肺容積の変化

図 8.18 吸息：肺の拡張

右肺（吸息）
Right lung (full inspiration)

Diaphragm
横隔膜

Costodiaphragmatic recess
肋骨横隔洞

図 8.19 呼息：肺の縮小

右肺（呼息）
Right lung (full expiration)

胸膜腔
Pleural space

Diaphragm
横隔膜

Costodiaphragmatic recess
肋骨横隔洞

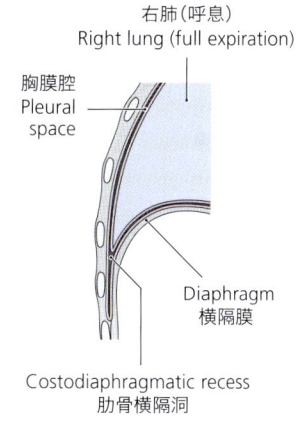

図 8.20 肺と気管支樹の運動
肺の大きさが胸膜腔と一緒に変化するのに応じて，気管支樹全体は肺の中を移動する．この構造的な動きは肺門から遠い気管支樹ほど顕著である．

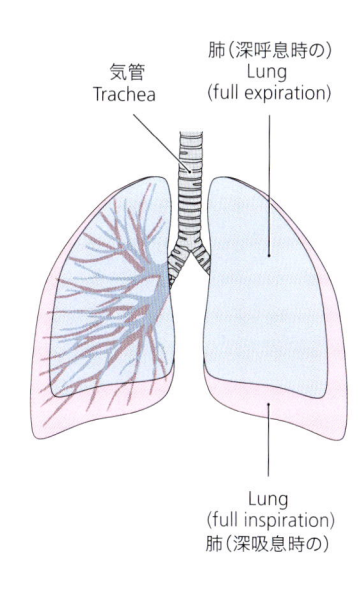

気管
Trachea

肺（深呼息時の）
Lung (full expiration)

Lung (full inspiration)
肺（深吸息時の）

臨床

気胸
　胸膜腔は通常は外界から閉ざされている．壁側胸膜，臓側胸膜，肺の損傷によって空気が胸膜腔に進入する（気胸）．肺は固有の弾性のために虚脱し，呼吸能が低下する．損傷を受けていない側の肺は正常な圧変化のもとで機能し続け，縦隔が吸息時に正常側に偏位し，呼息時に正中に戻る縦隔動揺が起こる．緊張性気胸（弁様気胸）は外傷によって剥離された組織が胸壁の内部から欠損部を覆うと起こる．この可動性の弁様の構造は空気を進入させるが，排出させないために，胸膜腔は圧が増加し続ける．縦隔は正常側に偏位し，大血管のねじれを起こし，静脈血の心臓への還流を阻害する．緊張性気胸は治療をしないと常に致死的となる．

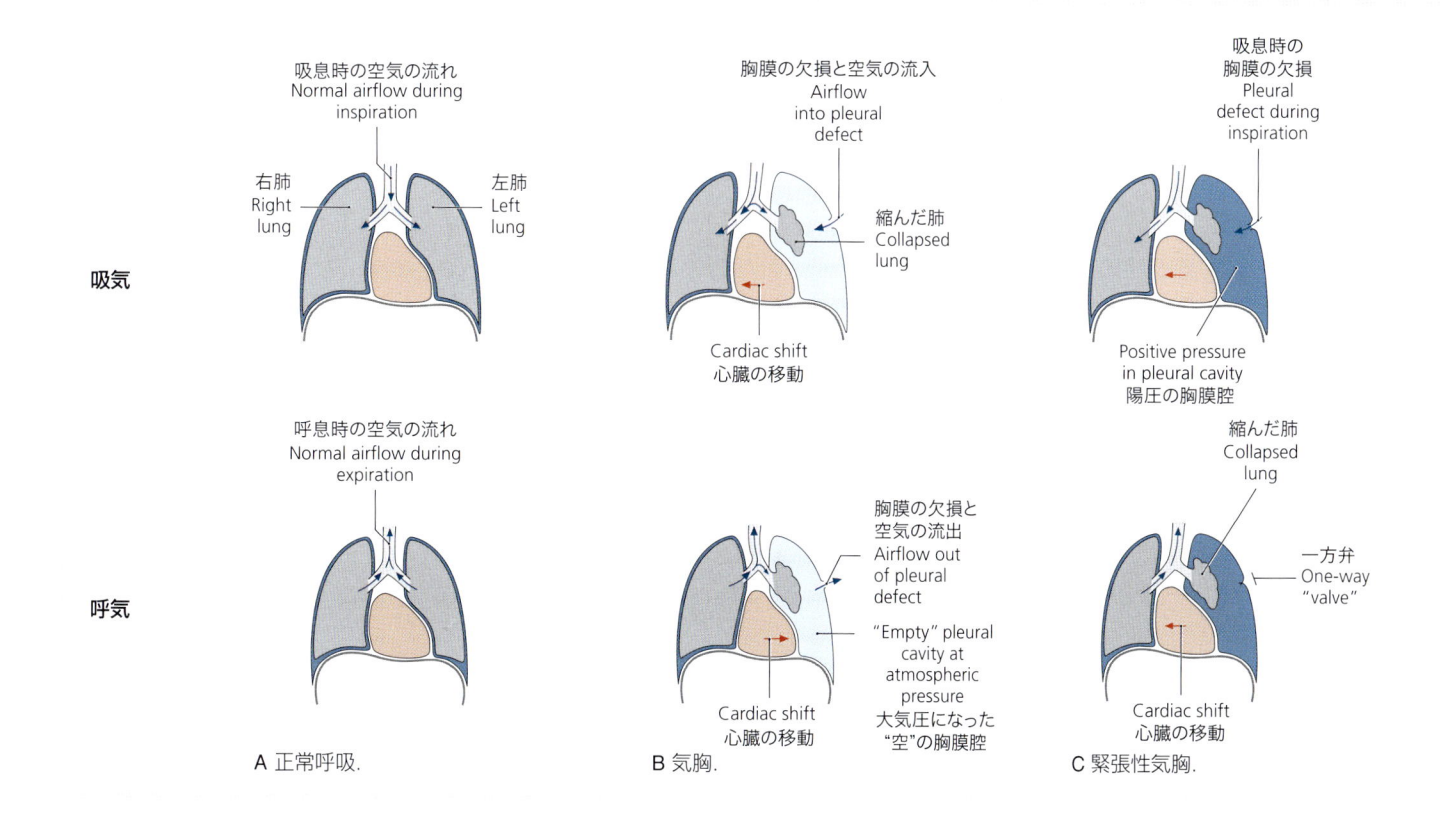

吸気

吸息時の空気の流れ
Normal airflow during inspiration

右肺　　左肺
Right lung　Left lung

胸膜の欠損と空気の流入
Airflow into pleural defect

縮んだ肺
Collapsed lung

Cardiac shift
心臓の移動

吸息時の胸膜の欠損
Pleural defect during inspiration

Positive pressure in pleural cavity
陽圧の胸膜腔

呼気

呼息時の空気の流れ
Normal airflow during expiration

胸膜の欠損と空気の流出
Airflow out of pleural defect

"Empty" pleural cavity at atmospheric pressure
大気圧になった"空"の胸膜腔

Cardiac shift
心臓の移動

縮んだ肺
Collapsed lung

一方弁
One-way "valve"

Cardiac shift
心臓の移動

A 正常呼吸．　　　B 気胸．　　　C 緊張性気胸．

肺動脈と肺静脈
Pulmonary Arteries & Veins

肺動脈幹は右心室から起こり，両肺への左右の肺動脈に分かれる．肺静脈は左右それぞれ2本ずつ両側から左心房に注ぐ．肺動脈は気管支樹に沿い，追随して分岐していくが，肺静脈は肺小葉の辺縁部にあり，気管支樹に随伴しない．

図 8.21 肺動脈と肺静脈
前方から見たところ．

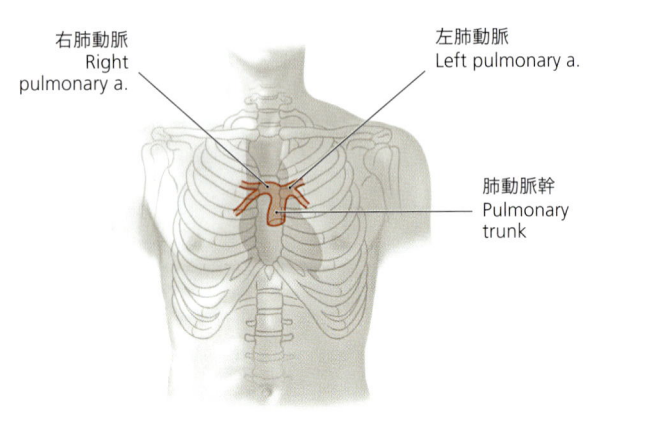

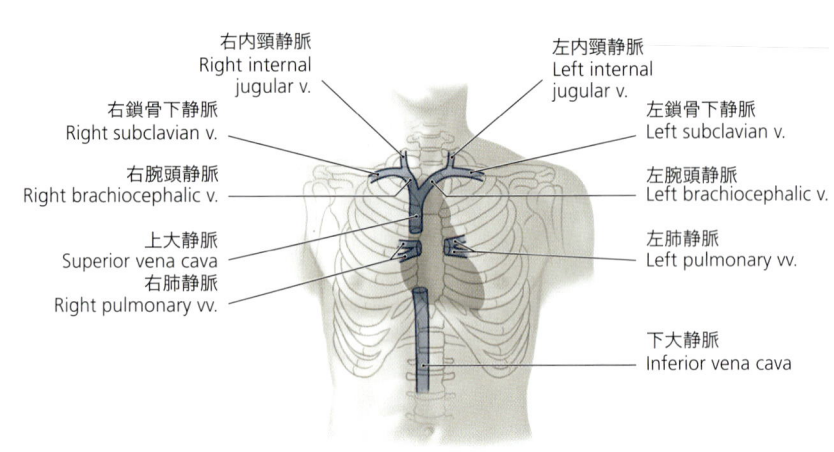

A 胸壁への肺動脈の投影．

ラベル:
- 右肺動脈 Right pulmonary a.
- 左肺動脈 Left pulmonary a.
- 肺動脈幹 Pulmonary trunk

B 胸壁への肺静脈の投影．

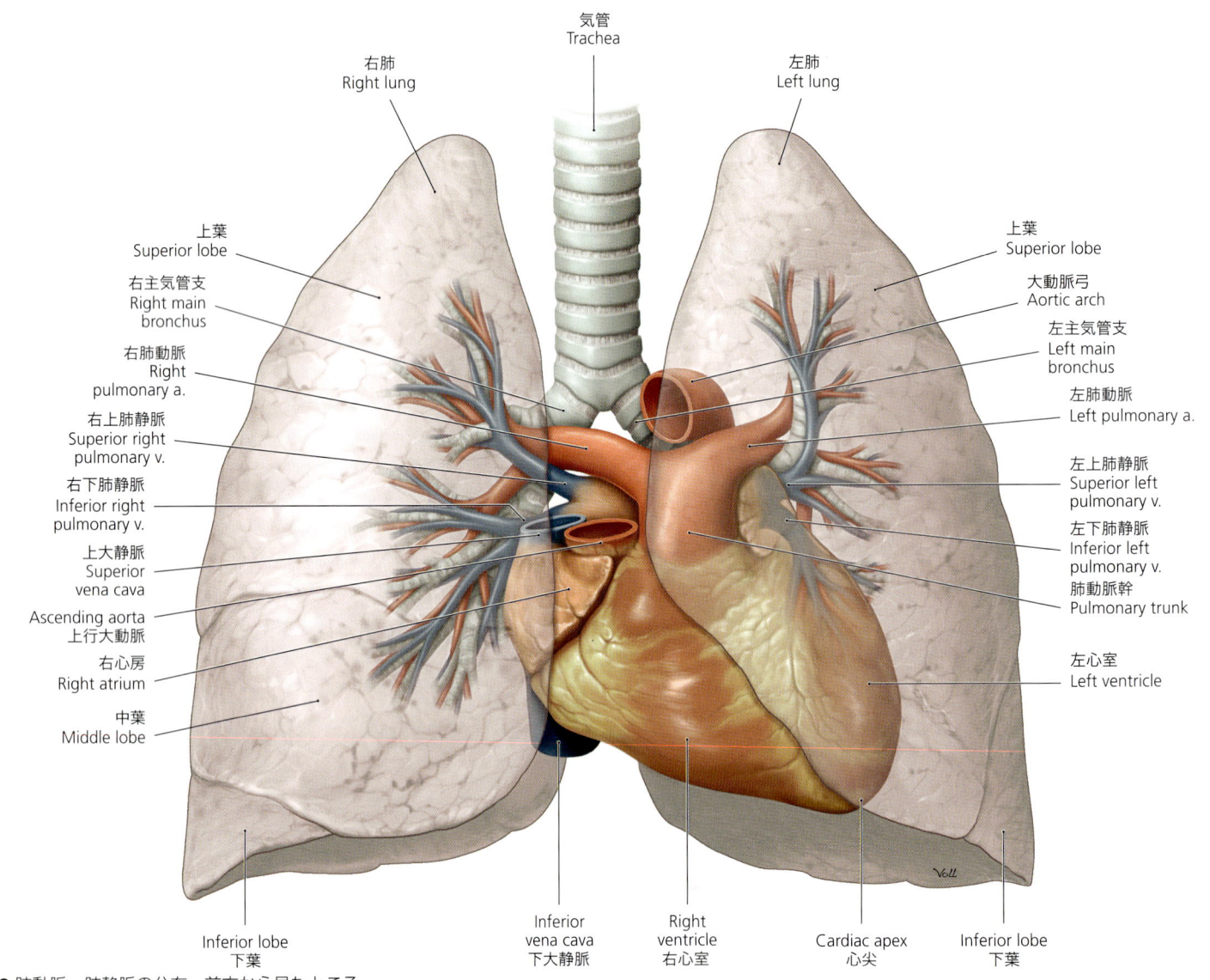

ラベル:
- 右内頸静脈 Right internal jugular v.
- 左内頸静脈 Left internal jugular v.
- 右鎖骨下静脈 Right subclavian v.
- 左鎖骨下静脈 Left subclavian v.
- 右腕頭静脈 Right brachiocephalic v.
- 左腕頭静脈 Left brachiocephalic v.
- 上大静脈 Superior vena cava
- 右肺静脈 Right pulmonary vv.
- 左肺静脈 Left pulmonary vv.
- 下大静脈 Inferior vena cava

C 肺動脈，肺静脈の分布，前方から見たところ．

ラベル:
- 気管 Trachea
- 右肺 Right lung
- 左肺 Left lung
- 上葉 Superior lobe
- 上葉 Superior lobe
- 右主気管支 Right main bronchus
- 大動脈弓 Aortic arch
- 右肺動脈 Right pulmonary a.
- 左主気管支 Left main bronchus
- 右上肺静脈 Superior right pulmonary v.
- 左肺動脈 Left pulmonary a.
- 右下肺静脈 Inferior right pulmonary v.
- 左上肺静脈 Superior left pulmonary v.
- 上大静脈 Superior vena cava
- 左下肺静脈 Inferior left pulmonary v.
- 上行大動脈 Ascending aorta
- 肺動脈幹 Pulmonary trunk
- 右心房 Right atrium
- 左心室 Left ventricle
- 中葉 Middle lobe
- 下葉 Inferior lobe
- 下大静脈 Inferior vena cava
- 右心室 Right ventricle
- 心尖 Cardiac apex
- 下葉 Inferior lobe

図8.22 肺動脈

腕頭動脈 Brachiocephalic trunk
左総頸動脈 Left common carotid a.
左鎖骨下動脈 Left subclavian a.
右肺動脈 Right pulmonary a.
大動脈弓 Aortic arch
中葉動脈 Middle lobe a.
動脈管索 Ligamentum arteriosum
左肺動脈 Left pulmonary a.
Pulmonary trunk 肺動脈幹

A 模式図.

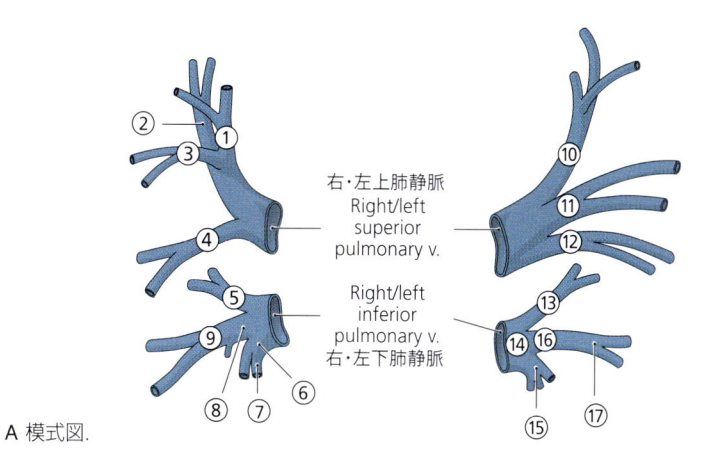

表8.3　肺動脈とその枝

	右肺動脈		左肺動脈
	上葉動脈		
①	肺尖動脈		⑪
②	後上葉動脈		⑫
③	前上葉動脈		⑬
	中葉動脈		
④	外側中葉動脈	肺舌動脈	⑭
⑤	内側中葉動脈		
	下葉動脈		
⑥	上-下葉動脈		⑮
⑦	前肺底動脈		⑯
⑧	外側肺底動脈		⑰
⑨	後肺底動脈		⑱
⑩	内側肺底動脈		⑲

B 肺血管造影像．動脈造影，前面．

図8.23　肺静脈

右・左上肺静脈 Right/left superior pulmonary v.
Right/left inferior pulmonary v. 右・左下肺静脈

A 模式図.

表8.4　肺静脈とその枝

	右肺静脈		左肺静脈
	上肺静脈		
①	肺尖静脈	肺尖後静脈	⑩
②	後上葉静脈		
③	前上葉静脈	前上葉静脈	⑪
④	中葉静脈	肺舌静脈	⑫
	下肺静脈		
⑤	上-下葉静脈		⑬
⑥	総肺底静脈		⑭
⑦	下肺底静脈		⑮
⑧	上肺底静脈		⑯
⑨	前肺底静脈		⑰

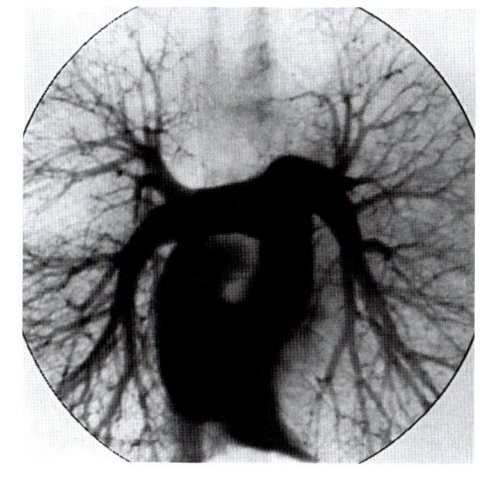

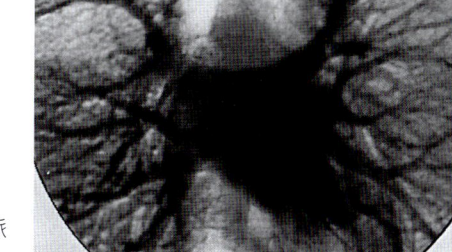

B 肺血管造影像．静脈造影，前面．

臨床

肺塞栓

潜在的に生命を脅かすような肺塞栓は，血栓が静脈系を通って移動して肺を栄養する動脈に入ったときに起こる．呼吸困難と頻拍が症候として見られる．

多くの肺塞栓は下肢と骨盤のよどんだ血液で生じる（静脈血栓塞栓症）．継続的な静止状態，異常な血液凝固，外傷が原因である．*Note*: 血栓塞栓とは血栓が移動して塞栓すること．

気管気管支樹の神経と血管
Neurovasculature of the Tracheobronchial Tree

図 8.24 肺の血管系

肺の血管系は肺内部でのガス交換を行う．肺動脈（青）は低酸素血を運び，気管支樹に伴行する．肺静脈（赤）は高酸素血を運ぶ唯一の静脈で，小葉末梢の肺胞毛細血管から酸素を受け取る．

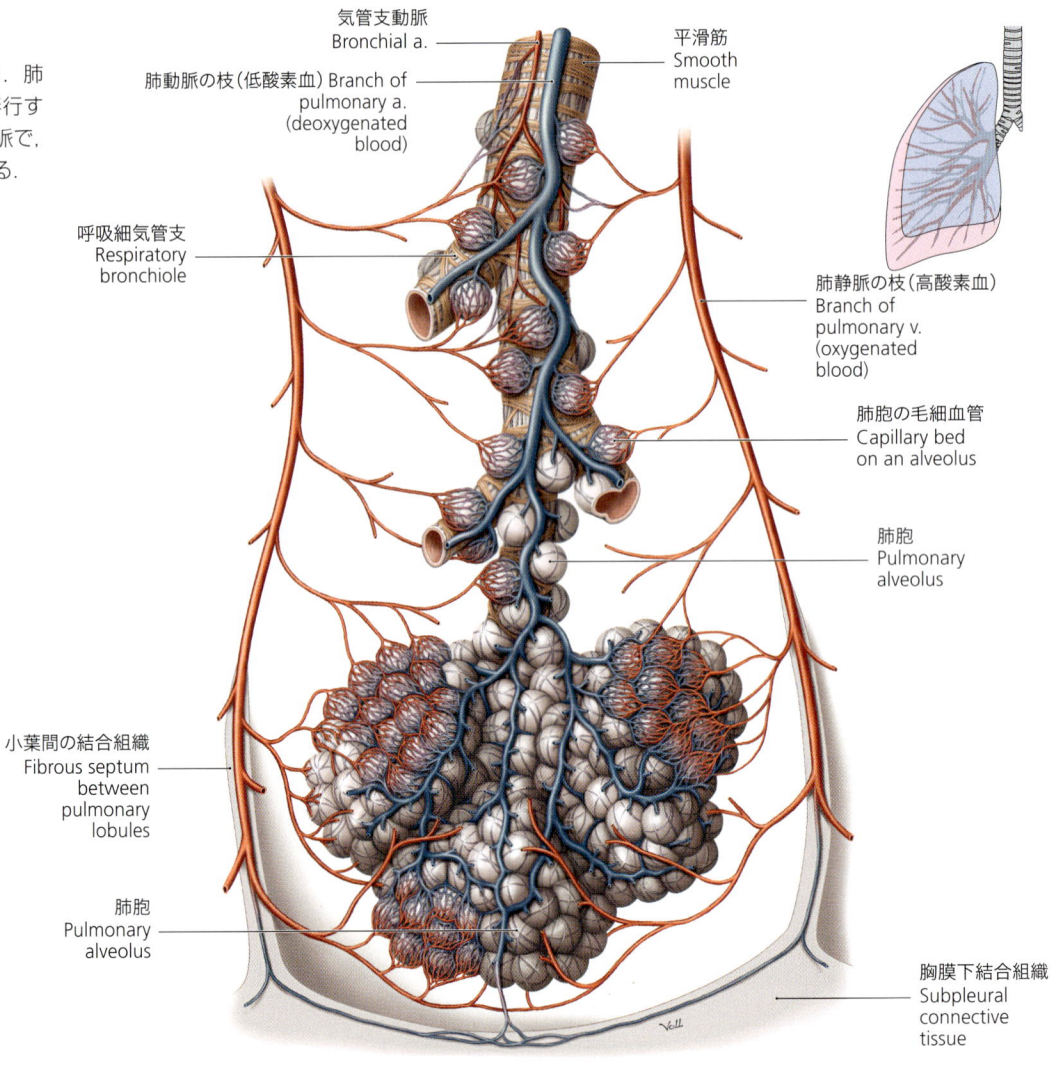

主な構造：
- 気管支動脈 Bronchial a.
- 肺動脈の枝（低酸素血）Branch of pulmonary a. (deoxygenated blood)
- 平滑筋 Smooth muscle
- 呼吸細気管支 Respiratory bronchiole
- 肺静脈の枝（高酸素血）Branch of pulmonary v. (oxygenated blood)
- 肺胞の毛細血管 Capillary bed on an alveolus
- 肺胞 Pulmonary alveolus
- 小葉間の結合組織 Fibrous septum between pulmonary lobules
- 肺胞 Pulmonary alveolus
- 胸膜下結合組織 Subpleural connective tissue

図 8.25 気管気管支樹の動脈

気管支樹は気道の外膜にある気管支動脈によって栄養される．一般的には1～3本の気管支動脈が大動脈から直接起こる．肋間動脈から起こることもある．

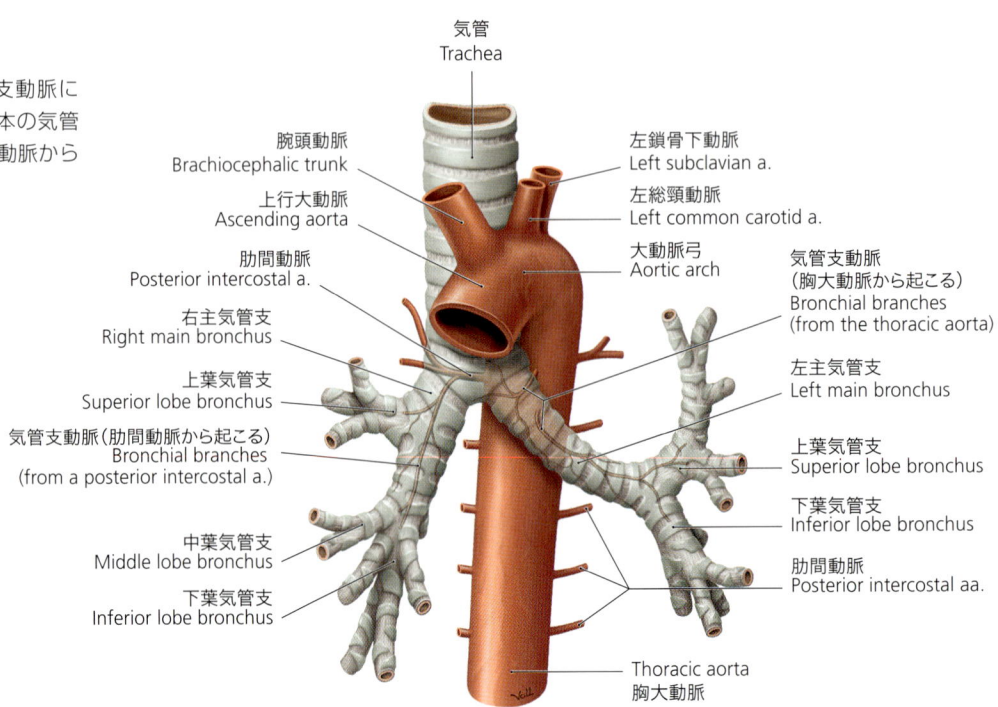

主な構造：
- 気管 Trachea
- 腕頭動脈 Brachiocephalic trunk
- 左鎖骨下動脈 Left subclavian a.
- 上行大動脈 Ascending aorta
- 左総頸動脈 Left common carotid a.
- 肋間動脈 Posterior intercostal a.
- 大動脈弓 Aortic arch
- 右主気管支 Right main bronchus
- 気管支動脈（胸大動脈から起こる）Bronchial branches (from the thoracic aorta)
- 上葉気管支 Superior lobe bronchus
- 左主気管支 Left main bronchus
- 気管支動脈（肋間動脈から起こる）Bronchial branches (from a posterior intercostal a.)
- 上葉気管支 Superior lobe bronchus
- 中葉気管支 Middle lobe bronchus
- 下葉気管支 Inferior lobe bronchus
- 下葉気管支 Inferior lobe bronchus
- 肋間動脈 Posterior intercostal aa.
- 胸大動脈 Thoracic aorta

図 8.26 気管気管支樹の静脈

- 気管 Trachea
- 下甲状腺静脈 Inferior thyroid v.
- 左腕頭静脈 Left brachiocephalic v.
- 右腕頭静脈 Right brachiocephalic v.
- 副半奇静脈 Accessory hemiazygos v.
- 上大静脈 Superior vena cava
- 左主気管支 Left main bronchus
- 気管支静脈(副半奇静脈へ) Bronchial vv. (opening into the accessory hemiazygos v.)
- 上葉気管支 Superior lobe bronchus
- 気管支静脈(奇静脈へ) Bronchial vv. (opening into the azygos v.)
- 上葉気管支 Superior lobe bronchus
- 中葉気管支 Middle lobe bronchus
- 下葉気管支 Inferior lobe bronchus
- 下葉気管支 Inferior lobe bronchus
- 奇静脈 Azygos v.
- 半奇静脈 Hemiazygos v.

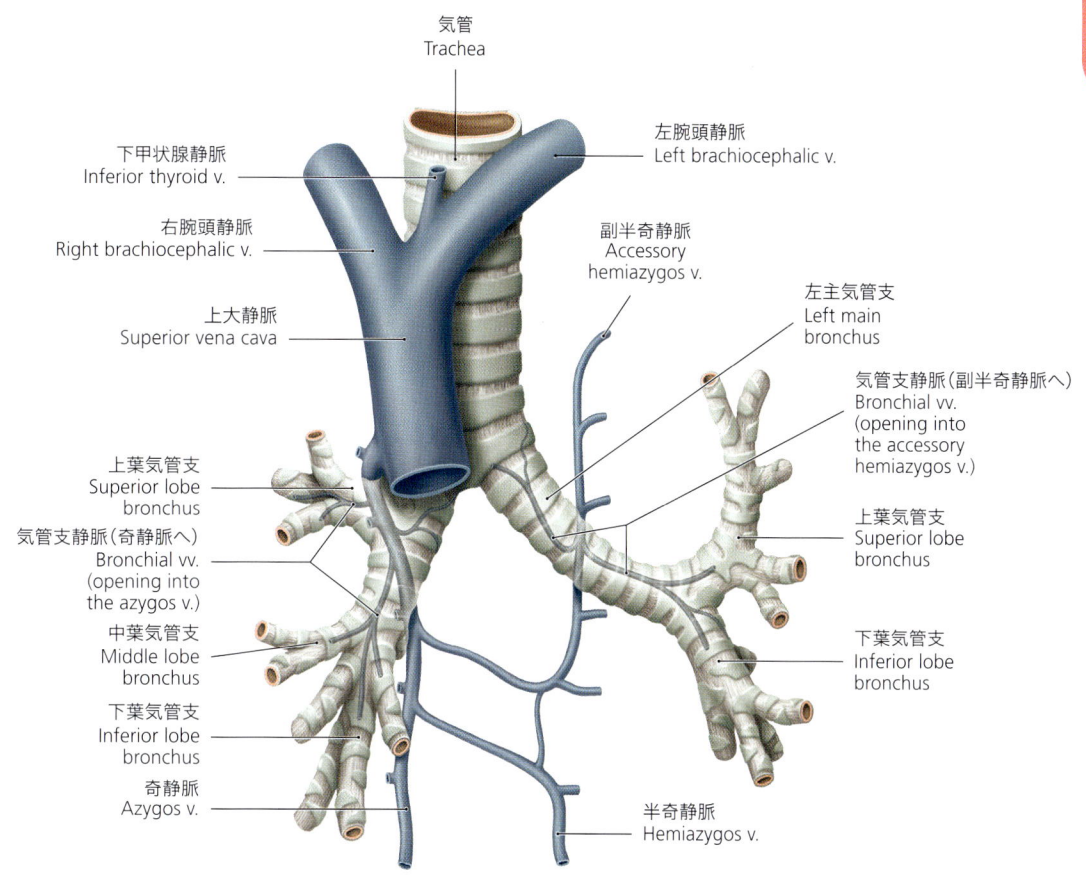

図 8.27 気管気管支樹の自律神経支配
交感神経支配(赤)，副交感神経支配(青)．

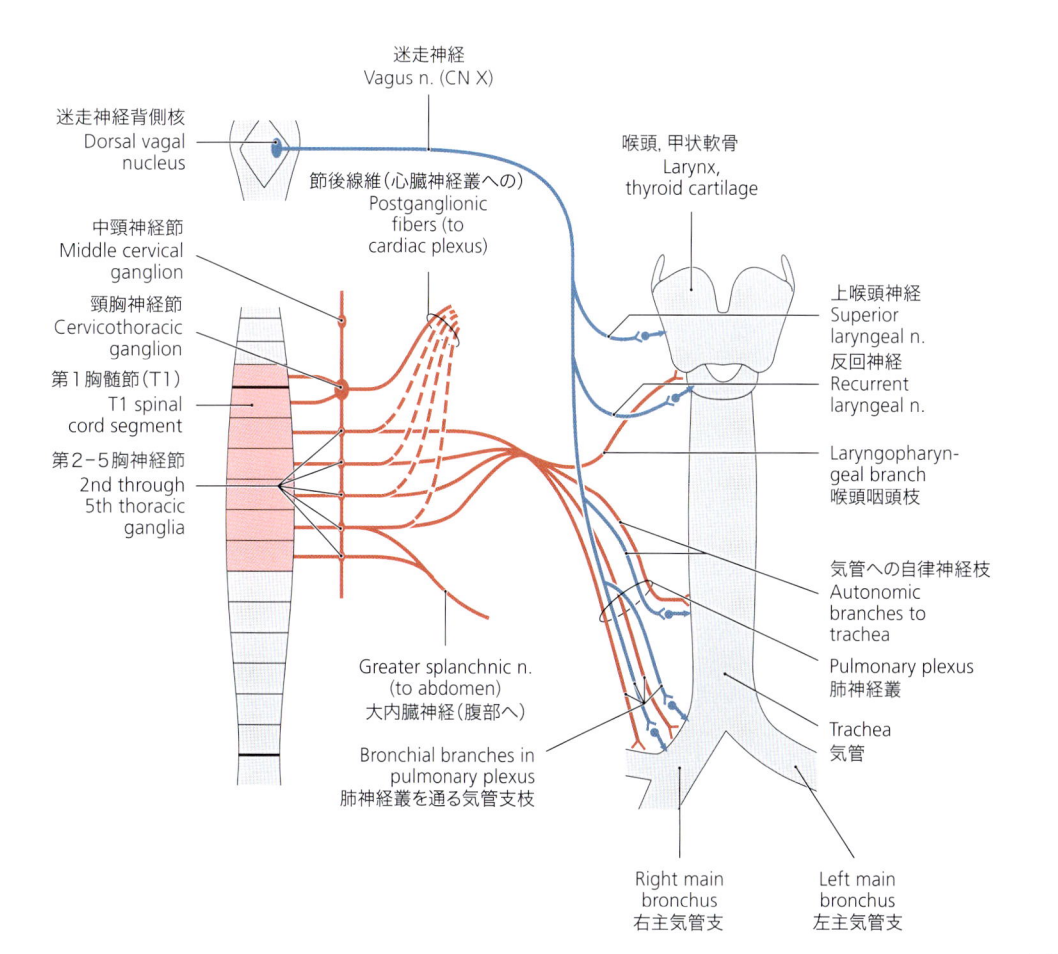

- 迷走神経 Vagus n. (CN X)
- 迷走神経背側核 Dorsal vagal nucleus
- 節後線維(心臓神経叢への) Postganglionic fibers (to cardiac plexus)
- 喉頭, 甲状軟骨 Larynx, thyroid cartilage
- 中頸神経節 Middle cervical ganglion
- 頸胸神経節 Cervicothoracic ganglion
- 第1胸髄節(T1) T1 spinal cord segment
- 第2-5胸神経節 2nd through 5th thoracic ganglia
- 上喉頭神経 Superior laryngeal n.
- 反回神経 Recurrent laryngeal n.
- Laryngopharyngeal branch 喉頭咽頭枝
- 気管への自律神経枝 Autonomic branches to trachea
- Pulmonary plexus 肺神経叢
- Trachea 気管
- Greater splanchnic n. (to abdomen) 大内臓神経(腹部へ)
- Bronchial branches in pulmonary plexus 肺神経叢を通る気管支枝
- Right main bronchus 右主気管支
- Left main bronchus 左主気管支

8 胸膜腔

胸膜腔のリンパ管
Lymphatics of the Pleural Cavity

肺と気管支は2つのリンパ系によってリンパが集められる．気管支周囲リンパ管叢は気管支樹にしたがって，気管支と肺の大部分からリンパを集める．胸膜下リンパ管叢は肺の末梢域と臓側胸膜からリンパを集める．

図8.28 胸膜腔のリンパ流路
水平断，下方から見たところ．

A 気管支周囲のリンパ管叢．冠状断．気管支樹周辺の肺内リンパ節は肺から気管支肺リンパ節にリンパを運ぶ．その後，下気管支気管支リンパ節，上気管支気管支リンパ節，気管傍リンパ節，気管支縦隔リンパ本幹，右リンパ本幹あるいは胸管へと順に運ばれる．*Note*: 左肺下葉からのリンパのかなりの量は右上気管気管支リンパ節に流入する．

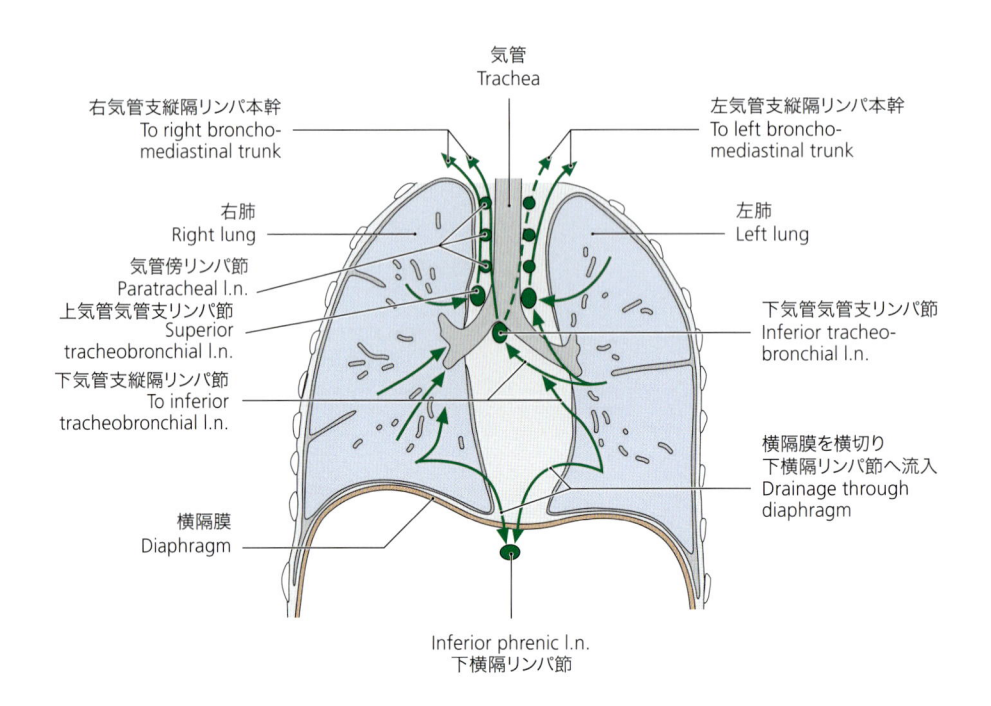

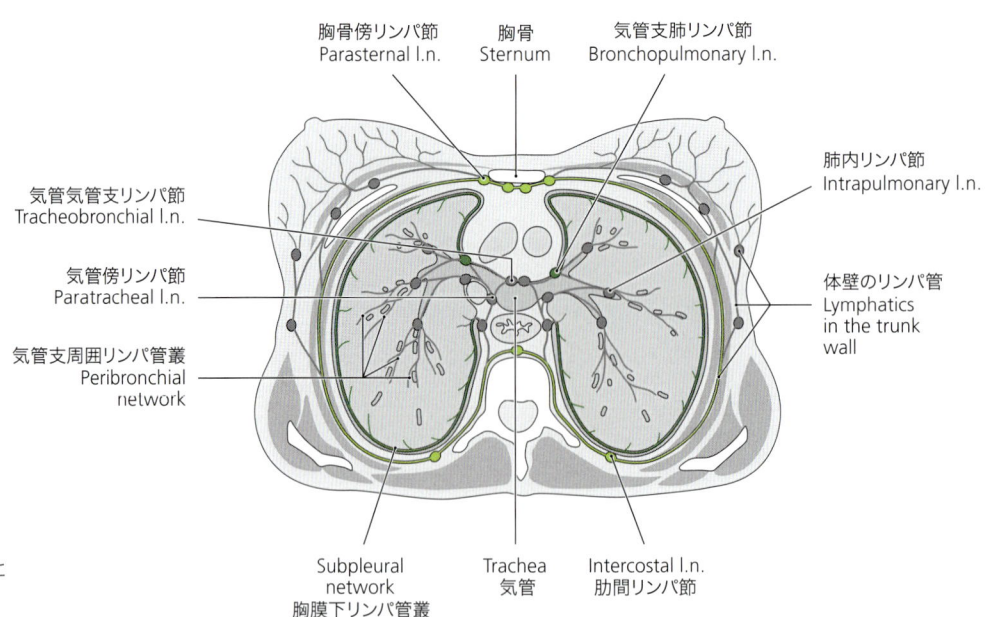

- 右気管支縦隔リンパ本幹 To right broncho-mediastinal trunk
- 気管 Trachea
- 左気管支縦隔リンパ本幹 To left broncho-mediastinal trunk
- 右肺 Right lung
- 左肺 Left lung
- 気管傍リンパ節 Paratracheal l.n.
- 上気管支気管支リンパ節 Superior tracheobronchial l.n.
- 下気管気管支リンパ節 Inferior tracheobronchial l.n.
- 下気管支縦隔リンパ節 To inferior tracheobronchial l.n.
- 横隔膜を横切り下横隔リンパ節へ流入 Drainage through diaphragm
- 横隔膜 Diaphragm
- 下横隔リンパ節 Inferior phrenic l.n.

B 胸膜下リンパ管叢．水平断，上方から見たところ．

- 胸骨傍リンパ節 Parasternal l.n.
- 胸骨 Sternum
- 気管支肺リンパ節 Bronchopulmonary l.n.
- 気管気管支リンパ節 Tracheobronchial l.n.
- 肺内リンパ節 Intrapulmonary l.n.
- 気管傍リンパ節 Paratracheal l.n.
- 体壁のリンパ管 Lymphatics in the trunk wall
- 気管支周囲リンパ管叢 Peribronchial network
- 胸膜下リンパ管叢 Subpleural network
- 気管 Trachea
- 肋間リンパ節 Intercostal l.n.

図 8.29　胸膜腔のリンパ節

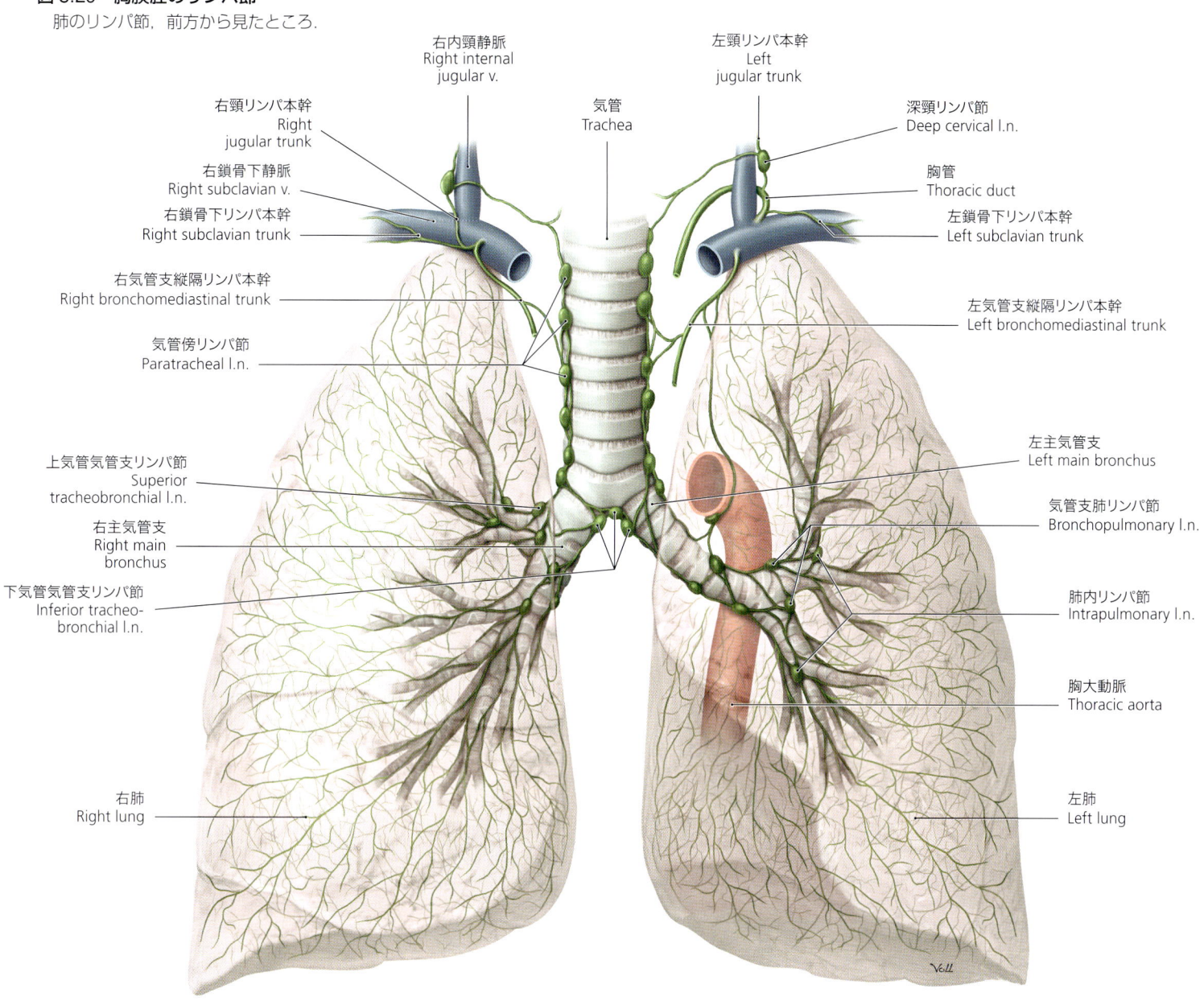

肺のリンパ節，前方から見たところ．

右内頸静脈	Right internal jugular v.
右頸リンパ本幹	Right jugular trunk
右鎖骨下静脈	Right subclavian v.
右鎖骨下リンパ本幹	Right subclavian trunk
右気管支縦隔リンパ本幹	Right bronchomediastinal trunk
気管傍リンパ節	Paratracheal l.n.
上気管気管支リンパ節	Superior tracheobronchial l.n.
右主気管支	Right main bronchus
下気管気管支リンパ節	Inferior tracheo-bronchial l.n.
右肺	Right lung
気管	Trachea
左頸リンパ本幹	Left jugular trunk
深頸リンパ節	Deep cervical l.n.
胸管	Thoracic duct
左鎖骨下リンパ本幹	Left subclavian trunk
左気管支縦隔リンパ本幹	Left bronchomediastinal trunk
左主気管支	Left main bronchus
気管支肺リンパ節	Bronchopulmonary l.n.
肺内リンパ節	Intrapulmonary l.n.
胸大動脈	Thoracic aorta
左肺	Left lung

体表解剖
Surface Anatomy

図 9.1 胸部の触知可能構造
前方から見たところ．背部の構造については pp.40-41 を参照．

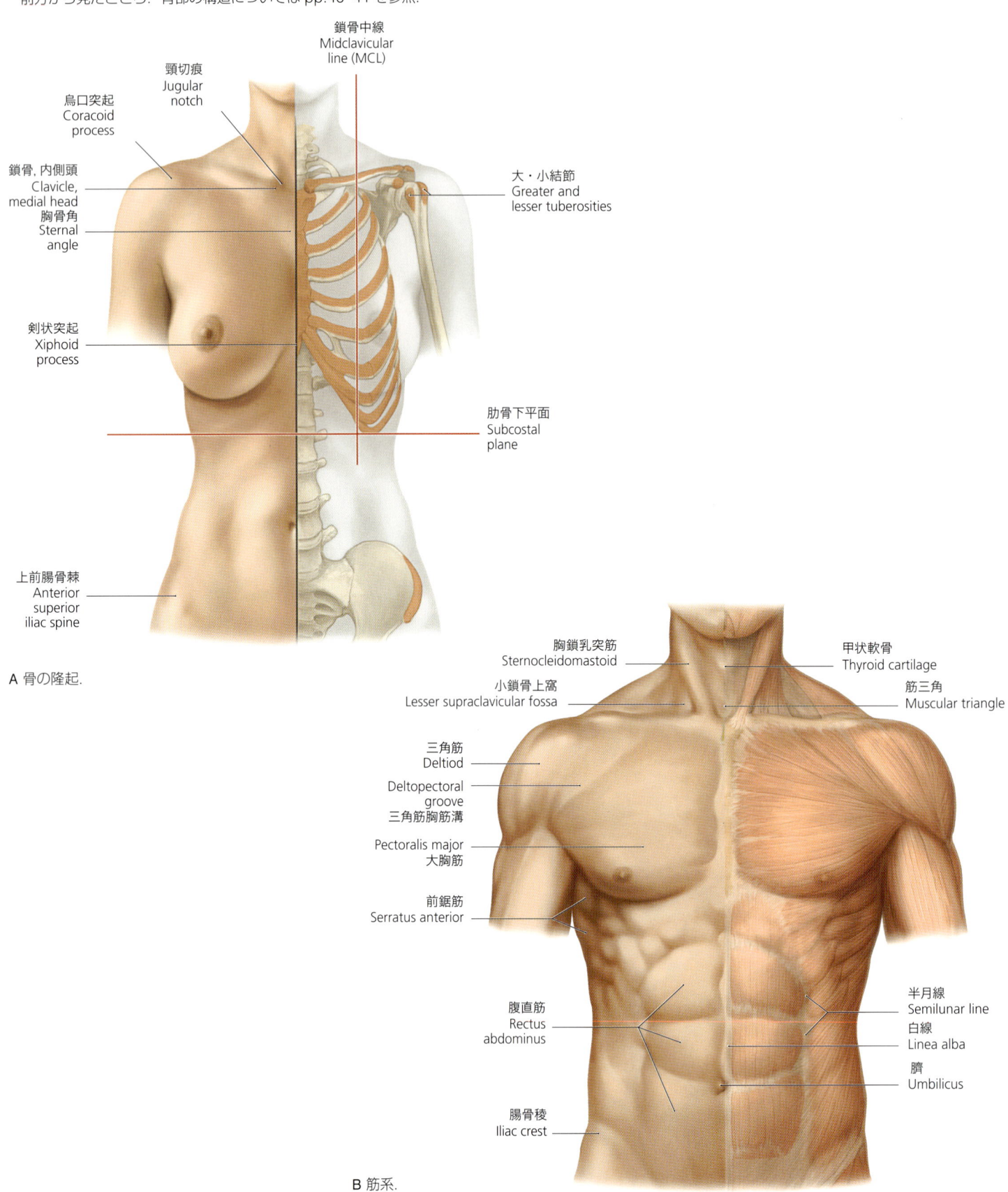

A 骨の隆起．

- 烏口突起 Coracoid process
- 頸切痕 Jugular notch
- 鎖骨中線 Midclavicular line (MCL)
- 鎖骨，内側頭 Clavicle, medial head
- 胸骨角 Sternal angle
- 大・小結節 Greater and lesser tuberosities
- 剣状突起 Xiphoid process
- 肋骨下平面 Subcostal plane
- 上前腸骨棘 Anterior superior iliac spine

B 筋系．

- 胸鎖乳突筋 Sternocleidomastoid
- 甲状軟骨 Thyroid cartilage
- 小鎖骨上窩 Lesser supraclavicular fossa
- 筋三角 Muscular triangle
- 三角筋 Deltiod
- 三角筋胸筋溝 Deltopectoral groove
- 大胸筋 Pectoralis major
- 前鋸筋 Serratus anterior
- 腹直筋 Rectus abdominus
- 半月線 Semilunar line
- 白線 Linea alba
- 臍 Umbilicus
- 腸骨稜 Iliac crest

図 9.2 胸部の体表解剖
前方から見たところ．背部の構造については pp.40-41 参照．

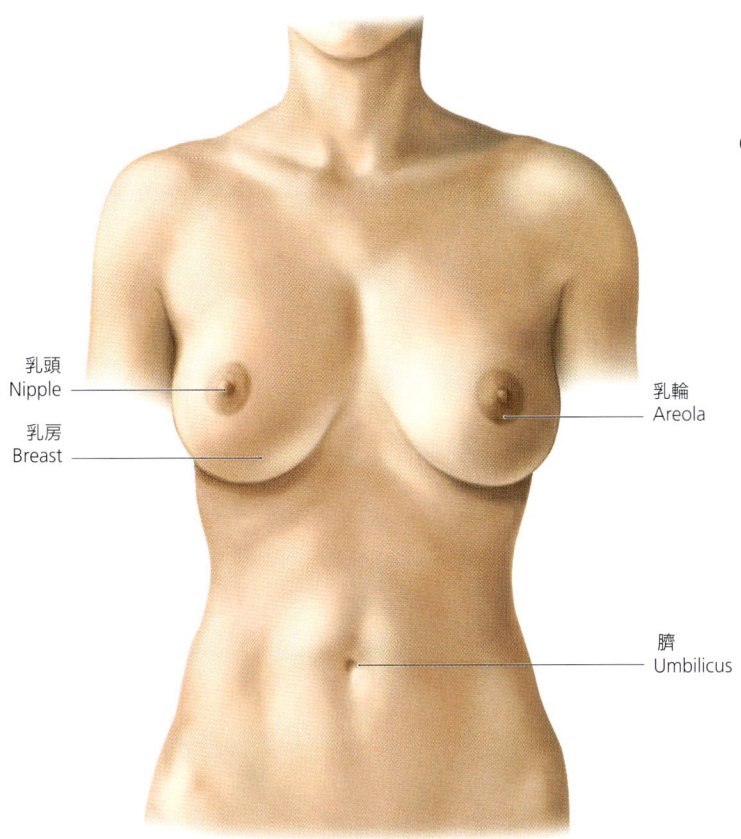

乳頭 Nipple
乳房 Breast
乳輪 Areola
臍 Umbilicus

A 女性の胸部．

Q1: 女性の患者．問診で自己検査によってしこりを発見したと告げられる．あなたはこの後何をしますか？どこでリンパ節を触診しますか？

Q2: あなたは病院で初めての患者の前胸部を前にしている．心臓の 4 つの弁の最適な検査をするためにどのような計画を立てますか？

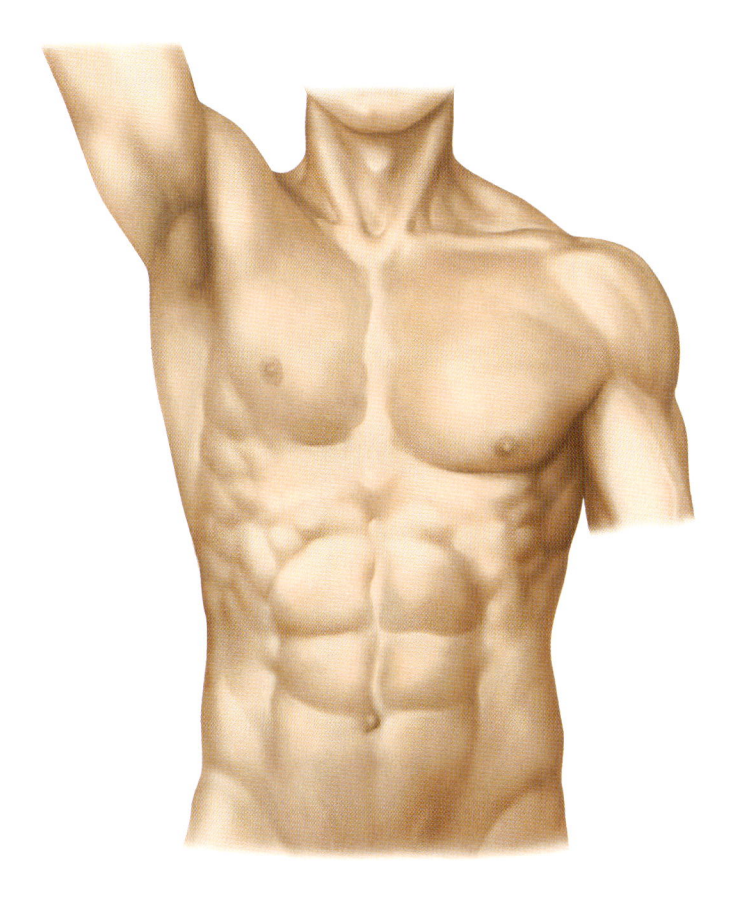

p.626 からの解答を参照．

B 男性の胸部．

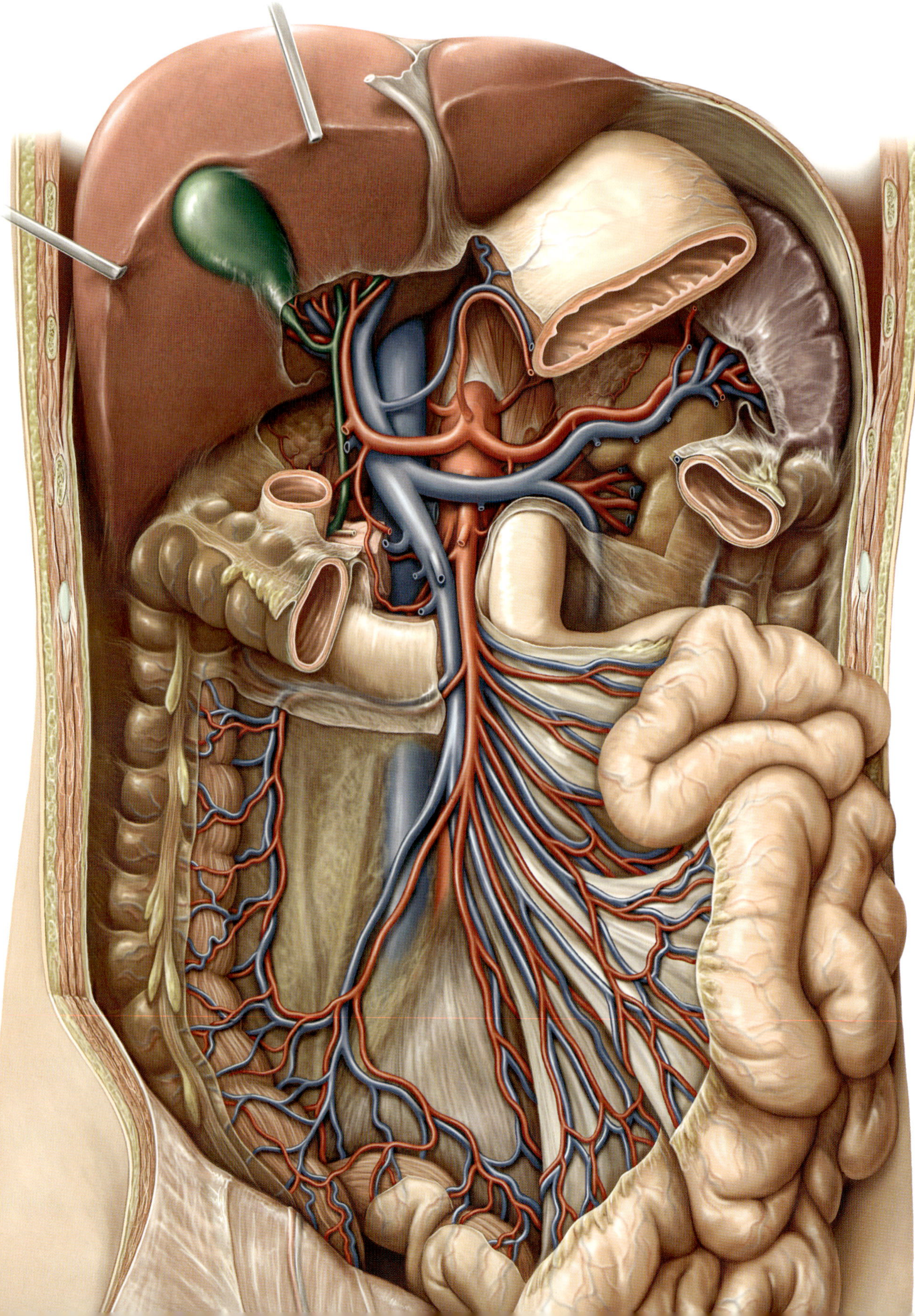

腹部・骨盤
Abdomen & Pelvis

10．骨，靱帯，関節
- 下肢帯……………………………………124
- 男性骨盤と女性骨盤……………………126
- 骨盤の靱帯………………………………128

11．腹壁
- 腹壁の筋…………………………………130
- 鼡径部と鼡径管…………………………132
- 腹壁と鼡径ヘルニア……………………134
- 会陰部……………………………………136
- 腹壁の筋…………………………………138
- 骨盤底の筋………………………………140

12．腹腔
- 腹腔・骨盤腔の区分……………………142
- 腹膜腔……………………………………144
- 網嚢………………………………………146
- 腸間膜と後壁……………………………148
- 骨盤の内容………………………………150
- 腹膜の位置関係…………………………152
- 骨盤と会陰………………………………154
- 水平断……………………………………156

13．内臓
- 胃…………………………………………158
- 十二指腸…………………………………160
- 空腸と回腸………………………………162
- 盲腸，虫垂，結腸………………………164
- 直腸と肛門管……………………………166
- 肝臓：概観………………………………168
- 肝臓：肝区域と肝葉……………………170
- 胆嚢と胆管………………………………172
- 膵臓と脾臓………………………………174
- 腎臓と副腎：概観………………………176
- 腎臓と副腎：詳説………………………178
- 尿管………………………………………180
- 膀胱………………………………………182
- 膀胱と尿道………………………………184

14．生殖器
- 生殖器の概観……………………………186
- 子宮と卵巣………………………………188
- 腟…………………………………………190
- 女性の外生殖器…………………………192
- 女性生殖器の神経と血管………………194
- 陰茎，陰嚢，精索………………………196
- 精巣と精巣上体…………………………198
- 男性の付属生殖腺………………………200
- 男性生殖器の神経と血管………………202
- 生殖器の発生……………………………204

15．動脈と静脈
- 腹部の動脈………………………………206
- 腹大動脈と腎動脈………………………208
- 腹腔動脈…………………………………210
- 上腸間膜動脈と下腸間膜動脈…………212
- 腹部の静脈………………………………214
- 下大静脈と腎静脈………………………216
- 門脈………………………………………218
- 上腸間膜静脈と下腸間膜静脈…………220
- 骨盤の動脈と静脈………………………222
- 直腸と生殖器の動脈と静脈……………224

16．リンパ系
- 腹部と骨盤部のリンパ節………………226
- 後腹壁のリンパ節………………………228
- 前腹部内臓のリンパ節…………………230
- 腸のリンパ節……………………………232
- 生殖器のリンパ節………………………234

17．神経系
- 自律神経叢………………………………236
- 腹部内臓の神経支配……………………238
- 腸の神経支配……………………………240
- 骨盤の神経支配…………………………242
- 自律神経支配：概観……………………244
- 自律神経支配：泌尿器と生殖器………246

18．体表解剖
- 体表解剖…………………………………248

下肢帯
Pelvic Girdle

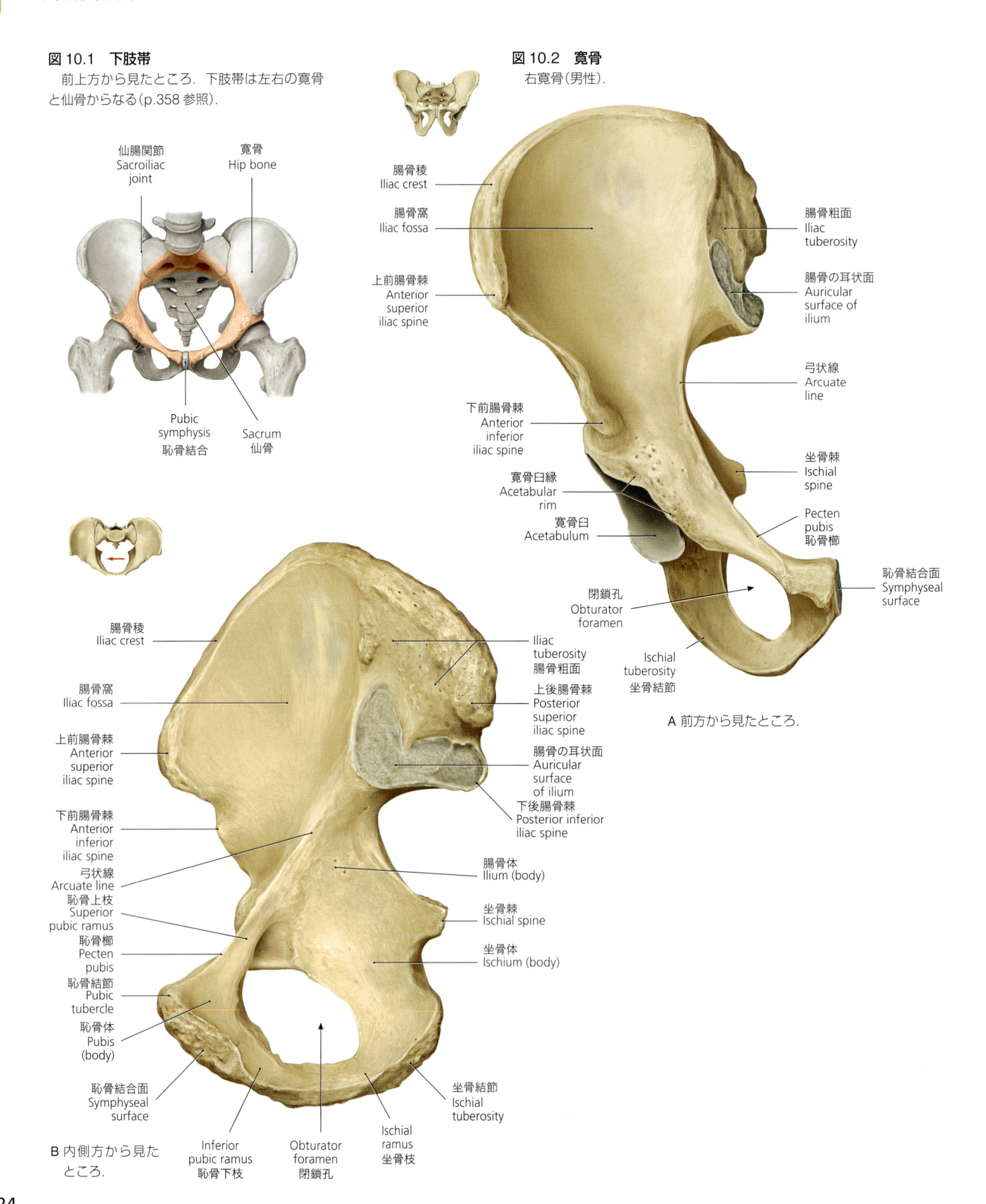

図 10.1　下肢帯
前上方から見たところ．下肢帯は左右の寛骨と仙骨からなる(p.358 参照)．

- 仙腸関節 Sacroiliac joint
- 寛骨 Hip bone
- Pubic symphysis 恥骨結合
- Sacrum 仙骨

図 10.2　寛骨
右寛骨(男性)．

A 前方から見たところ．

- 腸骨稜 Iliac crest
- 腸骨窩 Iliac fossa
- 上前腸骨棘 Anterior superior iliac spine
- 下前腸骨棘 Anterior inferior iliac spine
- 寛骨臼縁 Acetabular rim
- 寛骨臼 Acetabulum
- 閉鎖孔 Obturator foramen
- 腸骨粗面 Iliac tuberosity
- 腸骨の耳状面 Auricular surface of ilium
- 弓状線 Arcuate line
- 坐骨棘 Ischial spine
- Pecten pubis 恥骨櫛
- 恥骨結合面 Symphyseal surface
- Ischial tuberosity 坐骨結節

B 内側方から見たところ．

- 腸骨稜 Iliac crest
- 腸骨窩 Iliac fossa
- 上前腸骨棘 Anterior superior iliac spine
- 下前腸骨棘 Anterior inferior iliac spine
- 弓状線 Arcuate line
- 恥骨上枝 Superior pubic ramus
- 恥骨櫛 Pecten pubis
- 恥骨結節 Pubic tubercle
- 恥骨体 Pubis (body)
- 恥骨結合面 Symphyseal surface
- Inferior pubic ramus 恥骨下枝
- Obturator foramen 閉鎖孔
- Ischial ramus 坐骨枝
- 坐骨結節 Ischial tuberosity
- 坐骨体 Ischium (body)
- 坐骨棘 Ischial spine
- 腸骨体 Ilium (body)
- 下後腸骨棘 Posterior inferior iliac spine
- 腸骨の耳状面 Auricular surface of ilium
- 上後腸骨棘 Posterior superior iliac spine
- Iliac tuberosity 腸骨粗面

図10.3　寛骨のY軟骨

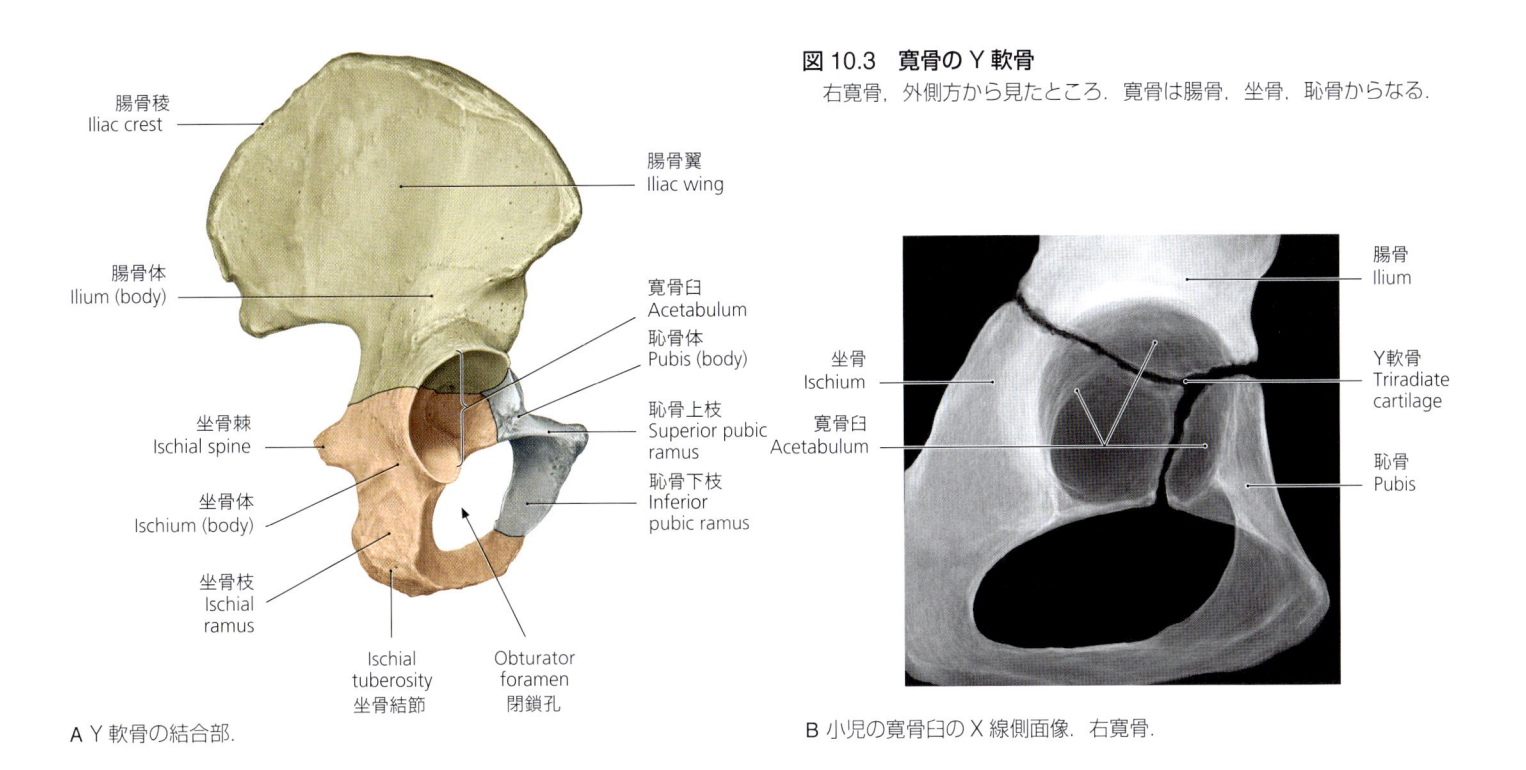

右寛骨，外側方から見たところ．寛骨は腸骨，坐骨，恥骨からなる．

A　Y軟骨の結合部．

B　小児の寛骨臼のX線側面像．右寛骨．

図10.4　寛骨：外側方から見たところ

右寛骨（男性）．

男性骨盤と女性骨盤
Male & Female Pelvis

図10.5 女性骨盤

A 前方から見たところ．

- 腸骨稜 Iliac crest
- 仙腸関節 Sacroiliac joint
- 仙骨 Sacrum
- 恥骨結節 Pubic tubercle
- 腸骨窩 Iliac fossa
- 上前腸骨棘 Anterior superior iliac spine
- 下前腸骨棘 Anterior inferior iliac spine
- 寛骨臼縁 Acetabular margin
- 恥骨上枝・下枝 Superior and inferior pubic rami
- 坐骨棘 Ischial spine
- 閉鎖孔 Obturator foramen
- Coccyx 尾骨
- 恥骨結合 Pubic symphysis
- Ischial ramus 坐骨枝

B 後方から見たところ．

- 腸骨稜 Iliac crest
- 仙骨管 Sacral canal
- 上後腸骨棘 Posterior superior iliac spine
- 下後腸骨棘 Posterior inferior iliac spine
- 恥骨上枝 Superior pubic ramus
- Ischial spine 坐骨棘
- Inferior pubic ramus 恥骨下枝
- Sacral hiatus 仙骨裂孔
- 腸骨翼 Iliac wing
- Median sacral crest 正中仙骨稜
- Greater sciatic notch 大坐骨切痕
- 小坐骨切痕 Lesser sciatic notch
- Ischial tuberosity 坐骨結節

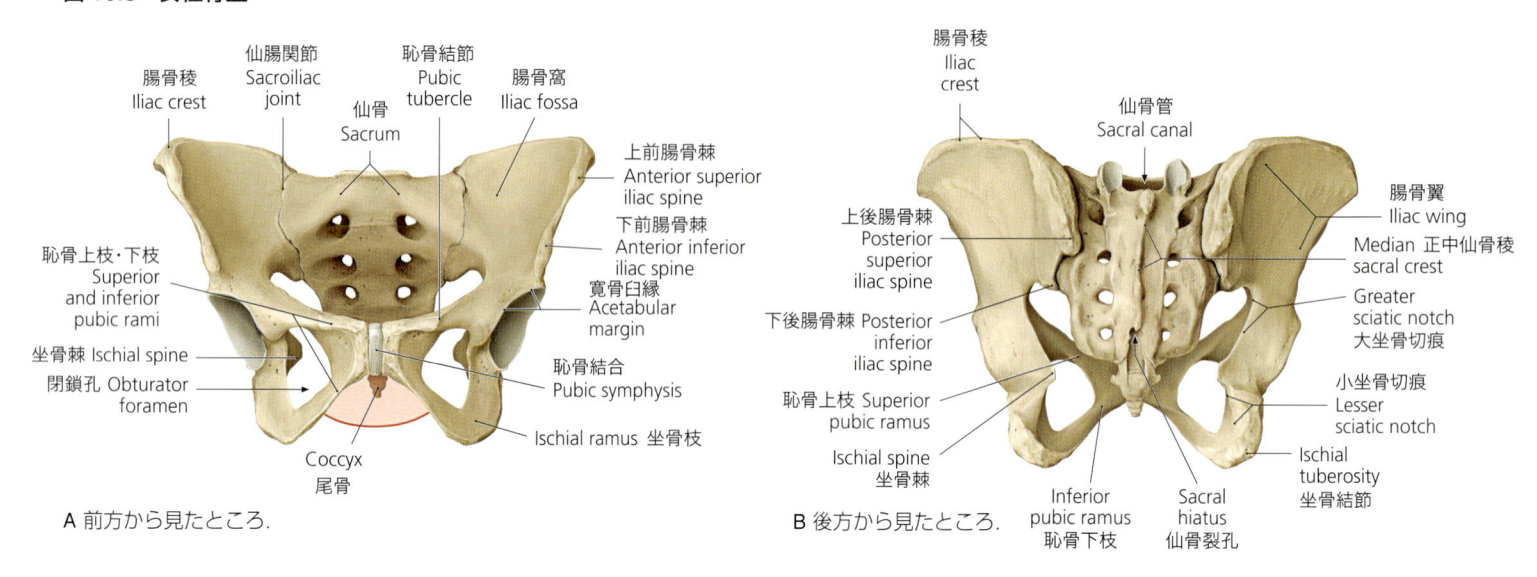

図10.6 男性骨盤

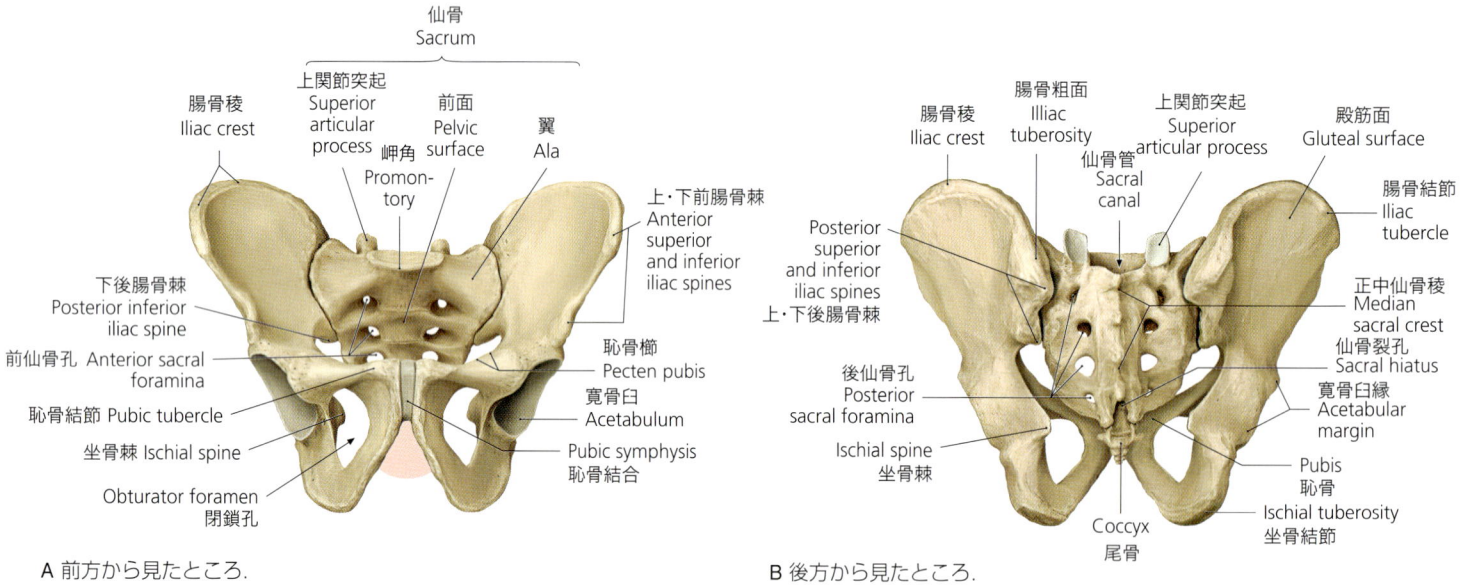

A 前方から見たところ．

- 腸骨稜 Iliac crest
- 仙骨 Sacrum
- 上関節突起 Superior articular process
- 前面 Pelvic surface
- 岬角 Promontory
- 翼 Ala
- 上・下前腸骨棘 Anterior superior and inferior iliac spines
- 下後腸骨棘 Posterior inferior iliac spine
- 前仙骨孔 Anterior sacral foramina
- 恥骨結節 Pubic tubercle
- 坐骨棘 Ischial spine
- Obturator foramen 閉鎖孔
- 恥骨櫛 Pecten pubis
- 寛骨臼 Acetabulum
- Pubic symphysis 恥骨結合

B 後方から見たところ．

- 腸骨稜 Iliac crest
- 腸骨粗面 Illiac tuberosity
- 上関節突起 Superior articular process
- 殿筋面 Gluteal surface
- 仙骨管 Sacral canal
- Posterior superior and inferior iliac spines 上・下後腸骨棘
- 後仙骨孔 Posterior sacral foramina
- Ischial spine 坐骨棘
- Coccyx 尾骨
- 腸骨結節 Iliac tubercle
- 正中仙骨稜 Median sacral crest
- 仙骨裂孔 Sacral hiatus
- 寛骨臼縁 Acetabular margin
- Pubis 恥骨
- Ischial tuberosity 坐骨結節

図 10.7　女性骨盤：上方から見たところ

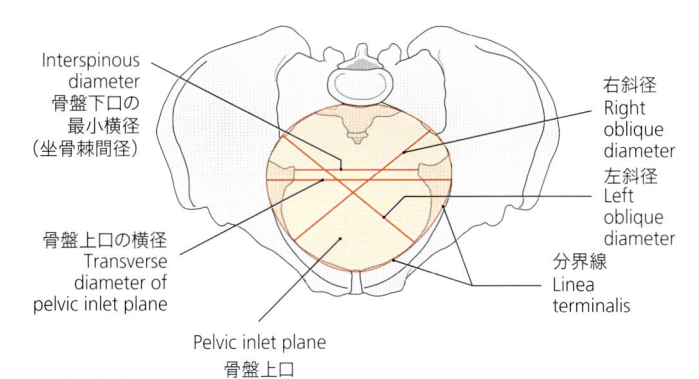

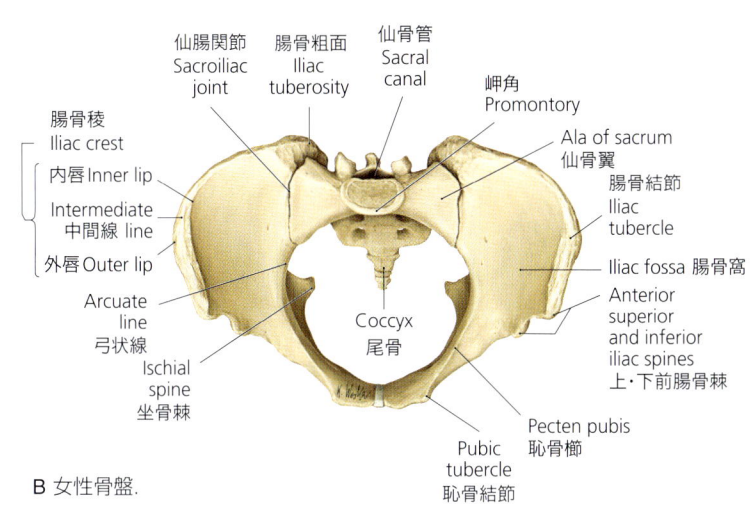

A　骨盤計測.
- Interspinous diameter 骨盤下口の最小横径（坐骨棘間径）
- 骨盤上口の横径 Transverse diameter of pelvic inlet plane
- Pelvic inlet plane 骨盤上口
- 右斜径 Right oblique diameter
- 左斜径 Left oblique diameter
- 分界線 Linea terminalis

B　女性骨盤.
- 腸骨稜 Iliac crest（内唇 Inner lip／中間線 Intermediate line／外唇 Outer lip）
- 仙腸関節 Sacroiliac joint
- 腸骨粗面 Iliac tuberosity
- 仙骨管 Sacral canal
- 岬角 Promontory
- Ala of sacrum 仙骨翼
- 腸骨結節 Iliac tubercle
- Iliac fossa 腸骨窩
- Anterior superior and inferior iliac spines 上・下前腸骨棘
- Pecten pubis 恥骨櫛
- Pubic tubercle 恥骨結節
- Arcuate line 弓状線
- Ischial spine 坐骨棘
- Coccyx 尾骨

図 10.8　男性骨盤：上方から見たところ

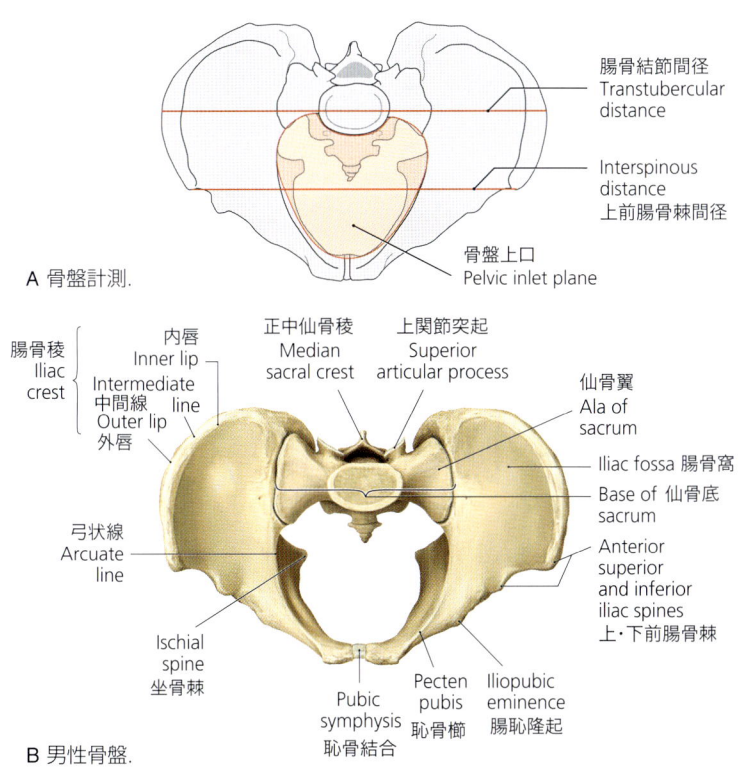

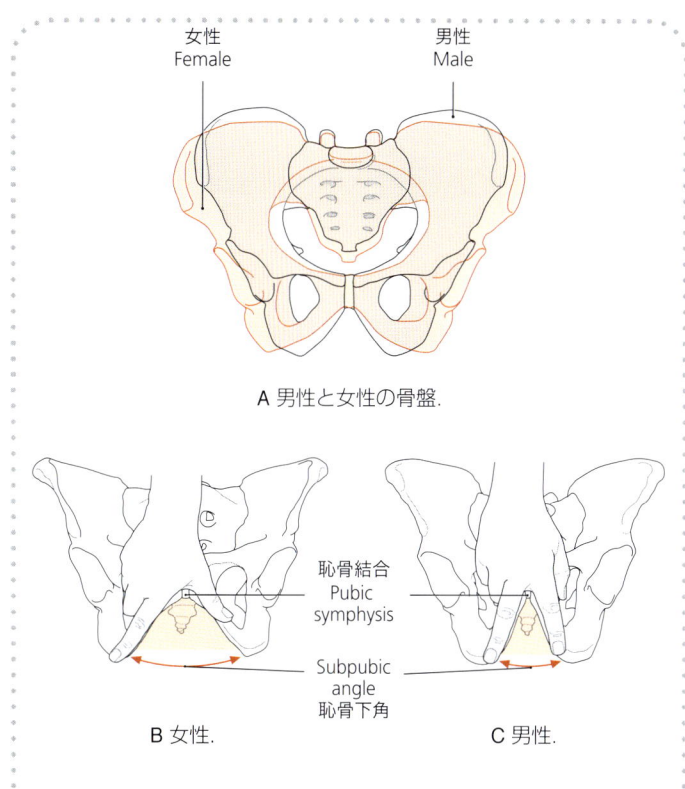

A　骨盤計測.
- 腸骨結節間径 Transtubercular distance
- Interspinous distance 上前腸骨棘間径
- 骨盤上口 Pelvic inlet plane

B　男性骨盤.
- 腸骨稜 Iliac crest（内唇 Inner lip／中間線 Intermediate line／外唇 Outer lip）
- 正中仙骨稜 Median sacral crest
- 上関節突起 Superior articular process
- 仙骨翼 Ala of sacrum
- Iliac fossa 腸骨窩
- Base of sacrum 仙骨底
- Anterior superior and inferior iliac spines 上・下前腸骨棘
- Pecten pubis 恥骨櫛
- Iliopubic eminence 腸恥隆起
- 弓状線 Arcuate line
- Ischial spine 坐骨棘
- Pubic symphysis 恥骨結合

A　男性と女性の骨盤.
- 女性 Female
- 男性 Male

B　女性.　C　男性.
- 恥骨結合 Pubic symphysis
- Subpubic angle 恥骨下角

表 10.1　骨盤の性差

構造	♀	♂
大骨盤	幅広く浅い	狭く深い
骨盤上口	横長楕円形	ハート型
骨盤下口	広く円い	狭く細長い
坐骨結節	外向き	内向き
骨盤腔	広く浅い	狭く深い
仙骨	短く，幅広く，平ら	長く，狭く，湾曲
恥骨下角	90-100°	70°

臨床

出産

母体の骨盤と胎児の頭部の大きさの関係が好ましくない場合は，出産時に合併症が起こる可能性があり，帝王切開が必要となる場合がある．母体側の原因には，初期の骨盤外傷や先天性奇形が含まれる．胎児側の原因には脳脊髄液の循環障害による脳の膨張と頭蓋の拡大を起こす水頭症が含まれる．

骨盤の靱帯
Pelvic Ligaments

腹部・骨盤

図 10.9　骨盤の靱帯
男性骨盤.

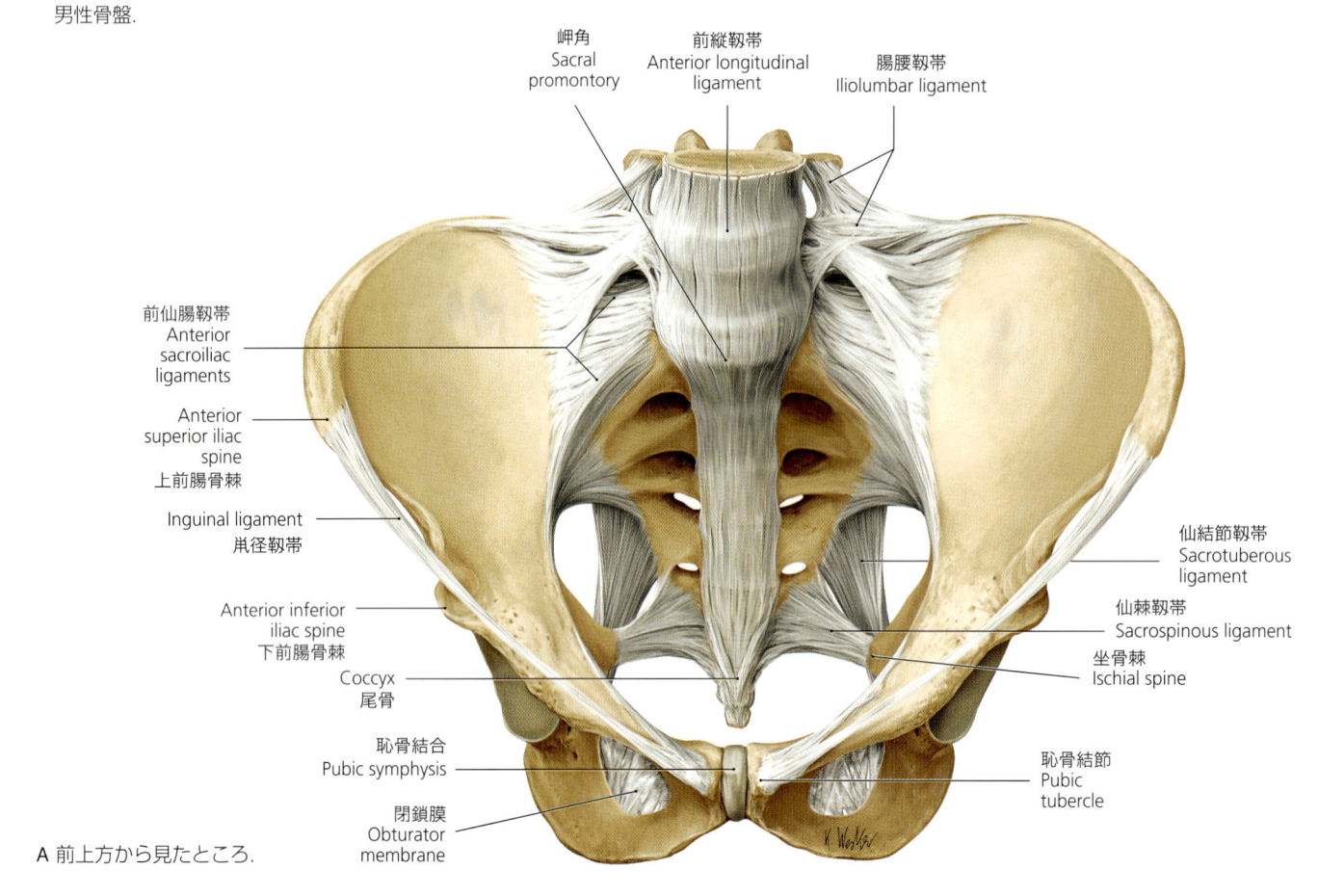

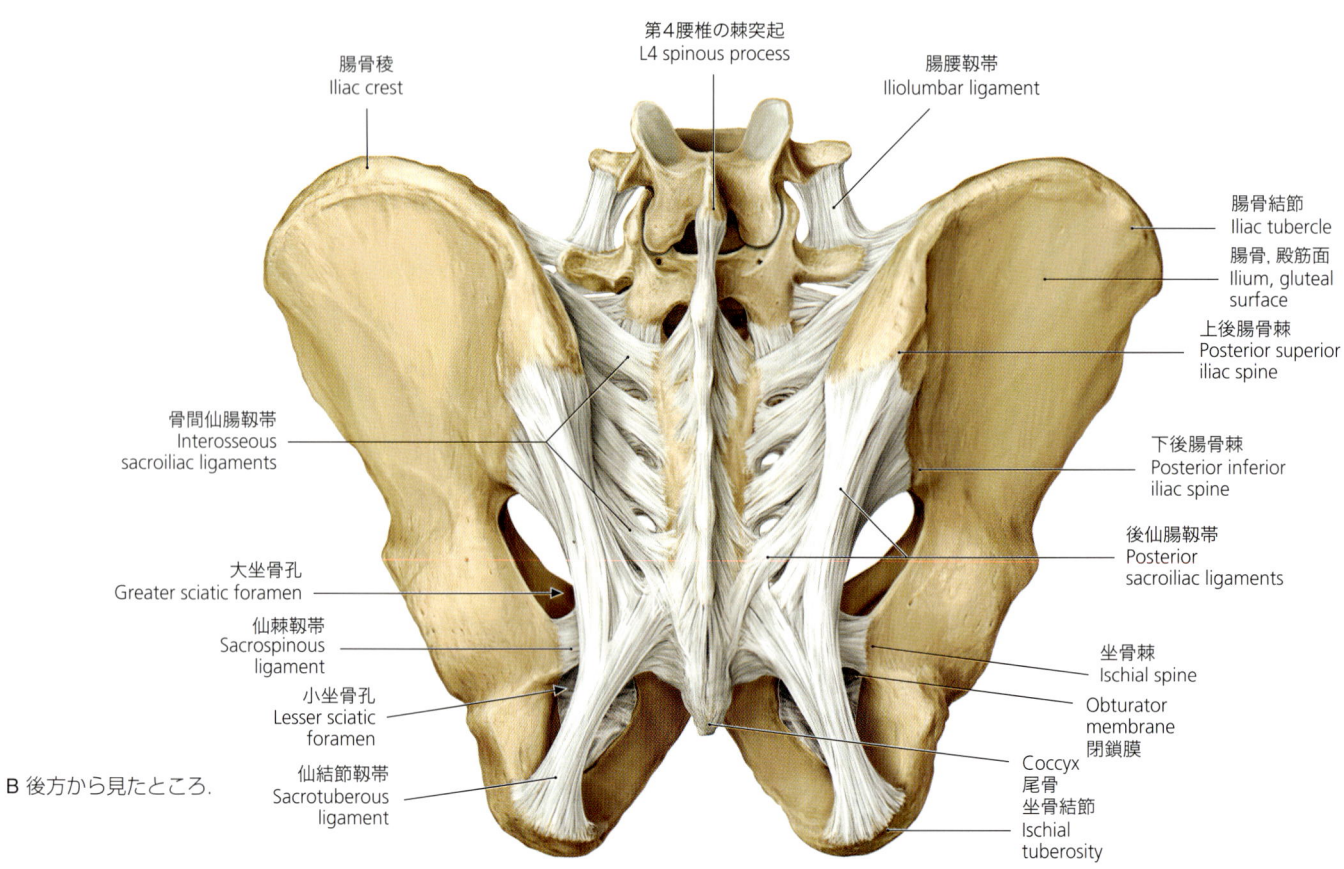

岬角　Sacral promontory
前縦靱帯　Anterior longitudinal ligament
腸腰靱帯　Iliolumbar ligament
前仙腸靱帯　Anterior sacroiliac ligaments
上前腸骨棘　Anterior superior iliac spine
鼠径靱帯　Inguinal ligament
下前腸骨棘　Anterior inferior iliac spine
尾骨　Coccyx
恥骨結合　Pubic symphysis
閉鎖膜　Obturator membrane
仙結節靱帯　Sacrotuberous ligament
仙棘靱帯　Sacrospinous ligament
坐骨棘　Ischial spine
恥骨結節　Pubic tubercle

A 前上方から見たところ.

第4腰椎の棘突起　L4 spinous process
腸骨稜　Iliac crest
腸腰靱帯　Iliolumbar ligament
腸骨結節　Iliac tubercle
腸骨，殿筋面　Ilium, gluteal surface
上後腸骨棘　Posterior superior iliac spine
骨間仙腸靱帯　Interosseous sacroiliac ligaments
下後腸骨棘　Posterior inferior iliac spine
後仙腸靱帯　Posterior sacroiliac ligaments
大坐骨孔　Greater sciatic foramen
仙棘靱帯　Sacrospinous ligament
小坐骨孔　Lesser sciatic foramen
仙結節靱帯　Sacrotuberous ligament
坐骨棘　Ischial spine
閉鎖膜　Obturator membrane
尾骨　Coccyx
坐骨結節　Ischial tuberosity

B 後方から見たところ.

図10.10 仙腸関節の靱帯
男性骨盤.

図10.11 骨盤の計測
女性骨盤の右半分，内側方から見たところ．
表10.1参照．

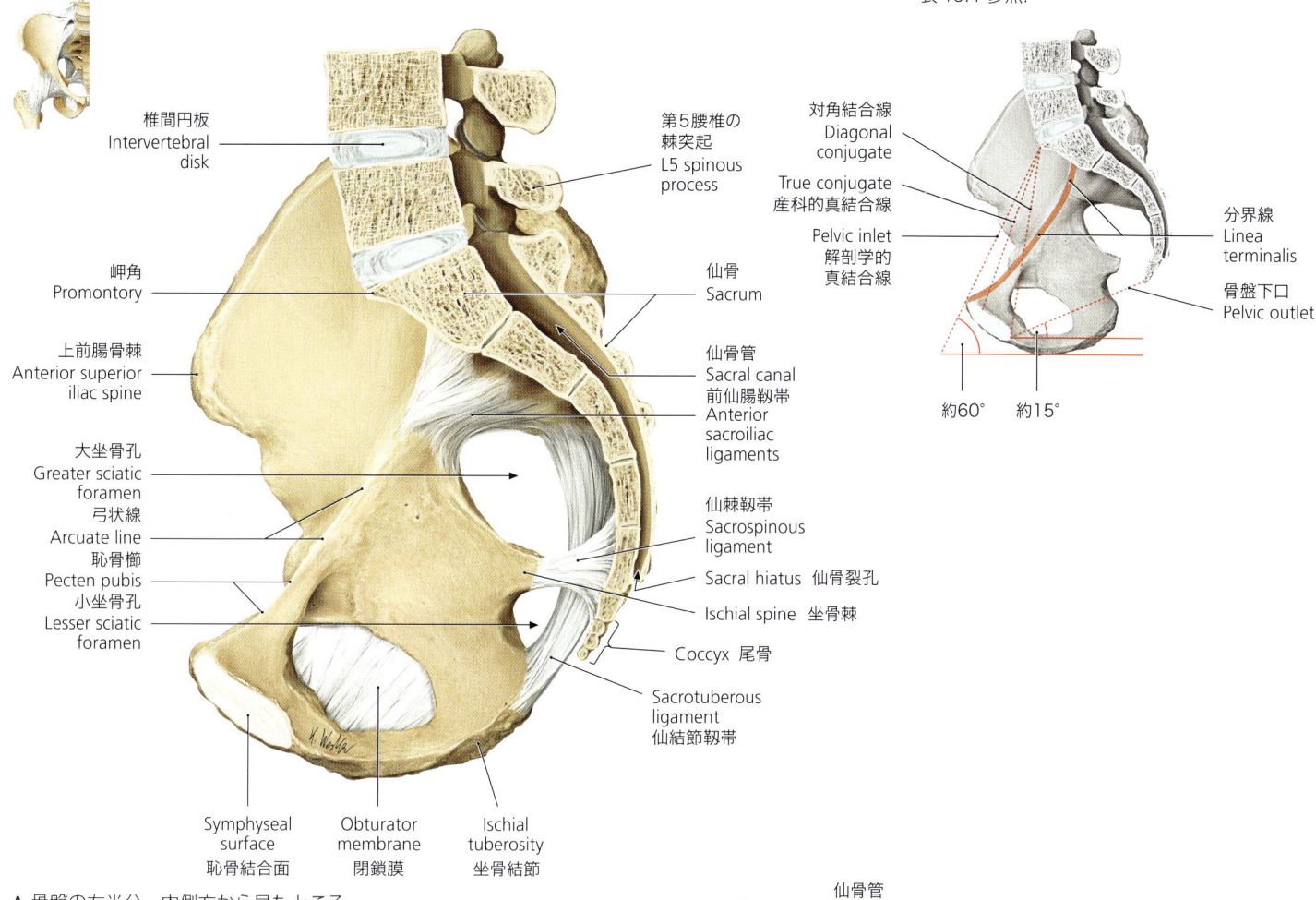

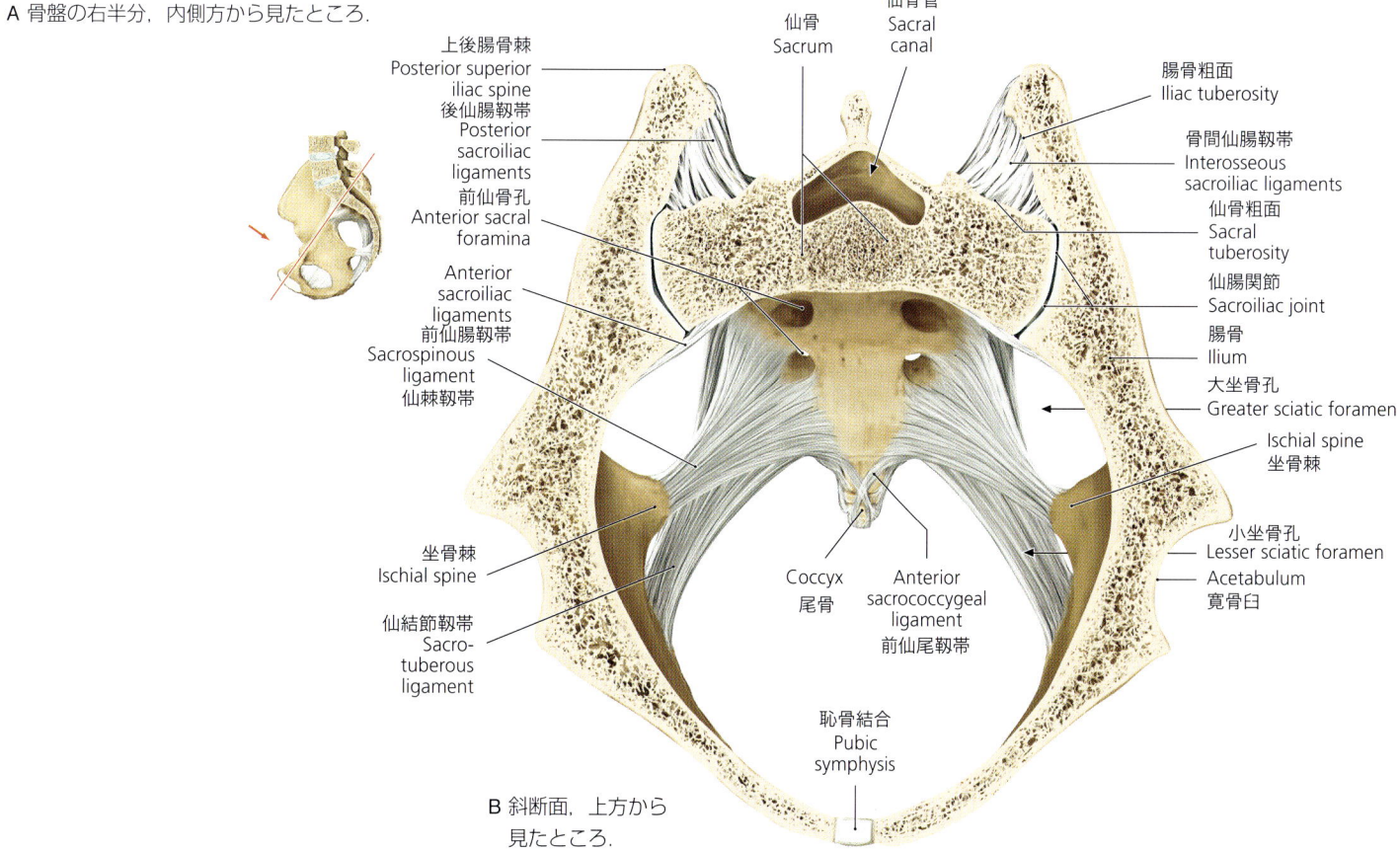

図10.10 ラベル（左図）:
- 椎間円板 Intervertebral disk
- 岬角 Promontory
- 上前腸骨棘 Anterior superior iliac spine
- 大坐骨孔 Greater sciatic foramen
- 弓状線 Arcuate line
- 恥骨櫛 Pecten pubis
- 小坐骨孔 Lesser sciatic foramen
- 第5腰椎の棘突起 L5 spinous process
- 仙骨 Sacrum
- 仙骨管 Sacral canal
- 前仙腸靱帯 Anterior sacroiliac ligaments
- 仙棘靱帯 Sacrospinous ligament
- 仙骨裂孔 Sacral hiatus
- 坐骨棘 Ischial spine
- 尾骨 Coccyx
- 仙結節靱帯 Sacrotuberous ligament
- 恥骨結合面 Symphyseal surface
- 閉鎖膜 Obturator membrane
- 坐骨結節 Ischial tuberosity

A 骨盤の右半分，内側方から見たところ．

図10.11 ラベル:
- 対角結合線 Diagonal conjugate
- 産科的真結合線 True conjugate
- 解剖学的真結合線 Pelvic inlet
- 分界線 Linea terminalis
- 骨盤下口 Pelvic outlet
- 約60°　約15°

下図 B ラベル:
- 上後腸骨棘 Posterior superior iliac spine
- 後仙腸靱帯 Posterior sacroiliac ligaments
- 前仙骨孔 Anterior sacral foramina
- 前仙腸靱帯 Anterior sacroiliac ligaments
- 仙棘靱帯 Sacrospinous ligament
- 坐骨棘 Ischial spine
- 仙結節靱帯 Sacrotuberous ligament
- 仙骨 Sacrum
- 仙骨管 Sacral canal
- 尾骨 Coccyx
- 前仙尾靱帯 Anterior sacrococcygeal ligament
- 恥骨結合 Pubic symphysis
- 腸骨粗面 Iliac tuberosity
- 骨間仙腸靱帯 Interosseous sacroiliac ligaments
- 仙骨粗面 Sacral tuberosity
- 仙腸関節 Sacroiliac joint
- 腸骨 Ilium
- 大坐骨孔 Greater sciatic foramen
- 坐骨棘 Ischial spine
- 小坐骨孔 Lesser sciatic foramen
- 寛骨臼 Acetabulum

B 斜断面，上方から見たところ．

腹壁の筋
Muscles of the Abdominal Wall

腹壁の斜筋は外腹斜筋と内腹斜筋，腹横筋からなる．大腰筋が代表する．腹壁後方の深腹筋は機能的には下肢帯の筋である（p.138 参照）

図 11.1　腹壁の筋
右側，前方から見たところ．

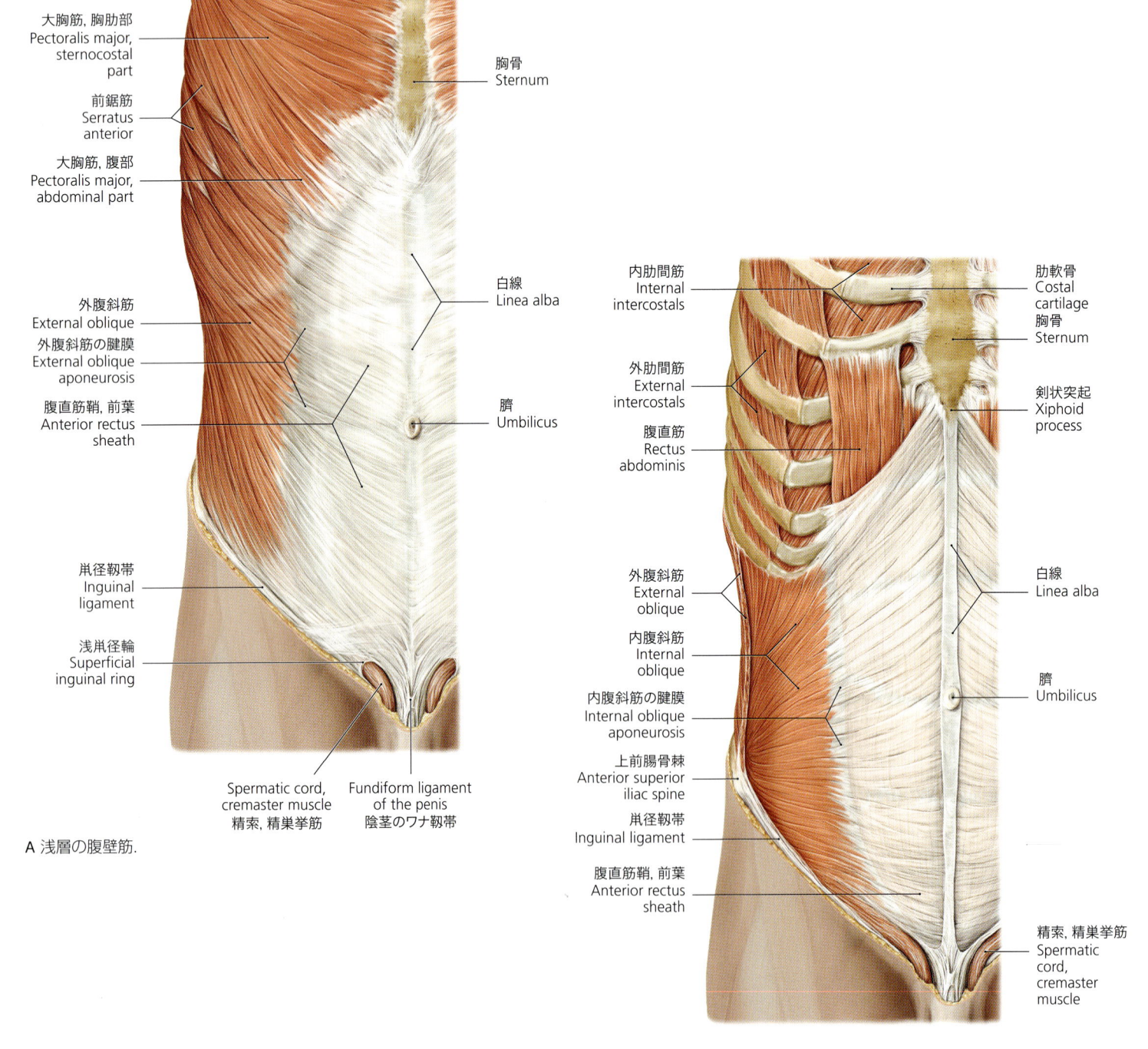

A 浅層の腹壁筋．

- 大胸筋, 胸肋部 Pectoralis major, sternocostal part
- 前鋸筋 Serratus anterior
- 大胸筋, 腹部 Pectoralis major, abdominal part
- 外腹斜筋 External oblique
- 外腹斜筋の腱膜 External oblique aponeurosis
- 腹直筋鞘, 前葉 Anterior rectus sheath
- 鼠径靱帯 Inguinal ligament
- 浅鼠径輪 Superficial inguinal ring
- 精索, 精巣挙筋 Spermatic cord, cremaster muscle
- 陰茎のワナ靱帯 Fundiform ligament of the penis
- 胸骨 Sternum
- 白線 Linea alba
- 臍 Umbilicus

B 外腹斜筋，大胸筋，前鋸筋は取り除いてある．

- 内肋間筋 Internal intercostals
- 外肋間筋 External intercostals
- 腹直筋 Rectus abdominis
- 外腹斜筋 External oblique
- 内腹斜筋 Internal oblique
- 内腹斜筋の腱膜 Internal oblique aponeurosis
- 上前腸骨棘 Anterior superior iliac spine
- 鼠径靱帯 Inguinal ligament
- 腹直筋鞘, 前葉 Anterior rectus sheath
- 肋軟骨 Costal cartilage
- 胸骨 Sternum
- 剣状突起 Xiphoid process
- 白線 Linea alba
- 臍 Umbilicus
- 精索, 精巣挙筋 Spermatic cord, cremaster muscle

C 内腹斜筋は取り除いてある.

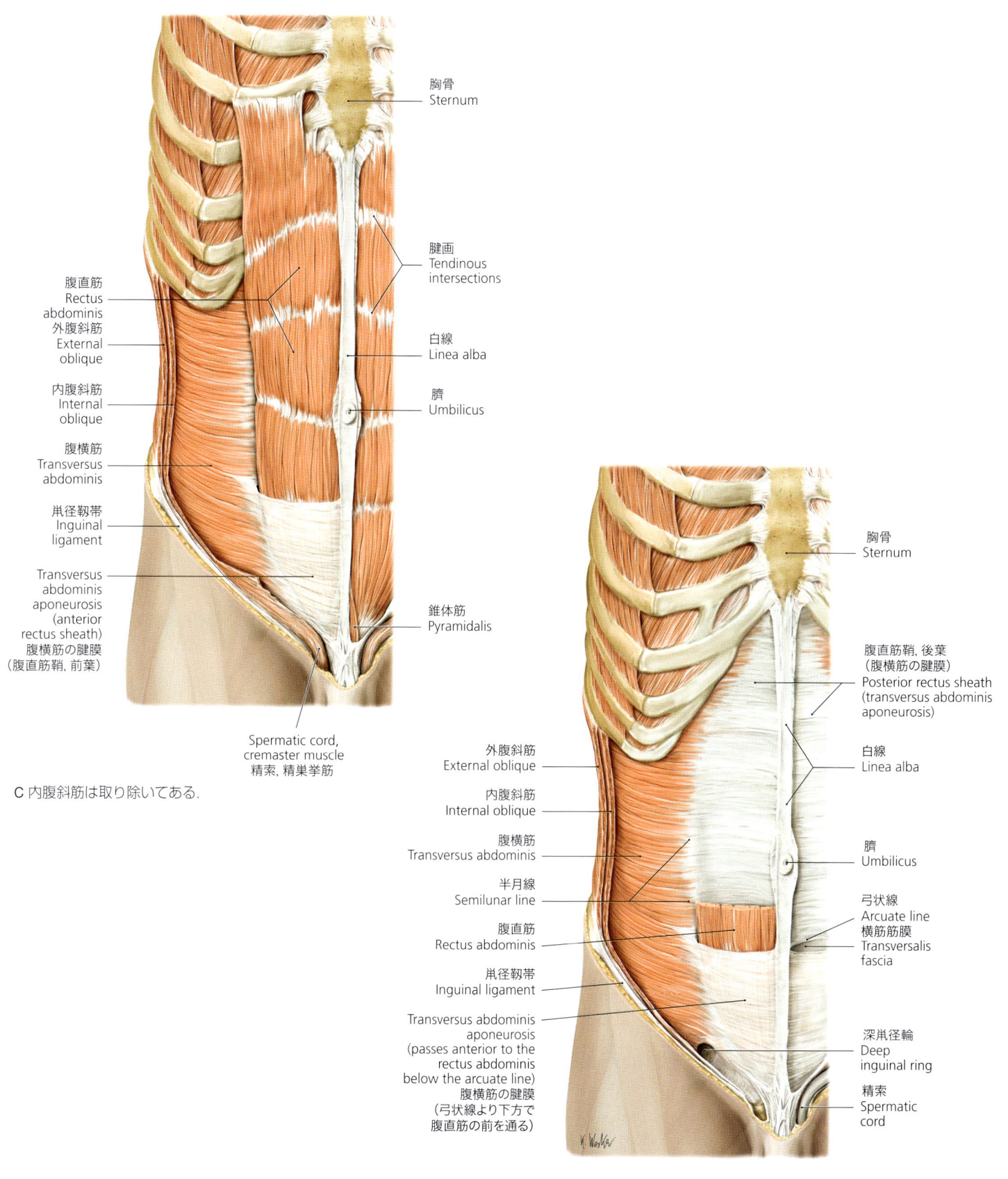

D 腹直筋は取り除いてある.

鼠径部と鼠径管
Inguinal Region & Canal

鼠径部は前腹壁と大腿前部の接合部である．鼠径管は腹腔へ構造（精索に含まれるものなど）が出入りするための重要な場所である．

図 11.2 鼠径部
右側，前方から見たところ．

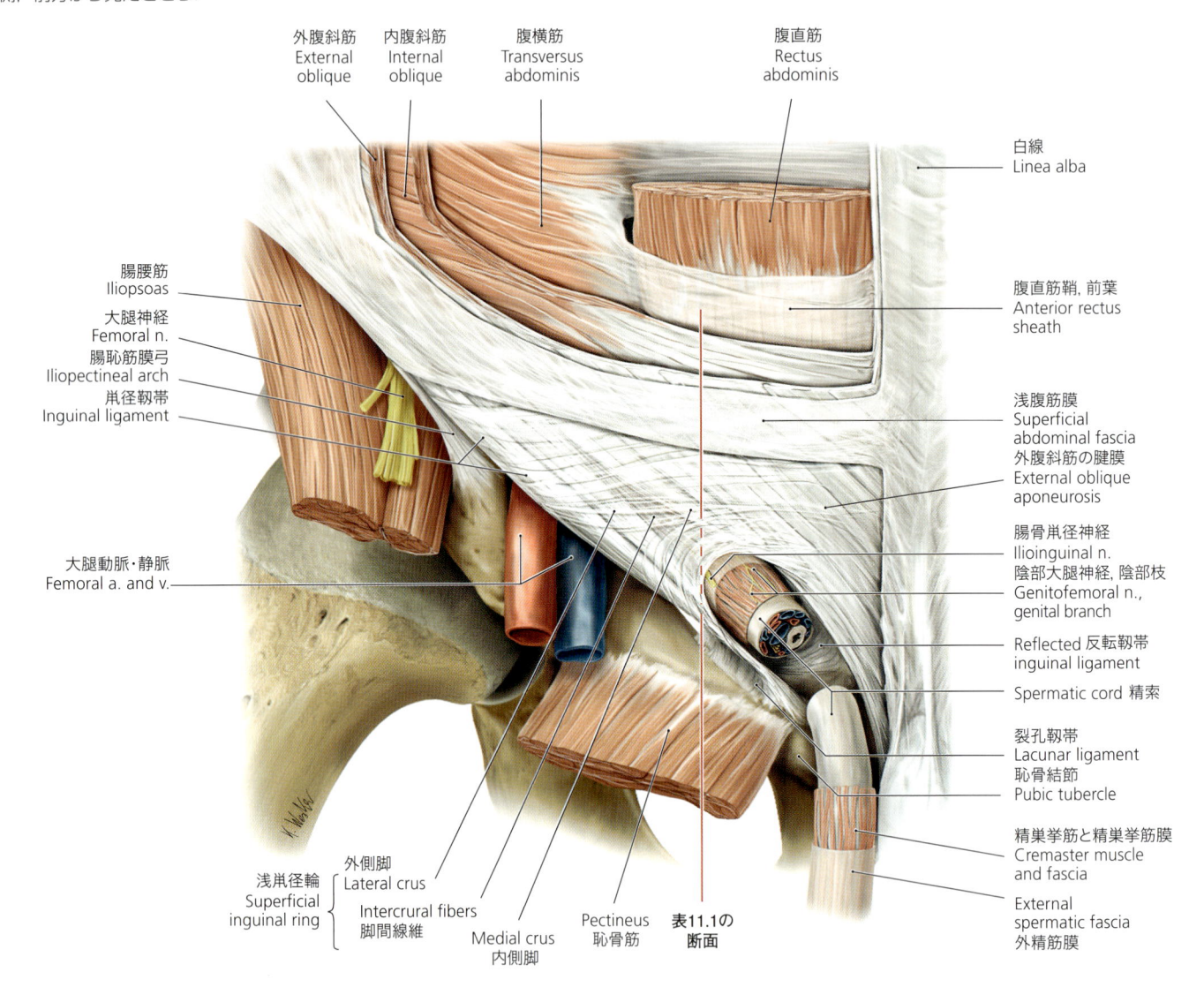

ラベル（上部、左から右）:
- 外腹斜筋 External oblique
- 内腹斜筋 Internal oblique
- 腹横筋 Transversus abdominis
- 腹直筋 Rectus abdominis

ラベル（左側）:
- 腸腰筋 Iliopsoas
- 大腿神経 Femoral n.
- 腸恥筋膜弓 Iliopectineal arch
- 鼠径靱帯 Inguinal ligament
- 大腿動脈・静脈 Femoral a. and v.

ラベル（下部）:
- 外側脚 Lateral crus
- 浅鼠径輪 Superficial inguinal ring
- 脚間線維 Intercrural fibers
- 内側脚 Medial crus
- 恥骨筋 Pectineus
- 表11.1の断面

ラベル（右側、上から下）:
- 白線 Linea alba
- 腹直筋鞘, 前葉 Anterior rectus sheath
- 浅腹筋膜 Superficial abdominal fascia
- 外腹斜筋の腱膜 External oblique aponeurosis
- 腸骨鼠径神経 Ilioinguinal n.
- 陰部大腿神経, 陰部枝 Genitofemoral n., genital branch
- 反転靱帯 Reflected inguinal ligament
- 精索 Spermatic cord
- 裂孔靱帯 Lacunar ligament
- 恥骨結節 Pubic tubercle
- 精巣挙筋と精巣挙筋膜 Cremaster muscle and fascia
- 外精筋膜 External spermatic fascia

表 11.1　鼠径管の構造

構造		構成
壁	前壁	① 外腹斜筋腱膜
	上壁	② 内腹斜筋
		③ 腹横筋
	後壁	④ 横筋筋膜
		⑤ 壁側腹膜
	下壁	⑥ 鼠径靱帯（外腹斜筋腱膜下部と付近の大腿筋膜の線維が密に絡み合っている）
開口部	浅鼠径輪	外腹斜筋腱膜に開口．内側脚と外側脚，脚間線維，反転靱帯に囲まれる
	深鼠径輪	外側臍ヒダ（下腹壁動静脈）の外側で横筋筋膜に開口．

図 11.2 の矢状断面．

図 11.3　鼠径管の切開
右側，前方から見たところ．

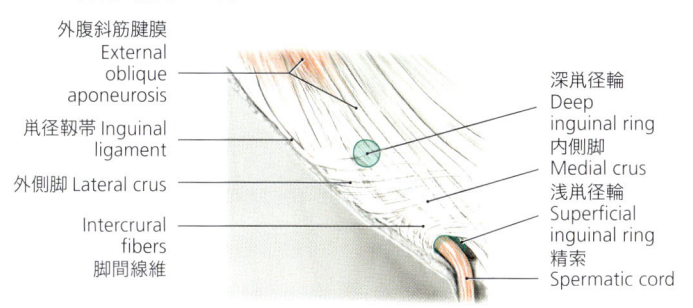

A 表層．

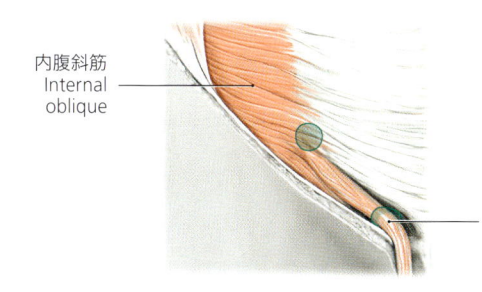

B 外腹斜筋腱膜は取り除いてある．

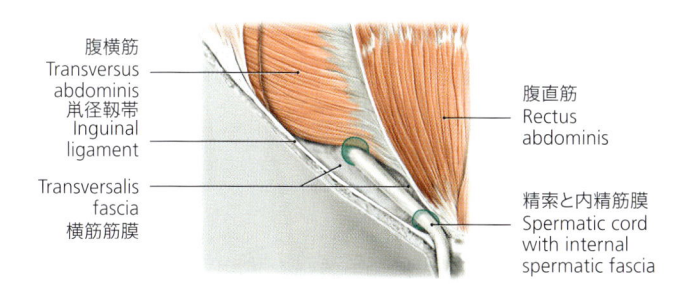

C 内腹斜筋は取り除いてある．

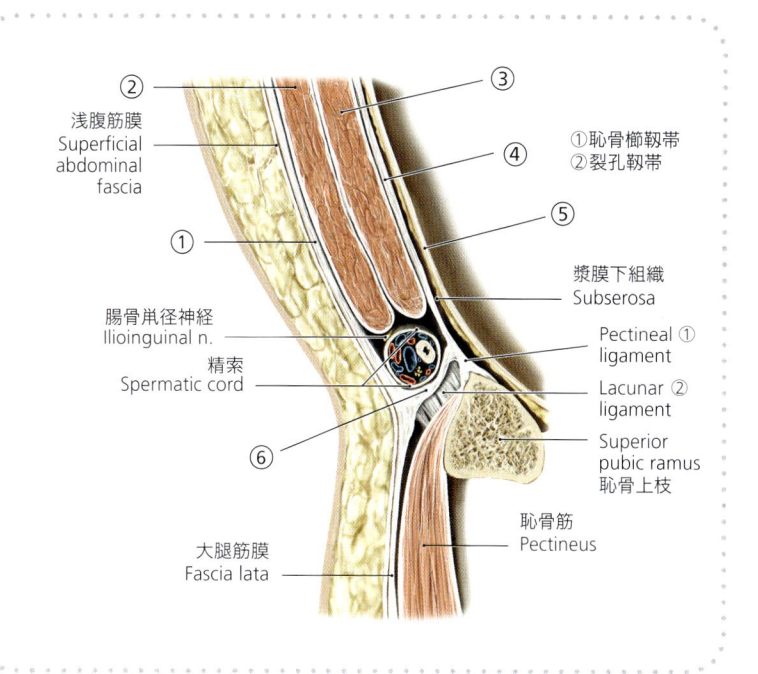

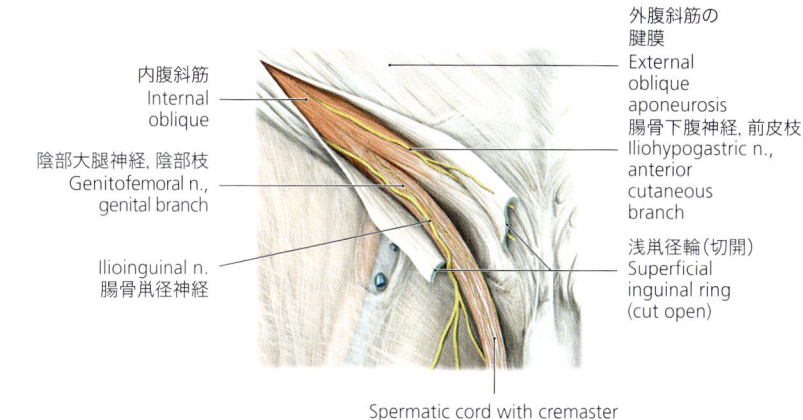

図 11.4　鼠径管の開口部
右側，前方から見たところ．

A 外腹斜筋腱膜を切開．

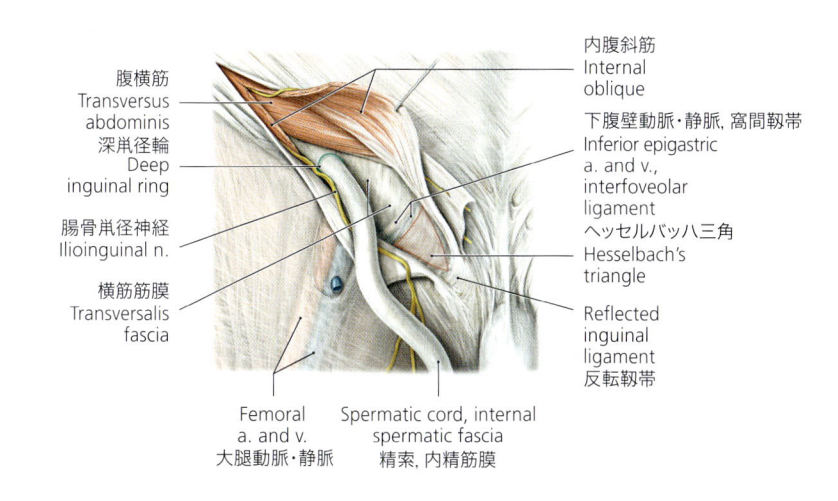

B 内腹斜筋と精巣挙筋を切開．

腹壁と鼠径ヘルニア
Abdominal Wall & Inguinal Hernias

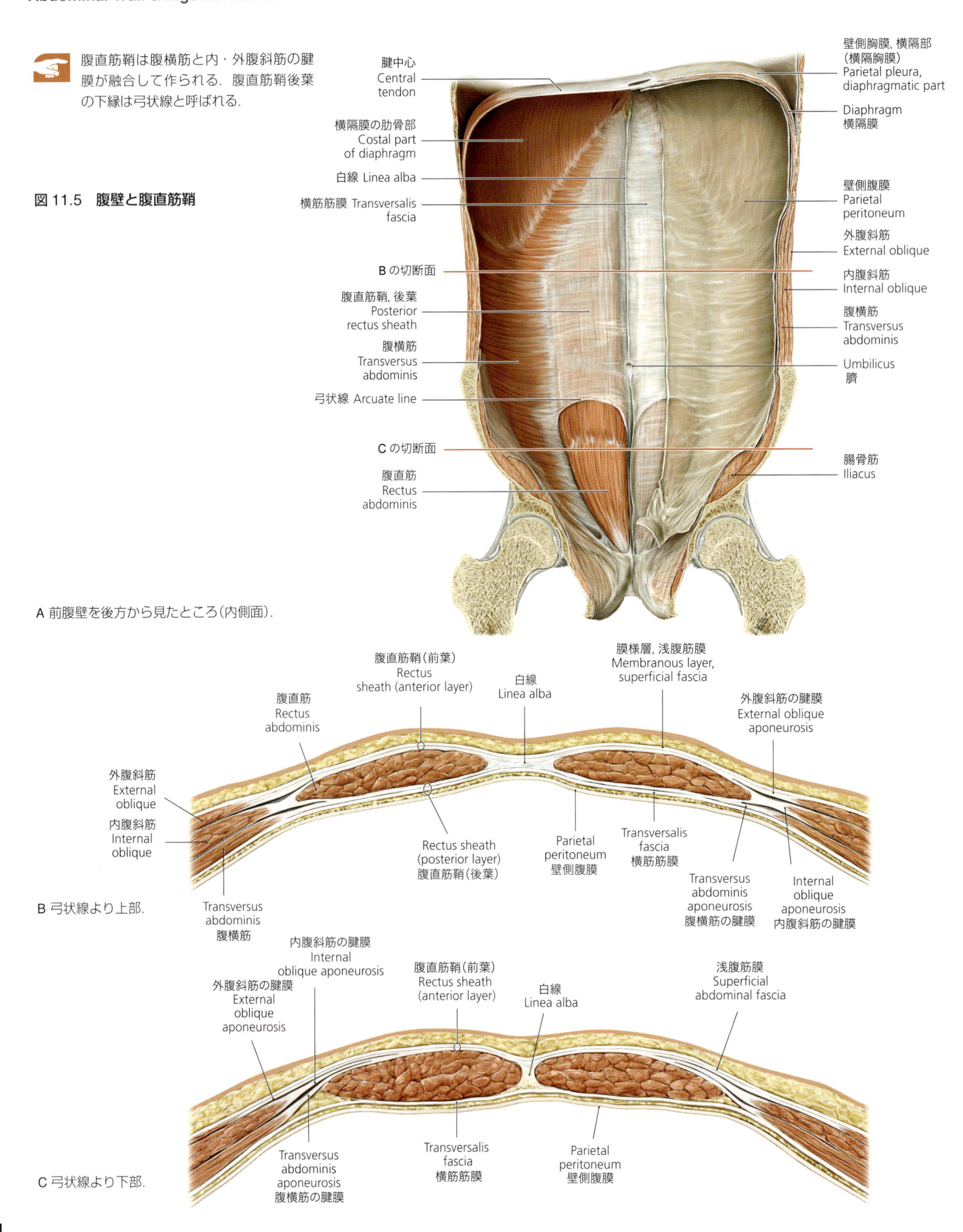

腹直筋鞘は腹横筋と内・外腹斜筋の腱膜が融合して作られる．腹直筋鞘後葉の下縁は弓状線と呼ばれる．

図11.5 腹壁と腹直筋鞘

腱中心 Central tendon
横隔膜の肋骨部 Costal part of diaphragm
白線 Linea alba
横筋筋膜 Transversalis fascia
Bの切断面
腹直筋鞘, 後葉 Posterior rectus sheath
腹横筋 Transversus abdominis
弓状線 Arcuate line
Cの切断面
腹直筋 Rectus abdominis

壁側胸膜, 横隔部（横隔胸膜）Parietal pleura, diaphragmatic part
横隔膜 Diaphragm
壁側腹膜 Parietal peritoneum
外腹斜筋 External oblique
内腹斜筋 Internal oblique
腹横筋 Transversus abdominis
臍 Umbilicus
腸骨筋 Iliacus

A 前腹壁を後方から見たところ（内側面）．

腹直筋鞘（前葉）Rectus sheath (anterior layer)
白線 Linea alba
膜様層, 浅腹筋膜 Membranous layer, superficial fascia
外腹斜筋の腱膜 External oblique aponeurosis
腹直筋 Rectus abdominis
外腹斜筋 External oblique
内腹斜筋 Internal oblique
Rectus sheath (posterior layer) 腹直筋鞘（後葉）
Parietal peritoneum 壁側腹膜
Transversalis fascia 横筋筋膜
Transversus abdominis aponeurosis 腹横筋の腱膜
Internal oblique aponeurosis 内腹斜筋の腱膜
Transversus abdominis 腹横筋

B 弓状線より上部．

内腹斜筋の腱膜 Internal oblique aponeurosis
外腹斜筋の腱膜 External oblique aponeurosis
腹直筋鞘（前葉）Rectus sheath (anterior layer)
白線 Linea alba
浅腹筋膜 Superficial abdominal fascia
Transversus abdominis aponeurosis 腹横筋の腱膜
Transversalis fascia 横筋筋膜
Parietal peritoneum 壁側腹膜

C 弓状線より下部．

図 11.6 腹壁：内側面の解剖

冠状断．後方から見たところ．円で示した前腹壁の3つの窩でヘルニアが起こる可能性がある．

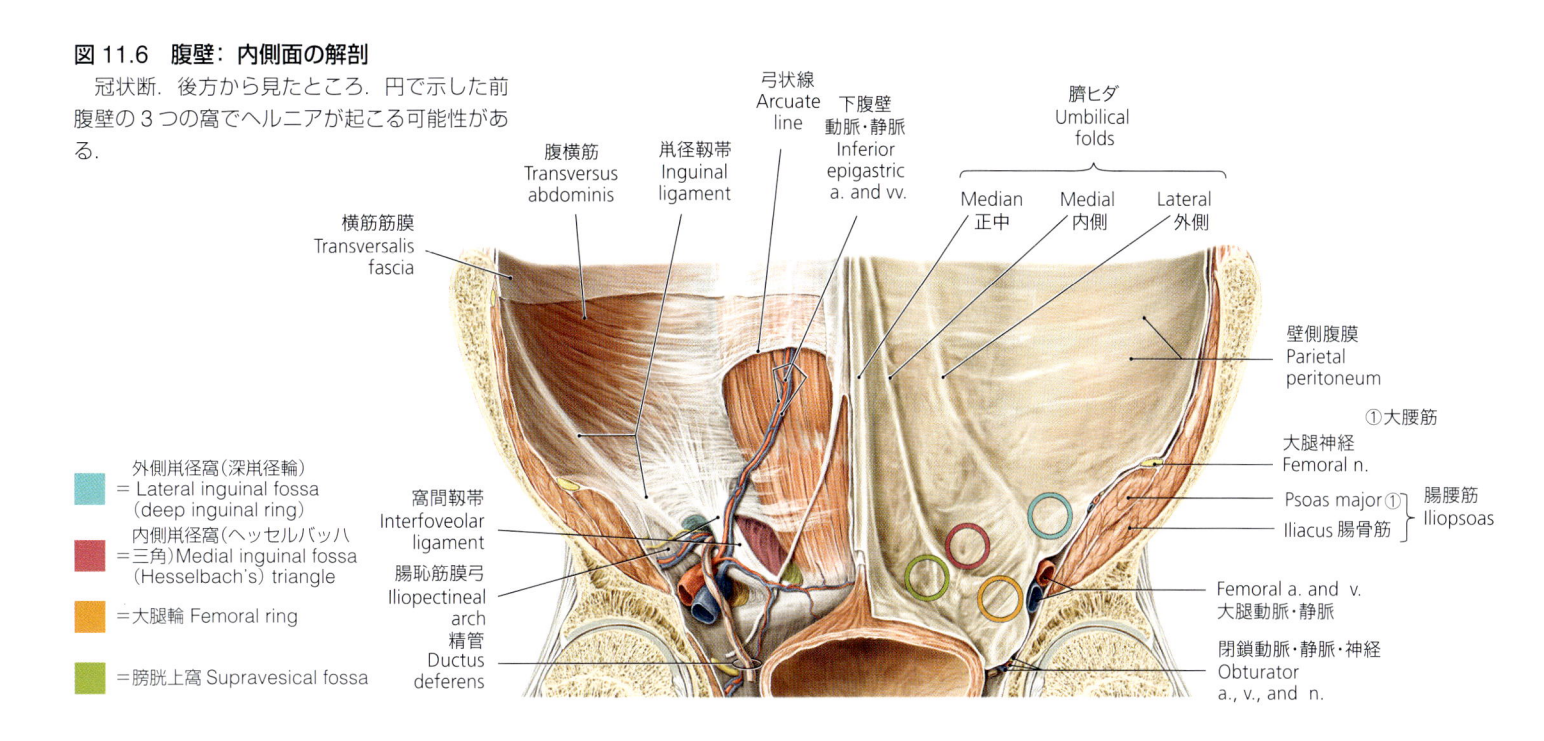

凡例:
- ■ 外側鼠径窩（深鼠径輪）= Lateral inguinal fossa (deep inguinal ring)
- ■ 内側鼠径窩（ヘッセルバッハ三角）Medial inguinal fossa (Hesselbach's) triangle
- ■ 大腿輪 Femoral ring
- ■ 膀胱上窩 Supravesical fossa

図中ラベル:
- 腹横筋 Transversus abdominis
- 鼠径靱帯 Inguinal ligament
- 弓状線 Arcuate line
- 下腹壁動脈・静脈 Inferior epigastric a. and vv.
- 臍ヒダ Umbilical folds
  - 正中 Median
  - 内側 Medial
  - 外側 Lateral
- 横筋筋膜 Transversalis fascia
- 壁側腹膜 Parietal peritoneum
- 大腰筋
- 大腿神経 Femoral n.
- Psoas major ① ┐ 腸腰筋 Iliopsoas
- Iliacus 腸骨筋 ┘
- 窩間靱帯 Interfoveolar ligament
- 腸恥筋膜弓 Iliopectineal arch
- 精管 Ductus deferens
- 大腿動脈・静脈 Femoral a. and v.
- 閉鎖動脈・静脈・神経 Obturator a., v., and n.

臨床

鼠径ヘルニア・大腿ヘルニア

間接鼠径ヘルニアは若い男性に起こり，先天性または後天性である．直接鼠径ヘルニアは常に後天性である．大腿ヘルニアは後天性で女性に多い．

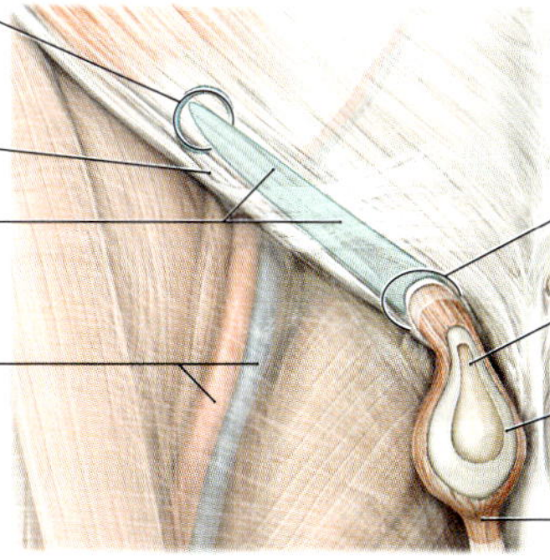

A 間接鼠径ヘルニア．
- 深鼠径輪 Deep inguinal ring
- 鼠径靱帯 Inguinal l.
- 鼠径管 Inguinal canal
- 大腿動脈・静脈 Femoral a. and vv.
- 浅鼠径輪 Superficial inguinal ring
- ヘルニア嚢の壁側腹膜 Peritoneum of hernial sac
- 横筋筋膜（=内精筋膜）Transversalis fascia (= internal spermatic fascia)
- 精巣挙筋と精索 Cremaster muscle and spermatic cord

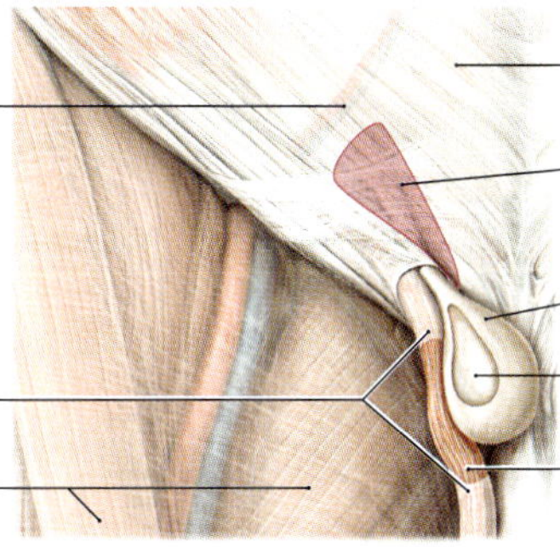

B 直接鼠径ヘルニア．
- 下腹壁動脈・静脈 Inferior epigastric a. and v.
- 精巣挙筋膜 Cremasteric fascia
- 縫工筋と恥骨筋，大腿筋膜 Sartorius and pectineus under fascia lata
- 外腹斜筋の腱膜 External oblique aponeurosis
- Location of ① Hesselbach's triangle
- 横筋筋膜 Transversalis fascia
- Peritoneum ② of hernial sac
- 精巣挙筋と精索 Cremaster muscle and spermatic cord
- ①ヘッセルバッハ三角の位置
- ②ヘルニア嚢の壁側腹膜

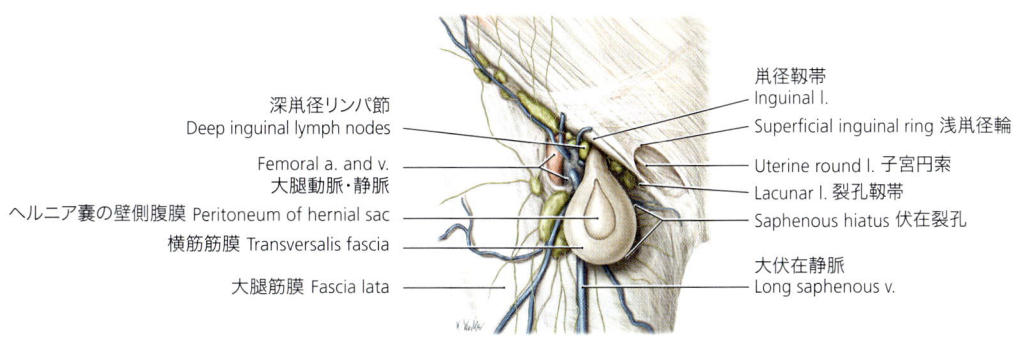

C 大腿ヘルニア．
- 深鼠径リンパ節 Deep inguinal lymph nodes
- 大腿動脈・静脈 Femoral a. and v.
- ヘルニア嚢の壁側腹膜 Peritoneum of hernial sac
- 横筋筋膜 Transversalis fascia
- 大腿筋膜 Fascia lata
- 鼠径靱帯 Inguinal l.
- 浅鼠径輪 Superficial inguinal ring
- 子宮円索 Uterine round l.
- 裂孔靱帯 Lacunar l.
- 伏在裂孔 Saphenous hiatus
- 大伏在静脈 Long saphenous v.

会陰部
Perineal Region

図 11.7 会陰と骨盤底：女性
切石位．尾側（下方）から見たところ．外生殖器については p.192 参照．

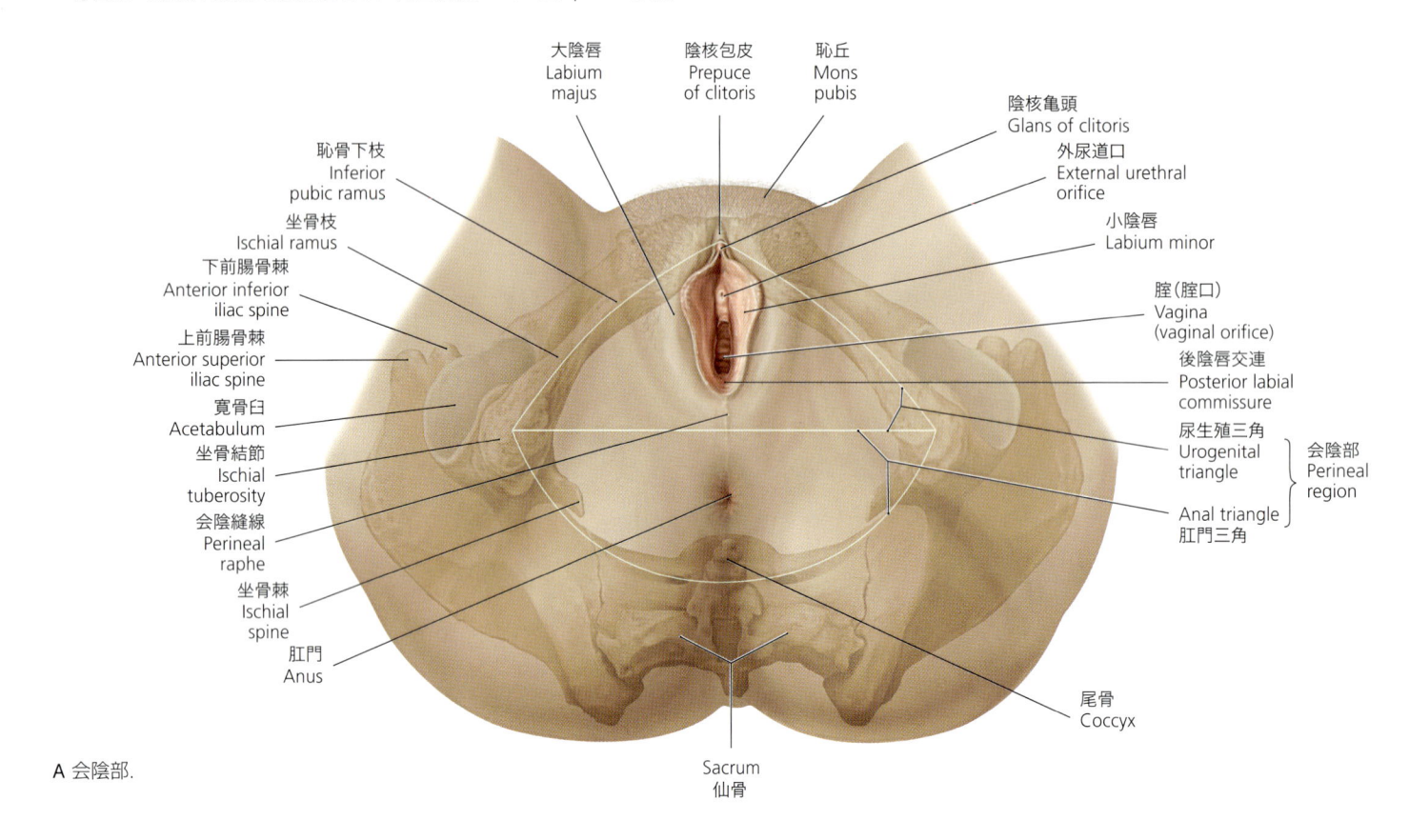

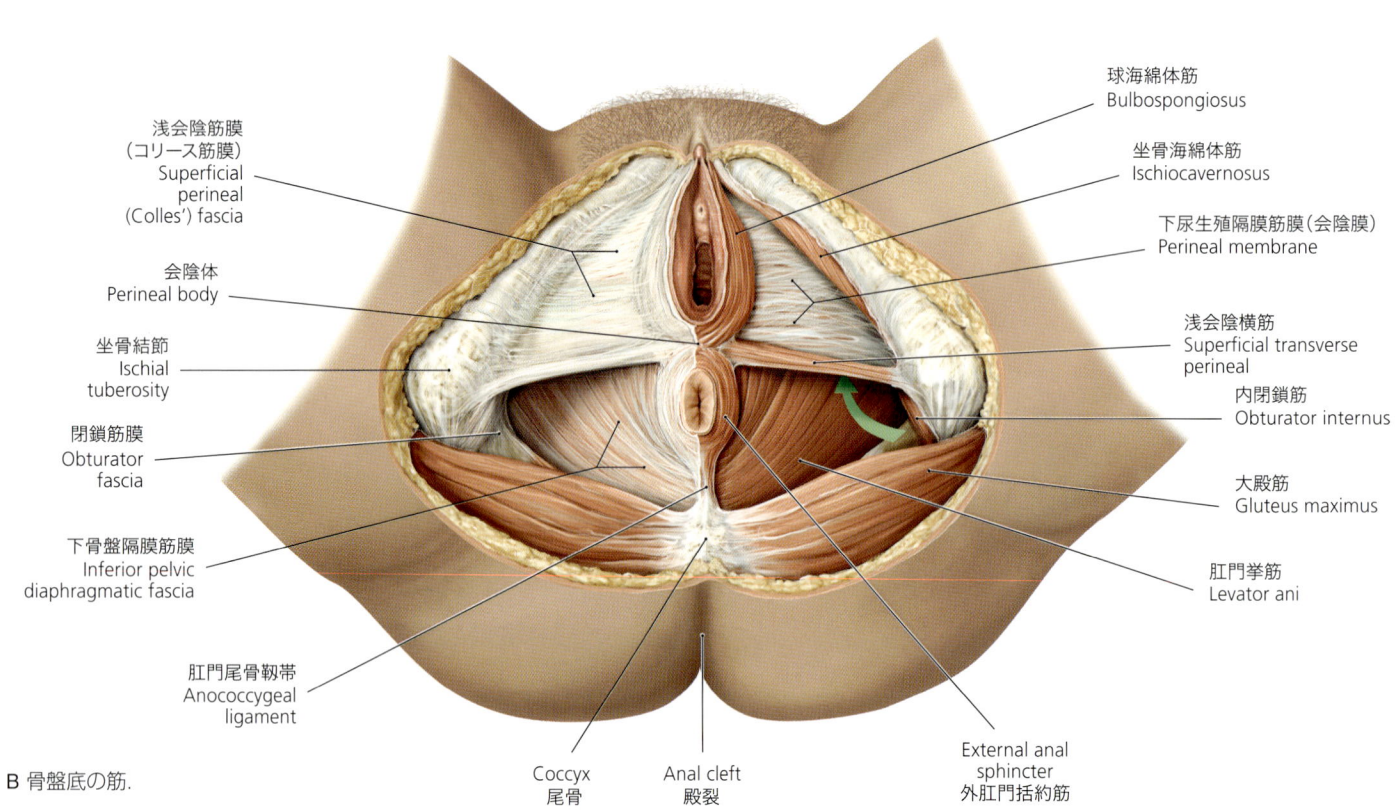

A 会陰部．

B 骨盤底の筋．

男女を問わず会陰の左右の境界は恥骨結節，坐骨恥骨枝，坐骨結節，仙結節靱帯，尾骨である．緑の矢印は，尿生殖隔膜上方の坐骨肛門窩の前方への陥凹を示している．

図11.8　会陰と骨盤底：男性

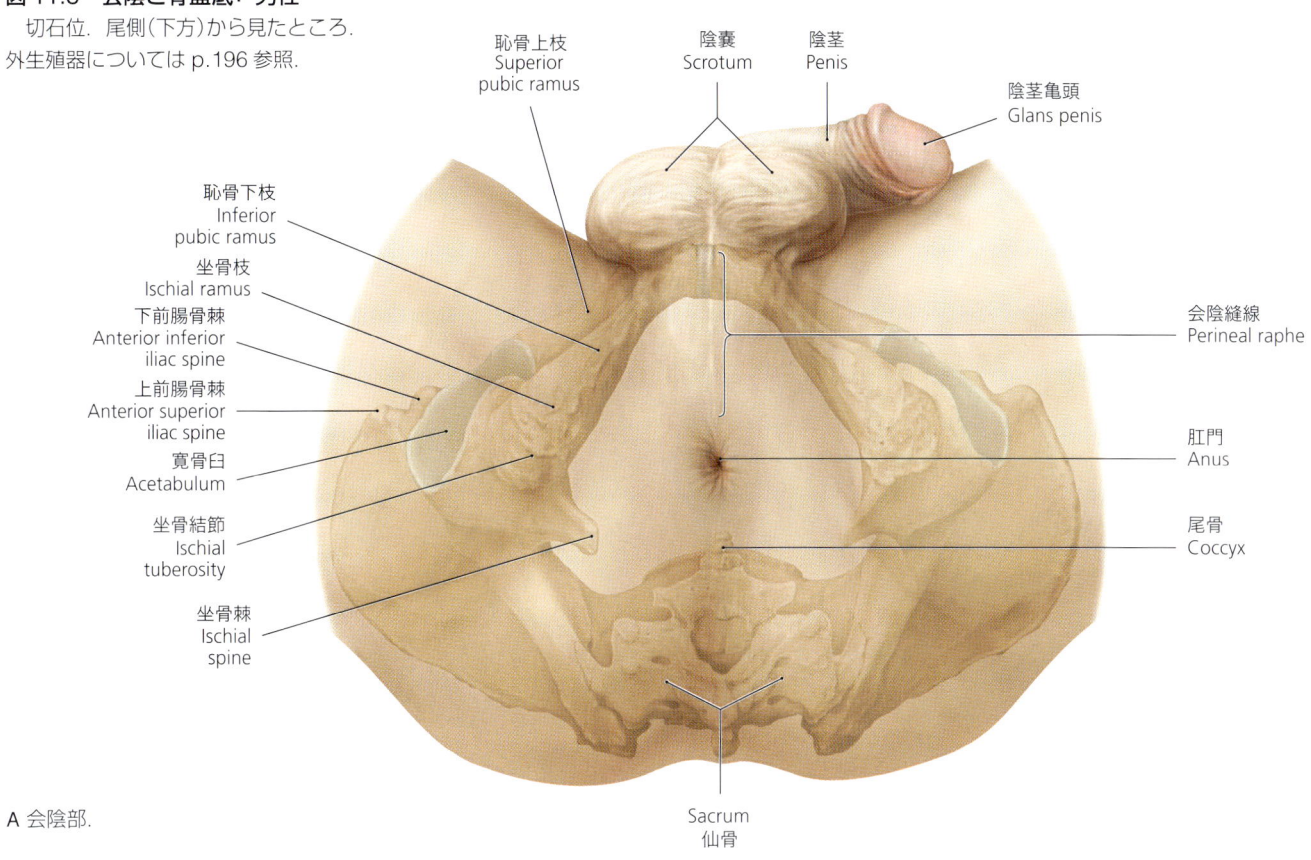

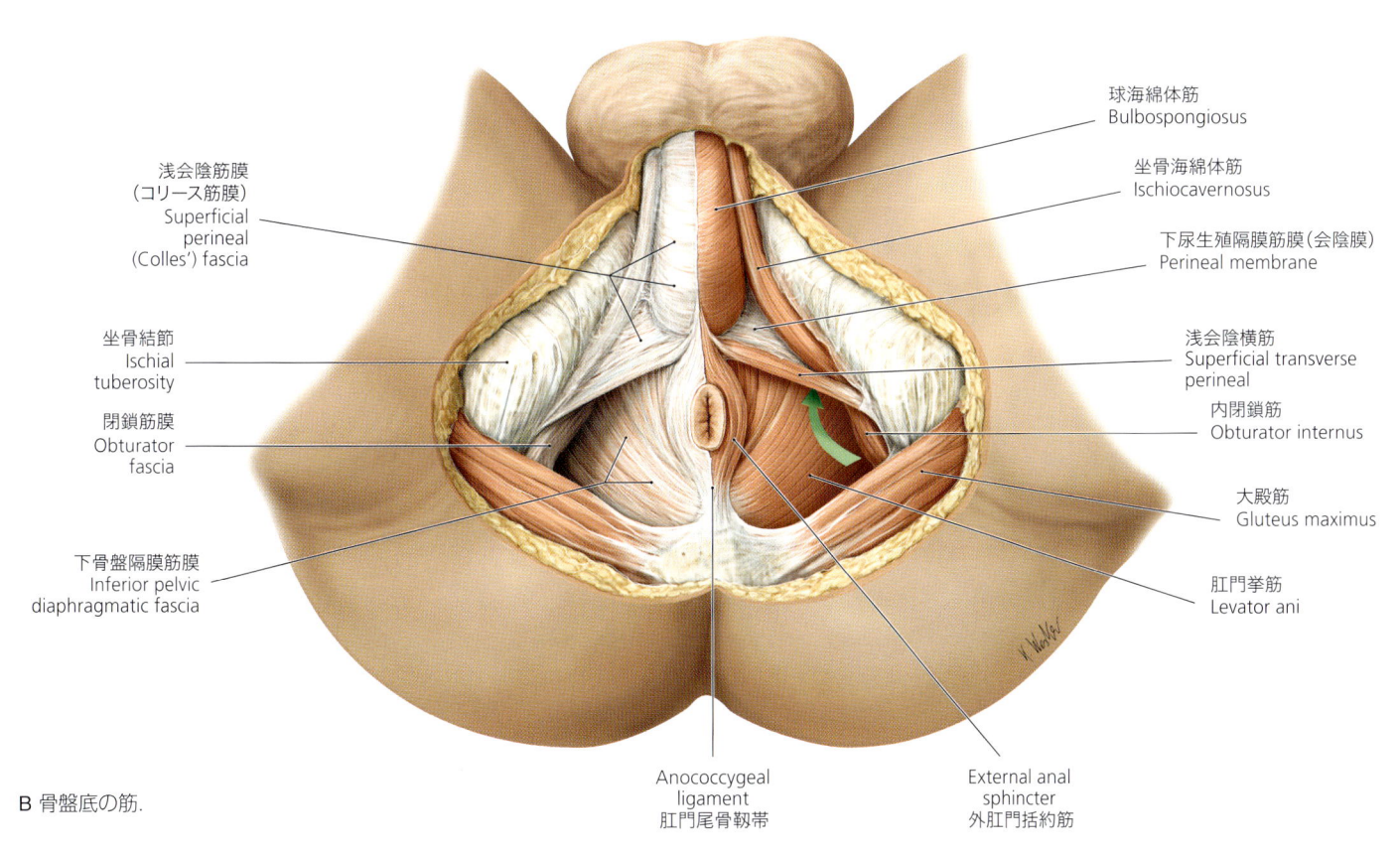

切石位．尾側（下方）から見たところ．
外生殖器については p.196 参照．

A 会陰部．

B 骨盤底の筋．

腹壁の筋
Abdominal Wall Muscle Facts

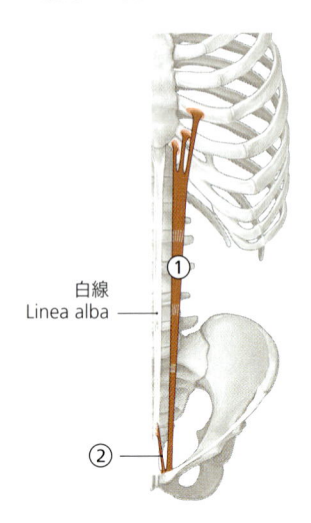

図 11.9　前筋
前方から見たところ.

白線
Linea alba

図 11.10　前外側筋
前方から見たところ.

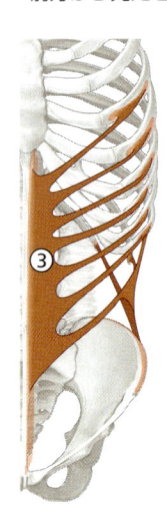

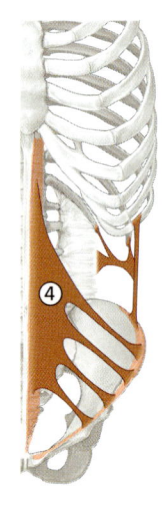

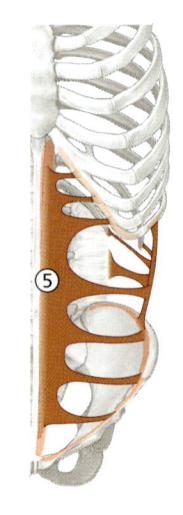

A 外腹斜筋.　　B 内腹斜筋.　　C 腹横筋.

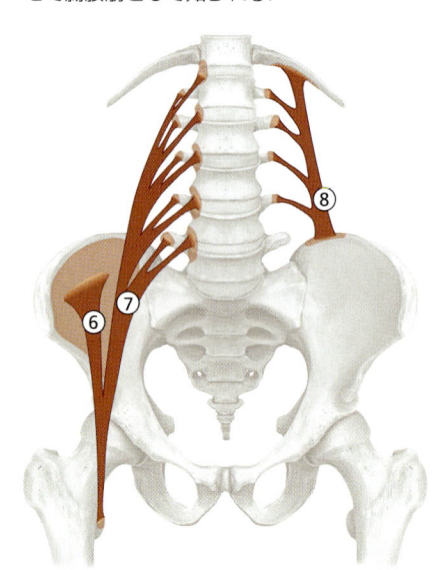

図 11.11　後筋
前方から見たところ. 大腰筋と腸骨筋は併せて腸腰筋として知られる.

表 11.2　腹壁の筋

筋		起始	停止	支配神経	作用
前腹壁の筋					
①腹直筋		恥骨(恥骨結節と恥骨結合の間)	第5-7肋軟骨, 胸骨剣状突起	肋間神経(T5-T12)	体幹の屈曲, 腹圧を高める, 骨盤の固定
②錐体筋		恥骨(腹直筋の前方)	白線(腹直筋鞘内を走る)	肋下神経(第12肋間神経)	白線の緊張
前外側腹壁の筋					
③外腹斜筋		第5-12肋骨(外側面)	白線, 恥骨結節, 前腸骨稜	肋間神経(T7-T12)	片側: 体幹を同側に曲げる, 体幹を反対側に回旋させる 両側: 体幹の屈曲, 腹圧を高める, 骨盤の固定
④内腹斜筋		胸腰筋膜(深層), 腸骨稜(中間線), 上前腸骨棘	第10-12肋骨(下縁), 白線(前・後層)	肋間神経(T7-T12), 腸骨下腹神経, 腸骨鼠径神経	
⑤腹横筋		第7-12肋軟骨(内側面), 胸腰筋膜(深層), 腸骨稜, 上前腸骨棘(内唇), 腸腰筋膜	白線, 恥骨稜		片側: 体幹を同側に曲げる 両側: 腹圧を高める
後腹壁の筋					
⑥腸骨筋		腸骨窩	大腿骨(小転子), 腸腰筋として停止	大腿神経(L2-L4)	股関節: 屈曲と外転 腰椎(大腿骨を固定した場合): 片側: 収縮によって体幹を外側に曲げる 両側: 収縮によって体幹を仰臥位から起こす
⑦大腰筋	浅層	第12胸椎-第4腰椎椎体と椎間板(外側面)		腰神経叢からの直接の枝(L2-L4)	
	深層	第1-5腰椎(肋骨突起)			
⑧腰方形筋		腸骨稜と腸腰靱帯(図には示されない)	第12肋骨, 第1-4腰椎(横突起)	第12肋間神経, 第1-4腰神経	片側: 体幹を同側に曲げる 両側: いきみ, 呼出, 第12肋骨の固定

図 11.12 腹壁の前筋と後筋
前方から見たところ.

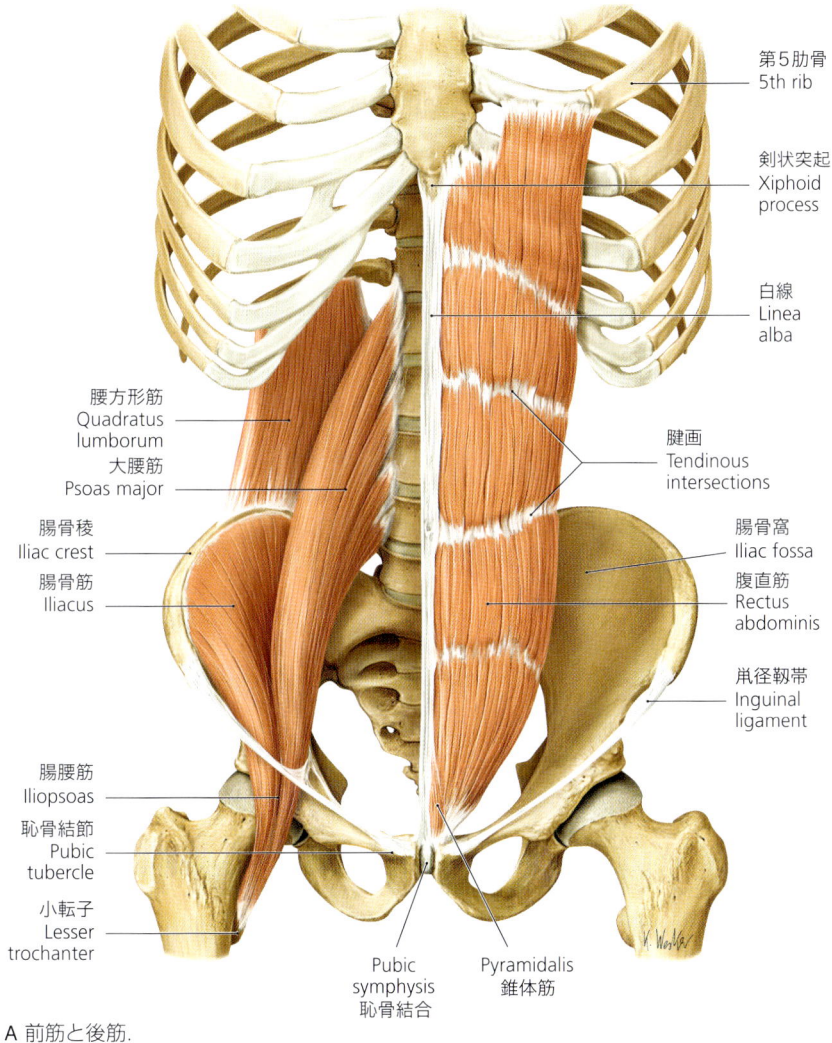

A 前筋と後筋.

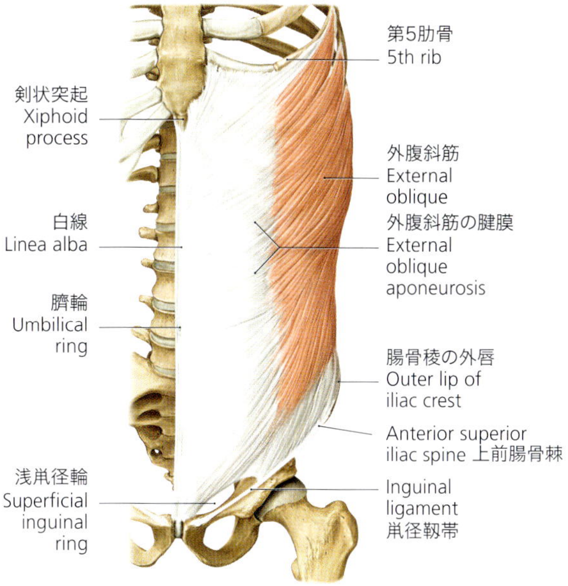

- 第5肋骨 / 5th rib
- 剣状突起 / Xiphoid process
- 白線 / Linea alba
- 腰方形筋 / Quadratus lumborum
- 大腰筋 / Psoas major
- 腱画 / Tendinous intersections
- 腸骨稜 / Iliac crest
- 腸骨筋 / Iliacus
- 腸骨窩 / Iliac fossa
- 腹直筋 / Rectus abdominis
- 鼠径靱帯 / Inguinal ligament
- 腸腰筋 / Iliopsoas
- 恥骨結節 / Pubic tubercle
- 小転子 / Lesser trochanter
- Pubic symphysis
- Pyramidalis 錐体筋

B 外腹斜筋.

- 第5肋骨 / 5th rib
- 剣状突起 / Xiphoid process
- 外腹斜筋 / External oblique
- 白線 / Linea alba
- 外腹斜筋の腱膜 / External oblique aponeurosis
- 臍輪 / Umbilical ring
- 腸骨稜の外唇 / Outer lip of iliac crest
- Anterior superior iliac spine 上前腸骨棘
- 浅鼠径輪 / Superficial inguinal ring
- Inguinal ligament 鼠径靱帯

C 内腹斜筋.

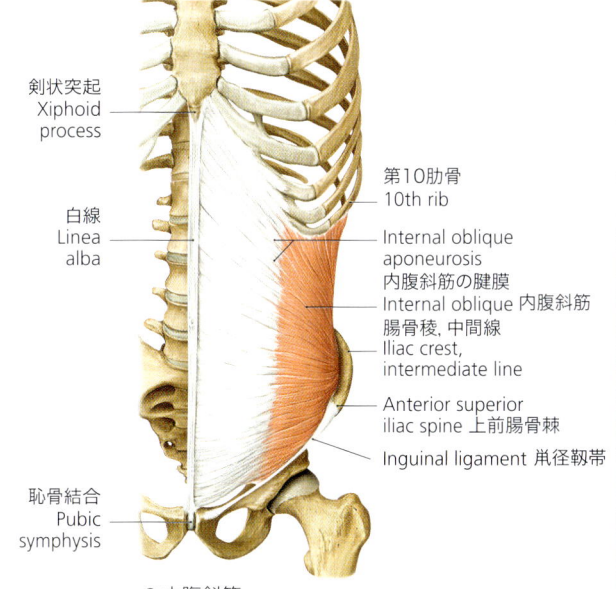

- 剣状突起 / Xiphoid process
- 第10肋骨 / 10th rib
- 白線 / Linea alba
- Internal oblique aponeurosis 内腹斜筋の腱膜
- Internal oblique 内腹斜筋
- 腸骨稜, 中間線 / Iliac crest, intermediate line
- Anterior superior iliac spine 上前腸骨棘
- Inguinal ligament 鼠径靱帯
- 恥骨結合 / Pubic symphysis

D 腹横筋.

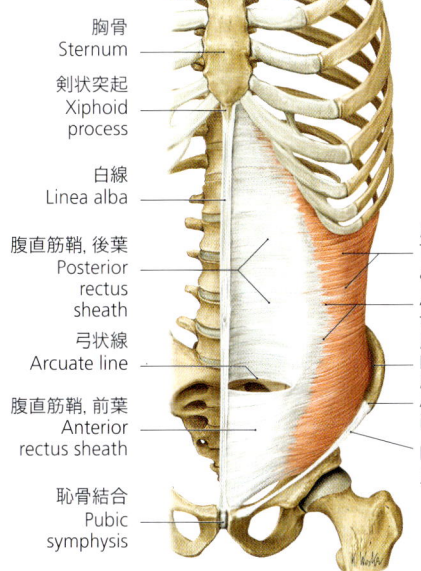

- 胸骨 / Sternum
- 剣状突起 / Xiphoid process
- 白線 / Linea alba
- 腹直筋鞘, 後葉 / Posterior rectus sheath
- 弓状線 / Arcuate line
- 腹直筋鞘, 前葉 / Anterior rectus sheath
- 腹横筋 / Transversus abdominis
- Aponeurosis of transversus abdominis 腹横筋の腱膜
- Inner lip of iliac crest 腸骨稜の内唇
- Anterior superior iliac spine 上前腸骨棘
- Inguinal ligament 鼠径靱帯
- 恥骨結合 / Pubic symphysis

骨盤底の筋
Pelvic Floor Muscle Facts

図 11.13　骨盤底の筋
上方から見たところ．

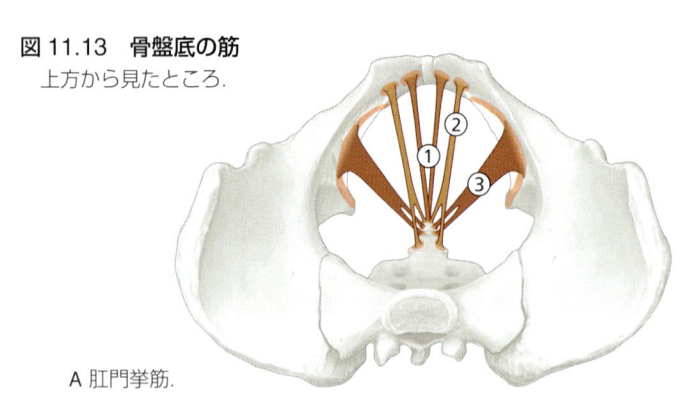

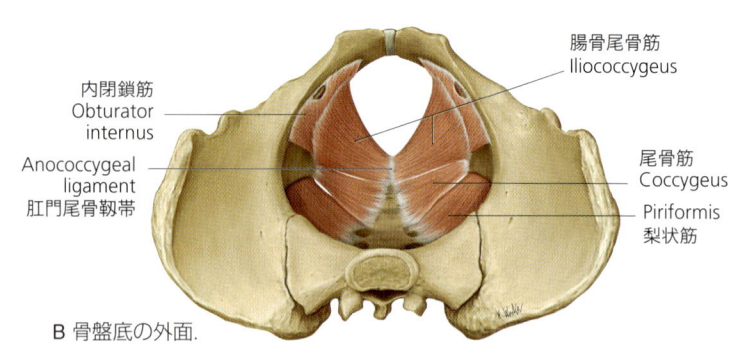

A 肛門挙筋．

B 骨盤底の外面．

内閉鎖筋 Obturator internus
肛門尾骨靱帯 Anococcygeal ligament
腸骨尾骨筋 Iliococcygeus
尾骨筋 Coccygeus
梨状筋 Piriformis

表 11.3　骨盤底の筋肉

筋		起始	停止	支配神経	作用
骨盤隔膜の筋					
肛門挙筋	①恥骨直腸筋	恥骨結合の両側の恥骨上枝	肛門尾骨靱帯	仙骨神経叢の枝(S4)，下直腸神経	骨盤隔膜：骨盤内臓の支持
	②恥骨尾骨筋	恥骨(恥骨直腸筋の起始の外側)	肛門尾骨靱帯，尾骨		
	③腸骨尾骨筋	肛門挙筋の内閉鎖筋筋膜の腱様弓			
尾骨筋		仙骨の下端	坐骨棘	仙骨神経叢(S4-5)の枝	骨盤内臓の支持，尾骨の屈曲
骨盤壁の筋(壁側筋)					
*梨状筋		仙骨の骨盤面	大腿骨の大転子の先端	仙骨神経叢(S1-2)の枝	股関節：外旋，安定，屈曲した股関節の外転
*内閉鎖筋		閉鎖膜と閉鎖孔の外周の内側面	大腿骨の大転子の内側面	仙骨神経叢(L5-S1)の枝	股関節：外旋，屈曲した股関節の外転
括約筋と起立筋					
④外肛門括約筋		肛門を取り囲む(会陰体より肛門尾骨靱帯まで後方に走る)		陰部神経(S2-4)	肛門を閉める
⑤外尿道括約筋		尿道を取り囲む(深会陰横筋からの分束)			尿道を閉める
⑥球海綿体筋		会陰腱中心から前方へ，女性では陰核に，男性では陰茎縫線に至る．			女性：大前庭腺を収縮 男性：勃起の補助
⑦坐骨海綿体筋		坐骨枝	陰核脚または陰茎脚		陰核海綿体あるいは陰茎海綿体に血液を押し込めて勃起を持続

*梨状筋と内閉鎖筋は殿部の筋と見なされる(p.374参照)．
女性・男性の外生殖器は pp.194，203 で示される．

図 11.14　骨盤底の括約筋と挙筋
下方から見たところ．
pp.194，203 参照．

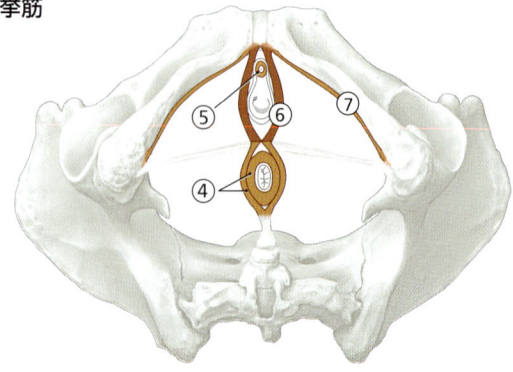

図 11.15 骨盤底
女性骨盤.

A 上方から見たところ.
- 挙筋門 Levator hiatus
- 閉鎖管 Obturator canal
- 閉鎖筋膜（内閉鎖筋）Obturator fascia (obturator internus muscle)
- 肛門挙筋腱弓 Tendinous arch of levator ani
- Anococcygeal raphe 肛門尾骨縫線
- 直腸前線維 Prerectal fibers
- 恥骨直腸筋① Puborectalis
- 恥骨尾骨筋② Pubococcygeus
- 腸骨尾骨筋③ Iliococcygeus
- 肛門挙筋 Levator ani
- 坐骨棘 Ischial spine
- 尾骨筋 Coccygeus
- 梨状筋 Piriformis
- Sacrum 仙骨

B 下方から見たところ.
- 恥骨結合 Pubic symphysis
- 恥骨弓靱帯 Pubic arcuate ligament
- 挙筋門 Levator hiatus
- 寛骨臼 Acetabulum
- 坐骨結節 Ischial tuberosity
- 尾骨 Coccyx
- 直腸前線維 Prerectal fibers
- 内閉鎖筋 Obturator internus
- 恥骨直腸筋 Puborectalis
- 恥骨尾骨筋 Pubococcygeus
- 腸骨尾骨筋 Iliococcygeus
- 肛門挙筋 Levator ani
- 梨状筋 Piriformis
- 尾骨筋 Coccygeus

C 右外側方から見たところ.
- 前仙腸靱帯 Anterior sacroiliac␣l.
- 弓状線 Arcuate line
- 内閉鎖筋筋膜 Obturator internus fascia
- 肛門挙筋腱弓 Tendinous arch of levator ani
- 恥骨結合 Pubic symphysis
- Deep transverse perineal 深会陰横筋
- 梨状筋 Piriformis
- Coccygeus 尾骨筋
- Ischial spine 坐骨棘
- 肛門尾骨靱帯 Anococcygeal␣l.
- ① Iliococcygeus 腸骨尾骨筋
- ② Pubococcygeus 恥骨尾骨筋
- ③ Puborectalis 恥骨直腸筋
- 肛門挙筋 Levator ani

D 骨盤右半分，内側方から見たところ.
- 上後腸骨棘 Posterior superior iliac spine
- 梨状筋 Piriformis
- 尾骨筋 Coccygeus
- 仙棘靱帯 Sacrospinous l.
- 仙結節靱帯 Sacrotuberous l.
- 尾骨 Coccyx
- Ischial spine 坐骨棘
- 恥骨結節 Pubic tubercle
- 閉鎖孔 Obturator foramen
- Levator ani 肛門挙筋

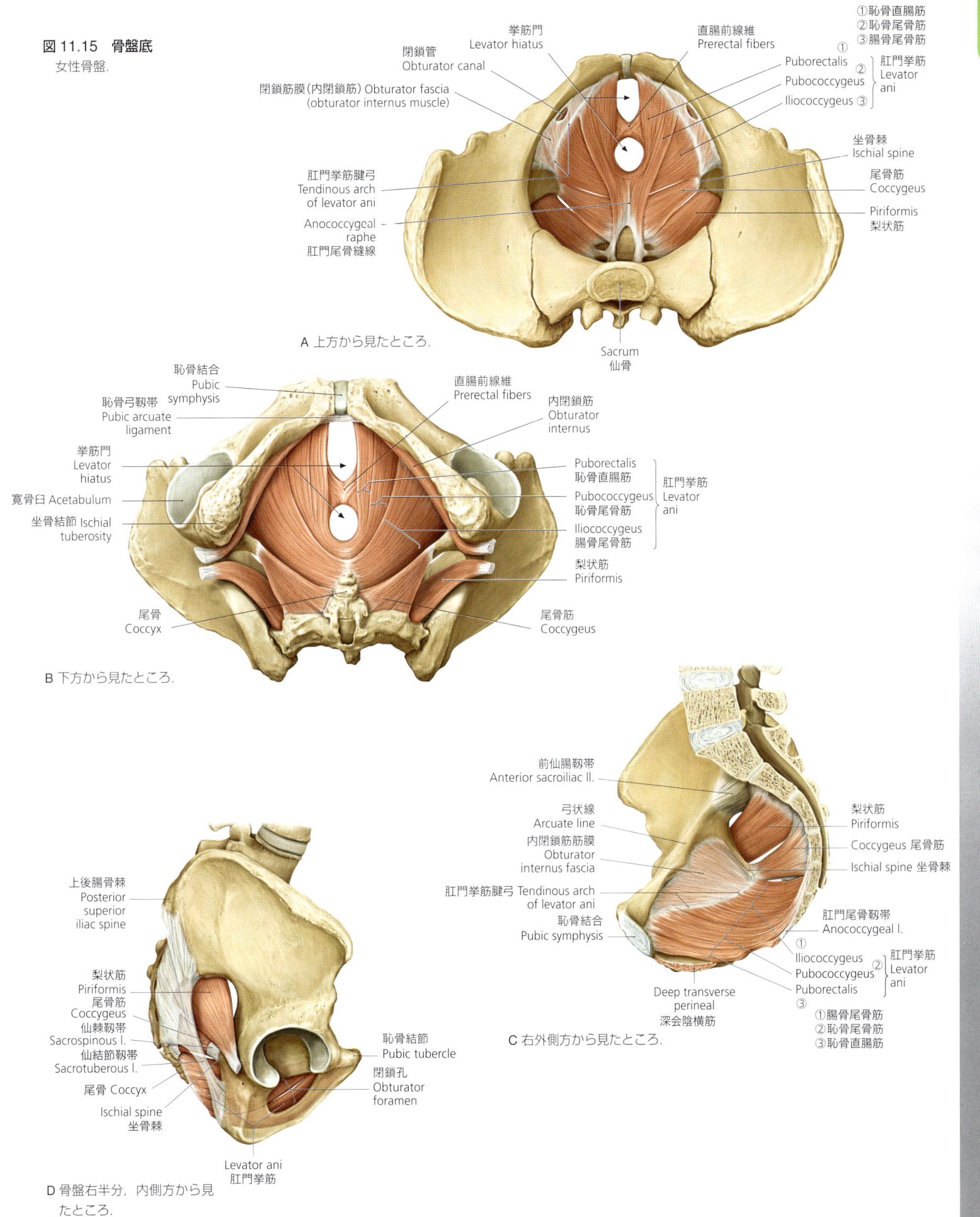

11 腹壁

腹腔・骨盤腔の区分
Divisions of the Abdominopelvic Cavity

図 12.1 内臓の層と 4 分円
前方から見たところ．腹部と骨盤の内臓の分類には，層によるもの，4 分円（第 4 腰椎の高さの臍を中心にする）によるもの，上下の位置によるもの（上腹部，下腹部，骨盤部），腸間膜の有無に関するものがある（表 12.1）．

肝臓 Liver
胃 Stomach
Transverse colon 横行結腸
Small intestine (jejunum and ileum) 小腸（空腸，回腸）

A 前層．

胆嚢 Gallbladder
脾臓 Spleen
Pancreas 膵臓
Duodenum 十二指腸
Descending colon 下行結腸
Ascending colon with cecum and vermiform appendix 上行結腸，盲腸，虫垂

B 中間層．

副腎 Suprarenal glands
腎臓 Kidneys
Abdominal aorta 腹大動脈
Ureters 尿管
Urinary bladder 膀胱

C 後層．

図 12.2 腹膜と腸間膜

腸間膜 Mesentery
腹膜腔 Peritoneal cavity
壁側板 Parietal layer
臓側板 Visceral layer
腹膜 Peritoneum
Intraperitoneal organ 腹膜内器官

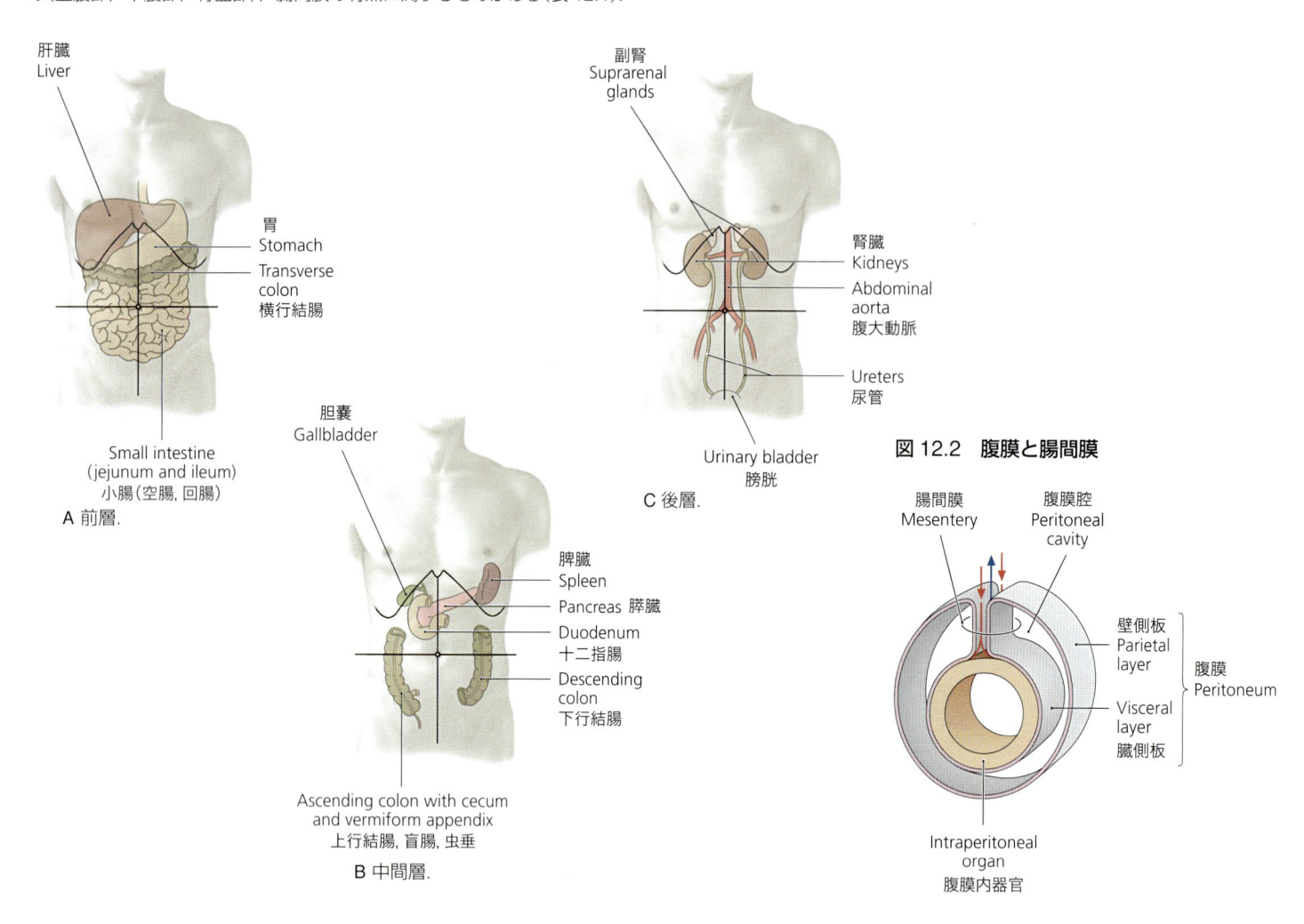

表 12.1　腹部・骨盤の器官

位置		器官		
腹膜内器官：腸間膜を持ち，完全に腹膜に覆われる．				
腹部腹膜腔		・胃 ・小腸（空腸，回腸，十二指腸上部の一部） ・脾臓 ・肝臓	・胆嚢 ・盲腸と虫垂（個体差があるが一部は腹膜後域に存在する） ・大腸（横行結腸と S 状結腸）	
骨盤腔		・子宮（子宮底と子宮体）	・卵巣	・卵管
腹膜外器官：腸間膜をまったく持たないか，発生過程で失っている．				
腹膜後器官	一次性	・腎臓	・副腎	・子宮頸
	二次性	・十二指腸（下行部，水平部，上部） ・上行結腸，下行結腸	・膵臓 ・直腸の上部 2/3	
腹膜下器官		・膀胱 ・精嚢 ・直腸の下部 1/3	・尿管遠位部 ・子宮頸	・前立腺 ・腟

図12.3 腹膜の関係

男性骨盤の正中矢状断．左外側方から見たところ．

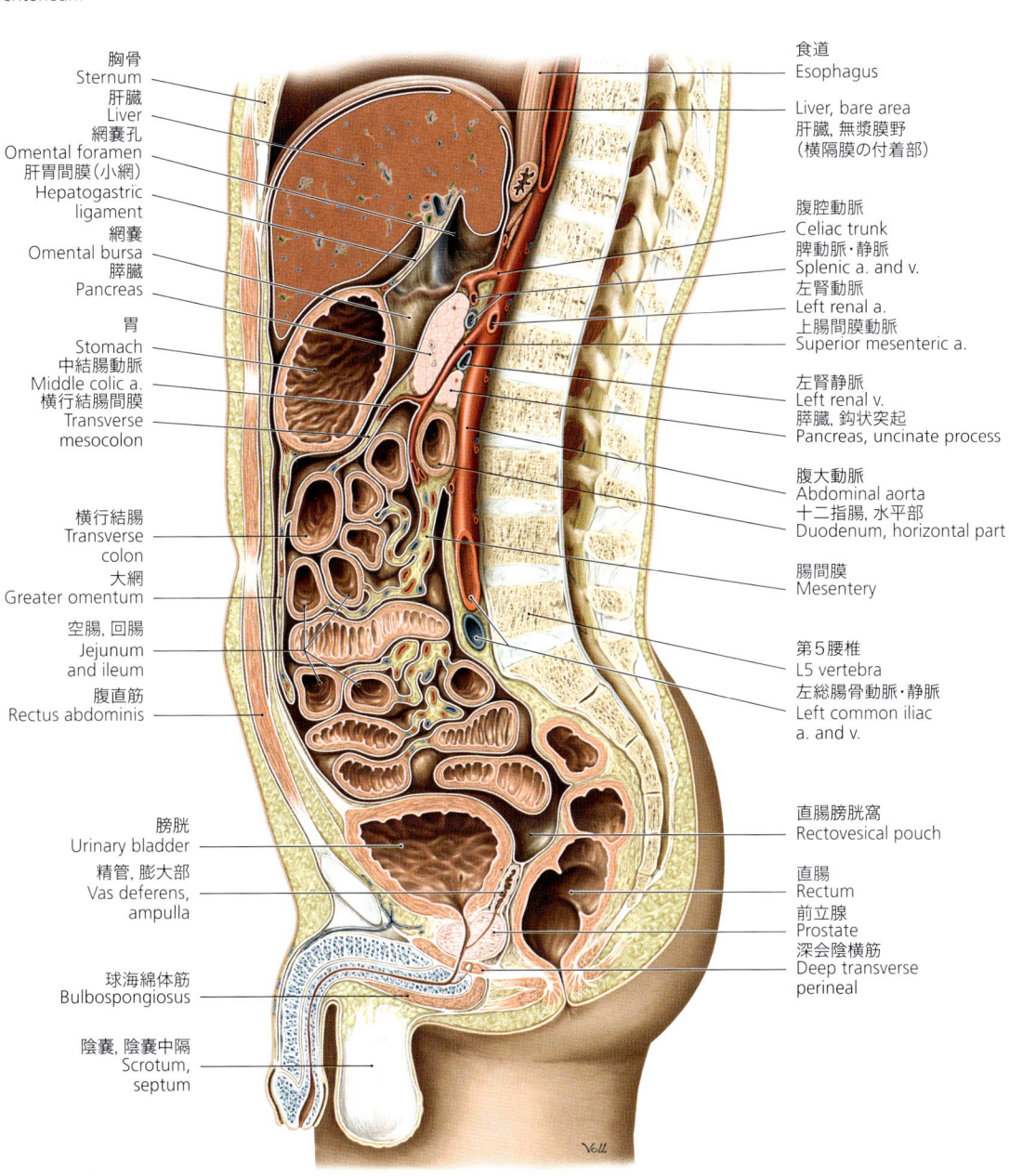

A 腹膜腔．腹膜は赤で示される．

ラベル（図A）:
- 壁側腹膜 Parietal peritoneum
- 網嚢 Lesser sac (omental bursa)
- 大網 Greater omentum
- 壁側腹膜 Parietal peritoneum
- 臓側腹膜 Visceral peritoneum

B 腹部と骨盤の内臓．

ラベル（図B 左側）:
- 胸骨 Sternum
- 肝臓 Liver
- 網嚢孔 Omental foramen
- 肝胃間膜（小網）Hepatogastric ligament
- 網嚢 Omental bursa
- 膵臓 Pancreas
- 胃 Stomach
- 中結腸動脈 Middle colic a.
- 横行結腸間膜 Transverse mesocolon
- 横行結腸 Transverse colon
- 大網 Greater omentum
- 空腸, 回腸 Jejunum and ileum
- 腹直筋 Rectus abdominis
- 膀胱 Urinary bladder
- 精管, 膨大部 Vas deferens, ampulla
- 球海綿体筋 Bulbospongiosus
- 陰嚢, 陰嚢中隔 Scrotum, septum

ラベル（図B 右側）:
- 食道 Esophagus
- 肝臓, 無漿膜野 Liver, bare area（横隔膜の付着部）
- 腹腔動脈 Celiac trunk
- 脾動脈・静脈 Splenic a. and v.
- 左腎動脈 Left renal a.
- 上腸間膜動脈 Superior mesenteric a.
- 左腎静脈 Left renal v.
- 膵臓, 鉤状突起 Pancreas, uncinate process
- 腹大動脈 Abdominal aorta
- 十二指腸, 水平部 Duodenum, horizontal part
- 腸間膜 Mesentery
- 第5腰椎 L5 vertebra
- 左総腸骨動脈・静脈 Left common iliac a. and v.
- 直腸膀胱窩 Rectovesical pouch
- 直腸 Rectum
- 前立腺 Prostate
- 深会陰横筋 Deep transverse perineal

臨床

急性腹痛

急性腹痛（急性腹症）は，重篤な場合には腹壁が極端に刺激に敏感になり（"防御"），腸が機能停止する．虫垂炎のような器官の炎症，胃潰瘍による胃穿孔（p.159参照），結石や腫瘍などによる器官の閉塞などが原因に含まれる．女性では，婦人病や異所性妊娠が重度の腹痛を引き起こすことがある．

腹膜腔
Peritoneal Cavity

> 大網は胃の大弯から垂れ下がり，横行結腸の前面を覆っているエプロン状の腹膜のヒダである．横行結腸は腹腔を上結腸区画（肝臓，胆嚢，胃）と下結腸区画（腸）に分ける．

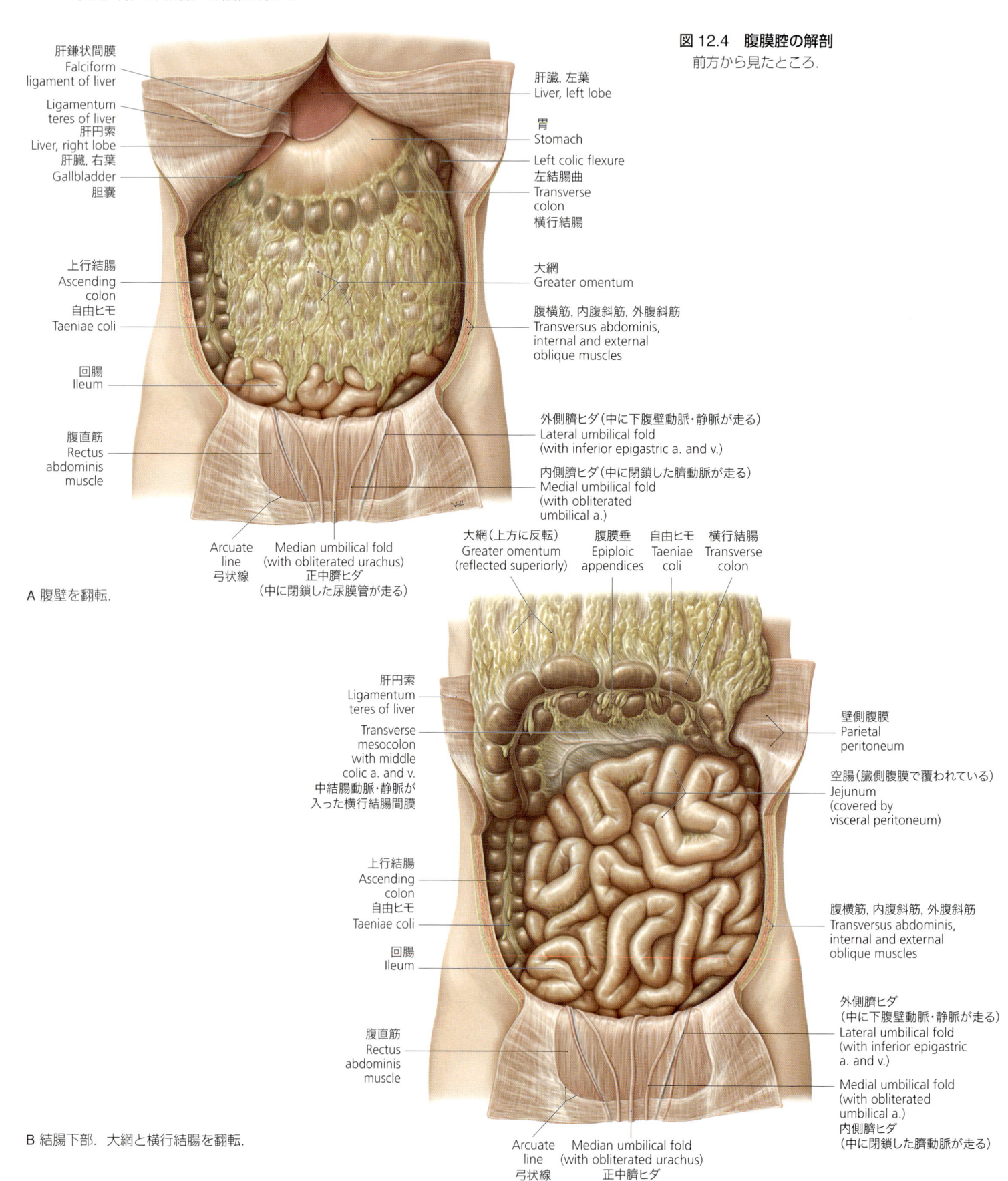

図 12.4　腹膜腔の解剖
前方から見たところ．

肝鎌状間膜　Falciform ligament of liver
Ligamentum teres of liver　肝円索
Liver, right lobe　肝臓，右葉
Gallbladder　胆嚢
上行結腸　Ascending colon
自由ヒモ　Taeniae coli
回腸　Ileum
腹直筋　Rectus abdominis muscle
Arcuate line　弓状線
Median umbilical fold (with obliterated urachus)　正中臍ヒダ（中に閉鎖した尿膜管が走る）

肝臓，左葉　Liver, left lobe
胃　Stomach
Left colic flexure　左結腸曲
Transverse colon　横行結腸
大網　Greater omentum
腹横筋，内腹斜筋，外腹斜筋　Transversus abdominis, internal and external oblique muscles
外側臍ヒダ（中に下腹壁動脈・静脈が走る）　Lateral umbilical fold (with inferior epigastric a. and v.)
内側臍ヒダ（中に閉鎖した臍動脈が走る）　Medial umbilical fold (with obliterated umbilical a.)

A　腹壁を翻転．

大網（上方に反転）Greater omentum (reflected superiorly)
腹膜垂　Epiploic appendices
自由ヒモ　Taeniae coli
横行結腸　Transverse colon

肝円索　Ligamentum teres of liver
Transverse mesocolon with middle colic a. and v.　中結腸動脈・静脈が入った横行結腸間膜
上行結腸　Ascending colon
自由ヒモ　Taeniae coli
回腸　Ileum
腹直筋　Rectus abdominis muscle
Arcuate line　弓状線
Median umbilical fold (with obliterated urachus)　正中臍ヒダ（中に閉鎖した尿膜管が走る）

壁側腹膜　Parietal peritoneum
空腸（臓側腹膜で覆われている）　Jejunum (covered by visceral peritoneum)
腹横筋，内腹斜筋，外腹斜筋　Transversus abdominis, internal and external oblique muscles
外側臍ヒダ（中に下腹壁動脈・静脈が走る）　Lateral umbilical fold (with inferior epigastric a. and v.)
Medial umbilical fold (with obliterated umbilical a.)　内側臍ヒダ（中に閉鎖した臍動脈が走る）

B　結腸下部．大網と横行結腸を翻転．

肝円索	Ligamentum teres of liver
	Epiploic appendices
腹膜垂	
横行結腸間膜	Transverse mesocolon
右結腸曲	Right colic flexure
腸間膜（断端）	Mesentery (cut)
自由ヒモ	Taeniae coli
上行結腸	Ascending colon
回腸	Ileum
盲腸	Cecum
直腸	Rectum
腹直筋	Rectus abdominis muscle
正中臍ヒダ（中に閉鎖した尿膜管が走る）	Median umbilical fold (with obliterated urachus)
大網（上方に反転）	Greater omentum (reflected superiorly)
横行結腸	Transverse colon
壁側腹膜	Parietal peritoneum
左結腸曲	Left colic flexure
空腸	Jejunum
下行結腸	Descending colon
腹横筋, 内腹斜筋, 外腹斜筋	Transversus abdominis, internal and external oblique muscles
S状結腸間膜	Sigmoid mesocolon
S状結腸	Sigmoid colon
外側臍ヒダ（中に下腹壁動脈・静脈が走る）	Lateral umbilical fold (with inferior epigastric a. and v.)
内側臍ヒダ（中に閉鎖した臍動脈が走る）	Medial umbilical fold (with obliterated umbilical a.)

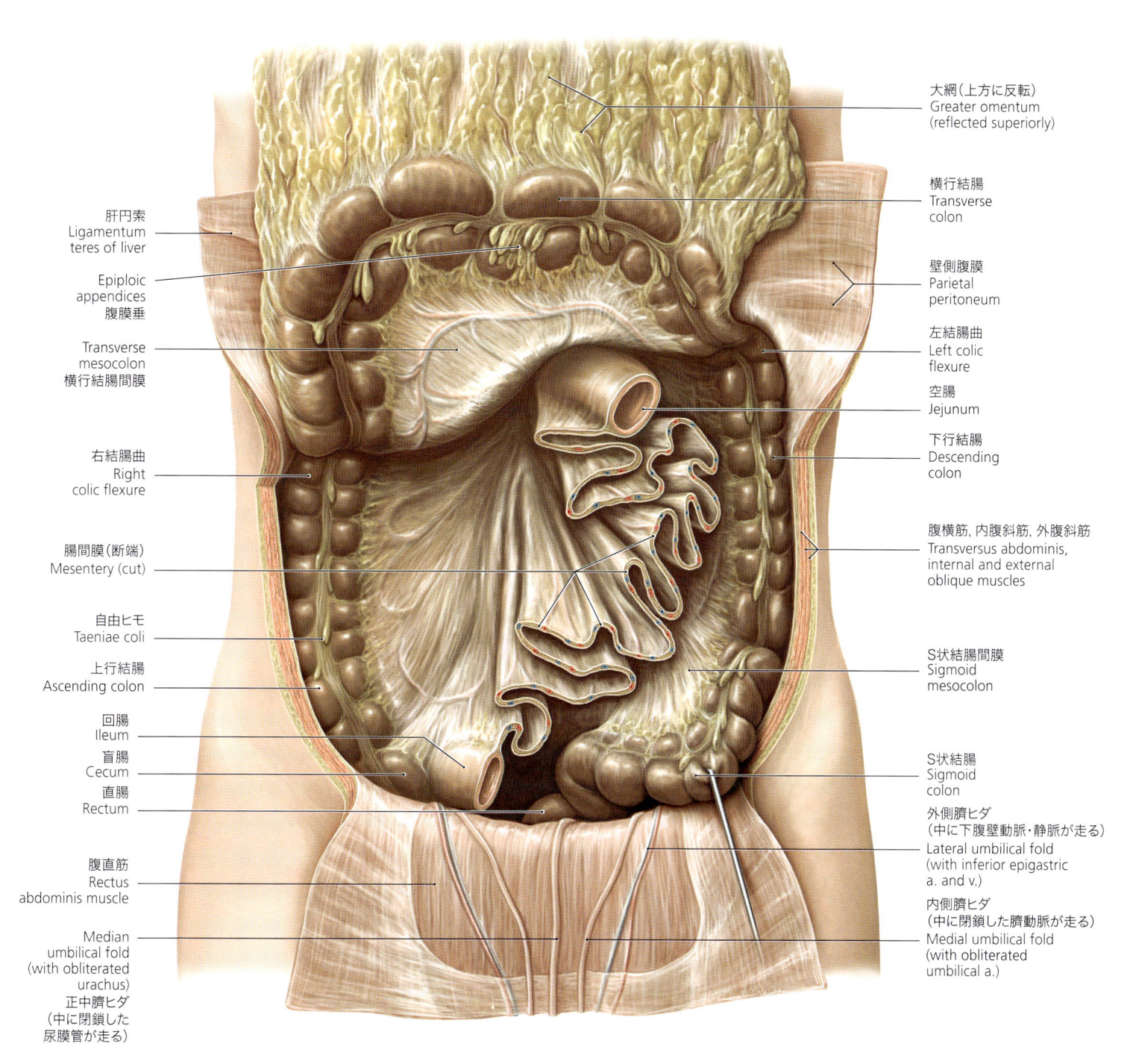

C 腸間膜，大網と横行結腸を翻転．腹腔内の小腸を取り除く．

12 腹腔

145

網嚢
Lesser Sac

図 12.5　網嚢
前方から見たところ．網嚢は腹膜腔の一部で，小網と胃の後ろに位置する．

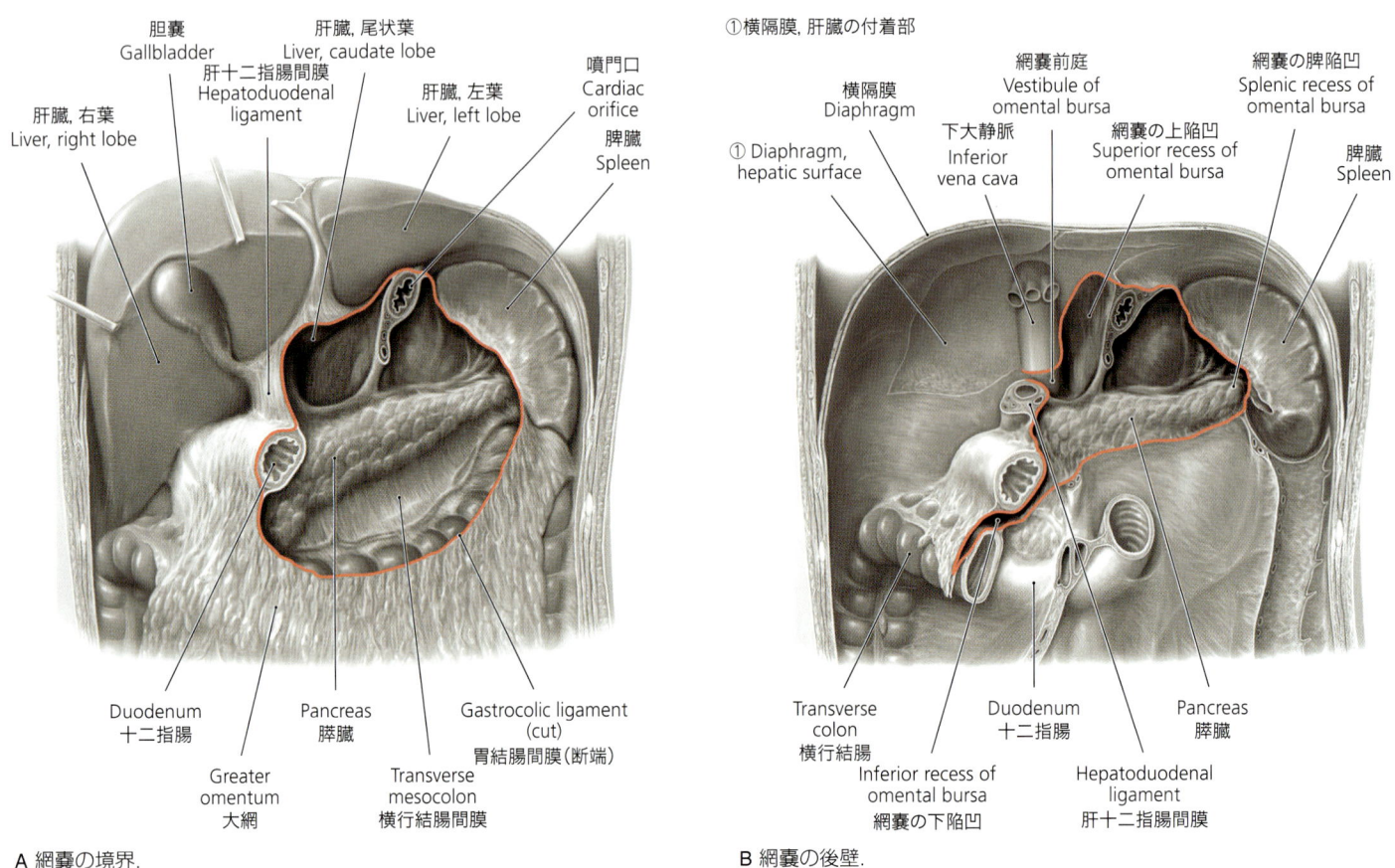

A　網嚢の境界．

ラベル：
- 胆嚢 Gallbladder
- 肝臓，尾状葉 Liver, caudate lobe
- 肝十二指腸間膜 Hepatoduodenal ligament
- 肝臓，右葉 Liver, right lobe
- 肝臓，左葉 Liver, left lobe
- 噴門口 Cardiac orifice
- 脾臓 Spleen
- Duodenum 十二指腸
- Pancreas 膵臓
- Gastrocolic ligament (cut) 胃結腸間膜（断端）
- Greater omentum 大網
- Transverse mesocolon 横行結腸間膜

B　網嚢の後壁．

ラベル：
- ①横隔膜，肝臓の付着部
- 横隔膜 Diaphragm
- ① Diaphragm, hepatic surface
- 網嚢前庭 Vestibule of omental bursa
- 網嚢の上陥凹 Superior recess of omental bursa
- 網嚢の脾陥凹 Splenic recess of omental bursa
- 下大静脈 Inferior vena cava
- 脾臓 Spleen
- Transverse colon 横行結腸
- Duodenum 十二指腸
- Pancreas 膵臓
- Inferior recess of omental bursa 網嚢の下陥凹
- Hepatoduodenal ligament 肝十二指腸間膜

図 12.6　網嚢の位置

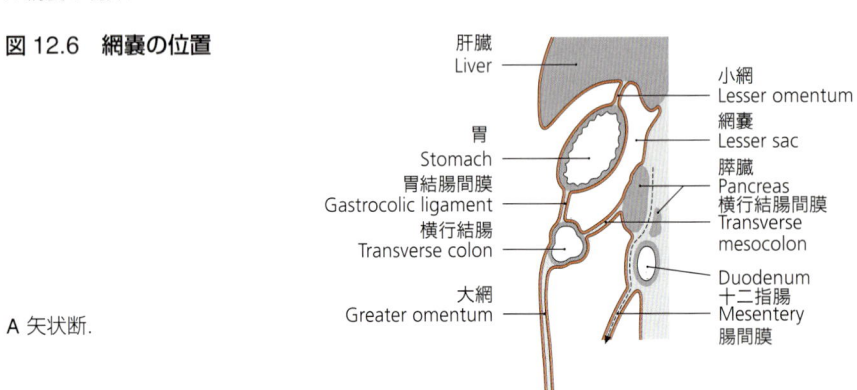

A　矢状断．

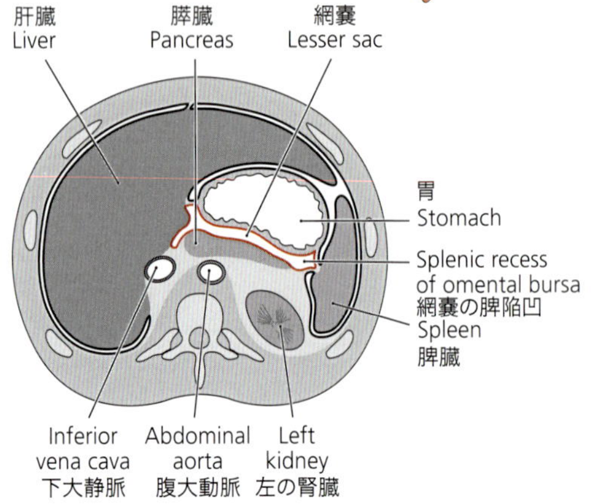

ラベル：
- 肝臓 Liver
- 小網 Lesser omentum
- 網嚢 Lesser sac
- 胃 Stomach
- 胃結腸間膜 Gastrocolic ligament
- 横行結腸 Transverse colon
- 大網 Greater omentum
- 膵臓 Pancreas
- 横行結腸間膜 Transverse mesocolon
- 十二指腸 Duodenum
- 腸間膜 Mesentery

B　水平断．

ラベル：
- 肝臓 Liver
- 膵臓 Pancreas
- 網嚢 Lesser sac
- 胃 Stomach
- 網嚢の脾陥凹 Splenic recess of omental bursa
- 脾臓 Spleen
- 下大静脈 Inferior vena cava
- 腹大動脈 Abdominal aorta
- 左の腎臓 Left kidney

表 12.2　網嚢の境界

方向	境界	陥部
前方	小網，胃結腸間膜	—
下方	横行結腸間膜	下陥凹
上方	肝臓（尾状葉を含む）	上陥凹
後方	膵臓，大動脈（腹大動脈），腹腔動脈，脾動脈・静脈，胃膵ヒダ，左の副腎，左の腎臓の上端	—
右方	肝臓，十二指腸球部	—
左方	脾臓，胃脾間膜	脾陥凹

図 12.7　原位置の網嚢
前方から見たところ．胃結腸間膜を切開し，肝臓を引っ張り，胃を翻転する．

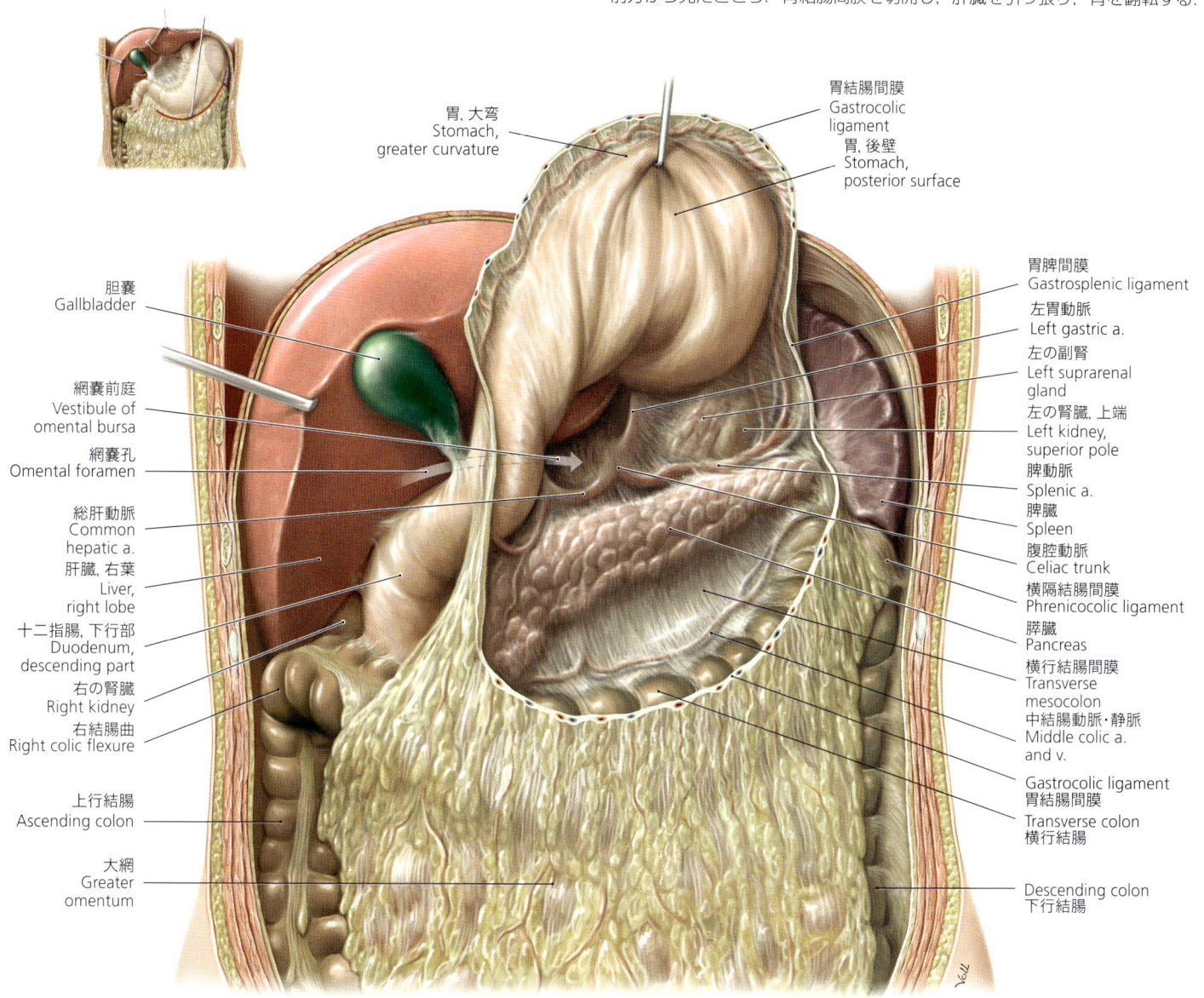

主なラベル：
- 胃, 大弯 Stomach, greater curvature
- 胃結腸間膜 Gastrocolic ligament
- 胃, 後壁 Stomach, posterior surface
- 胆嚢 Gallbladder
- 胃脾間膜 Gastrosplenic ligament
- 左胃動脈 Left gastric a.
- 網嚢前庭 Vestibule of omental bursa
- 左の副腎 Left suprarenal gland
- 網嚢孔 Omental foramen
- 左の腎臓, 上端 Left kidney, superior pole
- 総肝動脈 Common hepatic a.
- 脾動脈 Splenic a.
- 肝臓, 右葉 Liver, right lobe
- 脾臓 Spleen
- 十二指腸, 下行部 Duodenum, descending part
- 腹腔動脈 Celiac trunk
- 右の腎臓 Right kidney
- 横隔結腸間膜 Phrenicocolic ligament
- 右結腸曲 Right colic flexure
- 膵臓 Pancreas
- 上行結腸 Ascending colon
- 横行結腸間膜 Transverse mesocolon
- 中結腸動脈・静脈 Middle colic a. and v.
- Gastrocolic ligament 胃結腸間膜
- 大網 Greater omentum
- Transverse colon 横行結腸
- Descending colon 下行結腸

表 12.3　網嚢孔の境界

腹膜腔と網嚢は網嚢孔で連絡する（図 12.7 の矢印参照）．

方向	境界
前方	門脈・固有肝動脈・胆管を含む肝十二指腸間膜
下方	十二指腸上部
後方	下大静脈，横隔膜右脚
上方	肝臓の尾状葉

腸間膜と後壁
Mesenteries & Posterior Wall

図 12.8　腸間膜と腹膜腔の臓器
前方から見たところ．胃，空腸，回腸を取り除く．肝臓を翻転．

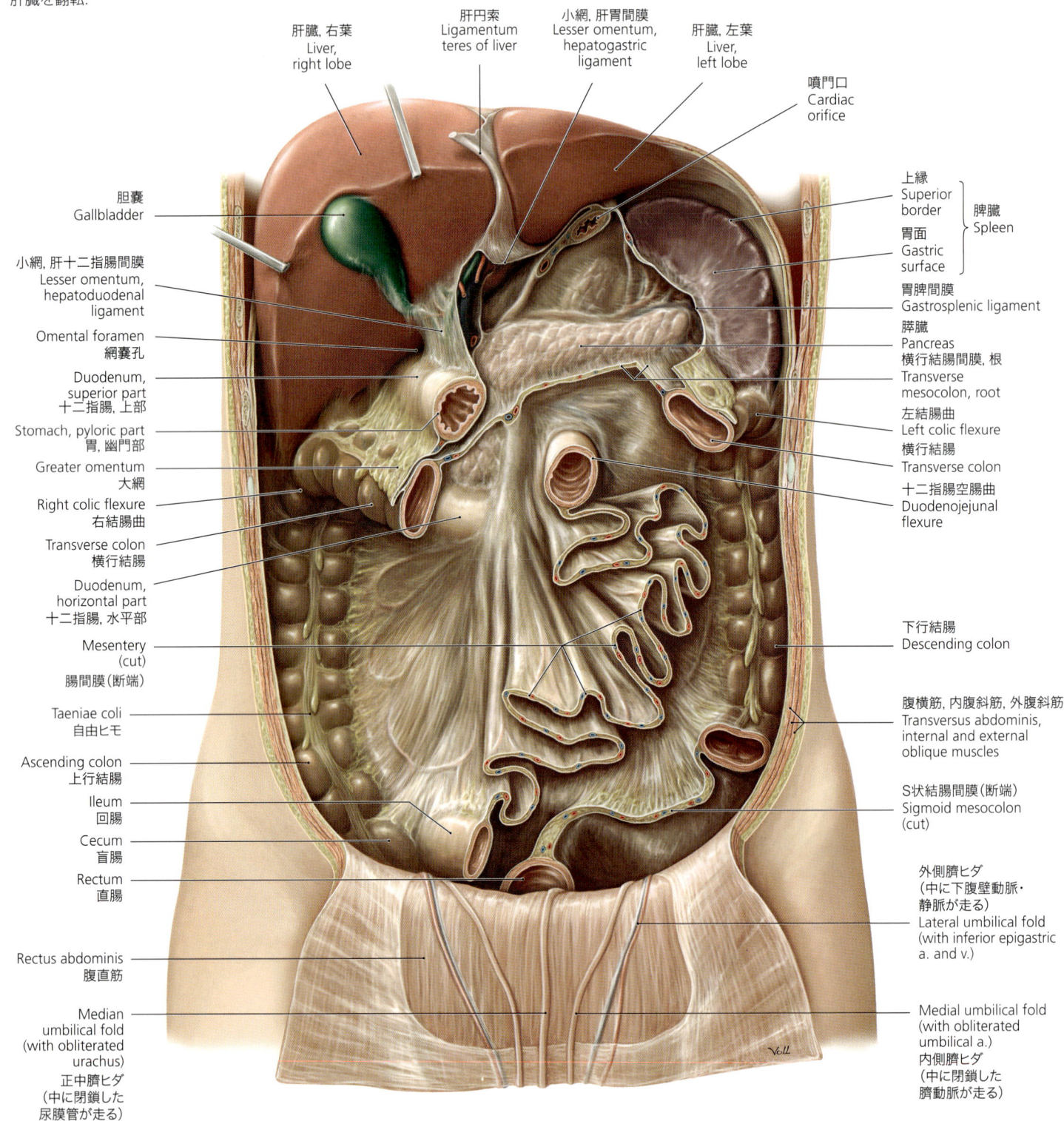

- 肝臓, 右葉 / Liver, right lobe
- 肝円索 / Ligamentum teres of liver
- 小網, 肝胃間膜 / Lesser omentum, hepatogastric ligament
- 肝臓, 左葉 / Liver, left lobe
- 噴門口 / Cardiac orifice
- 胆嚢 / Gallbladder
- 上縁 / Superior border ─ 脾臓 / Spleen
- 胃面 / Gastric surface
- 小網, 肝十二指腸間膜 / Lesser omentum, hepatoduodenal ligament
- 胃脾間膜 / Gastrosplenic ligament
- Omental foramen / 網嚢孔
- 膵臓 / Pancreas
- Duodenum, superior part / 十二指腸, 上部
- 横行結腸間膜, 根 / Transverse mesocolon, root
- Stomach, pyloric part / 胃, 幽門部
- 左結腸曲 / Left colic flexure
- Greater omentum / 大網
- 横行結腸 / Transverse colon
- Right colic flexure / 右結腸曲
- 十二指腸空腸曲 / Duodenojejunal flexure
- Transverse colon / 横行結腸
- Duodenum, horizontal part / 十二指腸, 水平部
- 下行結腸 / Descending colon
- Mesentery (cut) / 腸間膜 (断端)
- 腹横筋, 内腹斜筋, 外腹斜筋 / Transversus abdominis, internal and external oblique muscles
- Taeniae coli / 自由ヒモ
- S状結腸間膜 (断端) / Sigmoid mesocolon (cut)
- Ascending colon / 上行結腸
- Ileum / 回腸
- Cecum / 盲腸
- 外側臍ヒダ (中に下腹壁動脈・静脈が走る) / Lateral umbilical fold (with inferior epigastric a. and v.)
- Rectum / 直腸
- Rectus abdominis / 腹直筋
- Medial umbilical fold (with obliterated umbilical a.) / 内側臍ヒダ (中に閉鎖した臍動脈が走る)
- Median umbilical fold (with obliterated urachus) / 正中臍ヒダ (中に閉鎖した尿膜管が走る)

図12.9 腹膜腔の後壁

前方から見たところ．腹膜内器官をすべて取り除く．腹膜後器官が見える（表12.4とp.180を参照）．

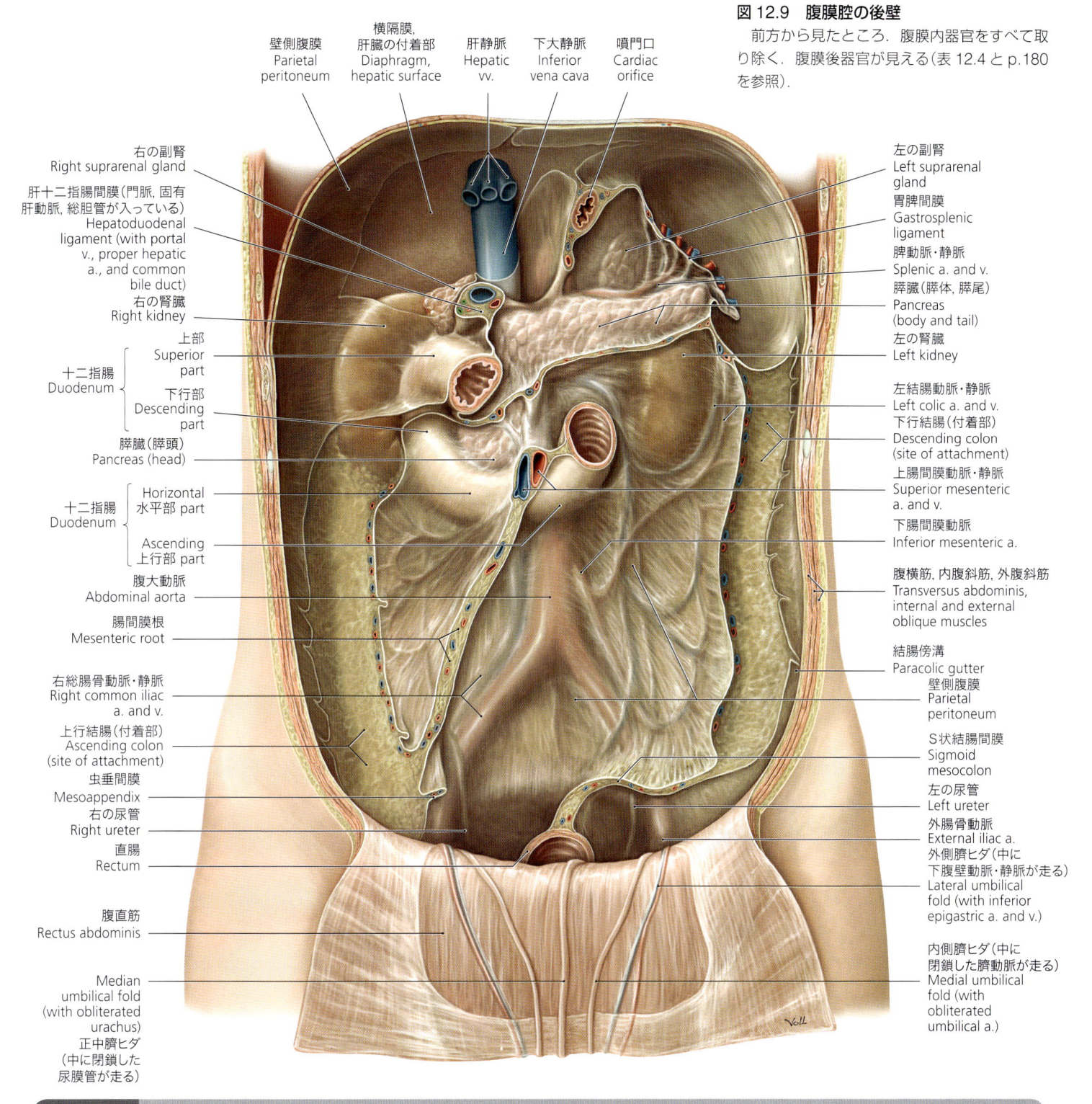

図中のラベル：

- 壁側腹膜 Parietal peritoneum
- 横隔膜，肝臓の付着部 Diaphragm, hepatic surface
- 肝静脈 Hepatic vv.
- 下大静脈 Inferior vena cava
- 噴門口 Cardiac orifice
- 右の副腎 Right suprarenal gland
- 肝十二指腸間膜（門脈，固有肝動脈，総胆管が入っている）Hepatoduodenal ligament (with portal v., proper hepatic a., and common bile duct)
- 右の腎臓 Right kidney
- 十二指腸 Duodenum
  - 上部 Superior part
  - 下行部 Descending part
- 膵臓（膵頭）Pancreas (head)
- 十二指腸 Duodenum
  - 水平部 Horizontal part
  - 上行部 Ascending part
- 腹大動脈 Abdominal aorta
- 腸間膜根 Mesenteric root
- 右総腸骨動脈・静脈 Right common iliac a. and v.
- 上行結腸（付着部）Ascending colon (site of attachment)
- 虫垂間膜 Mesoappendix
- 右の尿管 Right ureter
- 直腸 Rectum
- 腹直筋 Rectus abdominis
- 正中臍ヒダ（中に閉鎖した尿膜管が走る）Median umbilical fold (with obliterated urachus)
- 左の副腎 Left suprarenal gland
- 胃脾間膜 Gastrosplenic ligament
- 脾動脈・静脈 Splenic a. and v.
- 膵臓（膵体，膵尾）Pancreas (body and tail)
- 左の腎臓 Left kidney
- 左結腸動脈・静脈 Left colic a. and v.
- 下行結腸（付着部）Descending colon (site of attachment)
- 上腸間膜動脈・静脈 Superior mesenteric a. and v.
- 下腸間膜動脈 Inferior mesenteric a.
- 腹横筋，内腹斜筋，外腹斜筋 Transversus abdominis, internal and external oblique muscles
- 結腸傍溝 Paracolic gutter
- 壁側腹膜 Parietal peritoneum
- S状結腸間膜 Sigmoid mesocolon
- 左の尿管 Left ureter
- 外腸骨動脈 External iliac a.
- 外側臍ヒダ（中に下腹壁動脈・静脈が走る）Lateral umbilical fold (with inferior epigastric a. and v.)
- 内側臍ヒダ（中に閉鎖した臍動脈が走る）Medial umbilical fold (with obliterated umbilical a.)

表12.4 腹膜後部の構造

腹膜後部の脈管系についてはpp.216，228，239 参照．

分類	器官	血管	神経
一次性腹膜後器官（形成時から腹膜後器官）	・腎臓 ・副腎 ・尿管	・大動脈 ・下大静脈とその枝 ・上行腰静脈 ・門脈とその枝 ・腰リンパ節，仙骨リンパ節，腸骨リンパ節 ・腰リンパ本幹，乳び槽	・腰神経叢の枝 　◦腸骨下腹神経 　◦腸骨鼠径神経 　◦陰部大腿神経 　◦外側大腿皮神経 　◦大腿神経 　◦閉鎖神経 ・交感神経幹 ・自律神経節と自律神経叢
二次性腹膜後器官（形成過程で腸間膜を失う）	・膵臓 ・十二指腸（下行部と水平部，上行部の一部） ・上行結腸と下行結腸 ・盲腸（部分的，不定） ・直腸（上2/3）		

骨盤の内容
Contents of the Pelvis

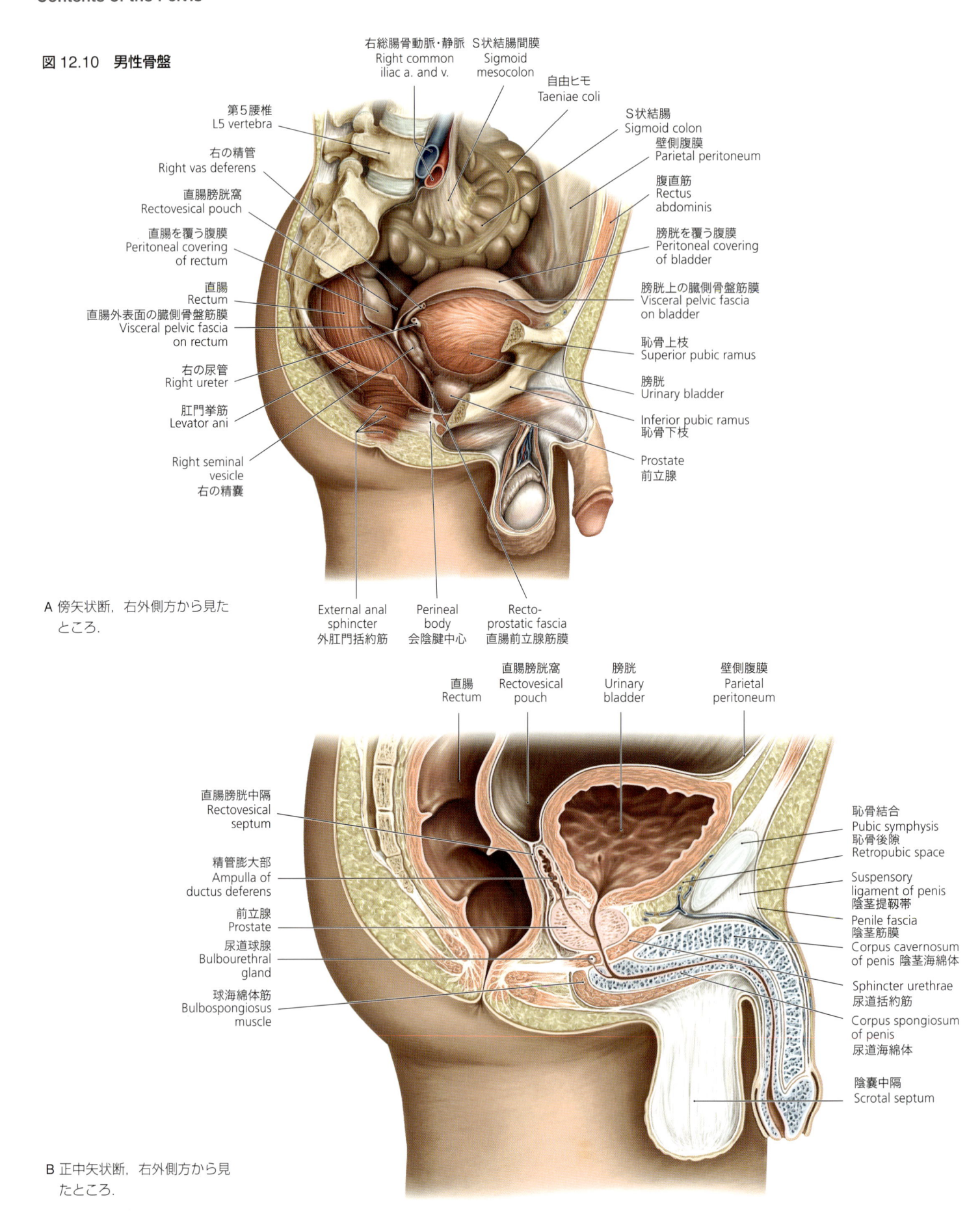

図 12.10　男性骨盤

A　傍矢状断，右外側方から見たところ．

B　正中矢状断，右外側方から見たところ．

図 12.11　女性骨盤

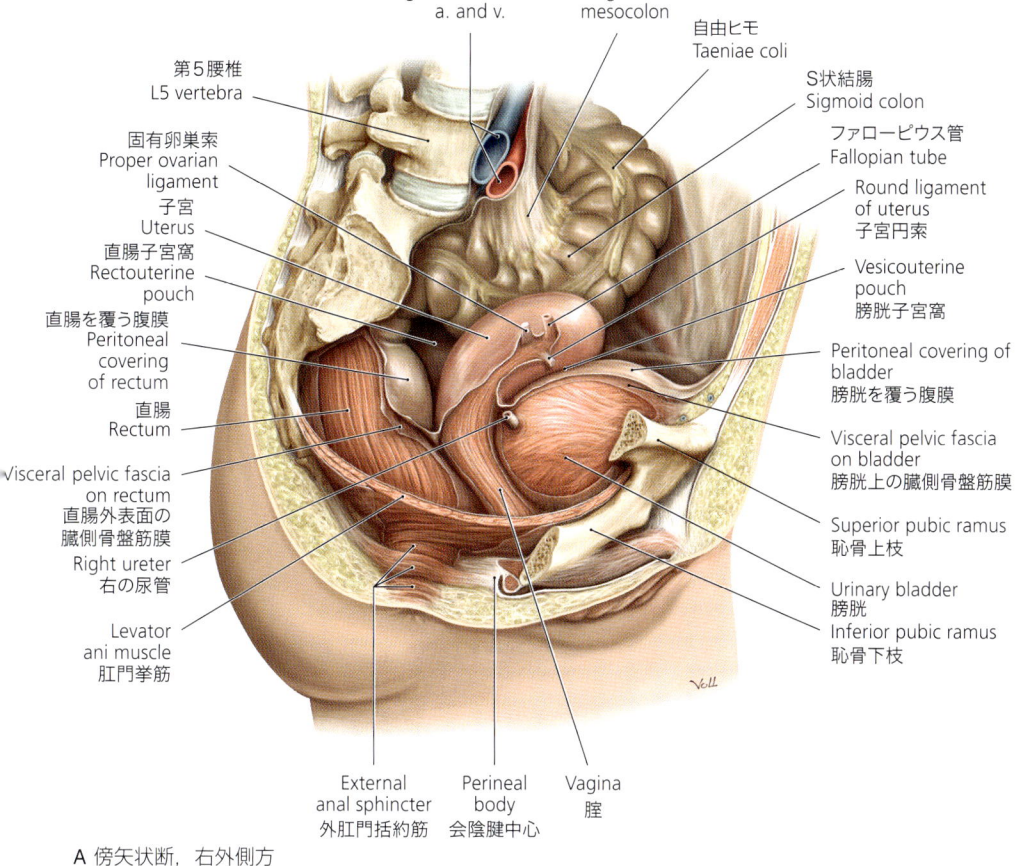

A　傍矢状断，右外側方から見たところ．

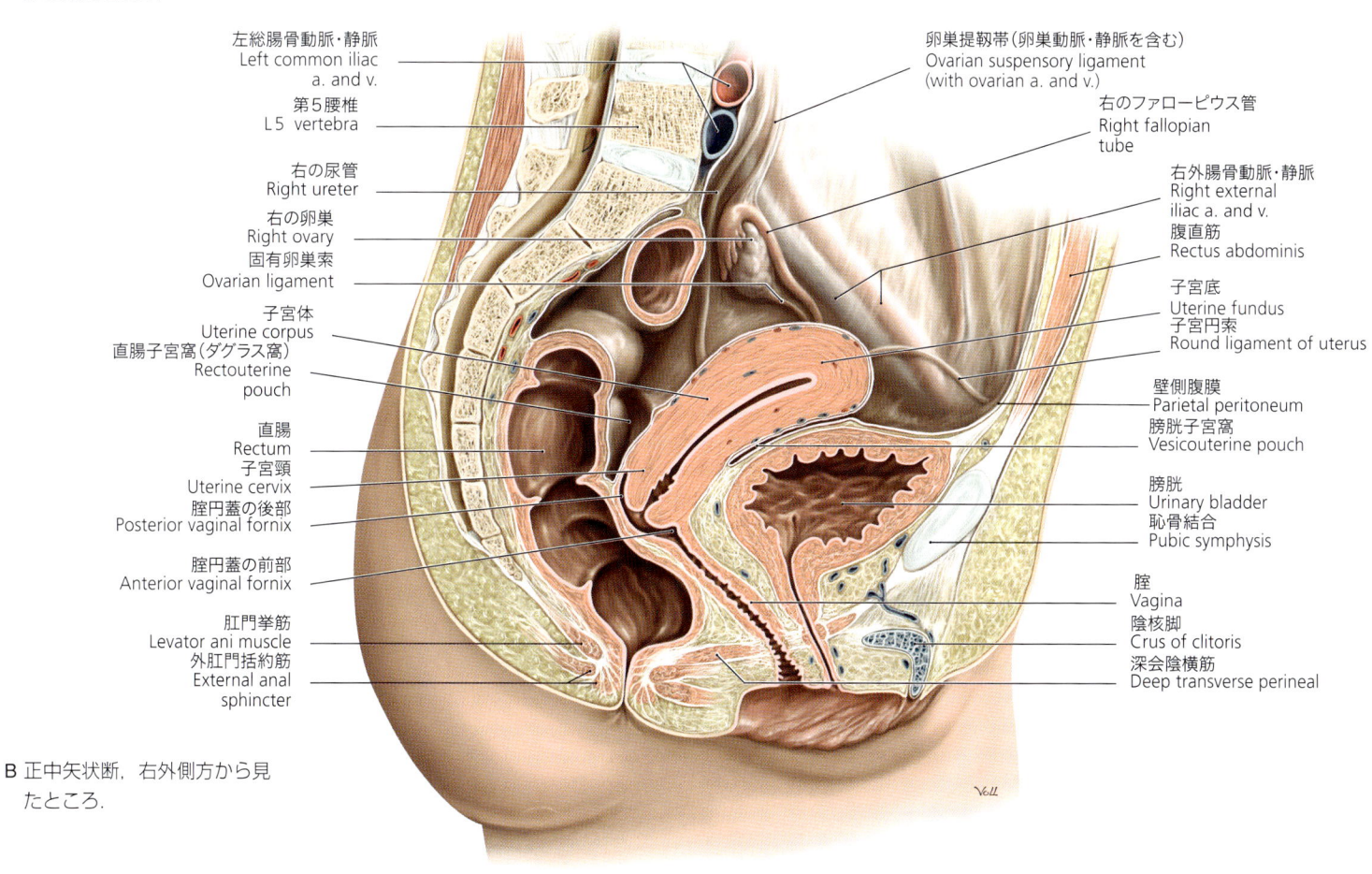

B　正中矢状断，右外側方から見たところ．

腹膜の位置関係
Peritoneal Relationships

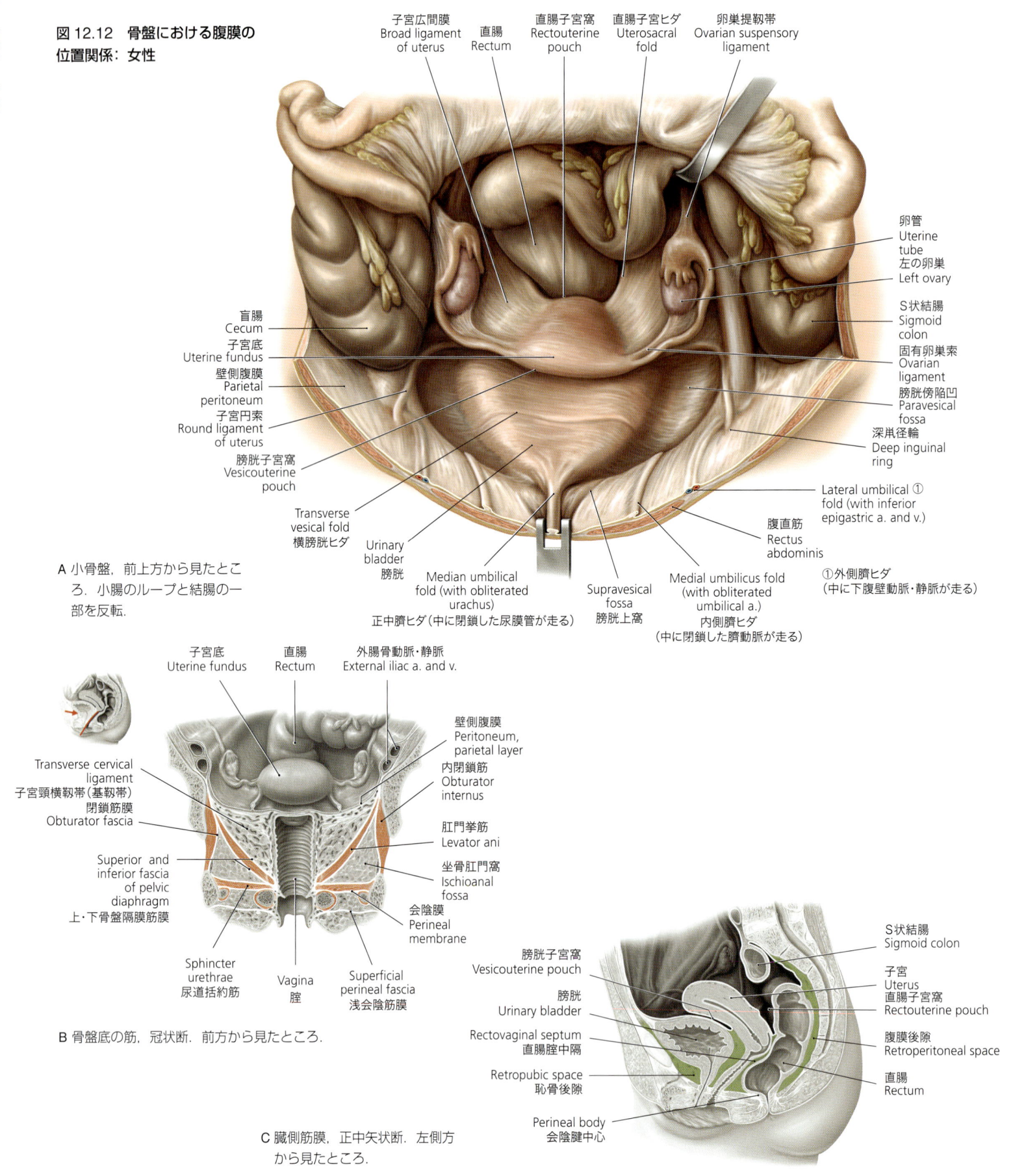

図 12.12 骨盤における腹膜の位置関係：女性

A 小骨盤．前上方から見たところ．小腸のループと結腸の一部を反転．

Labels (clockwise):
- 子宮広間膜 Broad ligament of uterus
- 直腸 Rectum
- 直腸子宮窩 Rectouterine pouch
- 直腸子宮ヒダ Uterosacral fold
- 卵巣提靱帯 Ovarian suspensory ligament
- 卵管 Uterine tube
- 左の卵巣 Left ovary
- S状結腸 Sigmoid colon
- 固有卵巣索 Ovarian ligament
- 膀胱傍陥凹 Paravesical fossa
- 深鼠径輪 Deep inguinal ring
- Lateral umbilical fold (with inferior epigastric a. and v.) ①外側臍ヒダ（中に下腹壁動脈・静脈が走る）
- 腹直筋 Rectus abdominis
- Medial umbilicus fold (with obliterated umbilical a.) 内側臍ヒダ（中に閉鎖した臍動脈が走る）
- 膀胱上窩 Supravesical fossa
- Median umbilical fold (with obliterated urachus) 正中臍ヒダ（中に閉鎖した尿膜管が走る）
- 膀胱 Urinary bladder
- 横膀胱ヒダ Transverse vesical fold
- 膀胱子宮窩 Vesicouterine pouch
- 子宮円索 Round ligament of uterus
- 壁側腹膜 Parietal peritoneum
- 子宮底 Uterine fundus
- 盲腸 Cecum

B 骨盤底の筋．冠状断．前方から見たところ．

Labels:
- 子宮底 Uterine fundus
- 直腸 Rectum
- 外腸骨動脈・静脈 External iliac a. and v.
- 壁側腹膜 Peritoneum, parietal layer
- 内閉鎖筋 Obturator internus
- 肛門挙筋 Levator ani
- 坐骨肛門窩 Ischioanal fossa
- 会陰膜 Perineal membrane
- 浅会陰筋膜 Superficial perineal fascia
- 膣 Vagina
- 尿道括約筋 Sphincter urethrae
- 上・下骨盤隔膜筋膜 Superior and inferior fascia of pelvic diaphragm
- 閉鎖筋膜 Obturator fascia
- 子宮頸横靱帯（基靱帯） Transverse cervical ligament

C 臓側筋膜．正中矢状断．左側方から見たところ．

Labels:
- S状結腸 Sigmoid colon
- 子宮 Uterus
- 直腸子宮窩 Rectouterine pouch
- 腹膜後隙 Retroperitoneal space
- 直腸 Rectum
- 会陰腱中心 Perineal body
- 恥骨後隙 Retropubic space
- 直腸腟中隔 Rectovaginal septum
- 膀胱 Urinary bladder
- 膀胱子宮窩 Vesicouterine pouch

図 12.13 骨盤における腹膜の位置関係：男性

A 小骨盤，前上方から見たところ．小腸のループと結腸の一部を翻転．

- 回腸 Ileum
- 直腸 Rectum
- 直腸膀胱窩 Rectovesical pouch
- 横膀胱ヒダ Transverse vesical fold
- 盲腸 Cecum
- 壁側腹膜 Parietal peritoneum
- 精管 Vas deferens
- Vermiform appendix 虫垂
- Lateral inguinal fossa 外側鼡径窩
- Urinary bladder 膀胱
- Median umbilical fold (with underlying obliterated urachus) 正中臍ヒダ（中に閉鎖した尿膜管が走る）
- Rectus abdominis 腹直筋
- Medial umbilicus fold (with underlying obliterated umbilical a.) 内側臍ヒダ（中に閉鎖した臍動脈が走る）
- S状結腸 Sigmoid colon
- 外側臍ヒダ（中に下腹壁動脈・静脈が走る）Lateral umbilical fold (with inferior epigastric a. and v.)

B 骨盤底の筋，冠状断，前方から見たところ．

- 膀胱 Urinary bladder
- 壁側腹膜 Peritoneum, parietal layer
- 精管 Vas deferens
- 膀胱傍結合組織 Paravesicular fascia
- 内閉鎖筋 Obturator internus
- 肛門挙筋 Levator ani
- 坐骨肛門窩（前陥凹）Ischioanal fossa (anterior recess)
- 尿道括約筋 Sphincter urethrae
- 会陰膜 Perineal membrane
- Bulb of penis 尿道球
- Crus of penis 陰茎脚
- 上・下骨盤隔膜筋膜 Superior and inferior fascia of pelvic diaphragm
- 前立腺 Prostate
- 恥骨下枝 Inferior pubic ramus

C 臓側筋膜，正中矢状断．左側方から見たところ．

- 膀胱 Urinary bladder
- 直腸膀胱中隔 Rectovesical septum
- 恥骨後隙 Retropubic space
- 会陰腱中心 Perineal body
- S状結腸間膜 Sigmoid mesocolon
- S状結腸 Sigmoid colon
- 直腸膀胱窩 Rectovesical pouch
- 腹膜後隙 Retroperitoneal space
- 直腸 Rectum

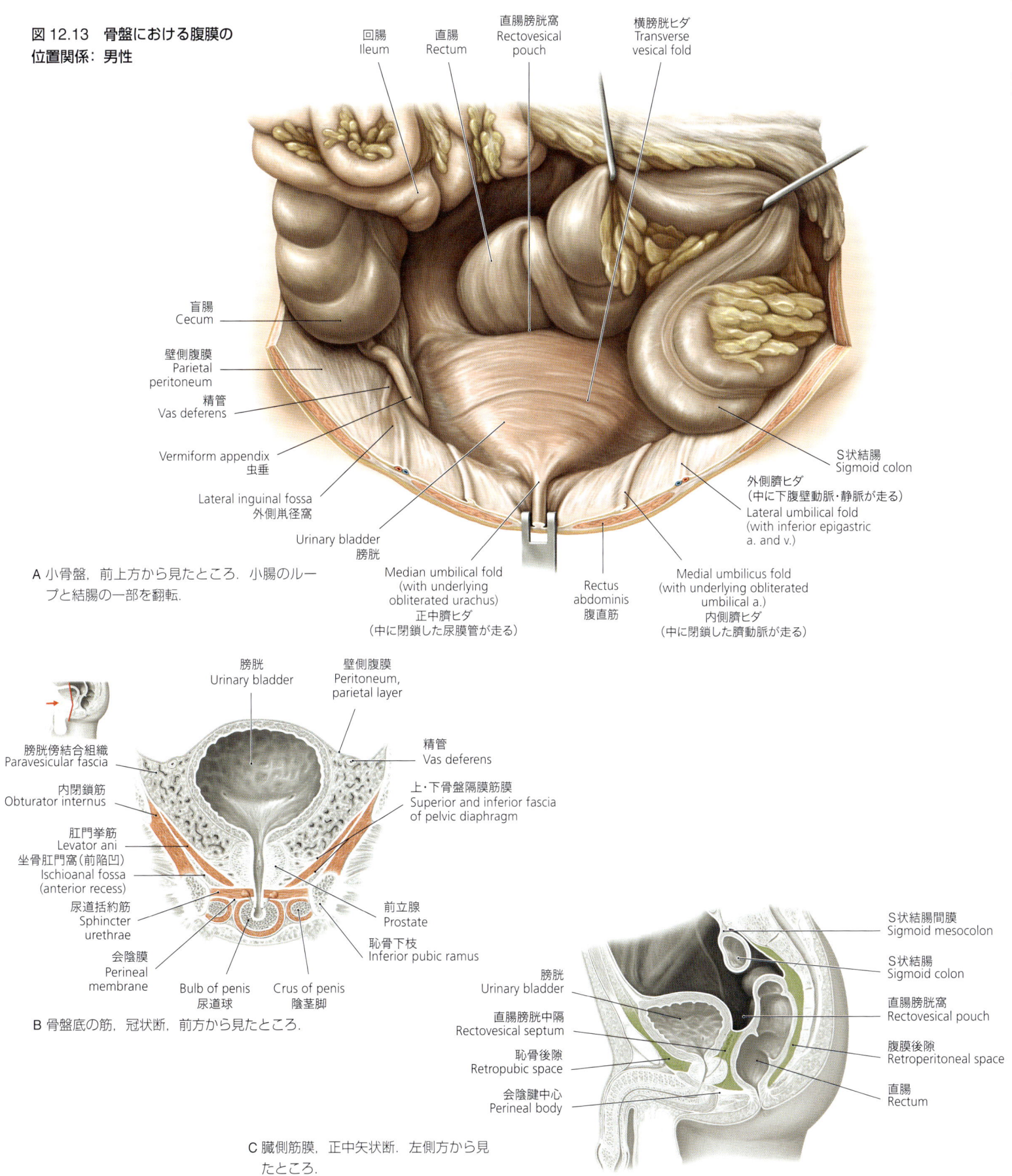

骨盤と会陰
Pelvis & Perineum

表 12.5　骨盤と会陰の区分

骨盤の高さは骨の確認点（腸骨陵と骨盤上口，p.126 参照）で決定される．
会陰の各構造は骨盤隔膜と 2 層の筋膜によって区分される．

腸骨陵		
骨盤	大骨盤	・回腸（coils）
		・盲腸と虫垂
		・S 状結腸
		・総腸骨動脈・静脈と外腸骨動脈・静脈
		・腰神経叢とその枝
	骨盤上口	
	骨盤	・尿管遠位部
		・膀胱
		・直腸
		♀：腟，子宮，卵管，卵巣
		♂：精管，精嚢，前立腺
		・内腸骨動脈・静脈とその枝
		・仙骨神経叢
		・下下腹神経叢
骨盤隔膜（肛門挙筋と浅・下骨盤隔膜筋膜）		
会陰	深会陰隙	・尿道括約筋と深会陰横筋
		・尿道隔膜部
		・腟
		・直腸
		・尿道球腺
		・坐骨直腸窩
		・内陰部動脈・静脈，陰部神経とその枝
	会陰膜	
	浅会陰隙	・坐骨海綿体筋，球海綿体筋，浅会陰横筋
		・尿道陰茎部
		・陰核と陰茎
		・内陰部動脈・静脈，陰部神経とその枝
	浅会陰筋膜（コリース筋膜）	
	皮下会陰隙	・脂肪
皮膚		

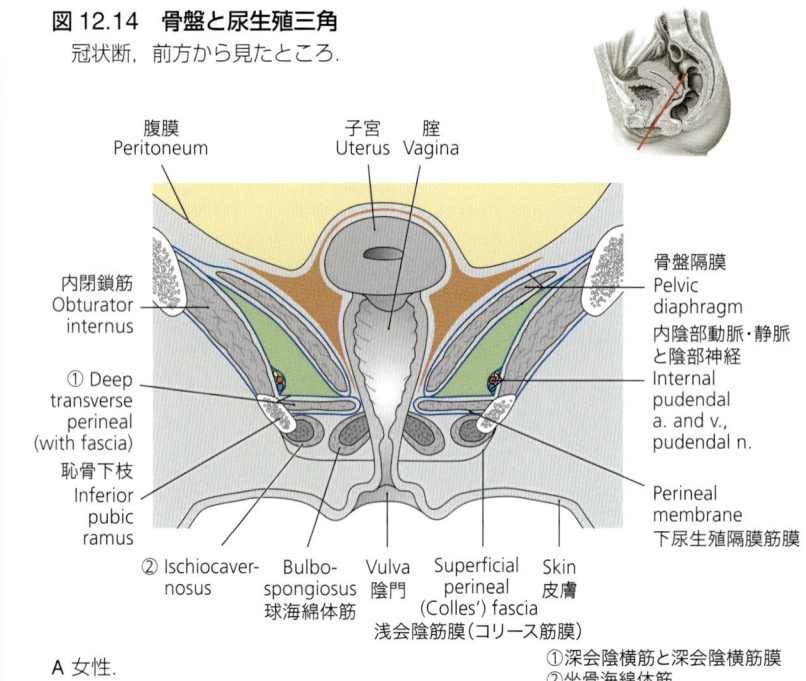

図 12.14　骨盤と尿生殖三角
冠状断，前方から見たところ．

A 女性．

①深会陰横筋と深会陰横筋膜
②坐骨海綿体筋

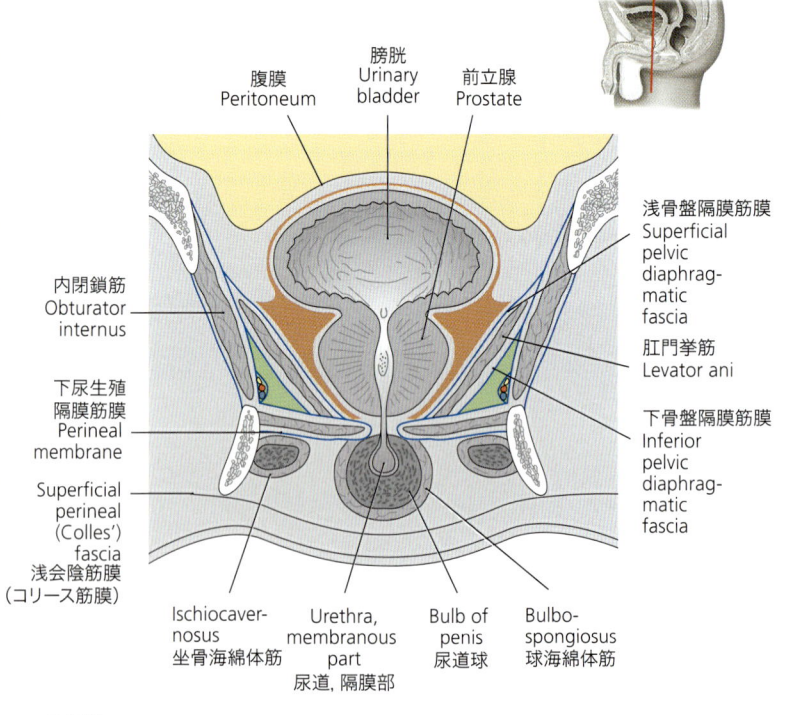

B 男性．

- 腹膜腔 Peritoneal cavity
- 腹膜下隙 Subperitoneal space
- 坐骨肛門窩（坐骨直腸窩） Ischioanal fossa
- 臓側骨盤筋膜 Visceral pelvic fascia
- 壁側骨盤筋膜 Parietal pelvic fascia

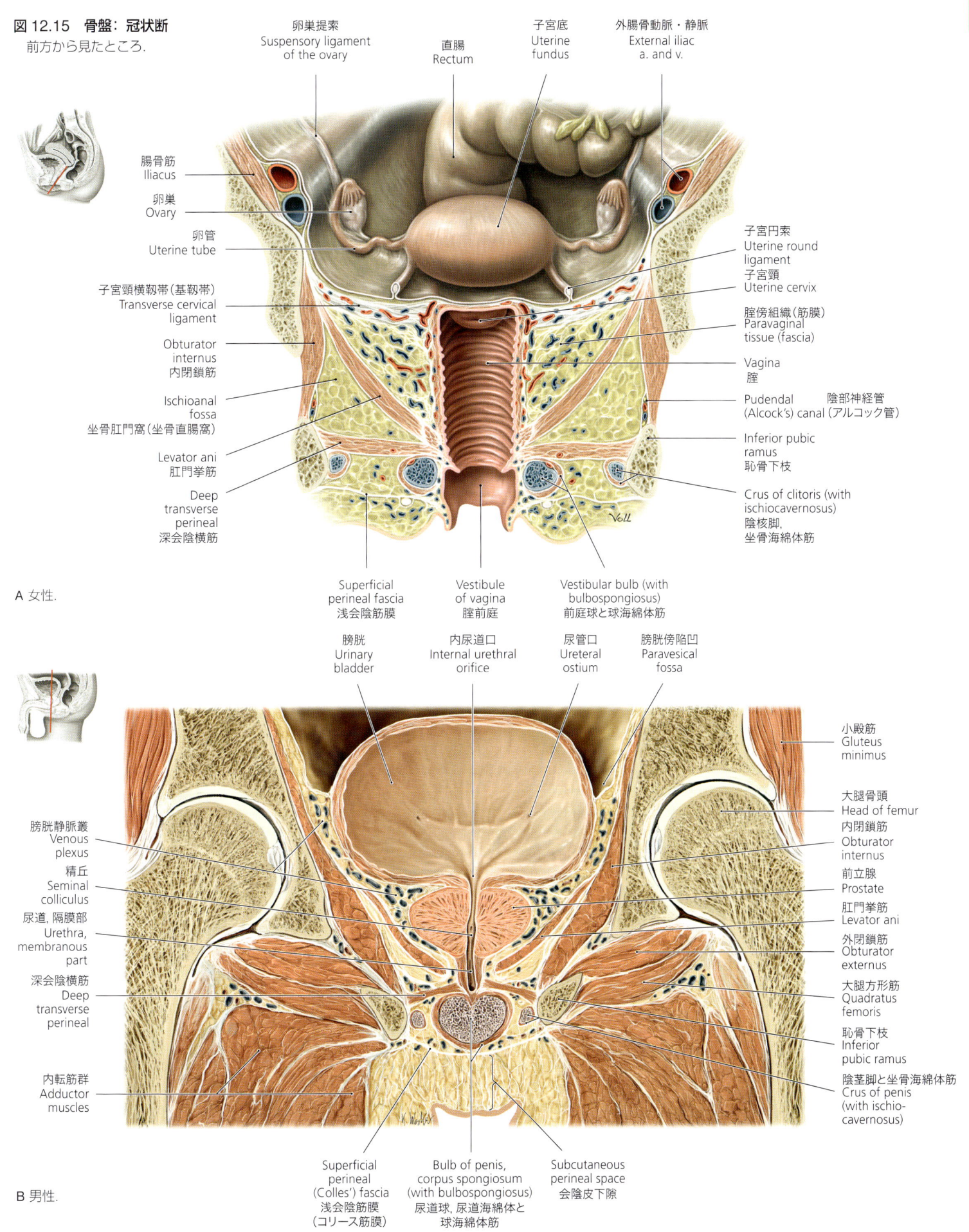

図 12.15　骨盤：冠状断
前方から見たところ．

A 女性．

- 卵巣提索 Suspensory ligament of the ovary
- 直腸 Rectum
- 子宮底 Uterine fundus
- 外腸骨動脈・静脈 External iliac a. and v.
- 腸骨筋 Iliacus
- 卵巣 Ovary
- 卵管 Uterine tube
- 子宮頸横靱帯（基靱帯） Transverse cervical ligament
- Obturator internus 内閉鎖筋
- Ischioanal fossa 坐骨肛門窩（坐骨直腸窩）
- Levator ani 肛門挙筋
- Deep transverse perineal 深会陰横筋
- 子宮円索 Uterine round ligament
- 子宮頸 Uterine cervix
- 腟傍組織（筋膜） Paravaginal tissue (fascia)
- Vagina 腟
- Pudendal (Alcock's) canal 陰部神経管（アルコック管）
- Inferior pubic ramus 恥骨下枝
- Crus of clitoris (with ischiocavernosus) 陰核脚, 坐骨海綿体筋
- Superficial perineal fascia 浅会陰筋膜
- Vestibule of vagina 腟前庭
- Vestibular bulb (with bulbospongiosus) 前庭球と球海綿体筋

B 男性．

- 膀胱 Urinary bladder
- 内尿道口 Internal urethral orifice
- 尿管口 Ureteral ostium
- 膀胱傍陥凹 Paravesical fossa
- 小殿筋 Gluteus minimus
- 大腿骨頭 Head of femur
- 内閉鎖筋 Obturator internus
- 前立腺 Prostate
- 肛門挙筋 Levator ani
- 外閉鎖筋 Obturator externus
- 大腿方形筋 Quadratus femoris
- 恥骨下枝 Inferior pubic ramus
- 陰茎脚と坐骨海綿体筋 Crus of penis (with ischiocavernosus)
- 膀胱静脈叢 Venous plexus
- 精丘 Seminal colliculus
- 尿道, 隔膜部 Urethra, membranous part
- 深会陰横筋 Deep transverse perineal
- 内転筋群 Adductor muscles
- Superficial perineal (Colles') fascia 浅会陰筋膜（コリース筋膜）
- Bulb of penis, corpus spongiosum (with bulbospongiosus) 尿道球, 尿道海綿体と球海綿体筋
- Subcutaneous perineal space 会陰皮下隙

12　腹腔

155

水平断
Transverse Sections

図 12.16　腹部：水平断
下方から見たところ．

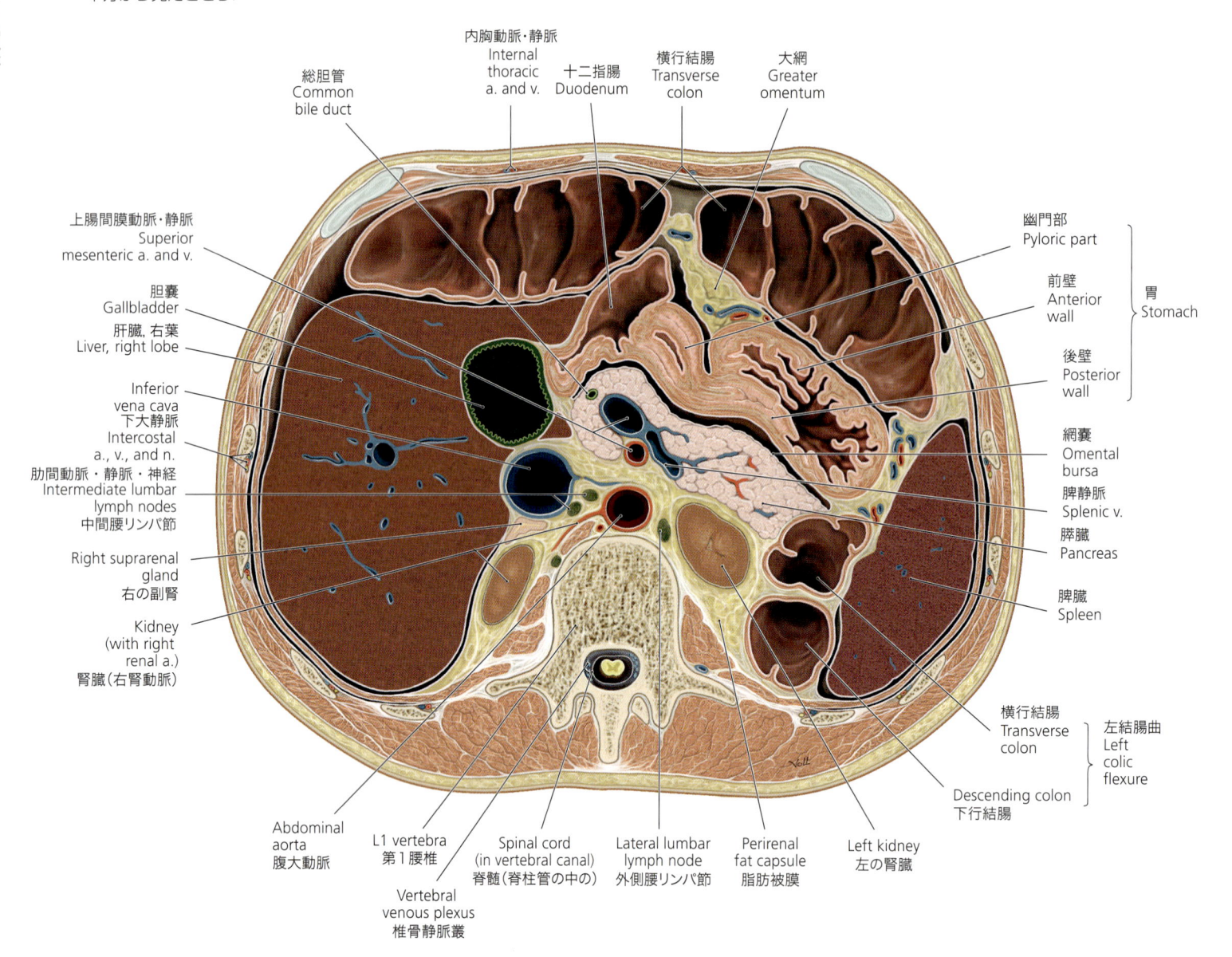

- 総胆管 / Common bile duct
- 内胸動脈・静脈 / Internal thoracic a. and v.
- 十二指腸 / Duodenum
- 横行結腸 / Transverse colon
- 大網 / Greater omentum
- 幽門部 / Pyloric part
- 前壁 / Anterior wall ｝胃 / Stomach
- 後壁 / Posterior wall
- 上腸間膜動脈・静脈 / Superior mesenteric a. and v.
- 胆嚢 / Gallbladder
- 肝臓, 右葉 / Liver, right lobe
- Inferior vena cava / 下大静脈
- 肋間動脈・静脈・神経 / Intercostal a., v., and n.
- Intermediate lumbar lymph nodes / 中間腰リンパ節
- Right suprarenal gland / 右の副腎
- Kidney (with right renal a.) / 腎臓（右腎動脈）
- 網嚢 / Omental bursa
- 脾静脈 / Splenic v.
- 膵臓 / Pancreas
- 脾臓 / Spleen
- 横行結腸 / Transverse colon ｝左結腸曲 / Left colic flexure
- Descending colon / 下行結腸
- Abdominal aorta / 腹大動脈
- L1 vertebra / 第1腰椎
- Spinal cord (in vertebral canal) / 脊髄（脊柱管の中の）
- Vertebral venous plexus / 椎骨静脈叢
- Lateral lumbar lymph node / 外側腰リンパ節
- Perirenal fat capsule / 脂肪被膜
- Left kidney / 左の腎臓

図 12.17　骨盤：水平断
下方から見たところ．

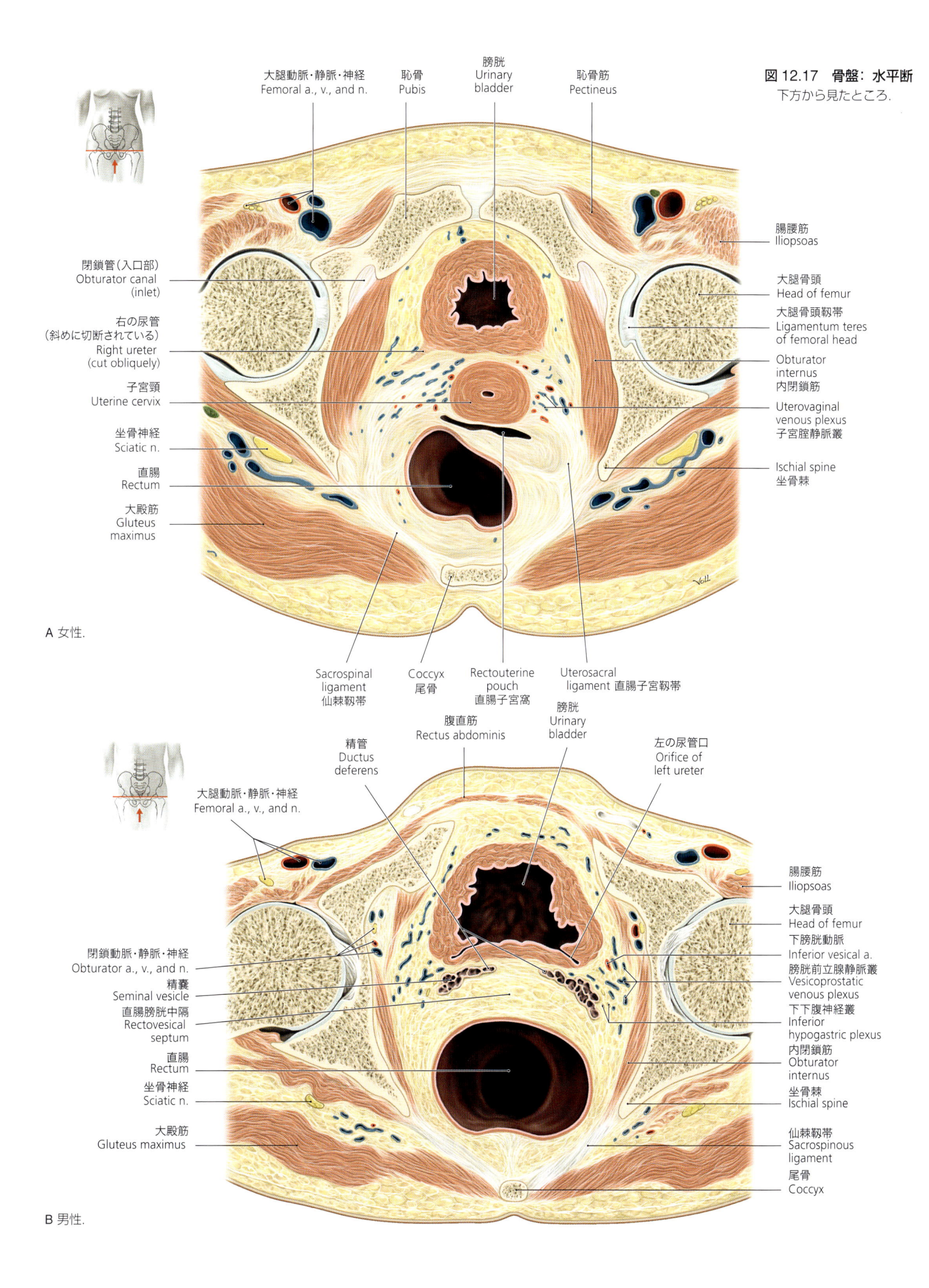

A 女性．

- 大腿動脈・静脈・神経 Femoral a., v., and n.
- 恥骨 Pubis
- 膀胱 Urinary bladder
- 恥骨筋 Pectineus
- 閉鎖管（入口部）Obturator canal (inlet)
- 右の尿管（斜めに切断されている）Right ureter (cut obliquely)
- 子宮頸 Uterine cervix
- 坐骨神経 Sciatic n.
- 直腸 Rectum
- 大殿筋 Gluteus maximus
- 腸腰筋 Iliopsoas
- 大腿骨頭 Head of femur
- 大腿骨頭靱帯 Ligamentum teres of femoral head
- 内閉鎖筋 Obturator internus
- 子宮腟静脈叢 Uterovaginal venous plexus
- 坐骨棘 Ischial spine
- Sacrospinal ligament 仙棘靱帯
- Coccyx 尾骨
- Rectouterine pouch 直腸子宮窩
- Uterosacral ligament 直腸子宮靱帯

B 男性．

- 腹直筋 Rectus abdominis
- 膀胱 Urinary bladder
- 左の尿管口 Orifice of left ureter
- 精管 Ductus deferens
- 大腿動脈・静脈・神経 Femoral a., v., and n.
- 閉鎖動脈・静脈・神経 Obturator a., v., and n.
- 精嚢 Seminal vesicle
- 直腸膀胱中隔 Rectovesical septum
- 直腸 Rectum
- 坐骨神経 Sciatic n.
- 大殿筋 Gluteus maximus
- 腸腰筋 Iliopsoas
- 大腿骨頭 Head of femur
- 下膀胱動脈 Inferior vesical a.
- 膀胱前立腺静脈叢 Vesicoprostatic venous plexus
- 下下腹神経叢 Inferior hypogastric plexus
- 内閉鎖筋 Obturator internus
- 坐骨棘 Ischial spine
- 仙棘靱帯 Sacrospinous ligament
- 尾骨 Coccyx

胃
Stomach

図 13.1 胃：位置

右上腹部 RUQ　左上腹部 LUQ

幽門平面
Transpyloric plane

A 前方から見たところ.

小網（肝胃間膜）
Lesser omentum (hepatogastric ligament)
膵臓 Pancreas
肝臓 Liver
胃 Stomach
網嚢 Omental bursa
脾臓 Spleen
下大静脈 Inferior vena cava
腹大動脈 Abdominal aorta
左の腎臓 Left kidney

B 水平断, 下方から見たところ.

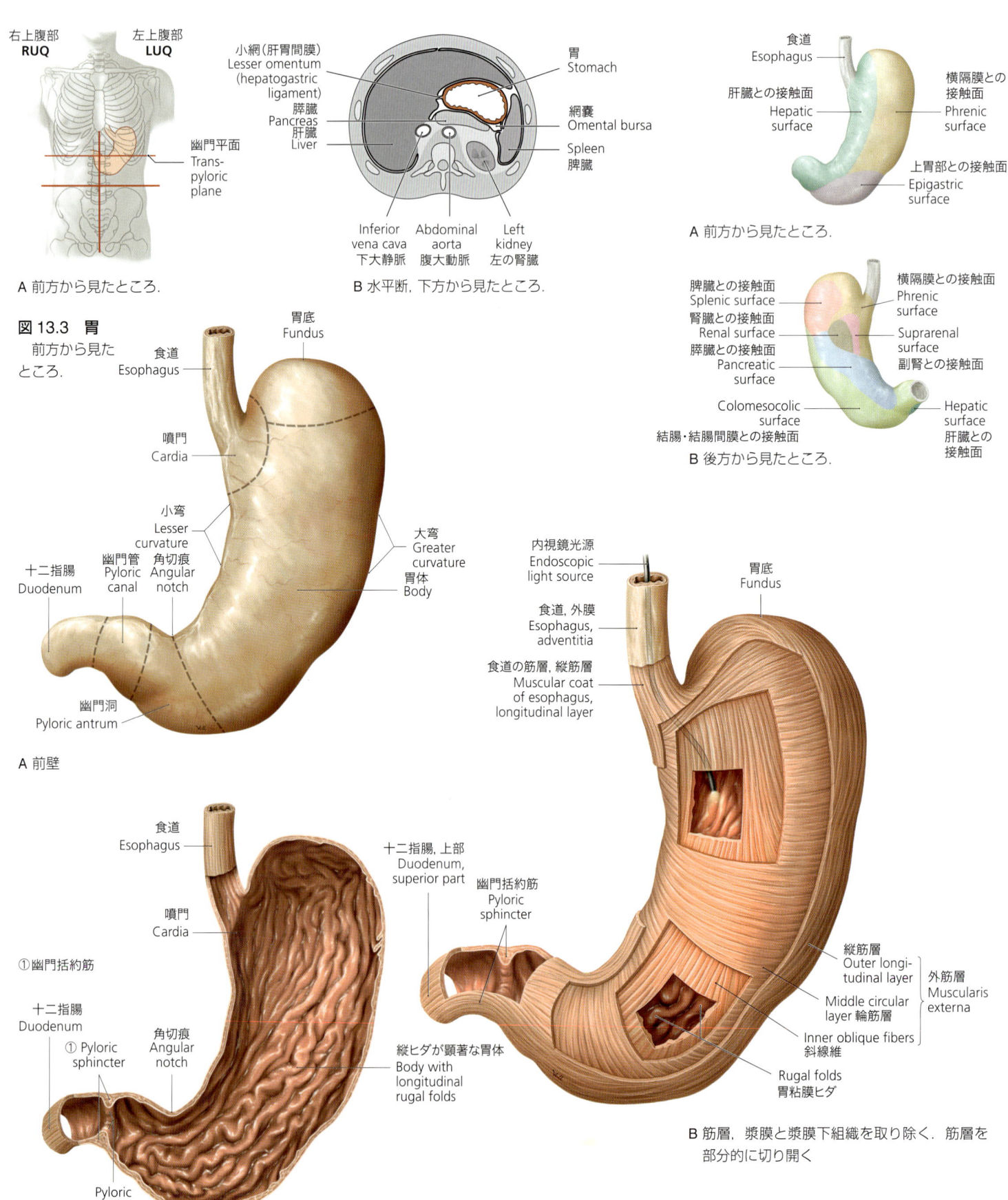

図 13.2 胃の表面

食道 Esophagus
肝臓との接触面 Hepatic surface
横隔膜との接触面 Phrenic surface
上胃部との接触面 Epigastric surface

A 前方から見たところ.

脾臓との接触面 Splenic surface
腎臓との接触面 Renal surface
膵臓との接触面 Pancreatic surface
横隔膜との接触面 Phrenic surface
副腎との接触面 Suprarenal surface
肝臓との接触面 Hepatic surface
結腸・結腸間膜との接触面 Colomesocolic surface

B 後方から見たところ.

図 13.3 胃

前方から見たところ.

胃底 Fundus
食道 Esophagus
噴門 Cardia
小弯 Lesser curvature
大弯 Greater curvature
胃体 Body
十二指腸 Duodenum
幽門管 Pyloric canal
角切痕 Angular notch
幽門洞 Pyloric antrum

A 前壁

食道 Esophagus
噴門 Cardia
①幽門括約筋 Pyloric sphincter
十二指腸 Duodenum
①角切痕 Angular notch
十二指腸, 上部 Duodenum, superior part
幽門括約筋 Pyloric sphincter
縦ヒダが顕著な胃体 Body with longitudinal rugal folds
幽門口 Pyloric orifice

C 内面, 前壁を取り除く

内視鏡光源 Endoscopic light source
胃底 Fundus
食道, 外膜 Esophagus, adventitia
食道の筋層, 縦筋層 Muscular coat of esophagus, longitudinal layer
縦筋層 Outer longitudinal layer
輪筋層 Middle circular layer
斜線維 Inner oblique fibers
外筋層 Muscularis externa
胃粘膜ヒダ Rugal folds

B 筋層, 漿膜と漿膜下組織を取り除く. 筋層を部分的に切り開く

胃は右・左上腹部にある．胃は腹膜内器官で，その腸間膜は小網と大網である．

図13.4　原位置の胃
開腹した上腹部を前方から見たところ．矢印は網嚢孔を示す．

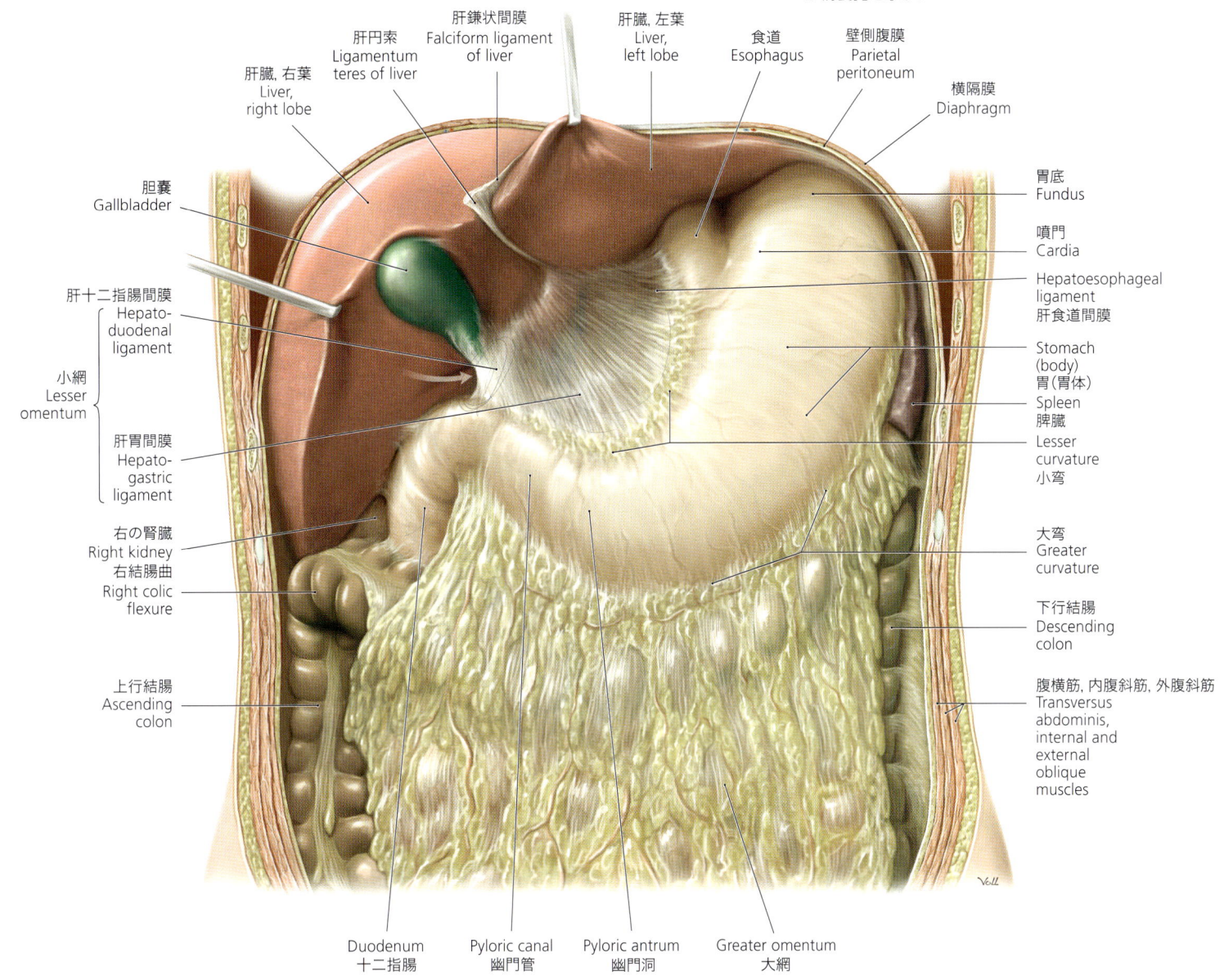

図中ラベル：
- 肝臓，右葉 Liver, right lobe
- 肝円索 Ligamentum teres of liver
- 肝鎌状間膜 Falciform ligament of liver
- 肝臓，左葉 Liver, left lobe
- 食道 Esophagus
- 壁側腹膜 Parietal peritoneum
- 横隔膜 Diaphragm
- 胆嚢 Gallbladder
- 胃底 Fundus
- 噴門 Cardia
- 肝十二指腸間膜 Hepatoduodenal ligament
- 小網 Lesser omentum
- 肝胃間膜 Hepatogastric ligament
- Hepatoesophageal ligament 肝食道間膜
- Stomach (body) 胃（胃体）
- Spleen 脾臓
- Lesser curvature 小弯
- 右の腎臓 Right kidney
- 右結腸曲 Right colic flexure
- 大弯 Greater curvature
- 下行結腸 Descending colon
- 上行結腸 Ascending colon
- 腹横筋，内腹斜筋，外腹斜筋 Transversus abdominis, internal and external oblique muscles
- Duodenum 十二指腸
- Pyloric canal 幽門管
- Pyloric antrum 幽門洞
- Greater omentum 大網

臨床

胃炎と胃潰瘍

胃のよく知られた疾患である胃炎と胃潰瘍は胃酸酸性過多と関連づけられるが，アルコールやアスピリンなどの薬物，細菌のヘリコバクターピロリが原因となる．食欲減退，胃痛，黒色便や吐瀉物中の暗褐色の物質などが症状として現れる．胃炎は胃壁の内側面に限られるが，胃潰瘍は胃壁に及ぶ．Cの胃潰瘍ではフィブリンで覆われ，ヘマチンの斑点が見られる．

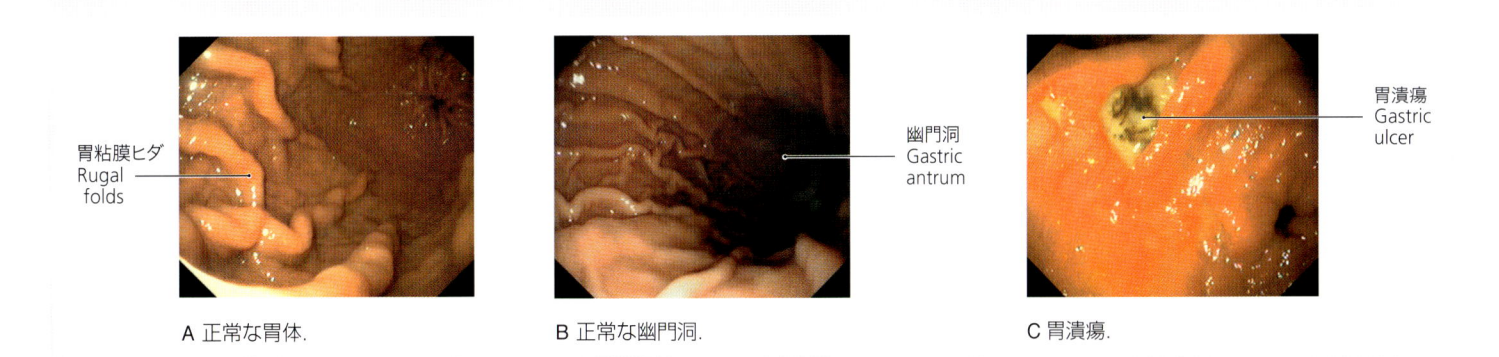

A 正常な胃体．
- 胃粘膜ヒダ Rugal folds

B 正常な幽門洞．
- 幽門洞 Gastric antrum

C 胃潰瘍．
- 胃潰瘍 Gastric ulcer

十二指腸
Duodenum

小腸は十二指腸，空腸，回腸からなる（p.162参照）．十二指腸は主として腹膜後器官で，上部，下行部，水平部，上行部の4部に分けられる．

図 13.5　十二指腸：位置
前方から見たところ．

- 右上腹部 RUQ
- 左上腹部 LUQ
- 十二指腸 Duodenum
- 十二指腸空腸曲 Duodeno-jejunal flexure
- 空腸と回腸 Jejunum and ileum

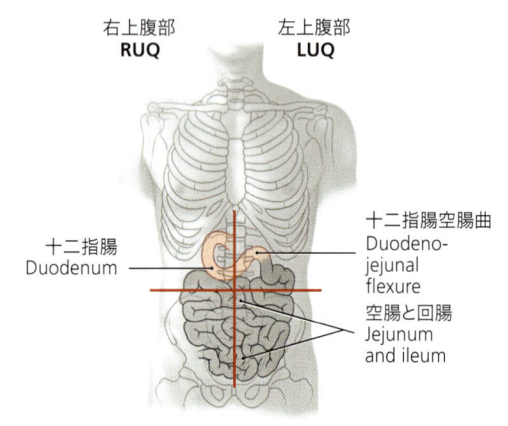

図 13.6　十二指腸の部分
前方から見たところ．

- 十二指腸球部 Duodenal bulb
- 下大静脈 Inferior vena cava
- 腹腔動脈 Celiac trunk
- 十二指腸提筋 Suspensory ligament of duodenum
- 上部 Superior part
- 上十二指腸曲 Superior duodenal flexure
- 上腸間膜動脈 Superior mesenteric a.
- 左腎静脈 Left renal v.
- 下行部 Descending part
- 空腸 Jejunum
- 下十二指腸曲 Inferior duodenal flexure
- 上行部 Ascending part
- 水平部 Horizontal part

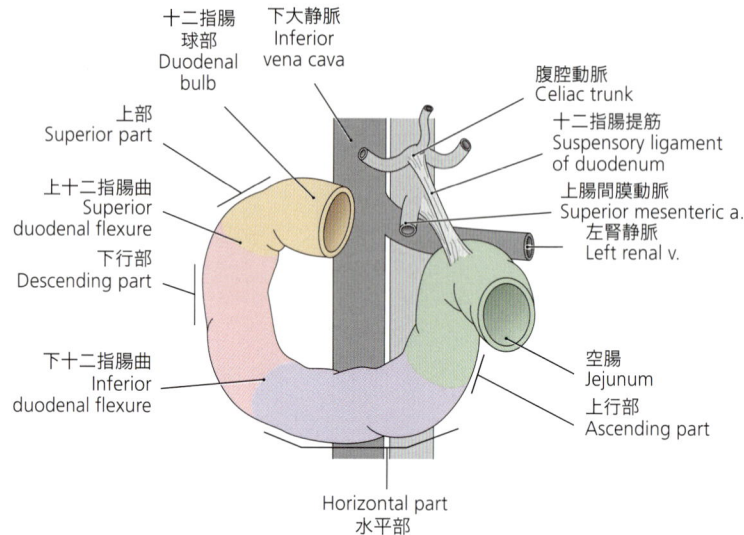

図 13.7　十二指腸
前方から見たところ．前壁を開く．

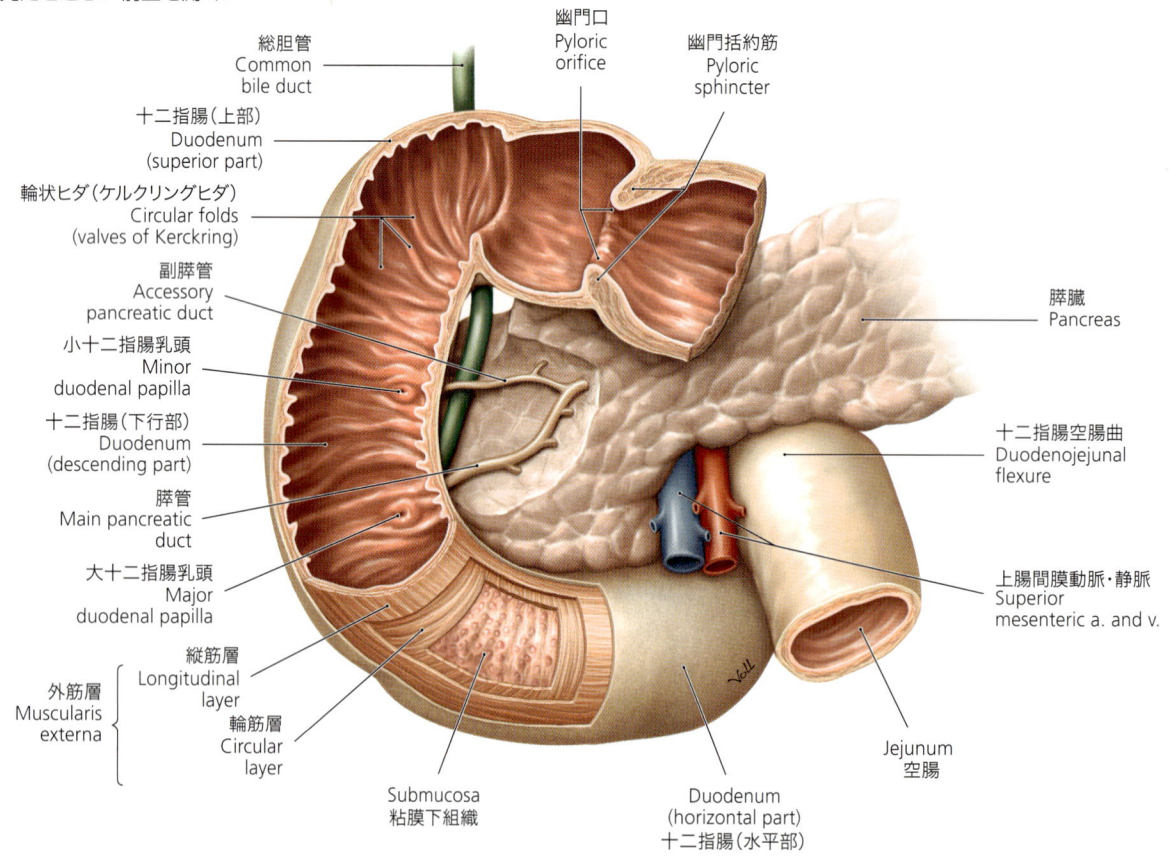

- 総胆管 Common bile duct
- 幽門口 Pyloric orifice
- 幽門括約筋 Pyloric sphincter
- 十二指腸（上部）Duodenum (superior part)
- 輪状ヒダ（ケルクリングヒダ）Circular folds (valves of Kerckring)
- 副膵管 Accessory pancreatic duct
- 小十二指腸乳頭 Minor duodenal papilla
- 十二指腸（下行部）Duodenum (descending part)
- 膵管 Main pancreatic duct
- 大十二指腸乳頭 Major duodenal papilla
- 外筋層 Muscularis externa
  - 縦筋層 Longitudinal layer
  - 輪筋層 Circular layer
- 粘膜下組織 Submucosa
- 十二指腸（水平部）Duodenum (horizontal part)
- 膵臓 Pancreas
- 十二指腸空腸曲 Duodenojejunal flexure
- 上腸間膜動脈・静脈 Superior mesenteric a. and v.
- 空腸 Jejunum

図 13.8 原位置の十二指腸

前方から見たところ．胃，肝臓，小腸，横行結腸の大部分を取り除く．
腹膜後部の脂肪と結合組織も取り除く．

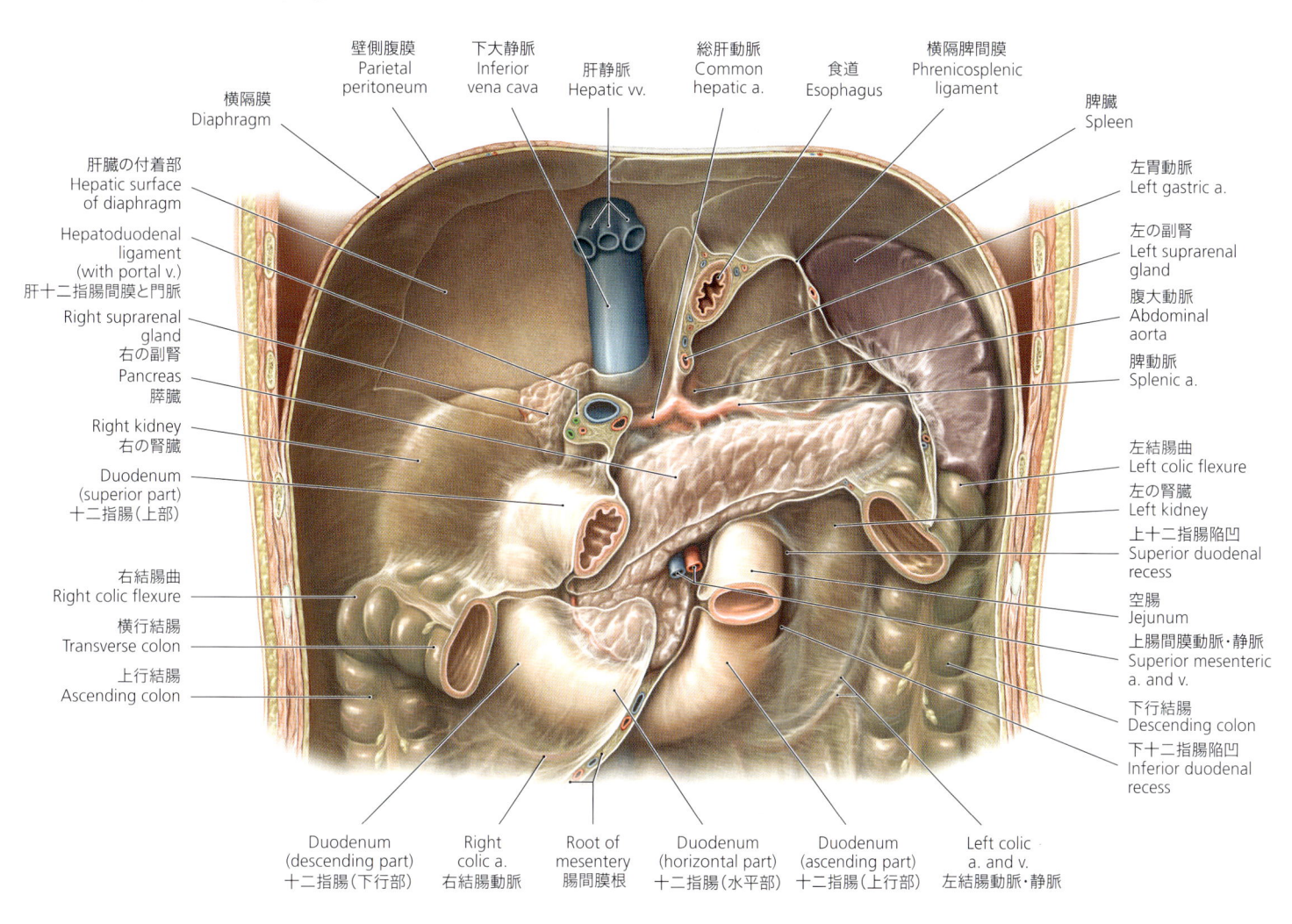

(図の主なラベル)
- 横隔膜 Diaphragm
- 壁側腹膜 Parietal peritoneum
- 下大静脈 Inferior vena cava
- 肝静脈 Hepatic vv.
- 総肝動脈 Common hepatic a.
- 食道 Esophagus
- 横隔脾間膜 Phrenicosplenic ligament
- 脾臓 Spleen
- 肝臓の付着部 Hepatic surface of diaphragm
- 肝十二指腸間膜と門脈 Hepatoduodenal ligament (with portal v.)
- 左胃動脈 Left gastric a.
- 左の副腎 Left suprarenal gland
- 腹大動脈 Abdominal aorta
- 右の副腎 Right suprarenal gland
- 膵臓 Pancreas
- 脾動脈 Splenic a.
- 右の腎臓 Right kidney
- 十二指腸（上部）Duodenum (superior part)
- 左結腸曲 Left colic flexure
- 左の腎臓 Left kidney
- 上十二指腸陥凹 Superior duodenal recess
- 右結腸曲 Right colic flexure
- 空腸 Jejunum
- 横行結腸 Transverse colon
- 上腸間膜動脈・静脈 Superior mesenteric a. and v.
- 上行結腸 Ascending colon
- 下行結腸 Descending colon
- 下十二指腸陥凹 Inferior duodenal recess
- 十二指腸（下行部）Duodenum (descending part)
- 右結腸動脈 Right colic a.
- 腸間膜根 Root of mesentery
- 十二指腸（水平部）Duodenum (horizontal part)
- 十二指腸（上行部）Duodenum (ascending part)
- 左結腸動脈・静脈 Left colic a. and v.

🏥 臨床

乳頭領域

十二指腸には総胆管と膵管（図 13.7 を参照）の 2 つの重要な導管が乳頭領域に開口している．この管は十二指腸乳頭に内視鏡で色素を注入する内視鏡的逆行性胆道膵管造影（ERCP）によって X 線撮影で確かめられる．十二指腸憩室は一般には無害であるが，この撮影を難しくする．

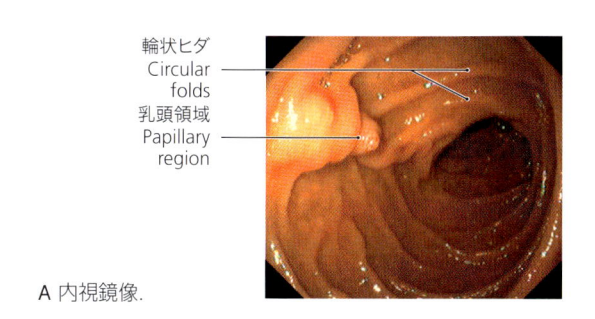

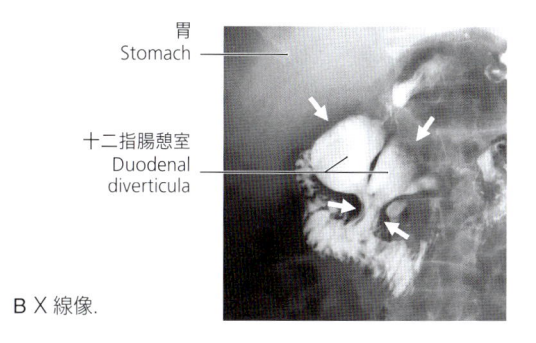

(図ラベル)
- 輪状ヒダ Circular folds
- 乳頭領域 Papillary region
- 胃 Stomach
- 十二指腸憩室 Duodenal diverticula

A 内視鏡像．
B X 線像．

空腸と回腸
Jejunum & Ileum

図 13.9 空腸と回腸：位置
前方から見たところ．空腸と回腸は腹膜内にあり，腸間膜で包まれる．

- 右上腹部 RUQ
- 左上腹部 LUQ
- 十二指腸空腸曲 Duodeno-jejunal flexure
- 上行結腸 Ascending colon
- Jejunum and ileum 空腸と回腸
- 右下腹部 RLQ
- LLQ 左下腹部
- Rectum 直腸

図 13.10 小腸壁の構造

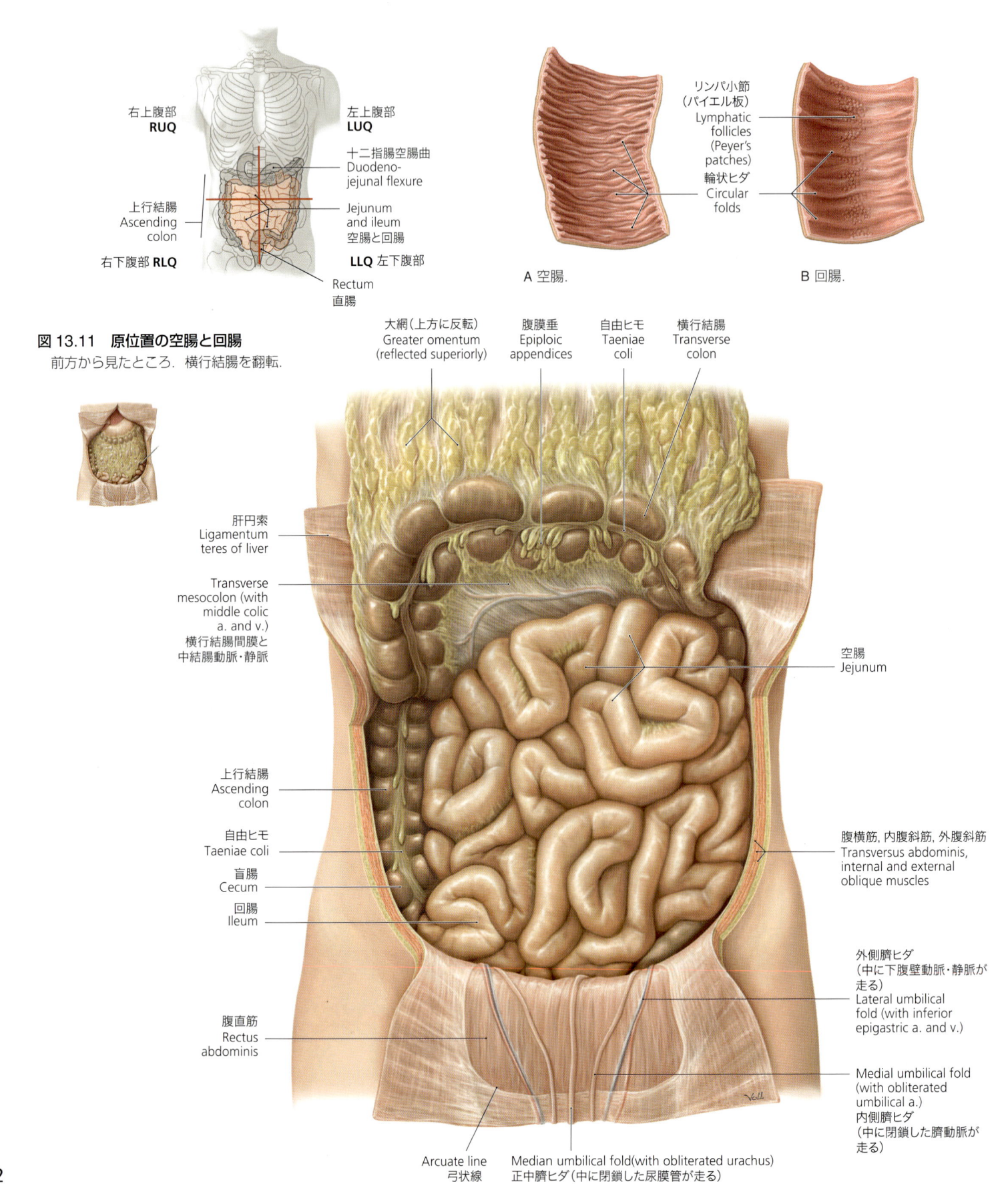

- リンパ小節（パイエル板）Lymphatic follicles (Peyer's patches)
- 輪状ヒダ Circular folds

A 空腸．

B 回腸．

図 13.11 原位置の空腸と回腸
前方から見たところ．横行結腸を翻転．

- 大網（上方に反転）Greater omentum (reflected superiorly)
- 腹膜垂 Epiploic appendices
- 自由ヒモ Taeniae coli
- 横行結腸 Transverse colon
- 肝円索 Ligamentum teres of liver
- Transverse mesocolon (with middle colic a. and v.) 横行結腸間膜と中結腸動脈・静脈
- 空腸 Jejunum
- 上行結腸 Ascending colon
- 自由ヒモ Taeniae coli
- 盲腸 Cecum
- 回腸 Ileum
- 腹横筋, 内腹斜筋, 外腹斜筋 Transversus abdominis, internal and external oblique muscles
- 外側臍ヒダ（中に下腹壁動脈・静脈が走る）Lateral umbilical fold (with inferior epigastric a. and v.)
- 内側臍ヒダ（中に閉鎖した臍動脈が走る）Medial umbilical fold (with obliterated umbilical a.)
- 腹直筋 Rectus abdominis
- Arcuate line 弓状線
- Median umbilical fold (with obliterated urachus) 正中臍ヒダ（中に閉鎖した尿膜管が走る）

臨床

クローン病
消化管の慢性炎症であるクローン病は結腸末端でよく見られる（約30％）．一般的に若者に起こり，腹痛，吐気，体温上昇，下痢が見られる．初期症状は虫垂炎と混同しやすい．クローン病の合併症に瘻孔も含まれる（B）．

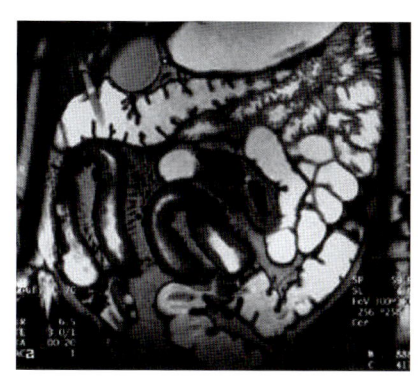

A　MR像．結腸末端の壁が肥厚している．

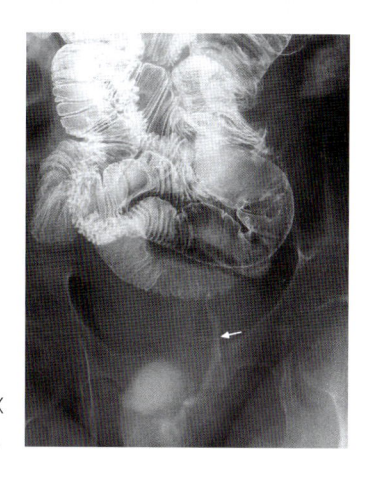

B　二重造影によるX線像．矢印は瘻孔．

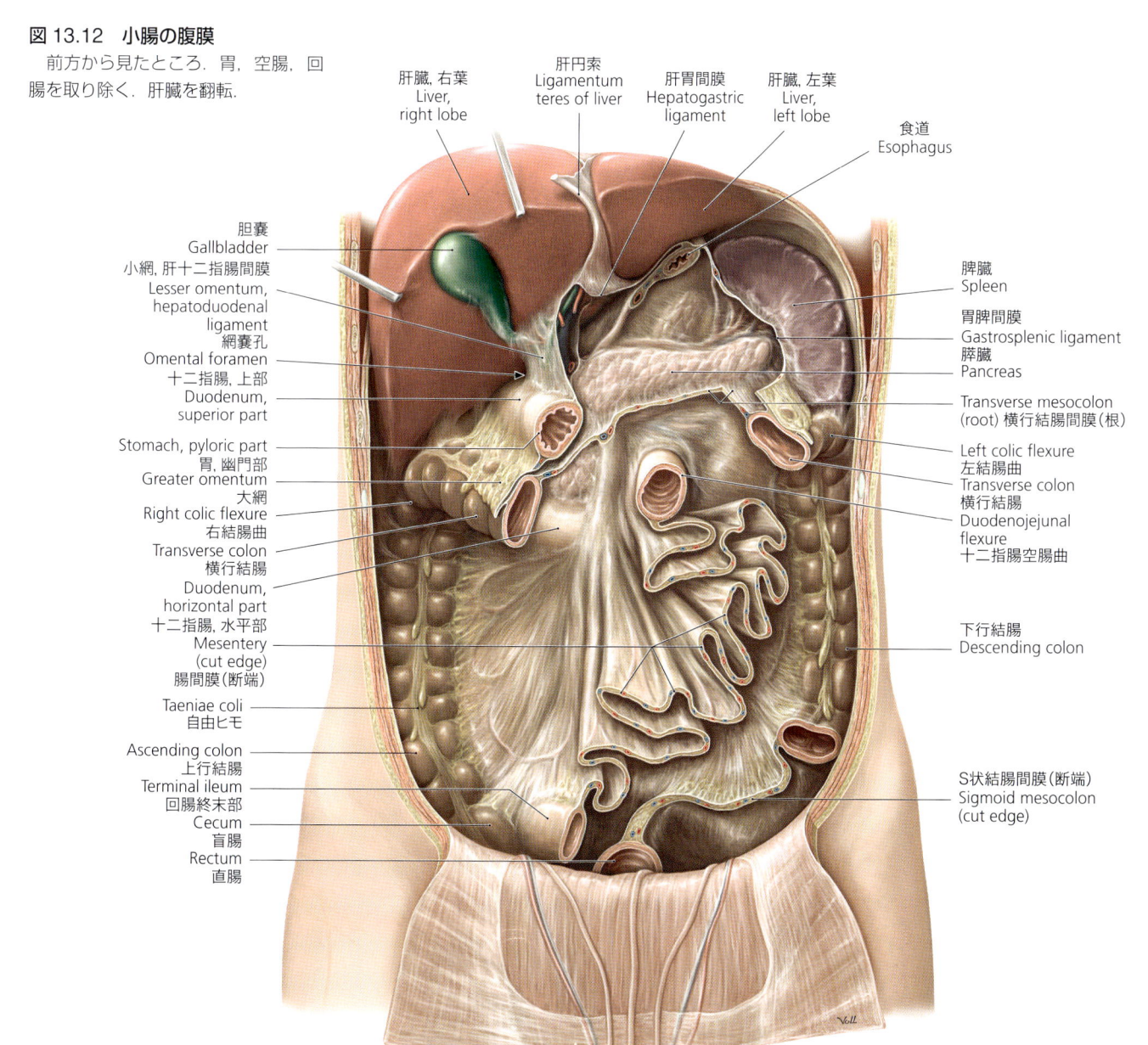

図13.12　小腸の腹膜

前方から見たところ．胃，空腸，回腸を取り除く．肝臓を翻転．

盲腸，虫垂，結腸
Cecum, Appendix & Colon

大腸は盲腸，虫垂，結腸，直腸（p.166 参照）からなる．結腸は上行結腸，横行結腸，下行結腸，S 状結腸の 4 部に分けられる．虫垂，横行結腸，S 状結腸は腹膜内器官であり，それぞれ虫垂間膜，横行結腸間膜，S 状結腸間膜が付着する．

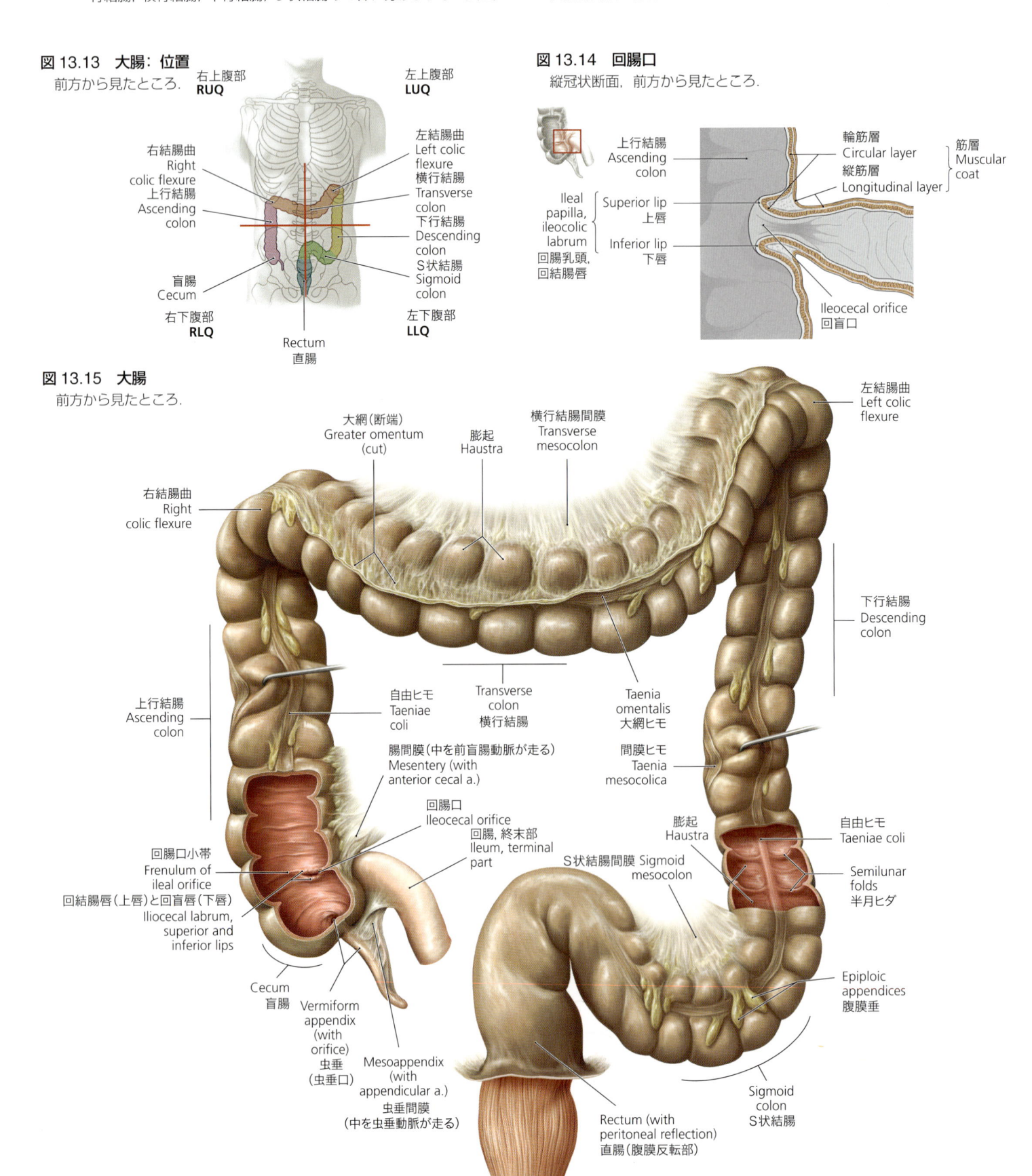

図 13.13　大腸：位置
前方から見たところ．

- 右上腹部 RUQ
- 左上腹部 LUQ
- 右結腸曲 Right colic flexure
- 上行結腸 Ascending colon
- 左結腸曲 Left colic flexure
- 横行結腸 Transverse colon
- 下行結腸 Descending colon
- 盲腸 Cecum
- S 状結腸 Sigmoid colon
- 右下腹部 RLQ
- 左下腹部 LLQ
- 直腸 Rectum

図 13.14　回腸口
縦冠状断面，前方から見たところ．

- 上行結腸 Ascending colon
- 輪筋層 Circular layer
- 縦筋層 Longitudinal layer
- 筋層 Muscular coat
- 回腸乳頭，回結腸唇 Ileal papilla, ileocolic labrum
- 上唇 Superior lip
- 下唇 Inferior lip
- 回盲口 Ileocecal orifice

図 13.15　大腸
前方から見たところ．

- 右結腸曲 Right colic flexure
- 大網（断端）Greater omentum (cut)
- 膨起 Haustra
- 横行結腸間膜 Transverse mesocolon
- 左結腸曲 Left colic flexure
- 上行結腸 Ascending colon
- 自由ヒモ Taeniae coli
- 横行結腸 Transverse colon
- 大網ヒモ Taenia omentalis
- 下行結腸 Descending colon
- 腸間膜（中を前盲腸動脈が走る）Mesentery (with anterior cecal a.)
- 間膜ヒモ Taenia mesocolica
- 回腸口小帯 Frenulum of ileal orifice
- 回盲口 Ileocecal orifice
- 回腸，終末部 Ileum, terminal part
- 回結腸唇（上唇）と回盲唇（下唇）Iliocecal labrum, superior and inferior lips
- 膨起 Haustra
- 自由ヒモ Taeniae coli
- 半月ヒダ Semilunar folds
- 盲腸 Cecum
- 虫垂（虫垂口）Vermiform appendix (with orifice)
- S 状結腸間膜 Sigmoid mesocolon
- 腹膜垂 Epiploic appendices
- 虫垂間膜（中を虫垂動脈が走る）Mesoappendix (with appendicular a.)
- S 状結腸 Sigmoid colon
- 直腸（腹膜反転部）Rectum (with peritoneal reflection)

図 13.16 原位置の大腸

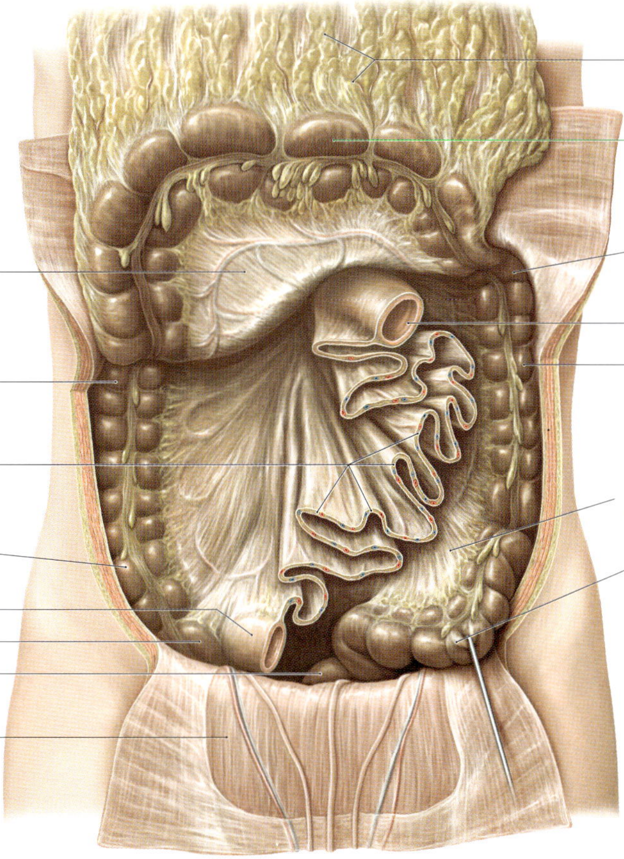

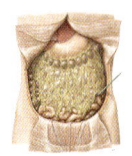

大網 Greater omentum
横行結腸 Transverse colon
左結腸曲 Left colic (splenic) flexure
空腸 Jejunum
Descending colon 下行結腸
S状結腸間膜 Sigmoid mesocolon
S状結腸 Sigmoid colon

横行結腸間膜 Transverse mesocolon
右結腸曲 Right colic (hepatic) flexure
腸間膜（断端） Mesentery (cut)
上行結腸 Ascending colon
回腸 Ileum
盲腸 Cecum
直腸 Rectum
腹直筋 Rectus abdominis

A 前方から見たところ．横行結腸と大網を翻転．腹膜内の小腸を取り除く．

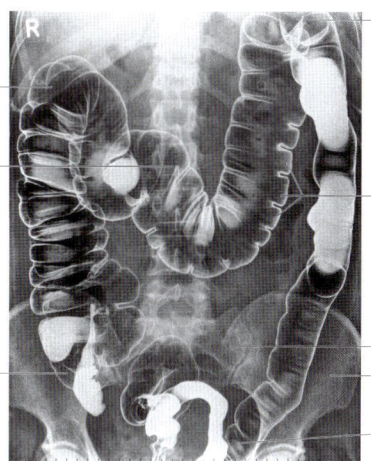

右結腸曲 Right colic flexure
横行結腸 Transverse colon
盲腸 Cecum
左結腸曲 Left colic flexure
結腸膨起 Colonic haustra
仙骨 Sacrum
腸骨 Ilium
Sigmoid colon S状結腸

B 正常な大腸の X 線正面像．二重造影．

臨床

大腸炎

潰瘍性大腸炎は，多くは直腸以下の大腸に起こる慢性の炎症である．典型的症候には下痢（しばしば血便），腹痛，体重減少，他臓器の炎症が含まれる．患者は結腸直腸癌の危険性も高い．

大腸癌

結腸と直腸の悪性腫瘍は最頻発の固形腫瘍の一つである．90% 以上が 50 歳以上の人に起こる．初期の腫瘍は無症候性であるが，後に食欲喪失，腸運動の変化，体重減少が見られる．便中の血液は特に重要な症候で，徹底的な検査が必要である．結腸鏡を含む他のすべてのテストが陰性でない限り，便中の血液を痔で説明することはできない．

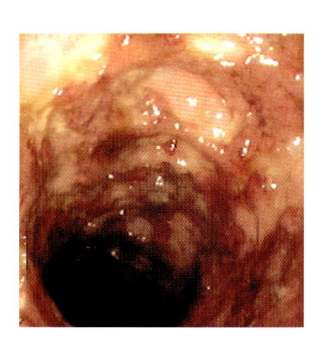

A 結腸鏡で見た潰瘍性大腸炎．

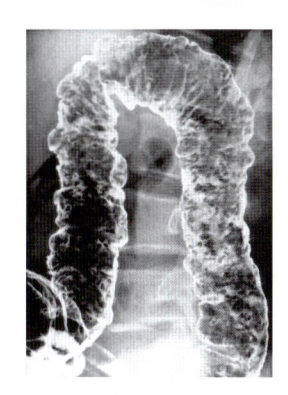

B 初期の大腸炎．残存した正常粘膜が偽ポリープのように見える．

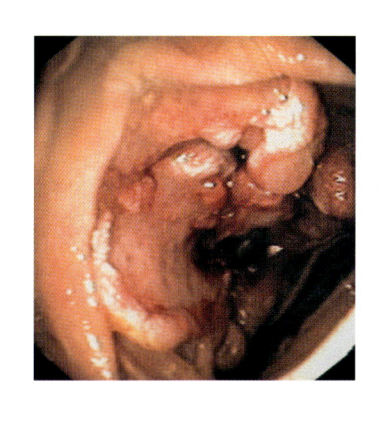

C 結腸鏡で見た大腸癌．腫瘍が結腸管腔を部分的に塞いでいる．

直腸と肛門管
Rectum & Anal Canal

図 13.17 直腸：位置

A 前方から見たところ．

- S状結腸 Sigmoid colon
- 直腸 Rectum
- RLQ 右下腹部
- LLQ 左下腹部

B 左前外側方から見たところ．

- 腸骨 Ilium
- 恥骨 Pubis
- 坐骨 Ischium
- 仙骨 Sacrum
- 仙骨曲 Sacral flexure
- 会陰曲 Perineal flexure
- 直腸 Rectum

図 13.18 直腸の閉鎖

左外側方から見たところ．恥骨直腸筋は肛門直腸移行部を曲げる筋肉の吊り糸として働き、排便抑制を維持する．

- 尾骨 Coccyx
- 恥骨尾骨筋 Pubococcygeus
- 会陰曲 Perineal flexure
- Pubis 恥骨
- Puborectalis 恥骨直腸筋

図 13.19 原位置の直腸

冠状断．女性骨盤を前方から見たところ．直腸の上 1/3 は前面と外側面が臓側腹膜で覆われる．中 1/3 は前面だけ臓側腹膜で覆われ、下 1/3 は壁側腹膜の下に位置する．

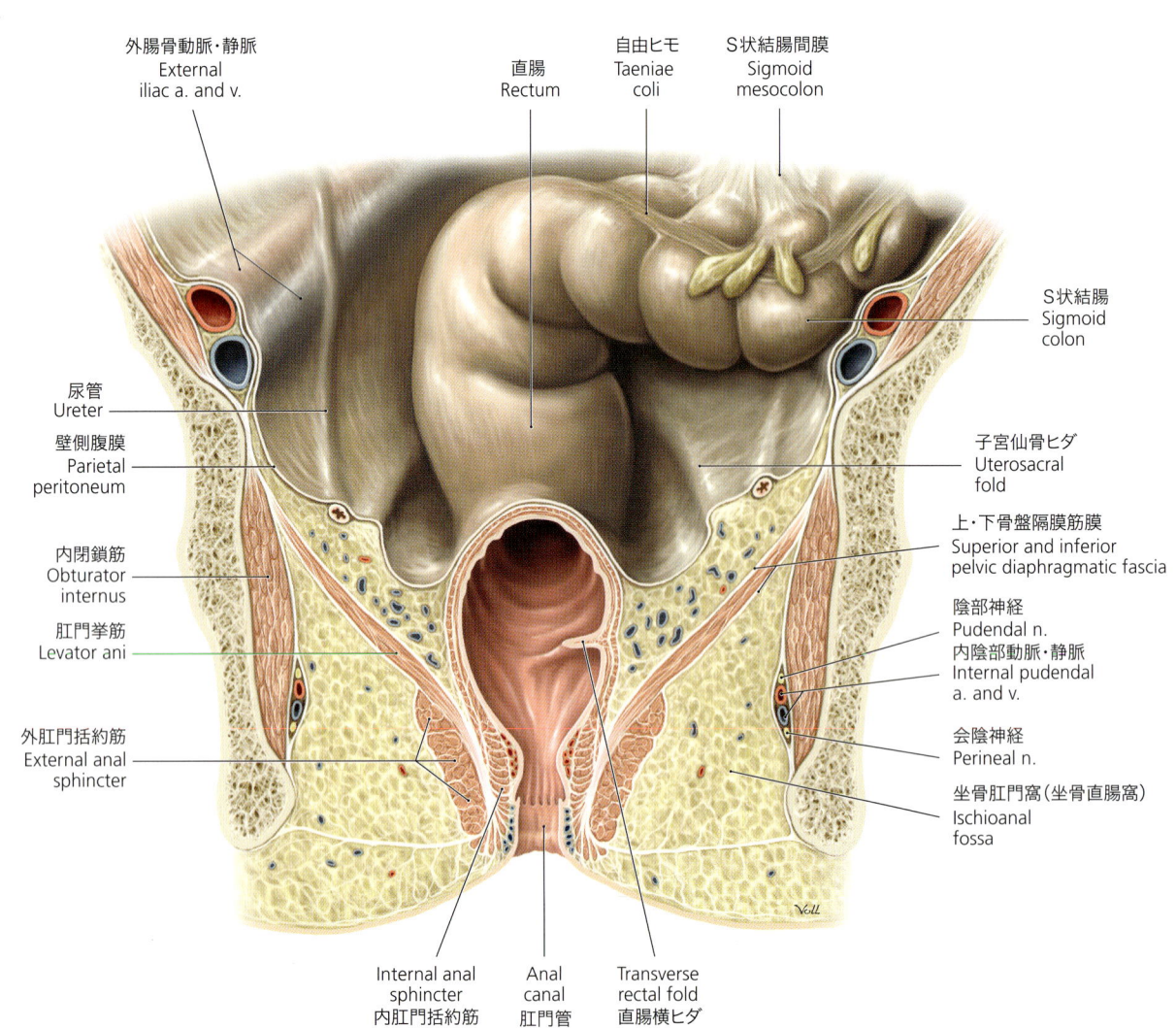

- 外腸骨動脈・静脈 External iliac a. and v.
- 直腸 Rectum
- 自由ヒモ Taeniae coli
- S状結腸間膜 Sigmoid mesocolon
- S状結腸 Sigmoid colon
- 尿管 Ureter
- 壁側腹膜 Parietal peritoneum
- 内閉鎖筋 Obturator internus
- 肛門挙筋 Levator ani
- 外肛門括約筋 External anal sphincter
- 子宮仙骨ヒダ Uterosacral fold
- 上・下骨盤隔膜筋膜 Superior and inferior pelvic diaphragmatic fascia
- 陰部神経 Pudendal n.
- 内陰部動脈・静脈 Internal pudendal a. and v.
- 会陰神経 Perineal n.
- 坐骨肛門窩（坐骨直腸窩）Ischioanal fossa
- 内肛門括約筋 Internal anal sphincter
- 肛門管 Anal canal
- 直腸横ヒダ Transverse rectal fold

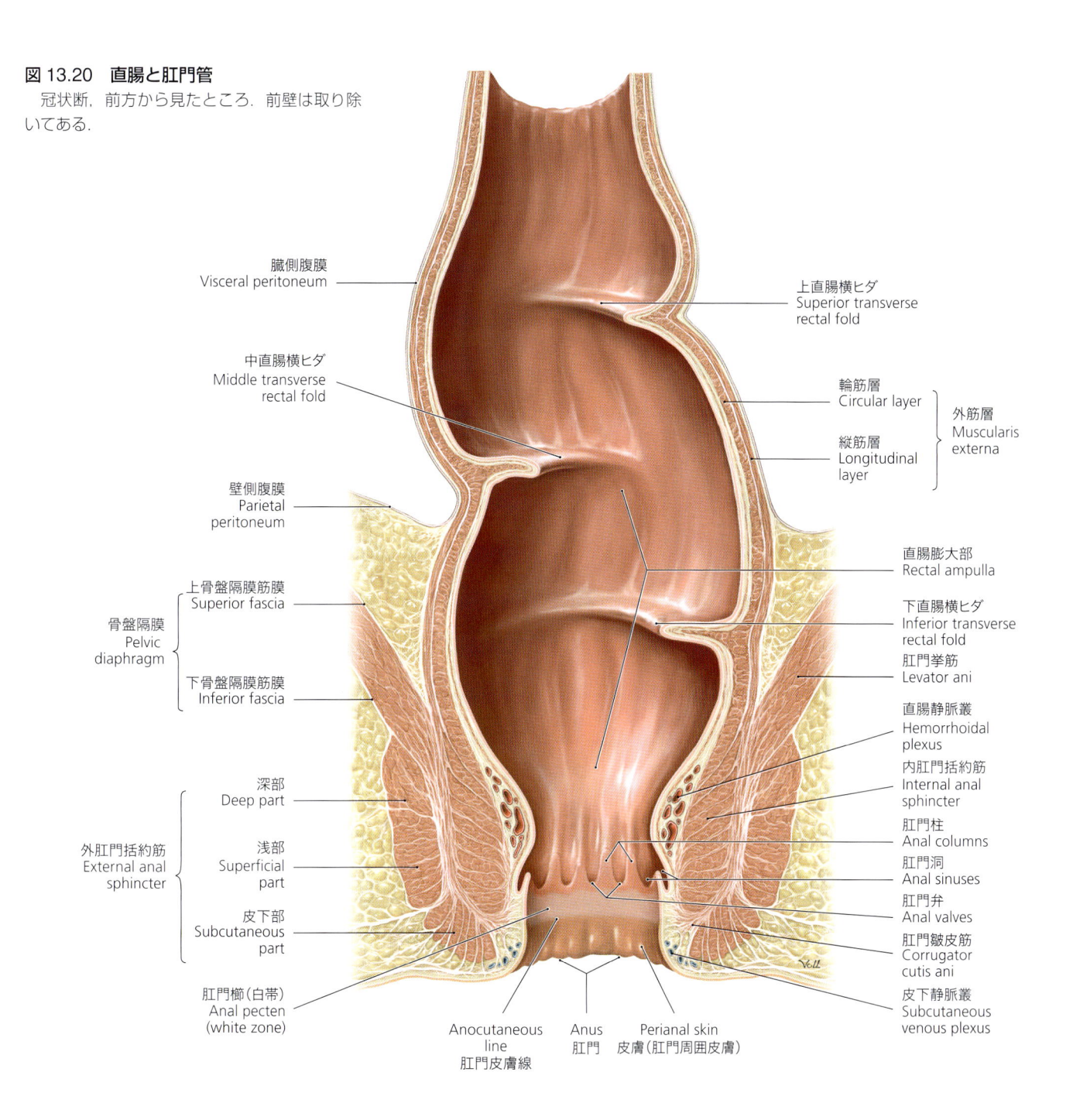

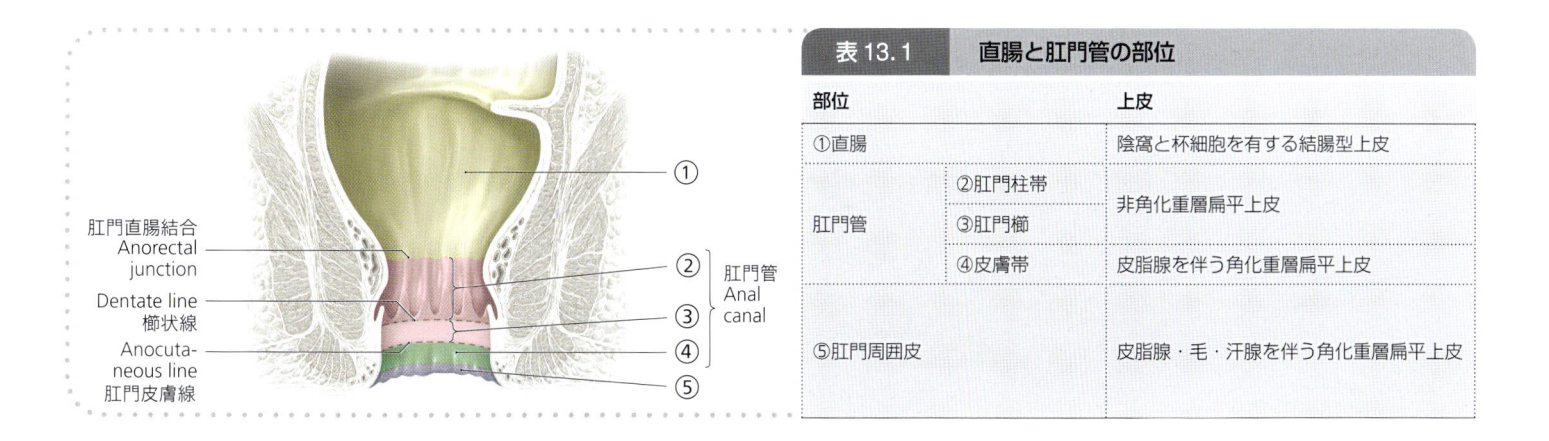

図 13.20 **直腸と肛門管**
冠状断，前方から見たところ．前壁は取り除いてある．

表 13.1		直腸と肛門管の部位
部位		上皮
①直腸		陰窩と杯細胞を有する結腸型上皮
肛門管	②肛門柱帯	非角化重層扁平上皮
	③肛門櫛	
	④皮膚帯	皮脂腺を伴う角化重層扁平上皮
⑤肛門周囲皮		皮脂腺・毛・汗腺を伴う角化重層扁平上皮

肝臓：概観
Liver: Overview

図 13.21　肝臓：位置

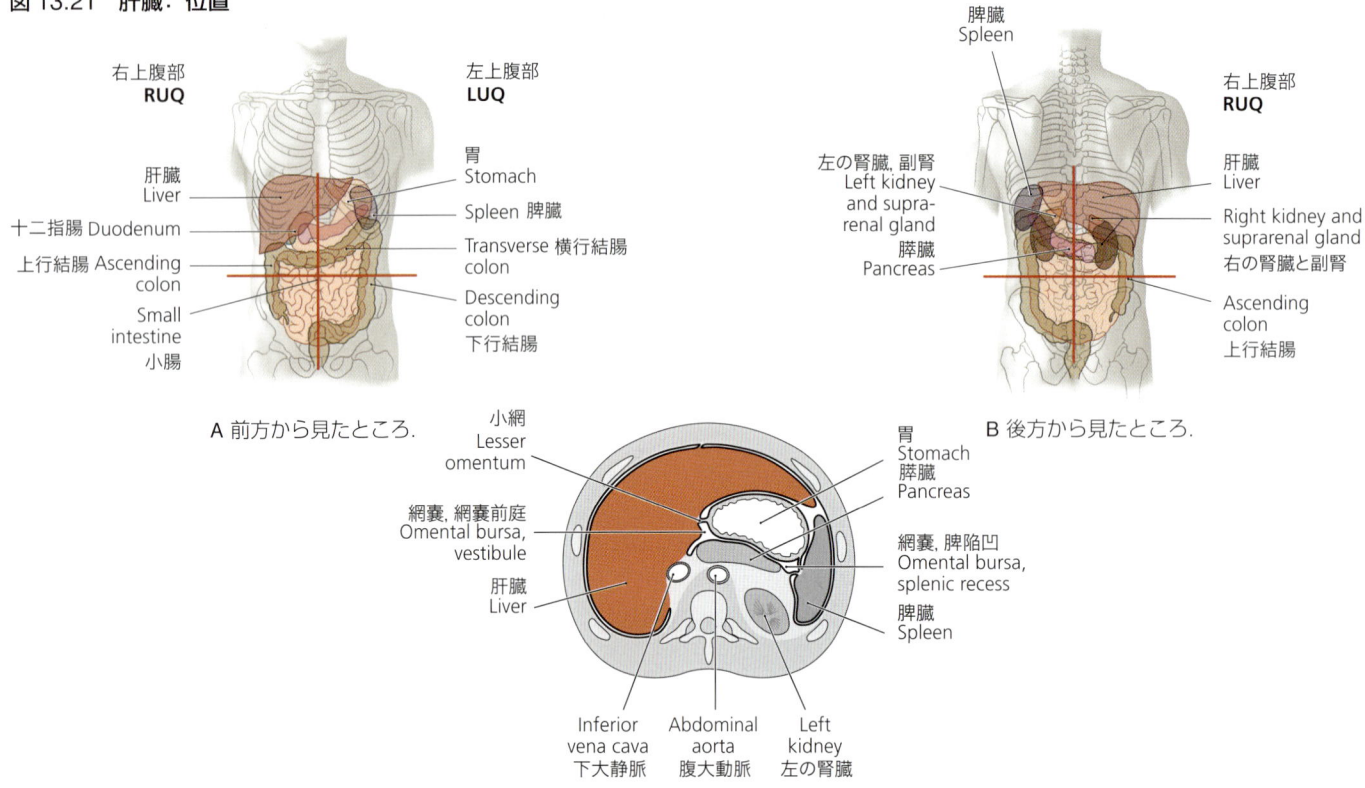

A 前方から見たところ．

- 右上腹部 **RUQ**
- 左上腹部 **LUQ**
- 肝臓 Liver
- 胃 Stomach
- 十二指腸 Duodenum
- Spleen 脾臓
- 上行結腸 Ascending colon
- Transverse 横行結腸 colon
- Small intestine 小腸
- Descending colon 下行結腸

B 後方から見たところ．

- 脾臓 Spleen
- 右上腹部 **RUQ**
- 左の腎臓, 副腎 Left kidney and suprarenal gland
- 肝臓 Liver
- 膵臓 Pancreas
- Right kidney and suprarenal gland 右の腎臓と副腎
- Ascending colon 上行結腸

C 水平断，下方から見たところ．

- 小網 Lesser omentum
- 胃 Stomach
- 膵臓 Pancreas
- 網嚢, 網嚢前庭 Omental bursa, vestibule
- 網嚢, 脾陥凹 Omental bursa, splenic recess
- 肝臓 Liver
- 脾臓 Spleen
- Inferior vena cava 下大静脈
- Abdominal aorta 腹大動脈
- Left kidney 左の腎臓

図 13.22　原位置の肝臓

前方から見たところ．肝臓を翻転．胃，空腸，回腸は取り除いてある．肝臓の無漿膜野（図13.26 参照）以外の部分では腹膜内にあり，その間膜には肝鎌状間膜，冠状間膜，三角間膜が含まれる（図 13.27 参照）．

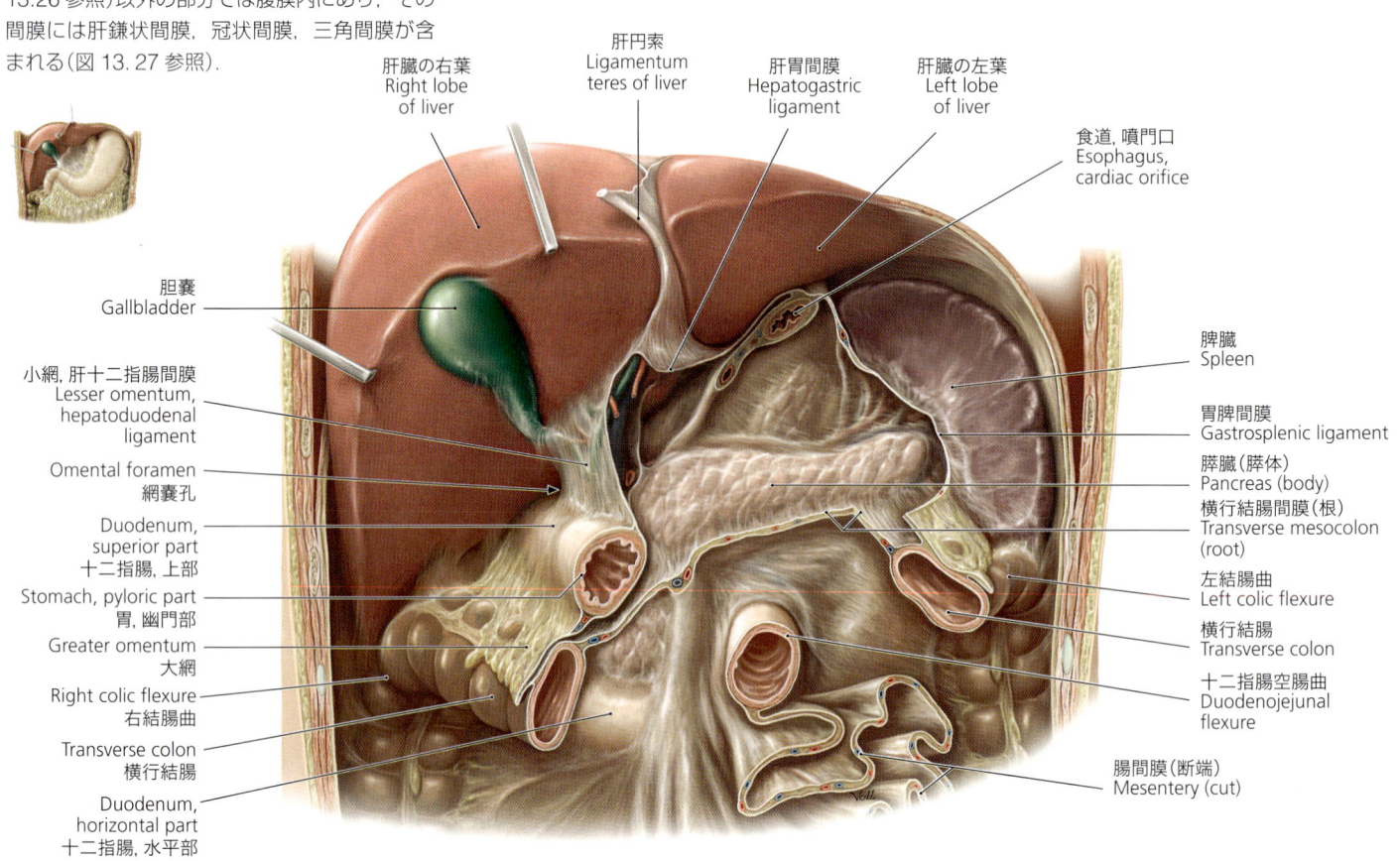

- 肝臓の右葉 Right lobe of liver
- 肝円索 Ligamentum teres of liver
- 肝胃間膜 Hepatogastric ligament
- 肝臓の左葉 Left lobe of liver
- 食道, 噴門口 Esophagus, cardiac orifice
- 胆嚢 Gallbladder
- 脾臓 Spleen
- 小網, 肝十二指腸間膜 Lesser omentum, hepatoduodenal ligament
- 胃脾間膜 Gastrosplenic ligament
- Omental foramen 網嚢孔
- 膵臓（膵体）Pancreas (body)
- Duodenum, superior part 十二指腸, 上部
- 横行結腸間膜（根）Transverse mesocolon (root)
- Stomach, pyloric part 胃, 幽門部
- 左結腸曲 Left colic flexure
- Greater omentum 大網
- 横行結腸 Transverse colon
- Right colic flexure 右結腸曲
- 十二指腸空腸曲 Duodenojejunal flexure
- Transverse colon 横行結腸
- 腸間膜（断端）Mesentery (cut)
- Duodenum, horizontal part 十二指腸, 水平部

図 13.23 腹部の MR 像
下方から見たところ.

A 第 12 胸椎の高さの水平断.

- 肝臓の右葉 Right lobe of liver
- 肝門脈 Hepatic portal v.
- 肝臓の左葉 Left lobe of liver
- 胃, 左胃動脈 Stomach (with left gastric a.)
- 腹直筋 Rectus abdominis
- 外腹斜筋 External oblique
- 左結腸曲 Left colic flexure
- 脾臓 Spleen
- 肝臓の尾状葉 Caudate lobe of liver
- 下大動脈 Inferior vena cava
- Right lung 右肺
- Azygos v. 奇静脈
- Spinal cord (in vertebral canal) 脊髄(脊柱管を通る)
- Abdominal aorta 腹大動脈
- Diaphragm 横隔膜
- Left lung 左肺

B 第 2 腰椎の高さの水平断.

- 胆嚢 Gallbladder
- 十二指腸, 下行部 Duodenum, descending part
- 膵臓, 膵頭 Pancreas, head
- 上腸間膜動脈 Superior mesenteric a. and v.
- 横行結腸 Transverse colon
- 肝臓の右葉 Right lobe of liver
- 左腎静脈 Left renal v.
- 空腸 Jejunum
- 下行結腸 Descending colon
- 外腹斜筋 External oblique
- 腎洞 Renal sinus
- Renal pyramids ①
- Renal cortex 腎皮質
- 左の腎臓 Left kidney
- 下大静脈 Inferior vena cava
- Diaphragm, right crus 横隔膜, 右脚
- Right kidney 右の腎臓
- 広背筋 Latissimus dorsi
- Iliocostalis 腸肋筋
- Quadratus lumborum 腰方形筋
- Longissimus thoracis 胸最長筋
- Spinal cord (in vertebral canal) 脊髄(脊柱管を通る)
- Abdominal aorta 腹大動脈
- Psoas major 大腰筋

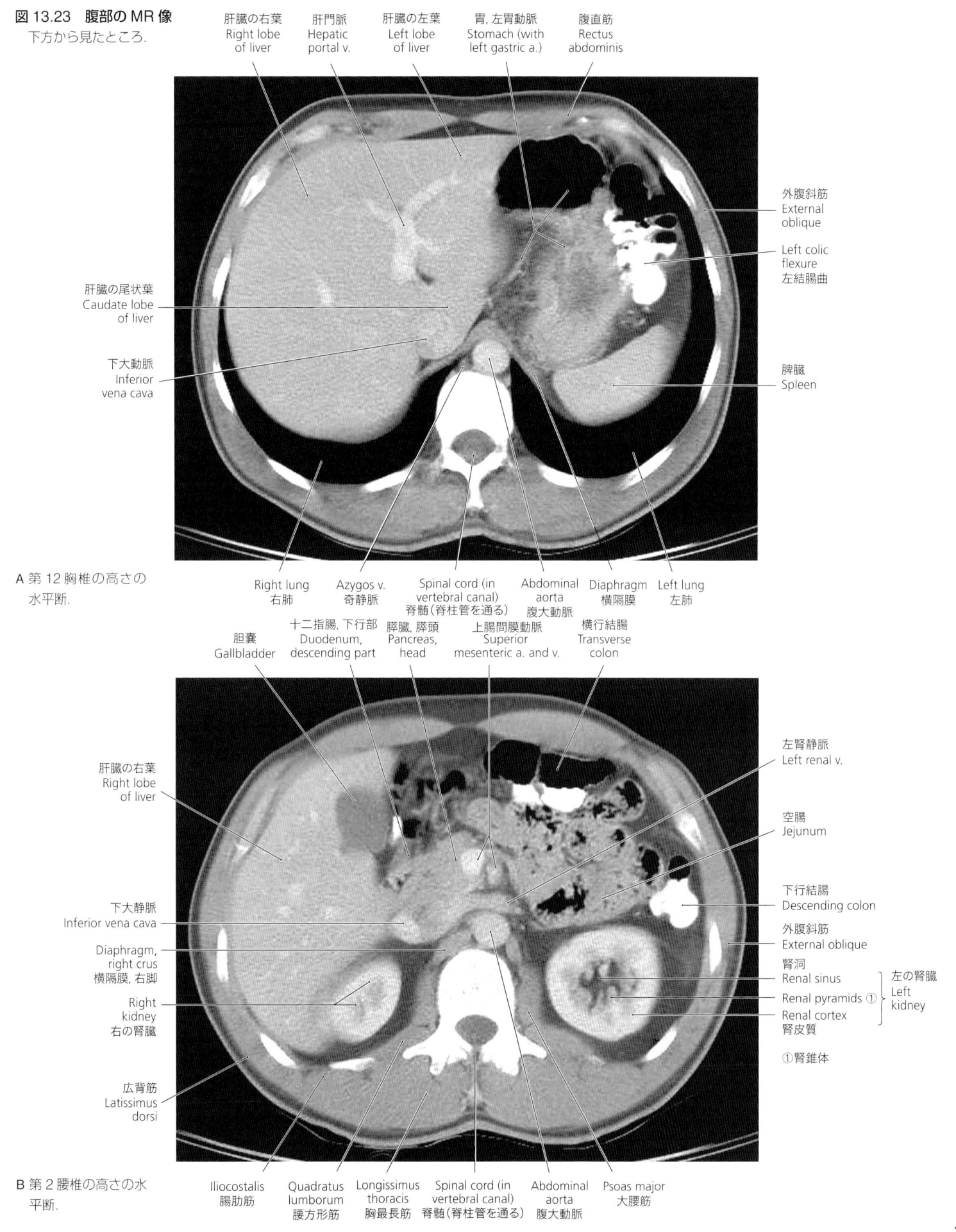

①腎錐体

肝臓：肝区域と肝葉
Liver: Segments & Lobes

図 13.24 肝区域
前方から見たところ．門脈3つ組(固有肝動脈，門脈，総肝管．pp.172, 219参照)は肝臓を肝区域に区分する(表13-2)．

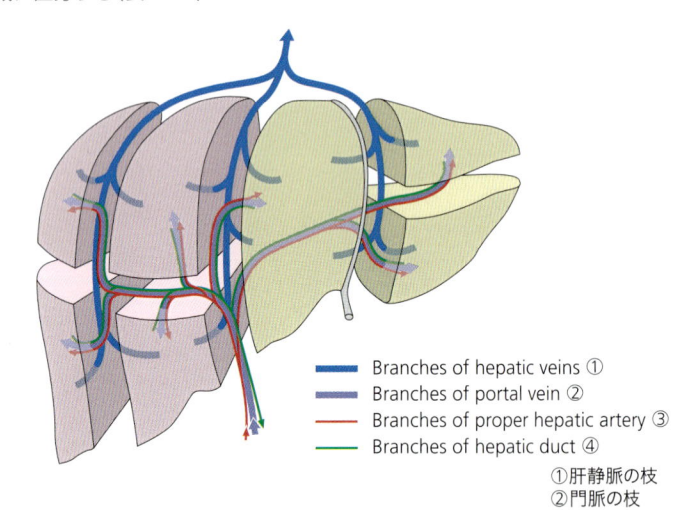

- Branches of hepatic veins ①
- Branches of portal vein ②
- Branches of proper hepatic artery ③
- Branches of hepatic duct ④

①肝静脈の枝
②門脈の枝
③固有肝動脈の枝
④肝管の枝

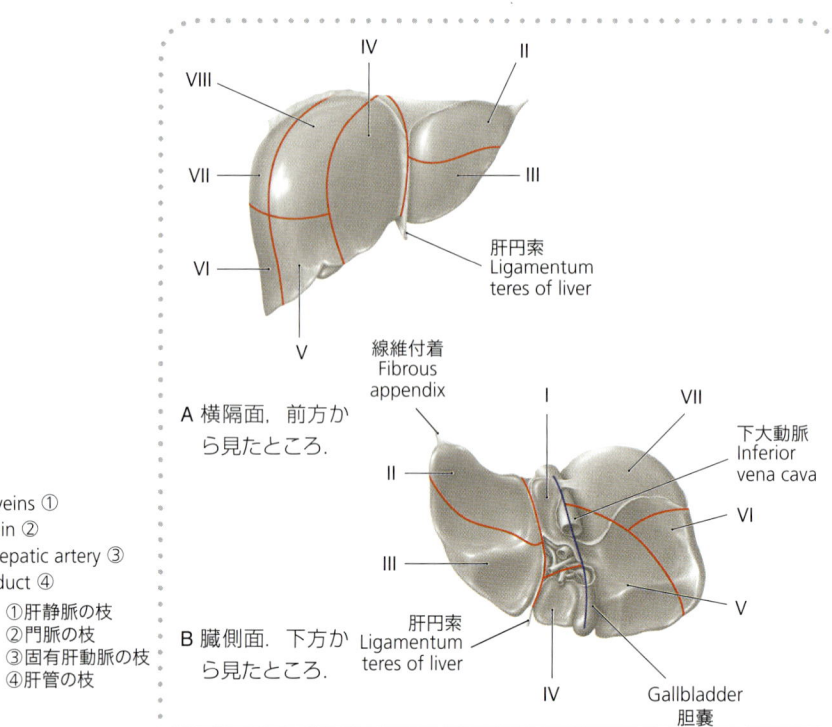

A 横隔面，前方から見たところ．

- 肝円索 Ligamentum teres of liver
- 線維付着 Fibrous appendix
- 下大動脈 Inferior vena cava
- 胆嚢 Gallbladder

B 臓側面．下方から見たところ．

図 13.25 肝臓：臓器と接触する領域
臓側面，下方から見たところ．

- 副腎圧痕 Suprarenal impression
- 腎圧痕 Renal impression
- 胃圧痕 Gastric impression
- 十二指腸圧痕 Duodenal impression
- 結腸圧痕 Colic impression

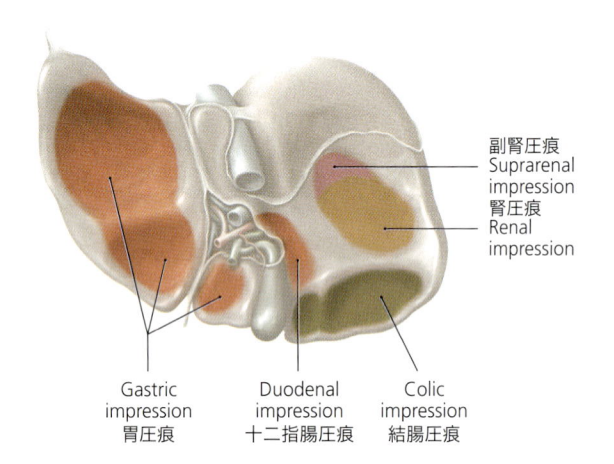

表 13.2　肝臓の区域

部位	区分	区域	
左肝部	肝後部	I	尾状葉
	左外側区	II	左外側後区域
		III	左外側前区域
	左内側区	IV	左内側区域
右肝部	右内側区	V	右内側前区域
		VIII	右内側後区域
	右外側区	VI	右外側前区域
		VII	右外側後区域

図 13.26 肝臓の横隔膜への付着

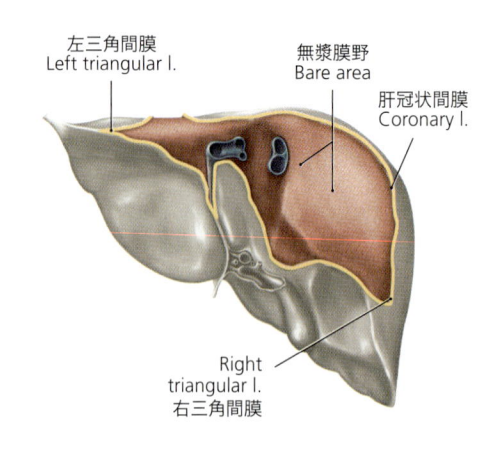

- 左三角間膜 Left triangular l.
- 無漿膜野 Bare area
- 肝冠状間膜 Coronary l.
- 右三角間膜 Right triangular l.

A 肝臓の横隔面，後方から見たところ．

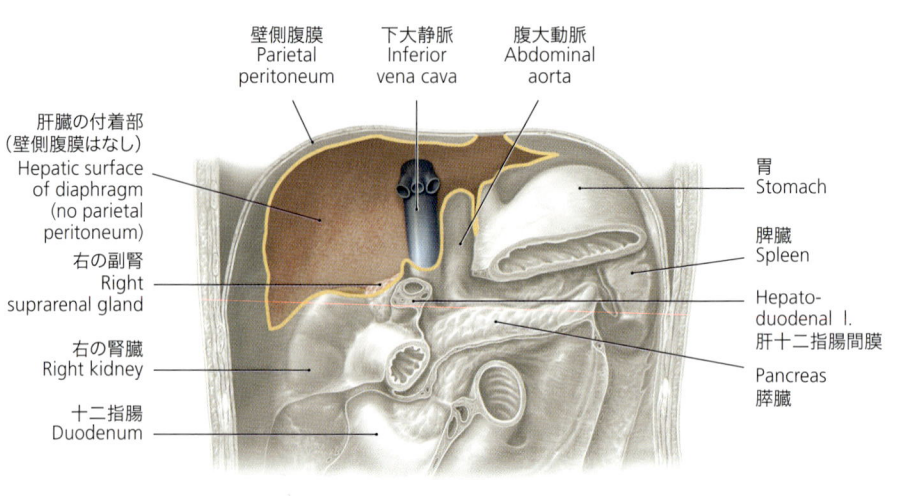

- 壁側腹膜 Parietal peritoneum
- 下大静脈 Inferior vena cava
- 腹大動脈 Abdominal aorta
- 肝臓の付着部（壁側腹膜はなし）Hepatic surface of diaphragm (no parietal peritoneum)
- 右の副腎 Right suprarenal gland
- 右の腎臓 Right kidney
- 十二指腸 Duodenum
- 胃 Stomach
- 脾臓 Spleen
- 肝十二指腸間膜 Hepato-duodenal l.
- 膵臓 Pancreas

B 横隔膜の肝臓面，前方から見たところ．

図 13.27 肝臓の表面

肝臓は間膜によって右葉，左葉，尾状葉，方形葉の4葉に区分される．

A 前方から見たところ．

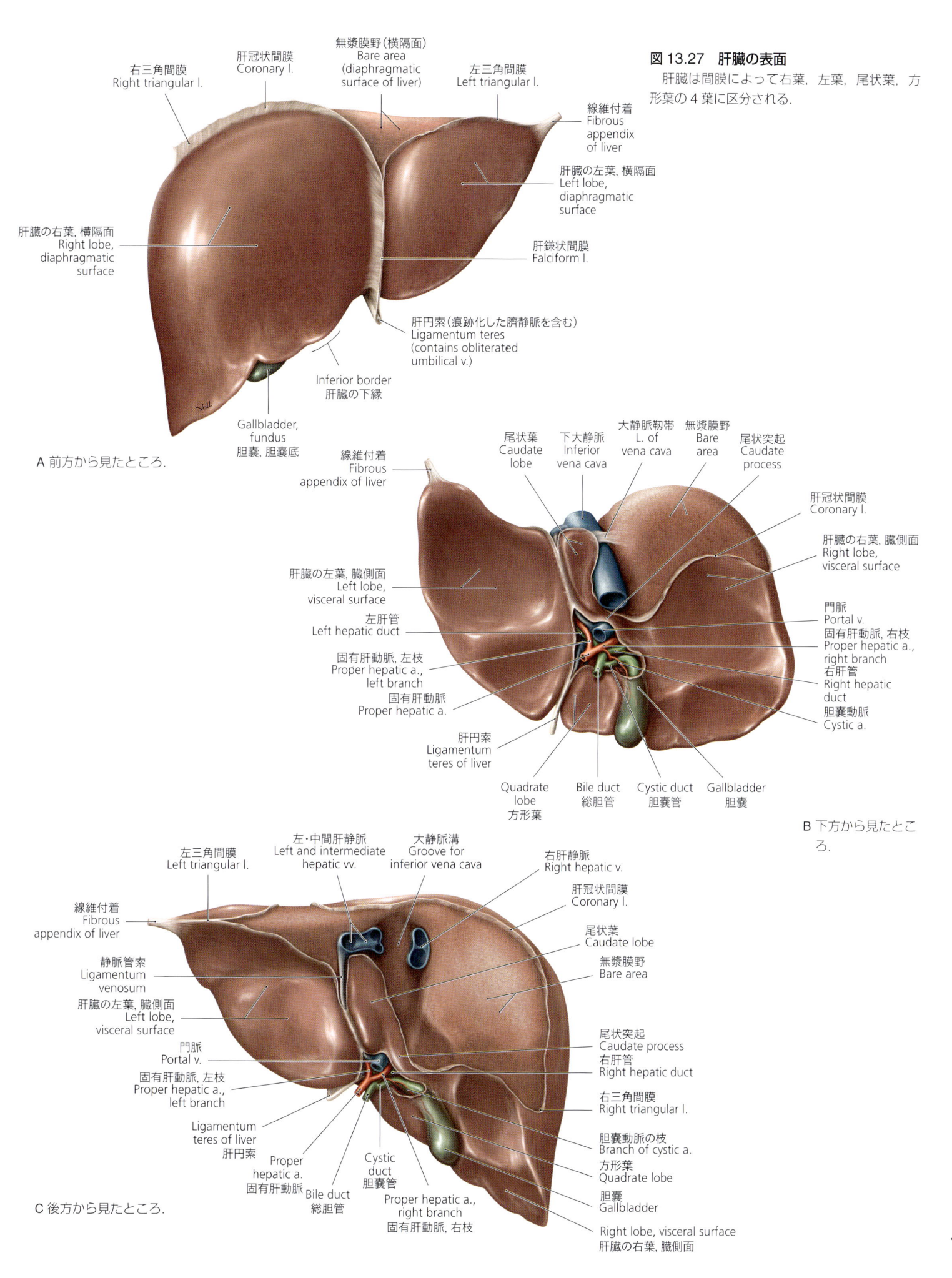

- 右三角間膜 Right triangular l.
- 肝冠状間膜 Coronary l.
- 無漿膜野(横隔面) Bare area (diaphragmatic surface of liver)
- 左三角間膜 Left triangular l.
- 線維付着 Fibrous appendix of liver
- 肝臓の左葉，横隔面 Left lobe, diaphragmatic surface
- 肝臓の右葉，横隔面 Right lobe, diaphragmatic surface
- 肝鎌状間膜 Falciform l.
- 肝円索(痕跡化した臍静脈を含む) Ligamentum teres (contains obliterated umbilical v.)
- 肝臓の下縁 Inferior border
- 胆嚢，胆嚢底 Gallbladder, fundus

B 下方から見たところ．

- 線維付着 Fibrous appendix of liver
- 尾状葉 Caudate lobe
- 下大静脈 Inferior vena cava
- 大静脈靱帯 L. of vena cava
- 無漿膜野 Bare area
- 尾状突起 Caudate process
- 肝冠状間膜 Coronary l.
- 肝臓の右葉，臓側面 Right lobe, visceral surface
- 肝臓の左葉，臓側面 Left lobe, visceral surface
- 左肝管 Left hepatic duct
- 門脈 Portal v.
- 固有肝動脈，左枝 Proper hepatic a., left branch
- 固有肝動脈，右枝 Proper hepatic a., right branch
- 右肝管 Right hepatic duct
- 固有肝動脈 Proper hepatic a.
- 胆嚢動脈 Cystic a.
- 肝円索 Ligamentum teres of liver
- 方形葉 Quadrate lobe
- 総胆管 Bile duct
- 胆嚢管 Cystic duct
- 胆嚢 Gallbladder

C 後方から見たところ．

- 左三角間膜 Left triangular l.
- 左・中間肝静脈 Left and intermediate hepatic vv.
- 大静脈溝 Groove for inferior vena cava
- 右肝静脈 Right hepatic v.
- 肝冠状間膜 Coronary l.
- 線維付着 Fibrous appendix of liver
- 尾状葉 Caudate lobe
- 静脈管索 Ligamentum venosum
- 無漿膜野 Bare area
- 肝臓の左葉，臓側面 Left lobe, visceral surface
- 尾状突起 Caudate process
- 右肝管 Right hepatic duct
- 門脈 Portal v.
- 右三角間膜 Right triangular l.
- 固有肝動脈，左枝 Proper hepatic a., left branch
- 胆嚢動脈の枝 Branch of cystic a.
- 肝円索 Ligamentum teres of liver
- 固有肝動脈 Proper hepatic a.
- 胆嚢管 Cystic duct
- 方形葉 Quadrate lobe
- 総胆管 Bile duct
- 固有肝動脈，右枝 Proper hepatic a., right branch
- 胆嚢 Gallbladder
- 肝臓の右葉，臓側面 Right lobe, visceral surface

胆嚢と胆管
Gallbladder & Bile Ducts

図 13.28　胆嚢：位置

右上腹部　RUQ

- 右肝管　Right hepatic duct
- 胆嚢管　Cystic duct
- 胆嚢　Gallbladder
- 左肝管　Left hepatic duct
- 総肝管　Common hepatic duct
- 総胆管　Bile duct

A 前方から見たところ．

- 左肝静脈　Left hepatic v.
- 尾状葉　Caudate lobe
- 左葉　Left lobe
- 左肝管　Left hepatic duct
- 総胆管　Bile duct
- 方形葉　Quadrate lobe
- 肝円索　Ligamentum teres of liver
- 無漿膜野　Bare area
- 大静脈靱帯　Ligament of vena cava
- 下大静脈　Inferior vena cava
- 門脈　Portal v.
- 右肝管　Right hepatic duct
- 総肝管　Common hepatic duct
- 胆嚢管　Cystic duct
- 胆嚢　Gallbladder

B 下方から見たところ．

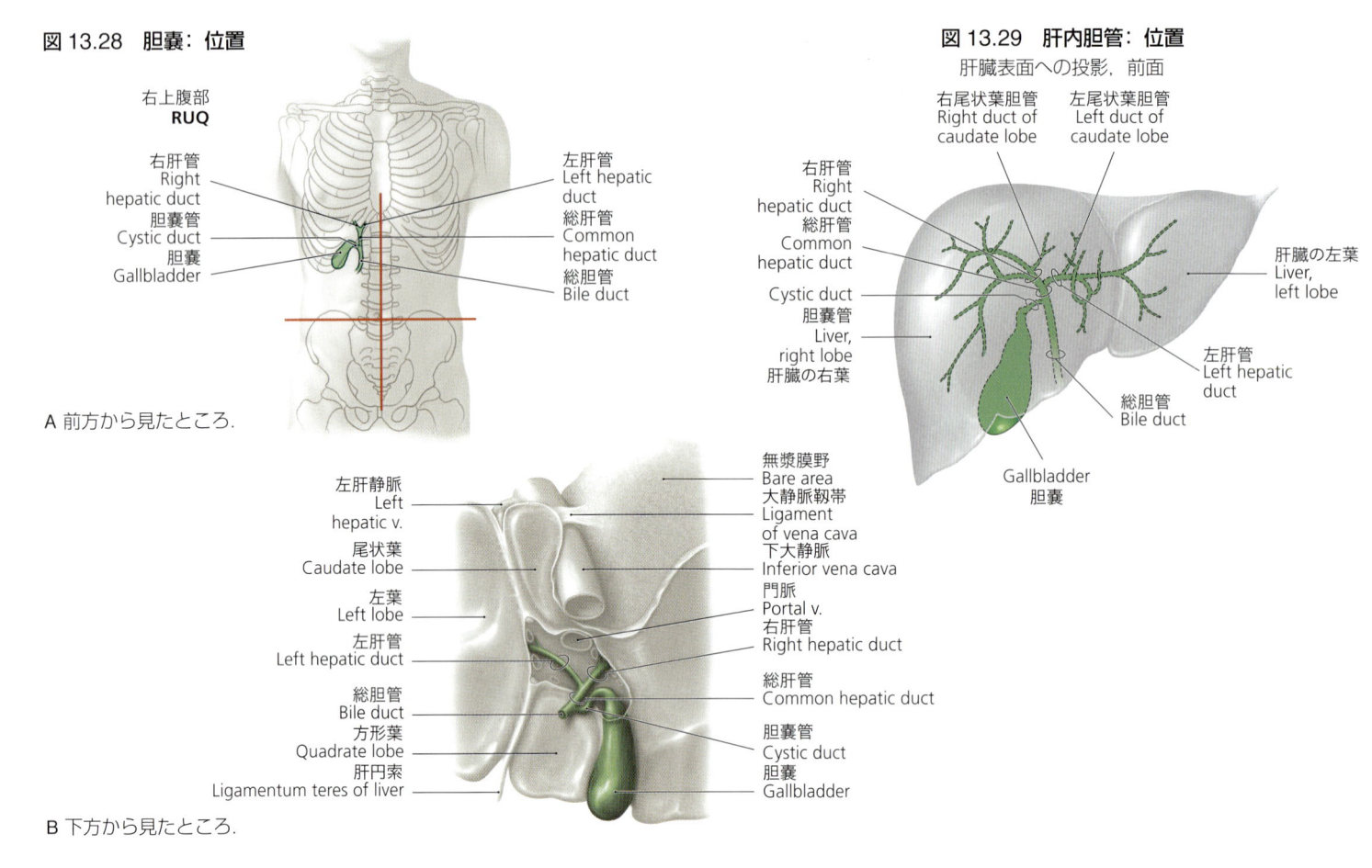

図 13.29　肝内胆管：位置
肝臓表面への投影．前面

- 右尾状葉胆管　Right duct of caudate lobe
- 左尾状葉胆管　Left duct of caudate lobe
- 右肝管　Right hepatic duct
- 総肝管　Common hepatic duct
- 胆嚢管　Cystic duct
- 肝臓の右葉　Liver, right lobe
- 肝臓の左葉　Liver, left lobe
- 左肝管　Left hepatic duct
- 総胆管　Bile duct
- 胆嚢　Gallbladder

図 13.30　胆管括約筋系

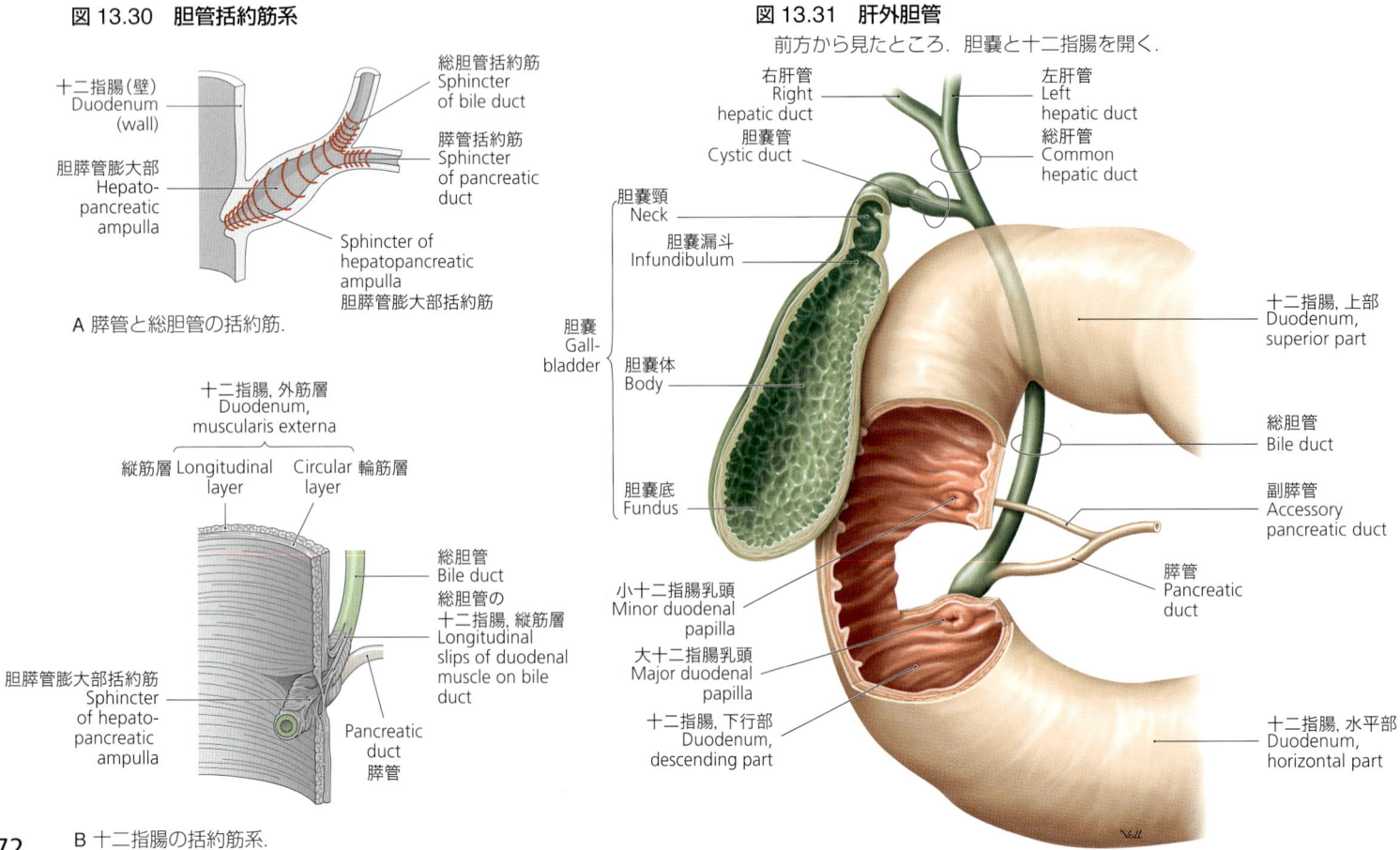

- 十二指腸（壁）　Duodenum (wall)
- 胆膵管膨大部　Hepato-pancreatic ampulla
- 総胆管括約筋　Sphincter of bile duct
- 膵管括約筋　Sphincter of pancreatic duct
- Sphincter of hepatopancreatic ampulla　胆膵管膨大部括約筋

A 膵管と総胆管の括約筋．

- 十二指腸, 外筋層　Duodenum, muscularis externa
- 縦筋層　Longitudinal layer
- 輪筋層　Circular layer
- 胆膵管膨大部括約筋　Sphincter of hepatopancreatic ampulla
- 総胆管　Bile duct
- 総胆管の十二指腸, 縦筋層　Longitudinal slips of duodenal muscle on bile duct
- 膵管　Pancreatic duct

B 十二指腸の括約筋系．

図 13.31　肝外胆管
前方から見たところ．胆嚢と十二指腸を開く．

- 右肝管　Right hepatic duct
- 胆嚢管　Cystic duct
- 胆嚢頸　Neck
- 胆嚢漏斗　Infundibulum
- 胆嚢　Gallbladder
  - 胆嚢体　Body
  - 胆嚢底　Fundus
- 小十二指腸乳頭　Minor duodenal papilla
- 大十二指腸乳頭　Major duodenal papilla
- 十二指腸, 下行部　Duodenum, descending part
- 左肝管　Left hepatic duct
- 総肝管　Common hepatic duct
- 十二指腸, 上部　Duodenum, superior part
- 総胆管　Bile duct
- 副膵管　Accessory pancreatic duct
- 膵管　Pancreatic duct
- 十二指腸, 水平部　Duodenum, horizontal part

図 13.32　原位置の胆路

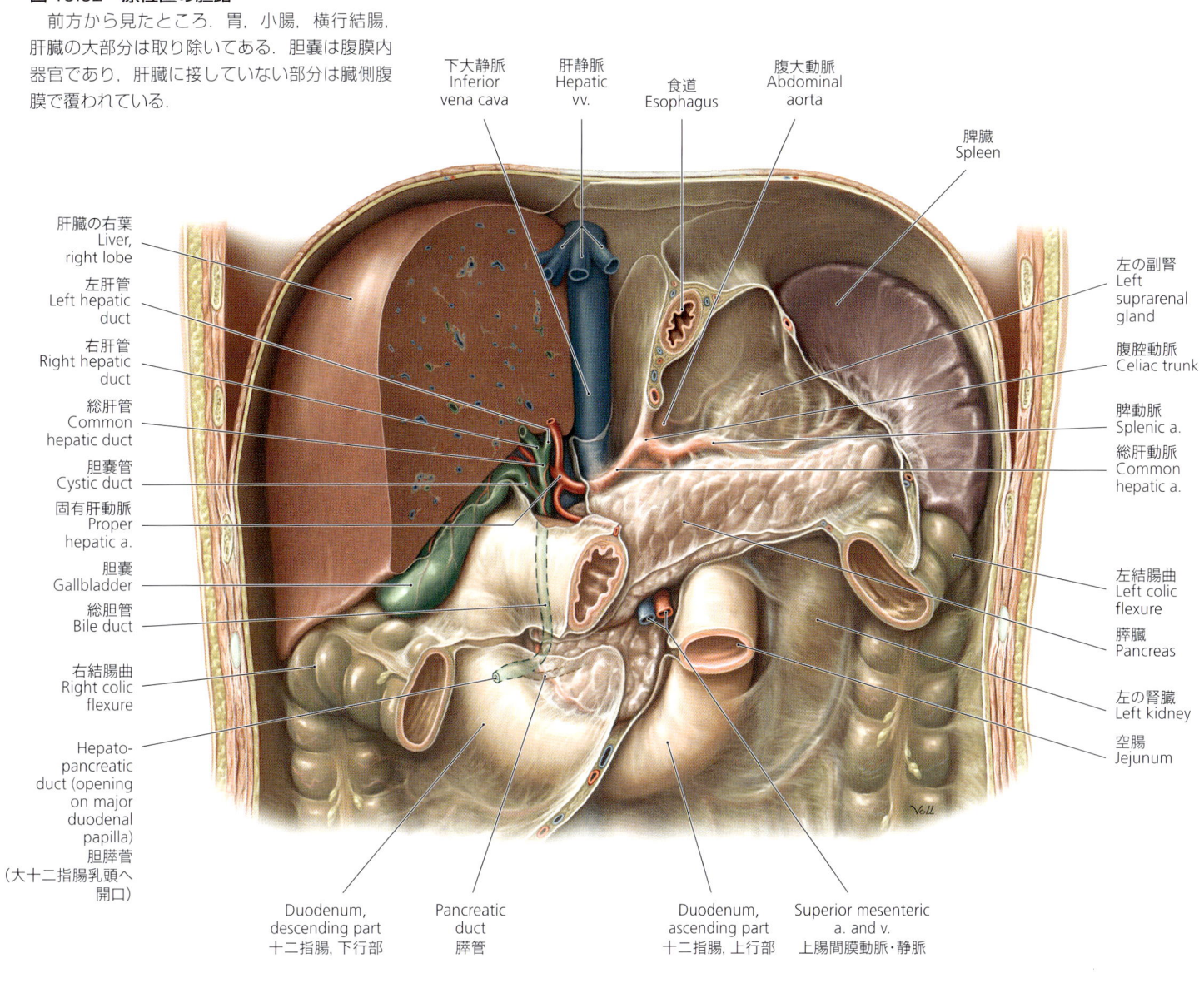

前方から見たところ．胃，小腸，横行結腸，肝臓の大部分は取り除いてある．胆嚢は腹膜内器官であり，肝臓に接していない部分は臓側腹膜で覆われている．

ラベル（図中）:
- 下大静脈 Inferior vena cava
- 肝静脈 Hepatic vv.
- 食道 Esophagus
- 腹大動脈 Abdominal aorta
- 脾臓 Spleen
- 肝臓の右葉 Liver, right lobe
- 左肝管 Left hepatic duct
- 右肝管 Right hepatic duct
- 総肝管 Common hepatic duct
- 胆嚢管 Cystic duct
- 固有肝動脈 Proper hepatic a.
- 胆嚢 Gallbladder
- 総胆管 Bile duct
- 右結腸曲 Right colic flexure
- Hepato-pancreatic duct (opening on major duodenal papilla) 胆膵菅（大十二指腸乳頭へ開口）
- 左の副腎 Left suprarenal gland
- 腹腔動脈 Celiac trunk
- 脾動脈 Splenic a.
- 総肝動脈 Common hepatic a.
- 左結腸曲 Left colic flexure
- 膵臓 Pancreas
- 左の腎臓 Left kidney
- 空腸 Jejunum
- Duodenum, descending part 十二指腸，下行部
- Pancreatic duct 膵管
- Duodenum, ascending part 十二指腸，上行部
- Superior mesenteric a. and v. 上腸間膜動脈・静脈

臨床

胆道閉鎖

胆汁が胆嚢で貯蔵・濃縮される間に，コレステロールなどの物質は結晶化して胆石となる．胆石が胆管に移動すると激しい痛み（疝痛）を起こす．胆石は乳頭領域で膵管の閉塞を起こすことがあり，激しい痛みと命を脅かす膵炎を発症させることがある．

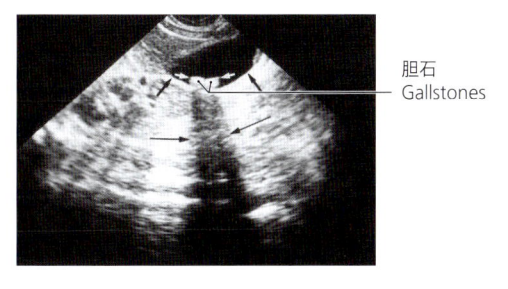

胆石 Gallstones

超音波で見られた 2 つの胆石．黒の矢印は胆石の背側の無エコー域．

膵臓と脾臓
Pancreas & Spleen

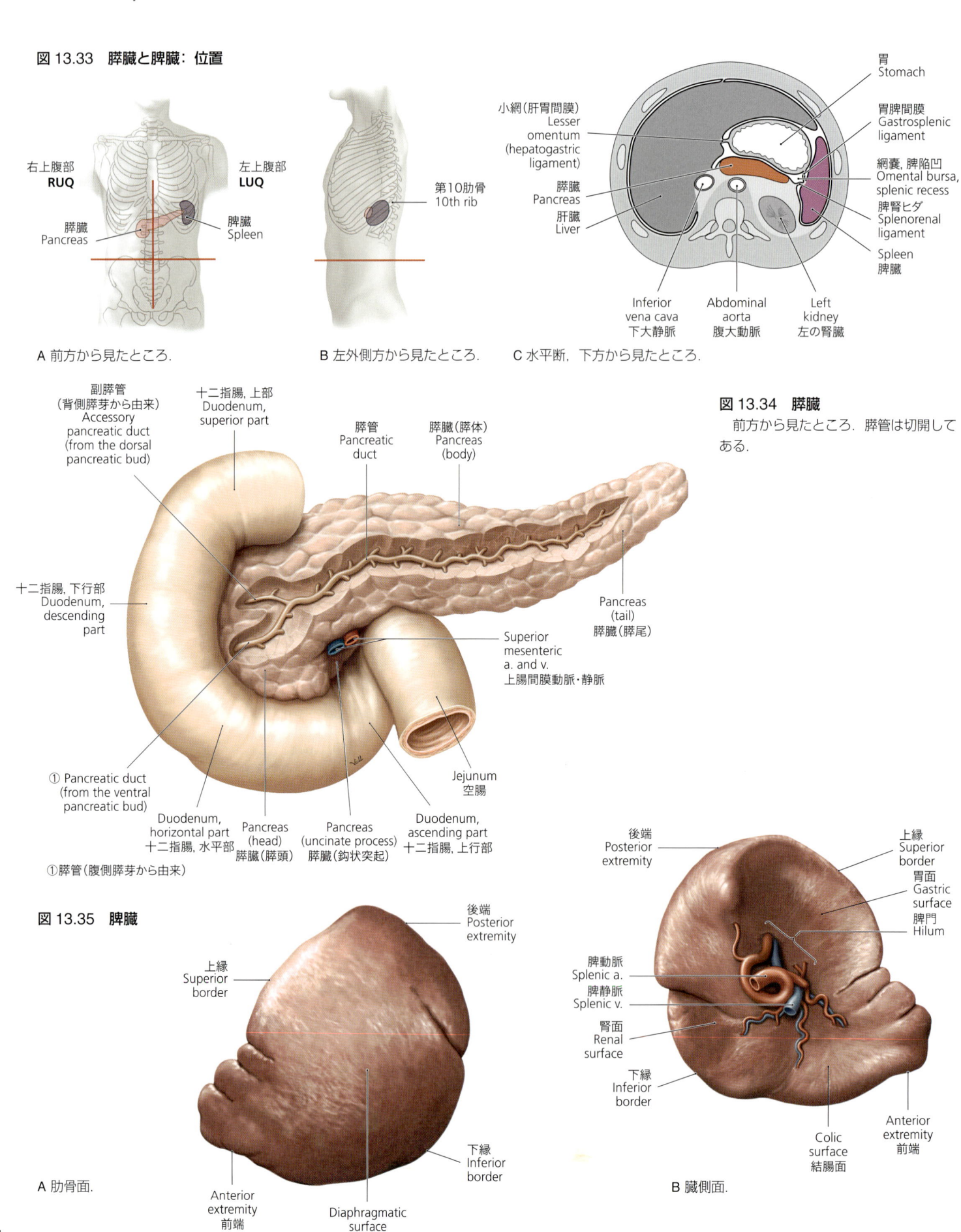

図 13.33 膵臓と脾臓：位置

A 前方から見たところ．
B 左外側方から見たところ．
C 水平断，下方から見たところ．

図 13.34 膵臓
前方から見たところ．膵管は切開してある．

図 13.35 脾臓

A 肋骨面．
B 臓側面．

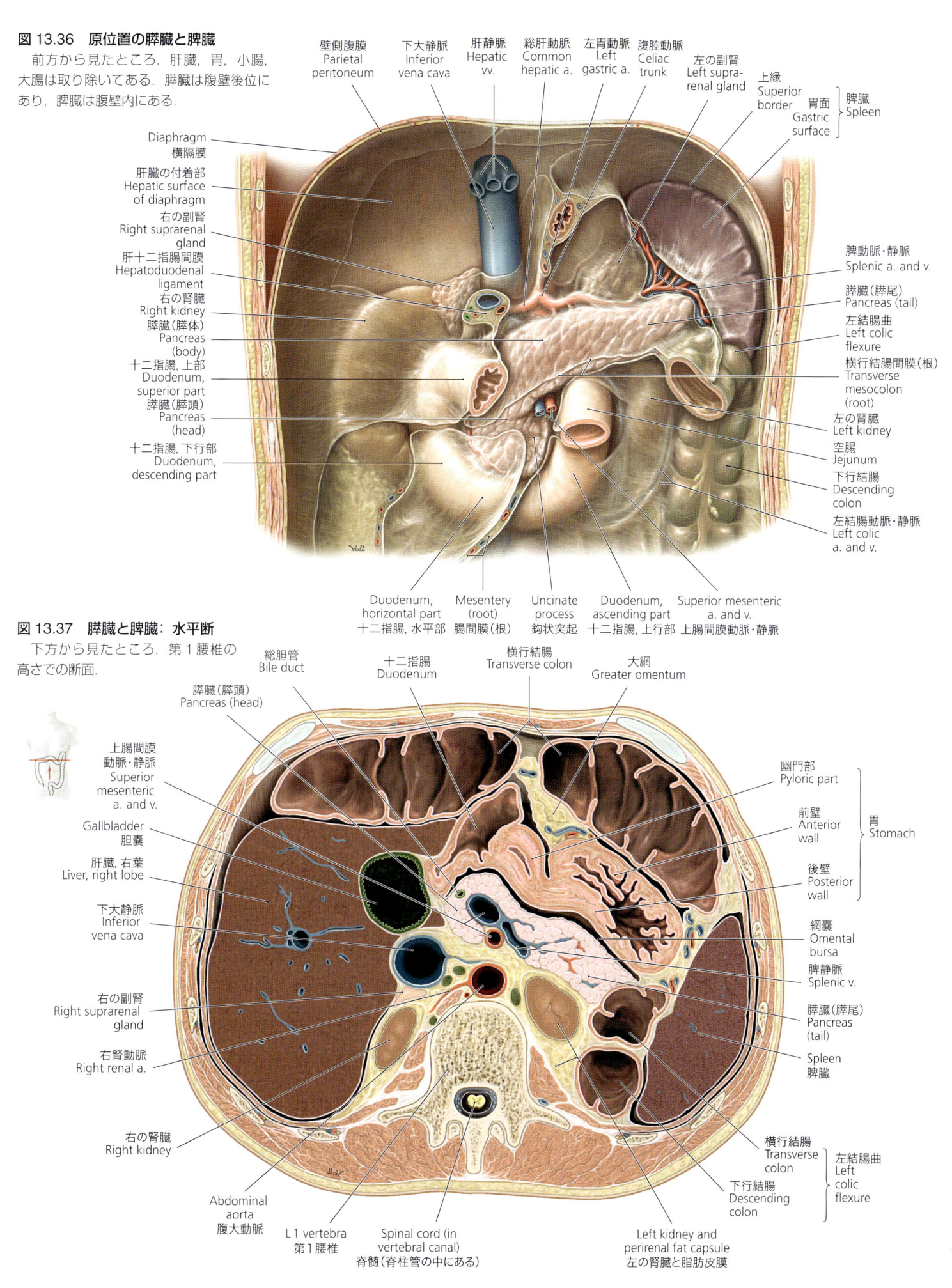

図 13.36 原位置の膵臓と脾臓
前方から見たところ．肝臓，胃，小腸，大腸は取り除いてある．膵臓は腹壁後位にあり，脾臓は腹壁内にある．

図 13.37 膵臓と脾臓：水平断
下方から見たところ．第1腰椎の高さでの断面．

腎臓と副腎：概観
Kidneys & Suprarenal Glands: Overview

図 13.38　腎臓と副腎：位置

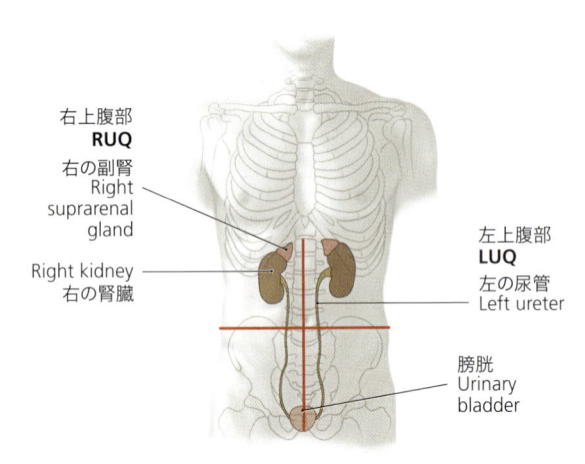

- 右上腹部 RUQ
- 右の副腎 Right suprarenal gland
- Right kidney 右の腎臓
- 左上腹部 LUQ
- 左の尿管 Left ureter
- 膀胱 Urinary bladder

A 前方から見たところ．

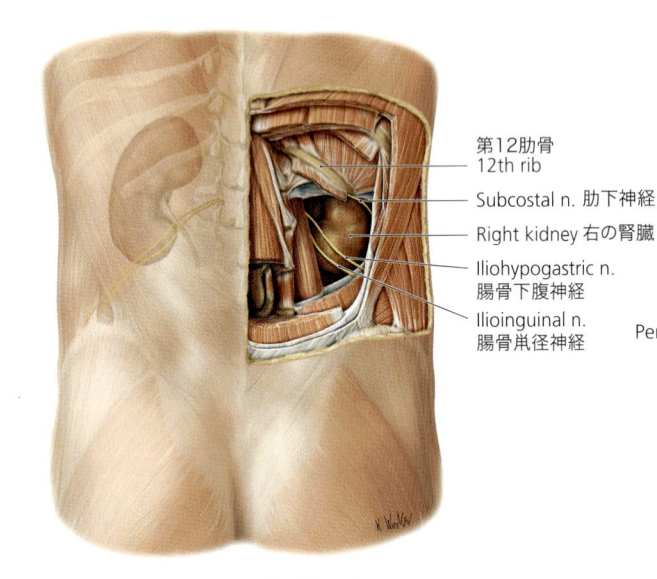

図 13.39　腎臓：臓器と接触する領域
前方から見たところ．

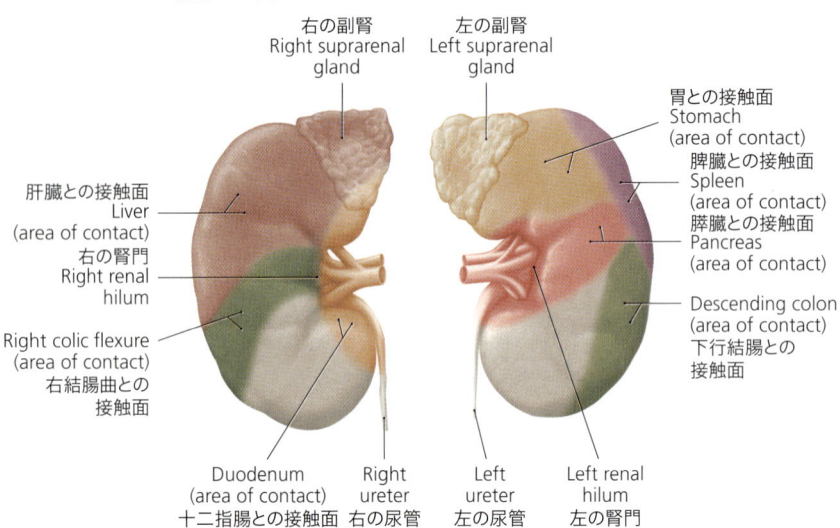

- 右の副腎 Right suprarenal gland
- 左の副腎 Left suprarenal gland
- 肝臓との接触面 Liver (area of contact)
- 胃との接触面 Stomach (area of contact)
- 脾臓との接触面 Spleen (area of contact)
- 膵臓との接触面 Pancreas (area of contact)
- 右の腎門 Right renal hilum
- Descending colon (area of contact) 下行結腸との接触面
- 右結腸曲との接触面 Right colic flexure (area of contact)
- Duodenum (area of contact) 十二指腸との接触面
- Right ureter 右の尿管
- Left ureter 左の尿管
- Left renal hilum 左の腎門

- 第12肋骨 12th rib
- Subcostal n. 肋下神経
- Right kidney 右の腎臓
- Iliohypogastric n. 腸骨下腹神経
- Ilioinguinal n. 腸骨鼡径神経

B 後方から見たところ．体壁を開く．

図 13.40　腎床での右腎
右の腎床での矢状断．

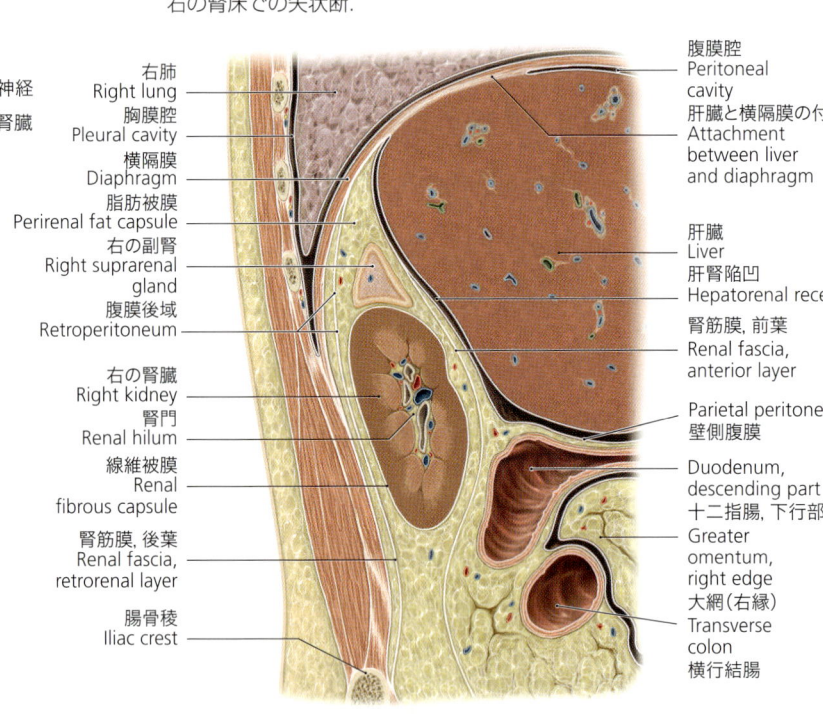

- 右肺 Right lung
- 胸膜腔 Pleural cavity
- 横隔膜 Diaphragm
- 脂肪被膜 Perirenal fat capsule
- 右の副腎 Right suprarenal gland
- 腹膜後域 Retroperitoneum
- 右の腎臓 Right kidney
- 腎門 Renal hilum
- 線維被膜 Renal fibrous capsule
- 腎筋膜, 後葉 Renal fascia, retrorenal layer
- 腸骨稜 Iliac crest
- 腹膜腔 Peritoneal cavity
- 肝臓と横隔膜の付着部 Attachment between liver and diaphragm
- 肝臓 Liver
- 肝腎陥凹 Hepatorenal recess
- 腎筋膜, 前葉 Renal fascia, anterior layer
- 壁側腹膜 Parietal peritoneum
- 十二指腸, 下行部 Duodenum, descending part
- 大網（右縁）Greater omentum, right edge
- 横行結腸 Transverse colon

図 13.41　副腎
前方から見たところ．

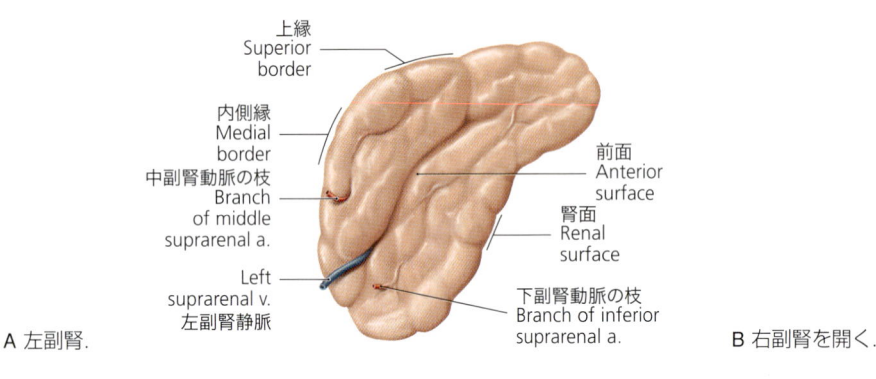

- 上縁 Superior border
- 内側縁 Medial border
- 中副腎動脈の枝 Branch of middle suprarenal a.
- 左副腎静脈 Left suprarenal v.
- 前面 Anterior surface
- 腎面 Renal surface
- 下副腎動脈の枝 Branch of inferior suprarenal a.

A 左副腎．

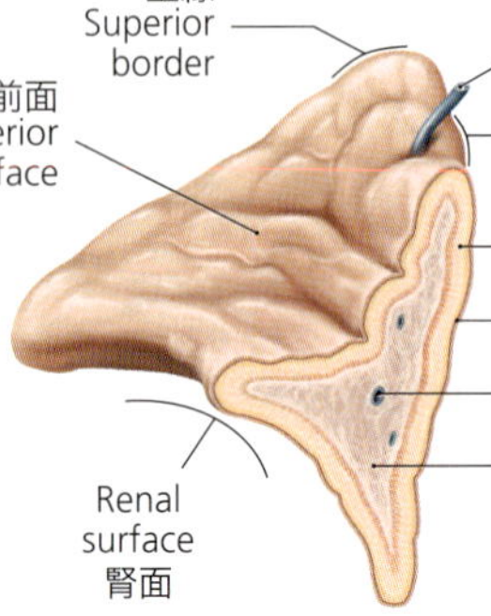

- 上縁 Superior border
- 前面 Anterior surface
- 右副腎静脈 Right suprarenal v.
- 内側縁 Medial border
- 皮質 Cortex
- 線維被膜 Fibrous capsule
- 中心静脈 Central v.
- 髄質 Medulla
- 腎面 Renal surface

B 右副腎を開く．

図 13.42 腹膜後域における腎臓と副腎

前方から見たところ．腎臓と副腎は腹膜後器官である．

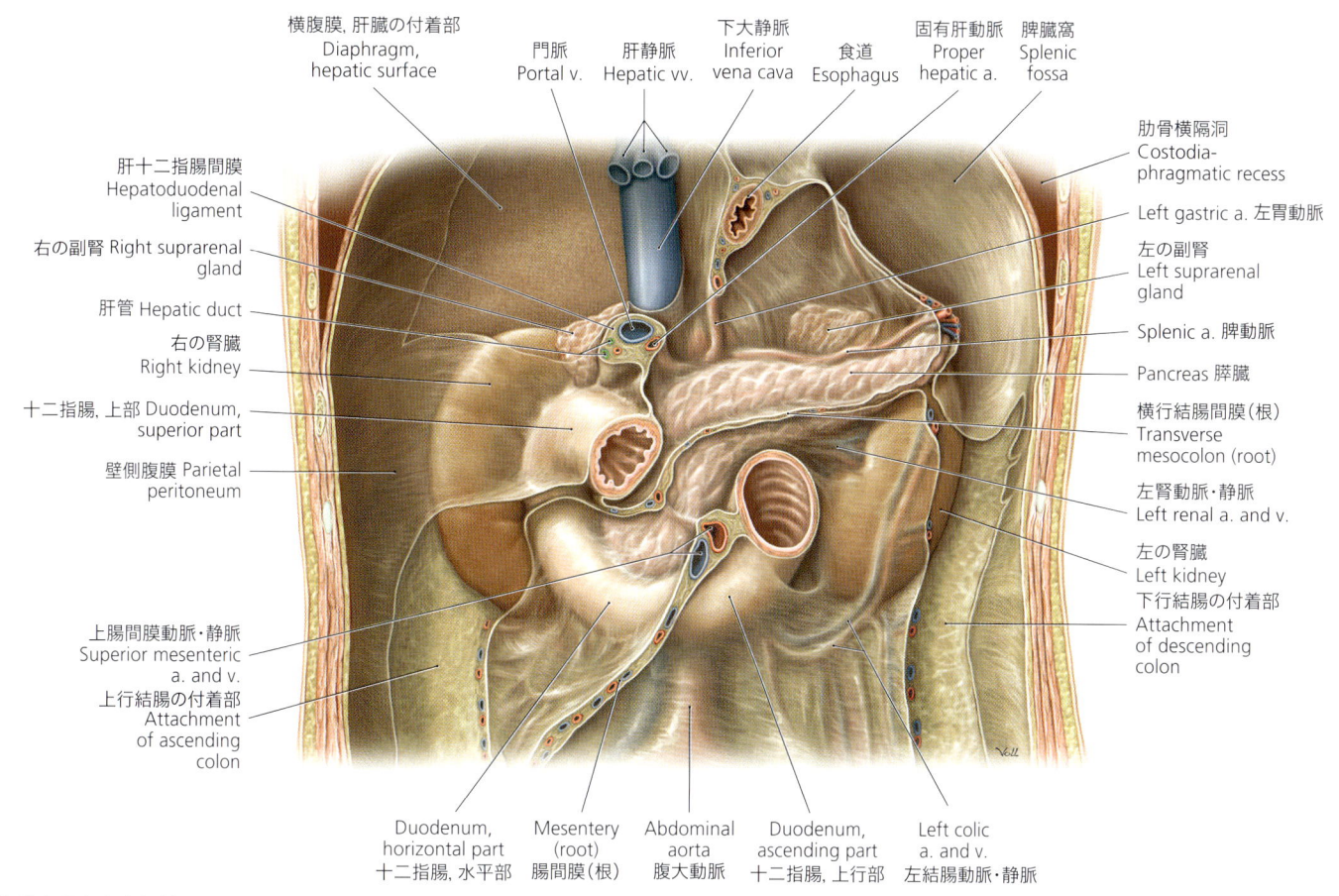

A 腹膜内器官と上行結腸，下行結腸は取り除いてある．

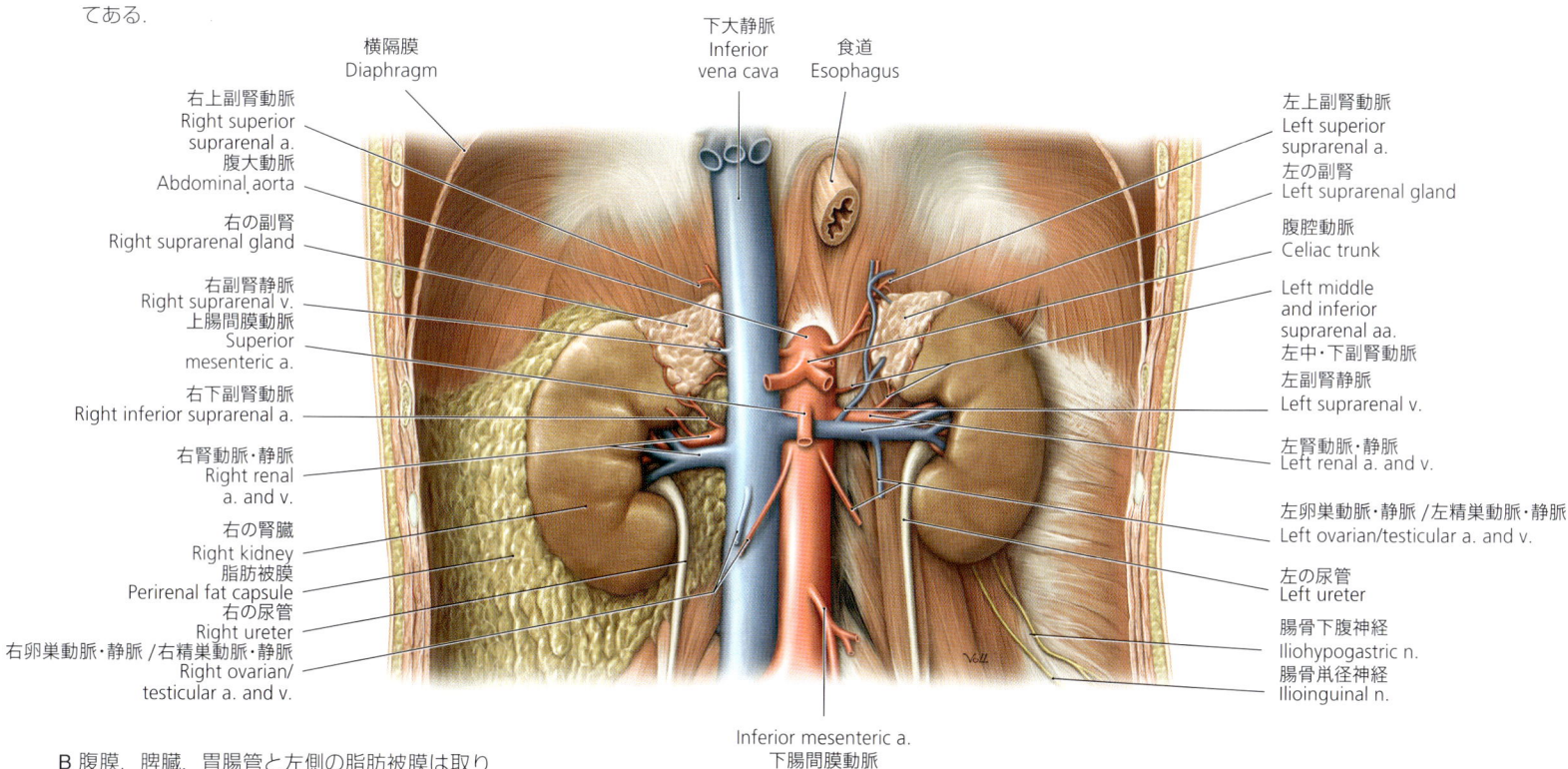

B 腹膜，脾臓，胃腸管と左側の脂肪被膜は取り除いてある．食道を引き出す．

腎臓と副腎：詳説
Kidneys & Suprarenal Glands: Features

図 13.43　右腎と副腎
前方から見たところ．腎臓周囲の脂肪被膜は取り除いてある．下大静脈を左側に引く．

ラベル（左側）：
- 横隔膜 Diaphragm
- 下横隔動脈・静脈 Inferior phrenic a. and v.
- 上副腎動脈 Superior suprarenal aa.
- 右の副腎 Right suprarenal gland
- 肋下神経（第12肋間神経）Subcostal n. (12th intercostal n.)
- 右の腎臓 Right kidney
- 右の尿管 Right ureter
- 腸骨下腹神経 Iliohypogastric n.
- 腸骨鼡径神経 Ilioinguinal n.

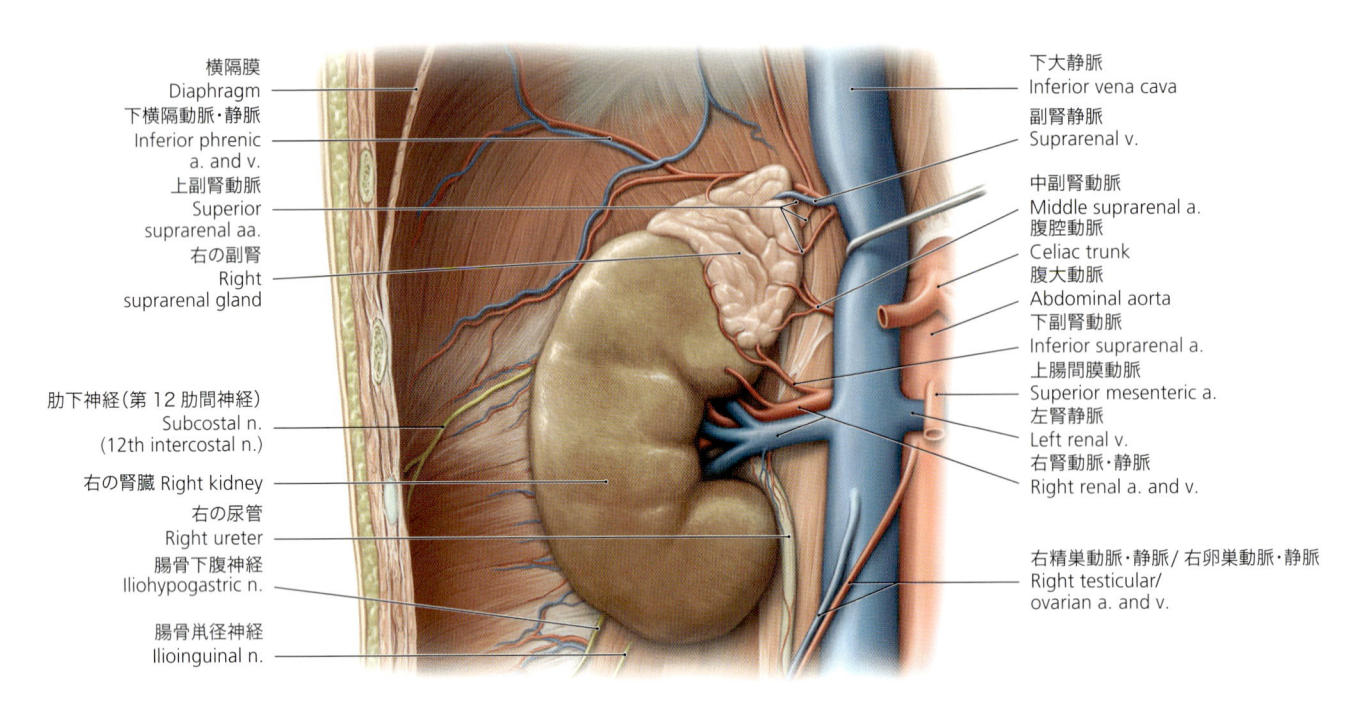

ラベル（右側）：
- 下大静脈 Inferior vena cava
- 副腎静脈 Suprarenal v.
- 中副腎動脈 Middle suprarenal a.
- 腹腔動脈 Celiac trunk
- 腹大動脈 Abdominal aorta
- 下副腎動脈 Inferior suprarenal a.
- 上腸間膜動脈 Superior mesenteric a.
- 左腎静脈 Left renal v.
- 右腎動脈・静脈 Right renal a. and v.
- 右精巣動脈・静脈／右卵巣動脈・静脈 Right testicular/ovarian a. and v.

図 13.45　腎臓：構造
右腎と副腎．

ラベル（A）：
- 脂肪被膜 Pararenal fat pad
- 上端 Superior pole
- 右の副腎 Right suprarenal gland
- 前面 Anterior surface
- 外側縁 Lateral border
- 腎門 Renal hilum

ラベル（中央）：
- 上副腎動脈 Superior suprarenal aa.
- 中副腎動脈 Middle suprarenal a.
- 右副腎静脈 Right suprarenal v.
- 下副腎動脈 Inferior suprarenal a.
- 内側縁 Medial border
- 右腎動脈・静脈 Right renal a. and v.
- 腎盂（腎盤）Renal pelvis
- 右の尿管 Right ureter
- 下端 Inferior pole

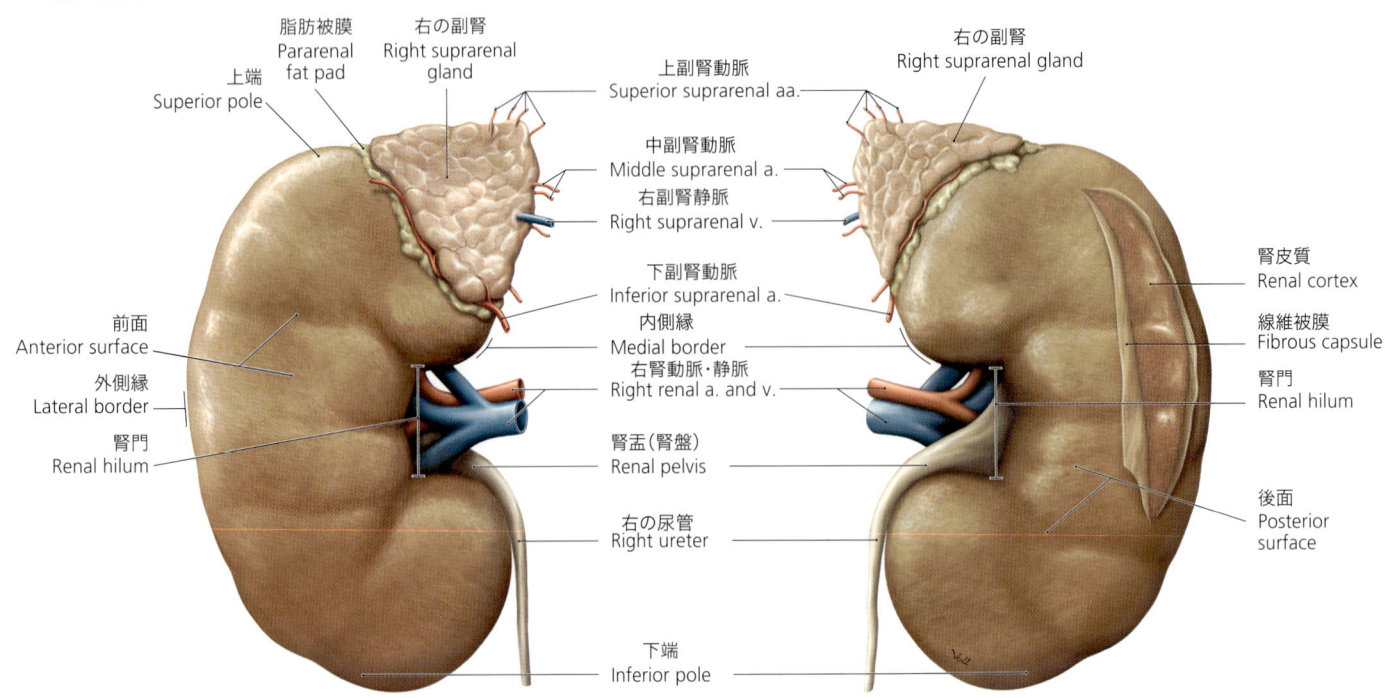

ラベル（B）：
- 右の副腎 Right suprarenal gland
- 腎皮質 Renal cortex
- 線維被膜 Fibrous capsule
- 腎門 Renal hilum
- 後面 Posterior surface

A 前方から見たところ．　　B 後方から見たところ．

図 13.44 左腎と副腎
前方から見たところ．腎臓周囲の脂肪被膜は取り除いてある．膵臓を下に引く．

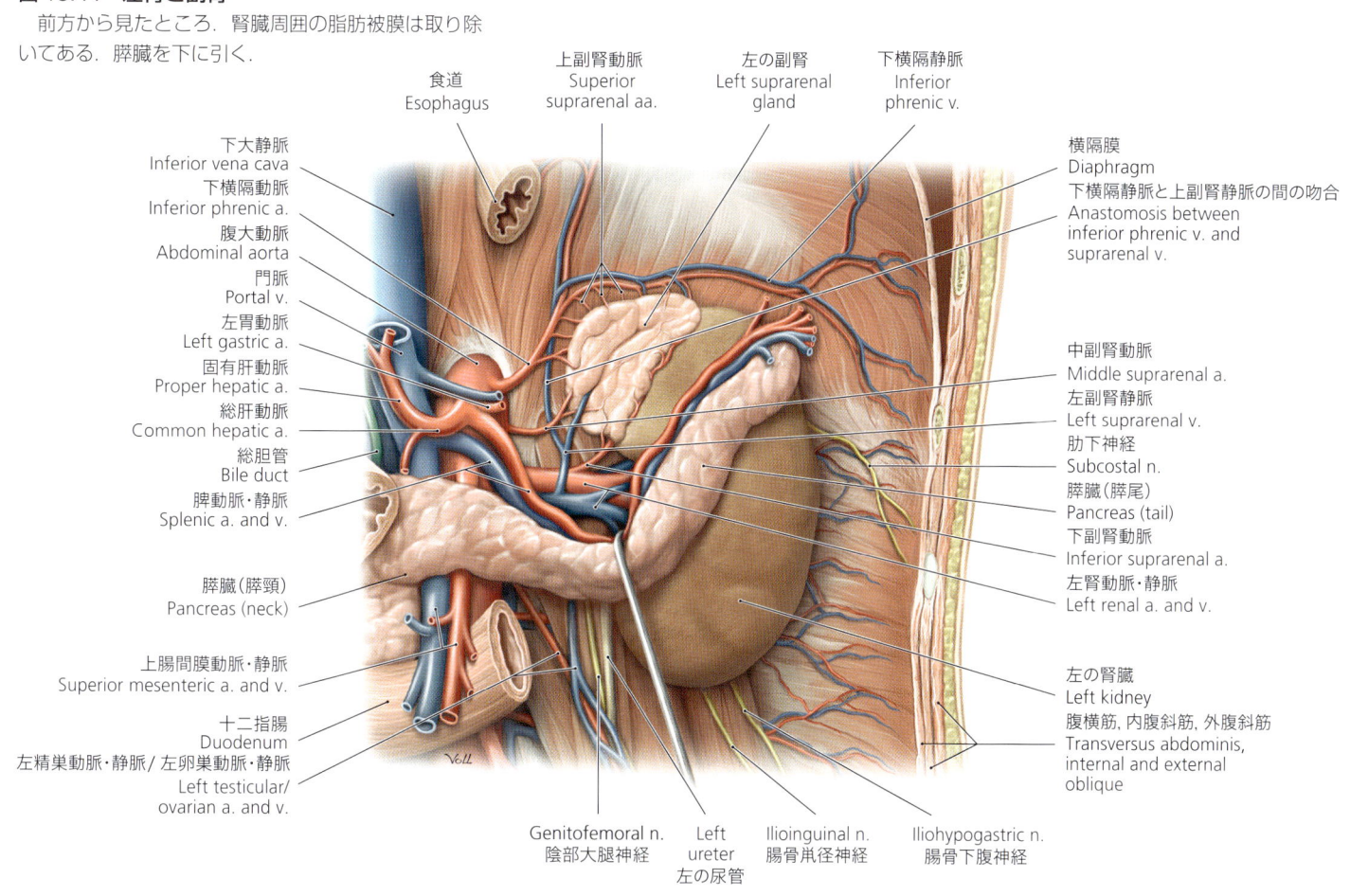

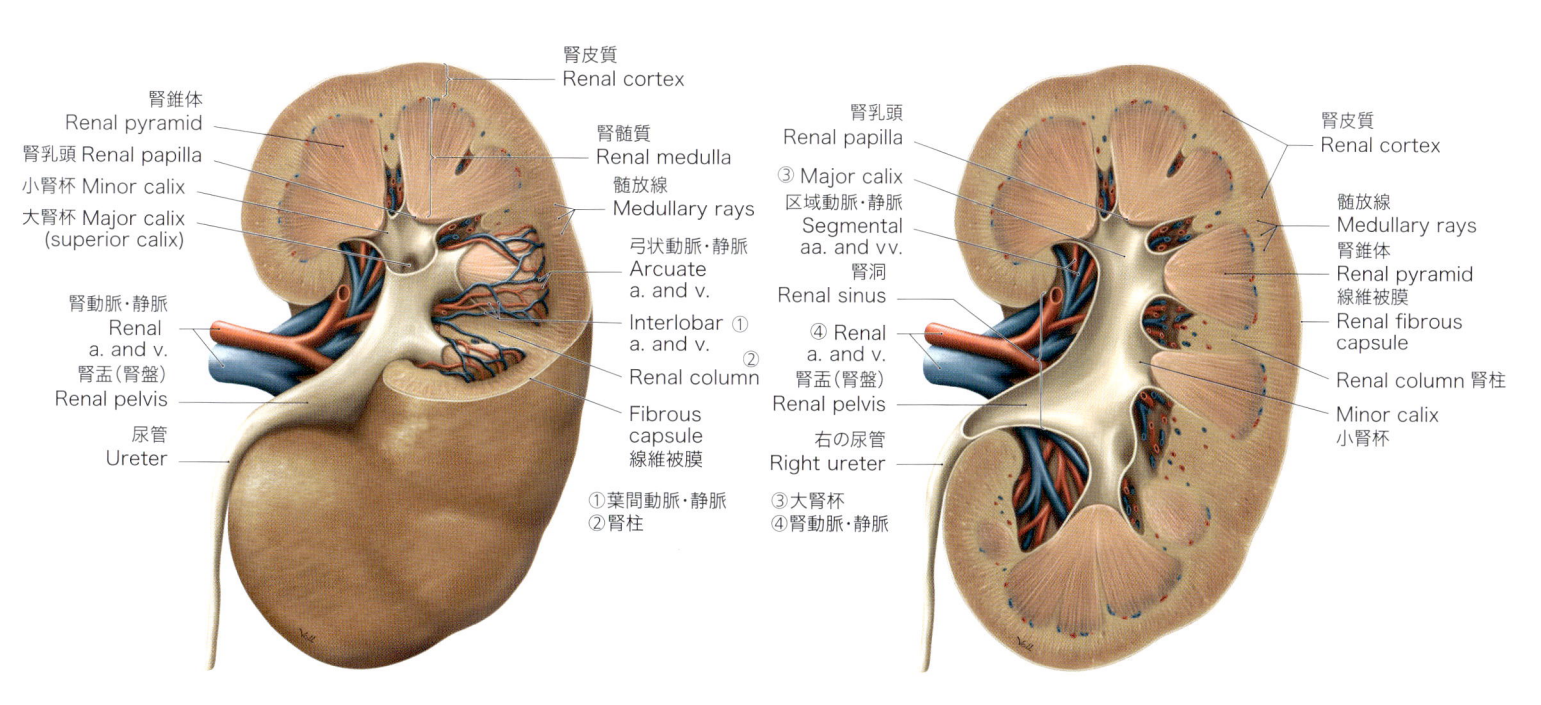

C 後方から見たところ．上半分の一部は部分的に取り除いてある．

D 中央縦断，後方から見たところ．

尿管
Ureter

図 13.46 尿管：位置
前方から見たところ．

尿管は外腸骨動脈と内腸骨動脈との分岐部で総腸骨動脈と交差する．

図 13.47 原位置の尿管
男性の腹部．前方から見たところ．泌尿器官以外の臓器と直腸断端は取り除いてある．尿管は腹膜後器官である．

- 左の副腎と腎臓 / Left suprarenal gland and kidney
- 右の尿管 / Right ureter
- 膀胱 / Urinary bladder
- 左中副腎動脈 / Left middle suprarenal a.
- 左下横隔動脈・静脈 / Left inferior phrenic a. and v.
- 左上副腎動脈 / Left superior suprarenal a.
- 腹大動脈 / Abdominal aorta
- 腹腔動脈 / Celiac trunk
- 下大静脈 / Inferior vena cava
- 左の副腎，左副腎静脈 / Left suprarenal gland and v.
- 右の副腎，右副腎静脈 / Right suprarenal gland and v.
- 右の腎臓 / Right kidney
- 左下副腎動脈 / Left inferior suprarenal a.
- 左腎動脈・静脈 / Left renal a. and v.
- 上腸間膜動脈 / Superior mesenteric a.
- 脂肪被膜 / Perirenal fat capsule
- 左精巣動脈・静脈 / Left testicular a. and v.
- 左の腎臓 / Left kidney
- 尿管(腹部) / Ureter (abdominal part)
- 下腸間膜動脈 / Inferior mesenteric a.
- 右精巣動脈・静脈 / Right testicular a. and v.
- 右総腸骨動脈 / Right common iliac a.
- 大腰筋 / Psoas major
- 腸骨筋 / Iliacus
- 左内腸骨動脈・静脈 / Left internal iliac a. and v.
- 正中仙骨動脈・静脈 / Median sacral a. and v.
- 左上殿動脈 / Left superior gluteal a.
- 内腸骨動脈・静脈の前枝 / Anterior trunk of internal iliac a. and v.
- 仙骨神経叢 / Sacral plexus
- 左外腸骨動脈・静脈 / Left external iliac a. and v.
- 下腹壁動脈・静脈 / Inferior epigastric a. and v.
- 右の精管 / Right ductus deferens
- 尿管(骨盤部) / Ureter (pelvic part)
- 直腸 / Rectum
- 膀胱 / Urinary bladder
- 恥骨結合 / Pubic symphysis
- 正中臍索 / Median umbilical ligament

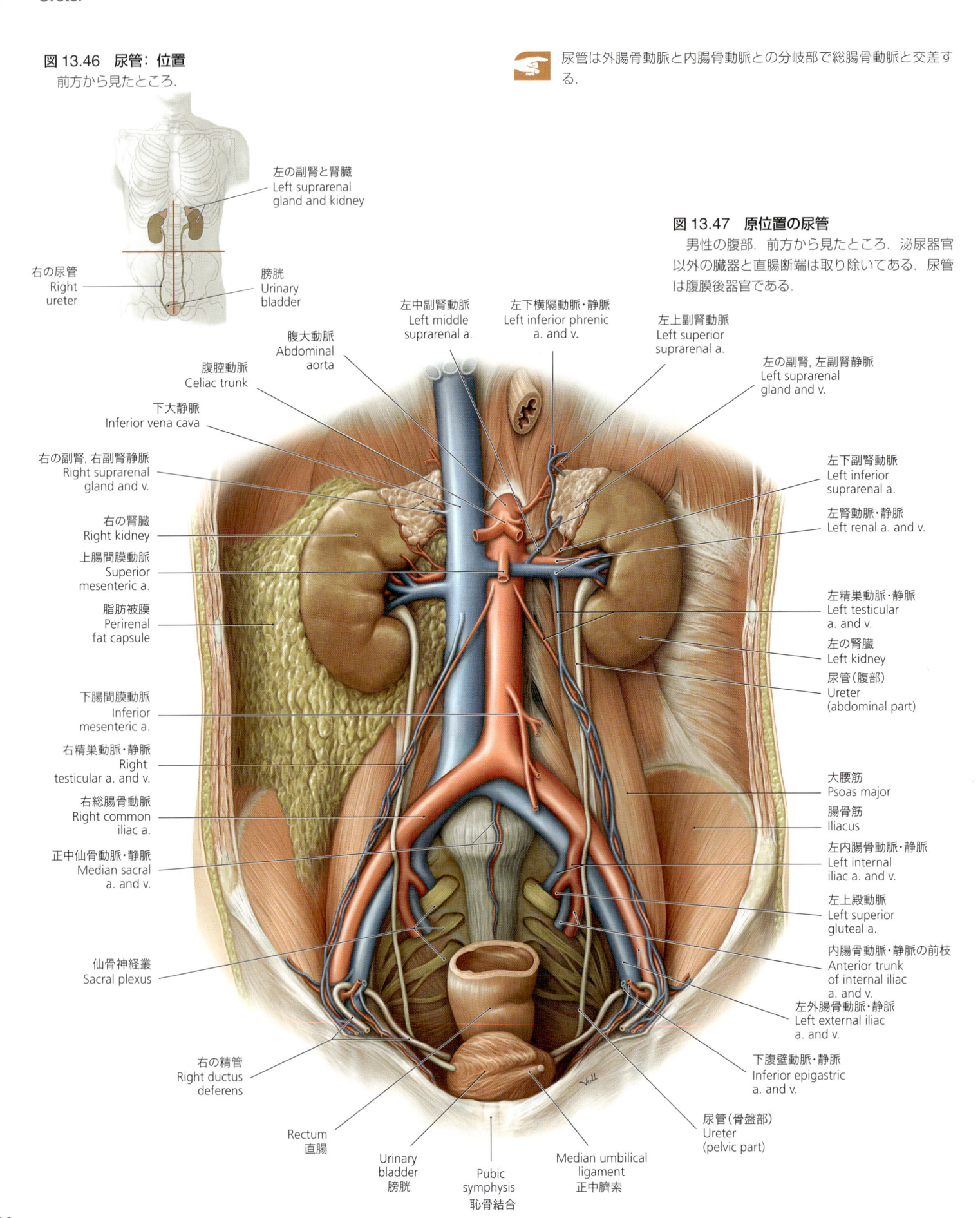

図 13.48　男性骨盤内の尿管
上方から見たところ．

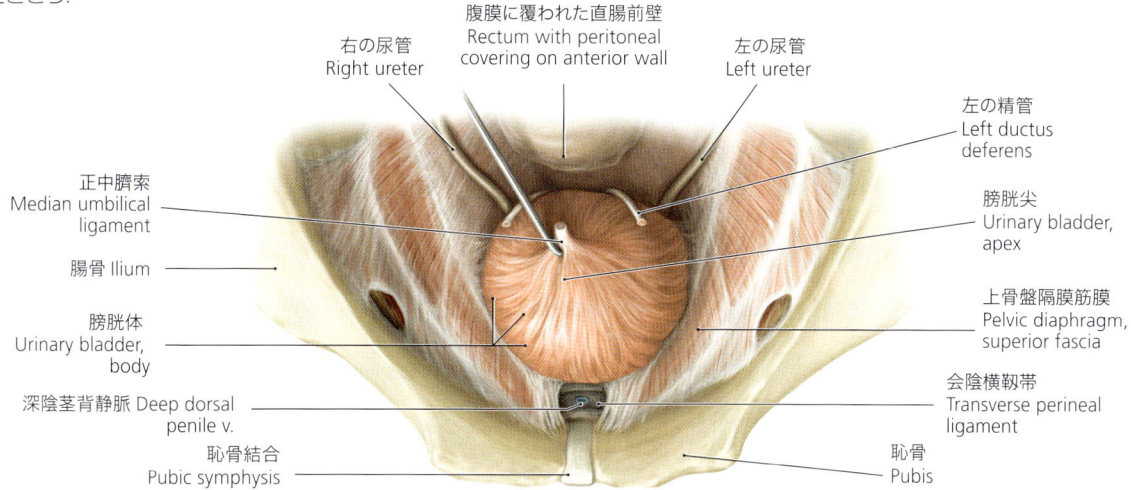

- 右の尿管 Right ureter
- 腹膜に覆われた直腸前壁 Rectum with peritoneal covering on anterior wall
- 左の尿管 Left ureter
- 左の精管 Left ductus deferens
- 膀胱尖 Urinary bladder, apex
- 正中臍索 Median umbilical ligament
- 腸骨 Ilium
- 膀胱体 Urinary bladder, body
- 上骨盤隔膜筋膜 Pelvic diaphragm, superior fascia
- 深陰茎背静脈 Deep dorsal penile v.
- 会陰横靱帯 Transverse perineal ligament
- 恥骨結合 Pubic symphysis
- 恥骨 Pubis

図 13.49　女性骨盤内の尿管
上方から見たところ．

- 右の尿管 Right ureter
- 直腸 Rectum
- 仙骨岬角（中に正中仙骨動脈・静脈が走る）Sacral promontory (with median sacral a. and v.)
- 直腸子宮窩 Rectouterine pouch
- 左卵巣動脈・静脈（卵巣提靱帯の中の）Left ovarian a. and v. (in ovarian suspensory ligament)
- 右の卵巣 Right ovary
- 直腸子宮ヒダと直腸子宮靱帯 Uterosacral fold (with uterosacral ligament)
- 右の卵管 Right uterine tube
- 子宮広間膜内を走る右の尿管 Passage of left ureter through broad ligament of uterus
- 子宮広間膜 Broad ligament of uterus
- 子宮, 後面 Uterus, posterior surface
- 子宮円索 Round ligament of uterus
- 子宮底 Uterine fundus
- 右外腸骨動脈・静脈 Right external iliac a. and v.
- 膀胱, 膀胱体 Urinary bladder, body
- 壁側腹膜 Parietal peritoneum
- 膀胱子宮窩 Vesicouterine pouch
- 内側臍ヒダ（臍動脈の閉塞部）Medial umbilical fold (obliterated umbilical a.)
- 横膀胱ヒダ Transverse vesical fold
- 恥骨結合 Pubic symphysis
- 正中臍索 Median umbilical ligament

膀胱
Urinary Bladder

図 13.50　男性の膀胱

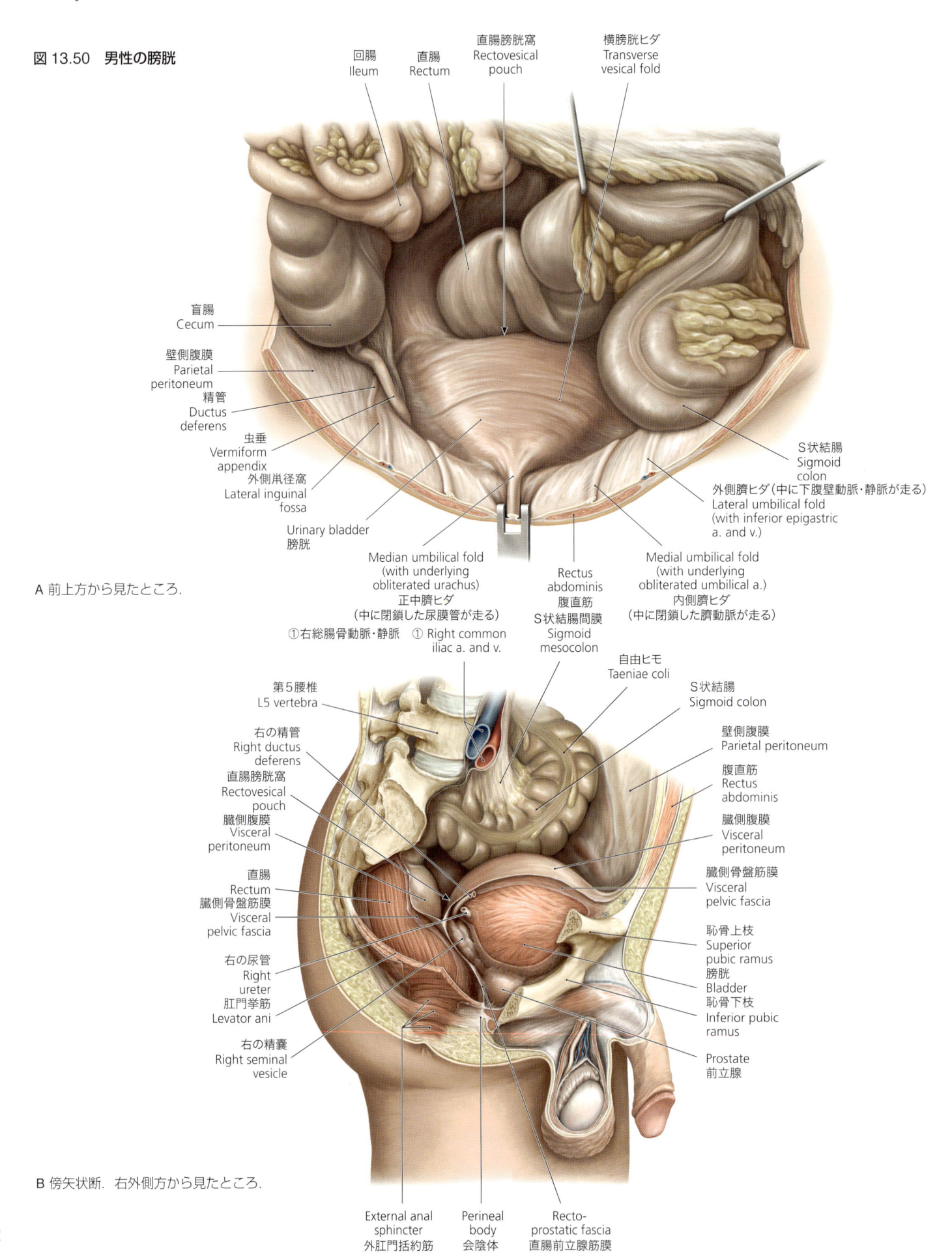

A 前上方から見たところ.

B 傍矢状断. 右外側方から見たところ.

👉 膀胱の位置は恥骨後方で腹膜後域にある.

図 13.51　女性の膀胱

- 子宮広間膜 Broad ligament of uterus
- 直腸 Rectum
- 直腸子宮窩 Rectouterine pouch
- 直腸子宮ヒダ Uterosacral fold
- 卵巣提靱帯 Ovarian suspensory ligament
- 卵管 Uterine tube
- 左の卵巣 Left ovary
- S状結腸 Sigmoid colon
- 固有卵巣索 Ovarian ligament
- 膀胱傍陥凹 Paravesical fossa
- 深鼠径輪 Deep inguinal ring
- 外側臍ヒダ（中に下腹壁動脈・静脈が走る）Lateral umbilical fold (with inferior epigastric a. and v.)
- 腹直筋 Rectus abdominis
- 内側臍ヒダ（中に閉鎖した臍動脈が走る）Medial umbilical fold (with obliterated umbilical a.)
- 膀胱上窩 Supravesical fossa
- 正中臍ヒダ（中に閉鎖した尿膜管が走る）Median umbilical fold (with obliterated urachus)
- 膀胱 Urinary bladder
- 横膀胱ヒダ Transverse vesical fold
- 膀胱子宮窩 Vesicouterine pouch
- 子宮円索 Round ligament of uterus
- 壁側腹膜 Parietal peritoneum
- 子宮 Uterus
- 盲腸 Cecum

A 前上方から見たところ.

- S状結腸とS状結腸間膜 Sigmoid colon and mesocolon
- 卵管 Uterine tube
- 子宮円索 Round ligament of uterus
- 膀胱子宮窩 Vesicouterine pouch
- 臓側腹膜 Visceral peritoneum
- 臓側骨盤筋膜 Visceral pelvic fascia
- 膀胱 Urinary bladder
- 膣 Vagina
- 会陰腱中心 Perineal body
- 外肛門括約筋 External anal sphincter
- 肛門挙筋 Levator ani
- 右の尿管 Right ureter
- 臓側骨盤筋膜 Visceral pelvic fascia
- 直腸 Rectum
- 臓側腹膜 Visceral peritoneum
- 直腸子宮窩 Rectouterine pouch
- 子宮 Uterus
- 固有卵巣索 Proper ovarian ligament

B 傍矢状断. 右外側方から見たところ.

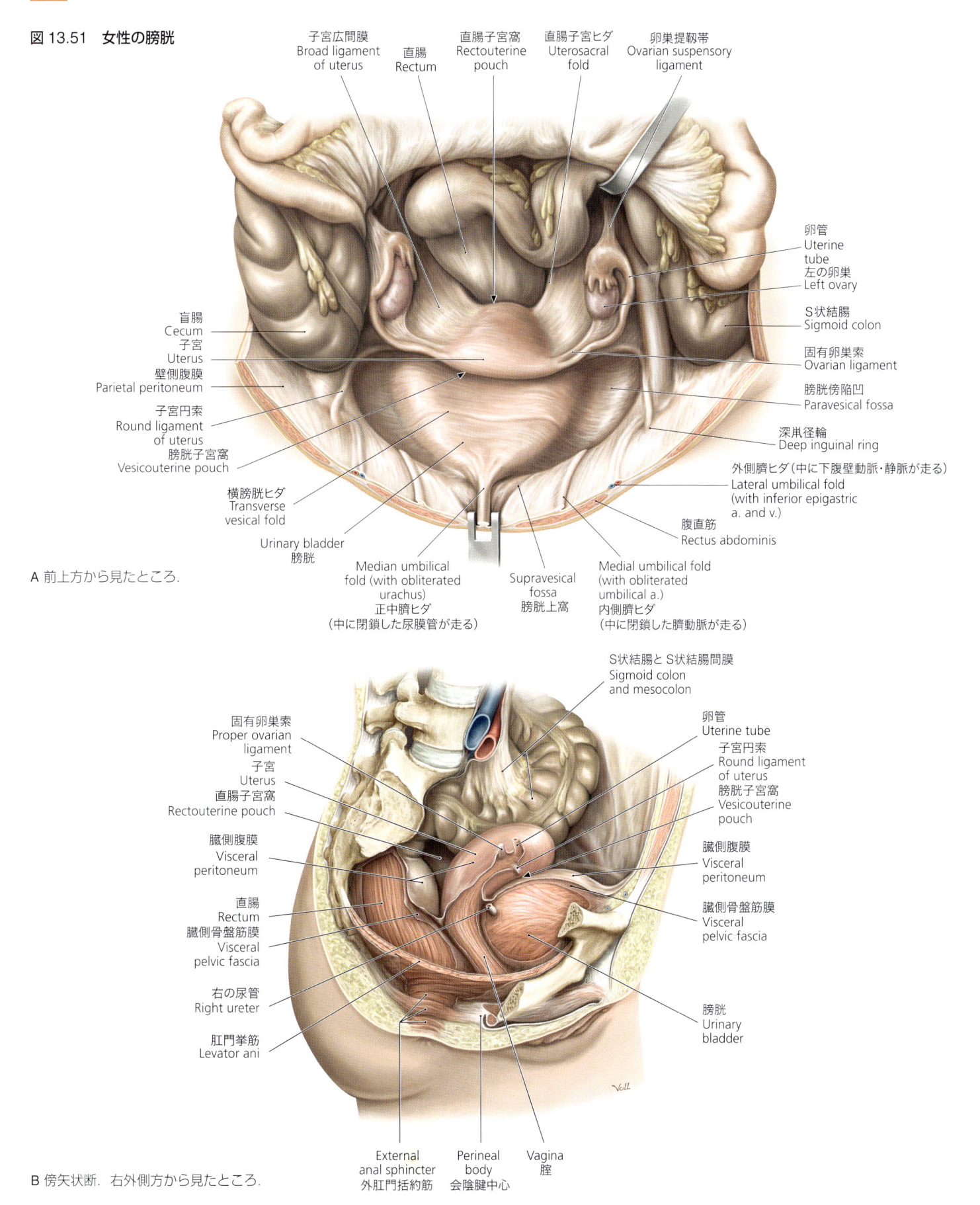

膀胱と尿道
Urinary Bladder & Urethra

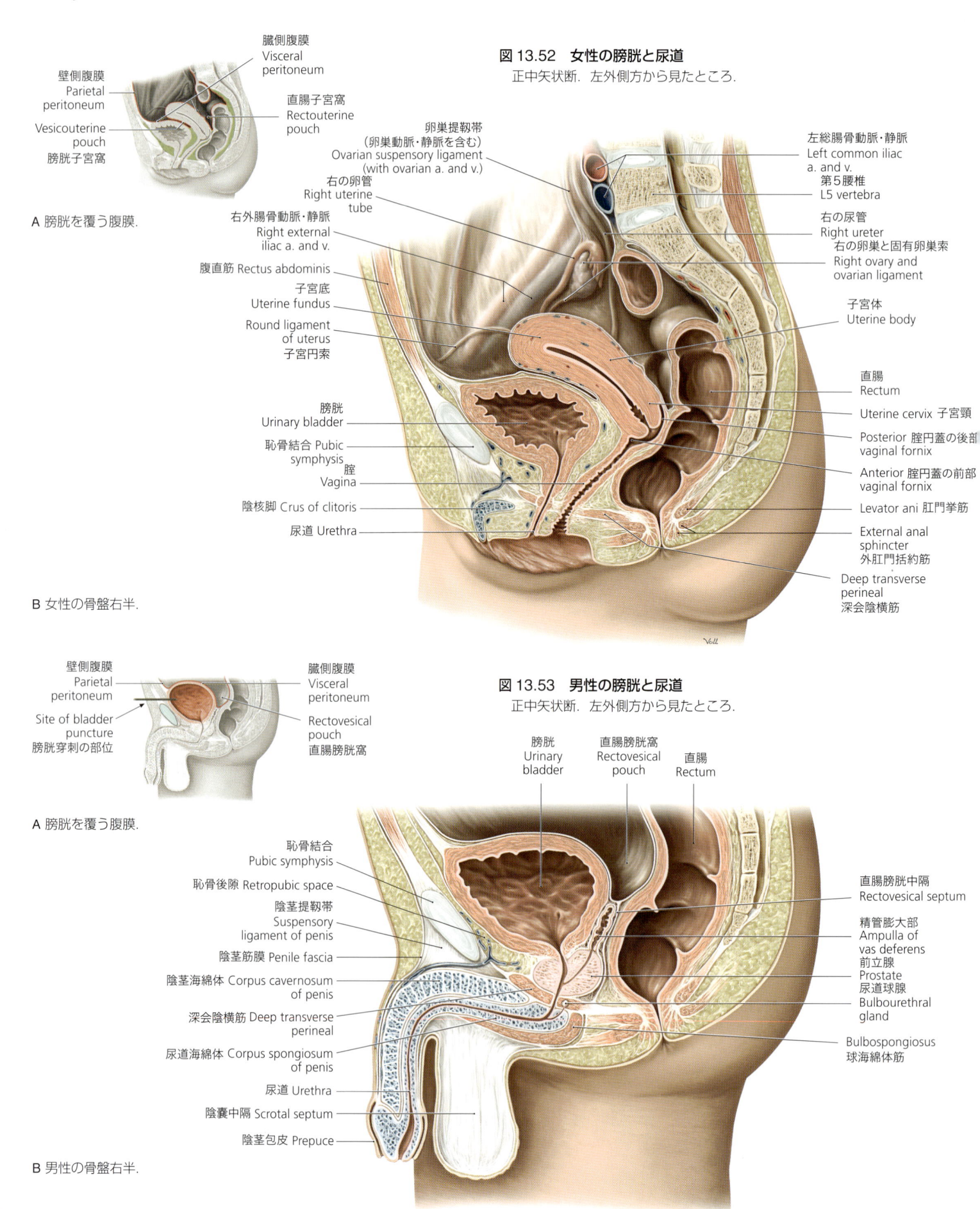

図 13.52 女性の膀胱と尿道
正中矢状断．左外側方から見たところ．

A 膀胱を覆う腹膜．
- 壁側腹膜 Parietal peritoneum
- 臓側腹膜 Visceral peritoneum
- 膀胱子宮窩 Vesicouterine pouch
- 直腸子宮窩 Rectouterine pouch

B 女性の骨盤右半．
- 卵巣提靭帯（卵巣動脈・静脈を含む） Ovarian suspensory ligament (with ovarian a. and v.)
- 右の卵管 Right uterine tube
- 右外腸骨動脈・静脈 Right external iliac a. and v.
- 腹直筋 Rectus abdominis
- 子宮底 Uterine fundus
- 子宮円索 Round ligament of uterus
- 膀胱 Urinary bladder
- 恥骨結合 Pubic symphysis
- 腟 Vagina
- 陰核脚 Crus of clitoris
- 尿道 Urethra
- 左総腸骨動脈・静脈 Left common iliac a. and v.
- 第5腰椎 L5 vertebra
- 右の尿管 Right ureter
- 右の卵巣と固有卵巣索 Right ovary and ovarian ligament
- 子宮体 Uterine body
- 直腸 Rectum
- 子宮頸 Uterine cervix
- 腟円蓋の後部 Posterior vaginal fornix
- 腟円蓋の前部 Anterior vaginal fornix
- 肛門挙筋 Levator ani
- 外肛門括約筋 External anal sphincter
- 深会陰横筋 Deep transverse perineal

図 13.53 男性の膀胱と尿道
正中矢状断．左外側方から見たところ．

A 膀胱を覆う腹膜．
- 壁側腹膜 Parietal peritoneum
- 膀胱穿刺の部位 Site of bladder puncture
- 臓側腹膜 Visceral peritoneum
- 直腸膀胱窩 Rectovesical pouch

B 男性の骨盤右半．
- 恥骨結合 Pubic symphysis
- 恥骨後隙 Retropubic space
- 陰茎提靭帯 Suspensory ligament of penis
- 陰茎筋膜 Penile fascia
- 陰茎海綿体 Corpus cavernosum of penis
- 深会陰横筋 Deep transverse perineal
- 尿道海綿体 Corpus spongiosum of penis
- 尿道 Urethra
- 陰嚢中隔 Scrotal septum
- 陰茎包皮 Prepuce
- 膀胱 Urinary bladder
- 直腸膀胱窩 Rectovesical pouch
- 直腸 Rectum
- 直腸膀胱中隔 Rectovesical septum
- 精管膨大部 Ampulla of vas deferens
- 前立腺 Prostate
- 尿道球腺 Bulbourethral gland
- 球海綿体筋 Bulbospongiosus

図 13.54 壁の構造
冠状断，前方から見たところ．

- 尿管間ヒダ Interureteric fold
- 膀胱（膀胱体）Urinary bladder (body)
- 右の尿管，壁内部 Right ureter, intramural part
- Ureteral orifice 尿管口
- 粘膜 Mucosa
- 筋層（＝排尿筋）Muscularis (= detrusor vesicae)
- Adventitia with visceral pelvic fascia 外膜と臓側骨盤筋膜
- 内尿道口と膀胱垂 Internal urethral orifice with bladder uvula
- Orifices of urethral glands 尿道腺の開口部
- 膀胱三角 Bladder trigone
- 膀胱頚 Neck
- 粘膜と縦走ヒダ Mucosa with longitudinal folds
- Submucosa 粘膜下組織
- Muscularis 筋層
- 尿道 Urethra

図 13.55 膀胱と尿道
前方から見たところ．

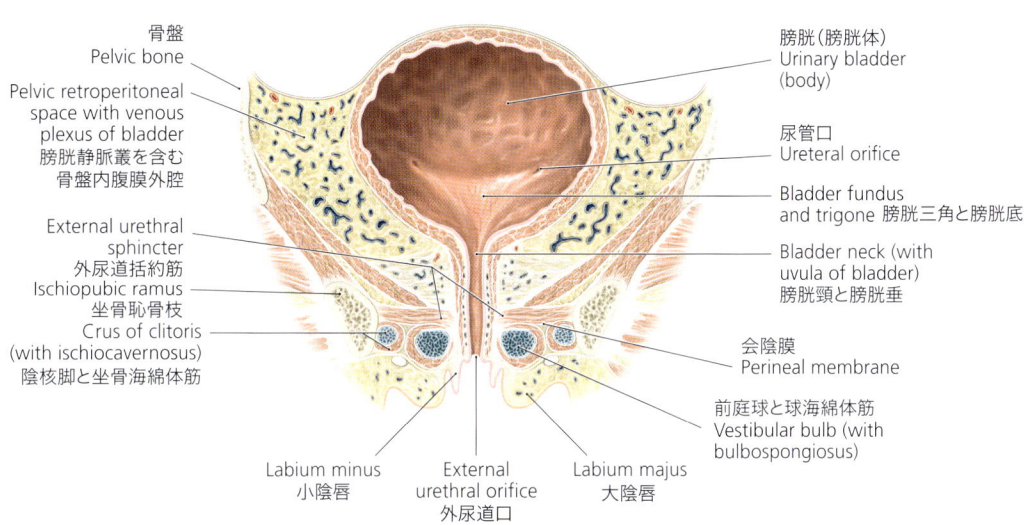

A 女性骨盤の冠状断．

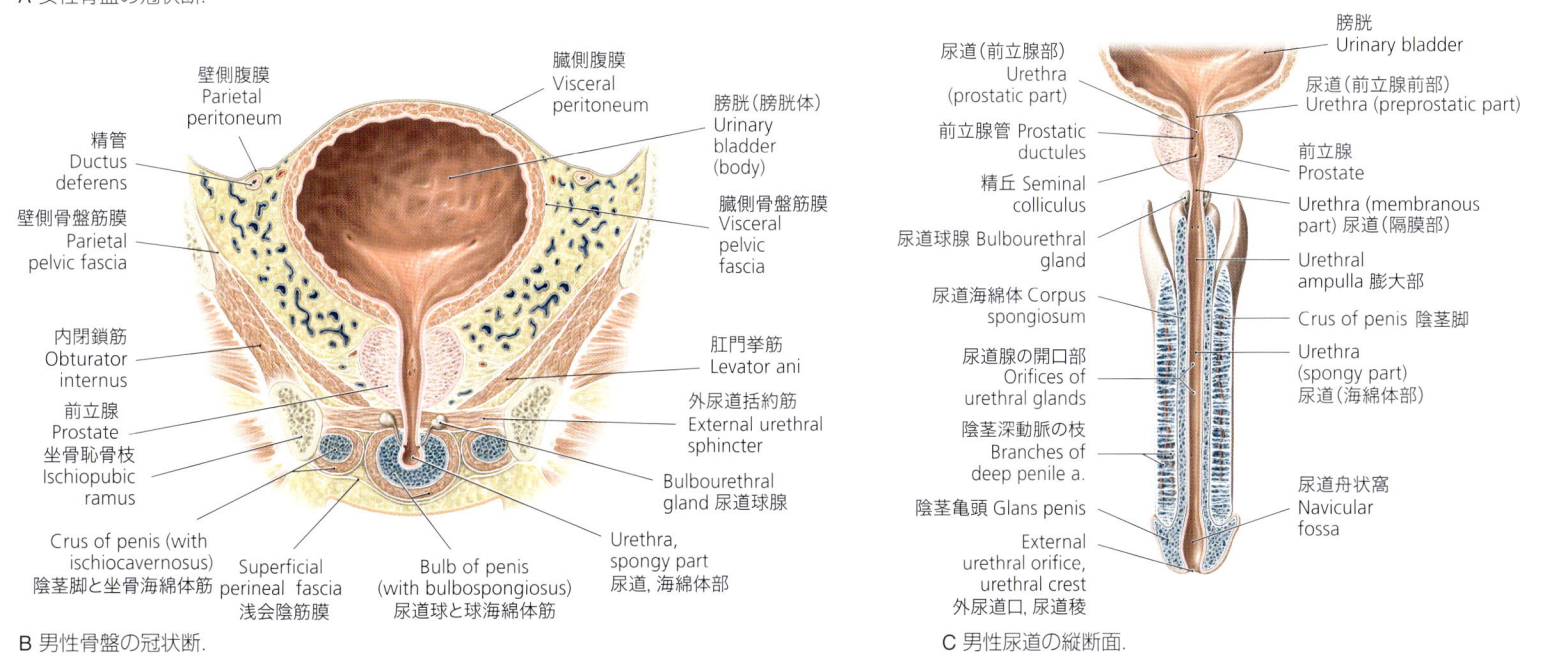

- 骨盤 Pelvic bone
- Pelvic retroperitoneal space with venous plexus of bladder 膀胱静脈叢を含む骨盤内腹膜外腔
- External urethral sphincter 外尿道括約筋
- Ischiopubic ramus 坐骨恥骨枝
- Crus of clitoris (with ischiocavernosus) 陰核脚と坐骨海綿体筋
- Labium minus 小陰唇
- External urethral orifice 外尿道口
- Labium majus 大陰唇
- 膀胱（膀胱体）Urinary bladder (body)
- 尿管口 Ureteral orifice
- Bladder fundus and trigone 膀胱三角と膀胱底
- Bladder neck (with uvula of bladder) 膀胱頚と膀胱垂
- 会陰膜 Perineal membrane
- 前庭球と球海綿体筋 Vestibular bulb (with bulbospongiosus)

B 男性骨盤の冠状断．

- 壁側腹膜 Parietal peritoneum
- 精管 Ductus deferens
- 壁側骨盤筋膜 Parietal pelvic fascia
- 内閉鎖筋 Obturator internus
- 前立腺 Prostate
- 坐骨恥骨枝 Ischiopubic ramus
- Crus of penis (with ischiocavernosus) 陰茎脚と坐骨海綿体筋
- Superficial perineal fascia 浅会陰筋膜
- Bulb of penis (with bulbospongiosus) 尿道球と球海綿体筋
- 臓側腹膜 Visceral peritoneum
- 膀胱（膀胱体）Urinary bladder (body)
- 臓側骨盤筋膜 Visceral pelvic fascia
- 肛門挙筋 Levator ani
- 外尿道括約筋 External urethral sphincter
- Bulbourethral gland 尿道球腺
- Urethra, spongy part 尿道，海綿体部

C 男性尿道の縦断面．

- 膀胱 Urinary bladder
- 尿道（前立腺部）Urethra (prostatic part)
- 前立腺管 Prostatic ductules
- 精丘 Seminal colliculus
- 尿道球腺 Bulbourethral gland
- 尿道海綿体 Corpus spongiosum
- 尿道腺の開口部 Orifices of urethral glands
- 陰茎深動脈の枝 Branches of deep penile a.
- 陰茎亀頭 Glans penis
- External urethral orifice, urethral crest 外尿道口，尿道稜
- 尿道（前立腺前部）Urethra (preprostatic part)
- 前立腺 Prostate
- Urethra (membranous part) 尿道（隔膜部）
- Urethral ampulla 膨大部
- Crus of penis 陰茎脚
- Urethra (spongy part) 尿道（海綿体部）
- 尿道舟状窩 Navicular fossa

生殖器の概観
Overview of the Genital Organs

生殖器は，局所解剖学的には内生殖器と外生殖器に分類され，他には機能によって（表14.1と表14.2），もしくは個体発生学的に（p.204 参照）分類される．

表14.1　女性生殖器

	器官		機能
内生殖器	卵巣		生殖細胞とホルモンの産生
	卵管		受精の場，接合子の運搬
	子宮		胎児の発育と分娩の器官
	腟（上部）		交接と分娩の器官
外生殖器	外陰部	腟（前庭）	
		大・小陰唇	交接器官
		陰核	
		大・小前庭腺	分泌液の産生
		恥丘	恥骨の保護

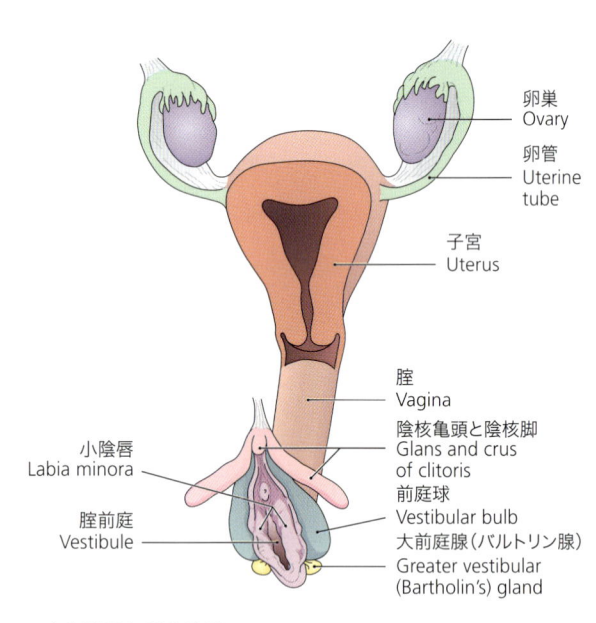

図14.1　女性生殖器

A 内生殖器と外生殖器．

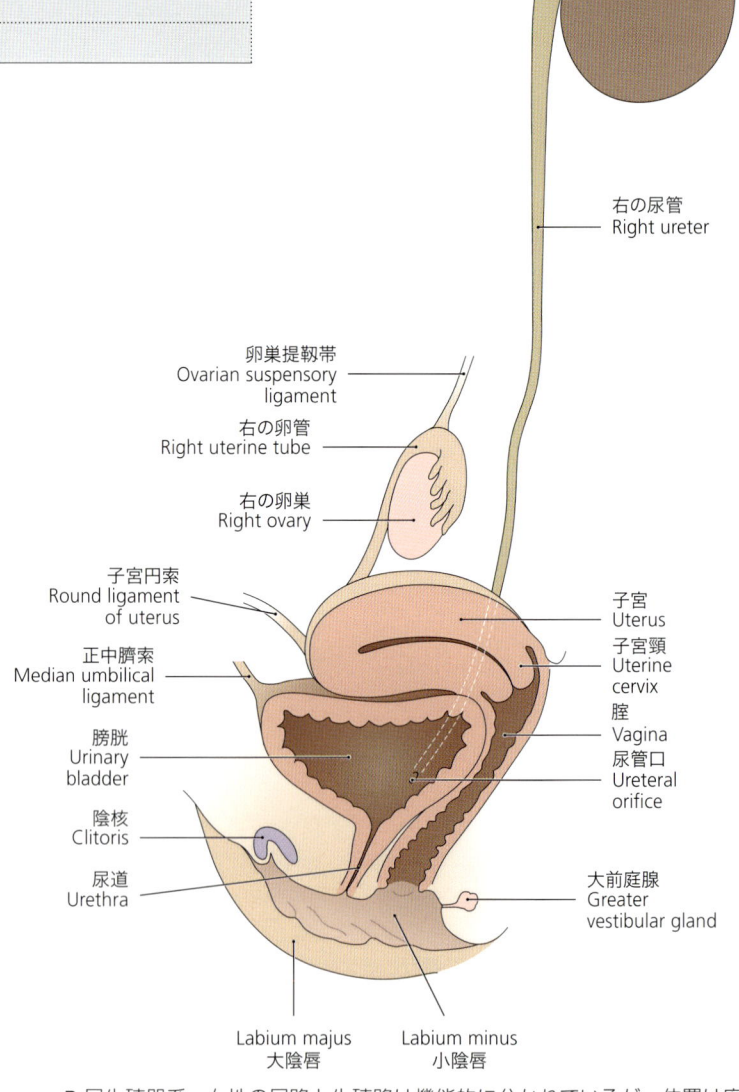

B 尿生殖器系．女性の尿路と生殖路は機能的に分かれているが，位置は密接している．

表14.2　男性生殖器

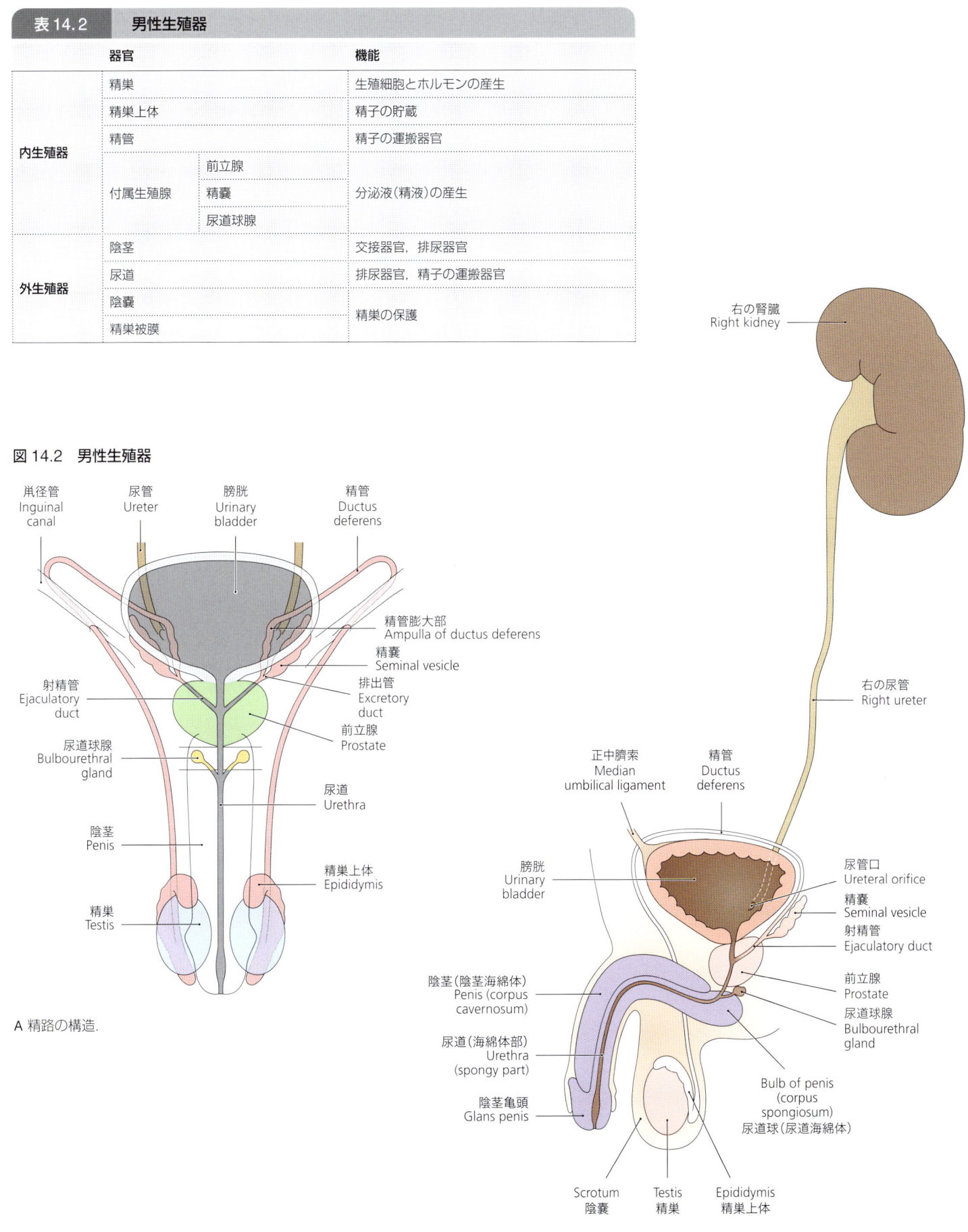

	器官		機能
内生殖器	精巣		生殖細胞とホルモンの産生
	精巣上体		精子の貯蔵
	精管		精子の運搬器官
	付属生殖腺	前立腺	分泌液（精液）の産生
		精嚢	
		尿道球腺	
外生殖器	陰茎		交接器官，排尿器官
	尿道		排尿器官，精子の運搬器官
	陰嚢		精巣の保護
	精巣被膜		

図14.2　男性生殖器

A　精路の構造．

B　尿生殖器系．男性の尿道は尿路と生殖路の共通の通路となっている．

子宮と卵巣
Uterus & Ovaries

図 14.3　女性の内生殖器
子宮と卵巣は卵巣間膜と子宮間膜（子宮広間膜の一部）で覆われる．

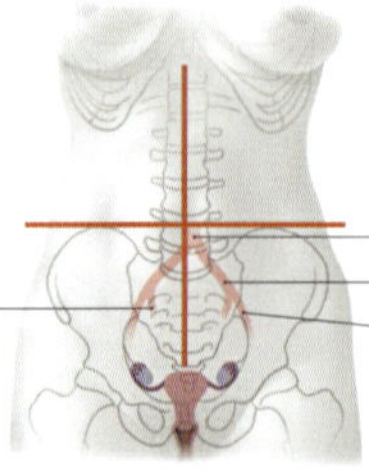

A　位置，前方から見たところ．

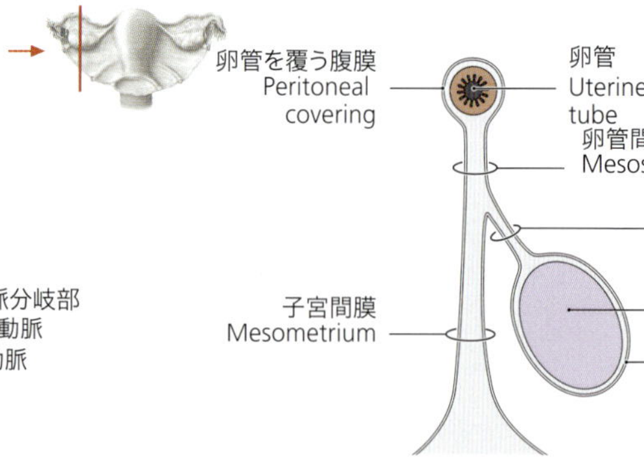

- 内腸骨動脈 Internal iliac a.
- Aortic bifurcation 大動脈分岐部
- Common iliac a. 総腸骨動脈
- External iliac a. 外腸骨動脈

- 卵管を覆う腹膜 Peritoneal covering
- 卵管 Uterine tube
- 卵管間膜 Mesosalpinx
- 卵巣間膜 Mesovarium
- 子宮間膜 Mesometrium
- 卵巣 Ovary
- Germinal epithelial covering 卵巣を覆う胚上皮

B　間膜，矢状断．子宮広間膜は卵管間膜と卵巣間膜と子宮間膜を合わせたものである．

図 14.4　卵巣
右卵巣，後方から見たところ．

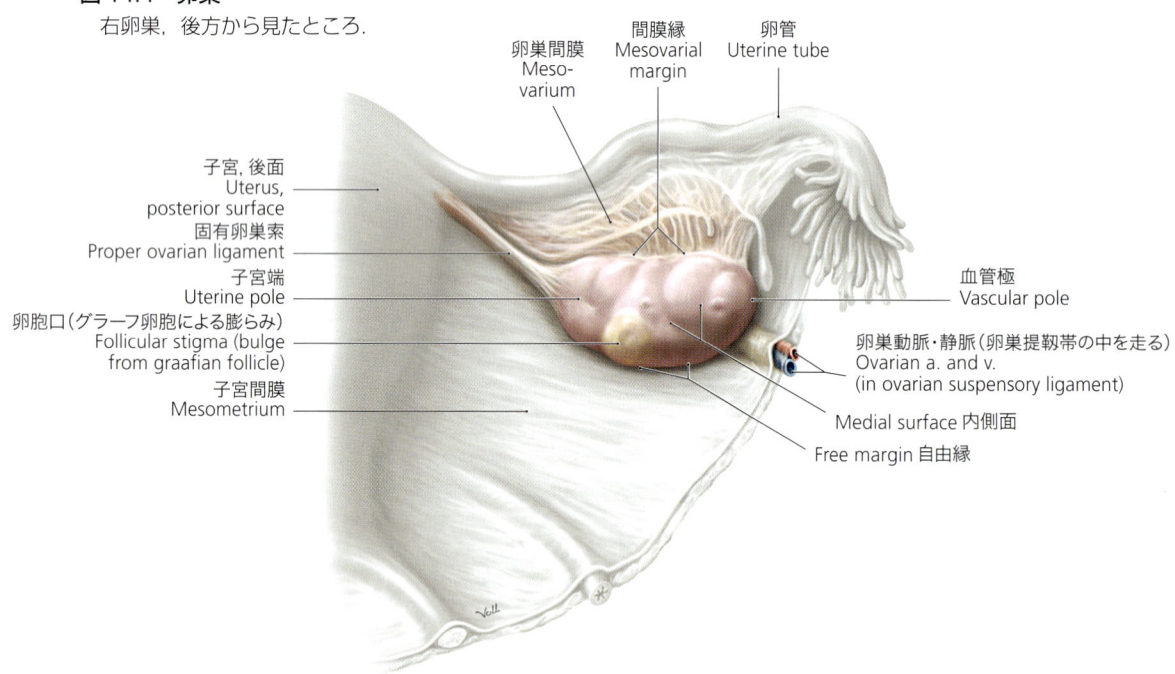

- 卵巣間膜 Mesovarium
- 間膜縁 Mesovarial margin
- 卵管 Uterine tube
- 子宮，後面 Uterus, posterior surface
- 固有卵巣索 Proper ovarian ligament
- 子宮端 Uterine pole
- 卵胞口（グラーフ卵胞による膨らみ） Follicular stigma (bulge from graafian follicle)
- 子宮間膜 Mesometrium
- 血管極 Vascular pole
- 卵巣動脈・静脈（卵巣提靱帯の中を走る） Ovarian a. and v. (in ovarian suspensory ligament)
- Medial surface 内側面
- Free margin 自由縁

図 14.5　子宮の弯曲
正中矢状断．左外側方から見たところ．子宮の位置は①屈曲と②傾斜で記述される．

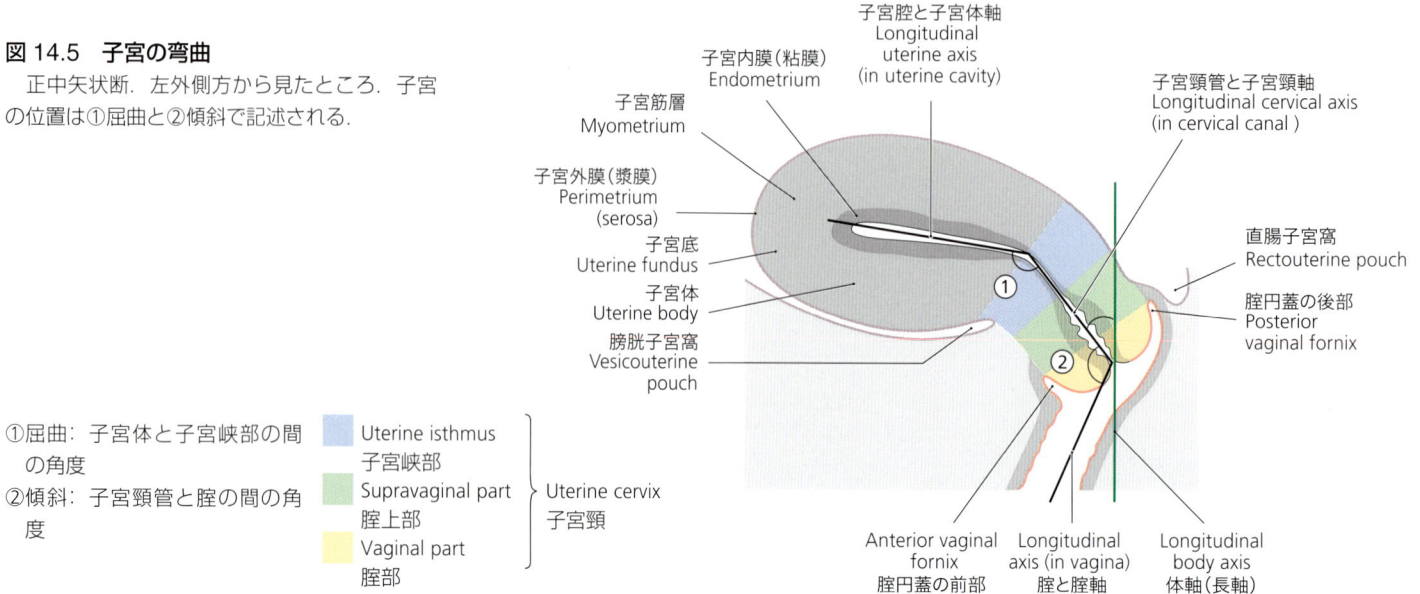

- 子宮内膜（粘膜） Endometrium
- 子宮腔と子宮体軸 Longitudinal uterine axis (in uterine cavity)
- 子宮筋層 Myometrium
- 子宮頸管と子宮頸軸 Longitudinal cervical axis (in cervical canal)
- 子宮外膜（漿膜） Perimetrium (serosa)
- 子宮底 Uterine fundus
- 直腸子宮窩 Rectouterine pouch
- 子宮体 Uterine body
- 腟円蓋の後部 Posterior vaginal fornix
- 膀胱子宮窩 Vesicouterine pouch

①屈曲：子宮体と子宮峡部の間の角度
②傾斜：子宮頸管と腟の間の角度

- Uterine isthmus 子宮峡部
- Supravaginal part 腟上部
- Vaginal part 腟部
} Uterine cervix 子宮頸

- Anterior vaginal fornix 腟円蓋の前部
- Longitudinal axis (in vagina) 腟と腟軸
- Longitudinal body axis 体軸（長軸）

図14.6 子宮と卵管

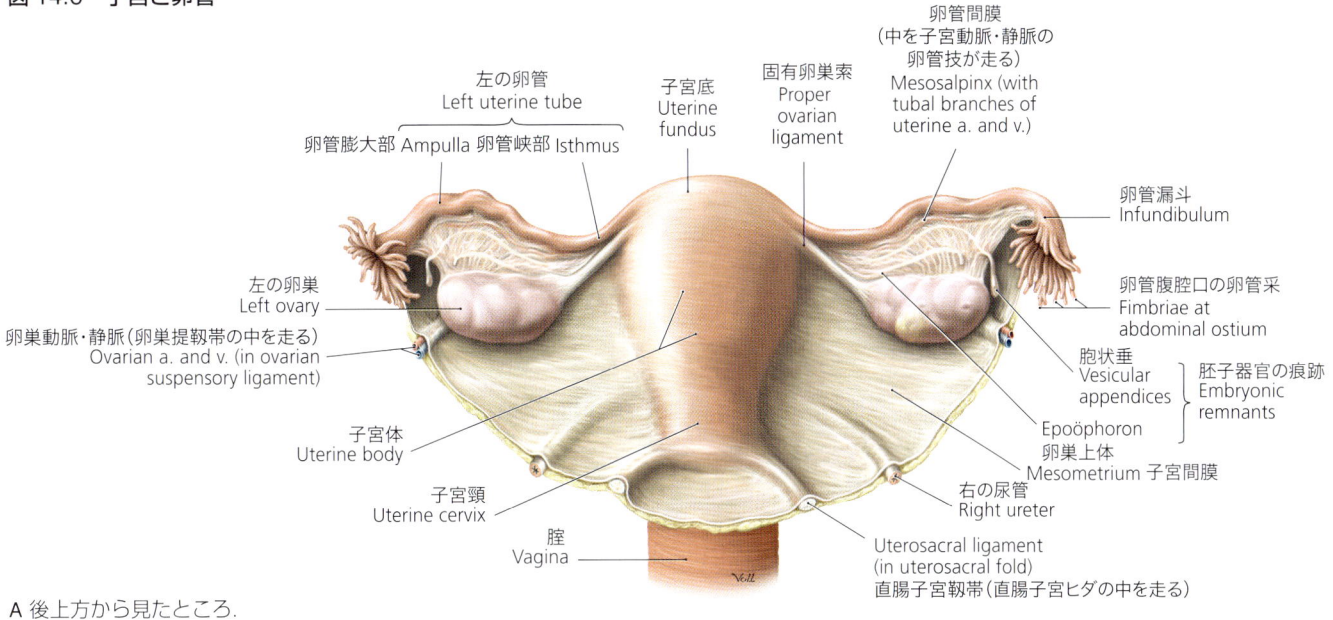

A 後上方から見たところ.

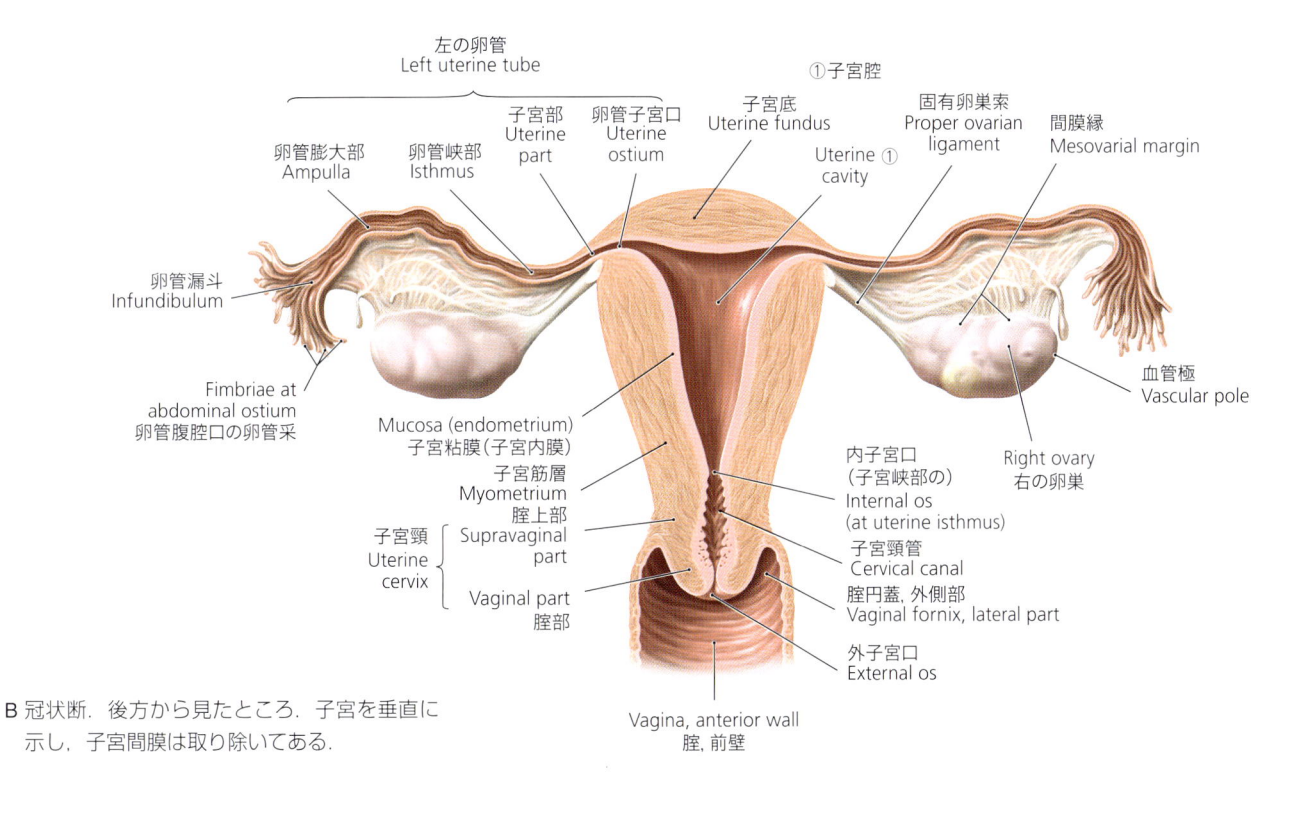

B 冠状断. 後方から見たところ. 子宮を垂直に示し, 子宮間膜は取り除いてある.

臨床

異所性妊娠

通常, 卵子は受精後に子宮腔の壁に着床するが, 他の場所 (卵管や場合によっては腹膜腔) に着床することもある. 最も一般的な異所性妊娠である卵管妊娠では卵管壁が破裂し, 腹膜腔内に出血することで生命の危機に陥る可能性がある. 卵管妊娠の多くは炎症の後に卵管粘膜に癒着が生じることにより起こる.

腟
Vagina

図14.7 位置
正中矢状断．左外側方から見たところ．

図14.8 構造
後方に向かっての冠状断．後方から見たところ．

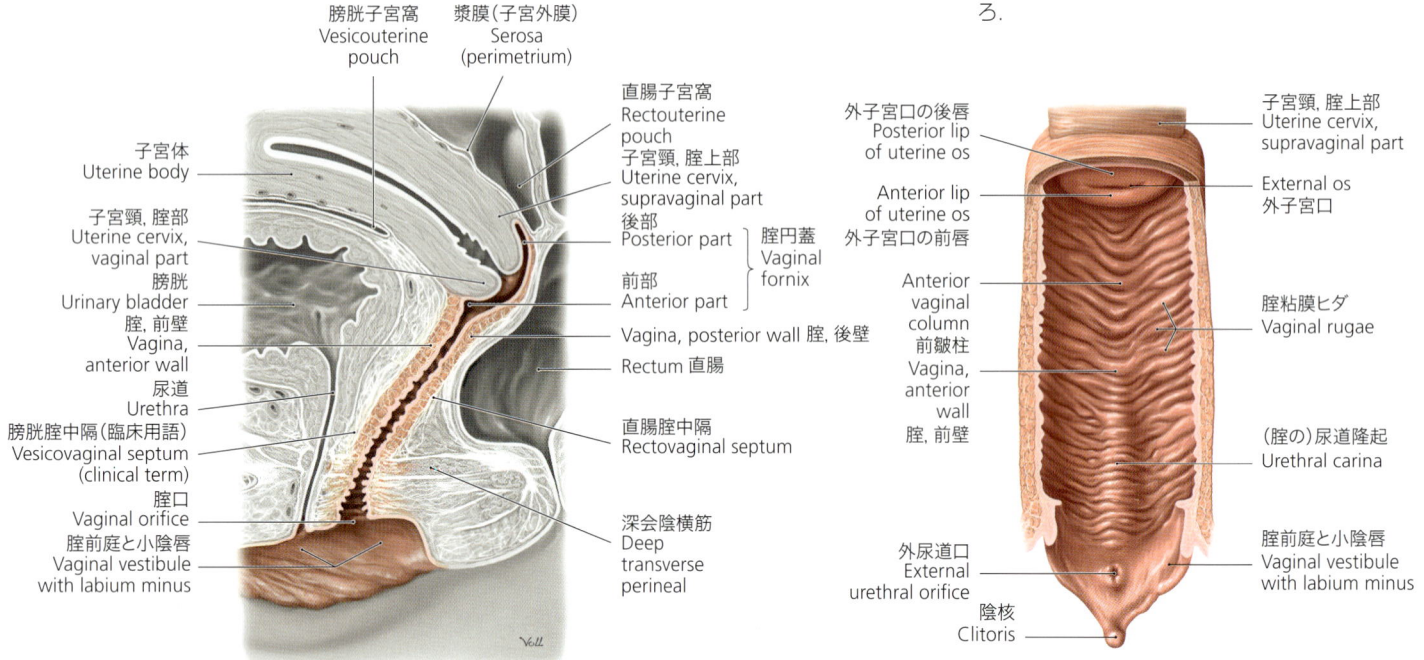

図14.9 子宮頸：水平断
下方から見たところ．

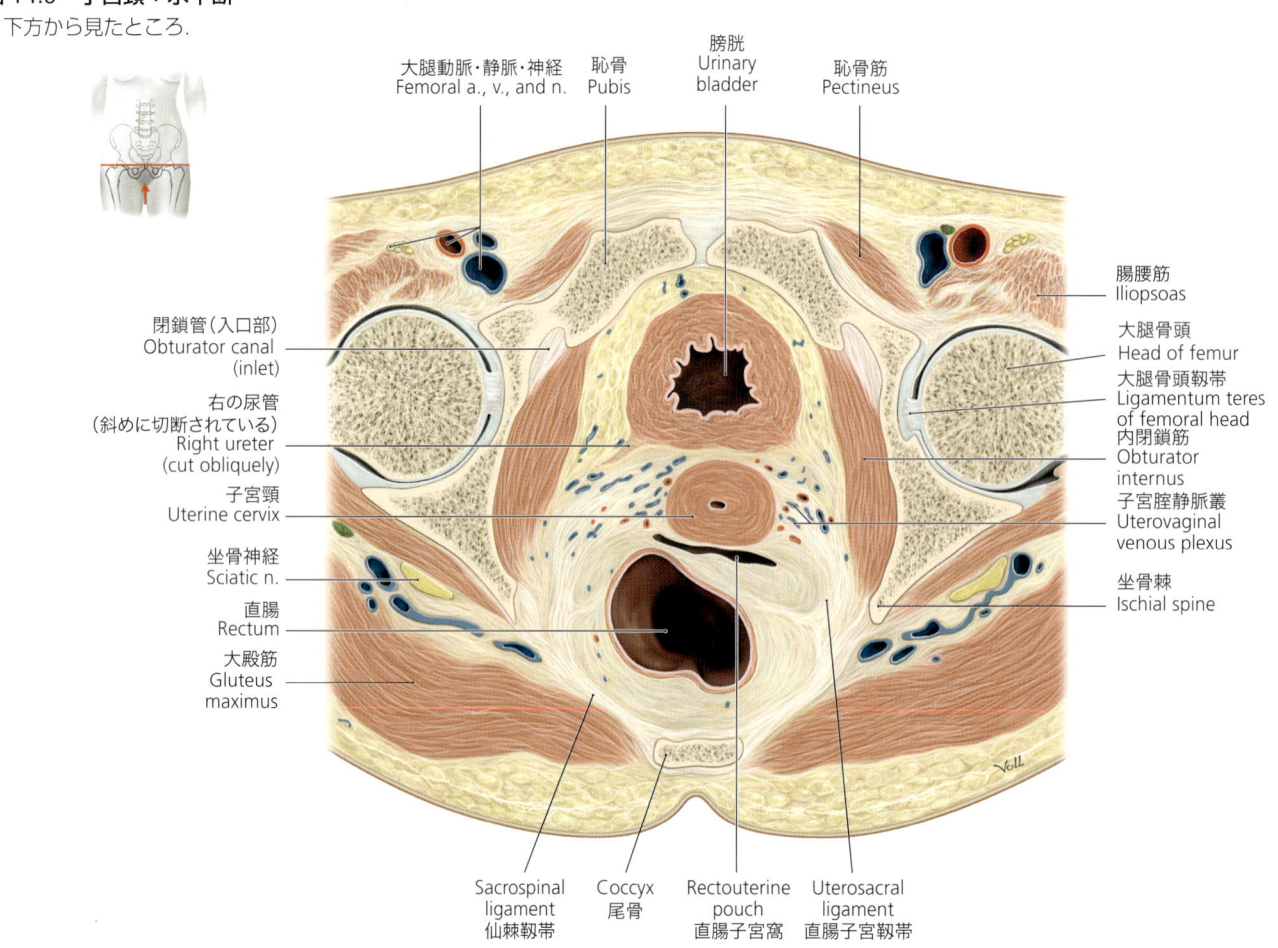

図 14.10 女性生殖器：冠状断

前方から見たところ．腟は骨盤内と会陰に位置し，腹膜後器官である．

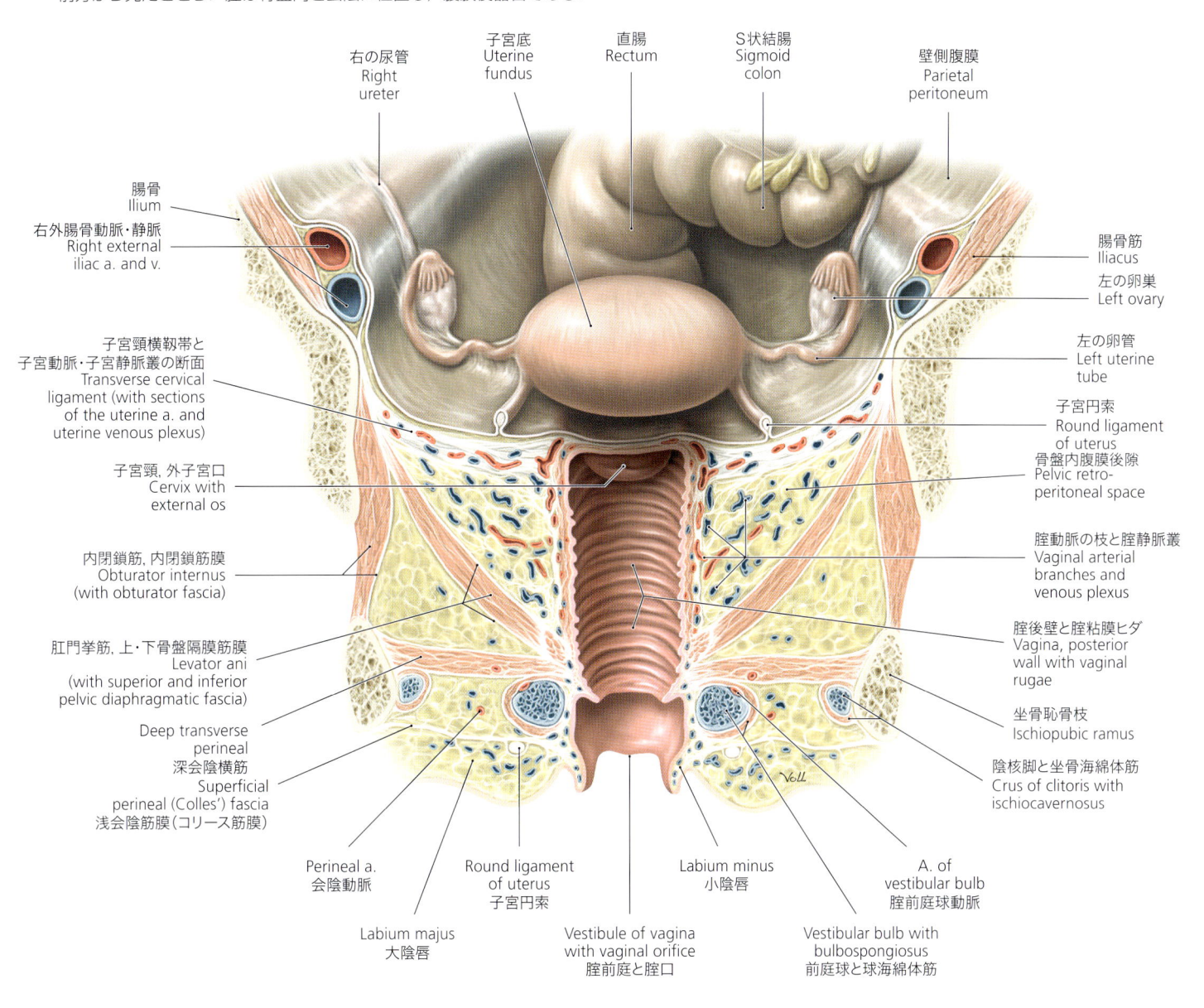

- 右の尿管 Right ureter
- 子宮底 Uterine fundus
- 直腸 Rectum
- S状結腸 Sigmoid colon
- 壁側腹膜 Parietal peritoneum
- 腸骨 Ilium
- 右外腸骨動脈・静脈 Right external iliac a. and v.
- 腸骨筋 Iliacus
- 左の卵巣 Left ovary
- 子宮頸横靱帯と子宮動脈・子宮静脈叢の断面 Transverse cervical ligament (with sections of the uterine a. and uterine venous plexus)
- 左の卵管 Left uterine tube
- 子宮円索 Round ligament of uterus
- 骨盤内腹膜後隙 Pelvic retro-peritoneal space
- 子宮頸, 外子宮口 Cervix with external os
- 内閉鎖筋, 内閉鎖筋膜 Obturator internus (with obturator fascia)
- 腟動脈の枝と腟静脈叢 Vaginal arterial branches and venous plexus
- 肛門挙筋, 上・下骨盤隔膜筋膜 Levator ani (with superior and inferior pelvic diaphragmatic fascia)
- 腟後壁と腟粘膜ヒダ Vagina, posterior wall with vaginal rugae
- 坐骨恥骨枝 Ischiopubic ramus
- Deep transverse perineal 深会陰横筋
- 陰核脚と坐骨海綿体筋 Crus of clitoris with ischiocavernosus
- Superficial perineal (Colles') fascia 浅会陰筋膜（コリース筋膜）
- Perineal a. 会陰動脈
- Round ligament of uterus 子宮円索
- Labium minus 小陰唇
- A. of vestibular bulb 腟前庭球動脈
- Labium majus 大陰唇
- Vestibule of vagina with vaginal orifice 腟前庭と腟口
- Vestibular bulb with bulbospongiosus 前庭球と球海綿体筋

図 14.11 腟：骨盤底での位置

下方から見たところ．

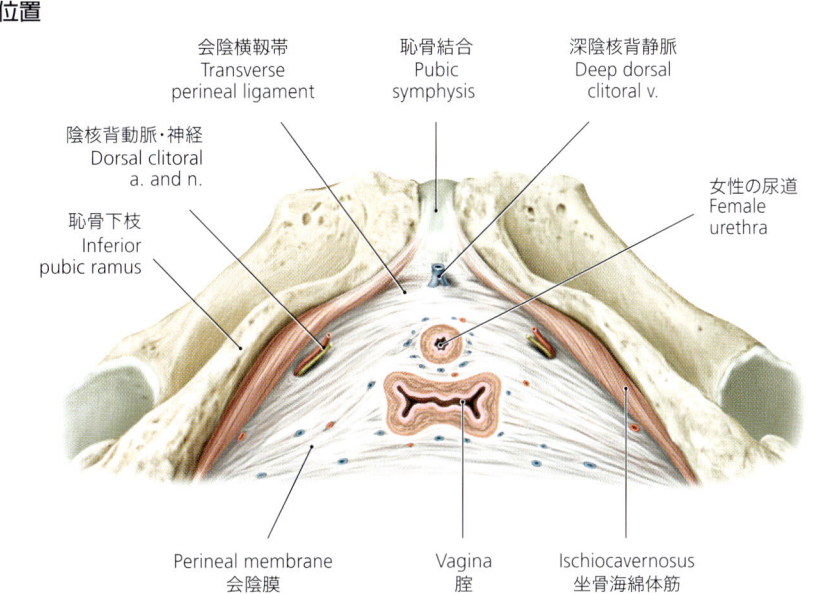

- 会陰横靱帯 Transverse perineal ligament
- 恥骨結合 Pubic symphysis
- 深陰核背静脈 Deep dorsal clitoral v.
- 陰核背動脈・神経 Dorsal clitoral a. and n.
- 女性の尿道 Female urethra
- 恥骨下枝 Inferior pubic ramus
- Perineal membrane 会陰膜
- Vagina 腟
- Ischiocavernosus 坐骨海綿体筋

女性の外生殖器
Female External Genitalia

図 14.12 女性の外生殖器
切石位. 小陰唇を開く.

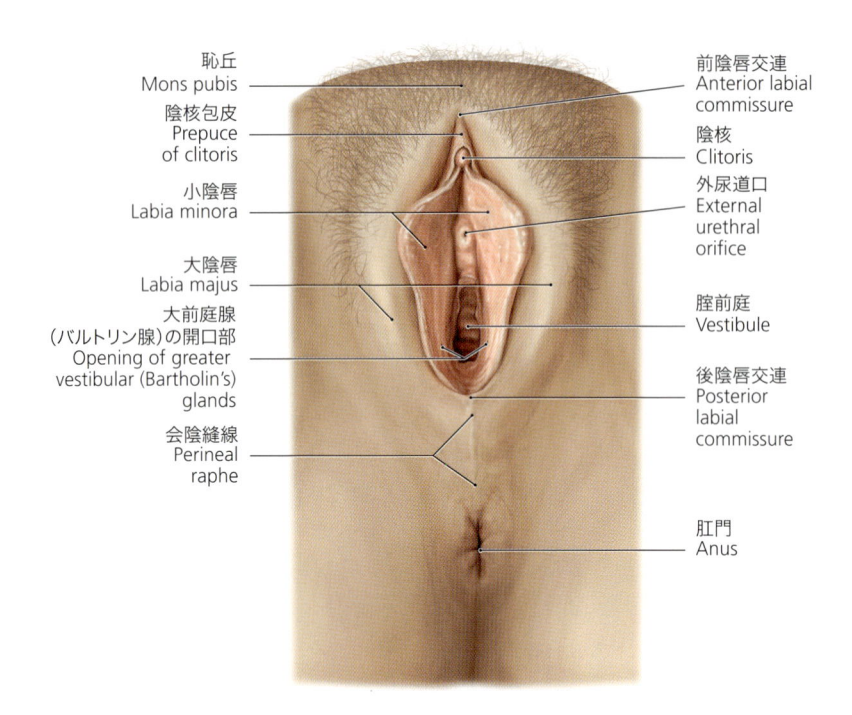

恥丘 Mons pubis
陰核包皮 Prepuce of clitoris
小陰唇 Labia minora
大陰唇 Labia majus
大前庭腺（バルトリン腺）の開口部 Opening of greater vestibular (Bartholin's) glands
会陰縫線 Perineal raphe
前陰唇交連 Anterior labial commissure
陰核 Clitoris
外尿道口 External urethral orifice
腟前庭 Vestibule
後陰唇交連 Posterior labial commissure
肛門 Anus

図 14.13 腟前庭と前庭腺
切石位. 小陰唇を開く.

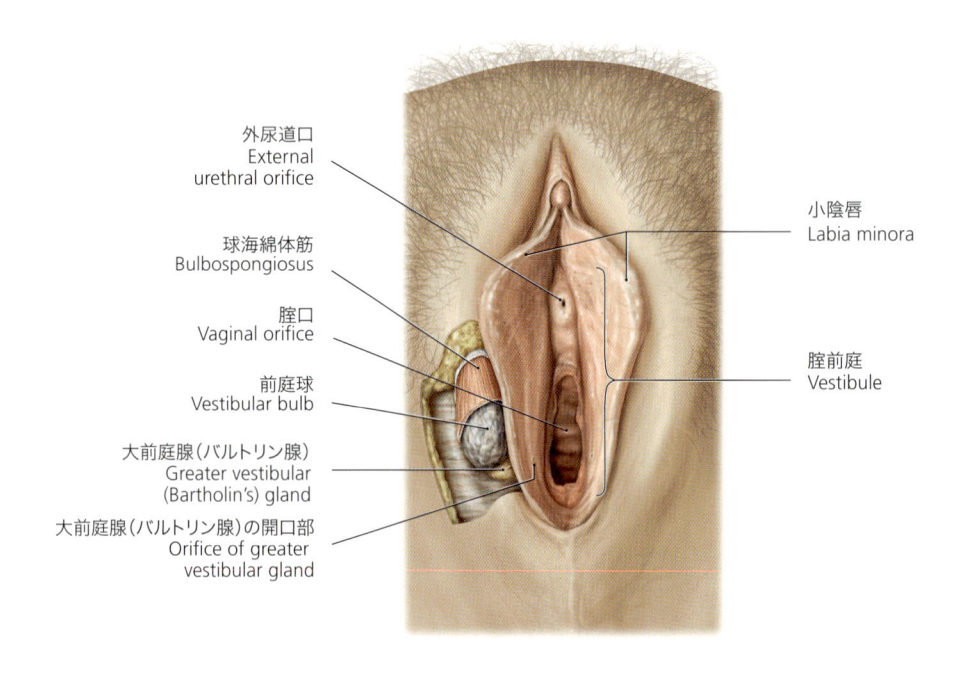

外尿道口 External urethral orifice
球海綿体筋 Bulbospongiosus
腟口 Vaginal orifice
前庭球 Vestibular bulb
大前庭腺（バルトリン腺） Greater vestibular (Bartholin's) gland
大前庭腺（バルトリン腺）の開口部 Orifice of greater vestibular gland
小陰唇 Labia minora
腟前庭 Vestibule

図 14.14 勃起協力筋と勃起組織：女性

切石位．大陰唇，小陰唇，会陰膜は取り除いてある．勃起筋（左側）．

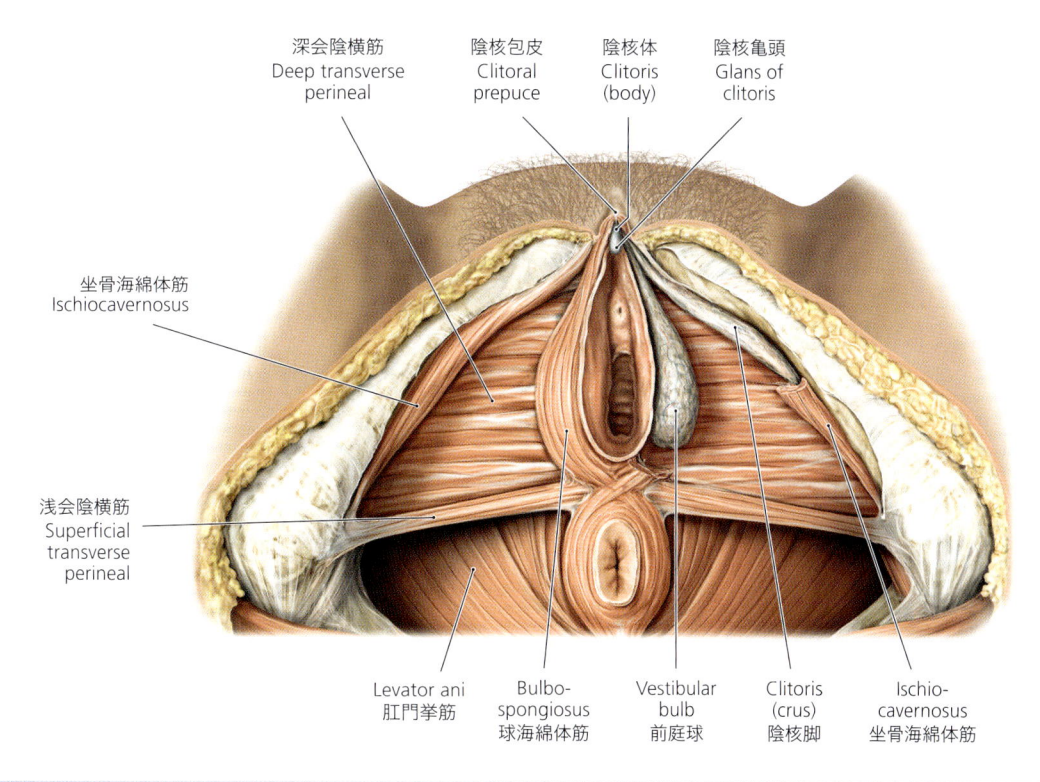

深会陰横筋 Deep transverse perineal
陰核包皮 Clitoral prepuce
陰核体 Clitoris (body)
陰核亀頭 Glans of clitoris
坐骨海綿体筋 Ischiocavernosus
浅会陰横筋 Superficial transverse perineal

Levator ani 肛門挙筋
Bulbo-spongiosus 球海綿体筋
Vestibular bulb 前庭球
Clitoris (crus) 陰核脚
Ischio-cavernosus 坐骨海綿体筋

臨床

会陰切開術

会陰切開術は分娩の娩出期に産道を拡大する産科的手技である．この手技は一般には娩出期の低酸素症を防ぎ娩出を早めるために用いられる．そのほか，会陰の皮膚が白色になった（血流の低下を表す）場合，会陰裂傷の危険が切迫しており，会陰切開術がしばしば行われる．側切開が切開の幅を最も広くとれるが，回復は難しくなる．

側切開 Lateral episiotomy
正中切開 Midline episiotomy
会陰 Perineum 肛門 Anus
Mediolateral episiotomy 正中側切開

A 切開術の各型．

後陰唇交連 Posterior commissure

B 子宮収縮最強時の正中側切開．

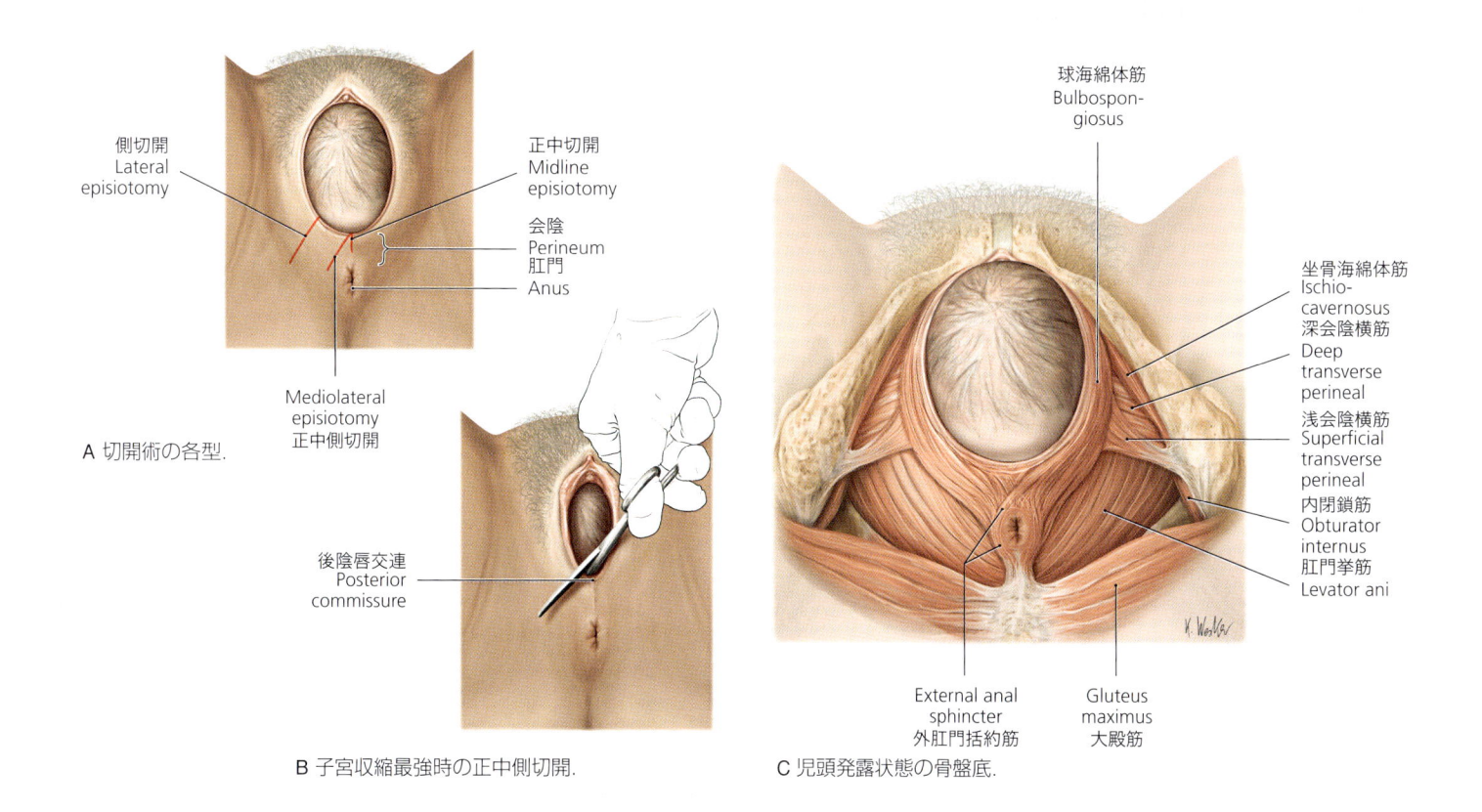

球海綿体筋 Bulbospongiosus
坐骨海綿体筋 Ischiocavernosus
深会陰横筋 Deep transverse perineal
浅会陰横筋 Superficial transverse perineal
内閉鎖筋 Obturator internus
肛門挙筋 Levator ani
External anal sphincter 外肛門括約筋
Gluteus maximus 大殿筋

C 児頭発露状態の骨盤底．

女性生殖器の神経と血管
Neurovasculature of the Female Genitalia

図 14.15　女性の会陰と生殖器の神経

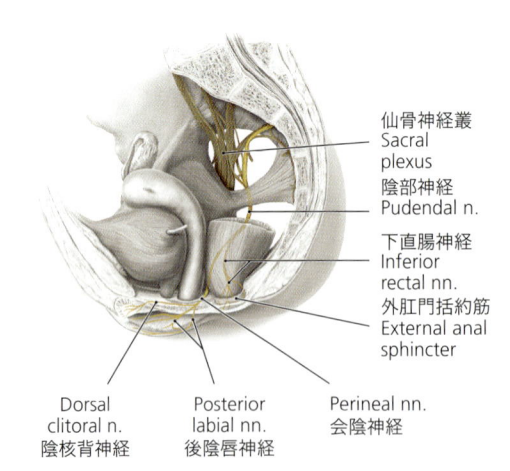

A　女性の外生殖器への神経分布．小骨盤を左外側方から見たところ．

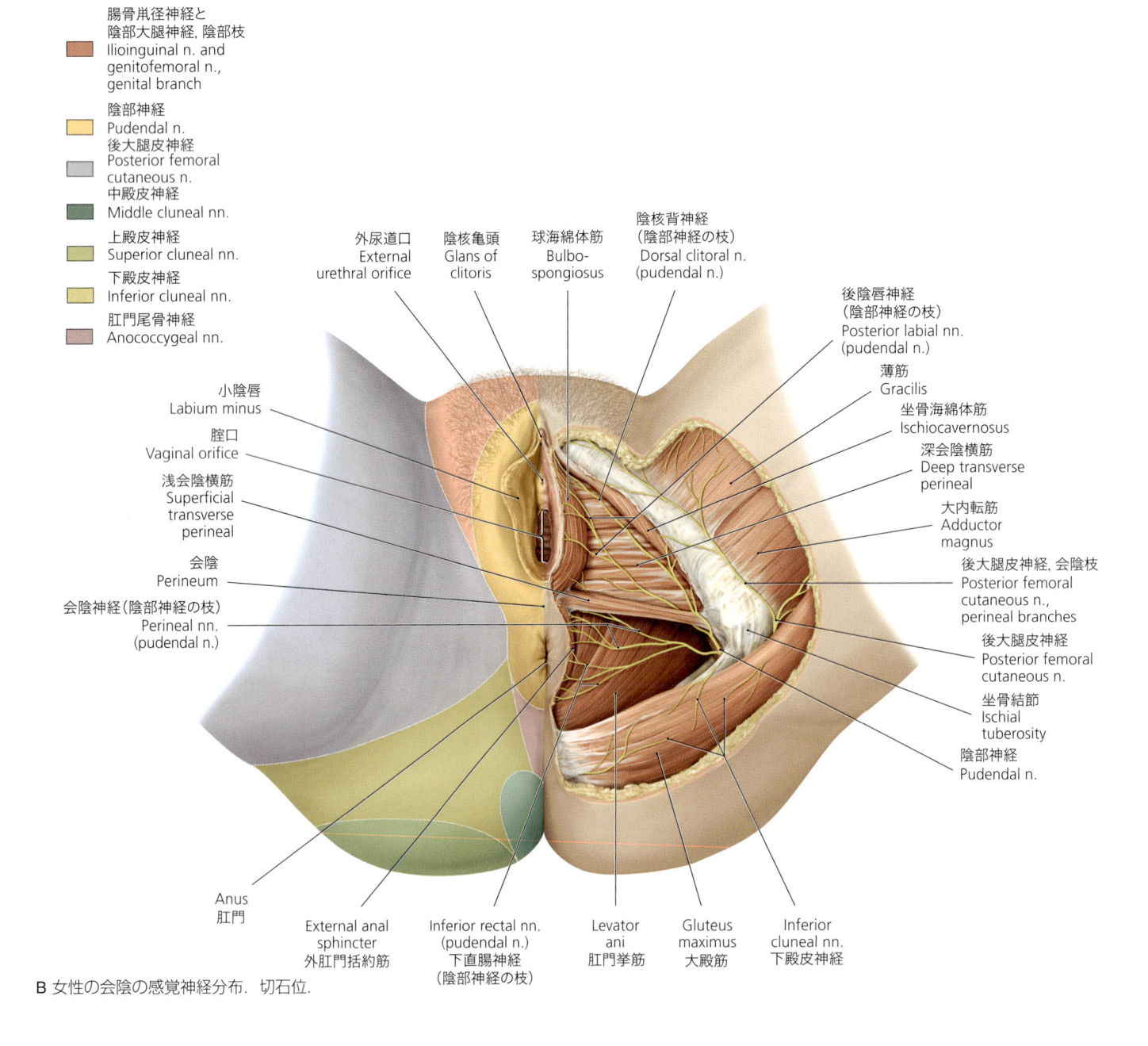

B　女性の会陰の感覚神経分布．切石位．

図 14.16 女性外生殖器の血管
下方から見たところ.

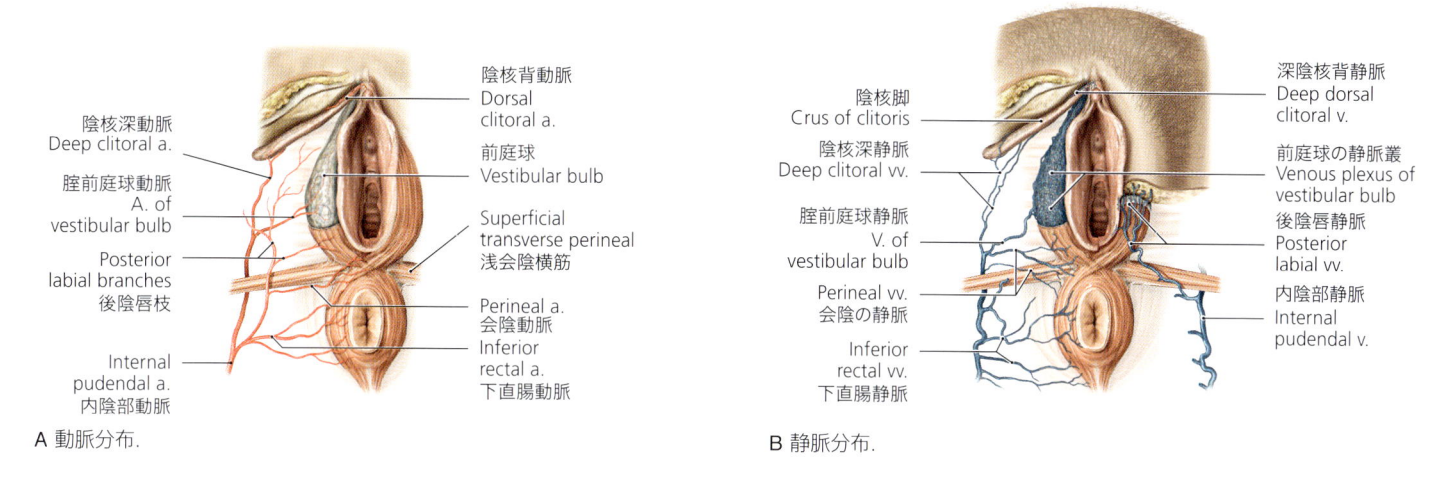

A 動脈分布.

- 陰核深動脈 Deep clitoral a.
- 腟前庭球動脈 A. of vestibular bulb
- Posterior labial branches 後陰唇枝
- Internal pudendal a. 内陰部動脈
- 陰核背動脈 Dorsal clitoral a.
- 前庭球 Vestibular bulb
- Superficial transverse perineal 浅会陰横筋
- Perineal a. 会陰動脈
- Inferior rectal a. 下直腸動脈

B 静脈分布.

- 陰核脚 Crus of clitoris
- 陰核深静脈 Deep clitoral vv.
- 腟前庭球静脈 V. of vestibular bulb
- Perineal vv. 会陰の静脈
- Inferior rectal vv. 下直腸静脈
- 深陰核背静脈 Deep dorsal clitoral v.
- 前庭球の静脈叢 Venous plexus of vestibular bulb
- 後陰唇静脈 Posterior labial vv.
- 内陰部静脈 Internal pudendal v.

図 14.17 女性会陰の神経・血管
切石位.

- 球海綿体筋 Bulbo-spongiosus
- 坐骨海綿体筋 Ischio-cavernosus
- 浅会陰横筋 Superficial transverse perineal
- 前庭球 Vestibular bulb
- 陰核背動脈・神経 Dorsal clitoral a. and n.
- 前陰唇神経 Anterior labial nn.
- 陰核深動脈 Deep clitoral a.
- 腟前庭球動脈 A. of vestibular bulb
- 後陰唇神経（陰部神経の枝） Posterior labial nn. (pudendal n.)
- 坐骨結節 Ischial tuberosity
- 下直腸動脈・静脈 Inferior rectal a. and v.
- 陰部神経 Pudendal n.
- 内陰部動脈・静脈 Internal pudendal a. and v.
- Deep transverse perineal 深会陰横筋
- Perineal nn. 会陰神経
- Inferior rectal nn. 下直腸神経
- Levator ani 肛門挙筋

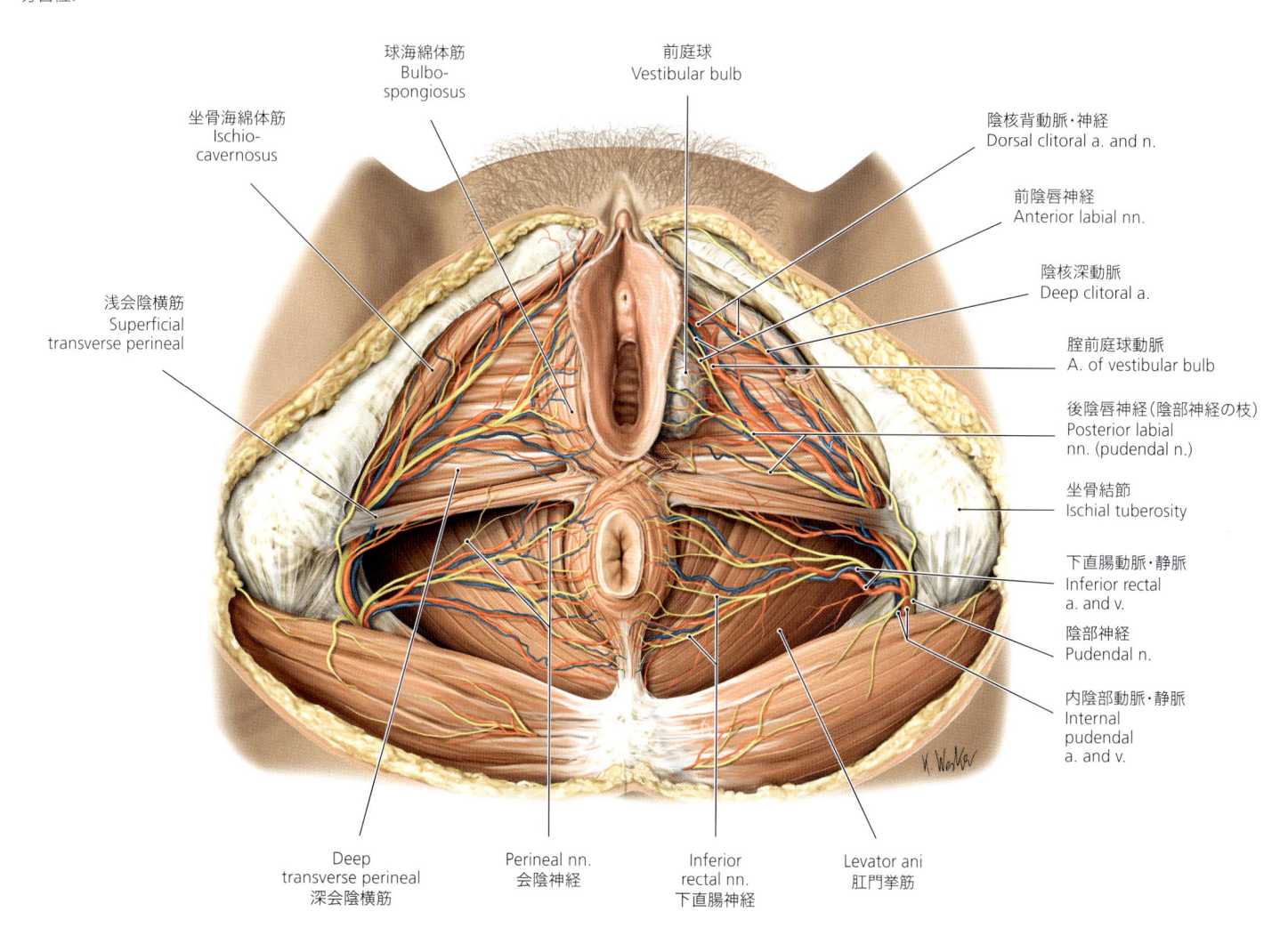

陰茎，陰嚢，精索
Penis, Scrotum & Spermatic Cord

図 14.18 陰茎，陰嚢，精索
前方から見たところ．陰嚢と精索の皮膚は取り除いてある．

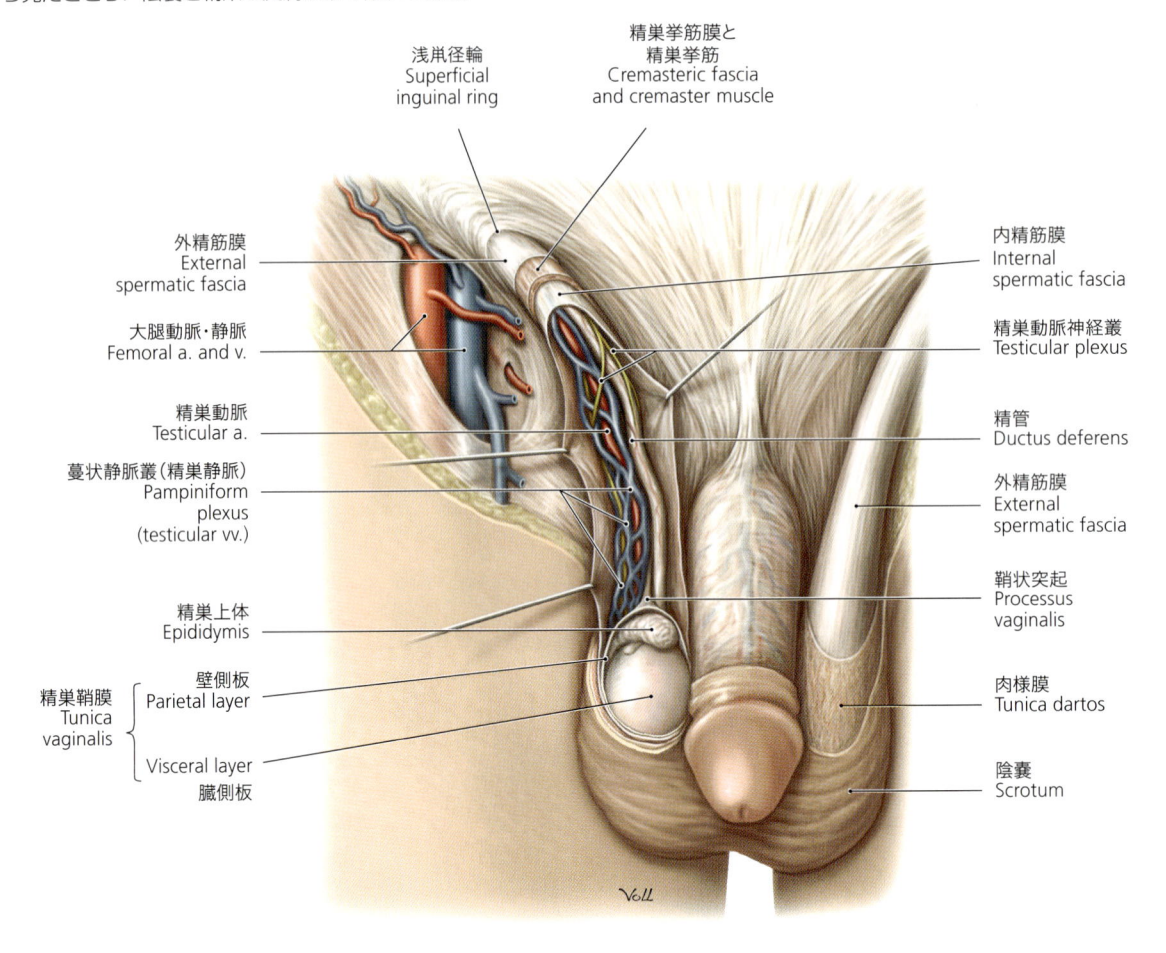

主な名称：
- 浅鼠径輪 Superficial inguinal ring
- 精巣挙筋膜と精巣挙筋 Cremasteric fascia and cremaster muscle
- 外精筋膜 External spermatic fascia
- 大腿動脈・静脈 Femoral a. and v.
- 精巣動脈 Testicular a.
- 蔓状静脈叢（精巣静脈）Pampiniform plexus (testicular vv.)
- 精巣上体 Epididymis
- 精巣鞘膜 Tunica vaginalis（壁側板 Parietal layer／臓側板 Visceral layer）
- 内精筋膜 Internal spermatic fascia
- 精巣動脈神経叢 Testicular plexus
- 精管 Ductus deferens
- 外精筋膜 External spermatic fascia
- 鞘状突起 Processus vaginalis
- 肉様膜 Tunica dartos
- 陰嚢 Scrotum

図 14.19 精索：内容
横断面．

主な名称：
- 精管動脈・静脈 A. and v. of ductus deferens
- 腸骨鼡経神経 Ilioinguinal n.
- 精管 Ductus deferens
- 陰部大腿神経，陰部枝 Genitofemoral n., genital branch
- 精巣動脈 Testicular a.
- 線維性間質 Fibrous stroma
- 精巣挙筋 Cremaster
- 精巣挙筋動脈・静脈 Cremasteric a. and v.
- 閉鎖した鞘状突起 Obliterated processus vaginalis
- 自律神経（精巣動脈神経叢）Autonomic nn. (testicular plexus)
- 精巣静脈（＝蔓状静脈叢）Testicular vv. (= pampiniform plexus)
- 外精筋膜 External spermatic fascia
- 精巣挙筋膜 Cremasteric fascia
- 内精筋膜 Internal spermatic fascia

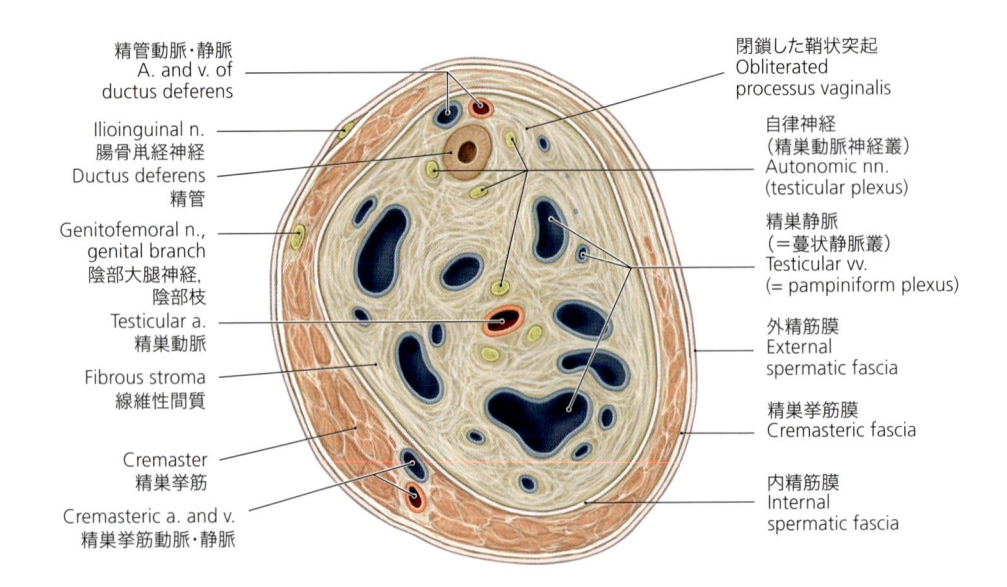

図 14.20　陰茎

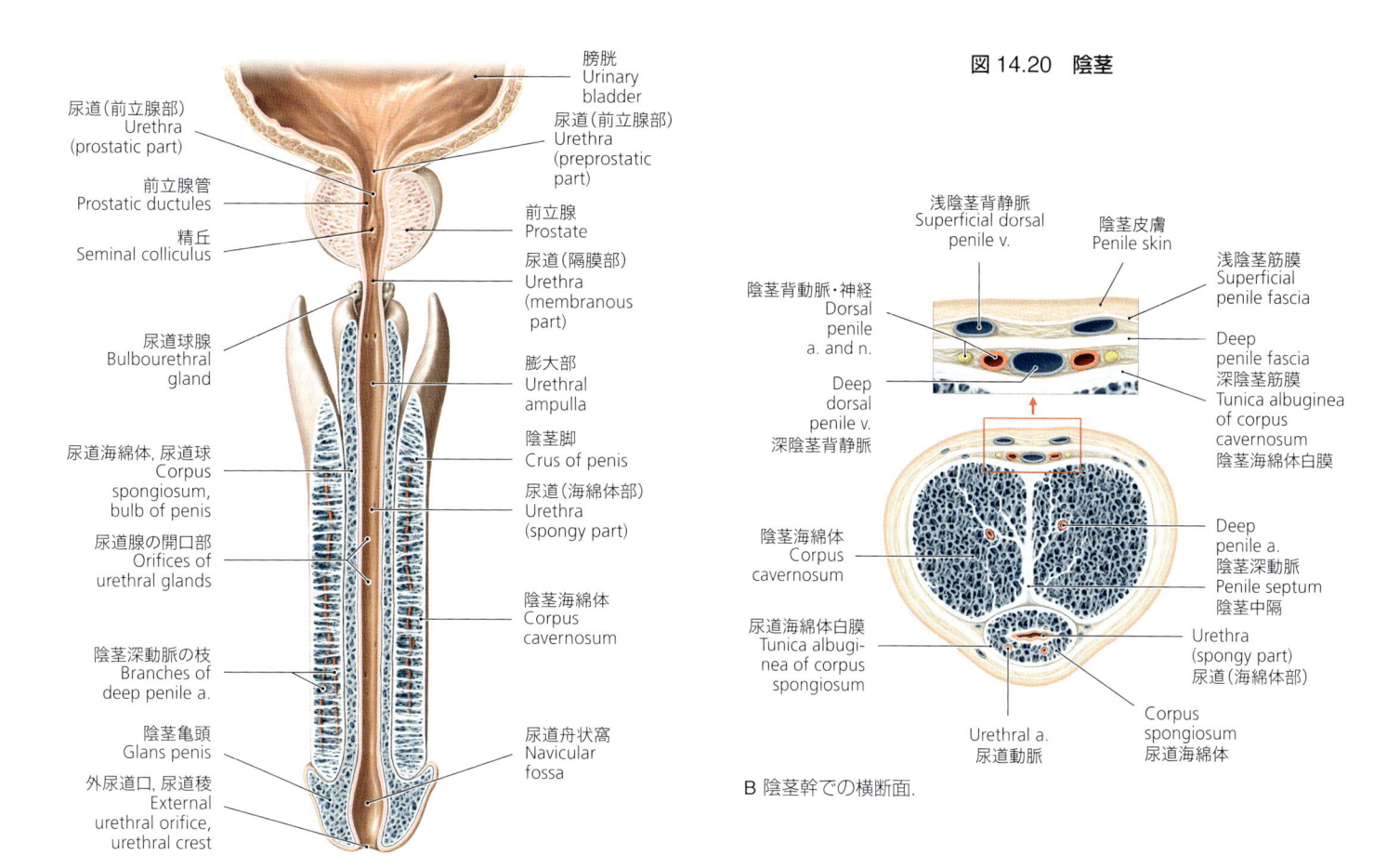

A 縦断面.

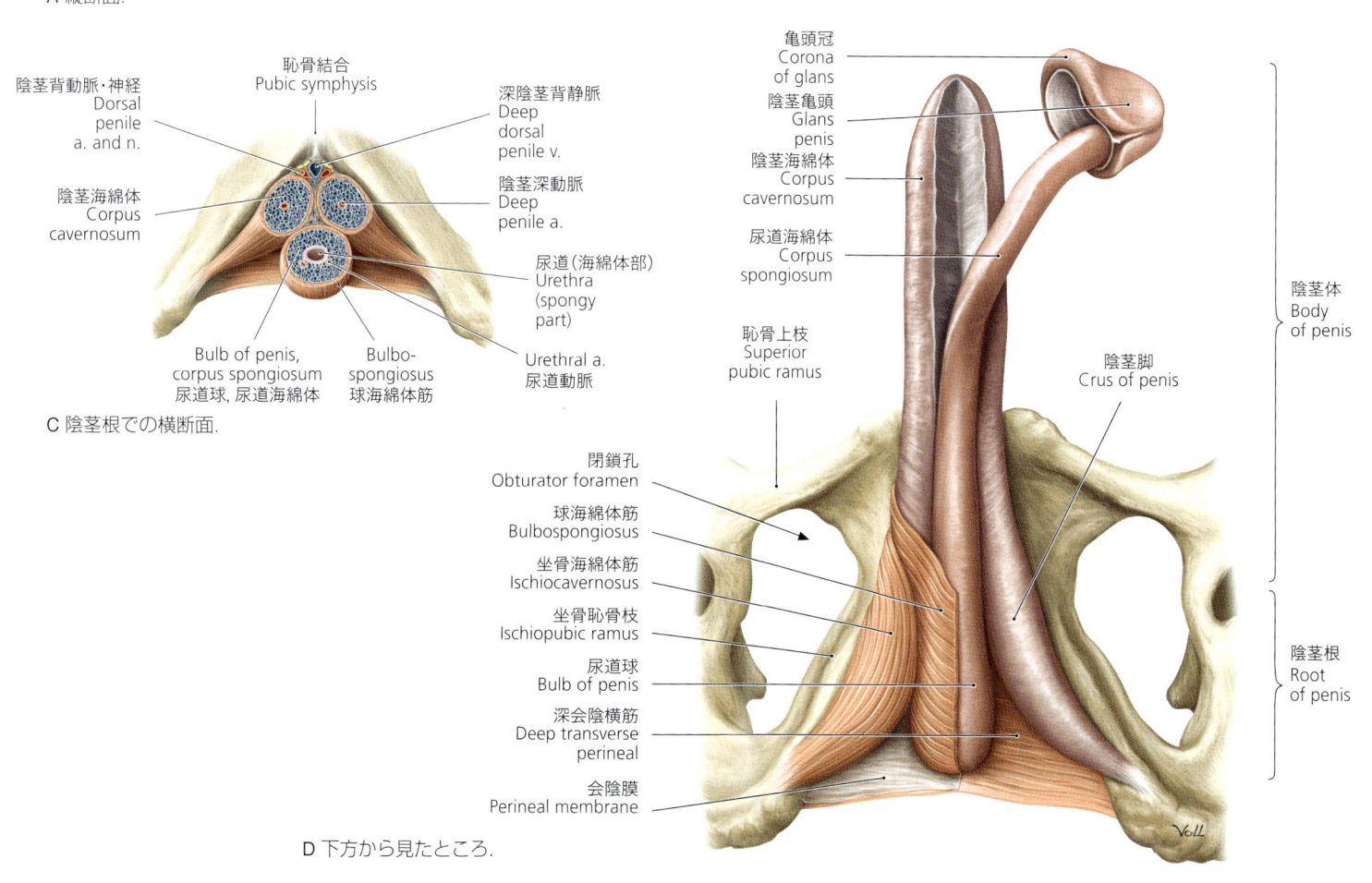

- 尿道（前立腺部）Urethra (prostatic part)
- 前立腺管 Prostatic ductules
- 精丘 Seminal colliculus
- 尿道球腺 Bulbourethral gland
- 尿道海綿体, 尿道球 Corpus spongiosum, bulb of penis
- 尿道腺の開口部 Orifices of urethral glands
- 陰茎深動脈の枝 Branches of deep penile a.
- 陰茎亀頭 Glans penis
- 外尿道口, 尿道稜 External urethral orifice, urethral crest
- 膀胱 Urinary bladder
- 尿道（前立腺部）Urethra (preprostatic part)
- 前立腺 Prostate
- 尿道（隔膜部）Urethra (membranous part)
- 膨大部 Urethral ampulla
- 陰茎脚 Crus of penis
- 尿道（海綿体部）Urethra (spongy part)
- 陰茎海綿体 Corpus cavernosum
- 尿道舟状窩 Navicular fossa

B 陰茎幹での横断面.

- 浅陰茎背静脈 Superficial dorsal penile v.
- 陰茎背動脈・神経 Dorsal penile a. and n.
- 深陰茎背静脈 Deep dorsal penile v.
- 陰茎海綿体 Corpus cavernosum
- 尿道海綿体白膜 Tunica albuginea of corpus spongiosum
- 尿道動脈 Urethral a.
- 陰茎皮膚 Penile skin
- 浅陰茎筋膜 Superficial penile fascia
- 深陰茎筋膜 Deep penile fascia
- 陰茎海綿体白膜 Tunica albuginea of corpus cavernosum
- 陰茎深動脈 Deep penile a.
- 陰茎中隔 Penile septum
- 尿道（海綿体部）Urethra (spongy part)
- 尿道海綿体 Corpus spongiosum

C 陰茎根での横断面.

- 陰茎背動脈・神経 Dorsal penile a. and n.
- 陰茎海綿体 Corpus cavernosum
- 恥骨結合 Pubic symphysis
- 深陰茎背静脈 Deep dorsal penile v.
- 陰茎深動脈 Deep penile a.
- 尿道（海綿体部）Urethra (spongy part)
- 尿道動脈 Urethral a.
- 尿道球, 尿道海綿体 Bulb of penis, corpus spongiosum
- 球海綿体筋 Bulbospongiosus

D 下方から見たところ.

- 亀頭冠 Corona of glans
- 陰茎亀頭 Glans penis
- 陰茎海綿体 Corpus cavernosum
- 尿道海綿体 Corpus spongiosum
- 恥骨上枝 Superior pubic ramus
- 閉鎖孔 Obturator foramen
- 球海綿体筋 Bulbospongiosus
- 坐骨海綿体筋 Ischiocavernosus
- 坐骨恥骨枝 Ischiopubic ramus
- 尿道球 Bulb of penis
- 深会陰横筋 Deep transverse perineal
- 会陰膜 Perineal membrane
- 陰茎脚 Crus of penis
- 陰茎体 Body of penis
- 陰茎根 Root of penis

生殖器

精巣と精巣上体
Testis & Epididymis

図 14.21 精巣と精巣上体
左外側方から見たところ．

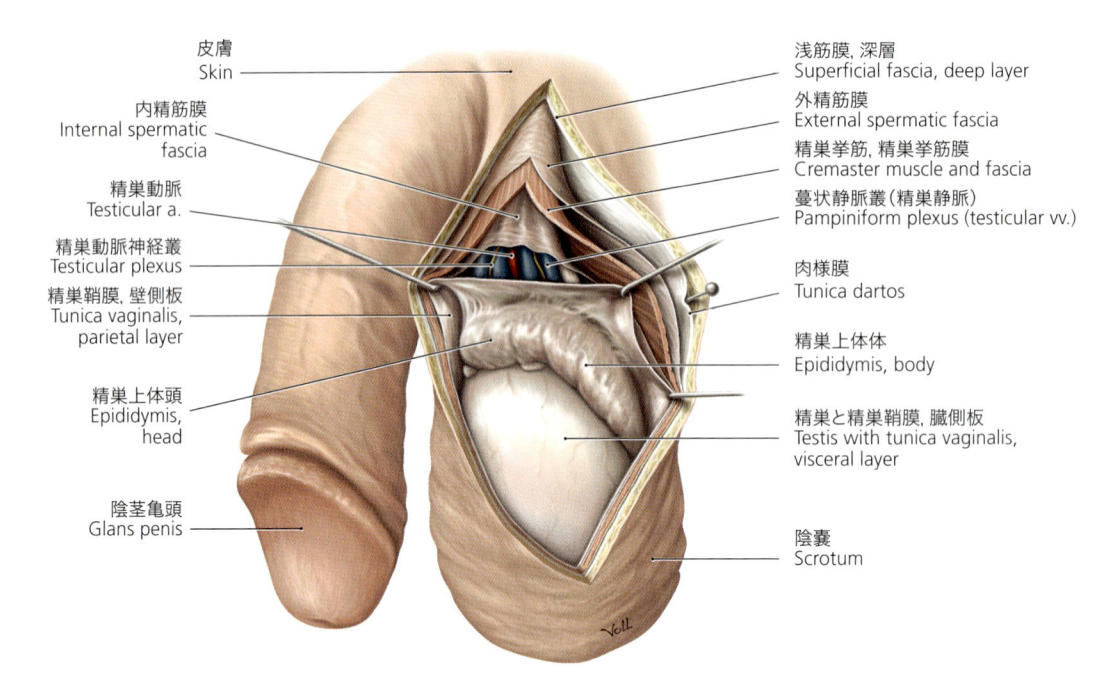

- 皮膚 Skin
- 内精筋膜 Internal spermatic fascia
- 精巣動脈 Testicular a.
- 精巣動脈神経叢 Testicular plexus
- 精巣鞘膜, 壁側板 Tunica vaginalis, parietal layer
- 精巣上体頭 Epididymis, head
- 陰茎亀頭 Glans penis
- 浅筋膜, 深層 Superficial fascia, deep layer
- 外精筋膜 External spermatic fascia
- 精巣挙筋, 精巣挙筋膜 Cremaster muscle and fascia
- 蔓状静脈叢（精巣静脈） Pampiniform plexus (testicular vv.)
- 肉様膜 Tunica dartos
- 精巣上体体 Epididymis, body
- 精巣と精巣鞘膜, 臓側板 Testis with tunica vaginalis, visceral layer
- 陰嚢 Scrotum

A 原位置の精巣と精巣上体．

- 精巣上体垂 Appendix epididymis
- 精巣垂 Appendix testis
- 精巣縦隔 Mediastinum testis
- 精巣上体頭 Epididymis (head)
- 精巣上体体 Epididymis (body)
- 精管 Ductus deferens
- 精巣上体尾 Epididymis (tail)

B 精巣と精巣上体の表面．

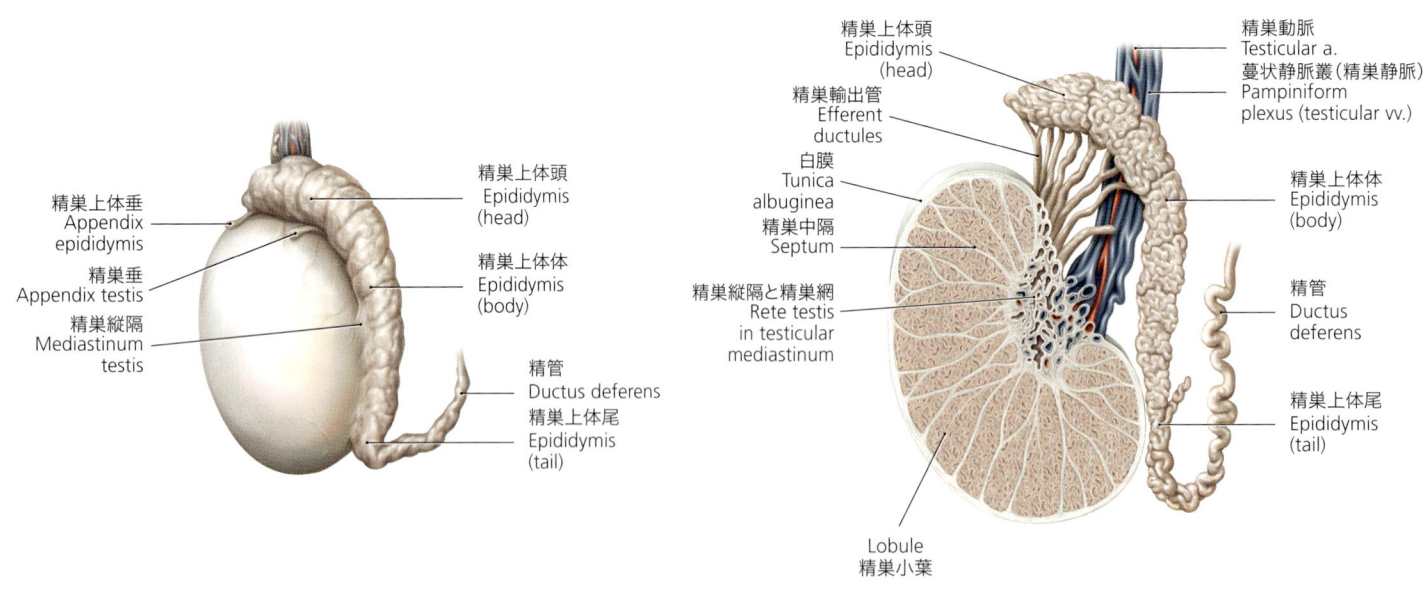

- 精巣上体頭 Epididymis (head)
- 精巣輸出管 Efferent ductules
- 白膜 Tunica albuginea
- 精巣中隔 Septum
- 精巣縦隔と精巣網 Rete testis in testicular mediastinum
- 精巣動脈 Testicular a.
- 蔓状静脈叢（精巣静脈） Pampiniform plexus (testicular vv.)
- 精巣上体体 Epididymis (body)
- 精管 Ductus deferens
- 精巣上体尾 Epididymis (tail)
- Lobule 精巣小葉

C 矢状断．

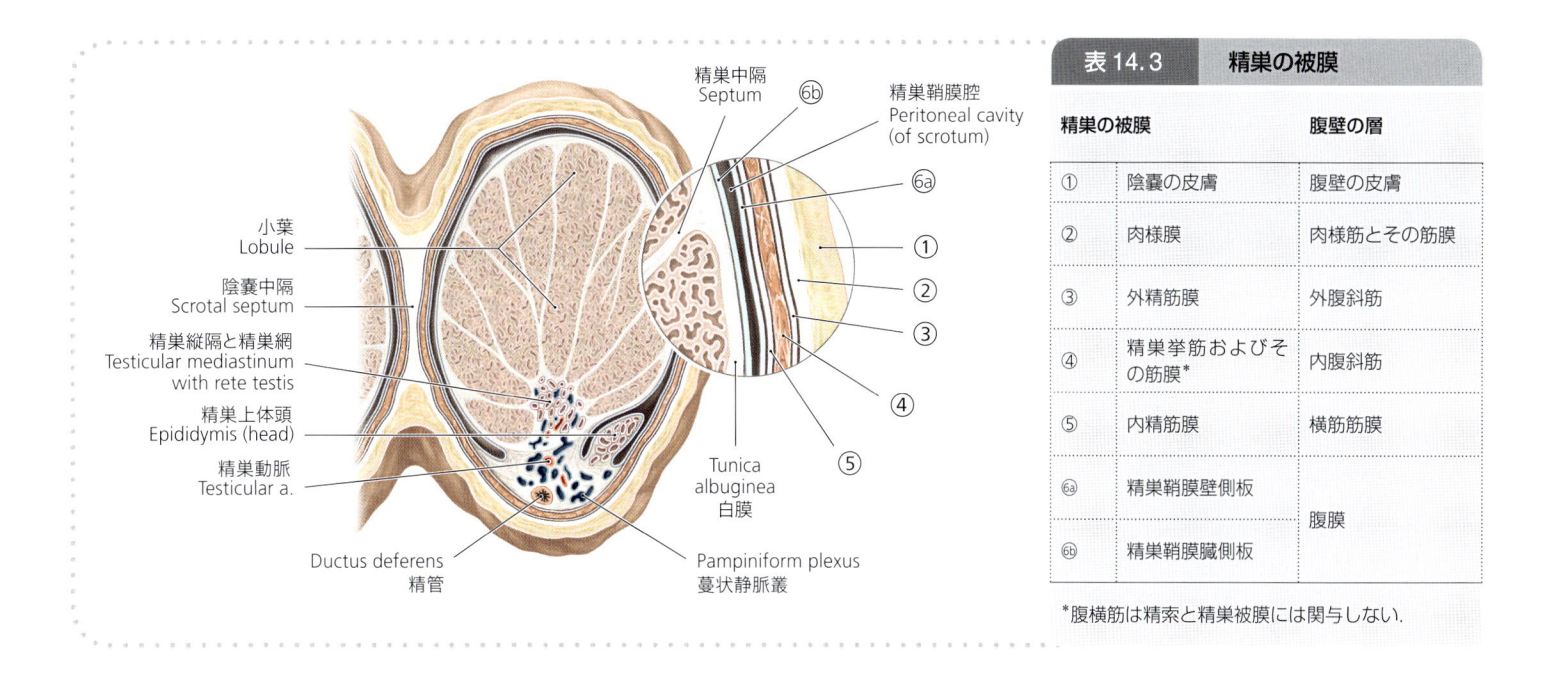

精巣中隔 Septum
精巣鞘膜腔 Peritoneal cavity (of scrotum)
小葉 Lobule
陰嚢中隔 Scrotal septum
精巣縦隔と精巣網 Testicular mediastinum with rete testis
精巣上体頭 Epididymis (head)
精巣動脈 Testicular a.
Ductus deferens 精管
Tunica albuginea 白膜
Pampiniform plexus 蔓状静脈叢

表 14.3 精巣の被膜

精巣の被膜		腹壁の層
①	陰嚢の皮膚	腹壁の皮膚
②	肉様膜	肉様筋とその筋膜
③	外精筋膜	外腹斜筋
④	精巣挙筋およびその筋膜*	内腹斜筋
⑤	内精筋膜	横筋筋膜
⑥a	精巣鞘膜壁側板	腹膜
⑥b	精巣鞘膜臓側板	

*腹横筋は精索と精巣被膜には関与しない.

図 14.22 精巣の血管
左外側方から見たところ.

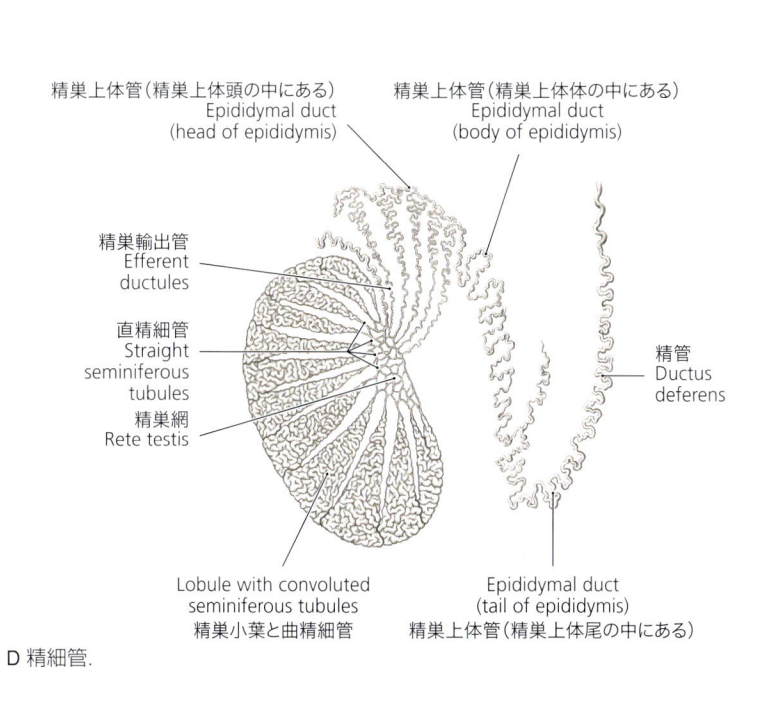

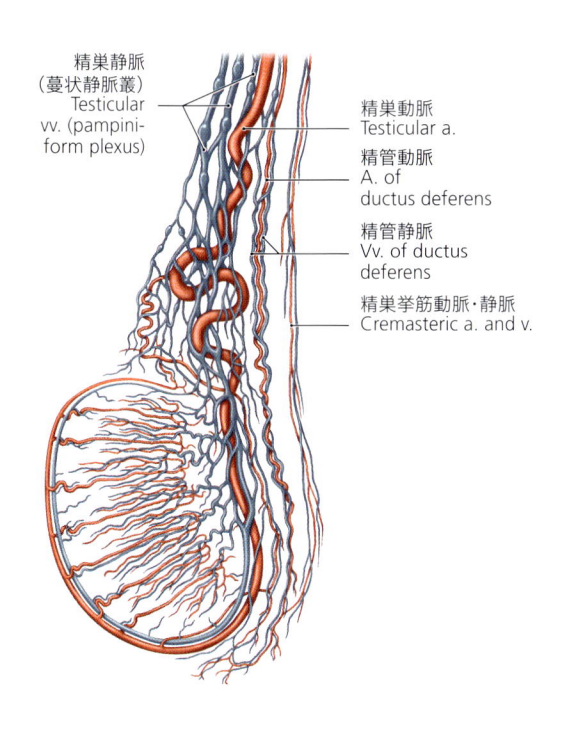

精巣静脈（蔓状静脈叢）Testicular vv. (pampiniform plexus)
精巣動脈 Testicular a.
精管動脈 A. of ductus deferens
精管静脈 Vv. of ductus deferens
精巣挙筋動脈・静脈 Cremasteric a. and v.

精巣上体管（精巣上体頭の中にある）Epididymal duct (head of epididymis)
精巣上体管（精巣上体体の中にある）Epididymal duct (body of epididymis)
精巣輸出管 Efferent ductules
直精細管 Straight seminiferous tubules
精巣網 Rete testis
精管 Ductus deferens
Lobule with convoluted seminiferous tubules 精巣小葉と曲精細管
Epididymal duct (tail of epididymis) 精巣上体管（精巣上体尾の中にある）

D 精細管.

男性の付属生殖腺
Male Accessory Sex Glands

図 14.23 付属生殖腺

① Urinary bladder 膀胱	⑤ Seminal vesicle 精嚢
② Ureter 尿管	⑥ Prostate 前立腺
③ Ductus deferens 精管	⑦ Bulbourethral gland
④ Urethra 尿道	尿道球腺

精管膨大部
Ampulla of ductus deferens

A 後方から見たところ．

射精管 Ejaculatory duct*
恥骨 Pubis
Corpus cavernosum 陰茎海綿体
Corpus spongiosum 尿道海綿体
Ischio-cavernosus 坐骨海綿体筋
中心領域 Central zone
辺縁領域 Peripheral zone
Prostatic capsule 前立腺被膜
尿道括約筋 Urethral sphincter

*精嚢の導管と精管は合流して射精管となる．

B MR 像．冠状断，前方から見たところ．

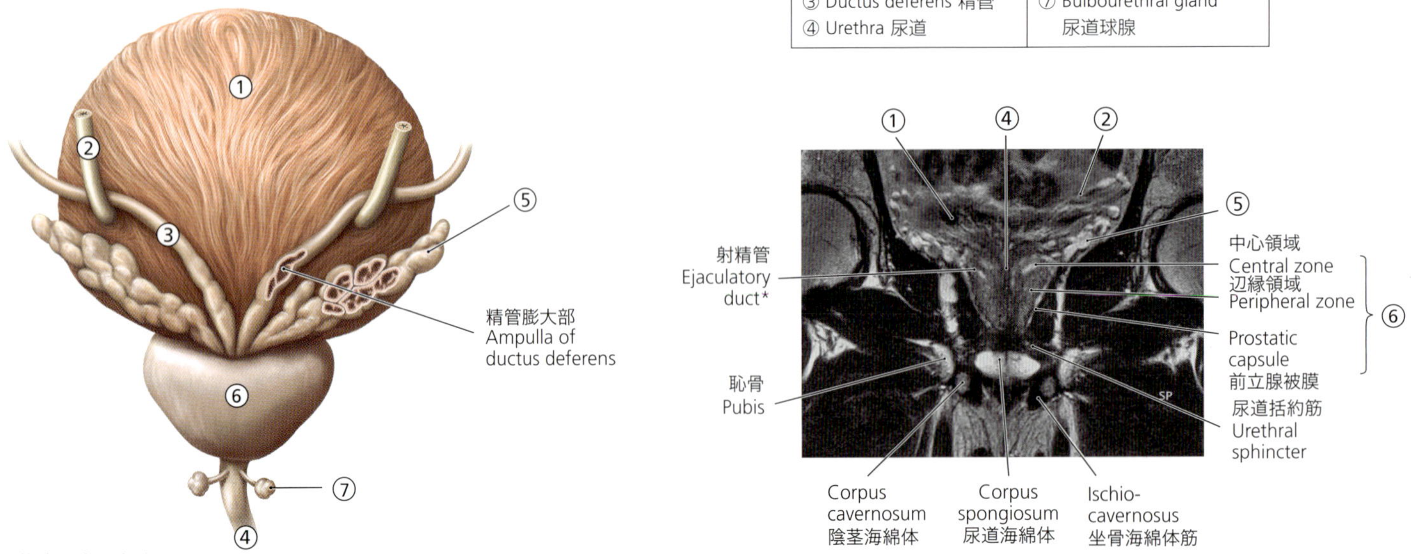

図 14.24 前立腺
前立腺の区分には解剖学的区分（上段）と臨床的区分（下段）がある．

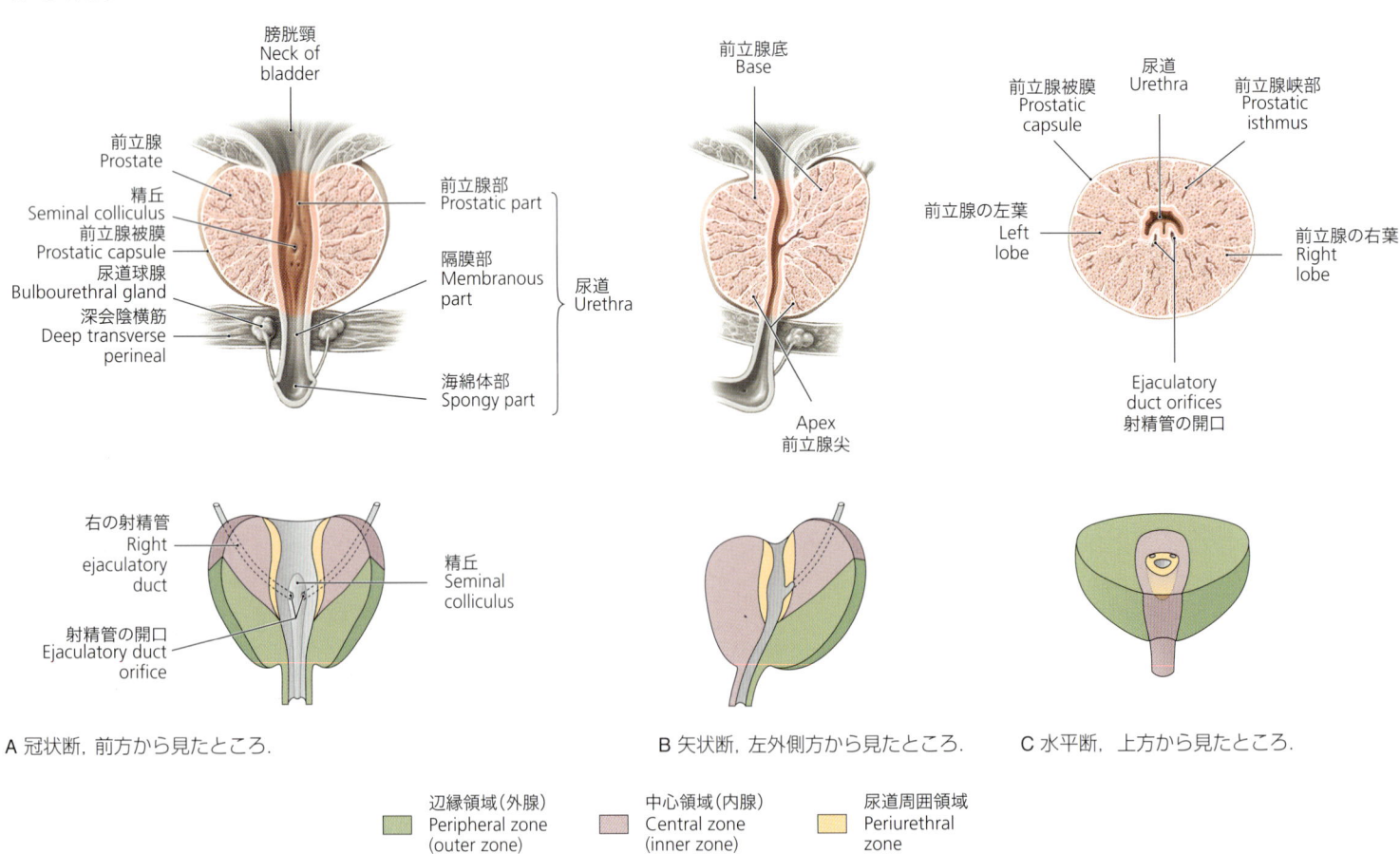

膀胱頸 Neck of bladder
前立腺 Prostate
精丘 Seminal colliculus
前立腺被膜 Prostatic capsule
尿道球腺 Bulbourethral gland
深会陰横筋 Deep transverse perineal
前立腺部 Prostatic part
隔膜部 Membranous part
海綿体部 Spongy part
尿道 Urethra

前立腺底 Base
前立腺尖 Apex

前立腺被膜 Prostatic capsule
前立腺の左葉 Left lobe
尿道 Urethra
前立腺峡部 Prostatic isthmus
前立腺の右葉 Right lobe
射精管の開口 Ejaculatory duct orifices

右の射精管 Right ejaculatory duct
射精管の開口 Ejaculatory duct orifice
精丘 Seminal colliculus

A 冠状断，前方から見たところ．
B 矢状断，左外側方から見たところ．
C 水平断，上方から見たところ．

辺縁領域（外腺）Peripheral zone (outer zone)
中心領域（内腺）Central zone (inner zone)
尿道周囲領域 Periurethral zone

図 14.25　原位置の前立腺
男性骨盤の矢状断．左外側方から見たところ．

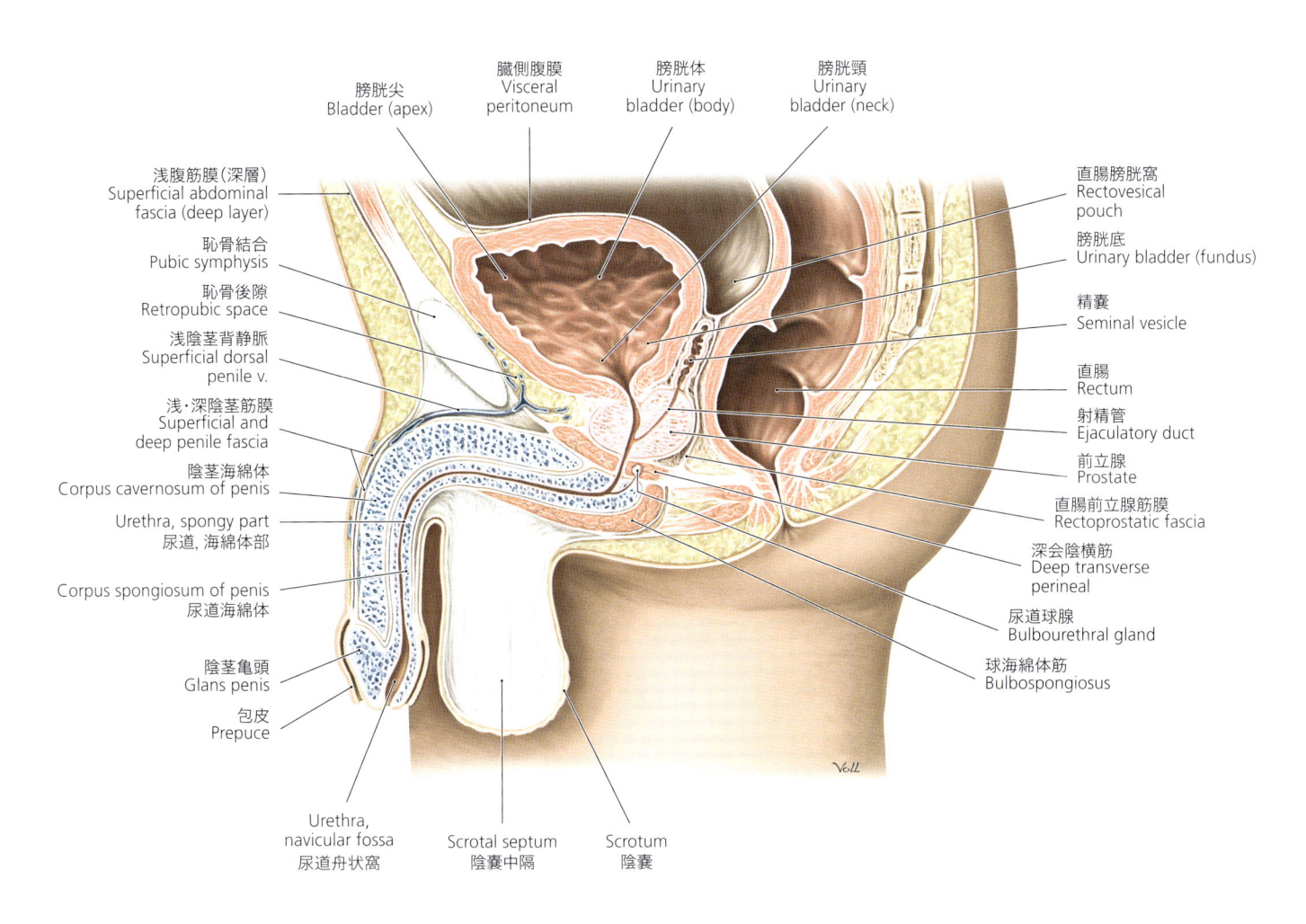

臨床

前立腺癌と前立腺肥大

前立腺癌は，高齢の男性において最もよくみられる悪性腫瘍の1つで，前立腺の辺縁領域の被膜下に増殖する．良性の前立腺肥大が中心領域で生じるのとは対照的に，前立腺癌は早期では尿路を閉塞しない．辺縁領域にある腫瘍は直腸内診では直腸の前壁を通して硬い塊として触知される．

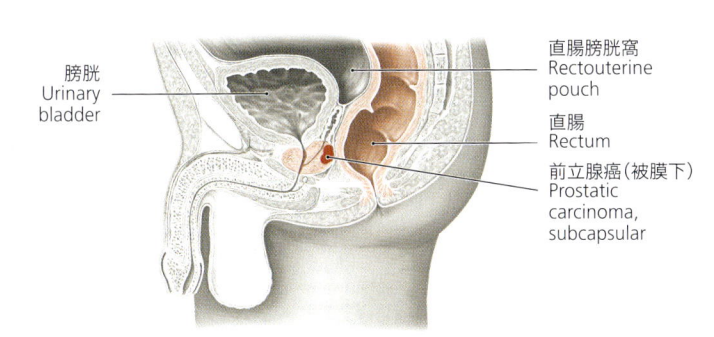

A　前立腺癌の頻発部位．

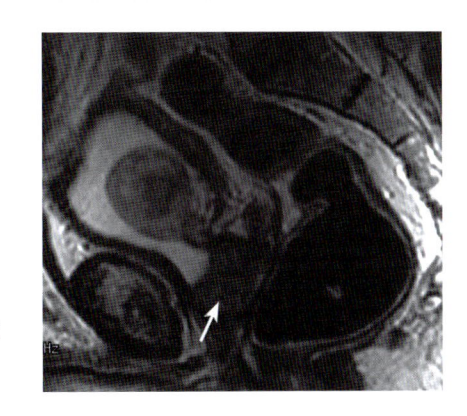

B　膀胱浸潤を伴う前立腺癌（矢印）．

前立腺疾患，特に前立腺癌では前立腺特異抗原 prostate-specific antigen（PSA）と呼ばれる蛋白質の量が増加する．この蛋白質は簡単な血液検査で測定できる．

男性生殖器の神経と血管
Neurovasculature of the Male Genitalia

図 14.26 男性生殖器の神経・血管
左外側方から見たところ.

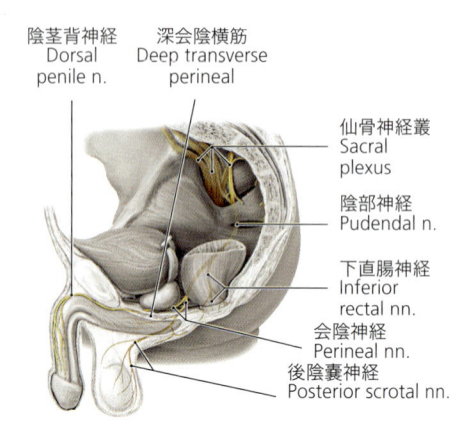

陰茎背神経 Dorsal penile n.
深会陰横筋 Deep transverse perineal
仙骨神経叢 Sacral plexus
陰部神経 Pudendal n.
下直腸神経 Inferior rectal nn.
会陰神経 Perineal nn.
後陰囊神経 Posterior scrotal nn.

A 神経分布.

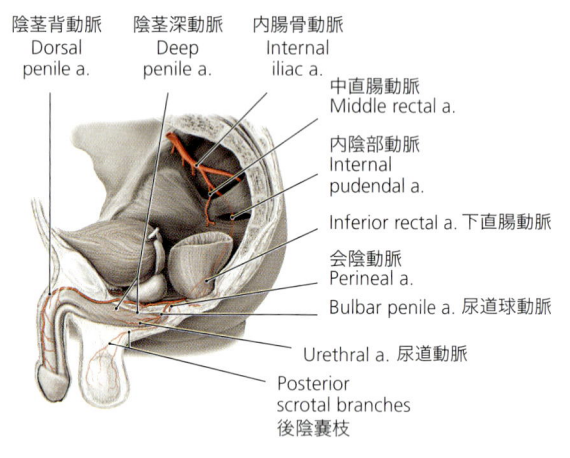

陰茎背動脈 Dorsal penile a.
陰茎深動脈 Deep penile a.
内腸骨動脈 Internal iliac a.
中直腸動脈 Middle rectal a.
内陰部動脈 Internal pudendal a.
Inferior rectal a. 下直腸動脈
会陰動脈 Perineal a.
Bulbar penile a. 尿道球動脈
Urethral a. 尿道動脈
Posterior scrotal branches 後陰囊枝

B 動脈分布.

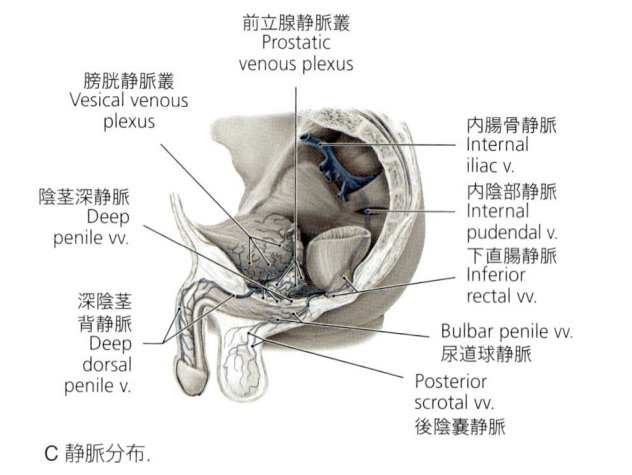

前立腺静脈叢 Prostatic venous plexus
膀胱静脈叢 Vesical venous plexus
内腸骨静脈 Internal iliac v.
内陰部静脈 Internal pudendal v.
下直腸静脈 Inferior rectal vv.
陰茎深静脈 Deep penile vv.
Bulbar penile vv. 尿道球静脈
深陰茎背静脈 Deep dorsal penile v.
Posterior scrotal vv. 後陰囊静脈

C 静脈分布.

図 14.27 陰茎と陰囊の神経・血管

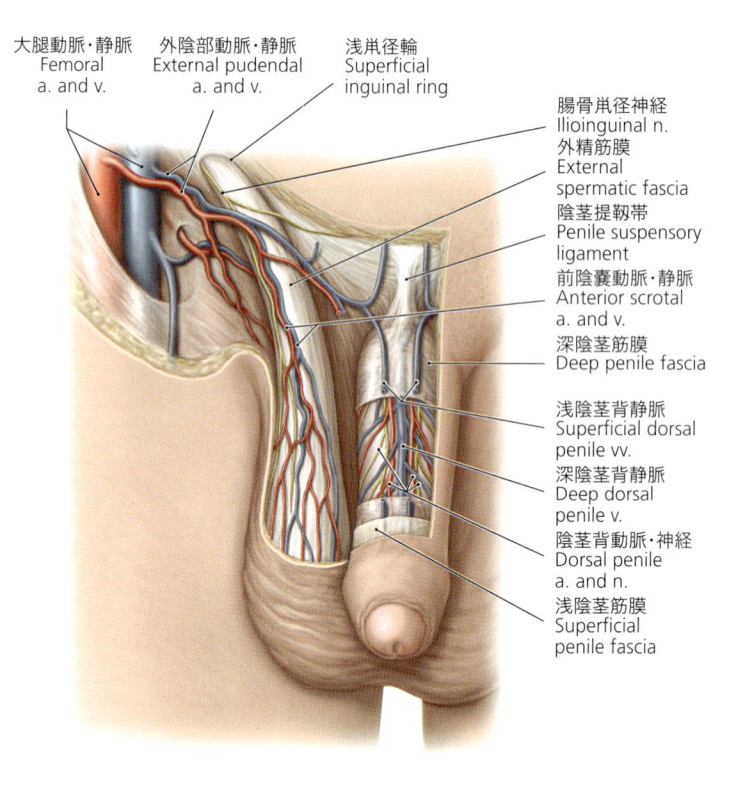

大腿動脈・静脈 Femoral a. and v.
外陰部動脈・静脈 External pudendal a. and v.
浅鼠径輪 Superficial inguinal ring
腸骨鼠径神経 Ilioinguinal n.
外精筋膜 External spermatic fascia
陰茎提靱帯 Penile suspensory ligament
前陰囊動脈・静脈 Anterior scrotal a. and v.
深陰茎筋膜 Deep penile fascia
浅陰茎背静脈 Superficial dorsal penile vv.
深陰茎背静脈 Deep dorsal penile v.
陰茎背動脈・神経 Dorsal penile a. and n.
浅陰茎筋膜 Superficial penile fascia

A 前方から見たところ. 皮膚と筋膜の一部は取り除いてある.

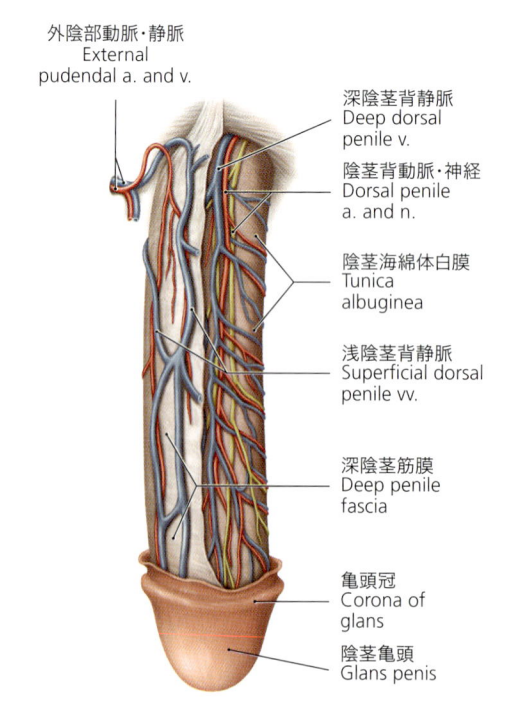

外陰部動脈・静脈 External pudendal a. and v.
深陰茎背静脈 Deep dorsal penile v.
陰茎背動脈・神経 Dorsal penile a. and n.
陰茎海綿体白膜 Tunica albuginea
浅陰茎背静脈 Superficial dorsal penile vv.
深陰茎筋膜 Deep penile fascia
亀頭冠 Corona of glans
陰茎亀頭 Glans penis

B 陰茎背側の血管.

図 14.28 男性の会陰と生殖器の神経
砕石位.

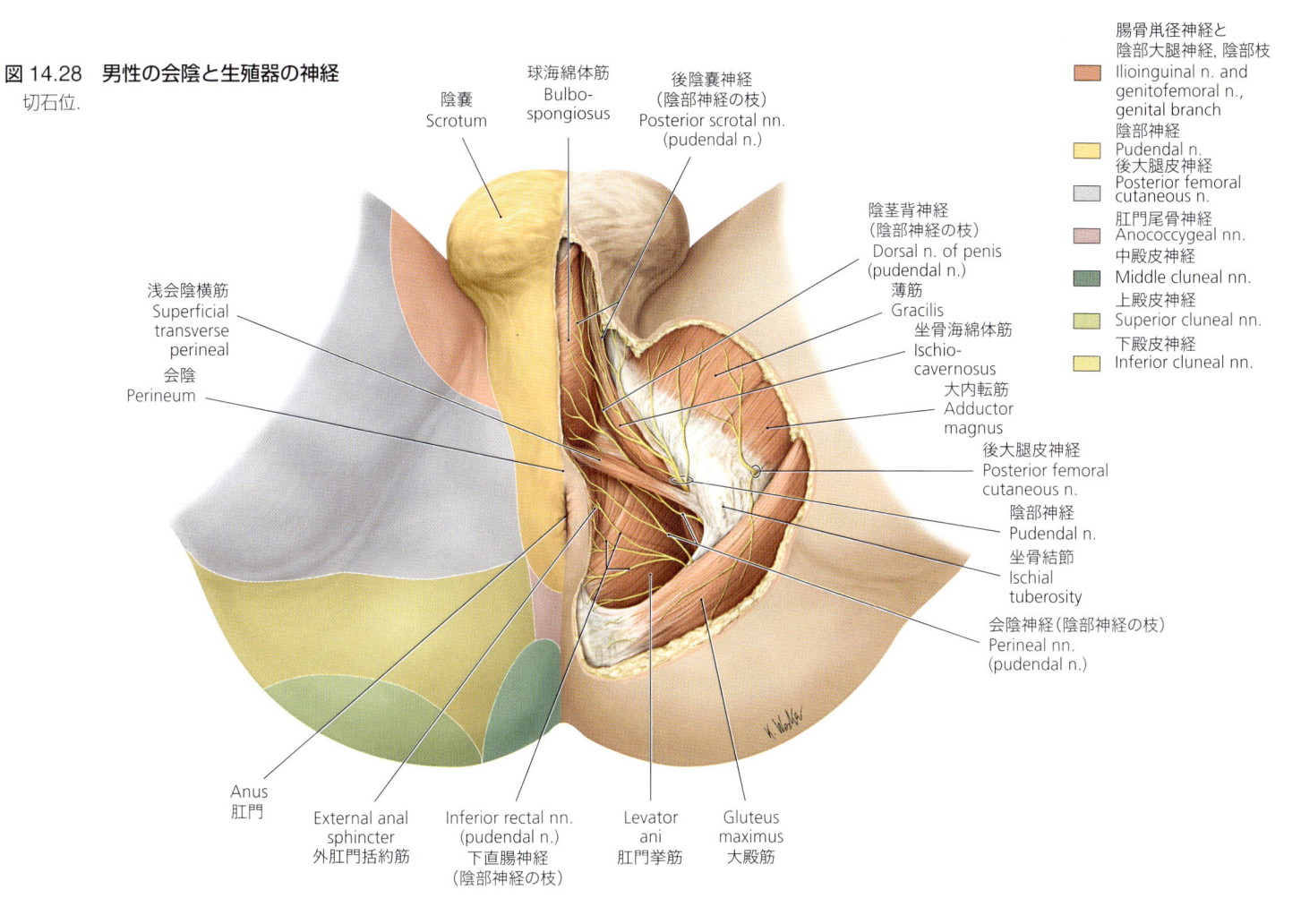

凡例:
- 腸骨鼠径神経と陰部大腿神経, 陰部枝 / Ilioinguinal n. and genitofemoral n., genital branch
- 陰部神経 / Pudendal n.
- 後大腿皮神経 / Posterior femoral cutaneous n.
- 肛門尾骨神経 / Anococcygeal nn.
- 中殿皮神経 / Middle cluneal nn.
- 上殿皮神経 / Superior cluneal nn.
- 下殿皮神経 / Inferior cluneal nn.

ラベル:
- 陰嚢 / Scrotum
- 球海綿体筋 / Bulbo-spongiosus
- 後陰嚢神経（陰部神経の枝）/ Posterior scrotal nn. (pudendal n.)
- 陰茎背神経（陰部神経の枝）/ Dorsal n. of penis (pudendal n.)
- 薄筋 / Gracilis
- 坐骨海綿体筋 / Ischio-cavernosus
- 大内転筋 / Adductor magnus
- 後大腿皮神経 / Posterior femoral cutaneous n.
- 陰部神経 / Pudendal n.
- 坐骨結節 / Ischial tuberosity
- 会陰神経（陰部神経の枝）/ Perineal nn. (pudendal n.)
- 浅会陰横筋 / Superficial transverse perineal
- 会陰 / Perineum
- 肛門 / Anus
- 外肛門括約筋 / External anal sphincter
- 下直腸神経（陰部神経の枝）/ Inferior rectal nn. (pudendal n.)
- 肛門挙筋 / Levator ani
- 大殿筋 / Gluteus maximus

図 14.29 男性の会陰と神経血管
砕石位.

ラベル:
- 陰茎海綿体 / Corpora cavernosa
- 深陰茎背静脈 / Deep dorsal penile v.
- 恥骨弓靱帯 / Arcuate pubic ligament
- 会陰横靱帯 / Transverse perineal ligament
- 陰茎背動脈 / Dorsal penile a.
- 陰茎背神経 / Dorsal penile n.
- 筋枝 / Muscular branches
- 尿道球腺 / Bulbourethral gland
- 坐骨結節 / Ischial tuberosity
- 内陰部動脈・静脈 / Internal pudendal a. and v.
- 陰部神経 / Pudendal n.
- 下直腸動脈・静脈 / Inferior rectal a. and v.
- 尿道海綿体 / Corpus spongiosum
- 精索 / Spermatic cord
- 球海綿体筋 / Bulbo-spongiosus
- 後陰嚢神経 / Posterior scrotal nn.
- 会陰神経 / Perineal nn.
- 肛門 / Anus
- 下直腸神経 / Inferior rectal nn.
- 外肛門括約筋 / External anal sphincter
- 大殿筋 / Gluteus maximus

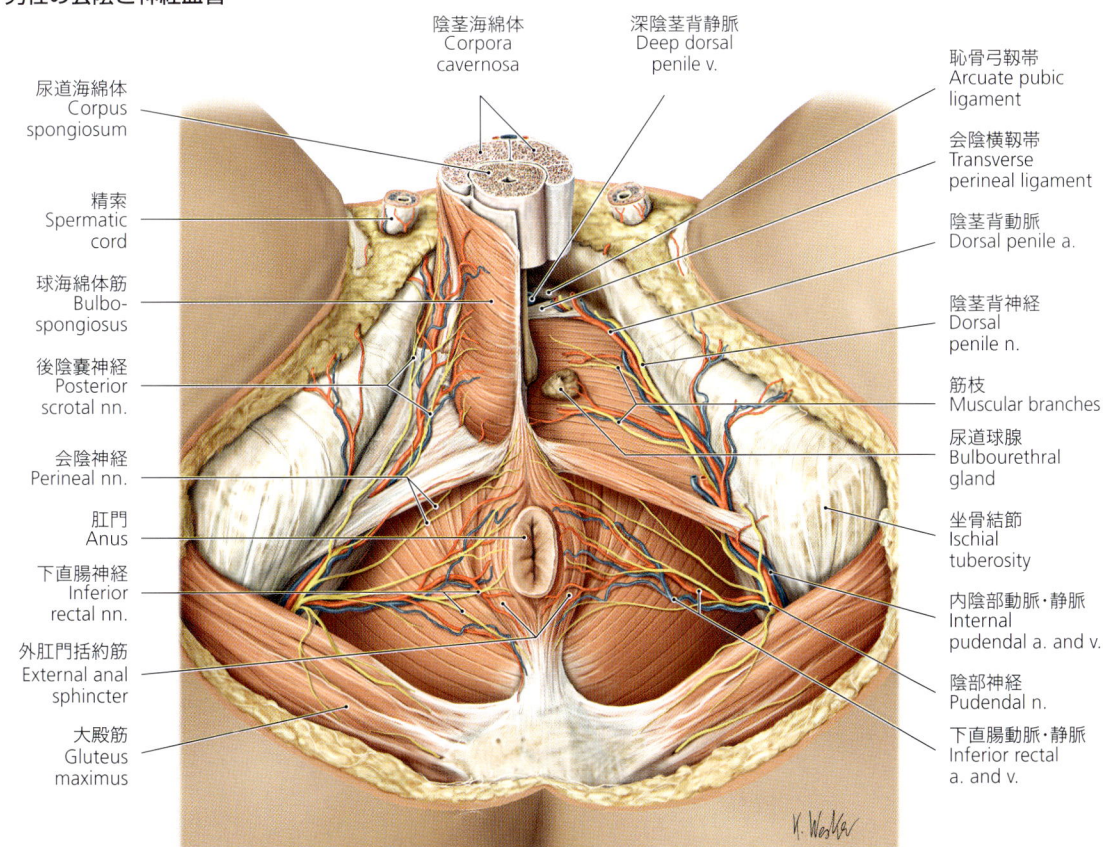

生殖器の発生
Development of the Genitalia

👉 生殖器は男性・女性ともに共通の性腺原基から発生する．

図 14.30　外生殖器の発生

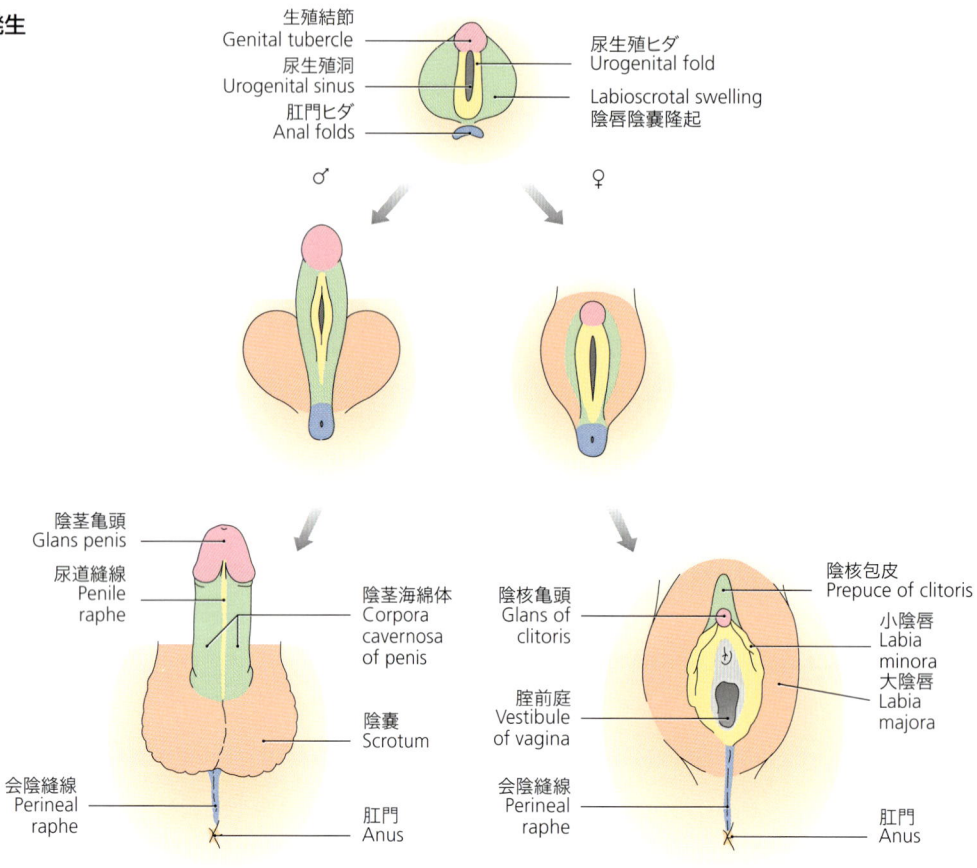

- 生殖結節 Genital tubercle
- 尿生殖ヒダ Urogenital fold
- 尿生殖洞 Urogenital sinus
- 陰唇陰嚢隆起 Labioscrotal swelling
- 肛門ヒダ Anal folds

♂
- 陰茎亀頭 Glans penis
- 尿道縫線 Penile raphe
- 陰茎海綿体 Corpora cavernosa of penis
- 陰嚢 Scrotum
- 会陰縫線 Perineal raphe
- 肛門 Anus

♀
- 陰核亀頭 Glans of clitoris
- 陰核包皮 Prepuce of clitoris
- 小陰唇 Labia minora
- 大陰唇 Labia majora
- 腟前庭 Vestibule of vagina
- 会陰縫線 Perineal raphe
- 肛門 Anus

図 14.31　精巣下行

左外側方から見たところ．

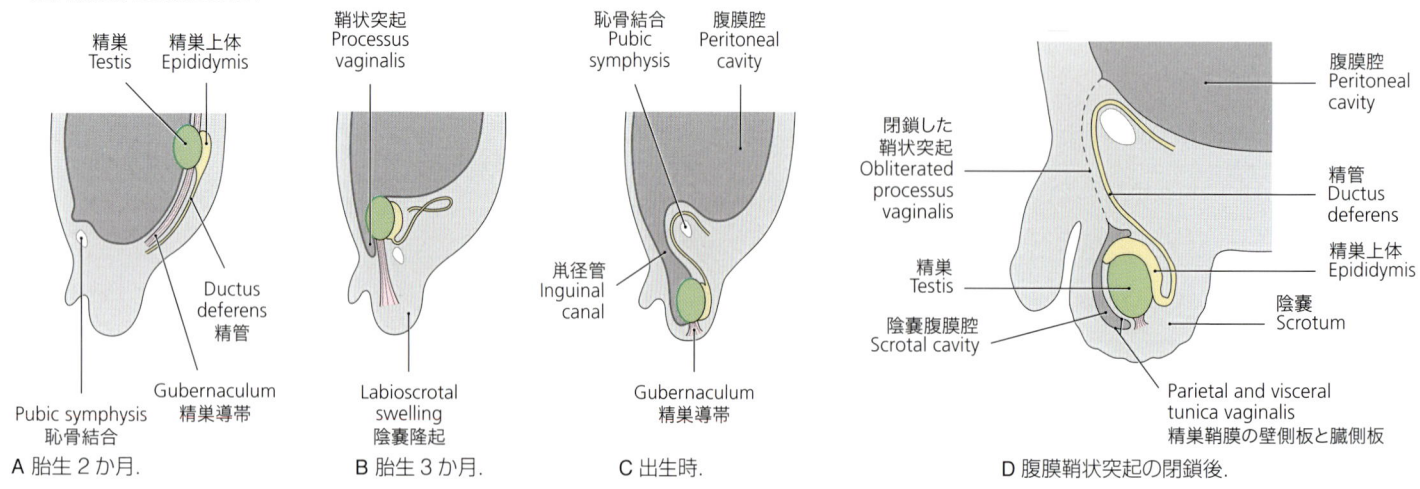

A　胎生2か月．
- 精巣 Testis
- 精巣上体 Epididymis
- 精管 Ductus deferens
- 精巣導帯 Gubernaculum
- 恥骨結合 Pubic symphysis

B　胎生3か月．
- 鞘状突起 Processus vaginalis
- 陰嚢隆起 Labioscrotal swelling

C　出生時．
- 恥骨結合 Pubic symphysis
- 腹膜腔 Peritoneal cavity
- 鼠径管 Inguinal canal
- 精巣導帯 Gubernaculum

D　腹膜鞘状突起の閉鎖後．
- 閉鎖した鞘状突起 Obliterated processus vaginalis
- 精管 Ductus deferens
- 精巣上体 Epididymis
- 陰嚢 Scrotum
- 精巣 Testis
- 陰嚢腹膜腔 Scrotal cavity
- 精巣鞘膜の壁側板と臓側板 Parietal and visceral tunica vaginalis
- 腹膜腔 Peritoneal cavity

図 14.32　内生殖器の発生
前方から見たところ．

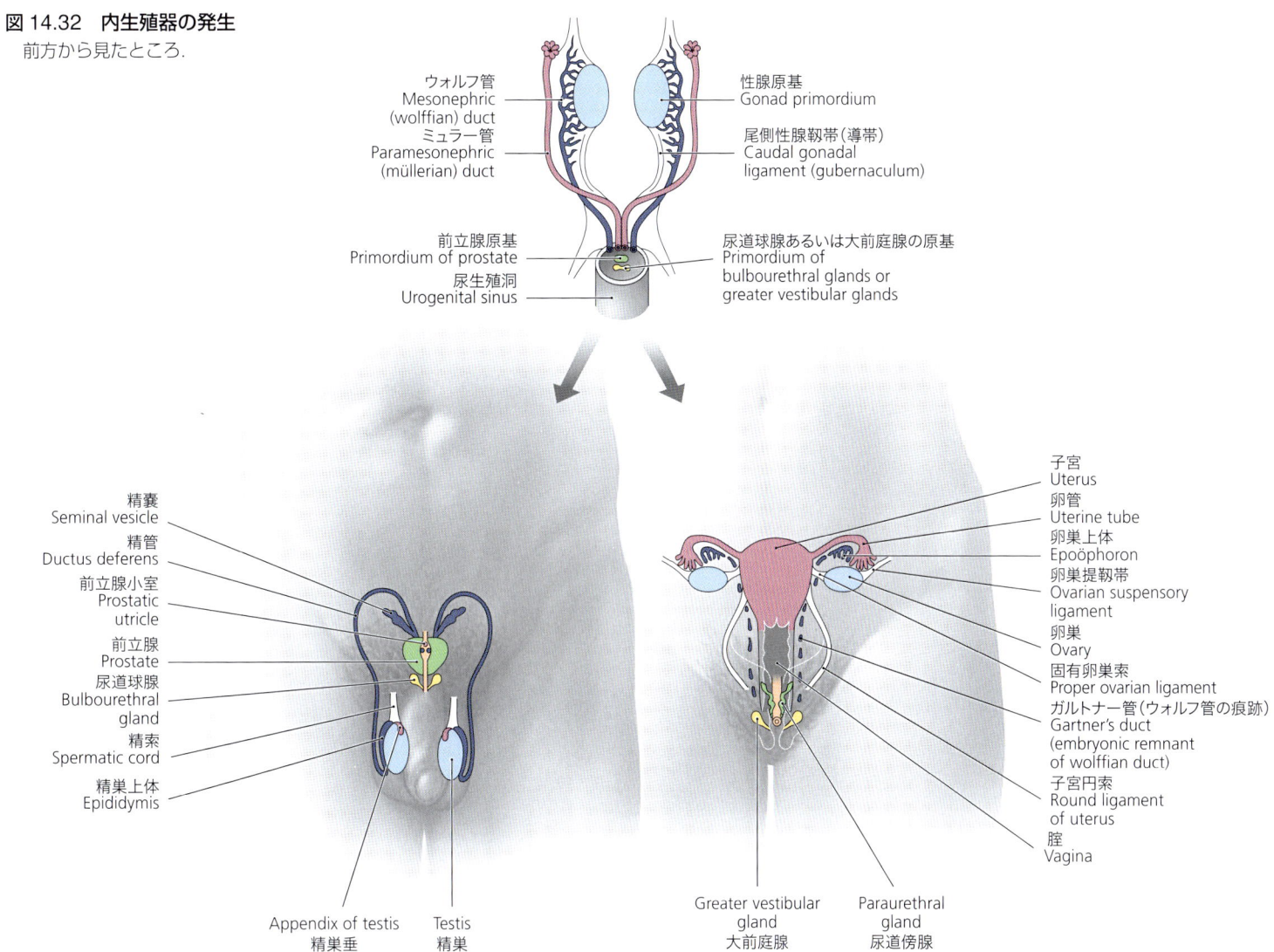

A　遺伝的男性胚子（精巣原基）．

B　遺伝的女性胚子（卵巣原基）．

表14.4	胚子の泌尿生殖構造からの派生物	

機能しない遺残物は斜体．両性に共通な構造は太字．

遺残物	男性での構造	女性での構造
未分化性腺	精巣	卵巣
皮質	精細管	卵胞
髄質	精巣網	卵巣支質
中腎細管	精巣輸出管，*精巣傍体*	*卵巣上体，卵巣傍体*
中腎管（ウォルフ管）	**尿管，腎盂，腎杯，集合管**	
	精巣上体管，精管，射精管，精嚢	―
中腎傍管（ミュラー管）	*精巣垂*	卵管，子宮，腟（上部），*モルガニー水胞体*
尿生殖洞	**膀胱，尿道**	
	前立腺，尿道球腺，*前立腺小室*	腟（下部），大・小前庭腺
生殖結節	陰茎海綿体	陰核，陰核亀頭
尿生殖ヒダ	陰茎亀頭，*陰茎縫線*	小陰唇，前庭球
陰唇陰嚢隆起	陰嚢	大陰唇
導帯	*精巣導帯*	固有卵巣索，子宮円索
性器結節（ミュラー結節）	*精丘*	*処女膜*

腹部の動脈
Arteries of the Abdomen

図 15.1　腹大動脈とその主枝
前方から見たところ．腹大動脈は第 12 胸椎の高さで横隔膜の大動脈裂孔(p.54 参照)を通って腹部に入る．第 4 腰椎の高さで 2 分岐して総腸骨動脈となる前に，腹大動脈は腎動脈(p.209 参照)と消化器系を栄養する 3 つの主枝を出す．

腹腔動脈：消化管の前部である前腸の構造に分布する．前腸は食道の遠位半，胃，十二指腸の近位半，肝臓，胆嚢，膵臓の上部からなる．

上腸間膜動脈：中腸の構造に分布する．中腸は十二指腸の遠位半，空腸，回腸，盲腸，虫垂，上行結腸，横行結腸，右結腸曲からなる．

下腸間膜動脈：後腸の構造に分布する．後腸は横行結腸の遠位 1/3，左結腸曲，下行結腸，S 状結腸，直腸，肛門管上部からなる．

上腸間膜動脈(第1腰椎)
Superior mesenteric a.
(L1)

下腸間膜動脈(第3腰椎)
Inferior mesenteric a.
(L3)

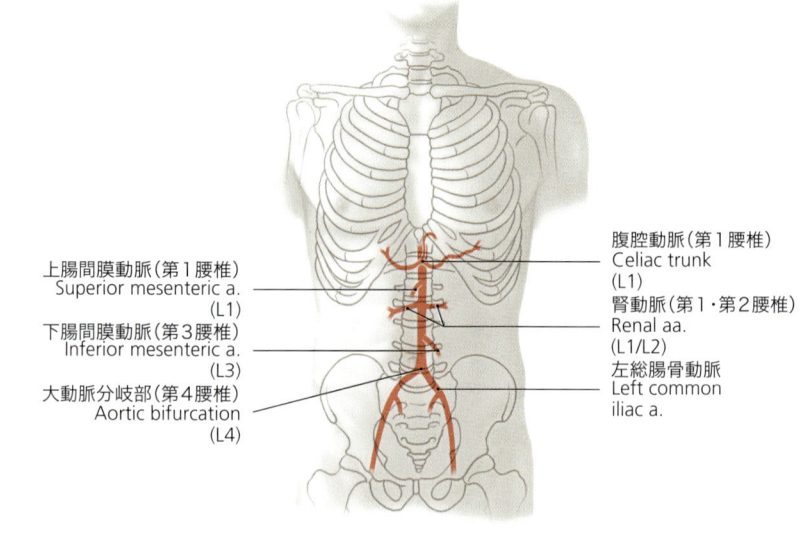

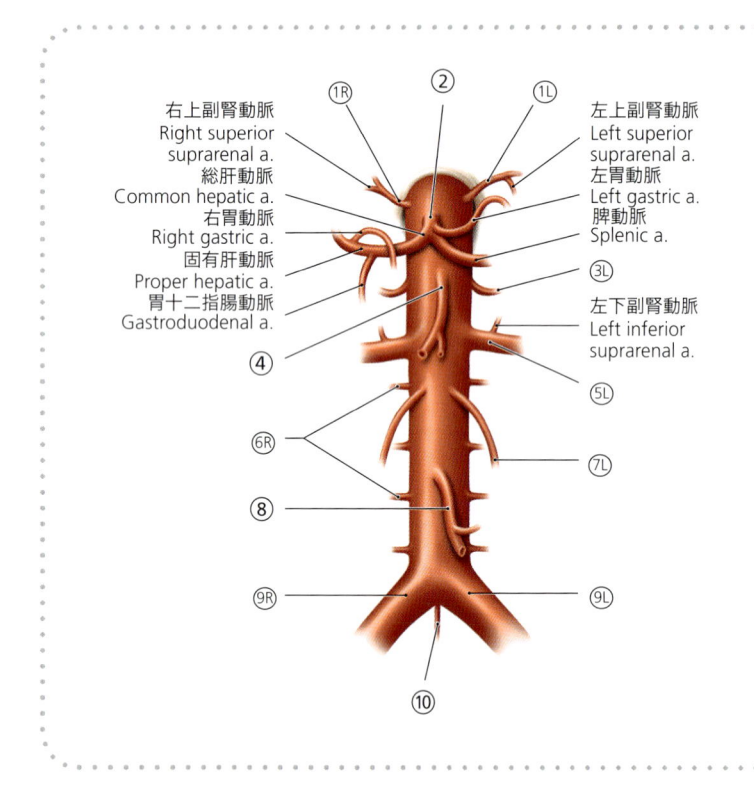

大動脈分岐部(第4腰椎)
Aortic bifurcation
(L4)

腹腔動脈(第1腰椎)
Celiac trunk
(L1)

腎動脈(第1・第2腰椎)
Renal aa.
(L1/L2)

左総腸骨動脈
Left common iliac a.

右上副腎動脈　Right superior suprarenal a.
総肝動脈　Common hepatic a.
右胃動脈　Right gastric a.
固有肝動脈　Proper hepatic a.
胃十二指腸動脈　Gastroduodenal a.

左上副腎動脈　Left superior suprarenal a.
左胃動脈　Left gastric a.
脾動脈　Splenic a.
左下副腎動脈　Left inferior suprarenal a.

表 15.1　腹大動脈の枝

腹大動脈は 3 つの不対の大きな動脈(太字)，不対の正中仙骨動脈，6 つの有対の動脈を出す．

大動脈からの枝		枝		
①R	①L	下横隔動脈(有対)	上副腎動脈	
②		**腹腔動脈**	左胃動脈	
			脾動脈	
			総肝動脈	固有肝動脈
				右胃動脈
				胃十二指腸動脈
③R	③L	中副腎動脈(有対)		
④		**上腸間膜動脈**		
⑤R	⑤L	腎動脈(有対)	下副腎動脈	
⑥R	⑥L	腰動脈(第1-4，有対)		
⑦R	⑦L	精巣・卵巣動脈(有対)		
⑧		**下腸間膜動脈**		
⑨R	⑨L	総腸骨動脈(有対)	外腸骨動脈	
			内腸骨動脈	
⑩		正中仙骨動脈		

図 15.2　腹腔動脈

A 位置，前方から見たところ．

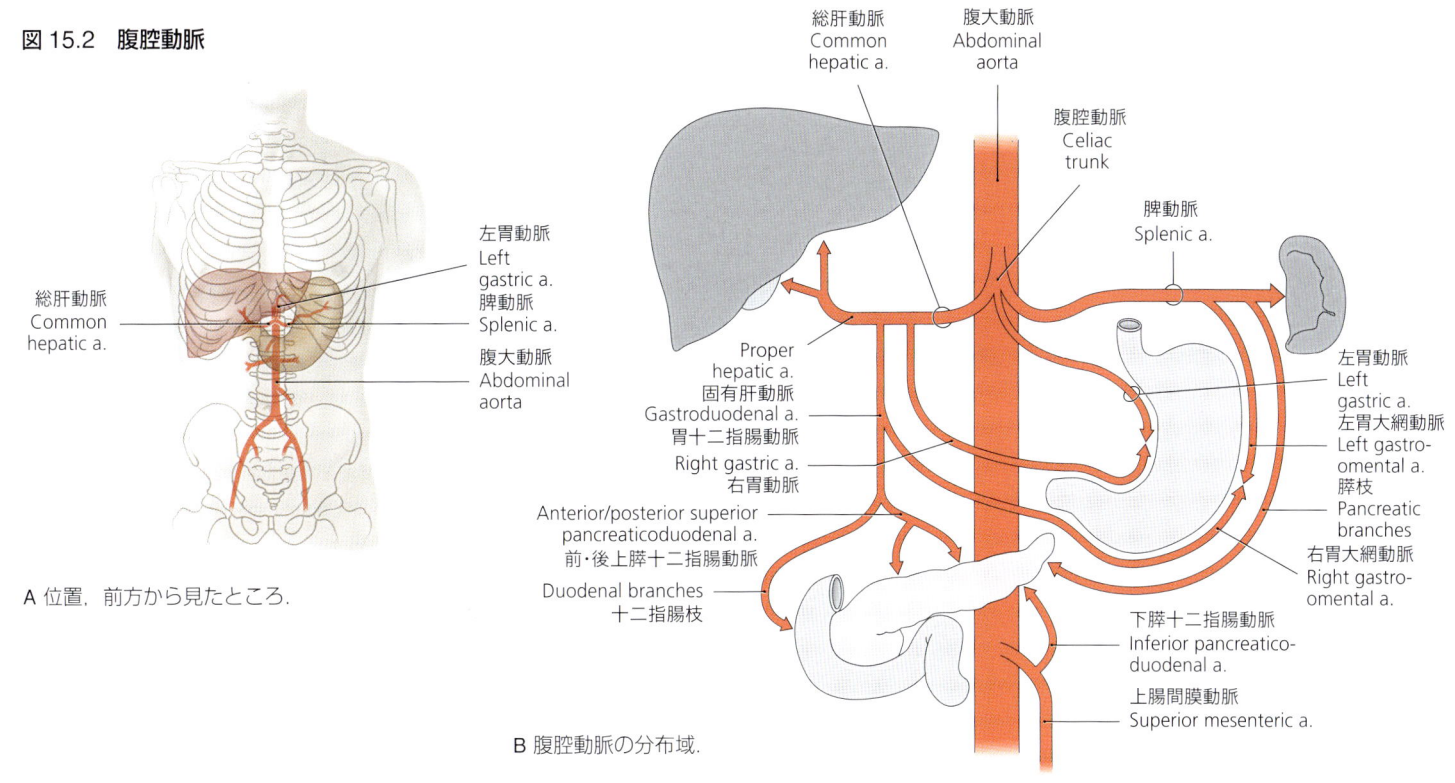

- 総肝動脈 Common hepatic a.
- 左胃動脈 Left gastric a.
- 脾動脈 Splenic a.
- 腹大動脈 Abdominal aorta

B 腹腔動脈の分布域．

- 総肝動脈 Common hepatic a.
- 腹大動脈 Abdominal aorta
- 腹腔動脈 Celiac trunk
- 脾動脈 Splenic a.
- 固有肝動脈 Proper hepatic a.
- 胃十二指腸動脈 Gastroduodenal a.
- 右胃動脈 Right gastric a.
- 前・後上膵十二指腸動脈 Anterior/posterior superior pancreaticoduodenal a.
- 十二指腸枝 Duodenal branches
- 左胃動脈 Left gastric a.
- 左胃大網動脈 Left gastro-omental a.
- 膵枝 Pancreatic branches
- 右胃大網動脈 Right gastro-omental a.
- 下膵十二指腸動脈 Inferior pancreaticoduodenal a.
- 上腸間膜動脈 Superior mesenteric a.

図 15.3　上腸間膜動脈
前方から見たところ．

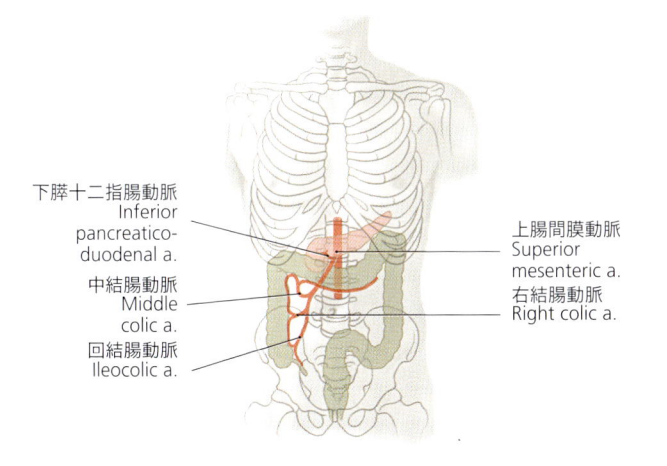

- 下膵十二指腸動脈 Inferior pancreaticoduodenal a.
- 中結腸動脈 Middle colic a.
- 回結腸動脈 Ileocolic a.
- 上腸間膜動脈 Superior mesenteric a.
- 右結腸動脈 Right colic a.

図 15.4　下腸間膜動脈
前方から見たところ．

- 下腸間膜動脈 Inferior mesenteric a.
- 上直腸動脈 Superior rectal a.
- S状結腸動脈 Sigmoid aa.
- 左結腸動脈 Left colic a.

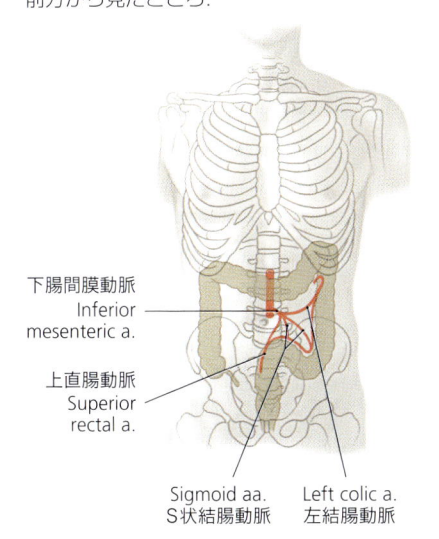

図 15.5　腹部の動脈間吻合
腹部の3つの主枝の吻合は正常な血液供給が失われた腸領域に血液を運ぶ．

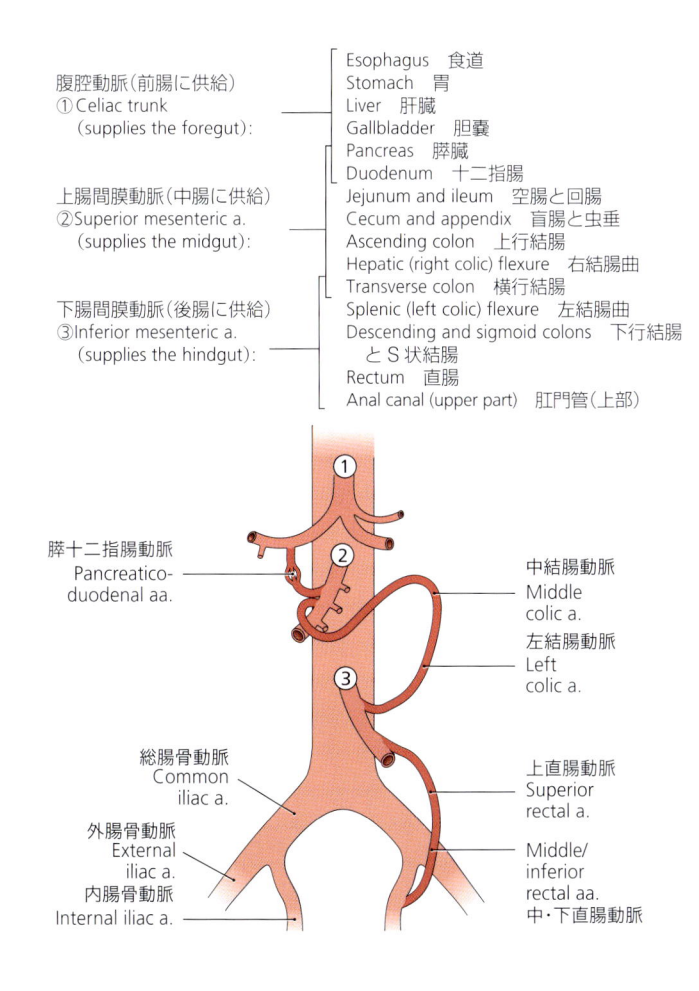

腹腔動脈（前腸に供給）
①Celiac trunk（supplies the foregut）:
- Esophagus 食道
- Stomach 胃
- Liver 肝臓
- Gallbladder 胆嚢
- Pancreas 膵臓
- Duodenum 十二指腸

上腸間膜動脈（中腸に供給）
②Superior mesenteric a.（supplies the midgut）:
- Jejunum and ileum 空腸と回腸
- Cecum and appendix 盲腸と虫垂
- Ascending colon 上行結腸
- Hepatic (right colic) flexure 右結腸曲
- Transverse colon 横行結腸

下腸間膜動脈（後腸に供給）
③Inferior mesenteric a.（supplies the hindgut）:
- Splenic (left colic) flexure 左結腸曲
- Descending and sigmoid colons 下行結腸とS状結腸
- Rectum 直腸
- Anal canal (upper part) 肛門管（上部）

- 膵十二指腸動脈 Pancreaticoduodenal aa.
- 総腸骨動脈 Common iliac a.
- 外腸骨動脈 External iliac a.
- 内腸骨動脈 Internal iliac a.
- 中結腸動脈 Middle colic a.
- 左結腸動脈 Left colic a.
- 上直腸動脈 Superior rectal a.
- 中・下直腸動脈 Middle/inferior rectal aa.

腹大動脈と腎動脈
Abdominal Aorta & Renal Arteries

図15.6 腹大動脈
女性の大動脈．前方から見たところ．腹部内臓と腹膜は取り除いてある．腹大動脈は胸大動脈（p.68参照）の遠位方向への延長である．腹大動脈は第12胸椎の高さで腹部に入り，第4腰椎の高さで2分岐して総腸骨動脈となる．

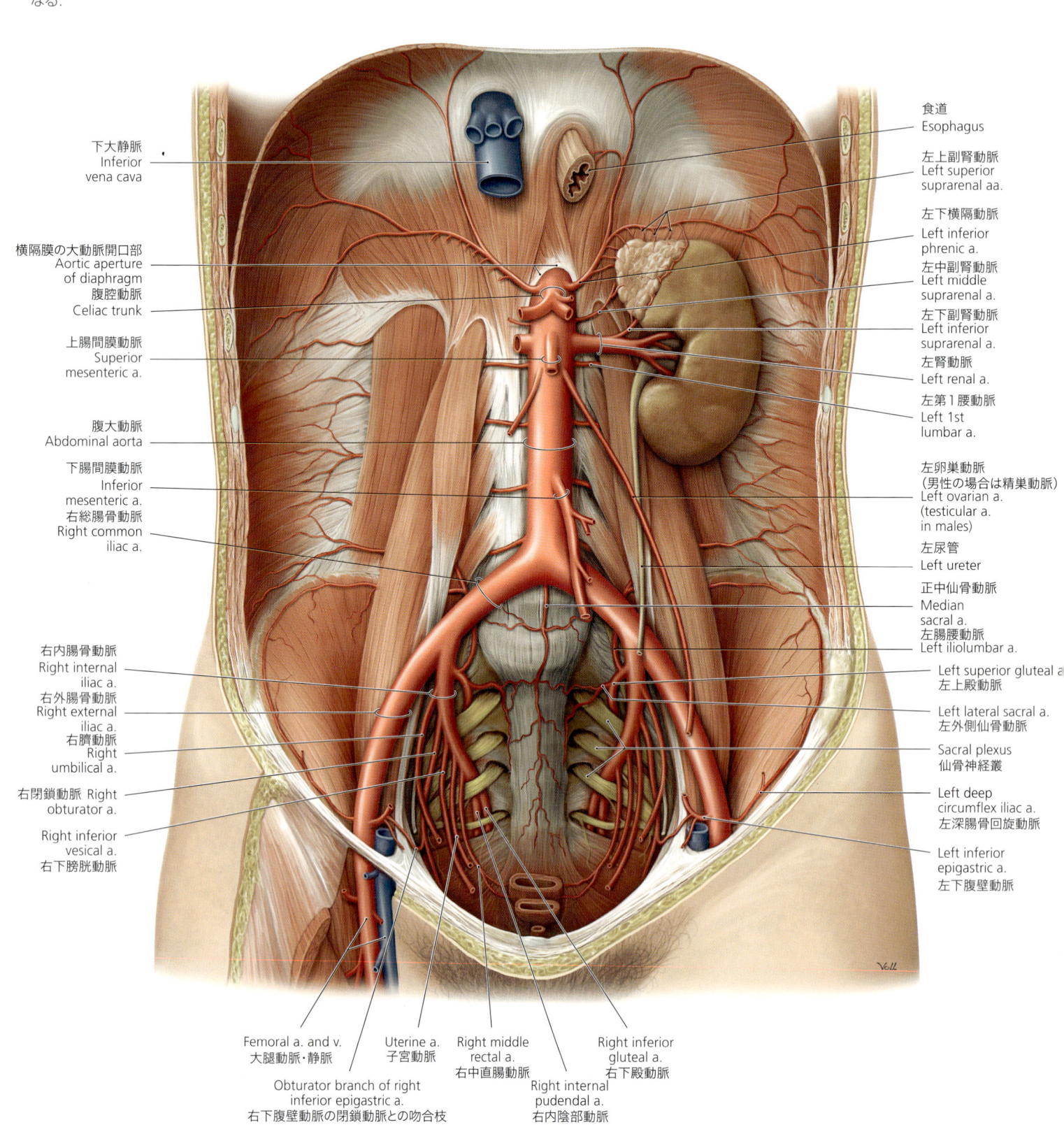

図15.7 腎動脈

左の腎臓．前方から見たところ．腎動脈はほぼ第2腰椎の高さから起こる．各腎動脈は前枝と後枝に分かれる．前枝はさらに4つの区動脈（丸で囲まれている）に分かれる．

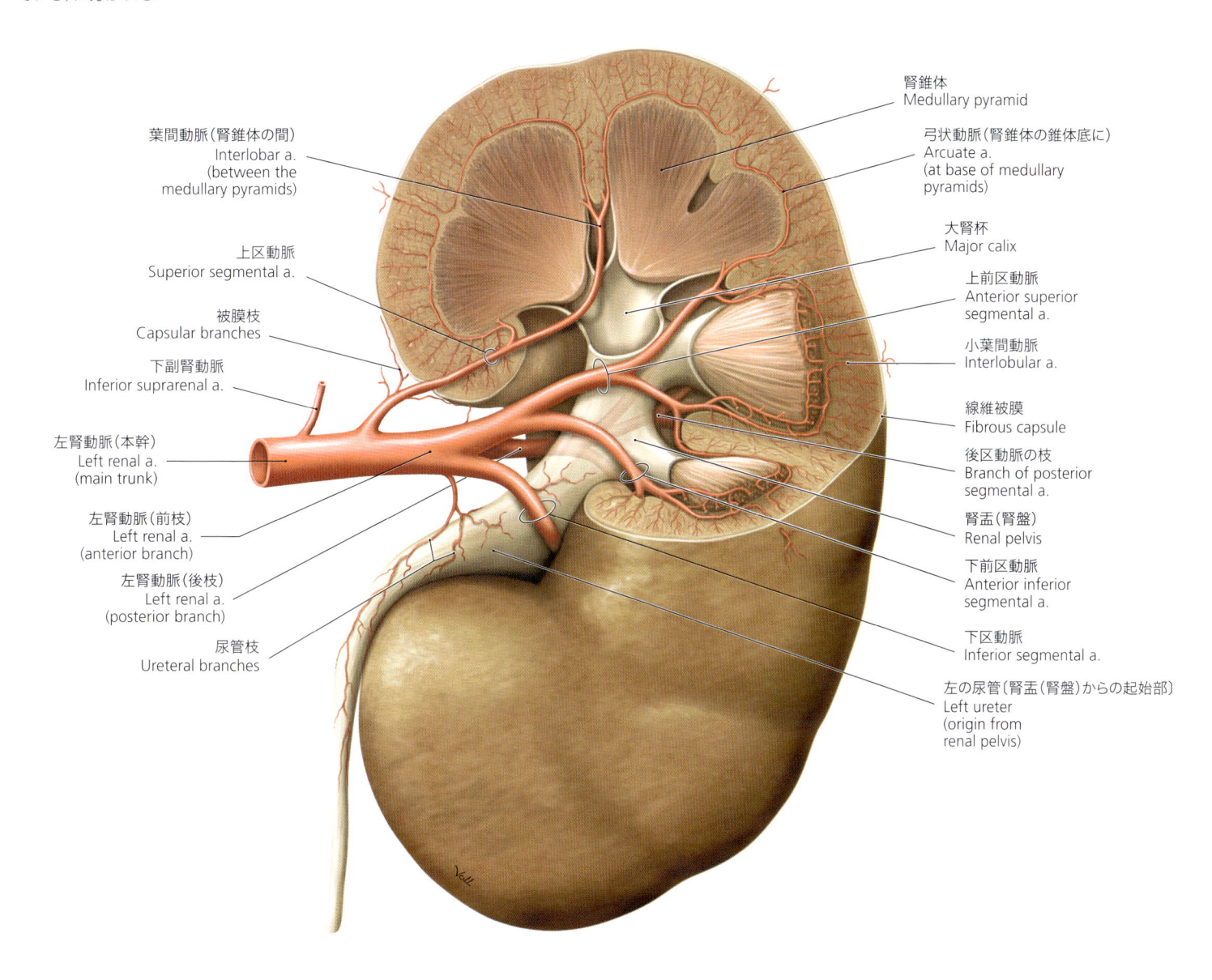

葉間動脈（腎錐体の間）
Interlobar a.
(between the medullary pyramids)

上区動脈
Superior segmental a.

被膜枝
Capsular branches

下副腎動脈
Inferior suprarenal a.

左腎動脈（本幹）
Left renal a.
(main trunk)

左腎動脈（前枝）
Left renal a.
(anterior branch)

左腎動脈（後枝）
Left renal a.
(posterior branch)

尿管枝
Ureteral branches

腎錐体
Medullary pyramid

弓状動脈（腎錐体の錐体底に）
Arcuate a.
(at base of medullary pyramids)

大腎杯
Major calix

上前区動脈
Anterior superior segmental a.

小葉間動脈
Interlobular a.

線維被膜
Fibrous capsule

後区動脈の枝
Branch of posterior segmental a.

腎盂（腎盤）
Renal pelvis

下前区動脈
Anterior inferior segmental a.

下区動脈
Inferior segmental a.

左の尿管（腎盂（腎盤）からの起始部）
Left ureter (origin from renal pelvis)

臨床

腎性高血圧

腎臓は血圧を感知して制御する重要な器官である．腎動脈の狭窄によって腎臓の血流量が減少すると，アンギオテンシノゲンを開裂させてアンギオテンシンⅠを遊離させるレニン分泌が促進される．さらに開裂すると，血管収縮を促進して血圧を高めるアンギオテンシンⅡが生じる．腎性高血圧は高血圧の診断において除外されるか，確定される必要がある．

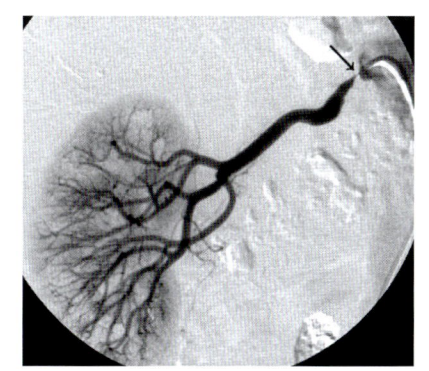

動脈造影によって可視化された右腎動脈（矢印）．

動脈と静脈

腹腔動脈
Celiac Trunk

> 腹腔動脈の分布域は p.207 に示されている．

図 15.8 腹腔動脈：胃，肝臓，胆嚢
前方から見たところ．小網は開いてある．大網は切開してある．腹腔動脈は第 1 腰椎の高さで腹大動脈から起こる．

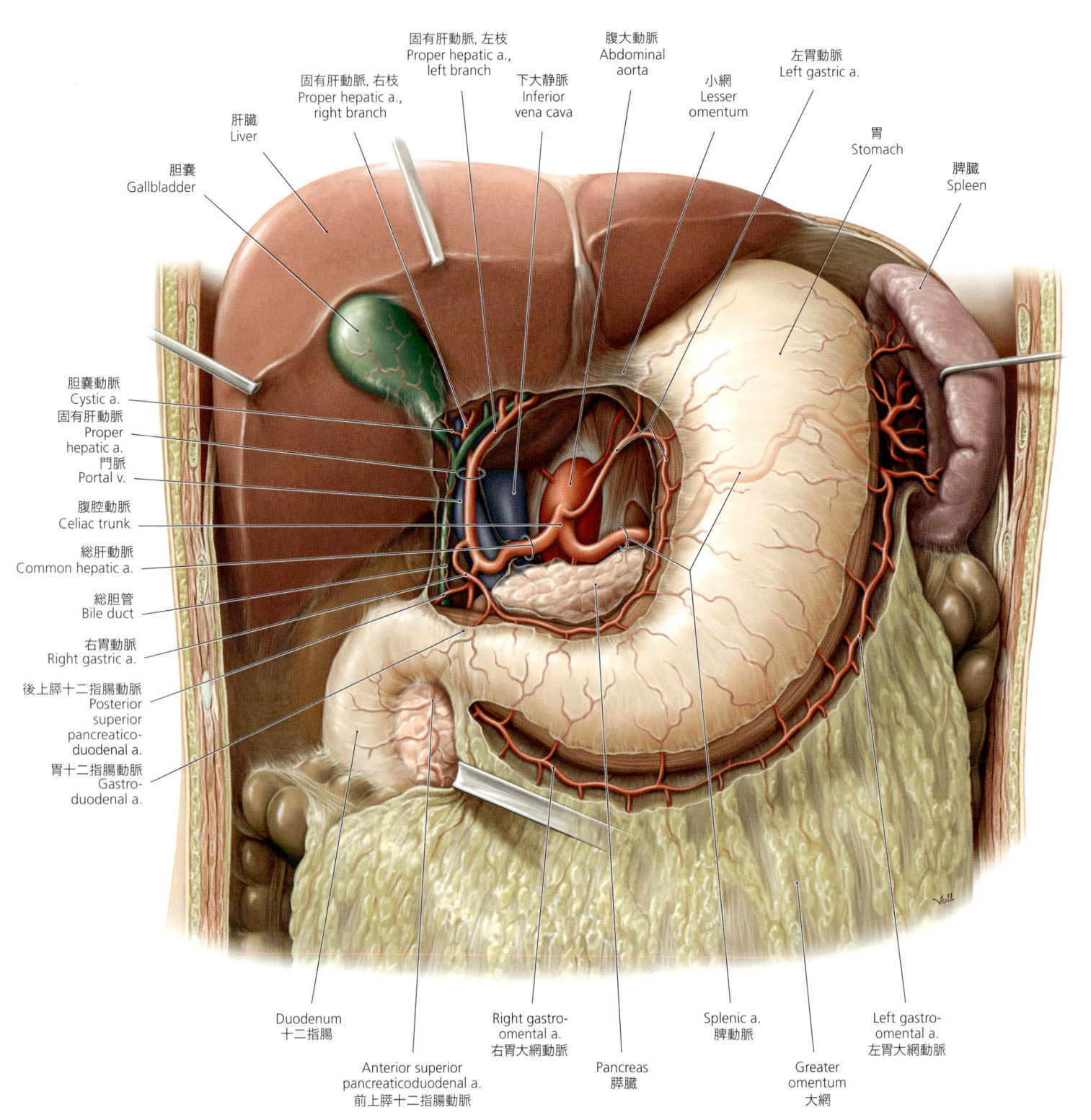

Labels:
- 固有肝動脈, 左枝 / Proper hepatic a., left branch
- 固有肝動脈, 右枝 / Proper hepatic a., right branch
- 肝臓 / Liver
- 胆嚢 / Gallbladder
- 下大静脈 / Inferior vena cava
- 腹大動脈 / Abdominal aorta
- 小網 / Lesser omentum
- 左胃動脈 / Left gastric a.
- 胃 / Stomach
- 脾臓 / Spleen
- 胆嚢動脈 / Cystic a.
- 固有肝動脈 / Proper hepatic a.
- 門脈 / Portal v.
- 腹腔動脈 / Celiac trunk
- 総肝動脈 / Common hepatic a.
- 総胆管 / Bile duct
- 右胃動脈 / Right gastric a.
- 後上膵十二指腸動脈 / Posterior superior pancreaticoduodenal a.
- 胃十二指腸動脈 / Gastroduodenal a.
- Duodenum 十二指腸
- Anterior superior pancreaticoduodenal a. 前上膵十二指腸動脈
- Right gastro-omental a. 右胃大網動脈
- Pancreas 膵臓
- Splenic a. 脾動脈
- Greater omentum 大網
- Left gastro-omental a. 左胃大網動脈

図 15.9 腹腔動脈：膵臓，十二指腸，脾臓
前方から見たところ．胃体と小網は取り除いてある．

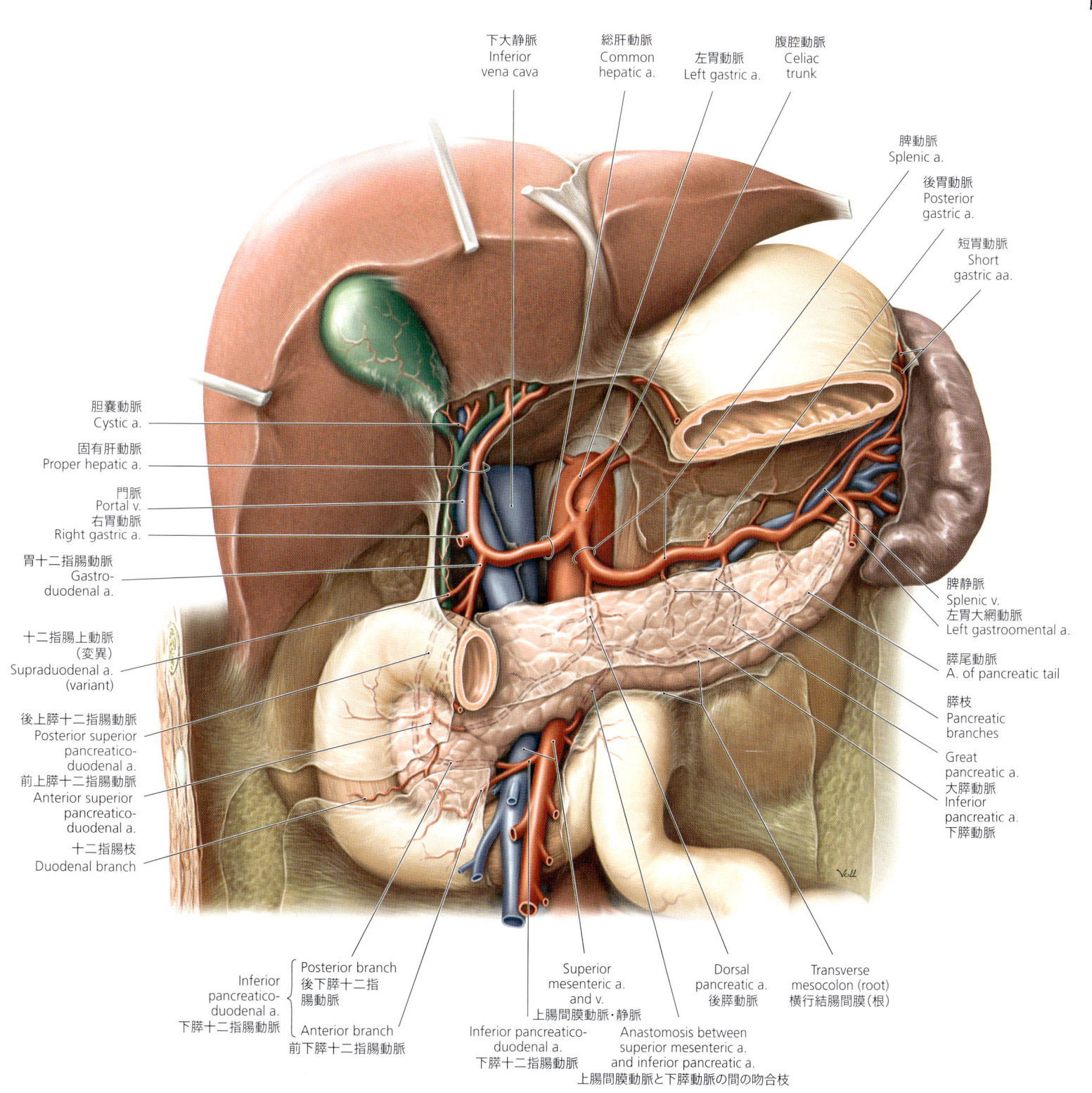

上腸間膜動脈と下腸間膜動脈
Superior & Inferior Mesenteric Arteries

図 15.10　上腸間膜動脈
前方から見たところ．胃と腹膜の一部は取り除いてある．
Note：中結腸動脈は切ってある（図 15.11 参照）．上腸間膜動脈と下腸間膜動脈はそれぞれ第 2 腰椎と第 3 腰椎の高さで腹大動脈から起こる．

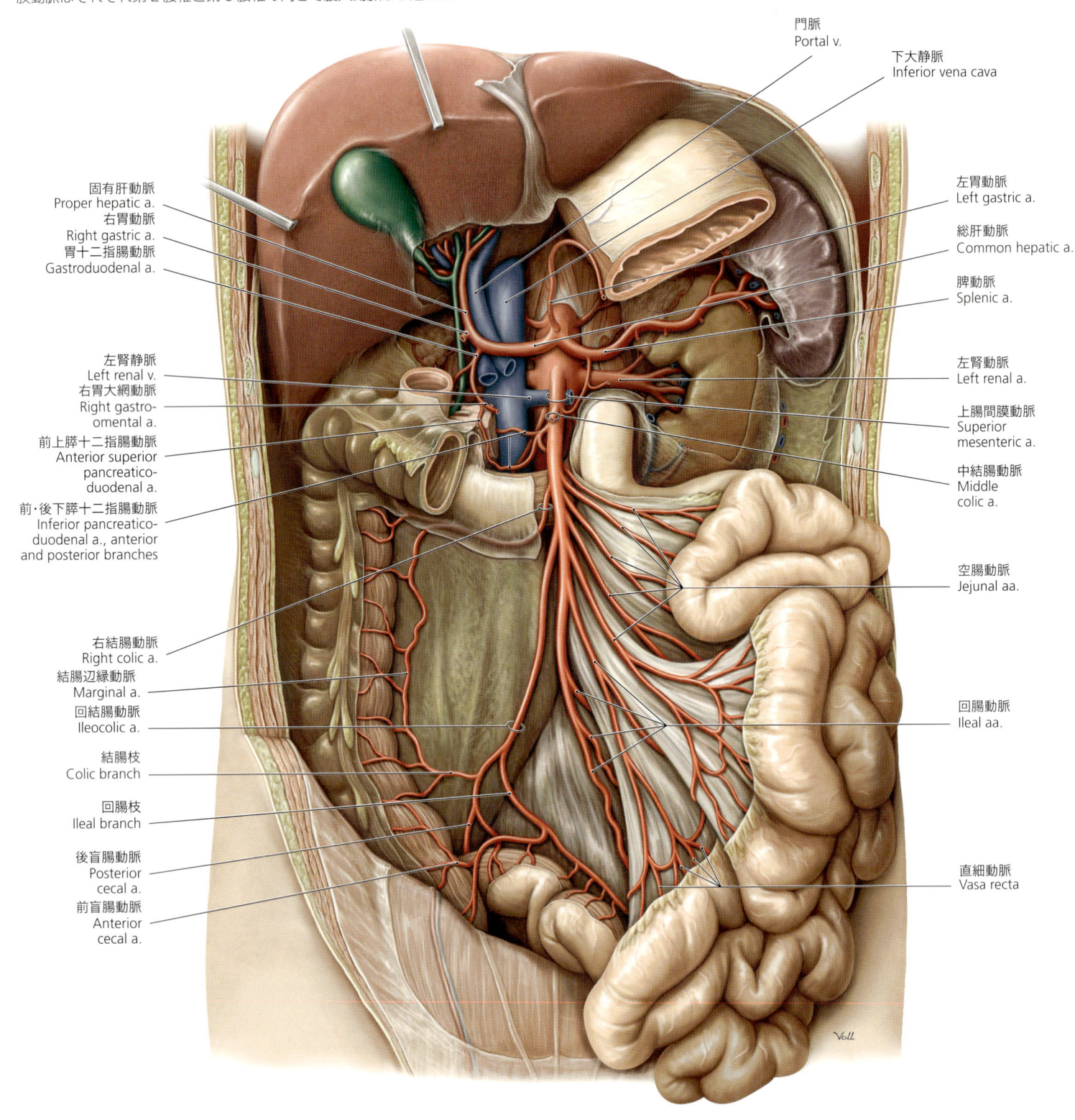

- 固有肝動脈 Proper hepatic a.
- 右胃動脈 Right gastric a.
- 胃十二指腸動脈 Gastroduodenal a.
- 左腎静脈 Left renal v.
- 右胃大網動脈 Right gastro-omental a.
- 前上膵十二指腸動脈 Anterior superior pancreaticoduodenal a.
- 前・後下膵十二指腸動脈 Inferior pancreaticoduodenal a., anterior and posterior branches
- 右結腸動脈 Right colic a.
- 結腸辺縁動脈 Marginal a.
- 回結腸動脈 Ileocolic a.
- 結腸枝 Colic branch
- 回腸枝 Ileal branch
- 後盲腸動脈 Posterior cecal a.
- 前盲腸動脈 Anterior cecal a.
- 門脈 Portal v.
- 下大静脈 Inferior vena cava
- 左胃動脈 Left gastric a.
- 総肝動脈 Common hepatic a.
- 脾動脈 Splenic a.
- 左腎動脈 Left renal a.
- 上腸間膜動脈 Superior mesenteric a.
- 中結腸動脈 Middle colic a.
- 空腸動脈 Jejunal aa.
- 回腸動脈 Ileal aa.
- 直細動脈 Vasa recta

図 15.11　下腸間膜動脈
前方から見たところ．空腸と回腸は取り除いてある．横行結腸を翻転してある．

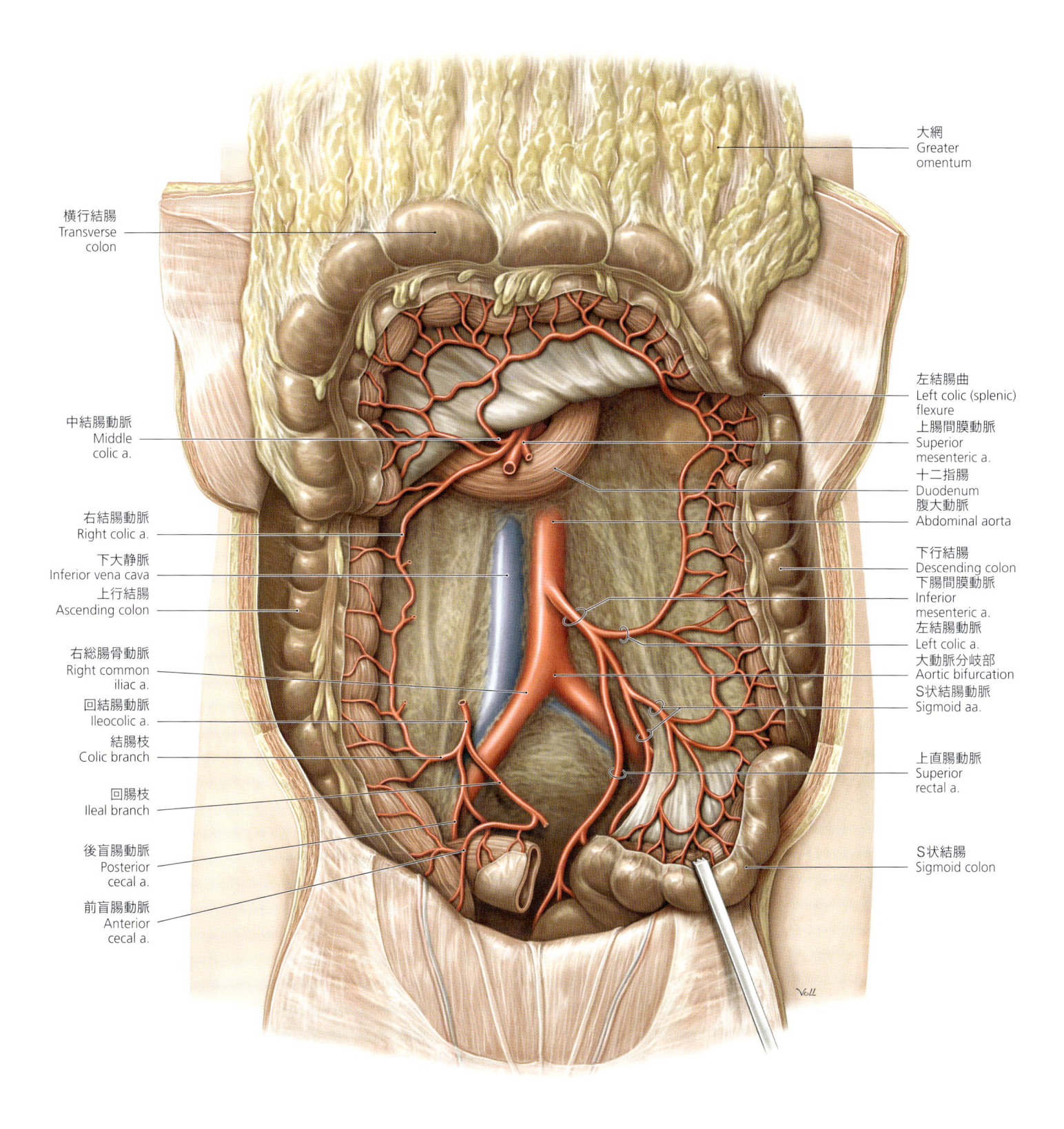

腹部の静脈
Veins of the Abdomen

図 15.12 下大静脈：位置
前方から見たところ．

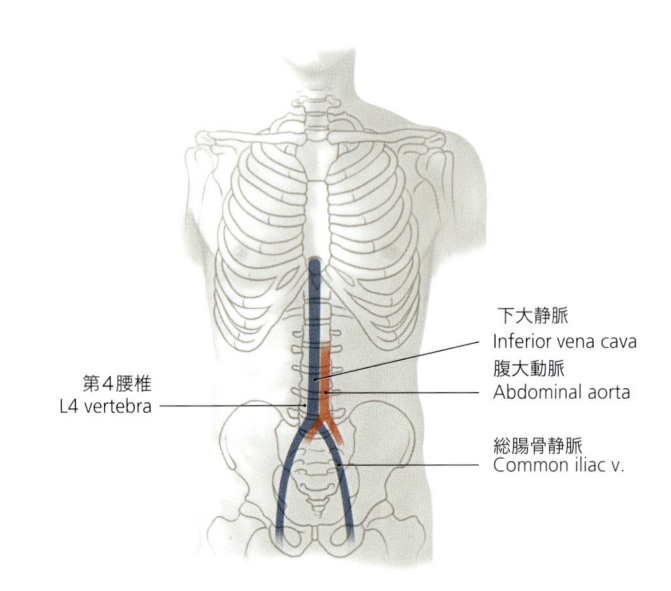

- 下大静脈 Inferior vena cava
- 第4腰椎 L4 vertebra
- 腹大動脈 Abdominal aorta
- 総腸骨静脈 Common iliac v.

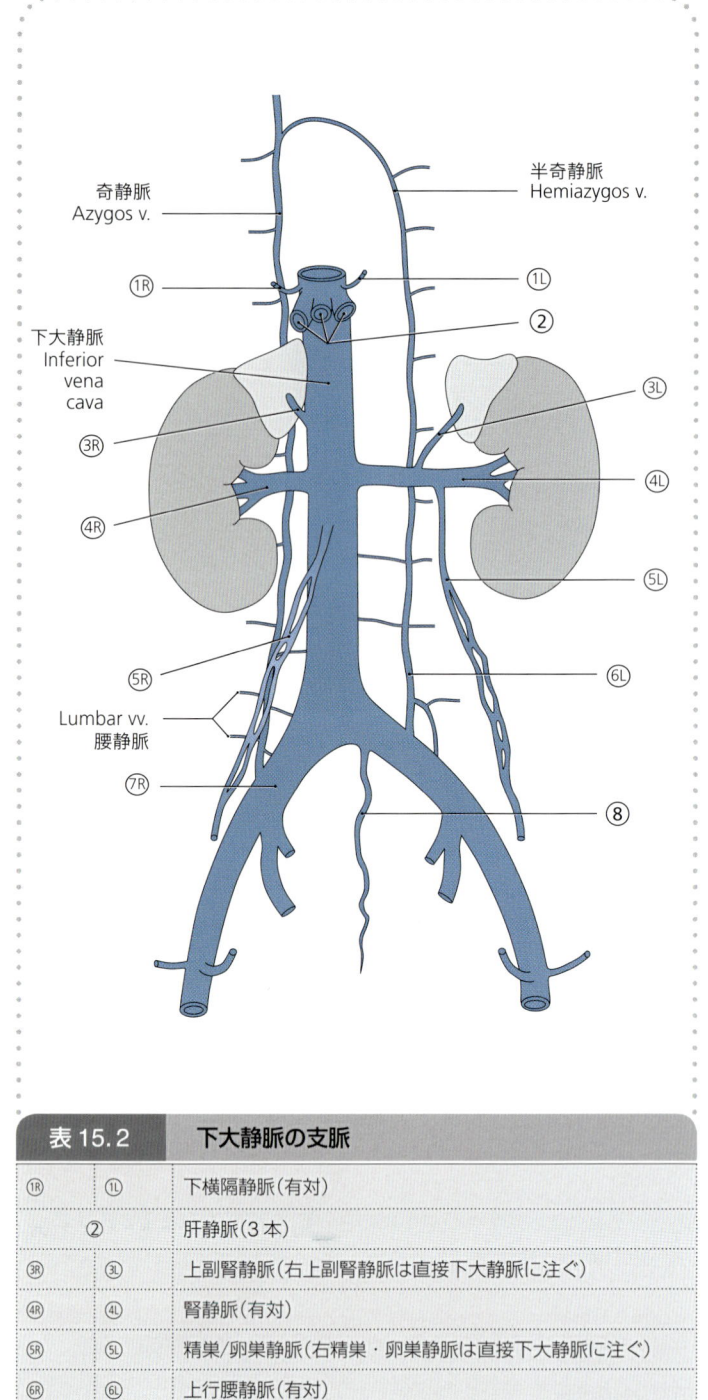

図右側：
- 奇静脈 Azygos v.
- 半奇静脈 Hemiazygos v.
- 下大静脈 Inferior vena cava
- 腰静脈 Lumbar vv.
- ①R, ①L, ②, ③R, ③L, ④R, ④L, ⑤R, ⑤L, ⑥R, ⑥L, ⑦R, ⑧

図 15.13 腎静脈の枝
前方から見たところ．

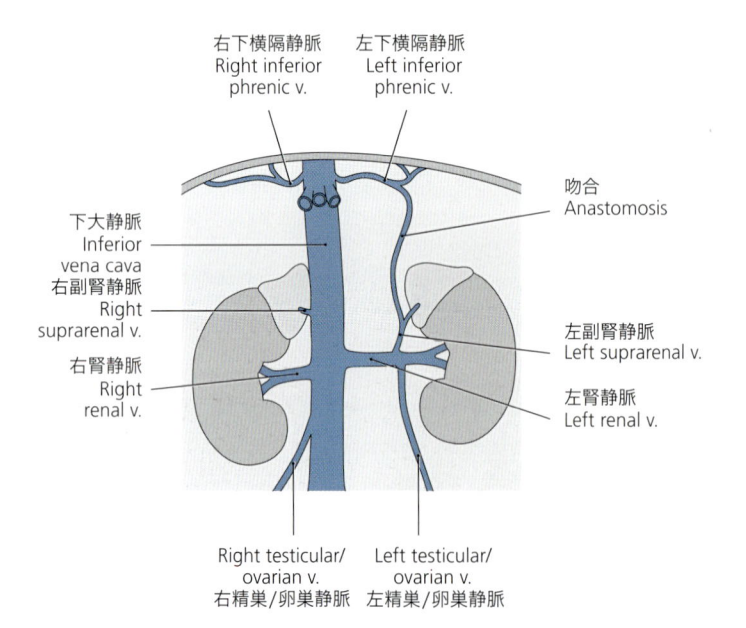

- 右下横隔静脈 Right inferior phrenic v.
- 左下横隔静脈 Left inferior phrenic v.
- 吻合 Anastomosis
- 下大静脈 Inferior vena cava
- 右副腎静脈 Right suprarenal v.
- 左副腎静脈 Left suprarenal v.
- 右腎静脈 Right renal v.
- 左腎静脈 Left renal v.
- 右精巣/卵巣静脈 Right testicular/ovarian v.
- 左精巣/卵巣静脈 Left testicular/ovarian v.

表 15.2　下大静脈の支脈

①R	①L	下横隔静脈（有対）
	②	肝静脈（3本）
③R	③L	上副腎静脈（右上副腎静脈は直接下大静脈に注ぐ）
④R	④L	腎静脈（有対）
⑤R	⑤L	精巣/卵巣静脈（右精巣・卵巣静脈は直接下大静脈に注ぐ）
⑥R	⑥L	上行腰静脈（有対）
⑦R	⑦L	総腸骨静脈（有対）
	⑧	正中仙骨静脈

図 15.14 門脈

門脈（p.218 参照）には腹腔動脈，上腸間膜動脈，下腸間膜動脈が分布する腹部と骨盤部の器官からの静脈血が注ぐ．

A 位置，前から見たところ．

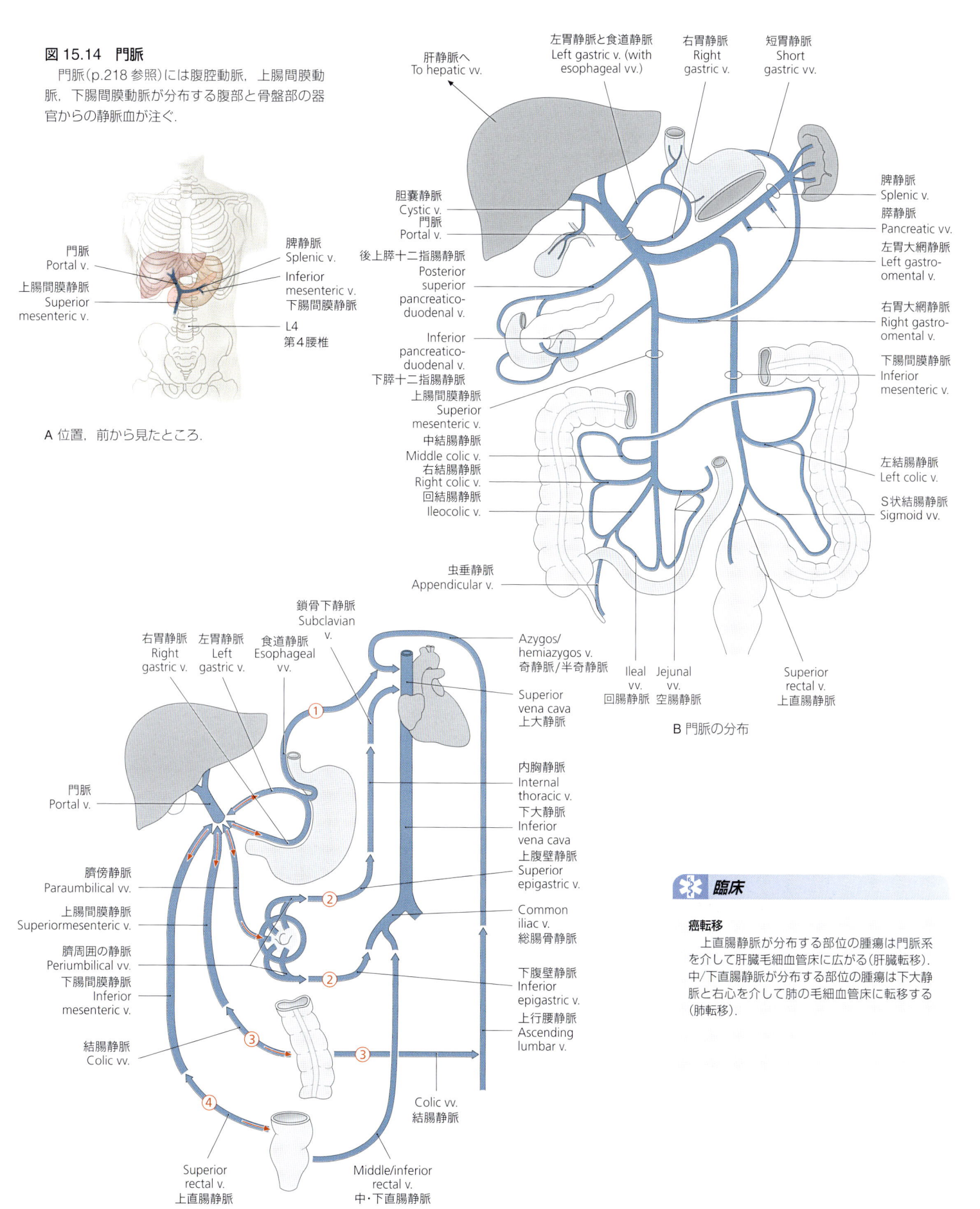

B 門脈の分布

C 側副路（門脈体循環側副路）．門脈系が閉塞したときは，栄養に富む血液は，肝臓を通らずに大静脈から心臓に運ばれ，赤の矢印の方向に逆流する．

臨床

癌転移

上直腸静脈が分布する部位の腫瘍は門脈系を介して肝臓毛細血管床に広がる（肝臓転移）．中／下直腸静脈が分布する部位の腫瘍は下大静脈と右心を介して肺の毛細血管床に転移する（肺転移）．

下大静脈と腎静脈
Inferior Vena Cava & Renal Veins

図 15.15　下大静脈
女性腹部，前方から見たところ．左の腎臓と副腎以外の全臓器は取り除いてある．

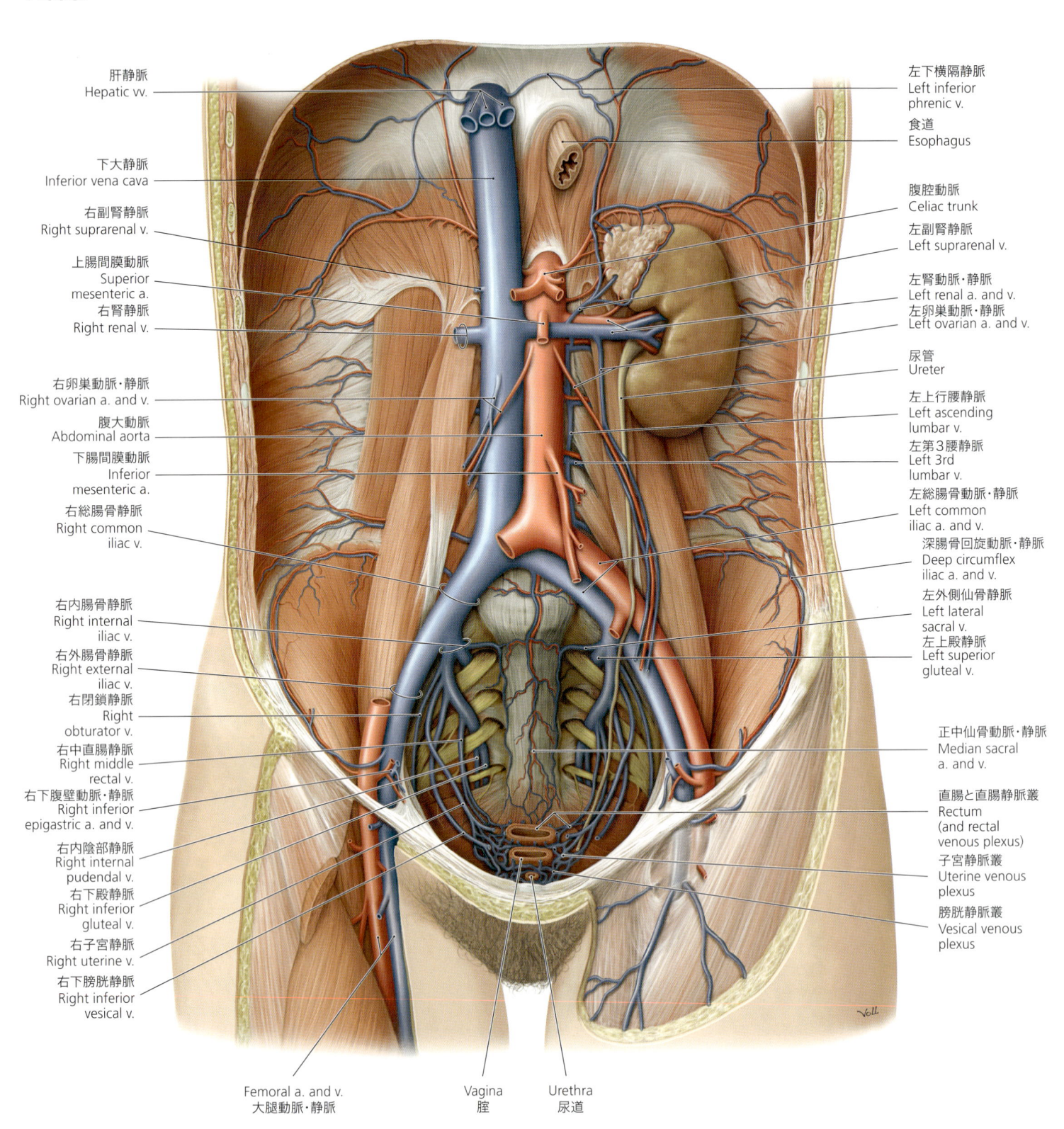

ラベル（左側，上から下）:
- 肝静脈　Hepatic vv.
- 下大静脈　Inferior vena cava
- 右副腎静脈　Right suprarenal v.
- 上腸間膜動脈　Superior mesenteric a.
- 右腎静脈　Right renal v.
- 右卵巣動脈・静脈　Right ovarian a. and v.
- 腹大動脈　Abdominal aorta
- 下腸間膜動脈　Inferior mesenteric a.
- 右総腸骨静脈　Right common iliac v.
- 右内腸骨静脈　Right internal iliac v.
- 右外腸骨静脈　Right external iliac v.
- 右閉鎖静脈　Right obturator v.
- 右中直腸静脈　Right middle rectal v.
- 右下腹壁動脈・静脈　Right inferior epigastric a. and v.
- 右内陰部静脈　Right internal pudendal v.
- 右下殿静脈　Right inferior gluteal v.
- 右子宮静脈　Right uterine v.
- 右下膀胱静脈　Right inferior vesical v.

ラベル（右側，上から下）:
- 左下横隔静脈　Left inferior phrenic v.
- 食道　Esophagus
- 腹腔動脈　Celiac trunk
- 左副腎静脈　Left suprarenal v.
- 左腎動脈・静脈　Left renal a. and v.
- 左卵巣動脈・静脈　Left ovarian a. and v.
- 尿管　Ureter
- 左上行腰静脈　Left ascending lumbar v.
- 左第3腰静脈　Left 3rd lumbar v.
- 左総腸骨動脈・静脈　Left common iliac a. and v.
- 深腸骨回旋動脈・静脈　Deep circumflex iliac a. and v.
- 左外側仙骨静脈　Left lateral sacral v.
- 左上殿静脈　Left superior gluteal v.
- 正中仙骨動脈・静脈　Median sacral a. and v.
- 直腸と直腸静脈叢　Rectum (and rectal venous plexus)
- 子宮静脈叢　Uterine venous plexus
- 膀胱静脈叢　Vesical venous plexus

下部ラベル:
- Femoral a. and v.　大腿動脈・静脈
- Vagina　腟
- Urethra　尿道

図 15.16　腎静脈
前方から見たところ．腎動脈については p.209 参照．

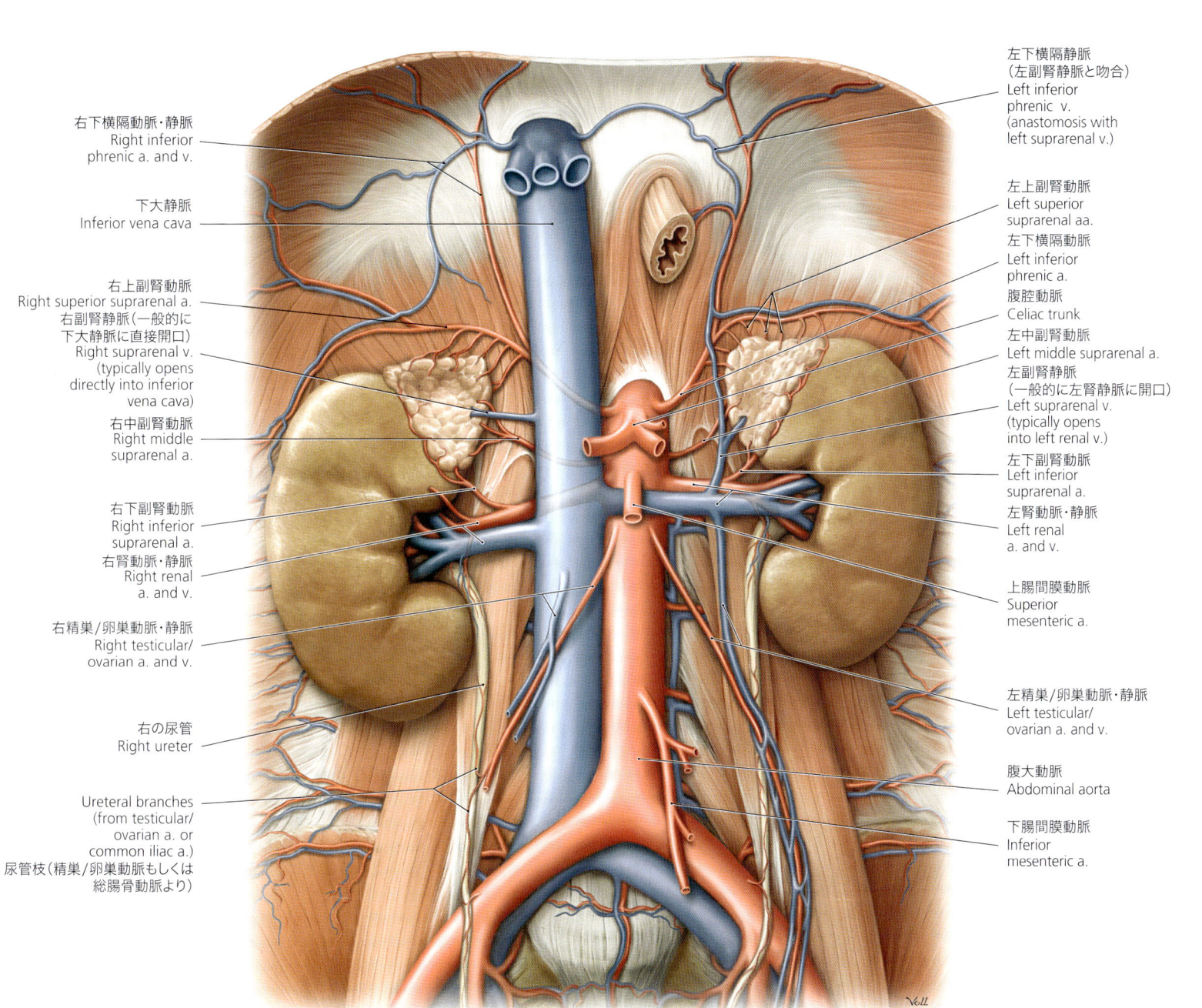

- 右下横隔動脈・静脈 Right inferior phrenic a. and v.
- 下大静脈 Inferior vena cava
- 右上副腎動脈 Right superior suprarenal a.
- 右副腎静脈（一般的に下大静脈に直接開口） Right suprarenal v. (typically opens directly into inferior vena cava)
- 右中副腎動脈 Right middle suprarenal a.
- 右下副腎動脈 Right inferior suprarenal a.
- 右腎動脈・静脈 Right renal a. and v.
- 右精巣／卵巣動脈・静脈 Right testicular/ovarian a. and v.
- 右の尿管 Right ureter
- Ureteral branches (from testicular/ovarian a. or common iliac a.)
- 尿管枝（精巣／卵巣動脈もしくは総腸骨動脈より）

- 左下横隔静脈（左副腎静脈と吻合） Left inferior phrenic v. (anastomosis with left suprarenal v.)
- 左上副腎動脈 Left superior suprarenal aa.
- 左下横隔動脈 Left inferior phrenic a.
- 腹腔動脈 Celiac trunk
- 左中副腎動脈 Left middle suprarenal a.
- 左副腎静脈（一般的に左腎静脈に開口） Left suprarenal v. (typically opens into left renal v.)
- 左下副腎動脈 Left inferior suprarenal a.
- 左腎動脈・静脈 Left renal a. and v.
- 上腸間膜動脈 Superior mesenteric a.
- 左精巣／卵巣動脈・静脈 Left testicular/ovarian a. and v.
- 腹大動脈 Abdominal aorta
- 下腸間膜動脈 Inferior mesenteric a.

15　動脈と静脈

門脈
Portal Vein

門脈は典型例では膵頸後方で上腸間静脈と脾静脈が合流して作られる．門脈の分布はp.215で示した．

図15.17 門脈：胃と十二指腸
前方から見たところ．肝臓，小網，腹膜は取り除いてある．大網は切り開いてある．

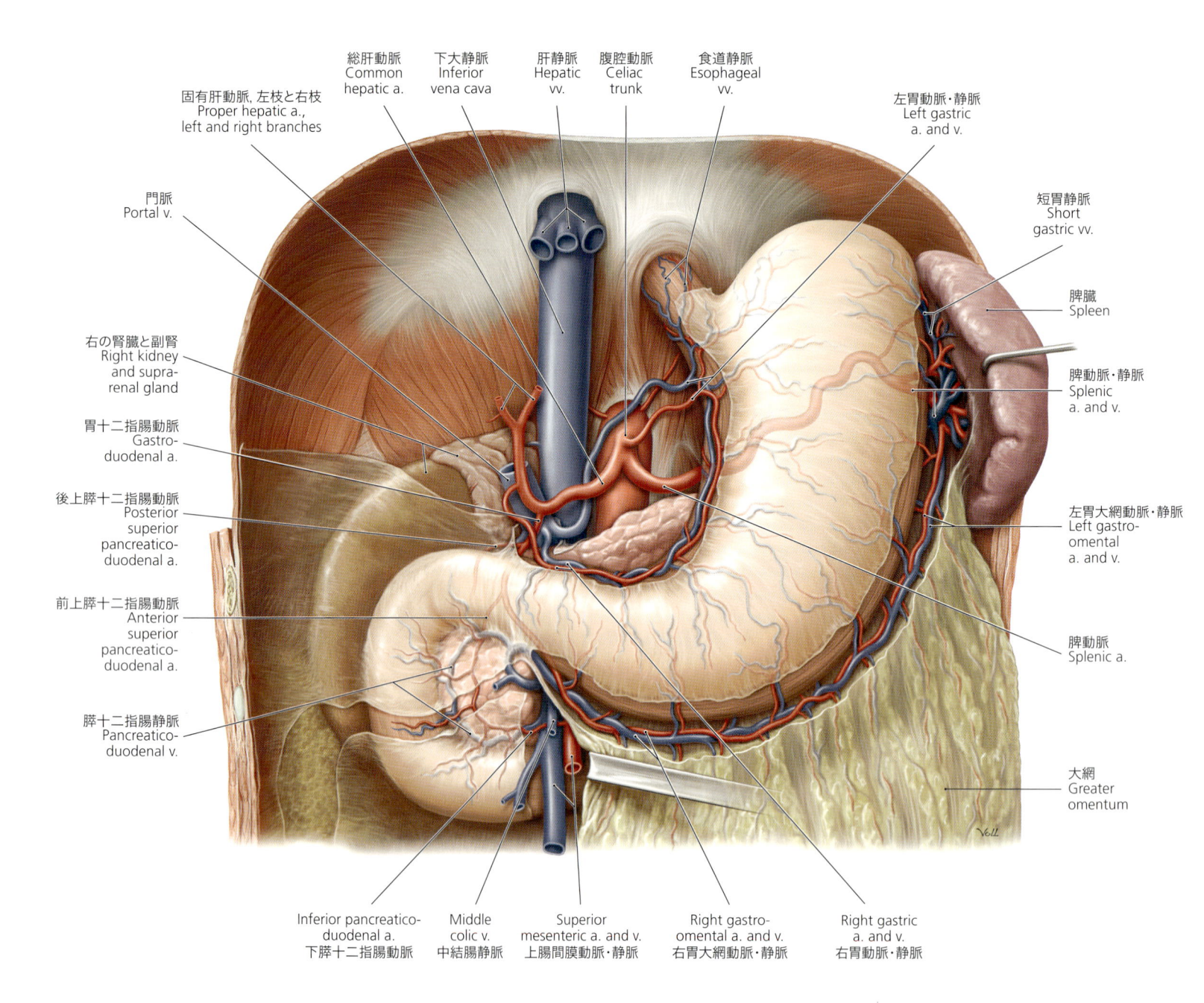

図 15.18　門脈：膵臓と脾臓

前方から見たところ．胃，膵臓，腹膜は一部取り除いてある．

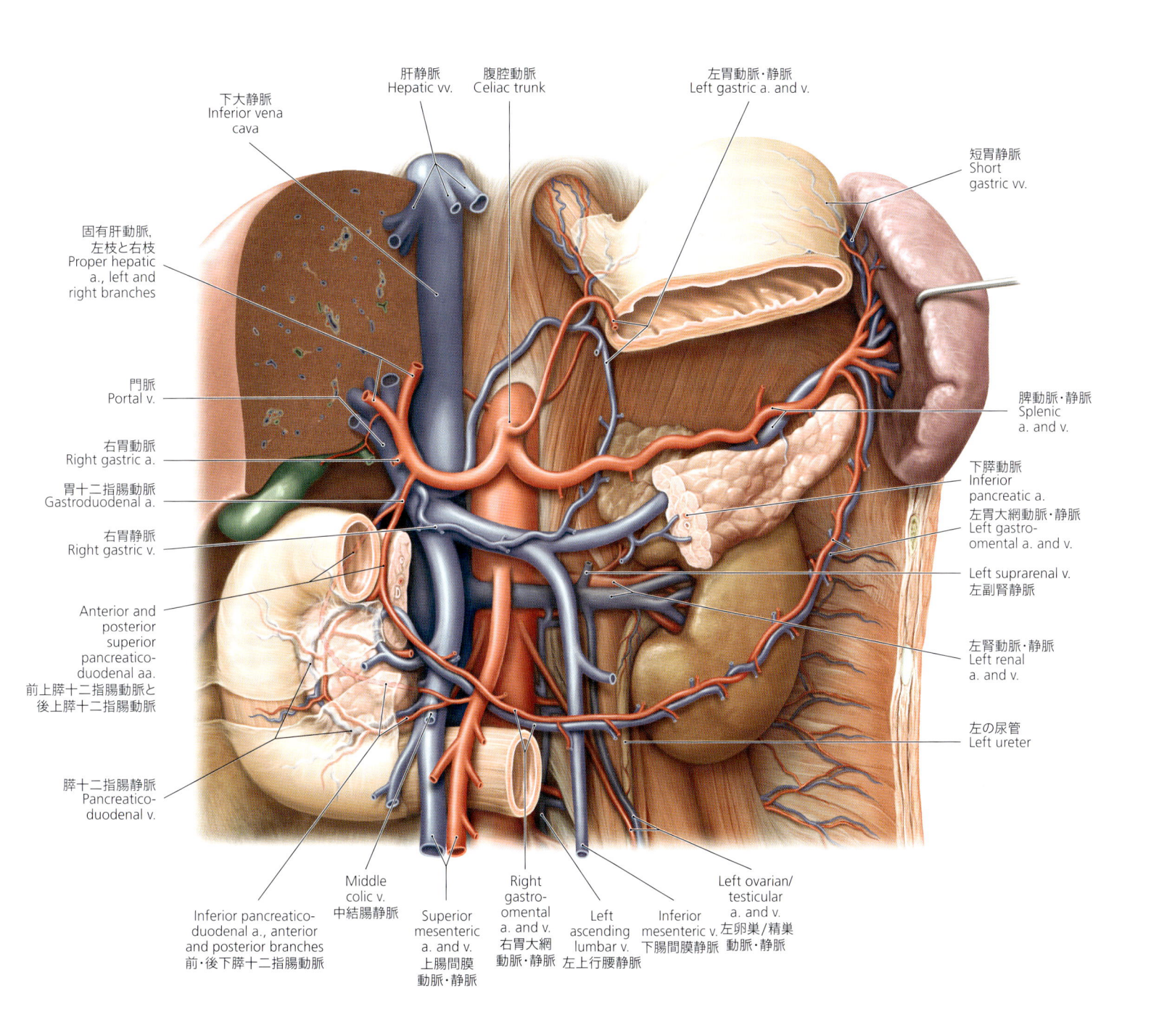

- 肝静脈 Hepatic vv.
- 腹腔動脈 Celiac trunk
- 左胃動脈・静脈 Left gastric a. and v.
- 下大静脈 Inferior vena cava
- 短胃静脈 Short gastric vv.
- 固有肝動脈，左枝と右枝 Proper hepatic a., left and right branches
- 脾動脈・静脈 Splenic a. and v.
- 門脈 Portal v.
- 右胃動脈 Right gastric a.
- 下膵動脈 Inferior pancreatic a.
- 胃十二指腸動脈 Gastroduodenal a.
- 左胃大網動脈・静脈 Left gastro-omental a. and v.
- 右胃静脈 Right gastric v.
- Left suprarenal v. 左副腎静脈
- Anterior and posterior superior pancreatico-duodenal aa. 前上膵十二指腸動脈と後上膵十二指腸動脈
- 左腎動脈・静脈 Left renal a. and v.
- 左の尿管 Left ureter
- 膵十二指腸静脈 Pancreatico-duodenal v.
- Inferior pancreatico-duodenal a., anterior and posterior branches 前・後下膵十二指腸動脈
- Middle colic v. 中結腸静脈
- Superior mesenteric a. and v. 上腸間膜動脈・静脈
- Right gastro-omental a. and v. 右胃大網動脈・静脈
- Left ascending lumbar v. 左上行腰静脈
- Inferior mesenteric v. 下腸間膜静脈
- Left ovarian/testicular a. and v. 左卵巣／精巣動脈・静脈

219

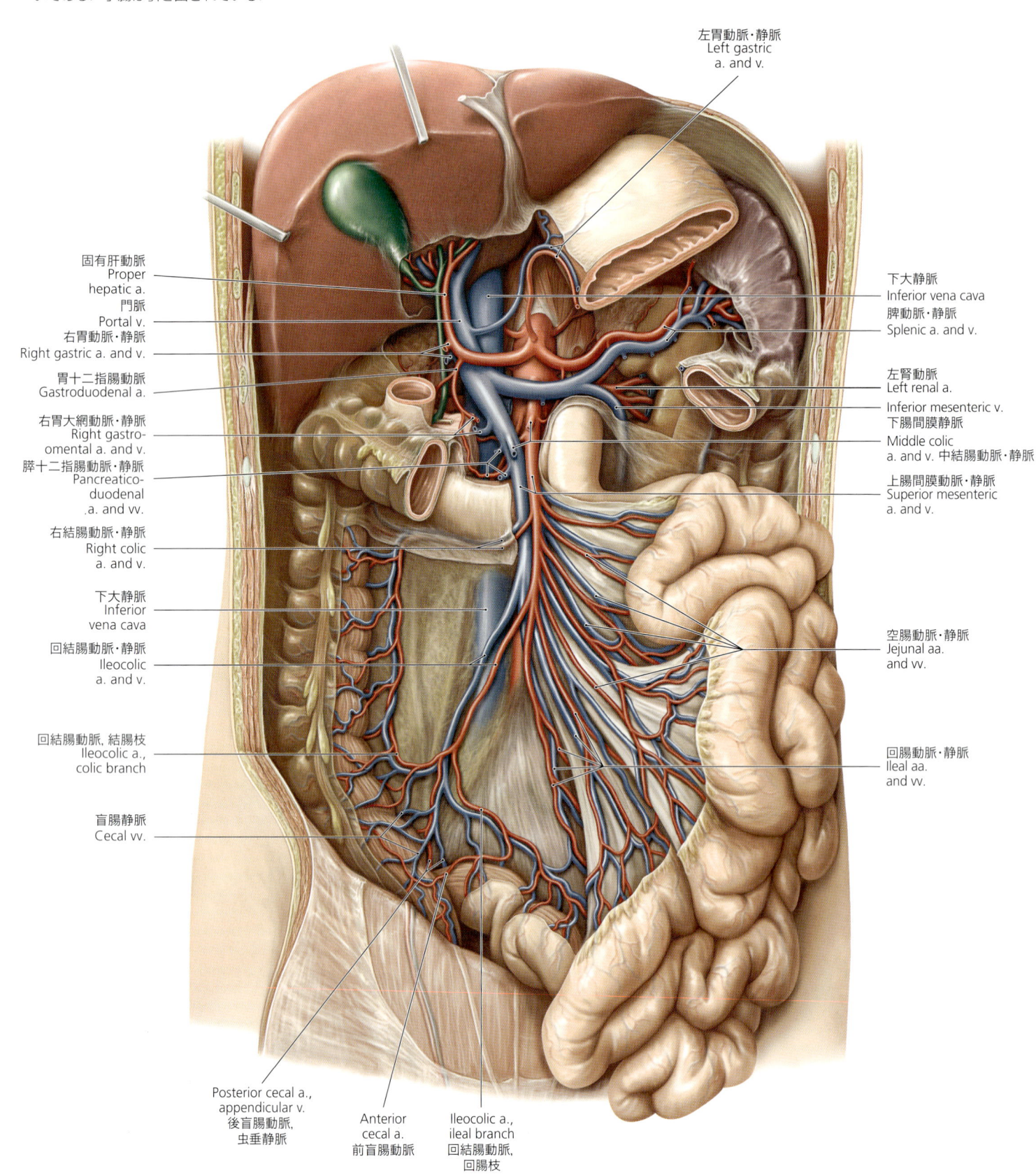

上腸間膜静脈と下腸間膜静脈
Superior & Inferior Mesenteric Veins

図 15.19　上腸間膜静脈
前方から見たところ．胃，膵臓，腹膜，腸間膜，横行結腸は一部取り除いてある．小腸は引き出されている．

Labels:
- 固有肝動脈 Proper hepatic a.
- 門脈 Portal v.
- 右胃動脈・静脈 Right gastric a. and v.
- 胃十二指腸動脈 Gastroduodenal a.
- 右胃大網動脈・静脈 Right gastro-omental a. and v.
- 膵十二指腸動脈・静脈 Pancreaticoduodenal a. and vv.
- 右結腸動脈・静脈 Right colic a. and v.
- 下大静脈 Inferior vena cava
- 回結腸動脈・静脈 Ileocolic a. and v.
- 回結腸動脈，結腸枝 Ileocolic a., colic branch
- 盲腸静脈 Cecal vv.
- 後盲腸動脈，虫垂静脈 Posterior cecal a., appendicular v.
- 前盲腸動脈 Anterior cecal a.
- 回結腸動脈，回腸枝 Ileocolic a., ileal branch
- 左胃動脈・静脈 Left gastric a. and v.
- 下大静脈 Inferior vena cava
- 脾動脈・静脈 Splenic a. and v.
- 左腎動脈 Left renal a.
- 下腸間膜静脈 Inferior mesenteric v.
- 中結腸動脈・静脈 Middle colic a. and v.
- 上腸間膜動脈・静脈 Superior mesenteric a. and v.
- 空腸動脈・静脈 Jejunal aa. and vv.
- 回腸動脈・静脈 Ileal aa. and vv.

図 15.20　下腸間膜静脈
前方から見たところ．胃，膵臓，小腸，腹膜は取り除いてある．

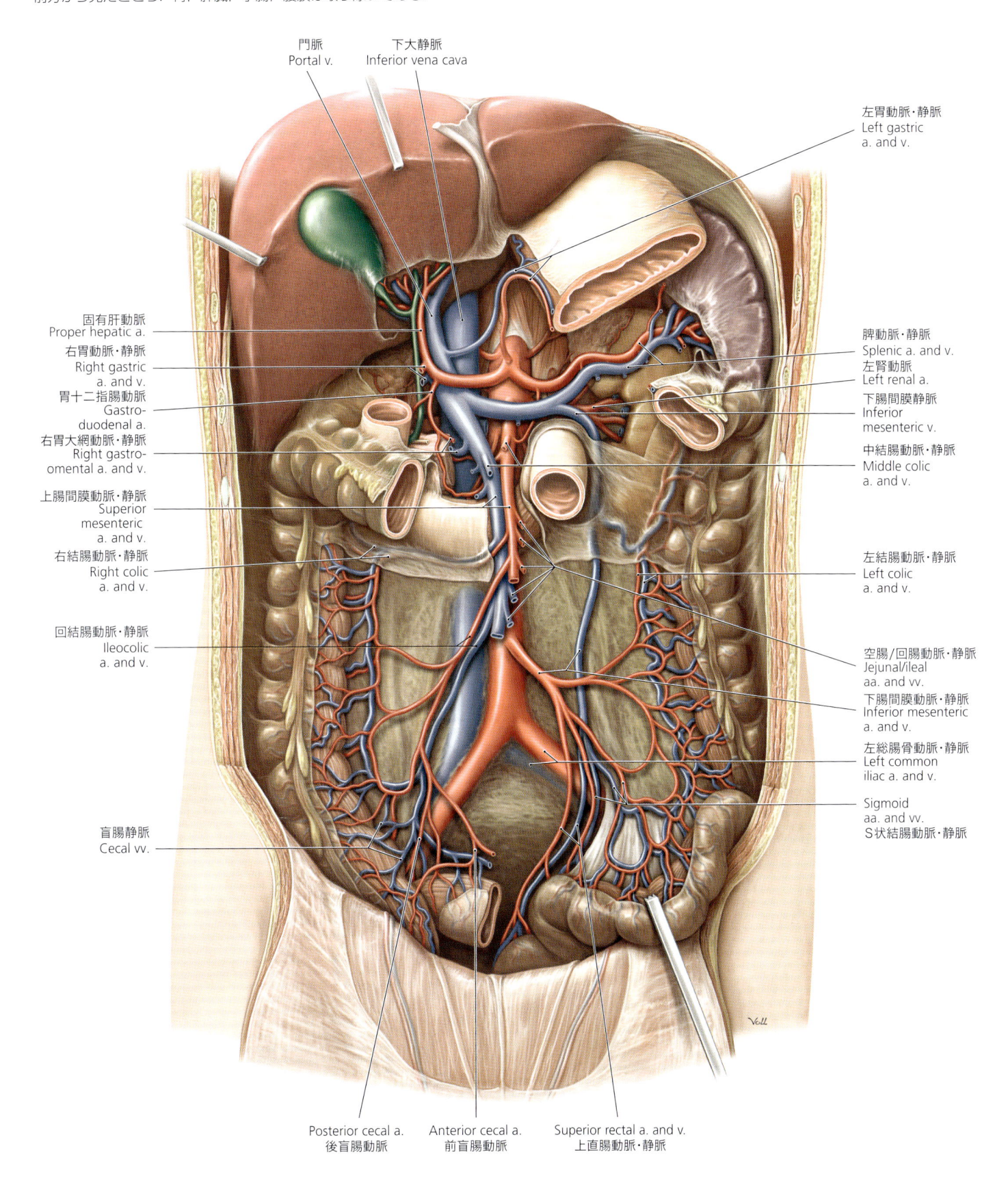

門脈 Portal v.
下大静脈 Inferior vena cava
左胃動脈・静脈 Left gastric a. and v.
固有肝動脈 Proper hepatic a.
右胃動脈・静脈 Right gastric a. and v.
胃十二指腸動脈 Gastroduodenal a.
右胃大網動脈・静脈 Right gastro-omental a. and v.
上腸間膜動脈・静脈 Superior mesenteric a. and v.
右結腸動脈・静脈 Right colic a. and v.
回結腸動脈・静脈 Ileocolic a. and v.
盲腸静脈 Cecal vv.
脾動脈・静脈 Splenic a. and v.
左腎動脈 Left renal a.
下腸間膜静脈 Inferior mesenteric v.
中結腸動脈・静脈 Middle colic a. and v.
左結腸動脈・静脈 Left colic a. and v.
空腸／回腸動脈・静脈 Jejunal/ileal aa. and vv.
下腸間膜動脈・静脈 Inferior mesenteric a. and v.
左総腸骨動脈・静脈 Left common iliac a. and v.
Sigmoid aa. and vv. S状結腸動脈・静脈

Posterior cecal a. 後盲腸動脈
Anterior cecal a. 前盲腸動脈
Superior rectal a. and v. 上直腸動脈・静脈

骨盤の動脈と静脈
Arteries & Veins of the Pelvis

A 男性骨盤.

B 女性骨盤.

A 男性骨盤.

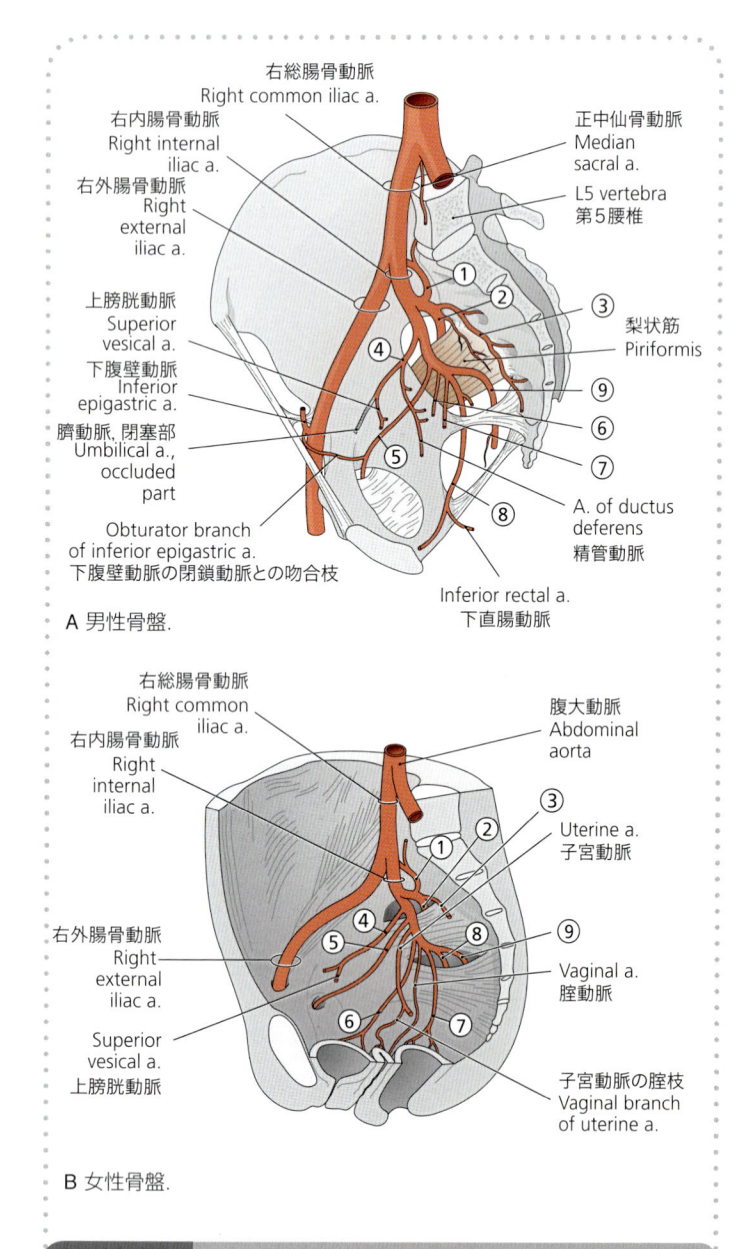

B 女性骨盤.

表 15.3	内腸骨動脈の枝	
内腸骨動脈は5本の骨盤への壁側枝と4本の骨盤内臓への内臓枝を出す*．壁側枝は斜体で示す．		
枝		
①	腸腰動脈	
②	上殿動脈	
③	外側仙骨動脈	
④	臍動脈	精管動脈
		上膀胱動脈
⑤	閉鎖動脈	
⑥	下膀胱動脈	
⑦	中直腸動脈	
⑧	内陰部動脈	下直腸動脈
⑨	下殿動脈	

*女性骨盤では子宮動脈と腟動脈が内腸骨動脈から直接起こる．

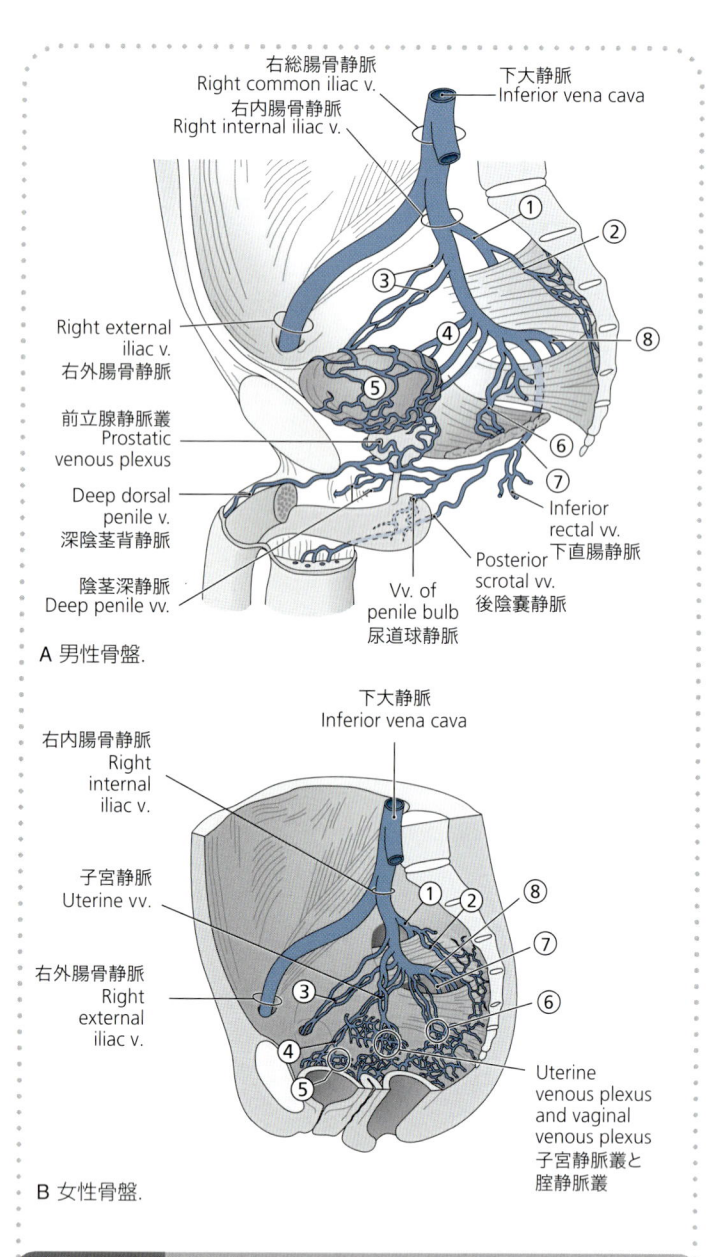

表 15.4	骨盤の静脈分布
支脈	
①	上殿静脈
②	外側仙骨静脈
③	閉鎖静脈
④	膀胱静脈
⑤	膀胱静脈叢
⑥	中直腸静脈（直腸静脈叢）（上・下直腸静脈は図には示されていない）
⑦	内陰部静脈
⑧	下殿静脈

男性骨盤には前立腺静脈叢と陰茎と陰嚢に分布する静脈がある．女性骨盤には子宮静脈叢と腟静脈叢がある．

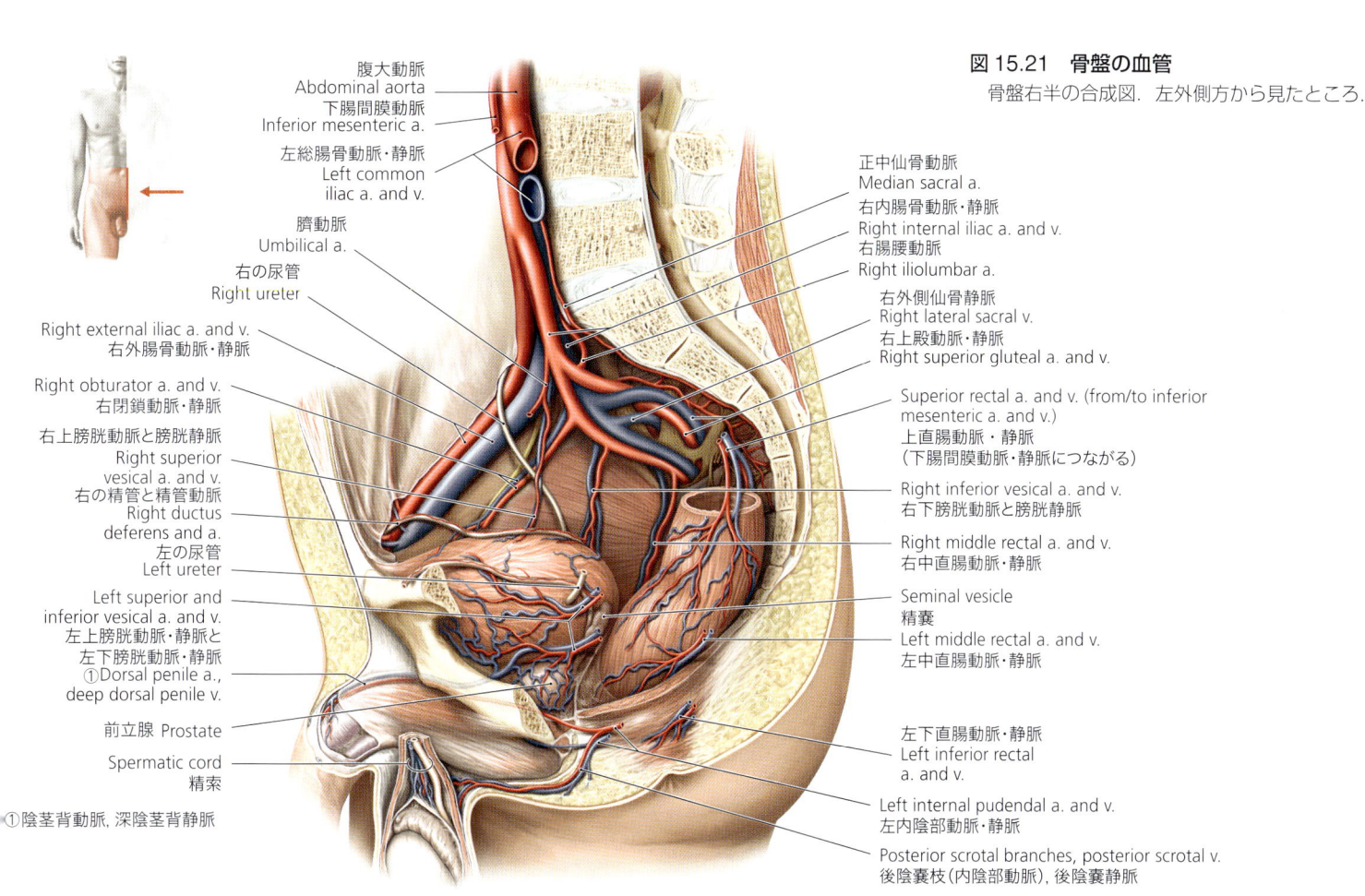

図 15.21 骨盤の血管
骨盤右半の合成図．左外側方から見たところ．

A 男性骨盤．

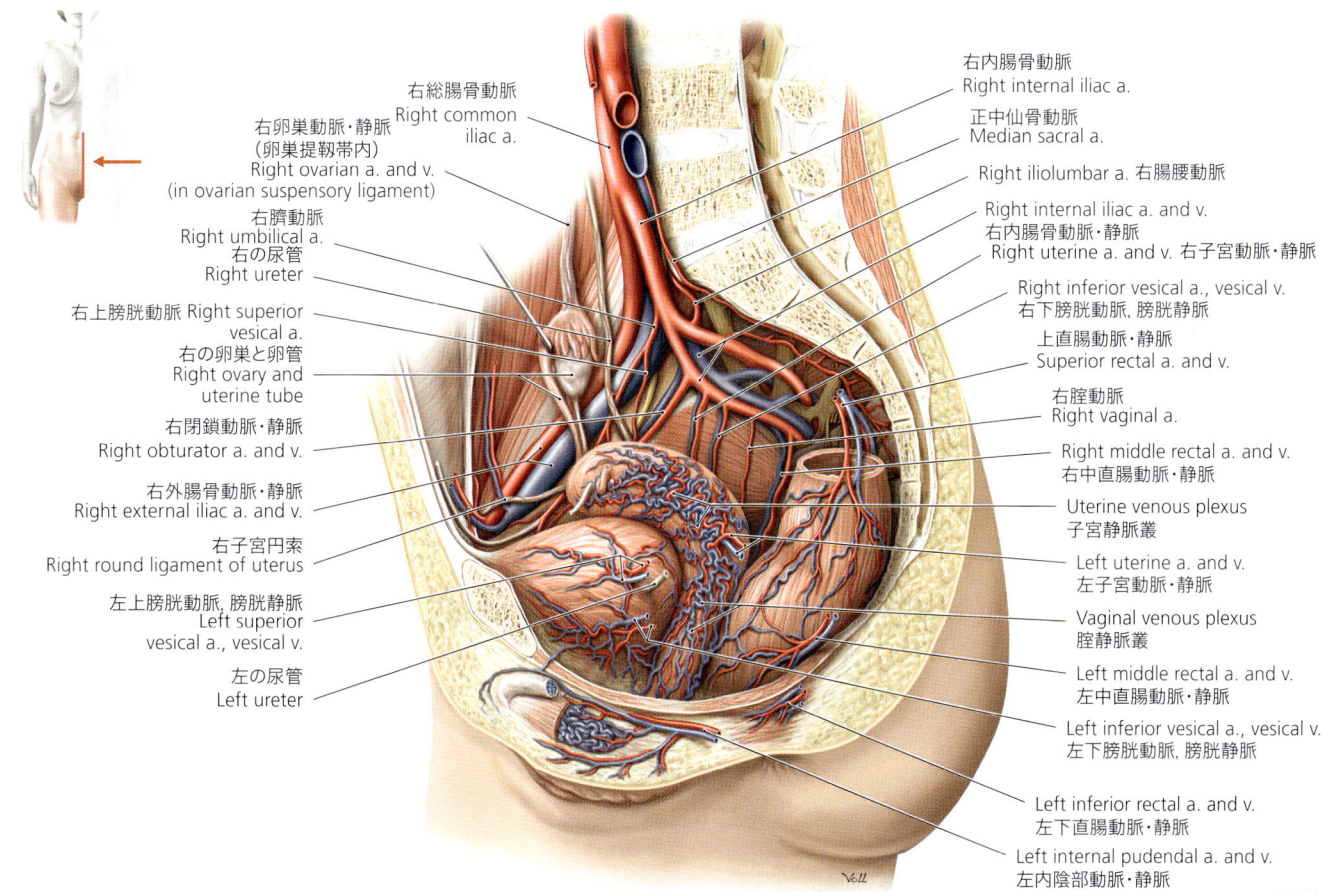

B 女性骨盤．

直腸と生殖器の動脈と静脈
Arteries & Veins of the Rectum & Genitalia

図 15.22　直腸の血管
後方から見たところ．主に直腸に分布するのは上直腸動脈である．中直腸動脈は上直腸動脈と下直腸動脈との間の吻合路となっている．

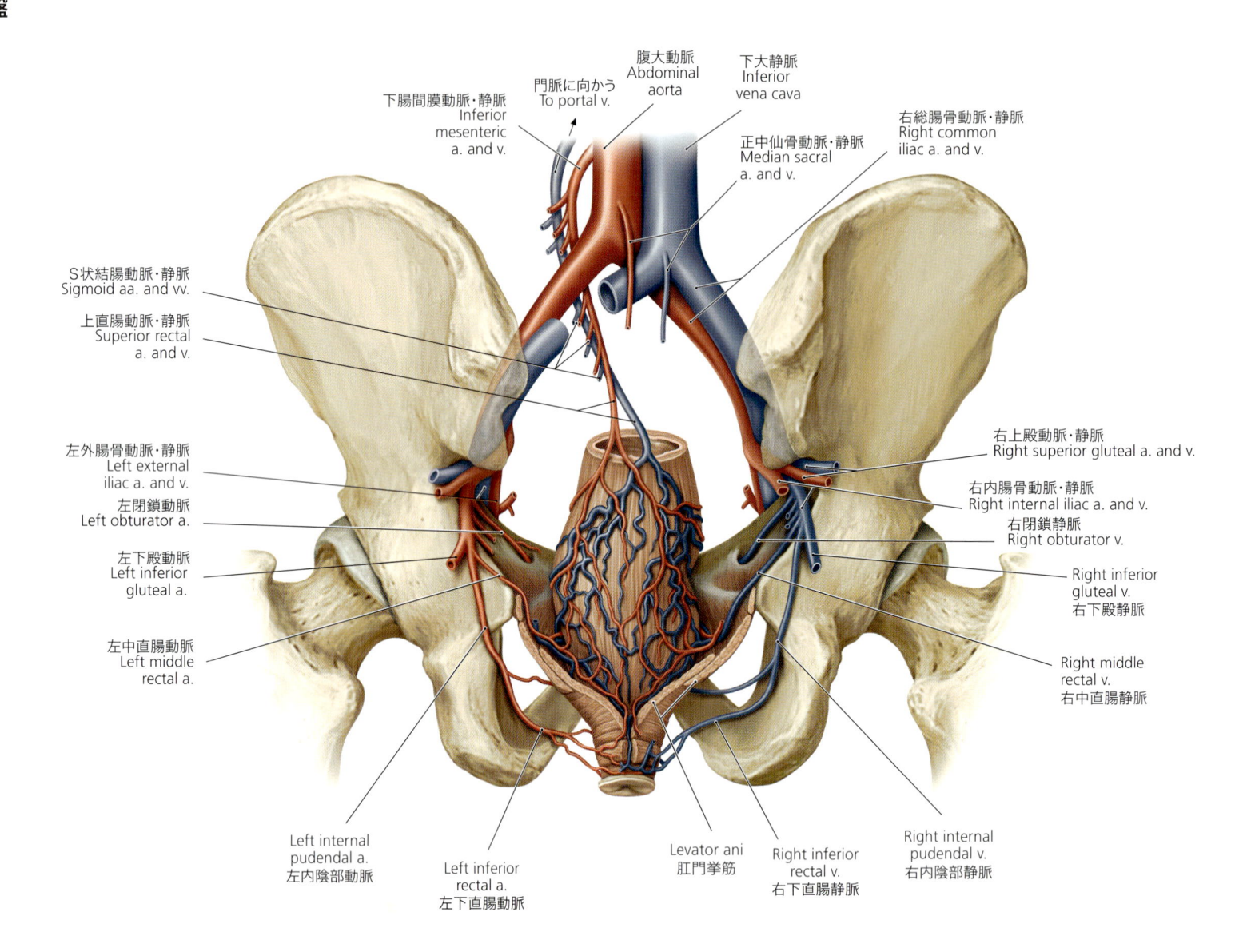

- 下腸間膜動脈・静脈 Inferior mesenteric a. and v.
- 門脈に向かう To portal v.
- 腹大動脈 Abdominal aorta
- 下大静脈 Inferior vena cava
- 正中仙骨動脈・静脈 Median sacral a. and v.
- 右総腸骨動脈・静脈 Right common iliac a. and v.
- S状結腸動脈・静脈 Sigmoid aa. and vv.
- 上直腸動脈・静脈 Superior rectal a. and v.
- 左外腸骨動脈・静脈 Left external iliac a. and v.
- 左閉鎖動脈 Left obturator a.
- 左下殿動脈 Left inferior gluteal a.
- 左中直腸動脈 Left middle rectal a.
- 右上殿動脈・静脈 Right superior gluteal a. and v.
- 右内腸骨動脈・静脈 Right internal iliac a. and v.
- 右閉鎖静脈 Right obturator v.
- 右下殿静脈 Right inferior gluteal v.
- 右中直腸静脈 Right middle rectal v.
- Left internal pudendal a. 左内陰部動脈
- Left inferior rectal a. 左下直腸動脈
- Levator ani 肛門挙筋
- Right inferior rectal v. 右下直腸静脈
- Right internal pudendal v. 右内陰部静脈

図 15.23 生殖器の血管
前方から見たところ．

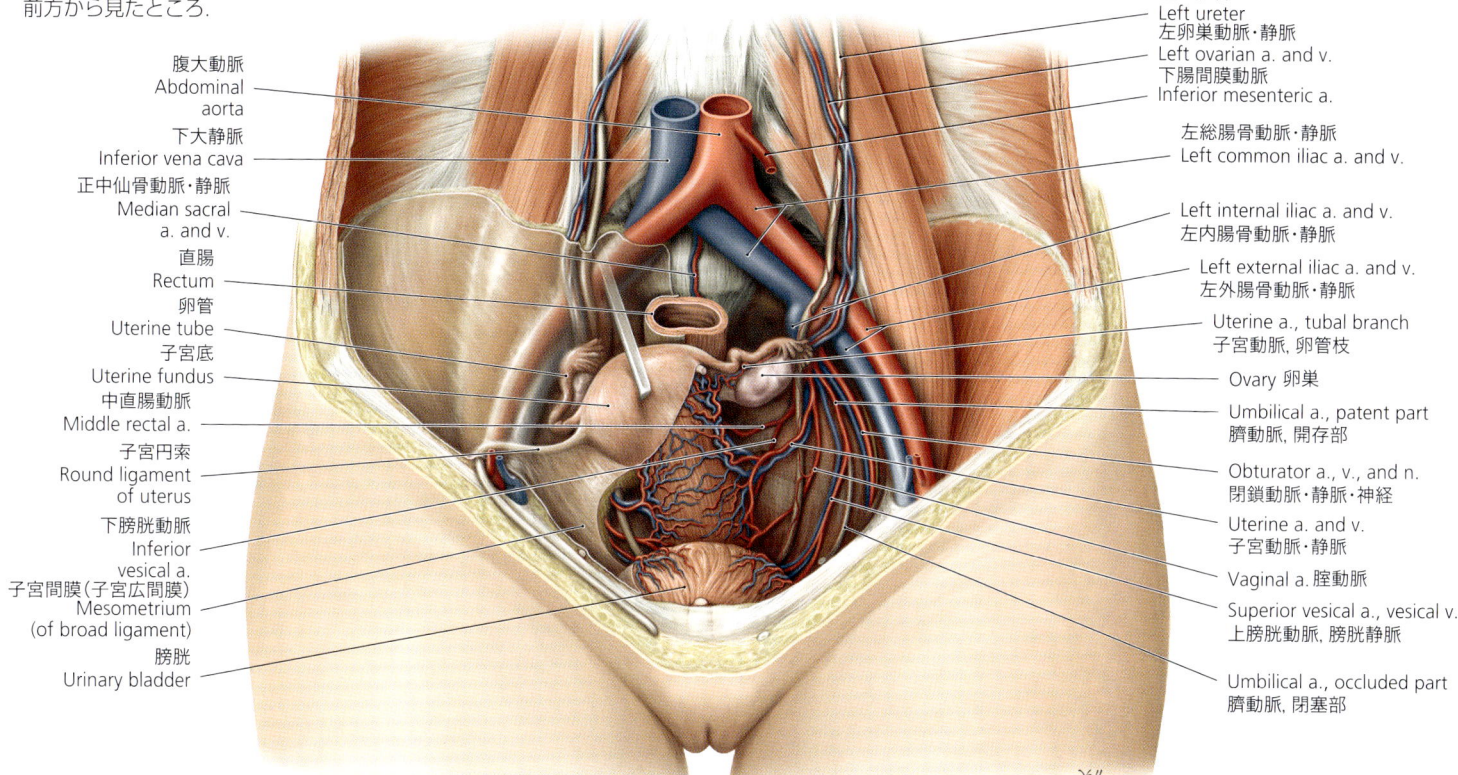

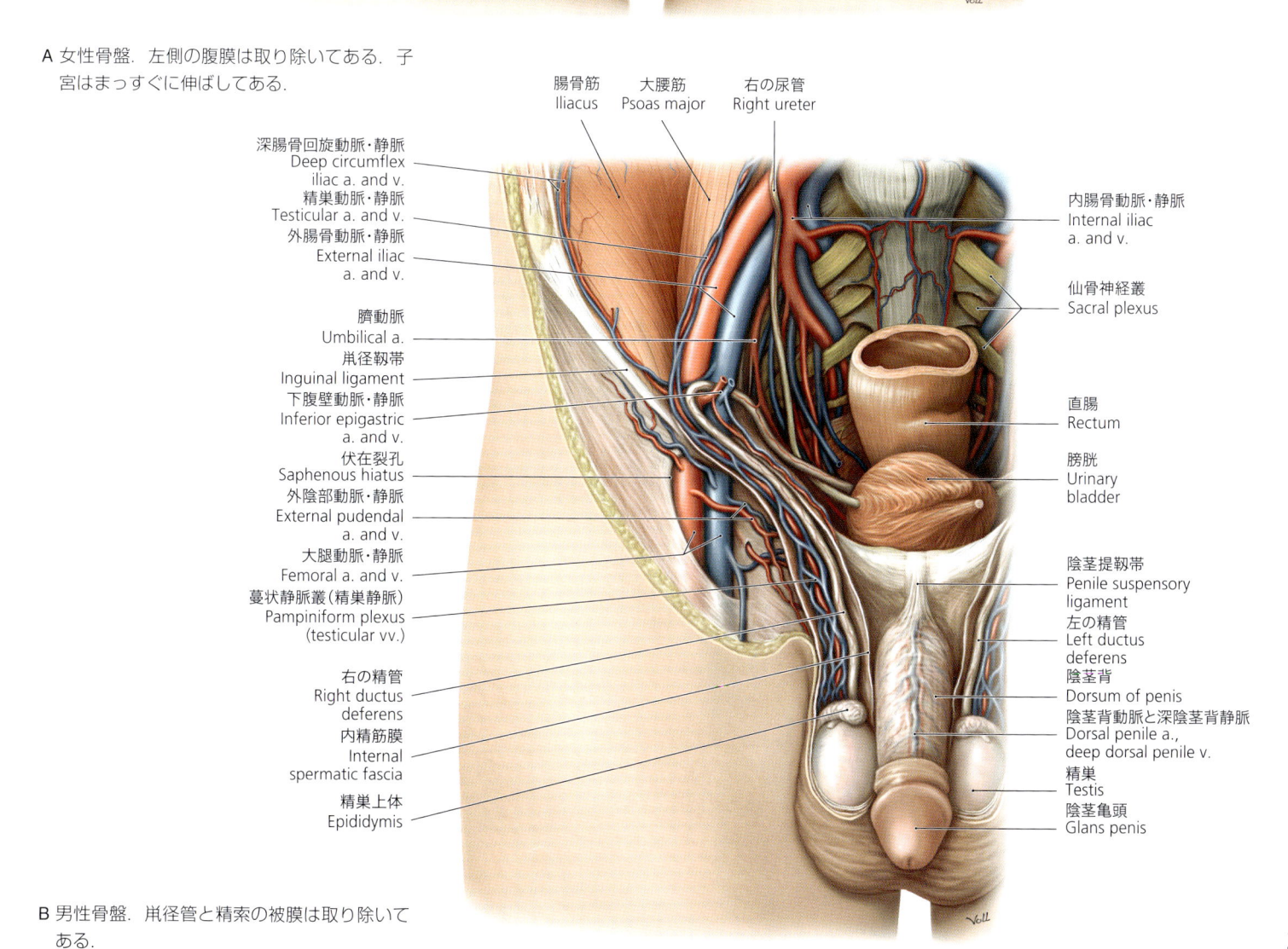

図Aラベル（女性骨盤）：
- 腹大動脈 / Abdominal aorta
- 下大静脈 / Inferior vena cava
- 正中仙骨動脈・静脈 / Median sacral a. and v.
- 直腸 / Rectum
- 卵管 / Uterine tube
- 子宮底 / Uterine fundus
- 中直腸動脈 / Middle rectal a.
- 子宮円索 / Round ligament of uterus
- 下膀胱動脈 / Inferior vesical a.
- 子宮間膜（子宮広間膜）/ Mesometrium (of broad ligament)
- 膀胱 / Urinary bladder
- 左の尿管 / Left ureter
- 左卵巣動脈・静脈 / Left ovarian a. and v.
- 下腸間膜動脈 / Inferior mesenteric a.
- 左総腸骨動脈・静脈 / Left common iliac a. and v.
- 左内腸骨動脈・静脈 / Left internal iliac a. and v.
- 左外腸骨動脈・静脈 / Left external iliac a. and v.
- 子宮動脈，卵管枝 / Uterine a., tubal branch
- 卵巣 / Ovary
- 臍動脈，開存部 / Umbilical a., patent part
- 閉鎖動脈・静脈・神経 / Obturator a., v., and n.
- 子宮動脈・静脈 / Uterine a. and v.
- 腟動脈 / Vaginal a.
- 上膀胱動脈，膀胱静脈 / Superior vesical a., vesical v.
- 臍動脈，閉塞部 / Umbilical a., occluded part

A 女性骨盤．左側の腹膜は取り除いてある．子宮はまっすぐに伸ばしてある．

図Bラベル（男性骨盤）：
- 深腸骨回旋動脈・静脈 / Deep circumflex iliac a. and v.
- 精巣動脈・静脈 / Testicular a. and v.
- 外腸骨動脈・静脈 / External iliac a. and v.
- 臍動脈 / Umbilical a.
- 鼠径靱帯 / Inguinal ligament
- 下腹壁動脈・静脈 / Inferior epigastric a. and v.
- 伏在裂孔 / Saphenous hiatus
- 外陰部動脈・静脈 / External pudendal a. and v.
- 大腿動脈・静脈 / Femoral a. and v.
- 蔓状静脈叢（精巣静脈）/ Pampiniform plexus (testicular vv.)
- 右の精管 / Right ductus deferens
- 内精筋膜 / Internal spermatic fascia
- 精巣上体 / Epididymis
- 腸骨筋 / Iliacus
- 大腰筋 / Psoas major
- 右の尿管 / Right ureter
- 内腸骨動脈・静脈 / Internal iliac a. and v.
- 仙骨神経叢 / Sacral plexus
- 直腸 / Rectum
- 膀胱 / Urinary bladder
- 陰茎提靱帯 / Penile suspensory ligament
- 左の精管 / Left ductus deferens
- 陰茎背 / Dorsum of penis
- 陰茎背動脈と深陰茎背静脈 / Dorsal penile a., deep dorsal penile v.
- 精巣 / Testis
- 陰茎亀頭 / Glans penis

B 男性骨盤．鼠径管と精索の被膜は取り除いてある．

腹部と骨盤部のリンパ節
Lymph Nodes of the Abdomen & Pelvis

図 16.1　内臓のリンパ流路

図中の番号については表 16.1 を参照．腹部，骨盤部，下肢からリンパは最終的には腰リンパ節（臨床では大動脈リンパ節と呼ばれる）を通過する．腰リンパ節は右外側大動脈（大静脈）リンパ節，左外側大動脈リンパ節，大動脈前リンパ節，大動脈後リンパ節からなる．腰リンパ節と大動脈前リンパ節からのリンパ管は，それぞれ腰リンパ本幹と腸リンパ本幹となる．腰リンパ本幹と腸リンパ本幹は乳ビ槽に至る．

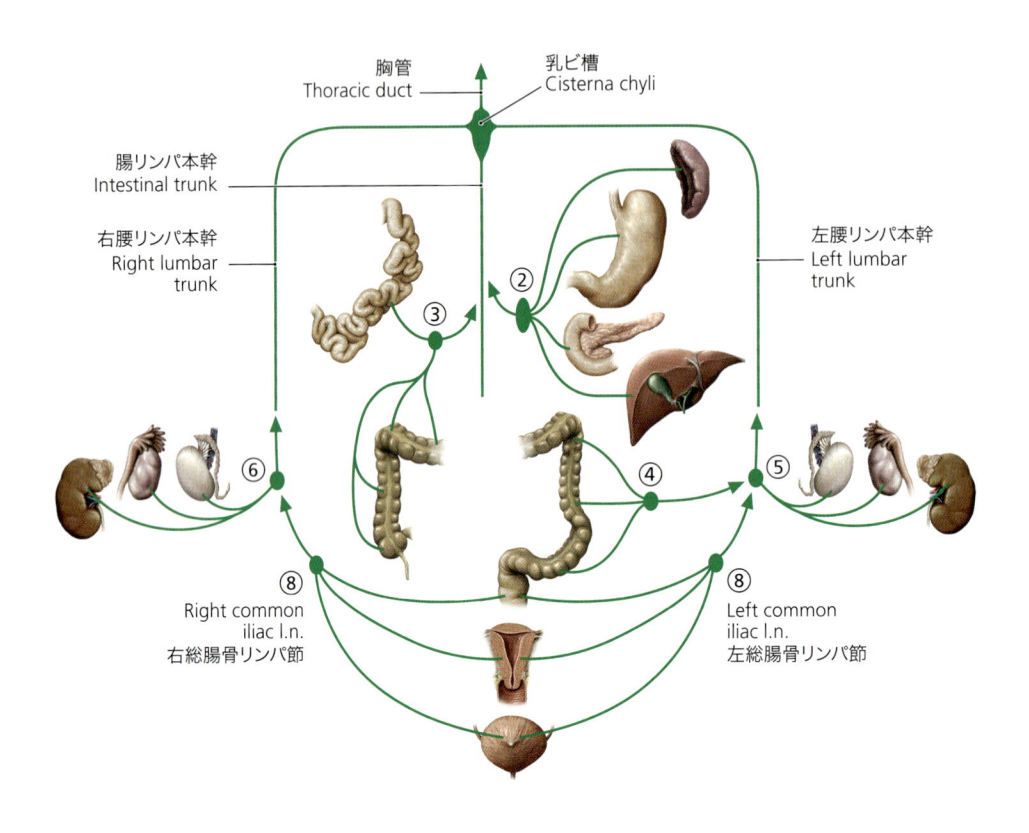

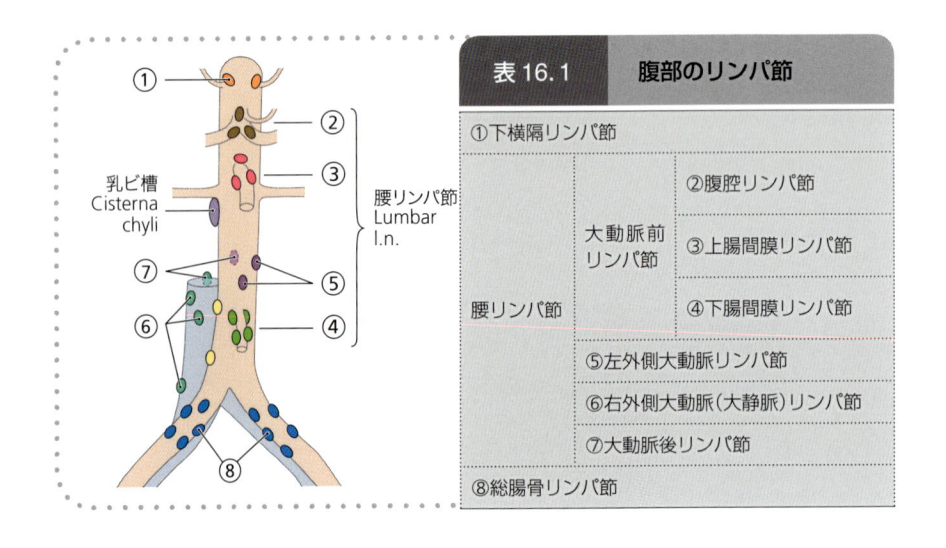

表 16.1	腹部のリンパ節		
①下横隔リンパ節			
腰リンパ節	大動脈前リンパ節	②腹腔リンパ節	
		③上腸間膜リンパ節	
		④下腸間膜リンパ節	
	⑤左外側大動脈リンパ節		
	⑥右外側大動脈（大静脈）リンパ節		
	⑦大動脈後リンパ節		
⑧総腸骨リンパ節			

図16.2　直腸のリンパ流路
前方から見たところ.

- 腹大動脈 Abdominal aorta
- 下腸間膜動脈, 下腸間膜リンパ節 Inferior mesenteric a. and l.n.
- 総腸骨動脈 Common iliac a.
- Superior rectal a. 上直腸動脈
- 内腸骨動脈, 内腸骨リンパ節 Internal iliac a. and l.n.
- 浅鼠径リンパ節 Superficial inguinal l.n.

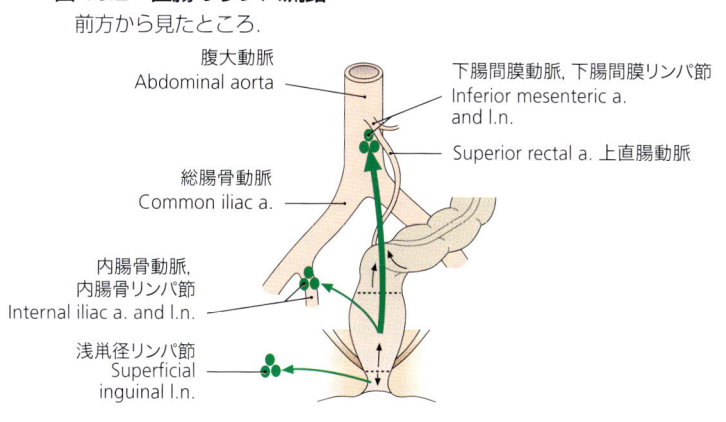

図16.3　膀胱と尿道のリンパ流路
前方から見たところ.

- 総腸骨リンパ節 Common iliac l.n.
- 内腸骨リンパ節 Internal iliac l.n.
- 浅・深鼠径リンパ節 Superficial and deep inguinal l.n.
- 外腸骨リンパ節 External iliac l.n.

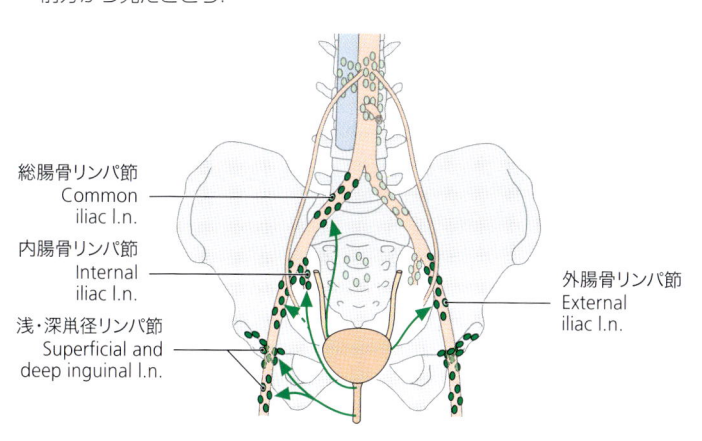

図16.4　男性生殖器のリンパ流路
前方から見たところ.

- 外側大動脈リンパ節 Lateral aortic l.n.
- 内腸骨リンパ節 Internal iliac l.n.
- 外腸骨リンパ節 External iliac l.n.
- 仙骨リンパ節 Sacral l.n.

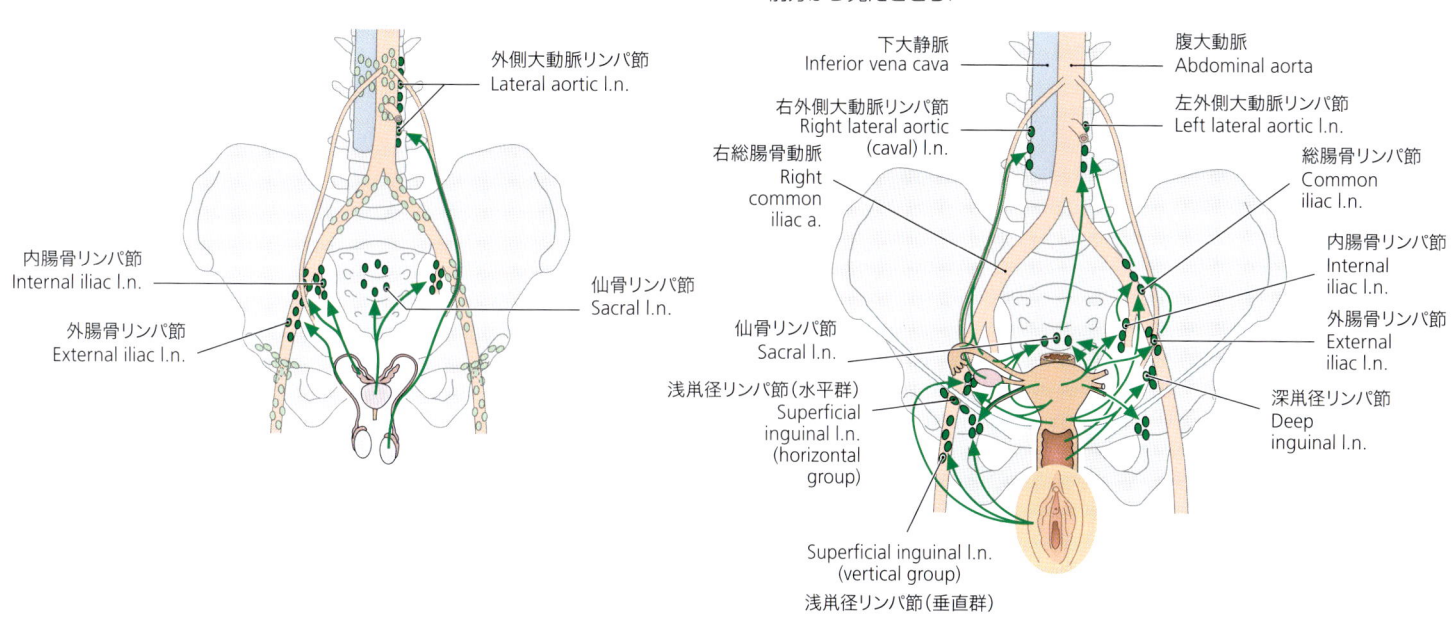

図16.5　女性生殖器のリンパ流路
前方から見たところ.

- 下大静脈 Inferior vena cava
- 腹大動脈 Abdominal aorta
- 右外側大動脈リンパ節 Right lateral aortic (caval) l.n.
- 左外側大動脈リンパ節 Left lateral aortic l.n.
- 右総腸骨動脈 Right common iliac a.
- 総腸骨リンパ節 Common iliac l.n.
- 内腸骨リンパ節 Internal iliac l.n.
- 外腸骨リンパ節 External iliac l.n.
- 仙骨リンパ節 Sacral l.n.
- 浅鼠径リンパ節（水平群） Superficial inguinal l.n. (horizontal group)
- 深鼠径リンパ節 Deep inguinal l.n.
- Superficial inguinal l.n. (vertical group) 浅鼠径リンパ節（垂直群）

水平群 Horizontal group
垂直群 Vertical group ⑪

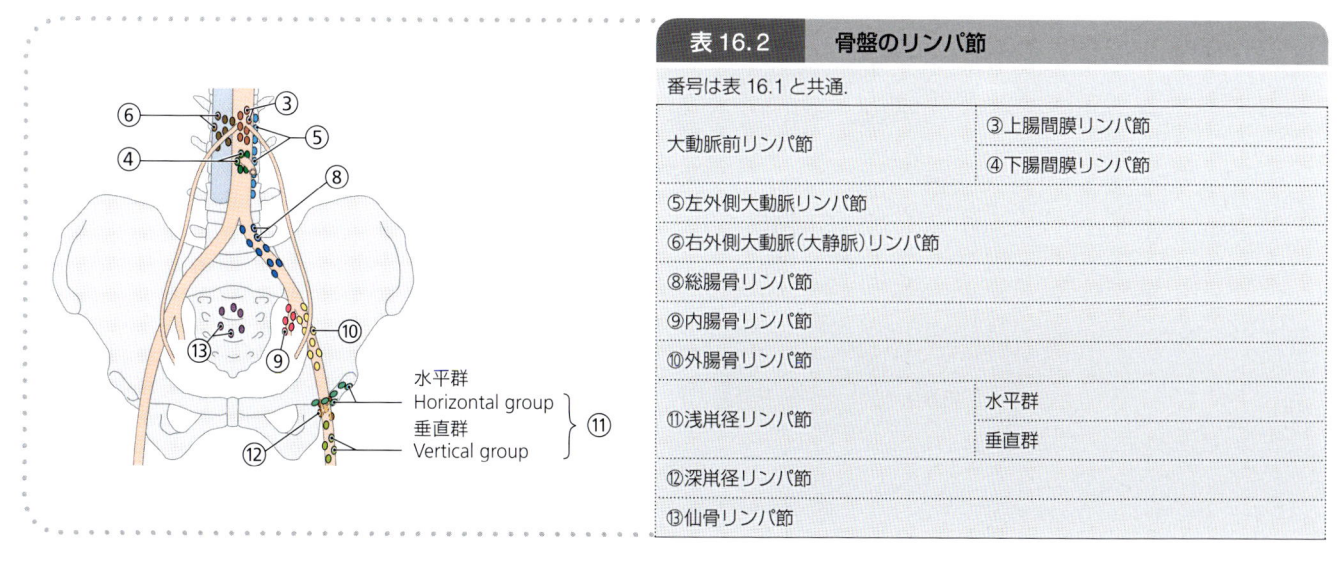

表16.2　骨盤のリンパ節

番号は表16.1と共通.

大動脈前リンパ節	③上腸間膜リンパ節
	④下腸間膜リンパ節
⑤左外側大動脈リンパ節	
⑥右外側大動脈（大静脈）リンパ節	
⑧総腸骨リンパ節	
⑨内腸骨リンパ節	
⑩外腸骨リンパ節	
⑪浅鼠径リンパ節	水平群
	垂直群
⑫深鼠径リンパ節	
⑬仙骨リンパ節	

後腹壁のリンパ節
Lymph Nodes of the Posterior Abdominal Wall

腹部と骨盤部のリンパ節は壁側と臓側に分類される．壁側リンパ節の大部分は後腹壁に位置する．

図 16.6 腹部と骨盤部の壁側リンパ節
前方から見たところ．血管以外の内臓はすべて取り除いてある．

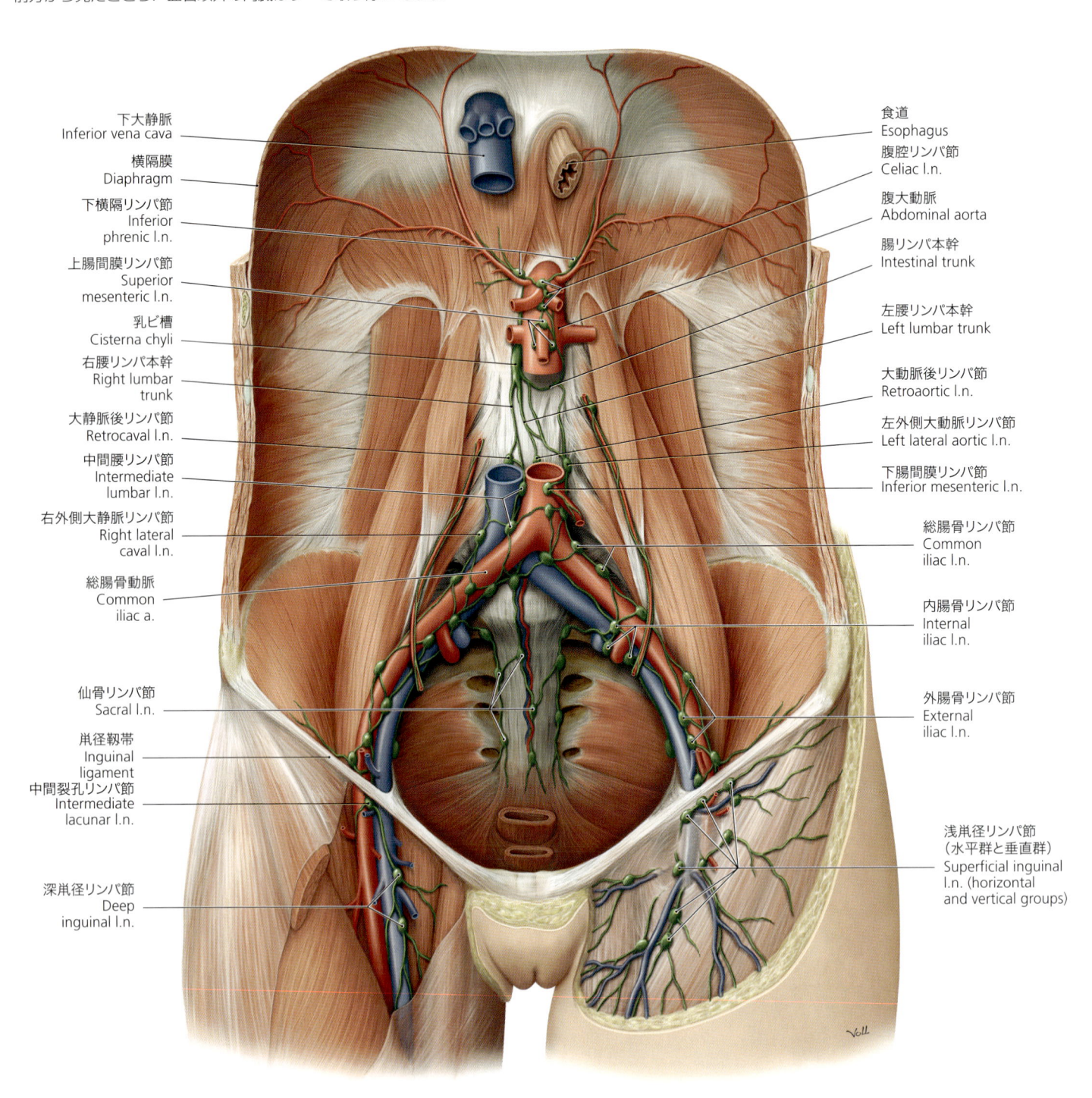

下大静脈 Inferior vena cava
横隔膜 Diaphragm
下横隔リンパ節 Inferior phrenic l.n.
上腸間膜リンパ節 Superior mesenteric l.n.
乳ビ槽 Cisterna chyli
右腰リンパ本幹 Right lumbar trunk
大静脈後リンパ節 Retrocaval l.n.
中間腰リンパ節 Intermediate lumbar l.n.
右外側大静脈リンパ節 Right lateral caval l.n.
総腸骨動脈 Common iliac a.
仙骨リンパ節 Sacral l.n.
鼠径靱帯 Inguinal ligament
中間裂孔リンパ節 Intermediate lacunar l.n.
深鼠径リンパ節 Deep inguinal l.n.

食道 Esophagus
腹腔リンパ節 Celiac l.n.
腹大動脈 Abdominal aorta
腸リンパ本幹 Intestinal trunk
左腰リンパ本幹 Left lumbar trunk
大動脈後リンパ節 Retroaortic l.n.
左外側大動脈リンパ節 Left lateral aortic l.n.
下腸間膜リンパ節 Inferior mesenteric l.n.
総腸骨リンパ節 Common iliac l.n.
内腸骨リンパ節 Internal iliac l.n.
外腸骨リンパ節 External iliac l.n.
浅鼠径リンパ節（水平群と垂直群）Superficial inguinal l.n. (horizontal and vertical groups)

図 16.7 泌尿器のリンパ節
前方から見たところ．

大静脈後リンパ節
Retrocaval l.n.

右外側大静脈リンパ節
Right lateral caval l.n.

中間腰リンパ節
Intermediate lumbar l.n.

岬角リンパ節
Promontory l.n.

下横隔リンパ節
Inferior phrenic l.n.

左外側大動脈リンパ節
Left lateral aortic l.n.

大動脈前リンパ節
Preaortic l.n.

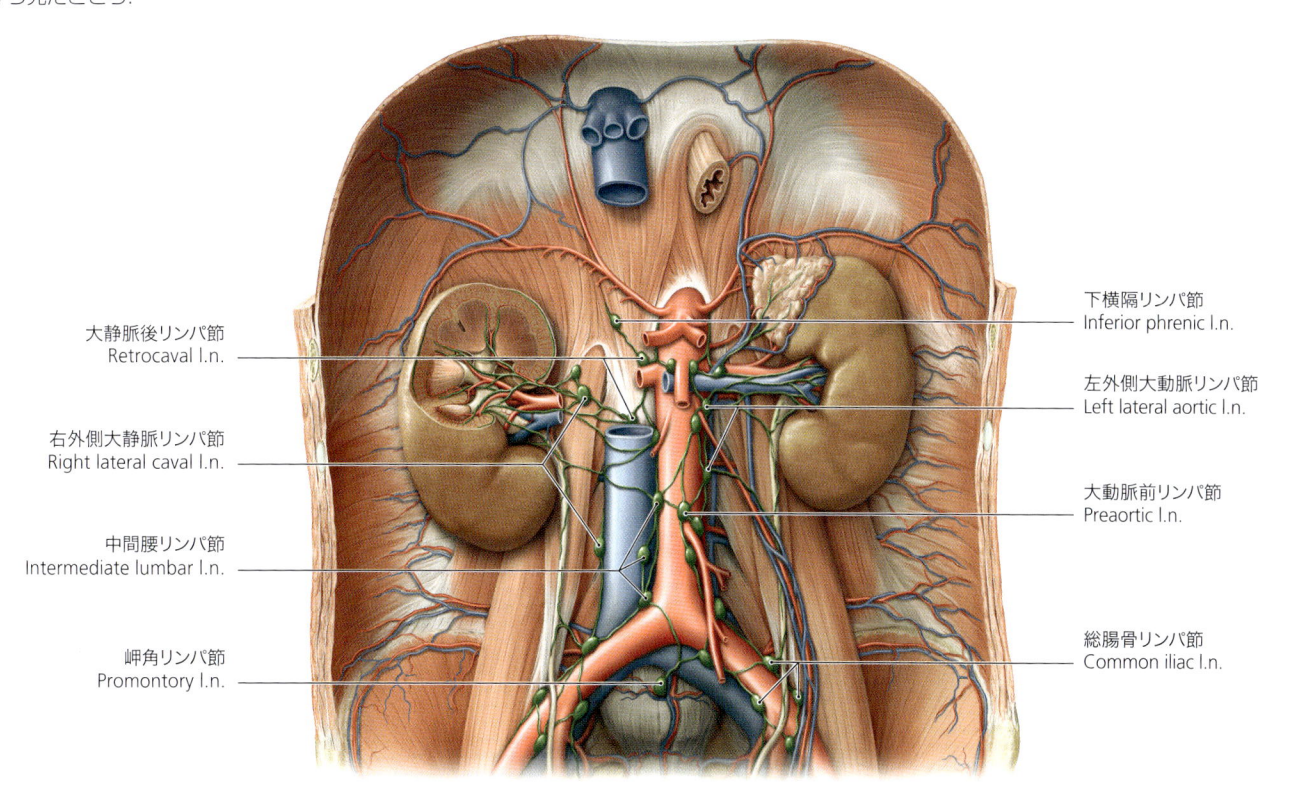

総腸骨リンパ節
Common iliac l.n.

図 16.8 腎臓と骨盤内臓のリンパ流路

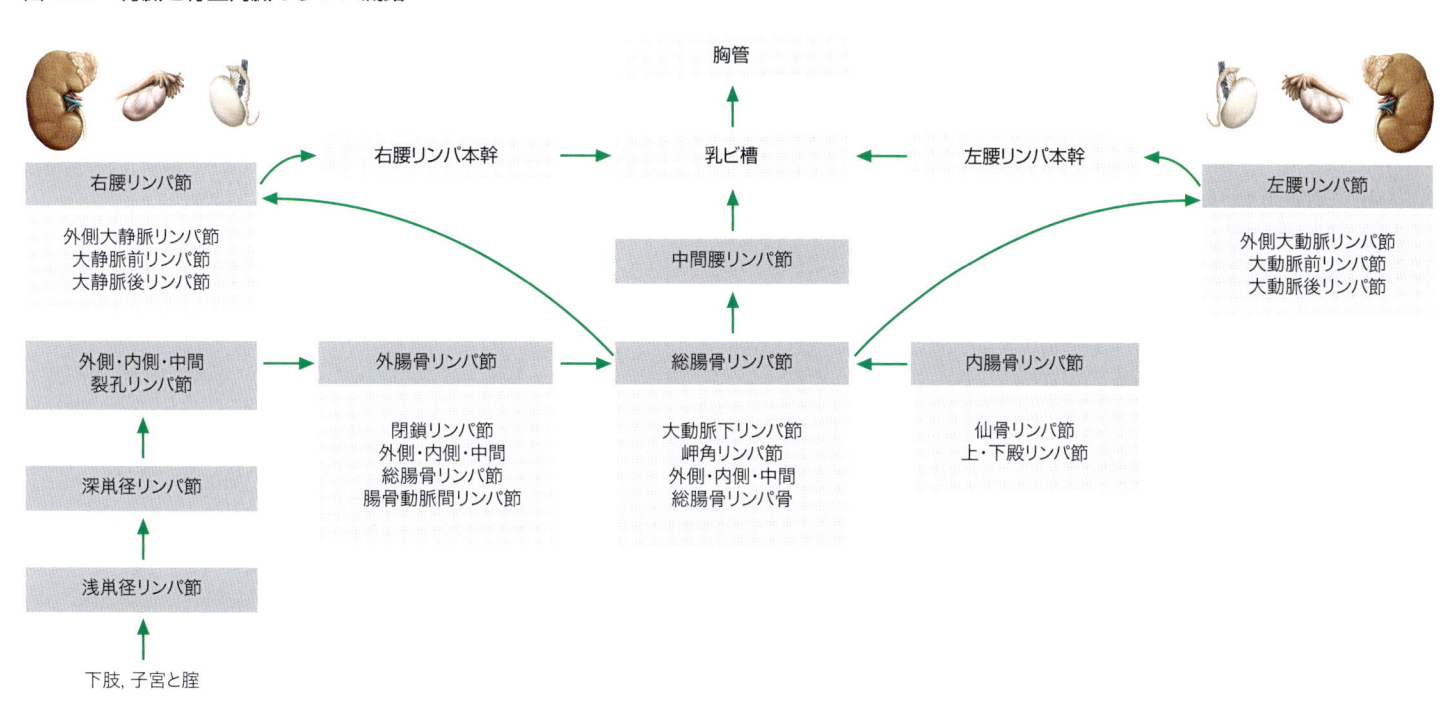

胸管 ← 乳ビ槽

右腰リンパ本幹 / 左腰リンパ本幹

右腰リンパ節
- 外側大静脈リンパ節
- 大静脈前リンパ節
- 大静脈後リンパ節

左腰リンパ節
- 外側大動脈リンパ節
- 大動脈前リンパ節
- 大動脈後リンパ節

中間腰リンパ節

外側・内側・中間 裂孔リンパ節 → 外腸骨リンパ節 → 総腸骨リンパ節 ← 内腸骨リンパ節

外腸骨リンパ節配下:
- 閉鎖リンパ節
- 外側・内側・中間総腸骨リンパ節
- 腸骨動脈間リンパ節

総腸骨リンパ節配下:
- 大動脈下リンパ節
- 岬角リンパ節
- 外側・内側・中間総腸骨リンパ骨

内腸骨リンパ節配下:
- 仙骨リンパ節
- 上・下殿リンパ節

深鼡径リンパ節 ← 浅鼡径リンパ節 ← 下肢, 子宮と腟

前腹部内臓のリンパ節
Lymph Nodes of the Anterior Abdominal Organs

図 16.9 胃と肝臓のリンパ節
前方から見たところ．小網は取り除いてある．大網は切り開いてある．
矢印はリンパ流路の方向を示す．

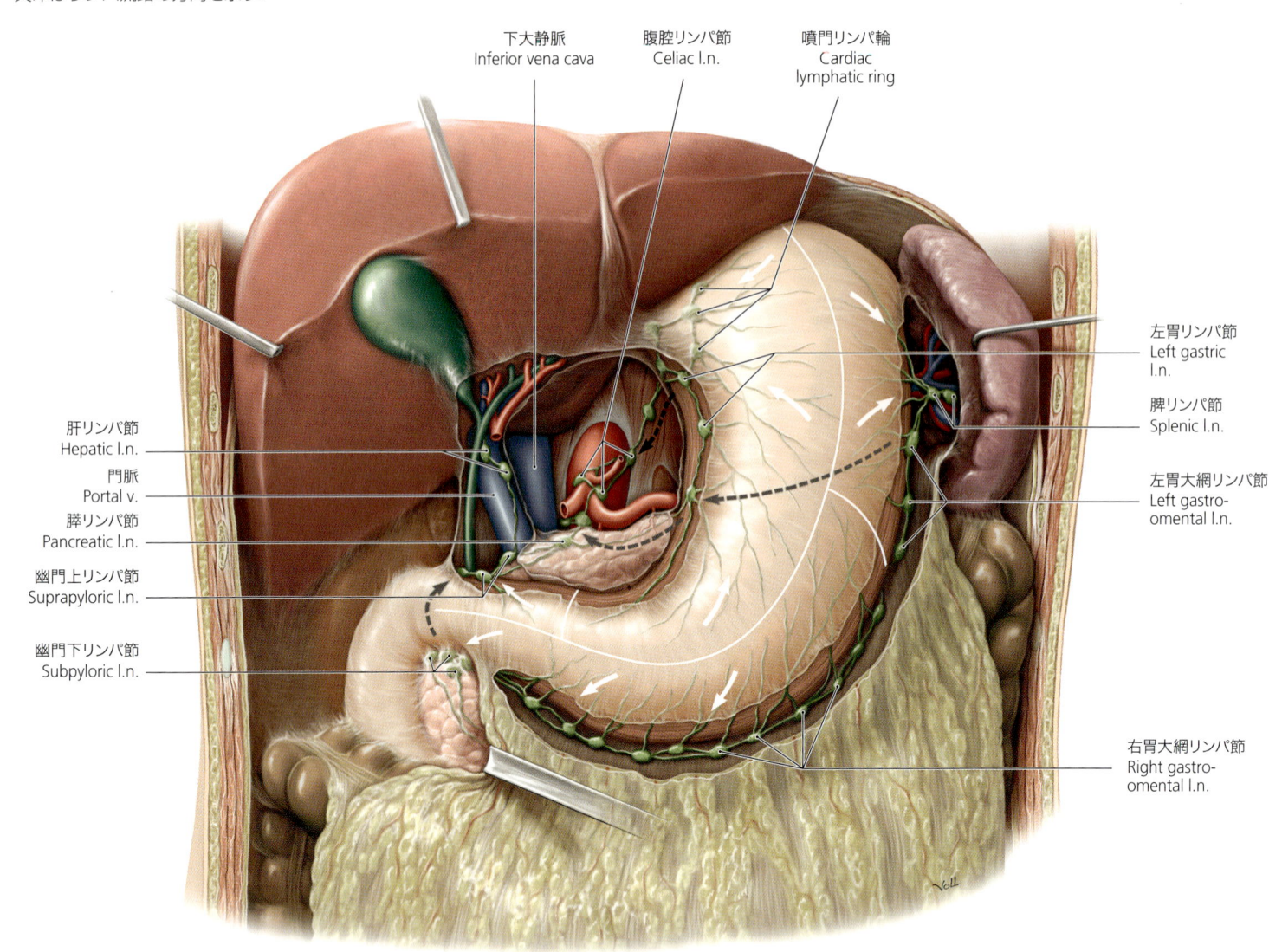

- 下大静脈 Inferior vena cava
- 腹腔リンパ節 Celiac l.n.
- 噴門リンパ輪 Cardiac lymphatic ring
- 左胃リンパ節 Left gastric l.n.
- 脾リンパ節 Splenic l.n.
- 左胃大網リンパ節 Left gastro-omental l.n.
- 肝リンパ節 Hepatic l.n.
- 門脈 Portal v.
- 膵リンパ節 Pancreatic l.n.
- 幽門上リンパ節 Suprapyloric l.n.
- 幽門下リンパ節 Subpyloric l.n.
- 右胃大網リンパ節 Right gastro-omental l.n.

図16.10 脾臓，膵臓，十二指腸のリンパ節
前方から見たところ．胃と結腸は取り除いてある．

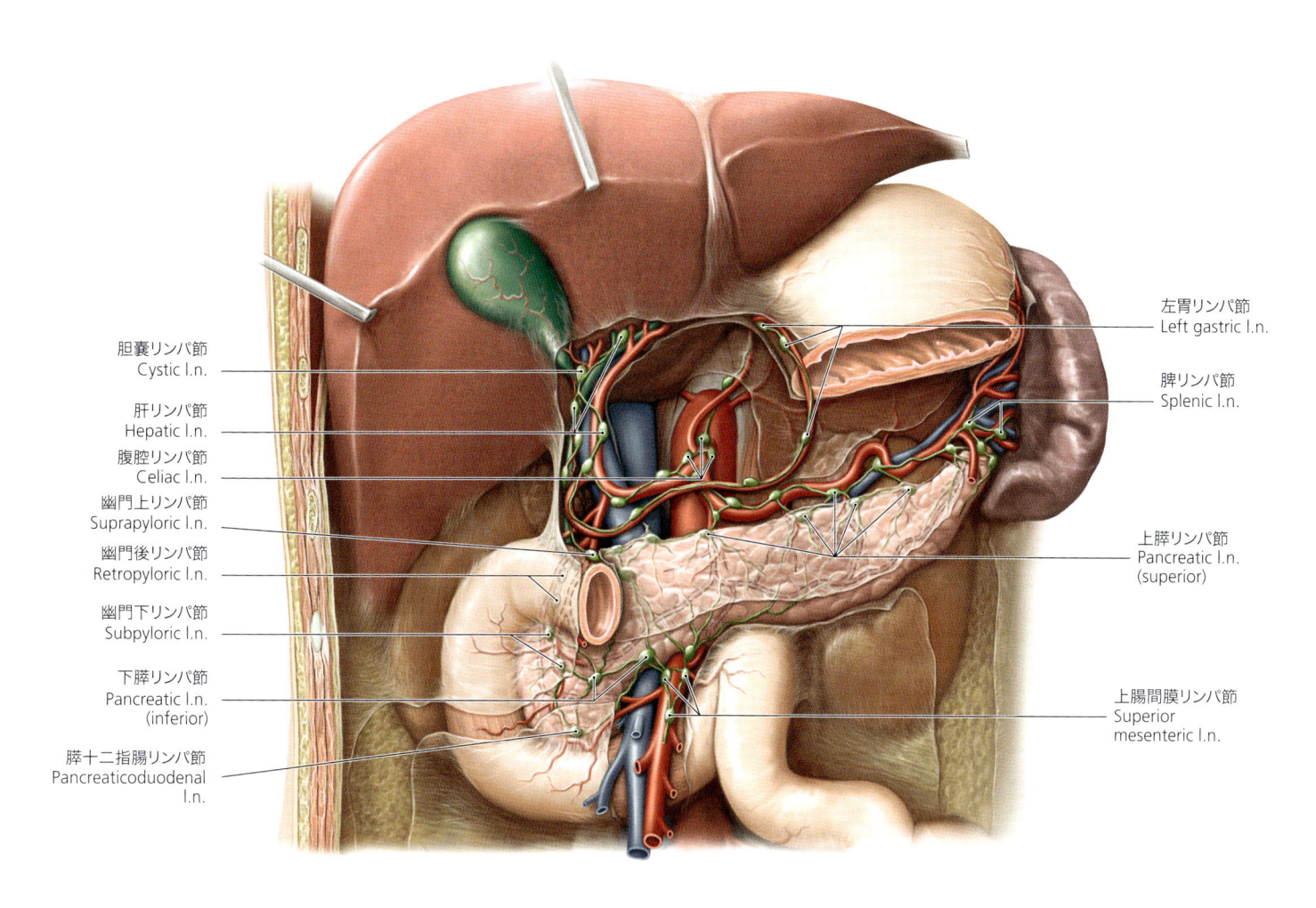

- 胆嚢リンパ節 Cystic l.n.
- 肝リンパ節 Hepatic l.n.
- 腹腔リンパ節 Celiac l.n.
- 幽門上リンパ節 Suprapyloric l.n.
- 幽門後リンパ節 Retropyloric l.n.
- 幽門下リンパ節 Subpyloric l.n.
- 下膵リンパ節 Pancreatic l.n. (inferior)
- 膵十二指腸リンパ節 Pancreaticoduodenal l.n.
- 左胃リンパ節 Left gastric l.n.
- 脾リンパ節 Splenic l.n.
- 上膵リンパ節 Pancreatic l.n. (superior)
- 上腸間膜リンパ節 Superior mesenteric l.n.

図16.11 胃，肝臓，脾臓，膵臓，十二指腸のリンパ流路

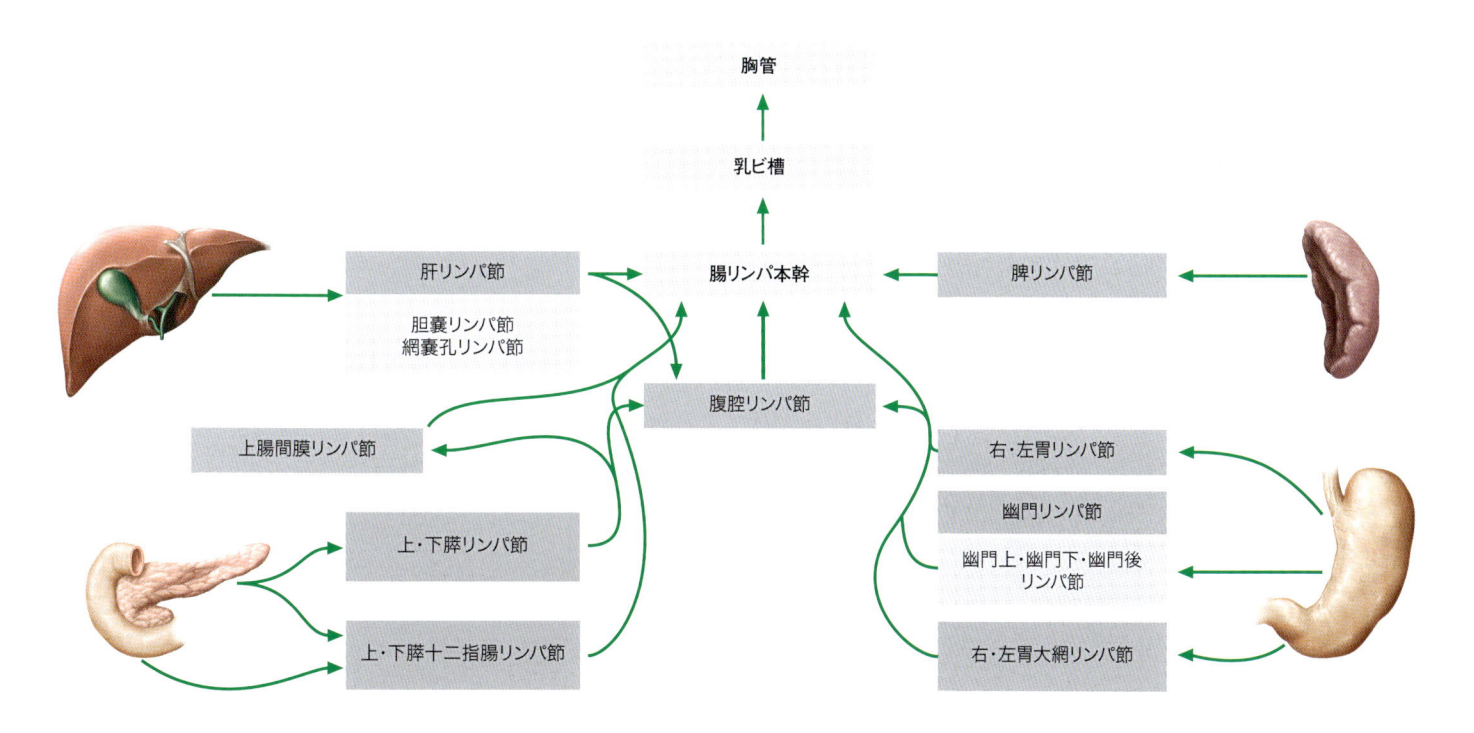

胸管 ← 乳ビ槽 ← 腸リンパ本幹

- 肝リンパ節（胆嚢リンパ節，網嚢孔リンパ節）
- 脾リンパ節
- 腹腔リンパ節
- 上腸間膜リンパ節
- 上・下膵リンパ節
- 上・下膵十二指腸リンパ節
- 右・左胃リンパ節
- 幽門リンパ節
- 幽門上・幽門下・幽門後リンパ節
- 右・左胃大網リンパ節

腸のリンパ節
Lymph Nodes of the Intestines

図 16.12　空腸と回腸のリンパ節
前方から見たところ．胃，肝臓，膵臓，結腸は取り除いてある．

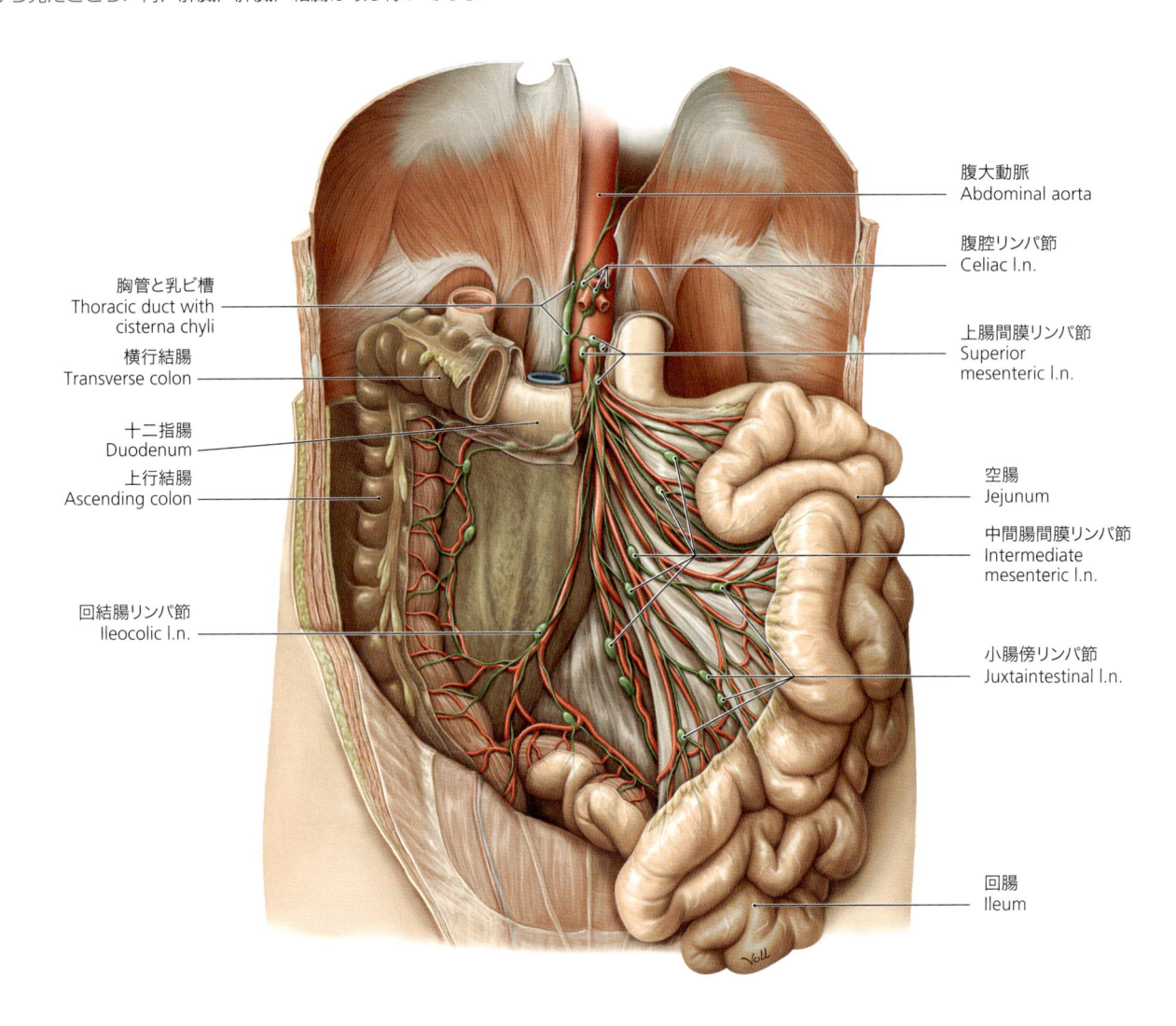

- 胸管と乳ビ槽　Thoracic duct with cisterna chyli
- 横行結腸　Transverse colon
- 十二指腸　Duodenum
- 上行結腸　Ascending colon
- 回結腸リンパ節　Ileocolic l.n.
- 腹大動脈　Abdominal aorta
- 腹腔リンパ節　Celiac l.n.
- 上腸間膜リンパ節　Superior mesenteric l.n.
- 空腸　Jejunum
- 中間腸間膜リンパ節　Intermediate mesenteric l.n.
- 小腸傍リンパ節　Juxtaintestinal l.n.
- 回腸　Ileum

図 16.13　腸のリンパ流路

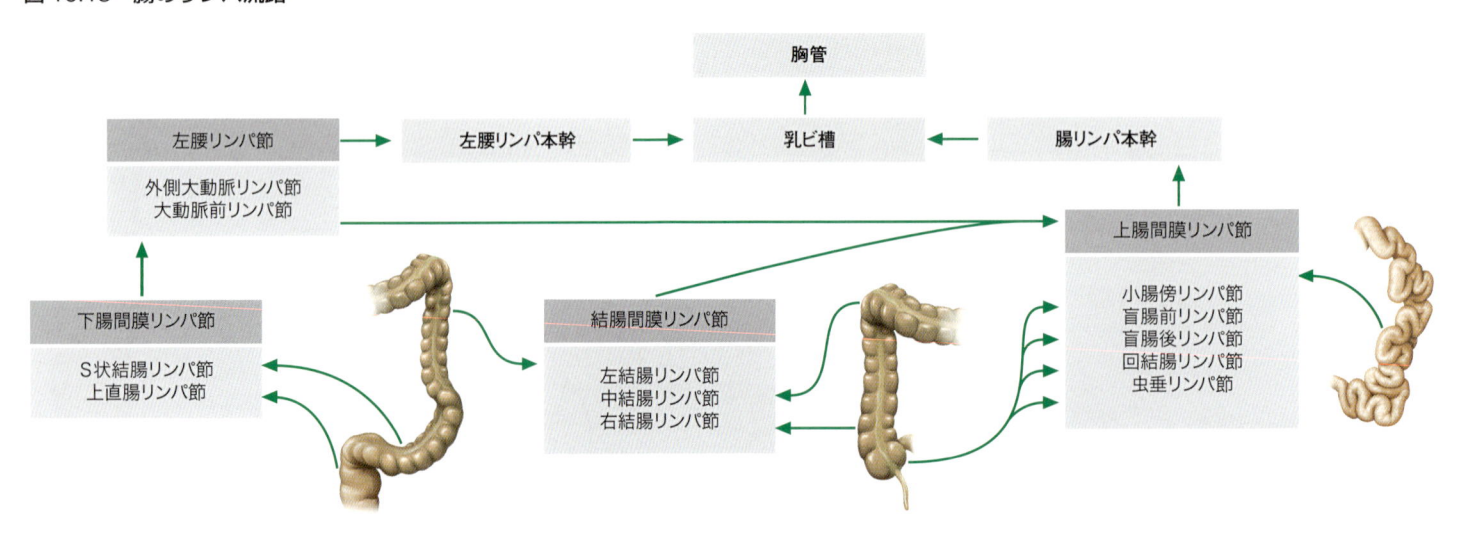

左腰リンパ節 → 左腰リンパ本幹 → 乳ビ槽 ← 腸リンパ本幹 → 胸管

- 外側大動脈リンパ節
- 大動脈前リンパ節

↑

- 下腸間膜リンパ節
  - S状結腸リンパ節
  - 上直腸リンパ節

→ 結腸間膜リンパ節
  - 左結腸リンパ節
  - 中結腸リンパ節
  - 右結腸リンパ節

→ 上腸間膜リンパ節
  - 小腸傍リンパ節
  - 盲腸前リンパ節
  - 盲腸後リンパ節
  - 回結腸リンパ節
  - 虫垂リンパ節

図 16.14　大腸のリンパ節
前方から見たところ．横行結腸と大網は翻転．

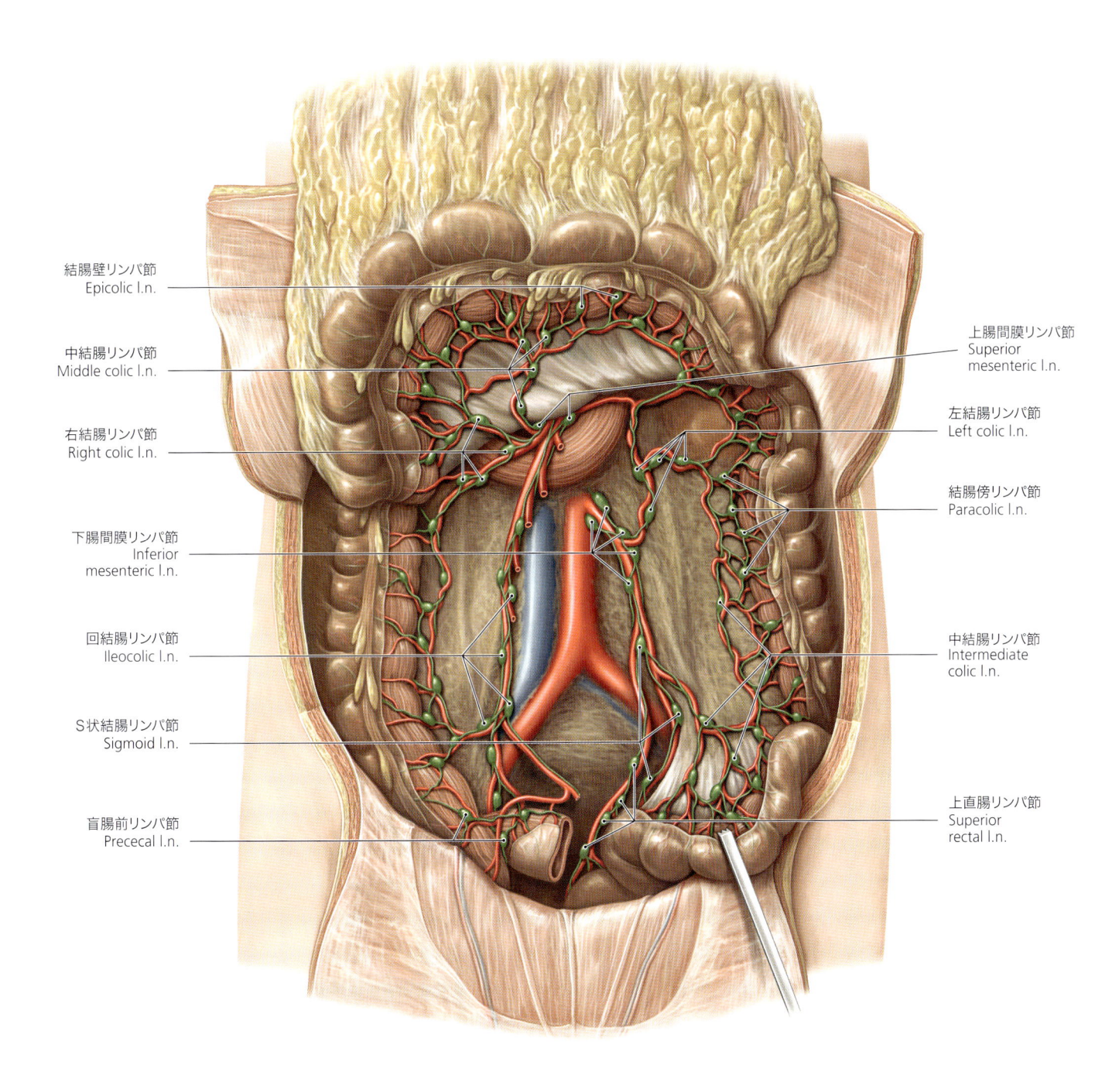

- 結腸壁リンパ節 Epicolic l.n.
- 中結腸リンパ節 Middle colic l.n.
- 右結腸リンパ節 Right colic l.n.
- 下腸間膜リンパ節 Inferior mesenteric l.n.
- 回結腸リンパ節 Ileocolic l.n.
- S状結腸リンパ節 Sigmoid l.n.
- 盲腸前リンパ節 Prececal l.n.
- 上腸間膜リンパ節 Superior mesenteric l.n.
- 左結腸リンパ節 Left colic l.n.
- 結腸傍リンパ節 Paracolic l.n.
- 中結腸リンパ節 Intermediate colic l.n.
- 上直腸リンパ節 Superior rectal l.n.

生殖器のリンパ節
Lymph Nodes of the Genitalia

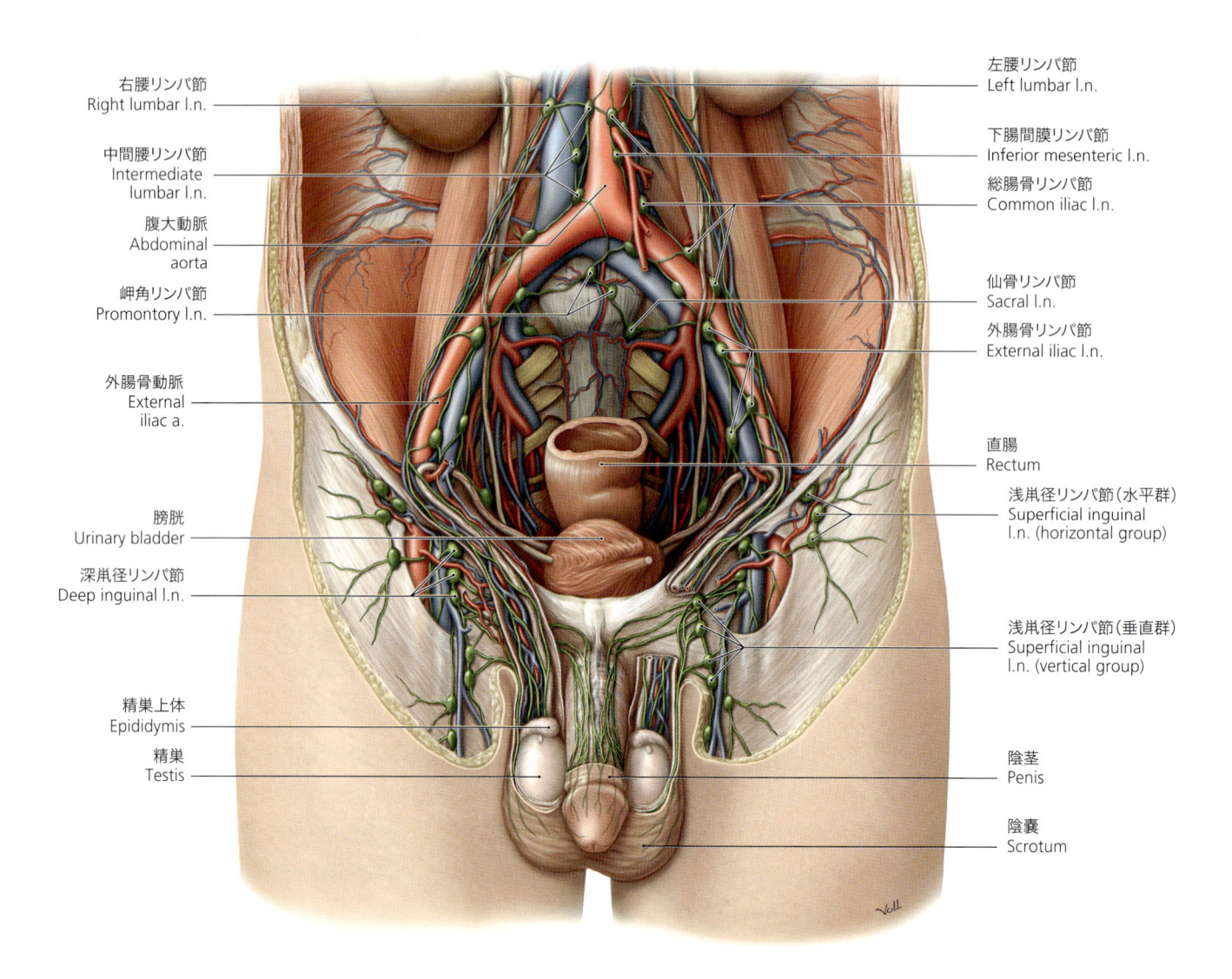

図 16.15　男性生殖器のリンパ節
前方から見たところ．直腸断端を除く消化管と腹膜は取り除いてある．

- 右腰リンパ節 / Right lumbar l.n.
- 中間腰リンパ節 / Intermediate lumbar l.n.
- 腹大動脈 / Abdominal aorta
- 岬角リンパ節 / Promontory l.n.
- 外腸骨動脈 / External iliac a.
- 膀胱 / Urinary bladder
- 深鼠径リンパ節 / Deep inguinal l.n.
- 精巣上体 / Epididymis
- 精巣 / Testis
- 左腰リンパ節 / Left lumbar l.n.
- 下腸間膜リンパ節 / Inferior mesenteric l.n.
- 総腸骨リンパ節 / Common iliac l.n.
- 仙骨リンパ節 / Sacral l.n.
- 外腸骨リンパ節 / External iliac l.n.
- 直腸 / Rectum
- 浅鼠径リンパ節（水平群）/ Superficial inguinal l.n. (horizontal group)
- 浅鼠径リンパ節（垂直群）/ Superficial inguinal l.n. (vertical group)
- 陰茎 / Penis
- 陰嚢 / Scrotum

図 16.16　女性生殖器のリンパ節

前方から見たところ．直腸断端を除く消化管と腹膜は取り除いてある．子宮は右方へ引いてある．

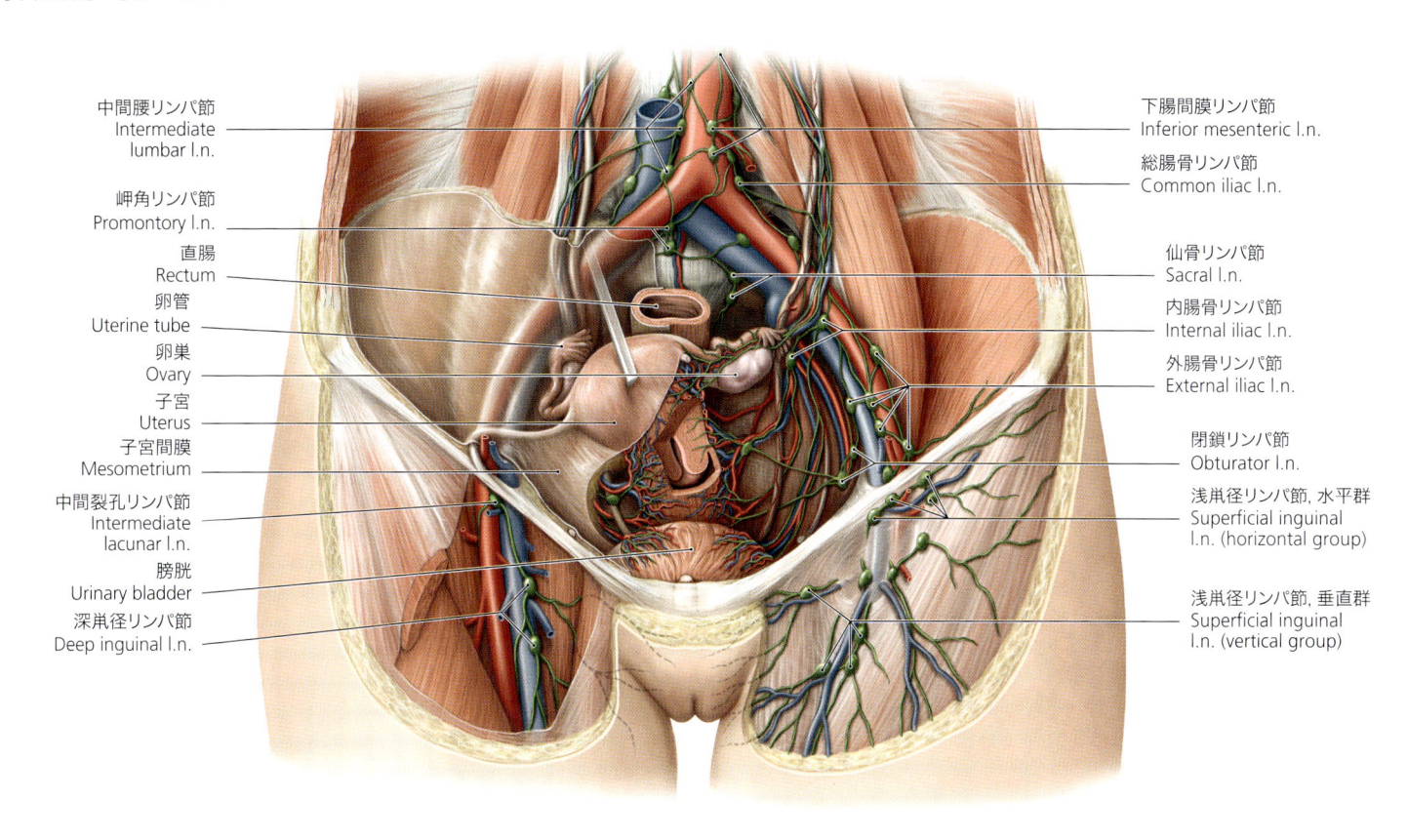

ラベル（左側）：
- 中間腰リンパ節 Intermediate lumbar l.n.
- 岬角リンパ節 Promontory l.n.
- 直腸 Rectum
- 卵管 Uterine tube
- 卵巣 Ovary
- 子宮 Uterus
- 子宮間膜 Mesometrium
- 中間裂孔リンパ節 Intermediate lacunar l.n.
- 膀胱 Urinary bladder
- 深鼠径リンパ節 Deep inguinal l.n.

ラベル（右側）：
- 下腸間膜リンパ節 Inferior mesenteric l.n.
- 総腸骨リンパ節 Common iliac l.n.
- 仙骨リンパ節 Sacral l.n.
- 内腸骨リンパ節 Internal iliac l.n.
- 外腸骨リンパ節 External iliac l.n.
- 閉鎖リンパ節 Obturator l.n.
- 浅鼠径リンパ節，水平群 Superficial inguinal l.n. (horizontal group)
- 浅鼠径リンパ節，垂直群 Superficial inguinal l.n. (vertical group)

図 16.17　骨盤内臓のリンパ流路

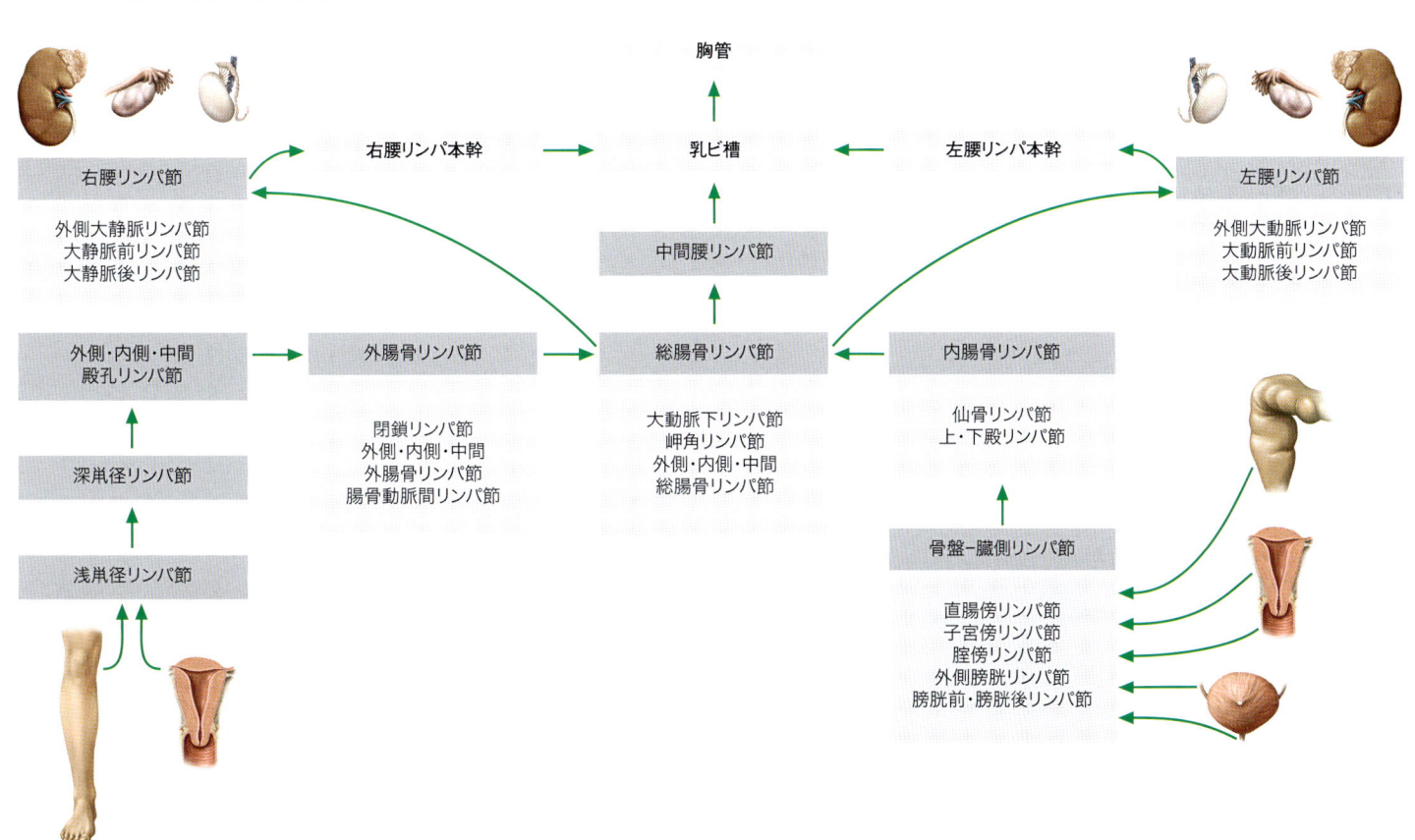

胸管
↑
右腰リンパ本幹 → 乳ビ槽 ← 左腰リンパ本幹

右腰リンパ節 ←→ 中間腰リンパ節 ←→ 左腰リンパ節
- 外側大静脈リンパ節
- 大静脈前リンパ節
- 大静脈後リンパ節

左腰リンパ節：
- 外側大動脈リンパ節
- 大動脈前リンパ節
- 大動脈後リンパ節

外側・内側・中間殿孔リンパ節 → 外腸骨リンパ節 → 総腸骨リンパ節 ← 内腸骨リンパ節

↑
深鼠径リンパ節
↑
浅鼠径リンパ節

外腸骨リンパ節：
- 閉鎖リンパ節
- 外側・内側・中間外腸骨リンパ節
- 腸骨動脈間リンパ節

総腸骨リンパ節：
- 大動脈下リンパ節
- 岬角リンパ節
- 外側・内側・中間総腸骨リンパ節

内腸骨リンパ節：
- 仙骨リンパ節
- 上・下殿リンパ節

骨盤-臓側リンパ節
- 直腸傍リンパ節
- 子宮傍リンパ節
- 腟傍リンパ節
- 外側膀胱リンパ節
- 膀胱前・膀胱後リンパ節

自律神経叢
Autonomous Plexuses

腹部・骨盤

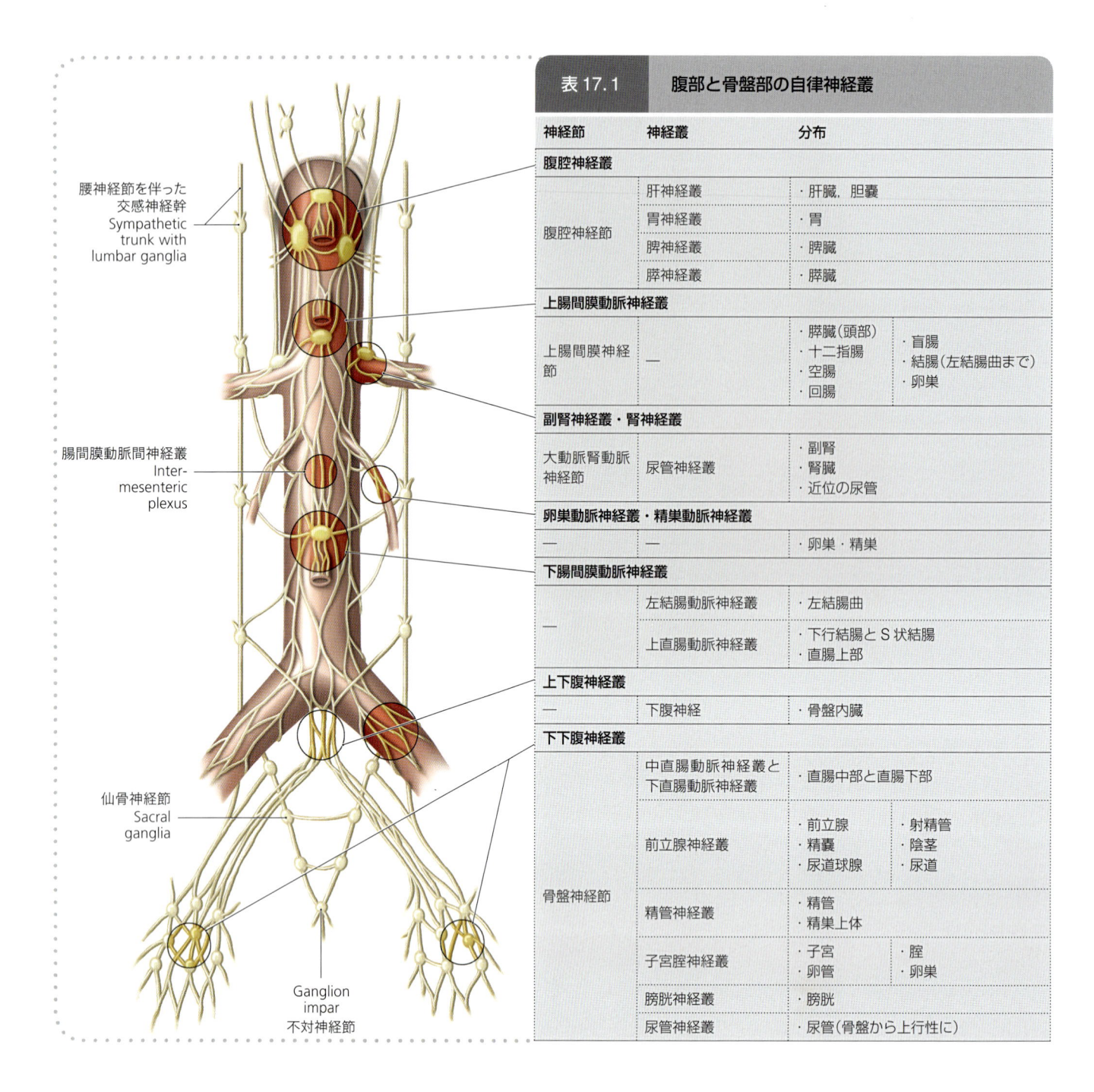

腰神経節を伴った交感神経幹
Sympathetic trunk with lumbar ganglia

腸間膜動脈間神経叢
Inter-mesenteric plexus

仙骨神経節
Sacral ganglia

Ganglion impar
不対神経節

表17.1 腹部と骨盤部の自律神経叢

神経節	神経叢	分布
腹腔神経叢		
腹腔神経節	肝神経叢	・肝臓, 胆嚢
	胃神経叢	・胃
	脾神経叢	・脾臓
	膵神経叢	・膵臓
上腸間膜動脈神経叢		
上腸間膜神経節	—	・膵臓（頭部）・盲腸 ・十二指腸・結腸（左結腸曲まで） ・空腸・卵巣 ・回腸
副腎神経叢・腎神経叢		
大動脈腎動脈神経節	尿管神経叢	・副腎 ・腎臓 ・近位の尿管
卵巣動脈神経叢・精巣動脈神経叢		
—	—	・卵巣・精巣
下腸間膜動脈神経叢		
—	左結腸動脈神経叢	・左結腸曲
	上直腸動脈神経叢	・下行結腸とS状結腸 ・直腸上部
上下腹神経叢		
—	下腹神経	・骨盤内臓
下下腹神経叢		
骨盤神経節	中直腸動脈神経叢と下直腸動脈神経叢	・直腸中部と直腸下部
	前立腺神経叢	・前立腺・射精管 ・精嚢・陰茎 ・尿道球腺・尿道
	精管神経叢	・精管 ・精巣上体
	子宮腟神経叢	・子宮・腟 ・卵管・卵巣
	膀胱神経叢	・膀胱
	尿管神経叢	・尿管（骨盤から上行性に）

図 17.1 腹部と骨盤部の自律神経叢

男性腹部を前方から見たところ．腹膜と胃の大部分は取り除いてある．

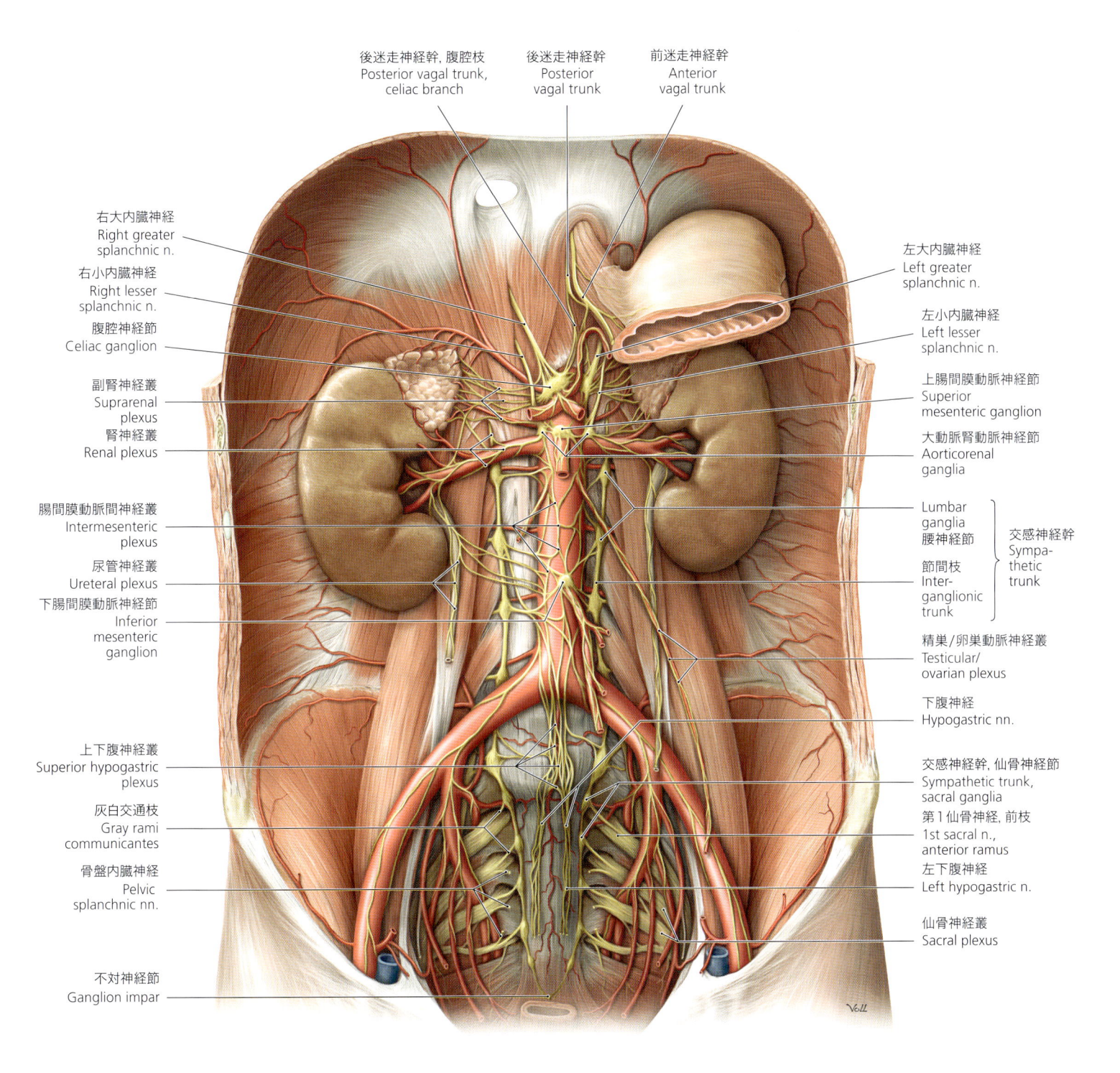

17 神経系

ラベル（左側、上から下へ）:
- 右大内臓神経 Right greater splanchnic n.
- 右小内臓神経 Right lesser splanchnic n.
- 腹腔神経節 Celiac ganglion
- 副腎神経叢 Suprarenal plexus
- 腎神経叢 Renal plexus
- 腸間膜動脈間神経叢 Intermesenteric plexus
- 尿管神経叢 Ureteral plexus
- 下腸間膜動脈神経節 Inferior mesenteric ganglion
- 上下腹神経叢 Superior hypogastric plexus
- 灰白交通枝 Gray rami communicantes
- 骨盤内臓神経 Pelvic splanchnic nn.
- 不対神経節 Ganglion impar

ラベル（上部）:
- 後迷走神経幹, 腹腔枝 Posterior vagal trunk, celiac branch
- 後迷走神経幹 Posterior vagal trunk
- 前迷走神経幹 Anterior vagal trunk

ラベル（右側、上から下へ）:
- 左大内臓神経 Left greater splanchnic n.
- 左小内臓神経 Left lesser splanchnic n.
- 上腸間膜動脈神経節 Superior mesenteric ganglion
- 大動脈腎動脈神経節 Aorticorenal ganglia
- 交感神経幹 Sympathetic trunk
  - Lumbar ganglia 腰神経節
  - 節間枝 Interganglionic trunk
- 精巣/卵巣動脈神経叢 Testicular/ovarian plexus
- 下腹神経 Hypogastric nn.
- 交感神経幹, 仙骨神経節 Sympathetic trunk, sacral ganglia
- 第1仙骨神経, 前枝 1st sacral n., anterior ramus
- 左下腹神経 Left hypogastric n.
- 仙骨神経叢 Sacral plexus

237

腹部内臓の神経支配
Innervation of the Abdominal Organs

図 17.2　前腹部内臓の神経支配
　前方から見たところ．小網，上行結腸，横行結腸の一部は取り除いてある．
網嚢は開いてある．前迷走神経幹と後迷走神経幹は腹腔枝，肝枝，幽門枝，
胃神経叢を出す．模式図は p.245 参照．

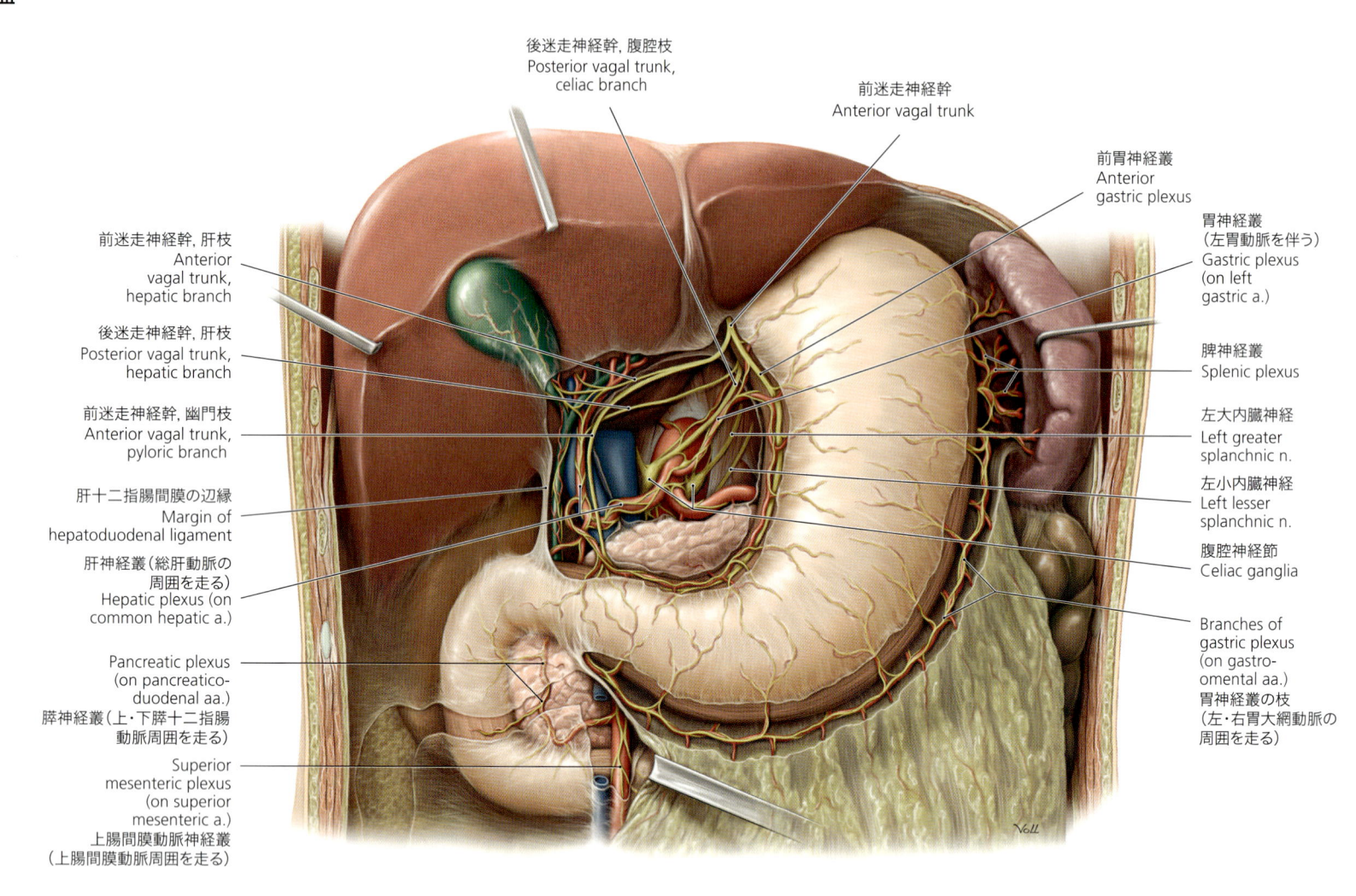

図 17.3 泌尿器の神経支配

男性腹部と骨盤を前方から見たところ．腹部内臓と腹膜は取り除いてある．模式図は p.246 参照．

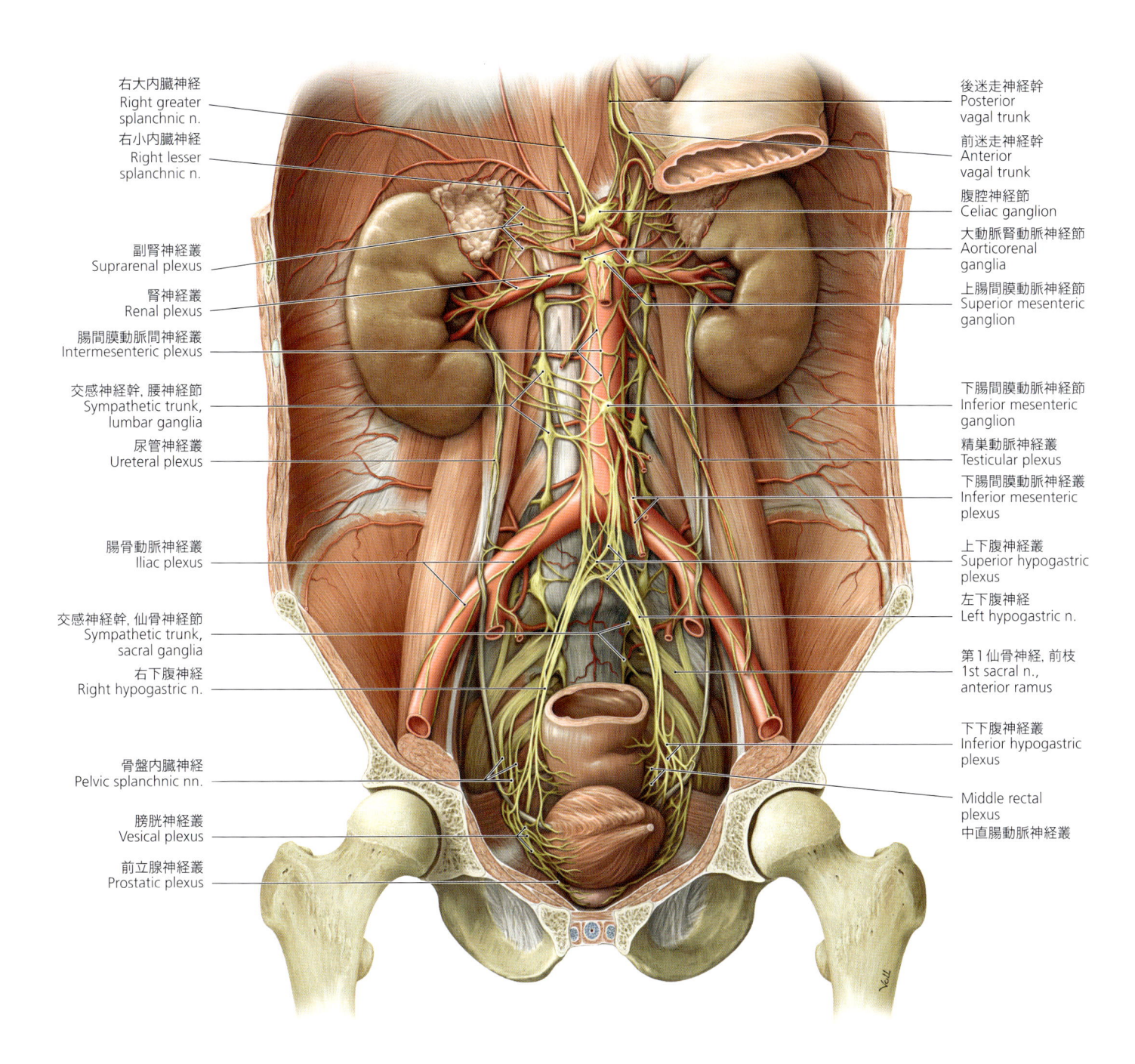

右大内臓神経 Right greater splanchnic n.
右小内臓神経 Right lesser splanchnic n.
副腎神経叢 Suprarenal plexus
腎神経叢 Renal plexus
腸間膜動脈間神経叢 Intermesenteric plexus
交感神経幹, 腰神経節 Sympathetic trunk, lumbar ganglia
尿管神経叢 Ureteral plexus
腸骨動脈神経叢 Iliac plexus
交感神経幹, 仙骨神経節 Sympathetic trunk, sacral ganglia
右下腹神経 Right hypogastric n.
骨盤内臓神経 Pelvic splanchnic nn.
膀胱神経叢 Vesical plexus
前立腺神経叢 Prostatic plexus

後迷走神経幹 Posterior vagal trunk
前迷走神経幹 Anterior vagal trunk
腹腔神経節 Celiac ganglion
大動脈腎動脈神経節 Aorticorenal ganglia
上腸間膜動脈神経節 Superior mesenteric ganglion
下腸間膜動脈神経節 Inferior mesenteric ganglion
精巣動脈神経叢 Testicular plexus
下腸間膜動脈神経叢 Inferior mesenteric plexus
上下腹神経叢 Superior hypogastric plexus
左下腹神経 Left hypogastric n.
第1仙骨神経, 前枝 1st sacral n., anterior ramus
下下腹神経叢 Inferior hypogastric plexus
Middle rectal plexus 中直腸動脈神経叢

腸の神経支配
Innervation of the Intestines

図 17.4　小腸の神経支配
前方から見たところ．胃，膵臓，横行結腸の遠位部は一部取り除いてある．
模式図は p.245 参照．

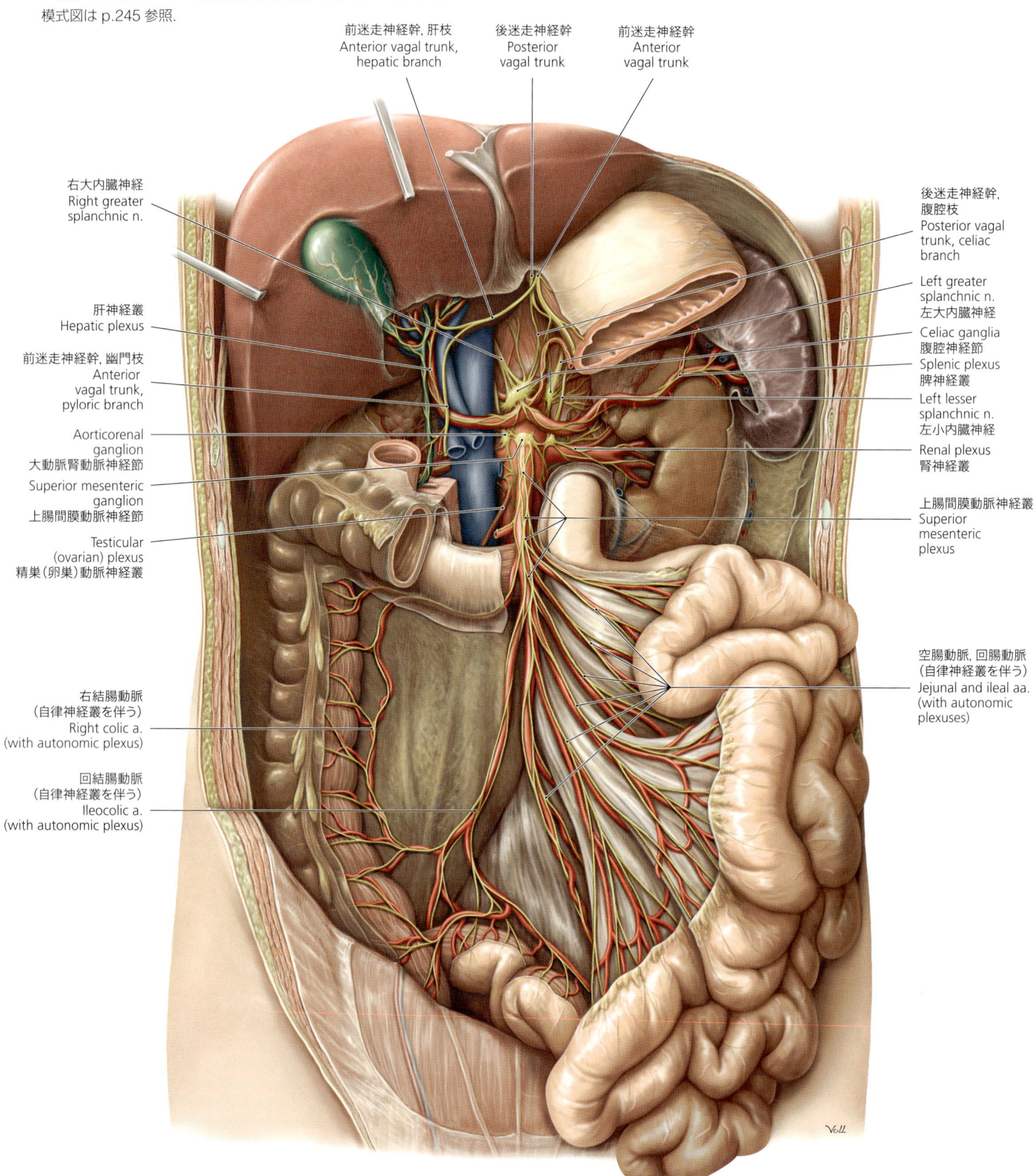

Labels:
- 前迷走神経幹, 肝枝 / Anterior vagal trunk, hepatic branch
- 後迷走神経幹 / Posterior vagal trunk
- 前迷走神経幹 / Anterior vagal trunk
- 右大内臓神経 / Right greater splanchnic n.
- 肝神経叢 / Hepatic plexus
- 前迷走神経幹, 幽門枝 / Anterior vagal trunk, pyloric branch
- Aorticorenal ganglion / 大動脈腎動脈神経節
- Superior mesenteric ganglion / 上腸間膜動脈神経節
- Testicular (ovarian) plexus / 精巣（卵巣）動脈神経叢
- 右結腸動脈（自律神経叢を伴う）/ Right colic a. (with autonomic plexus)
- 回結腸動脈（自律神経叢を伴う）/ Ileocolic a. (with autonomic plexus)
- 後迷走神経幹, 腹腔枝 / Posterior vagal trunk, celiac branch
- Left greater splanchnic n. / 左大内臓神経
- Celiac ganglia / 腹腔神経節
- Splenic plexus / 脾神経叢
- Left lesser splanchnic n. / 左小内臓神経
- Renal plexus / 腎神経叢
- 上腸間膜動脈神経叢 / Superior mesenteric plexus
- 空腸動脈, 回腸動脈（自律神経叢を伴う）/ Jejunal and ileal aa. (with autonomic plexuses)

図 17.5 大腸の神経支配

前から見たところ．空腸と回腸は取り除いてある．横行結腸を上に，S状結腸を下に翻転．模式図は p.245 参照．

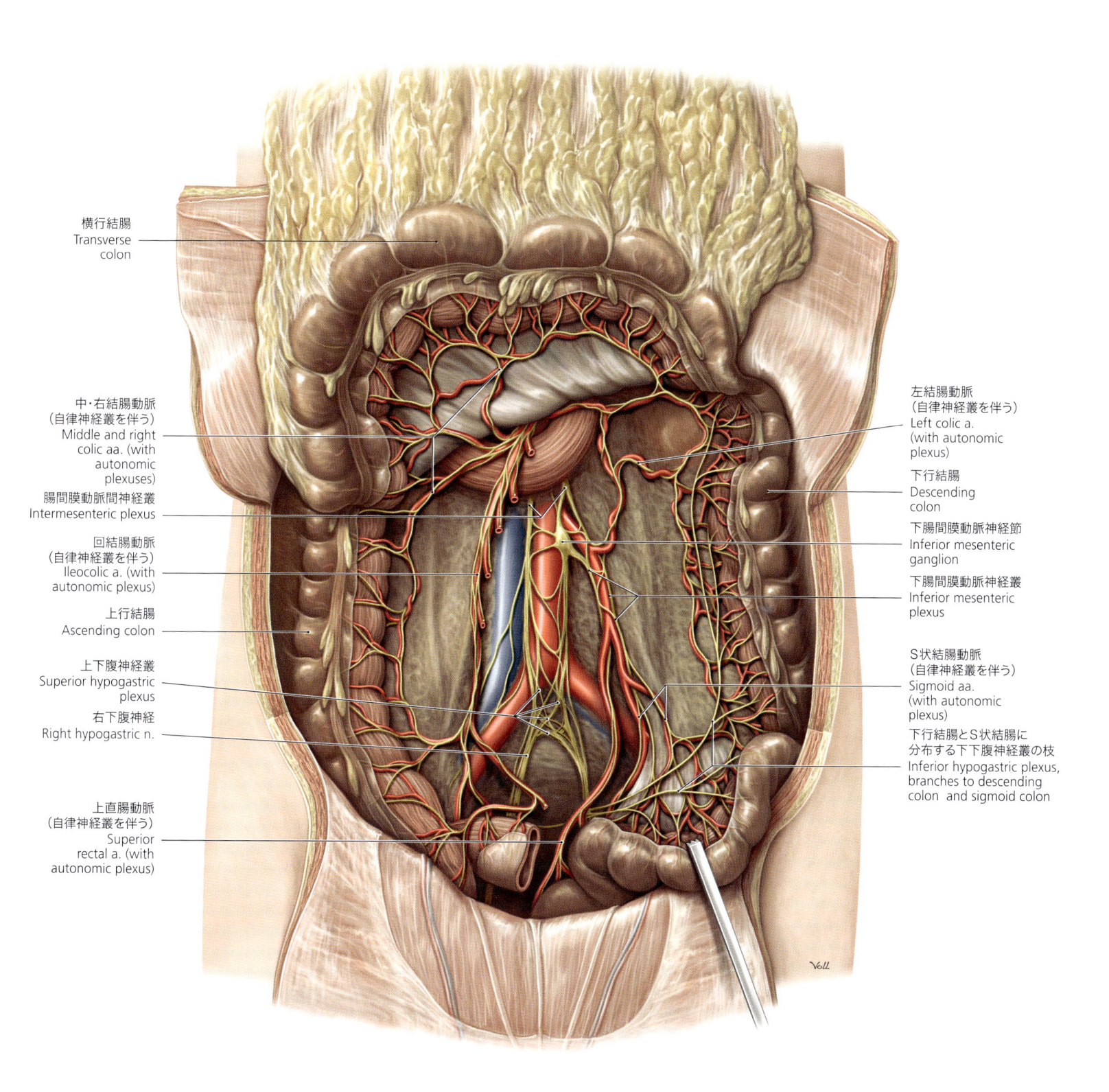

- 横行結腸 Transverse colon
- 中・右結腸動脈（自律神経叢を伴う）Middle and right colic aa. (with autonomic plexuses)
- 腸間膜動脈間神経叢 Intermesenteric plexus
- 回結腸動脈（自律神経叢を伴う）Ileocolic a. (with autonomic plexus)
- 上行結腸 Ascending colon
- 上下腹神経叢 Superior hypogastric plexus
- 右下腹神経 Right hypogastric n.
- 上直腸動脈（自律神経叢を伴う）Superior rectal a. (with autonomic plexus)
- 左結腸動脈（自律神経叢を伴う）Left colic a. (with autonomic plexus)
- 下行結腸 Descending colon
- 下腸間膜動脈神経節 Inferior mesenteric ganglion
- 下腸間膜動脈神経叢 Inferior mesenteric plexus
- S状結腸動脈（自律神経叢を伴う）Sigmoid aa. (with autonomic plexus)
- 下行結腸とS状結腸に分布する下下腹神経叢の枝 Inferior hypogastric plexus, branches to descending colon and sigmoid colon

骨盤の神経支配
Innervation of the Pelvis

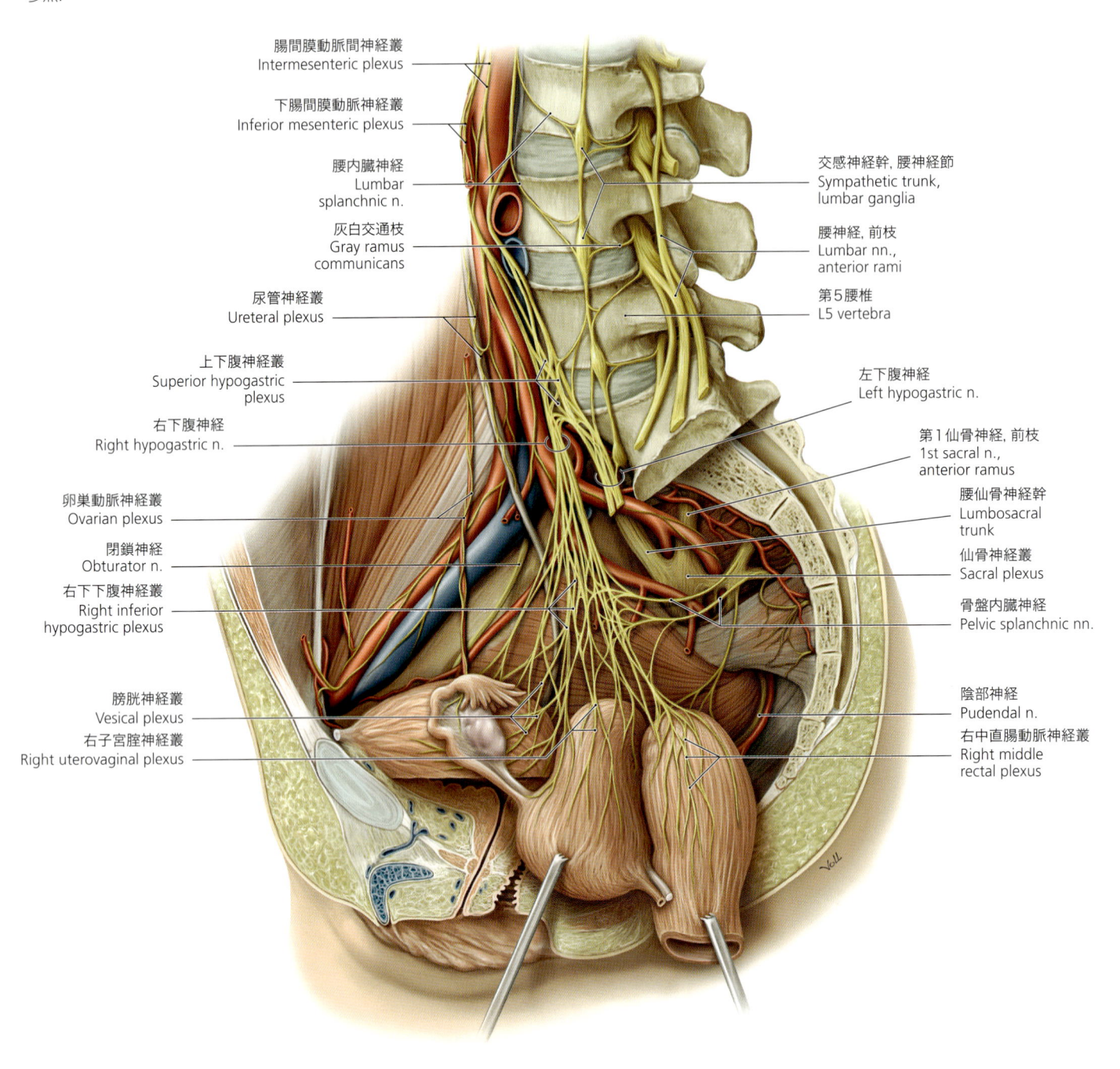

図 17.6 女性骨盤の神経支配
右骨盤．左外側方から見たところ．子宮と直腸を下に引く．模式図はp.247参照．

図 17.7　男性骨盤の神経支配
右骨盤．左外側方から見たところ．模式図は p.247 参照．

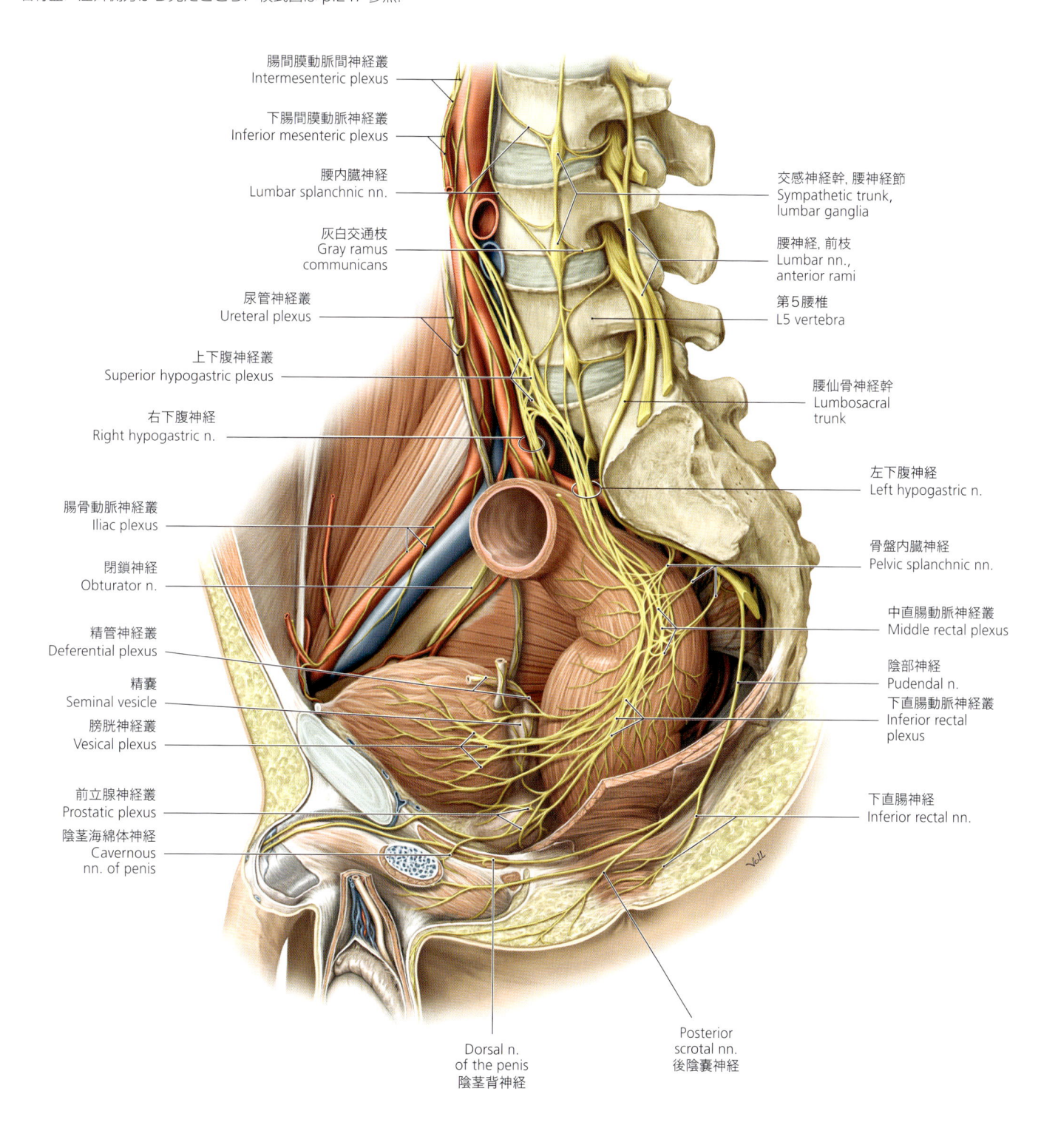

- 腸間膜動脈間神経叢 Intermesenteric plexus
- 下腸間膜動脈神経叢 Inferior mesenteric plexus
- 腰内臓神経 Lumbar splanchnic nn.
- 灰白交通枝 Gray ramus communicans
- 尿管神経叢 Ureteral plexus
- 上下腹神経叢 Superior hypogastric plexus
- 右下腹神経 Right hypogastric n.
- 腸骨動脈神経叢 Iliac plexus
- 閉鎖神経 Obturator n.
- 精管神経叢 Deferential plexus
- 精嚢 Seminal vesicle
- 膀胱神経叢 Vesical plexus
- 前立腺神経叢 Prostatic plexus
- 陰茎海綿体神経 Cavernous nn. of penis
- 交感神経幹, 腰神経節 Sympathetic trunk, lumbar ganglia
- 腰神経, 前枝 Lumbar nn., anterior rami
- 第5腰椎 L5 vertebra
- 腰仙骨神経幹 Lumbosacral trunk
- 左下腹神経 Left hypogastric n.
- 骨盤内臓神経 Pelvic splanchnic nn.
- 中直腸動脈神経叢 Middle rectal plexus
- 陰部神経 Pudendal n.
- 下直腸動脈神経叢 Inferior rectal plexus
- 下直腸神経 Inferior rectal nn.
- Dorsal n. of the penis 陰茎背神経
- Posterior scrotal nn. 後陰嚢神経

自律神経支配：概観
Autonomic Innervation: Overview

図 17.8　腹部と骨盤部の交感神経系と副交感神経系

交感神経系

- 交感神経幹 Sympathetic trunk
- C8, T1, T5, L1
- 交感神経節（椎傍神経節）Sympathetic (paravertebral) ganglia
- 腹腔神経節 Celiac ganglion
- 胸内臓神経 Thoracic splanchnic nn.
- 腰内臓神経 Lumbar splanchnic nn.
- 仙骨内臓神経 Sacral splanchnic nn.
- Superior and inferior mesenteric ganglia (with intermesenteric plexus) 上・下腸間膜動脈神経叢（腸間膜動脈間神経叢を伴う）
- Inferior hypogastric plexus 下下腹神経叢

A 交感神経系．

副交感神経系

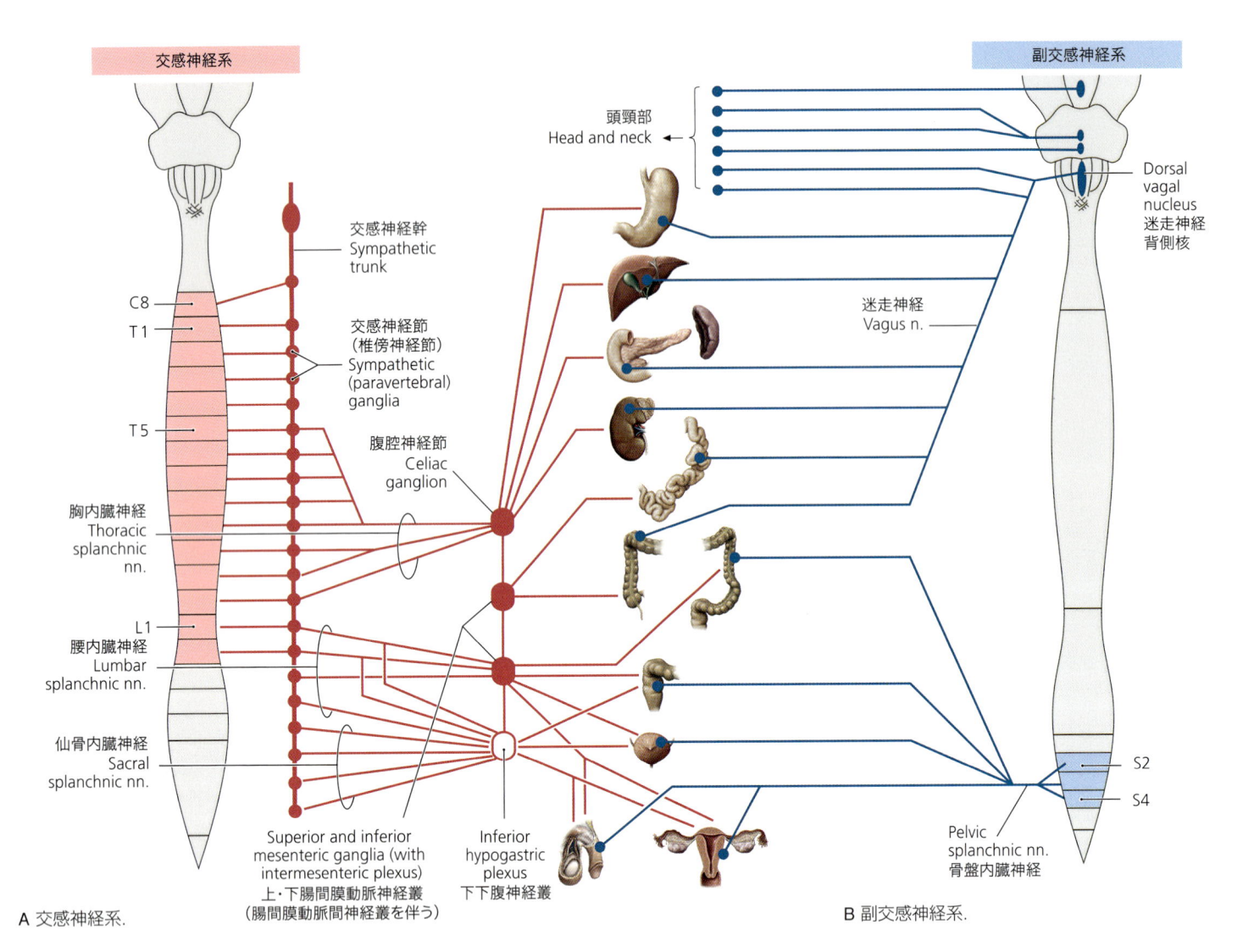

- 頭頸部 Head and neck
- Dorsal vagal nucleus 迷走神経背側核
- 迷走神経 Vagus n.
- S2, S4
- Pelvic splanchnic nn. 骨盤内臓神経

B 副交感神経系．

表 17.2　腹部と骨盤の自律神経節の作用

器官（器官系）		交感神経の作用	副交感神経の作用
胃腸管	縦走筋線維と輪走筋線維	↓運動性	↑運動性
	括約筋	収縮	弛緩
	腺	↓分泌	↑分泌
脾臓の被膜		収縮	
肝臓		↑糖原分解・糖新生	作用なし
膵臓	膵臓内分泌部	↓インスリン分泌	
	膵臓外分泌部	↓分泌	↑分泌
膀胱	排尿筋	弛緩	収縮
	機能的膀胱括約筋	収縮	収縮を抑制
精嚢と精管		収縮（射精）	作用なし
子宮		ホルモンの状態に応じて収縮あるいは弛緩	
動脈		血管収縮	陰茎動脈と陰核動脈の血管拡張（勃起）
副腎（髄質）		アドレナリン放出	作用なし
尿路	腎臓	血管収縮（↓尿生成）	血管拡張

図 17.9 腹膜内器官の自律神経支配

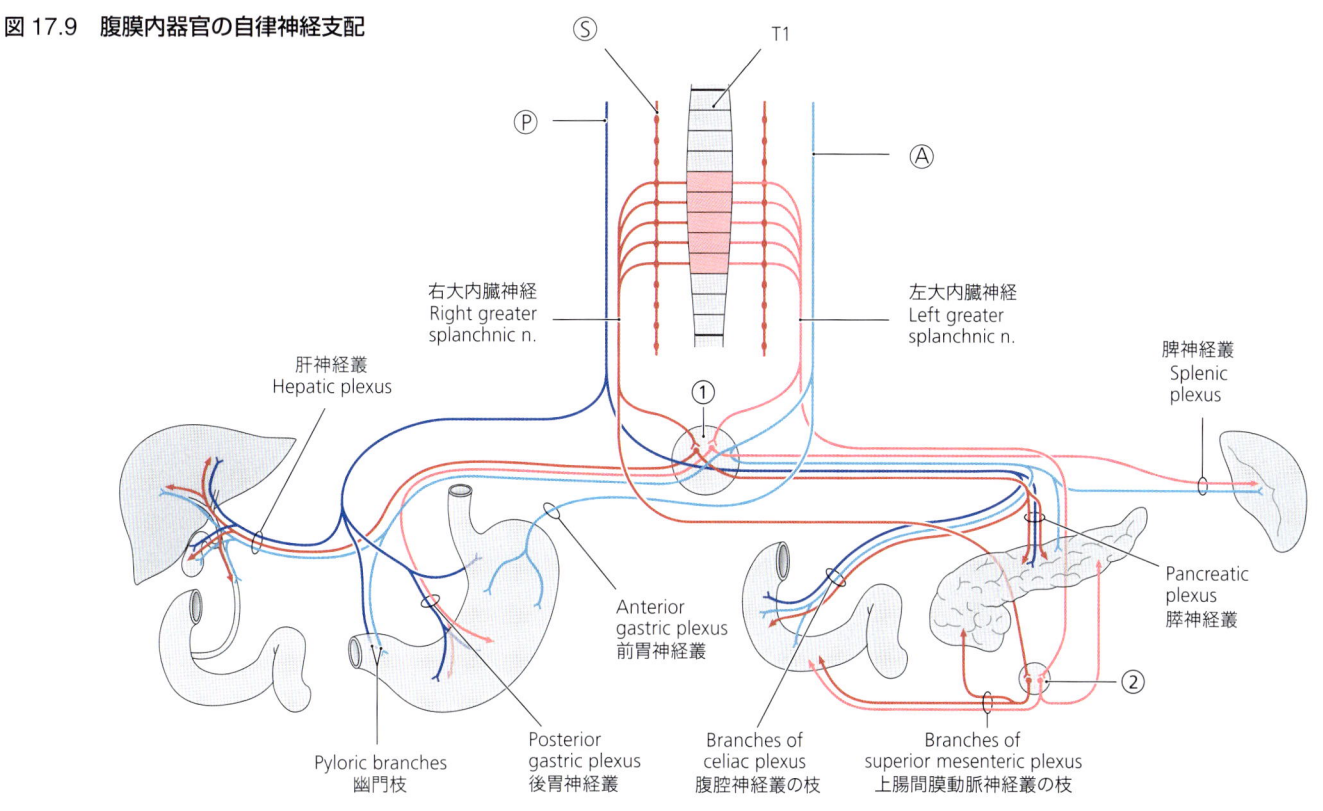

A 前腸の神経支配．左迷走神経と右迷走神経が食道に沿って下行し，それぞれ前迷走神経幹と後迷走神経幹になる．各迷走神経幹は腹腔枝，幽門枝，肝枝，胃神経叢を作る．

Ⓢ	交感神経幹
Ⓟ	後迷走神経幹（右迷走神経から）
Ⓐ	前迷走神経幹（左迷走神経から）
①	腹腔神経節
②	上腸間膜動脈神経節
③	下腸間膜動脈神経節
④	大内臓神経（T5-T9）
⑤	小内臓神経（T10-T11）
⑥	最下内臓神経（T12）
⑦	腰内臓神経（L1-L2）
⑧	腰内臓神経（第3-第5腰神経節）
⑨	仙骨内臓神経（第1-第3仙骨神経節）
⑩	骨盤内臓神経（S2-S4）

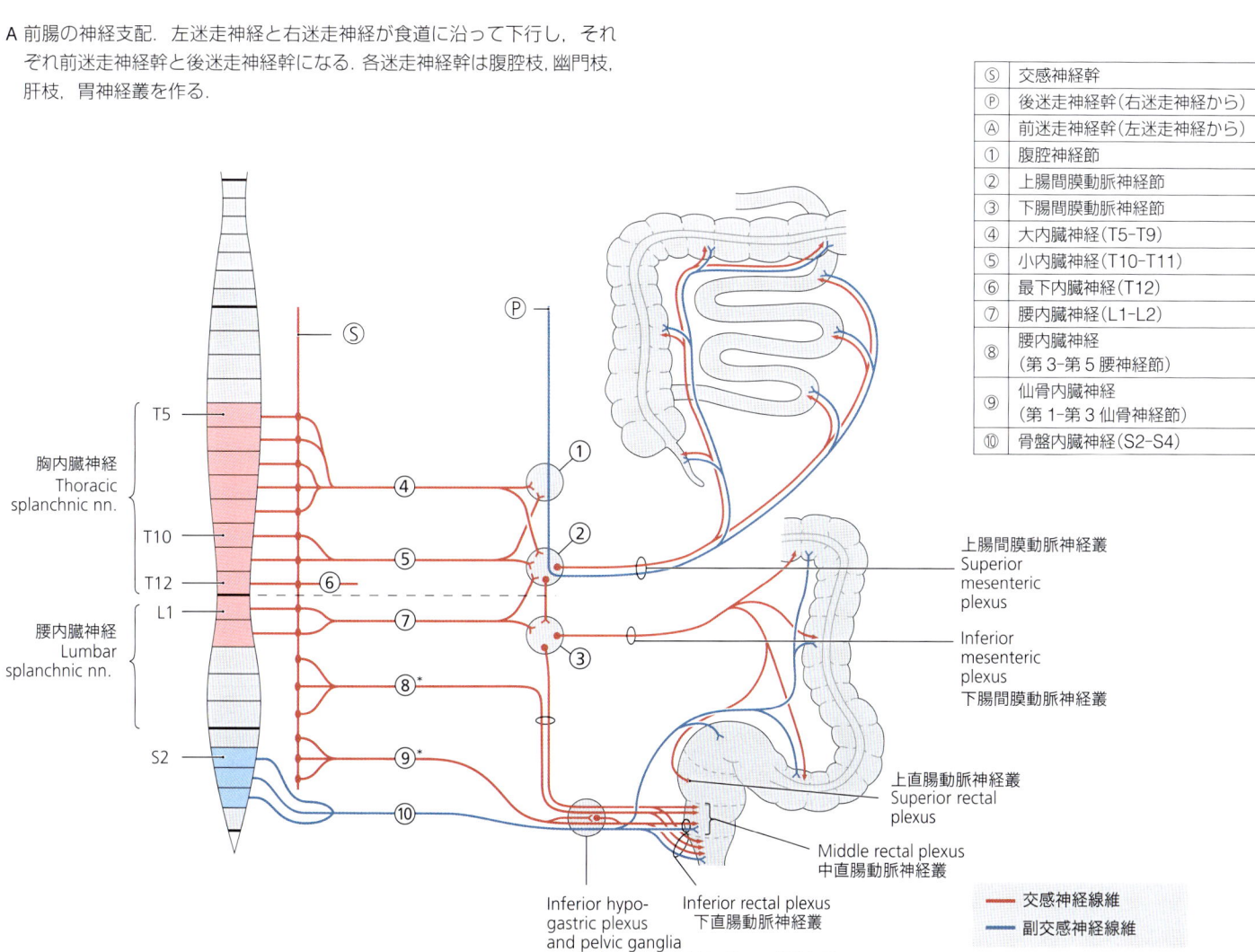

B 中腸と後腸の神経支配．
＊腰部の交感神経節でシナプスを作る．

自律神経支配：泌尿器と生殖器
Autonomic Innervation: Urinary & Genital Organs

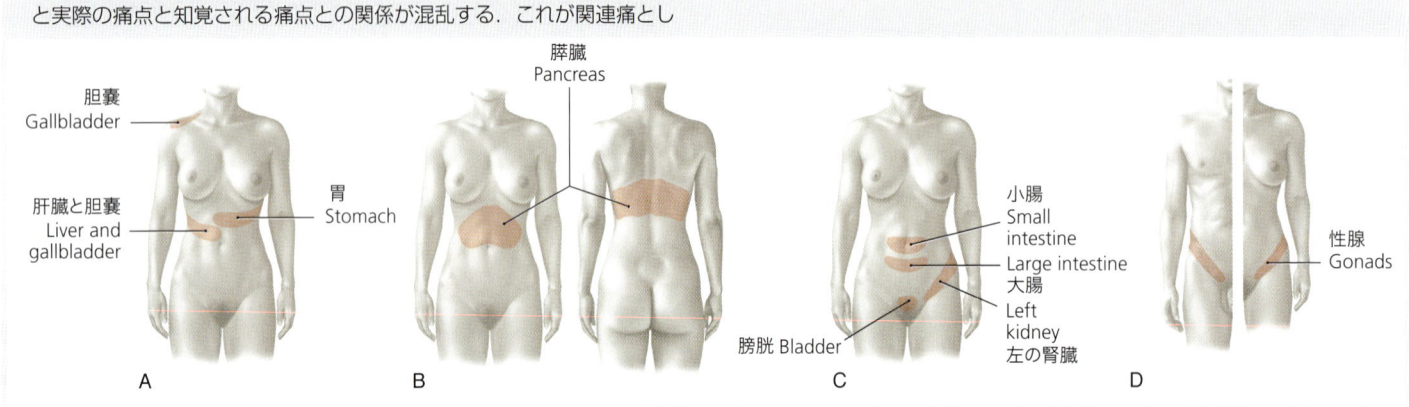

図 17.10　泌尿器の自律神経支配

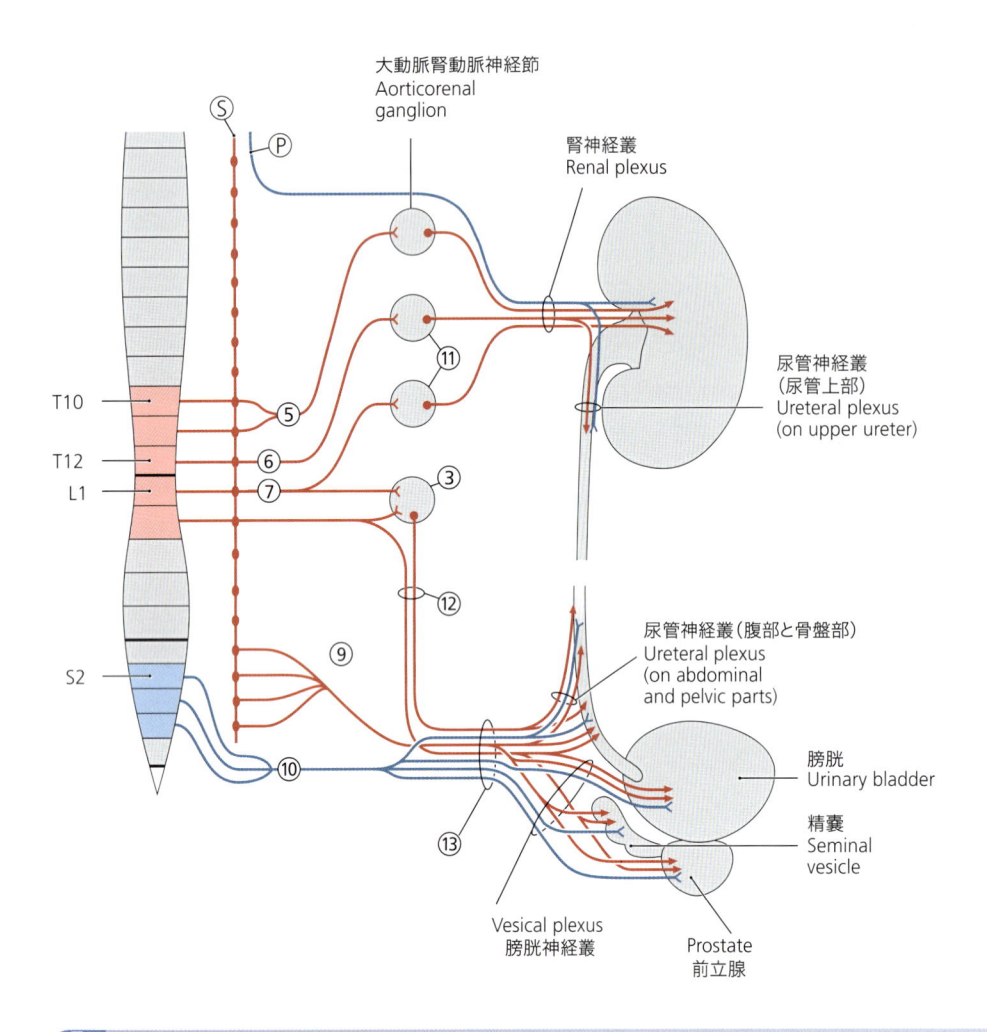

― 交感神経線維
― 副交感神経線維

大動脈腎動脈神経節
Aorticorenal ganglion

腎神経叢
Renal plexus

尿管神経叢（尿管上部）
Ureteral plexus (on upper ureter)

尿管神経叢（腹部と骨盤部）
Ureteral plexus (on abdominal and pelvic parts)

膀胱
Urinary bladder

精嚢
Seminal vesicle

前立腺
Prostate

膀胱神経叢
Vesical plexus

数字は p.245 と共通	
ⓢ	交感神経幹
ⓟ	後迷走神経幹（右迷走神経から）
③	下腸間膜動脈神経節
⑤	小内臓神経（T10-T11）
⑥	最下内臓神経（T12）
⑦	腰内臓神経（L1-L2）
⑨	仙骨内臓神経（第1-第3仙骨神経節）
⑩	骨盤内臓神経（S2-S4）
⑪	腎神経節
⑫	上下腹神経叢
⑬	下下腹神経叢

臨床

内臓の関連痛

体性求心性線維と内臓求心性線維が同じ高さの脊髄神経へと収束すると実際の痛点と知覚される痛点との関係が混乱する．これが関連痛として知られる現象である．ある臓器の痛みは特定の皮膚領域に常に放散する．

A：胆嚢 Gallbladder／肝臓と胆嚢 Liver and gallbladder／胃 Stomach

B：膵臓 Pancreas

C：小腸 Small intestine／大腸 Large intestine／膀胱 Bladder／左の腎臓 Left kidney

D：性腺 Gonads

図 17.11　生殖器の自律神経支配

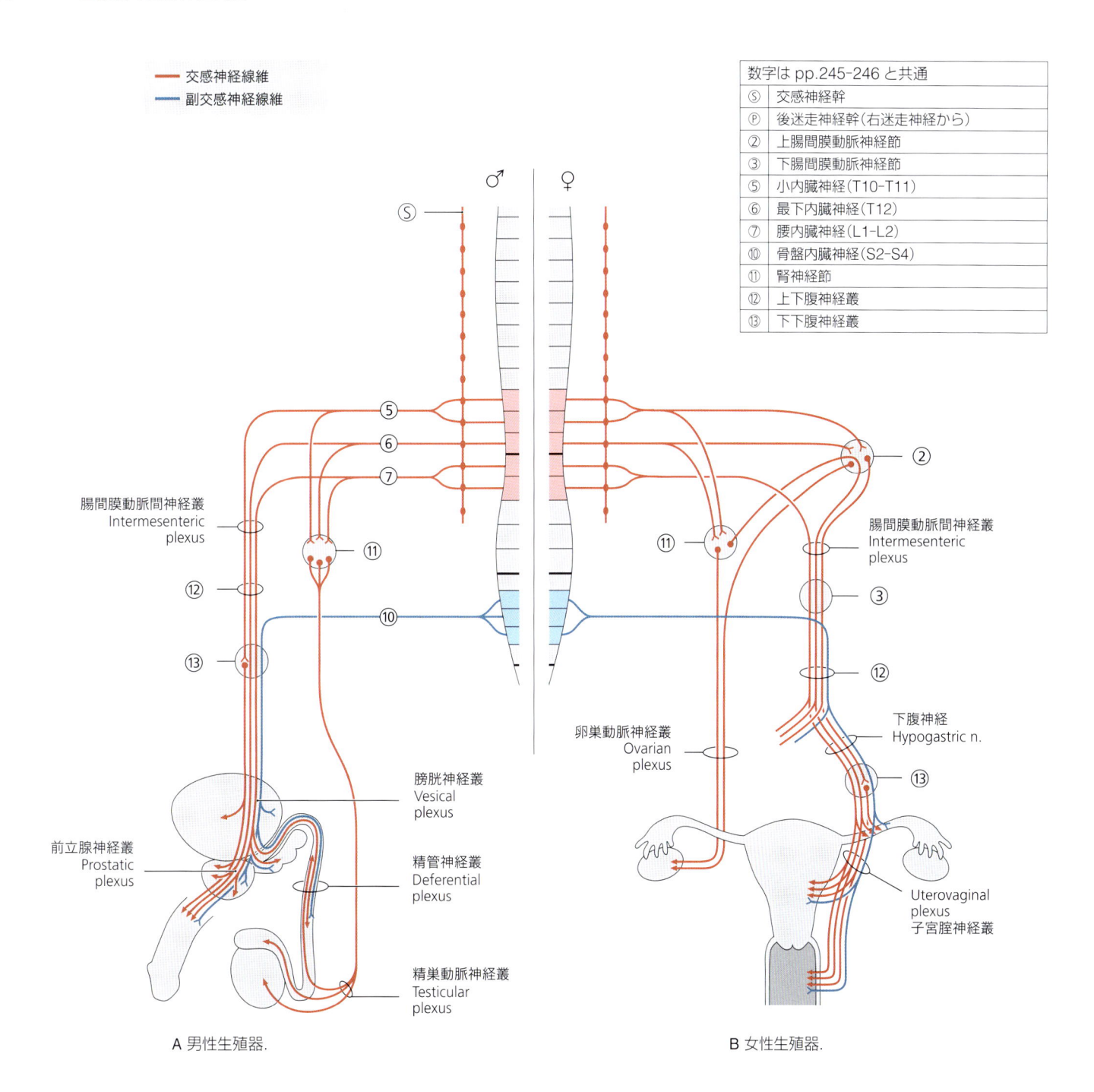

― 交感神経線維
― 副交感神経線維

数字は pp.245-246 と共通
Ⓢ 交感神経幹
Ⓟ 後迷走神経幹（右迷走神経から）
② 上腸間膜動脈神経節
③ 下腸間膜動脈神経節
⑤ 小内臓神経（T10-T11）
⑥ 最下内臓神経（T12）
⑦ 腰内臓神経（L1-L2）
⑩ 骨盤内臓神経（S2-S4）
⑪ 腎神経節
⑫ 上下腹神経叢
⑬ 下下腹神経叢

腸間膜動脈間神経叢
Intermesenteric plexus

腸間膜動脈間神経叢
Intermesenteric plexus

卵巣動脈神経叢
Ovarian plexus

下腹神経
Hypogastric n.

膀胱神経叢
Vesical plexus

前立腺神経叢
Prostatic plexus

精管神経叢
Deferential plexus

精巣動脈神経叢
Testicular plexus

Uterovaginal plexus
子宮腟神経叢

A 男性生殖器.

B 女性生殖器.

体表解剖
Surface Anatomy

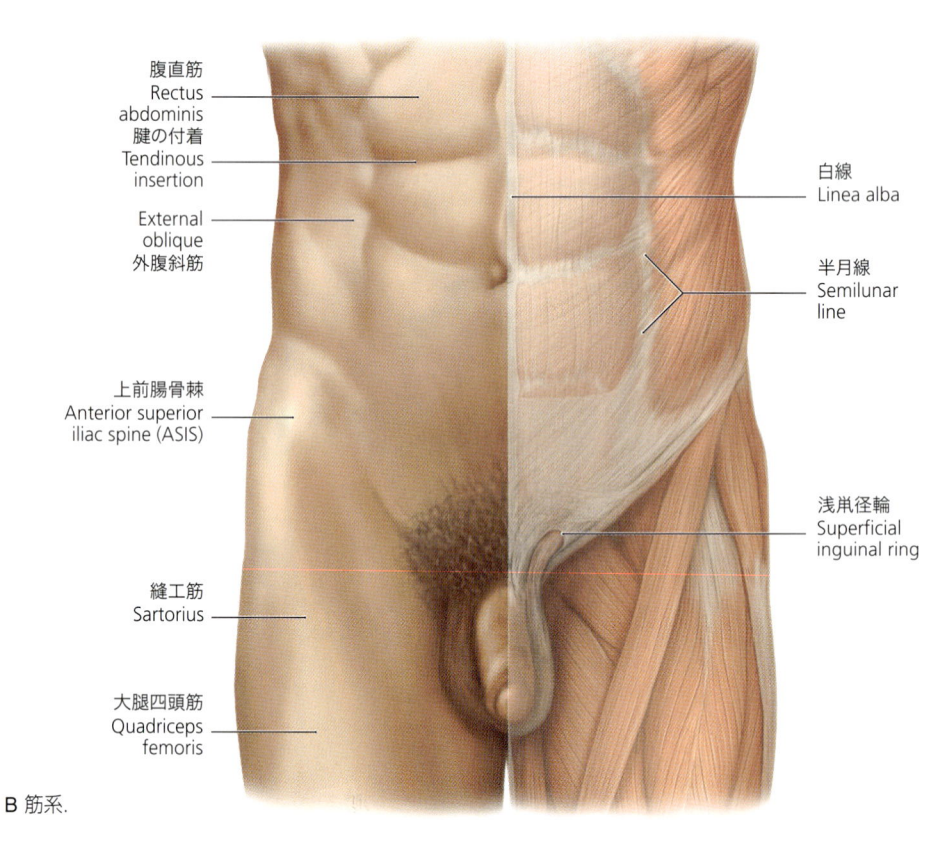

図 18.1　腹部と骨盤部の触知可能構造
前方から見たところ．背部の構造は pp.40-41 参照．

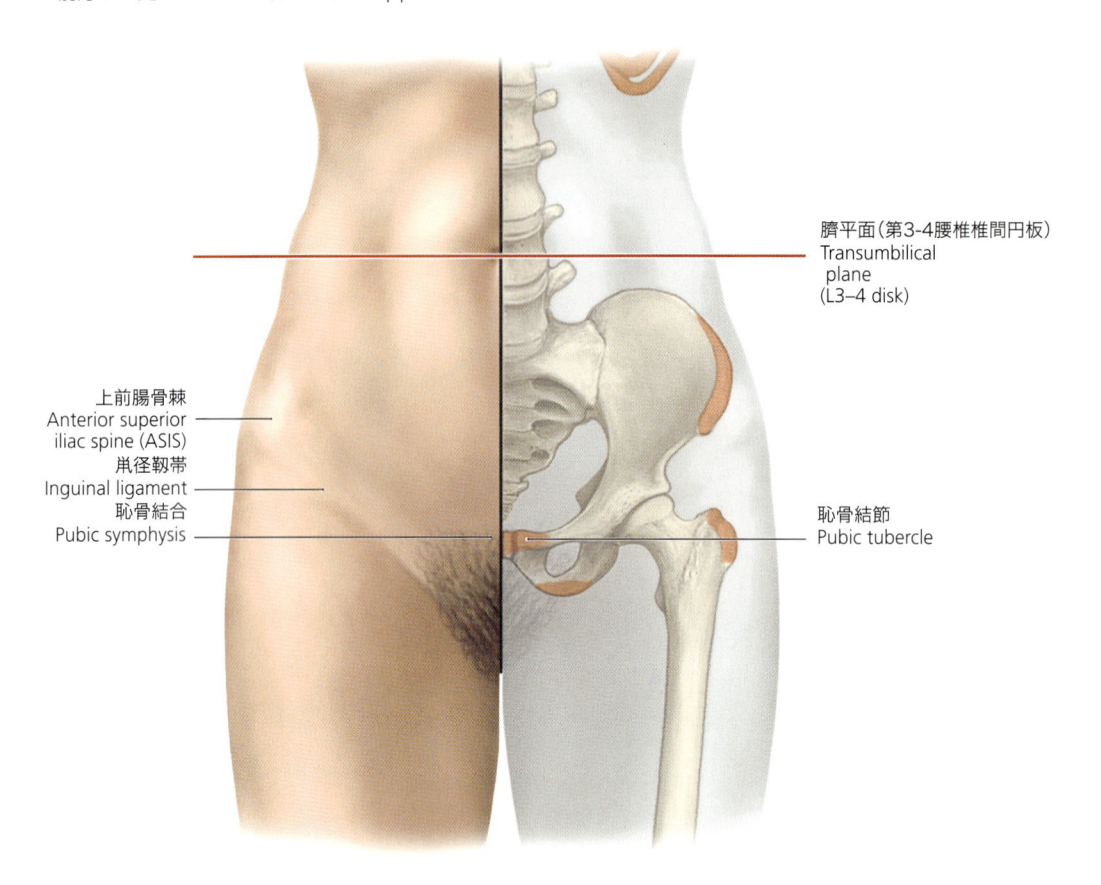

- 臍平面（第3-4腰椎椎間円板）
  Transumbilical plane (L3–4 disk)
- 上前腸骨棘　Anterior superior iliac spine (ASIS)
- 鼠径靱帯　Inguinal ligament
- 恥骨結合　Pubic symphysis
- 恥骨結節　Pubic tubercle

A 骨の隆起．

- 腹直筋　Rectus abdominis
- 腱の付着　Tendinous insertion
- External oblique 外腹斜筋
- 上前腸骨棘　Anterior superior iliac spine (ASIS)
- 縫工筋　Sartorius
- 大腿四頭筋　Quadriceps femoris
- 白線　Linea alba
- 半月線　Semilunar line
- 浅鼠径輪　Superficial inguinal ring

B 筋系．

図 18.2　**腹部と骨盤部の体表解剖**
前方から見たところ．背部の構造は pp.40-41 参照．

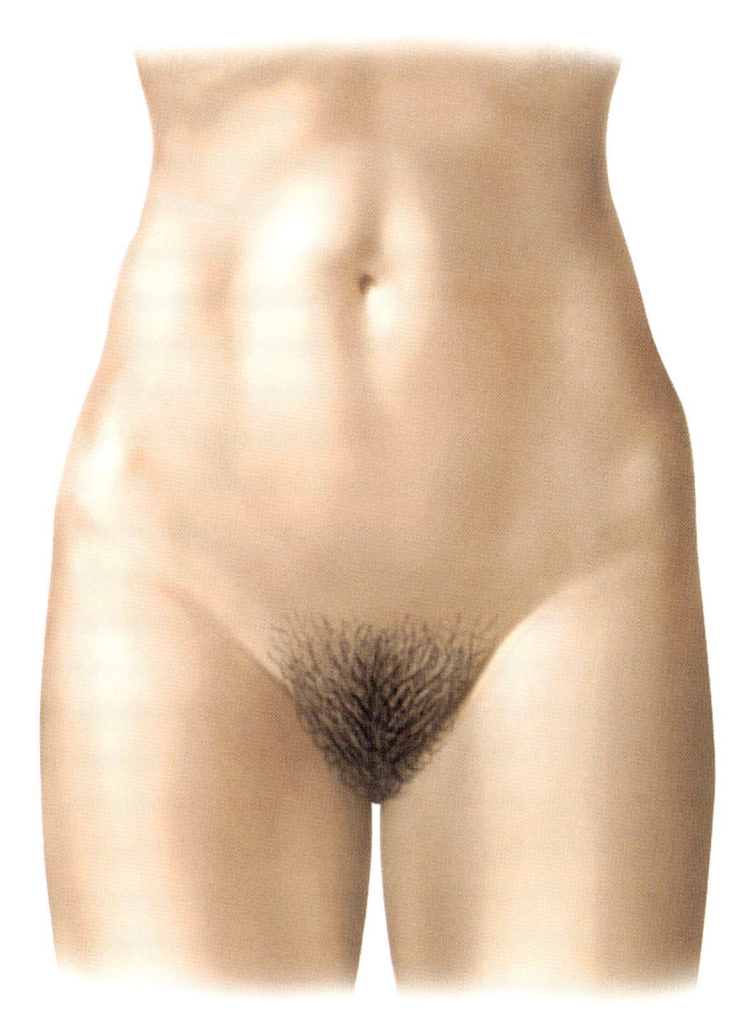

Q1：患者の腹部について4分円(右上腹部・右下腹部・左上腹部・左下腹部の4つの領域)を用いて記述するにはどのように区分されるか．4分円ごとに臓器を5つ挙げよ．

A　女性の腹部と骨盤部．

Q2：患者の鼡径部の中点の上方にわずかながら膨らみが見られる．直接鼡径ヘルニアか間接鼡径ヘルニアかを決定する際に有用な要素(解剖学的要因，年齢的要因)は何か．

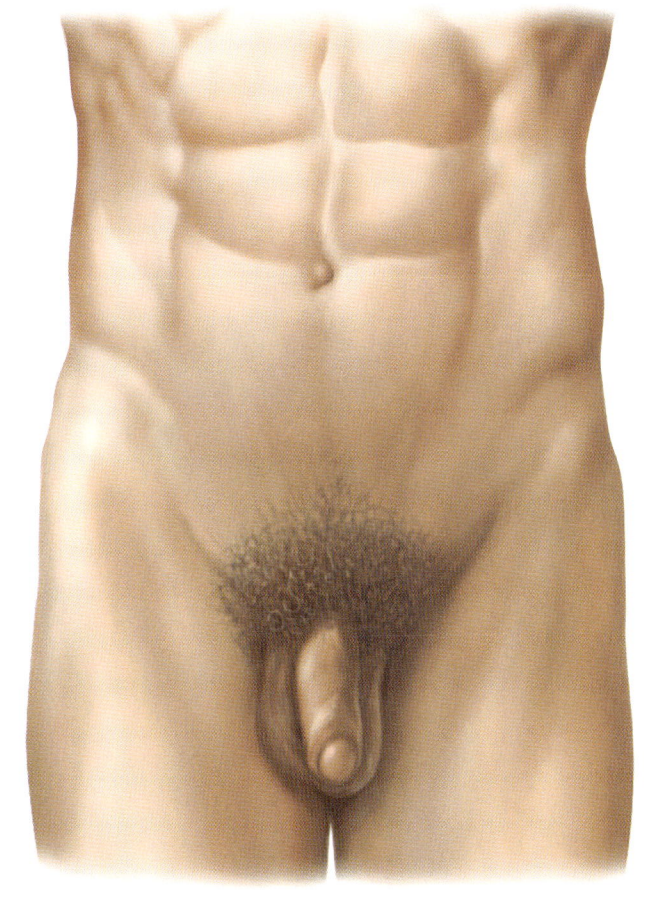

p.626 からの解答を参照．

B　男性の腹部と骨盤部．

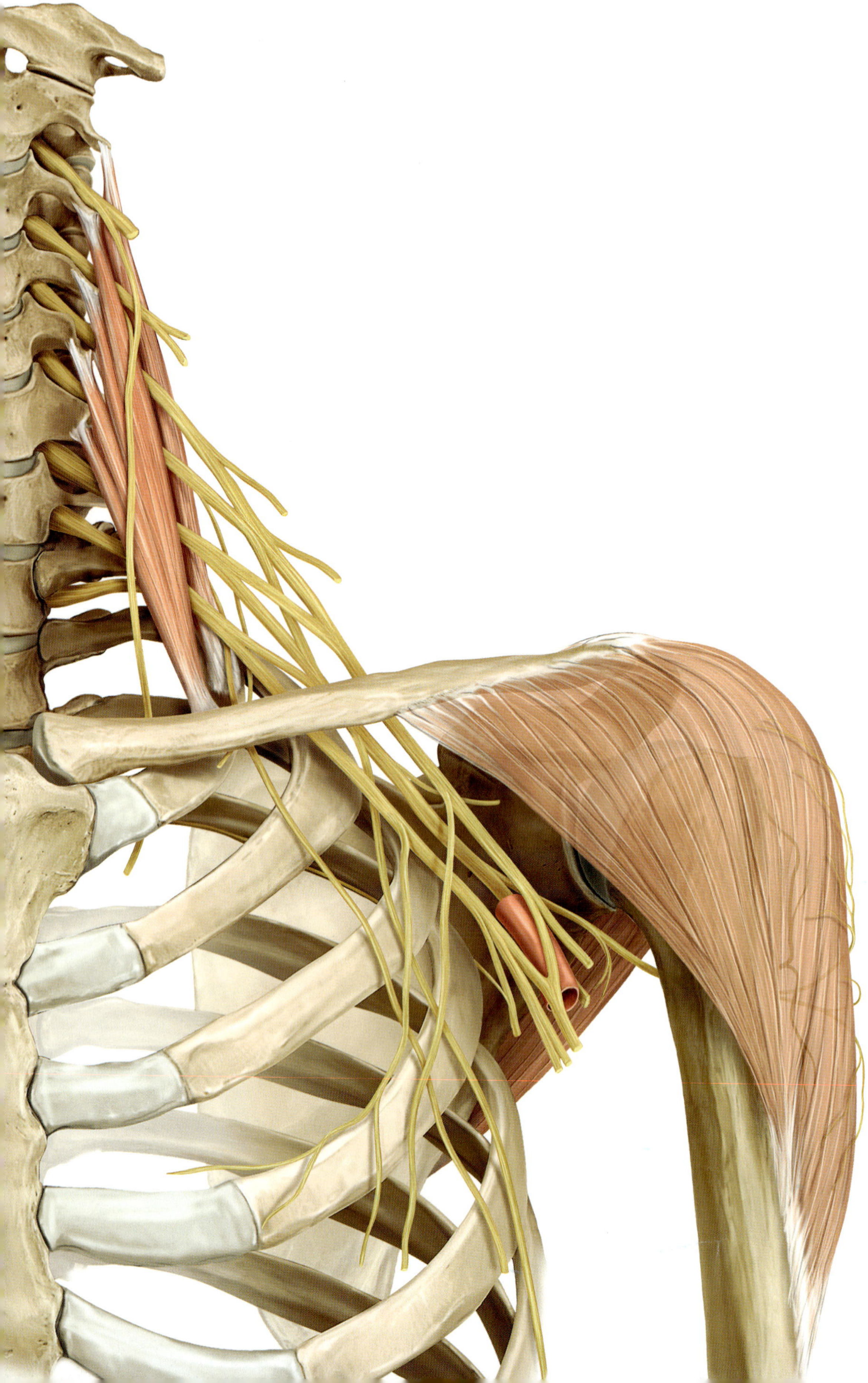

上 肢
Upper Limb

19. 肩と上腕
- 上肢の骨 252
- 鎖骨と肩甲骨 254
- 上腕骨 256
- 肩の関節 258
- 肩の関節：肩関節（肩甲上腕関節） 260
- 肩峰下腔と肩峰下包 262
- 肩と上腕の前面にある筋(1) 264
- 肩と上腕の前面にある筋(2) 266
- 肩と上腕の後面にある筋(1) 268
- 肩と上腕の後面にある筋(2) 270
- 個々の筋(1) 272
- 個々の筋(2) 274
- 個々の筋(3) 276
- 個々の筋(4) 278

20. 肘と前腕
- 橈骨と尺骨 280
- 肘関節 282
- 肘関節の靱帯 284
- 橈尺関節 286
- 前腕の筋(1) 288
- 前腕の筋(2) 290
- 個々の筋(1) 292
- 個々の筋(2) 294
- 個々の筋(3) 296

21. 手首と手
- 手首と手の骨 298
- 手首と手の関節 300
- 手首と手の靱帯 302
- 指の靱帯 304
- 手の筋：浅層と中間層 306
- 手の筋：中間層と深層 308
- 手背 310
- 個々の筋(1) 312
- 個々の筋(2) 314

22. 神経と脈管
- 上肢の動脈 316
- 上肢の静脈とリンパ管 318
- 腕神経叢とその枝 320
- 腕神経叢の鎖骨上部からの枝，後神経束 322
- 後神経束：橈骨神経と腋窩神経 324
- 内側・外側神経束 326
- 正中神経，尺骨神経 328
- 上肢の皮静脈，皮神経 330
- 肩と腋窩の後部 332
- 肩の前面 334
- 腋窩の局所解剖 336
- 上腕と肘の局所解剖 338
- 前腕の局所解剖 340
- 手根の局所解剖 342
- 手掌の局所解剖 344
- 手背の局所解剖 346
- 断面解剖 348

23. 体表解剖
- 体表解剖(1) 350
- 体表解剖(2) 352

上肢の骨
Bones of the Upper Limb

図 19.1 上肢の骨格
右上肢．上肢は上肢帯と自由上肢からなり，自由上肢はさらに上腕，前腕，手に区分される．上肢帯（鎖骨と肩甲骨）は自由上肢を胸鎖関節によって胸郭に連結している．

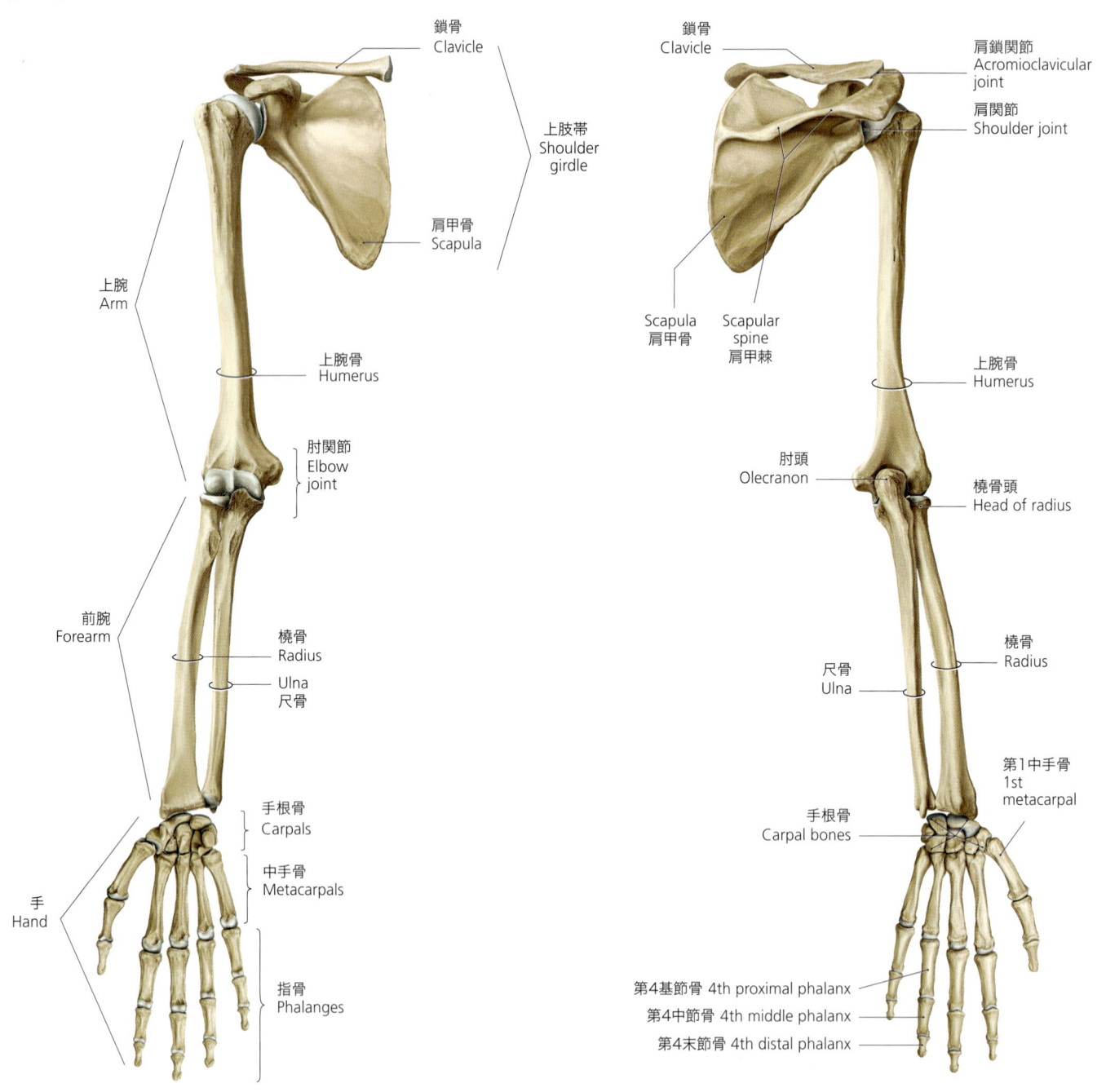

A 前方から見たところ．

B 後方から見たところ．

図 19.2 体表から触知できる骨の隆起

月状骨と小菱形骨を除く上肢の全ての骨は皮膚や軟部組織を介して触知できる.

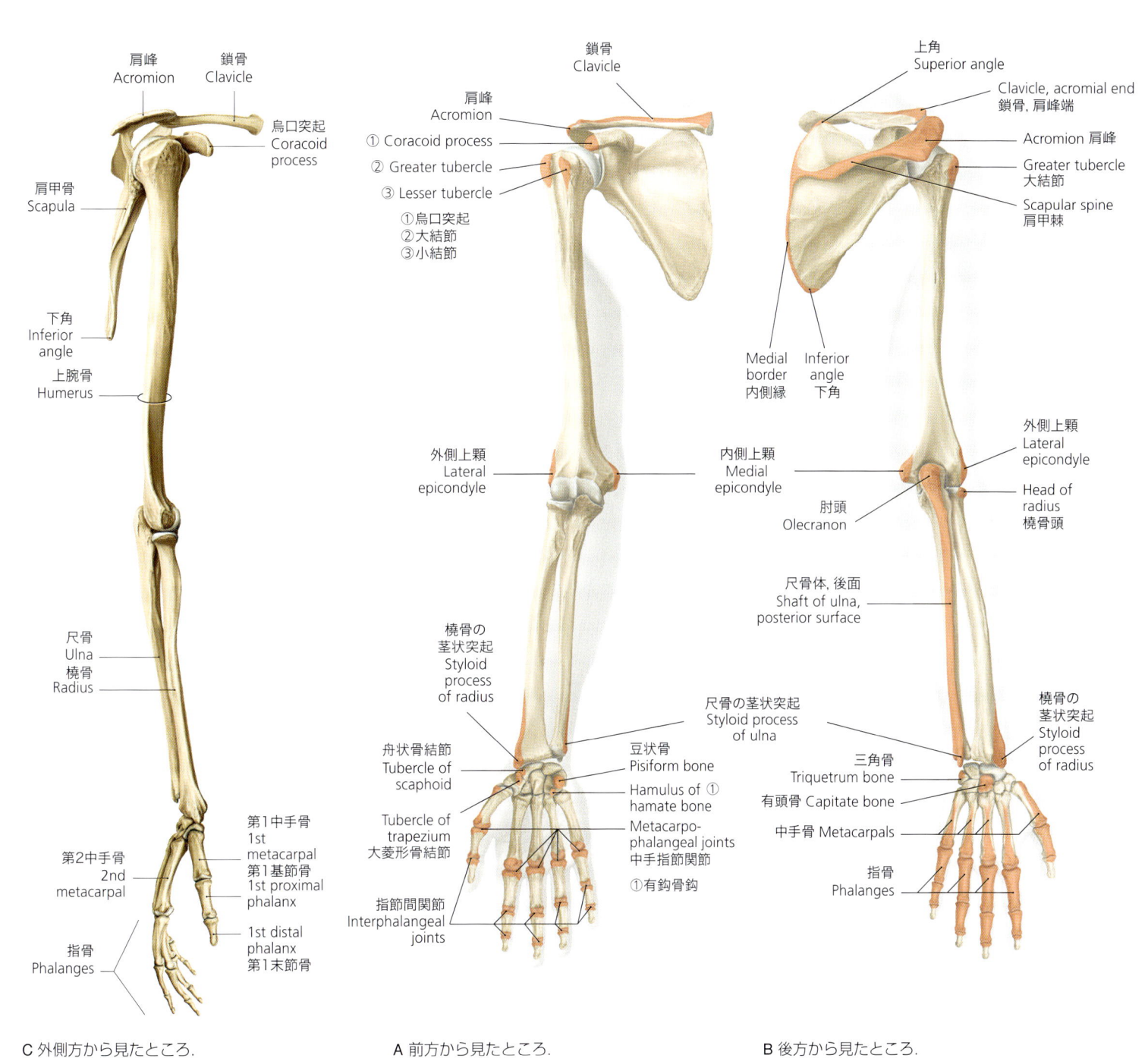

C 外側方から見たところ.

- 肩峰 Acromion
- 鎖骨 Clavicle
- 烏口突起 Coracoid process
- 肩甲骨 Scapula
- 下角 Inferior angle
- 上腕骨 Humerus
- 尺骨 Ulna
- 橈骨 Radius
- 第1中手骨 1st metacarpal
- 第2中手骨 2nd metacarpal
- 第1基節骨 1st proximal phalanx
- 第1末節骨 1st distal phalanx
- 指骨 Phalanges

A 前方から見たところ.

- 鎖骨 Clavicle
- 肩峰 Acromion
- ① Coracoid process
- ② Greater tubercle
- ③ Lesser tubercle
- ①烏口突起
- ②大結節
- ③小結節
- 外側上顆 Lateral epicondyle
- 内側上顆 Medial epicondyle
- 橈骨の茎状突起 Styloid process of radius
- 尺骨の茎状突起 Styloid process of ulna
- 舟状骨結節 Tubercle of scaphoid
- 大菱形骨結節 Tubercle of trapezium
- 豆状骨 Pisiform bone
- Hamulus of ①
- ①有鈎骨鈎
- 中手指節関節 Metacarpophalangeal joints
- 指節間関節 Interphalangeal joints

B 後方から見たところ.

- 上角 Superior angle
- 鎖骨, 肩峰端 Clavicle, acromial end
- 肩峰 Acromion
- 大結節 Greater tubercle
- 肩甲棘 Scapular spine
- 内側縁 Medial border
- 下角 Inferior angle
- 外側上顆 Lateral epicondyle
- 肘頭 Olecranon
- 橈骨頭 Head of radius
- 尺骨体, 後面 Shaft of ulna, posterior surface
- 橈骨の茎状突起 Styloid process of radius
- 三角骨 Triquetrum bone
- 有頭骨 Capitate bone
- 中手骨 Metacarpals
- 指骨 Phalanges

鎖骨と肩甲骨
Clavicle & Scapula

> 上肢帯(鎖骨と肩甲骨)は自由上肢を胸郭に連結する．下肢帯(一対の寛骨)は中軸骨格と一体化しているのに対し(p.358 参照)，上肢帯は可動性が極めて大きい．

図 19.3　鎖骨

右鎖骨．鎖骨は S 字型の骨で，皮下にその全長を見ることができる(全長は 12-15 cm)．鎖骨の内側端(胸骨端)は胸骨との間に胸鎖関節を形成する(p.258 参照)．外側端(肩峰端)は肩甲骨との間に肩鎖関節を形成する(p.259 参照)．

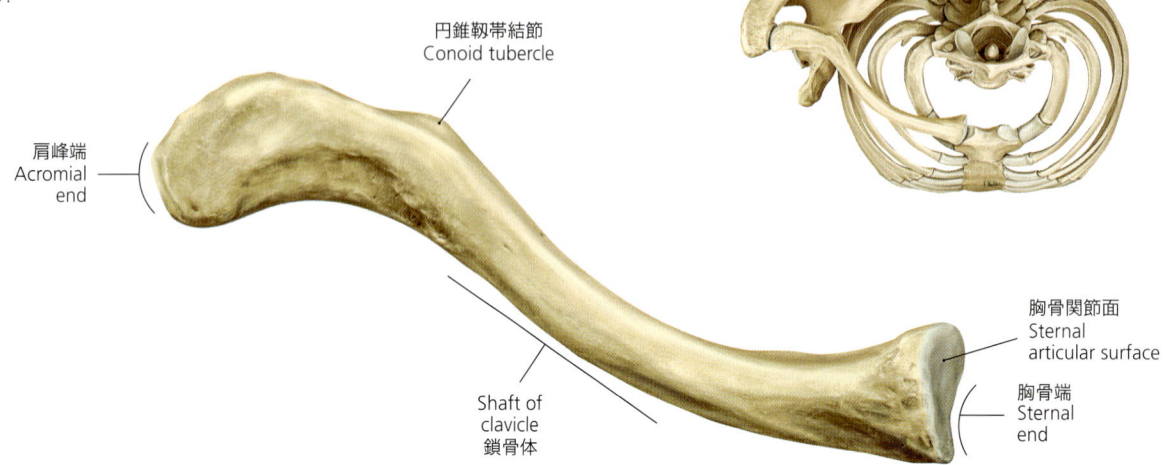

- 円錐靱帯結節　Conoid tubercle
- 肩峰端　Acromial end
- Shaft of clavicle　鎖骨体
- 胸骨関節面　Sternal articular surface
- 胸骨端　Sternal end

A　上方から見たところ．

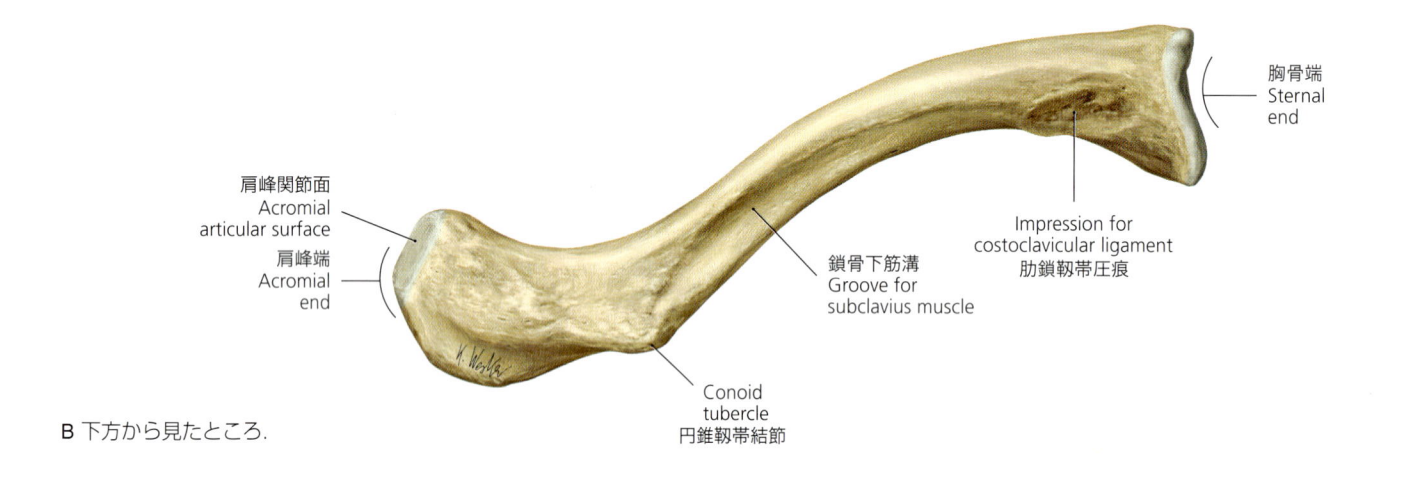

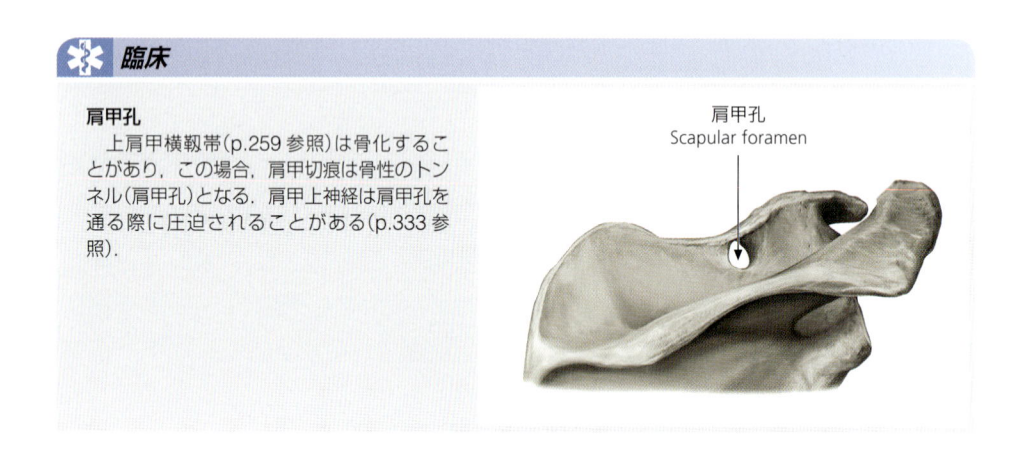

- 胸骨端　Sternal end
- Impression for costoclavicular ligament　肋鎖靱帯圧痕
- 鎖骨下筋溝　Groove for subclavius muscle
- 肩峰関節面　Acromial articular surface
- 肩峰端　Acromial end
- Conoid tubercle　円錐靱帯結節

B　下方から見たところ．

臨床

肩甲孔

上肩甲横靱帯(p.259 参照)は骨化することがあり，この場合，肩甲切痕は骨性のトンネル(肩甲孔)となる．肩甲上神経は肩甲孔を通る際に圧迫されることがある(p.333 参照)．

- 肩甲孔　Scapular foramen

図 19.4　肩甲骨
右肩甲骨．解剖学的正位において，肩甲骨は第 2-7 肋骨の高さに存在する．

A 前方から見たところ．

B 外側方から見たところ．

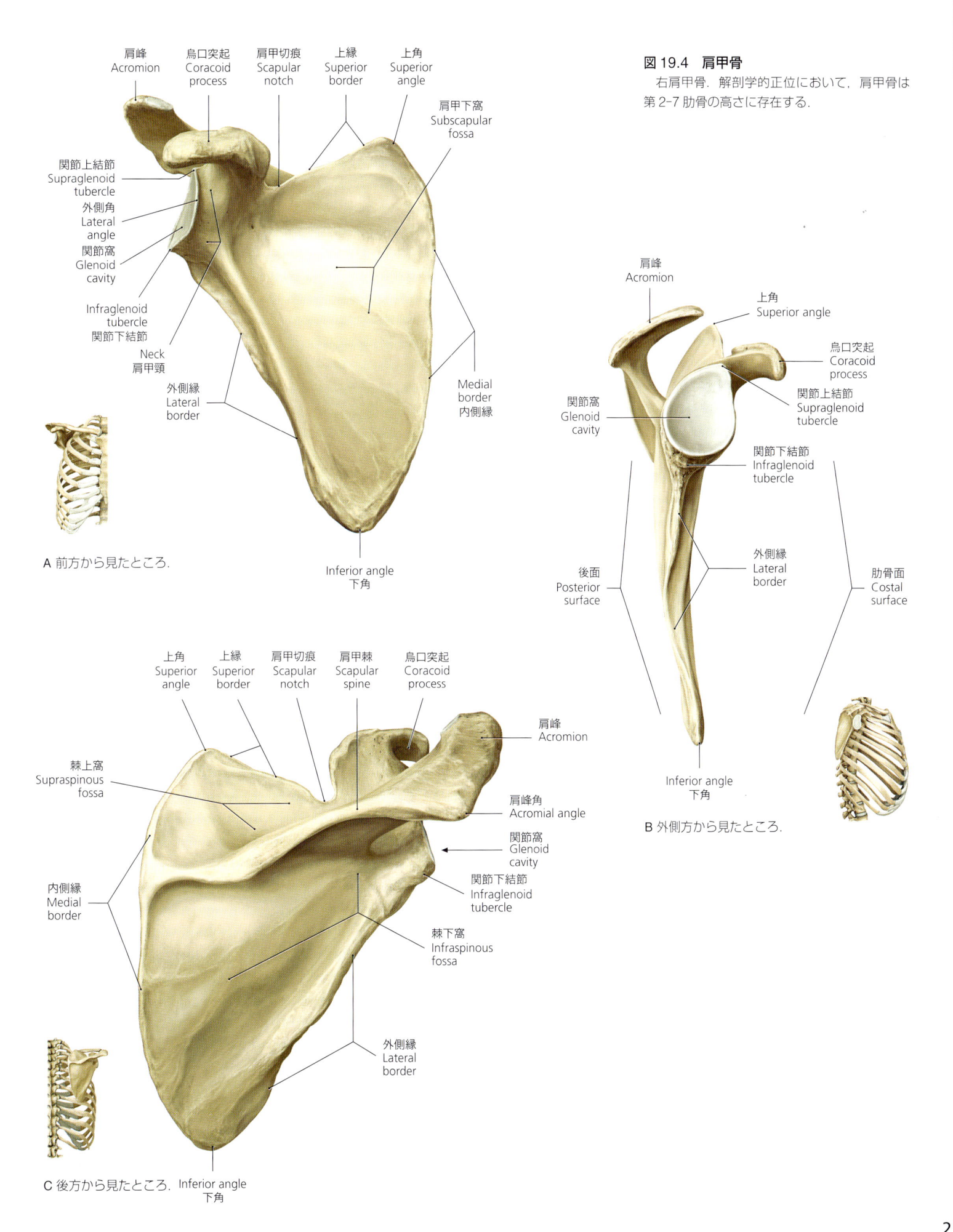

C 後方から見たところ．

上腕骨
Humerus

図 19.5 上腕骨
右上腕骨．上腕骨頭は肩甲骨との間に肩関節（肩甲上腕関節）を形成する（p.258 参照）．上腕骨小頭および上腕骨滑車は，橈骨および尺骨との間にそれぞれ関節を形成する（p.282 参照）．

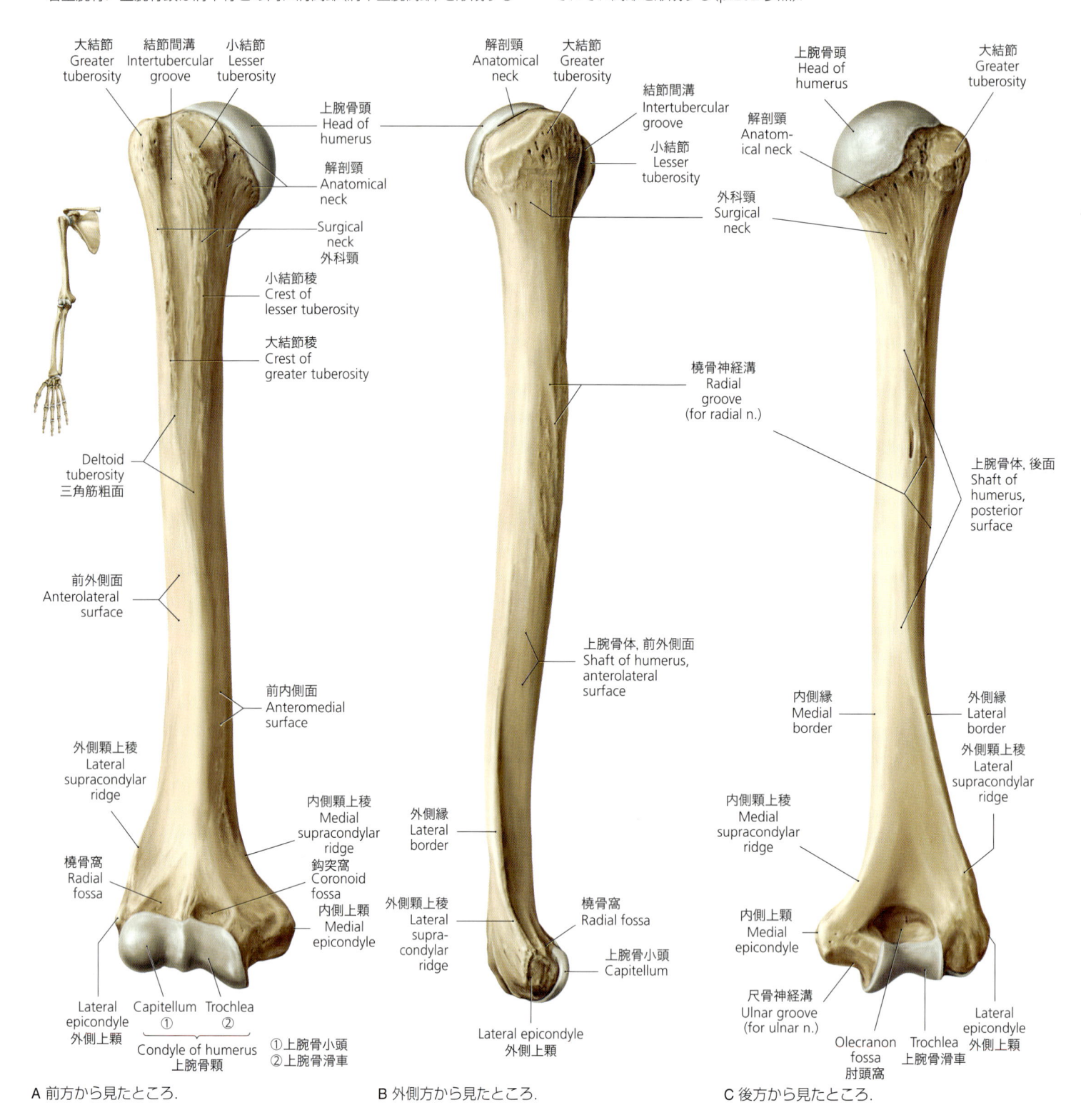

A 前方から見たところ．

B 外側方から見たところ．

C 後方から見たところ．

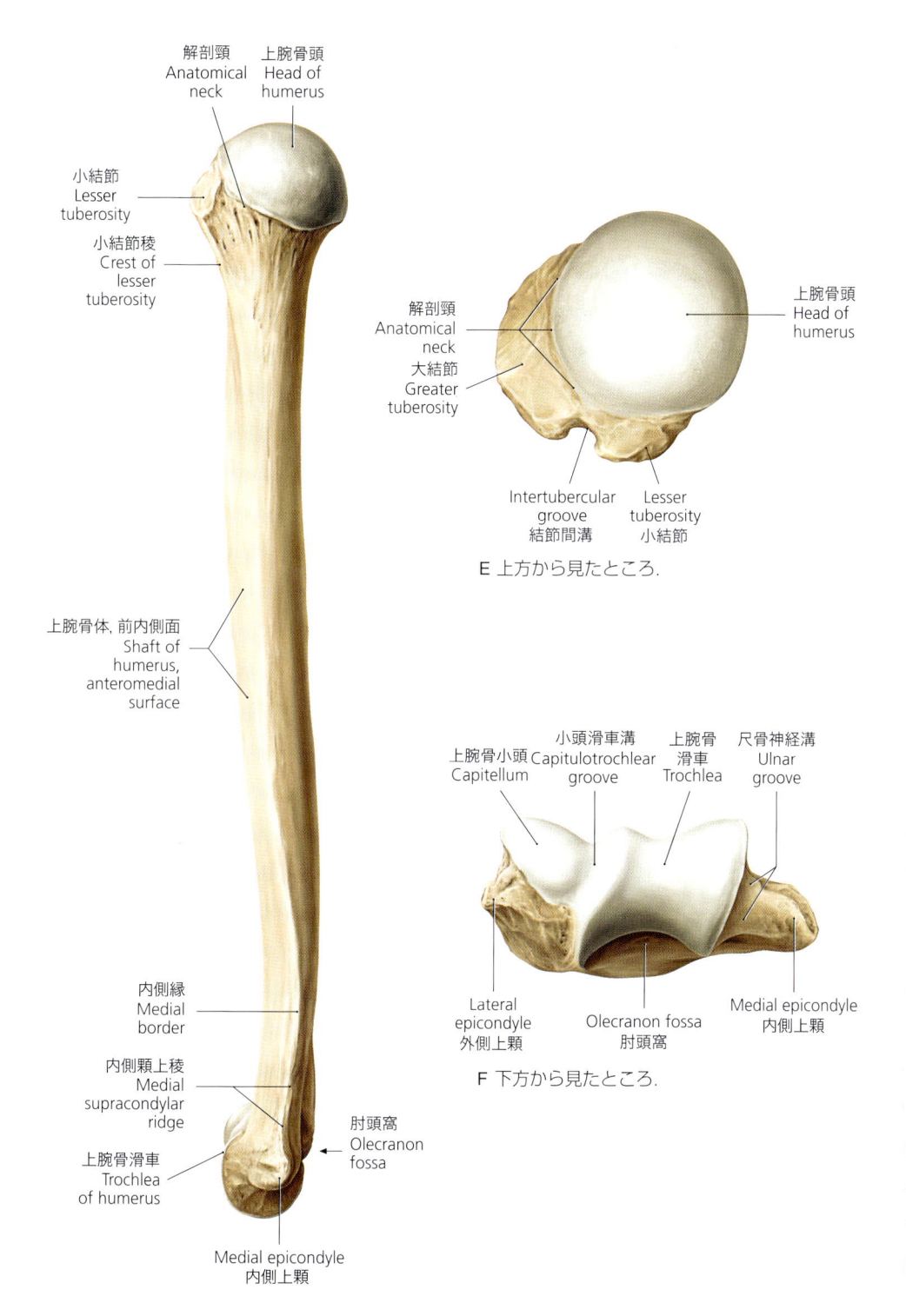

臨床

上腕骨骨折

前面．上腕骨近位端の骨折はよく見られる骨折のひとつである．ほとんどが高齢者で起こり，転倒した際に伸ばした腕で体を支えたり，肩から直接倒れたりした場合に生じる．3つの主要なタイプに分類される．

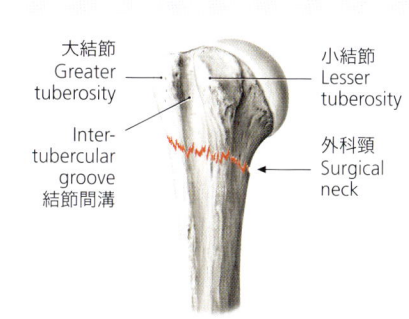

A 関節外骨折．

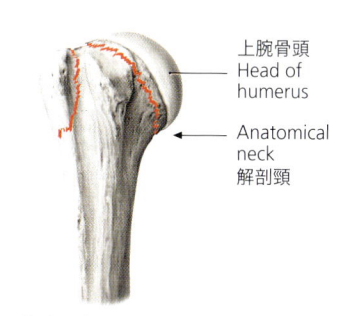

B 関節内骨折．

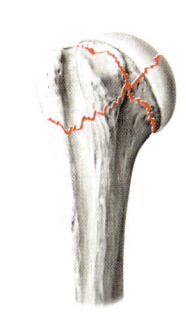

C 粉砕骨折．

関節外骨折と関節内骨折は，上腕骨頭に分布する動脈（前・後上腕回旋動脈の枝）の損傷をしばしば合併する．この動脈が損傷された場合，外傷後の無血管性骨壊死を生じる危険がある．

上腕骨体と遠位端の骨折は，しばしば橈骨神経の損傷を伴う．

D 内側方から見たところ．

E 上方から見たところ．

F 下方から見たところ．

19 肩と上腕

肩の関節
Joints of the Shoulder

図 19.6 肩の関節：概観
右肩，前方から見たところ．

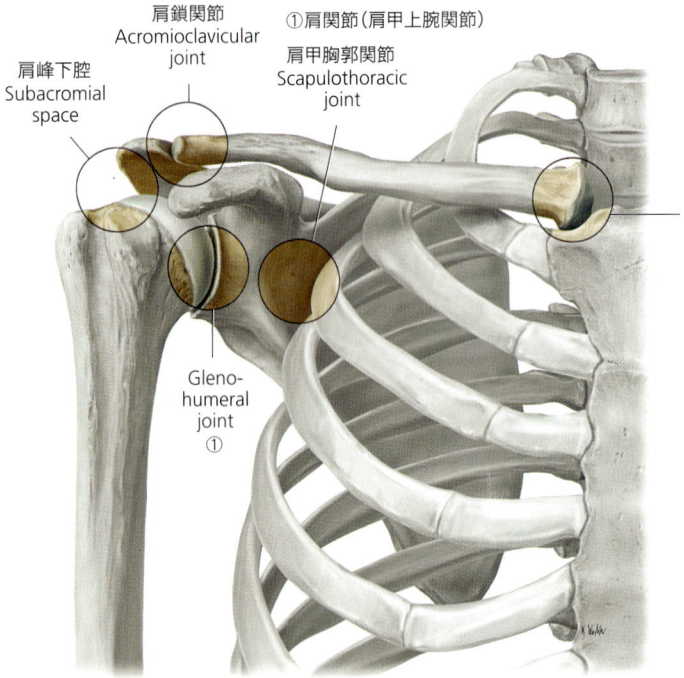

- 肩峰下腔 Subacromial space
- 肩鎖関節 Acromioclavicular joint
- ①肩関節（肩甲上腕関節）
- 肩甲胸郭関節 Scapulothoracic joint
- 胸鎖関節 Sternoclavicular joint
- Glenohumeral joint ①

図 19.7 上肢帯の関節
右肩，上方から見たところ．

- 肩鎖関節（肩鎖靱帯）Acromioclavicular joint (with acromioclavicular l.)
- 烏口肩峰靱帯 Coracoacromial l.
- 肩関節（肩甲上腕関節）Glenohumeral joint
- Scapulothoracic joint 肩甲胸郭関節
- Posterior sternoclavicular l. 後胸鎖靱帯
- Sternoclavicular joint (with anterior sternoclavicular l.) 胸鎖関節と前胸鎖靱帯

図 19.8 肩甲胸郭関節
右肩，上方から見たところ．上肢帯の全ての運動時において，肩甲骨は前鋸筋と肩甲下筋の間にある疎性結合組織の表面を滑る．この面がいわゆる肩甲胸郭関節である．

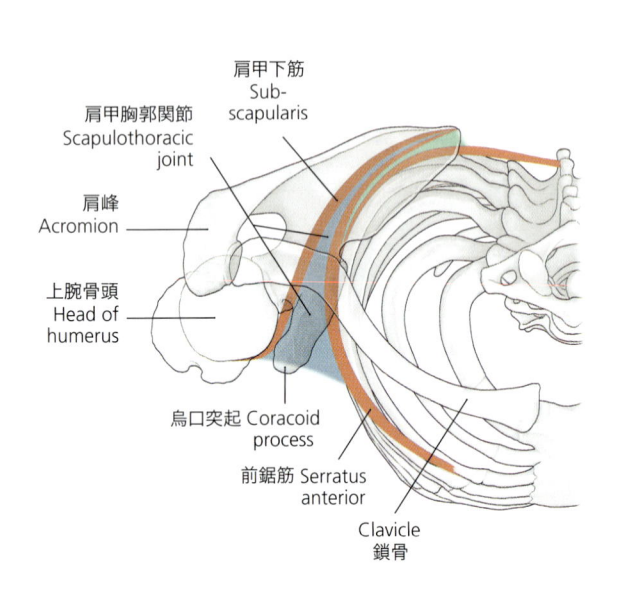

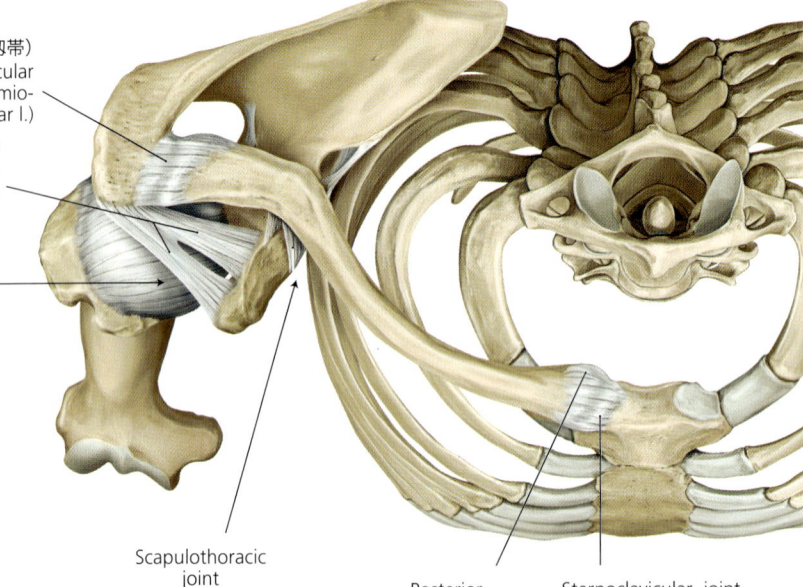

- 肩甲胸郭関節 Scapulothoracic joint
- 肩甲下筋 Subscapularis
- 肩峰 Acromion
- 上腕骨頭 Head of humerus
- 烏口突起 Coracoid process
- 前鋸筋 Serratus anterior
- Clavicle 鎖骨

図 19.9 胸鎖関節

前方から見たところ．胸骨の左半部は前額方向に切断されている．*Note*：線維軟骨からなる関節円板は，鎖骨と胸骨柄の2つの鞍状の関節面の間にできる表面の不整合を解消する．

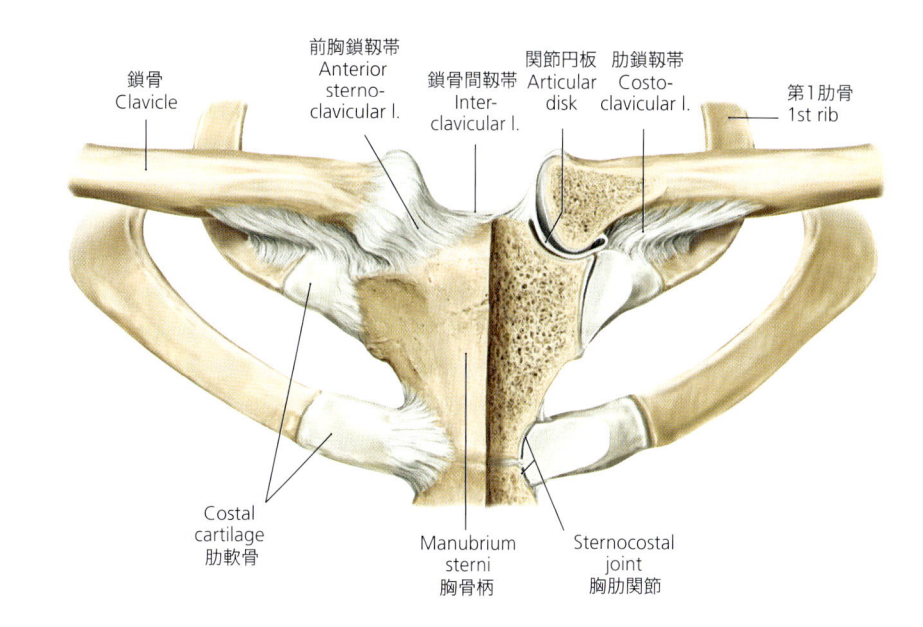

- 鎖骨 Clavicle
- 前胸鎖靱帯 Anterior sternoclavicular l.
- 鎖骨間靱帯 Interclavicular l.
- 関節円板 Articular disk
- 肋鎖靱帯 Costoclavicular l.
- 第1肋骨 1st rib
- Costal cartilage 肋軟骨
- Manubrium sterni 胸骨柄
- Sternocostal joint 胸肋関節

図 19.10 肩鎖関節

前方から見たところ．肩鎖関節は平面関節の一種である．関節面が平坦であり，なおかつ強力な靱帯によって固定されている．したがって，肩鎖関節の可動性は大きく制限される．

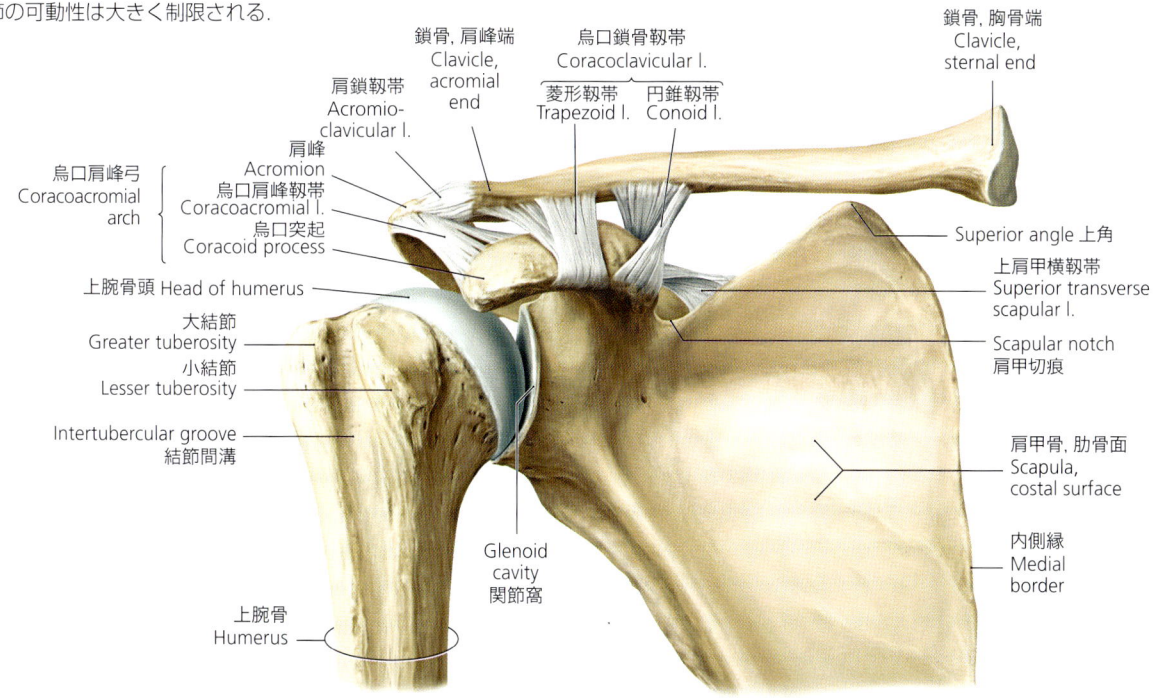

- 鎖骨, 肩峰端 Clavicle, acromial end
- 烏口鎖骨靱帯 Coracoclavicular l.
- 菱形靱帯 Trapezoid l.
- 円錐靱帯 Conoid l.
- 鎖骨, 胸骨端 Clavicle, sternal end
- 肩鎖靱帯 Acromioclavicular l.
- 烏口肩峰弓 Coracoacromial arch
- 肩峰 Acromion
- 烏口肩峰靱帯 Coracoacromial l.
- 烏口突起 Coracoid process
- 上腕骨頭 Head of humerus
- 大結節 Greater tuberosity
- 小結節 Lesser tuberosity
- Intertubercular groove 結節間溝
- Glenoid cavity 関節窩
- 上腕骨 Humerus
- Superior angle 上角
- 上肩甲横靱帯 Superior transverse scapular l.
- Scapular notch 肩甲切痕
- 肩甲骨, 肋骨面 Scapula, costal surface
- 内側縁 Medial border

臨床

肩鎖関節の外傷

転倒した際に伸ばした腕で体重を支えたり，肩から転倒した場合に，肩鎖関節の脱臼と烏口鎖骨靱帯の損傷がしばしば生じる．

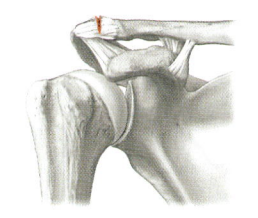

A 靱帯の過伸展．

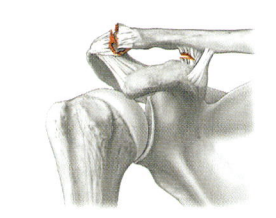

B 肩鎖靱帯の断裂．

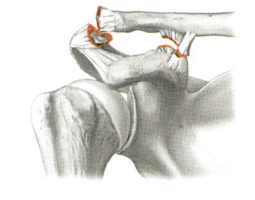

C 肩鎖関節の完全脱臼．

肩の関節：肩関節（肩甲上腕関節）
Joints of the Shoulder: Glenohumeral Joint

図 19.11　肩関節（肩甲上腕関節）：骨
右肩．

主なラベル（図A 前方から見たところ）：
- 烏口突起 Coracoid process
- 関節上結節 Supraglenoid tubercle
- 鎖骨 Clavicle
- 肩甲切痕 Scapular notch
- 肩峰 Acromion
- 上腕骨頭 Head of humerus
- 小結節 Lesser tuberosity
- 大結節 Greater tuberosity
- 関節窩 Glenoid cavity
- 結節間溝 Intertubercular groove
- 関節下結節 Infraglenoid tubercle
- 外側縁 Lateral border

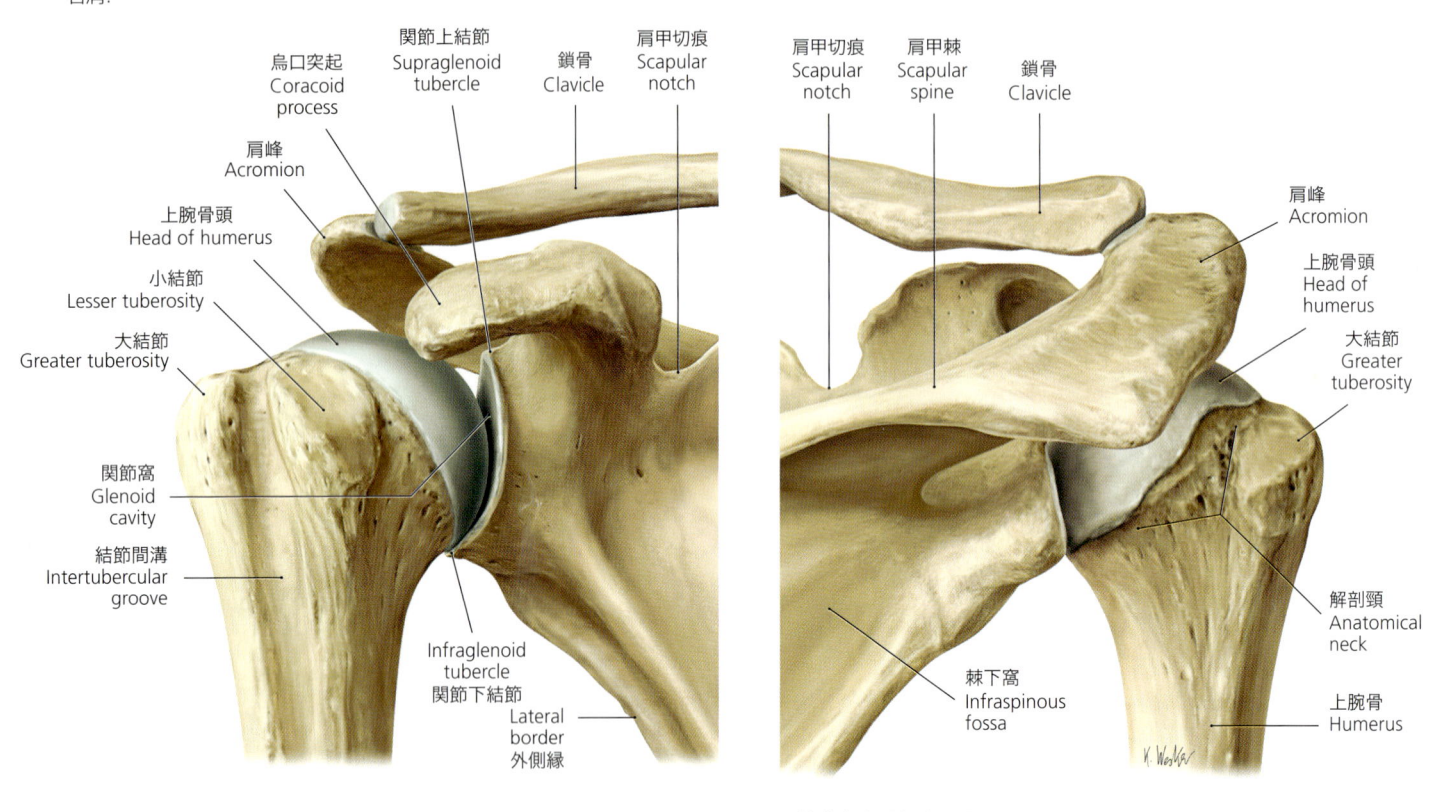

主なラベル（図B 後方から見たところ）：
- 肩甲切痕 Scapular notch
- 肩甲棘 Scapular spine
- 鎖骨 Clavicle
- 肩峰 Acromion
- 上腕骨頭 Head of humerus
- 大結節 Greater tuberosity
- 解剖頸 Anatomical neck
- 上腕骨 Humerus
- 棘下窩 Infraspinous fossa

A　前方から見たところ．
B　後方から見たところ．

図 19.12　肩の X 線写真
前後像．

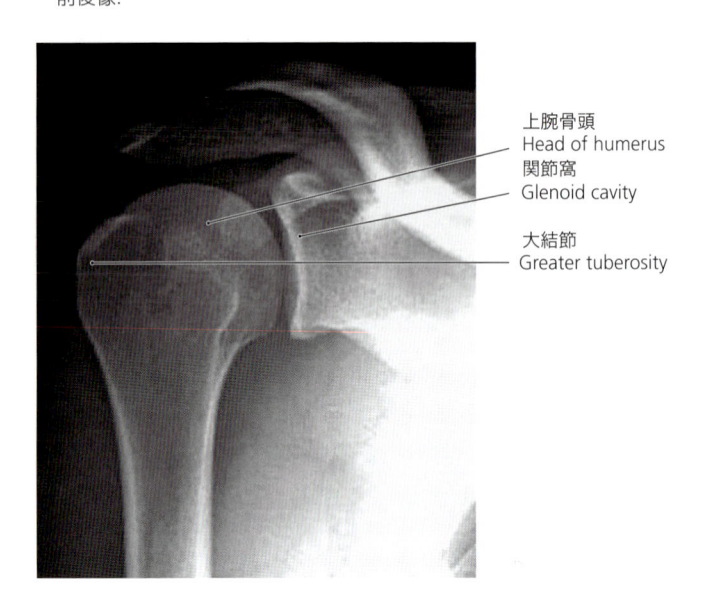

- 上腕骨頭 Head of humerus
- 関節窩 Glenoid cavity
- 大結節 Greater tuberosity

図 19.13 肩関節（肩甲上腕関節）：関節包と靱帯

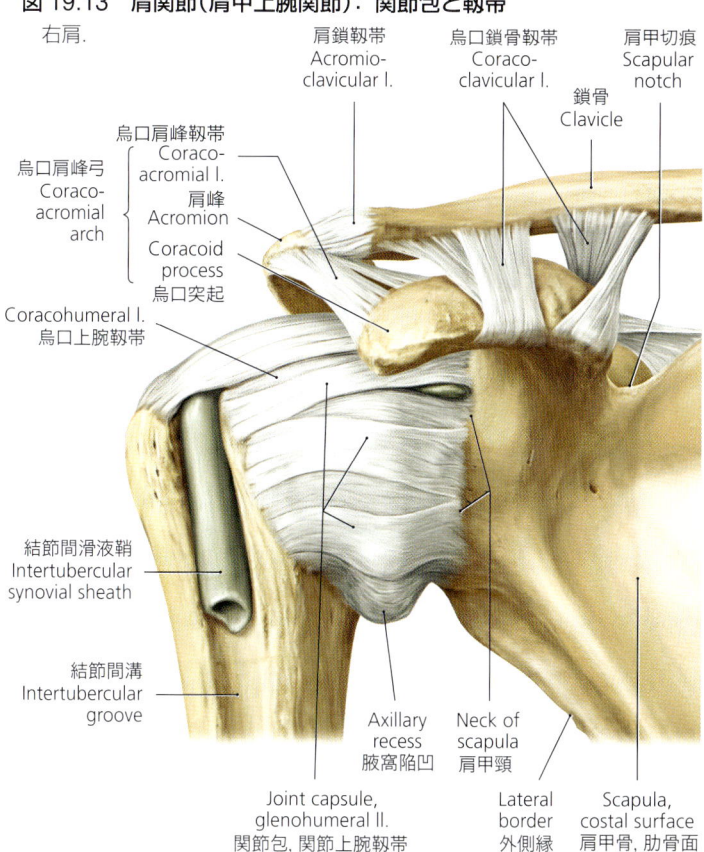

右肩．

A 前方から見たところ．

- 肩鎖靱帯 Acromio-clavicular l.
- 烏口鎖骨靱帯 Coraco-clavicular l.
- 肩甲切痕 Scapular notch
- 鎖骨 Clavicle
- 烏口肩峰靱帯 Coraco-acromial l.
- 烏口肩峰弓 Coraco-acromial arch
- 肩峰 Acromion
- 烏口突起 Coracoid process
- 烏口上腕靱帯 Coracohumeral l.
- 結節間滑液鞘 Intertubercular synovial sheath
- 結節間溝 Intertubercular groove
- 関節包, 関節上腕靱帯 Joint capsule, glenohumeral ll.
- 腋窩陥凹 Axillary recess
- 肩甲頸 Neck of scapula
- 外側縁 Lateral border
- 肩甲骨, 肋骨面 Scapula, costal surface

B 後方から見たところ．

- 上肩甲横靱帯 Superior transverse scapular l.
- 烏口鎖骨靱帯 Coraco-clavicular l.
- 鎖骨 Clavicle
- 肩鎖靱帯 Acromio-clavicular l.
- ①肩甲切痕 ① Scapular notch
- 肩峰 Acromion
- 大結節 Greater tuberosity
- 上腕骨 Humerus
- 関節包 Joint capsule
- 肩甲棘 Scapular spine
- 棘下窩 Infraspinous fossa
- 腋窩陥凹 Axillary recess

図 19.14 肩関節の関節腔

前方から見たところ．

- 肩鎖靱帯 Acromio-clavicular l.
- 烏口鎖骨靱帯 Coraco-clavicular l.
- 上肩甲横靱帯 Superior transverse scapular l.
- 烏口肩峰靱帯 Coraco-acromial l.
- 烏口突起 Coracoid process
- 鎖骨 Clavicle
- 肩峰 Acromion
- 烏口腕筋包 Subcoracoid bursa
- 上腕横靱帯 Transverse l. of humerus
- 上腕二頭筋, 長頭の腱 Tendon of biceps brachii, long head
- 結節間溝 Intertubercular groove
- 結節間滑液鞘 Intertubercular synovial sheath
- 肩甲下筋の腱下包 Subtendinous bursa of subscapularis
- 腋窩陥凹 Axillary recess

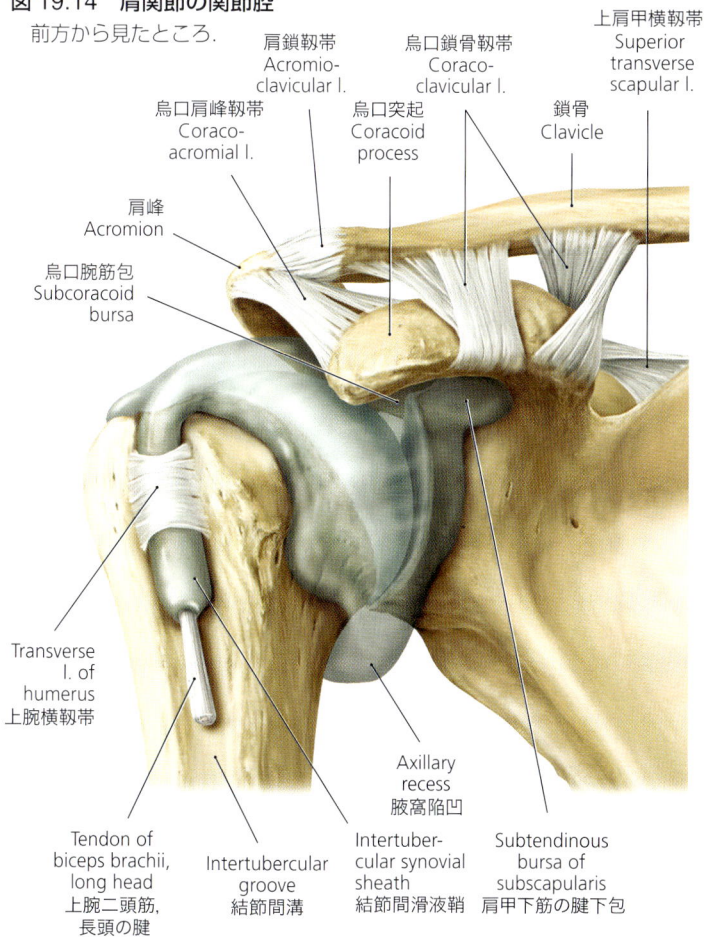

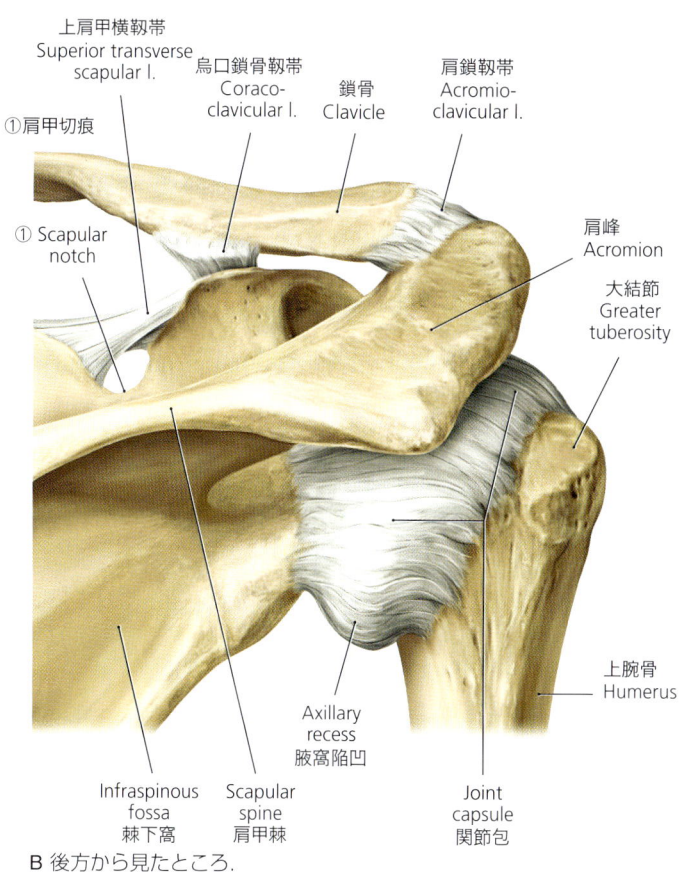

図 19.15 肩の MR 像

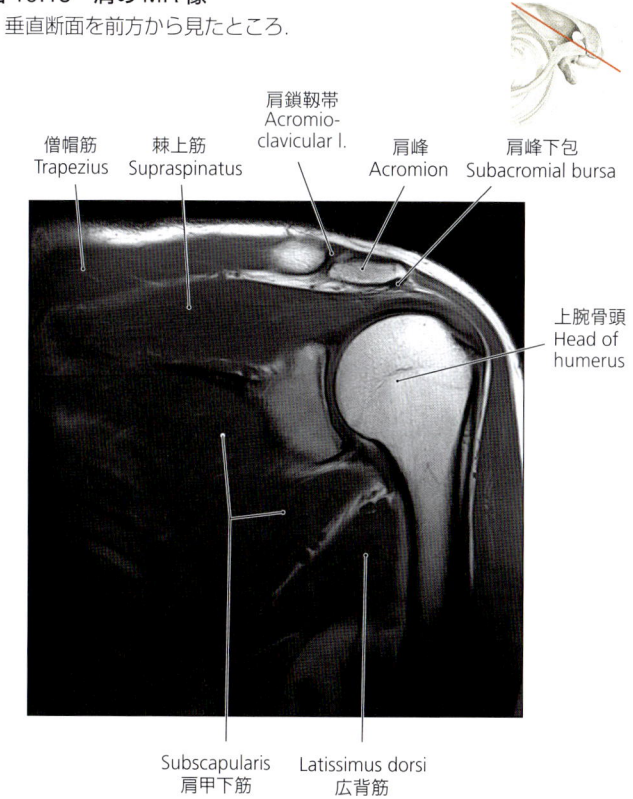

垂直断面を前方から見たところ．

- 僧帽筋 Trapezius
- 棘上筋 Supraspinatus
- 肩鎖靱帯 Acromio-clavicular l.
- 肩峰 Acromion
- 肩峰下包 Subacromial bursa
- 上腕骨頭 Head of humerus
- 肩甲下筋 Subscapularis
- 広背筋 Latissimus dorsi

肩峰下腔と肩峰下包
Subacromial Space & Bursae

図 19.16 肩峰下腔
右肩.

- 烏口肩峰弓 Coracoacromial arch
- 肩峰 Acromion
- 烏口肩峰靱帯 Coracoacromial ligament
- 烏口突起 Coracoid process
- 肩峰下包 Subacromial bursa
- 肩甲下筋の腱下包 Subtendinous bursa of subscapularis
- Subdeltoid bursa 三角筋下包
- 大結節 Greater tuberosity
- 上腕横靱帯 Transverse ligament of humerus
- 棘下筋 Infraspinatus
- 結節間の腱鞘 Intertubercular tendon sheath
- 小円筋 Teres minor
- 上腕二頭筋, 短頭 Biceps brachii, short head
- 上腕骨 Humerus
- 上腕二頭筋, 長頭 Biceps brachii, long head

A 外側方から見たところ.

図 19.17 肩峰下包と関節腔
右肩. 矢状断を外側方から見たところ. 上腕骨を取り除いてある.

- 烏口肩峰弓 Coracoacromial arch
- ①烏口肩峰靱帯
- 肩峰 Acromion
- Coracoacromial ligament ①
- Coracoid process 烏口突起
- 棘上筋 Supraspinatus
- 肩峰下包 Subacromial bursa
- 肩甲下筋の腱下包 Subtendinous bursa of subscapularis
- 棘下筋 Infraspinatus
- 関節窩 Glenoid cavity
- 上腕二頭筋, 長頭の腱 Tendon of biceps brachii, long head
- 関節唇 Glenoid labrum
- 関節包 Joint capsule
- Subscapularis 肩甲下筋
- 小円筋 Teres minor
- 腋窩陥凹 Axillary recess
- 棘下筋 Infraspinatus
- 肩甲下筋 Subscapularis
- 肩甲骨, 外側縁 Scapula, lateral border

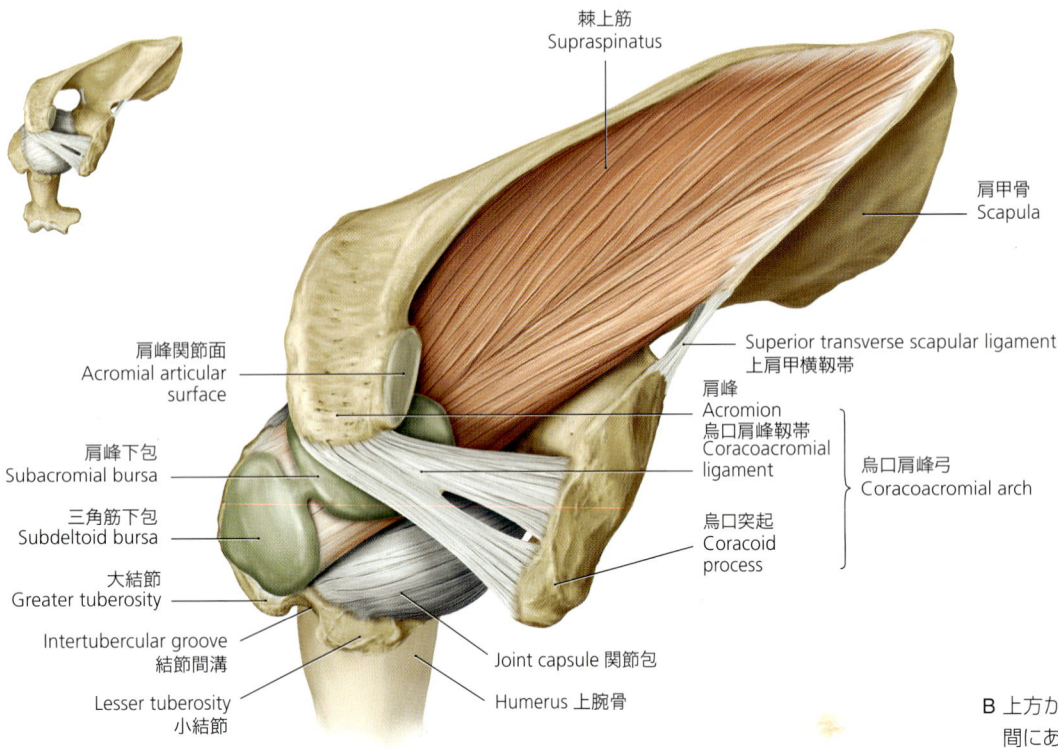

- 棘上筋 Supraspinatus
- 肩甲骨 Scapula
- 肩峰関節面 Acromial articular surface
- Superior transverse scapular ligament 上肩甲横靱帯
- 肩峰 Acromion
- 肩峰下包 Subacromial bursa
- 烏口肩峰靱帯 Coracoacromial ligament
- 三角筋下包 Subdeltoid bursa
- 烏口肩峰弓 Coracoacromial arch
- 大結節 Greater tuberosity
- 烏口突起 Coracoid process
- Intertubercular groove 結節間溝
- Joint capsule 関節包
- Lesser tuberosity 小結節
- Humerus 上腕骨

B 上方から見たところ. 棘上筋と烏口肩峰弓の間にある肩峰下包に注目.

図 19.18 肩峰下包と三角筋下包
右肩，前方から見たところ．

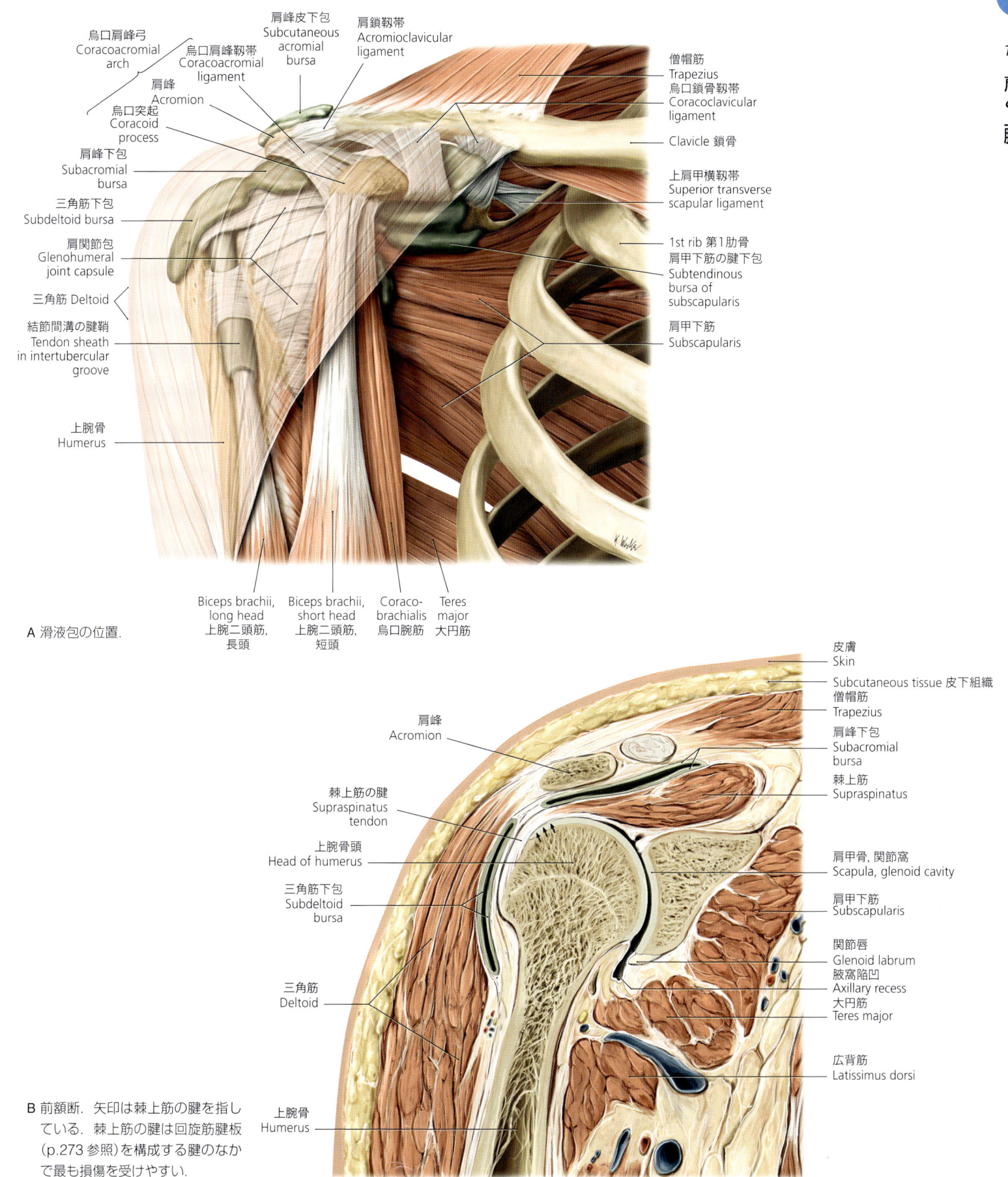

烏口肩峰弓
Coracoacromial arch

烏口肩峰靱帯
Coracoacromial ligament

肩峰
Acromion

烏口突起
Coracoid process

肩峰下包
Subacromial bursa

三角筋下包
Subdeltoid bursa

肩関節包
Glenohumeral joint capsule

三角筋 Deltoid

結節間溝の腱鞘
Tendon sheath in intertubercular groove

上腕骨
Humerus

肩峰皮下包
Subcutaneous acromial bursa

肩鎖靱帯
Acromioclavicular ligament

僧帽筋
Trapezius

烏口鎖骨靱帯
Coracoclavicular ligament

Clavicle 鎖骨

上肩甲横靱帯
Superior transverse scapular ligament

1st rib 第1肋骨

肩甲下筋の腱下包
Subtendinous bursa of subscapularis

肩甲下筋
Subscapularis

Biceps brachii, long head
上腕二頭筋, 長頭

Biceps brachii, short head
上腕二頭筋, 短頭

Coraco-brachialis
烏口腕筋

Teres major
大円筋

A 滑液包の位置．

皮膚
Skin

Subcutaneous tissue 皮下組織

僧帽筋
Trapezius

肩峰
Acromion

肩峰下包
Subacromial bursa

棘上筋
Supraspinatus

棘上筋の腱
Supraspinatus tendon

上腕骨頭
Head of humerus

肩甲骨, 関節窩
Scapula, glenoid cavity

三角筋下包
Subdeltoid bursa

肩甲下筋
Subscapularis

関節唇
Glenoid labrum

腋窩陥凹
Axillary recess

三角筋
Deltoid

大円筋
Teres major

広背筋
Latissimus dorsi

上腕骨
Humerus

B 前額断．矢印は棘上筋の腱を指している．棘上筋の腱は回旋筋腱板（p.273 参照）を構成する腱のなかで最も損傷を受けやすい．

肩と上腕の前面にある筋 (1)
Anterior Muscles of the Shoulder & Arm (I)

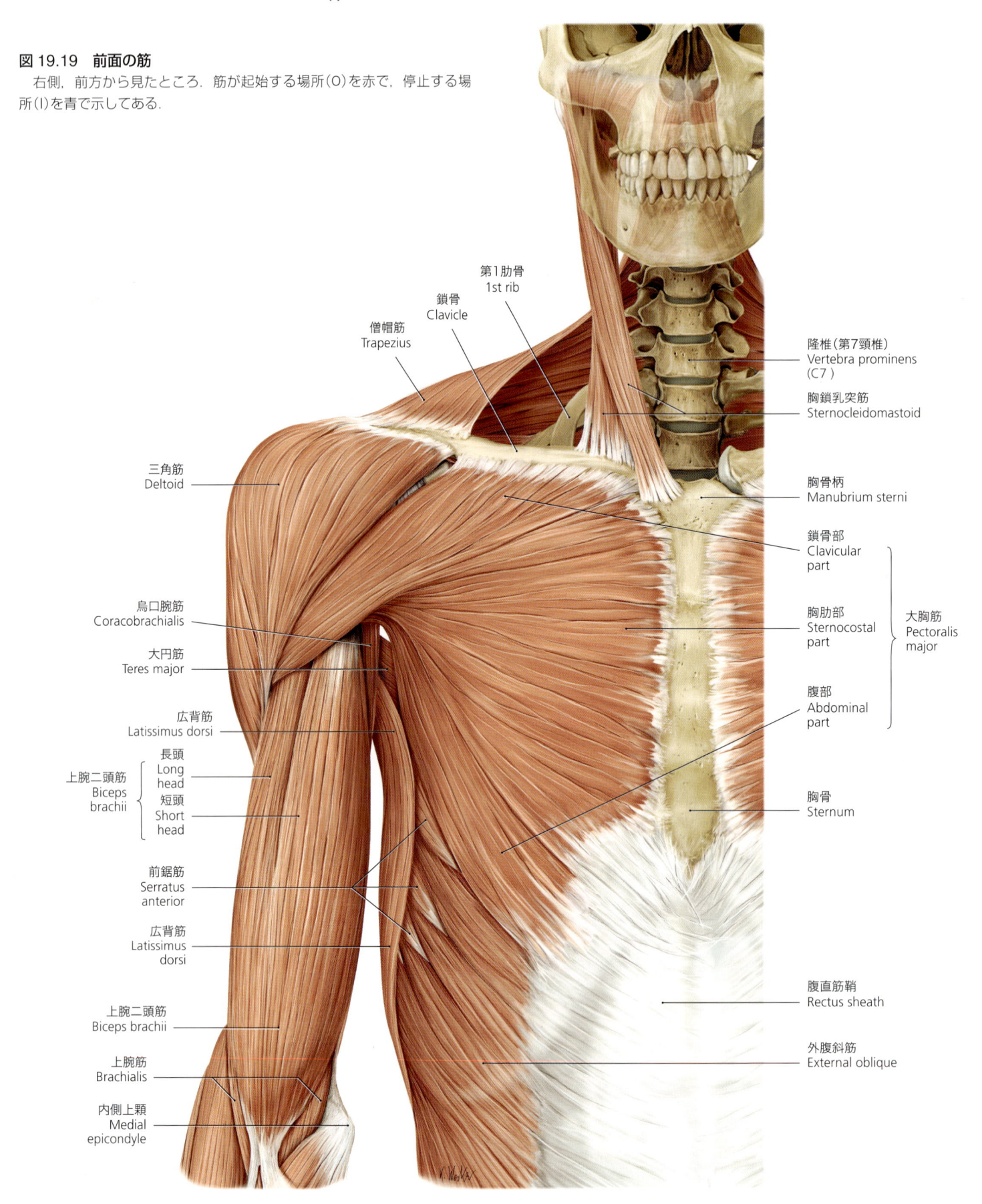

図 19.19 前面の筋
右側，前方から見たところ．筋が起始する場所(O)を赤で，停止する場所(I)を青で示してある．

主なラベル：
- 僧帽筋 Trapezius
- 鎖骨 Clavicle
- 第1肋骨 1st rib
- 隆椎（第7頸椎）Vertebra prominens (C7)
- 胸鎖乳突筋 Sternocleidomastoid
- 三角筋 Deltoid
- 胸骨柄 Manubrium sterni
- 烏口腕筋 Coracobrachialis
- 大円筋 Teres major
- 大胸筋 Pectoralis major
  - 鎖骨部 Clavicular part
  - 胸肋部 Sternocostal part
  - 腹部 Abdominal part
- 広背筋 Latissimus dorsi
- 胸骨 Sternum
- 上腕二頭筋 Biceps brachii
  - 長頭 Long head
  - 短頭 Short head
- 前鋸筋 Serratus anterior
- 広背筋 Latissimus dorsi
- 腹直筋鞘 Rectus sheath
- 上腕二頭筋 Biceps brachii
- 上腕筋 Brachialis
- 外腹斜筋 External oblique
- 内側上顆 Medial epicondyle

A 表層の筋．

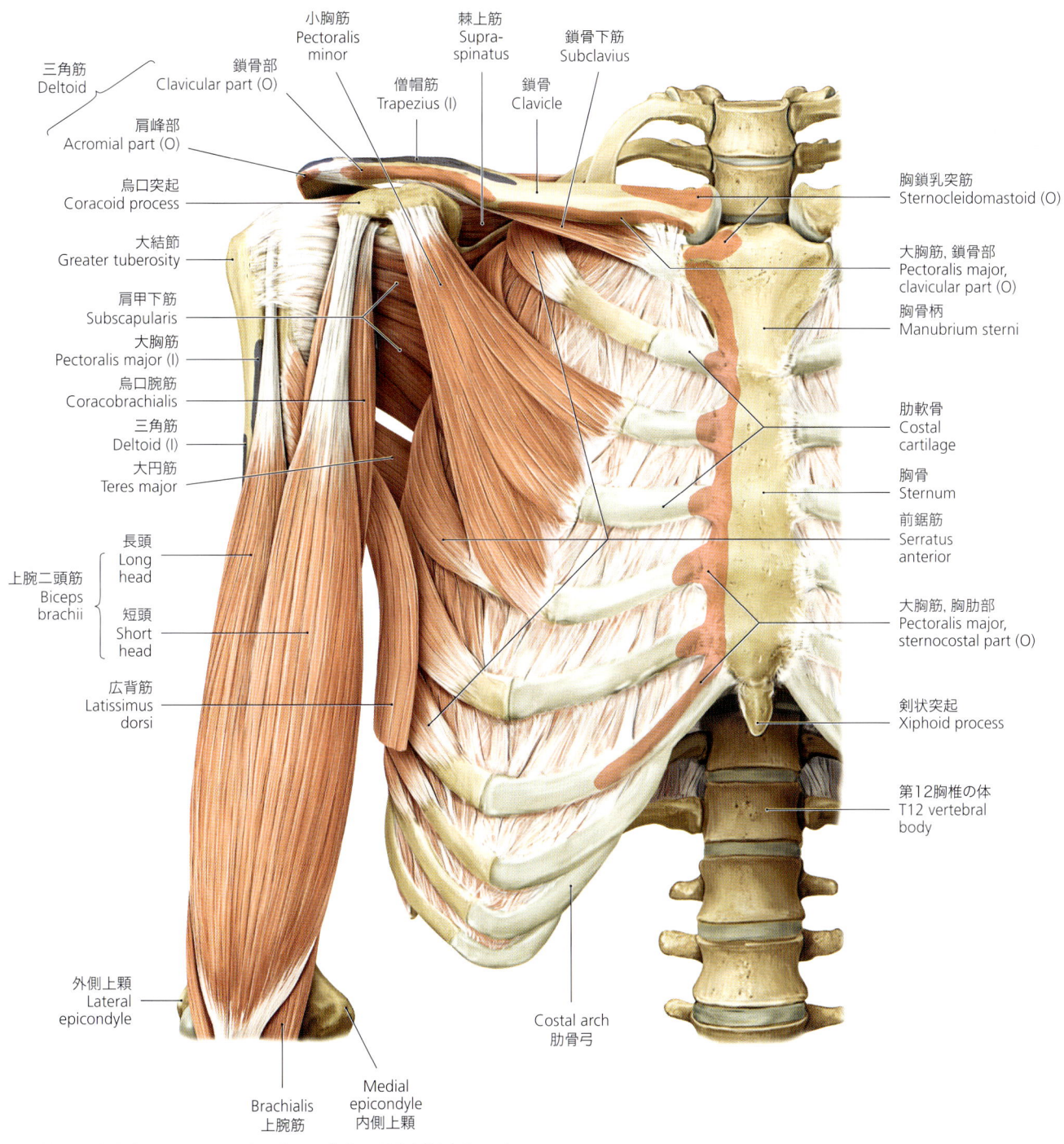

B 深層の筋．胸鎖乳突筋，僧帽筋，大胸筋，三角筋，外腹斜筋を取り除いてある．

肩と上腕の前面にある筋（2）
Anterior Muscles of the Shoulder & Arm (II)

図 19.20　前方からの剖出
右上肢．前方から見たところ．筋が起始する場所（O）を赤で，停止する場所（I）を青で示してある．

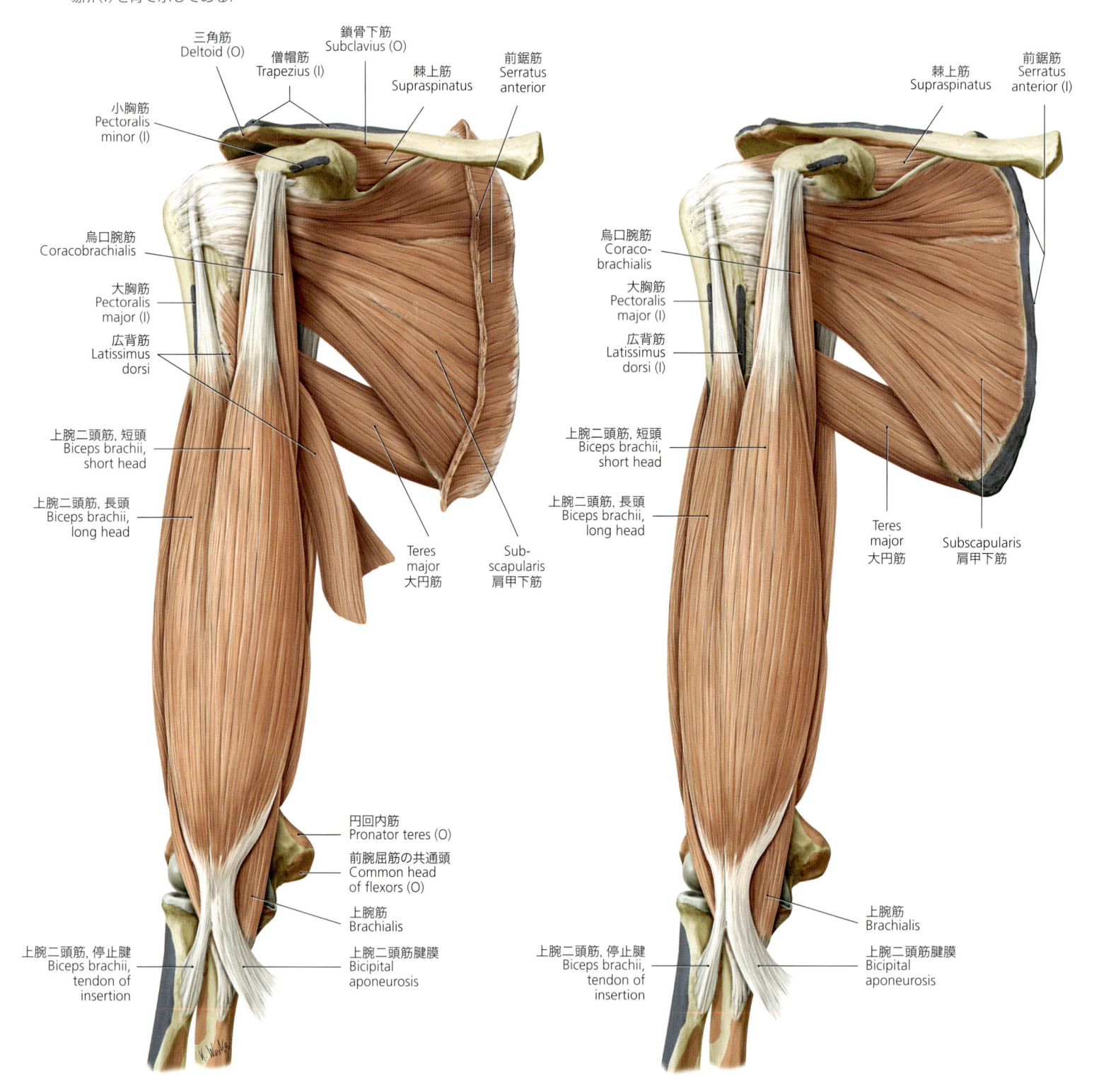

A 胸郭の骨格を取り除いてある．また，広背筋と前鋸筋を部分的に取り除いてある．

B 広背筋と前鋸筋を取り除いたところ．

主な標識：
- 三角筋 Deltoid (O)
- 僧帽筋 Trapezius (I)
- 鎖骨下筋 Subclavius (O)
- 棘上筋 Supraspinatus
- 前鋸筋 Serratus anterior
- 小胸筋 Pectoralis minor (I)
- 烏口腕筋 Coracobrachialis
- 大胸筋 Pectoralis major (I)
- 広背筋 Latissimus dorsi (I)
- 上腕二頭筋, 短頭 Biceps brachii, short head
- 上腕二頭筋, 長頭 Biceps brachii, long head
- 大円筋 Teres major
- 肩甲下筋 Subscapularis
- 円回内筋 Pronator teres (O)
- 前腕屈筋の共通頭 Common head of flexors (O)
- 上腕筋 Brachialis
- 上腕二頭筋, 停止腱 Biceps brachii, tendon of insertion
- 上腕二頭筋腱膜 Bicipital aponeurosis

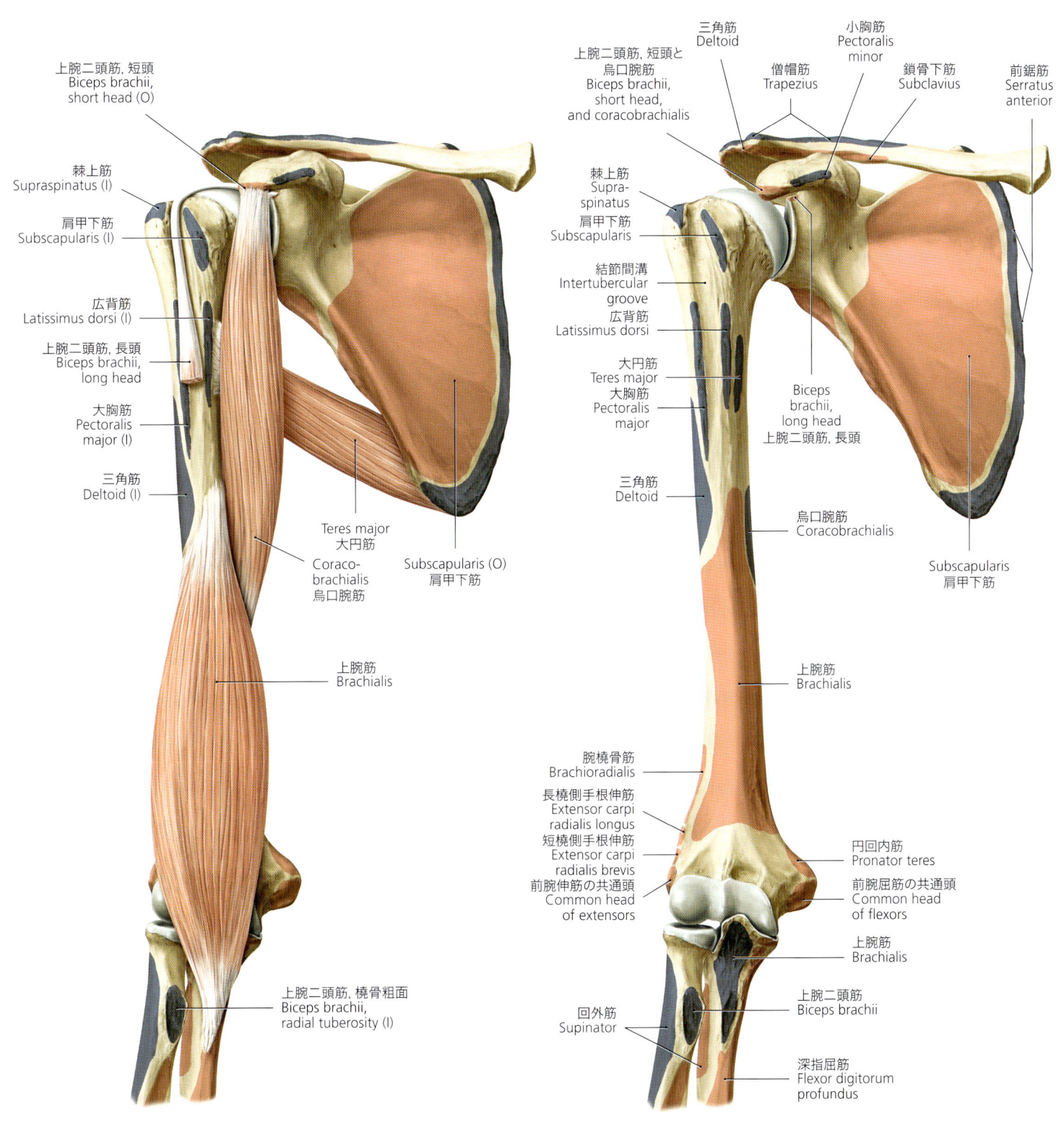

C 肩甲下筋と棘上筋を取り除いたところ．また，上腕二頭筋を部分的に取り除いてある．

D 上腕二頭筋，烏口腕筋，上腕筋，大円筋を取り除いたところ．

肩と上腕の後面にある筋 (1)
Posterior Muscles of the Shoulder & Arm (I)

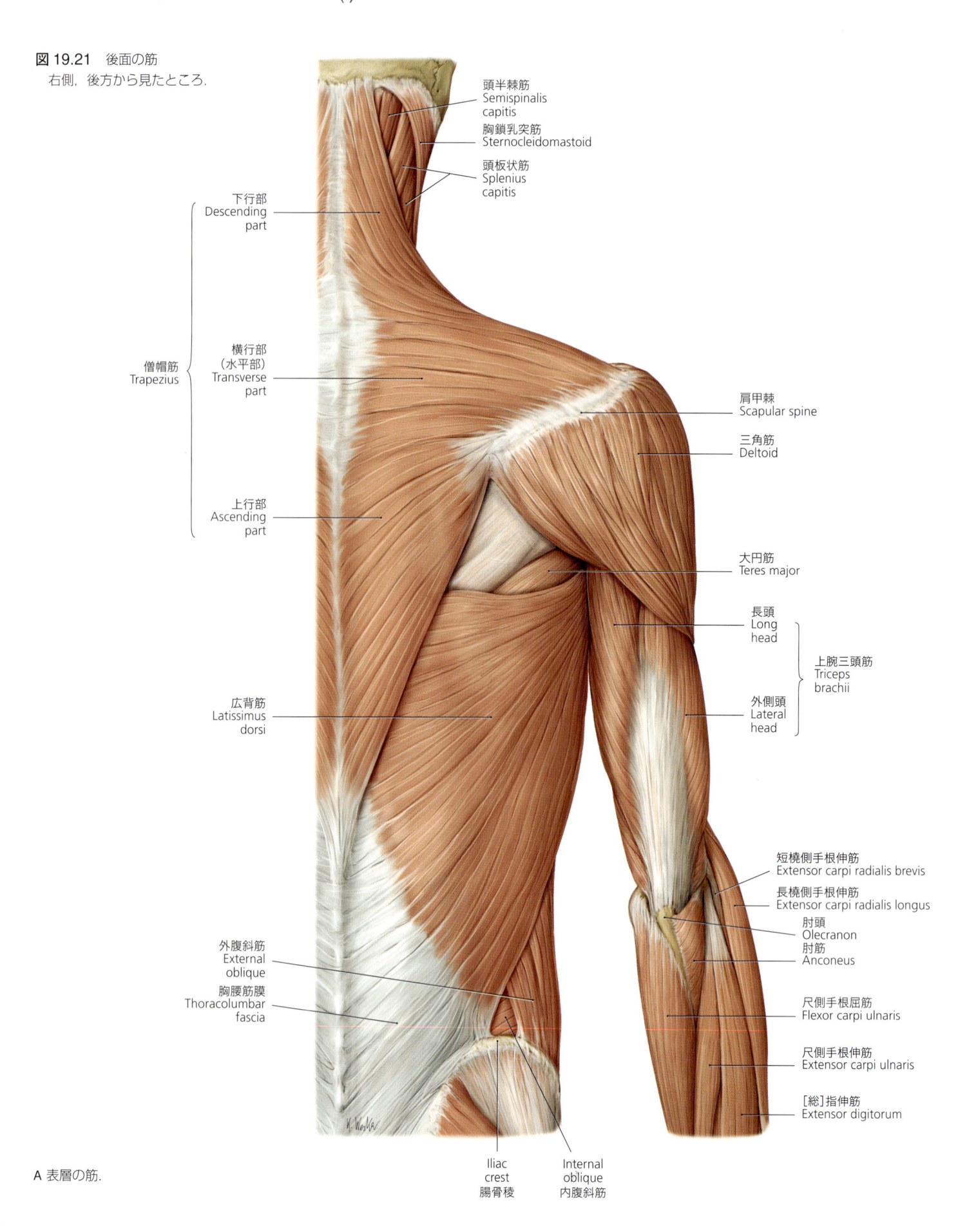

図 19.21　後面の筋
右側，後方から見たところ．

僧帽筋 Trapezius
- 下行部 Descending part
- 横行部（水平部） Transverse part
- 上行部 Ascending part

頭半棘筋 Semispinalis capitis
胸鎖乳突筋 Sternocleidomastoid
頭板状筋 Splenius capitis
肩甲棘 Scapular spine
三角筋 Deltoid
大円筋 Teres major

上腕三頭筋 Triceps brachii
- 長頭 Long head
- 外側頭 Lateral head

広背筋 Latissimus dorsi
短橈側手根伸筋 Extensor carpi radialis brevis
長橈側手根伸筋 Extensor carpi radialis longus
肘頭 Olecranon
肘筋 Anconeus
尺側手根屈筋 Flexor carpi ulnaris
尺側手根伸筋 Extensor carpi ulnaris
［総］指伸筋 Extensor digitorum
外腹斜筋 External oblique
胸腰筋膜 Thoracolumbar fascia
腸骨稜 Iliac crest
内腹斜筋 Internal oblique

A 表層の筋．

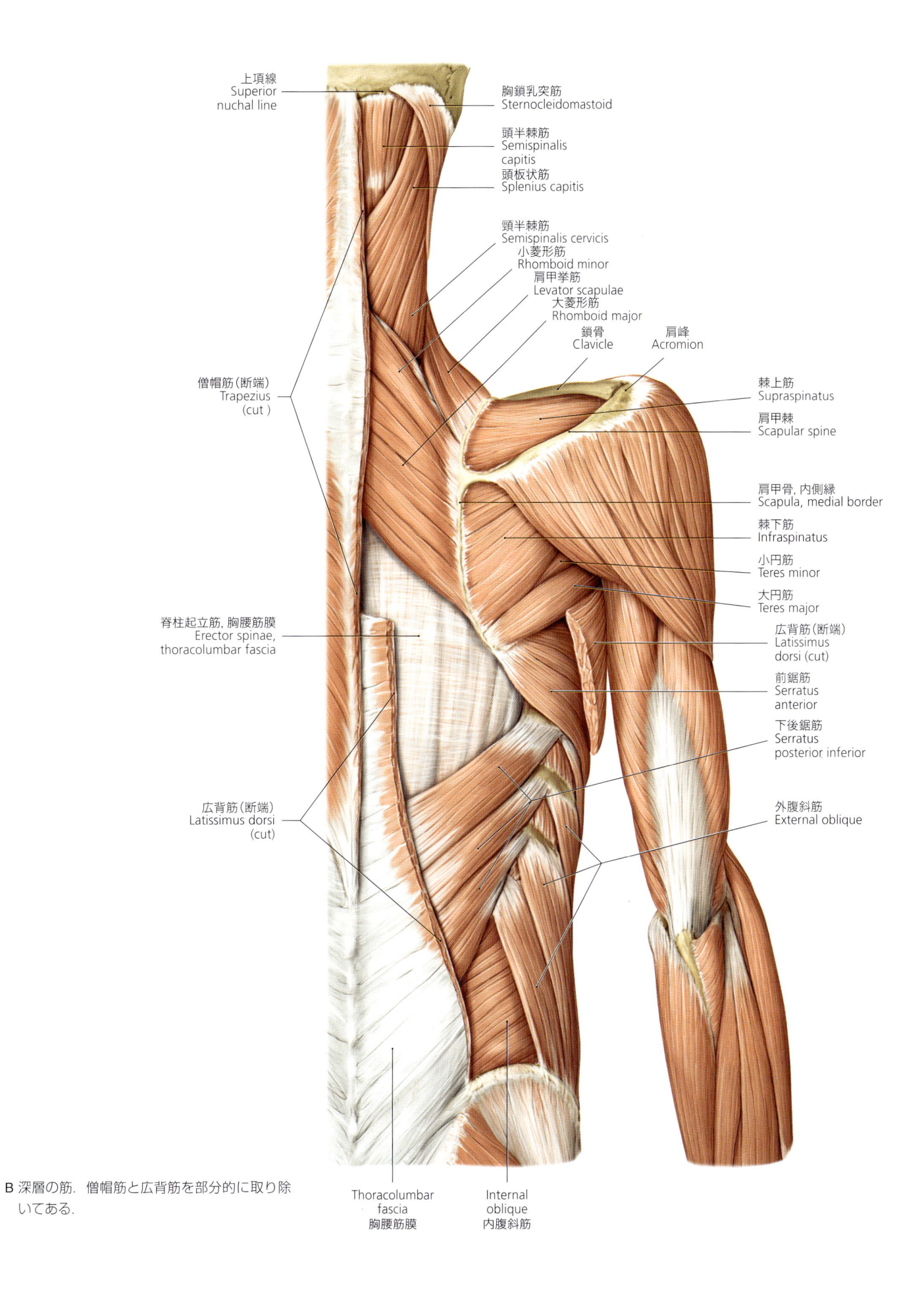

B 深層の筋．僧帽筋と広背筋を部分的に取り除いてある．

肩と上腕の後面にある筋 (2)
Posterior Muscles of the Shoulder & Arm (II)

図 19.22 後方からの剖出
右上肢，後方から見たところ．筋が起始する場所(O)を赤で，停止する場所(I)を青で示してある．

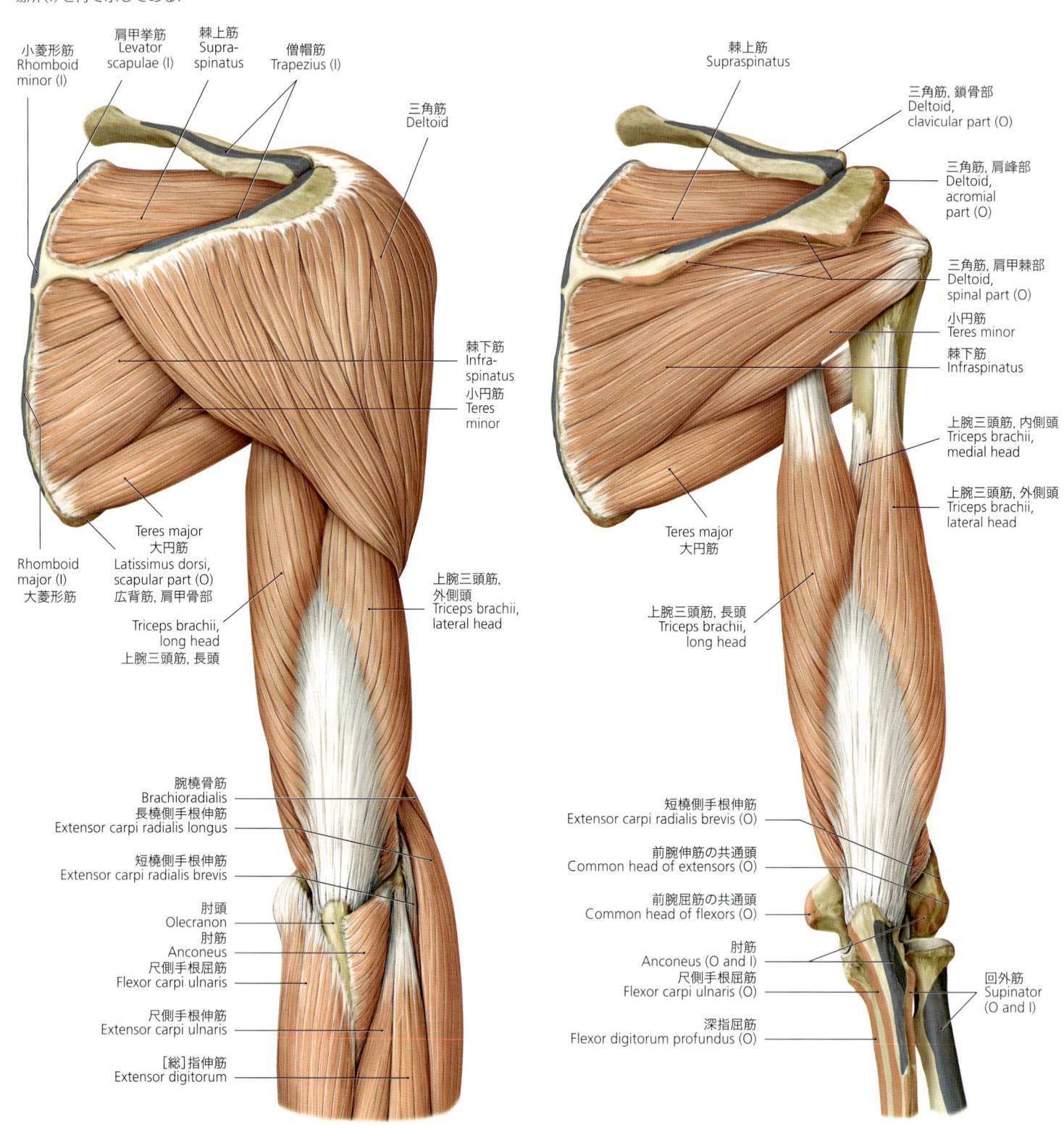

A 大菱形筋，小菱形筋，前鋸筋，肩甲挙筋を取り除いてある．

B 三角筋と前腕の筋を取り除いたところ．

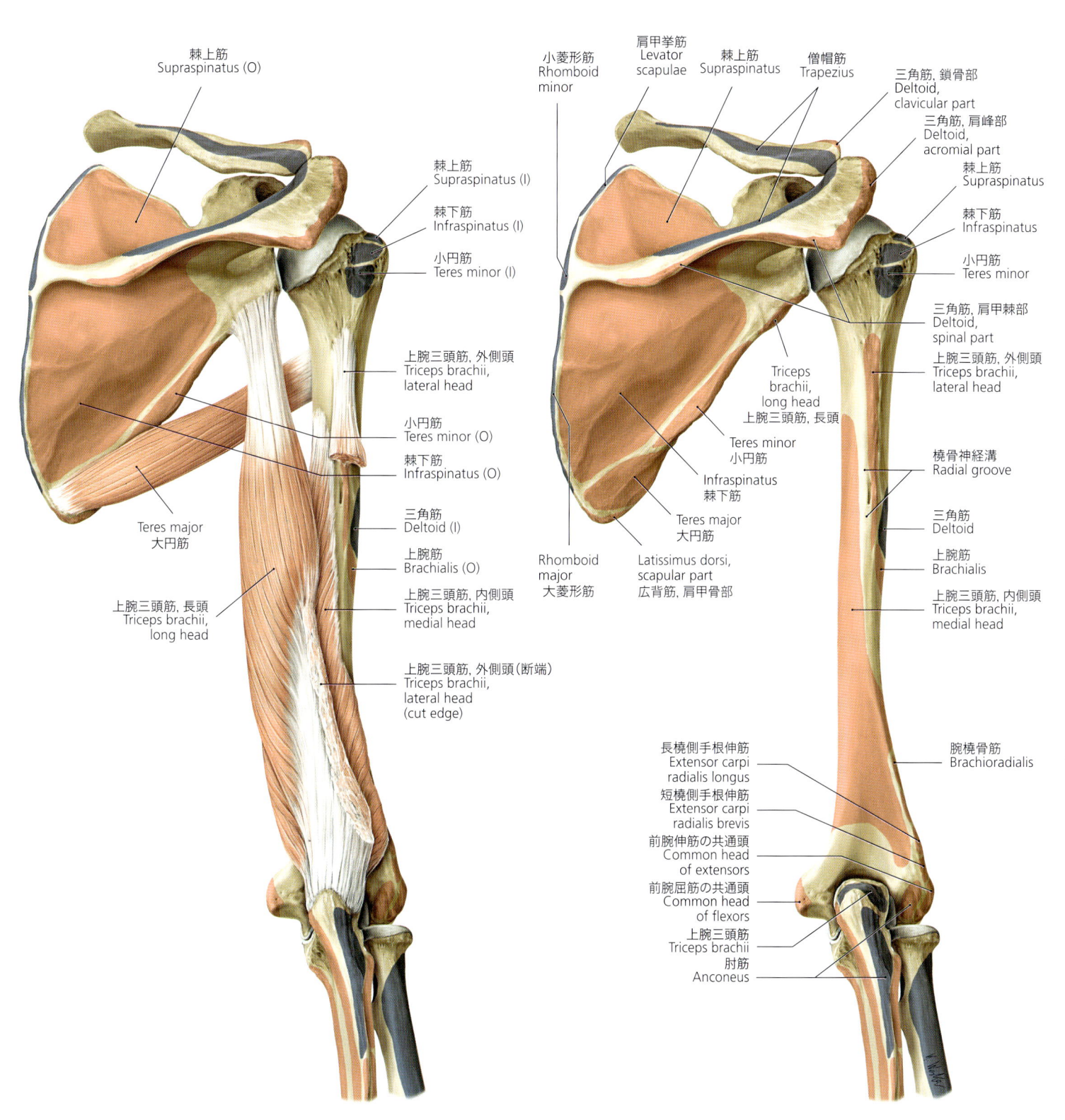

C 棘上筋，棘下筋，小円筋を取り除いたところ．また，上腕三頭筋も部分的に取り除いてある．

D 上腕三頭筋と大円筋を取り除いたところ．

個々の筋（1）
Muscle Facts (I)

> 三角筋の3つの部分の作用は，筋と上腕骨の位置関係，あるいは筋と運動軸との関係によって決まる．三角筋（鎖骨部と肩甲棘部）は60°以下の外転位では内転筋として，60°以上の外転位では外転筋として作用する．つまりこれらの部位は拮抗的にも，協調的にも作用することができる．

図 19.23　三角筋
右肩．

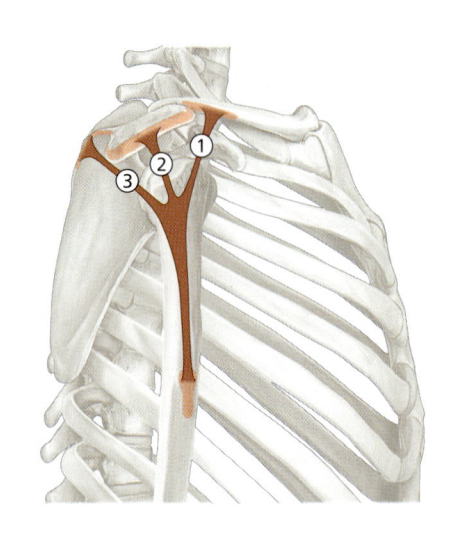

A 三角筋の各部，右外側方から見たところ．

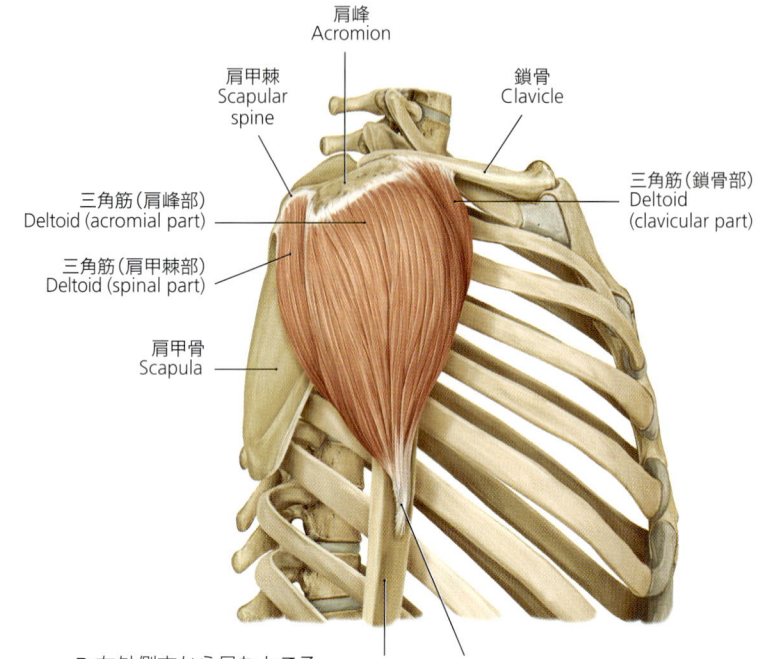

B 右外側方から見たところ．

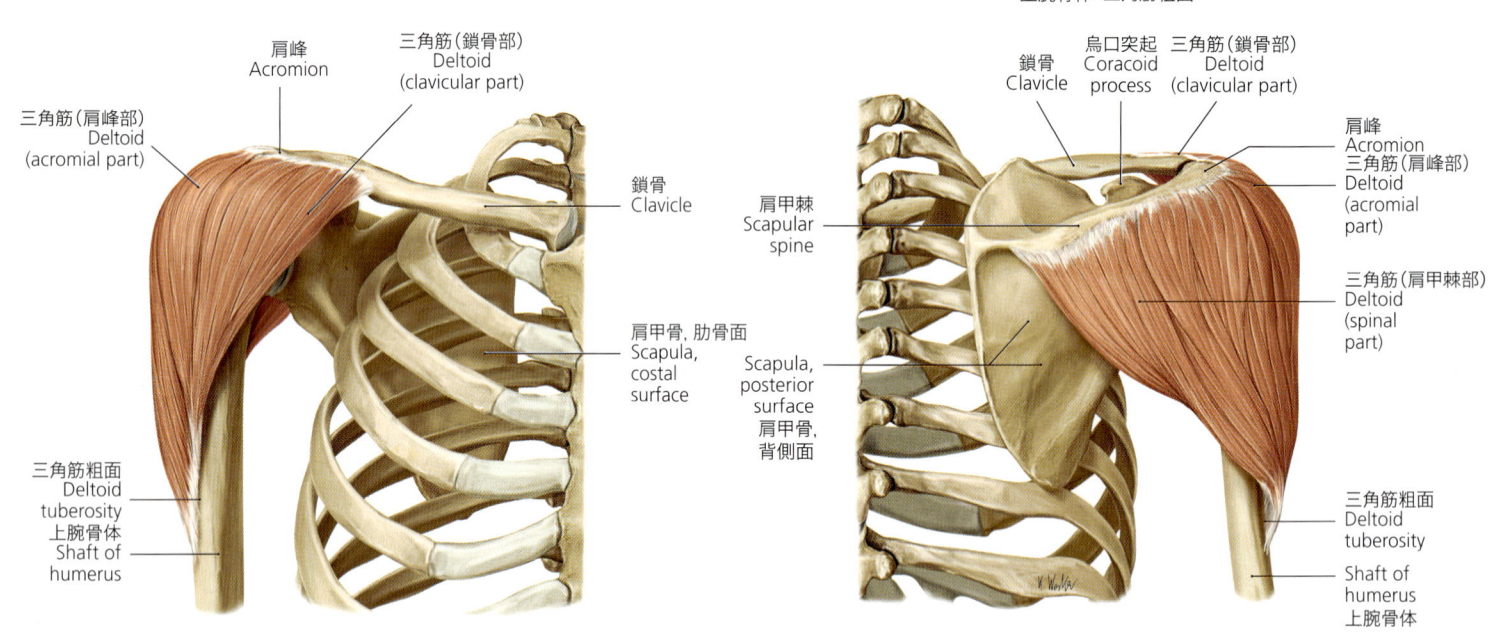

C 前方から見たところ．

D 後方から見たところ．

表 19.2　三角筋の各部

筋		起始	停止	神経支配	作用*
三角筋	①鎖骨部	鎖骨の外側3分の1	上腕骨（三角筋粗面）	腋窩神経（C5, C6）	上腕の前方挙上，内旋，内転
	②肩峰部	肩峰			上腕の外転
	③肩甲棘部	肩甲棘			上腕の後方挙上，外旋，内転

*60°〜90°の外転位では，鎖骨部と肩甲棘部は肩峰部の外転作用を補助する．

図 19.24 回旋筋腱板

右肩．回旋筋腱板は4つの筋（棘上筋，棘下筋，小円筋，肩甲下筋）によって形成される．

A 後方から見たところ．

B 前方から見たところ．

C 前方から見たところ．

D 外側方から見たところ．

E 後方から見たところ．

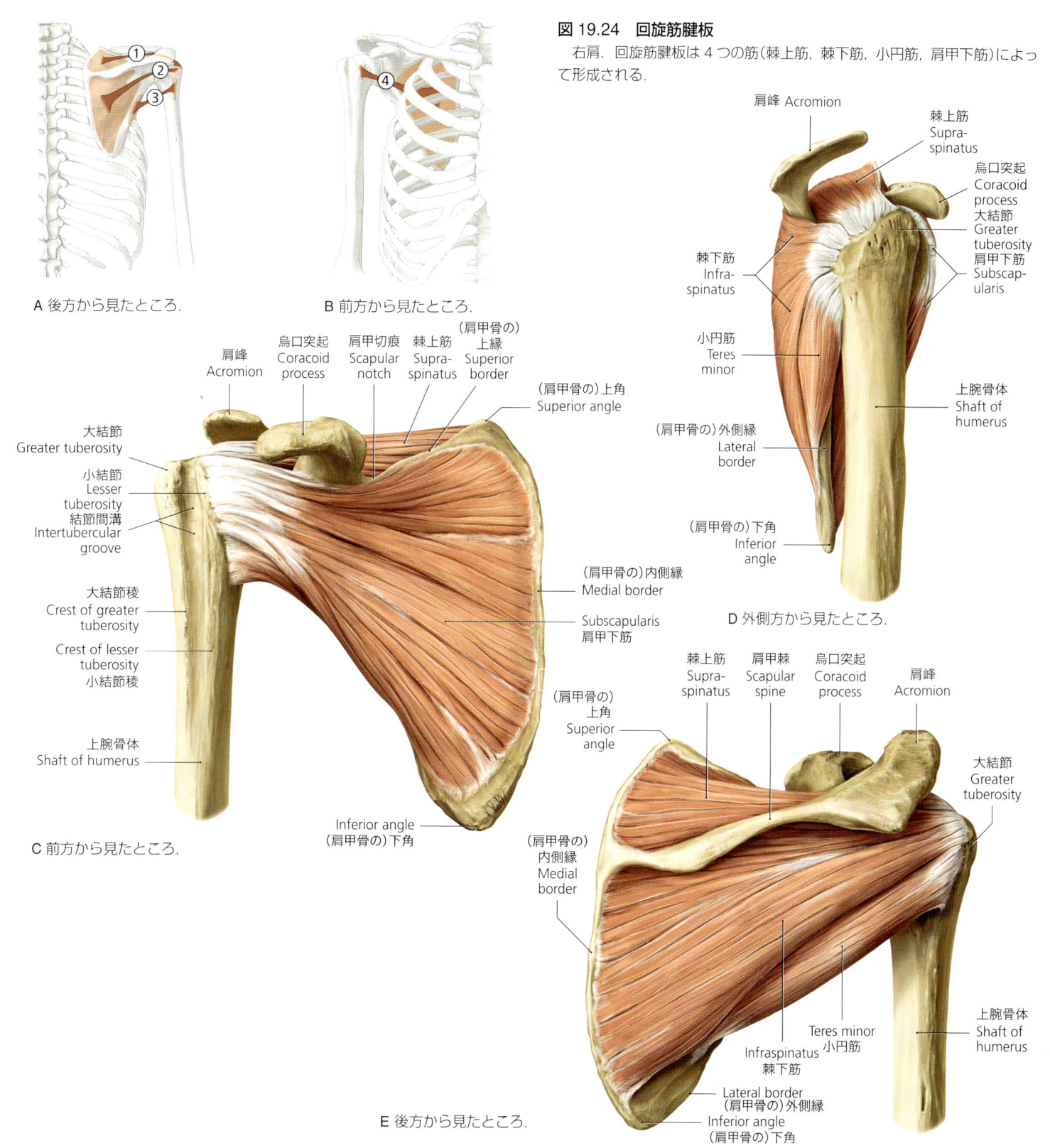

表 19.3	回旋筋腱板を構成する筋				
筋	起始	停止		神経支配	作用
①棘上筋	肩甲骨	棘上窩	上腕骨 大結節	肩甲上神経（C4-C6）	上腕の外転
②棘下筋		棘下窩			上腕の外旋
③小円筋		外側縁		腋窩神経（C5, C6）	上腕の外旋，弱い内転作用もある
④肩甲下筋		肩甲下窩	小結節	肩甲下神経（C5, C6）	上腕の内旋

個々の筋 (2)
Muscle Facts (II)

図 19.25　大胸筋と烏口腕筋
前方から見たところ.

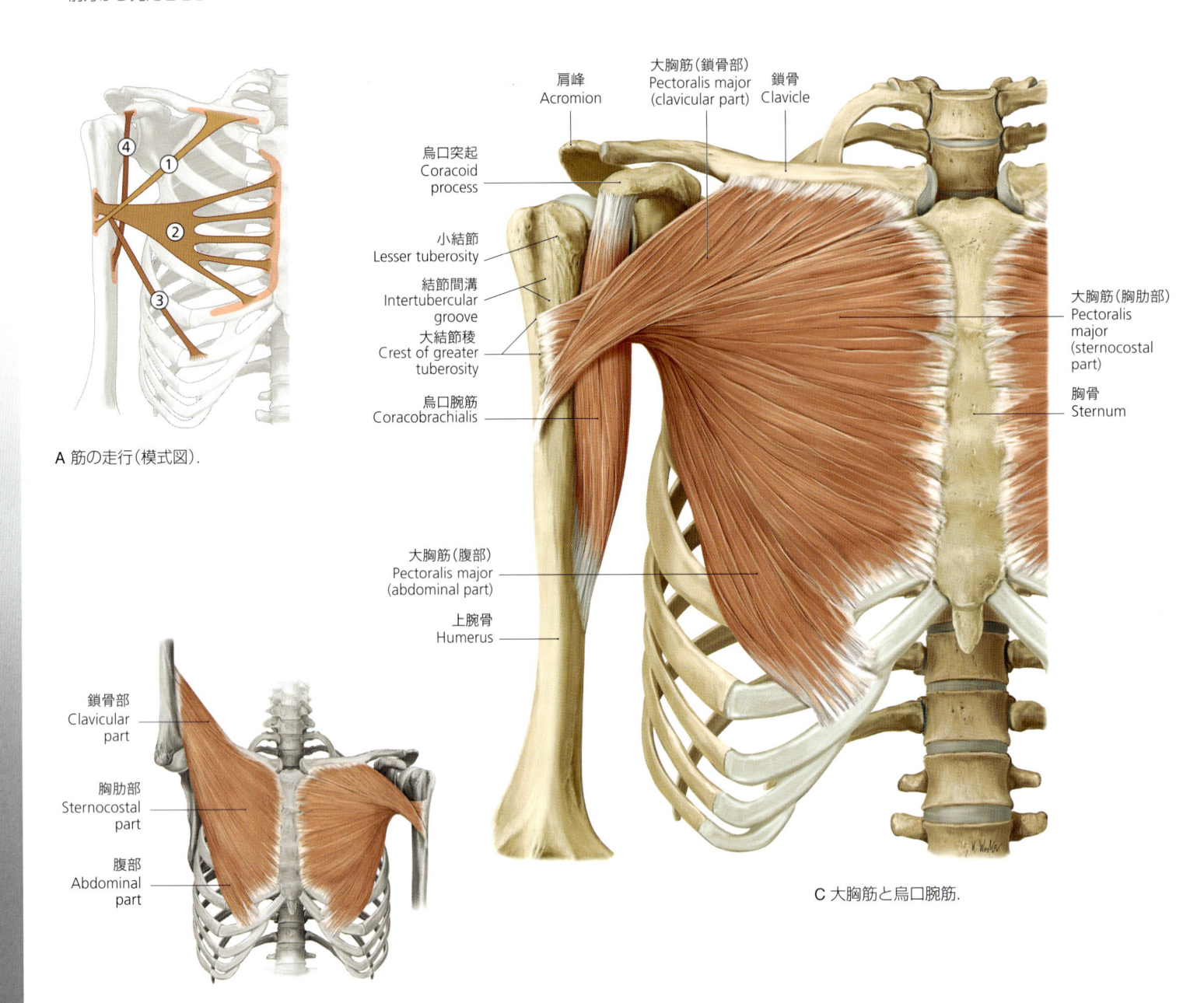

A 筋の走行 (模式図).

B 大胸筋, 解剖学的正位 (左) と上肢を挙上した場合 (右).

- 鎖骨部　Clavicular part
- 胸肋部　Sternocostal part
- 腹部　Abdominal part

C 大胸筋と烏口腕筋.

- 肩峰　Acromion
- 大胸筋 (鎖骨部)　Pectoralis major (clavicular part)
- 鎖骨　Clavicle
- 烏口突起　Coracoid process
- 小結節　Lesser tuberosity
- 結節間溝　Intertubercular groove
- 大結節稜　Crest of greater tuberosity
- 烏口腕筋　Coracobrachialis
- 大胸筋 (胸肋部)　Pectoralis major (sternocostal part)
- 胸骨　Sternum
- 大胸筋 (腹部)　Pectoralis major (abdominal part)
- 上腕骨　Humerus

表 19.4　大胸筋と烏口腕筋

筋		起始	停止	神経支配	作用
大胸筋	①鎖骨部	鎖骨 (内側半分)	上腕骨 (大結節稜)	内側・外側胸筋神経 (C5-T1)	筋全体: 上腕の内転・内旋 鎖骨部と胸肋部: 上腕の前方挙上, 肩が固定されている場合には呼吸 (吸息) を補助する
	②胸肋部	胸骨と第1-6肋軟骨			
	③腹部	腹直筋鞘 (前葉)			
④烏口腕筋		肩甲骨 (烏口突起)	上腕骨 (小結節稜の下方に続く線)	筋皮神経 (C6, C7)	上腕の前方挙上, 内転, 内旋

図 19.26 鎖骨下筋と小胸筋
右側，前方から見たところ．

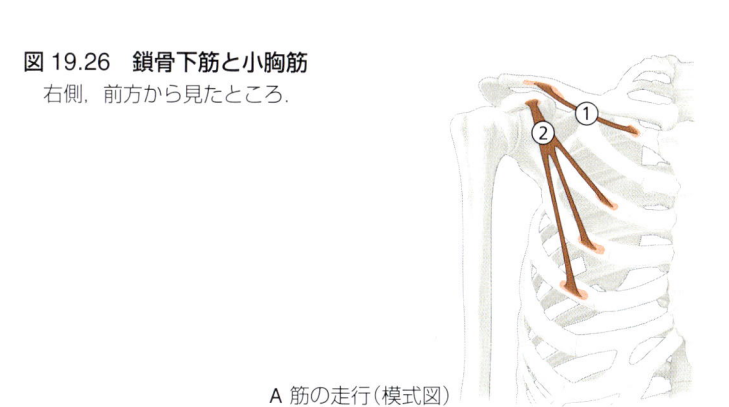

A 筋の走行（模式図）

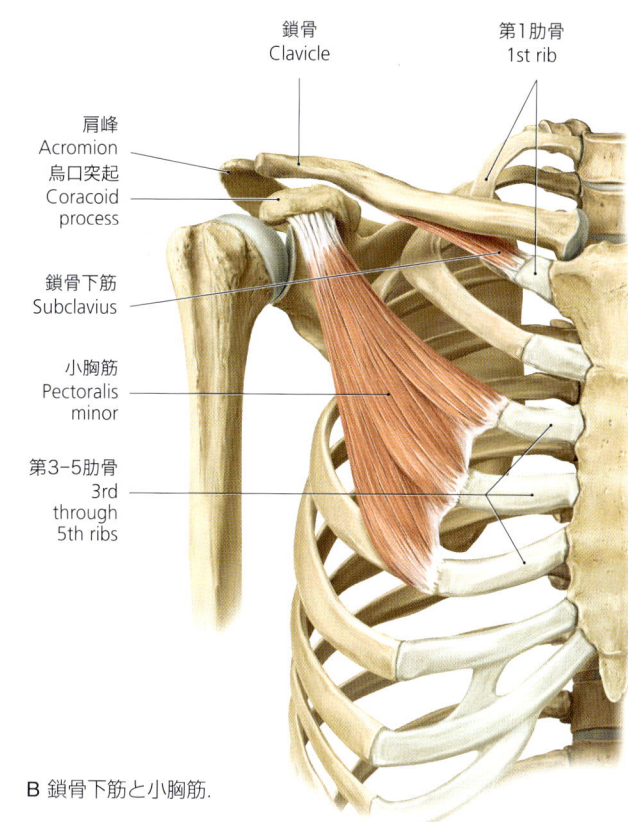

B 鎖骨下筋と小胸筋．

図 19.27 前鋸筋
右側，外側方から見たところ．

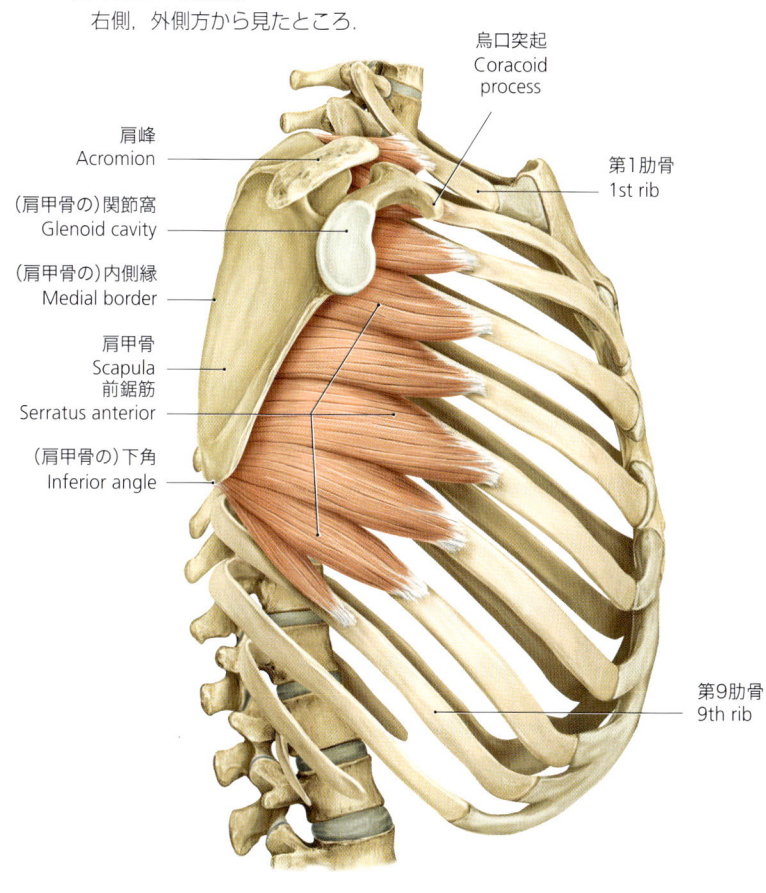

A 前鋸筋．

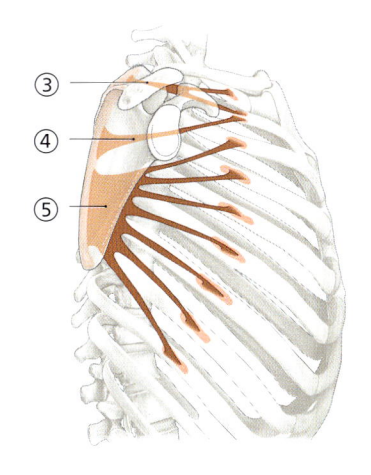

B 前鋸筋の走行（模式図）．

表 19.5　鎖骨下筋，小胸筋，前鋸筋

筋		起始	停止	神経支配	作用
①鎖骨下筋		第1肋骨	鎖骨（下面）	鎖骨下筋神経（C5，C6）	胸鎖関節において鎖骨を安定に保つ
②小胸筋		第3-5肋骨	烏口突起	内側・外側胸筋神経（C6-T1）	肩甲骨を引き下げ，下角を後内側に引く　関節窩を下方に回す，吸息の補助
前鋸筋	③上部	第1-9肋骨	肩甲骨（内側縁）	長胸神経（C5-C7）	上部：挙上した上腕を下げる
	④中間部				筋全体：肩甲骨を前外側に引く，肩が固定されている場合には肋骨を挙上する（吸息の補助）
	⑤下部				下部：肩甲骨の下角を前外側に引く

個々の筋(3)
Muscle Facts (III)

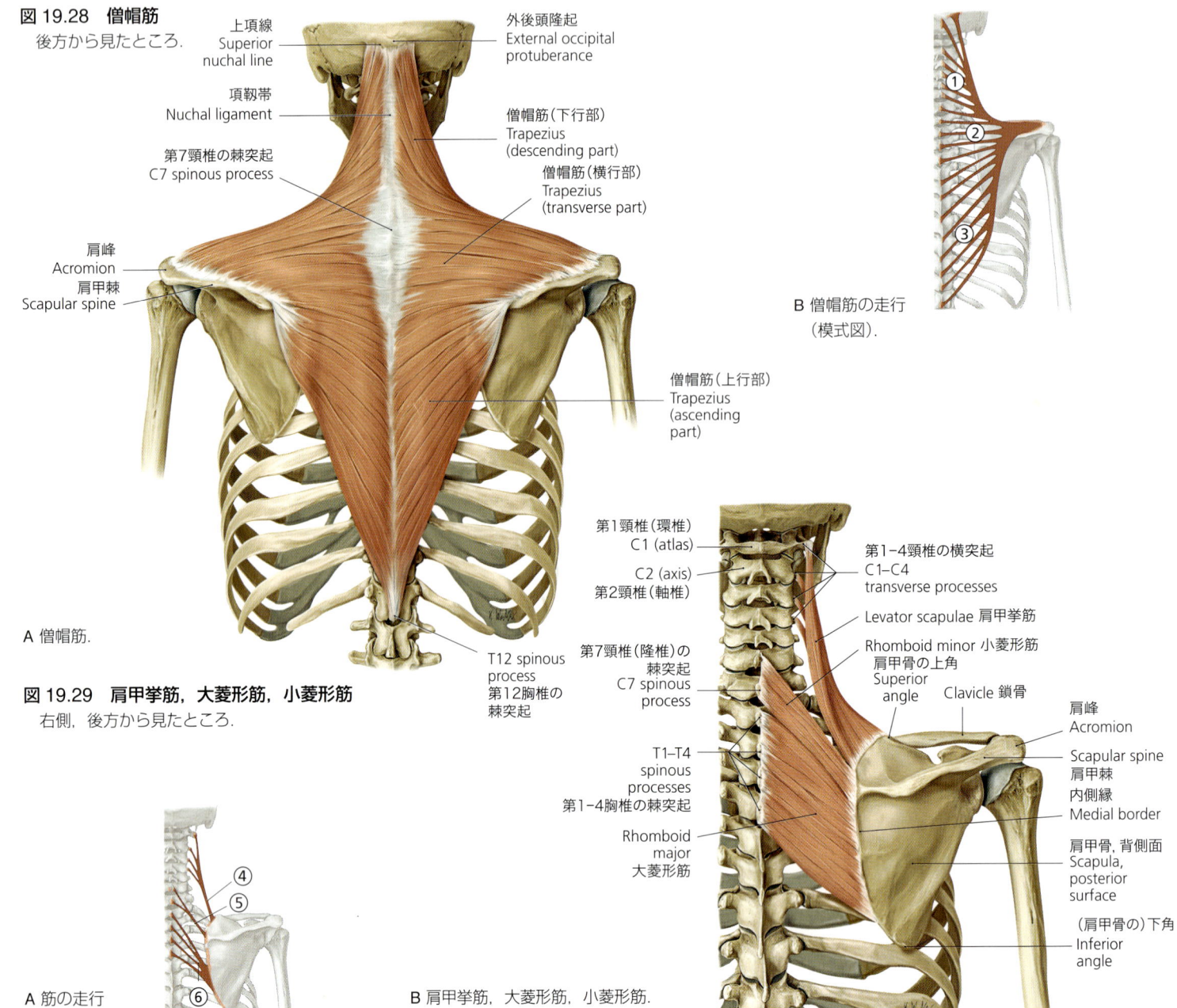

図 19.28 僧帽筋
後方から見たところ．

A 僧帽筋．

B 僧帽筋の走行（模式図）．

図 19.29 肩甲挙筋，大菱形筋，小菱形筋
右側，後方から見たところ．

A 筋の走行（模式図）．

B 肩甲挙筋，大菱形筋，小菱形筋．

表 19.6　僧帽筋，肩甲挙筋，大菱形筋，小菱形筋

筋		起始	停止	神経支配	作用
僧帽筋	①下行部	後頭骨：C1-C7 の棘突起	鎖骨（外側 3 分の 1）	副神経（CN XI），頸神経叢（C3, C4）	肩甲骨を上内側に引き，関節窩を上方に回す　頭を同側に傾け，対側に回旋する
	②水平部（横行部）	T1-T4 の高さの腱膜	肩峰		肩甲骨を内側に引く
	③上行部	T5-T12 の棘突起	肩甲棘		肩甲骨を下内側に引く
④肩甲挙筋		C1-C4 の横突起	肩甲骨（上角）	肩甲背神経（C4, C5）	肩甲骨を上内側に引き，下角を内側に動かす
⑤小菱形筋		C6, C7 の棘突起	肩甲骨の内側縁（肩甲棘より上の部分）		肩甲骨を安定させる，肩甲骨を上内側に引く
⑥大菱形筋		T1-T4 の棘突起	肩甲骨の内側縁（肩甲棘より下の部分）		

CN＝脳神経．

図 19.30　広背筋と大円筋
後方から見たところ．

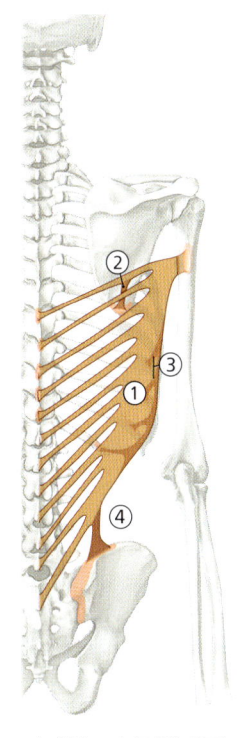

A　広背筋の走行（模式図）．

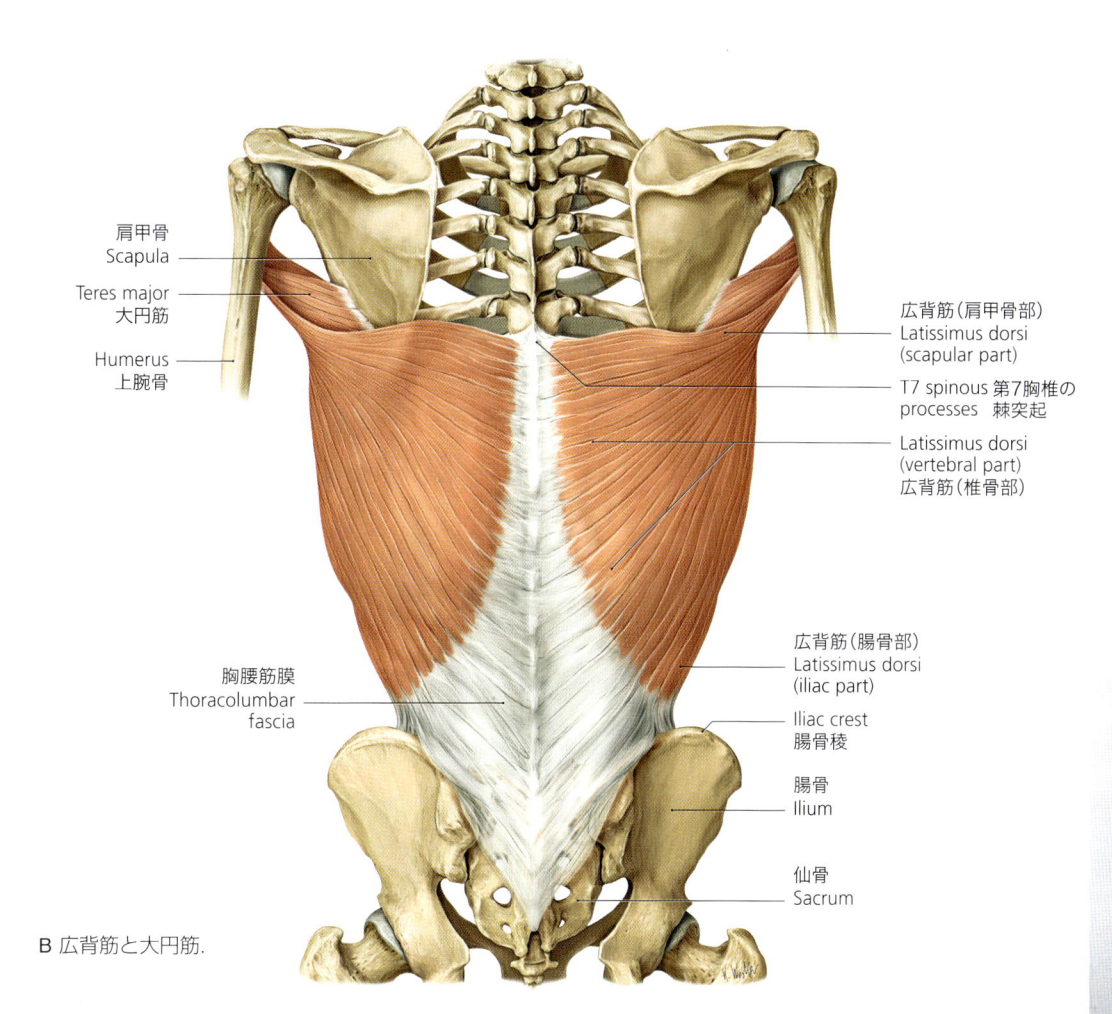

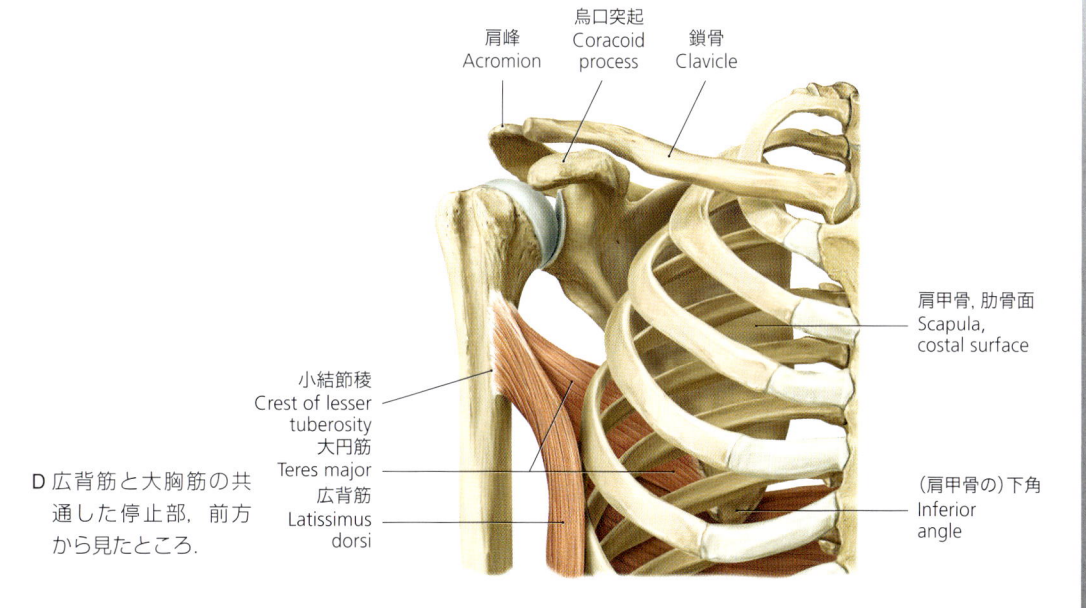

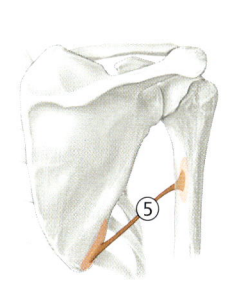

B　広背筋と大円筋．

C　大円筋の走行（模式図）．

D　広背筋と大胸筋の共通した停止部，前方から見たところ．

表 19.7		広背筋と大円筋			
筋		起始	停止	神経支配	作用
広背筋	①椎骨部	T7-T12 の棘突起，胸腰筋膜	上腕骨の小結節稜	胸背神経（C6-C8）	上腕の内旋，内転，後方挙上，呼息の補助（咳嗽筋）
	②肩甲骨部	肩甲骨（下角）			
	③肋骨部	第 9-12 肋骨			
	④腸骨部	腸骨稜（後 3 分の 1）			
⑤大円筋		肩甲骨（下角）		下位の肩甲下神経（C5-C7）	上腕の内旋，内転，後方挙上

個々の筋 (4)
Muscle Facts (IV)

上腕の前面と後面の筋は，肘関節に対する作用に基づき，それぞれ屈筋および伸筋と総称される．烏口腕筋は局所解剖学的には上腕前方の筋であるが，機能的には肩の筋に含まれる（p.274 参照）．

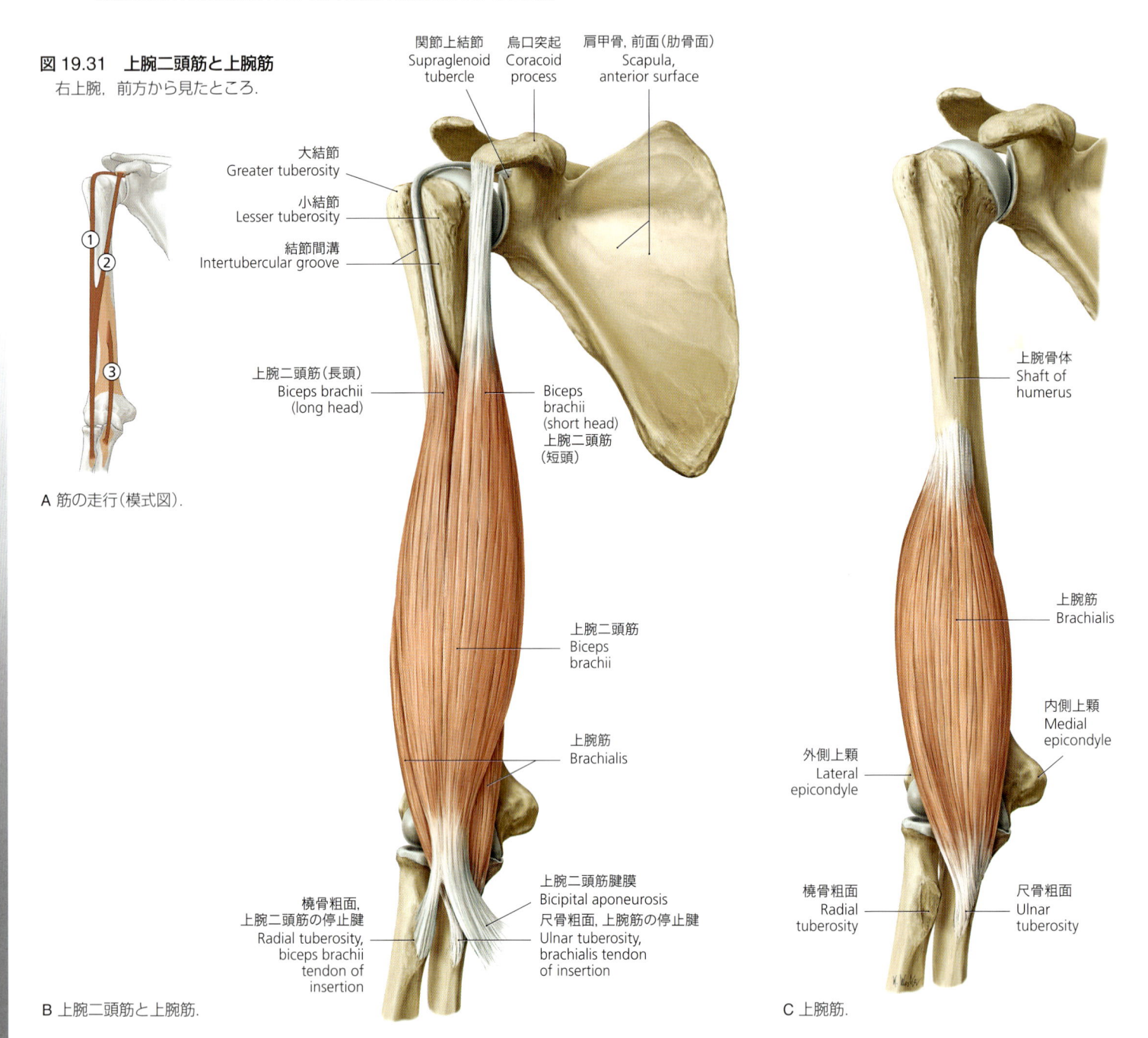

図 19.31 上腕二頭筋と上腕筋
右上腕，前方から見たところ．

A 筋の走行（模式図）．

B 上腕二頭筋と上腕筋．

C 上腕筋．

表 19.8 上腕前面の筋：上腕二頭筋と上腕筋

筋		起始	停止	神経支配	作用
上腕二頭筋	①長頭	肩甲骨の関節上結節	橈骨粗面	筋皮神経（C5，C6）	肘関節：屈曲と回外* 肩関節：上腕の前方挙上，三角筋が収縮している際に上腕骨頭を安定に保つ，上腕骨の外転と内旋
	②短頭	肩甲骨の烏口突起			
③上腕筋		上腕骨（前面の遠位半分）	尺骨粗面	筋皮神経（C5，C6），橈骨神経（C7，一部の筋束のみ）	肘関節の屈曲

*肘が屈曲している場合，上腕二頭筋は強力な回外筋として働く．というのも，屈曲時には，てこの役割をする上腕二頭筋の腱が回内/回外軸に対してほとんど垂直だからである．

図 19.32 上腕三頭筋と肘筋
右上腕，後方から見たところ．

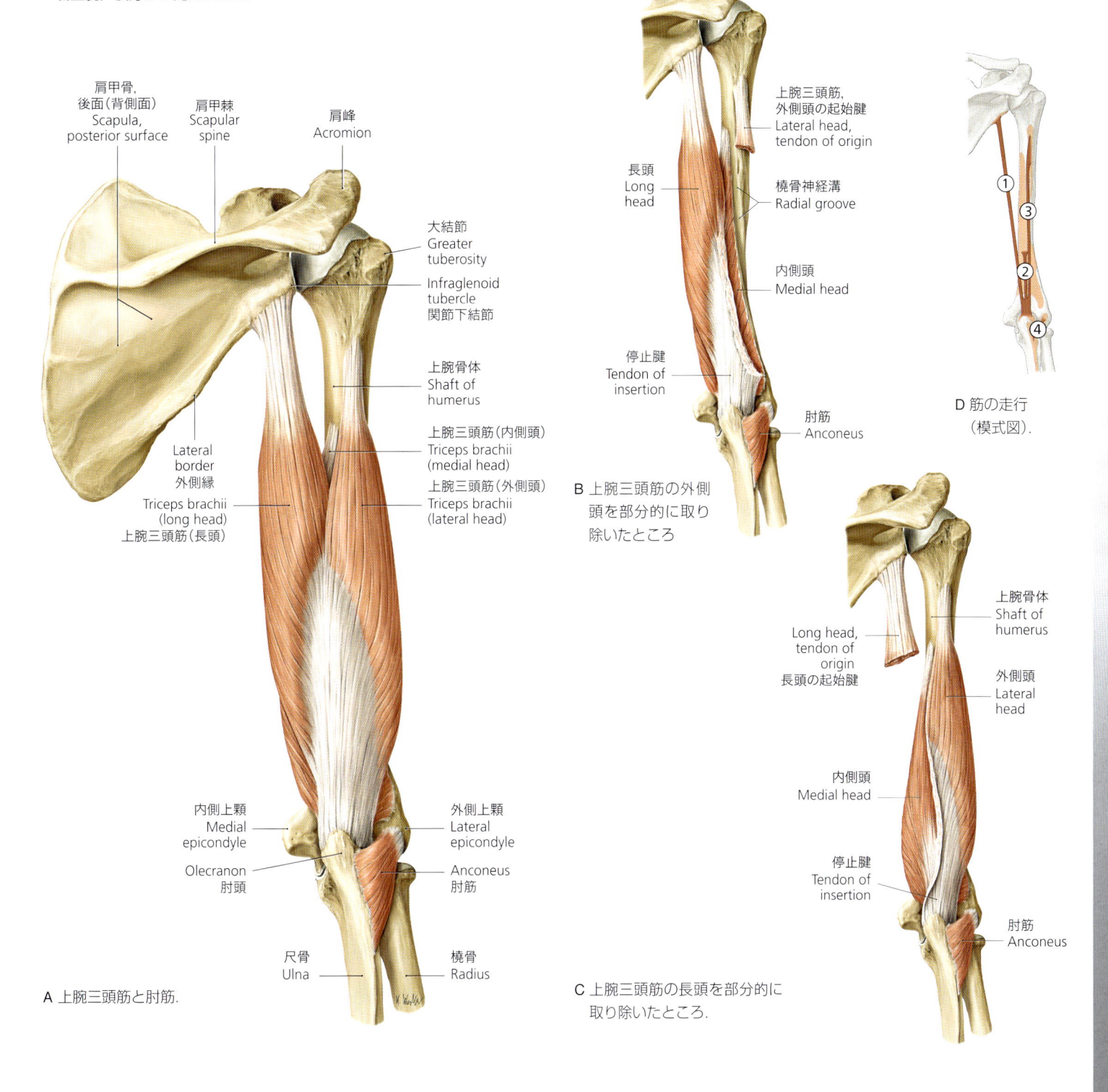

A 上腕三頭筋と肘筋．

B 上腕三頭筋の外側頭を部分的に取り除いたところ

C 上腕三頭筋の長頭を部分的に取り除いたところ．

D 筋の走行（模式図）．

表 19.9		上腕後面の筋：上腕三頭筋と肘筋			
筋		起始	停止	神経支配	作用
上腕三頭筋	①長頭	肩甲骨（関節下結節）	尺骨の肘頭	橈骨神経（C6-C8）	肘関節：伸展 肩関節（長頭の作用）：上腕の後方挙上と内転
	②内側頭	上腕骨の後面（橈骨神経溝の遠位），内側筋間中隔			
	③外側頭	上腕骨の後面（橈骨神経溝の近位），外側筋間中隔			
④肘筋		上腕骨の外側上顆（肘関節包の後部から起始することもある）	尺骨の肘頭（橈側面）		肘関節の伸展と安定化

橈骨と尺骨
Radius & Ulna

図 20.1　橈骨と尺骨
右前腕.

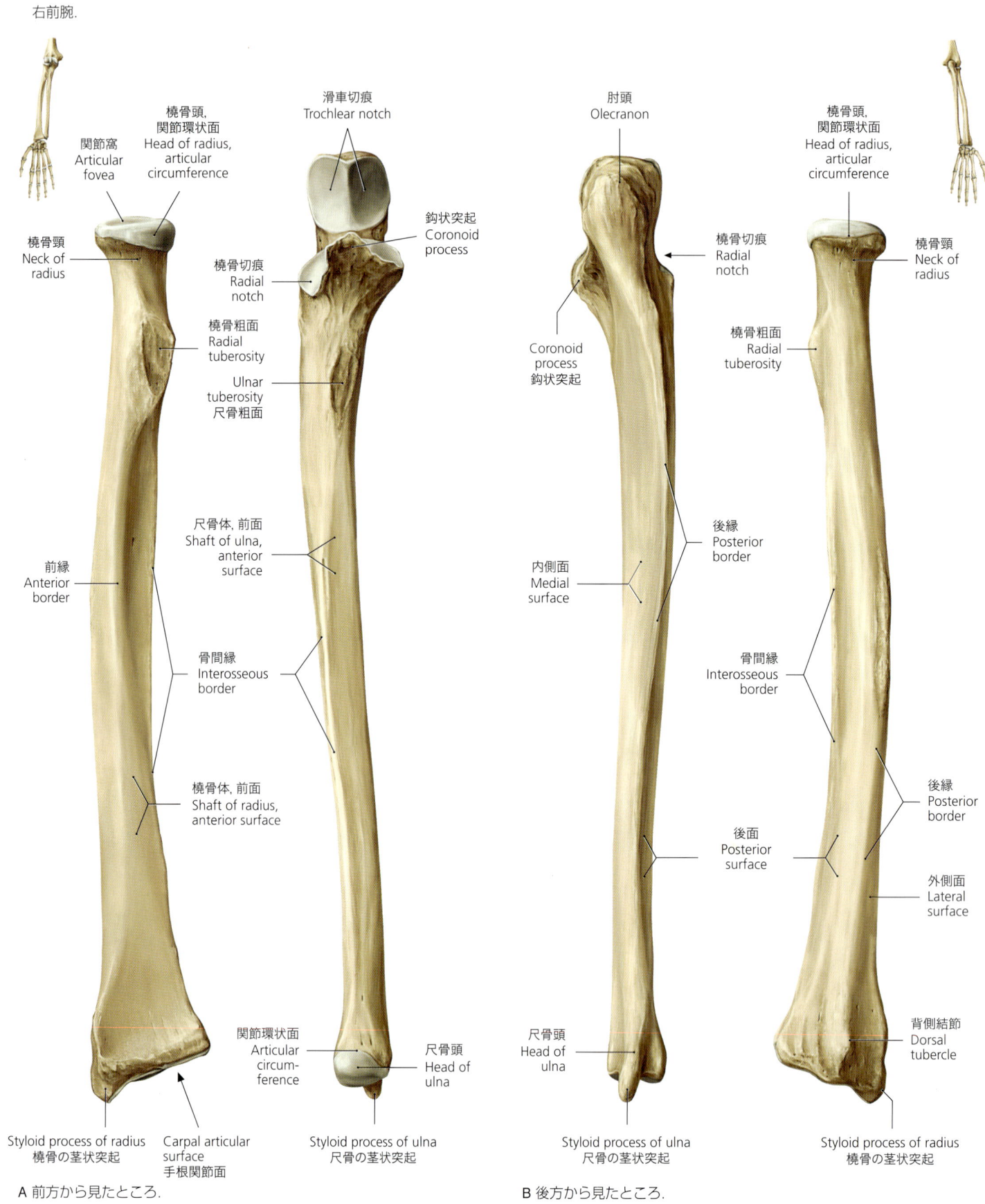

A 前方から見たところ.

B 後方から見たところ.

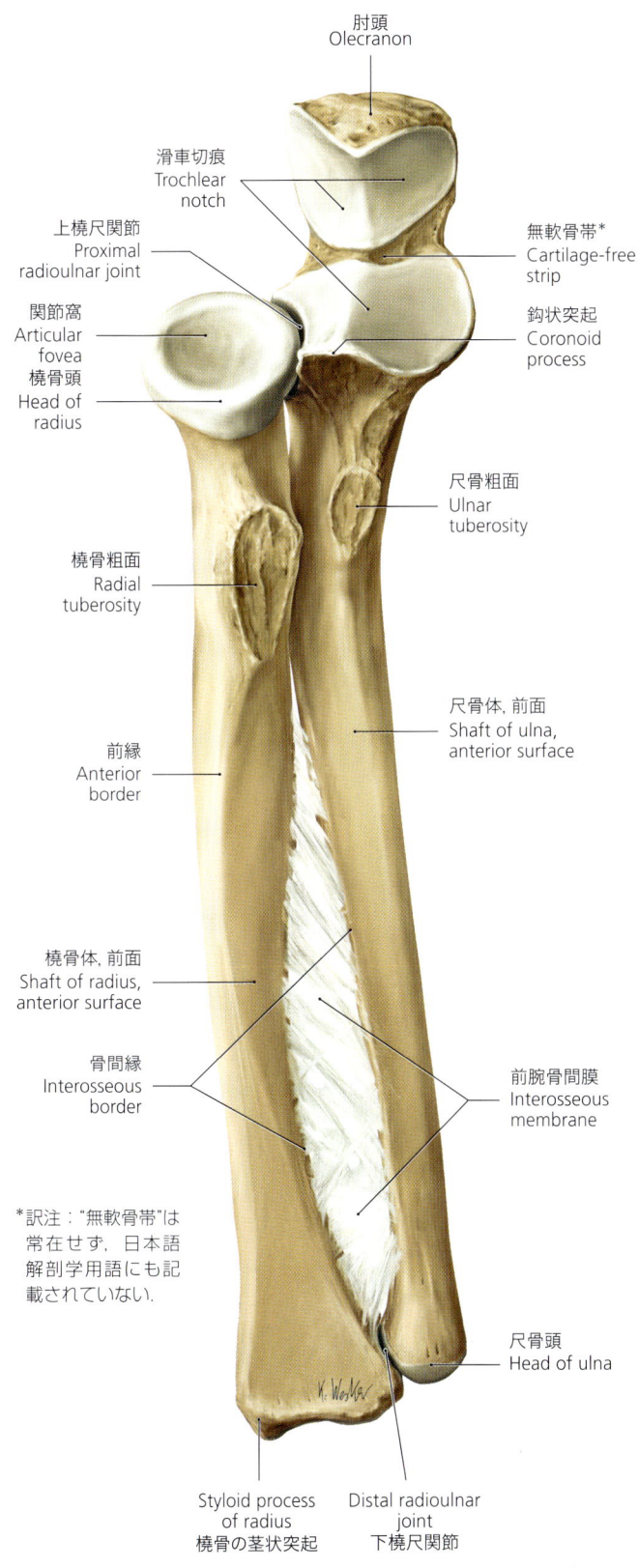

C 前上方から見たところ.

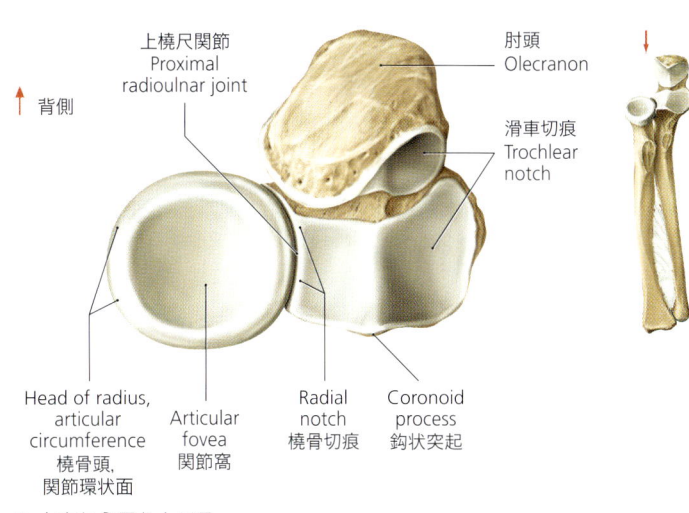

- 肘頭 Olecranon
- 滑車切痕 Trochlear notch
- 上橈尺関節 Proximal radioulnar joint
- 関節窩 Articular fovea
- 橈骨頭 Head of radius
- 無軟骨帯* Cartilage-free strip
- 鈎状突起 Coronoid process
- 尺骨粗面 Ulnar tuberosity
- 橈骨粗面 Radial tuberosity
- 尺骨体, 前面 Shaft of ulna, anterior surface
- 前縁 Anterior border
- 橈骨体, 前面 Shaft of radius, anterior surface
- 骨間縁 Interosseous border
- 前腕骨間膜 Interosseous membrane
- 尺骨頭 Head of ulna
- 橈骨の茎状突起 Styloid process of radius
- 下橈尺関節 Distal radioulnar joint

*訳注:"無軟骨帯"は常在せず, 日本語解剖学用語にも記載されていない.

D 上方から見たところ.

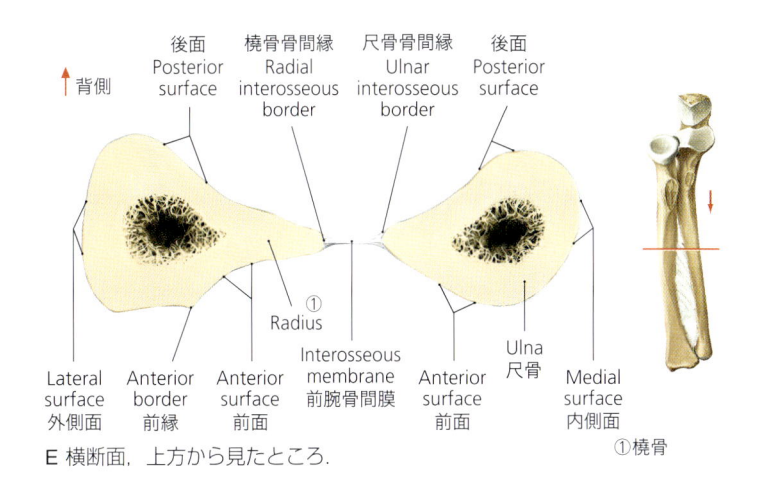

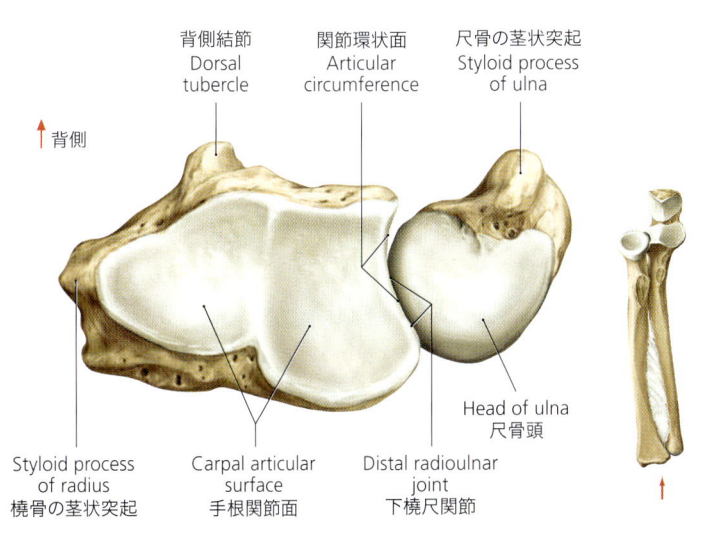

- 肘頭 Olecranon
- 上橈尺関節 Proximal radioulnar joint
- 滑車切痕 Trochlear notch
- 橈骨頭, 関節環状面 Head of radius, articular circumference
- 関節窩 Articular fovea
- 橈骨切痕 Radial notch
- 鈎状突起 Coronoid process

E 横断面, 上方から見たところ.

- 後面 Posterior surface
- 橈骨骨間縁 Radial interosseous border
- 尺骨骨間縁 Ulnar interosseous border
- 後面 Posterior surface
- 外側面 Lateral surface
- 前縁 Anterior border
- 前面 Anterior surface
- ① Radius
- 前腕骨間膜 Interosseous membrane
- 前面 Anterior surface
- 尺骨 Ulna
- 内側面 Medial surface

① 橈骨

F 下方から見たところ.

- 背側結節 Dorsal tubercle
- 関節環状面 Articular circumference
- 尺骨の茎状突起 Styloid process of ulna
- 橈骨の茎状突起 Styloid process of radius
- 手根関節面 Carpal articular surface
- 尺骨頭 Head of ulna
- 下橈尺関節 Distal radioulnar joint

肘関節
Elbow Joint

図 20.2 肘関節
右上肢．肘関節は上腕骨，尺骨，橈骨のそれぞれの間にできる3つの関節（腕尺関節，腕橈関節，上橈尺関節）からなる．

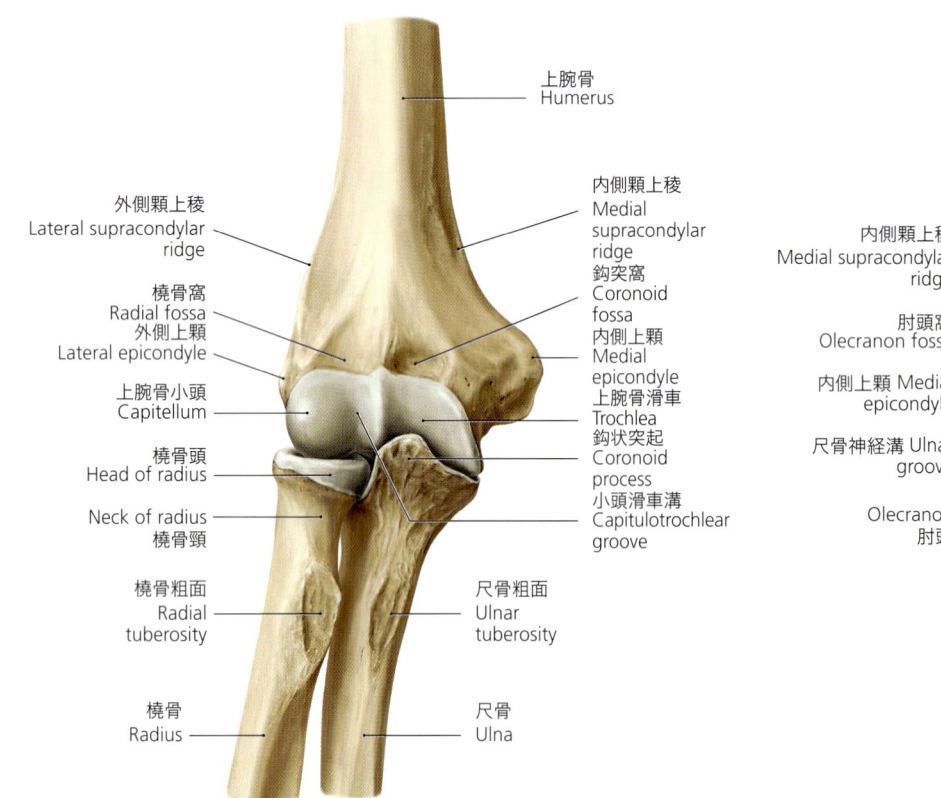

A 前方から見たところ．

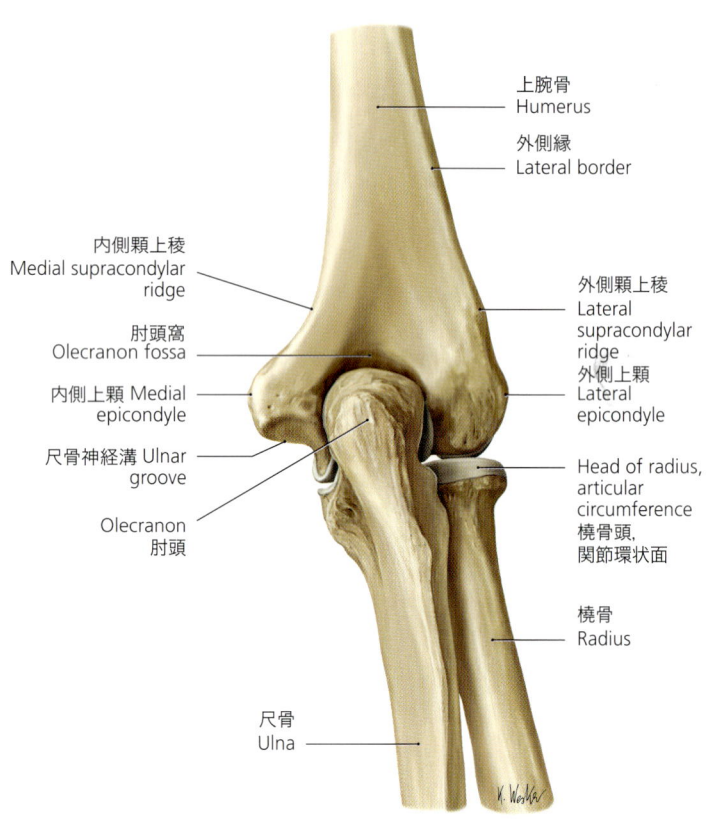

B 後方から見たところ．

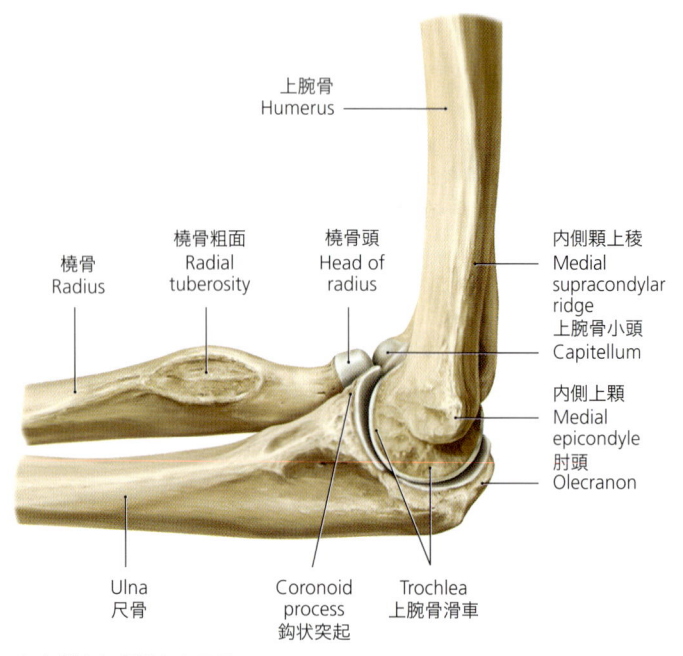

C 内側方から見たところ．

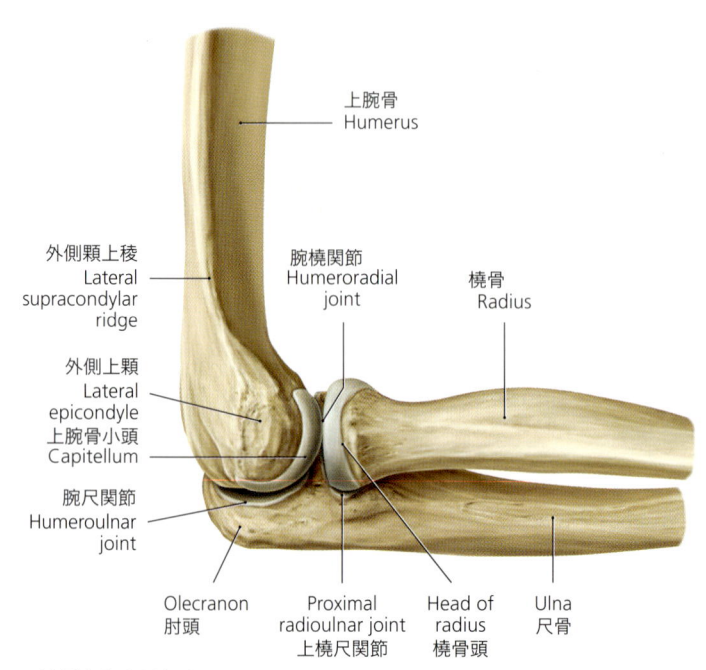

D 外側方から見たところ．

図 20.3　肘関節のMR像
矢状断面.

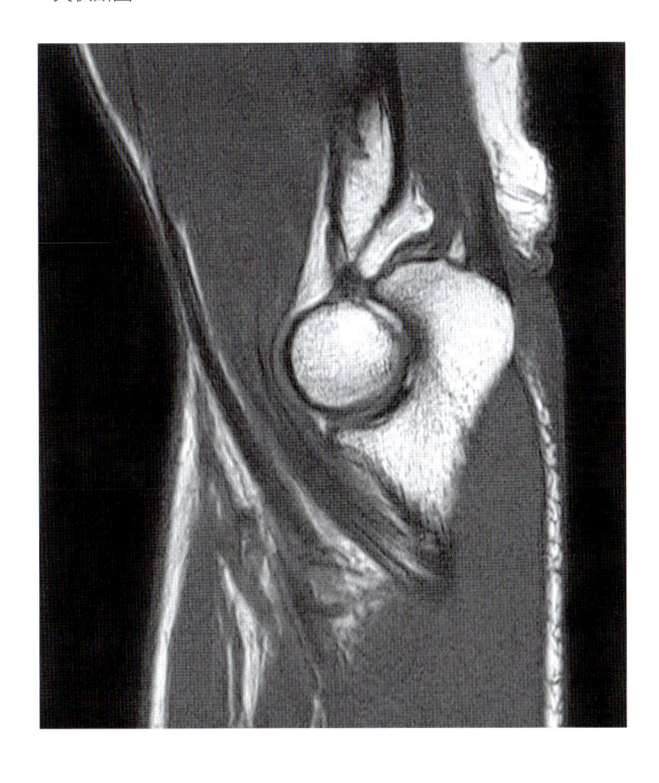

図 20.4　腕尺関節
腕尺関節を通る矢状断面，内側方から見たところ.

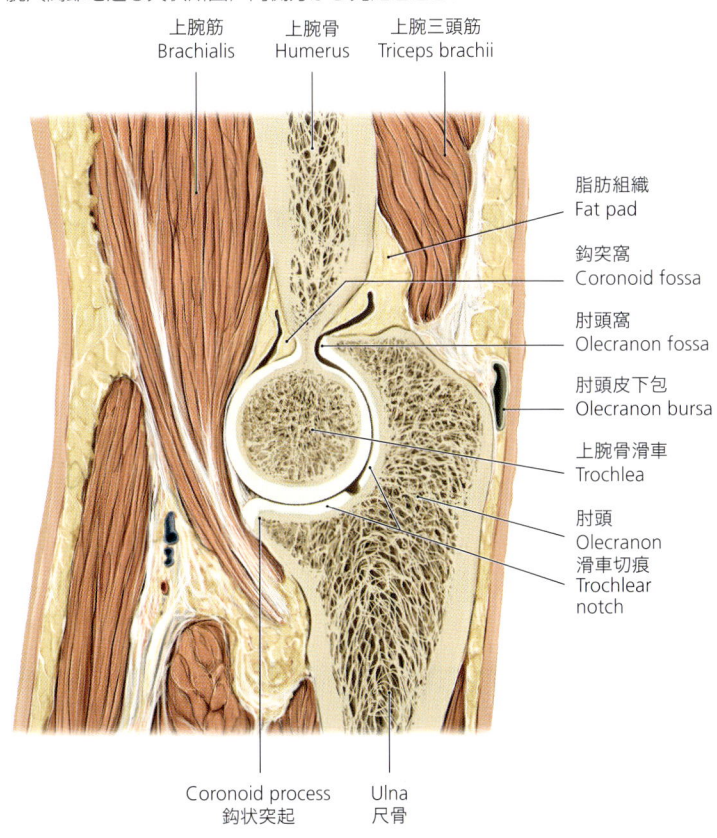

上腕筋 Brachialis
上腕骨 Humerus
上腕三頭筋 Triceps brachii
脂肪組織 Fat pad
鈎突窩 Coronoid fossa
肘頭窩 Olecranon fossa
肘頭皮下包 Olecranon bursa
上腕骨滑車 Trochlea
肘頭 Olecranon
滑車切痕 Trochlear notch
Coronoid process 鈎状突起
Ulna 尺骨

臨床

肘外傷の評価

正常な肘関節を見ると，関節包の線維被膜と滑膜の間に脂肪塊が存在する．前面にある脂肪塊は矢状断のMR像で簡単に見ることができるが，後面にある脂肪塊はしばしば骨の窪み（肘頭窩）の中に隠れている（図20.3）．関節腔に浸出液が溜まると，液が前方の脂肪塊を圧迫し，脂肪塊の下縁が上方に凹んで見える．圧迫された脂肪塊は形が船の帆に似るので，画像上のこのような徴候を帆徴候 sail sign と呼ぶ．また，肘における隆起部の配列をみることは，骨折や脱臼を診断するうえで参考となる．

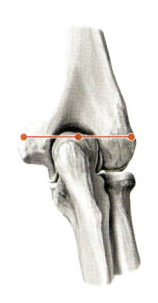

A 伸展した肘を後方から見たところ．内側上顆，肘頭，外側上顆が一直線上に並ぶ．

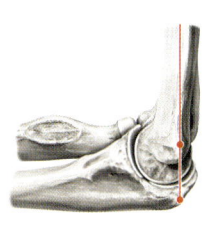

B 屈曲した肘を外側方から見たところ．内側（もしくは外側）上顆と肘頭が一直線上に並ぶ．

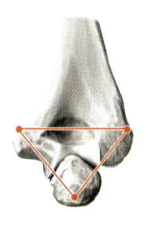

C 屈曲した肘を後方から見たところ．内側上顆，外側上顆，肘頭の先端が二等辺三角形を形成する．骨折や脱臼によってこの三角形は変形する．

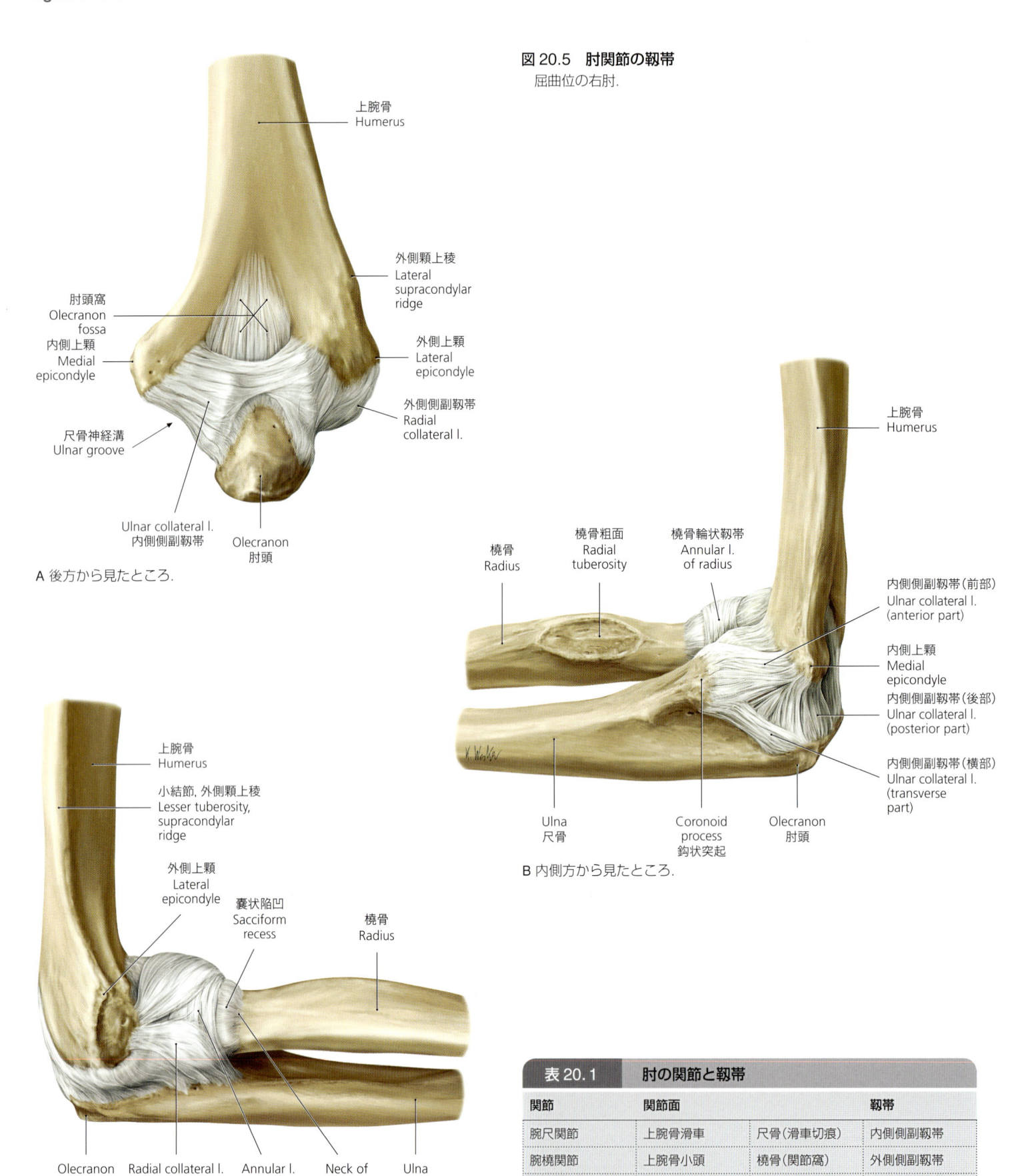

肘関節の靱帯
Ligaments of the Elbow Joint

図 20.5　肘関節の靱帯
屈曲位の右肘.

A 後方から見たところ.

B 内側方から見たところ.

C 外側方から見たところ.

表 20.1	肘の関節と靱帯		
関節	関節面		靱帯
腕尺関節	上腕骨滑車	尺骨（滑車切痕）	内側側副靱帯
腕橈関節	上腕骨小頭	橈骨（関節窩）	外側側副靱帯
上橈尺関節	橈骨（関節環状面）	尺骨（橈骨切痕）	橈骨輪状靱帯

図 20.6 肘の関節包
伸展位の右肘,前方から見たところ.

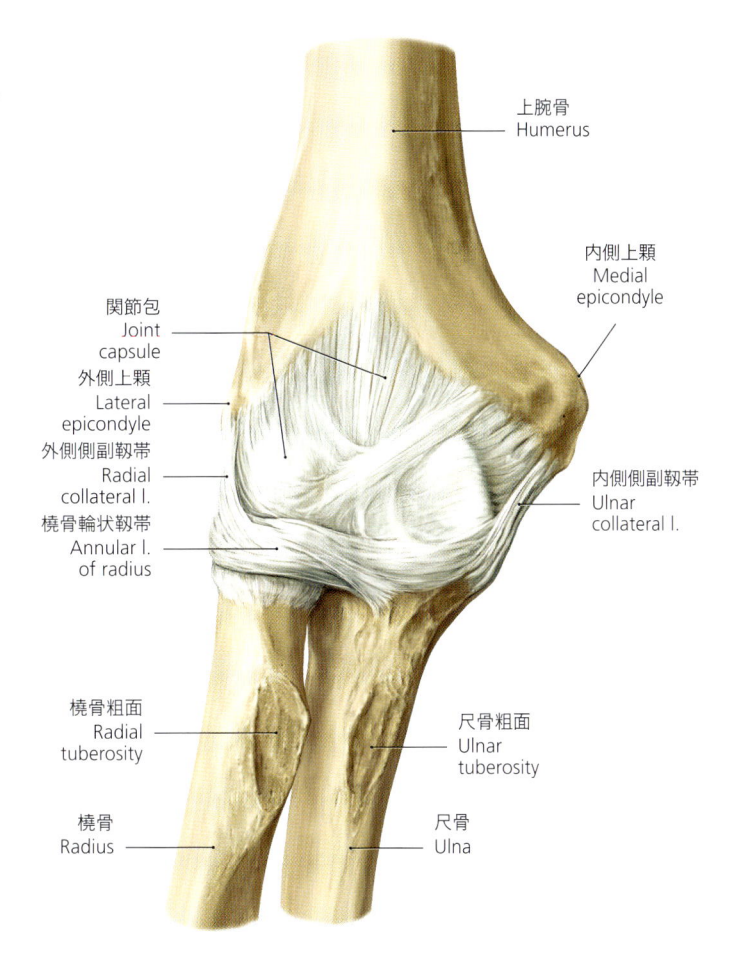

A 関節包.

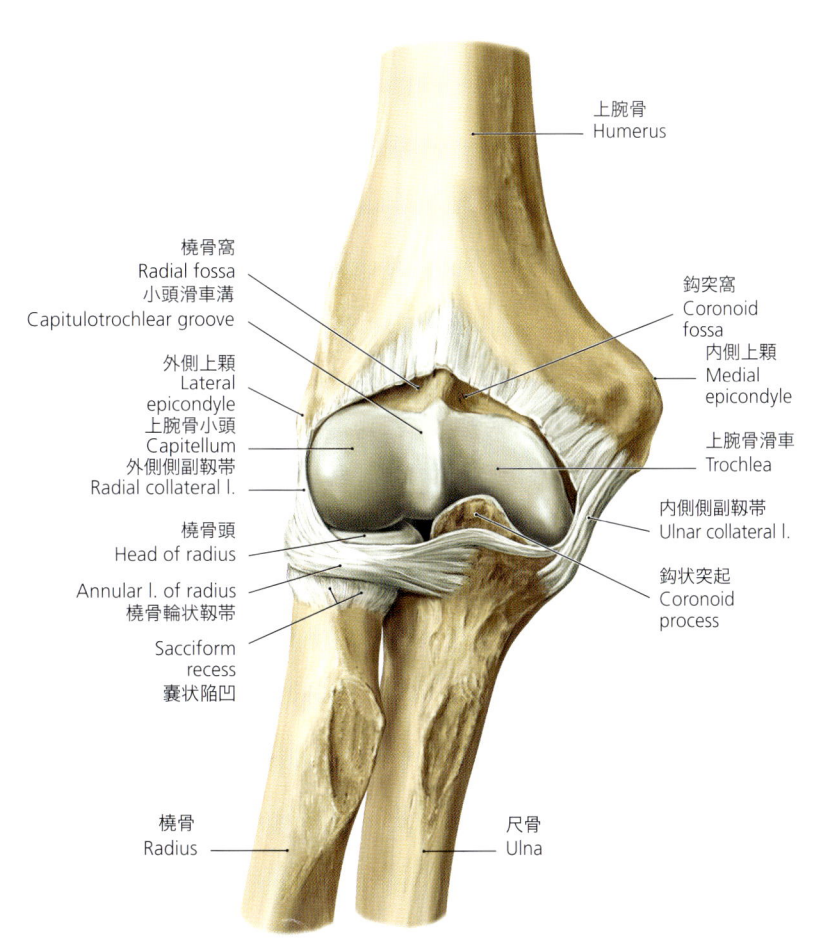

B 関節包を開いたところ.

橈尺関節
Radioulnar Joints

上・下橈尺関節は共同して働き，前腕の回内・回外運動を可能にする．この2つの関節は，骨間膜によって，機能的に連結されている．

回内・回外軸は斜めに走っており，上腕骨小頭の中心から，橈骨頭の関節面の中心を通り，尺骨の茎状突起に達する．

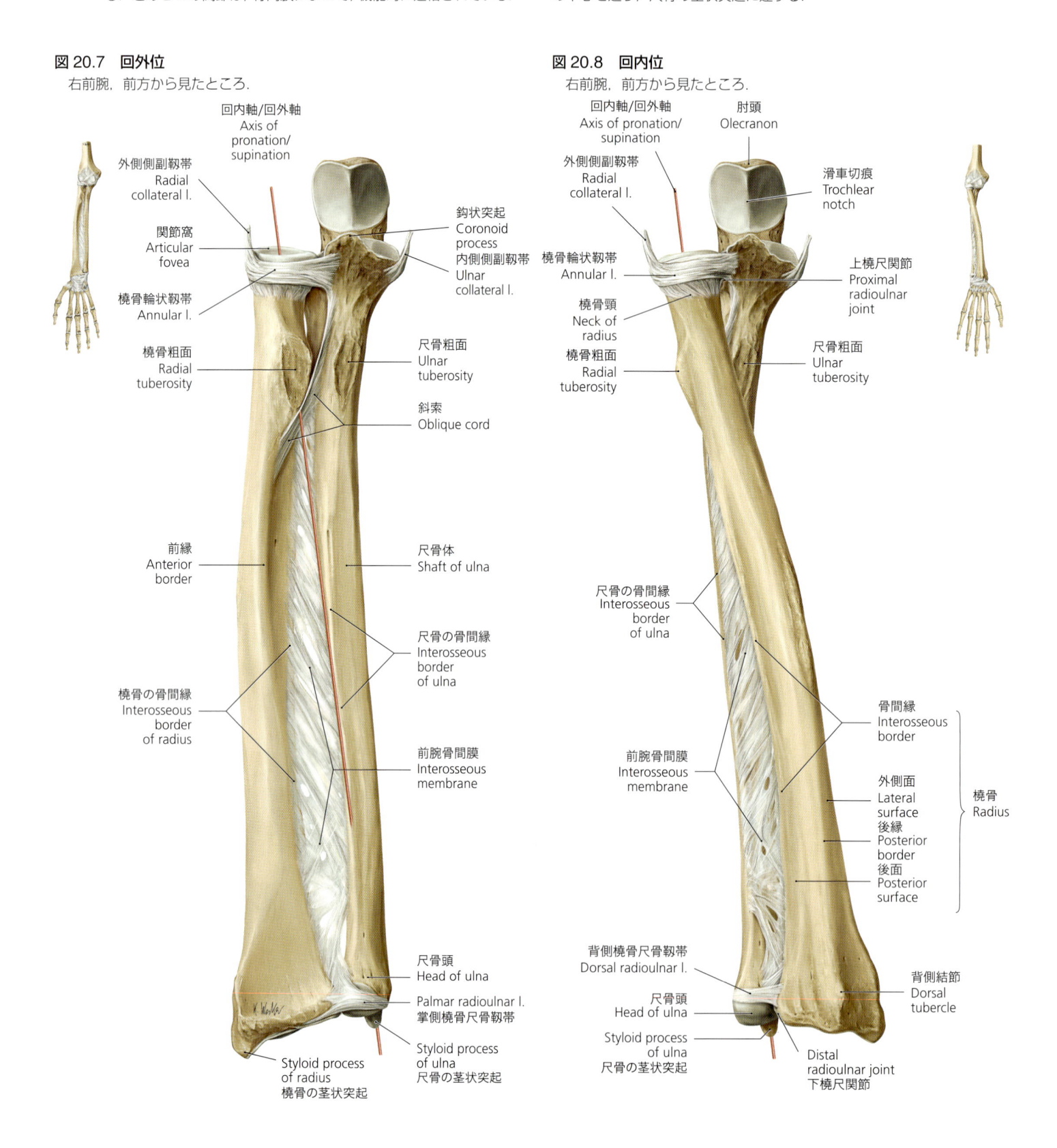

図 20.7 回外位
右前腕，前方から見たところ．

- 回内軸/回外軸 Axis of pronation/supination
- 外側側副靱帯 Radial collateral l.
- 関節窩 Articular fovea
- 橈骨輪状靱帯 Annular l.
- 橈骨粗面 Radial tuberosity
- 前縁 Anterior border
- 橈骨の骨間縁 Interosseous border of radius
- 鈎状突起 Coronoid process
- 内側側副靱帯 Ulnar collateral l.
- 尺骨粗面 Ulnar tuberosity
- 斜索 Oblique cord
- 尺骨体 Shaft of ulna
- 尺骨の骨間縁 Interosseous border of ulna
- 前腕骨間膜 Interosseous membrane
- 尺骨頭 Head of ulna
- 掌側橈骨尺骨靱帯 Palmar radioulnar l.
- 橈骨の茎状突起 Styloid process of radius
- 尺骨の茎状突起 Styloid process of ulna

図 20.8 回内位
右前腕，前方から見たところ．

- 回内軸/回外軸 Axis of pronation/supination
- 肘頭 Olecranon
- 外側側副靱帯 Radial collateral l.
- 滑車切痕 Trochlear notch
- 橈骨輪状靱帯 Annular l.
- 上橈尺関節 Proximal radioulnar joint
- 橈骨頭 Neck of radius
- 橈骨粗面 Radial tuberosity
- 尺骨粗面 Ulnar tuberosity
- 尺骨の骨間縁 Interosseous border of ulna
- 前腕骨間膜 Interosseous membrane
- 骨間縁 Interosseous border
- 外側面 Lateral surface
- 後縁 Posterior border
- 後面 Posterior surface
- 橈骨 Radius
- 背側橈骨尺骨靱帯 Dorsal radioulnar l.
- 尺骨頭 Head of ulna
- 背側結節 Dorsal tubercle
- 尺骨の茎状突起 Styloid process of ulna
- 下橈尺関節 Distal radioulnar joint

上肢

臨床

橈骨頭の亜脱臼（肘内障，子守肘 nursemaid's elbow）
子供が腕を急に引っ張られた場合，未熟な橈骨頭が橈骨輪状靱帯から脱臼することがある．患児は疼痛を訴え，前腕は回内位をとる．

図 20.9 上橈尺関節
右肘，上方から見たところ．

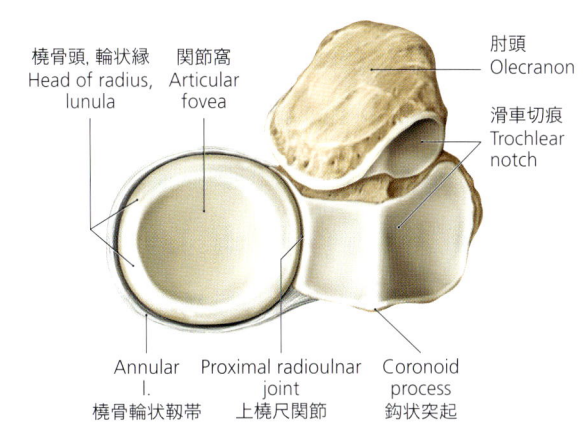

- 橈骨頭，輪縁 Head of radius, lunula
- 関節窩 Articular fovea
- 肘頭 Olecranon
- 滑車切痕 Trochlear notch
- Annular l. 橈骨輪状靱帯
- Proximal radioulnar joint 上橈尺関節
- Coronoid process 鉤状突起

A 橈骨と尺骨の上端にある関節面．

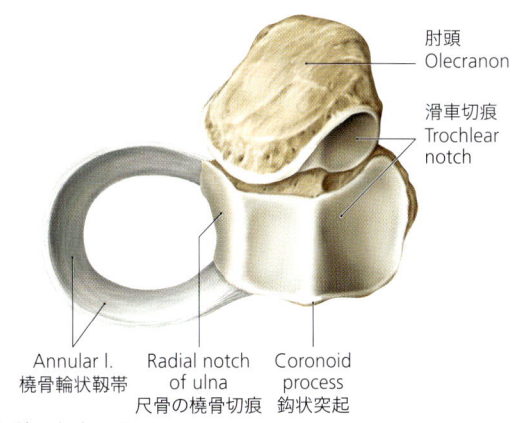

- 肘頭 Olecranon
- 滑車切痕 Trochlear notch
- Annular l. 橈骨輪状靱帯
- Radial notch of ulna 尺骨の橈骨切痕
- Coronoid process 鉤状突起

B 橈骨を取り除いたところ．

臨床

橈骨骨折
腕を伸ばしたままで，手のひらをついて転倒すると，しばしば橈骨遠位部が骨折する．コリース Colles 骨折では，遠位の骨片は手背側へ傾く．

- 背側への力
- Styloid process of radius 橈骨の茎状突起

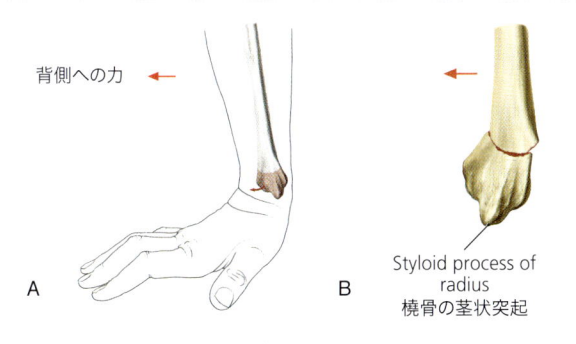

図 20.10 下橈尺関節
右肘，橈骨と尺骨の下端にある関節面．背側・掌側橈骨尺骨靱帯は下橈尺関節を安定させる．

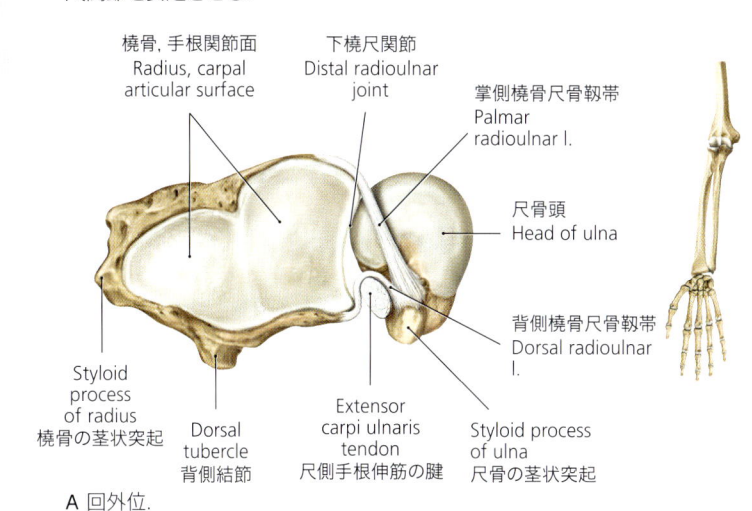

- 橈骨，手根関節面 Radius, carpal articular surface
- 下橈尺関節 Distal radioulnar joint
- 掌側橈骨尺骨靱帯 Palmar radioulnar l.
- 尺骨頭 Head of ulna
- 背側橈骨尺骨靱帯 Dorsal radioulnar l.
- Styloid process of radius 橈骨の茎状突起
- Dorsal tubercle 背側結節
- Extensor carpi ulnaris tendon 尺側手根伸筋の腱
- Styloid process of ulna 尺骨の茎状突起

A 回外位．

- 橈骨の茎状突起 Styloid process of radius
- Ulnar notch 尺骨切痕
- Articular circumference 関節環状面
- Styloid process of ulna 尺骨の茎状突起

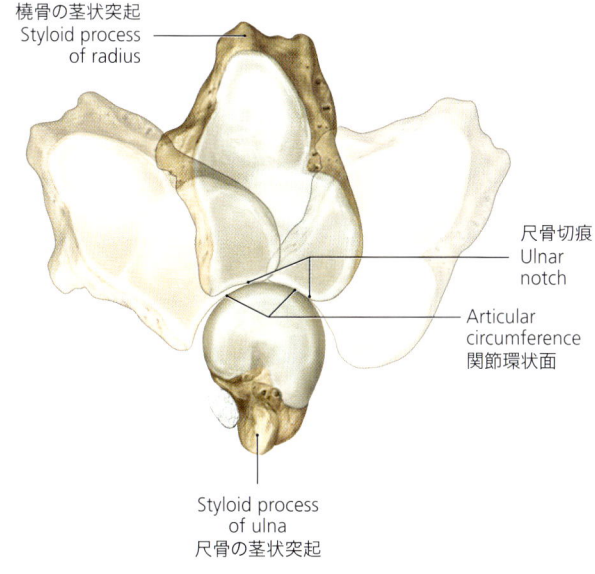

B 中間位．

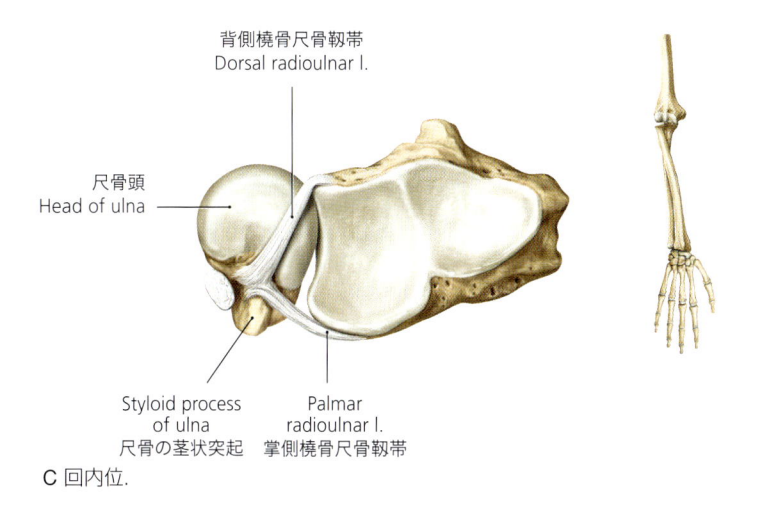

- 背側橈骨尺骨靱帯 Dorsal radioulnar l.
- 尺骨頭 Head of ulna
- Styloid process of ulna 尺骨の茎状突起
- Palmar radioulnar l. 掌側橈骨尺骨靱帯

C 回内位．

前腕の筋(1)
Muscles of the Forearm(I)

図 20.11　前腕前面の筋
右前腕，前方から見たところ．筋の起始(O)を赤，停止(I)を青で示してある．

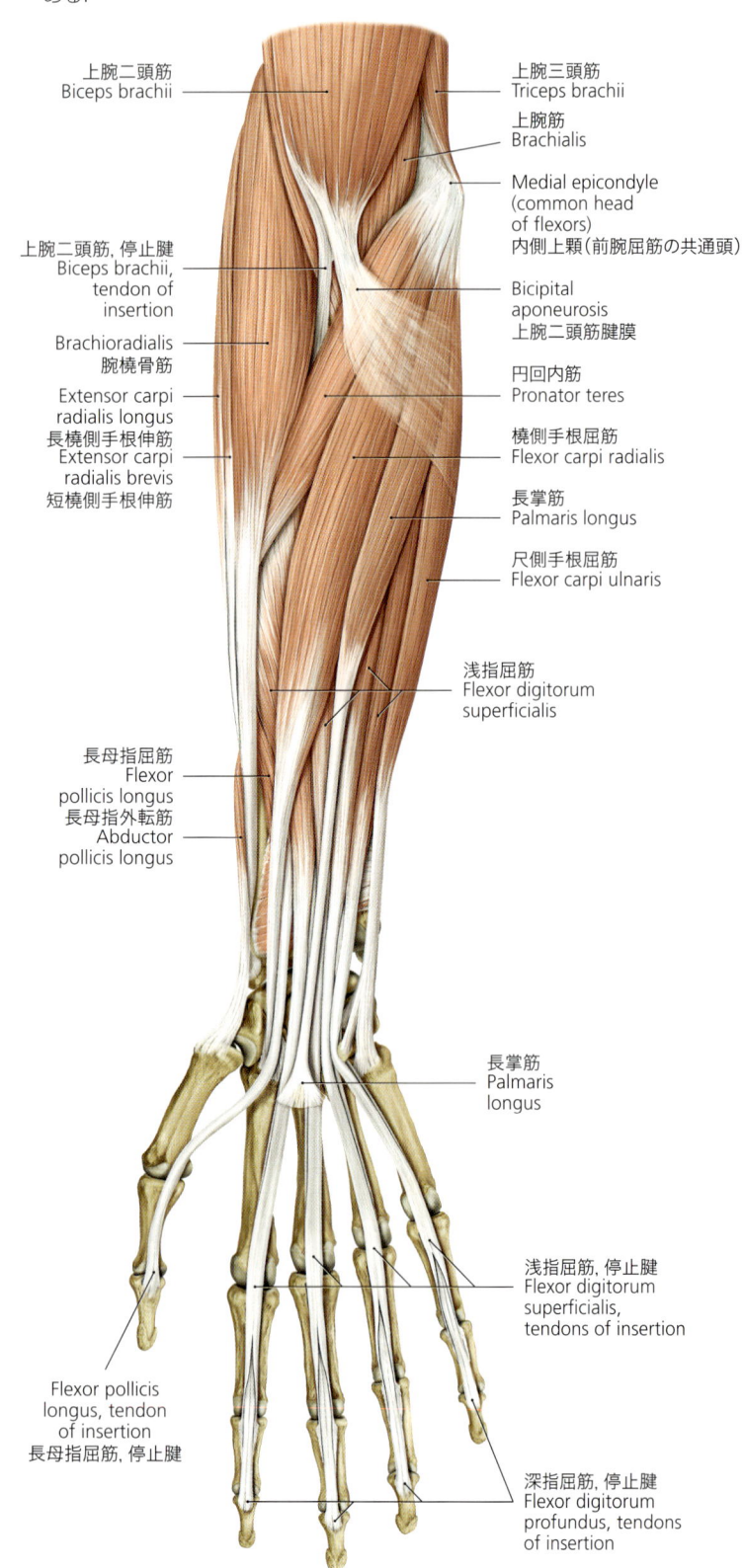

A 浅層の屈筋群と橈側筋群．

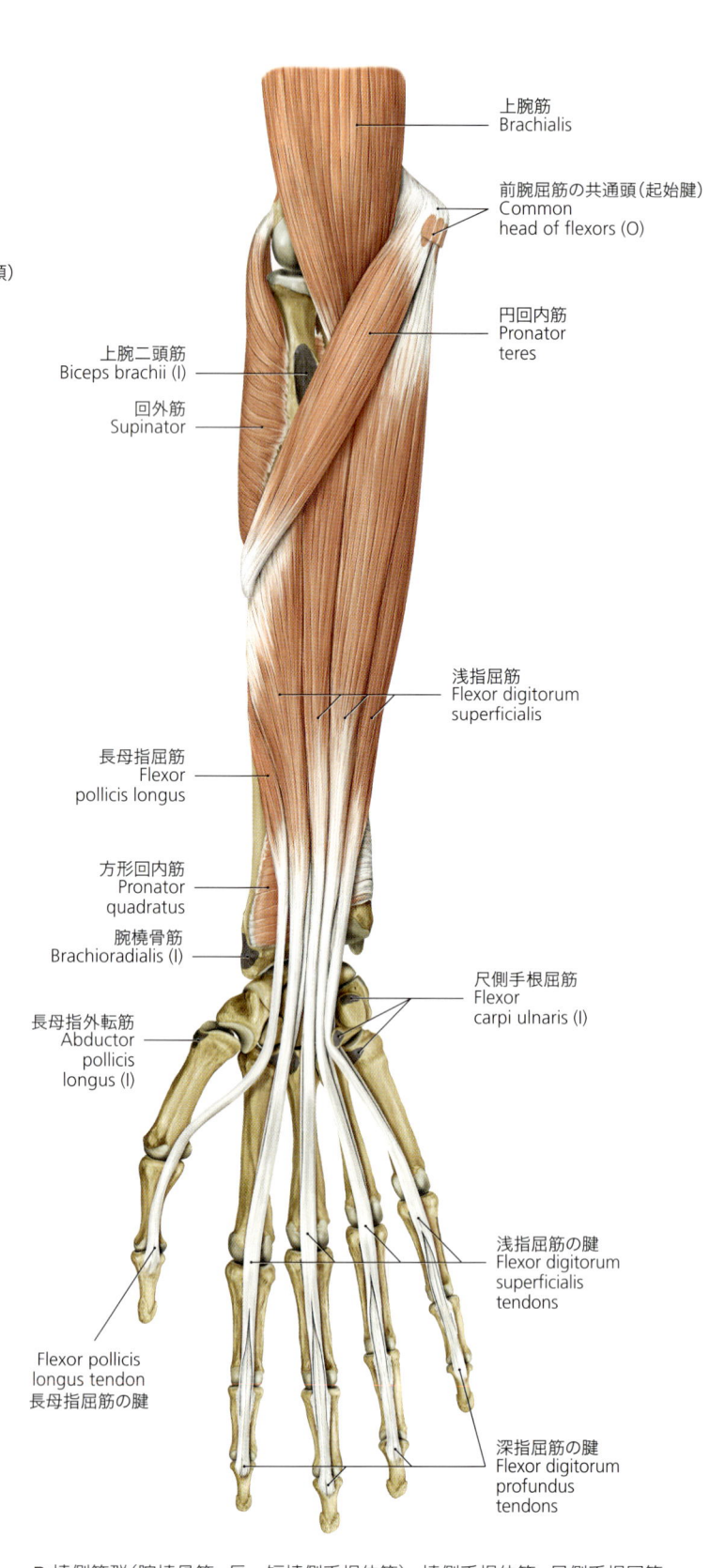

B 橈側筋群(腕橈骨筋，長・短橈側手根伸筋)，橈側手根伸筋，尺側手根屈筋，長母指外転筋，長掌筋，上腕二頭筋を取り除いたところ．

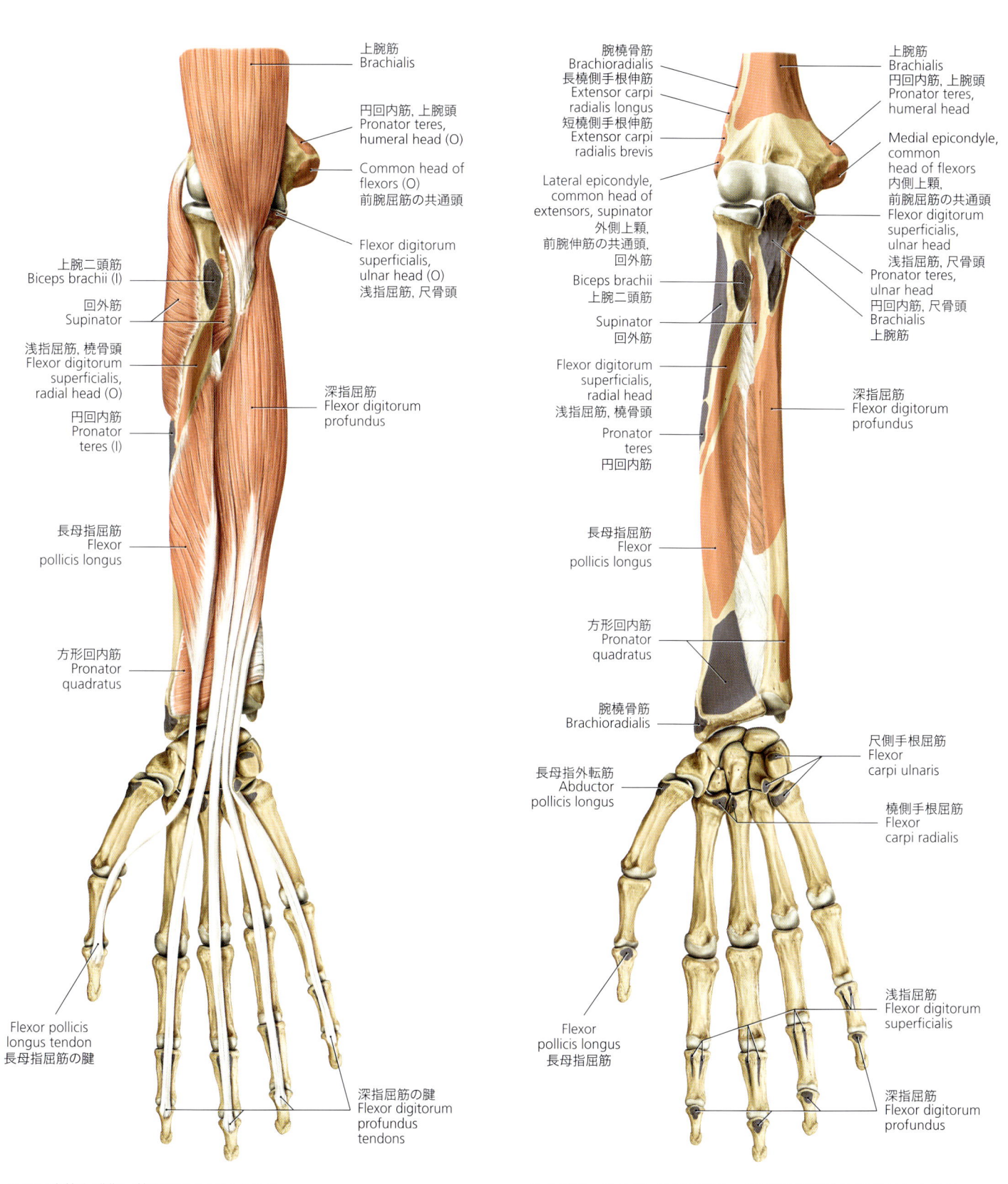

C 円回内筋と浅指屈筋を取り除いたところ．

D 上腕筋，回外筋，方形回内筋，深層の屈筋群を取り除いたところ．

前腕の筋(2)
Muscles of the Forearm(II)

図 20.12 前腕後面の筋
右前腕．後方から見たところ．筋の起始(O)を赤，停止(I)を青で示してある．

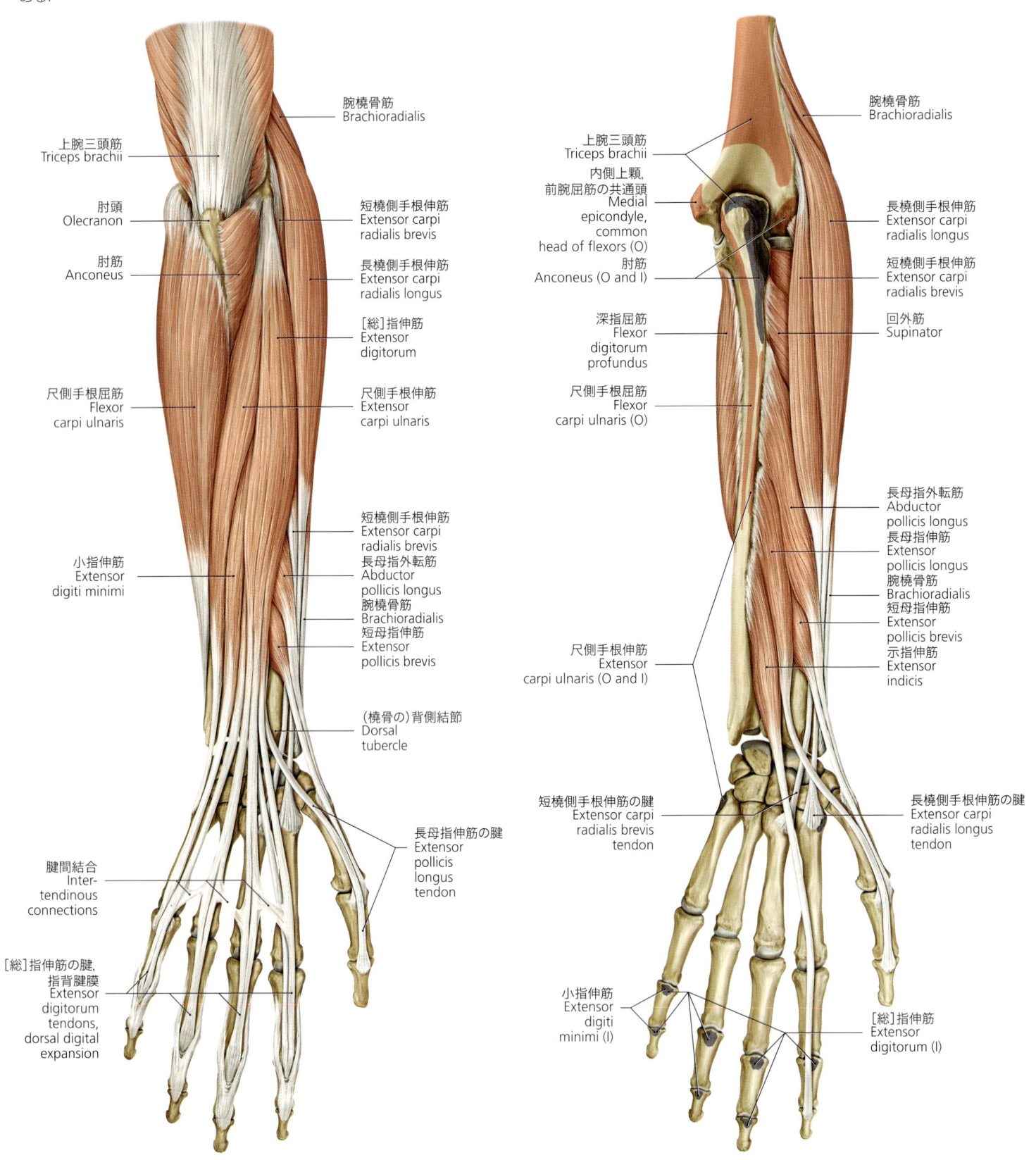

A 浅層の伸筋群と橈側筋群．

B 上腕三頭筋，肘筋，尺側手根伸筋，尺側手根屈筋，総指伸筋を取り除いたところ．

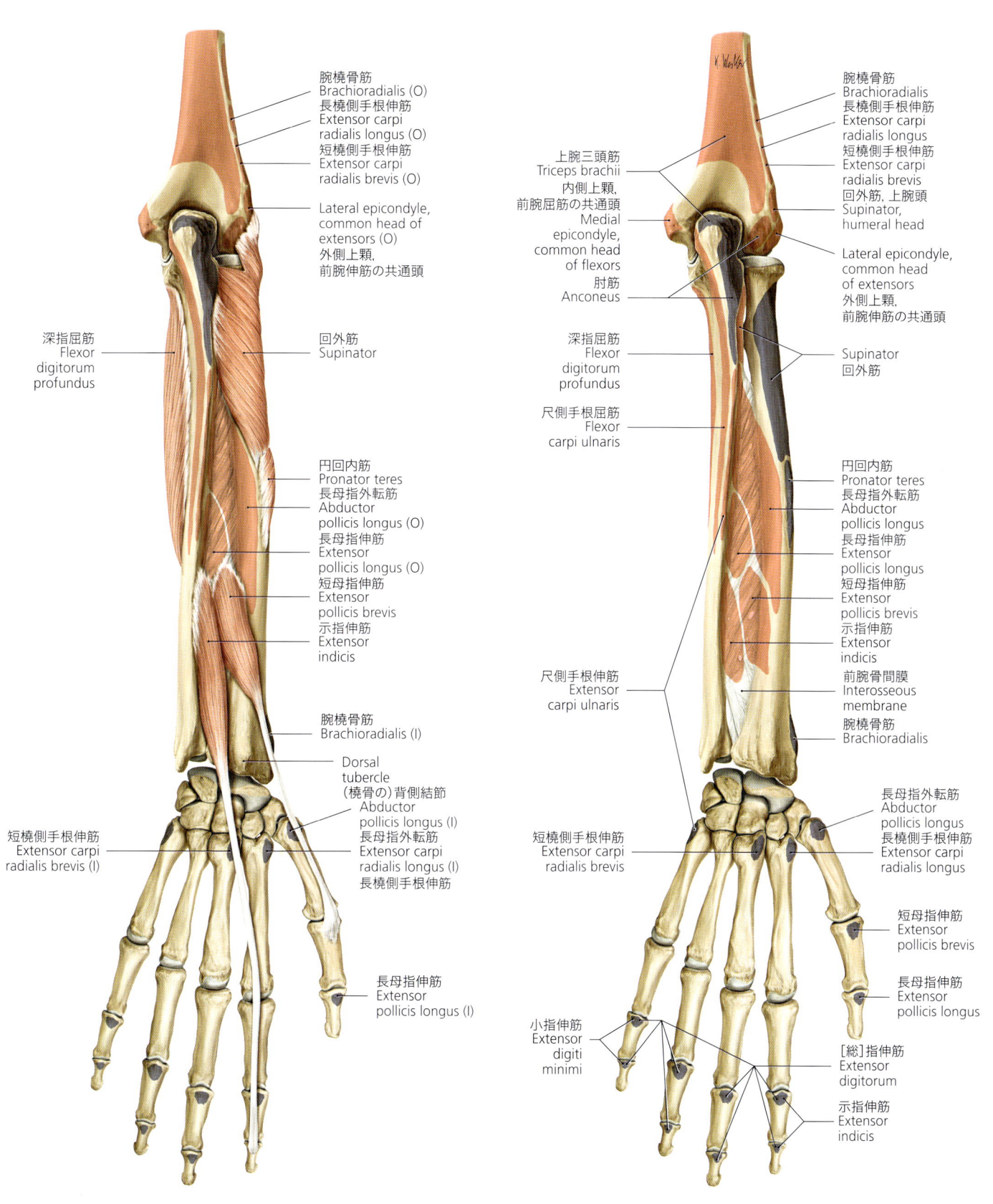

C 長母指外転筋，長母指伸筋，橈側筋群を取り除いたところ．

D 深指屈筋，回外筋，短母指伸筋，示指伸筋を取り除いたところ．

個々の筋(1)
Muscle Facts(I)

図 20.13 前腕前面の筋
右前腕，前方から見たところ．

前腕骨間膜
Interosseous membrane

浅指屈筋(上腕頭)
Flexor digitorum superficialis (humeral head)

浅指屈筋(尺骨頭)
Flexor digitorum superficialis (ulnar head)

A 浅層．　　B 中間層．　　C 深層．

表 20.2 前腕前面の筋

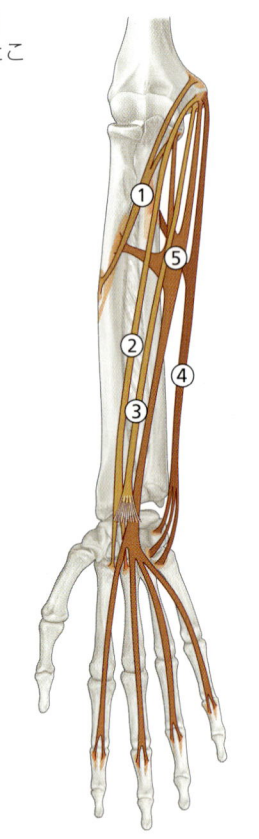

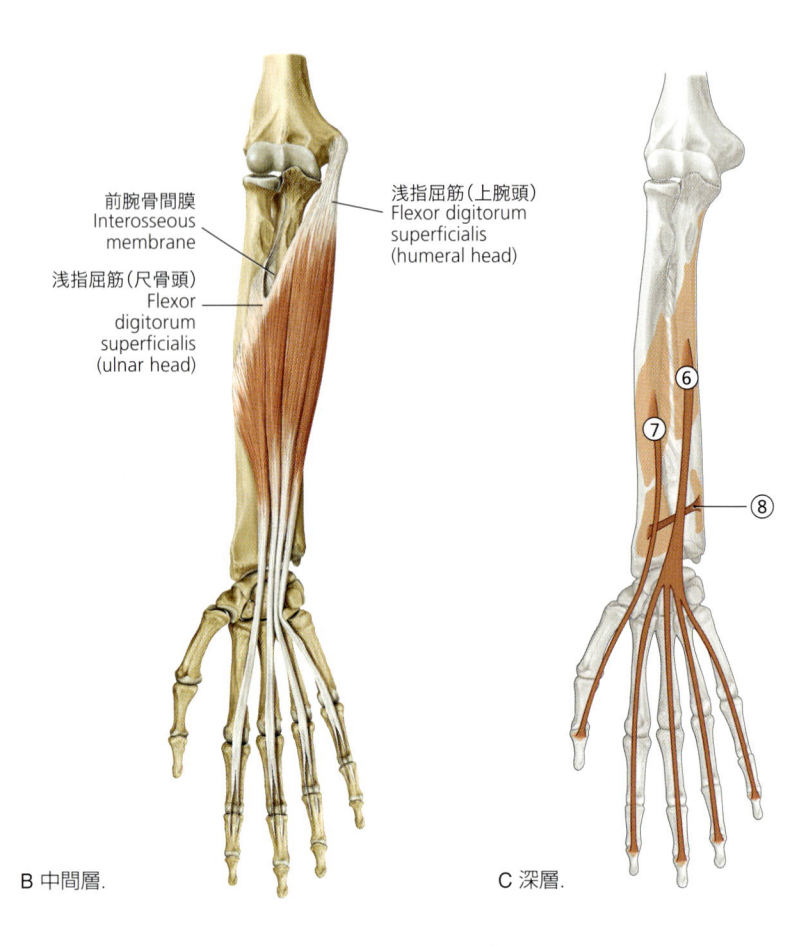

筋	起始	停止	神経支配	作用
浅層				
①円回内筋	上腕頭：上腕骨の内側上顆 尺骨頭：尺骨の鈎状突起	橈骨の外側面(回外筋の停止部よりも遠位)	正中神経(C6, C7)	肘：弱い屈曲作用 前腕：回内
②橈側手根屈筋	上腕骨の内側上顆	第2中手骨底(変異：第3中手骨底)	正中神経(C6, C7)	手首：屈曲・外転(橈側偏位)
③長掌筋	上腕骨の内側上顆	手掌腱膜	正中神経(C7, C8)	肘：弱い屈曲作用 手首：屈曲・手掌腱膜を緊張させる
④尺側手根屈筋	上腕頭：上腕骨の内側上顆 尺骨頭：尺骨の肘頭	豆状骨，有鈎骨鈎，第5中手骨底	尺骨神経(C7-T1)	手首：屈曲・内転(尺側偏位)
中間層				
⑤浅指屈筋	上腕頭：上腕骨の内側上顆 尺骨頭：尺骨の鈎状突起 橈骨頭：橈骨上部の前面(橈骨粗面より遠位)	第2-5指の中節骨(両縁)	正中神経(C8, T1)	肘：弱い屈曲作用 手首：屈曲 第2-5指のMCP関節・PIP関節：屈曲
深層				
⑥深指屈筋	尺骨前面(近位3分の2)と骨間膜	第2-5指の末節骨(掌側面)	正中神経(C8, T1), 尺骨神経(C8, T1)	手首：屈曲 第2-5指のMCP関節・PIP関節・DIP関節：屈曲
⑦長母指屈筋	橈骨前面(中央3分の1)と骨間膜	母指の末節骨(掌側面)	正中神経(C7, C8)	手首：屈曲・外転(橈側偏位) 母指の手根中手関節・MCP関節・IP関節：屈曲
⑧方形回内筋	尺骨前面(遠位4分の1)	橈骨前面(遠位4分の1)	正中神経(C7, C8)	前腕：回内，下橈尺関節の安定化

DIP関節＝遠位指節間関節，IP関節＝指節間関節，MCP関節＝中手指節関節，PIP関節＝近位指節間関節．

図 20.14 前腕前面の筋（表層と中間層）
右前腕，前方から見たところ．

- 内側上顆（前腕屈筋の共通頭） Medial epicondyle (common head of flexors)
- 橈骨粗面 Radial tuberosity
- 円回内筋 Pronator teres
- 橈側手根屈筋 Flexor carpi radialis
- 長掌筋 Palmaris longus
- 尺側手根屈筋 Flexor carpi ulnaris
- 浅指屈筋 Flexor digitorum superficialis
- 第2中手骨の底 Base of 2nd metacarpal
- 豆状骨 Pisiform bone
- 有鈎骨鈎 Hook of hamate
- 第5中手骨の底 Base of 5th metacarpal
- 手掌腱膜 Palmar aponeurosis
- 第2–5中節骨 2nd through 5th middle phalanges

図 20.15 前腕前面の筋（深層）
右前腕，前方から見たところ．

- 内側上顆 Medial epicondyle
- 鈎状突起 Coronoid process
- 橈骨粗面 Radial tuberosity
- 尺骨粗面 Ulnar tuberosity
- 前腕骨間膜 Interosseous membrane
- 橈骨 Radius
- 深指屈筋 Flexor digitorum profundus
- 長母指屈筋 Flexor pollicis longus
- 方形回内筋 Pronator quadratus
- 大菱形骨結節 Tubercle of trapezium
- 大菱形骨 Trapezium
- 豆状骨 Pisiform bone
- 有鈎骨鈎 Hook of hamate
- 1st distal phalanx, base 第1末節骨の底
- 第4末節骨 4th distal phalanx

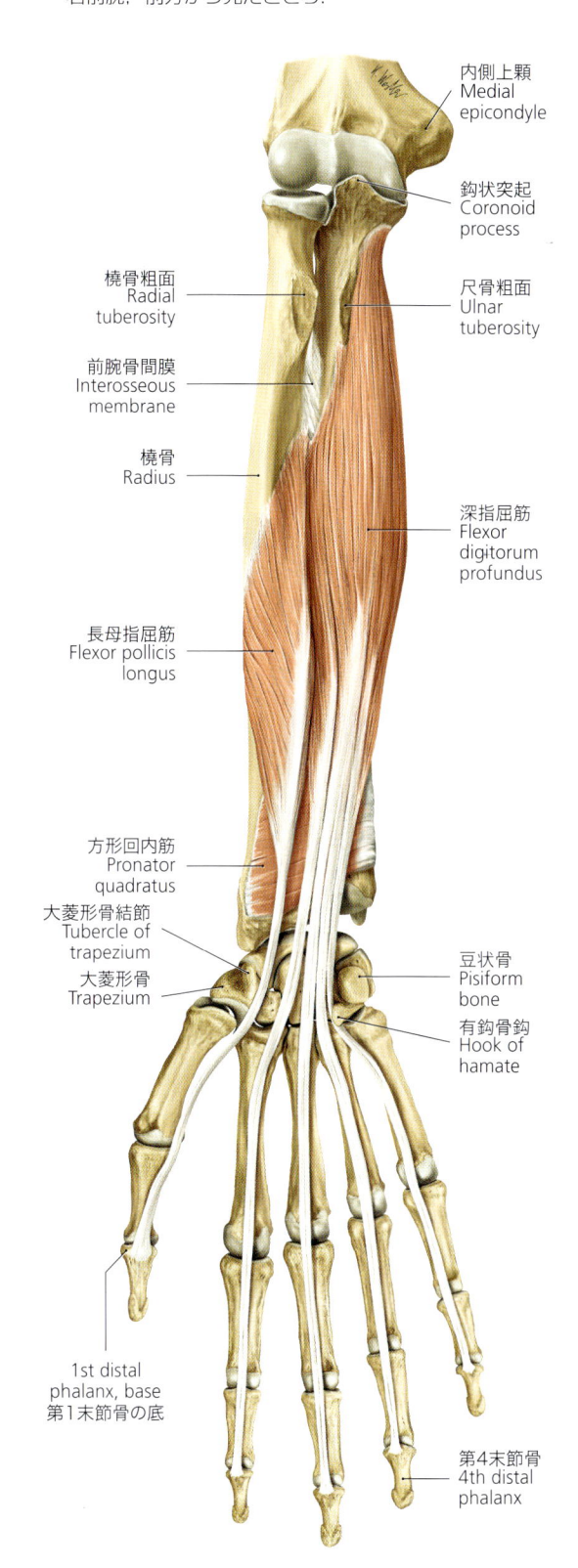

個々の筋（2）
Muscle Facts (II)

図 20.16　前腕橈側の筋
右前腕，後方から見たところ．

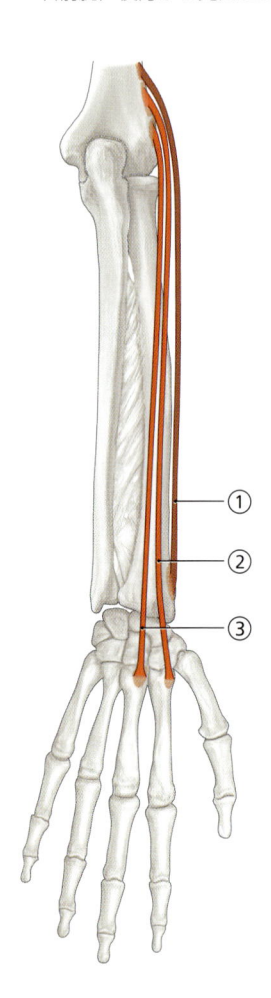

表 20.3	前腕橈側の筋			
筋	起始	停止	神経支配	作用
①腕橈骨筋	上腕骨遠位部（前外側面），外側筋間中隔	橈骨の茎状突起	橈骨神経（C5, C6）	肘：屈曲 前腕：半回内
②長橈側手根伸筋	上腕骨の外側上顆稜，外側筋間中隔	第2中手骨底	橈骨神経（C6, C7）	肘：弱い屈曲作用
③短橈側手根伸筋	上腕骨の外側上顆	第3中手骨底	橈骨神経（C7, C8）	手首：伸展・外転（橈側偏位）

図 20.17　前腕橈側の筋
右前腕.

A　外側(橈側)方から見たところ.

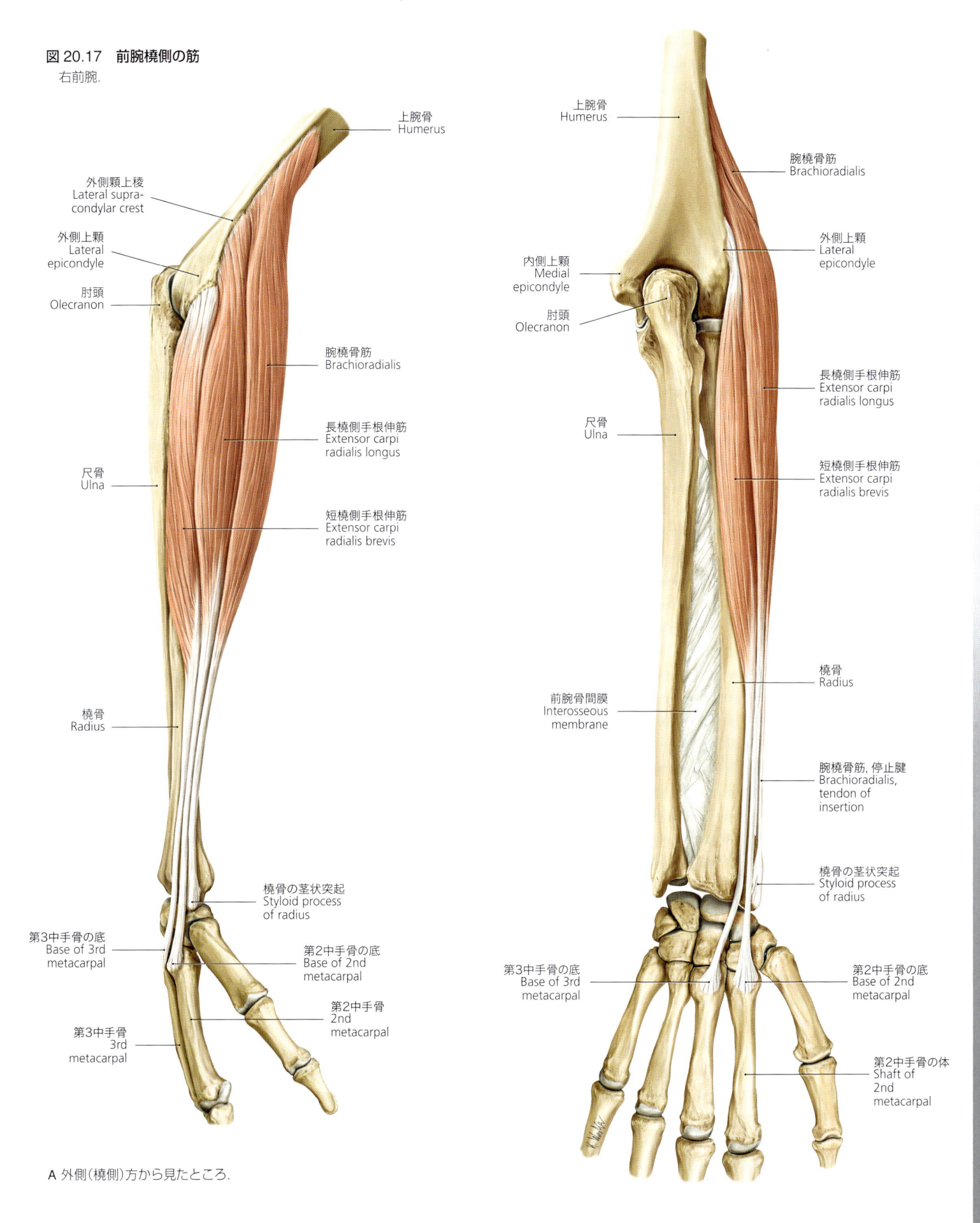

B　後方から見たところ.

個々の筋(3)
Muscle Facts(III)

図20.18　前腕後面の筋（浅層）
右前腕，後方から見たところ．

図20.19　前腕後面の筋（深層）
右前腕，後方から見たところ．

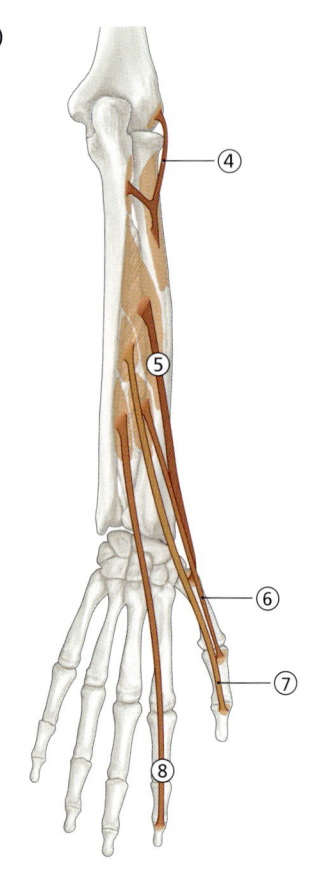

表20.4　前腕後面の筋

筋	起始	停止	神経支配	作用
浅層				
①総指伸筋	共通頭：上腕骨の外側上顆	第2-5指の指背腱膜	橈骨神経(C7, C8)	手首：伸展 第2-5指のMCP関節・PIP関節・DIP関節：伸展・外転
②小指伸筋		第5指の指背腱膜		手首：伸展・外転（橈側偏位） 第5指のMCP関節・PIP関節・DIP関節：伸展・外転
③尺側手根伸筋	共通頭：上腕骨の外側上顆，尺骨頭：尺骨の後面	第5中手骨底		手首：伸展・内転（尺側偏位）
深層				
④回外筋	肘頭，外側上顆，外側側副靱帯，橈骨輪状靱帯	橈骨（橈骨粗面と円回内筋停止部の間）	橈骨神経(C6, C7)	前腕：回外
⑤長母指外転筋	橈骨と尺骨の後面，骨間膜	第1中手骨底	橈骨神経(C7, C8)	手首：外転（橈側偏位） 母指の手根中手関節：外転
⑥短母指伸筋	橈骨の後面，骨間膜	母指の基節骨底		手首：外転（橈側偏位） 母指の手根中手関節・MCP関節：伸展
⑦長母指伸筋	尺骨の後面，骨間膜	母指の末節骨底		手首：伸展・外転（橈側偏位） 母指の手根中手関節：外転 母指のMCP関節・IP関節：伸展
⑧示指伸筋	尺骨の後面，骨間膜	示指の指背腱膜		手首：伸展 第2指のMCP関節・PIP関節・DIP関節：伸展

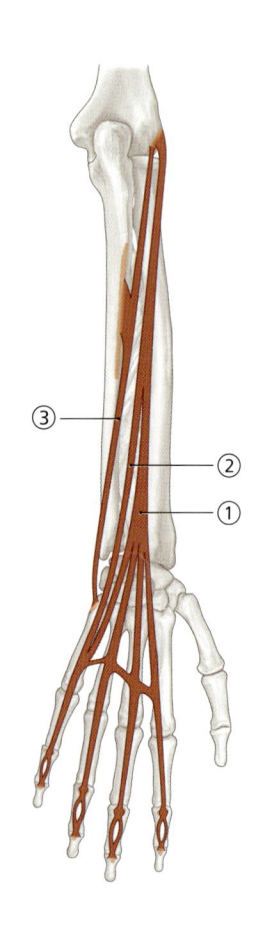

DIP関節＝遠位指節間関節，IP関節＝指節間関節，MCP関節＝中手指節関節，PIP関節＝近位指節間関節．

図 20.20 前腕後面の筋
右前腕，後方から見たところ．

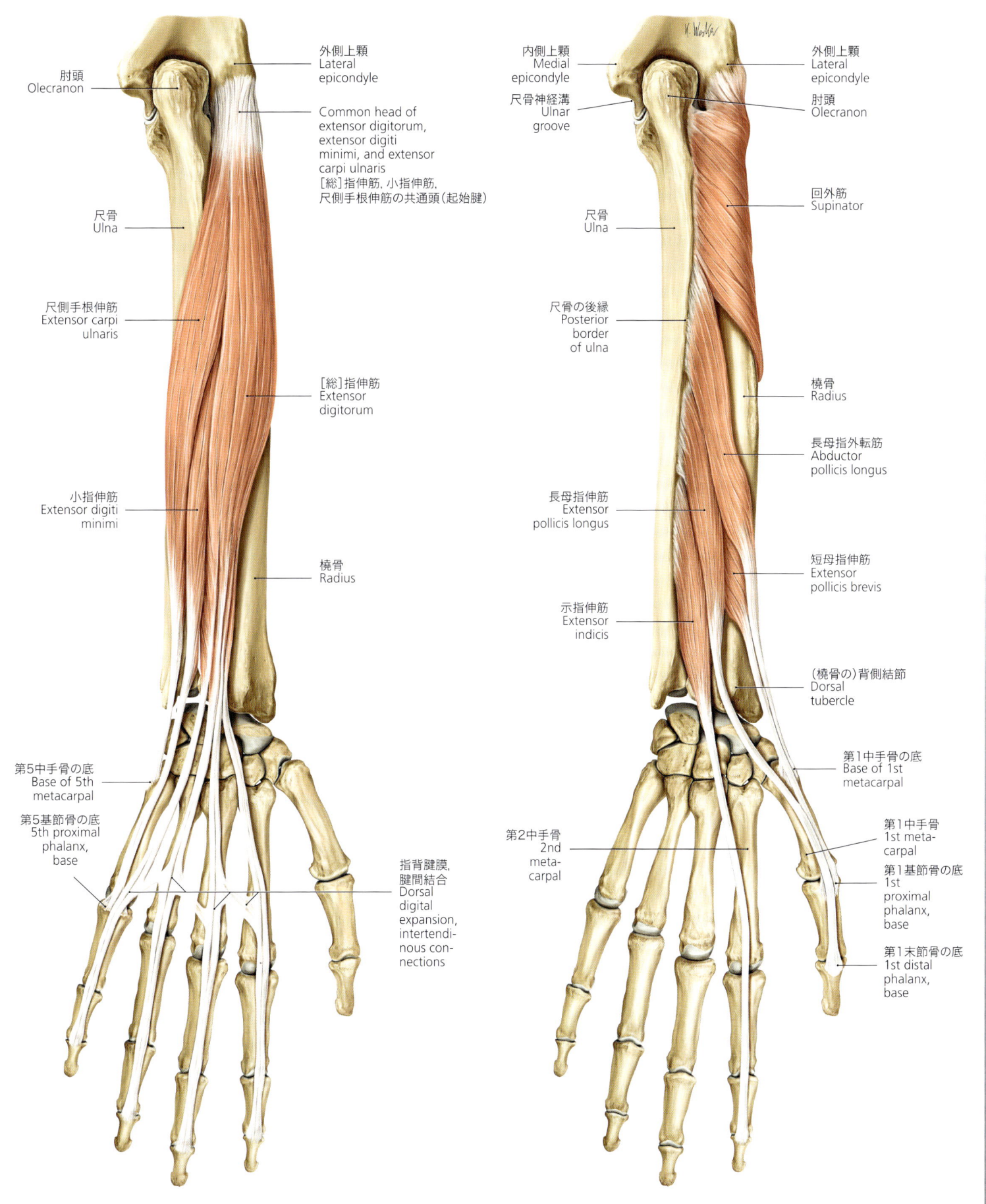

A 浅層の伸筋．

B 深層の伸筋と回外筋．

手首と手の骨
Bones of the Wrist & Hand

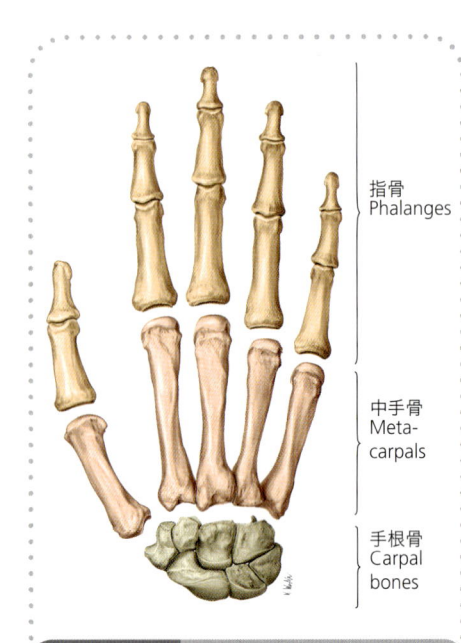

表 21.1	手首と手の骨	
指骨	第 1-5 基節骨	
	第 2-5 中節骨*	
	第 1-5 末節骨	
中手骨	第 1-5 中手骨	
手根骨	大菱形骨	舟状骨
	小菱形骨	月状骨
	有頭骨	三角骨
	有鈎骨	豆状骨

*ひとつの手にある中節骨は 4 個である（母指には基節骨と末節骨しかない）．

図 21.1　背側面（後方から見たところ）
右手．

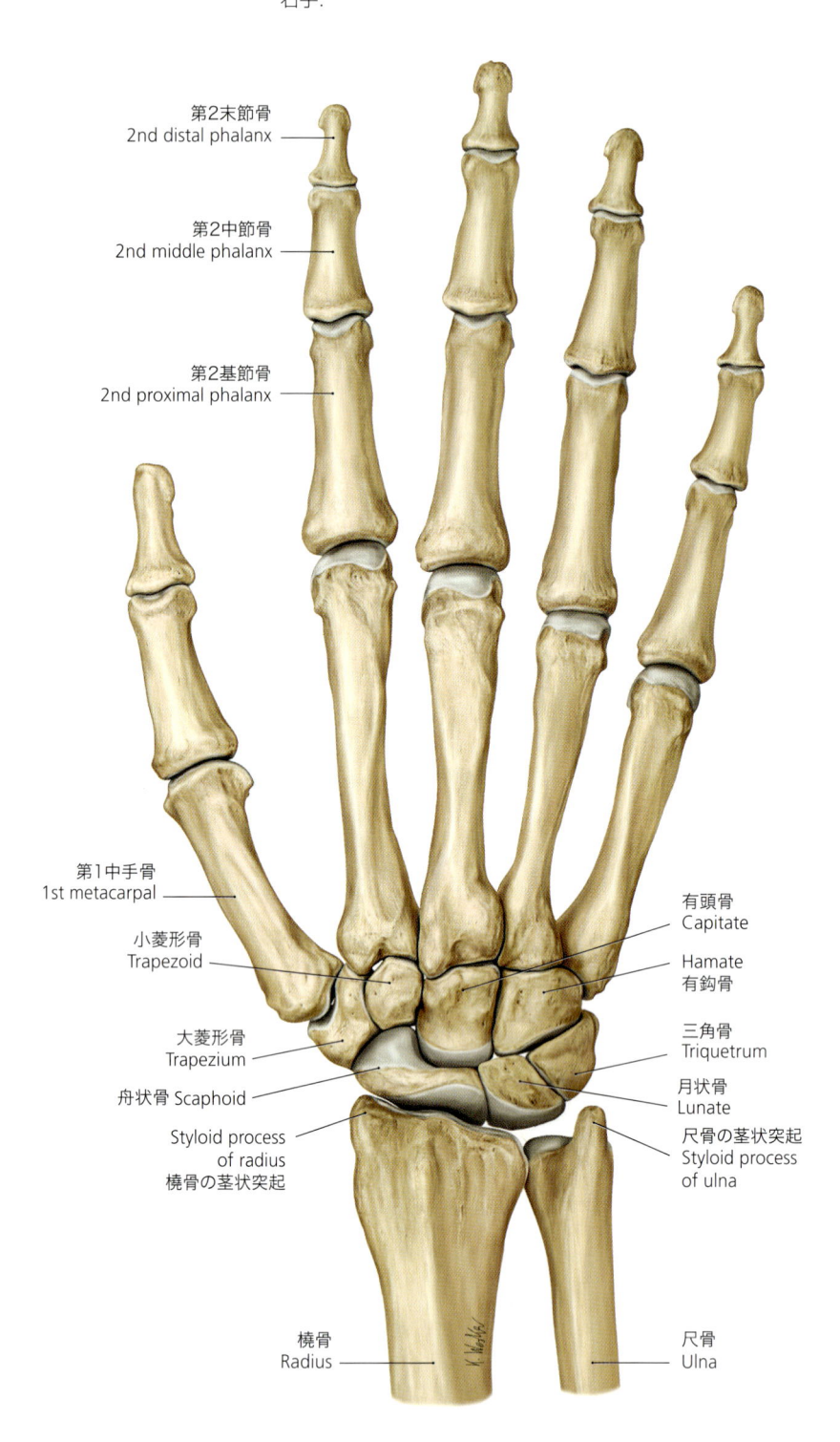

- 第2末節骨 2nd distal phalanx
- 第2中節骨 2nd middle phalanx
- 第2基節骨 2nd proximal phalanx
- 第1中手骨 1st metacarpal
- 小菱形骨 Trapezoid
- 大菱形骨 Trapezium
- 舟状骨 Scaphoid
- Styloid process of radius 橈骨の茎状突起
- 橈骨 Radius
- 有頭骨 Capitate
- Hamate 有鈎骨
- 三角骨 Triquetrum
- 月状骨 Lunate
- 尺骨の茎状突起 Styloid process of ulna
- 尺骨 Ulna

指骨 Phalanges
中手骨 Meta-carpals
手根骨 Carpal bones

図 21.2 掌側面（前方から見たところ）
右手．

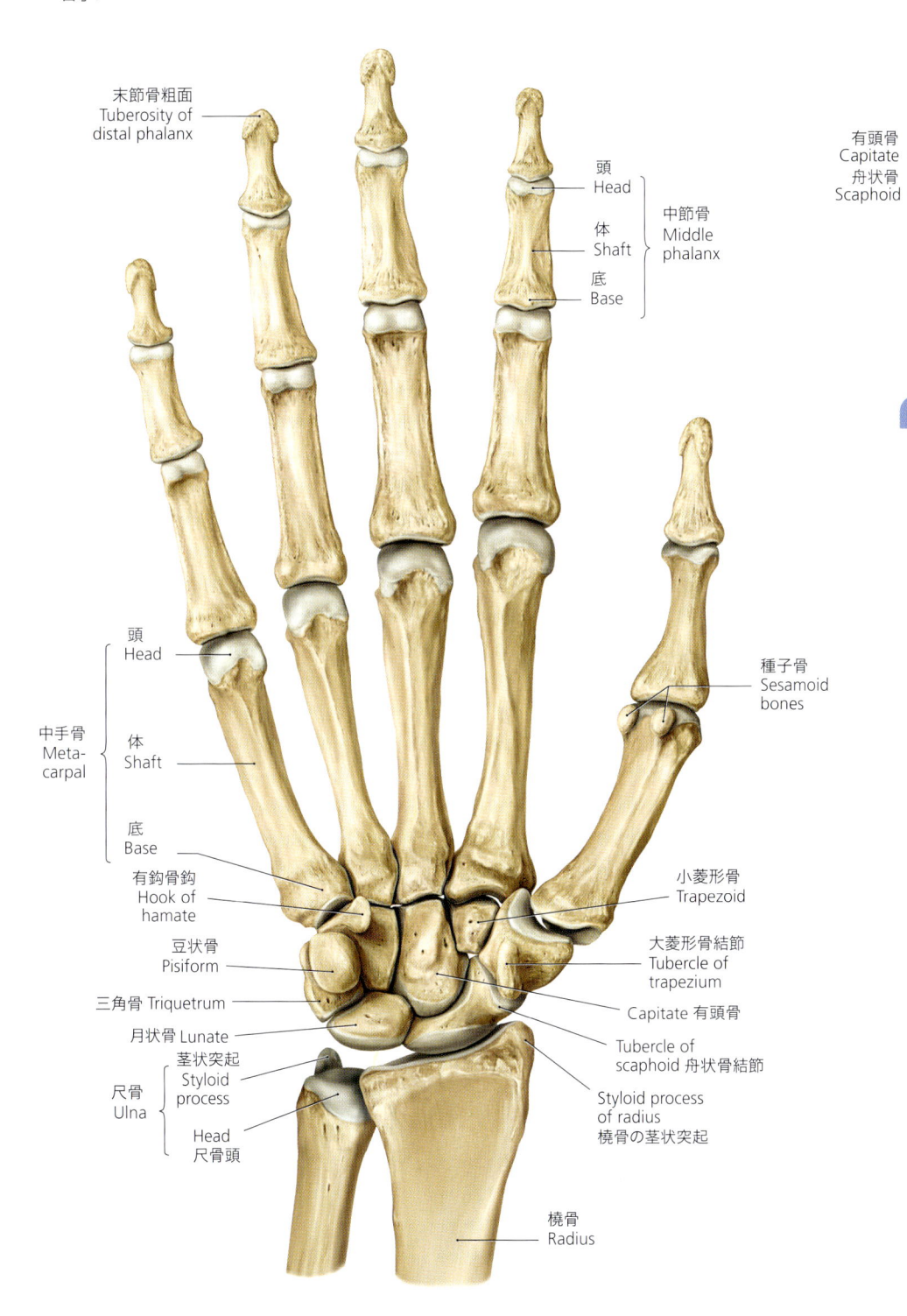

- 末節骨粗面 Tuberosity of distal phalanx
- 頭 Head
- 体 Shaft — 中節骨 Middle phalanx
- 底 Base
- 頭 Head
- 体 Shaft — 中手骨 Meta-carpal
- 底 Base
- 種子骨 Sesamoid bones
- 有鈎骨鈎 Hook of hamate
- 小菱形骨 Trapezoid
- 豆状骨 Pisiform
- 三角骨 Triquetrum
- 月状骨 Lunate
- 大菱形骨結節 Tuberacle of trapezium
- Capitate 有頭骨
- Tubercle of scaphoid 舟状骨結節
- 茎状突起 Styloid process
- Head 尺骨頭
- 尺骨 Ulna
- Styloid process of radius 橈骨の茎状突起
- 橈骨 Radius

図 21.3 手首の X 線写真
左手首の前後像．

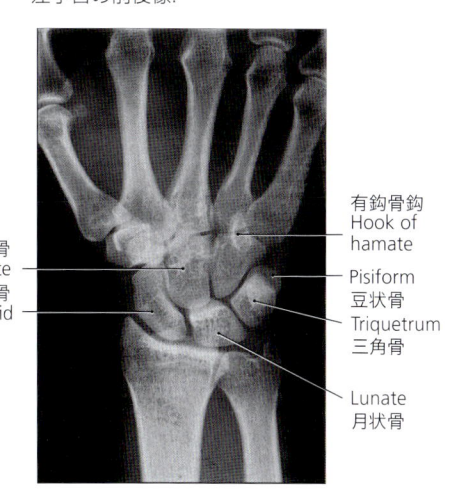

- 有頭骨 Capitate
- 舟状骨 Scaphoid
- 有鈎骨鈎 Hook of hamate
- 豆状骨 Pisiform
- 三角骨 Triquetrum
- 月状骨 Lunate

臨床

舟状骨骨折

舟状骨骨折は最もよく見られる手根骨の骨折であり，通常は近位端と遠位端の間にあるくびれた部位で起こる（A，右舟状骨）．舟状骨には通常は遠位端から動脈が入る．このため，くびれた部分で骨折が起こると（B の矢印），近位端の血流が減少し，しばしば骨の癒合が妨げられたり，近位端が無血管性壊死に陥る．

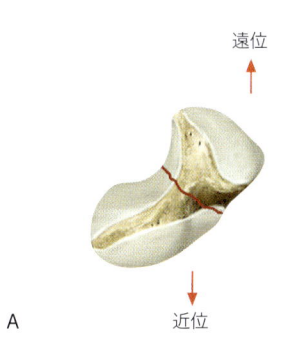

遠位

近位

A

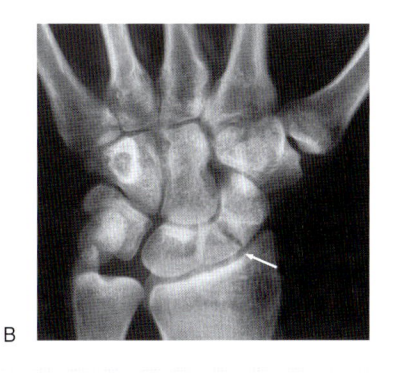

B

手首と手の関節
Joints of the Wrist & Hand

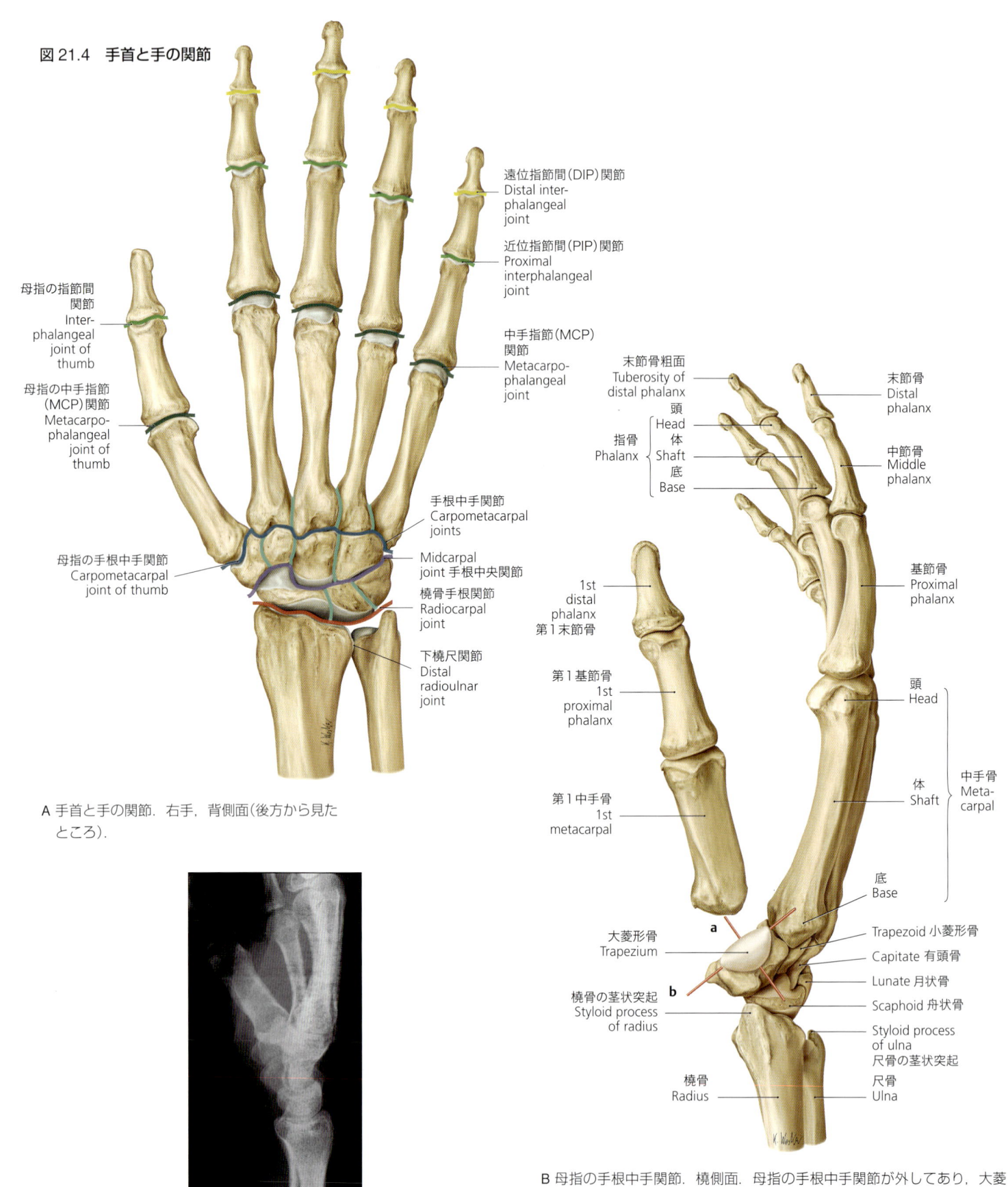

図 21.4　手首と手の関節

遠位指節間(DIP)関節
Distal interphalangeal joint

近位指節間(PIP)関節
Proximal interphalangeal joint

中手指節(MCP)関節
Metacarpophalangeal joint

母指の指節間関節
Interphalangeal joint of thumb

母指の中手指節(MCP)関節
Metacarpophalangeal joint of thumb

手根中手関節
Carpometacarpal joints

母指の手根中手関節
Carpometacarpal joint of thumb

Midcarpal joint 手根中央関節

橈骨手根関節
Radiocarpal joint

下橈尺関節
Distal radioulnar joint

末節骨粗面
Tuberosity of distal phalanx

指骨 Phalanx
　頭 Head
　体 Shaft
　底 Base

末節骨
Distal phalanx

中節骨
Middle phalanx

基節骨
Proximal phalanx

1st distal phalanx
第1末節骨

第1基節骨
1st proximal phalanx

第1中手骨
1st metacarpal

頭 Head

体 Shaft

中手骨 Metacarpal

底 Base

大菱形骨 Trapezium

Trapezoid 小菱形骨

Capitate 有頭骨

Lunate 月状骨

Scaphoid 舟状骨

橈骨の茎状突起
Styloid process of radius

Styloid process of ulna
尺骨の茎状突起

橈骨 Radius

尺骨 Ulna

A　手首と手の関節．右手，背側面（後方から見たところ）．

C　手首のX線写真．橈側面．

B　母指の手根中手関節．橈側面．母指の手根中手関節が外してあり，大菱形骨の関節面がみえている．この関節における動きの主軸（2本）が示してある：(a)屈曲/伸展軸，(b)外転/内転軸．

図 21.5 手首と手：前額断面
右手．

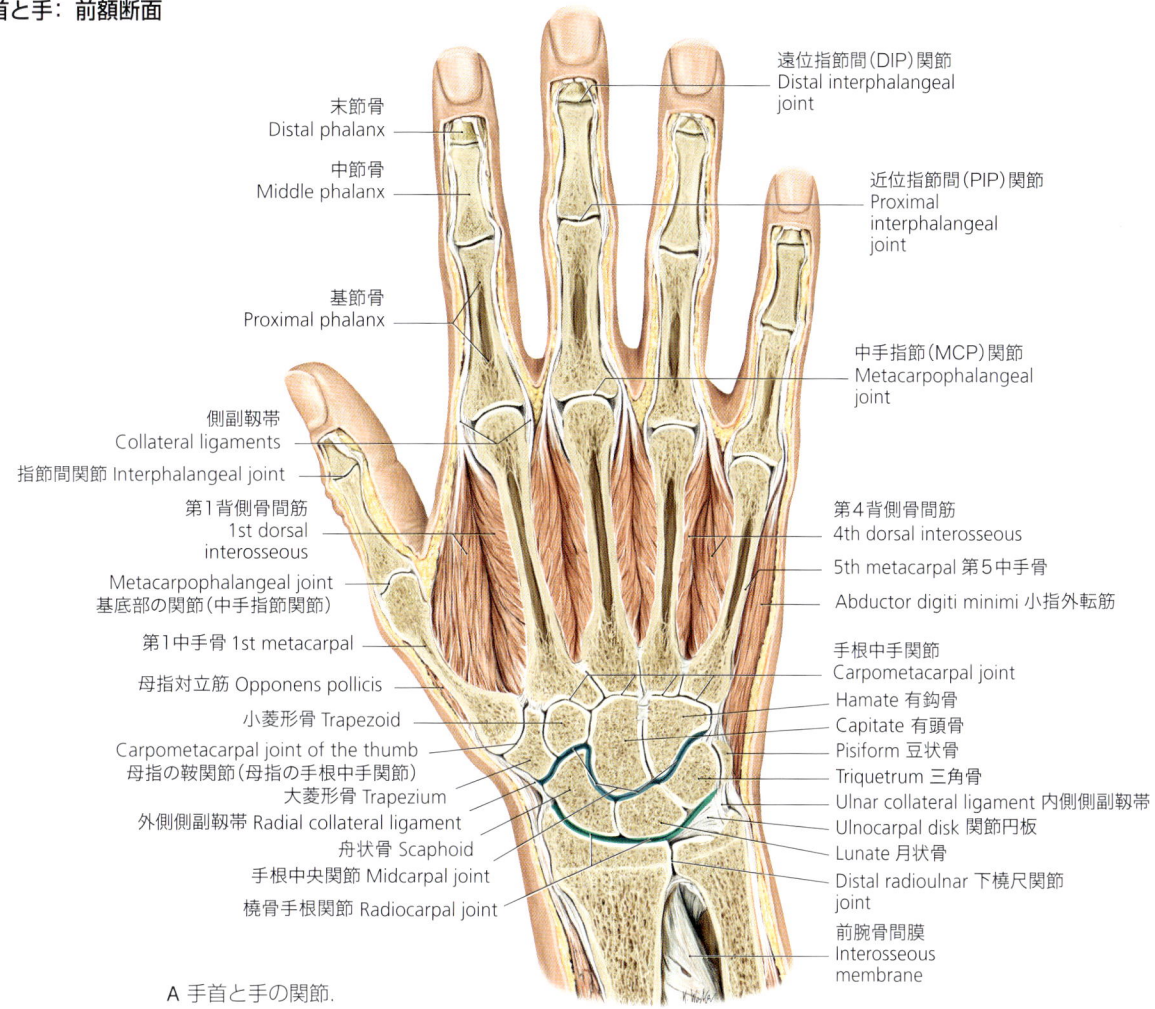

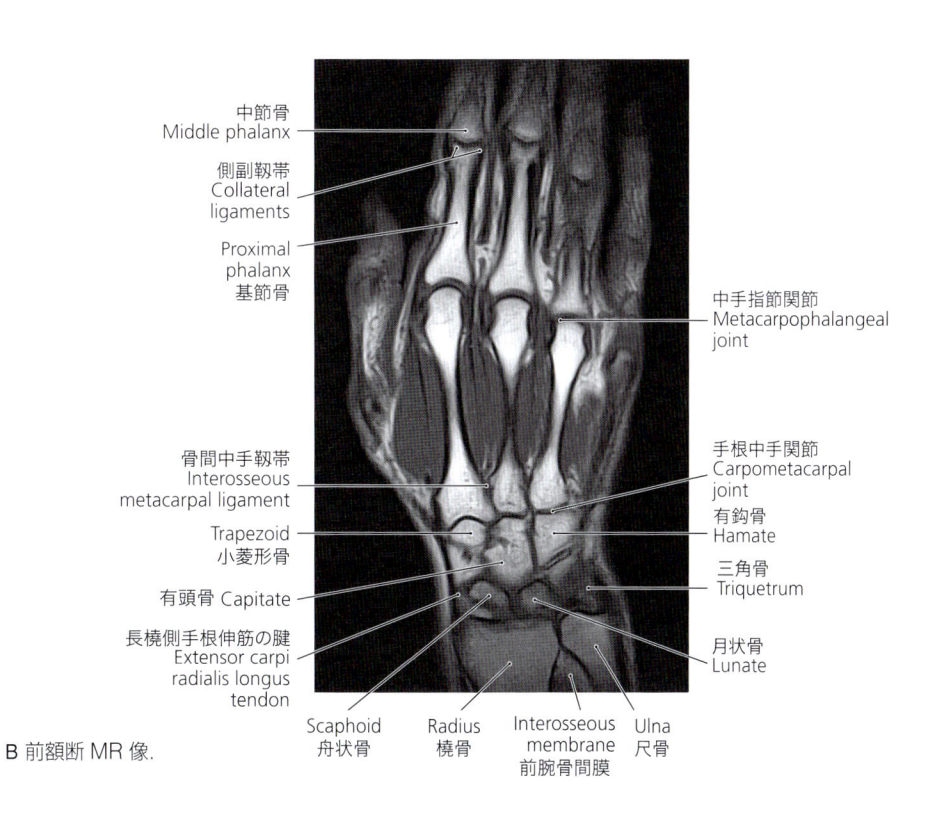

A 手首と手の関節．

B 前額断 MR 像．

手首と手の靱帯
Ligaments of the Wrist & Hand

図 21.6　手の靱帯
右手.

背側手根中手靱帯
Dorsal carpometacarpal ll.

背側手根間靱帯
Dorsal intercarpal ll.

外側手根側副靱帯
Radial carpal collateral l.

背側中手靱帯
Dorsal metacarpal ll.

内側手根側副靱帯
Ulnar carpal collateral l.

背側橈骨手根靱帯
Dorsal radiocarpal l.

背側橈骨尺骨靱帯
Dorsal radioulnar l.

遠位指節間(DIP)関節(側副靱帯)
Distal interphalangeal joint (collateral ll.)

近位指節間(PIP)関節(側副靱帯)
Proximal interphalangeal joint (collateral ll.)

中手指節(MCP)関節(側副靱帯)
Metacarpophalangeal joint (collateral ll.)

A 背側面(後方から見たところ).

遠位指節間(DIP)関節, 関節包
Distal interphalangeal joint capsule

近位指節間(PIP)関節, 関節包
Proximal interphalangeal joint capsule

深横中手靱帯
Deep transverse metacarpal ll.

中手指節(MCP)関節
Metacarpophalangeal joint capsule

掌側中手靱帯
Palmar metacarpal ll.

掌側手根間靱帯
Palmar intercarpal ll.

Flexor carpi ulnaris tendon
尺側手根屈筋の腱

Palmar ulnocarpal l.
掌側尺骨手根靱帯

掌側靱帯
Palmar ll.

掌側手根中手靱帯
Palmar carpometacarpal ll.

外側手根側副靱帯
Radial carpal collateral l.

掌側橈骨手根靱帯
Palmar radiocarpal l.

Palmar radioulnar l.
掌側橈骨尺骨靱帯

B 掌側面(前方から見たところ).

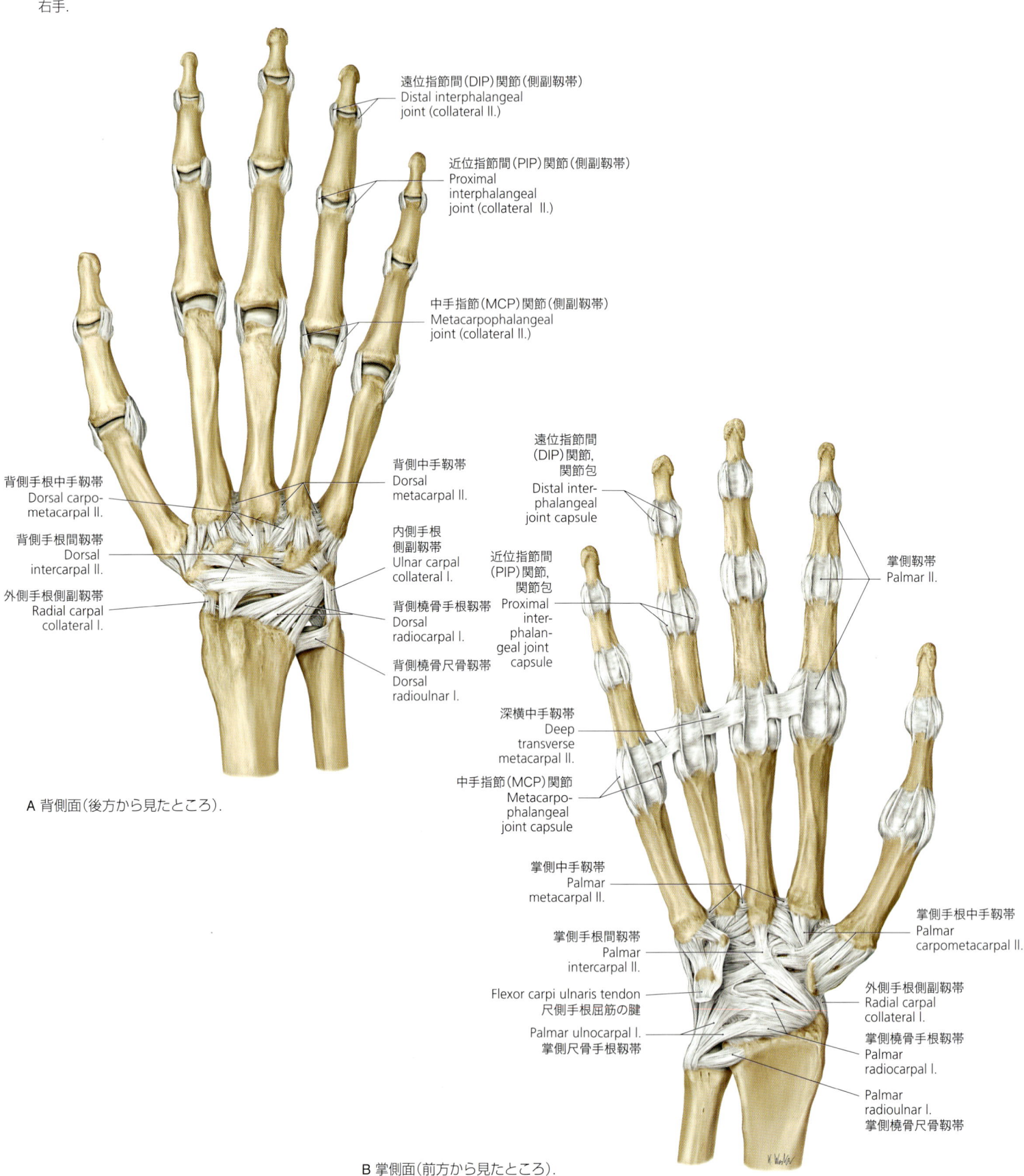

図 21.7　手根管の靭帯
右手．前方から見たところ．

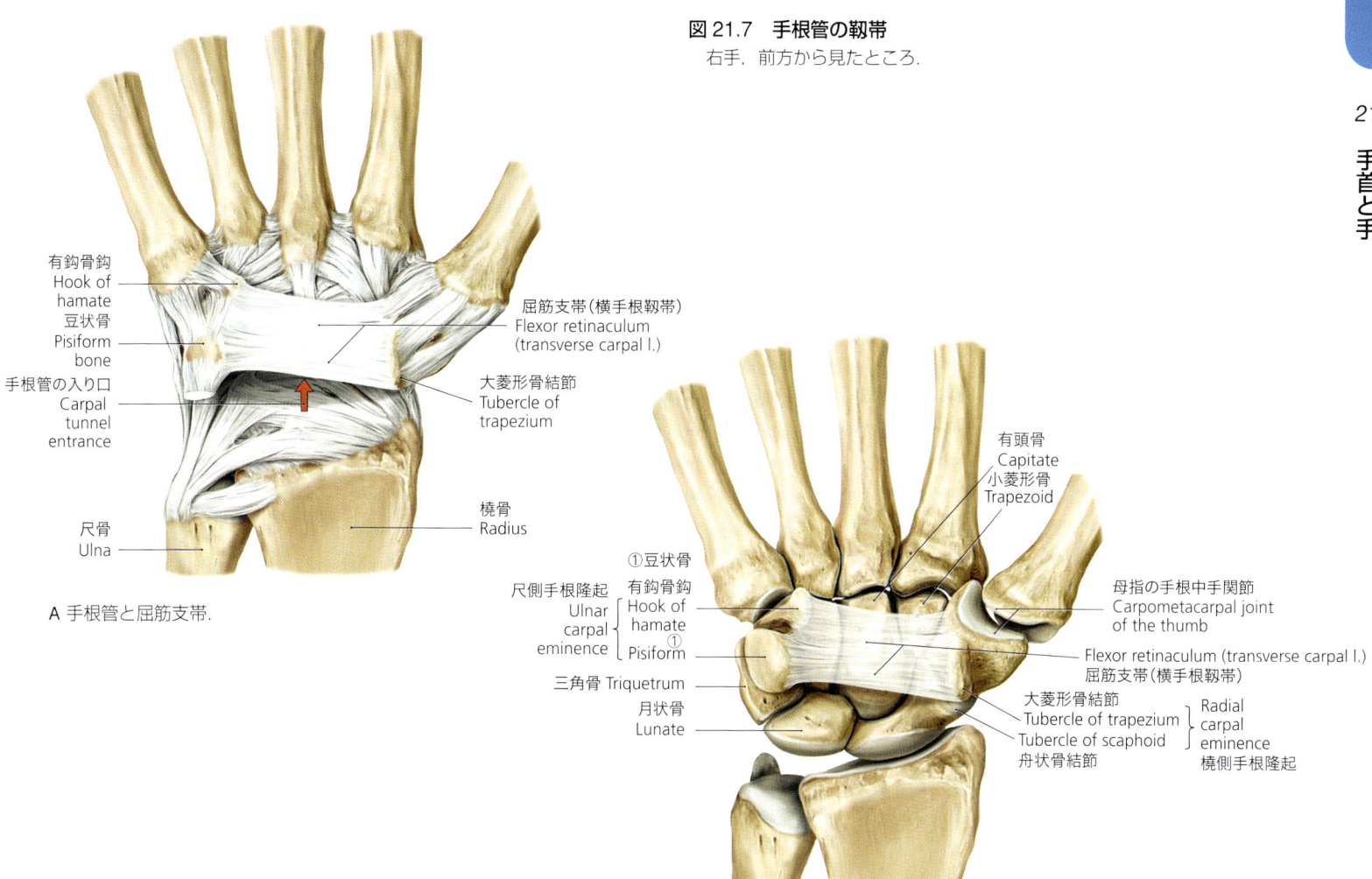

- 有鈎骨鈎 Hook of hamate
- 豆状骨 Pisiform bone
- 手根管の入り口 Carpal tunnel entrance
- 尺骨 Ulna
- 屈筋支帯（横手根靭帯）Flexor retinaculum (transverse carpal l.)
- 大菱形骨結節 Tubercle of trapezium
- 橈骨 Radius

A 手根管と屈筋支帯．

- 有頭骨 Capitate
- 小菱形骨 Trapezoid
- 母指の手根中手関節 Carpometacarpal joint of the thumb
- 屈筋支帯（横手根靭帯）Flexor retinaculum (transverse carpal l.)
- 尺側手根隆起 Ulnar carpal eminence
  - 有鈎骨鈎 Hook of hamate
  - ①豆状骨 Pisiform
- 三角骨 Triquetrum
- 月状骨 Lunate
- 大菱形骨結節 Tubercle of trapezium
- 舟状骨結節 Tubercle of scaphoid
- 橈側手根隆起 Radial carpal eminence

B 手根管を形成する各骨の境界．

図 21.8　手根管
横断面．手根管の内容については p.342 で扱う．尺骨神経管と掌側手根靭帯については p.343 参照．

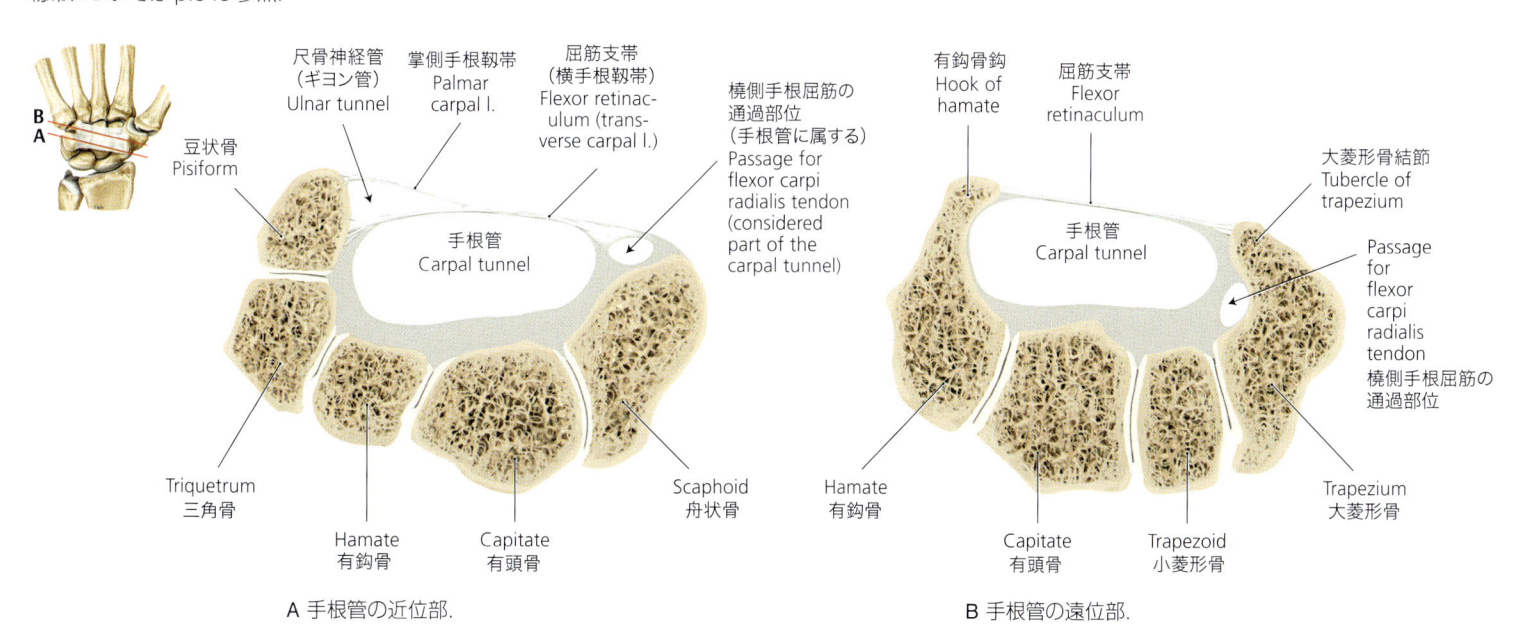

- 尺骨神経管（ギヨン管）Ulnar tunnel
- 掌側手根靭帯 Palmar carpal l.
- 屈筋支帯（横手根靭帯）Flexor retinaculum (transverse carpal l.)
- 橈側手根屈筋の通過部位（手根管に属する）Passage for flexor carpi radialis tendon (considered part of the carpal tunnel)
- 豆状骨 Pisiform
- 手根管 Carpal tunnel
- 三角骨 Triquetrum
- 有鈎骨 Hamate
- 有頭骨 Capitate
- 舟状骨 Scaphoid

A 手根管の近位部．

- 有鈎骨鈎 Hook of hamate
- 屈筋支帯 Flexor retinaculum
- 大菱形骨結節 Tubercle of trapezium
- 橈側手根屈筋の通過部位 Passage for flexor carpi radialis tendon
- 手根管 Carpal tunnel
- 有鈎骨 Hamate
- 有頭骨 Capitate
- 小菱形骨 Trapezoid
- 大菱形骨 Trapezium

B 手根管の遠位部．

指の靱帯
Ligaments of the Fingers

図 21.9　指の靱帯：外側面
右中指，外側方から見たところ．腱鞘の外層をなす線維鞘は，一部が肥厚して輪状部と十字部を形成する．この 2 種類の肥厚部は腱鞘を指骨の掌側面につなぎ留め，指の屈曲時に腱鞘が掌側に偏位するのを防ぐ．

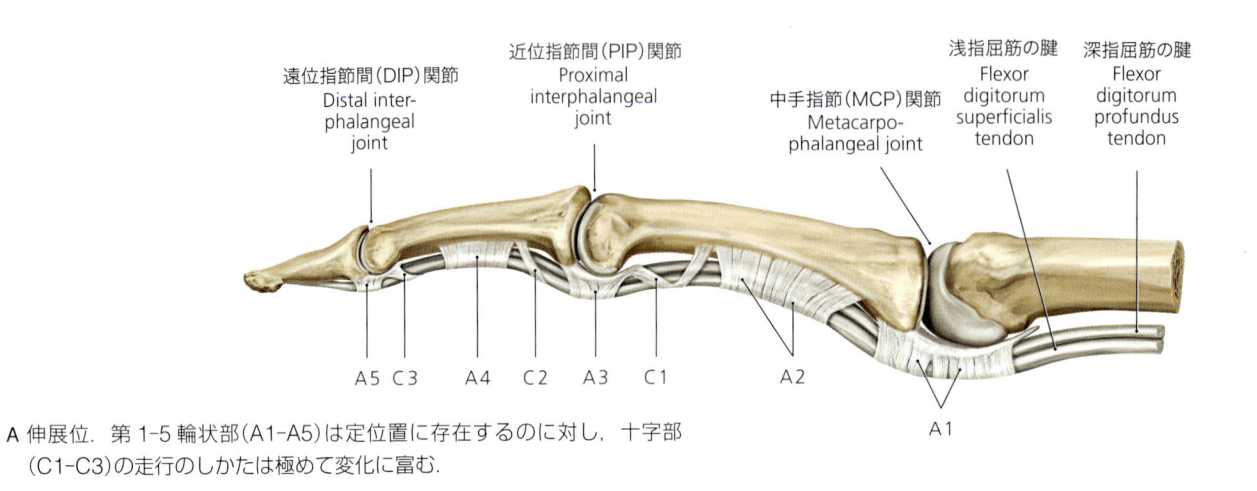

遠位指節間(DIP)関節　Distal interphalangeal joint
近位指節間(PIP)関節　Proximal interphalangeal joint
中手指節(MCP)関節　Metacarpophalangeal joint
浅指屈筋の腱　Flexor digitorum superficialis tendon
深指屈筋の腱　Flexor digitorum profundus tendon

A5　C3　A4　C2　A3　C1　A2　A1

A 伸展位．第 1-5 輪状部(A1-A5)は定位置に存在するのに対し，十字部(C1-C3)の走行のしかたは極めて変化に富む．

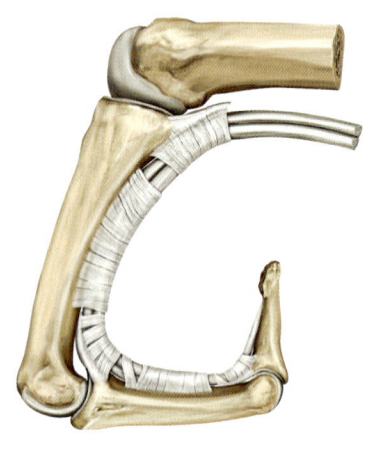

指節関節靱帯　Phalangoglenoid l.
側副靱帯　Collateral l.
基節骨　Proximal phalanx
中手骨　Metacarpal bone
A2　A1
副側副靱帯　Accessory collateral l.

B 屈曲位．

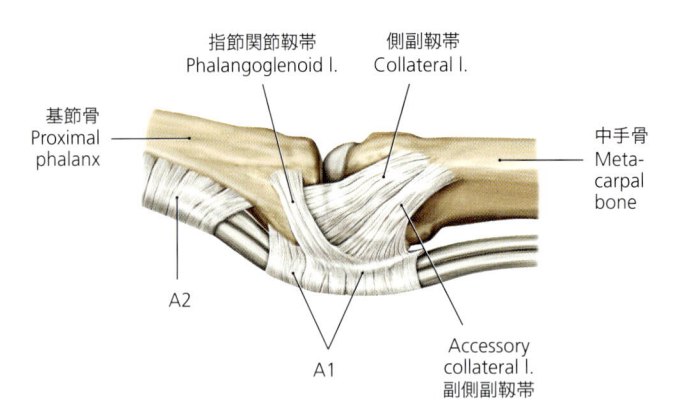

C 中手指節関節の伸展位．
Note：側副靱帯が緩んでいる．

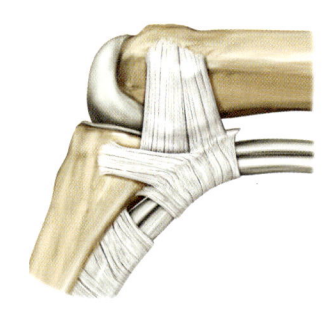

D 中手指節関節の屈曲位．
Note：側副靱帯が緊張している．

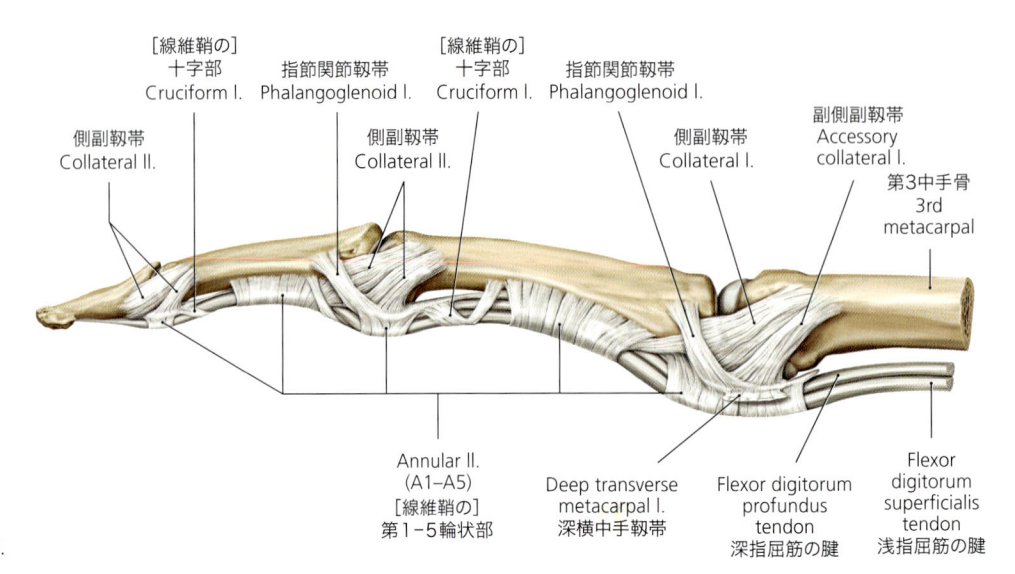

［線維鞘の］十字部　Cruciform l.
指節関節靱帯　Phalangoglenoid l.
側副靱帯　Collateral l.
副側副靱帯　Accessory collateral l.
第3中手骨　3rd metacarpal
Annular ll. (A1–A5) ［線維鞘の］第1-5輪状部
深横中手靱帯　Deep transverse metacarpal l.
深指屈筋の腱　Flexor digitorum profundus tendon
浅指屈筋の腱　Flexor digitorum superficialis tendon

E 関節包，靱帯，腱鞘．

図 21.10 指の靱帯：前方から見たところ（掌側面）
右中指．

- 深指屈筋の腱 Flexor digitorum profundus tendon
- 遠位指節間(DIP)関節（側副靱帯）Distal interphalangeal joints (collateral ll.)
- [線維鞘の]十字部 Cruciform ll.
- 中節骨 Middle phalanx
- 近位指節間(PIP)関節（側副靱帯）Proximal interphalangeal joints (collateral ll.)
- 浅指屈筋の腱 Flexor digitorum superficialis tendon
- [線維鞘の]十字部 Cruciform ll.
- Annular ll. (A1–A5) [線維鞘の]第1–5輪状部
- 基節骨 Proximal phalanx
- 深横中手靱帯 Deep transverse metacarpal l.
- 中手骨 Metacarpal bone
- Flexor digitorum superficialis tendon 浅指屈筋の腱
- Flexor digitorum profundus tendon 深指屈筋の腱
- 中手指節(MCP)関節（側副靱帯）Metacarpophalangeal joint (collateral ll.)

A 浅層の靱帯．
B 深層の靱帯，腱鞘と腱を取り除いたところ．

図 21.11 第3中手骨：横断面
近位方向から見たところ．

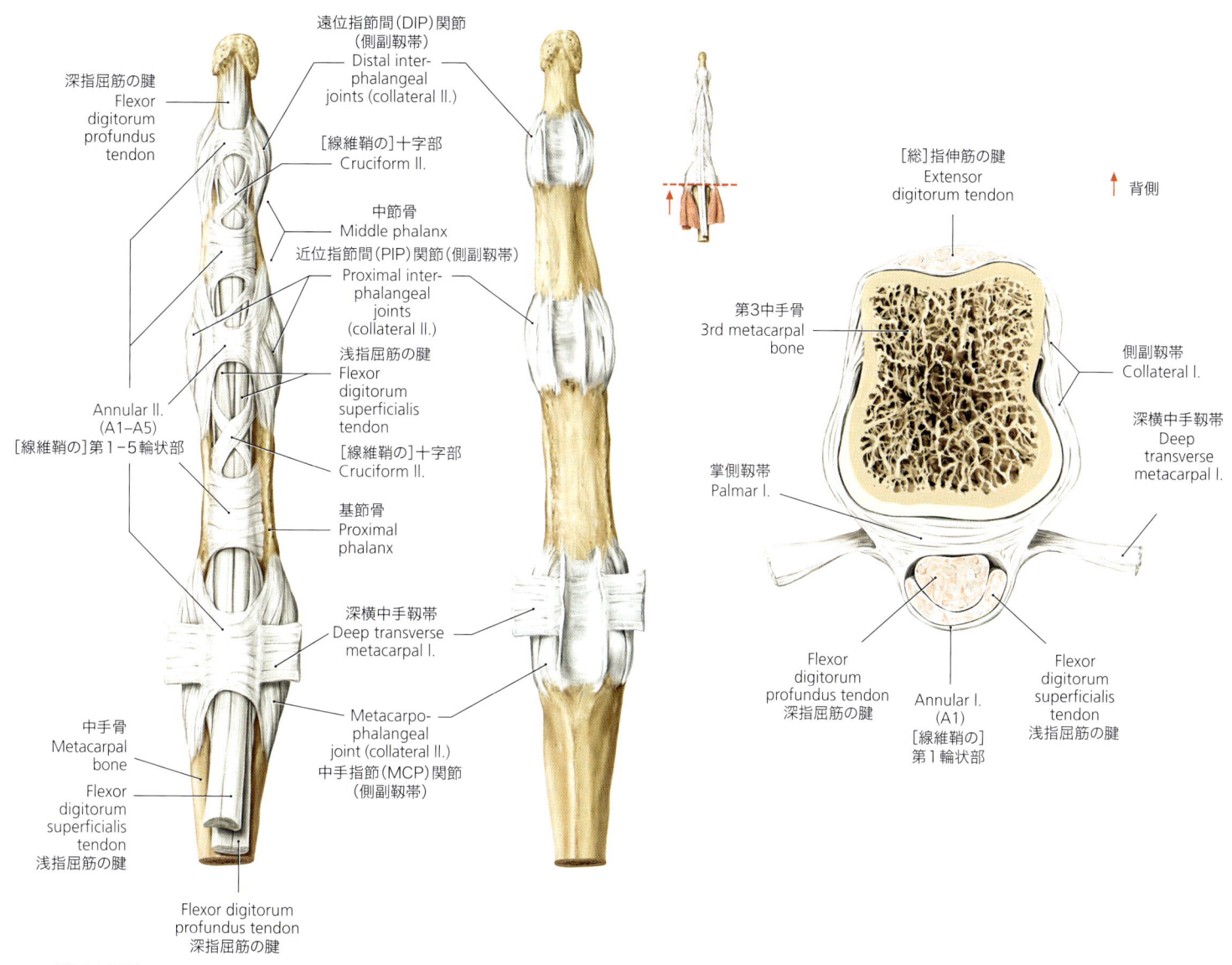

- [総]指伸筋の腱 Extensor digitorum tendon
- 背側
- 第3中手骨 3rd metacarpal bone
- 側副靱帯 Collateral l.
- 深横中手靱帯 Deep transverse metacarpal l.
- 掌側靱帯 Palmar l.
- Flexor digitorum profundus tendon 深指屈筋の腱
- Annular l. (A1) [線維鞘の]第1輪状部
- Flexor digitorum superficialis tendon 浅指屈筋の腱

図 21.12 指先：縦断面
指の関節では，近位側の関節面が掌側に広がっている．線維軟骨の板からなる掌側靱帯（掌側板）は関節面の広がった部分と接しており，腱鞘の床となる．

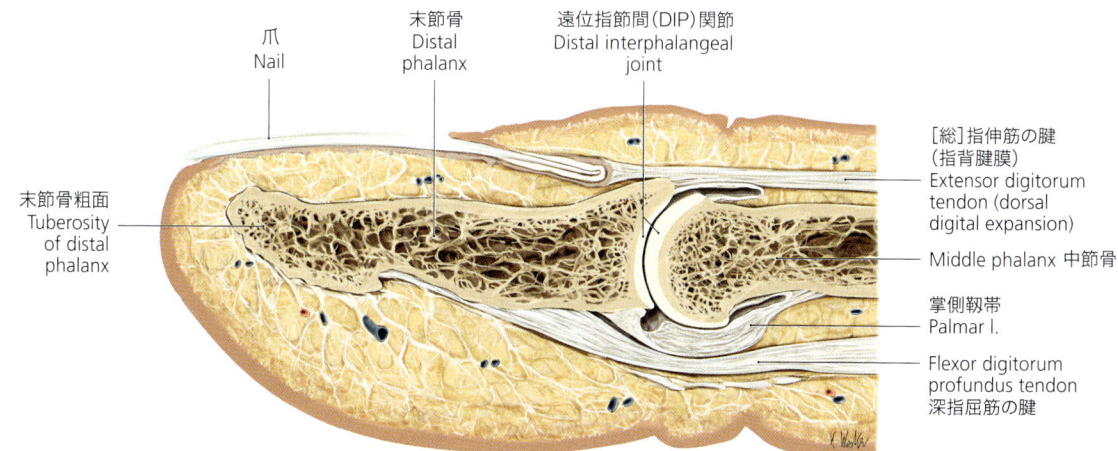

- 爪 Nail
- 末節骨 Distal phalanx
- 遠位指節間(DIP)関節 Distal interphalangeal joint
- 末節骨粗面 Tuberosity of distal phalanx
- [総]指伸筋の腱（指背腱膜）Extensor digitorum tendon (dorsal digital expansion)
- Middle phalanx 中節骨
- 掌側靱帯 Palmar l.
- Flexor digitorum profundus tendon 深指屈筋の腱

手の筋：浅層と中間層
Muscles of the Hand: Superficial & Middle Layers

図21.13 手内筋：表層と中間層
右手，掌側面．

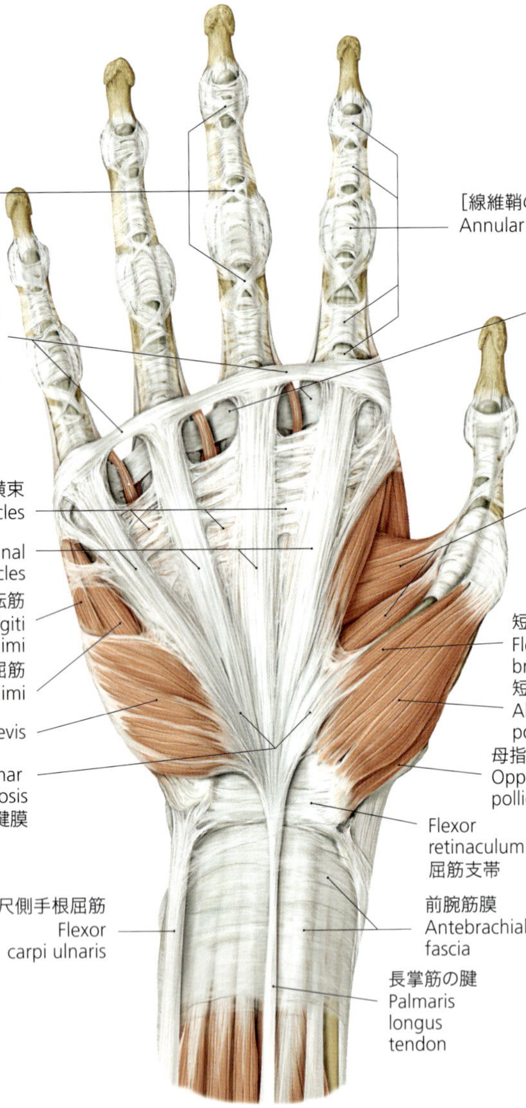

臨床

デュピイトラン拘縮

手掌腱膜が徐々に萎縮すると，それに伴って手掌筋膜も短縮し，主に第4・5指に機能障害が現れる．1年以上放置すると拘縮は極めて重症化し，指先が手掌に触れるほどの屈曲位をとるようになり，物を握る機能が著しく損なわれる．デュピイトラン拘縮の原因はよくわかっていないが，慢性肝疾患（例えば肝硬変症）を有する40歳以上の男性においてよくみられる．一般的な治療法は，肥厚した手掌腱膜を外科的に完全に除去することである．

図中ラベル（左図 A）：
- [線維鞘の]十字部 Cruciform ll.
- [線維鞘の]第1-5輪状部 Annular ll. (A1–A5)
- 浅横中手靱帯 Superficial transverse metacarpal l.
- 深横中手靱帯 Deep transverse metacarpal l.
- 横束 Transverse fascicles
- 縦束 Longitudinal fascicles
- 小指外転筋 Abductor digiti minimi
- 短小指屈筋 Flexor digiti minimi
- 短掌筋 Palmaris brevis
- Palmar aponeurosis 手掌腱膜
- 母指内転筋 Adductor pollicis
- 短母指屈筋 Flexor pollicis brevis
- 短母指外転筋 Abductor pollicis brevis
- 母指対立筋 Opponens pollicis
- Flexor retinaculum* 屈筋支帯
- 前腕筋膜 Antebrachial fascia
- 尺側手根屈筋 Flexor carpi ulnaris
- 長掌筋の腱 Palmaris longus tendon

A 手掌腱膜．
*横手根靱帯とも呼ばれる．

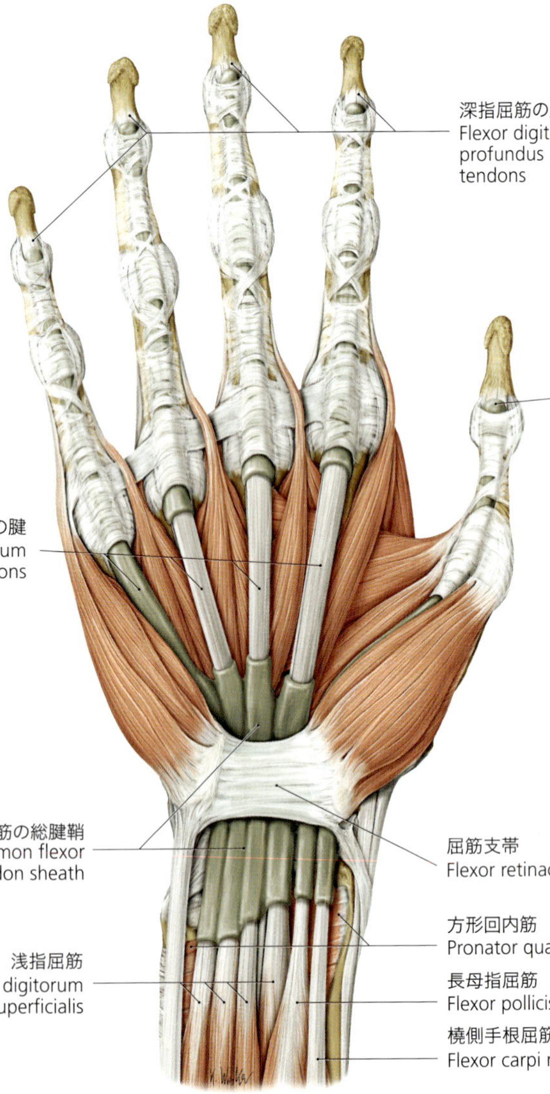

図中ラベル（右図 B）：
- 深指屈筋の腱 Flexor digitorum profundus tendons
- 長母指屈筋の腱 Flexor pollicis longus tendon
- 浅指屈筋の腱 Flexor digitorum superficialis tendons
- 指屈筋の総腱鞘 Common flexor tendon sheath
- 浅指屈筋 Flexor digitorum superficialis
- 屈筋支帯 Flexor retinaculum
- 方形回内筋 Pronator quadratus
- 長母指屈筋 Flexor pollicis longus
- 橈側手根屈筋 Flexor carpi radialis

B 手根部と指にある腱鞘．手掌腱膜，長掌筋，前腕筋膜，短掌筋を取り除いたところ．

21 手首と手

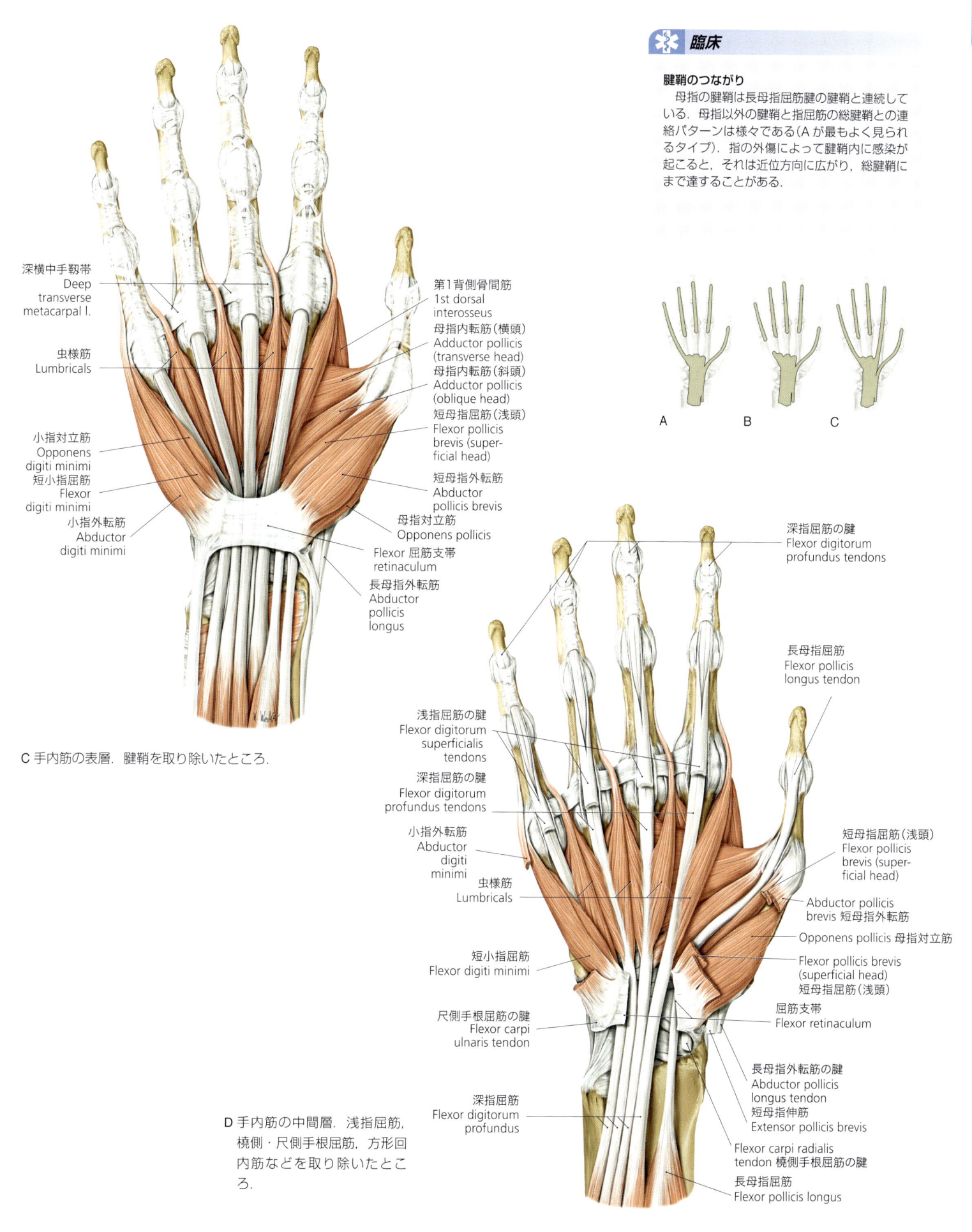

臨床

腱鞘のつながり

母指の腱鞘は長母指屈筋腱の腱鞘と連続している．母指以外の腱鞘と指屈筋の総腱鞘との連絡パターンは様々である（Aが最もよく見られるタイプ）．指の外傷によって腱鞘内に感染が起こると，それは近位方向に広がり，総腱鞘にまで達することがある．

A   B   C

C 手内筋の表層．腱鞘を取り除いたところ．

D 手内筋の中間層．浅指屈筋，橈側・尺側手根屈筋，方形回内筋などを取り除いたところ．

手の筋：中間層と深層
Muscles of the Hand: Middle & Deep Layers

図 21.14　手内筋：中間層と深層
右手，掌側面．

Labels (figure A, palmar view):
- 深指屈筋の腱 Flexor digitorum profundus tendons
- 長母指屈筋の腱 Flexor pollicis longus tendon
- 母指内転筋（横頭）Adductor pollicis (transverse head)
- 母指内転筋（斜頭）Adductor pollicis (oblique head)
- 短母指屈筋 Flexor pollicis brevis
- 短母指外転筋 Abductor pollicis brevis
- 母指対立筋 Opponens pollicis
- 屈筋支帯 Flexor retinaculum
- 浅指屈筋の腱 Flexor digitorum superficialis tendons
- 虫様筋 Lumbricals
- 小指外転筋 Abductor digiti minimi
- 短小指屈筋 Flexor digiti minimi
- 第2・3掌側骨間筋 2nd and 3rd palmar interossei
- 小指対立筋 Opponens digiti minimi
- 短小指屈筋 Flexor digiti minimi
- 小指外転筋 Abductor digiti minimi

A 手内筋の中間層．深指屈筋，虫様筋，長母指屈筋，短小指屈筋などを取り除いたところ．

Labels (figure B, deep layer):
- 掌側靭帯 Palmar ll.
- 母指内転筋 Adductor pollicis
- 短母指屈筋 Flexor pollicis brevis
- 短母指屈筋（深頭）Flexor pollicis brevis (deep head)
- 母指対立筋 Opponens pollicis
- 長母指外転筋の腱 Abductor pollicis longus tendon
- 短母指伸筋 Extensor pollicis brevis
- 橈側手根屈筋の腱 Flexor carpi radialis tendon
- 尺側手根屈筋の腱 Flexor carpi ulnaris tendon
- 第1〜3掌側骨間筋 1st through 3rd palmar interossei
- 小指外転筋 Opponens digiti minimi
- 第1〜4背側骨間筋 1st through 4th dorsal interossei

B 手内筋の深層．小指対立筋，母指対立筋，短母指屈筋，母指外転筋（横頭と斜頭）を取り除いたところ．

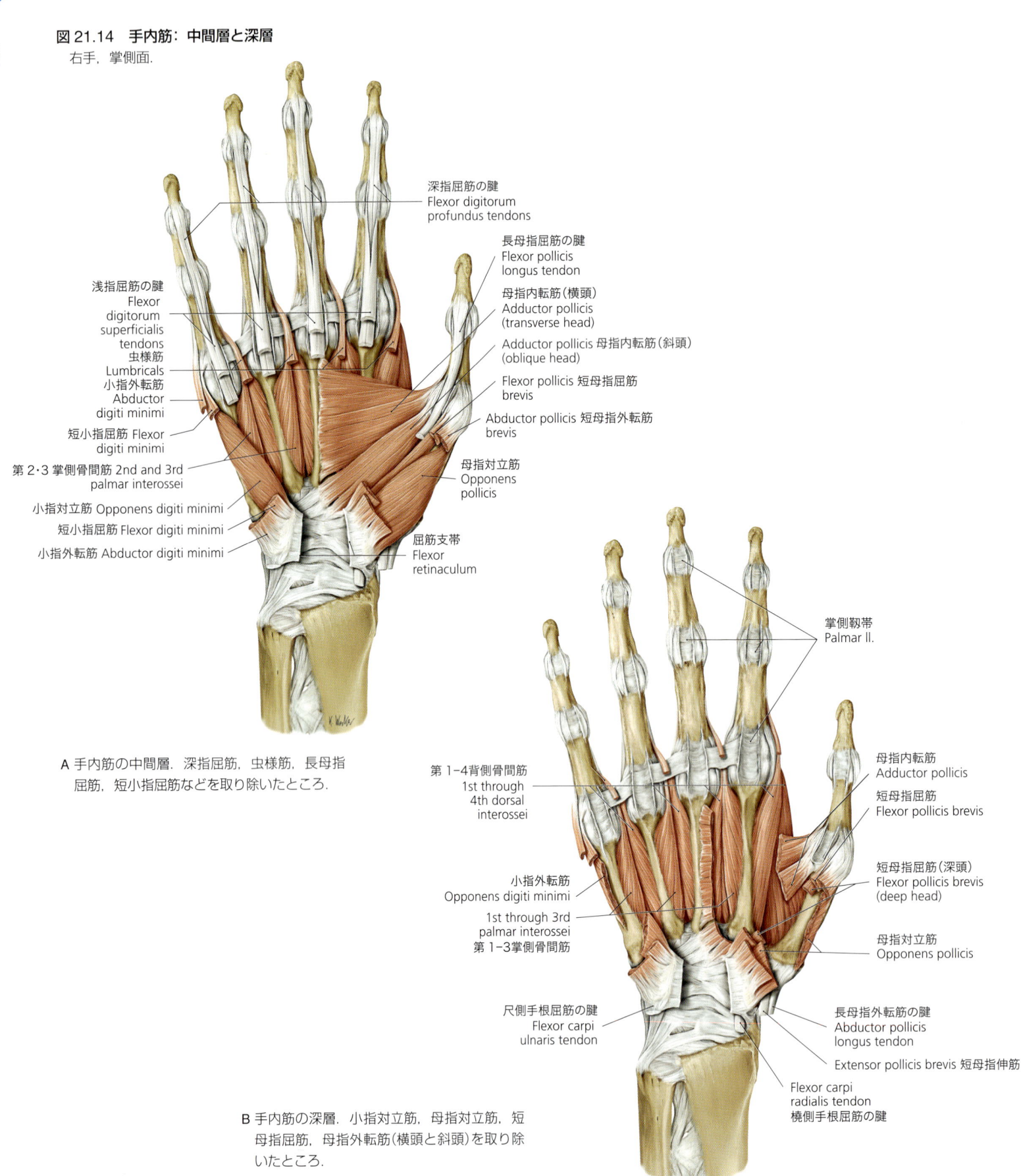

図21.15 手内筋の起始と停止
右手. 筋の起始を赤, 停止を青で示す.

示指伸筋 Extensor indicis
小指伸筋 Extensor digiti minimi
[総]指伸筋 Extensor digitorum
掌側・背側骨間筋 Palmar and dorsal interossei
Extensor pollicis longus 長母指伸筋
Extensor pollicis brevis 短母指伸筋
Adductor pollicis 母指内転筋
Abductor pollicis longus 長母指外転筋
Extensor carpi radialis longus 長橈側手根伸筋
Abductor digiti minimi 小指外転筋
Opponens digiti minimi 小指対立筋
Dorsal interossei 背側骨間筋
Extensor carpi ulnaris 尺側手根伸筋
Extensor carpi radialis brevis 短橈側手根伸筋

A 背側面（後方から見たところ）.

深指屈筋 Flexor digitorum profundus
浅指屈筋 Flexor digitorum superficialis
骨間筋 Interossei
長母指屈筋 Flexor pollicis longus
母指内転筋 Adductor pollicis
短母指屈筋, 短母指外転筋 Flexor pollicis brevis and abductor pollicis brevis
第1背側骨間筋 1st dorsal interosseus
橈側手根屈筋 Flexor carpi radialis
母指対立筋 Opponens pollicis
長母指外転筋 Abductor pollicis longus
短母指外転筋 Abductor pollicis brevis

小指外転筋 Abductor digiti minimi
短小指屈筋 Flexor digiti minimi
小指対立筋 Opponens digiti minimi
尺側手根伸筋 Extensor carpi ulnaris
小指外転筋 Abductor digiti minimi
尺側手根屈筋 Flexor carpi ulnaris
短母指屈筋 Flexor pollicis brevis

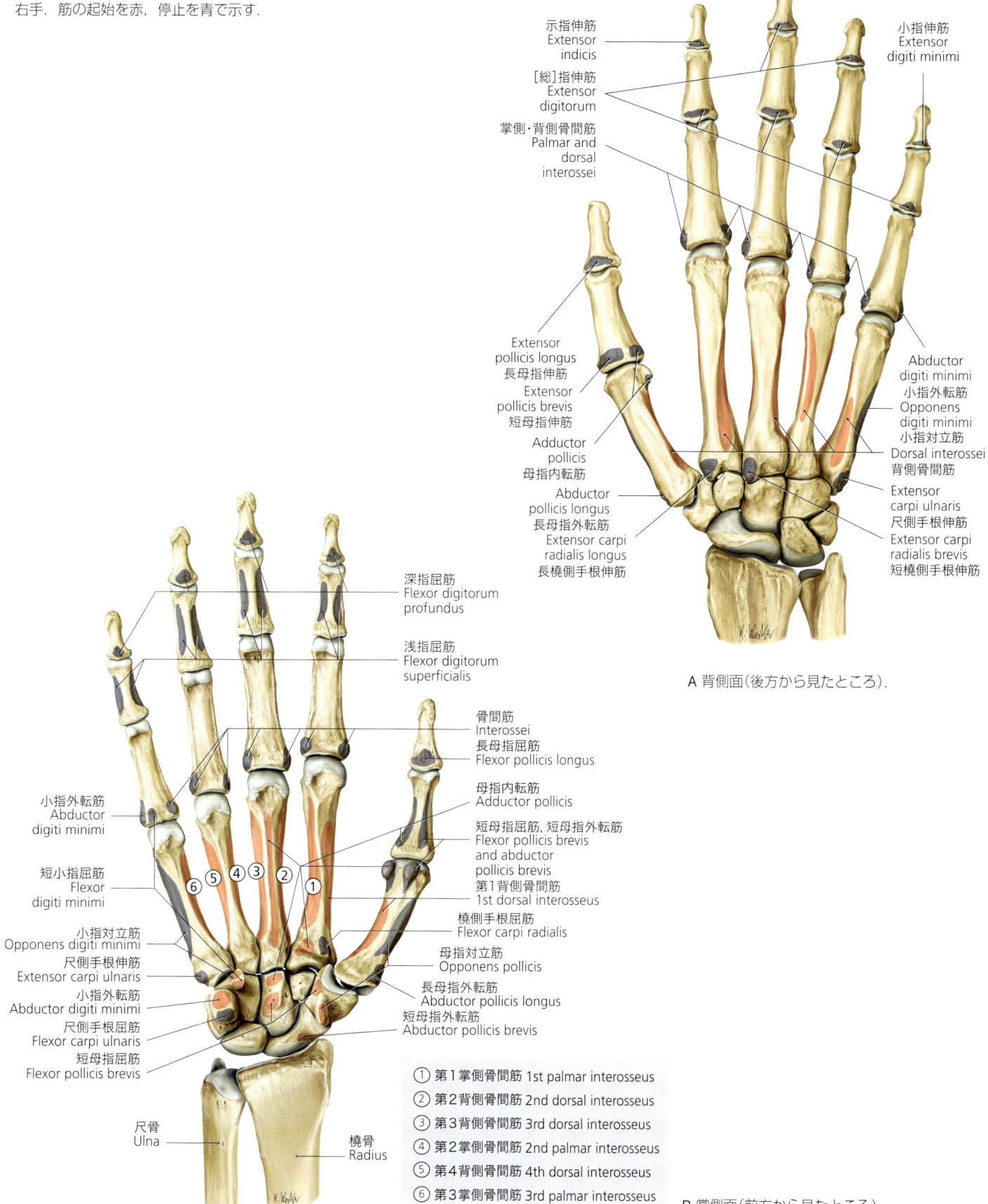

尺骨 Ulna
橈骨 Radius

① 第1掌側骨間筋 1st palmar interosseus
② 第2背側骨間筋 2nd dorsal interosseus
③ 第3背側骨間筋 3rd dorsal interosseus
④ 第2掌側骨間筋 2nd palmar interosseus
⑤ 第4背側骨間筋 4th dorsal interosseus
⑥ 第3掌側骨間筋 3rd palmar interosseus

B 掌側面（前方から見たところ）.

手背
Dorsum of the Hand

図 21.16 伸筋支帯と背側手根腱鞘
右手，背側面（後方から見たところ）．

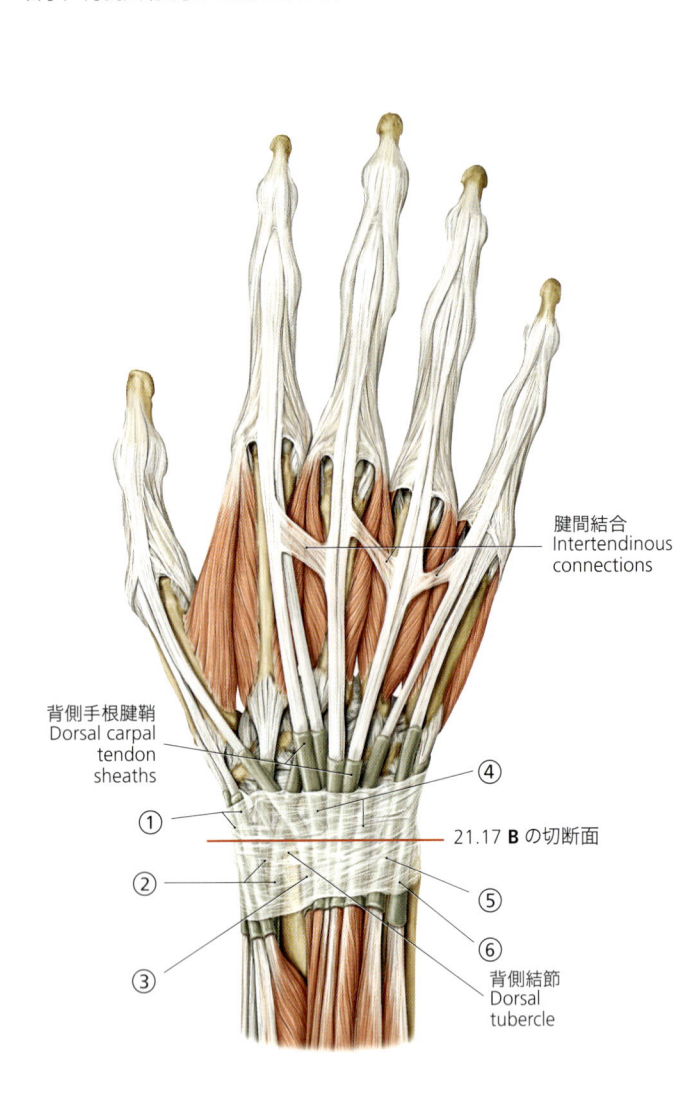

図 21.17 手背の筋と腱
右手．

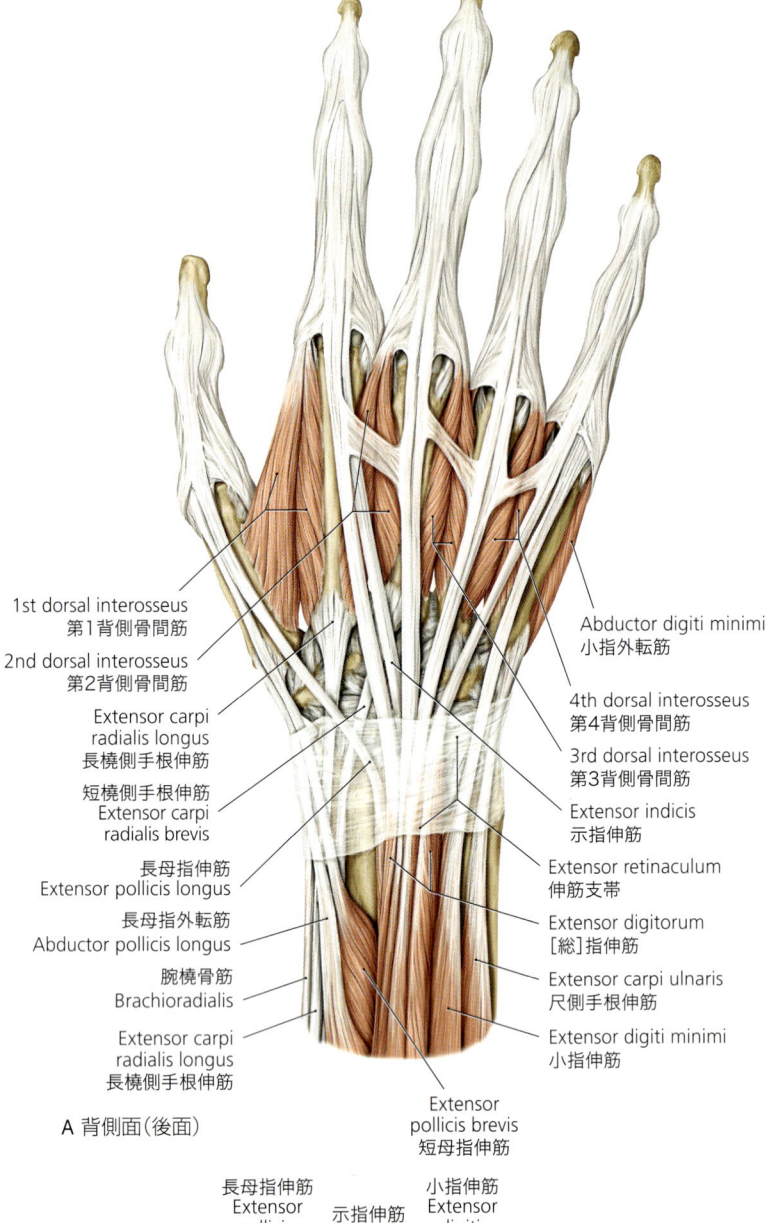

A 背側面（後面）

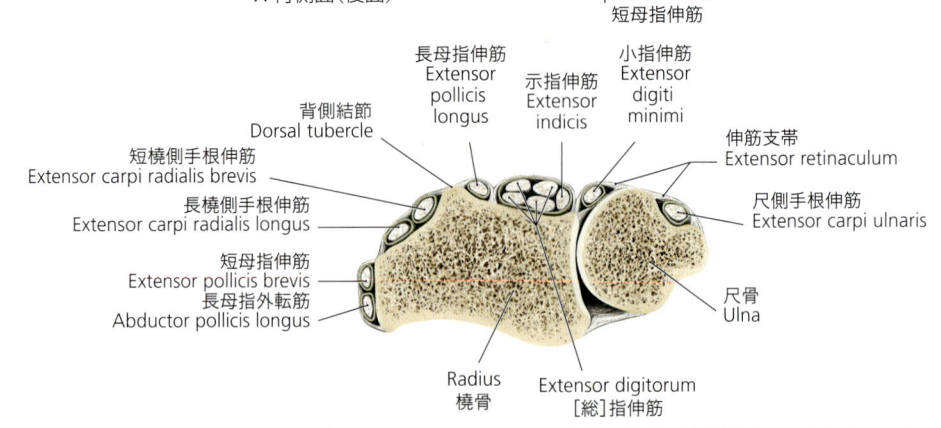

- 腱間結合 Intertendinous connections
- 背側手根腱鞘 Dorsal carpal tendon sheaths
- 21.17 B の切断面
- 背側結節 Dorsal tubercle
- 1st dorsal interosseus 第1背側骨間筋
- 2nd dorsal interosseus 第2背側骨間筋
- Extensor carpi radialis longus 長橈側手根伸筋
- 短橈側手根伸筋 Extensor carpi radialis brevis
- 長母指伸筋 Extensor pollicis longus
- 長母指外転筋 Abductor pollicis longus
- 腕橈骨筋 Brachioradialis
- Extensor carpi radialis longus 長橈側手根伸筋
- Extensor pollicis brevis 短母指伸筋
- Abductor digiti minimi 小指外転筋
- 4th dorsal interosseus 第4背側骨間筋
- 3rd dorsal interosseus 第3背側骨間筋
- Extensor indicis 示指伸筋
- Extensor retinaculum 伸筋支帯
- Extensor digitorum ［総］指伸筋
- Extensor carpi ulnaris 尺側手根伸筋
- Extensor digiti minimi 小指伸筋

B 背側腱区画，図 21.16 で示した位置の横断面を近位方向から見たところ．

- 長母指伸筋 Extensor pollicis longus
- 示指伸筋 Extensor indicis
- 小指伸筋 Extensor digiti minimi
- 背側結節 Dorsal tubercle
- 短橈側手根伸筋 Extensor carpi radialis brevis
- 長橈側手根伸筋 Extensor carpi radialis longus
- 短母指伸筋 Extensor pollicis brevis
- 長母指外転筋 Abductor pollicis longus
- 伸筋支帯 Extensor retinaculum
- 尺側手根伸筋 Extensor carpi ulnaris
- 尺骨 Ulna
- 橈骨 Radius
- Extensor digitorum ［総］指伸筋

表 21.2	伸筋腱の通路となる背側腱区画
①第1腱区画	長母指外転筋
	短母指伸筋
②第2腱区画	長橈側手根伸筋
	短橈側手根伸筋
③第3腱区画	長母指伸筋
④第4腱区画	［総］指伸筋
	示指伸筋
⑤第5腱区画	小指伸筋
⑥第6腱区画	尺側手根伸筋

図 21.18 指背腱膜

右手の中指．指に停止する長い伸筋や手内筋は，指背腱膜によって，指にある3つの関節すべてに作用することができる．

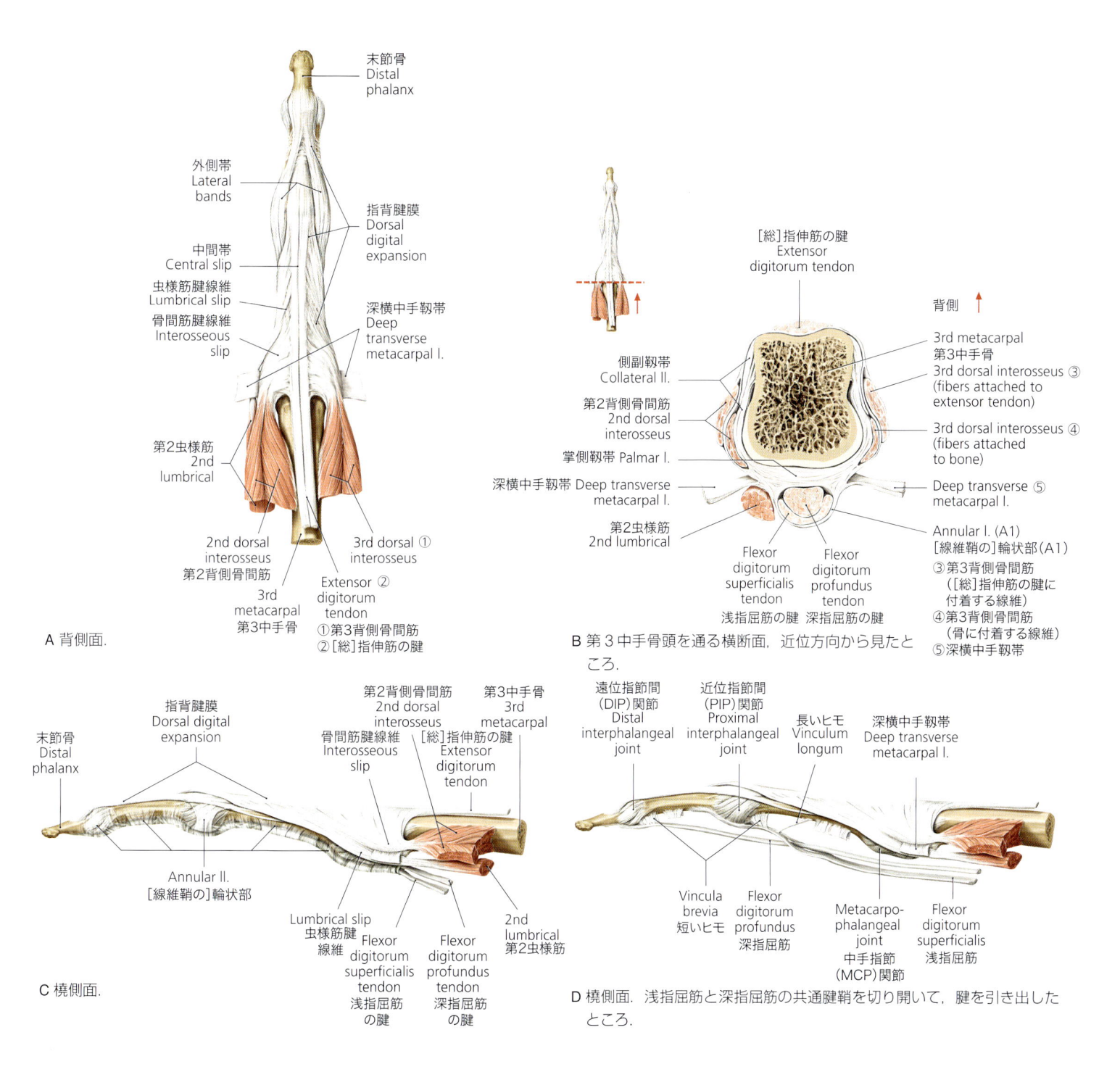

A 背側面．

- 末節骨 Distal phalanx
- 外側帯 Lateral bands
- 中間帯 Central slip
- 虫様筋腱線維 Lumbrical slip
- 骨間筋腱線維 Interosseous slip
- 指背腱膜 Dorsal digital expansion
- 深横中手靱帯 Deep transverse metacarpal l.
- 第2虫様筋 2nd lumbrical
- 2nd dorsal interosseus 第2背側骨間筋
- 3rd metacarpal 第3中手骨
- 3rd dorsal interosseus ①
- Extensor digitorum tendon ②
- ①第3背側骨間筋
- ②[総]指伸筋の腱

B 第3中手骨頭を通る横断面，近位方向から見たところ．

- [総]指伸筋の腱 Extensor digitorum tendon
- 背側 ↑
- 側副靱帯 Collateral ll.
- 第2背側骨間筋 2nd dorsal interosseus
- 掌側靱帯 Palmar l.
- 深横中手靱帯 Deep transverse metacarpal l.
- 第2虫様筋 2nd lumbrical
- Flexor digitorum superficialis tendon 浅指屈筋の腱
- Flexor digitorum profundus tendon 深指屈筋の腱
- 3rd metacarpal 第3中手骨
- 3rd dorsal interosseus ③ (fibers attached to extensor tendon)
- 3rd dorsal interosseus ④ (fibers attached to bone)
- Deep transverse ⑤ metacarpal l.
- Annular l. (A1) [線維鞘の]輪状部（A1）
- ③第3背側骨間筋（[総]指伸筋の腱に付着する線維）
- ④第3背側骨間筋（骨に付着する線維）
- ⑤深横中手靱帯

C 橈側面．

- 末節骨 Distal phalanx
- 指背腱膜 Dorsal digital expansion
- Annular ll. [線維鞘の]輪状部
- Lumbrical slip 虫様筋腱線維
- Flexor digitorum superficialis tendon 浅指屈筋の腱
- 第2背側骨間筋 2nd dorsal interosseus
- 骨間筋腱線維 Interosseous slip
- 第3中手骨 3rd metacarpal
- [総]指伸筋の腱 Extensor digitorum tendon
- Flexor digitorum profundus tendon 深指屈筋の腱
- 2nd lumbrical 第2虫様筋

D 橈側面．浅指屈筋と深指屈筋の共通腱鞘を切り開いて，腱を引き出したところ．

- 遠位指節間（DIP）関節 Distal interphalangeal joint
- 近位指節間（PIP）関節 Proximal interphalangeal joint
- 長いヒモ Vinculum longum
- 深横中手靱帯 Deep transverse metacarpal l.
- Vincula brevia 短いヒモ
- Flexor digitorum profundus 深指屈筋
- Metacarpo-phalangeal joint 中手指節（MCP）関節
- Flexor digitorum superficialis 浅指屈筋

個々の筋(1)
Muscle Facts(I)

手内筋は3つのグループ(母指球筋,小指球筋,中手筋)に分けられる(p.314参照).母指球筋は母指の運動にとって重要であり,同様に小指球筋は小指の運動に関与する.

表21.3　母指球筋

筋	起始		停止	神経支配		作用
①母指内転筋	横頭:第3中手骨(掌側面)		尺側の種子骨を介して	尺骨神経	C8, T1	母指のCMC関節:内転,母指のMCP関節:屈曲
	斜頭:有頭骨,第2・3中手骨底					
②短母指外転筋	舟状骨,大菱形骨,屈筋支帯		母指の基節骨底	正中神経		母指のCMC関節:外転
③短母指屈筋	浅頭:屈筋支帯		橈側の種子骨を介して	浅頭:正中神経		母指のCMC関節:屈曲
	深頭:有頭骨,大菱形骨			深頭:尺骨神経		
④母指対立筋	大菱形骨		第1中手骨(橈側縁)	正中神経		母指のCMC関節:対立

CMC関節=手根中手関節,MCP関節=中手指節関節.

図21.19　母指球筋と小指球筋
右手,掌側面(前方から見たところ).

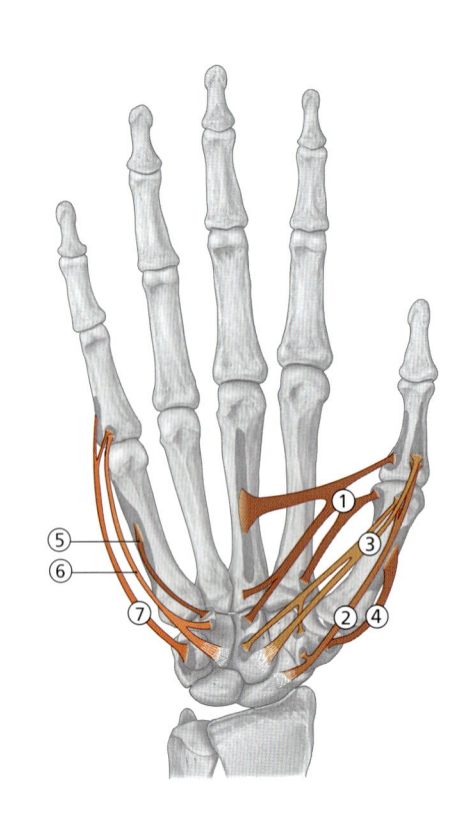

表21.4　小指球筋

筋	起始	停止	神経支配	作用
⑤小指対立筋	有鈎骨鈎,屈筋支帯	第5中手骨(尺側縁)	尺骨神経(C8, T1)	小指のMCP関節:対立
⑥短小指屈筋		第5基節骨底		小指のMCP関節:屈曲
⑦小指外転筋	豆状骨	第5基節骨底(尺側),小指の指背腱膜		小指のMCP関節:屈曲・外転,小指のPIP関節・DIP関節:伸展
短掌筋	手掌腱膜(尺側縁)	小指球の皮膚		手掌腱膜を緊張させる(保護的機能)

DIP関節=遠位指節間関節,MCP関節=中手指節関節,PIP関節=近位指節間関節.

図 21.20 母指球筋と小指球筋
右手，掌側面（前方から見たところ）.

- 第5基節骨 5th proximal phalanx
- 第1基節骨 1st proximal phalanx
- 第5中手骨 5th metacarpal
- 横頭 Transverse head ┐ 母指内転筋 Adductor pollicis
- 斜頭 Oblique head ┘
- 小指外転筋 Abductor digiti minimi
- 小指対立筋 Opponens digiti minimi
- 短母指外転筋 Abductor pollicis brevis
- 有頭骨 Capitate
- Hook of hamate 有鈎骨鈎
- 大菱形骨 Trapezium
- Pisiform 豆状骨
- 舟状骨 Scaphoid

A 短母指屈筋，母指対立筋，短小指屈筋を取り除いてある.

- 5th proximal phalanx 第5基節骨
- 第1基節骨 1st proximal phalanx
- Flexor digiti minimi 短小指屈筋
- 短母指屈筋 Flexor pollicis brevis
- 有鈎骨鈎 Hook of hamate
- 母指対立筋 Opponens pollicis
- 有頭骨 Capitate
- 大菱形骨 Trapezium

B 母指内転筋，短母指外転筋，小指外転筋，小指対立筋を取り除いてある.

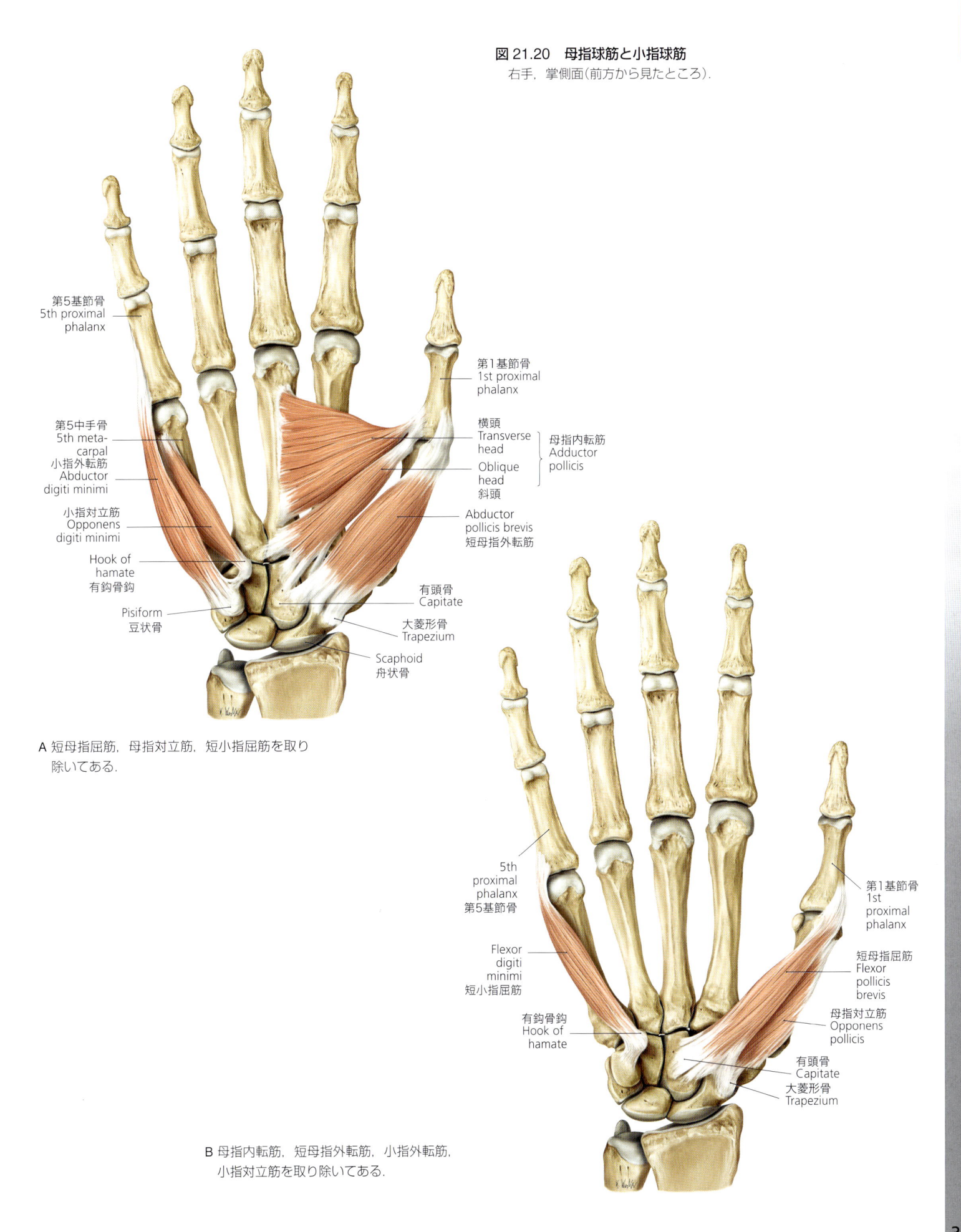

個々の筋(2)
Muscle Facts(II)

中手筋は虫様筋と骨間筋からなる．これらの筋は指の運動に重要な役割を果たす．

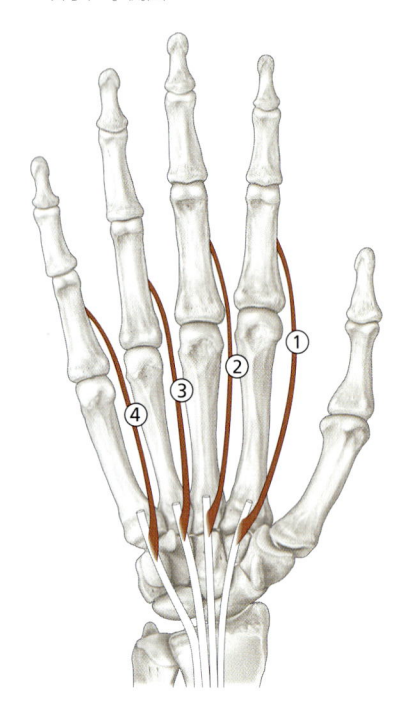

図 21.21　虫様筋
右手，掌側面．

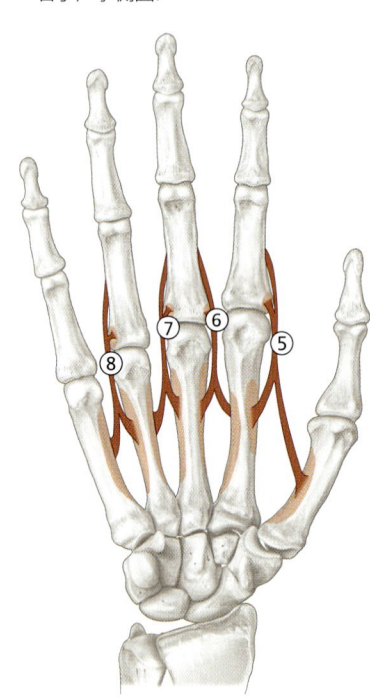

図 21.22　背側骨間筋
右手，掌側面．

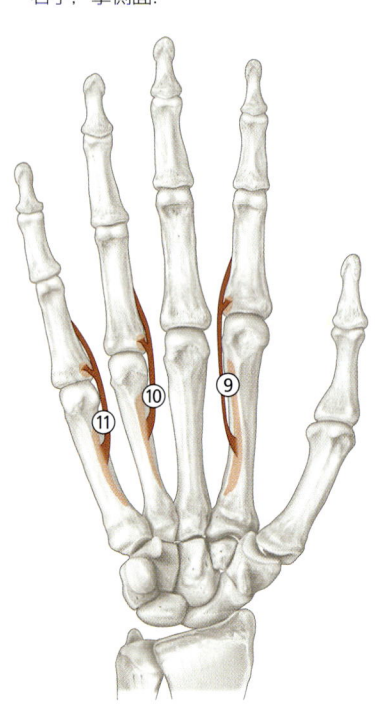

図 21.23　掌側骨間筋
右手，掌側面．

表 21.5　中手筋

筋群	筋	起始	停止	神経支配	作用
虫様筋	①第1虫様筋	深指屈筋腱（橈側縁）	第2指の指背腱膜	正中神経 (C8, T1)	第2-5指：・MCP関節の屈曲 ・PIP・DIP関節の伸展
	②第2虫様筋		第3指の指背腱膜		
	③第3虫様筋	深指屈筋腱（隣接する2腱の橈側縁と尺側縁から起始する，2頭）	第4指の指背腱膜	尺骨神経 (C8, T1)	
	④第4虫様筋		第5指の指背腱膜		
背側骨間筋	⑤第1背側骨間筋	第1・2中手骨（相対する面，2頭）	第2指の指背腱膜と基節骨底（橈側）		第2-4指：・MCP関節の屈曲 ・PIP・DIP関節の伸展，第3指を中心とした外転
	⑥第2背側骨間筋	第2・3中手骨（相対する面，2頭）	第3指の指背腱膜と基節骨底（橈側）		
	⑦第3背側骨間筋	第3・4中手骨（相対する面，2頭）	第3指の指背腱膜と基節骨底（尺側）		
	⑧第4背側骨間筋	第4・5中手骨（相対する面，2頭）	第4指の指背腱膜と基節骨底（尺側）		
掌側骨間筋	⑨第1掌側骨間筋	第2中手骨（尺側面）	第2指の指背腱膜と基節骨底		第2, 4, 5指：・MCP関節の屈曲，・PIP・DIP関節の伸展，第3指を中心とした内転
	⑩第2掌側骨間筋	第4中手骨（橈側面）	第4指の指背腱膜と基節骨底		
	⑪第3掌側骨間筋	第5中手骨（橈側面）	第5指の指背腱膜と基節骨底		

PIP・DIP＝近・遠位指節間関節，MCP関節＝中手指節関節．

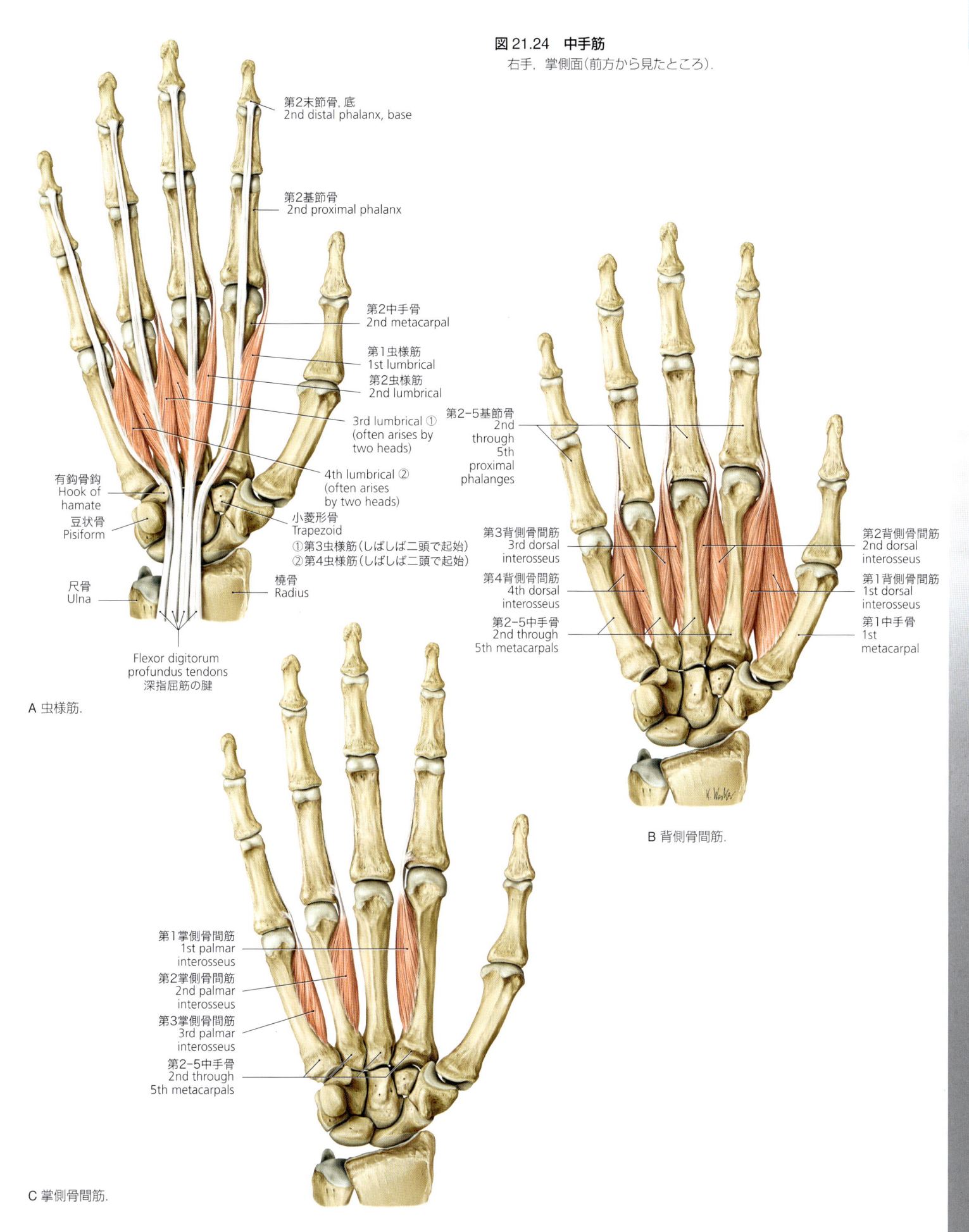

図 21.24 中手筋
右手，掌側面（前方から見たところ）.

A 虫様筋.

- 第2末節骨，底 / 2nd distal phalanx, base
- 第2基節骨 / 2nd proximal phalanx
- 第2中手骨 / 2nd metacarpal
- 第1虫様筋 / 1st lumbrical
- 第2虫様筋 / 2nd lumbrical
- 3rd lumbrical ① (often arises by two heads)
- 4th lumbrical ② (often arises by two heads)
- 小菱形骨 / Trapezoid
- ①第3虫様筋（しばしば二頭で起始）
- ②第4虫様筋（しばしば二頭で起始）
- 橈骨 / Radius
- 尺骨 / Ulna
- 豆状骨 / Pisiform
- 有鈎骨鈎 / Hook of hamate
- Flexor digitorum profundus tendons / 深指屈筋の腱

B 背側骨間筋.

- 第2-5基節骨 / 2nd through 5th proximal phalanges
- 第2背側骨間筋 / 2nd dorsal interosseus
- 第1背側骨間筋 / 1st dorsal interosseus
- 第1中手骨 / 1st metacarpal
- 第2-5中手骨 / 2nd through 5th metacarpals
- 第4背側骨間筋 / 4th dorsal interosseus
- 第3背側骨間筋 / 3rd dorsal interosseus

C 掌側骨間筋.

- 第1掌側骨間筋 / 1st palmar interosseus
- 第2掌側骨間筋 / 2nd palmar interosseus
- 第3掌側骨間筋 / 3rd palmar interosseus
- 第2-5中手骨 / 2nd through 5th metacarpals

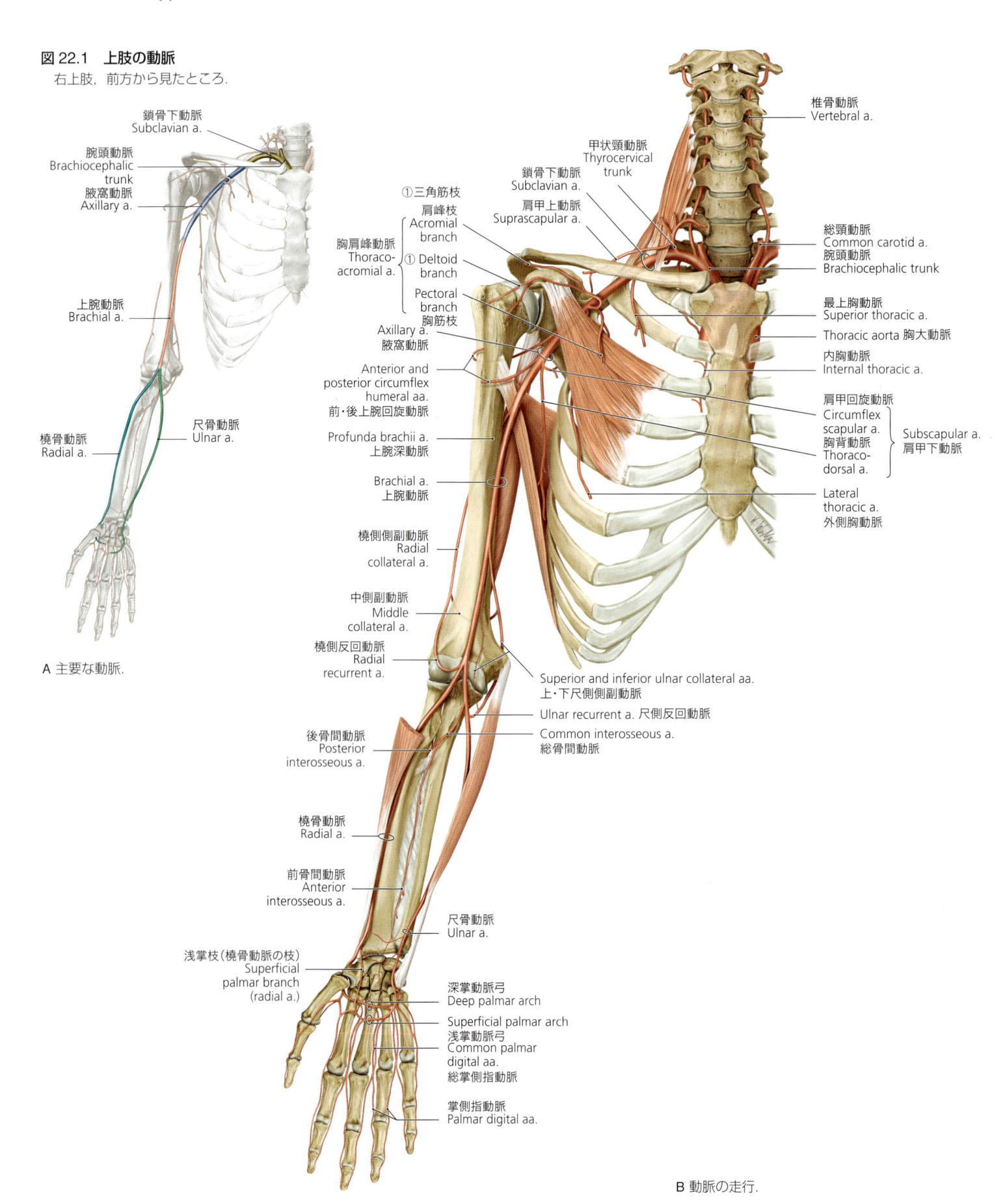

上肢の動脈
Arteries of the Upper Limb

図 22.1 上肢の動脈
右上肢，前方から見たところ．

A 主要な動脈．

B 動脈の走行．

図22.2 鎖骨下動脈の枝
右側，前方から見たところ．

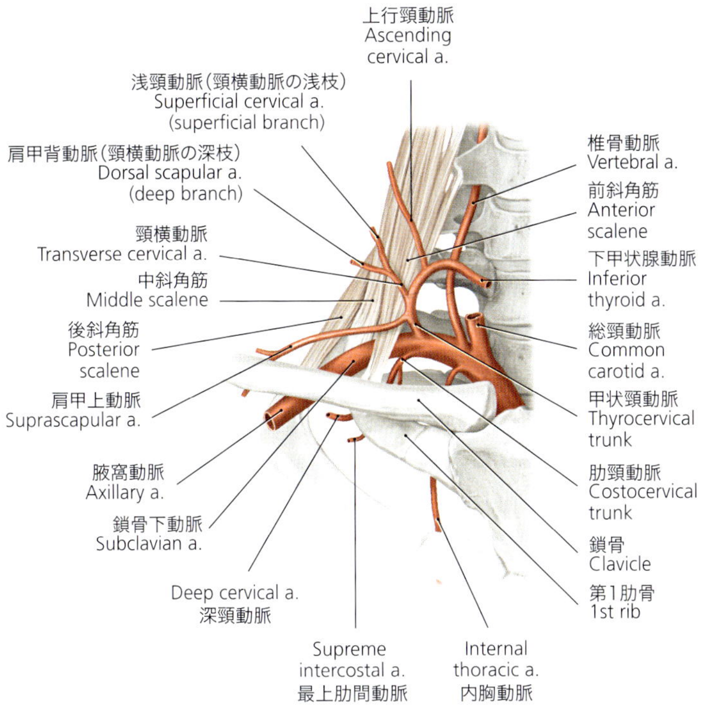

図22.3 肩甲アーケード
右側，後方から見たところ．

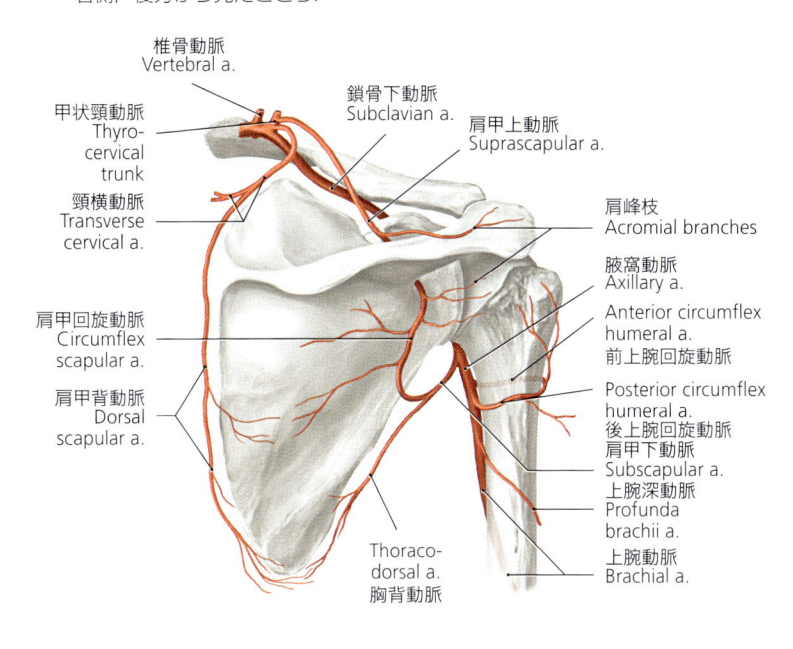

図22.4 前腕と手の動脈
右上肢．尺骨動脈と橈骨動脈は浅掌動脈弓，深掌動脈弓，貫通枝，手背手根動脈網によって交通している．

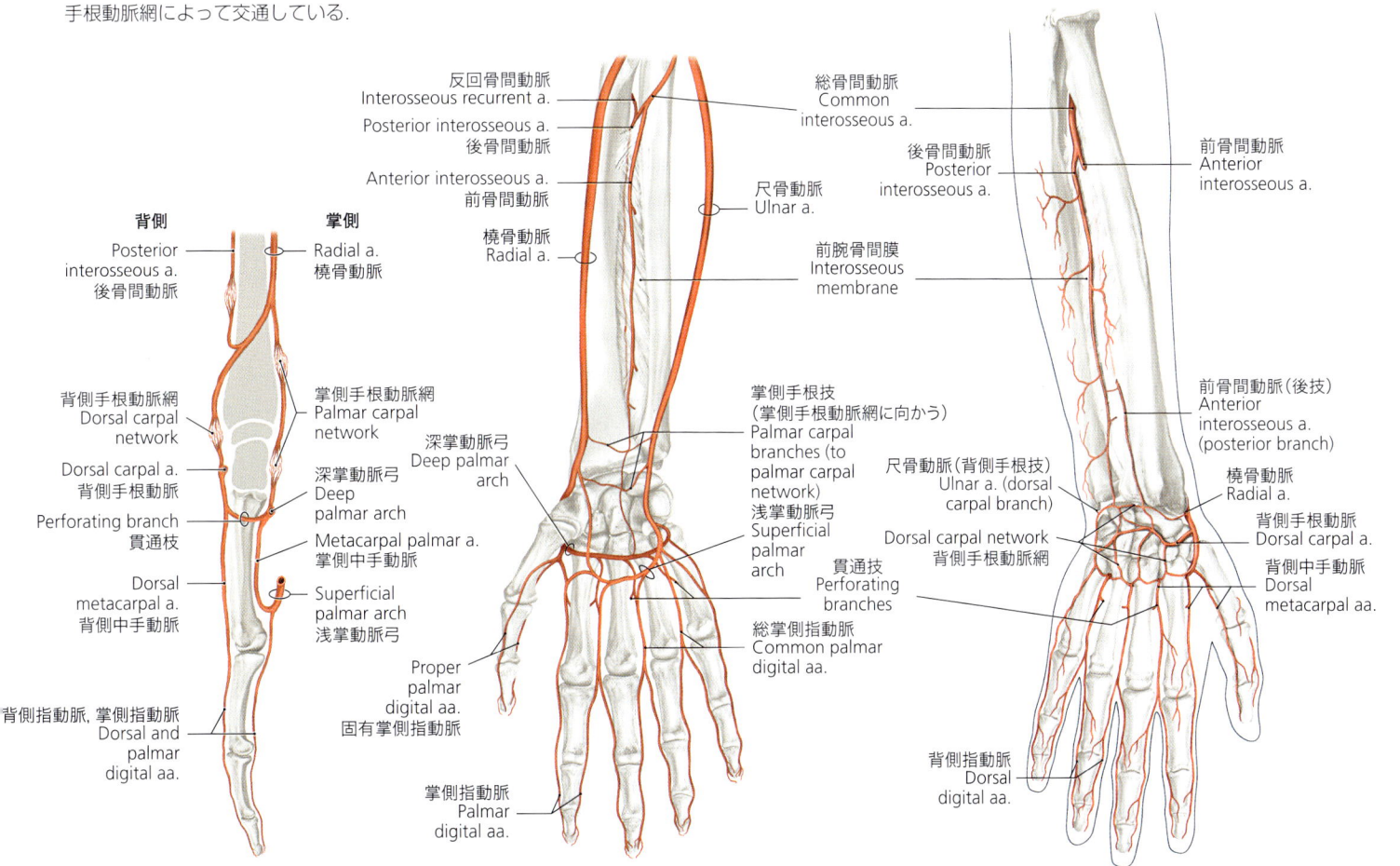

A 中指を外側方から見たところ．　　B 掌側面（前方から見たところ）．　　C 背面（後方から見たところ）．

上肢の静脈とリンパ管
Veins & Lymphatics of the Upper Limb

図 22.5 上肢の静脈
右上肢，前方から見たところ．

A 表層の静脈．

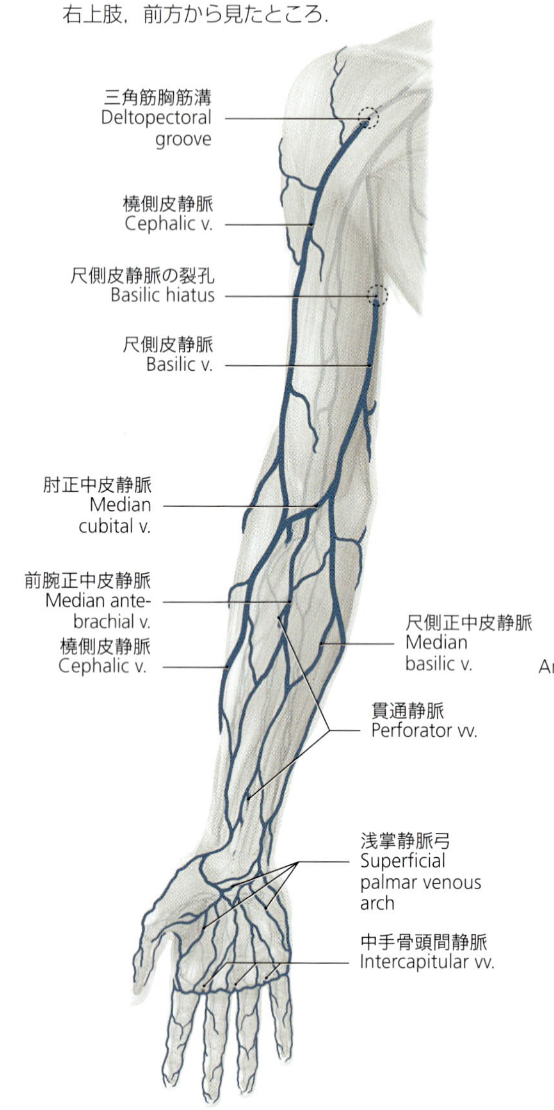

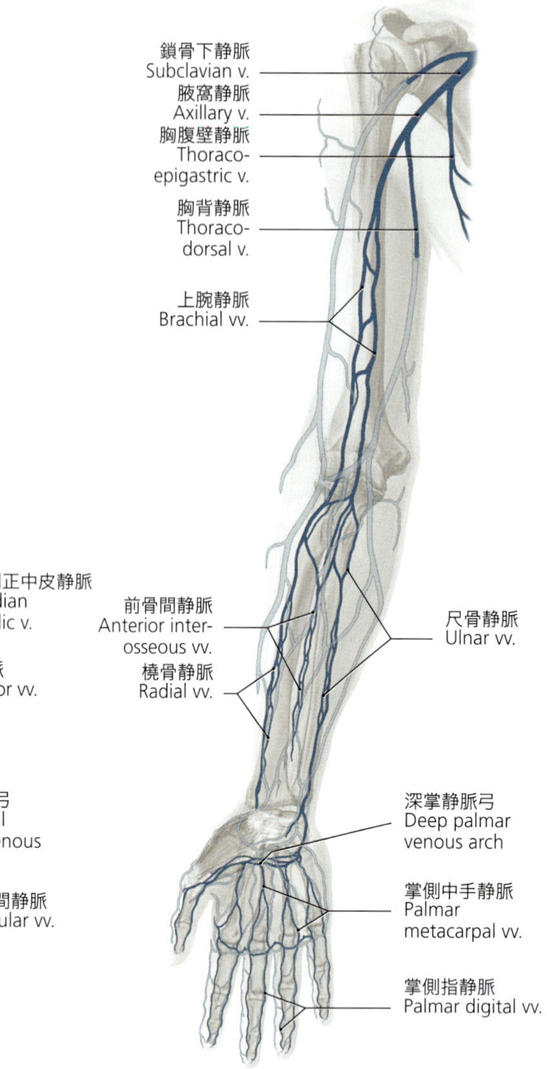

- 三角筋胸筋溝 Deltopectoral groove
- 橈側皮静脈 Cephalic v.
- 尺側皮静脈の裂孔 Basilic hiatus
- 尺側皮静脈 Basilic v.
- 肘正中皮静脈 Median cubital v.
- 前腕正中皮静脈 Median antebrachial v.
- 橈側皮静脈 Cephalic v.
- 尺側正中皮静脈 Median basilic v.
- 貫通静脈 Perforator vv.
- 浅掌静脈弓 Superficial palmar venous arch
- 中手骨頭間静脈 Intercapitular vv.

B 深部の静脈．

- 鎖骨下静脈 Subclavian v.
- 腋窩静脈 Axillary v.
- 胸腹壁静脈 Thoraco-epigastric v.
- 胸背静脈 Thoraco-dorsal v.
- 上腕静脈 Brachial vv.
- 前骨間静脈 Anterior interosseous vv.
- 橈骨静脈 Radial vv.
- 尺骨静脈 Ulnar vv.
- 深掌静脈弓 Deep palmar venous arch
- 掌側中手静脈 Palmar metacarpal vv.
- 掌側指静脈 Palmar digital vv.

図 22.6 手背の静脈
右手，背側面（後方から見たところ）．

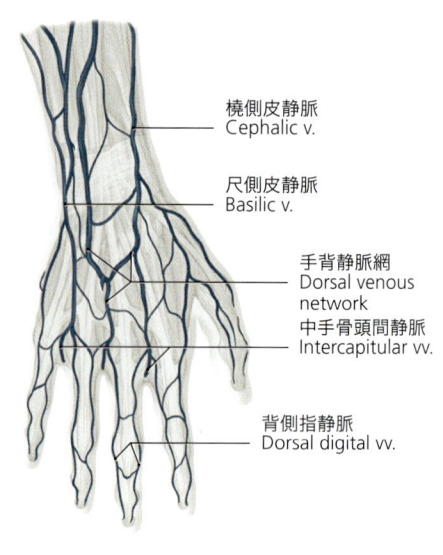

- 橈側皮静脈 Cephalic v.
- 尺側皮静脈 Basilic v.
- 手背静脈網 Dorsal venous network
- 中手骨頭間静脈 Intercapitular vv.
- 背側指静脈 Dorsal digital vv.

臨床

静脈穿刺

肘窩の皮静脈は採血の場所としてよく選ばれる．静脈穿刺の前処置として，上腕に駆血帯を巻く．駆血帯は動脈血の流れは妨げないが，静脈血の戻りを滞らせる．結果として静脈は膨らみ，より見えやすく，より触知しやすくなる．

図 22.7 肘窩の静脈
右上肢，前方から見たところ．肘窩の皮静脈は，その走行が極めて変化に富む．

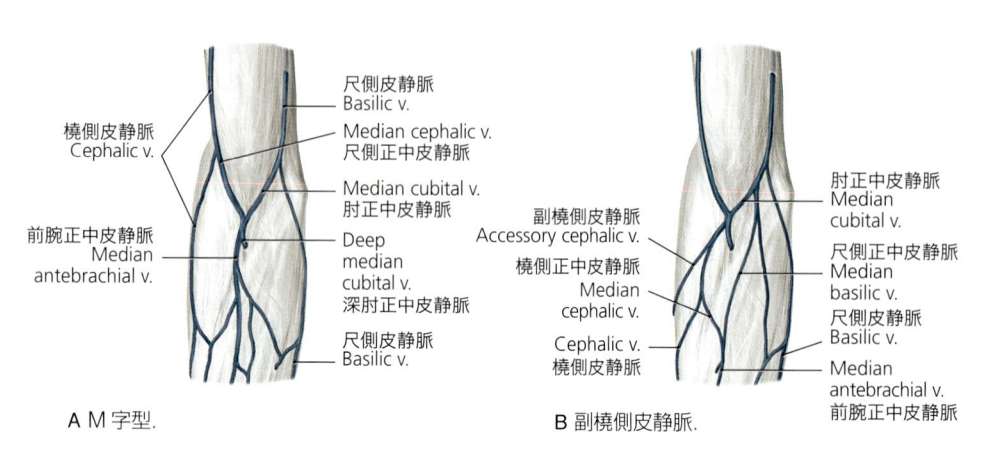

A M字型．

- 橈側皮静脈 Cephalic v.
- 尺側皮静脈 Basilic v.
- Median cephalic v. 尺側正中皮静脈
- Median cubital v. 肘正中皮静脈
- Deep median cubital v. 深肘正中皮静脈
- 前腕正中皮静脈 Median antebrachial v.
- 尺側皮静脈 Basilic v.

B 副橈側皮静脈．

- 副橈側皮静脈 Accessory cephalic v.
- 橈側正中皮静脈 Median cephalic v.
- Cephalic v. 橈側皮静脈
- 肘正中皮静脈 Median cubital v.
- 尺側正中皮静脈 Median basilic v.
- 尺側皮静脈 Basilic v.
- Median antebrachial v. 前腕正中皮静脈

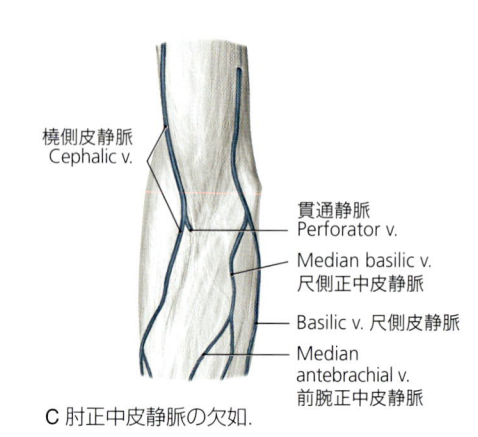

C 肘正中皮静脈の欠如．

- 橈側皮静脈 Cephalic v.
- 貫通静脈 Perforator v.
- Median basilic v. 尺側正中皮静脈
- Basilic v. 尺側皮静脈
- Median antebrachial v. 前腕正中皮静脈

上肢と乳房からのリンパは腋窩リンパ節に流れ込む．上肢の浅リンパ管は皮下組織の中に存在するが，深リンパ管は動脈や深部の静脈とともに走る．この2つのリンパ管の間には多くの交通枝が存在する．

図 22.8　上肢のリンパ管
右上肢．

- 上腕背外側領域 Dorsolateral arm territory
- 腋窩リンパ節 Axillary lymph nodes
- 上腕背内側領域 Dorsomedial arm territory
- 上腕中間領域 Middle arm territory
- 肘リンパ節 Cubital lymph nodes
- 橈側リンパ管束領域 Radial bundle territory
- 尺側リンパ管束領域 Ulnar bundle territory
- 前腕中間領域 Middle forearm territory
- 橈側リンパ管群 Radial group of lymphatics
- 尺側リンパ管群 Ulnar group of lymphatics
- 手背に回っていくリンパ管 Dorsal descending lymphatics

A 前方から見たところ．
B 後方から見たところ．

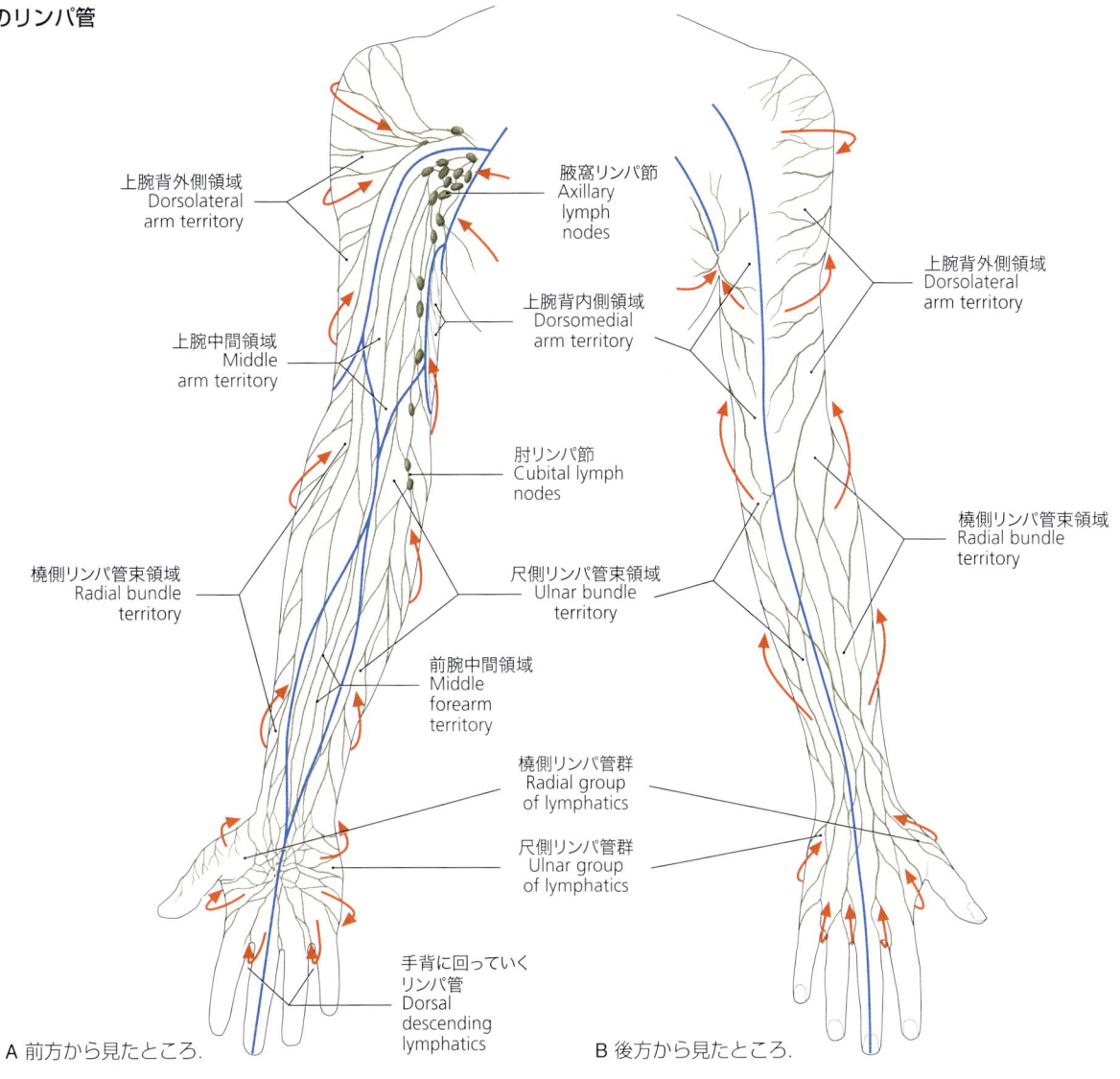

図 22.9　手のリンパ流路
右手，橈側面．手のリンパの大部分は肘窩リンパ節を経由して腋窩リンパ節に流れ込む．しかし，母指，示指，手背のリンパは直接腋窩リンパ節に流れ込む．

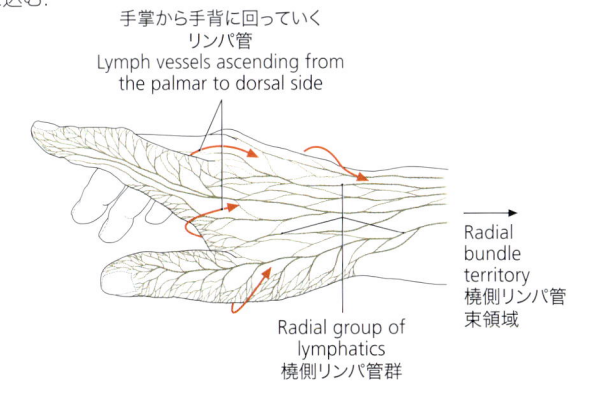

- 手掌から手背に回っていくリンパ管 Lymph vessels ascending from the palmar to dorsal side
- Radial bundle territory 橈側リンパ管束領域
- Radial group of lymphatics 橈側リンパ管群

図 22.10　腋窩リンパ節
右側，前方から見たところ．腋窩リンパ節は，小胸筋の位置に基づき，3つのレベルに分けられる．このリンパ節は乳癌の臨床において極めて重要である（p.65 参照）．

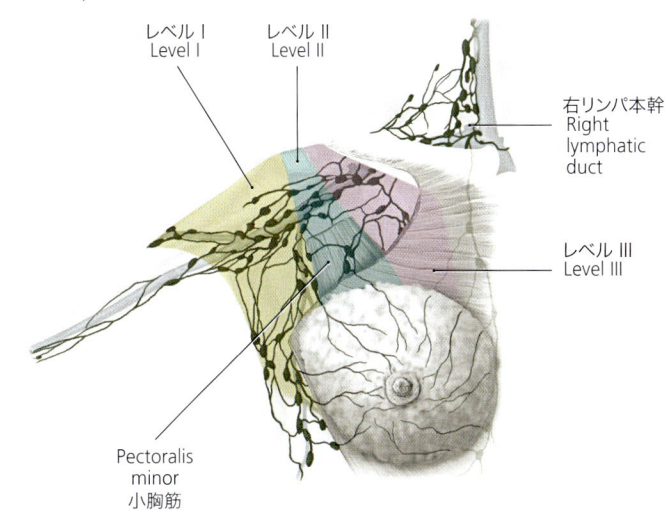

- レベル I　Level I
- レベル II　Level II
- レベル III　Level III
- 右リンパ本幹 Right lymphatic duct
- Pectoralis minor 小胸筋

腕神経叢とその枝
Nerves of the Brachial Plexus

上肢のほぼ全ての筋は腕神経叢から出る神経によって支配される．この神経叢を形成する神経は脊髄分節のC5-T1に由来する．腕神経叢の鎖骨上部では，脊髄神経前枝もしくは神経幹から直接枝が分枝される．また鎖骨上部では，5本の脊髄神経前枝が癒合して3本の神経幹となり，さらに6本の神経幹枝（3本の前神経幹枝と3本の後神経幹枝）を経て3本の神経束に再編成される．腕神経叢の鎖骨下部は，神経束から出る短い枝と上肢を縦断する長い枝（終枝）からなる．

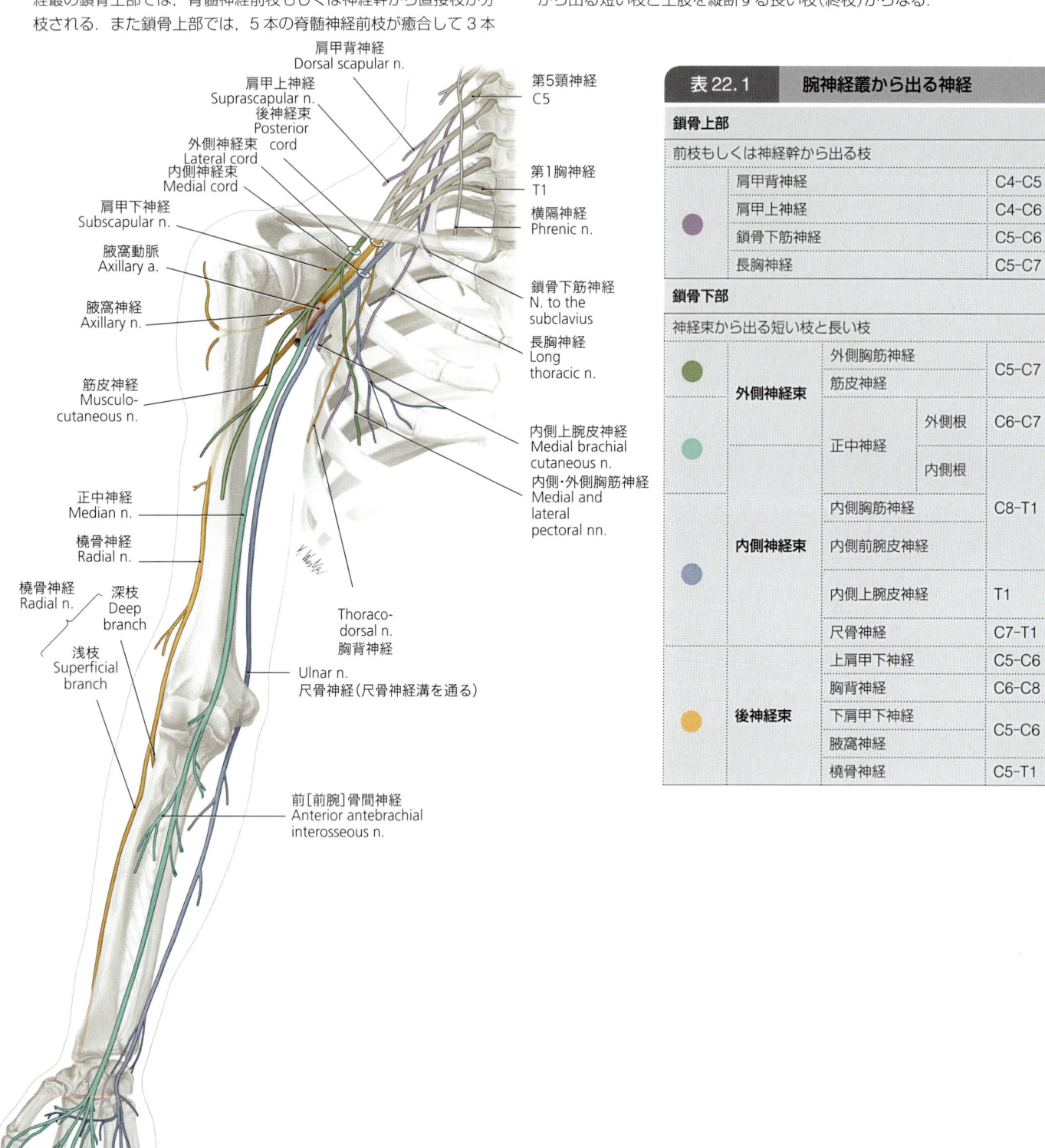

表22.1　腕神経叢から出る神経

鎖骨上部			
前枝もしくは神経幹から出る枝			
	肩甲背神経		C4-C5
	肩甲上神経		C4-C6
	鎖骨下筋神経		C5-C6
	長胸神経		C5-C7

鎖骨下部			
神経束から出る短い枝と長い枝			
外側神経束	外側胸筋神経		C5-C7
	筋皮神経		
	正中神経	外側根	C6-C7
		内側根	
内側神経束	内側胸筋神経		C8-T1
	内側前腕皮神経		
	内側上腕皮神経		T1
	尺骨神経		C7-T1
後神経束	上肩甲下神経		C5-C6
	胸背神経		C6-C8
	下肩甲下神経		C5-C6
	腋窩神経		
	橈骨神経		C5-T1

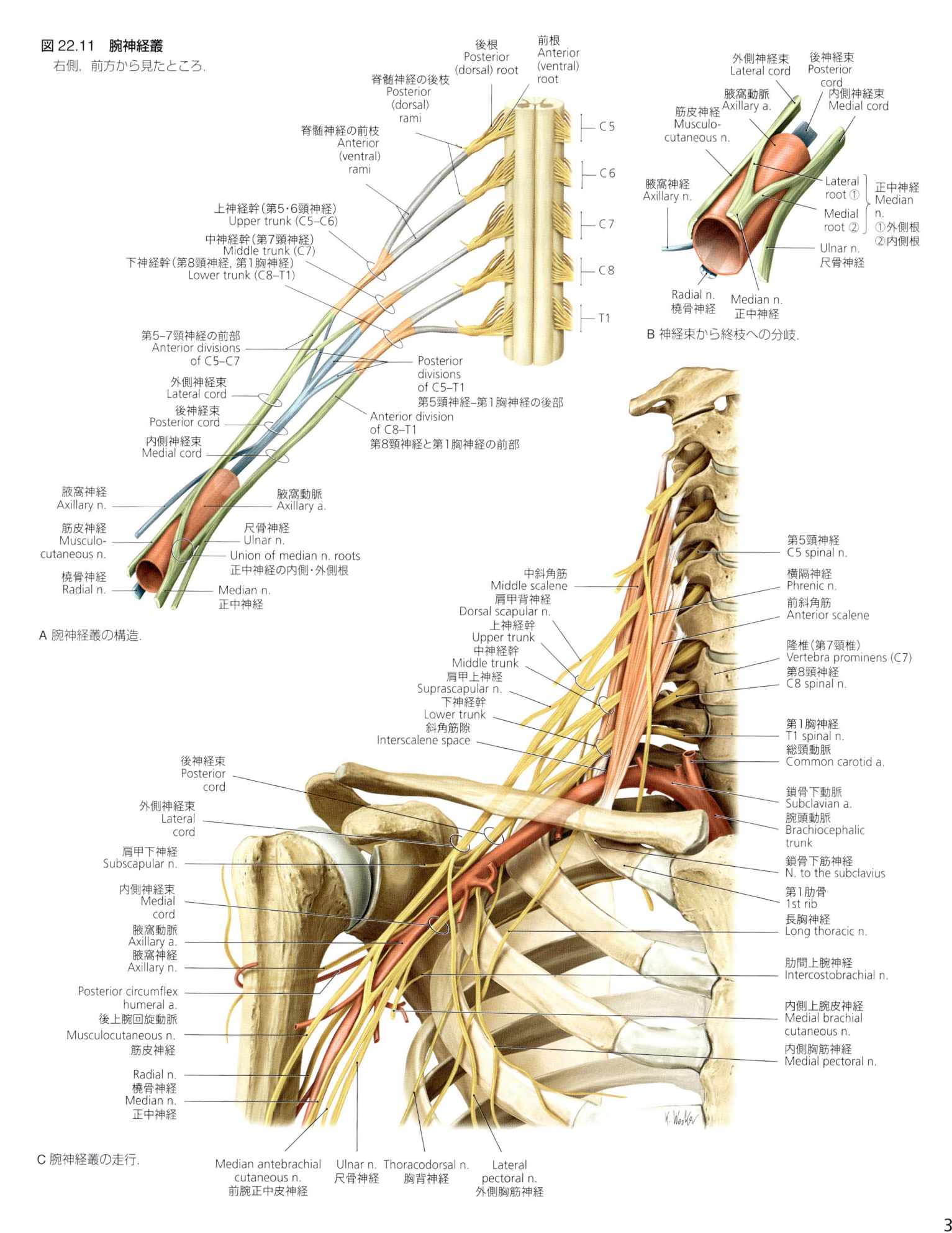

図 22.11 腕神経叢
右側，前方から見たところ．

A 腕神経叢の構造．

B 神経束から終枝への分岐．

C 腕神経叢の走行．

腕神経叢の鎖骨上部からの枝，後神経束
Supraclavicular Branches & Posterior Cord

図22.12 鎖骨上部の枝
右肩．

腕神経叢の鎖骨上部から出る枝（直接枝）は，外側頸三角において脊髄神経前枝もしくは神経幹から分枝される．

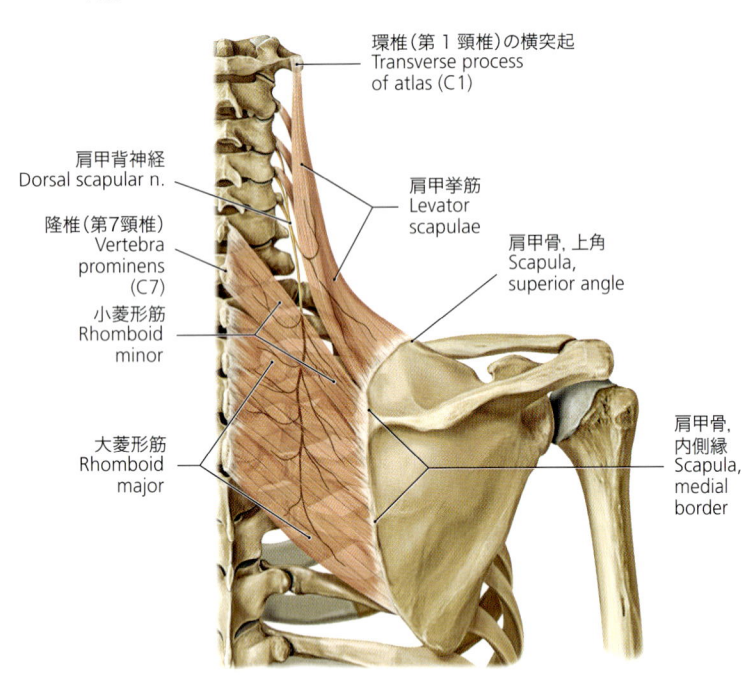

A 肩甲下神経，後方から見たところ．

- 環椎（第1頸椎）の横突起 Transverse process of atlas (C1)
- 肩甲背神経 Dorsal scapular n.
- 肩甲挙筋 Levator scapulae
- 隆椎（第7頸椎）Vertebra prominens (C7)
- 肩甲骨, 上角 Scapula, superior angle
- 小菱形筋 Rhomboid minor
- 大菱形筋 Rhomboid major
- 肩甲骨, 内側縁 Scapula, medial border

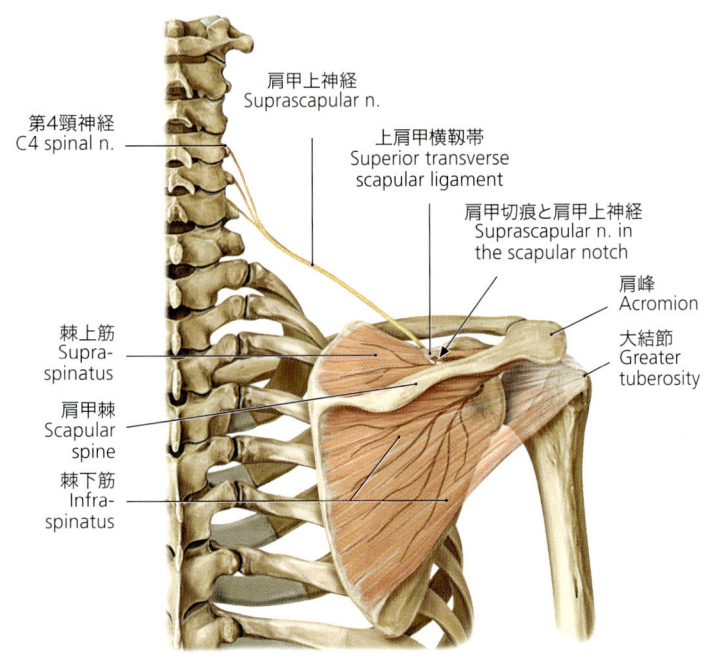

B 肩甲上神経，後方から見たところ．

- 肩甲上神経 Suprascapular n.
- 第4頸神経 C4 spinal n.
- 上肩甲横靱帯 Superior transverse scapular ligament
- 肩甲切痕と肩甲上神経 Suprascapular n. in the scapular notch
- 肩峰 Acromion
- 棘上筋 Supraspinatus
- 大結節 Greater tuberosity
- 肩甲棘 Scapular spine
- 棘下筋 Infraspinatus

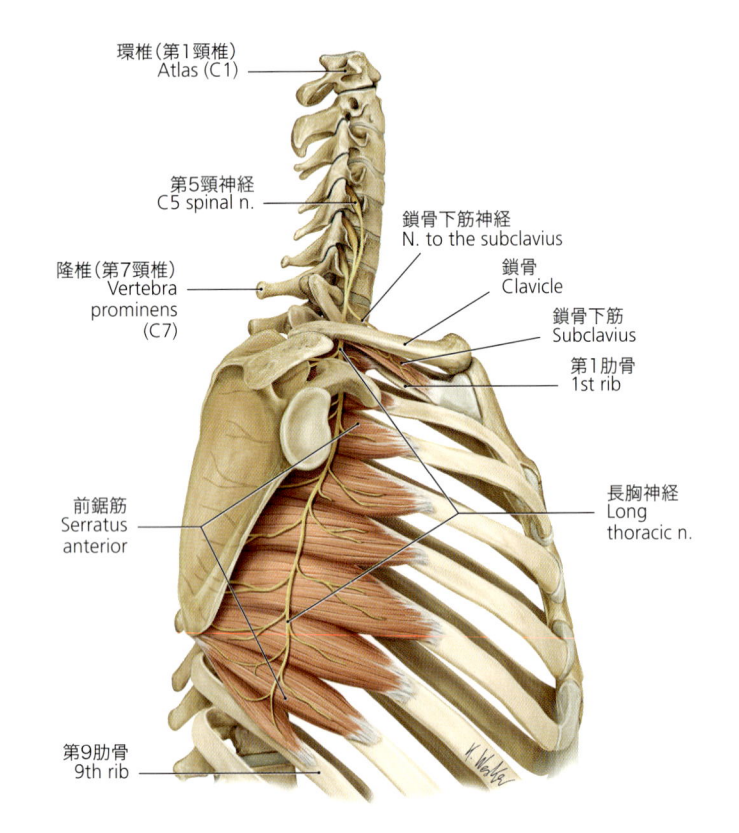

C 長胸神経と鎖骨下筋神経，右外側方から見たところ．

- 環椎（第1頸椎）Atlas (C1)
- 第5頸神経 C5 spinal n.
- 隆椎（第7頸椎）Vertebra prominens (C7)
- 鎖骨下筋神経 N. to the subclavius
- 鎖骨 Clavicle
- 鎖骨下筋 Subclavius
- 第1肋骨 1st rib
- 前鋸筋 Serratus anterior
- 長胸神経 Long thoracic n.
- 第9肋骨 9th rib

表22.2 鎖骨上部の枝

神経	脊髄分節	支配筋
肩甲背神経	C4–C5	肩甲挙筋，大菱形筋，小菱形筋
肩甲上神経	C4–C6	棘上筋，棘下筋
鎖骨下筋神経	C5–C6	鎖骨下筋
長胸神経	C5–C7	前鋸筋

図 22.13　後神経束：短い枝
右肩.

腕神経叢の後神経束は3種類の短い枝を出したのち，最終的には2本の長い枝（終枝，pp.324-325参照）となる．

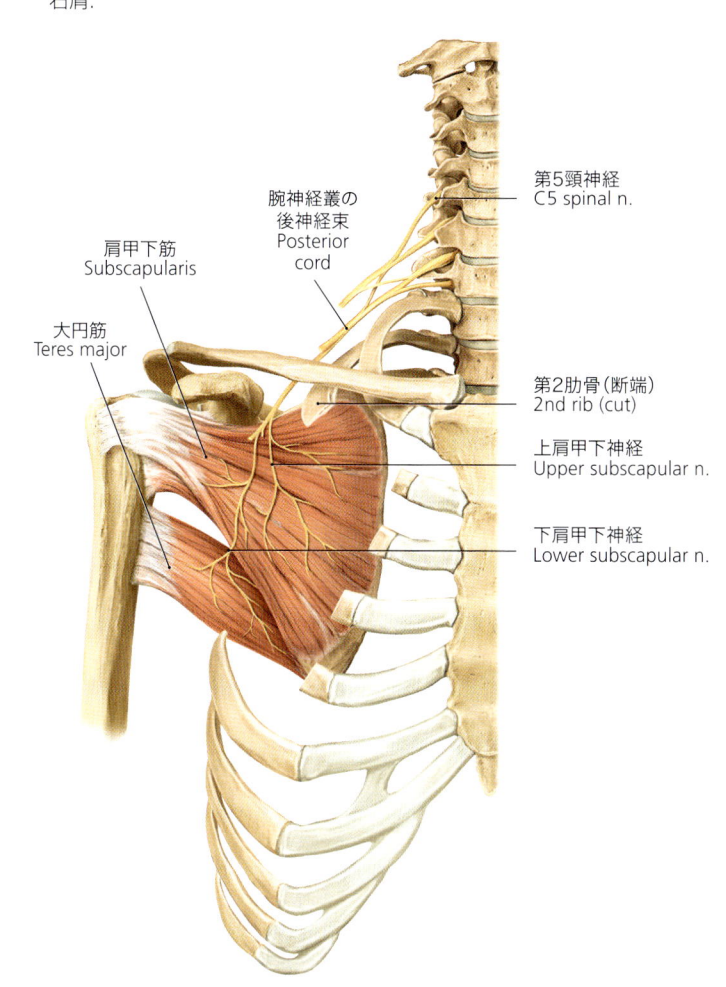

- 肩甲下筋 Subscapularis
- 大円筋 Teres major
- 腕神経叢の後神経束 Posterior cord
- 第5頸神経 C5 spinal n.
- 第2肋骨（断端）2nd rib (cut)
- 上肩甲下神経 Upper subscapular n.
- 下肩甲下神経 Lower subscapular n.

A　肩甲下神経，前方から見たところ．

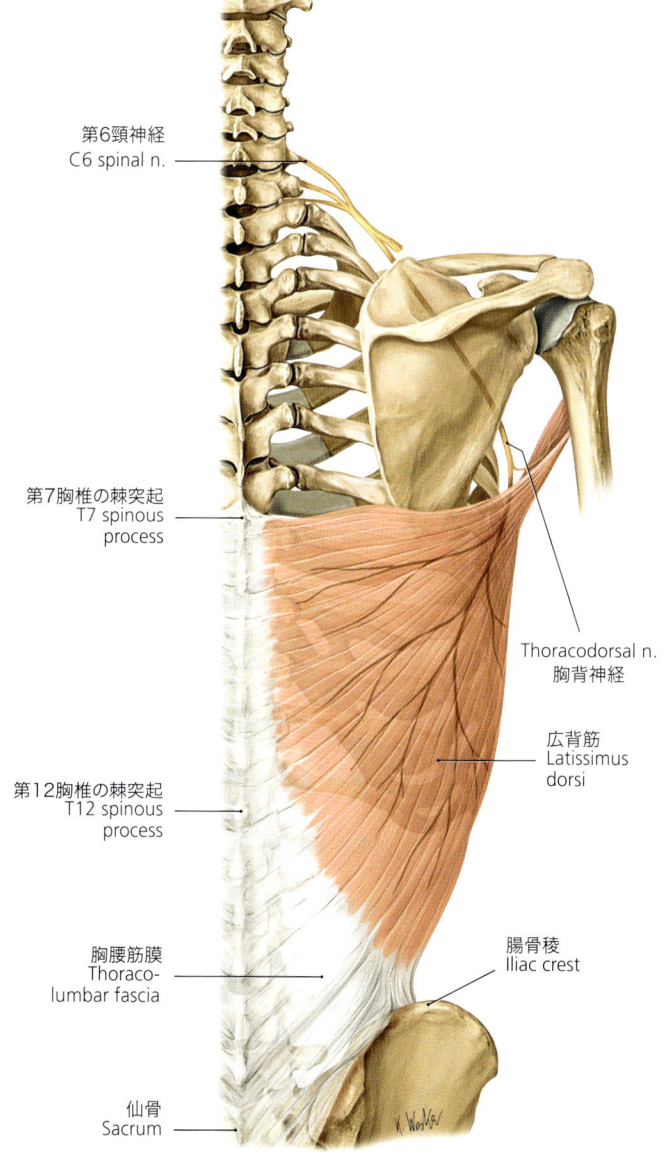

- 第6頸神経 C6 spinal n.
- 第7胸椎の棘突起 T7 spinous process
- 胸背神経 Thoracodorsal n.
- 広背筋 Latissimus dorsi
- 第12胸椎の棘突起 T12 spinous process
- 胸腰筋膜 Thoracolumbar fascia
- 腸骨稜 Iliac crest
- 仙骨 Sacrum

B　胸背神経，後方から見たところ．

表 22.3　後神経束の枝

神経	脊髄分節	支配筋
短い枝		
上肩甲下神経	C5-C6	肩甲下筋
下肩甲下神経	C5-C6	肩甲下筋，大円筋
胸背神経	C6-C8	広背筋
長い枝（終枝）		
腋窩神経	C5-C6	p. 324 参照
橈骨神経	C5-T1	p. 325 参照

後神経束：橈骨神経と腋窩神経
Posterior Cord: Axillary & Radial Nerves

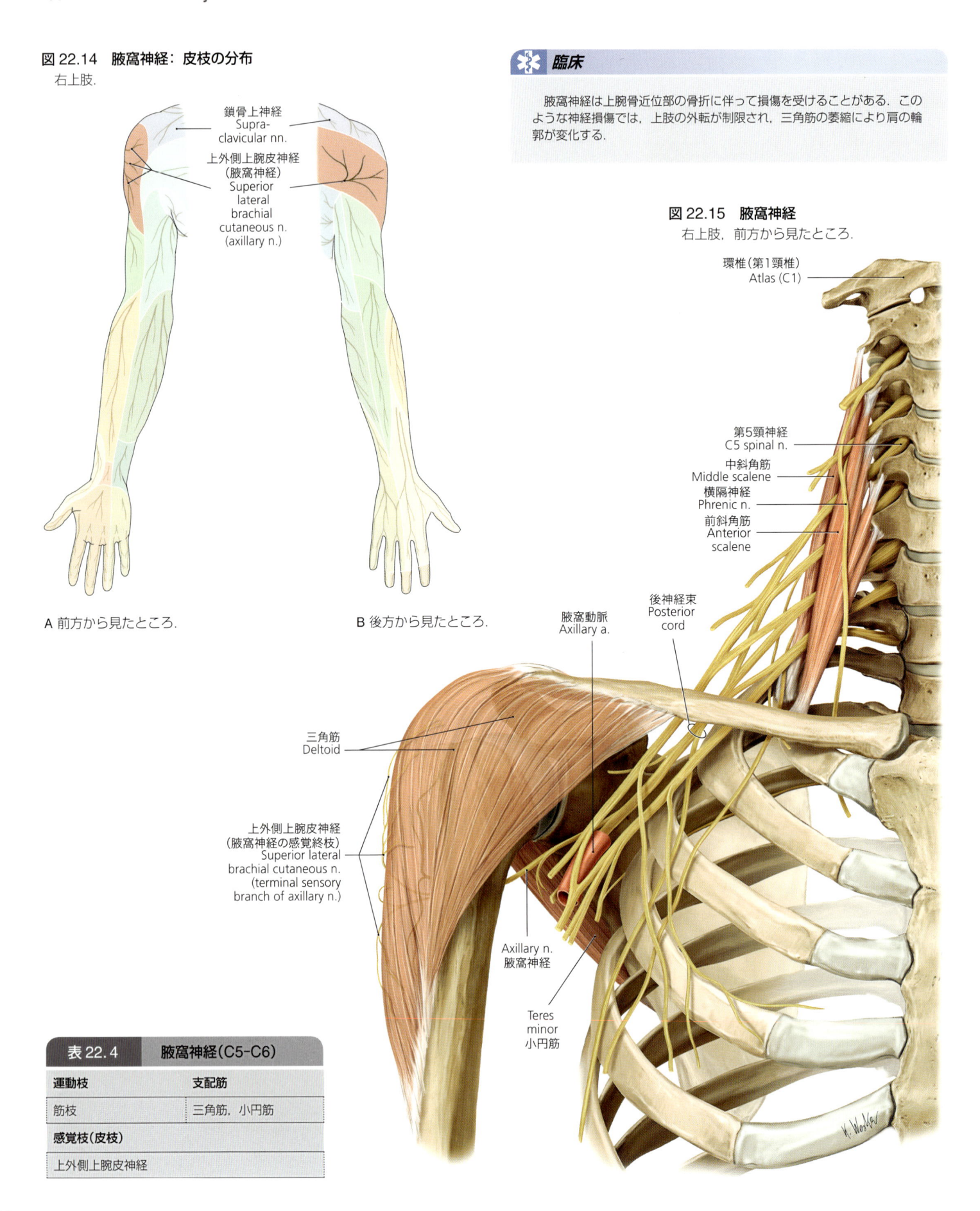

図 22.14　腋窩神経：皮枝の分布
右上肢．

- 鎖骨上神経　Supra-clavicular nn.
- 上外側上腕皮神経（腋窩神経）　Superior lateral brachial cutaneous n. (axillary n.)

A 前方から見たところ．
B 後方から見たところ．

臨床

腋窩神経は上腕骨近位部の骨折に伴って損傷を受けることがある．このような神経損傷では，上肢の外転が制限され，三角筋の萎縮により肩の輪郭が変化する．

図 22.15　腋窩神経
右上肢，前方から見たところ．

- 環椎（第1頸椎）　Atlas (C1)
- 第5頸神経　C5 spinal n.
- 中斜角筋　Middle scalene
- 横隔神経　Phrenic n.
- 前斜角筋　Anterior scalene
- 腋窩動脈　Axillary a.
- 後神経束　Posterior cord
- 三角筋　Deltoid
- 上外側上腕皮神経（腋窩神経の感覚終枝）　Superior lateral brachial cutaneous n. (terminal sensory branch of axillary n.)
- Axillary n.　腋窩神経
- Teres minor　小円筋

表 22.4	腋窩神経（C5-C6）
運動枝	支配筋
筋枝	三角筋，小円筋
感覚枝（皮枝）	
上外側上腕皮神経	

図 22.16　橈骨神経：皮枝の分布

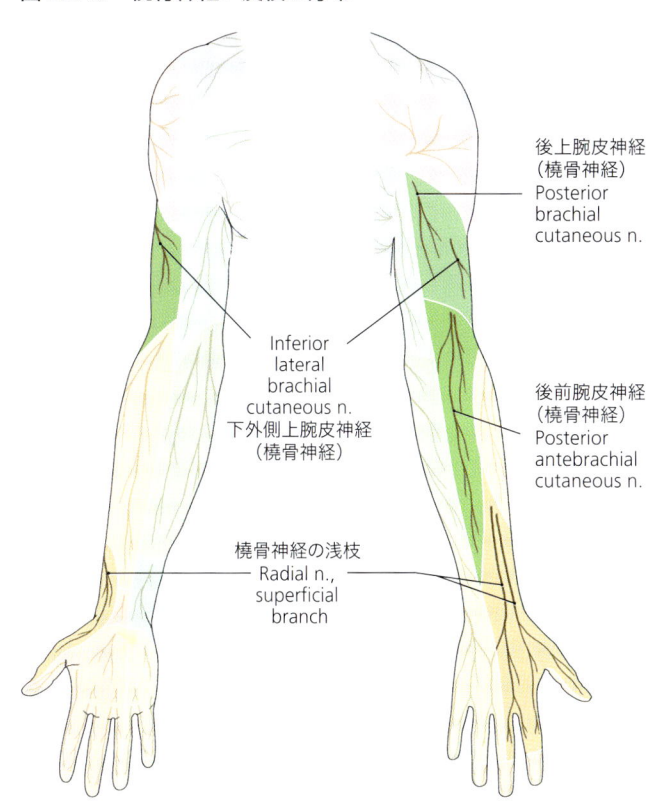

- 後上腕皮神経（橈骨神経）Posterior brachial cutaneous n.
- Inferior lateral brachial cutaneous n. 下外側上腕皮神経（橈骨神経）
- 後前腕皮神経（橈骨神経）Posterior antebrachial cutaneous n.
- 橈骨神経の浅枝 Radial n., superficial branch

A 前方から見たところ.　　B 後方から見たところ.

図 22.17　橈骨神経

右上肢．前方から見たところ．前腕は回内位．

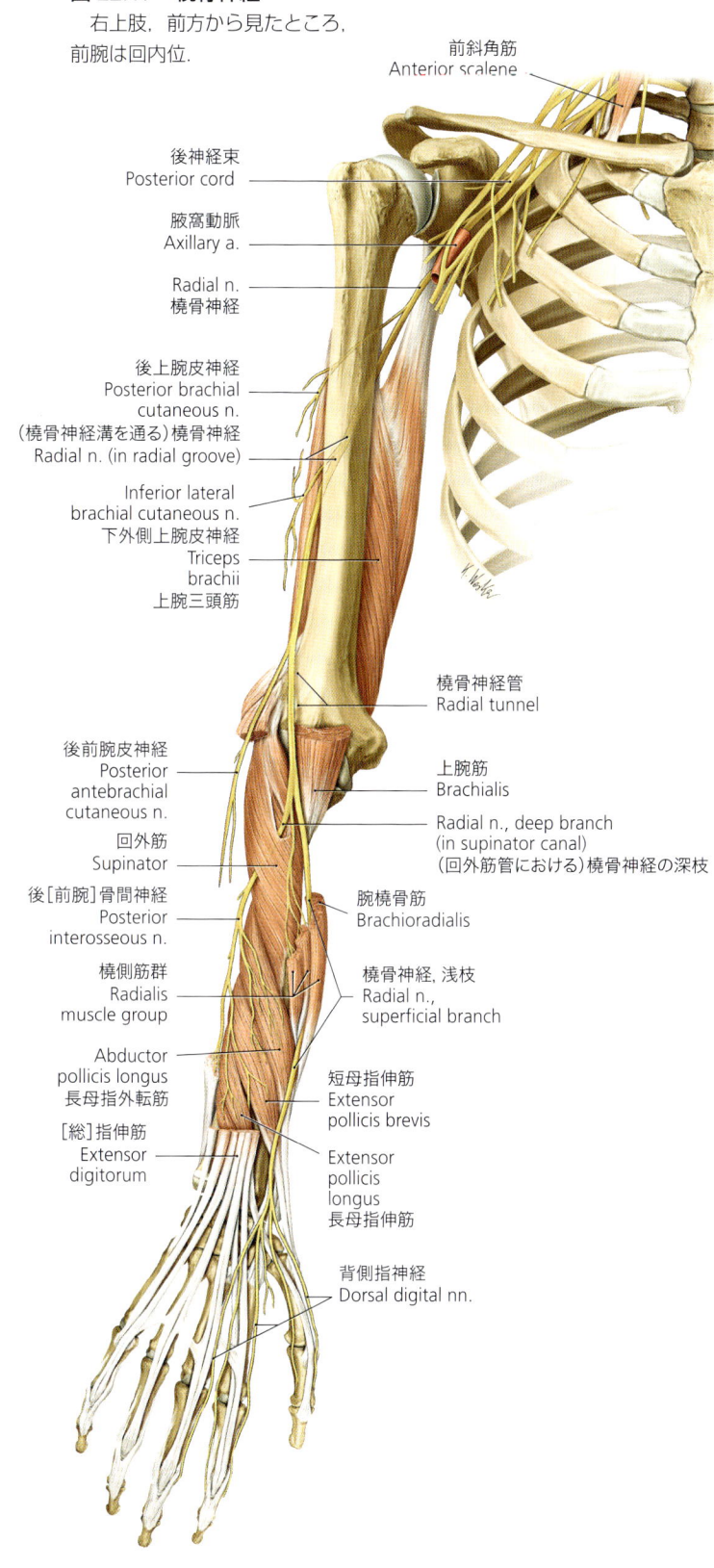

- 前斜角筋 Anterior scalene
- 後神経束 Posterior cord
- 腋窩動脈 Axillary a.
- Radial n. 橈骨神経
- 後上腕皮神経 Posterior brachial cutaneous n.
- （橈骨神経溝を通る）橈骨神経 Radial n. (in radial groove)
- Inferior lateral brachial cutaneous n. 下外側上腕皮神経
- Triceps brachii 上腕三頭筋
- 橈骨神経管 Radial tunnel
- 上腕筋 Brachialis
- Radial n., deep branch (in supinator canal) （回外筋管における）橈骨神経の深枝
- 後前腕皮神経 Posterior antebrachial cutaneous n.
- 回外筋 Supinator
- 腕橈骨筋 Brachioradialis
- 後[前腕]骨間神経 Posterior interosseous n.
- 橈側筋群 Radialis muscle group
- 橈骨神経, 浅枝 Radial n., superficial branch
- Abductor pollicis longus 長母指外転筋
- 短母指伸筋 Extensor pollicis brevis
- [総]指伸筋 Extensor digitorum
- Extensor pollicis longus 長母指伸筋
- 背側指神経 Dorsal digital nn.

表 22.5　橈骨神経（C5-T1）

運動枝	支配筋
橈骨神経（本幹）から出る筋枝	上腕筋（部分的）
	上腕三頭筋
	肘筋
	腕橈骨筋
	長・短橈側手根伸筋
深枝（橈骨神経の終枝である後骨間神経となる）	回外筋
	[総]指伸筋
	小指伸筋
	尺側手根伸筋
	長・短母指伸筋
	示指伸筋
	長母指外転筋
感覚枝	
橈骨神経から出る関節枝：肩関節の関節包	
後骨間神経から出る関節枝：手首の関節の関節包，第1-4中手指節関節の関節包	
後上腕皮神経	
下外側前腕皮神経	
後前腕皮神経	
浅枝	背側指神経
	尺骨神経との交通枝

臨床

腋窩における橈骨神経の慢性的な圧迫（例えば，長期にわたり松葉杖を不適切に使用した場合）により，手や前腕，上腕後面の感覚や運動が障害されることがある．橈骨神経の損傷がより遠位で生じた場合（例えば，麻酔中の不適切な肢位で生じる），麻痺する筋は少なくなり，上腕三頭筋の機能は正常だが下垂手が見られるといった状態になることもある．

内側・外側神経束
Medial & Lateral Cords

> 内側神経束と外側神経束は4本の短い神経を出す．ここでは肋間上腕神経は腕神経叢の短い枝に含めているが，実際にはこの神経は第2-3肋間神経の外側皮枝である．

表22.6　内側・外側神経束の枝

神経	脊髄分節	神経束	支配筋
短い枝			
外側胸筋神経	C5-C7	外側神経束	大胸筋と小胸筋
内側胸筋神経	C8-T1	内側神経束	
内側上腕皮神経	T1	内側神経束	―（皮膚に分布する感覚枝）
内側前腕皮神経	C8-T1		
肋間上腕神経	T2-T3		
長い枝（終枝）			
筋皮神経	C5-C7	外側神経束	烏口腕筋，上腕二頭筋，上腕筋
正中神経	C6-T1		p.328参照
尺骨神経	C7-T1	内側神経束	p.329参照

図22.18　内側・外側神経束：短い枝
右側，前方から見たところ．

A 内側・外側胸筋神経．

B 肋間上腕神経．

図22.19　短い枝：皮枝の分布

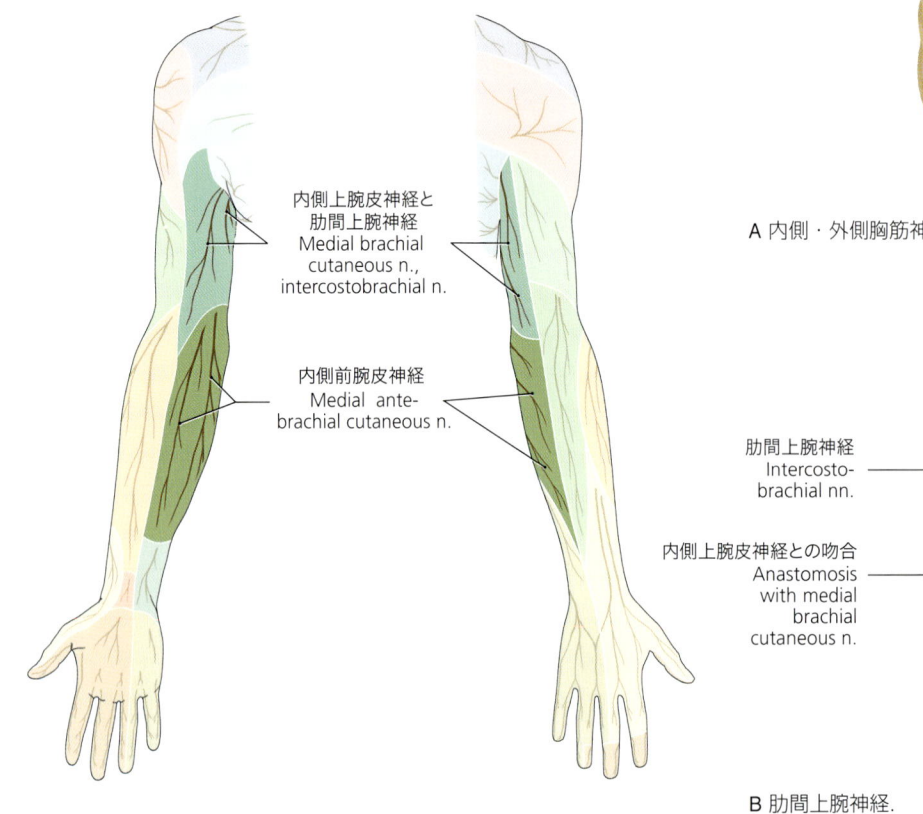

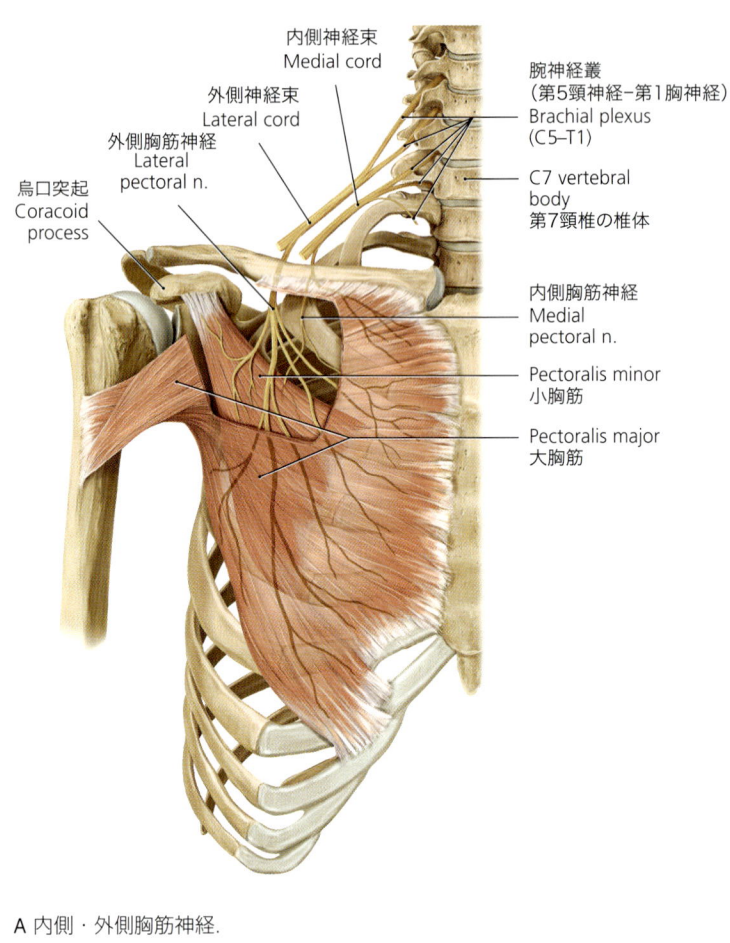

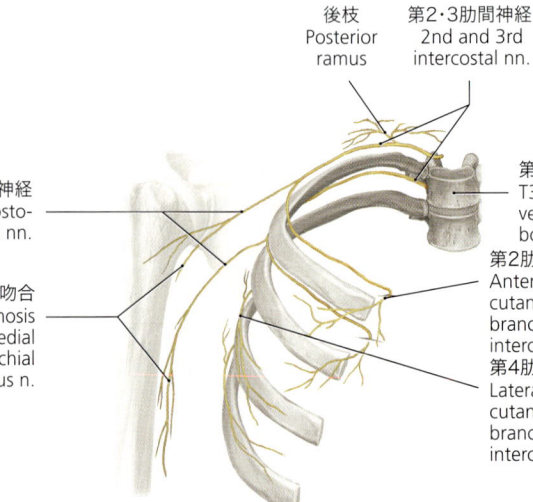

A 前方から見たところ．　　**B** 後方から見たところ．

図 22.20 筋皮神経
右上肢，前方から見たところ．

主な符号：
- 結節間溝 Intertubercular groove
- 烏口突起 Coracoid process
- 外側神経束 Lateral cord
- 前斜角筋 Anterior scalene
- 腋窩動脈 Axillary a.
- 筋皮神経 Musculocutaneous n.
- 上腕二頭筋, 短頭 Biceps brachii, short head
- 上腕二頭筋, 長頭 Biceps brachii, long head
- 烏口腕筋 Coracobrachialis
- 上腕筋 Brachialis
- 上腕二頭筋 Biceps brachii
- Musculocutaneous n. 筋皮神経
- 上腕筋 Brachialis
- 外側前腕皮神経 Lateral antebrachial cutaneous n.
- 尺骨 Ulna
- 橈骨 Radius

表 22.7	筋皮神経（C5-C7）
運動枝	支配筋
筋枝	烏口腕筋
	上腕二頭筋
	上腕筋
感覚枝	
外側前腕皮神経	
関節枝：肘関節の関節包（前面）	

筋皮神経は上腕では運動枝だけを出し，前腕（肘関節を含む）では感覚枝だけを出す．

図 22.21 筋皮神経：皮枝の分布

外側前腕皮神経 Lateral antebrachial cutaneous n.

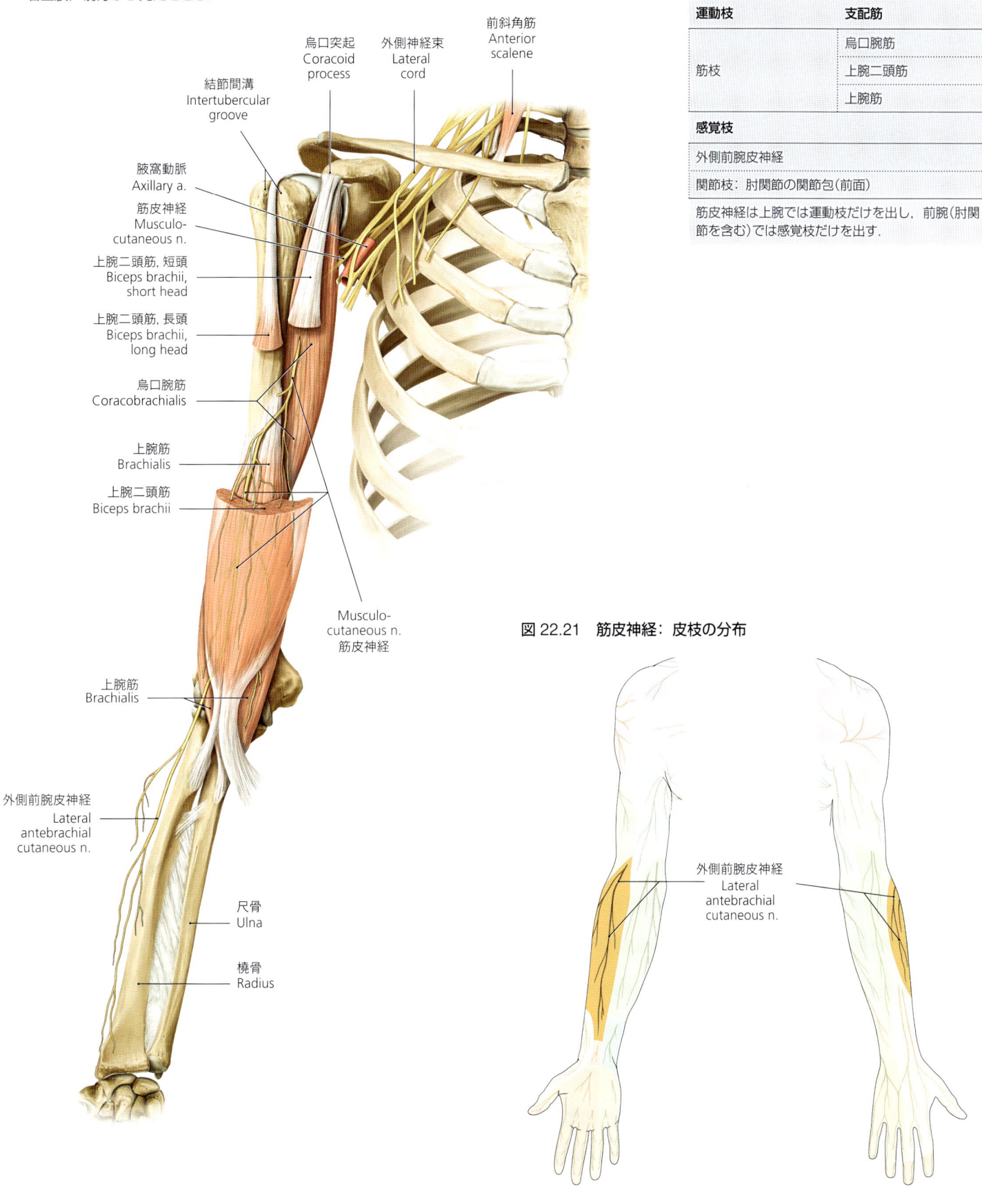

A 前方から見たところ．　　B 後方から見たところ．

22 神経と脈管

327

正中神経，尺骨神経
Median & Ulnar Nerves

正中神経は内側・外側神経束の両方に由来する終枝である．一方，尺骨神経は内側神経束だけに由来する終枝である．

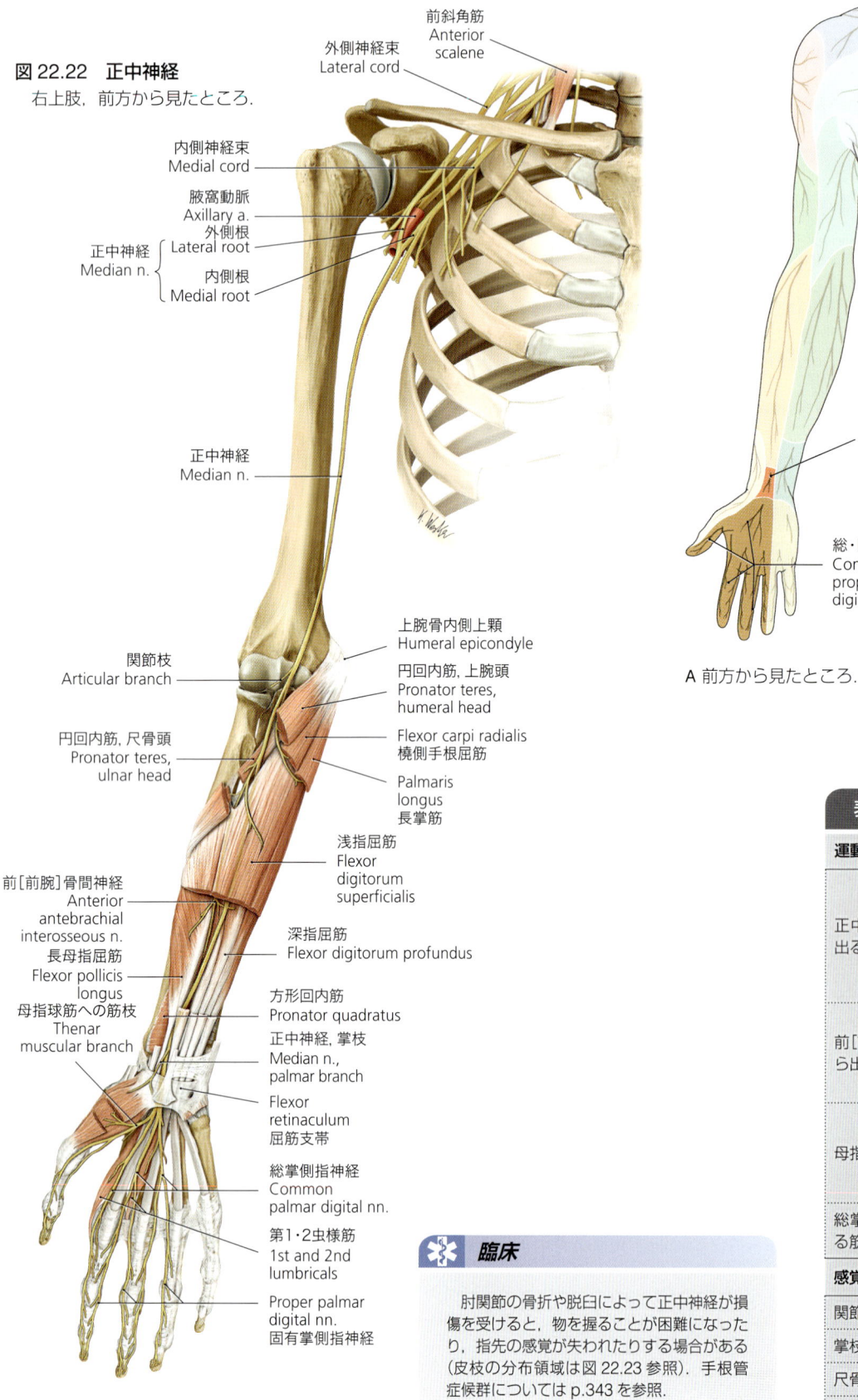

図22.22　正中神経
右上肢，前方から見たところ．

- 前斜角筋 Anterior scalene
- 外側神経束 Lateral cord
- 内側神経束 Medial cord
- 腋窩動脈 Axillary a.
- 外側根 Lateral root
- 正中神経 Median n.
- 内側根 Medial root
- 正中神経 Median n.
- 上腕骨内側上顆 Humeral epicondyle
- 関節枝 Articular branch
- 円回内筋，上腕頭 Pronator teres, humeral head
- 円回内筋，尺骨頭 Pronator teres, ulnar head
- 橈側手根屈筋 Flexor carpi radialis
- 長掌筋 Palmaris longus
- 浅指屈筋 Flexor digitorum superficialis
- 前[前腕]骨間神経 Anterior antebrachial interosseous n.
- 深指屈筋 Flexor digitorum profundus
- 長母指屈筋 Flexor pollicis longus
- 母指球筋への筋枝 Thenar muscular branch
- 方形回内筋 Pronator quadratus
- 正中神経，掌枝 Median n., palmar branch
- 屈筋支帯 Flexor retinaculum
- 総掌側指神経 Common palmar digital nn.
- 第1・2虫様筋 1st and 2nd lumbricals
- 固有掌側指神経 Proper palmar digital nn.

図22.23　正中神経：皮枝の分布

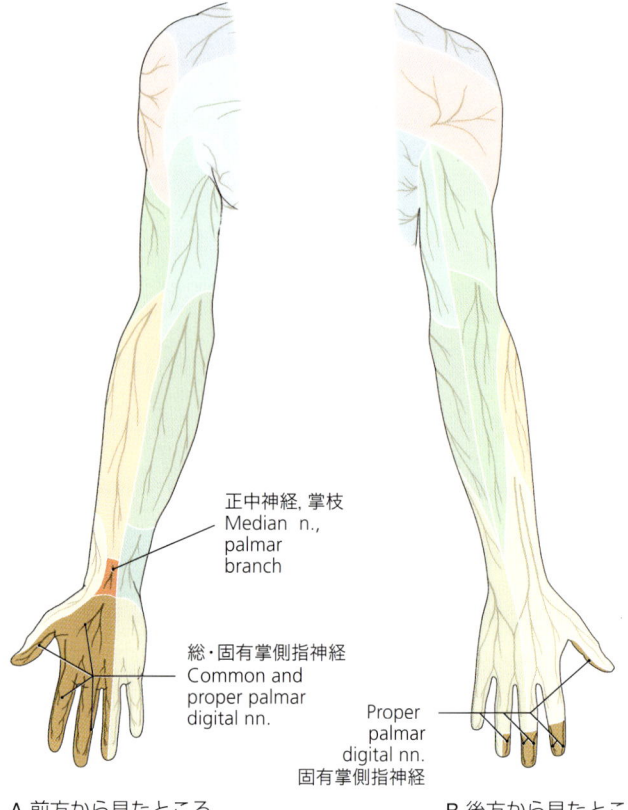

- 正中神経，掌枝 Median n., palmar branch
- 総・固有掌側指神経 Common and proper palmar digital nn.
- 固有掌側指神経 Proper palmar digital nn.

A　前方から見たところ．　　B　後方から見たところ．

臨床

肘関節の骨折や脱臼によって正中神経が損傷を受けると，物を握ることが困難になったり，指先の感覚が失われたりする場合がある（皮枝の分布領域は図22.23参照）．手根管症候群についてはp.343を参照．

表22.8　正中神経（C6-T1）

運動枝	支配筋
正中神経（本幹）から出る筋枝	円回内筋
	橈側手根屈筋
	長掌筋
	浅指屈筋
前[前腕]骨間神経から出る筋枝	方形回内筋
	長母指屈筋
	深指屈筋（橈側半）
母指球筋への筋枝	短母指外転筋
	短母指屈筋（浅頭）
	母指対立筋
総掌側指神経から出る筋枝	第1・2虫様筋
感覚枝	
関節枝：肘と手首の関節の関節包	
掌枝（母指球の皮膚に分布）	
尺骨神経との交通枝	
総掌側指神経	

図 22.24　尺骨神経：皮枝の分布

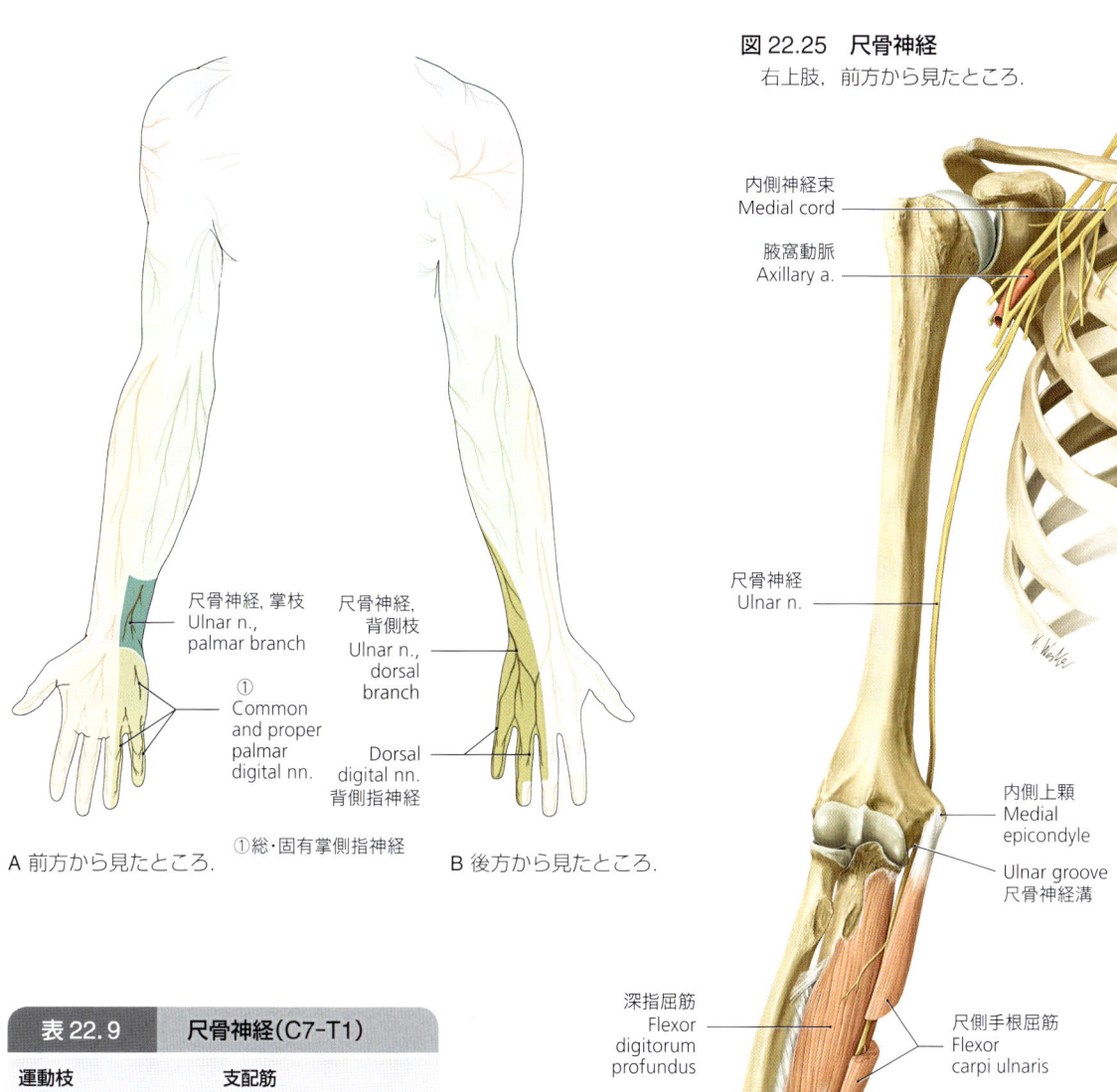

A　前方から見たところ．
- 尺骨神経, 掌枝 Ulnar n., palmar branch
- ① Common and proper palmar digital nn.
- ①総・固有掌側指神経

B　後方から見たところ．
- 尺骨神経, 背側枝 Ulnar n., dorsal branch
- Dorsal digital nn. 背側指神経

図 22.25　尺骨神経
右上肢，前方から見たところ．

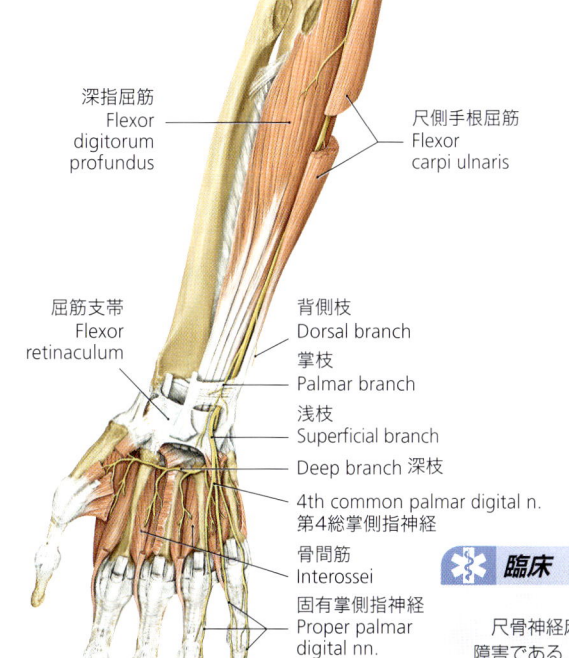

- 内側神経束 Medial cord
- 腋窩動脈 Axillary a.
- 尺骨神経 Ulnar n.
- 内側上顆 Medial epicondyle
- 尺骨神経溝 Ulnar groove
- 深指屈筋 Flexor digitorum profundus
- 尺側手根屈筋 Flexor carpi ulnaris
- 屈筋支帯 Flexor retinaculum
- 背側枝 Dorsal branch
- 掌枝 Palmar branch
- 浅枝 Superficial branch
- 深枝 Deep branch
- 第4総掌側指神経 4th common palmar digital n.
- 骨間筋 Interossei
- 固有掌側指神経 Proper palmar digital nn.

表 22.9	尺骨神経（C7–T1）
運動枝	**支配筋**
尺骨神経（本幹）から出る筋枝	尺側手根屈筋
	深指屈筋（尺側半）
浅枝から出る筋枝	短掌筋
深枝から出る筋枝	小指外転筋
	短小指屈筋
	小指対立筋
	第3・4虫様筋
	掌側・背側骨間筋
	母指内転筋
	短母指屈筋（深頭）
感覚枝	
関節枝：肘関節・手首の関節・中手指節関節の関節包	
手背枝（背側指神経となって終わる）	
掌枝	
総掌側指神経（浅枝から出る，固有掌側指神経となって終わる）	

臨床

尺骨神経麻痺は最もよくみられる末梢神経障害である．この神経は肘関節や尺骨神経管（p. 343 参照）における外傷や慢性的な圧迫により容易に損傷される．尺骨神経の損傷では，鷲手と骨間筋の萎縮がみられる．感覚障害は多くの場合，小指に限られる．

上肢の皮静脈，皮神経
Superficial Veins & Nerves of the Upper Limb

図 22.26 上肢における皮神経の分布：前方から見たところ

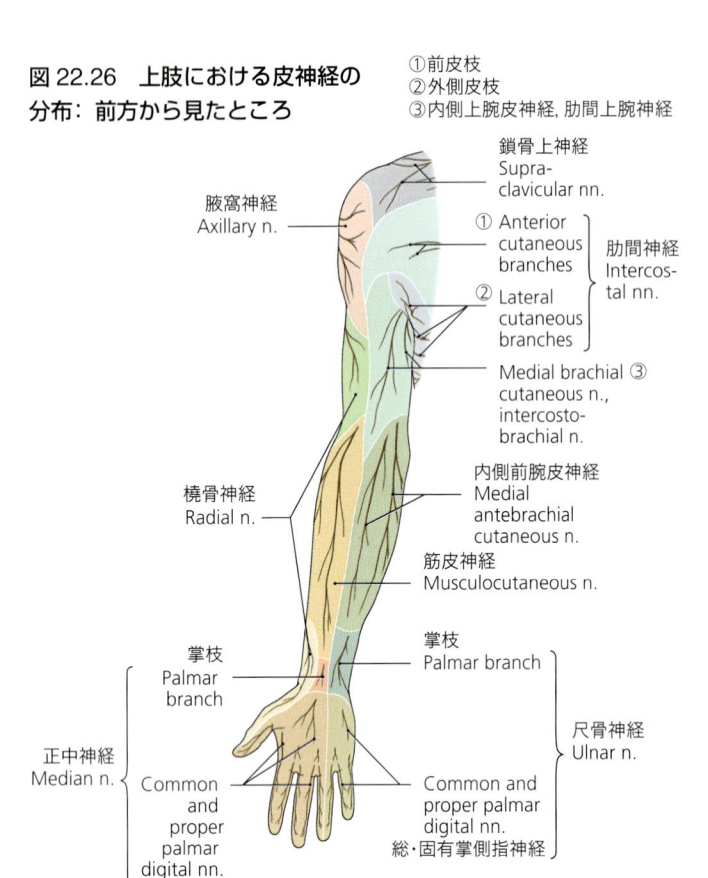

① 前皮枝
② 外側皮枝
③ 内側上腕皮神経，肋間上腕神経

- 鎖骨上神経 Supraclavicular nn.
- 腋窩神経 Axillary n.
- ① Anterior cutaneous branches
- ② Lateral cutaneous branches ｝肋間神経 Intercostal nn.
- 内側上腕皮神経 Medial brachial cutaneous n., intercostobrachial n. ③
- 橈骨神経 Radial n.
- 内側前腕皮神経 Medial antebrachial cutaneous n.
- 筋皮神経 Musculocutaneous n.
- 掌枝 Palmar branch
- 掌枝 Palmar branch
- 正中神経 Median n. ｛ Common and proper palmar digital nn. 総・固有掌側指神経
- 尺骨神経 Ulnar n. ｛ Common and proper palmar digital nn. 総・固有掌側指神経

A 皮神経の分布．

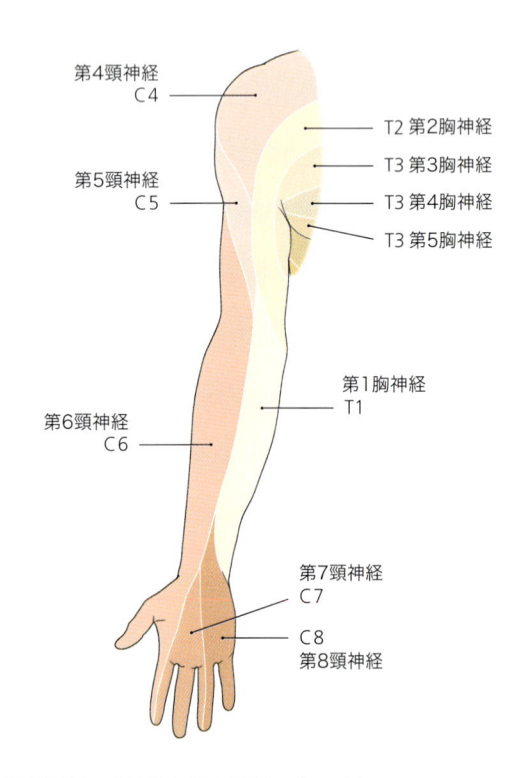

B 脊髄神経根の分節的な分布（デルマトーム）．
- 第4頸神経 C4
- 第5頸神経 C5
- 第6頸神経 C6
- 第7頸神経 C7
- 第8頸神経 C8
- 第1胸神経 T1
- T2 第2胸神経
- T3 第3胸神経
- T3 第4胸神経
- T3 第5胸神経

図 22.27 上肢における皮静脈と皮神経

- 鎖骨上神経 Supraclavicular nn.
- 上外側上腕皮神経（腋窩神経）Superior lateral brachial cutaneous n. (axillary n.)
- 肋間神経，前皮枝 Intercostal nn., anterior cutaneous branches
- 肋間上腕神経 Intercostobrachial n.
- 橈側皮静脈 Cephalic v.
- 内側上腕皮神経 Medial brachial cutaneous n.
- 下外側上腕皮神経（橈骨神経）Inferior lateral brachial cutaneous n. (radial n.)
- 尺側皮静脈の裂孔 Basilic hiatus
- 外側前腕皮神経（筋皮神経）Lateral antebrachial cutaneous n. (musculocutaneous n.)
- 尺側皮静脈 Basilic v.
- 内側前腕皮神経 Medial antebrachial cutaneous n.
- 肘正中皮静脈 Median cubital v.
- 橈側皮静脈 Cephalic v.
- 前腕正中皮静脈 Median antebrachial v.
- 貫通枝 Perforating branches
- 内側前腕皮神経 Medial antebrachial cutaneous n.
- 橈骨神経，浅枝 Radial n., superficial branch
- 尺骨神経，掌枝 Ulnar n., palmar branch
- 正中神経，掌枝 Median n., palmar branch
- 手掌腱膜 Palmar aponeurosis

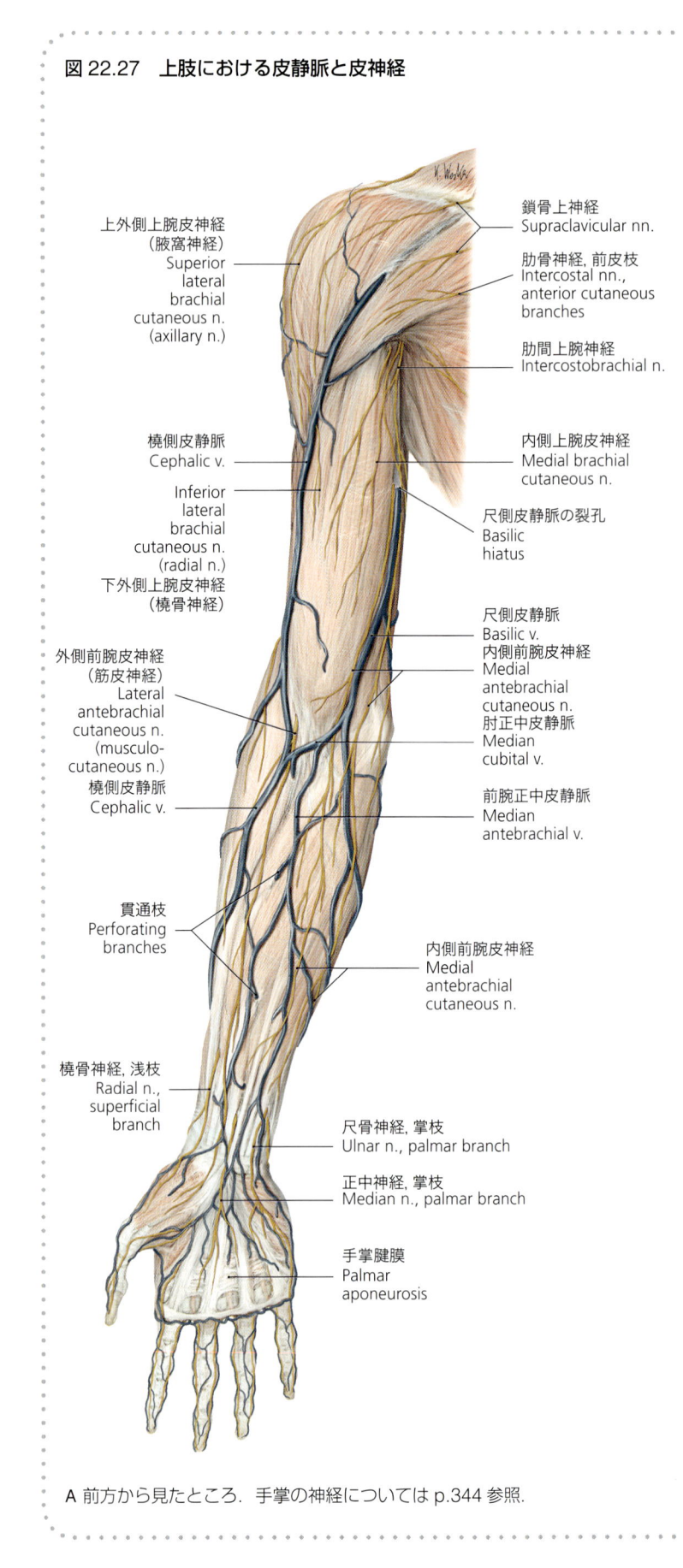

A 前方から見たところ．手掌の神経については p.344 参照．

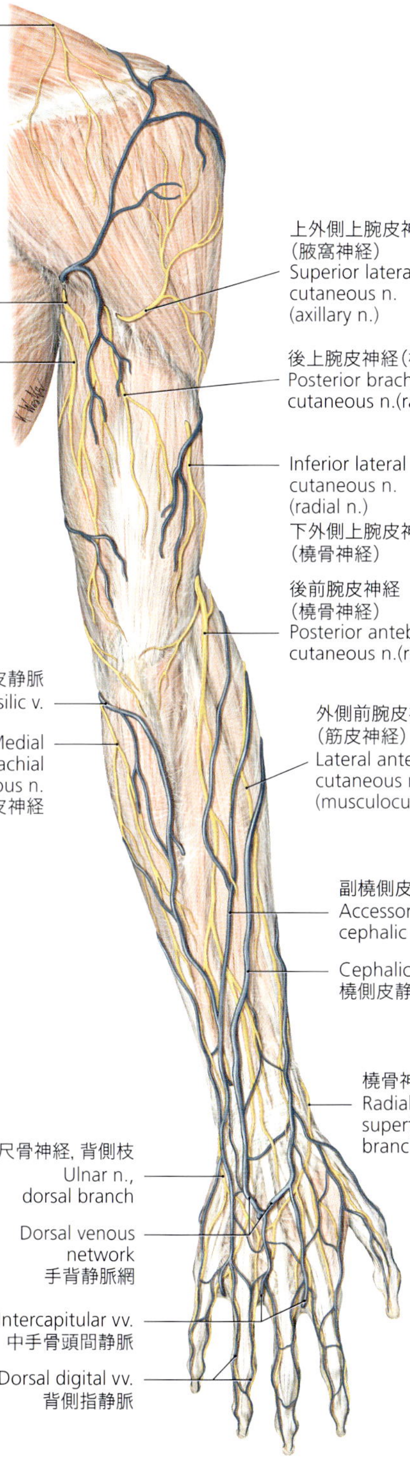

図 22.28　上肢における皮神経の分布：後方から見たところ

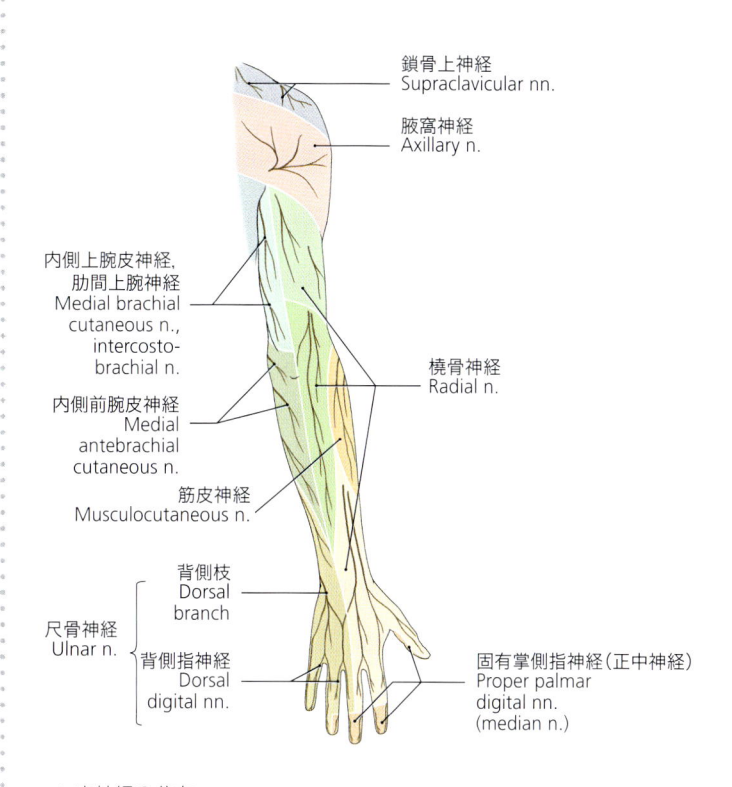

鎖骨上神経　Supra-clavicular nn.
肋間上腕神経　Intercosto-brachial n.
Medial brachial cutaneous n.　内側上腕皮神経
上外側上腕皮神経（腋窩神経）　Superior lateral brachial cutaneous n. (axillary n.)
後上腕皮神経（橈骨神経）　Posterior brachial cutaneous n. (radial n.)
Inferior lateral brachial cutaneous n. (radial n.)　下外側上腕皮神経（橈骨神経）
後前腕皮神経（橈骨神経）　Posterior antebrachial cutaneous n. (radial n.)
尺側皮静脈　Basilic v.
Medial antebrachial cutaneous n.　内側前腕皮神経
外側前腕皮神経（筋皮神経）　Lateral antebrachial cutaneous n. (musculocutaneous n.)
副橈側皮静脈　Accessory cephalic v.
Cephalic v.　橈側皮静脈
橈骨神経，浅枝　Radial n., superficial branch
尺骨神経，背側枝　Ulnar n., dorsal branch
Dorsal venous network　手背静脈網
Intercapitular vv.　中手骨頭間静脈
Dorsal digital vv.　背側指静脈

B 後方から見たところ．手背の神経については p.346 参照．

鎖骨上神経　Supraclavicular nn.
腋窩神経　Axillary n.
内側上腕皮神経，肋間上腕神経　Medial brachial cutaneous n., intercostobrachial n.
橈骨神経　Radial n.
内側前腕皮神経　Medial antebrachial cutaneous n.
筋皮神経　Musculocutaneous n.
尺骨神経　Ulnar n.
　背側枝　Dorsal branch
　背側指神経　Dorsal digital nn.
固有掌側指神経（正中神経）　Proper palmar digital nn. (median n.)

A 皮神経の分布．

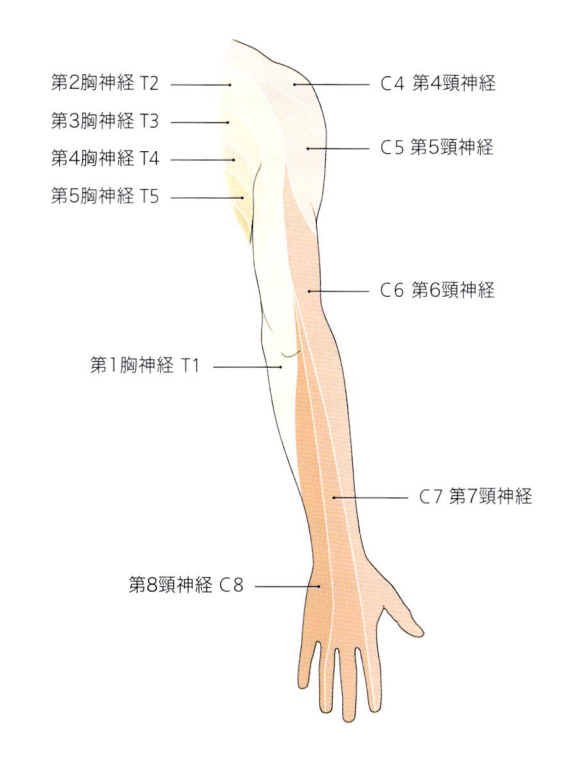

第2胸神経 T2
第3胸神経 T3
第4胸神経 T4
第5胸神経 T5
第1胸神経 T1
C4 第4頸神経
C5 第5頸神経
C6 第6頸神経
C7 第7頸神経
第8頸神経 C8

B 脊髄神経根の分節的な分布（デルマトーム）．

肩と腋窩の後部
Posterior Shoulder & Axilla

図 22.29 肩を後方から見たところ
右肩．僧帽筋（横行部）をめくり返し，棘上筋の一部を取り除いてある．
肩甲切痕の領域が現れている．

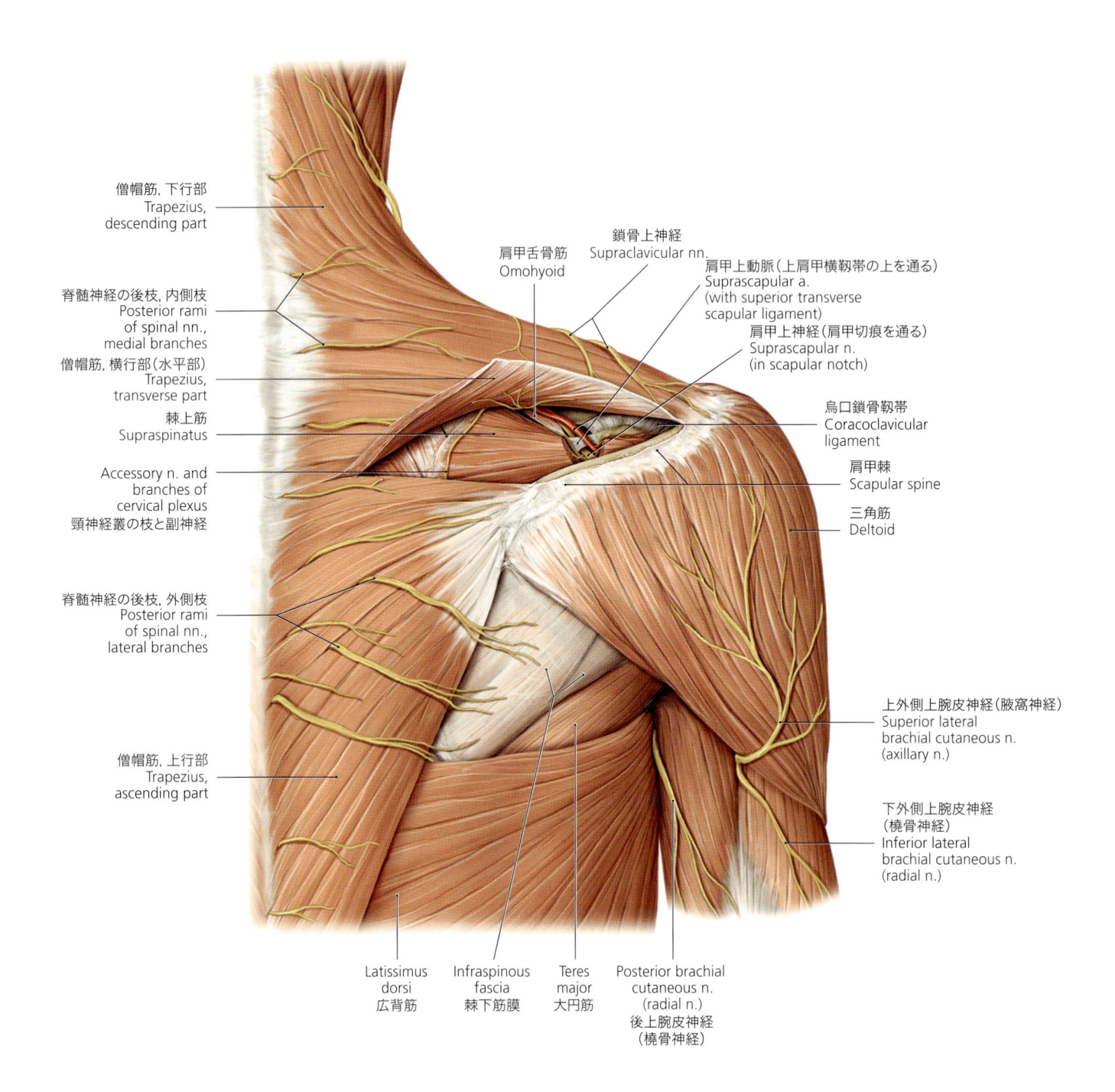

- 僧帽筋, 下行部 / Trapezius, descending part
- 脊髄神経の後枝, 内側枝 / Posterior rami of spinal nn., medial branches
- 僧帽筋, 横行部（水平部）/ Trapezius, transverse part
- 棘上筋 / Supraspinatus
- Accessory n. and branches of cervical plexus / 頸神経叢の枝と副神経
- 脊髄神経の後枝, 外側枝 / Posterior rami of spinal nn., lateral branches
- 僧帽筋, 上行部 / Trapezius, ascending part
- 肩甲舌骨筋 / Omohyoid
- 鎖骨上神経 / Supraclavicular nn.
- 肩甲上動脈（上肩甲横靱帯の上を通る）/ Suprascapular a. (with superior transverse scapular ligament)
- 肩甲上神経（肩甲切痕を通る）/ Suprascapular n. (in scapular notch)
- 烏口鎖骨靱帯 / Coracoclavicular ligament
- 肩甲棘 / Scapular spine
- 三角筋 / Deltoid
- 上外側上腕皮神経（腋窩神経）/ Superior lateral brachial cutaneous n. (axillary n.)
- 下外側上腕皮神経（橈骨神経）/ Inferior lateral brachial cutaneous n. (radial n.)
- Latissimus dorsi / 広背筋
- Infraspinous fascia / 棘下筋膜
- Teres major / 大円筋
- Posterior brachial cutaneous n. (radial n.) / 後上腕皮神経（橈骨神経）

上肢

表 22.10　肩甲骨周囲における神経・血管の通路

通路		通路を縁取る構造	通過する構造
①	肩甲切痕	上肩甲横靱帯, 肩甲骨	肩甲上動脈*・神経
②	肩甲骨の内側縁	肩甲骨	肩甲背動脈・神経
③	三角隙（内側腋窩隙）	大円筋, 小円筋, 上腕三頭筋の長頭	肩甲回旋動脈
④	上腕三頭筋裂孔	上腕三頭筋の長頭, 大円筋, 上腕骨	上腕深動脈, 橈骨神経
⑤	四角隙（外側腋窩隙）	大円筋, 小円筋, 上腕三頭筋の長頭, 上腕骨	後上腕回旋動脈, 腋窩神経

*訳注）　肩甲上動脈は上肩甲横靱帯の上方を走る.

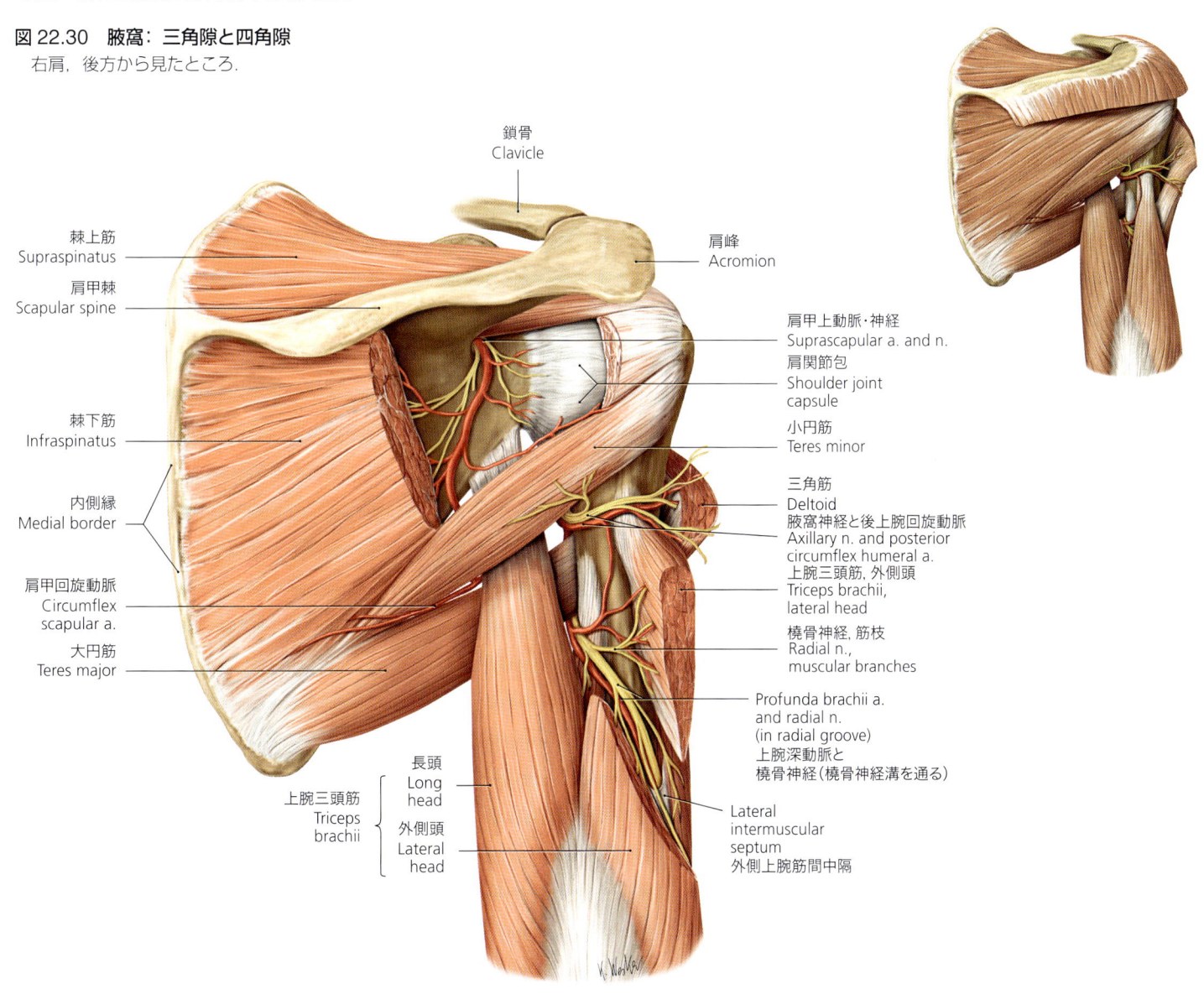

図 22.30　腋窩：三角隙と四角隙
右肩，後方から見たところ．

肩の前面
Anterior Shoulder

図 22.31 肩を前方から見たところ：表面
右肩．

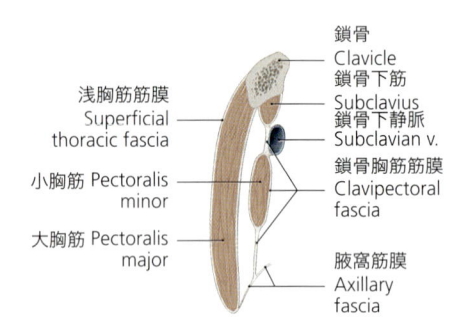

A 腋窩の前壁を通る矢状断面．

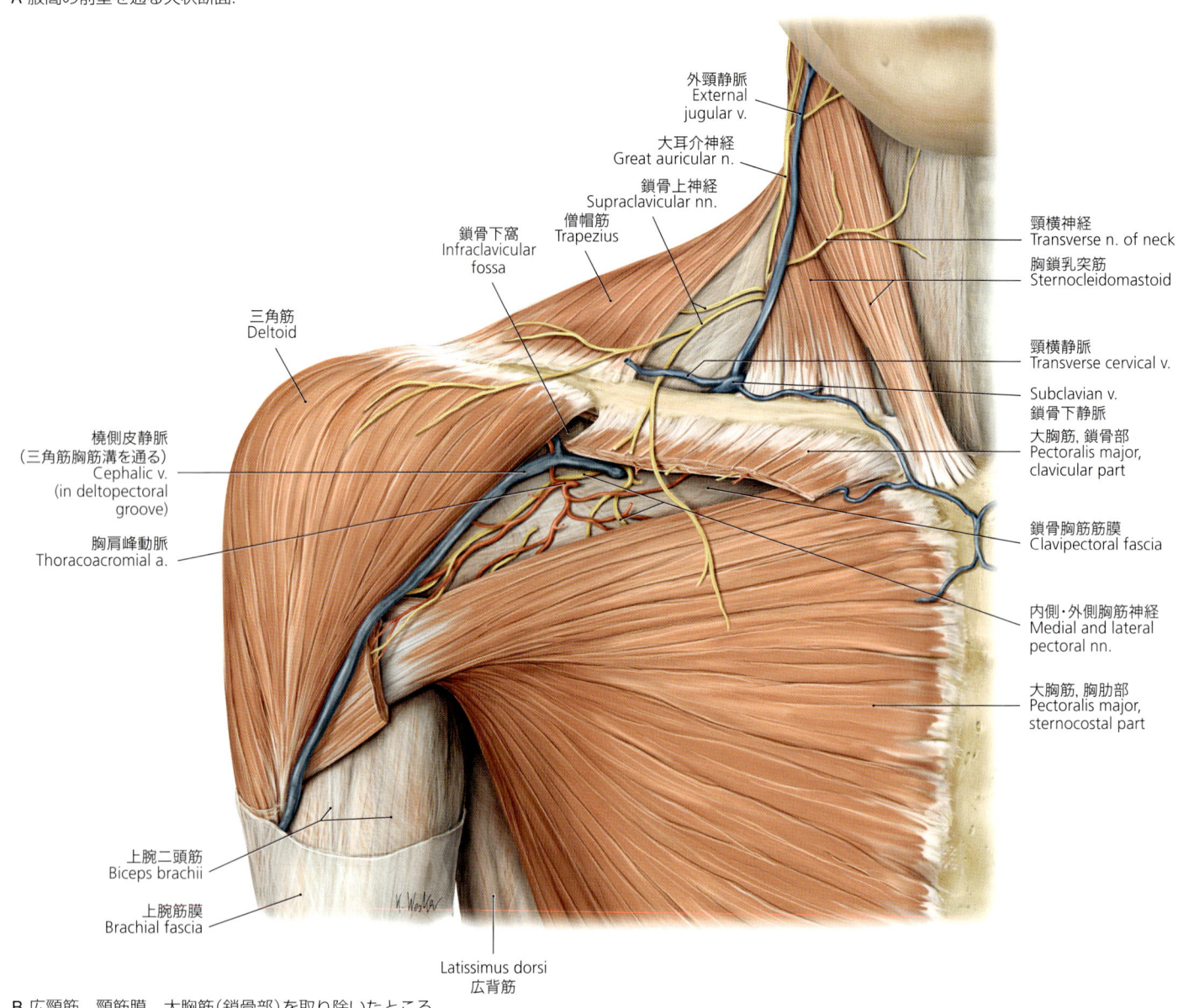

- 浅胸筋筋膜 Superficial thoracic fascia
- 小胸筋 Pectoralis minor
- 大胸筋 Pectoralis major
- 鎖骨 Clavicle
- 鎖骨下筋 Subclavius
- 鎖骨下静脈 Subclavian v.
- 鎖骨胸筋筋膜 Clavipectoral fascia
- 腋窩筋膜 Axillary fascia

- 三角筋 Deltoid
- 橈側皮静脈（三角筋胸筋溝を通る）Cephalic v. (in deltopectoral groove)
- 胸肩峰動脈 Thoracoacromial a.
- 上腕二頭筋 Biceps brachii
- 上腕筋膜 Brachial fascia
- 鎖骨下窩 Infraclavicular fossa
- 僧帽筋 Trapezius
- 広背筋 Latissimus dorsi
- 外頸静脈 External jugular v.
- 大耳介神経 Great auricular n.
- 鎖骨上神経 Supraclavicular nn.
- 頸横神経 Transverse n. of neck
- 胸鎖乳突筋 Sternocleidomastoid
- 頸横静脈 Transverse cervical v.
- 鎖骨下静脈 Subclavian v.
- 大胸筋, 鎖骨部 Pectoralis major, clavicular part
- 鎖骨胸筋筋膜 Clavipectoral fascia
- 内側・外側胸筋神経 Medial and lateral pectoral nn.
- 大胸筋, 胸肋部 Pectoralis major, sternocostal part

B 広頸筋，頸筋膜，大胸筋（鎖骨部）を取り除いたところ．鎖骨胸筋筋膜が見えている．

図 22.32 肩：横断面
右肩，下方から見たところ．

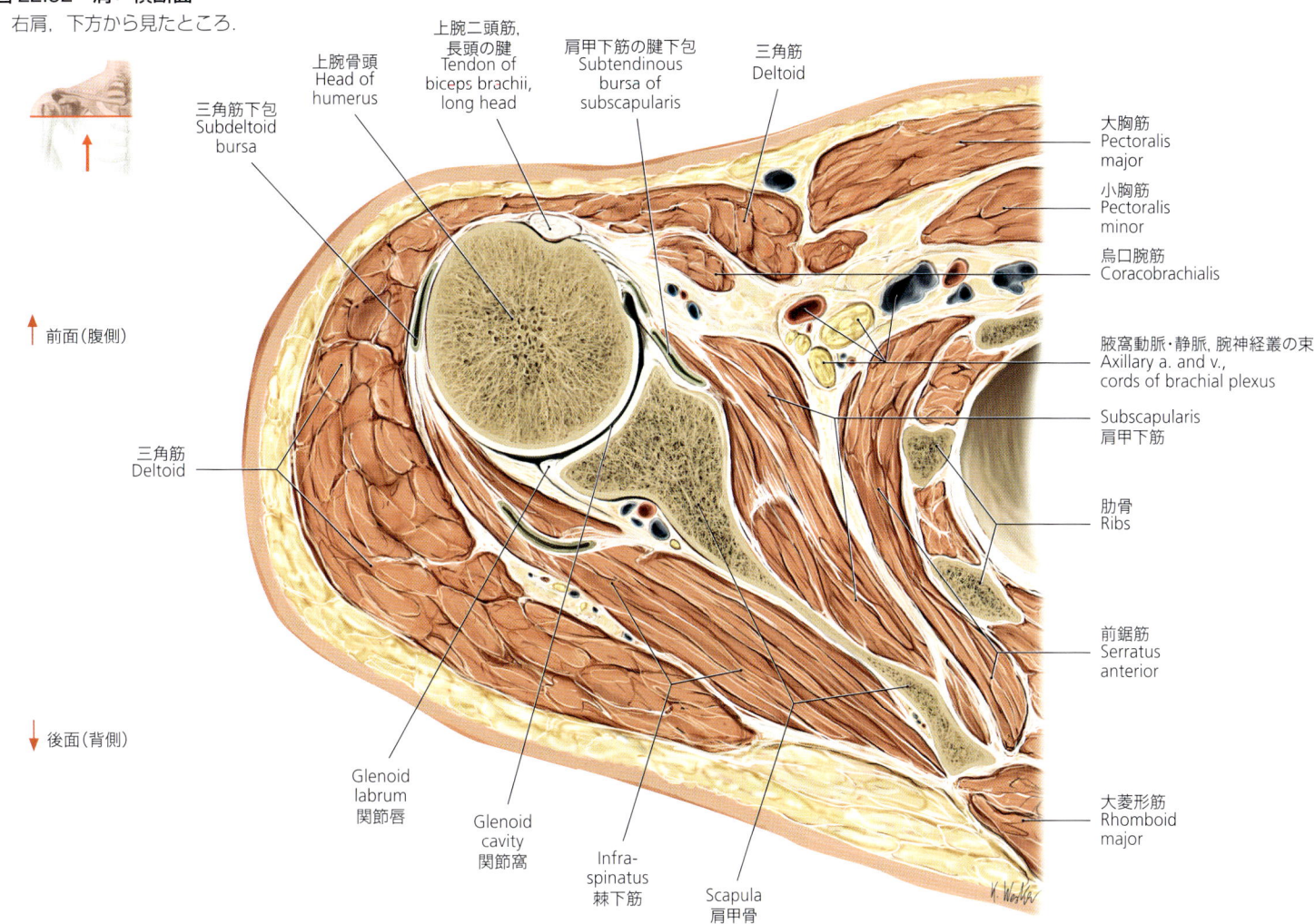

主要ラベル：
- 上腕骨頭 Head of humerus
- 上腕二頭筋，長頭の腱 Tendon of biceps brachii, long head
- 肩甲下筋の腱下包 Subtendinous bursa of subscapularis
- 三角筋 Deltoid
- 三角筋下包 Subdeltoid bursa
- 大胸筋 Pectoralis major
- 小胸筋 Pectoralis minor
- 烏口腕筋 Coracobrachialis
- 腋窩動脈・静脈，腕神経叢の束 Axillary a. and v., cords of brachial plexus
- 肩甲下筋 Subscapularis
- 肋骨 Ribs
- 前鋸筋 Serratus anterior
- 大菱形筋 Rhomboid major
- 三角筋 Deltoid
- 関節唇 Glenoid labrum
- 関節窩 Glenoid cavity
- 棘下筋 Infraspinatus
- 肩甲骨 Scapula

前面（腹側） ↑
後面（背側） ↓

図 22.33 肩を前方から見たところ：深部
右上肢．胸鎖乳突筋，肩甲舌骨筋，大胸筋を取り除き，外側頸三角（pp.580-581 参照）と腋窩（pp.336-337 参照）にある神経と血管を示している．

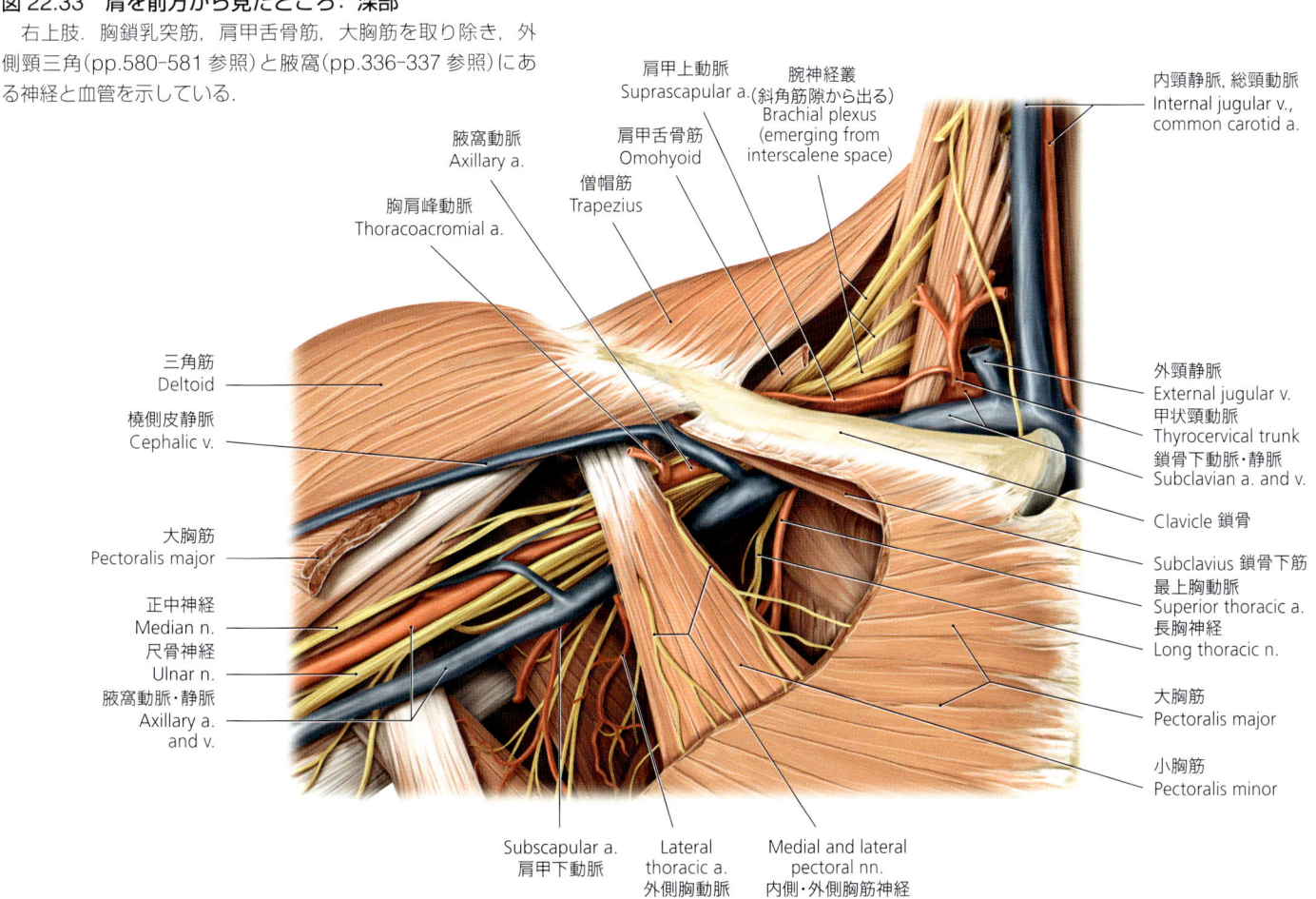

主要ラベル：
- 腋窩動脈 Axillary a.
- 胸肩峰動脈 Thoracoacromial a.
- 肩甲上動脈 Suprascapular a.
- 肩甲舌骨筋 Omohyoid
- 僧帽筋 Trapezius
- 腕神経叢（斜角筋隙から出る）Brachial plexus (emerging from interscalene space)
- 内頸静脈，総頸動脈 Internal jugular v., common carotid a.
- 外頸静脈 External jugular v.
- 甲状頸動脈 Thyrocervical trunk
- 鎖骨下動脈・静脈 Subclavian a. and v.
- 鎖骨 Clavicle
- 鎖骨下筋 Subclavius
- 最上胸動脈 Superior thoracic a.
- 長胸神経 Long thoracic n.
- 大胸筋 Pectoralis major
- 小胸筋 Pectoralis minor
- 三角筋 Deltoid
- 橈側皮静脈 Cephalic v.
- 大胸筋 Pectoralis major
- 正中神経 Median n.
- 尺骨神経 Ulnar n.
- 腋窩動脈・静脈 Axillary a. and v.
- 肩甲下動脈 Subscapular a.
- 外側胸動脈 Lateral thoracic a.
- 内側・外側胸筋神経 Medial and lateral pectoral nn.

22 神経と脈管

腋窩の局所解剖
Topography of the Axilla

図 22.34　腋窩
右肩，前方から見たところ．

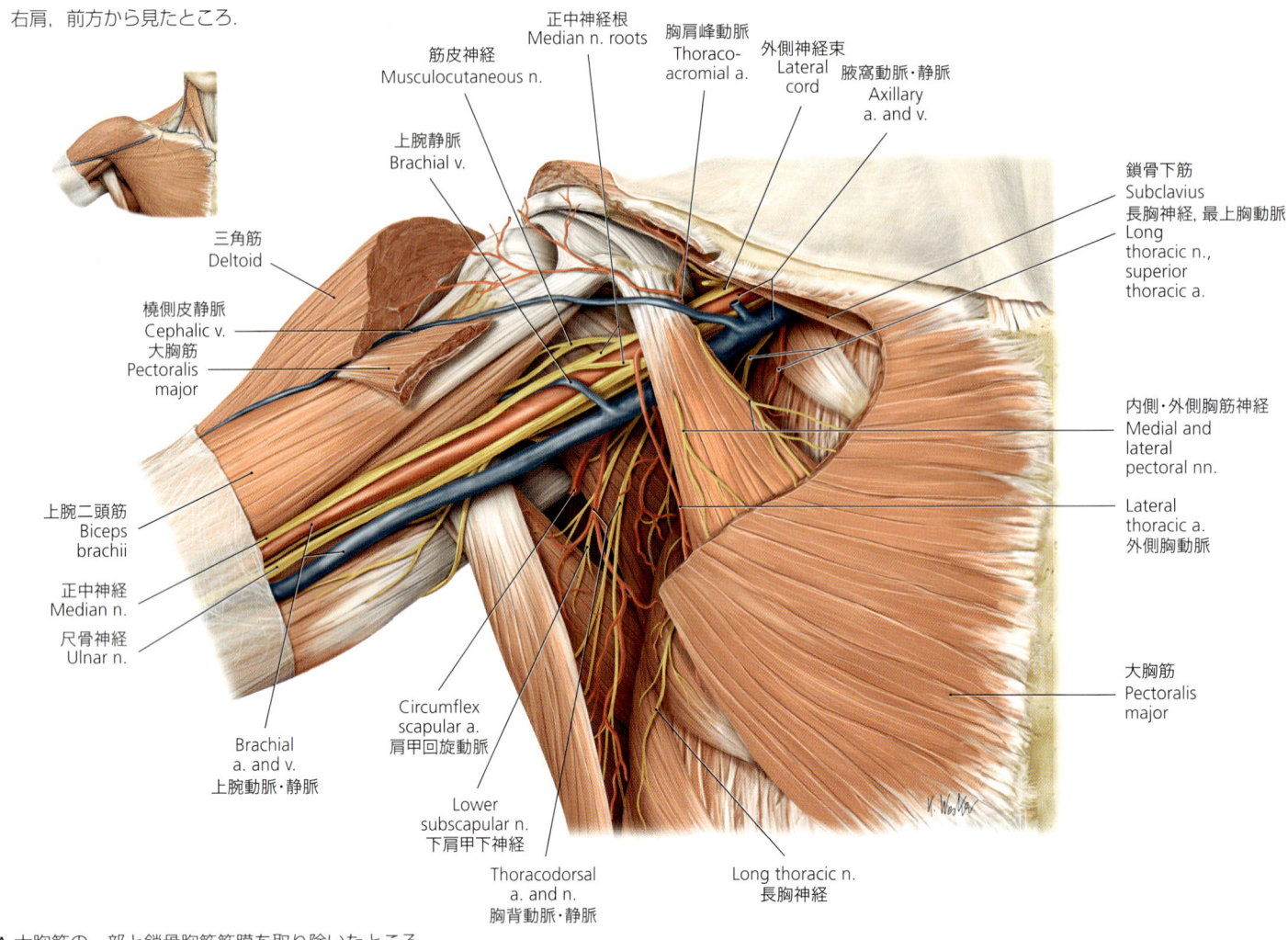

Labels:
- 筋皮神経 Musculocutaneous n.
- 正中神経根 Median n. roots
- 胸肩峰動脈 Thoraco-acromial a.
- 外側神経束 Lateral cord
- 腋窩動脈・静脈 Axillary a. and v.
- 上腕静脈 Brachial v.
- 三角筋 Deltoid
- 橈側皮静脈 Cephalic v.
- 大胸筋 Pectoralis major
- 上腕二頭筋 Biceps brachii
- 正中神経 Median n.
- 尺骨神経 Ulnar n.
- 上腕動脈・静脈 Brachial a. and v.
- 肩甲回旋動脈 Circumflex scapular a.
- 下肩甲下神経 Lower subscapular n.
- 胸背動脈・静脈 Thoracodorsal a. and n.
- 長胸神経 Long thoracic n.
- 鎖骨下筋 Subclavius
- 長胸神経, 最上胸動脈 Long thoracic n., superior thoracic a.
- 内側・外側胸筋神経 Medial and lateral pectoral nn.
- 外側胸動脈 Lateral thoracic a.
- 大胸筋 Pectoralis major

A 大胸筋の一部と鎖骨胸筋筋膜を取り除いたところ．

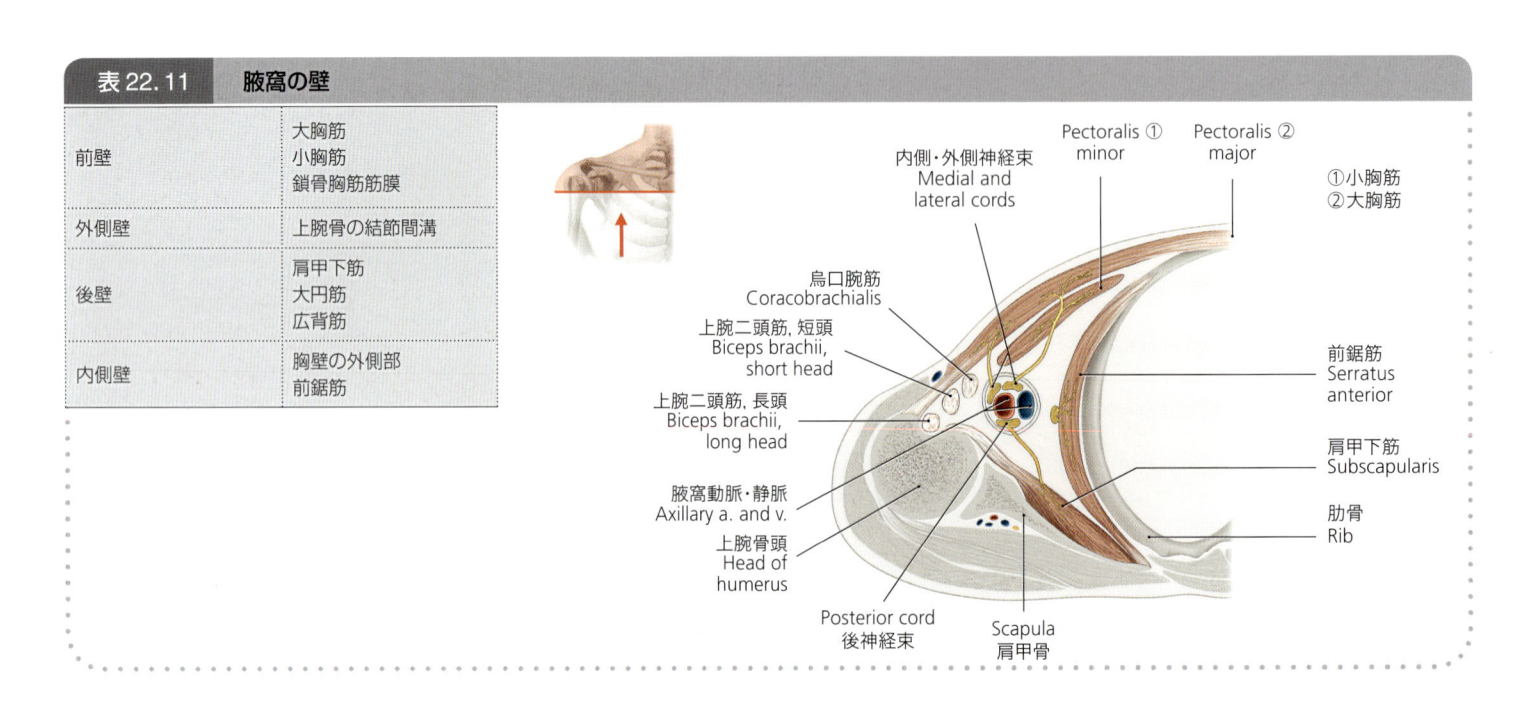

表 22.11　腋窩の壁

前壁	大胸筋 小胸筋 鎖骨胸筋筋膜
外側壁	上腕骨の結節間溝
後壁	肩甲下筋 大円筋 広背筋
内側壁	胸壁の外側部 前鋸筋

Cross-section labels:
- Pectoralis ① minor / Pectoralis ② major — ①小胸筋 ②大胸筋
- 内側・外側神経束 Medial and lateral cords
- 烏口腕筋 Coracobrachialis
- 上腕二頭筋, 短頭 Biceps brachii, short head
- 上腕二頭筋, 長頭 Biceps brachii, long head
- 腋窩動脈・静脈 Axillary a. and v.
- 上腕骨頭 Head of humerus
- 後神経束 Posterior cord
- 肩甲骨 Scapula
- 前鋸筋 Serratus anterior
- 肩甲下筋 Subscapularis
- 肋骨 Rib

B 腋窩の前壁（大胸筋，小胸筋，鎖骨胸筋筋膜）を取り除き，腕神経叢の内側・外側神経束を上方に引いたところ．

C 内側・外側神経束，腋窩動静脈を取り除いたところ．後神経束が見えている．

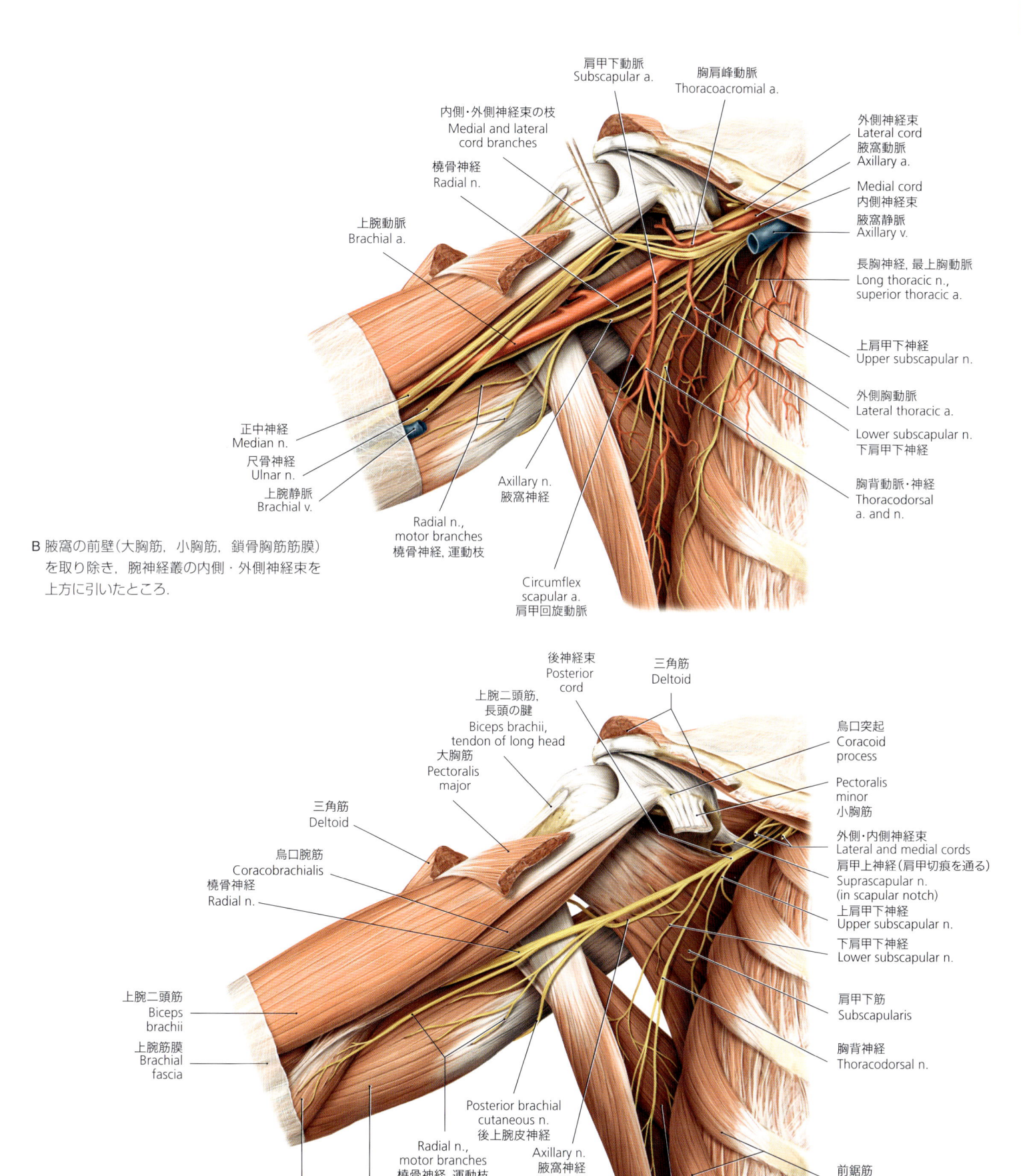

上腕と肘の局所解剖
Topography of the Brachial & Cubital Regions

図 22.35 上腕
右上腕，前方から見たところ．三角筋，大胸筋，小胸筋を取り除いたところ．内側二頭筋溝*にある構造が見えている．

*訳注）上腕二頭筋，上腕筋，内側上腕筋間中隔によって囲まれる溝で，上腕前面を走る主要な神経・血管がここを通る．

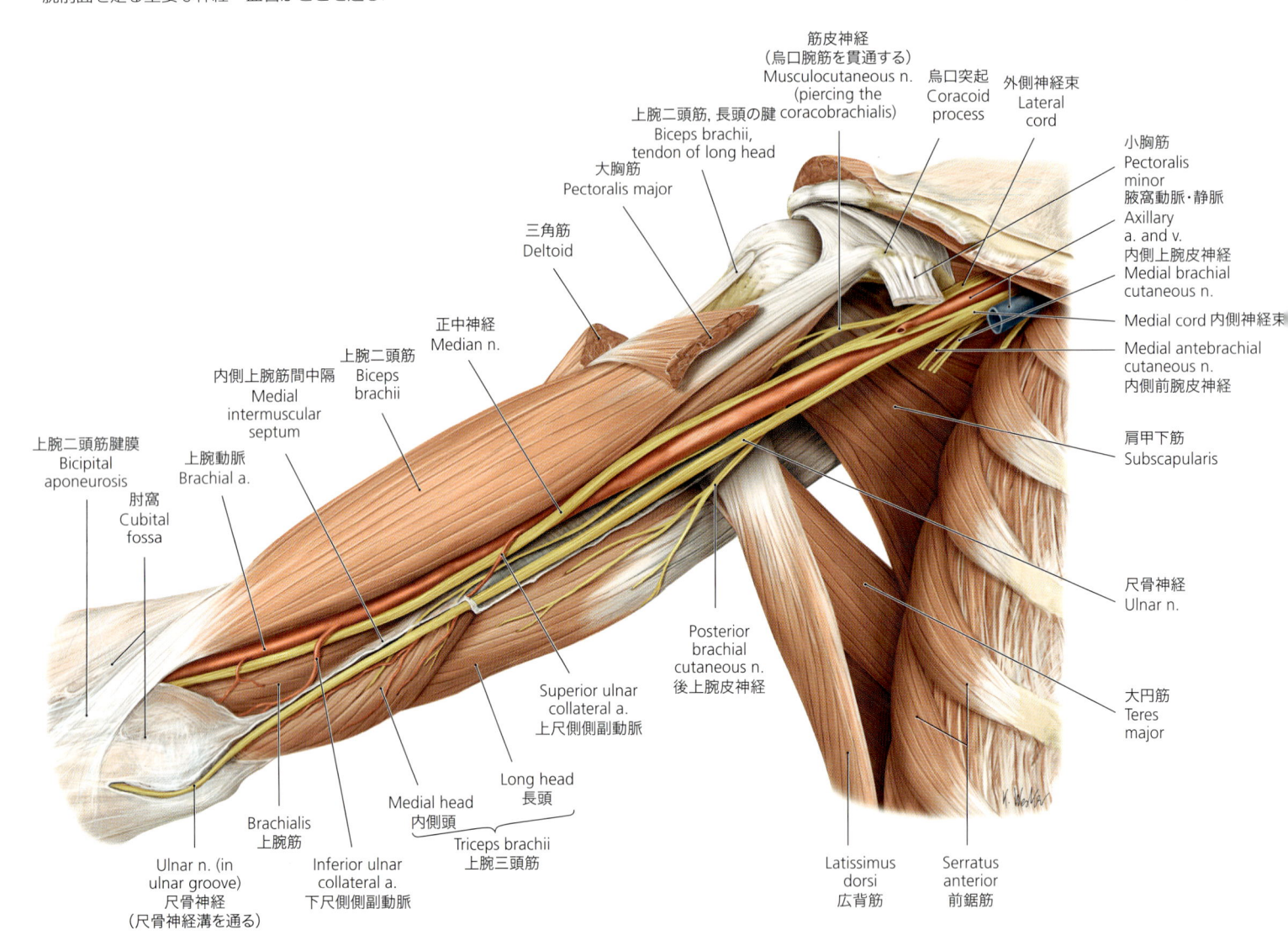

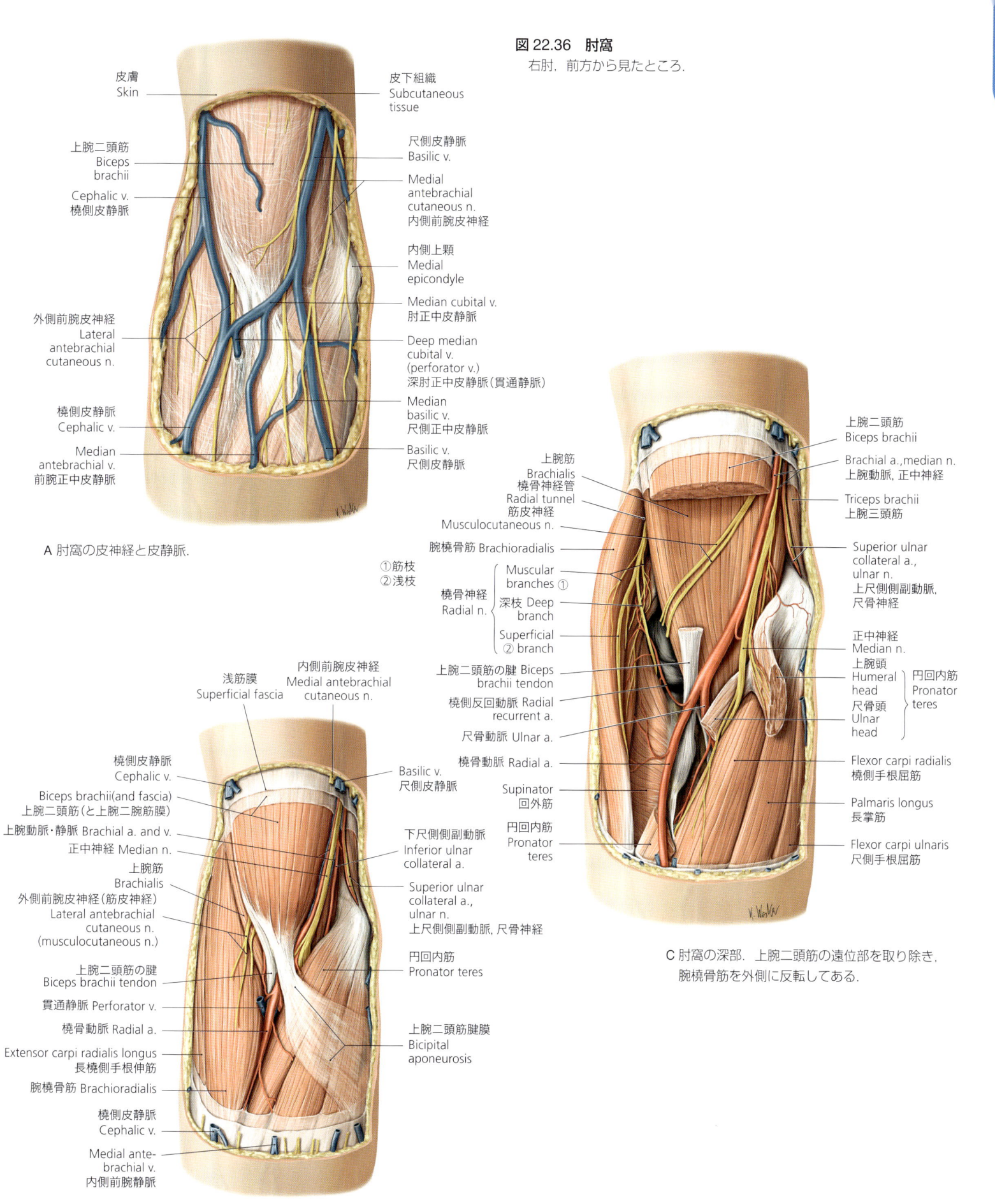

図 22.36 肘窩
右肘，前方から見たところ．

A 肘窩の皮神経と皮静脈．

B 肘窩の浅部．皮神経，皮静脈，上腕・前腕筋膜を取り除いたところ．

C 肘窩の深部．上腕二頭筋の遠位部を取り除き，腕橈骨筋を外側に反転してある．

前腕の局所解剖
Topography of the Forearm

図 22.37 前腕前部
右前腕，前方から見たところ．

A（左図）浅層．皮神経，皮静脈，前腕筋膜を取り除いたところ．

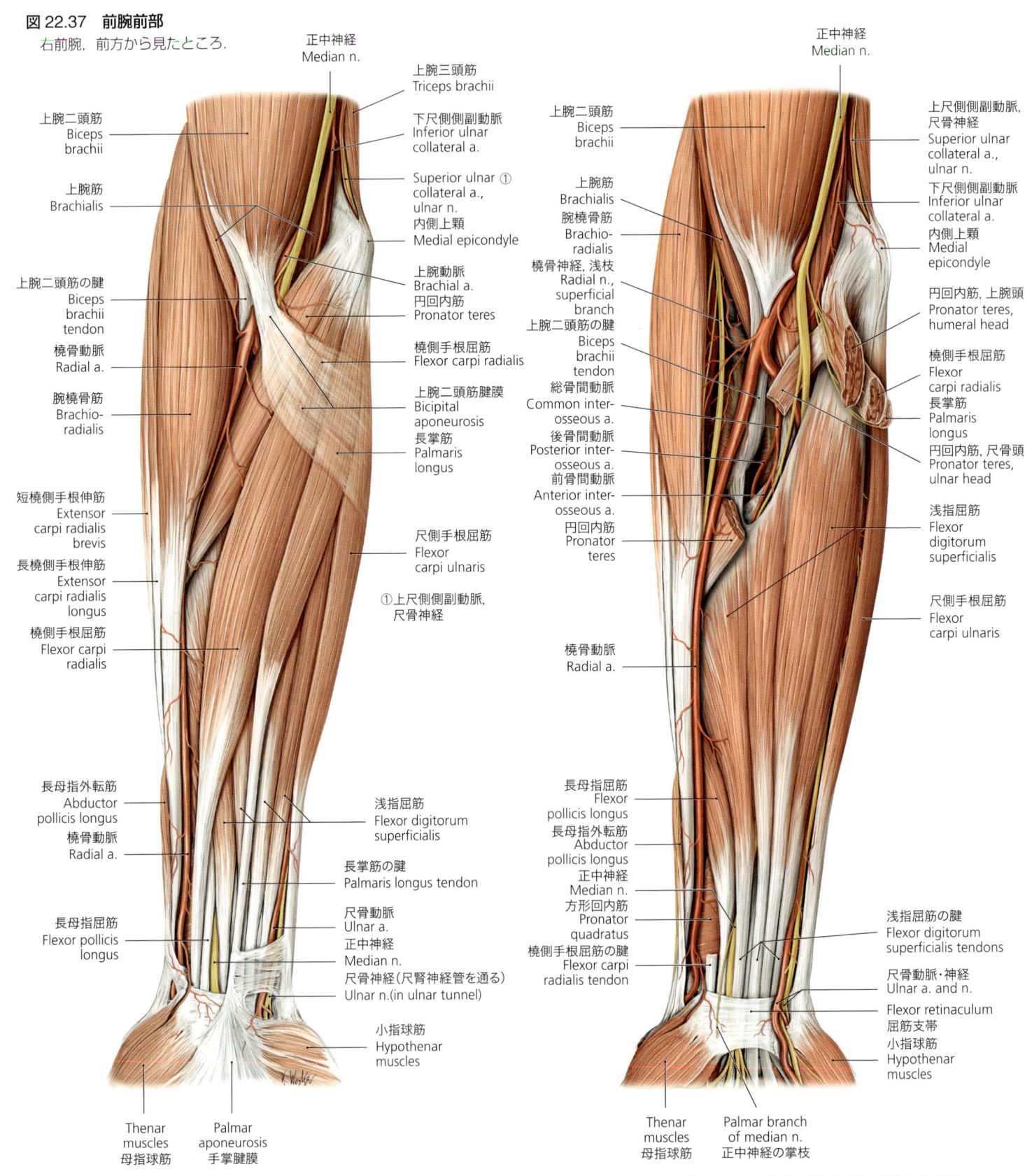

ラベル（上から下へ）：
- 正中神経 Median n.
- 上腕二頭筋 Biceps brachii
- 上腕筋 Brachialis
- 上腕二頭筋の腱 Biceps brachii tendon
- 橈骨動脈 Radial a.
- 腕橈骨筋 Brachioradialis
- 短橈側手根伸筋 Extensor carpi radialis brevis
- 長橈側手根伸筋 Extensor carpi radialis longus
- 橈側手根屈筋 Flexor carpi radialis
- 長母指外転筋 Abductor pollicis longus
- 橈骨動脈 Radial a.
- 長母指屈筋 Flexor pollicis longus
- 上腕三頭筋 Triceps brachii
- 下尺側側副動脈 Inferior ulnar collateral a.
- ①上尺側側副動脈, 尺骨神経 Superior ulnar collateral a., ulnar n.
- 内側上顆 Medial epicondyle
- 上腕動脈 Brachial a.
- 円回内筋 Pronator teres
- 橈側手根屈筋 Flexor carpi radialis
- 上腕二頭筋腱膜 Bicipital aponeurosis
- 長掌筋 Palmaris longus
- 尺側手根屈筋 Flexor carpi ulnaris
- ①上尺側側副動脈, 尺骨神経
- 浅指屈筋 Flexor digitorum superficialis
- 長掌筋の腱 Palmaris longus tendon
- 尺骨動脈 Ulnar a.
- 正中神経 Median n.
- 尺骨神経（尺骨神経管を通る）Ulnar n.(in ulnar tunnel)
- 小指球筋 Hypothenar muscles
- Thenar muscles 母指球筋
- Palmar aponeurosis 手掌腱膜

B（右図）中層．浅層の屈筋（円回内筋，長掌筋，橈側手根屈筋）を部分的に取り除いたところ．

ラベル：
- 正中神経 Median n.
- 上腕二頭筋 Biceps brachii
- 上腕筋 Brachialis
- 腕橈骨筋 Brachioradialis
- 橈骨神経，浅枝 Radial n., superficial branch
- 上腕二頭筋の腱 Biceps brachii tendon
- 総骨間動脈 Common interosseous a.
- 後骨間動脈 Posterior interosseous a.
- 前骨間動脈 Anterior interosseous a.
- 円回内筋 Pronator teres
- 橈骨動脈 Radial a.
- 長母指屈筋 Flexor pollicis longus
- 長母指外転筋 Abductor pollicis longus
- 正中神経 Median n.
- 方形回内筋 Pronator quadratus
- 橈側手根屈筋の腱 Flexor carpi radialis tendon
- Thenar muscles 母指球筋
- Palmar branch of median n. 正中神経の掌枝
- 上尺側側副動脈, 尺骨神経 Superior ulnar collateral a., ulnar n.
- 下尺側側副動脈 Inferior ulnar collateral a.
- 内側上顆 Medial epicondyle
- 円回内筋, 上腕頭 Pronator teres, humeral head
- 橈側手根屈筋 Flexor carpi radialis
- 長掌筋 Palmaris longus
- 円回内筋, 尺骨頭 Pronator teres, ulnar head
- 浅指屈筋 Flexor digitorum superficialis
- 尺側手根屈筋 Flexor carpi ulnaris
- 浅指屈筋の腱 Flexor digitorum superficialis tendons
- 尺骨動脈・神経 Ulnar a. and n.
- 屈筋支帯 Flexor retinaculum
- 小指球筋 Hypothenar muscles

図 22.38 前腕後部
回内位にある右前腕．前方から見たところ．肘筋と上腕三頭筋を反転し，尺側手根伸筋と[総]指伸筋を部分的に取り除いてある．

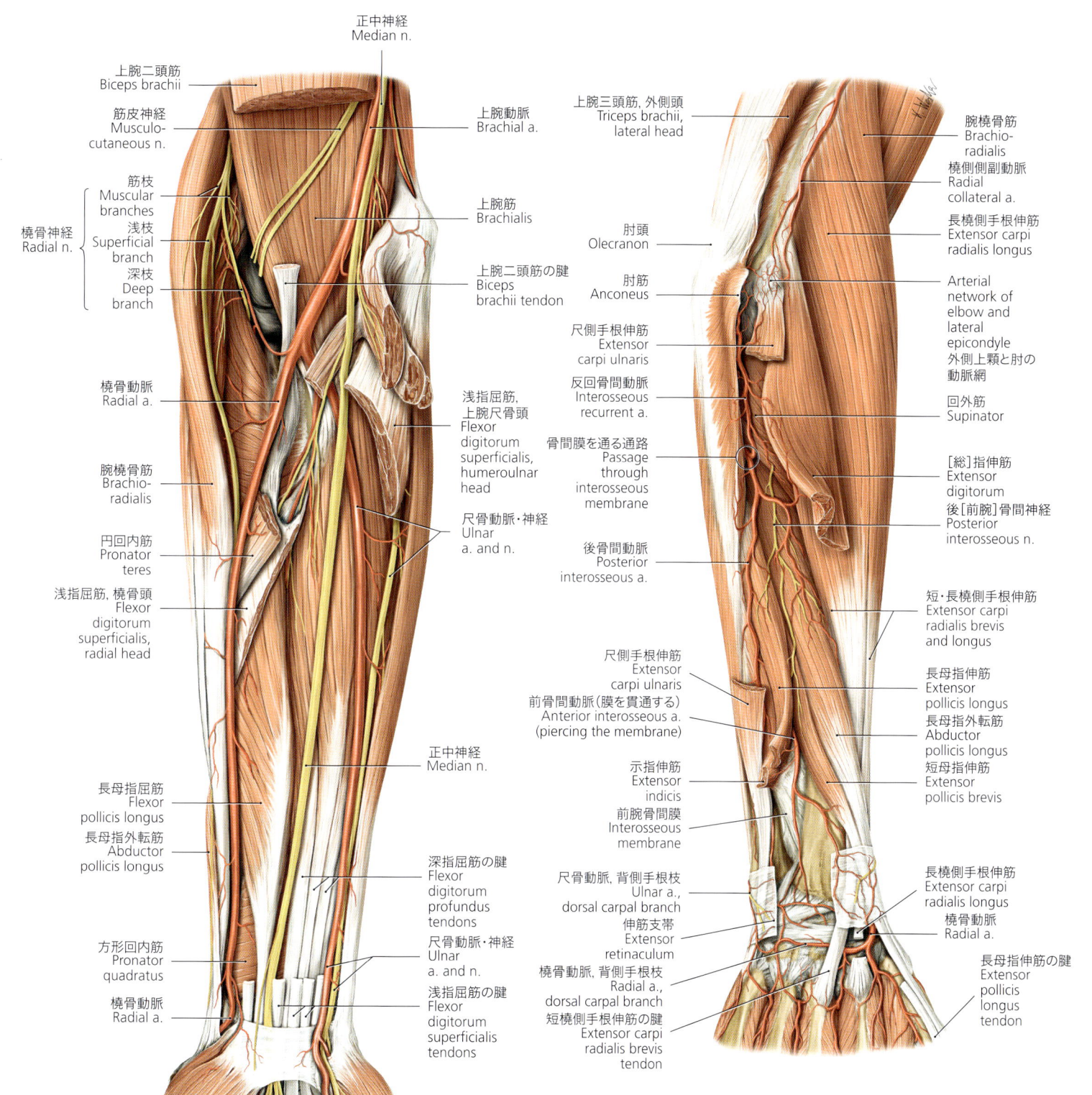

C 深層．浅指屈筋を部分的に取り除いたところ．

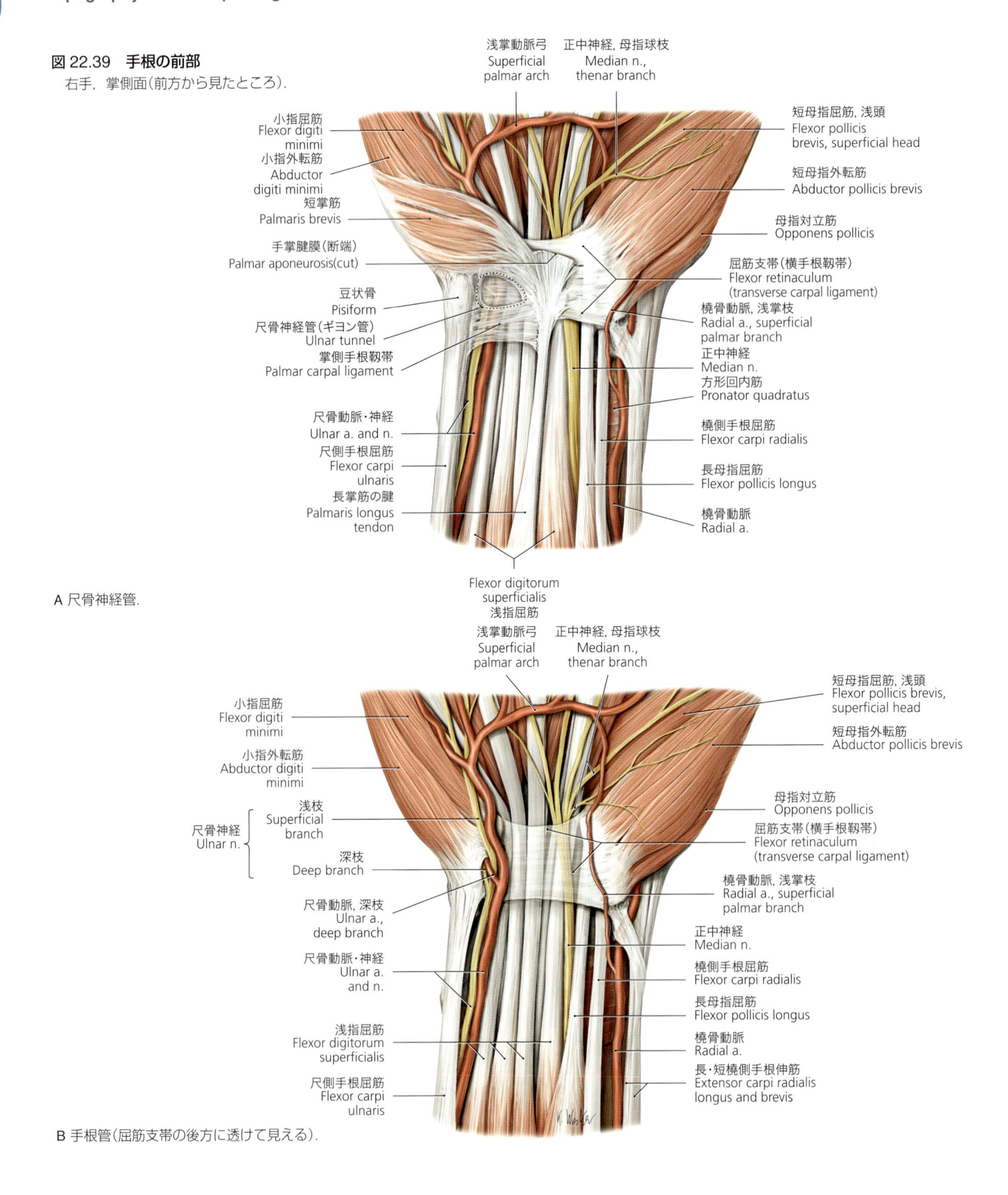

手根の局所解剖
Topography of the Carpal Region

図22.39 手根の前部
右手，掌側面（前方から見たところ）．

主なラベル（上図 A 尺骨神経管）：
- 浅掌動脈弓 Superficial palmar arch
- 正中神経, 母指球枝 Median n., thenar branch
- 小指屈筋 Flexor digiti minimi
- 小指外転筋 Abductor digiti minimi
- 短掌筋 Palmaris brevis
- 手掌腱膜（断端） Palmar aponeurosis (cut)
- 豆状骨 Pisiform
- 尺骨神経管（ギヨン管） Ulnar tunnel
- 掌側手根靱帯 Palmar carpal ligament
- 尺骨動脈・神経 Ulnar a. and n.
- 尺側手根屈筋 Flexor carpi ulnaris
- 長掌筋の腱 Palmaris longus tendon
- 浅指屈筋 Flexor digitorum superficialis
- 短母指屈筋, 浅頭 Flexor pollicis brevis, superficial head
- 短母指外転筋 Abductor pollicis brevis
- 母指対立筋 Opponens pollicis
- 屈筋支帯（横手根靱帯） Flexor retinaculum (transverse carpal ligament)
- 橈骨動脈, 浅掌枝 Radial a., superficial palmar branch
- 正中神経 Median n.
- 方形回内筋 Pronator quadratus
- 橈側手根屈筋 Flexor carpi radialis
- 長母指屈筋 Flexor pollicis longus
- 橈骨動脈 Radial a.

A 尺骨神経管.

主なラベル（下図 B 手根管）：
- 浅掌動脈弓 Superficial palmar arch
- 正中神経, 母指球枝 Median n., thenar branch
- 小指屈筋 Flexor digiti minimi
- 小指外転筋 Abductor digiti minimi
- 尺骨神経 Ulnar n.
  - 浅枝 Superficial branch
  - 深枝 Deep branch
- 尺骨動脈, 深枝 Ulnar a., deep branch
- 尺骨動脈・神経 Ulnar a. and n.
- 浅指屈筋 Flexor digitorum superficialis
- 尺側手根屈筋 Flexor carpi ulnaris
- 短母指屈筋, 浅頭 Flexor pollicis brevis, superficial head
- 短母指外転筋 Abductor pollicis brevis
- 母指対立筋 Opponens pollicis
- 屈筋支帯（横手根靱帯） Flexor retinaculum (transverse carpal ligament)
- 橈骨動脈, 浅掌枝 Radial a., superficial palmar branch
- 正中神経 Median n.
- 橈側手根屈筋 Flexor carpi radialis
- 長母指屈筋 Flexor pollicis longus
- 橈骨動脈 Radial a.
- 長・短橈側手根伸筋 Extensor carpi radialis longus and brevis

B 手根管（屈筋支帯の後方に透けて見える）．

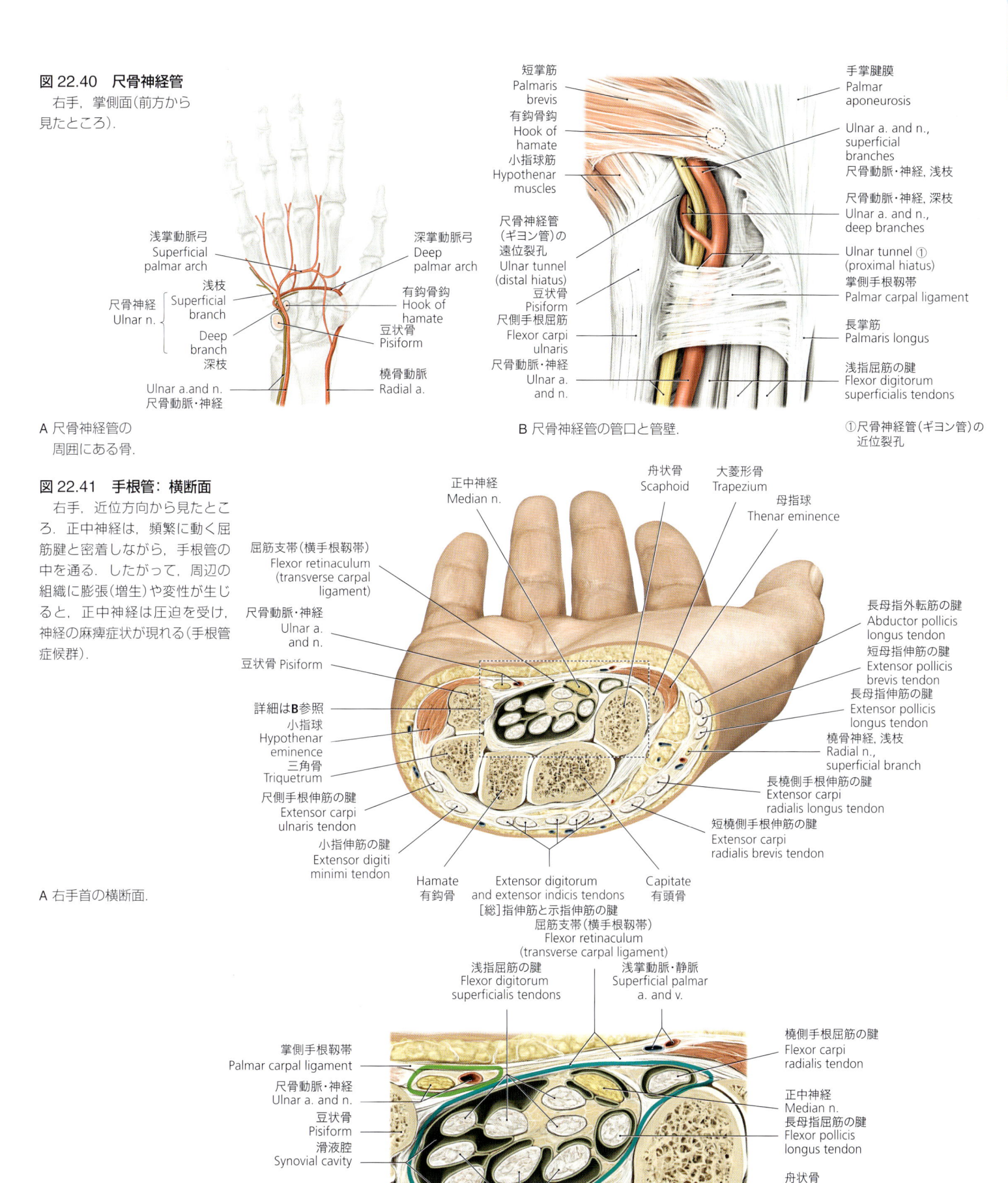

図 22.40 尺骨神経管
右手，掌側面（前方から見たところ）．

A 尺骨神経管の周囲にある骨．

- 浅掌動脈弓 Superficial palmar arch
- 深掌動脈弓 Deep palmar arch
- 尺骨神経 Ulnar n.
  - 浅枝 Superficial branch
  - 深枝 Deep branch
- 有鈎骨鈎 Hook of hamate
- 豆状骨 Pisiform
- 橈骨動脈 Radial a.
- Ulnar a. and n. 尺骨動脈・神経

B 尺骨神経管の管口と管壁．

- 短掌筋 Palmaris brevis
- 有鈎骨鈎 Hook of hamate
- 小指球筋 Hypothenar muscles
- 尺骨神経管（ギヨン管）の遠位裂孔 Ulnar tunnel (distal hiatus)
- 豆状骨 Pisiform
- 尺側手根屈筋 Flexor carpi ulnaris
- 尺骨動脈・神経 Ulnar a. and n.
- 手掌腱膜 Palmar aponeurosis
- 尺骨動脈・神経，浅枝 Ulnar a. and n., superficial branches
- 尺骨動脈・神経，深枝 Ulnar a. and n., deep branches
- Ulnar tunnel ① (proximal hiatus)
- 掌側手根靱帯 Palmar carpal ligament
- 長掌筋 Palmaris longus
- 浅指屈筋の腱 Flexor digitorum superficialis tendons

①尺骨神経管（ギヨン管）の近位裂孔

図 22.41 手根管：横断面
右手，近位方向から見たところ．正中神経は，頻繁に動く屈筋腱と密着しながら，手根管の中を通る．したがって，周辺の組織に膨張（増生）や変性が生じると，正中神経は圧迫を受け，神経の麻痺症状が現れる（手根管症候群）．

A 右手首の横断面．

- 正中神経 Median n.
- 舟状骨 Scaphoid
- 大菱形骨 Trapezium
- 母指球 Thenar eminence
- 屈筋支帯（横手根靱帯）Flexor retinaculum (transverse carpal ligament)
- 尺骨動脈・神経 Ulnar a. and n.
- 豆状骨 Pisiform
- 詳細はB参照
- 小指球 Hypothenar eminence
- 三角骨 Triquetrum
- 尺側手根屈筋の腱 Extensor carpi ulnaris tendon
- 小指伸筋の腱 Extensor digiti minimi tendon
- 有鈎骨 Hamate
- [総]指伸筋と示指伸筋の腱 Extensor digitorum and extensor indicis tendons
- 有頭骨 Capitate
- 短橈側手根伸筋の腱 Extensor carpi radialis brevis tendon
- 長橈側手根伸筋の腱 Extensor carpi radialis longus tendon
- 橈骨神経，浅枝 Radial n., superficial branch
- 長母指伸筋の腱 Extensor pollicis longus tendon
- 短母指伸筋の腱 Extensor pollicis brevis tendon
- 長母指外転筋の腱 Abductor pollicis longus tendon

B 尺骨神経管（緑）と手根管（青）を通る構造．

- 掌側手根靱帯 Palmar carpal ligament
- 尺骨動脈・神経 Ulnar a. and n.
- 豆状骨 Pisiform
- 滑液腔 Synovial cavity
- 三角骨 Triquetrum
- 有鈎骨 Hamate
- 深指屈筋の腱 Flexor digitorum profundus tendons
- 有頭骨 Capitate
- 浅指屈筋の腱 Flexor digitorum superficialis tendons
- 浅掌動脈・静脈 Superficial palmar a. and v.
- 橈側手根屈筋の腱 Flexor carpi radialis tendon
- 正中神経 Median n.
- 長母指屈筋の腱 Flexor pollicis longus tendon
- 舟状骨 Scaphoid

手掌の局所解剖
Topography of the Palm of the Hand

図 22.42 手掌浅層の神経と動脈
右手，前方から見たところ．

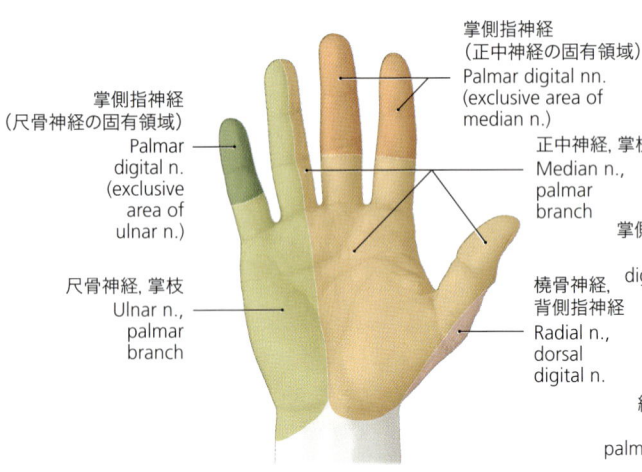

A 皮神経の分布領域．隣接する皮神経の分布領域は実際には広く重なっている．特定の皮神経だけが分布する領域（固有支配領域）を濃い色で示してある．

- 掌側指神経（尺骨神経の固有領域）Palmar digital n. (exclusive area of ulnar n.)
- 尺骨神経, 掌枝 Ulnar n., palmar branch
- 掌側指神経（正中神経の固有領域）Palmar digital nn. (exclusive area of median n.)
- 正中神経, 掌枝 Median n., palmar branch
- 橈骨神経, 背側指神経 Radial n., dorsal digital n.

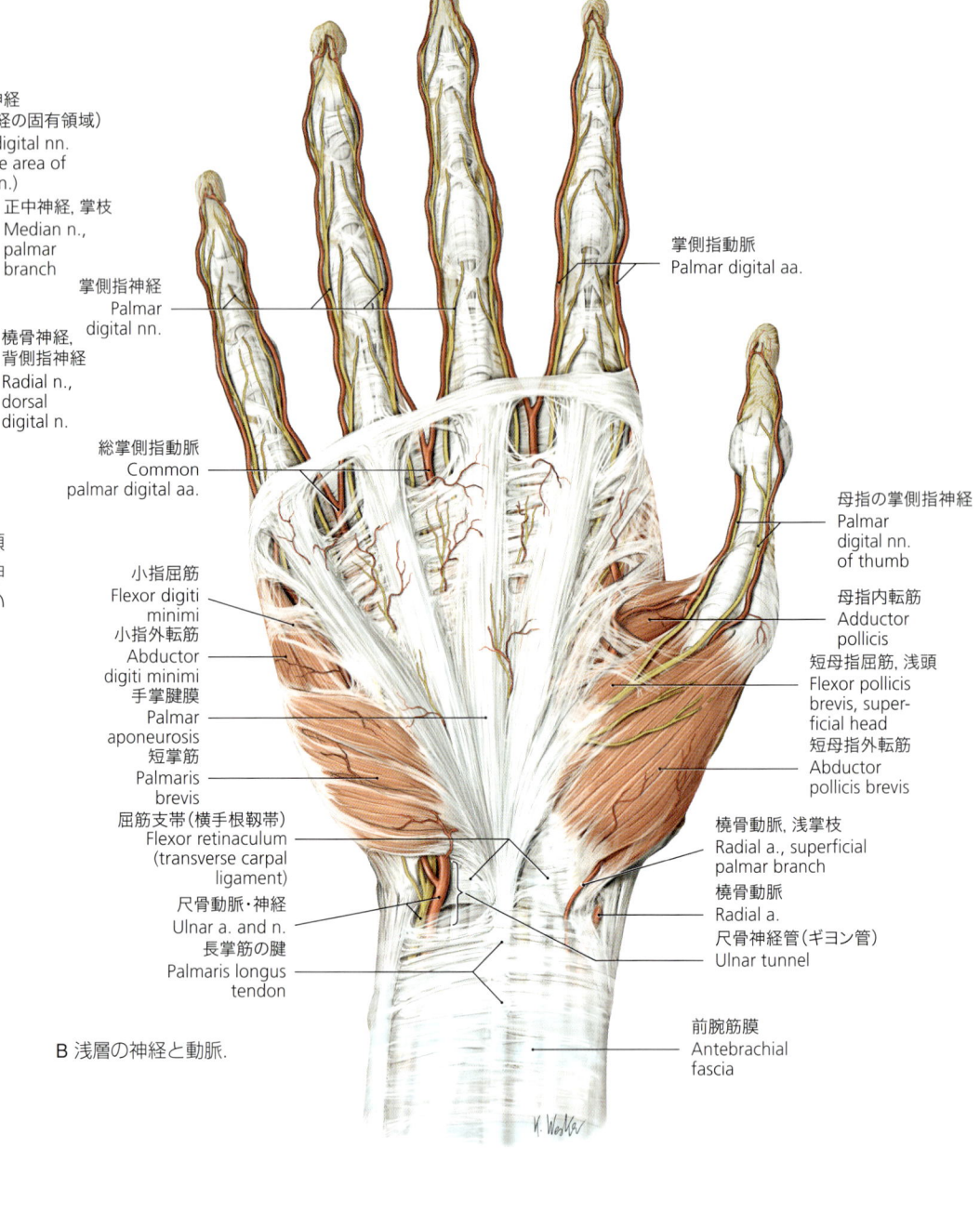

B 浅層の神経と動脈．

- 掌側指神経 Palmar digital nn.
- 掌側指動脈 Palmar digital aa.
- 総掌側指動脈 Common palmar digital aa.
- 母指の掌側指神経 Palmar digital nn. of thumb
- 小指屈筋 Flexor digiti minimi
- 小指外転筋 Abductor digiti minimi
- 手掌腱膜 Palmar aponeurosis
- 短掌筋 Palmaris brevis
- 屈筋支帯（横手根靱帯）Flexor retinaculum (transverse carpal ligament)
- 尺骨動脈・神経 Ulnar a. and n.
- 長掌筋の腱 Palmaris longus tendon
- 母指内転筋 Adductor pollicis
- 短母指屈筋, 浅頭 Flexor pollicis brevis, superficial head
- 短母指外転筋 Abductor pollicis brevis
- 橈骨動脈, 浅掌枝 Radial a., superficial palmar branch
- 橈骨動脈 Radial a.
- 尺骨神経管（ギヨン管）Ulnar tunnel
- 前腕筋膜 Antebrachial fascia

図 22.43 指の神経と動脈
右中指，外側方から見たところ．

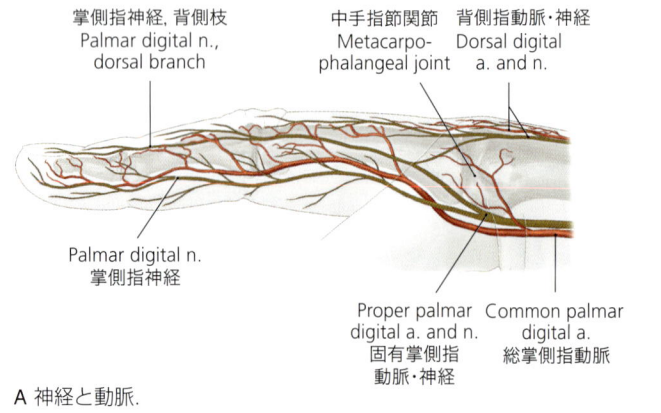

A 神経と動脈．

- 掌側指神経, 背側枝 Palmar digital n., dorsal branch
- 中手指節関節 Metacarpophalangeal joint
- 背側指動脈・神経 Dorsal digital a. and n.
- 掌側指神経 Palmar digital n.
- 固有掌側動脈・神経 Proper palmar digital a. and n.
- 総掌側指動脈 Common palmar digital a.

B 腱鞘内にある屈筋腱への動脈分布．

- 掌側指動脈 Palmar digital a.
- 掌側指枝 Digitopalmar branches
- 中手骨 Metacarpal
- 短いヒモ Vincula brevia
- 長いヒモ Vincula longa
- 深指屈筋 Flexor digitorum profundus
- 浅指屈筋 Flexor digitorum superficialis

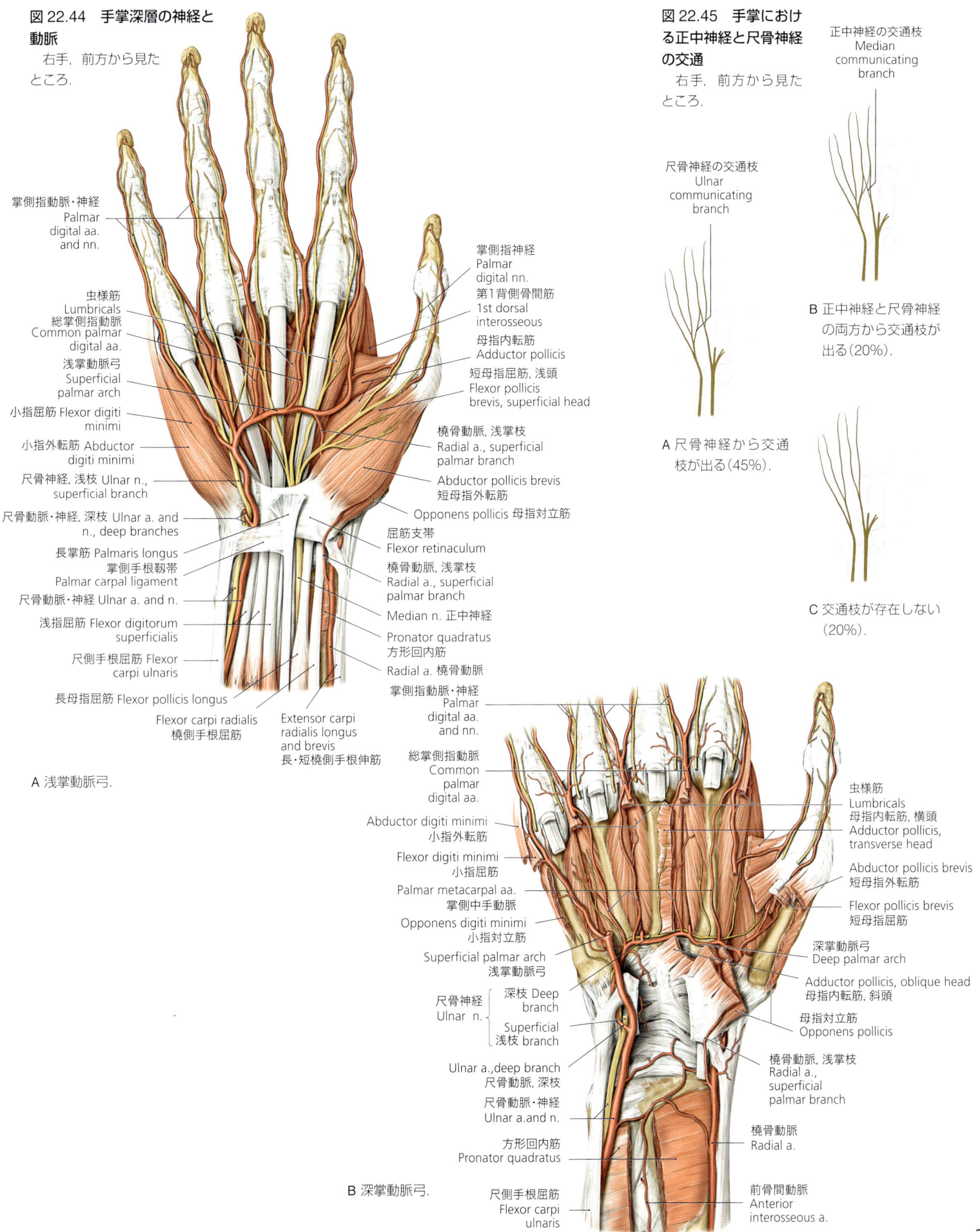

図 22.44 手掌深層の神経と動脈
右手，前方から見たところ．

- 掌側指動脈・神経 Palmar digital aa. and nn.
- 虫様筋 Lumbricals
- 総掌側指動脈 Common palmar digital aa.
- 浅掌動脈弓 Superficial palmar arch
- 小指屈筋 Flexor digiti minimi
- 小指外転筋 Abductor digiti minimi
- 尺骨神経，浅枝 Ulnar n., superficial branch
- 尺骨動脈・神経，深枝 Ulnar a. and n., deep branches
- 長掌筋 Palmaris longus
- 掌側手根靱帯 Palmar carpal ligament
- 尺骨動脈・神経 Ulnar a. and n.
- 浅指屈筋 Flexor digitorum superficialis
- 尺側手根屈筋 Flexor carpi ulnaris
- 長母指屈筋 Flexor pollicis longus
- Flexor carpi radialis 橈側手根屈筋
- Extensor carpi radialis longus and brevis 長・短橈側手根伸筋
- 掌側指神経 Palmar digital nn.
- 第1背側骨間筋 1st dorsal interosseous
- 母指内転筋 Adductor pollicis
- 短母指屈筋，浅頭 Flexor pollicis brevis, superficial head
- 橈骨動脈，浅掌枝 Radial a., superficial palmar branch
- Abductor pollicis brevis 短母指外転筋
- Opponens pollicis 母指対立筋
- 屈筋支帯 Flexor retinaculum
- 橈骨動脈，浅掌枝 Radial a., superficial palmar branch
- Median n. 正中神経
- Pronator quadratus 方形回内筋
- Radial a. 橈骨動脈

A 浅掌動脈弓．

図 22.45 手掌における正中神経と尺骨神経の交通
右手，前方から見たところ．

- 正中神経の交通枝 Median communicating branch
- 尺骨神経の交通枝 Ulnar communicating branch

A 尺骨神経から交通枝が出る (45%)．

B 正中神経と尺骨神経の両方から交通枝が出る (20%)．

C 交通枝が存在しない (20%)．

B 深掌動脈弓．

- 掌側指動脈・神経 Palmar digital aa. and nn.
- 総掌側指動脈 Common palmar digital aa.
- Abductor digiti minimi 小指外転筋
- Flexor digiti minimi 小指屈筋
- Palmar metacarpal aa. 掌側中手動脈
- Opponens digiti minimi 小指対立筋
- Superficial palmar arch 浅掌動脈弓
- 尺骨神経 Ulnar n. 深枝 Deep branch／浅枝 Superficial branch
- Ulnar a., deep branch 尺骨動脈，深枝
- 尺骨動脈・神経 Ulnar a. and n.
- 方形回内筋 Pronator quadratus
- 尺側手根屈筋 Flexor carpi ulnaris
- 虫様筋 Lumbricals
- 母指内転筋，横頭 Adductor pollicis, transverse head
- Abductor pollicis brevis 短母指外転筋
- Flexor pollicis brevis 短母指屈筋
- 深掌動脈弓 Deep palmar arch
- Adductor pollicis, oblique head 母指内転筋，斜頭
- 母指対立筋 Opponens pollicis
- 橈骨動脈，浅掌枝 Radial a., superficial palmar branch
- 橈骨動脈 Radial a.
- 前骨間動脈 Anterior interosseous a.

手背の局所解剖
Topography of the Dorsum of the Hand

図 22.46　手背における皮神経の分布
右手，背側面（後方から見たところ）．

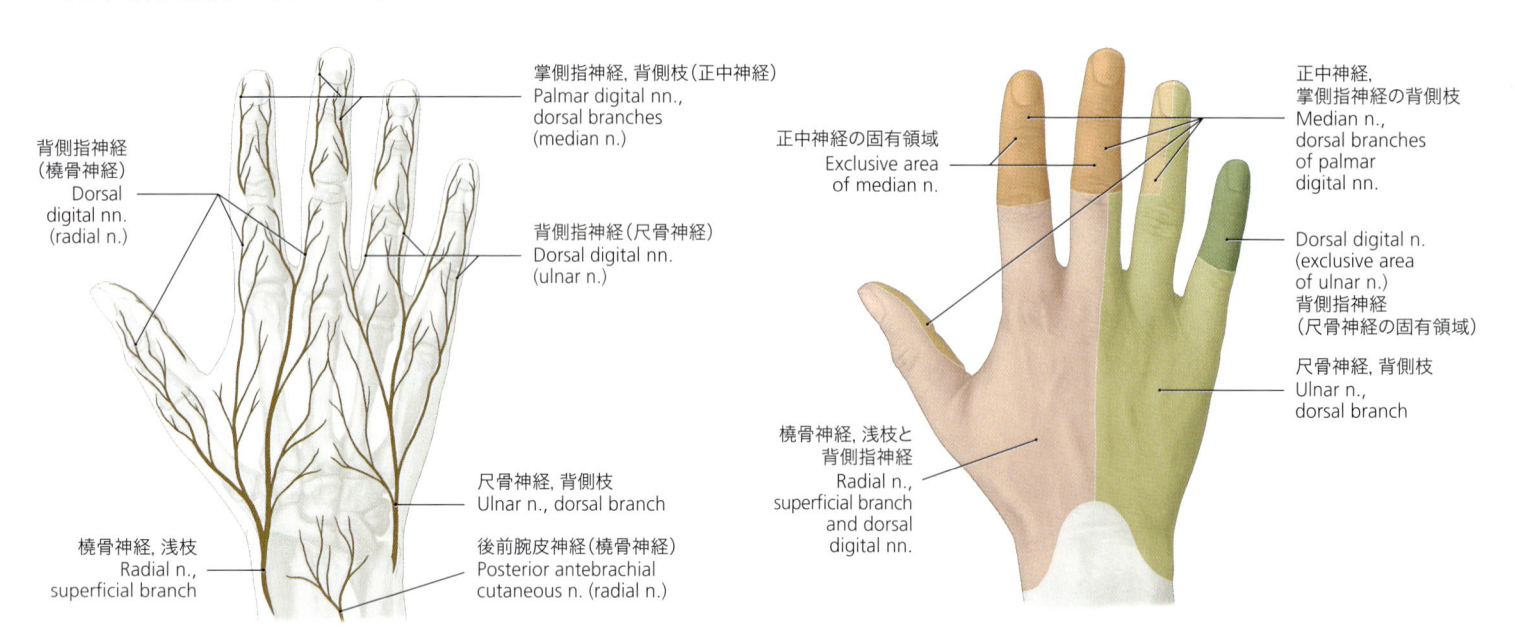

A 手背の皮神経．

- 背側指神経（橈骨神経）Dorsal digital nn. (radial n.)
- 掌側指神経, 背側枝（正中神経）Palmar digital nn., dorsal branches (median n.)
- 背側指神経（尺骨神経）Dorsal digital nn. (ulnar n.)
- 尺骨神経, 背側枝 Ulnar n., dorsal branch
- 橈骨神経, 浅枝 Radial n., superficial branch
- 後前腕皮神経（橈骨神経）Posterior antebrachial cutaneous n. (radial n.)

B 皮神経の分布領域．隣接する皮神経の分布領域は実際には広く重なっている．特定の皮神経だけが分布する領域（固有支配領域）を濃い色で示してある．

- 正中神経の固有領域 Exclusive area of median n.
- 正中神経, 掌側指神経の背側枝 Median n., dorsal branches of palmar digital nn.
- 背側指神経（尺骨神経の固有領域）Dorsal digital n. (exclusive area of ulnar n.)
- 尺骨神経, 背側枝 Ulnar n., dorsal branch
- 橈骨神経, 浅枝と背側指神経 Radial n., superficial branch and dorsal digital nn.

図 22.47　解剖学的嗅ぎタバコ入れ
右手，橈側面．"解剖学的嗅ぎタバコ入れ"は3方を囲まれたくぼみであり，背側の境界は長母指伸筋腱，掌側の境界は短母指伸筋腱と長母指外転筋腱によって作られる．

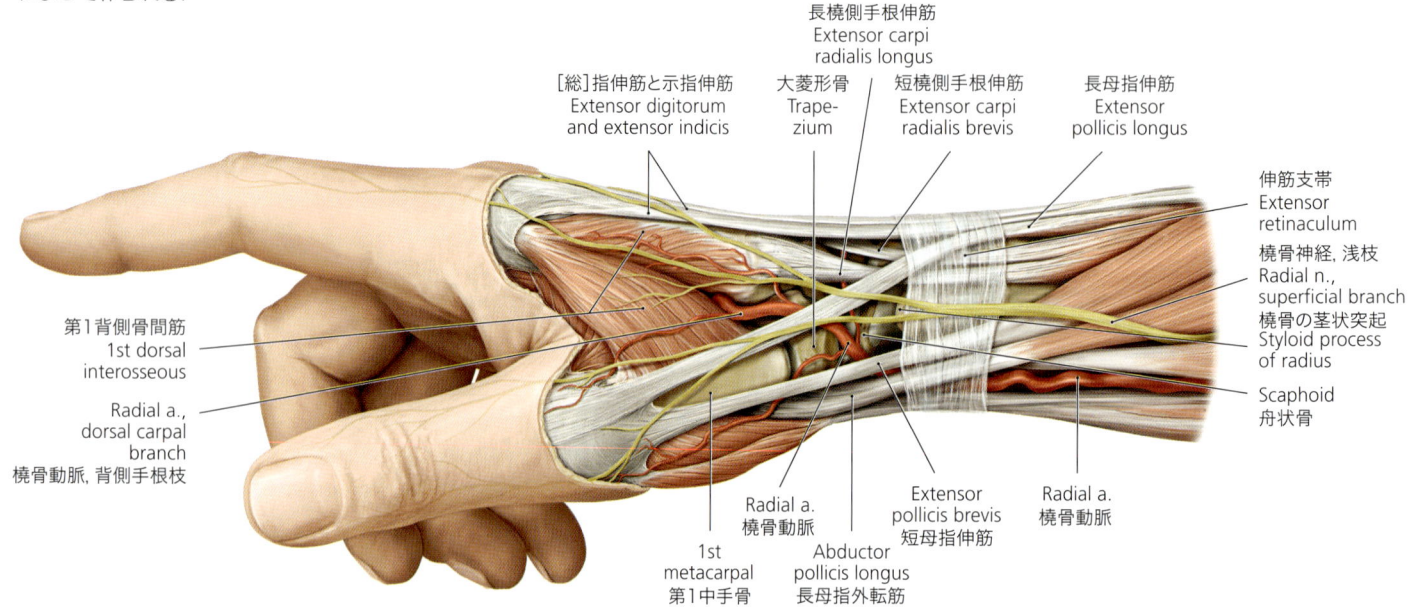

- [総]指伸筋と示指伸筋 Extensor digitorum and extensor indicis
- 長橈側手根伸筋 Extensor carpi radialis longus
- 大菱形骨 Trapezium
- 短橈側手根伸筋 Extensor carpi radialis brevis
- 長母指伸筋 Extensor pollicis longus
- 伸筋支帯 Extensor retinaculum
- 橈骨神経, 浅枝 Radial n., superficial branch
- 橈骨の茎状突起 Styloid process of radius
- 舟状骨 Scaphoid
- 橈骨動脈 Radial a.
- 短母指伸筋 Extensor pollicis brevis
- 長母指外転筋 Abductor pollicis longus
- 第1中手骨 1st metacarpal
- 橈骨動脈, 背側手根枝 Radial a., dorsal carpal branch
- 第1背側骨間筋 1st dorsal interosseous

図 22.48 手背の神経と動脈

A 浅層.

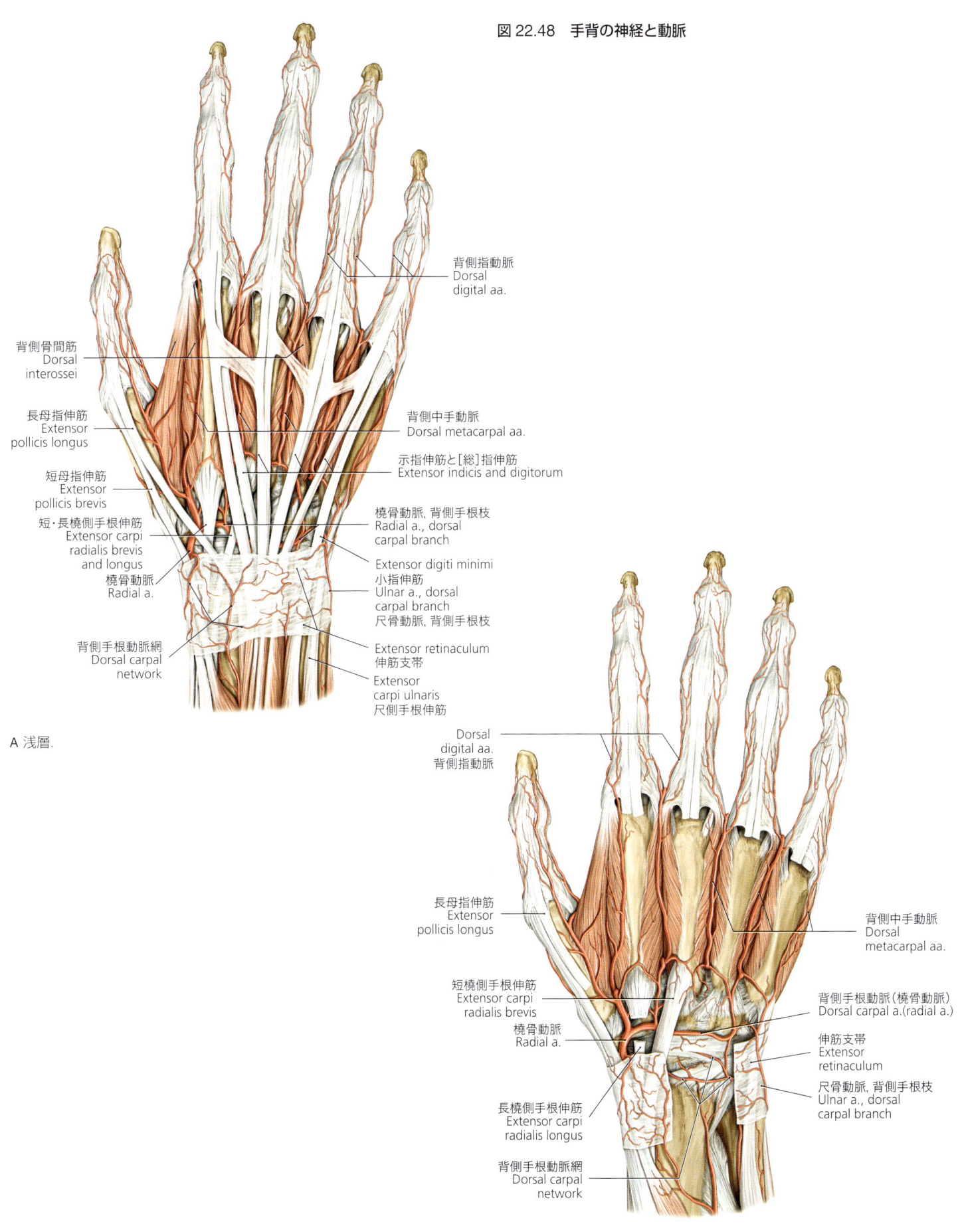

B 深層.

断面解剖
Transverse Sections

図 22.49 立体断面
右上肢，前方から見たところ．

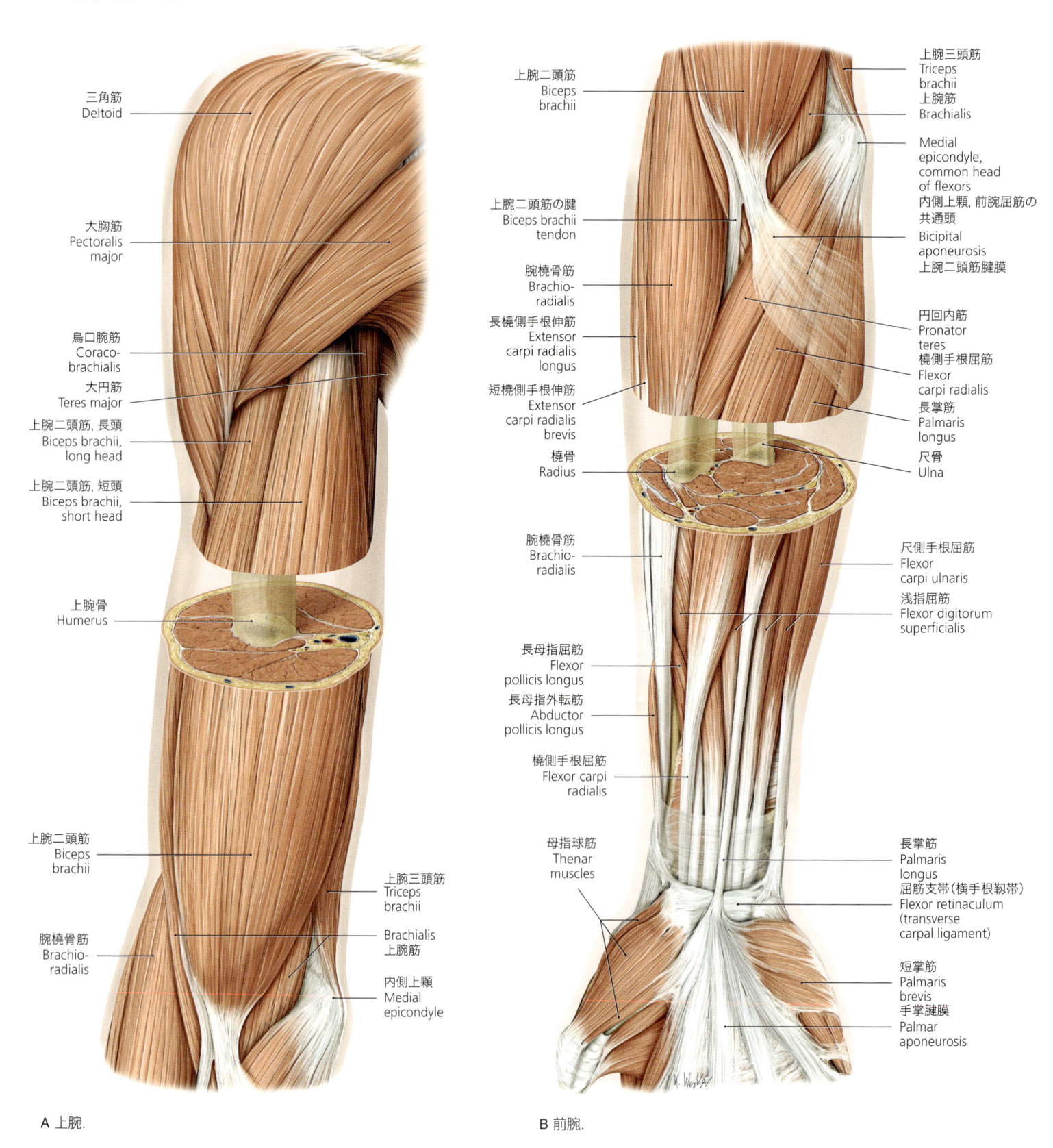

A 上腕．

- 三角筋 Deltoid
- 大胸筋 Pectoralis major
- 烏口腕筋 Coraco-brachialis
- 大円筋 Teres major
- 上腕二頭筋, 長頭 Biceps brachii, long head
- 上腕二頭筋, 短頭 Biceps brachii, short head
- 上腕骨 Humerus
- 上腕二頭筋 Biceps brachii
- 腕橈骨筋 Brachio-radialis
- 上腕三頭筋 Triceps brachii
- Brachialis 上腕筋
- 内側上顆 Medial epicondyle

B 前腕．

- 上腕二頭筋 Biceps brachii
- 上腕二頭筋の腱 Biceps brachii tendon
- 腕橈骨筋 Brachio-radialis
- 長橈側手根伸筋 Extensor carpi radialis longus
- 短橈側手根伸筋 Extensor carpi radialis brevis
- 橈骨 Radius
- 腕橈骨筋 Brachio-radialis
- 長母指屈筋 Flexor pollicis longus
- 長母指外転筋 Abductor pollicis longus
- 橈側手根屈筋 Flexor carpi radialis
- 母指球筋 Thenar muscles
- 上腕三頭筋 Triceps brachii
- 上腕筋 Brachialis
- 内側上顆, 前腕屈筋の共通頭 Medial epicondyle, common head of flexors
- 上腕二頭筋腱膜 Bicipital aponeurosis
- 円回内筋 Pronator teres
- 橈側手根屈筋 Flexor carpi radialis
- 長掌筋 Palmaris longus
- 尺骨 Ulna
- 尺側手根屈筋 Flexor carpi ulnaris
- 浅指屈筋 Flexor digitorum superficialis
- 長掌筋 Palmaris longus
- 屈筋支帯（横手根靱帯） Flexor retinaculum (transverse carpal ligament)
- 短掌筋 Palmaris brevis
- 手掌腱膜 Palmar aponeurosis

図 22.50 横断面
右上肢，近位方向（上方）から見たところ．

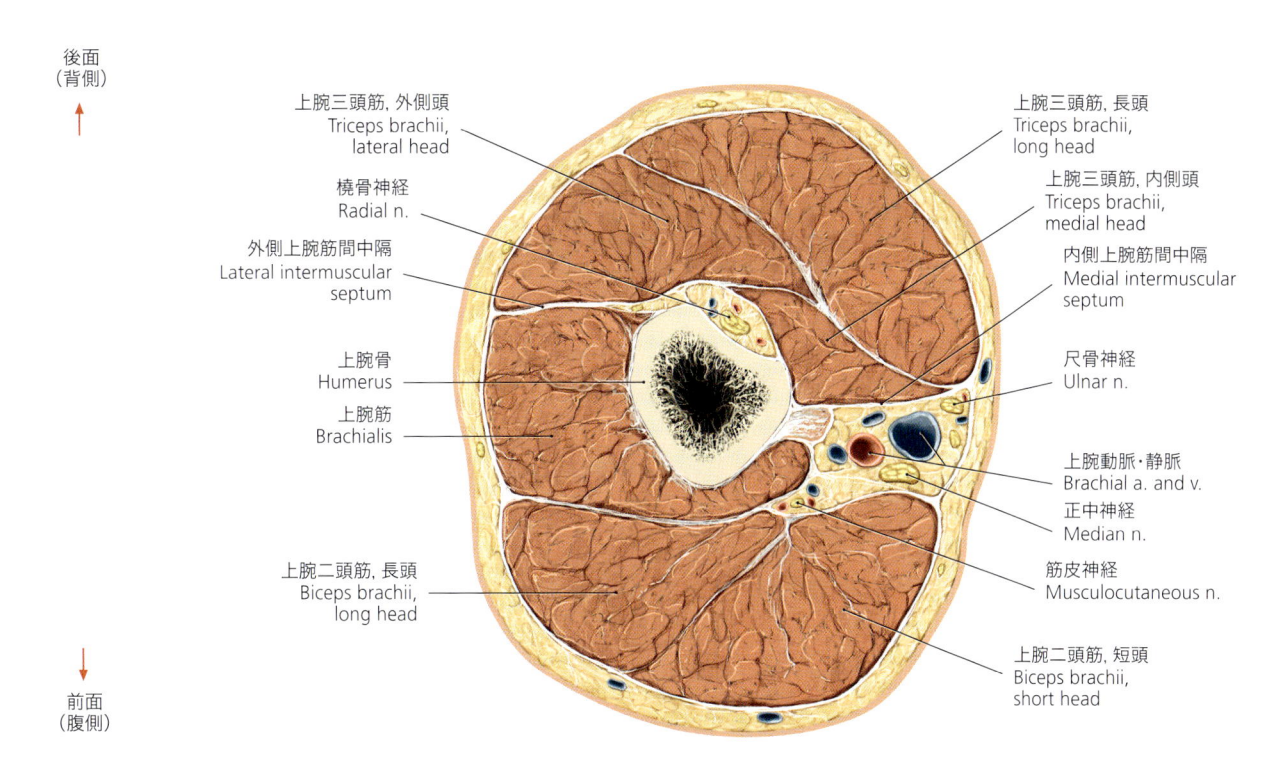

A 上腕（図 22.49A で示した断面）．

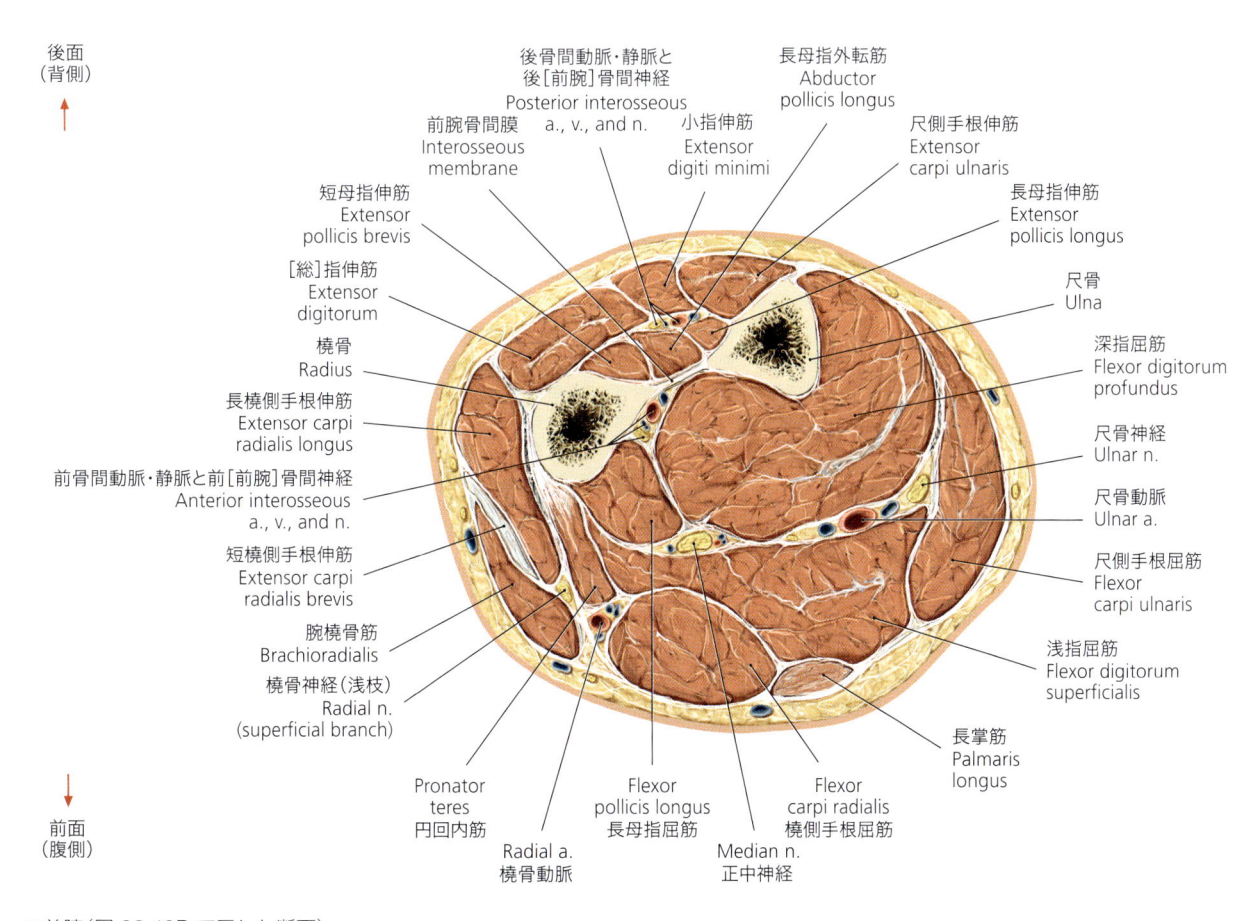

後面（背側）
前面（腹側）

上腕三頭筋，外側頭 Triceps brachii, lateral head
橈骨神経 Radial n.
外側上腕筋間中隔 Lateral intermuscular septum
上腕骨 Humerus
上腕筋 Brachialis
上腕二頭筋，長頭 Biceps brachii, long head
上腕三頭筋，長頭 Triceps brachii, long head
上腕三頭筋，内側頭 Triceps brachii, medial head
内側上腕筋間中隔 Medial intermuscular septum
尺骨神経 Ulnar n.
上腕動脈・静脈 Brachial a. and v.
正中神経 Median n.
筋皮神経 Musculocutaneous n.
上腕二頭筋，短頭 Biceps brachii, short head

B 前腕（図 22.49B で示した断面）．

後面（背側）
前面（腹側）

後骨間動脈・静脈と後［前腕］骨間神経 Posterior interosseous a., v., and n.
前腕骨間膜 Interosseous membrane
短母指伸筋 Extensor pollicis brevis
［総］指伸筋 Extensor digitorum
橈骨 Radius
長橈側手根伸筋 Extensor carpi radialis longus
前骨間動脈・静脈と前［前腕］骨間神経 Anterior interosseous a., v., and n.
短橈側手根伸筋 Extensor carpi radialis brevis
腕橈骨筋 Brachioradialis
橈骨神経（浅枝） Radial n. (superficial branch)
円回内筋 Pronator teres
橈骨動脈 Radial a.
長母指屈筋 Flexor pollicis longus
橈側手根屈筋 Flexor carpi radialis
正中神経 Median n.
小指伸筋 Extensor digiti minimi
長母指外転筋 Abductor pollicis longus
尺側手根伸筋 Extensor carpi ulnaris
長母指伸筋 Extensor pollicis longus
尺骨 Ulna
深指屈筋 Flexor digitorum profundus
尺骨神経 Ulnar n.
尺骨動脈 Ulnar a.
尺側手根屈筋 Flexor carpi ulnaris
浅指屈筋 Flexor digitorum superficialis
長掌筋 Palmaris longus

体表解剖 (1)
Surface Anatomy (I)

図 23.1 上肢：前方から見たところ

- 大胸筋 Pectoralis major
- 上腕二頭筋 Biceps brachii
- 尺側皮静脈 Basilic v.
- 肘正中皮静脈 Median cubital v.
- 尺側手根屈筋 Flexor carpi ulnaris
- 小指球 Hypothenar eminence
- 第1指（母指）1st digit (thumb)
- 手掌 Palm
- 第5指（小指）5th digit (little finger)

- 鎖骨 Clavicle
- 三角筋 Deltoid
- 橈側皮静脈（三角筋胸筋溝を通る）Cephalic v. (in deltopectoral groove)
- 上腕三頭筋, 外側頭 Triceps brachii, lateral head
- 橈側皮静脈 Cephalic v.
- 長橈側手根伸筋 Extensor carpi radialis longus
- Brachioradialis 腕橈骨筋
- 橈側手根屈筋 Flexor carpi radialis
- 長掌筋の腱 Palmaris longus tendon
- 母指球 Thenar eminence
- 手掌静脈網 Palmer venous network

A 体表解剖, 右上肢.

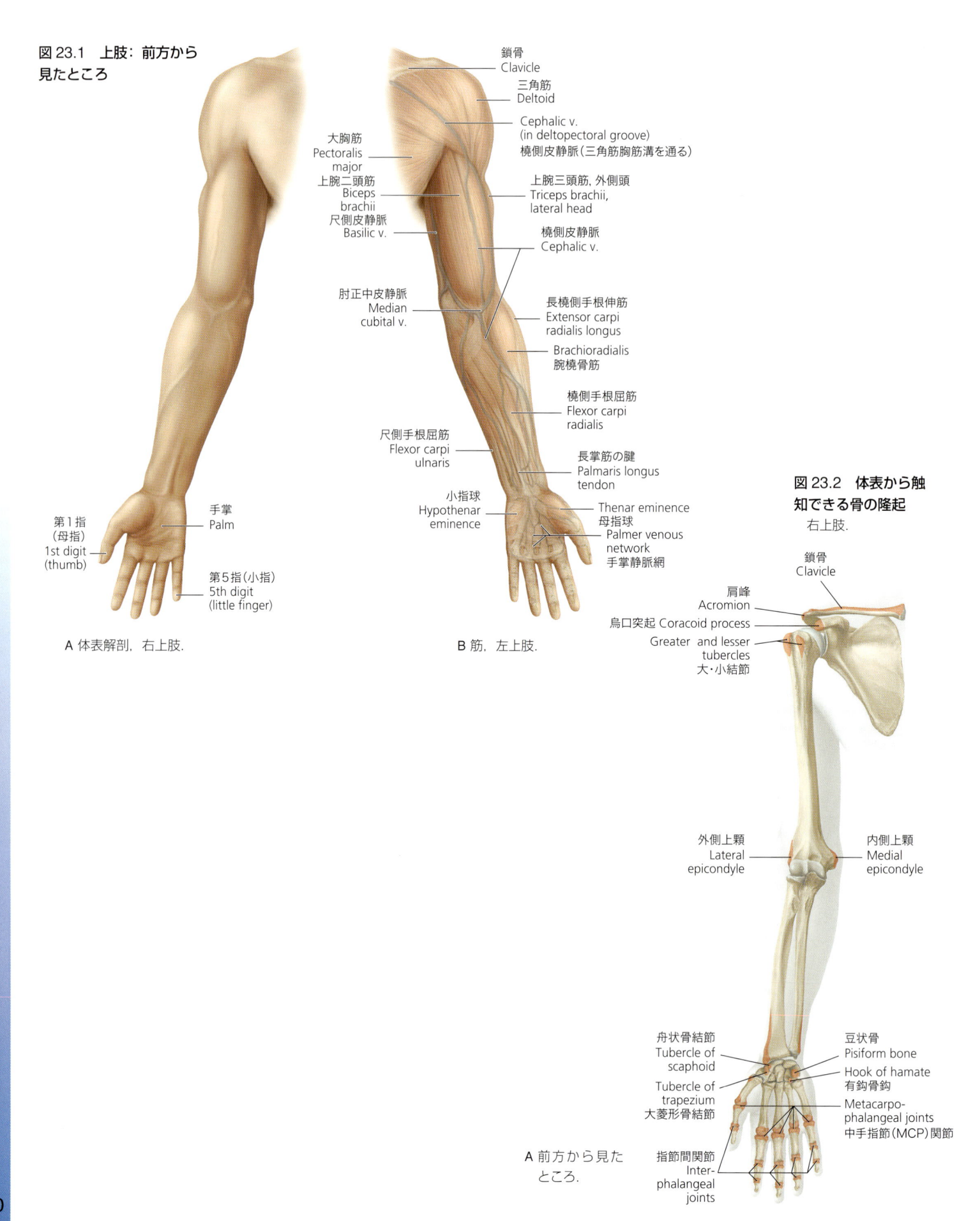

B 筋, 左上肢.

図 23.2 体表から触知できる骨の隆起
右上肢.

- 鎖骨 Clavicle
- 肩峰 Acromion
- 烏口突起 Coracoid process
- 大・小結節 Greater and lesser tubercles
- 外側上顆 Lateral epicondyle
- 内側上顆 Medial epicondyle
- 舟状骨結節 Tubercle of scaphoid
- 大菱形骨結節 Tubercle of trapezium
- 豆状骨 Pisiform bone
- 有鉤骨鉤 Hook of hamate
- 中手指節（MCP）関節 Metacarpophalangeal joints
- 指節間関節 Interphalangeal joints

A 前方から見たところ.

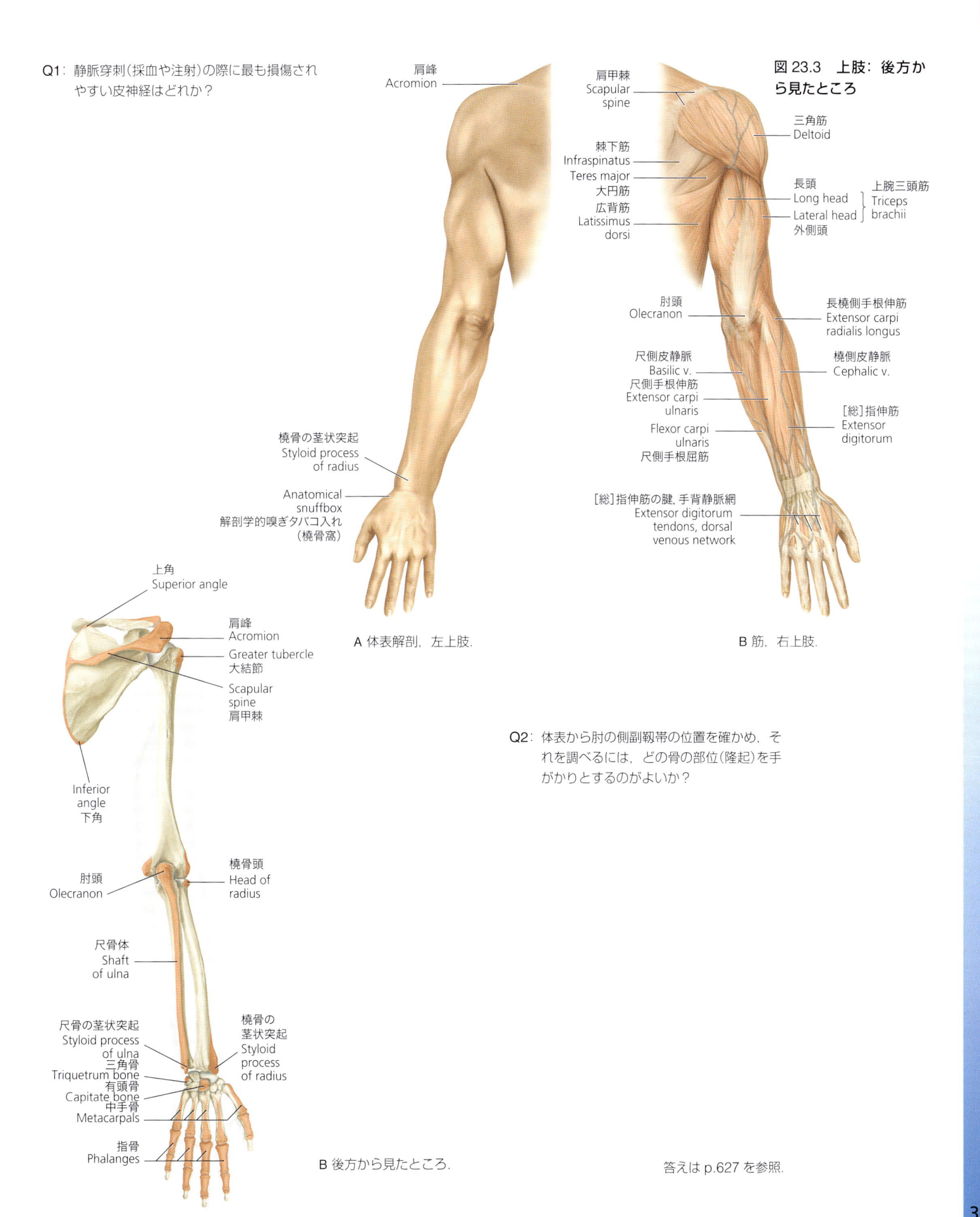

Q1: 静脈穿刺（採血や注射）の際に最も損傷されやすい皮神経はどれか？

図 23.3　上肢：後方から見たところ

肩峰 Acromion
肩甲棘 Scapular spine
三角筋 Deltoid
棘下筋 Infraspinatus
大円筋 Teres major
広背筋 Latissimus dorsi
長頭 Long head
外側頭 Lateral head
上腕三頭筋 Triceps brachii
肘頭 Olecranon
長橈側手根伸筋 Extensor carpi radialis longus
尺側皮静脈 Basilic v.
橈側皮静脈 Cephalic v.
尺側手根伸筋 Extensor carpi ulnaris
尺側手根屈筋 Flexor carpi ulnaris
[総]指伸筋 Extensor digitorum
橈骨の茎状突起 Styloid process of radius
解剖学的嗅ぎタバコ入れ（橈骨窩） Anatomical snuffbox
[総]指伸筋の腱，手背静脈網 Extensor digitorum tendons, dorsal venous network

A　体表解剖，左上肢．

B　筋，右上肢．

上角 Superior angle
肩峰 Acromion
大結節 Greater tubercle
肩甲棘 Scapular spine
下角 Inferior angle
肘頭 Olecranon
橈骨頭 Head of radius
尺骨体 Shaft of ulna
尺骨の茎状突起 Styloid process of ulna
橈骨の茎状突起 Styloid process of radius
三角骨 Triquetrum bone
有頭骨 Capitate bone
中手骨 Metacarpals
指骨 Phalanges

B　後方から見たところ．

Q2: 体表から肘の側副靭帯の位置を確かめ，それを調べるには，どの骨の部位（隆起）を手がかりとするのがよいか？

答えは p.627 を参照．

体表解剖(2)
Surface Anatomy (II)

図 23.4 体表から触知できる骨の隆起
左手.

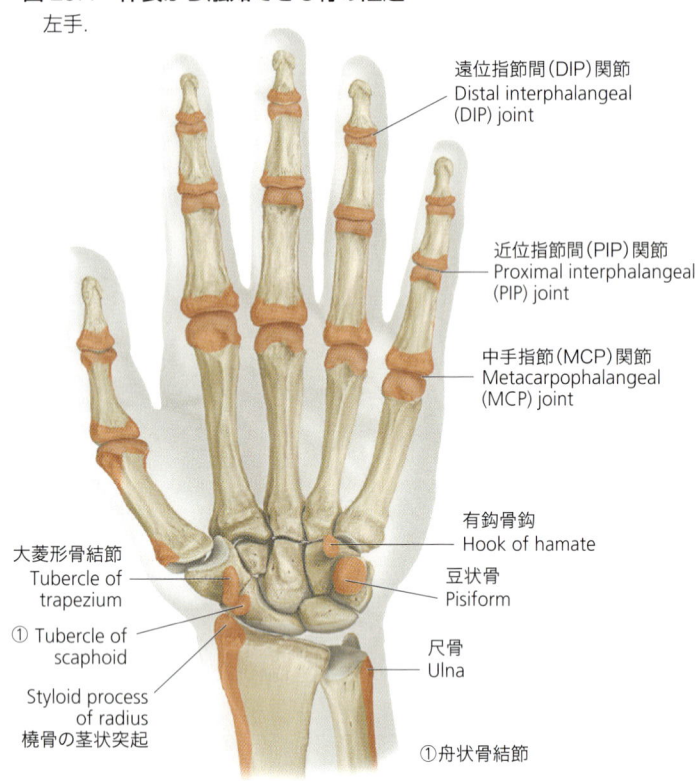

- 遠位指節間(DIP)関節 Distal interphalangeal (DIP) joint
- 近位指節間(PIP)関節 Proximal interphalangeal (PIP) joint
- 中手指節(MCP)関節 Metacarpophalangeal (MCP) joint
- 有鈎骨鈎 Hook of hamate
- 豆状骨 Pisiform
- 尺骨 Ulna
- ①舟状骨結節
- 大菱形骨結節 Tubercle of trapezium
- ①舟状骨結節 Tubercle of scaphoid
- 橈骨の茎状突起 Styloid process of radius

A 掌側面(前方から見たところ).

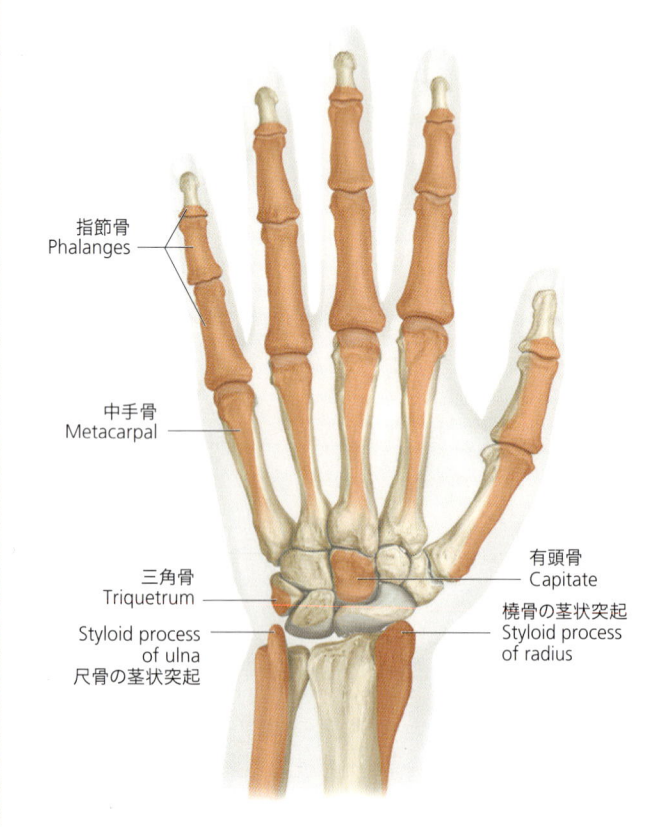

- 指節骨 Phalanges
- 中手骨 Metacarpal
- 三角骨 Triquetrum
- 尺骨の茎状突起 Styloid process of ulna
- 有頭骨 Capitate
- 橈骨の茎状突起 Styloid process of radius

B 背側面(後方から見たところ).

図 23.5 手首の体表解剖
左手首,前外側方から見たところ.

- 小指球 Hypothenar eminence
- 豆状骨 Pisiform
- 尺側手根屈筋の腱 Flexor carpi ulnaris tendon
- 母指球 Thenar eminence
- 長掌筋の腱 Palmaris longus tendon
- 橈側手根屈筋の腱 Flexor carpi radialis tendon

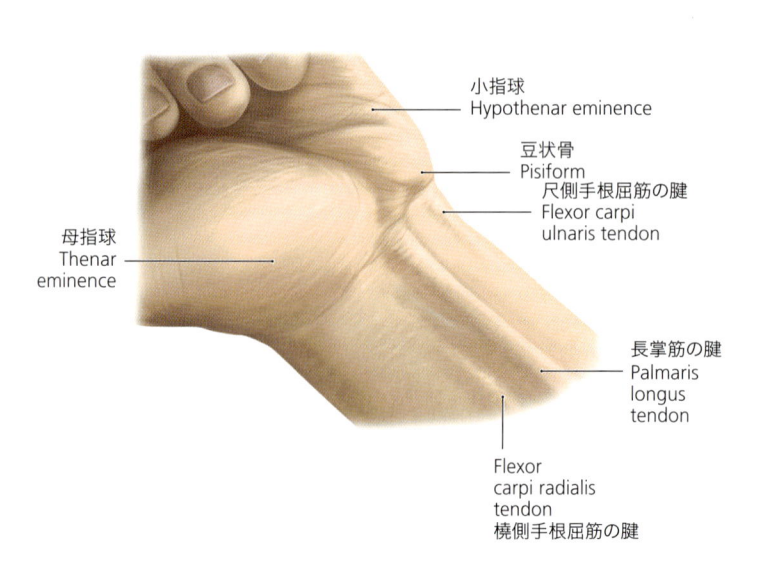

Q3:手首における重要な動脈や神経の位置を知るためには,手首で触知できる腱をどのように利用したらよいか?

図 23.6 解剖学的嗅ぎタバコ入れ
左手,後外側方から見たところ.

- [総]指伸筋の腱,手背静脈網 Extensor digitorum tendons, dorsal venous network
- 示指伸筋の腱 Extensor indicis tendon
- 第1背側骨間筋 1st dorsal interosseus
- 長母指伸筋 Extensor pollicis longus
- 第1中手骨頭 Head of 1st metacarpal
- 長母指伸筋 Extensor pollicis longus
- 橈骨の茎状突起 Styloid process of radius
- 解剖学的嗅ぎタバコ入れ(橈骨窩) Anatomic snuffbox

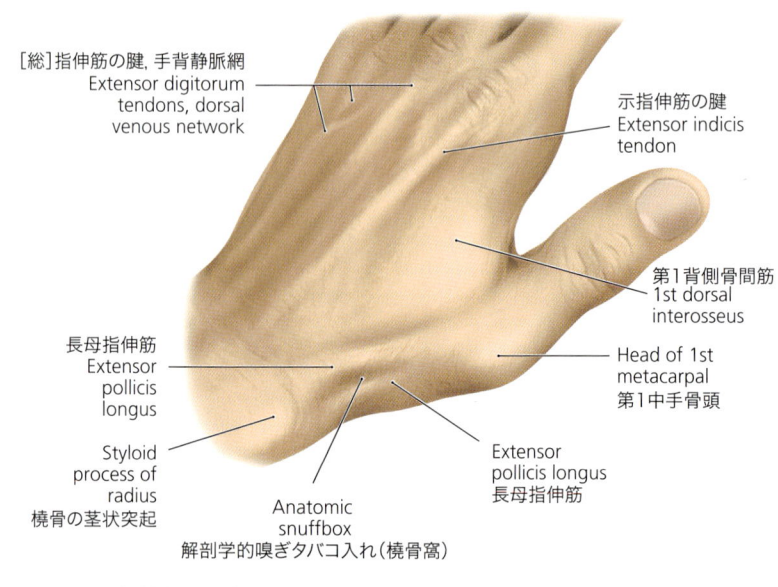

Q4:解剖学的嗅ぎタバコ入れの底に圧痛を感じる場合,どの手根骨の骨折が疑われるか?

答えは p.627 を参照.

図 23.7　手掌

- 遠位指節間関節線 DIP joint crease
- 近位指節間関節線 PIP joint crease
- 中手指節関節線 MCP joint crease
- 指節間関節線 IP joint crease
- 中手指節関節線 MCP joint crease
- 母指球 Thenar eminence
- Thenar crease ("life line") 母指線 ("生命線")
- 遠位横手掌線 Distal transverse crease
- 近位横手掌線 Proximal transverse crease
- 中位手掌線 Middle crease
- 小指球 Hypothenar eminence
- 遠位手根線 Distal wrist crease
- 近位手根線 Proximal wrist crease

- 手掌静脈網 Palmar venous network
- 短掌筋 Palmaris brevis
- 豆状骨 Pisiform
- 長掌筋の腱 Palmaris longus tendon
- 短母指屈筋 Flexor pollicis brevis
- 短母指外転筋 Abductor pollicis brevis
- 大菱形骨結節 Tubercle of trapezium

A 体表解剖，左手．　　B 筋，右手．

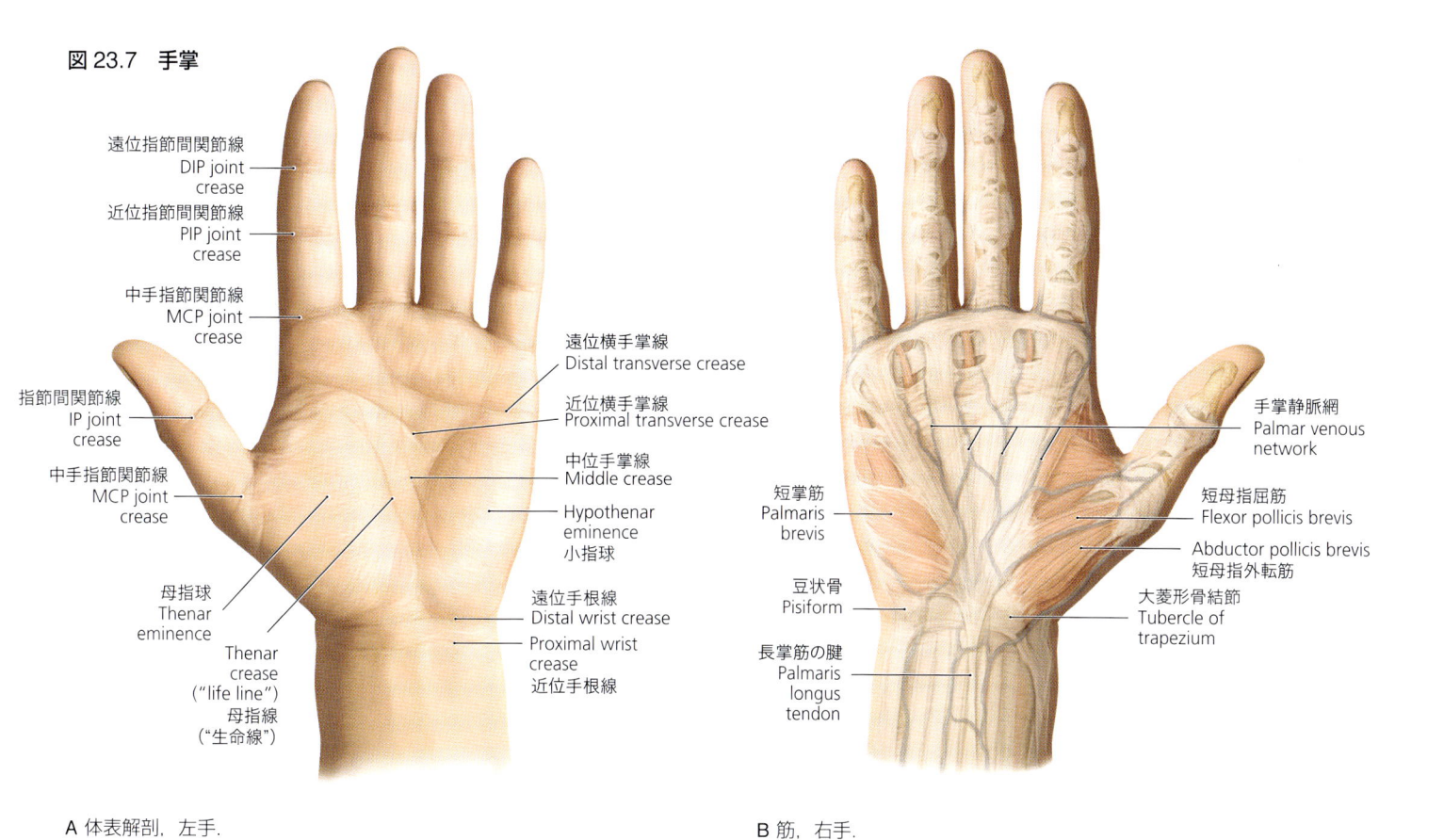

図 23.8　手背

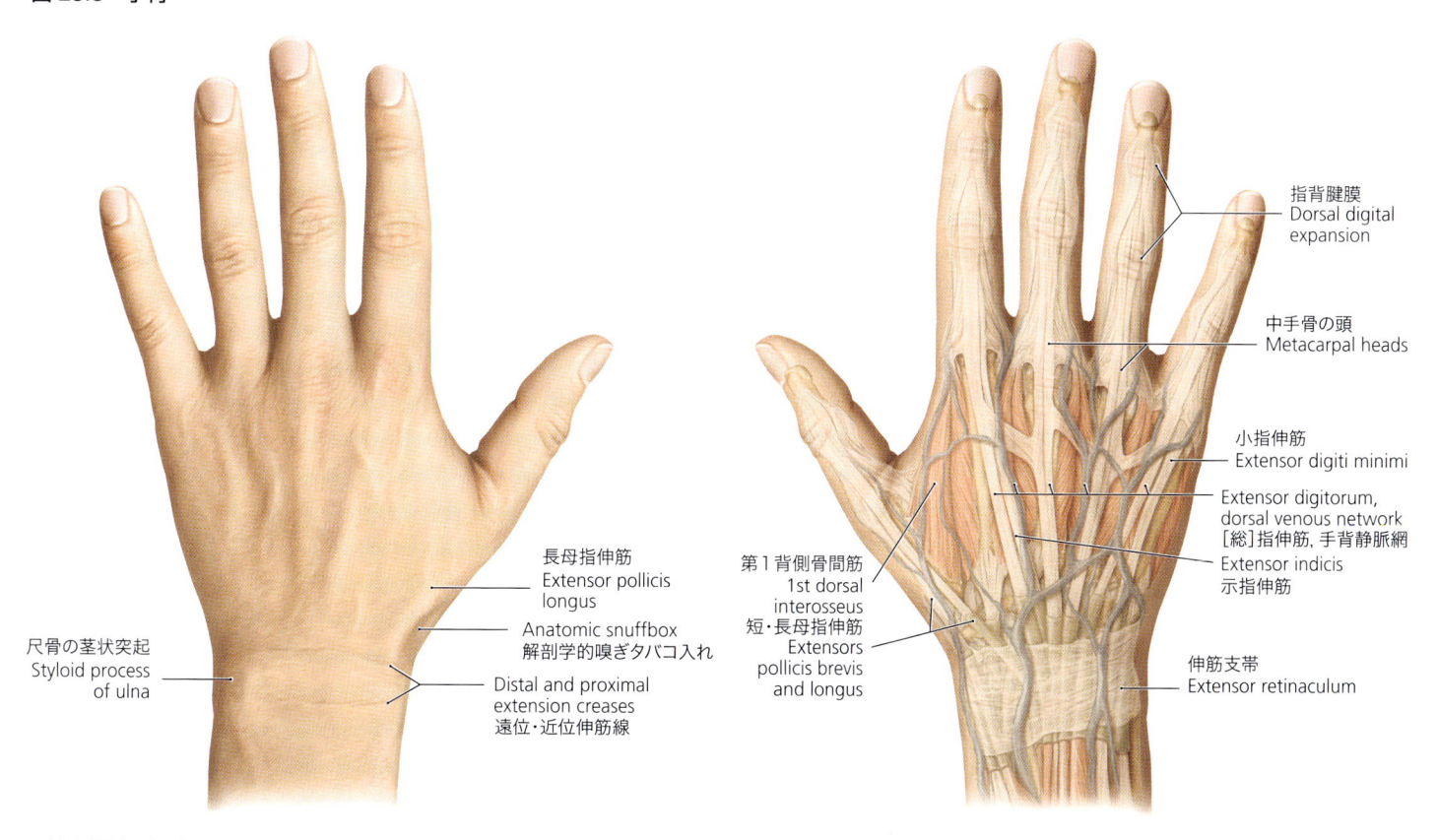

- 長母指伸筋 Extensor pollicis longus
- 解剖学的嗅ぎタバコ入れ Anatomic snuffbox
- 尺骨の茎状突起 Styloid process of ulna
- 遠位・近位伸筋線 Distal and proximal extension creases

- 指背腱膜 Dorsal digital expansion
- 中手骨の頭 Metacarpal heads
- 小指伸筋 Extensor digiti minimi
- [総]指伸筋, 手背静脈網 Extensor digitorum, dorsal venous network
- 示指伸筋 Extensor indicis
- 第1背側骨間筋 1st dorsal interosseus
- 短・長母指伸筋 Extensors pollicis brevis and longus
- 伸筋支帯 Extensor retinaculum

A 体表解剖，左手．　　B 筋，右手．

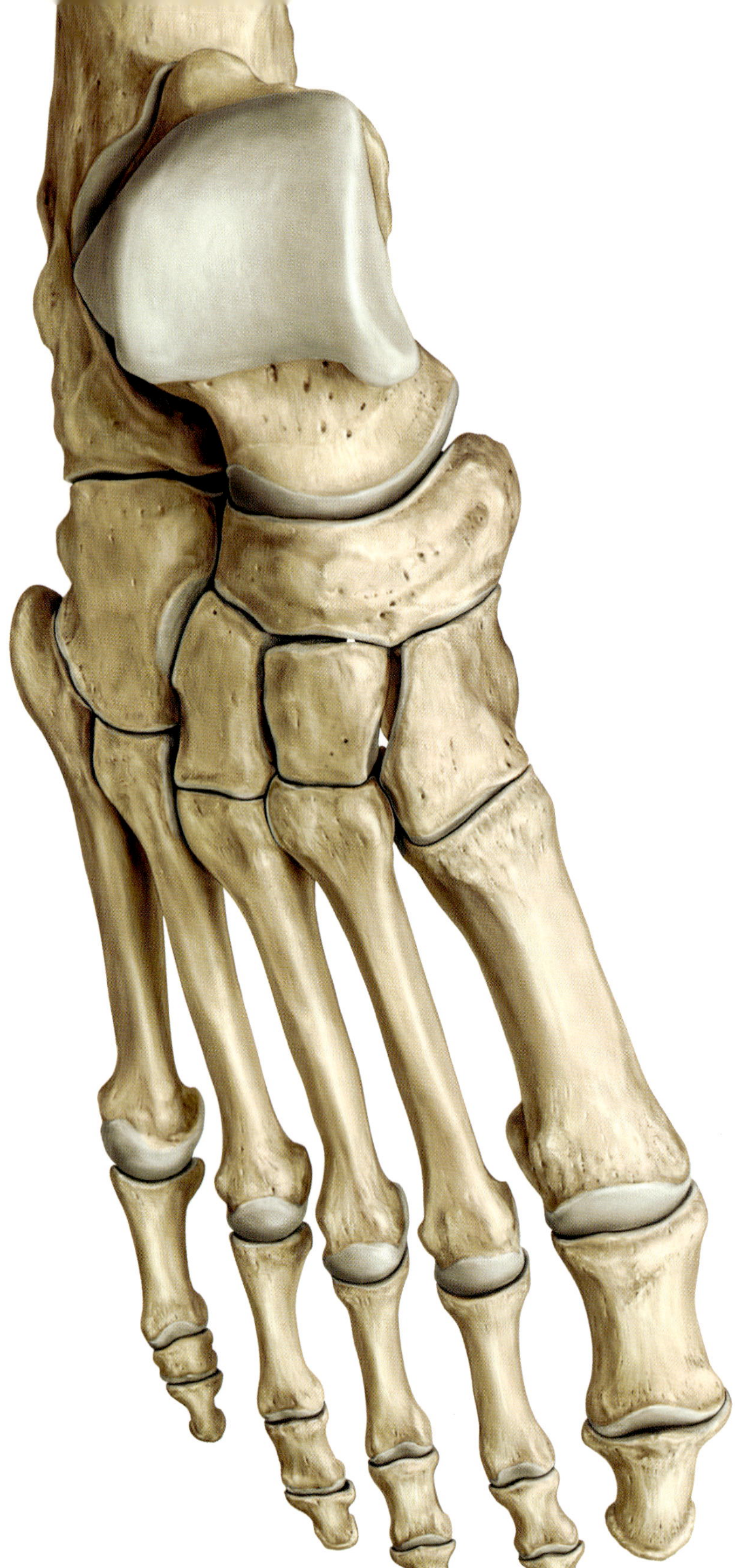

下 肢
Lower Limb

24. 骨盤と大腿
- 下肢の骨 …… 356
- 下肢帯と寛骨 …… 358
- 大腿骨 …… 360
- 股関節：概観 …… 362
- 股関節：靭帯と関節包 …… 364
- 骨盤部と大腿の前面にある筋(1) …… 366
- 骨盤部と大腿の前面にある筋(2) …… 368
- 骨盤部と大腿の後面にある筋(1) …… 370
- 骨盤部と大腿の後面にある筋(2) …… 372
- 個々の筋(1) …… 374
- 個々の筋(2) …… 376
- 個々の筋(3) …… 378

25. 膝と下腿
- 脛骨と腓骨 …… 380
- 膝関節：概観 …… 382
- 膝関節：靭帯，関節包，滑液包 …… 384
- 膝関節：靭帯と半月 …… 386
- 十字靭帯 …… 388
- 膝関節腔 …… 390
- 下腿の前面と外側面にある筋 …… 392
- 下腿の後面にある筋 …… 394
- 個々の筋(1) …… 396
- 個々の筋(2) …… 398

26. 足首と足
- 足の骨 …… 400
- 足の関節(1) …… 402
- 足の関節(2) …… 404
- 足の関節(3) …… 406
- 足首と足の靭帯 …… 408
- 土踏まずと足底弓 …… 410
- 足底の筋 …… 412
- 足の筋と腱鞘 …… 414
- 個々の筋(1) …… 416
- 個々の筋(2) …… 418

27. 神経と脈管
- 下肢の動脈 …… 420
- 下肢の静脈とリンパ管 …… 422
- 腰仙骨神経叢 …… 424
- 腰神経叢の枝 …… 426
- 腰神経叢の枝：閉鎖神経と大腿神経 …… 428
- 仙骨神経叢の枝 …… 430
- 仙骨神経叢の枝：坐骨神経 …… 432
- 下肢の皮神経と皮静脈 …… 434
- 鼡径部の局所解剖 …… 436
- 殿部の局所解剖 …… 438
- 大腿の前面と後面の局所解剖 …… 440
- 下腿の後面と内側面の局所解剖 …… 442
- 下腿の外側面と前面の局所解剖 …… 444
- 足底の局所解剖 …… 446
- 大腿と下腿の断面解剖 …… 448

28. 体表解剖
- 体表解剖 …… 450

下肢の骨
Bones of the Lower Limb

図 24.1　下肢の骨
右下肢．下肢の骨格は，下肢帯とそれに連結する自由下肢からなる．自由下肢は大腿（大腿骨），下腿（脛骨と腓骨），足に分かれる．自由下肢は股関節によって下肢帯と連結する．

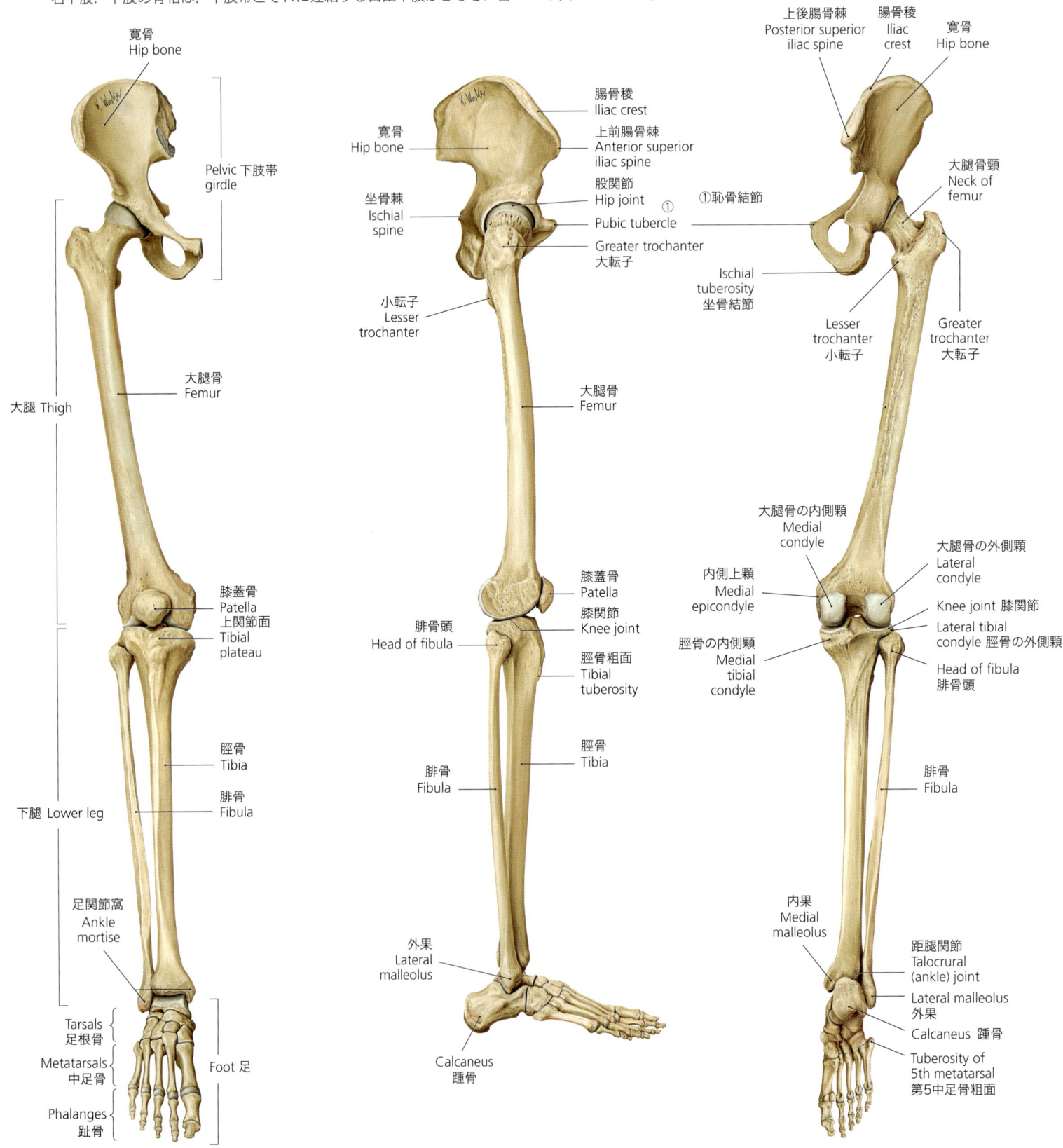

A 前方から見たところ．

B 右外側方から見たところ．

C 後方から見たところ．

図 24.2 重心線

右外側方から見たところ．重心線は重心から垂直に下り，特定の点を通過して地表面にいたる．

- 外耳道 External auditory canal
- 軸椎の歯突起（第2頸椎） Dens of axis (C2)
- 脊柱の弯曲点 Inflection points of vertebral column
- 重心 Center of gravity
- 股関節 Hip joint
- 膝関節 Knee joint
- 足関節 Ankle joint

図 24.3 体表から触知できる骨の隆起

下肢の骨の多くは，皮膚や軟部組織を介して触知できる隆起や縁，面（例えば，脛骨の内側面）を持っている．

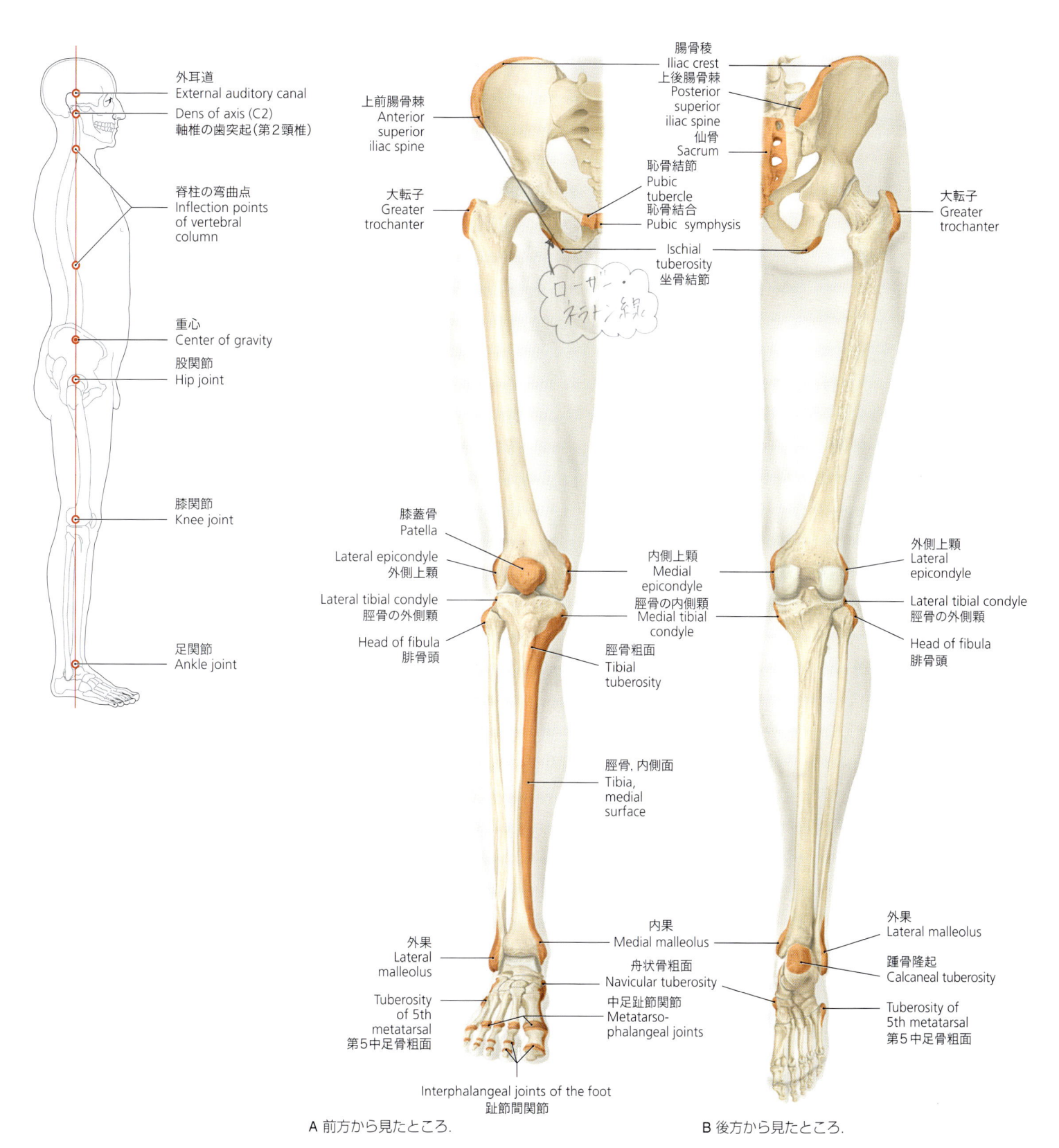

- 腸骨稜 Iliac crest
- 上前腸骨棘 Anterior superior iliac spine
- 上後腸骨棘 Posterior superior iliac spine
- 仙骨 Sacrum
- 恥骨結節 Pubic tubercle
- 恥骨結合 Pubic symphysis
- 大転子 Greater trochanter
- 坐骨結節 Ischial tuberosity
- 膝蓋骨 Patella
- 外側上顆 Lateral epicondyle
- 内側上顆 Medial epicondyle
- 脛骨の外側顆 Lateral tibial condyle
- 脛骨の内側顆 Medial tibial condyle
- 腓骨頭 Head of fibula
- 脛骨粗面 Tibial tuberosity
- 脛骨，内側面 Tibia, medial surface
- 外果 Lateral malleolus
- 内果 Medial malleolus
- 踵骨隆起 Calcaneal tuberosity
- 舟状骨粗面 Navicular tuberosity
- 中足趾節関節 Metatarso-phalangeal joints
- 第5中足骨粗面 Tuberosity of 5th metatarsal
- 趾節間関節 Interphalangeal joints of the foot

A 前方から見たところ．　　B 後方から見たところ．

下肢帯と寛骨
Pelvic Girdle & Hip Bone

図 24.4　下肢帯
前方から見たところ．骨盤輪を赤色で示してある．

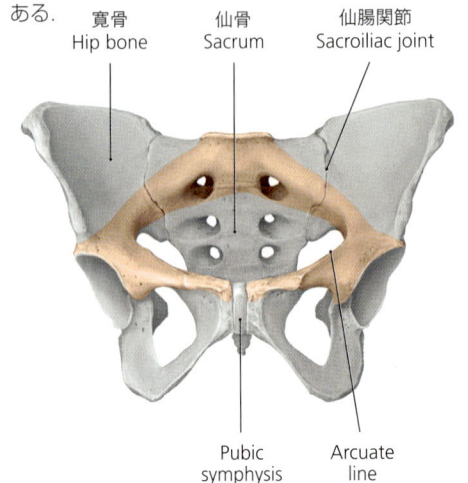

- 寛骨　Hip bone
- 仙骨　Sacrum
- 仙腸関節　Sacroiliac joint
- Pubic symphysis　恥骨結合
- Arcuate line　弓状線

個々の下肢帯はひとつの寛骨からなり，寛骨と大腿骨頭の間に股関節が形成される．上肢帯と異なり，下肢帯の骨は中軸骨格と強固に連結している．つまり，1対の寛骨は，前方では軟骨を介した恥骨結合によってお互いに連結し，後方では仙腸関節によって仙骨と連結している．

図 24.5　右寛骨

- 腸骨稜　Iliac crest
- 腸骨窩　Iliac fossa
- 上前腸骨棘　Anterior superior iliac spine
- 下前腸骨棘　Anterior inferior iliac spine
- 寛骨臼縁　Acetabular rim
- Acetabulum　寛骨臼
- 腸骨粗面　Iliac tuberosity
- 腸骨の耳状面　Auricular surface of ilium
- 弓状線　Arcuate line
- 坐骨棘　Ischial spine
- Pecten pubis　恥骨櫛
- 恥骨結合面　Symphyseal surface
- 閉鎖孔　Obturator foramen
- Ischial tuberosity　坐骨結節

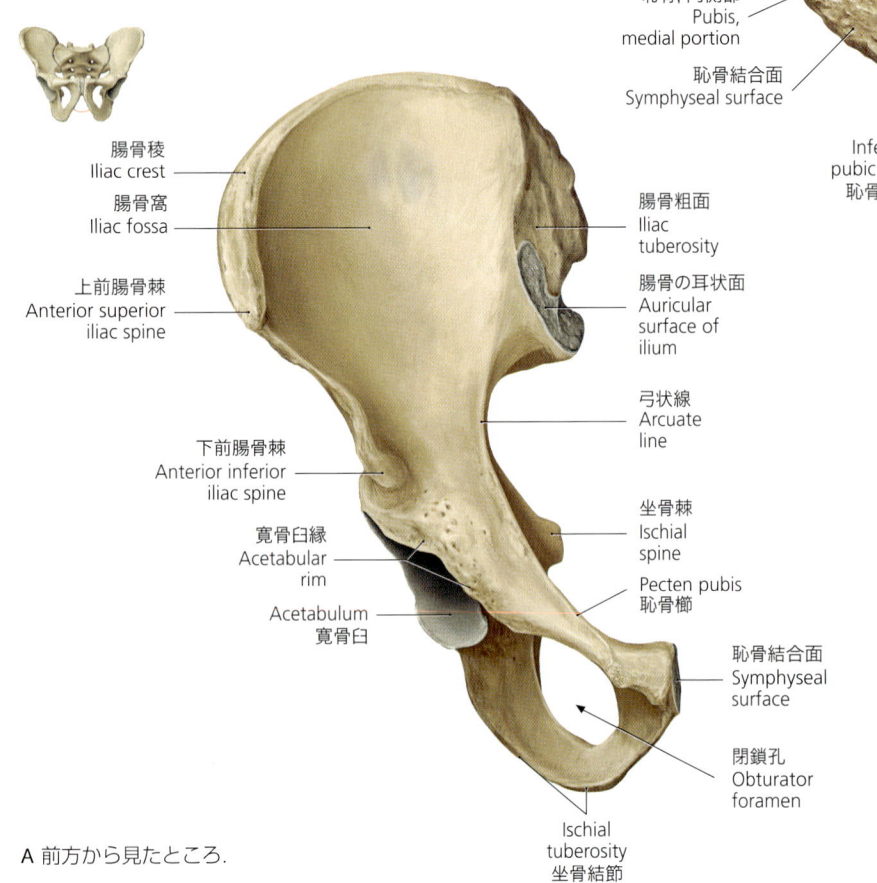

A　前方から見たところ．

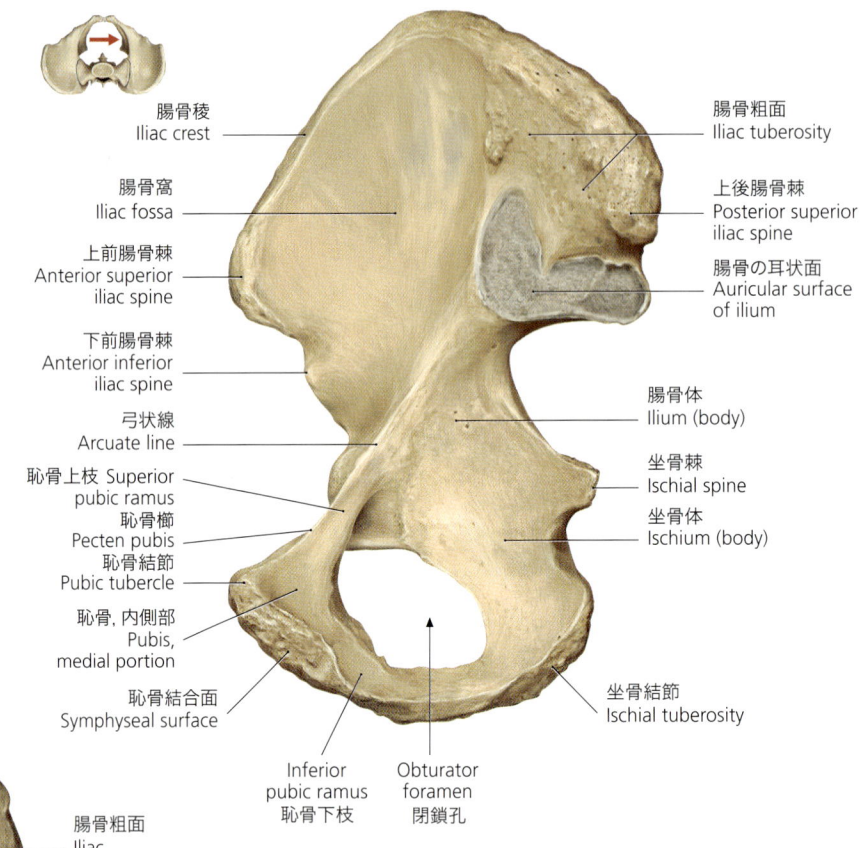

- 腸骨稜　Iliac crest
- 腸骨窩　Iliac fossa
- 上前腸骨棘　Anterior superior iliac spine
- 下前腸骨棘　Anterior inferior iliac spine
- 弓状線　Arcuate line
- 恥骨上枝　Superior pubic ramus
- 恥骨櫛　Pecten pubis
- 恥骨結節　Pubic tubercle
- 恥骨, 内側部　Pubis, medial portion
- 恥骨結合面　Symphyseal surface
- Inferior pubic ramus　恥骨下枝
- Obturator foramen　閉鎖孔
- 腸骨粗面　Iliac tuberosity
- 上後腸骨棘　Posterior superior iliac spine
- 腸骨の耳状面　Auricular surface of ilium
- 腸骨体　Ilium (body)
- 坐骨棘　Ischial spine
- 坐骨体　Ischium (body)
- 坐骨結節　Ischial tuberosity

B　内側方から見たところ．

図 24.6 寛骨の構成要素

右寛骨．寛骨を構成する3つの骨（腸骨，坐骨，恥骨）は寛骨臼の部分で接する．Y字型の隙間（Y軟骨）が閉じて，3つの骨が完全に癒合するのは14～16歳の間である．

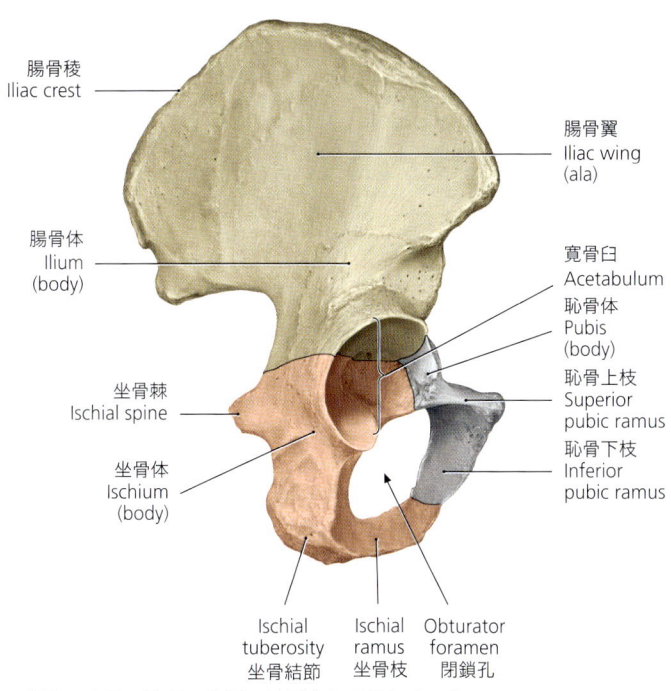

A 腸骨，坐骨，恥骨の位置．外側方から見たところ．

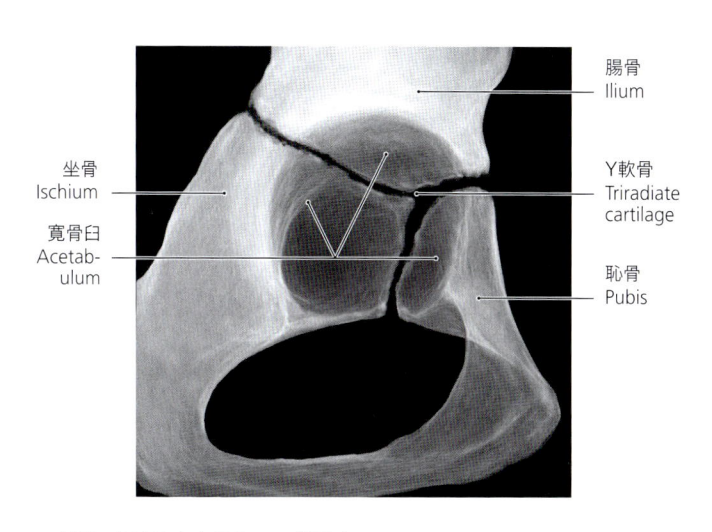

B 小児における右寛骨臼のX線写真．

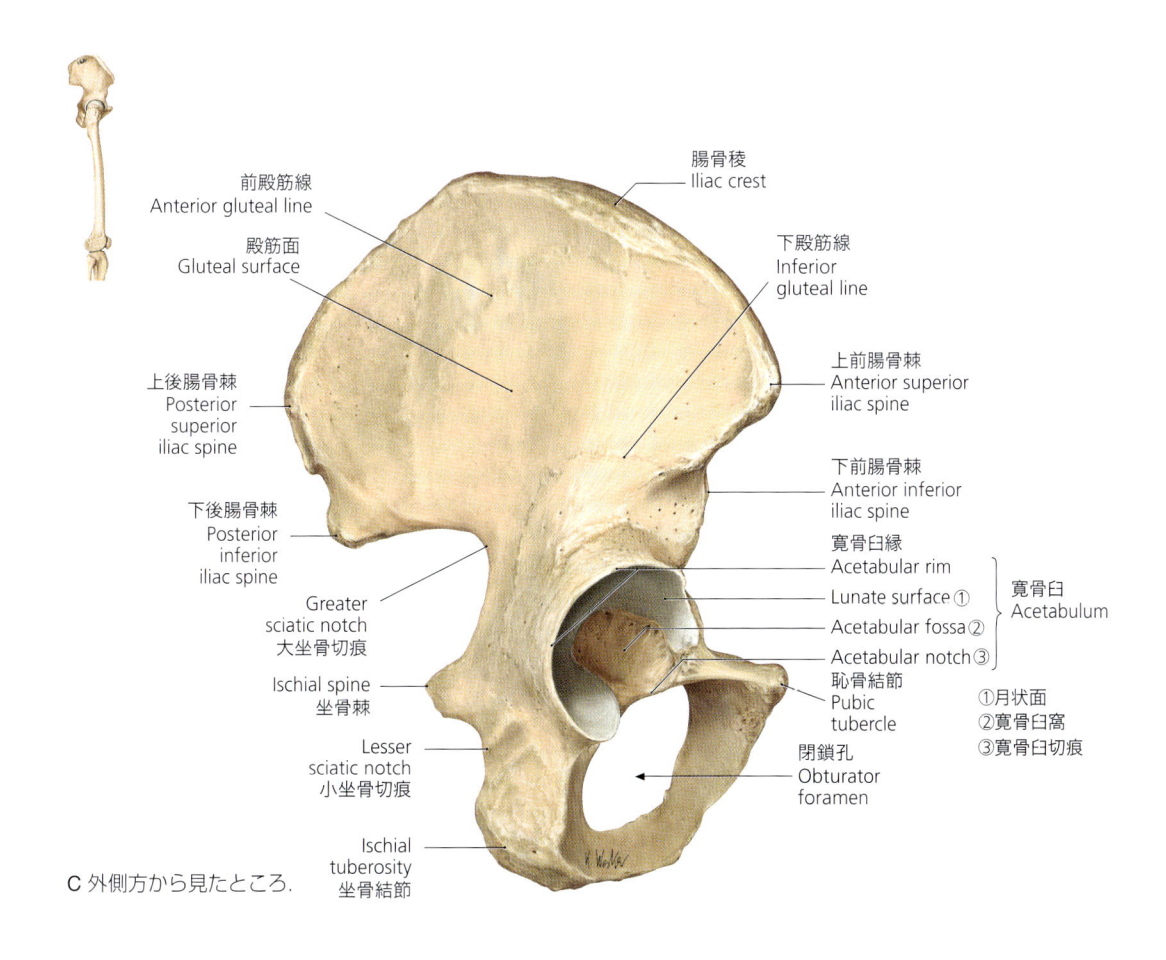

C 外側方から見たところ．

① 月状面
② 寛骨臼窩
③ 寛骨臼切痕

大腿骨
Femur

図 24.7　右大腿骨

日本語	English
大腿骨頭	Head
大腿骨頭窩	Fovea
転子窩	Trochanteric fossa
大転子	Greater trochanter
大腿骨頸	Neck
転子間稜	Intertrochanteric crest
転子間線	Intertrochanteric line
小転子	Lesser trochanter
恥骨筋線	Pectineal line
殿筋粗面	Gluteal tuberosity
大腿骨体	Shaft
外側唇	Lateral lip
内側唇	Medial lip
粗線	Linea aspera
内側顆上線	Medial supracondylar line
外側顆上線	Lateral supracondylar line
内転筋結節	Adductor tubercle
膝窩面	Popliteal surface
内側上顆	Medial epicondyle
顆間線	Intercondylar line
外側上顆	Lateral epicondyle
外側顆	Lateral condyle
膝蓋面	Patellar surface
内側顆	Medial condyle
顆間窩	Intercondylar notch

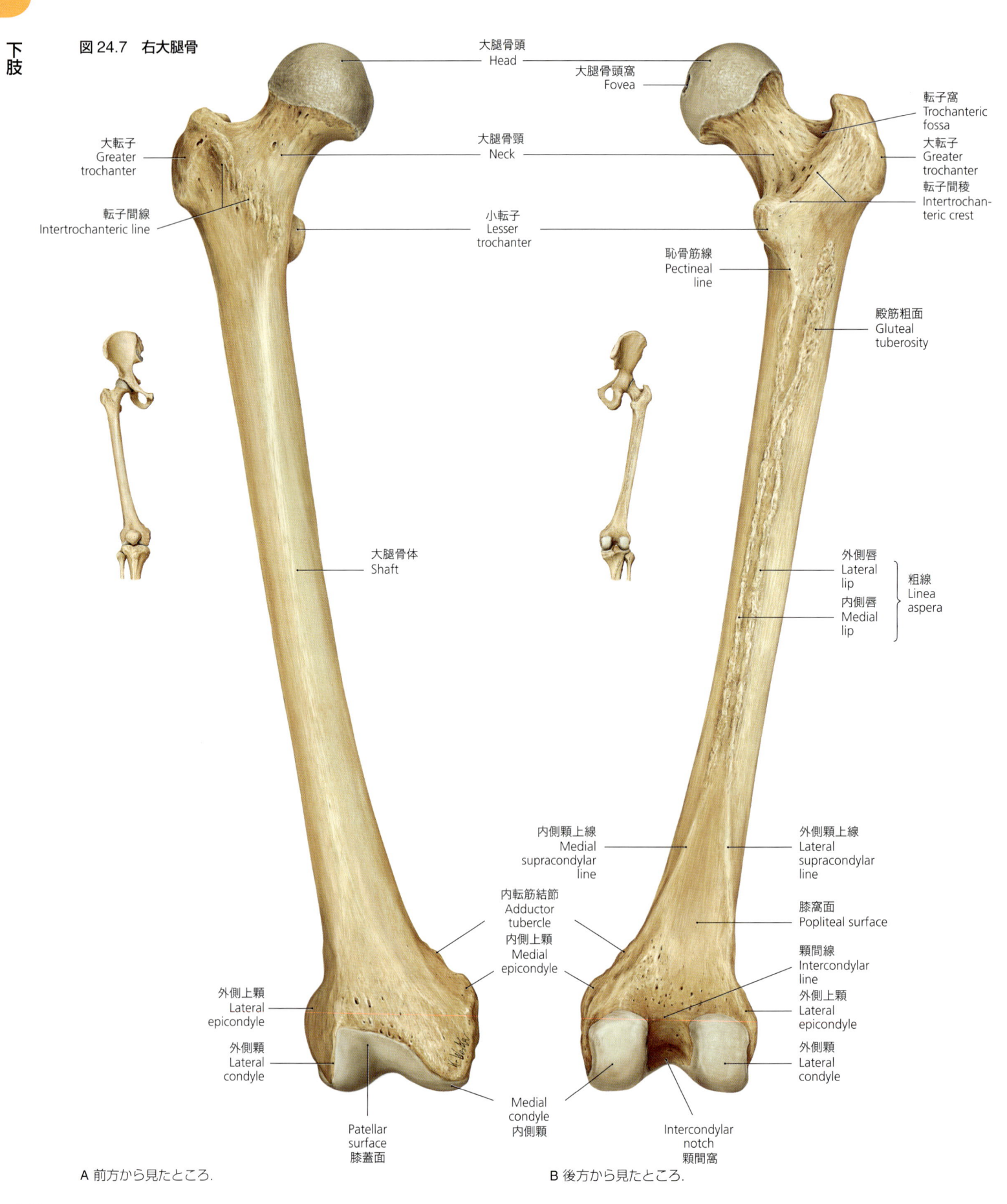

A　前方から見たところ．
B　後方から見たところ．

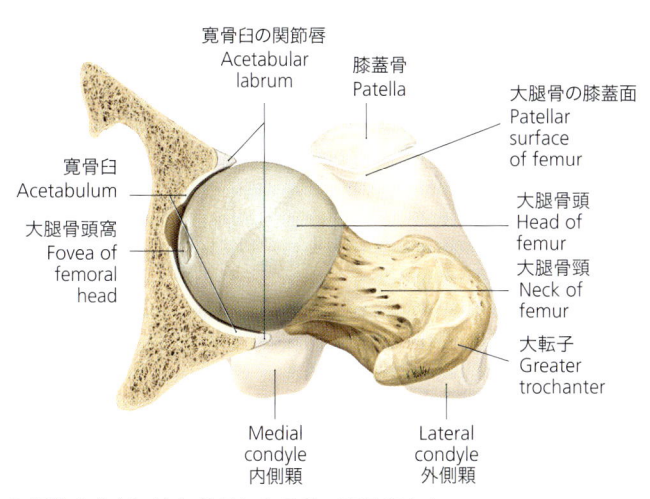

図 24.8 股関節における大腿骨頭
右股関節，上方から見たところ．

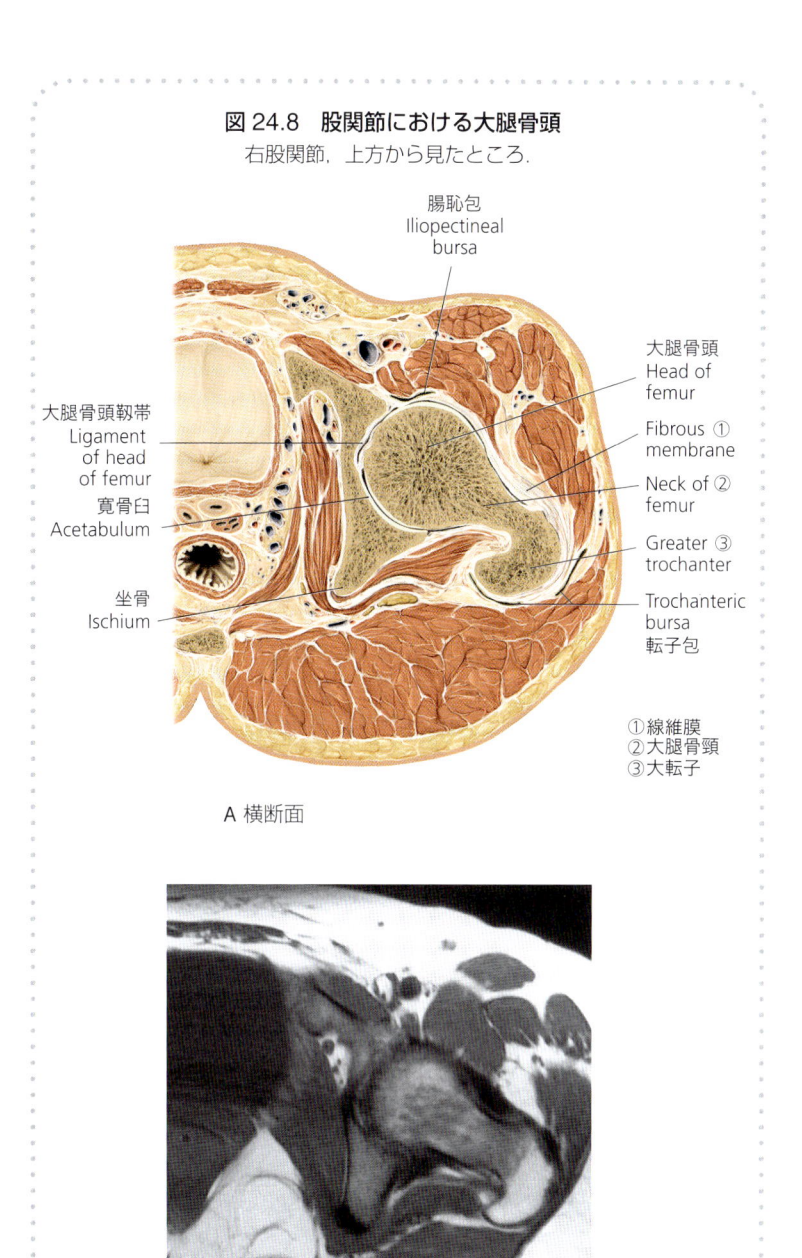

C 近位方向（上方）から見たところ．寛骨臼を水平断し，上半を取り除いてある．

ラベル（左上図 C）:
- 寛骨臼の関節唇 Acetabular labrum
- 膝蓋骨 Patella
- 大腿骨の膝蓋面 Patellar surface of femur
- 大腿骨頭 Head of femur
- 大腿骨頸 Neck of femur
- 大転子 Greater trochanter
- 内側顆 Medial condyle
- 外側顆 Lateral condyle
- 大腿骨頭窩 Fovea of femoral head
- 寛骨臼 Acetabulum

臨床

大腿骨骨折

骨粗鬆症患者が転倒し，大腿骨を骨折した場合，骨折の大部分は大腿骨頸に生じる．大腿骨体の骨折はずっと頻度が低く，通常は強い衝撃（例えば，自動車事故）によって生じる．

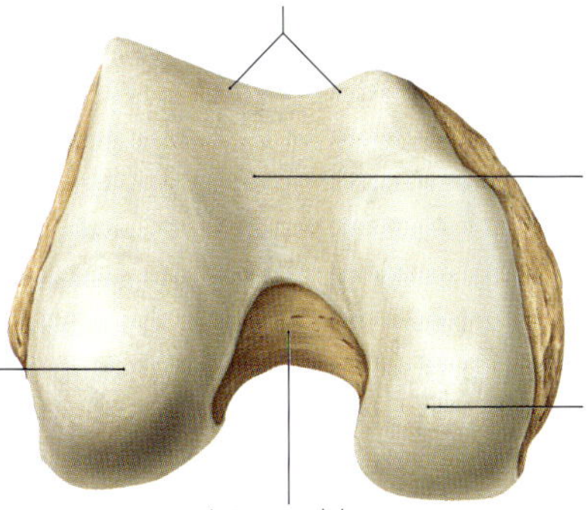

D 遠位方向（下方）から見たところ．膝関節については pp.382–383 を参照．

ラベル（左下図 D）:
- 大腿骨の膝蓋面（大腿骨滑車面）Patellar surface of femur (femoral trochlea)
- 大腿骨の膝蓋面 Patellar surface of femur
- 外側顆 Lateral condyle
- 内側顆 Medial condyle
- 顆間窩 Intercondylar notch

A 横断面

ラベル（A 横断面）:
- 腸恥包 Iliopectineal bursa
- 大腿骨頭 Head of femur
- 線維膜 Fibrous membrane ①
- 大腿骨頸 Neck of femur ②
- 大転子 Greater trochanter ③
- 転子包 Trochanteric bursa
- 大腿骨頭靱帯 Ligament of head of femur
- 寛骨臼 Acetabulum
- 坐骨 Ischium

①線維膜
②大腿骨頸
③大転子

B T1 強調 MR 像

股関節：概観
Hip Joint: Overview

図 24.9　右股関節

大腿骨頭は寛骨の寛骨臼と連結し，球関節の一種である股関節を形成する．大腿骨頭はほぼ球状であり（球の平均半径は約 2.5 cm），そのほとんどが寛骨臼の中に納まっている．

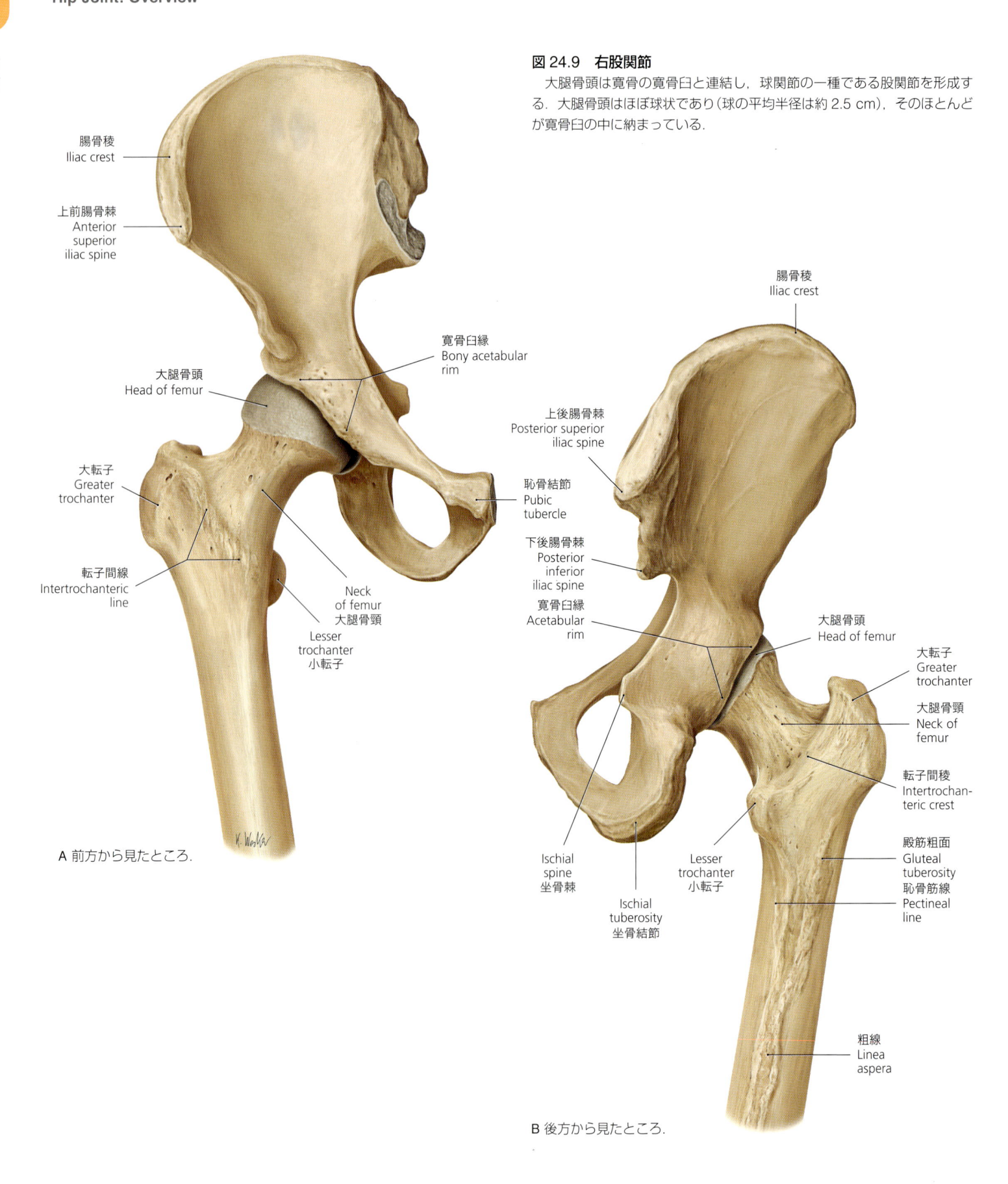

A　前方から見たところ．

B　後方から見たところ．

図 24.10　股関節：前額断面
右股関節，前方から見たところ．

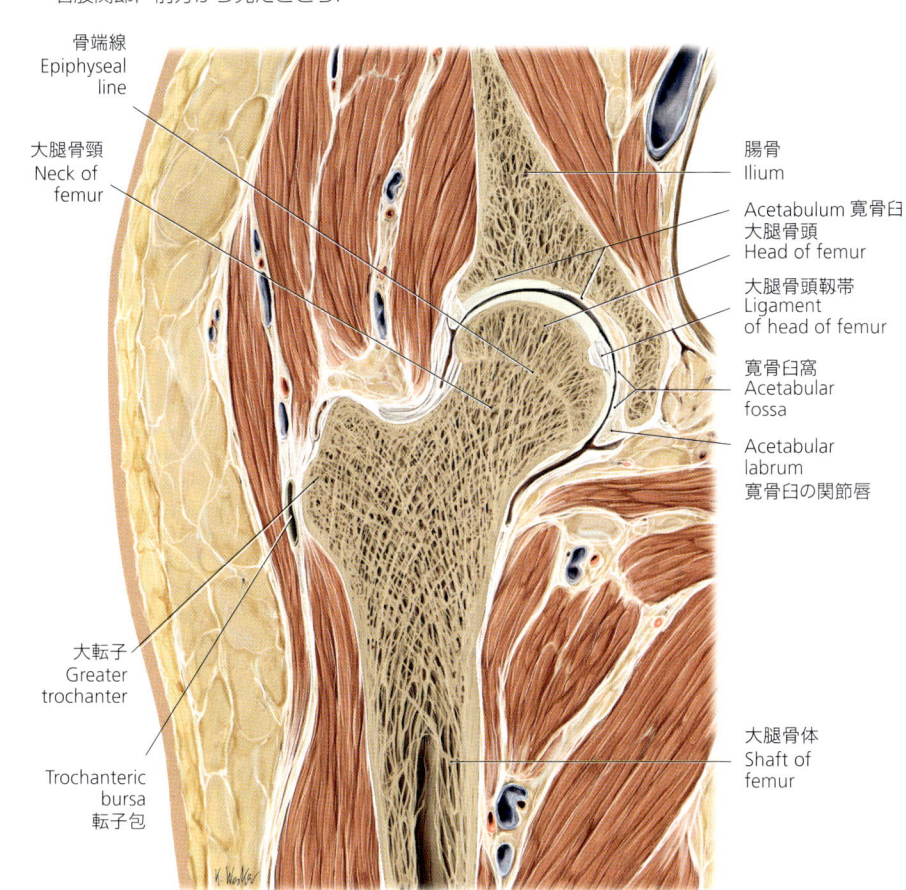

- 骨端線 Epiphyseal line
- 大腿骨頸 Neck of femur
- 腸骨 Ilium
- Acetabulum 寛骨臼
- 大腿骨頭 Head of femur
- 大腿骨頭靱帯 Ligament of head of femur
- 寛骨臼窩 Acetabular fossa
- Acetabular labrum 寛骨臼の関節唇
- 大転子 Greater trochanter
- Trochanteric bursa 転子包
- 大腿骨体 Shaft of femur

A 前額断面．

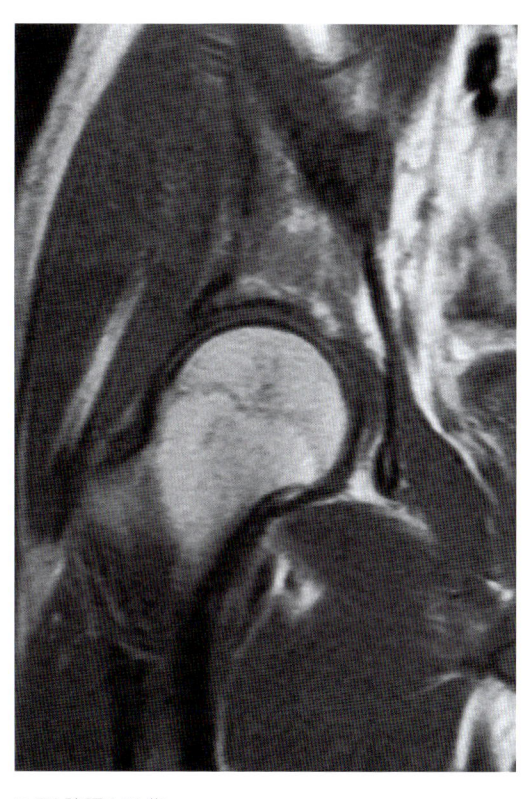

B T1 強調 MR 像．

臨床

乳児における寛骨臼低形成と股関節脱臼の診断

超音波断層法は乳児の股関節をスクリーニングするうえで，最も重要な画像診断法であり，寛骨臼の低形成や股関節脱臼といった形態的変化を見つけるのに使われる．先天性の股関節脱臼では，股関節の不安定性や外転制限がみられる．また，患側の下肢が短くなり，殿溝が左右非対称となる．

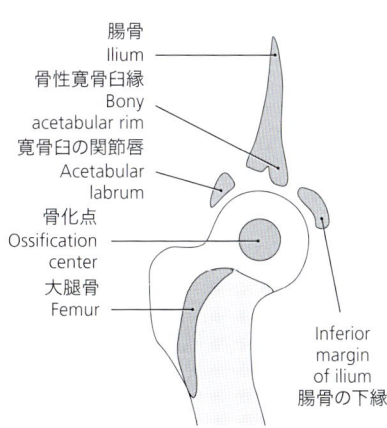

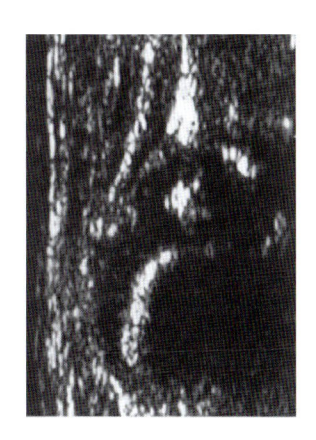

- 腸骨 Ilium
- 骨性寛骨臼縁 Bony acetabular rim
- 寛骨臼の関節唇 Acetabular labrum
- 骨化点 Ossification center
- 大腿骨 Femur
- Inferior margin of ilium 腸骨の下縁

A 5か月乳児の正常な股関節．

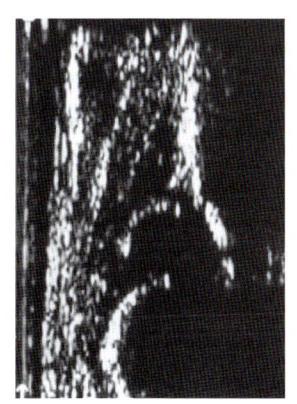

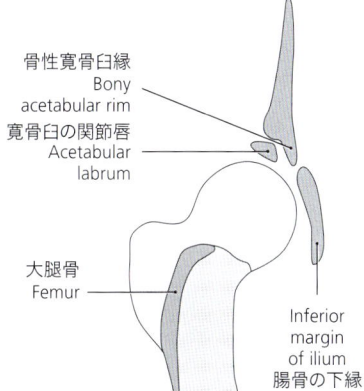

- 骨性寛骨臼縁 Bony acetabular rim
- 寛骨臼の関節唇 Acetabular labrum
- 大腿骨 Femur
- Inferior margin of ilium 腸骨の下縁

B 3か月乳児の股関節脱臼と寛骨臼の低形成．

股関節：靱帯と関節包
Hip Joint: Ligaments & Capsule

> 股関節は3つの主要な靱帯（腸骨大腿靱帯，恥骨大腿靱帯，坐骨大腿靱帯）によって補強されている．これらの靱帯の深層には輪帯が存在する（図示していない）．輪帯（輪状靱帯）は関節包の輪状線維が束になったもので，大腿骨頸をボタン穴のように取り囲んでいる．

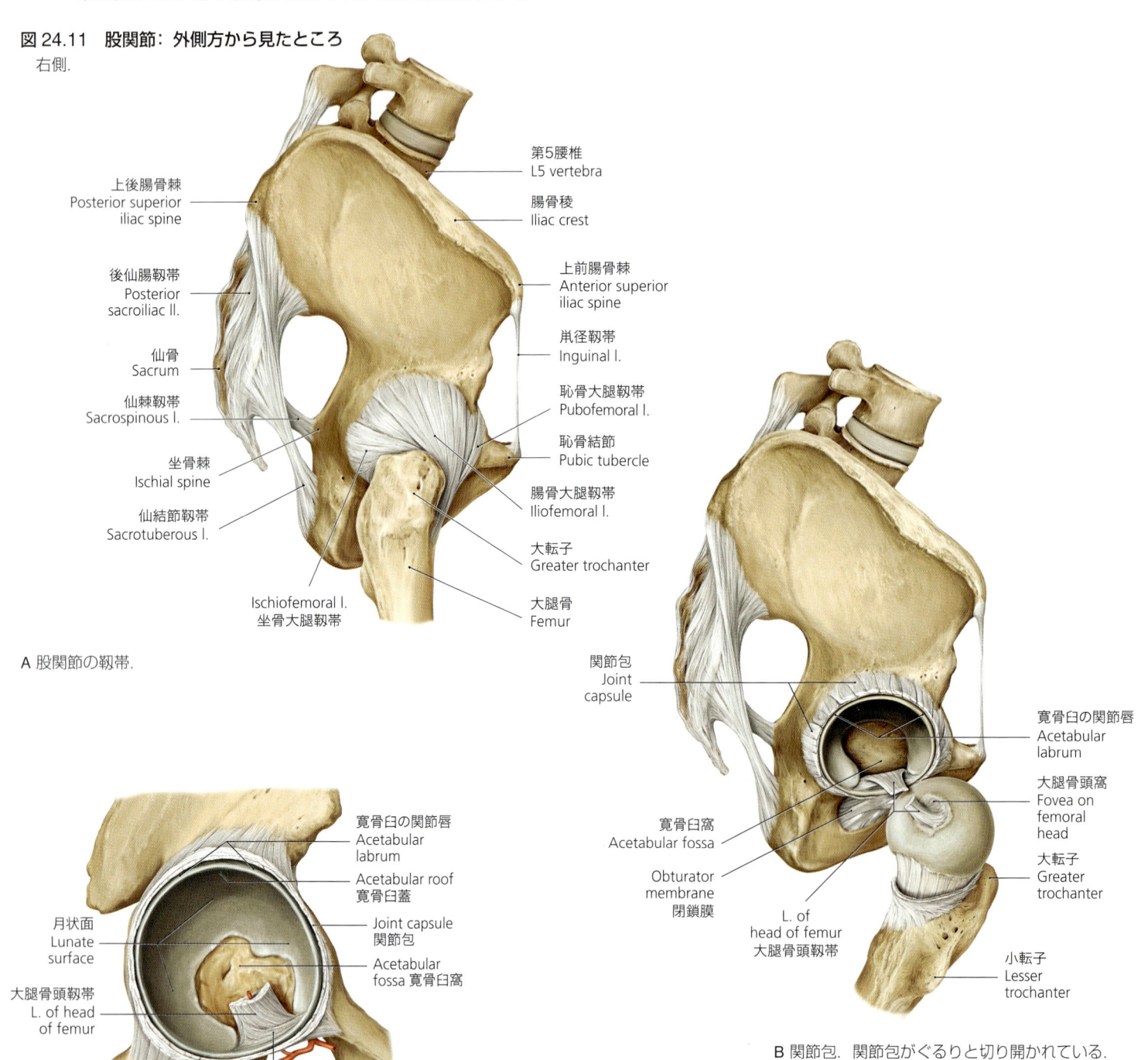

図 24.11　股関節：外側方から見たところ
右側．

A 股関節の靱帯．

ラベル：上後腸骨棘 Posterior superior iliac spine／第5腰椎 L5 vertebra／腸骨稜 Iliac crest／後仙腸靱帯 Posterior sacroiliac l.／上前腸骨棘 Anterior superior iliac spine／仙骨 Sacrum／鼡径靱帯 Inguinal l.／仙棘靱帯 Sacrospinous l.／恥骨大腿靱帯 Pubofemoral l.／坐骨棘 Ischial spine／恥骨結節 Pubic tubercle／仙結節靱帯 Sacrotuberous l.／腸骨大腿靱帯 Iliofemoral l.／大転子 Greater trochanter／大腿骨 Femur／Ischiofemoral l. 坐骨大腿靱帯

B 関節包．関節包がぐるりと切り開かれている．大腿骨頭が寛骨臼から外れ，切断された大腿骨頭靱帯が見えている．

ラベル：関節包 Joint capsule／寛骨臼の関節唇 Acetabular labrum／寛骨臼窩 Acetabular fossa／大腿骨頭窩 Fovea on femoral head／閉鎖膜 Obturator membrane／L. of head of femur 大腿骨頭靱帯／大転子 Greater trochanter／小転子 Lesser trochanter

C 寛骨臼．大腿骨頭靱帯（断端が見えている）の中に閉鎖動脈の枝が走っている．この動脈枝は大腿骨頭を栄養する（p.421 参照）．

ラベル：寛骨臼の関節唇 Acetabular labrum／Acetabular roof 寛骨臼蓋／月状面 Lunate surface／Joint capsule 関節包／大腿骨頭靱帯 L. of head of femur／Acetabular fossa 寛骨臼窩／Transverse l. of acetabulum 寛骨臼横靱帯

図 24.12 股関節: 前方から見たところ
右側.

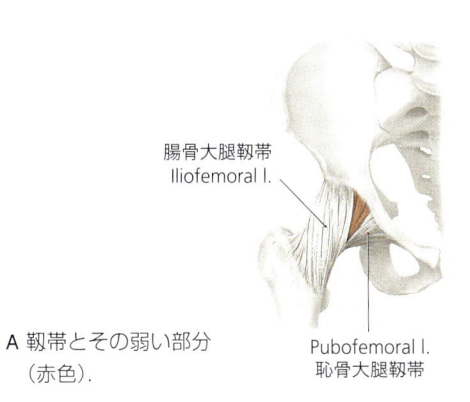

A 靱帯とその弱い部分（赤色）.
- 腸骨大腿靱帯 Iliofemoral l.
- 恥骨大腿靱帯 Pubofemoral l.

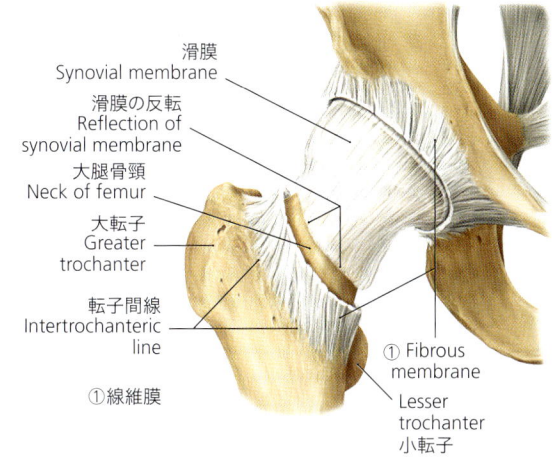

C 関節包. 大腿骨頸の部分で，股関節を取り巻く靱帯と関節包の線維膜を取り除いたところ. 滑膜が見えている.
- 滑膜 Synovial membrane
- 滑膜の反転 Reflection of synovial membrane
- 大腿骨頸 Neck of femur
- 大転子 Greater trochanter
- 転子間線 Intertrochanteric line
- ① 線維膜 Fibrous membrane
- 小転子 Lesser trochanter

B 股関節の靱帯.
- 腸腰靱帯 Iliolumbar l.
- 第4腰椎 L4 vertebra
- 前縦靱帯 Anterior longitudinal l.
- 第5腰椎 L5 vertebra
- 岬角 Sacral promontory
- 前仙腸靱帯 Anterior sacroiliac ll.
- 仙結節靱帯 Sacrotuberous l.
- 仙棘靱帯 Sacrospinous l.
- 坐骨棘 Ischial spine
- 恥骨結合 Pubic symphysis
- 腸骨稜 Iliac crest
- 上前腸骨棘 Anterior superior iliac spine
- 鼡径靱帯 Inguinal l.
- 腸骨大腿靱帯 Iliofemoral l.
- 大転子 Greater trochanter
- 転子間線 Intertrochanteric line
- 小転子 Lesser trochanter
- 恥骨大腿靱帯 Pubofemoral l.

図 24.13 股関節: 後方から見たところ
右側.

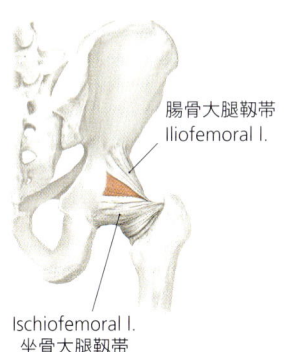

A 靱帯とその弱い部分（赤色）.
- 腸骨大腿靱帯 Iliofemoral l.
- 坐骨大腿靱帯 Ischiofemoral l.

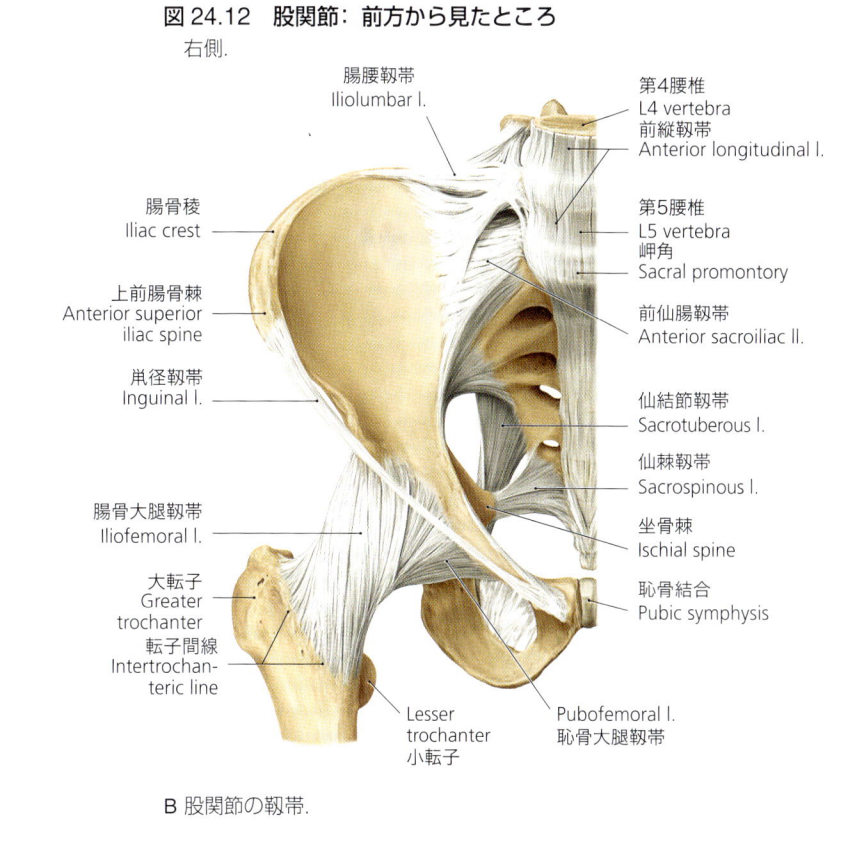

C 関節包.
- 線維膜 Fibrous membrane
- 滑膜 Synovial membrane

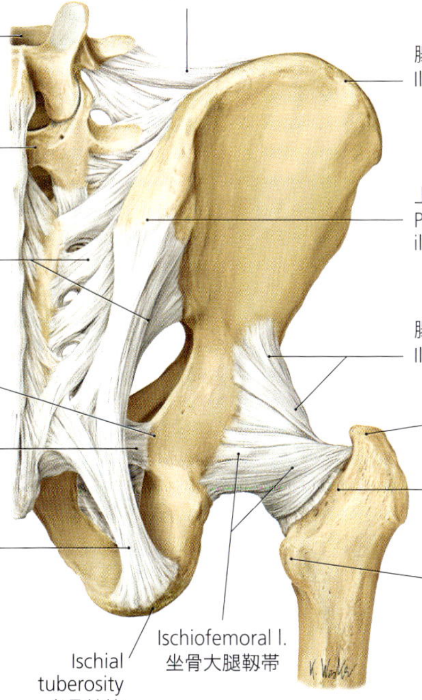

B 股関節の靱帯.
- 腸腰靱帯 Iliolumbar l.
- 第4腰椎 L4 vertebra
- 第5腰椎 L5 vertebra
- 後仙腸靱帯 Posterior sacroiliac ll.
- 坐骨棘 Ischial spine
- 仙棘靱帯 Sacrospinous l.
- 仙結節靱帯 Sacrotuberous l.
- 坐骨大腿靱帯 Ischiofemoral l.
- 坐骨結節 Ischial tuberosity
- 腸骨稜 Iliac crest
- 上後腸骨棘 Posterior superior iliac spine
- 腸骨大腿靱帯 Iliofemoral l.
- 大転子 Greater trochanter
- 転子間稜 Intertrochanteric crest
- 小転子 Lesser trochanter

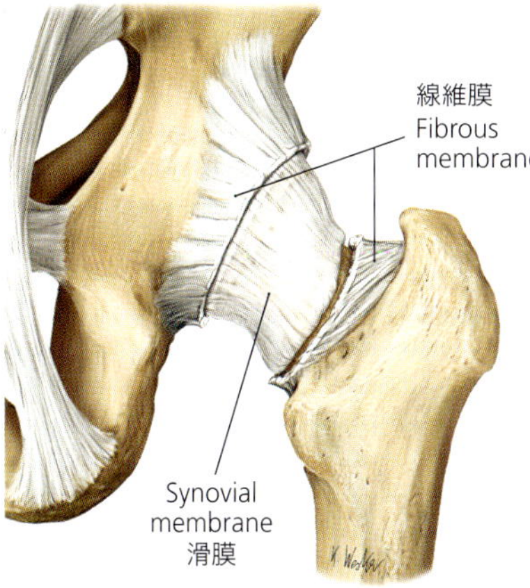

骨盤部と大腿の前面にある筋 (1)
Anterior Muscles of the Thigh, Hip & Gluteal Region (I)

図 24.14 骨盤と大腿の筋：前方から見たところ (1)
右下肢．筋の起始(O)を赤，停止(I)を青で示してある．

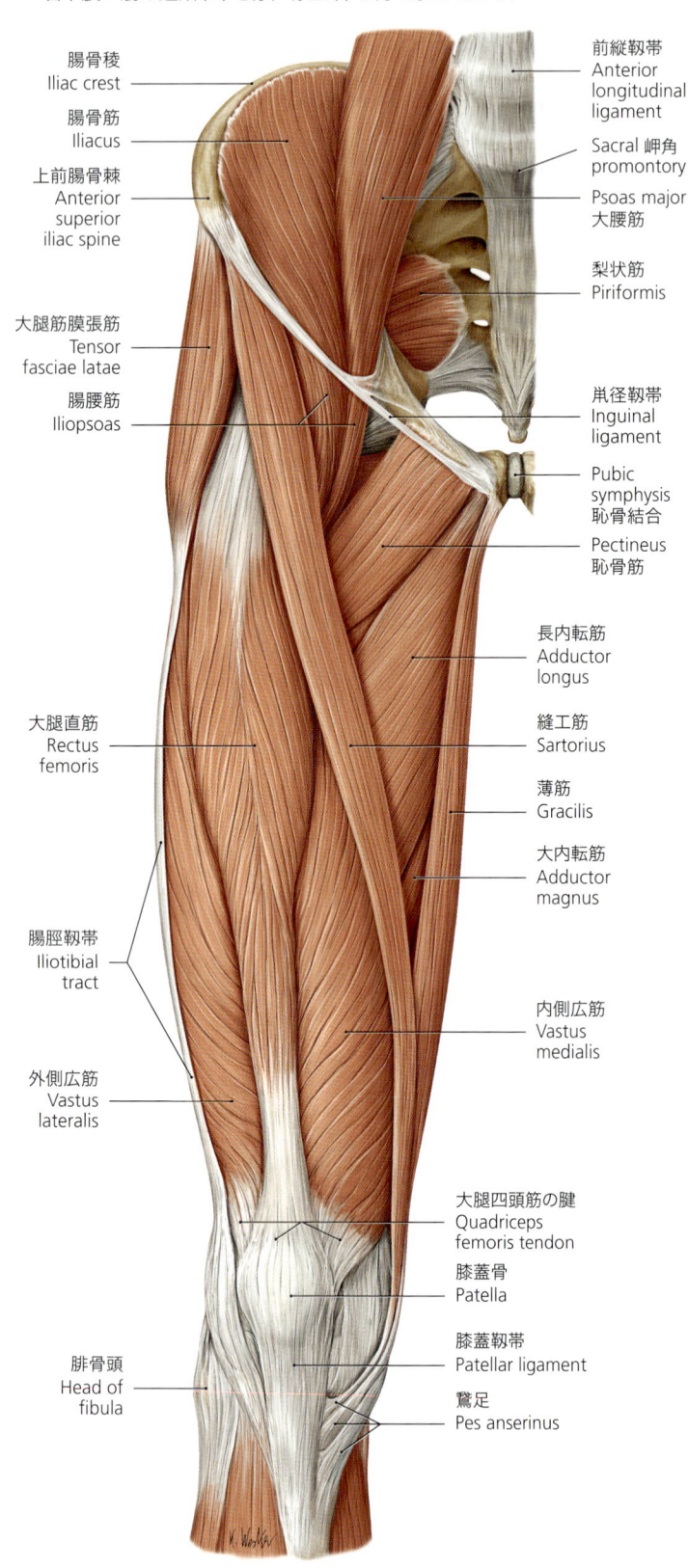

左図ラベル：
- 腸骨稜 Iliac crest
- 腸骨筋 Iliacus
- 上前腸骨棘 Anterior superior iliac spine
- 大腿筋膜張筋 Tensor fasciae latae
- 腸腰筋 Iliopsoas
- 大腿直筋 Rectus femoris
- 腸脛靱帯 Iliotibial tract
- 外側広筋 Vastus lateralis
- 腓骨頭 Head of fibula
- 前縦靱帯 Anterior longitudinal ligament
- 岬角 Sacral promontory
- 大腰筋 Psoas major
- 梨状筋 Piriformis
- 鼡径靱帯 Inguinal ligament
- 恥骨結合 Pubic symphysis
- 恥骨筋 Pectineus
- 長内転筋 Adductor longus
- 縫工筋 Sartorius
- 薄筋 Gracilis
- 大内転筋 Adductor magnus
- 内側広筋 Vastus medialis
- 大腿四頭筋の腱 Quadriceps femoris tendon
- 膝蓋骨 Patella
- 膝蓋靱帯 Patellar ligament
- 鵞足 Pes anserinus

右図ラベル：
- 縫工筋 Sartorius
- 大腿直筋 Rectus femoris
- 中間広筋 Vastus intermedius
- 縫工筋 Sartorius
- 薄筋 Gracilis
- 鵞足（共通の停止腱）Pes anserinus (common tendon of insertion)
- 半腱様筋 Semitendinosus

A 大腿筋膜を腸脛靱帯のところまで取り除いてある．

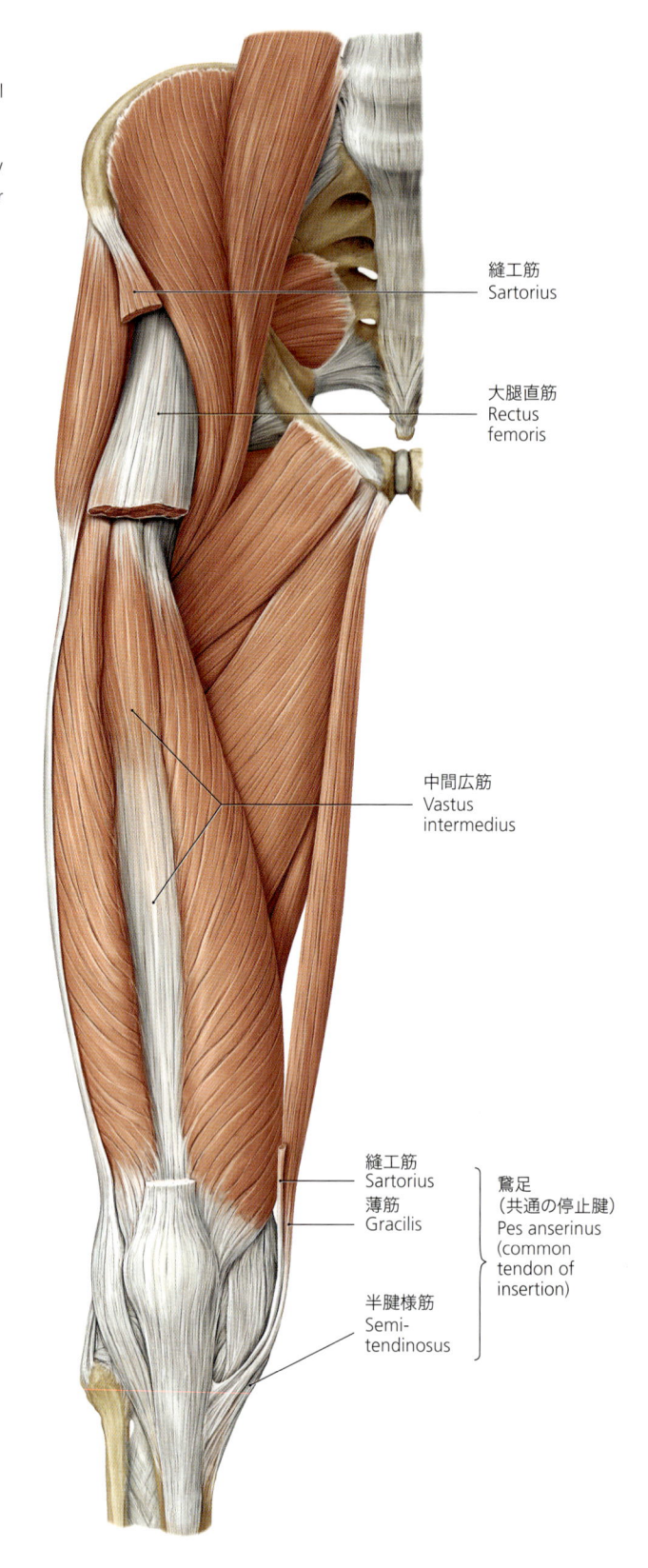

B 縫工筋と大腿直筋を取り除いたところ．

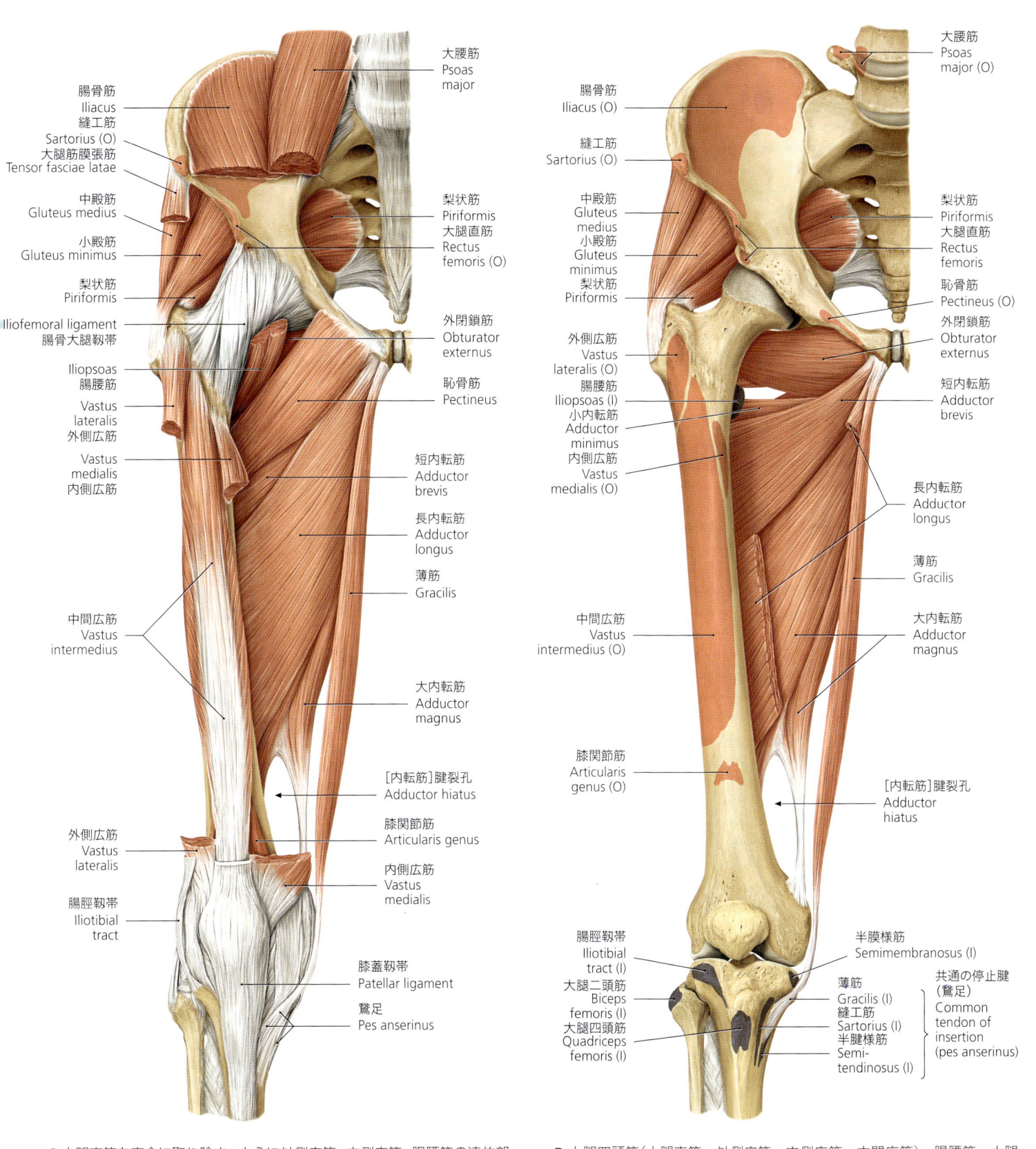

C 大腿直筋を完全に取り除き，さらに外側広筋，内側広筋，腸腰筋の遠位部，大腿筋膜張筋を取り除いたところ．

D 大腿四頭筋（大腿直筋，外側広筋，内側広筋，中間広筋），腸腰筋，大腿筋膜張筋，恥骨筋，長内転筋の中央部を取り除いたところ．

骨盤部と大腿の前面にある筋 (2)
Anterior Muscles of the Thigh, Hip & Gluteal Region (II)

図 24.15　骨盤と大腿の筋：前方から見たところ (2)
右下肢．筋の起始 (O) を赤，停止 (I) を青で示してある．

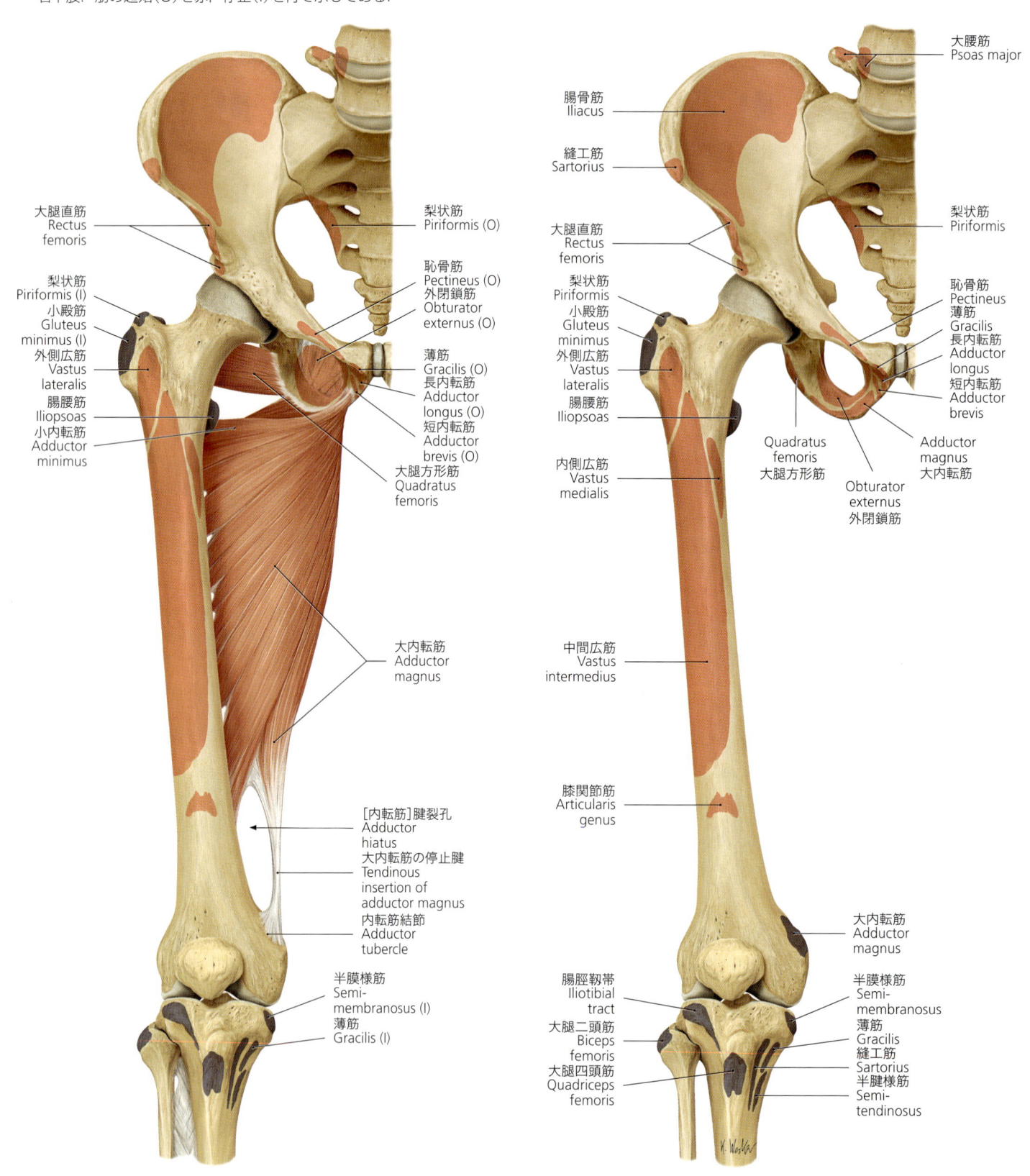

A 中殿筋，小殿筋，梨状筋，外閉鎖筋，長・短内転筋，薄筋を取り除いたところ．

B 全ての筋を取り除いたところ．

図 24.16 骨盤，殿部，大腿の筋：内側方から見たところ

右下肢．正中矢状断．

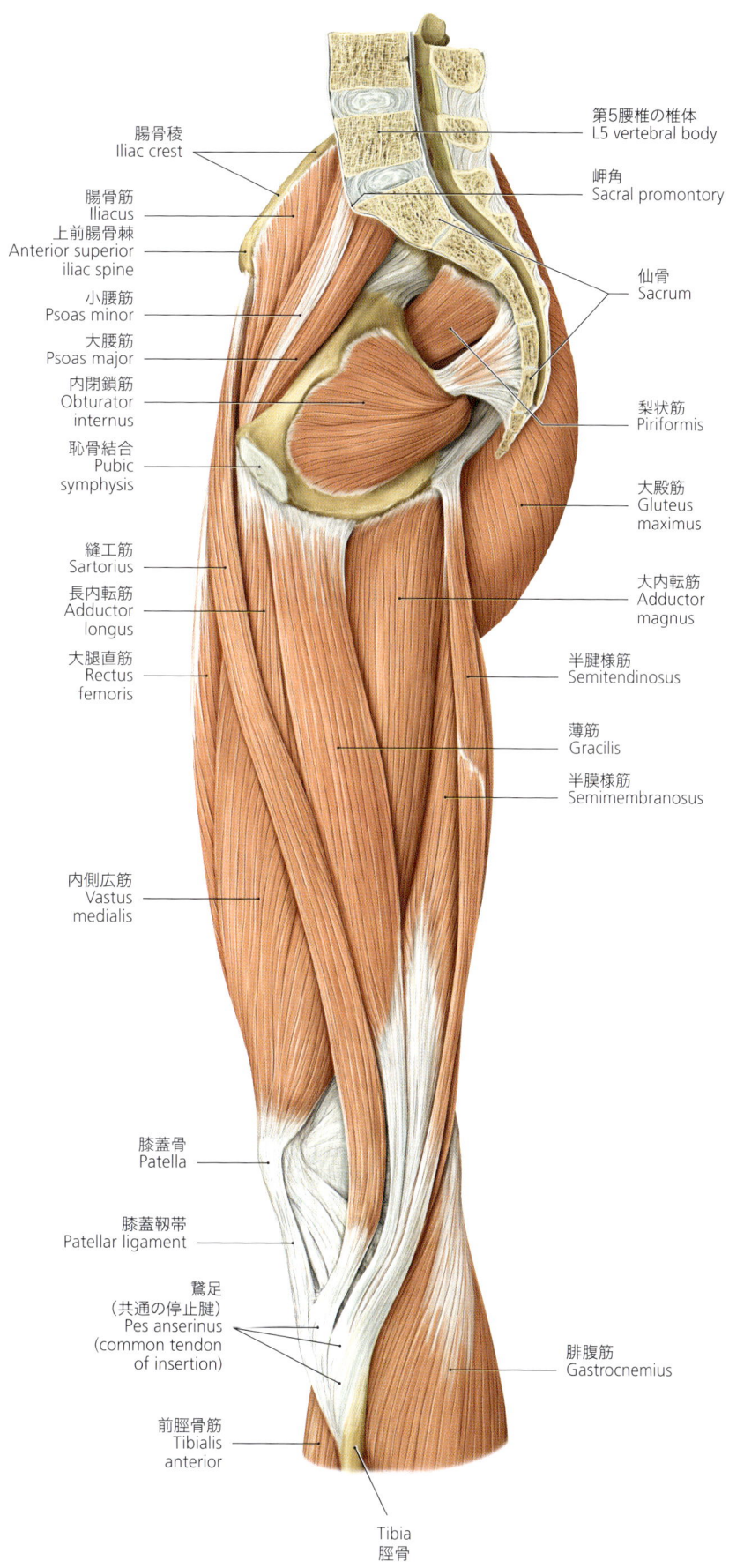

- 腸骨稜 Iliac crest
- 腸骨筋 Iliacus
- 上前腸骨棘 Anterior superior iliac spine
- 小腰筋 Psoas minor
- 大腰筋 Psoas major
- 内閉鎖筋 Obturator internus
- 恥骨結合 Pubic symphysis
- 縫工筋 Sartorius
- 長内転筋 Adductor longus
- 大腿直筋 Rectus femoris
- 内側広筋 Vastus medialis
- 膝蓋骨 Patella
- 膝蓋靱帯 Patellar ligament
- 鵞足（共通の停止腱） Pes anserinus (common tendon of insertion)
- 前脛骨筋 Tibialis anterior
- 第5腰椎の椎体 L5 vertebral body
- 岬角 Sacral promontory
- 仙骨 Sacrum
- 梨状筋 Piriformis
- 大殿筋 Gluteus maximus
- 大内転筋 Adductor magnus
- 半腱様筋 Semitendinosus
- 薄筋 Gracilis
- 半膜様筋 Semimembranosus
- 腓腹筋 Gastrocnemius
- 脛骨 Tibia

骨盤部と大腿の後面にある筋 (1)
Posterior Muscles of the Thigh, Hip & Gluteal Region (I)

図 24.17 骨盤，殿部，大腿の筋：後方から見たところ(1)
右下肢．筋の起始(O)を赤，停止(I)を青で示してある．

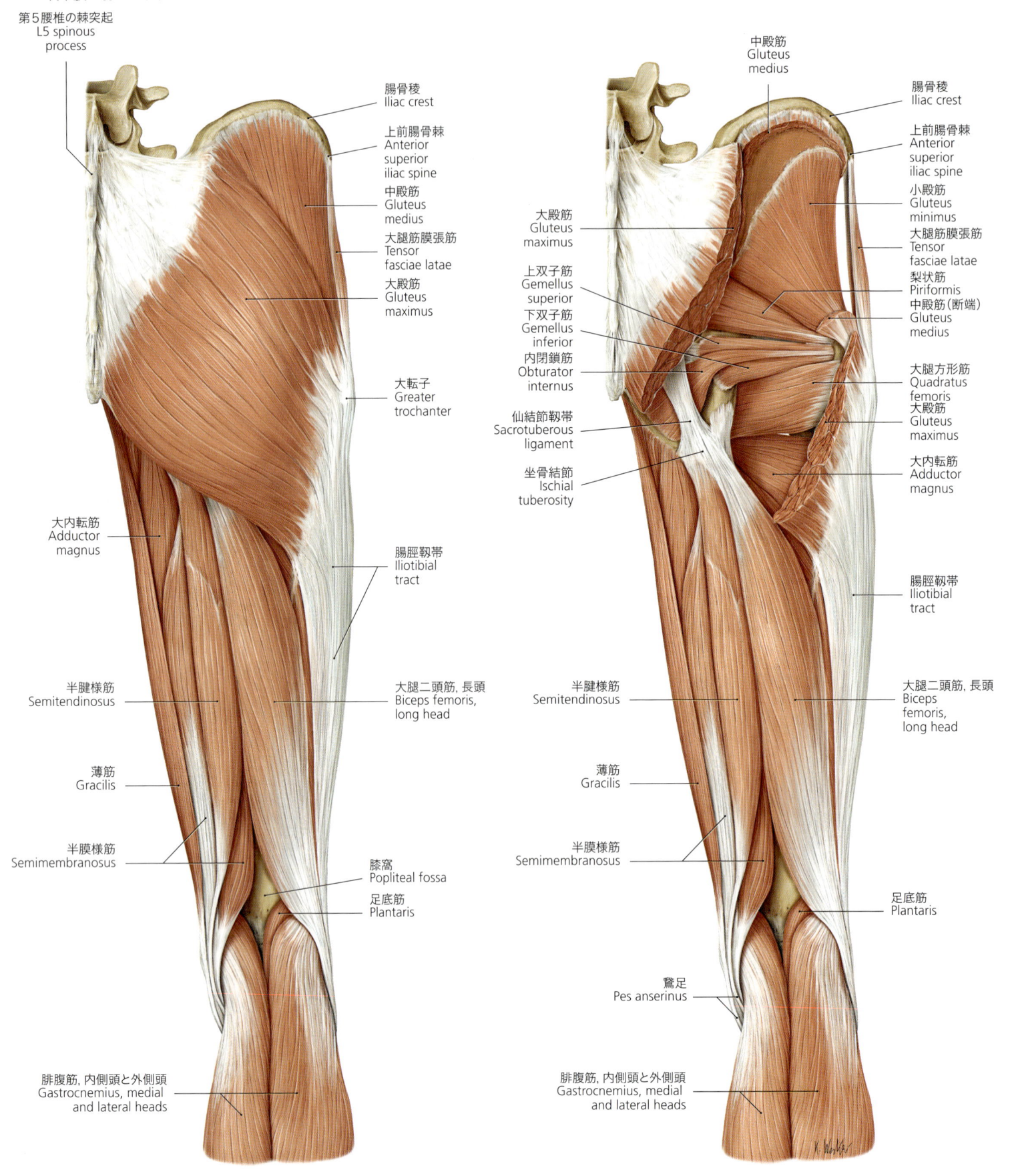

A 大腿筋膜を腸脛靱帯のところまで取り除いてある．

B 大殿筋（中央部）と中殿筋を取り除いたところ．

骨盤と大腿

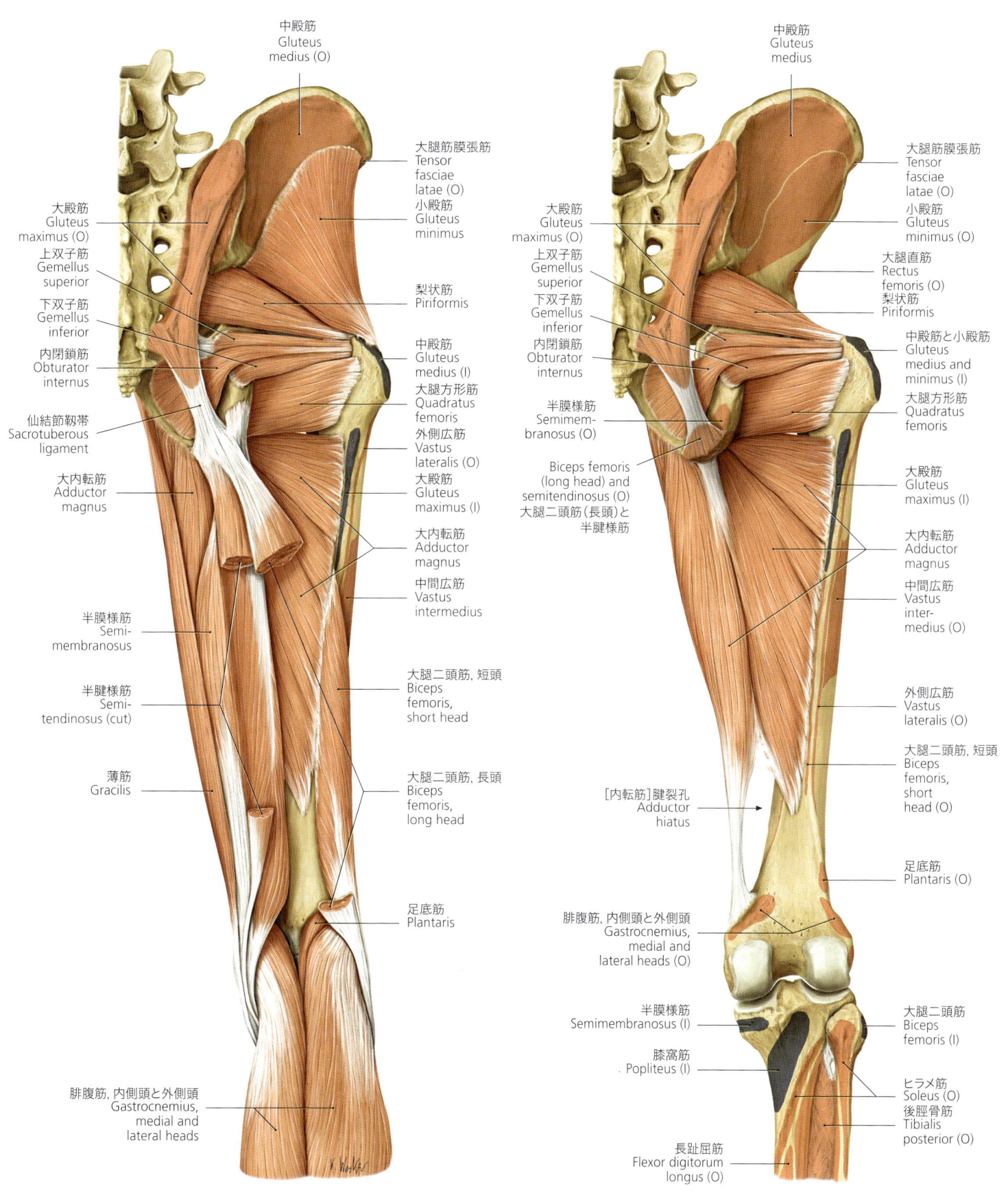

C 半腱様筋，大腿二頭筋を部分的に取り除いたところ．また，大殿筋と中殿筋を完全に取り除いてある．

D ハムストリングス（半腱様筋，半膜様筋，大腿二頭筋），小殿筋，下腿の筋（腓腹筋など）を完全に取り除いたところ．

骨盤部と大腿の後面にある筋 (2)
Posterior Muscles of the Thigh, Hip & Gluteal Region (II)

図 24.18 骨盤, 殿部, 大腿の筋: 後方から見たところ (1)
右下肢. 筋の起始 (O) を赤, 停止 (I) を青で示してある.

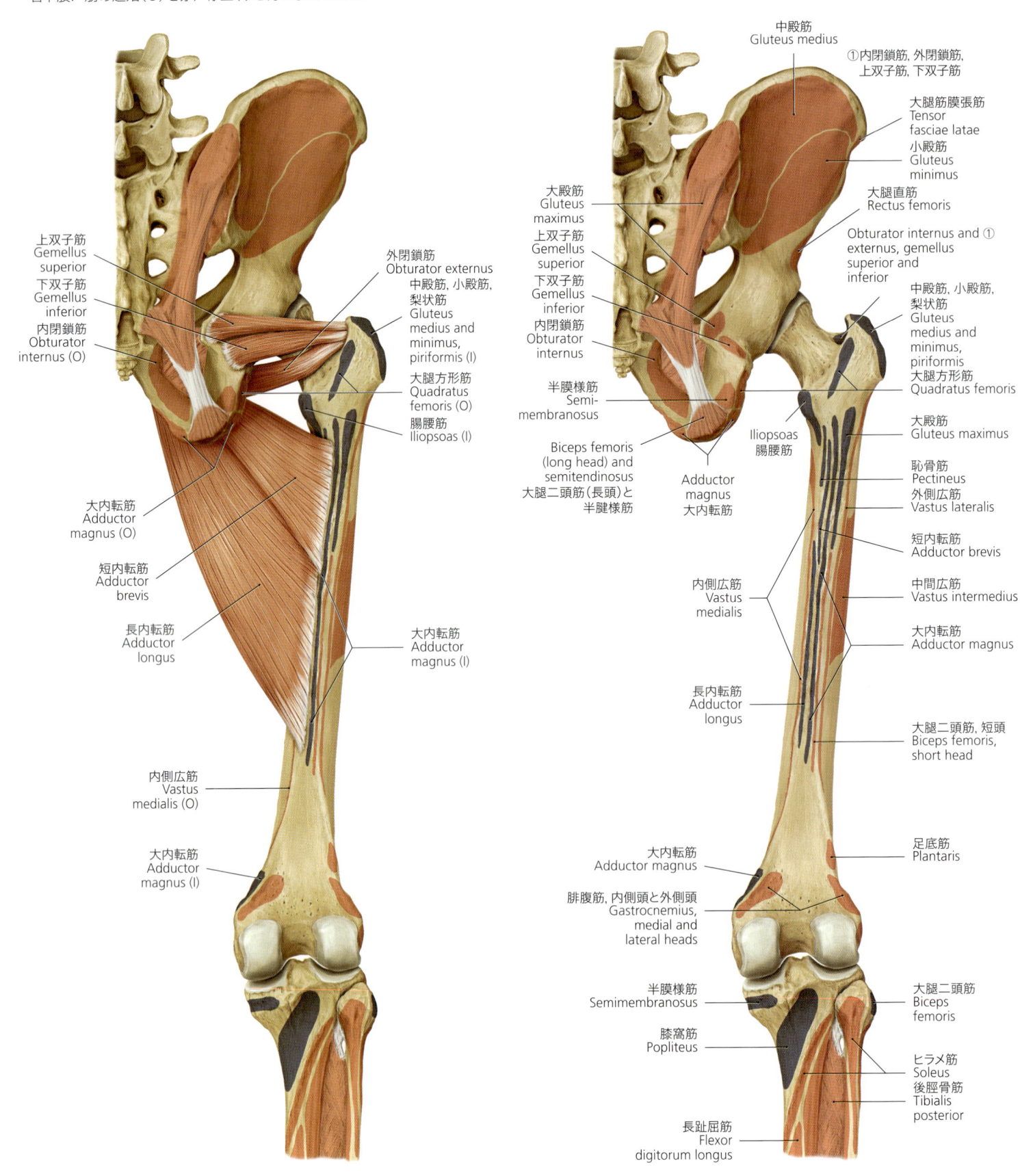

A 梨状筋, 内閉鎖筋, 大腿方形筋, 大内転筋を取り除いたところ.

B 全ての筋を取り除いたところ.

図 24.19 骨盤，殿部，大腿の筋：外側方から見たところ
腸脛靱帯（大腿筋膜の帯状に肥厚した部分）は，張力帯（引き綱）として働き，大腿骨近位部を曲げようとする力を軽減する．

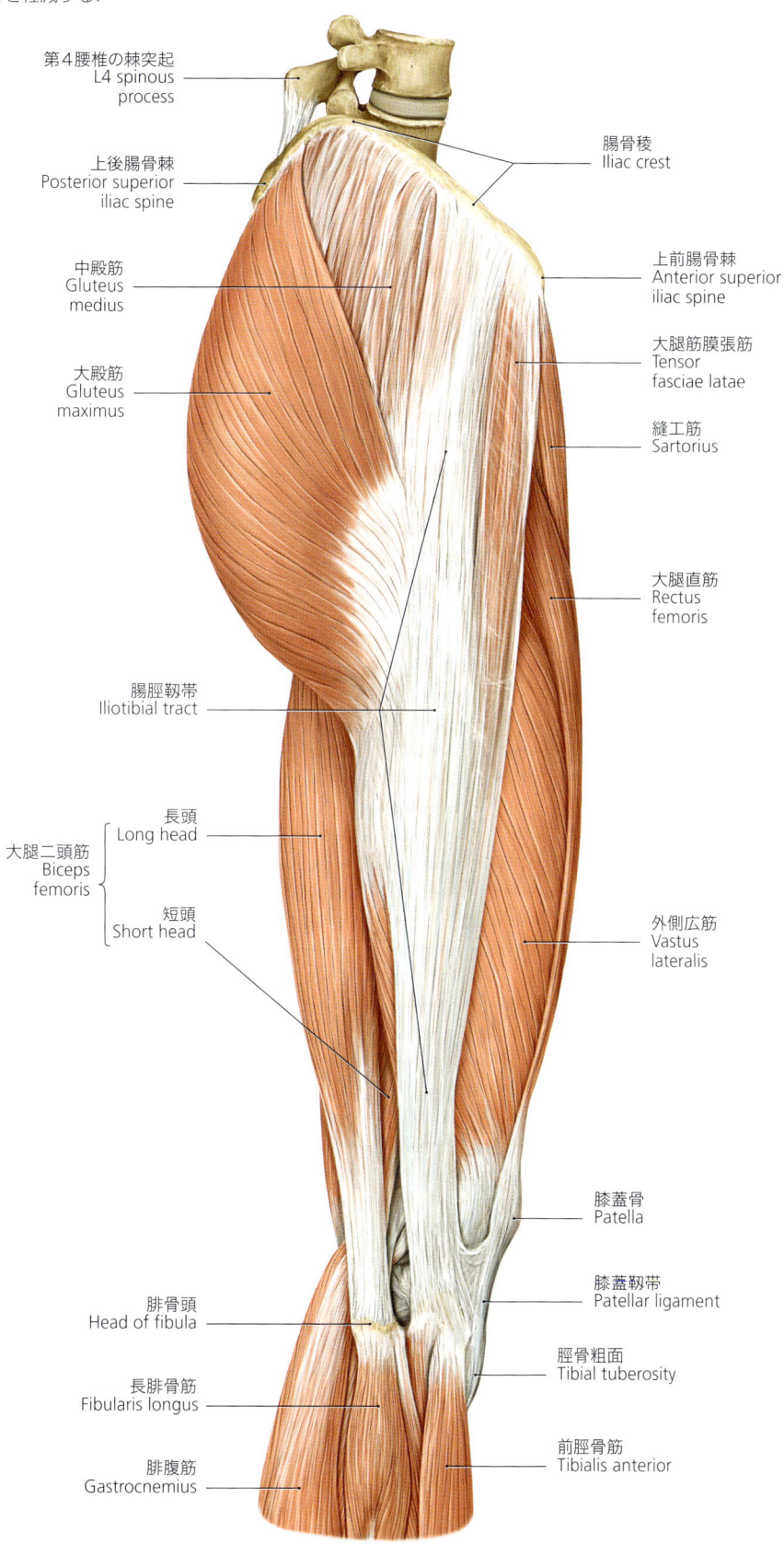

- 第4腰椎の棘突起 L4 spinous process
- 上後腸骨棘 Posterior superior iliac spine
- 中殿筋 Gluteus medius
- 大殿筋 Gluteus maximus
- 腸脛靱帯 Iliotibial tract
- 大腿二頭筋 Biceps femoris
  - 長頭 Long head
  - 短頭 Short head
- 腓骨頭 Head of fibula
- 長腓骨筋 Fibularis longus
- 腓腹筋 Gastrocnemius
- 腸骨稜 Iliac crest
- 上前腸骨棘 Anterior superior iliac spine
- 大腿筋膜張筋 Tensor fasciae latae
- 縫工筋 Sartorius
- 大腿直筋 Rectus femoris
- 外側広筋 Vastus lateralis
- 膝蓋骨 Patella
- 膝蓋靱帯 Patellar ligament
- 脛骨粗面 Tibial tuberosity
- 前脛骨筋 Tibialis anterior

個々の筋 (1)
Muscle Facts (I)

表 24.1　大腰筋, 小腰筋, 腸骨筋

筋		起始	停止	神経支配	作用
③腸腰筋	小腰筋	T12-L1 の椎骨と椎間円板 (外側面)	腸恥筋膜弓, 腸恥隆起	腰神経叢から直接出る枝 (L2-L4)	骨盤の上方への回旋を助ける
	①大腰筋	浅層: T12-L4 の椎骨と椎間円板 (外側面), 深層: L1-L5 の椎骨 (肋骨突起)	小転子		・股関節: 屈曲・外旋 ・腰部脊柱: 大腿を固定した状態で片側が収縮すると体幹を同側に曲げる, 仰臥位で両側が収縮すると体幹を引き起こす
	②腸骨筋	腸骨窩		大腿神経 (L2-L4)	

図 24.20　骨盤の筋
右側.

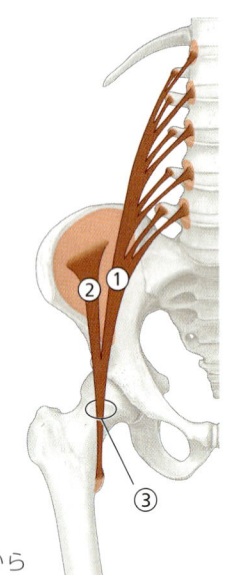

A 腸腰筋, 前方から見たところ.

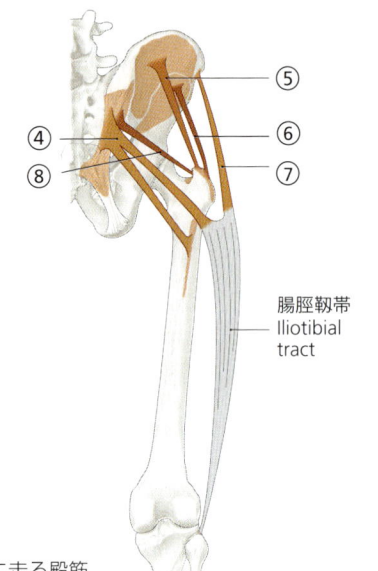

B 縦方向に走る殿筋群, 後方から見たところ. 腸脛靱帯 Iliotibial tract

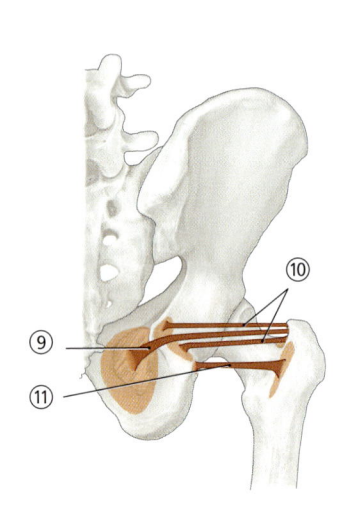

C 水平方向に走る殿筋群, 後方から見たところ.

表 24.2　殿部と骨盤の筋

筋	起始	停止	神経支配	作用
④大殿筋	仙骨 (後面の外側部), 腸骨 (殿筋面の後部), 胸腰筋膜, 仙結節靱帯	・上部の筋束: 腸脛靱帯 ・下部の筋束: 殿筋粗面	下殿神経 (L5-S2)	・筋全体: 股関節の伸展・外旋・矢状面および前額面における股関節の安定化 ・上部の筋束: 股関節の外転 ・下部の筋束: 股関節の内転
⑤中殿筋	腸骨 (殿筋面, 前・後殿筋線に挟まれた部分)	大腿骨の大転子 (外側面)	上殿神経 (L4-S1)	・筋全体: 股関節の外転・前額面における骨盤の安定化 ・外側部の筋束: 股関節の屈曲・内旋 ・内側部の筋束: 股関節の伸展と外旋
⑥小殿筋	腸骨 (殿筋面, 中殿筋の起始部よりも下方の部分)	大腿骨の大転子 (前外側面)		
⑦大腿筋膜張筋	上前腸骨棘	腸脛靱帯		・大腿筋膜の緊張 ・股関節の外転・伸展・内旋
⑧梨状筋	仙骨の前面 184.585 mm	大腿骨の大転子 (尖端)	仙骨神経叢から直接出る枝 (S1, S2)	・股関節の外旋・外転・伸展 ・股関節の安定化
⑨内閉鎖筋	閉鎖膜とこれを縁どる恥骨と坐骨の内面	大腿骨の大転子 (内側面)	仙骨神経叢から直接出る枝 (L5, S1)	股関節の外旋・内転・伸展 (関節の位置によっては外転作用も持つ)
⑩双子筋	・上双子筋: 坐骨棘 ・下双子筋: 坐骨結節	大腿骨の大転子 (内側面), 内閉鎖筋の腱と共に停止する		
⑪大腿方形筋	坐骨結節の外側縁	大腿骨の転子間稜		股関節の外旋・内転

図 24.21 大腰筋，小腰筋，腸骨筋
右側，前方から見たところ．

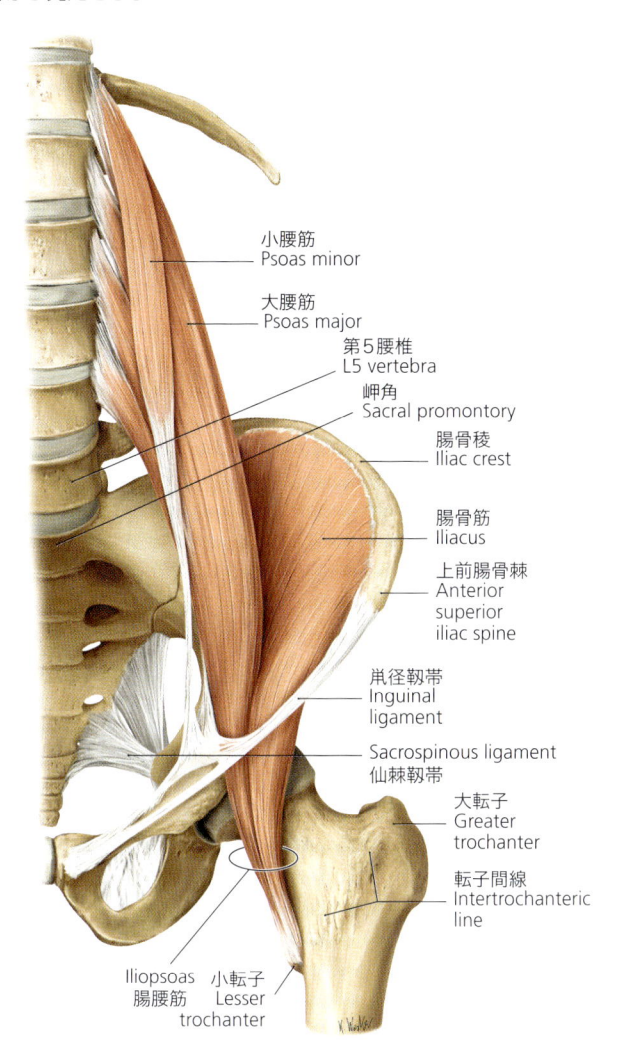

- 小腰筋 Psoas minor
- 大腰筋 Psoas major
- 第5腰椎 L5 vertebra
- 岬角 Sacral promontory
- 腸骨稜 Iliac crest
- 腸骨筋 Iliacus
- 上前腸骨棘 Anterior superior iliac spine
- 鼠径靱帯 Inguinal ligament
- Sacrospinous ligament 仙棘靱帯
- 大転子 Greater trochanter
- 転子間線 Intertrochanteric line
- Iliopsoas 腸腰筋
- 小転子 Lesser trochanter

図 24.22 殿部表層の筋
右側，後方から見たところ．

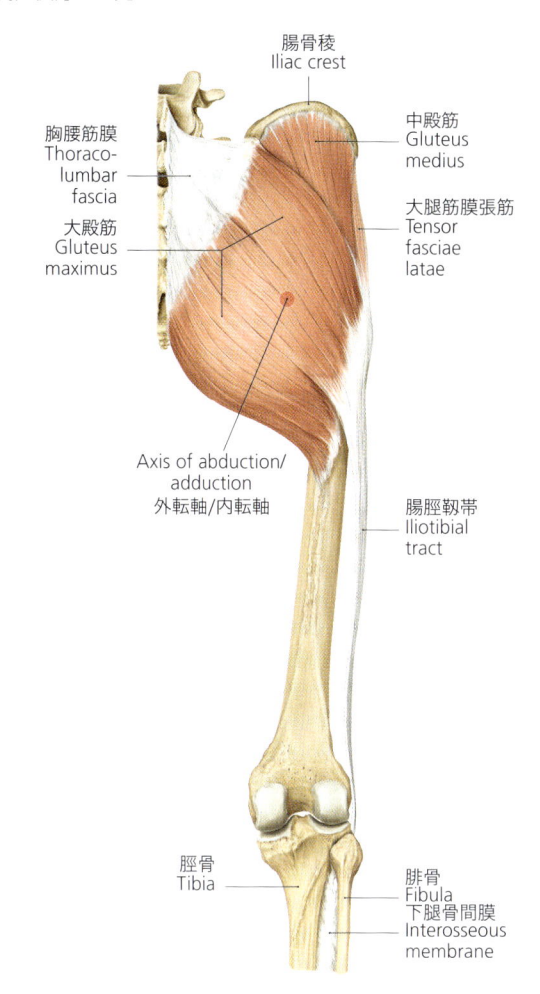

- 腸骨稜 Iliac crest
- 中殿筋 Gluteus medius
- 胸腰筋膜 Thoracolumbar fascia
- 大腿筋膜張筋 Tensor fasciae latae
- 大殿筋 Gluteus maximus
- Axis of abduction/adduction 外転軸/内転軸
- 腸脛靱帯 Iliotibial tract
- 脛骨 Tibia
- 腓骨 Fibula
- 下腿骨間膜 Interosseous membrane

図 24.23 殿部深層の筋
右側，後方から見たところ．

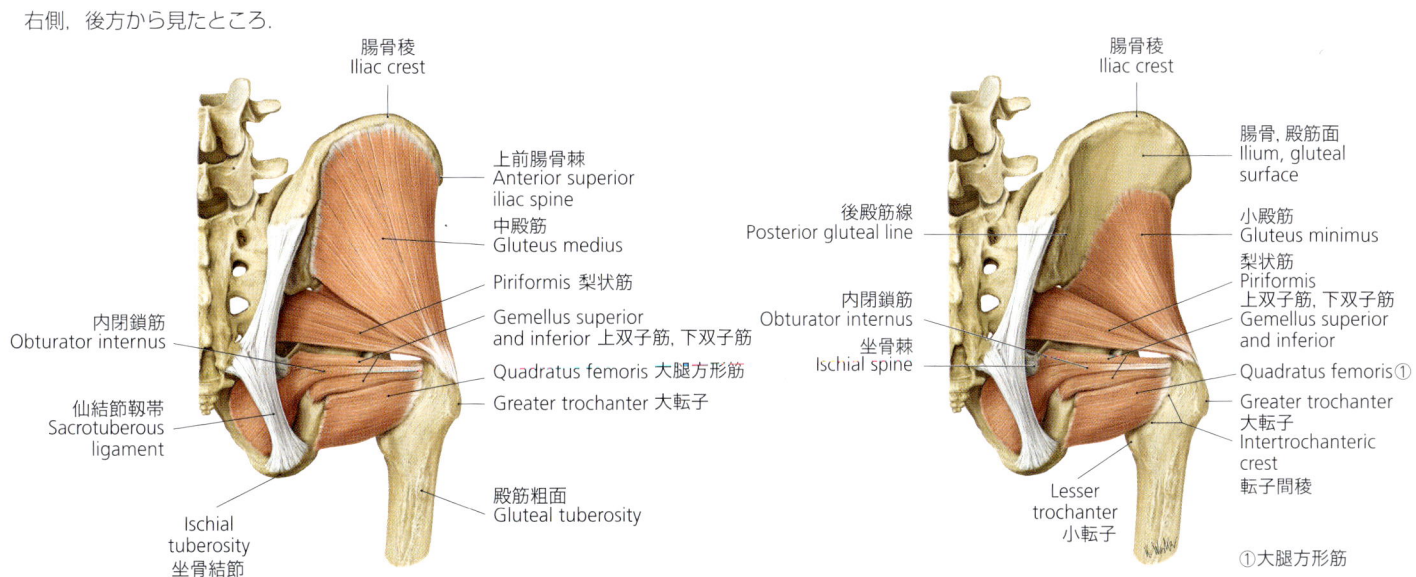

A 大殿筋を取り除いたところ．

- 腸骨稜 Iliac crest
- 上前腸骨棘 Anterior superior iliac spine
- 中殿筋 Gluteus medius
- Piriformis 梨状筋
- Gemellus superior and inferior 上双子筋，下双子筋
- Quadratus femoris 大腿方形筋
- Greater trochanter 大転子
- 殿筋粗面 Gluteal tuberosity
- 内閉鎖筋 Obturator internus
- 仙結節靱帯 Sacrotuberous ligament
- Ischial tuberosity 坐骨結節

B 中殿筋を取り除いたところ．

- 腸骨稜 Iliac crest
- 腸骨，殿筋面 Ilium, gluteal surface
- 小殿筋 Gluteus minimus
- 梨状筋 Piriformis
- 上双子筋，下双子筋 Gemellus superior and inferior
- Quadratus femoris ①
- Greater trochanter 大転子
- Intertrochanteric crest 転子間稜
- Lesser trochanter 小転子
- 後殿筋線 Posterior gluteal line
- 内閉鎖筋 Obturator internus
- 坐骨棘 Ischial spine

①大腿方形筋

個々の筋（2）
Muscle Facts (II)

大腿内側の筋は股関節の内転筋である．

図 24.24　大腿内側の筋：表層
前方から見たところ．

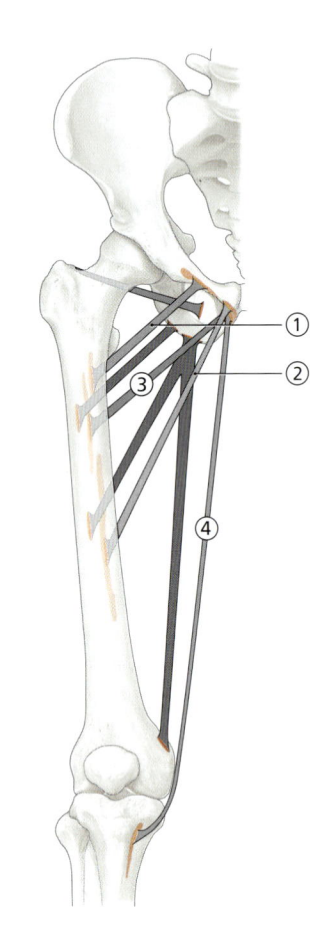

A 右側，概要．

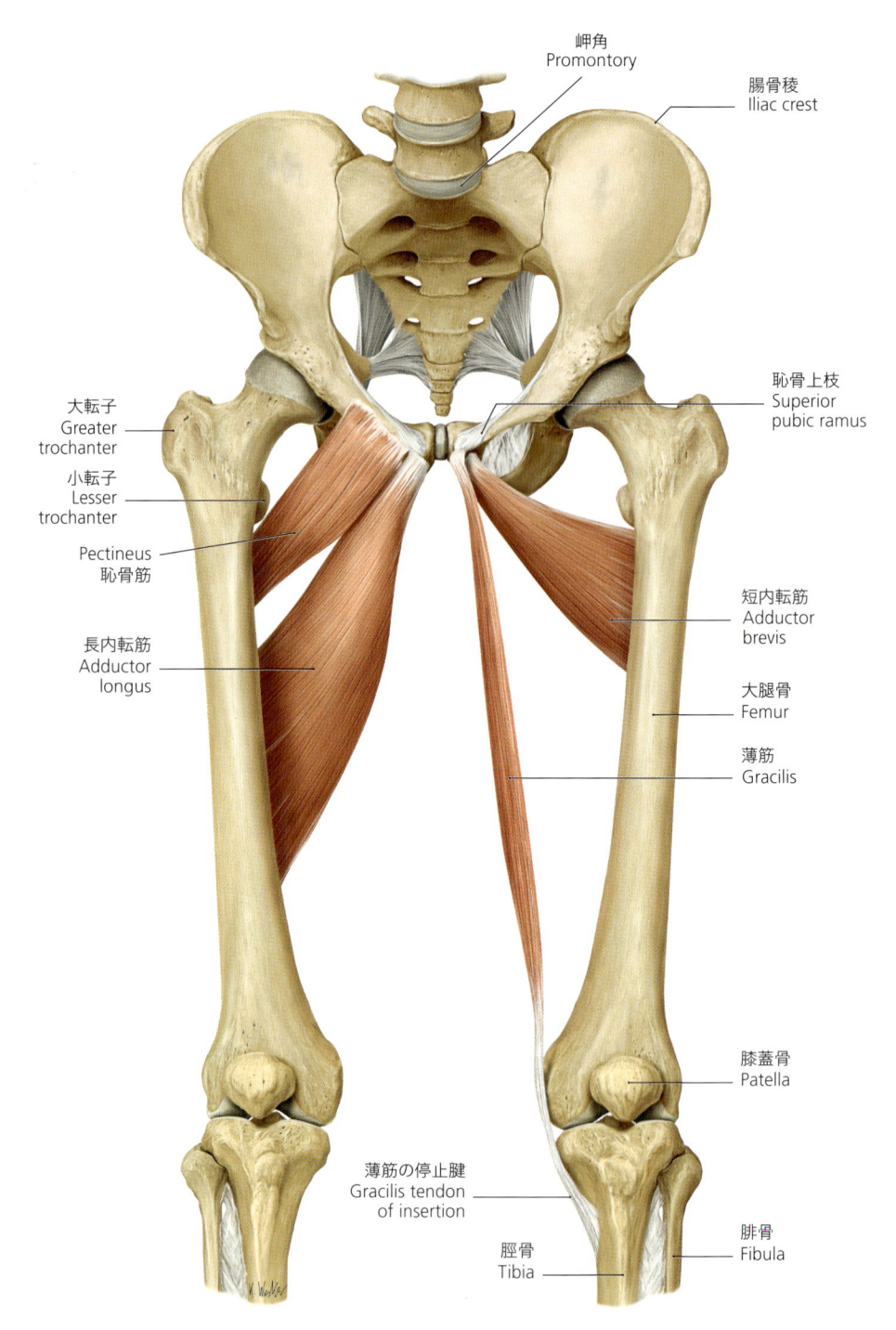

B 大腿の内転筋（表層）．

表 24.3　大腿内側の筋：表層

筋	起始	停止	神経支配	作用
①恥骨筋	恥骨櫛	大腿骨（恥骨筋線，粗線の近位部）	大腿神経，閉鎖神経（L2, L3）	・股関節：内転・外旋・わずかな屈曲 ・前額面と矢状面での骨盤の安定化
②長内転筋	恥骨上枝，恥骨結合の前面	大腿骨（粗線中央3分の1の内側唇）	閉鎖神経（L2-L4）	・股関節：内転・屈曲（70°までの屈曲位）・伸展（80°以上の屈曲位） ・前額面と矢状面での骨盤の安定化
③短内転筋	恥骨下枝			
④薄筋	恥骨下枝（恥骨結合より下方の部分）	脛骨粗面よりも内側の部分に停止する，停止腱は縫工筋腱や半腱様筋腱とともに鵞足を形成する	閉鎖神経（L2, L3）	・股関節：内転・屈曲 ・膝関節：屈曲と内旋

図 24.25 大腿内側の筋：深層
前方から見たところ．

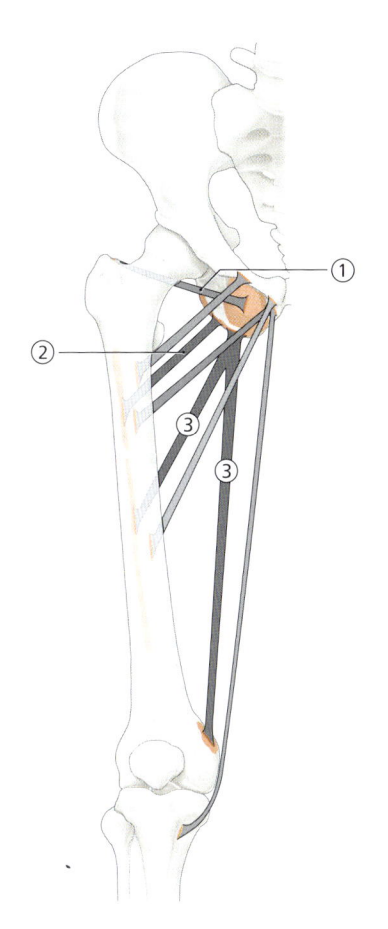

A 右側，概要．

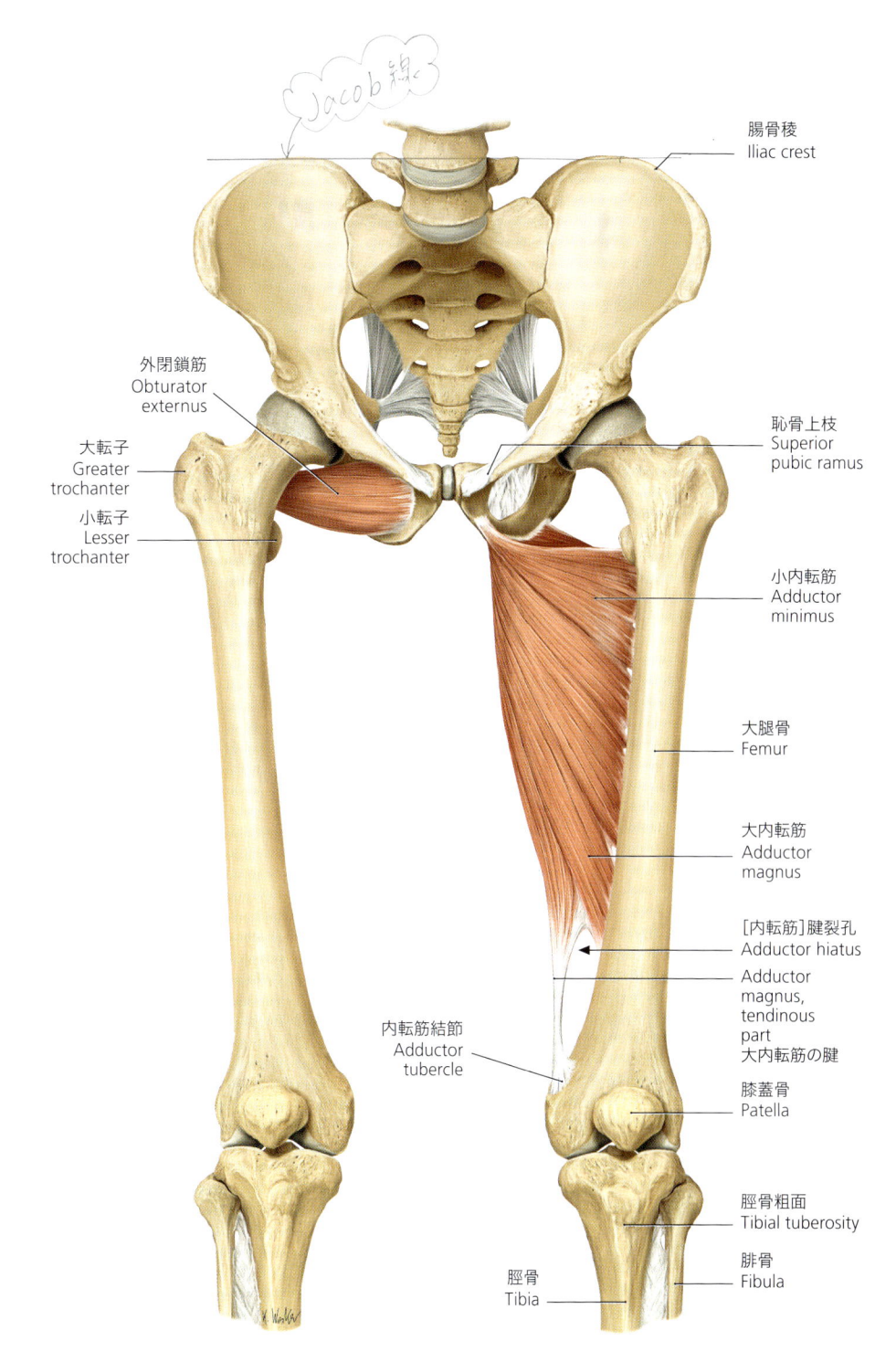

外閉鎖筋
Obturator externus

大転子
Greater trochanter

小転子
Lesser trochanter

腸骨稜
Iliac crest

恥骨上枝
Superior pubic ramus

小内転筋
Adductor minimus

大腿骨
Femur

大内転筋
Adductor magnus

[内転筋]腱裂孔
Adductor hiatus

大内転筋の腱
Adductor magnus, tendinous part

内転筋結節
Adductor tubercle

膝蓋骨
Patella

脛骨粗面
Tibial tuberosity

脛骨
Tibia

腓骨
Fibula

B 大腿の内転筋（深層）．

表 24.4　大腿内側の筋：深層

筋	起始	停止	神経支配	作用
①外閉鎖筋	閉鎖膜とこれを縁どる骨の外面	大腿骨の転子窩	閉鎖神経（L3, L4）	股関節：内転・外旋，矢状面での骨盤の安定化
②小内転筋	恥骨下枝	粗線の内側唇	閉鎖神経（L2-L4）	股関節：内転・外旋・わずかな屈曲
③大内転筋	恥骨下枝，坐骨枝，坐骨結節	・深部（筋性の停止部）：粗線の内側唇	・深部：閉鎖神経（L2-L4）	股関節：内転，外旋，わずかな屈曲（浅部は内旋作用もある），前額面と矢状面で骨盤を安定化する
		・浅部（腱性の停止部）：大腿骨の内転筋結節	・浅部：脛骨神経（L4）	

個々の筋(3)
Muscle Facts (III)

大腿の前面と後面の筋は，それぞれ膝関節に対する伸筋および屈筋として分類される．

図 24.26 大腿前面の筋
右側，前方から見たところ．

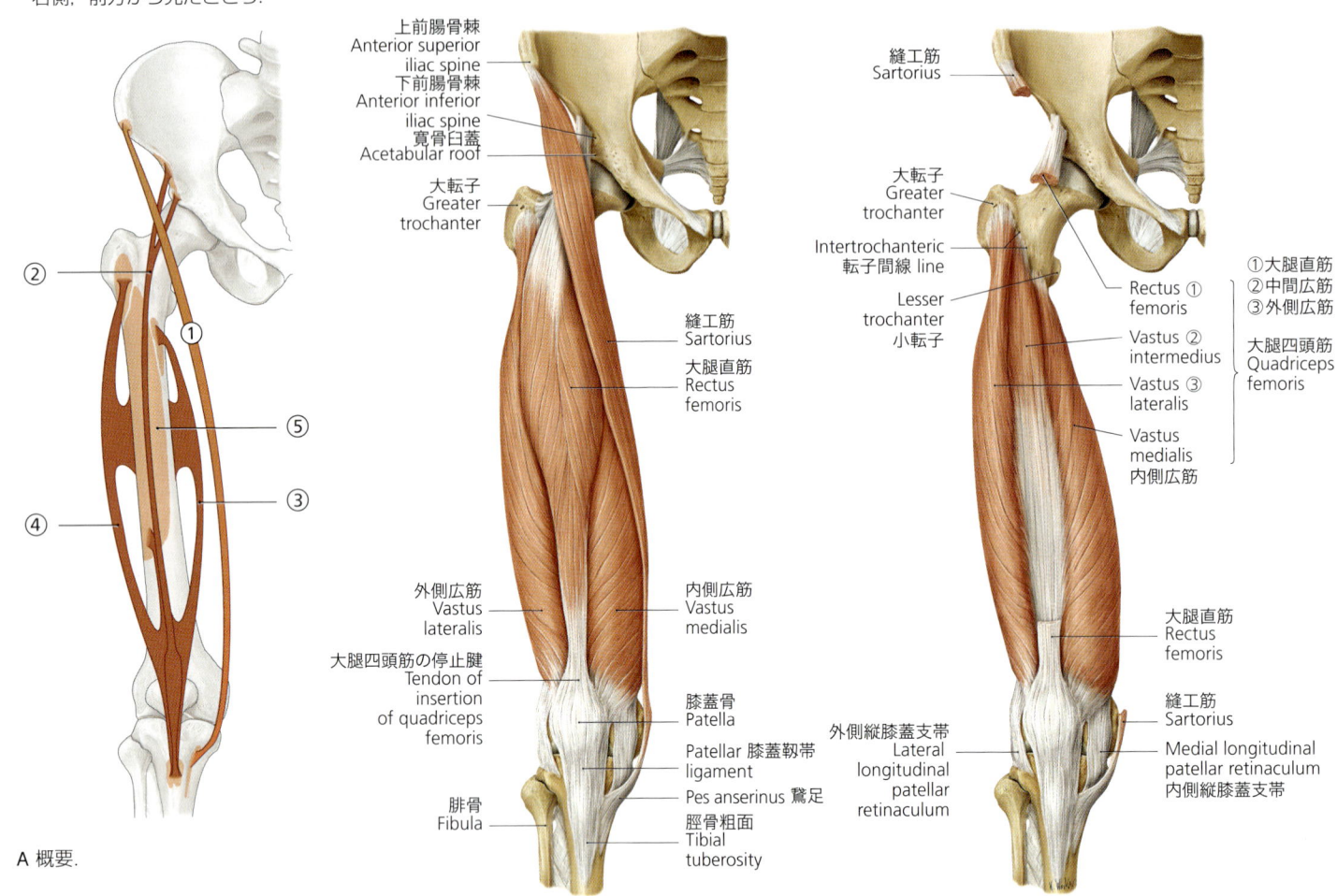

ラベル（B 浅層）:
- 上前腸骨棘 Anterior superior iliac spine
- 下前腸骨棘 Anterior inferior iliac spine
- 寛骨臼蓋 Acetabular roof
- 大転子 Greater trochanter
- 縫工筋 Sartorius
- 大腿直筋 Rectus femoris
- 外側広筋 Vastus lateralis
- 内側広筋 Vastus medialis
- 大腿四頭筋の停止腱 Tendon of insertion of quadriceps femoris
- 膝蓋骨 Patella
- 膝蓋靱帯 Patellar ligament
- 鵞足 Pes anserinus
- 腓骨 Fibula
- 脛骨粗面 Tibial tuberosity

ラベル（C 深層. 縫工筋と大腿直筋を取り除いてある）:
- 縫工筋 Sartorius
- 大転子 Greater trochanter
- 転子間線 Intertrochanteric line
- 小転子 Lesser trochanter
- ①大腿直筋 Rectus femoris
- ②中間広筋 Vastus intermedius
- ③外側広筋 Vastus lateralis
- 内側広筋 Vastus medialis
- 大腿四頭筋 Quadriceps femoris
- 大腿直筋 Rectus femoris
- 縫工筋 Sartorius
- 外側縦膝蓋支帯 Lateral longitudinal patellar retinaculum
- 内側縦膝蓋支帯 Medial longitudinal patellar retinaculum

A 概要．
B 浅層．
C 深層．縫工筋と大腿直筋を取り除いてある．

表 24.5 大腿前面の筋

筋		起始	停止	神経支配	作用
①縫工筋		上前腸骨棘	脛骨粗面よりも内側の部分（薄筋や半腱様筋とともに鵞足を形成して停止する）	大腿神経 (L2, L3)	・股関節：屈曲・外転・外旋 ・膝関節：屈曲・内旋
大腿四頭筋*	②大腿直筋	下前腸骨棘，寛骨臼上縁	脛骨粗面（膝蓋靱帯を介して停止する）	大腿神経 (L2–L4)	・股関節：屈曲 ・膝関節：伸展
	③内側広筋	粗線（内側唇），転子間線（遠位部）	脛骨粗面（内側・外側縦膝蓋支帯を介して停止する）		膝関節：伸展
	④外側広筋	粗線（外側唇），大転子（外側面）			
	⑤中間広筋	大腿骨体（前面）	脛骨粗面（膝蓋靱帯を介して停止する）		
膝関節筋（中間広筋の遠位筋束）		大腿骨体（前面，膝蓋上陥凹の高さ）	膝蓋上陥凹		膝関節：伸展．関節包が巻き込まれるのを防ぐ

*筋全体としては膝蓋靱帯を介して脛骨粗面に停止する．

図 24.27　大腿後面の筋
右側，後方から見たところ．

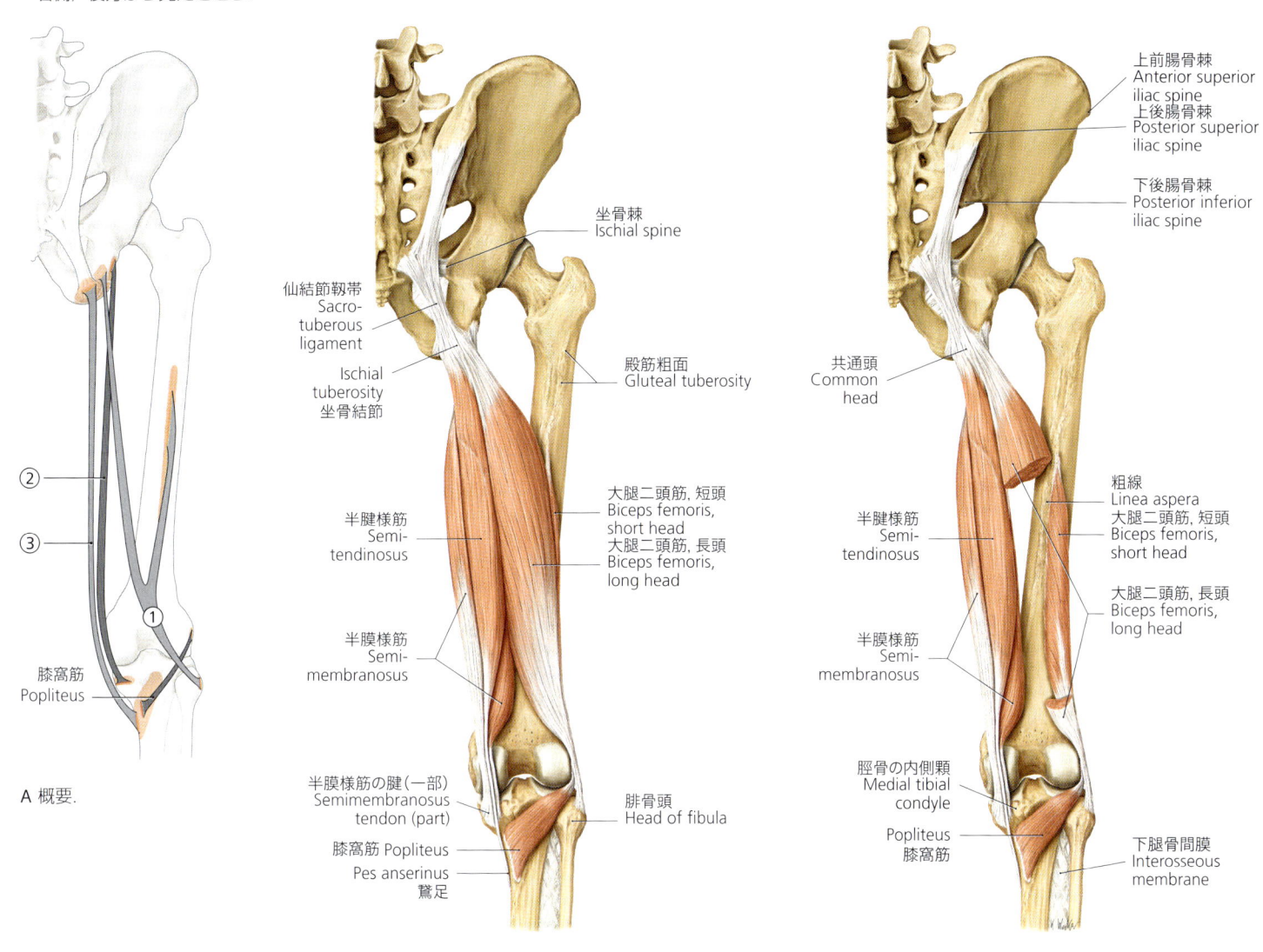

A 概要．

B 浅層．

C 深層．大腿二頭筋の長頭を部分的に取り除いてある．

表 24.6　大腿後面の筋

筋	起始	停止	神経支配	作用
①大腿二頭筋	長頭：坐骨結節，仙結節靱帯（半腱様筋と共通頭を形成する）	腓骨頭	脛骨神経（L5-S2）	・股関節（長頭）：伸展・矢状面で骨盤を安定化する ・膝関節：屈曲・外旋
	短頭：粗線外側唇の中央3分の1		総腓骨神経（L5-S2）	膝関節：屈曲・外旋
②半膜様筋	坐骨結節	脛骨の内側顆，斜膝窩靱帯，膝窩筋膜	脛骨神経（L5-S2）	・股関節：伸展・矢状面で骨盤を安定化する ・膝関節：屈曲・内旋
③半腱様筋	坐骨結節，仙結節靱帯（大腿二頭筋の長頭と共通頭を形成する）	脛骨粗面よりも内側の部分に薄筋や縫工筋とともに鵞足を形成して停止する		

膝窩筋については p.399 を参照．

脛骨と腓骨
Tibia & Fibula

下肢

👉 脛骨と腓骨の間には 2 つの関節が形成されるが，2 骨の間の運動（回旋）は制限されている．下腿骨間膜は丈夫な結合組織性のシートで，いくつかの下腿の筋がここから起始する．下腿骨間膜は脛腓靱帯結合と共にともに働き，足首の関節を安定に保つ．

図 25.1　脛骨と腓骨
右下腿．

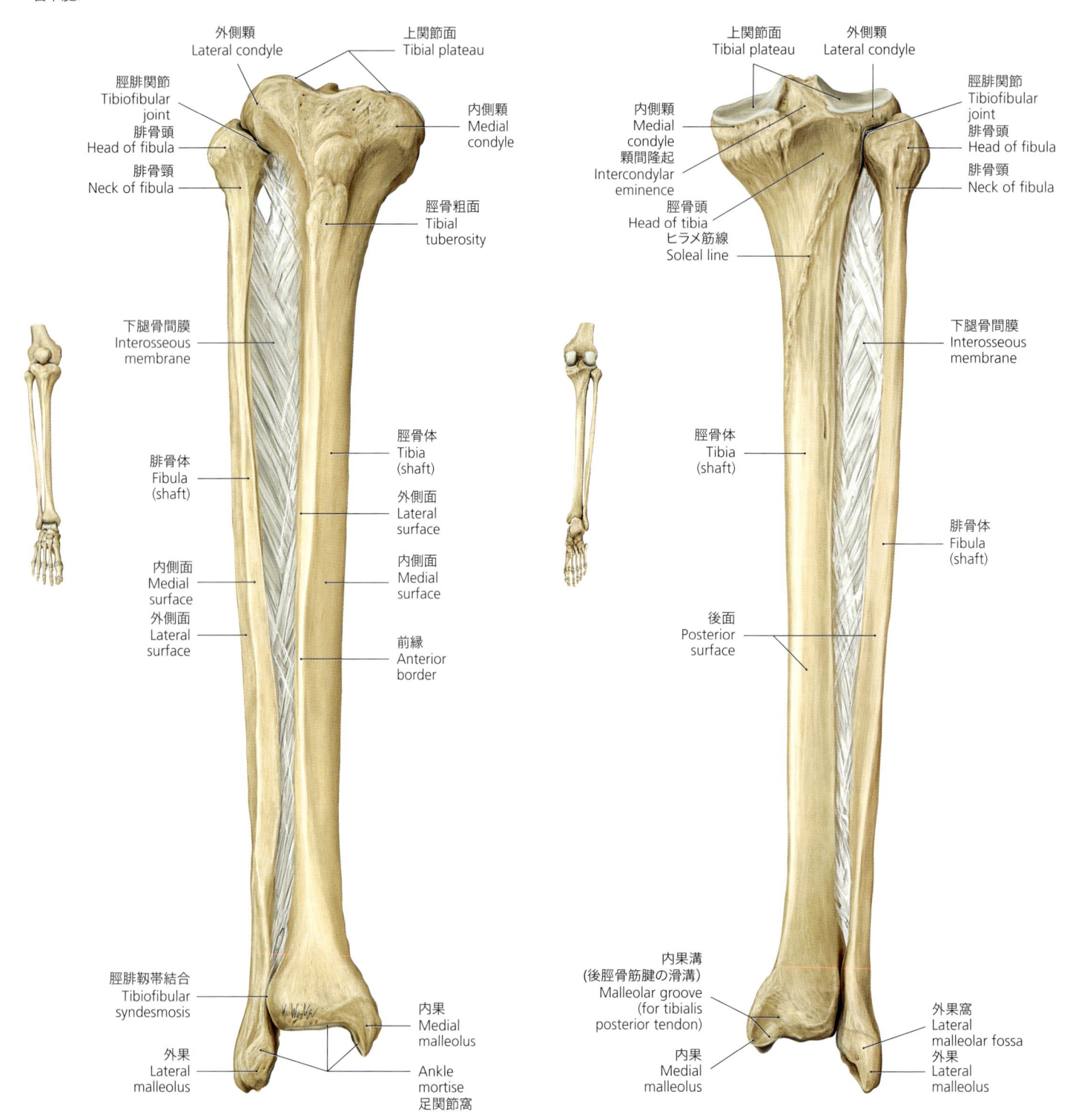

A 前方から見たところ．

- 外側顆 Lateral condyle
- 上関節面 Tibial plateau
- 脛腓関節 Tibiofibular joint
- 腓骨頭 Head of fibula
- 腓骨頸 Neck of fibula
- 内側顆 Medial condyle
- 脛骨粗面 Tibial tuberosity
- 下腿骨間膜 Interosseous membrane
- 腓骨体 Fibula (shaft)
- 内側面 Medial surface
- 外側面 Lateral surface
- 脛骨体 Tibia (shaft)
- 外側面 Lateral surface
- 内側面 Medial surface
- 前縁 Anterior border
- 脛腓靱帯結合 Tibiofibular syndesmosis
- 外果 Lateral malleolus
- 内果 Medial malleolus
- 足関節窩 Ankle mortise

B 後方から見たところ．

- 上関節面 Tibial plateau
- 外側顆 Lateral condyle
- 脛腓関節 Tibiofibular joint
- 腓骨頭 Head of fibula
- 腓骨頸 Neck of fibula
- 内側顆 Medial condyle
- 顆間隆起 Intercondylar eminence
- 脛骨頭 Head of tibia
- ヒラメ筋線 Soleal line
- 下腿骨間膜 Interosseous membrane
- 脛骨体 Tibia (shaft)
- 腓骨体 Fibula (shaft)
- 後面 Posterior surface
- 内果溝（後脛骨筋腱の滑溝） Malleolar groove (for tibialis posterior tendon)
- 内果 Medial malleolus
- 外果窩 Lateral malleolar fossa
- 外果 Lateral malleolus

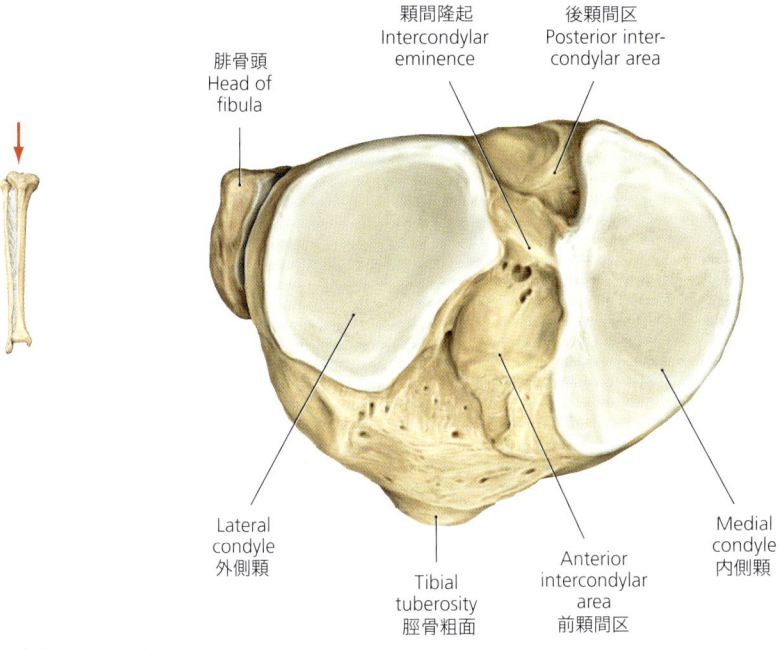

C 上方から見たところ.

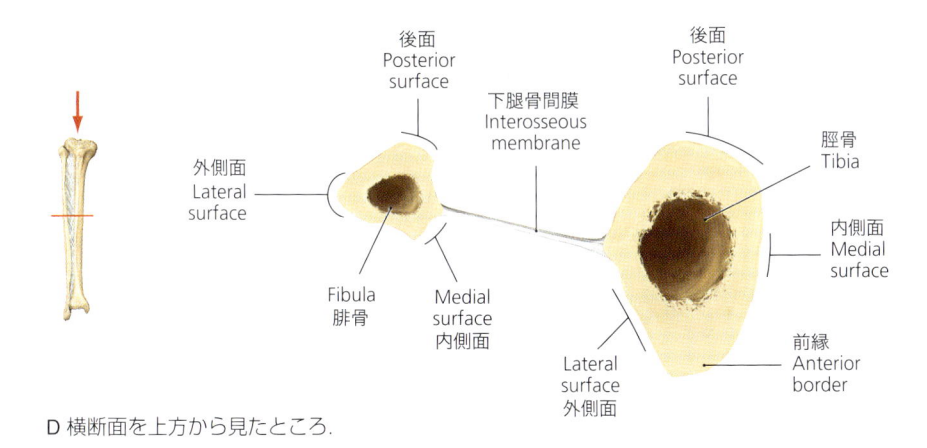

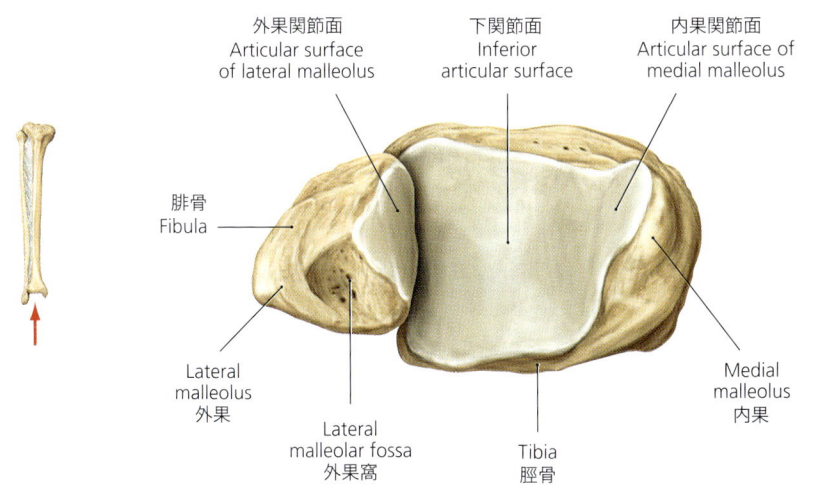

- 腓骨頭 Head of fibula
- 顆間隆起 Intercondylar eminence
- 後顆間区 Posterior intercondylar area
- Lateral condyle 外側顆
- Tibial tuberosity 脛骨粗面
- Anterior intercondylar area 前顆間区
- Medial condyle 内側顆

D 横断面を上方から見たところ.

- 後面 Posterior surface
- 下腿骨間膜 Interosseous membrane
- 後面 Posterior surface
- 外側面 Lateral surface
- 脛骨 Tibia
- Fibula 腓骨
- Medial surface 内側面
- 内側面 Medial surface
- Lateral surface 外側面
- 前縁 Anterior border

E 下方から見たところ.

- 外果関節面 Articular surface of lateral malleolus
- 下関節面 Inferior articular surface
- 内果関節面 Articular surface of medial malleolus
- 腓骨 Fibula
- Lateral malleolus 外果
- Lateral malleolar fossa 外果窩
- Tibia 脛骨
- Medial malleolus 内果

臨床

腓骨骨折

腓骨骨折と診断された場合，脛腓靱帯結合（p. 380参照）が損傷されているかどうかを判定する必要がある．腓骨骨折は脛腓靱帯結合を基準にして，遠位，同じ高さ，近位で起こりうる．同じ高さもしくは近位での腓骨骨折は，しばしば脛腓靱帯結合の断裂を伴う．

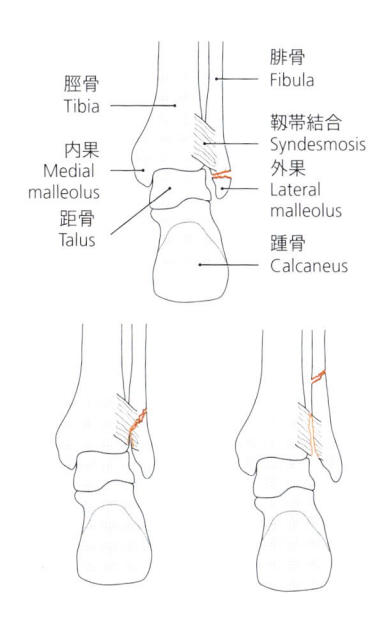

- 脛骨 Tibia
- 腓骨 Fibula
- 靱帯結合 Syndesmosis
- 内果 Medial malleolus
- 外果 Lateral malleolus
- 距骨 Talus
- 踵骨 Calcaneus

下のX線写真では，近位での腓骨骨折がみられる（矢印）．また，距腿関節の内側の関節腔が外側よりも広がっていることから（p.405参照），脛腓靱帯結合が断裂していることもわかる．

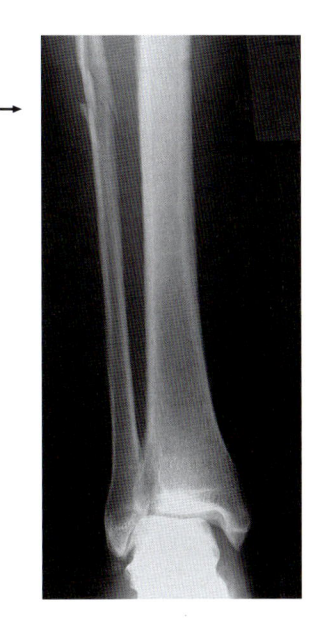

25 膝と下腿

膝関節：概観
Knee Joint: Overview

膝関節において，大腿骨は脛骨および膝蓋骨との間に2つの関節を形成する．両方の関節は共通の関節包で包まれ，関節腔はつながっている．Note：腓骨は膝関節に加わっていない（肘関節における尺骨と対比すること，p.282参照）．その代わり，腓骨は脛骨との間で別の強固な関節を形成する．

図25.2 右膝関節

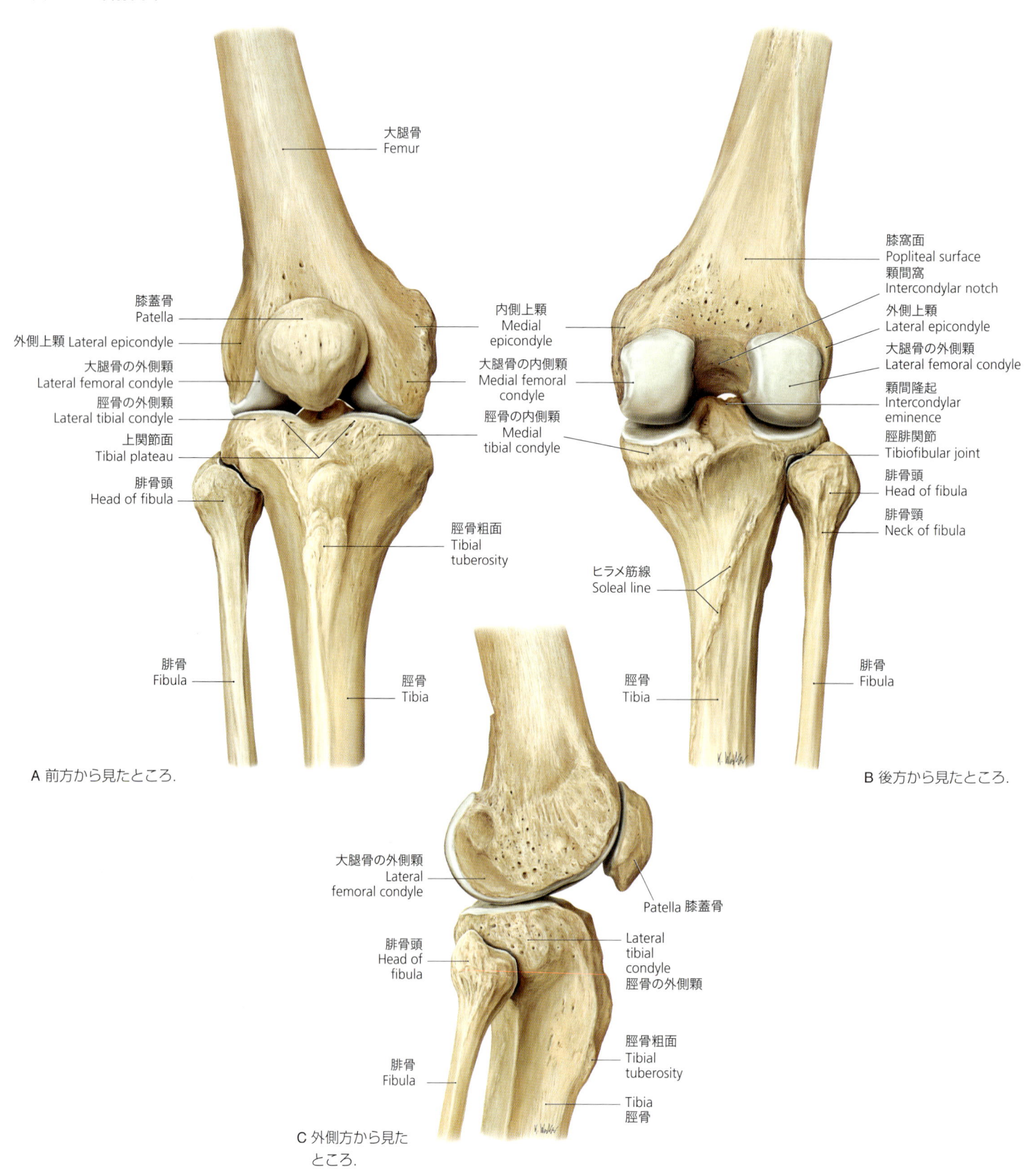

A 前方から見たところ．

B 後方から見たところ．

C 外側方から見たところ．

図 25.4 右膝蓋骨

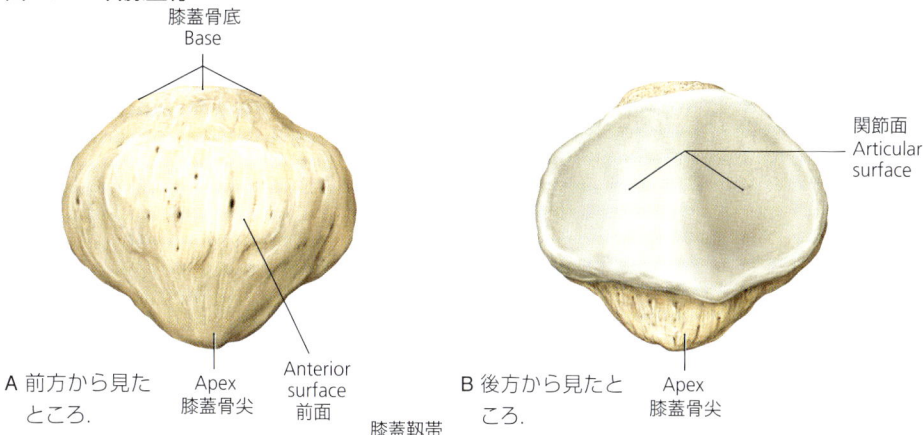

膝蓋骨底
Base

関節面
Articular surface

Apex
膝蓋骨尖

Anterior surface
前面

A 前方から見たところ．

B 後方から見たところ．

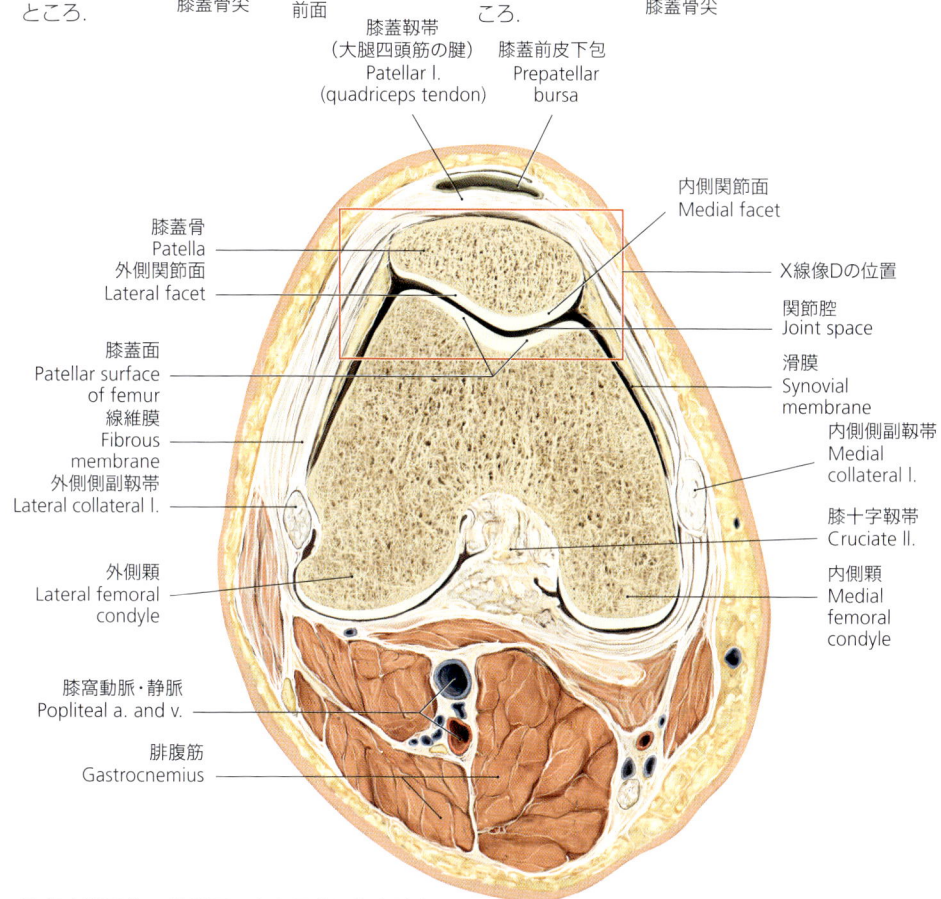

Apex
膝蓋骨尖

図 25.3 膝関節のX線像

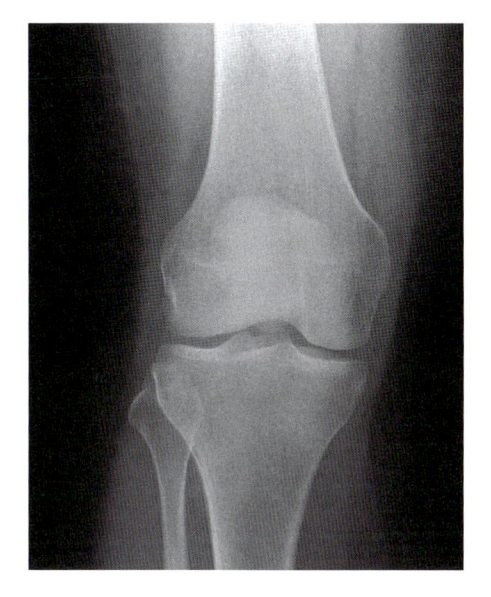

A 前後像

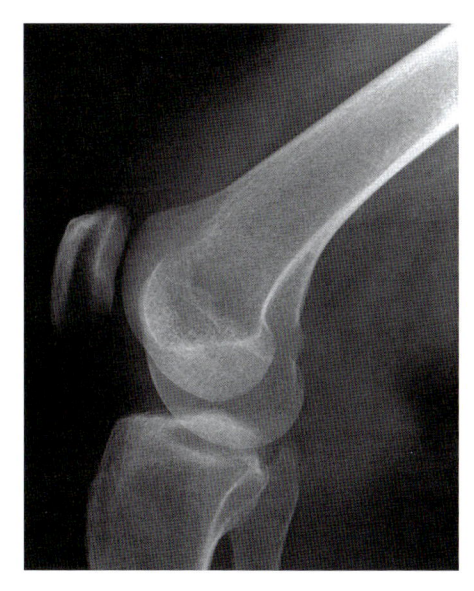

B 側面像

膝蓋靱帯（大腿四頭筋の腱）
Patellar l. (quadriceps tendon)

膝蓋前皮下包
Prepatellar bursa

内側関節面
Medial facet

膝蓋骨
Patella

外側関節面
Lateral facet

X線像Dの位置

関節腔
Joint space

膝蓋面
Patellar surface of femur

滑膜
Synovial membrane

線維膜
Fibrous membrane

内側側副靱帯
Medial collateral l.

外側側副靱帯
Lateral collateral l.

膝十字靱帯
Cruciate ll.

外側顆
Lateral femoral condyle

内側顆
Medial femoral condyle

膝窩動脈・静脈
Popliteal a. and v.

腓腹筋
Gastrocnemius

C 膝蓋大腿関節の横断面．やや屈曲した右膝を遠位方向から見たところ．

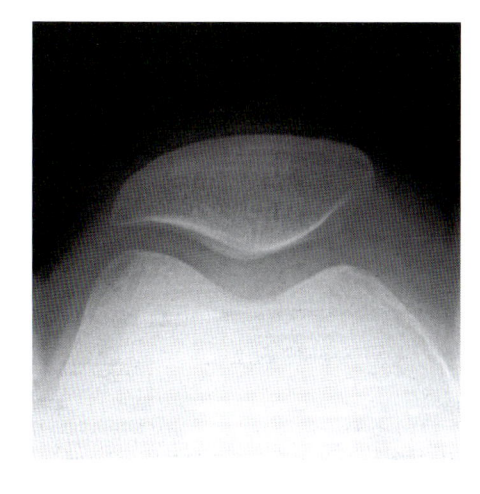

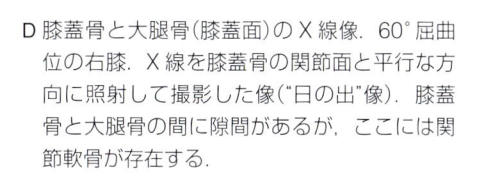

D 膝蓋骨と大腿骨（膝蓋面）のX線像．60°屈曲位の右膝．X線を膝蓋骨の関節面と平行な方向に照射して撮影した像（"日の出"像）．膝蓋骨と大腿骨の間に隙間があるが，ここには関節軟骨が存在する．

膝関節：靭帯，関節包，滑液包
Knee Joint: Capsule, Ligaments & Bursae

表 25.1　膝関節の靭帯

関節外靭帯		
前面	膝蓋靭帯
	内側縦膝蓋支帯
	外側縦膝蓋支帯
	内側横膝蓋支帯
	外側横膝蓋支帯
内側・外側面	内側側副靭帯
	外側側副靭帯
後面	斜膝窩靭帯
	弓状膝窩靭帯
関節内靭帯		
前十字靭帯		
後十字靭帯		
膝横靭帯		
後半月大腿靭帯		

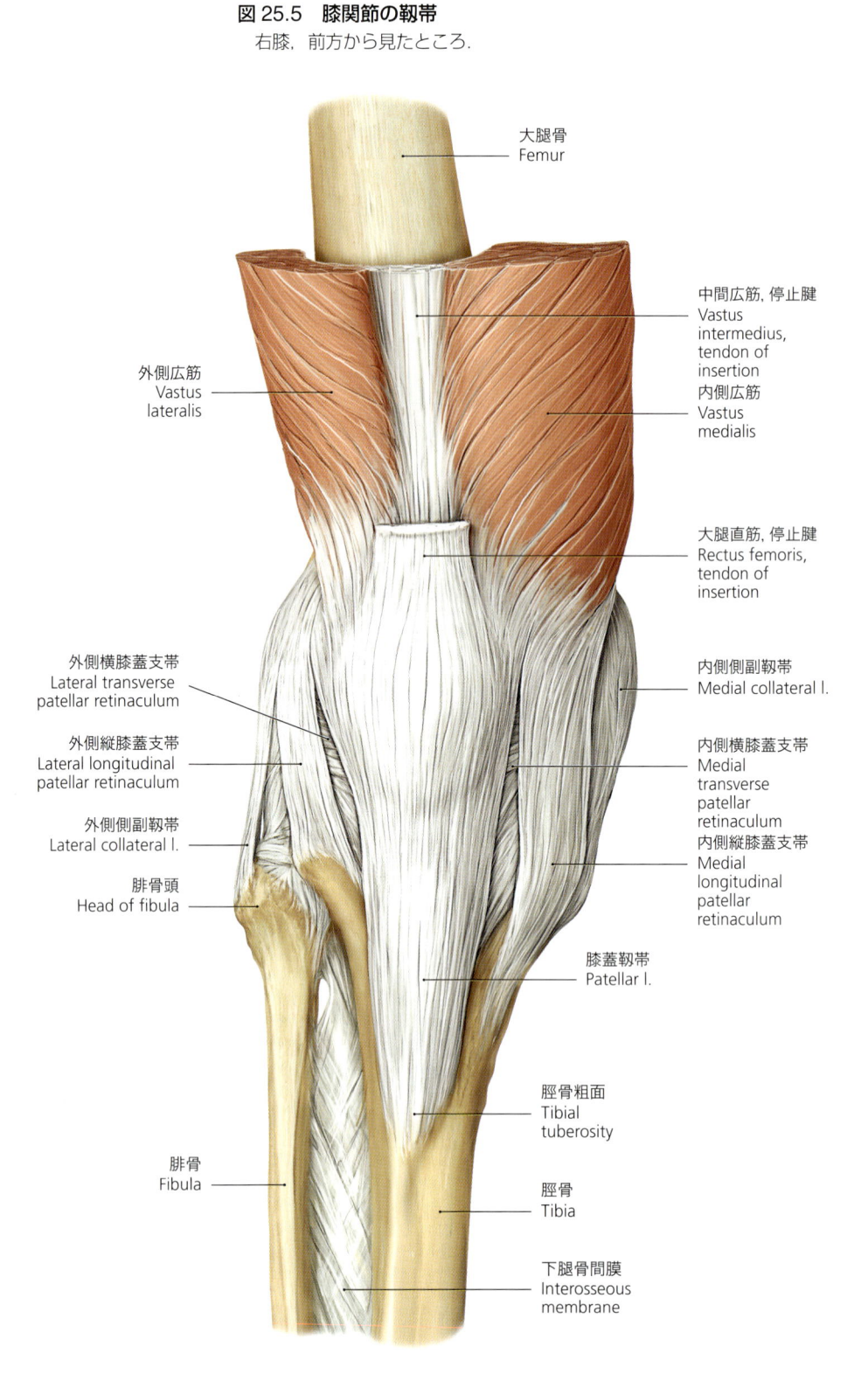

図 25.5　膝関節の靭帯
右膝，前方から見たところ．

ラベル：
- 大腿骨 Femur
- 中間広筋, 停止腱 Vastus intermedius, tendon of insertion
- 外側広筋 Vastus lateralis
- 内側広筋 Vastus medialis
- 大腿直筋, 停止腱 Rectus femoris, tendon of insertion
- 外側横膝蓋支帯 Lateral transverse patellar retinaculum
- 内側側副靭帯 Medial collateral l.
- 外側縦膝蓋支帯 Lateral longitudinal patellar retinaculum
- 内側横膝蓋支帯 Medial transverse patellar retinaculum
- 外側側副靭帯 Lateral collateral l.
- 内側縦膝蓋支帯 Medial longitudinal patellar retinaculum
- 腓骨頭 Head of fibula
- 膝蓋靭帯 Patellar l.
- 脛骨粗面 Tibial tuberosity
- 腓骨 Fibula
- 脛骨 Tibia
- 下腿骨間膜 Interosseous membrane

図 25.6 膝関節の関節包，靱帯，滑液包

右膝，後方から見たところ．膝関節の関節腔は関節周辺にある滑液包（膝窩筋下陥凹，半膜様筋の滑液包，腓腹筋の内側・外側腱下包）とつながっている．

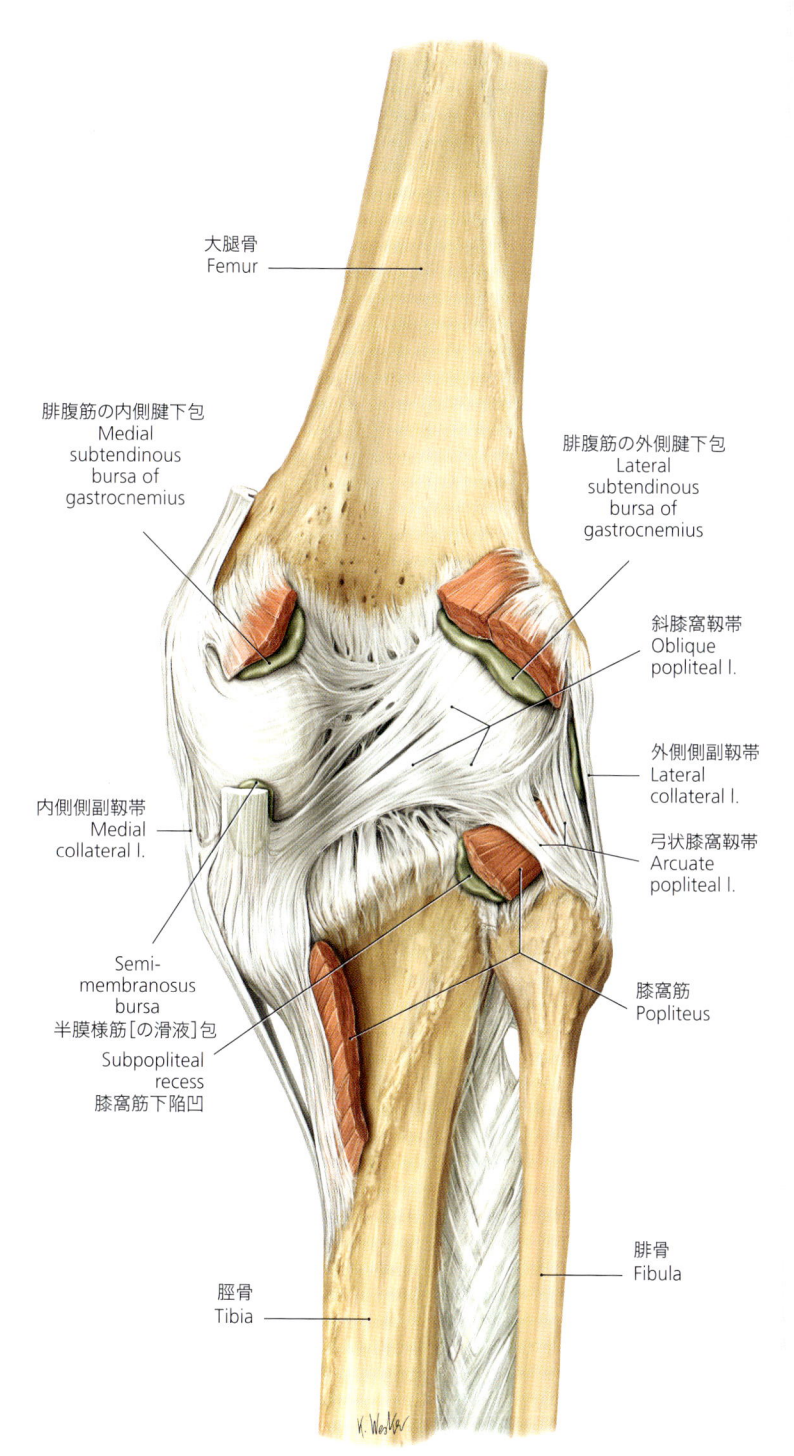

- 大腿骨 Femur
- 腓腹筋の内側腱下包 Medial subtendinous bursa of gastrocnemius
- 腓腹筋の外側腱下包 Lateral subtendinous bursa of gastrocnemius
- 斜膝窩靱帯 Oblique popliteal l.
- 内側側副靱帯 Medial collateral l.
- 外側側副靱帯 Lateral collateral l.
- 弓状膝窩靱帯 Arcuate popliteal l.
- Semi-membranosus bursa 半膜様筋［の滑液］包
- Subpopliteal recess 膝窩筋下陥凹
- 膝窩筋 Popliteus
- 脛骨 Tibia
- 腓骨 Fibula

臨床

腓腹筋-半膜様筋包（ベイカー Baker 嚢胞）

膝窩の痛みを伴った腫脹は，関節包が嚢胞状に膨れ出たことに起因する場合がある．このような嚢胞状の膨らみは，関節腔内の圧が高まった場合（例えば，関節リウマチ）においてよく生じる．

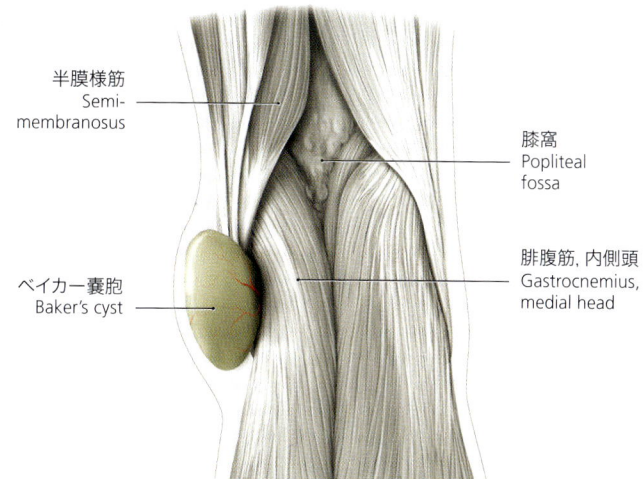

- 半膜様筋 Semi-membranosus
- 膝窩 Popliteal fossa
- ベイカー嚢胞 Baker's cyst
- 腓腹筋，内側頭 Gastrocnemius, medial head

A 右膝窩のベイカー嚢胞．この嚢胞は膝窩の内側部に見られることが多く，大腿骨の内側顆の高さで，半膜様筋腱と腓腹筋内側頭の間に生じる．

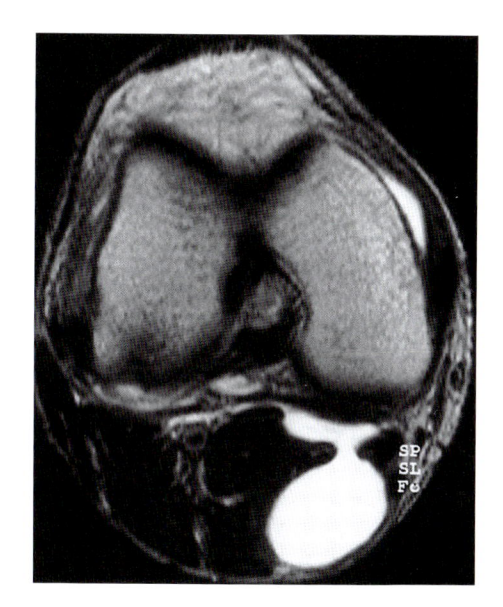

B 膝窩におけるベイカー嚢胞の横断 MR 像，下方から見たところ．

膝関節：靭帯と半月
Knee Joint: Ligaments & Menisci

図 25.7 膝関節の側副靭帯と膝蓋靭帯

右膝関節．膝関節は内側・外側側副靭帯によって補強される．内側側副靭帯は関節包と内側半月の両方と接着するが，外側側副靭帯は関節包や外側半月とは直接に接することはない．膝関節が伸展し，前額面内で安定している場合には，どちらの側副靭帯も緊張している．

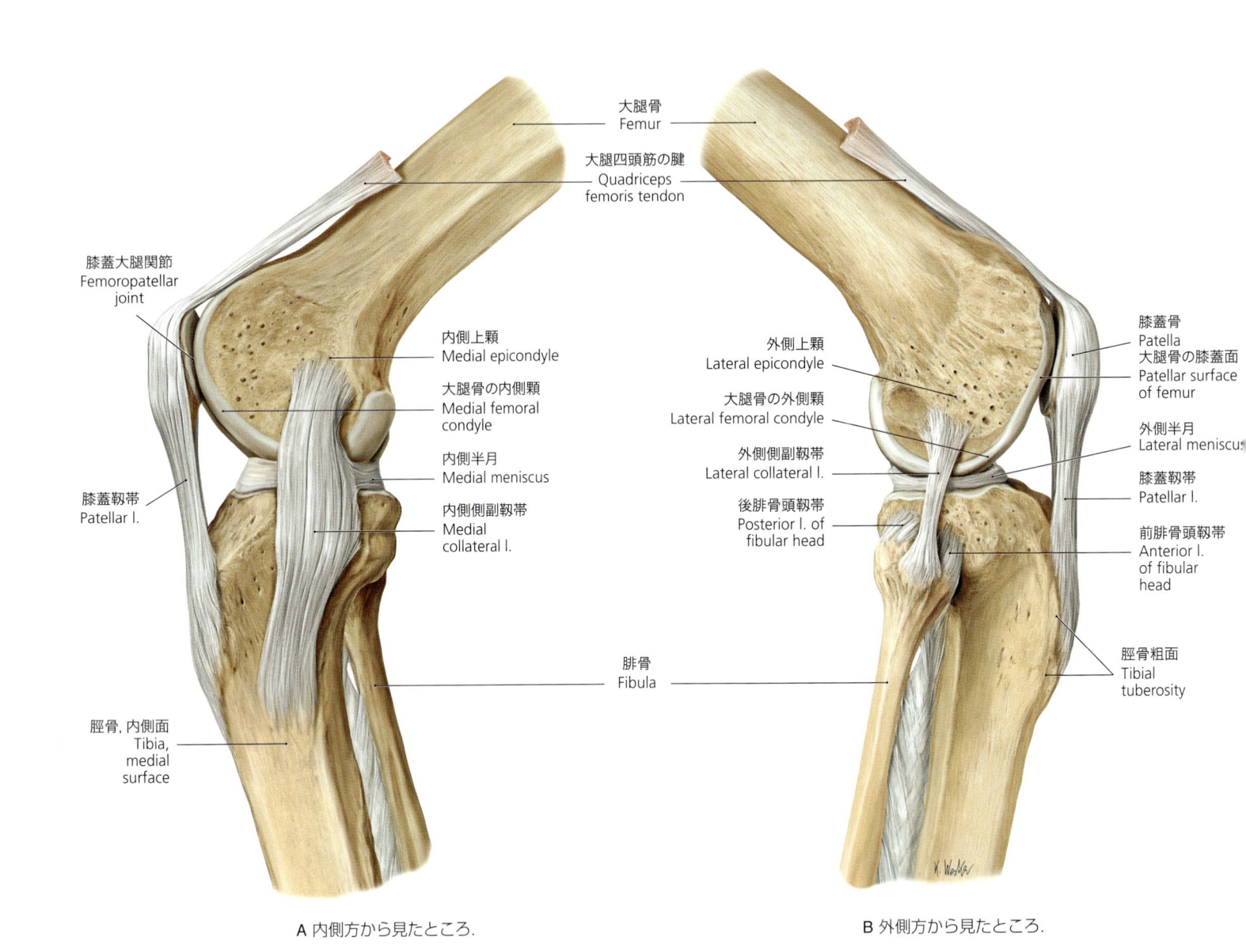

A 内側方から見たところ．

B 外側方から見たところ．

図 25.8 膝関節の半月
右脛骨の上関節面，近位方向から見たところ．

- 前十字靱帯 Anterior cruciate l.
- 内側半月 Medial meniscus
- 膝蓋靱帯 Patellar l.
- 膝横靱帯 Transverse l. of knee
- 脛腓関節 Tibiofibular joint
- 内側側副靱帯 Medial collateral l.
- 後十字靱帯 Posterior cruciate l.
- 後半月大腿靱帯 Posterior meniscofemoral l.
- 外側半月 Lateral meniscus
- 腓骨頭 Head of fibula
- 外側側副靱帯 Lateral collateral l.

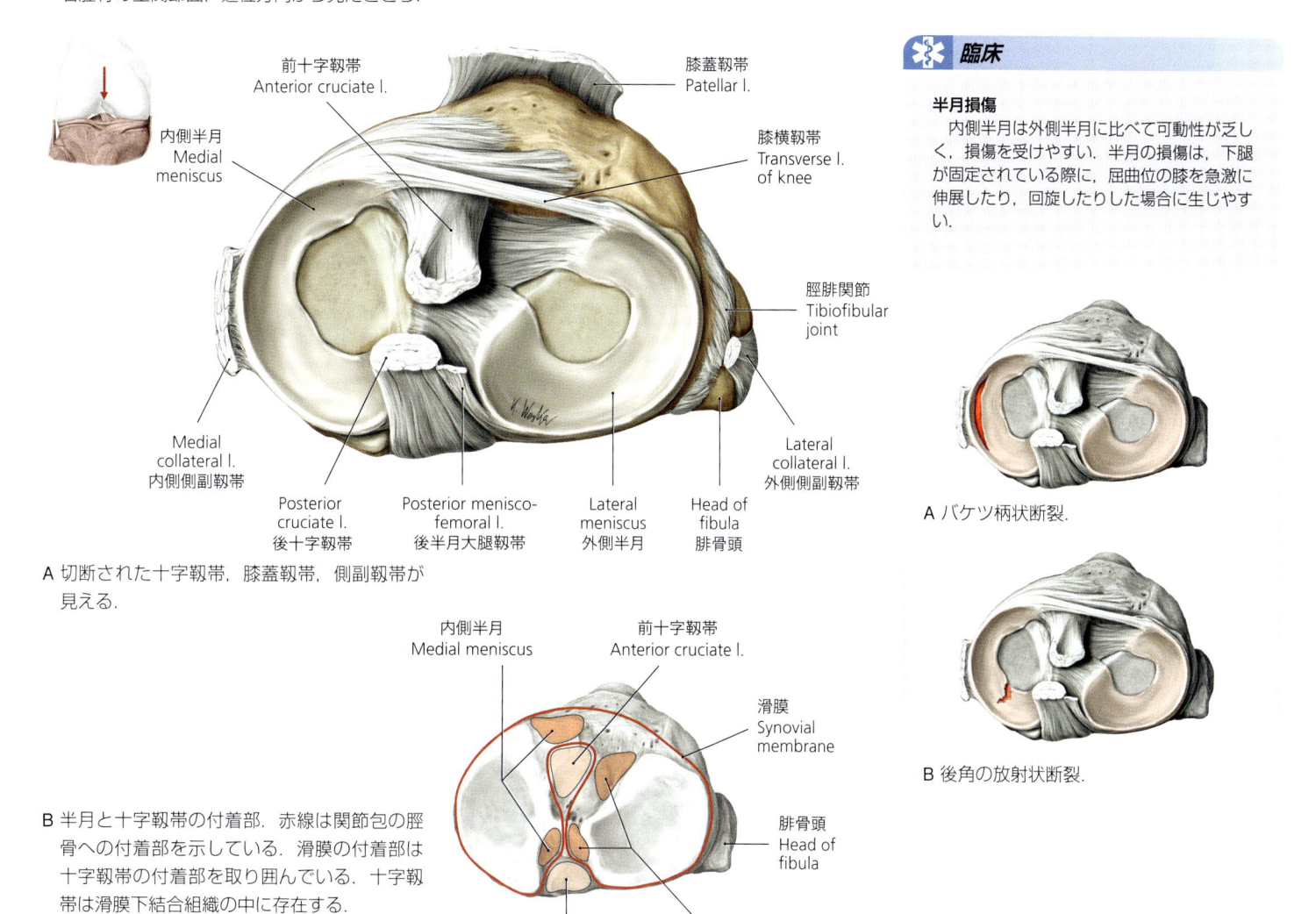

A 切断された十字靱帯，膝蓋靱帯，側副靱帯が見える．

- 内側半月 Medial meniscus
- 前十字靱帯 Anterior cruciate l.
- 滑膜 Synovial membrane
- 腓骨頭 Head of fibula
- 後十字靱帯 Posterior cruciate l.
- 外側半月 Lateral meniscus

B 半月と十字靱帯の付着部．赤線は関節包の脛骨への付着部を示している．滑膜の付着部は十字靱帯の付着部を取り囲んでいる．十字靱帯は滑膜下結合組織の中に存在する．

臨床

半月損傷

内側半月は外側半月に比べて可動性が乏しく，損傷を受けやすい．半月の損傷は，下腿が固定されている際に，屈曲位の膝を急激に伸展したり，回旋したりした場合に生じやすい．

A バケツ柄状断裂．

B 後角の放射状断裂．

図 25.9 半月の運動
右膝関節．

- 膝蓋骨 Patella
- 膝蓋靱帯 Patellar ligament
- 外側側副靱帯 Lateral collateral ligament
- 伸展 Extension
- 屈曲 Flexion

A 伸展位．
B 屈曲位．
C 脛骨の上関節面，近位方向から見たところ．

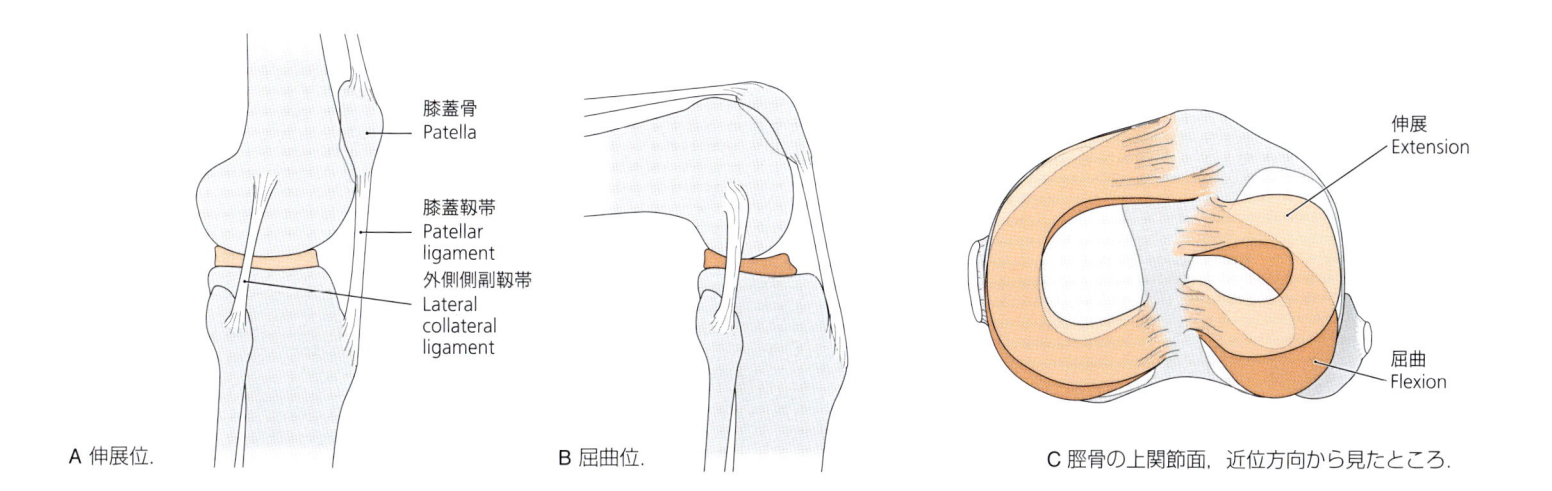

十字靱帯
Cruciate Ligaments

図 25.10　十字靱帯と側副靱帯
右膝関節．十字靱帯は大腿骨と脛骨の関節面を接触させた状態に保ち，脛骨が前後方向にずれるのを防いでいる．主に矢状面内において膝関節を安定にする．どちらの十字靱帯も全ての肢位において緊張している．

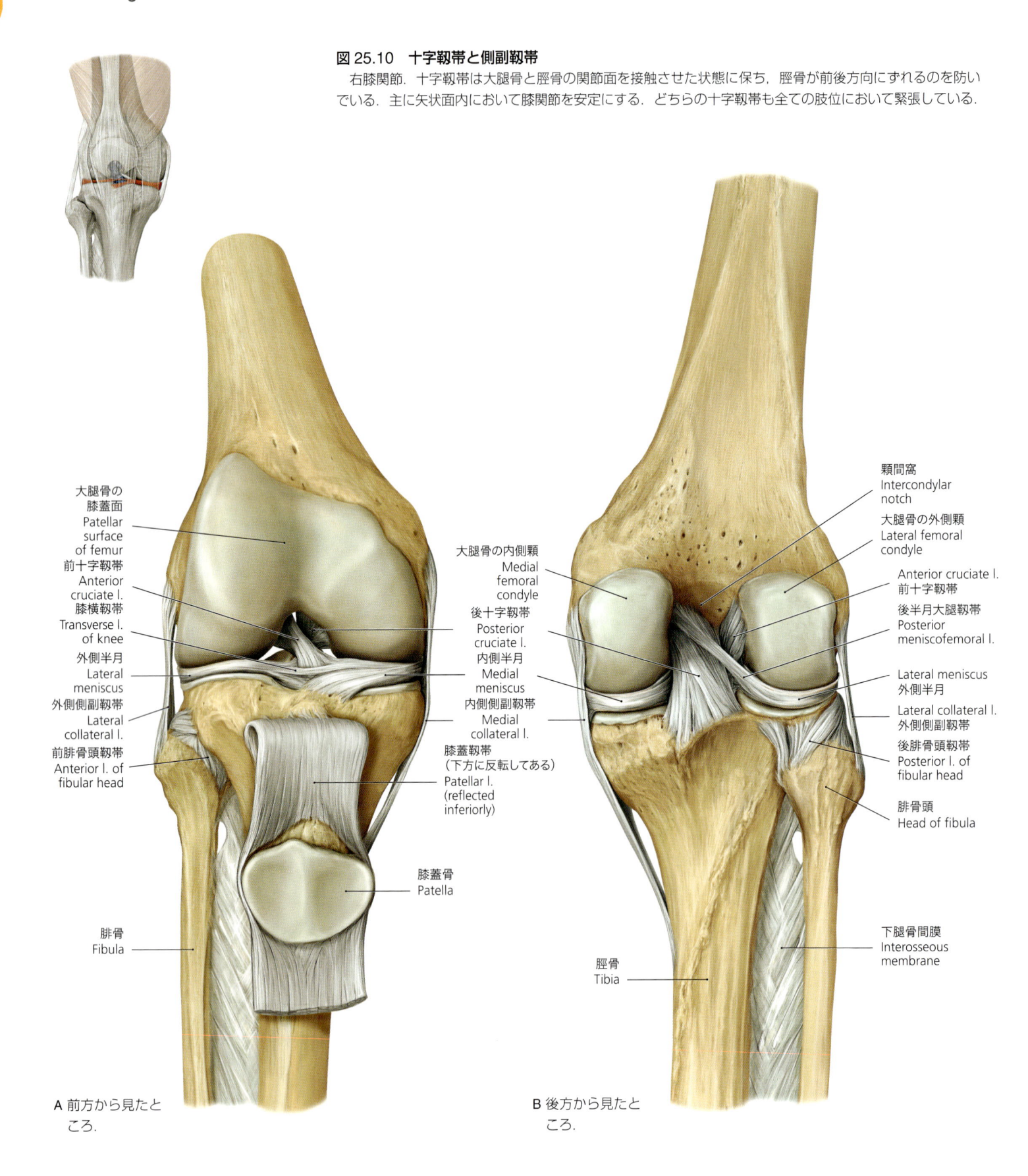

A 前方から見たところ．

- 大腿骨の膝蓋面 Patellar surface of femur
- 前十字靱帯 Anterior cruciate l.
- 膝横靱帯 Transverse l. of knee
- 外側半月 Lateral meniscus
- 外側側副靱帯 Lateral collateral l.
- 前腓骨頭靱帯 Anterior l. of fibular head
- 腓骨 Fibula
- 大腿骨の内側顆 Medial femoral condyle
- 後十字靱帯 Posterior cruciate l.
- 内側半月 Medial meniscus
- 内側側副靱帯 Medial collateral l.
- 膝蓋靱帯（下方に反転してある）Patellar l. (reflected inferiorly)
- 膝蓋骨 Patella

B 後方から見たところ．

- 顆間窩 Intercondylar notch
- 大腿骨の外側顆 Lateral femoral condyle
- 前十字靱帯 Anterior cruciate l.
- 後半月大腿靱帯 Posterior meniscofemoral l.
- 外側半月 Lateral meniscus
- 外側側副靱帯 Lateral collateral l.
- 後腓骨頭靱帯 Posterior l. of fibular head
- 腓骨頭 Head of fibula
- 下腿骨間膜 Interosseous membrane
- 脛骨 Tibia

図 25.11 屈曲位の右膝関節
前方から見たところ．関節包と膝蓋靱帯を取り除いてある．

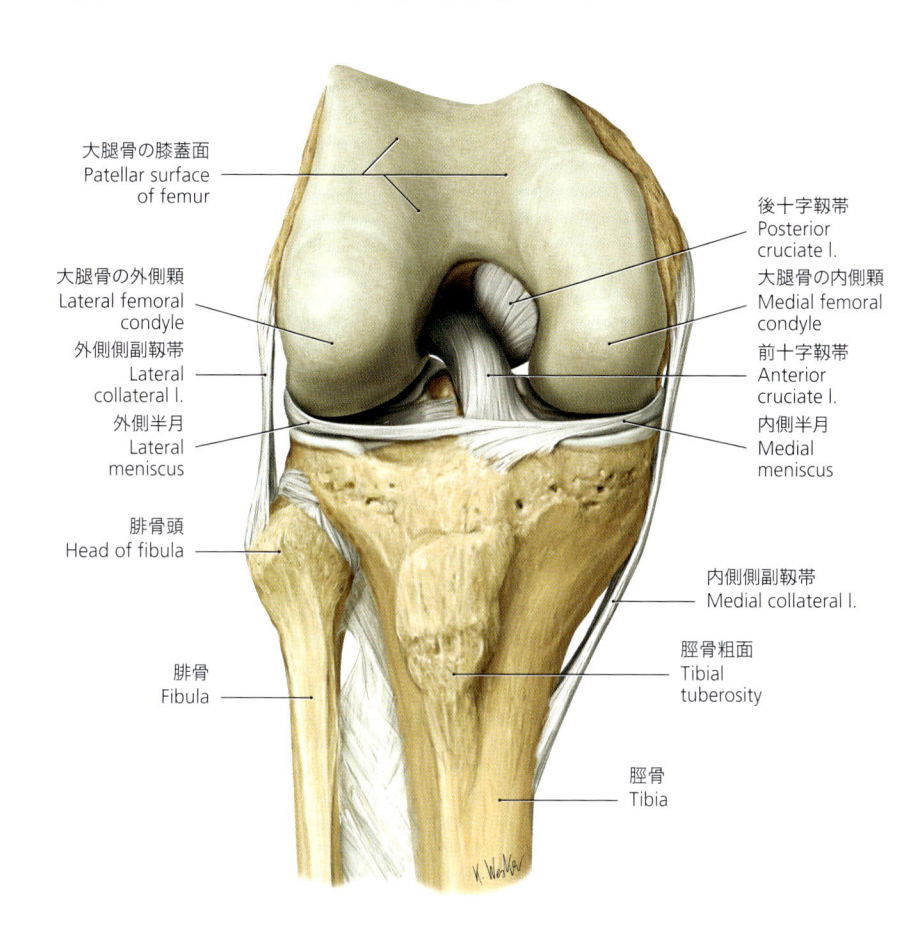

- 大腿骨の膝蓋面 Patellar surface of femur
- 大腿骨の外側顆 Lateral femoral condyle
- 外側側副靱帯 Lateral collateral l.
- 外側半月 Lateral meniscus
- 腓骨頭 Head of fibula
- 腓骨 Fibula
- 後十字靱帯 Posterior cruciate l.
- 大腿骨の内側顆 Medial femoral condyle
- 前十字靱帯 Anterior cruciate l.
- 内側半月 Medial meniscus
- 内側側副靱帯 Medial collateral l.
- 脛骨粗面 Tibial tuberosity
- 脛骨 Tibia

臨床

十字靱帯の断裂

十字靱帯の断裂により膝関節は不安定になり，脛骨が大腿骨に対して前方あるいは後方に動くようになる（前方・後方引き出し徴候）．前十字靱帯の断裂は後十字靱帯のそれよりも約10倍の頻度で発生する．前十字靱帯の損傷は，下腿を固定した状態で，膝を内旋した場合に最もよくみられる．また，足を地面に着けたまま，膝を完全に屈曲した状態で外側から膝に強い衝撃を受けると，前十字靱帯と内側側副靱帯が断裂し，さらに内側側副靱帯と接着している内側半月も断裂することが多い．

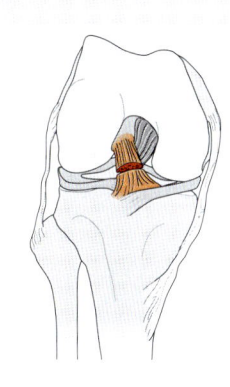

A 前十字靱帯の断裂．前方から見たところ．

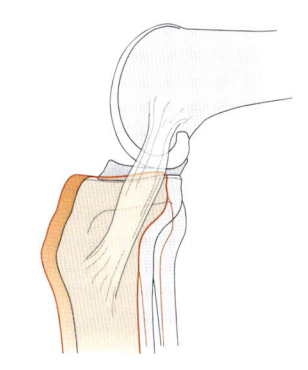

B "前方引き出し徴候"．内側方から見たところ．

右膝（屈曲位）．

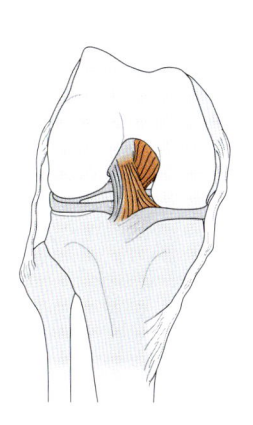

図 25.12 屈曲位と伸展位における十字靱帯と側副靱帯
右膝，前方から見たところ．緊張している線維を赤色で示してある．

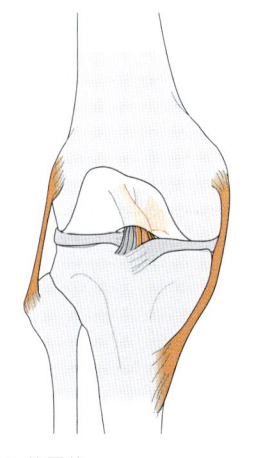

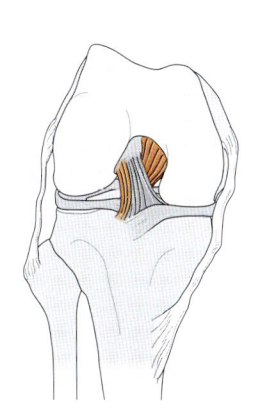

A 伸展位．   B 屈曲位．   C 屈曲・内旋位．

膝関節腔
Knee Joint Cavity

図 25.13 関節腔
右膝，外側方から見たところ．関節腔に樹脂を注入し，硬化させた後に関節包を取り除いてある．

- 大腿四頭筋の腱 Quadriceps tendon
- 膝蓋上陥凹 Suprapatellar pouch
- 大腿骨 Femur
- 膝蓋骨 Patella
- 外側側副靱帯 Lateral collateral l.
- 外側半月 Lateral meniscus
- 膝蓋靱帯 Patellar l.
- 膝窩筋下陥凹 Subpopliteal recess
- 深膝蓋下包 Infrapatellar bursa
- 腓骨 Fibula
- 脛骨 Tibia

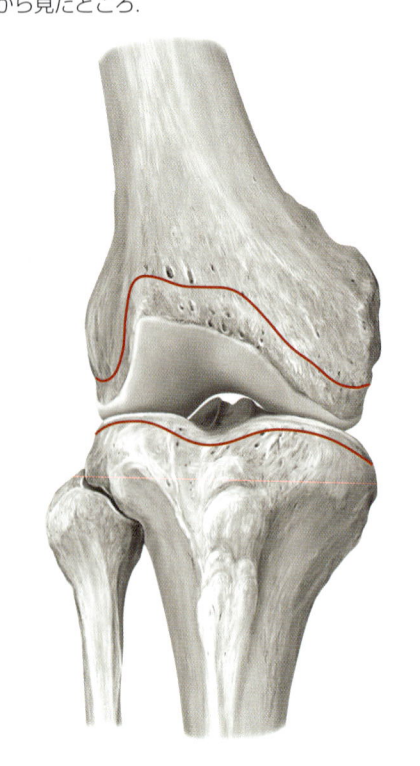

図 25.14 切り開かれた関節包
右膝，前方から見たところ．膝蓋骨を下方に反転してある．

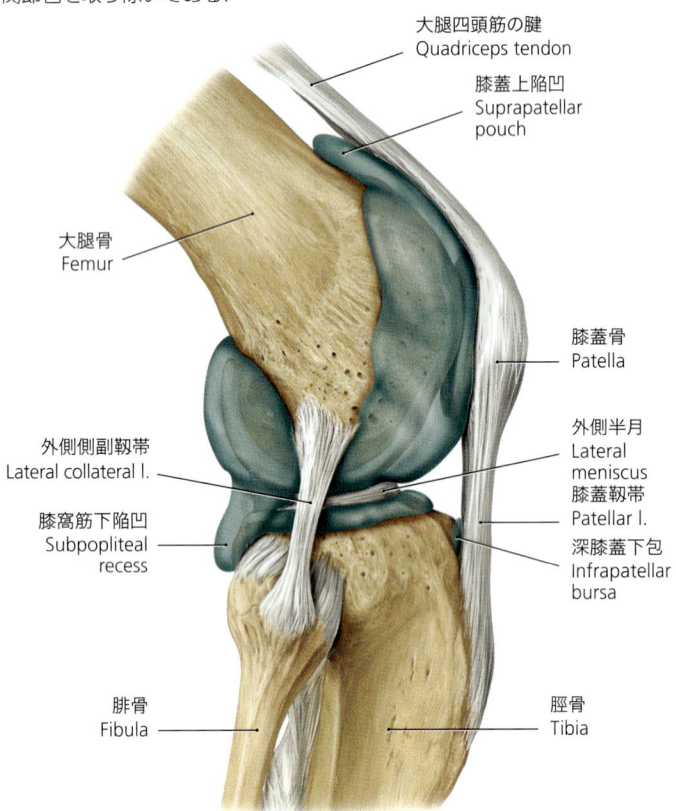

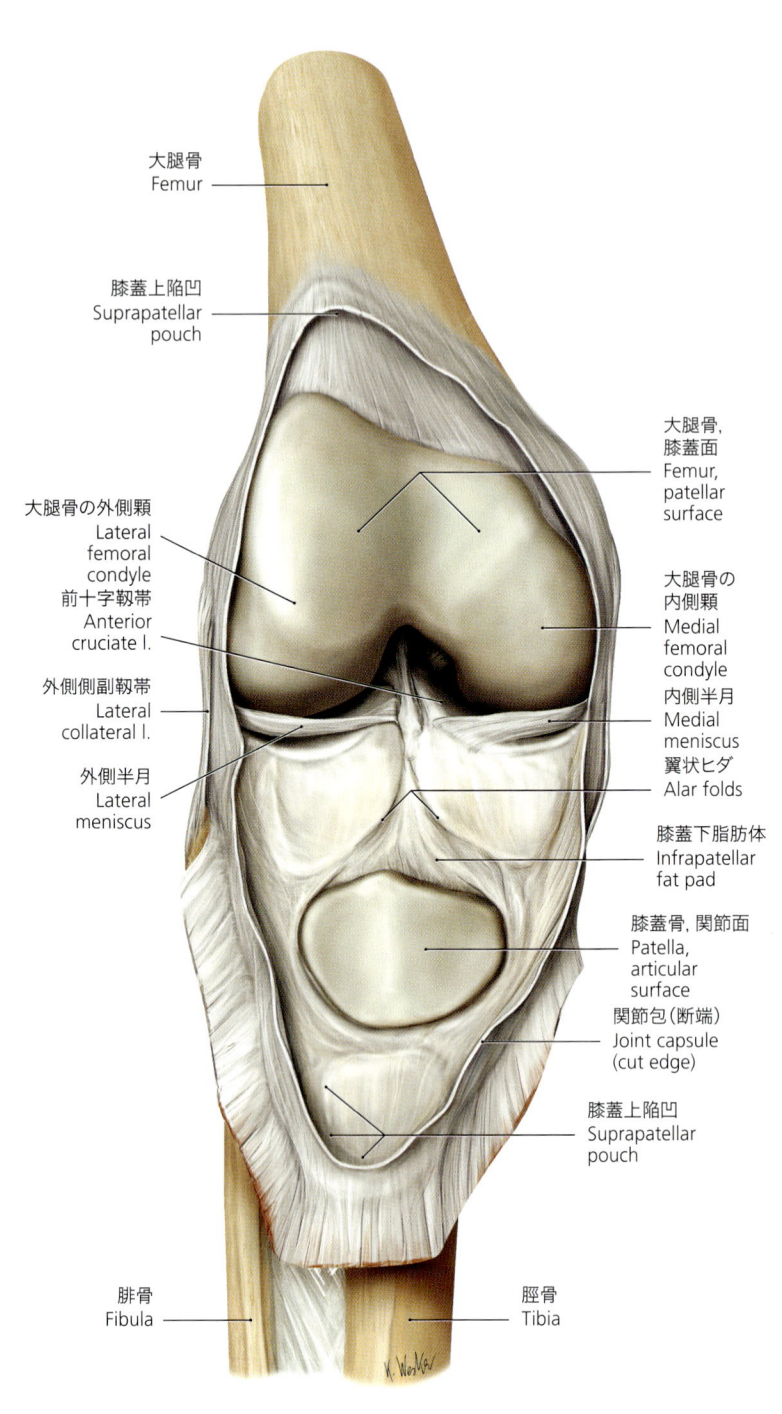

- 大腿骨 Femur
- 膝蓋上陥凹 Suprapatellar pouch
- 大腿骨，膝蓋面 Femur, patellar surface
- 大腿骨の外側顆 Lateral femoral condyle
- 前十字靱帯 Anterior cruciate l.
- 外側側副靱帯 Lateral collateral l.
- 外側半月 Lateral meniscus
- 大腿骨の内側顆 Medial femoral condyle
- 内側半月 Medial meniscus
- 翼状ヒダ Alar folds
- 膝蓋下脂肪体 Infrapatellar fat pad
- 膝蓋骨，関節面 Patella, articular surface
- 関節包（断端） Joint capsule (cut edge)
- 膝蓋上陥凹 Suprapatellar pouch
- 腓骨 Fibula
- 脛骨 Tibia

図 25.15 関節包の付着部
右膝，前方から見たところ．

図 25.16 屈曲時の膝蓋上陥凹
右膝関節，内側方から見たところ．

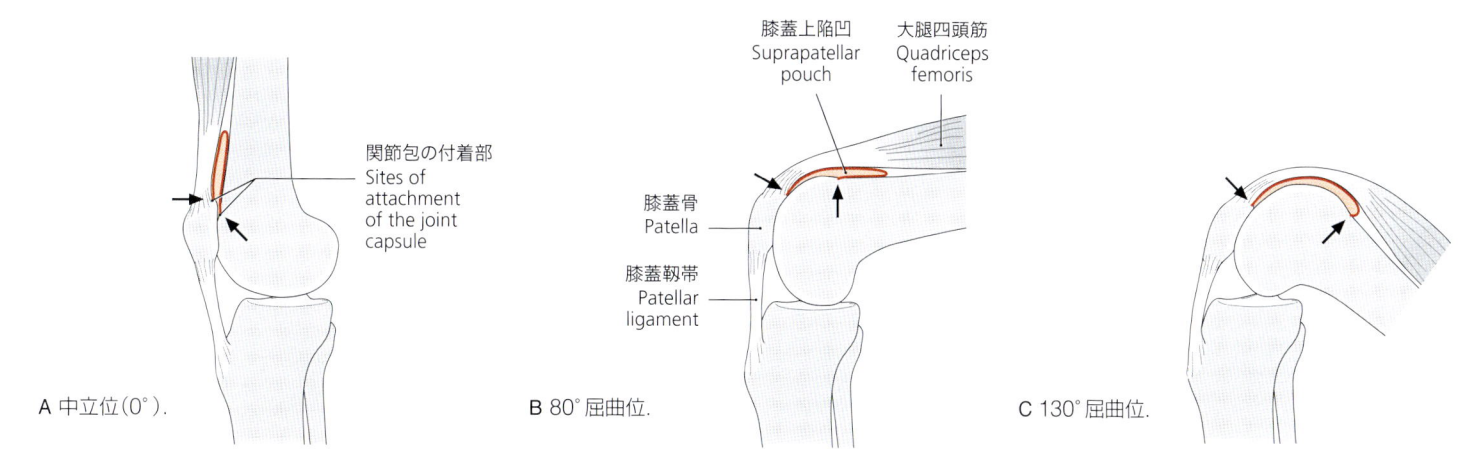

関節包の付着部
Sites of attachment of the joint capsule

膝蓋上陥凹
Suprapatellar pouch

大腿四頭筋
Quadriceps femoris

膝蓋骨
Patella

膝蓋靱帯
Patellar ligament

A 中立位（0°）．

B 80°屈曲位．

C 130°屈曲位．

図 25.17 右膝関節：正中矢状断面

大腿骨
Femur

膝蓋上陥凹
Suprapatellar pouch

大腿四頭筋の腱
Quadriceps tendon

膝蓋骨
Patella

膝蓋前皮下包
Prepatellar bursa

膝蓋靱帯
Patellar l.

膝蓋下脂肪体
Infrapatellar fat pad

前顆間区
Anterior intercondylar area

深膝蓋下包
Infrapatellar bursa

脛骨
Tibia

前十字靱帯
Anterior cruciate l.

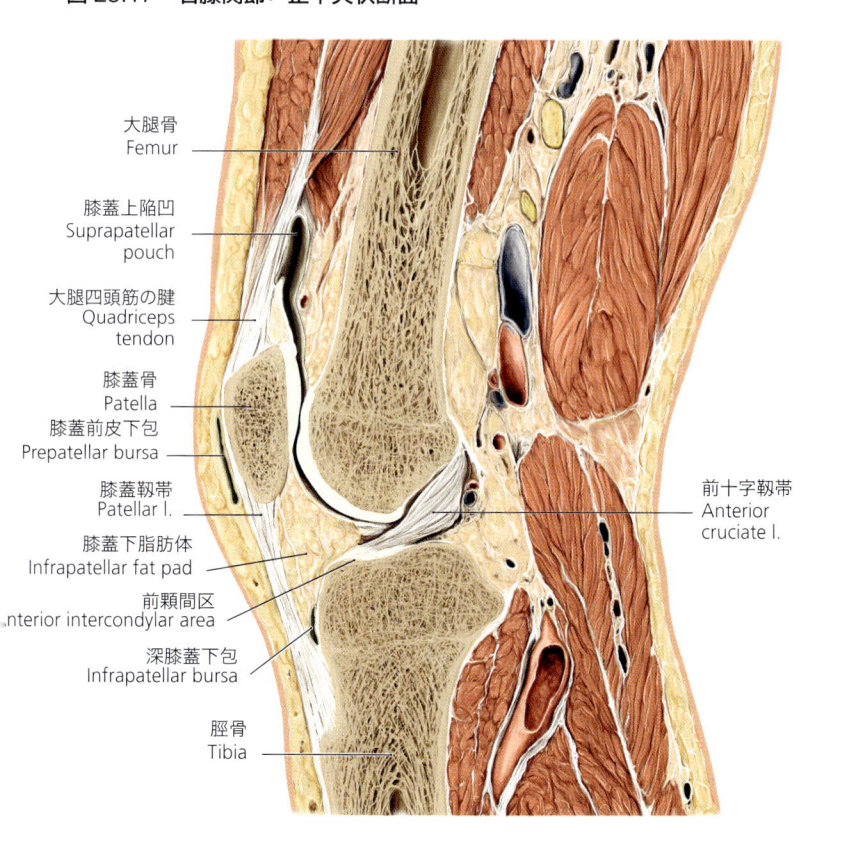

図 25.18 膝関節のMR像
矢状断T2強調MR像．

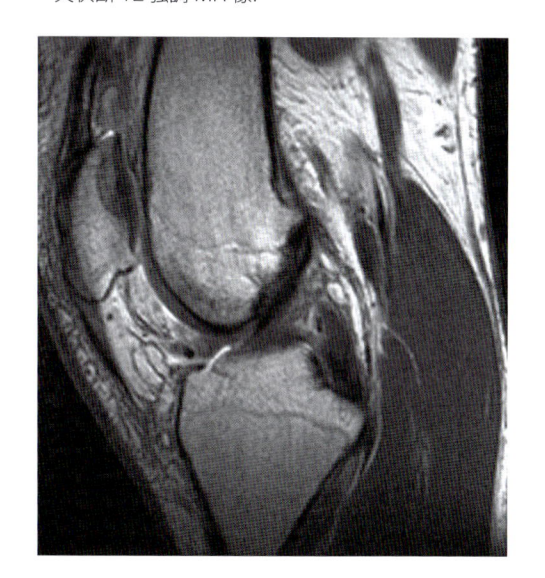

下腿の前面と外側面にある筋
Muscles of the Leg: Anterior & Lateral Views

図 25.19　下腿の筋：前方から見たところ
右下腿．筋の起始(O)を赤，停止(I)を青で示してある．

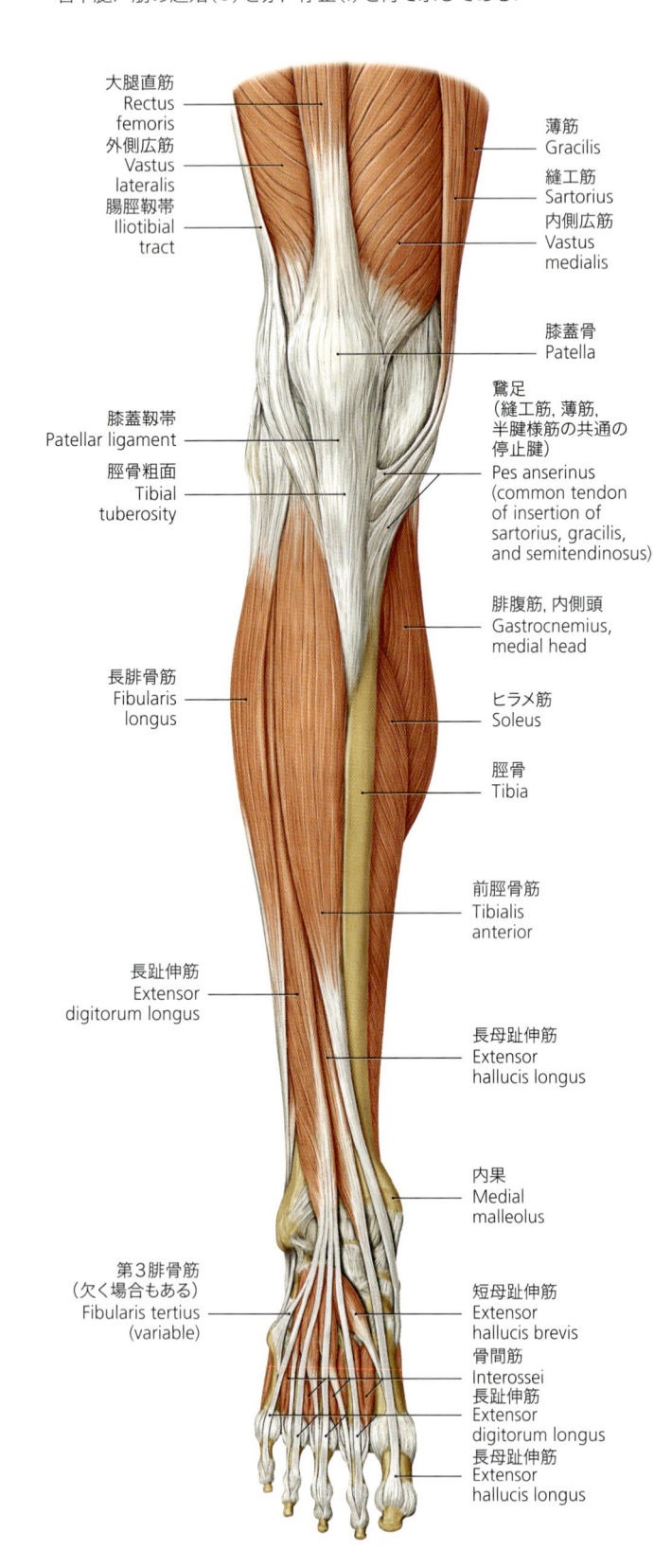

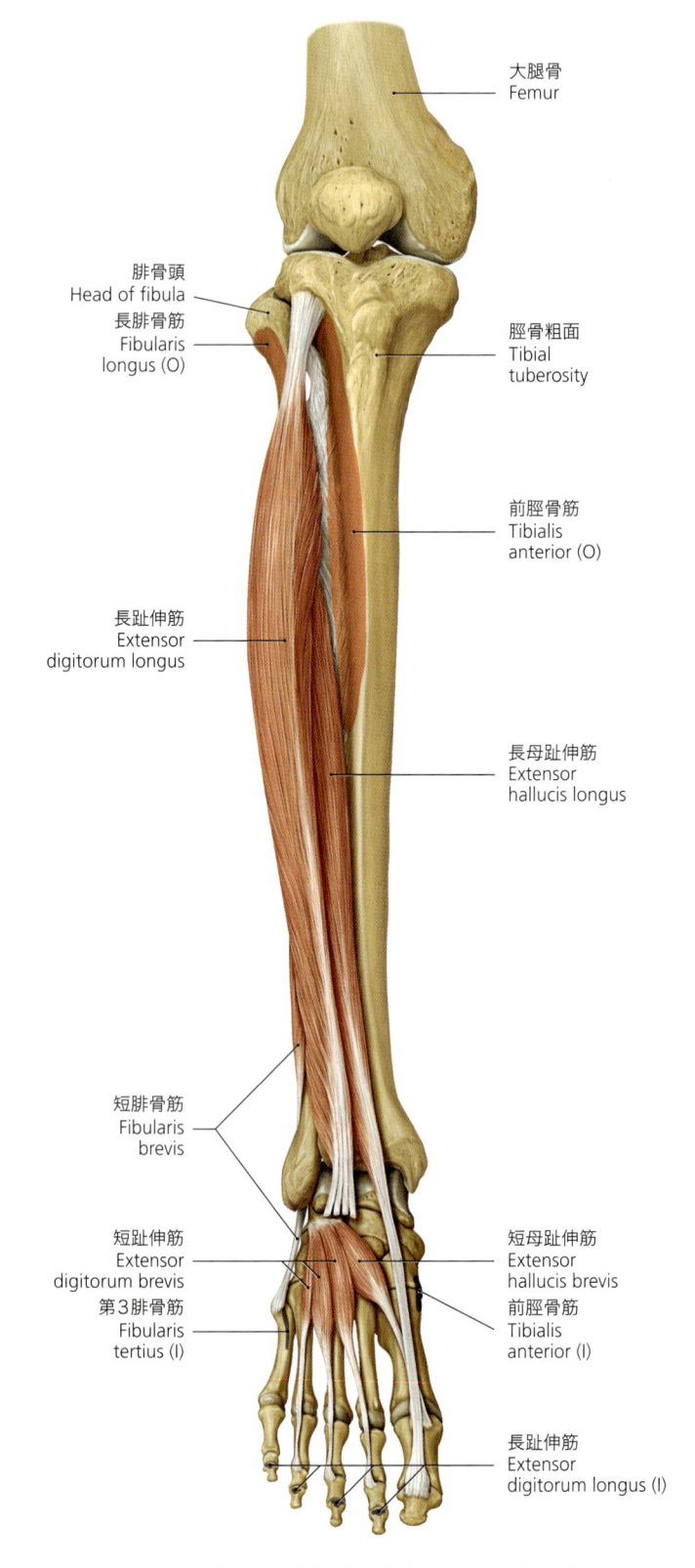

A 全ての筋．

B 前脛骨筋，長腓骨筋，長趾伸筋の腱（遠位部）を取り除いてある．
Note: 第3腓骨筋は長趾伸筋の分束である．

図 25.20　下腿の筋: 外側方から見たところ
右下腿.

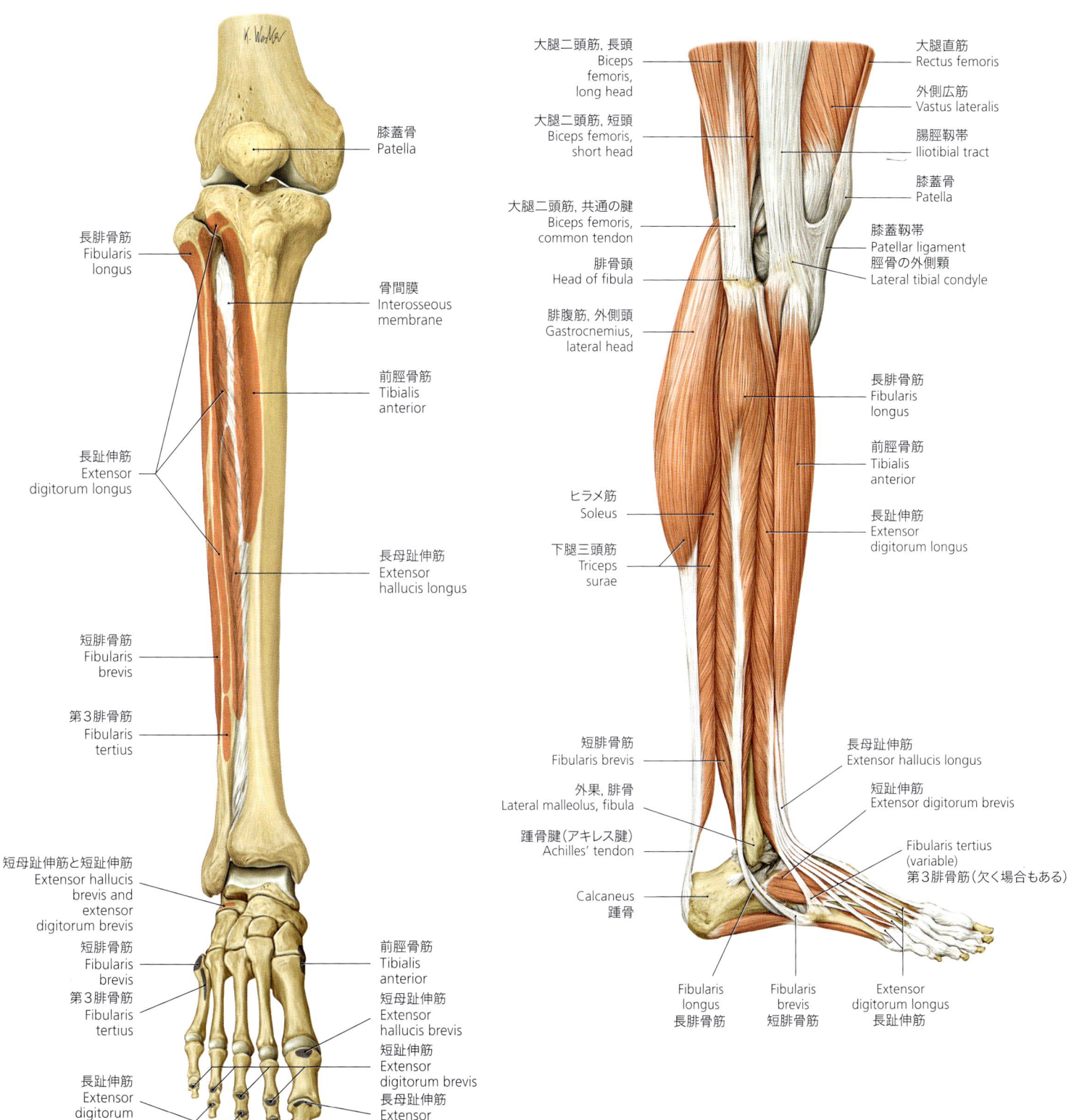

C 全ての筋を取り除いたところ.

下腿の後面にある筋
Muscles of the Leg: Posterior View

図 25.21 下腿の筋：後方から見たところ
右下腿．筋の起始（O）を赤，停止（I）を青で示してある．

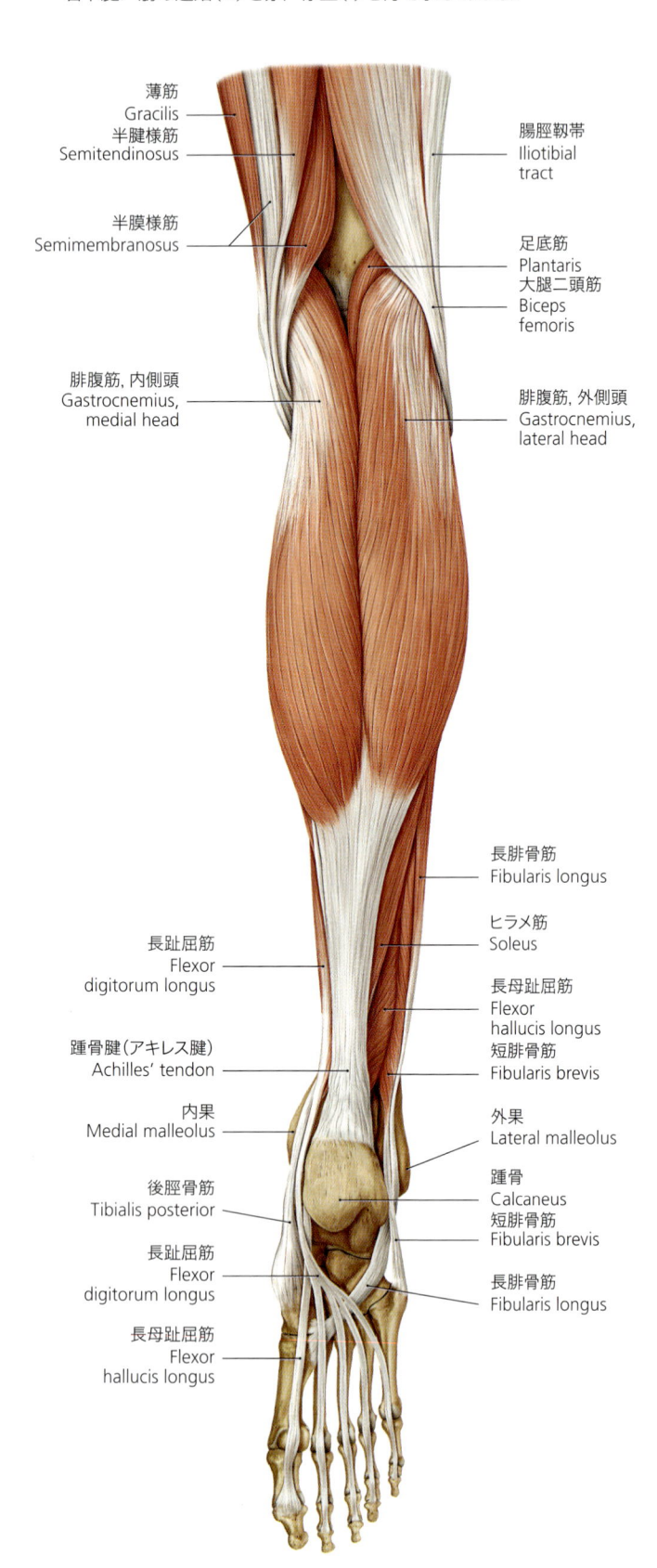

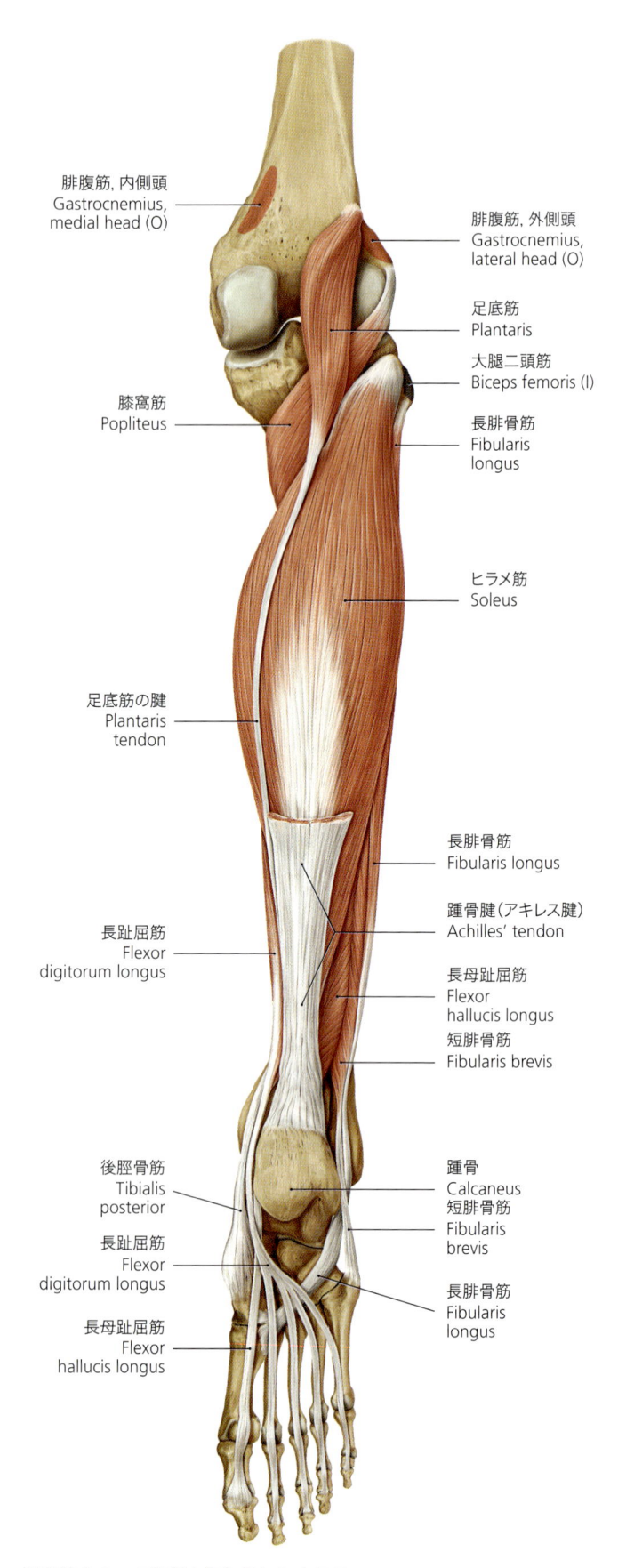

左図ラベル（A）:
- 薄筋 Gracilis
- 半腱様筋 Semitendinosus
- 半膜様筋 Semimembranosus
- 腓腹筋, 内側頭 Gastrocnemius, medial head
- 腸脛靱帯 Iliotibial tract
- 足底筋 Plantaris
- 大腿二頭筋 Biceps femoris
- 腓腹筋, 外側頭 Gastrocnemius, lateral head
- 長腓骨筋 Fibularis longus
- ヒラメ筋 Soleus
- 長母趾屈筋 Flexor hallucis longus
- 短腓骨筋 Fibularis brevis
- 長趾屈筋 Flexor digitorum longus
- 踵骨腱（アキレス腱）Achilles' tendon
- 内果 Medial malleolus
- 外果 Lateral malleolus
- 踵骨 Calcaneus
- 後脛骨筋 Tibialis posterior
- 短腓骨筋 Fibularis brevis
- 長趾屈筋 Flexor digitorum longus
- 長腓骨筋 Fibularis longus
- 長母趾屈筋 Flexor hallucis longus

右図ラベル（B）:
- 腓腹筋, 内側頭 Gastrocnemius, medial head (O)
- 腓腹筋, 外側頭 Gastrocnemius, lateral head (O)
- 足底筋 Plantaris
- 大腿二頭筋 Biceps femoris (I)
- 膝窩筋 Popliteus
- 長腓骨筋 Fibularis longus
- ヒラメ筋 Soleus
- 足底筋の腱 Plantaris tendon
- 長腓骨筋 Fibularis longus
- 踵骨腱（アキレス腱）Achilles' tendon
- 長趾屈筋 Flexor digitorum longus
- 長母趾屈筋 Flexor hallucis longus
- 短腓骨筋 Fibularis brevis
- 後脛骨筋 Tibialis posterior
- 踵骨 Calcaneus
- 短腓骨筋 Fibularis brevis
- 長趾屈筋 Flexor digitorum longus
- 長腓骨筋 Fibularis longus
- 長母趾屈筋 Flexor hallucis longus

A Note：ふくらはぎの膨らみは主に下腿三頭筋（腓腹筋の2つの筋頭とヒラメ筋）によって形成される．

B 腓腹筋の2つの筋頭を取り除いたところ．

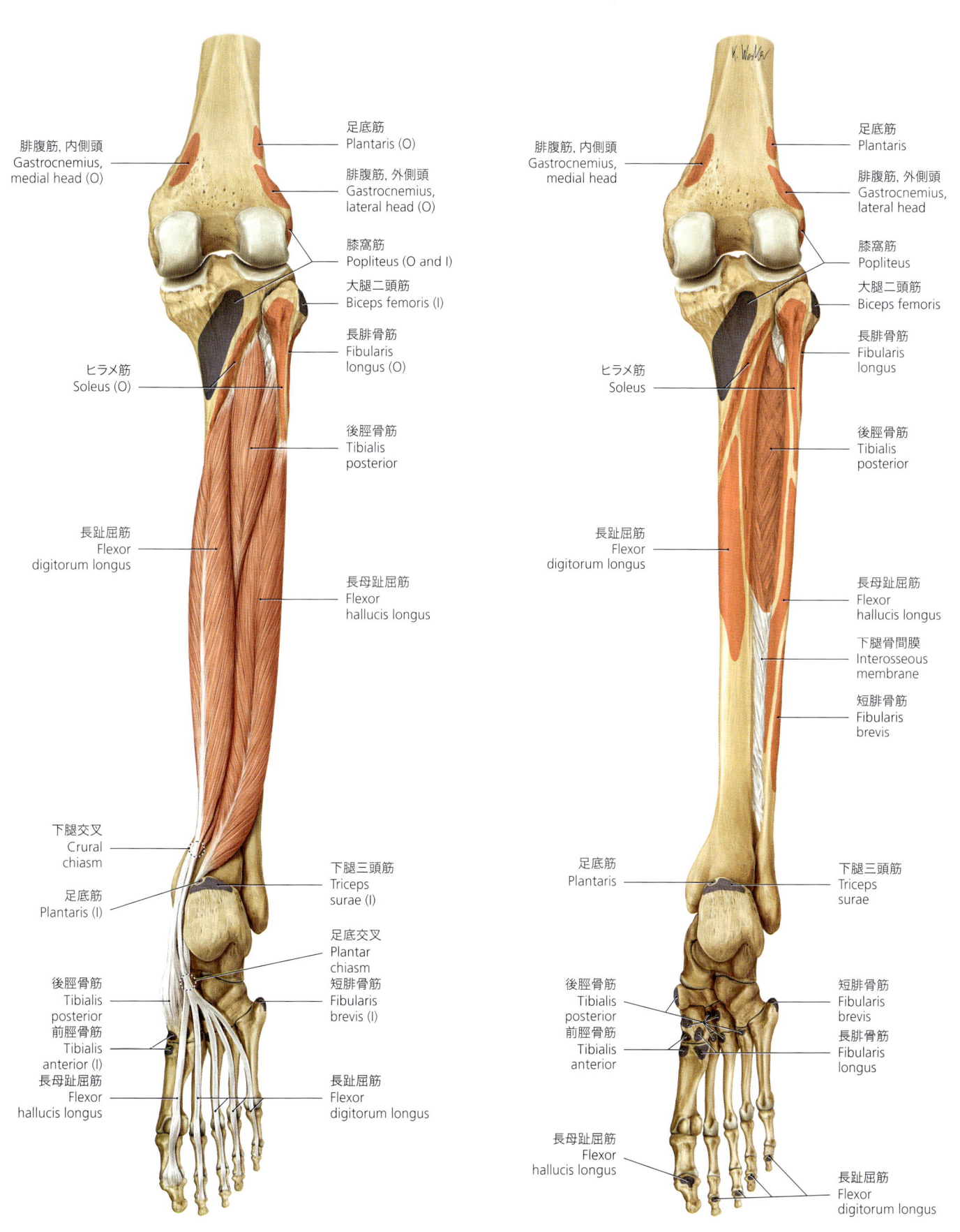

C 下腿三頭筋，足底筋，膝窩筋，長腓骨筋を取り除いたところ．

D 全ての筋を取り除いたところ．

個々の筋（1）
Muscle Facts (I)

> 下腿の筋により，足の屈曲・伸展や外反・内反が行われる．

図 25.22　下腿外側の筋
右の下腿と足．

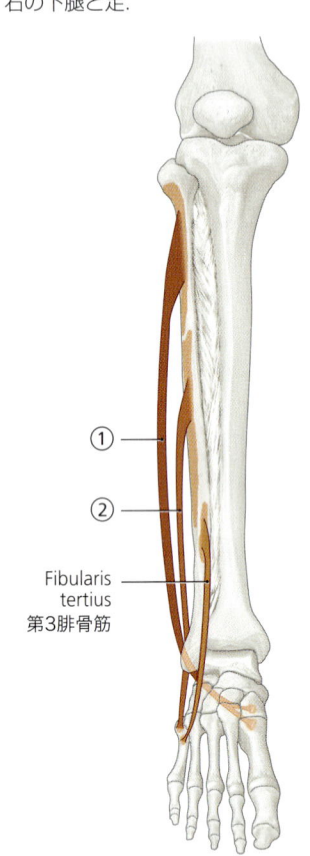

A　模式図，前方から見たところ．第3腓骨筋も描いてある．

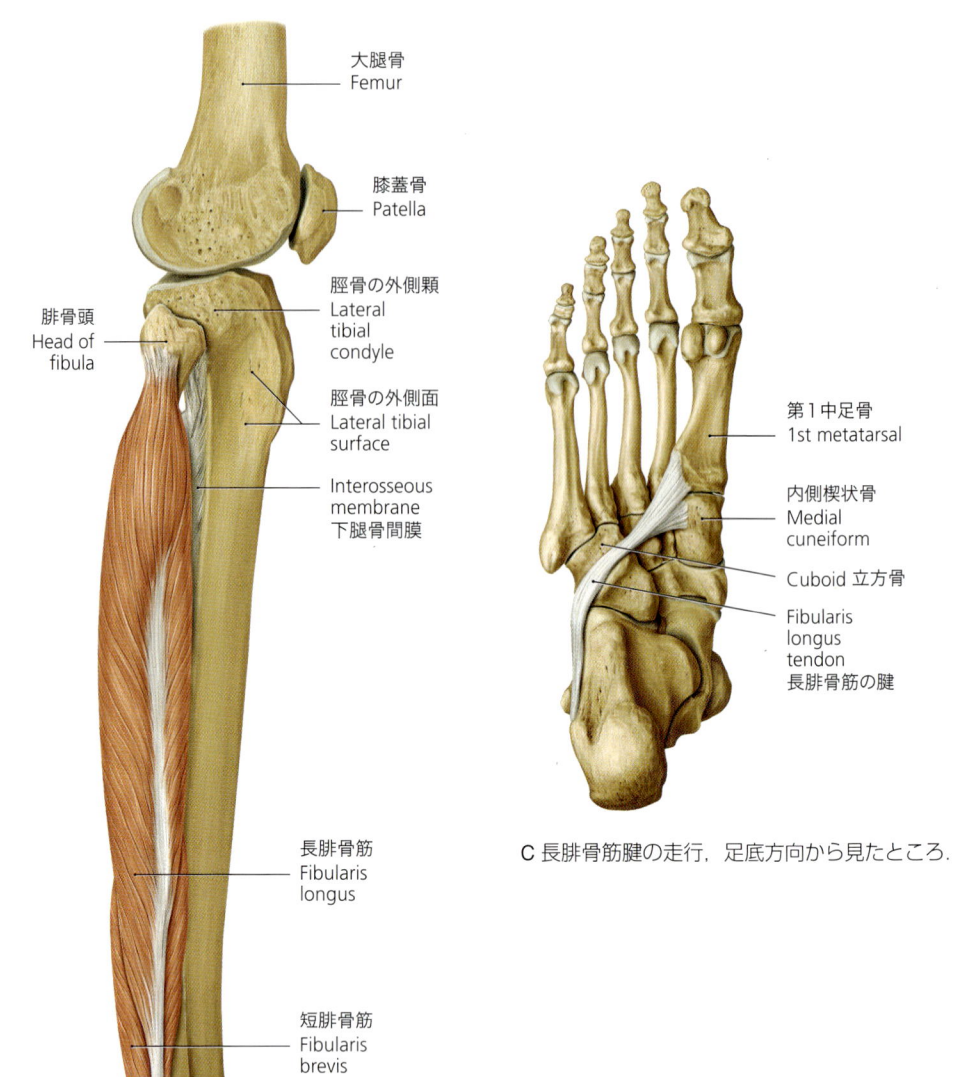

B　下腿外側の筋，外側方から見たところ．

C　長腓骨筋腱の走行，足底方向から見たところ．

表 25.2　下腿外側の筋

筋	起始	停止	神経支配	作用
①長腓骨筋	腓骨（頭，外側面の近位3分の2，一部は筋間中隔からも起始する）	内側楔状骨（足底面），第1中足骨底	浅腓骨神経 (L5, S1)	・距腿関節：底屈 ・距骨下関節：外反 ・横足弓の保持
②短腓骨筋	腓骨（外側面の遠位半分），筋間中隔	第5中足骨粗面（場合によっては第5趾の指背腱膜へ分岐腱を伸ばす）		・距腿関節：底屈 ・距骨下関節：外反

図 25.23 下腿前面の筋
右の下腿と足，前方から見たところ．

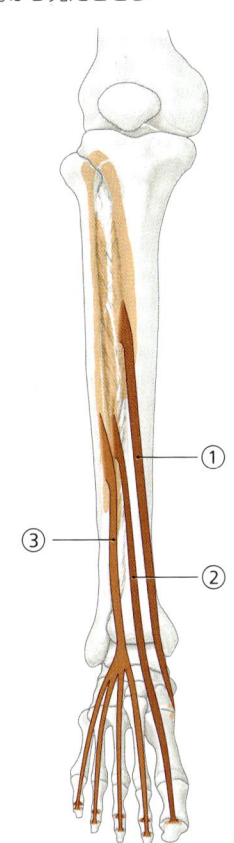

A 模式図．

B 下腿前面の筋．

図中ラベル（B）：
- 大腿骨 Femur
- 外側上顆 Lateral epicondyle
- 脛骨の外側顆 Lateral tibial condyle
- 腓骨頭 Head of fibula
- 脛骨粗面 Tibial tuberosity
- 脛骨体 Shaft of tibia
- 前脛骨筋 Tibialis anterior
- 長趾伸筋 Extensor digitorum longus
- 長母趾伸筋 Extensor hallucis longus
- 第3腓骨筋 Fibularis tertius
- 外果 Lateral malleolus
- 内果 Medial malleolus
- 長趾伸筋の腱 Extensor digitorum longus tendon
- 第3腓骨筋の腱 Fibularis tertius tendon
- 長母趾伸筋の腱 Extensor hallucis longus tendon
- 1st through 5th distal phalanges 第1-5末節骨

表 25.3 下腿前面の筋

筋	起始	停止	神経支配	作用
①前脛骨筋	脛骨（外側面の近位3分の2），骨間膜，下腿筋膜（最上部）	内側楔状骨（内側面，足底面），第1中足骨底（内側面）	深腓骨神経（L4, L5）	・距腿関節：背屈 ・距腿下関節：内反
②長母趾伸筋	腓骨（内側面の中間3分の1），骨間膜	第1趾（指背腱膜，末節骨底）	深腓骨神経（L5）	・距腿関節：背屈 ・距腿下関節：足の位置に応じ，内反と外反の両方に働く ・第1趾のMTP関節とIP関節：伸展
③長趾伸筋	腓骨（頭と前縁），脛骨（外側顆），骨間膜	第2-5趾（指背腱膜，末節骨底）	深腓骨神経（L5, S1）	・距腿関節：背屈 ・距腿下関節：外反 ・第2-5趾のMTP関節とIP関節：伸展
第3腓骨筋（図25.22参照）	腓骨（前縁）の遠位部	第5中足骨底	深腓骨神経（L5, S1）	・距腿関節：背屈 ・距腿下関節：外反

IP関節＝趾節間関節，MTP関節＝中足趾節関節．

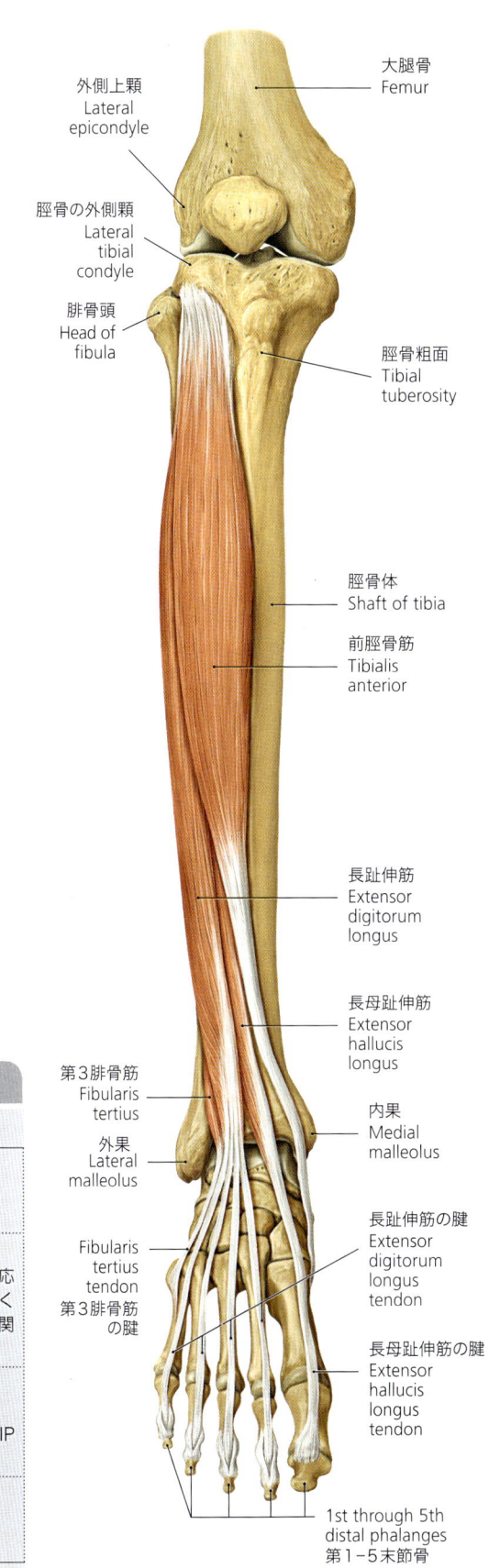

個々の筋（2）
Muscle Facts (II)

> 下腿後面の筋は2つのグループ（浅層と深層の屈筋）に分けられる．
> この2つの筋群の間には横筋間中隔が存在する．

図 25.24 浅層の屈筋
右下腿，後方から見たところ．

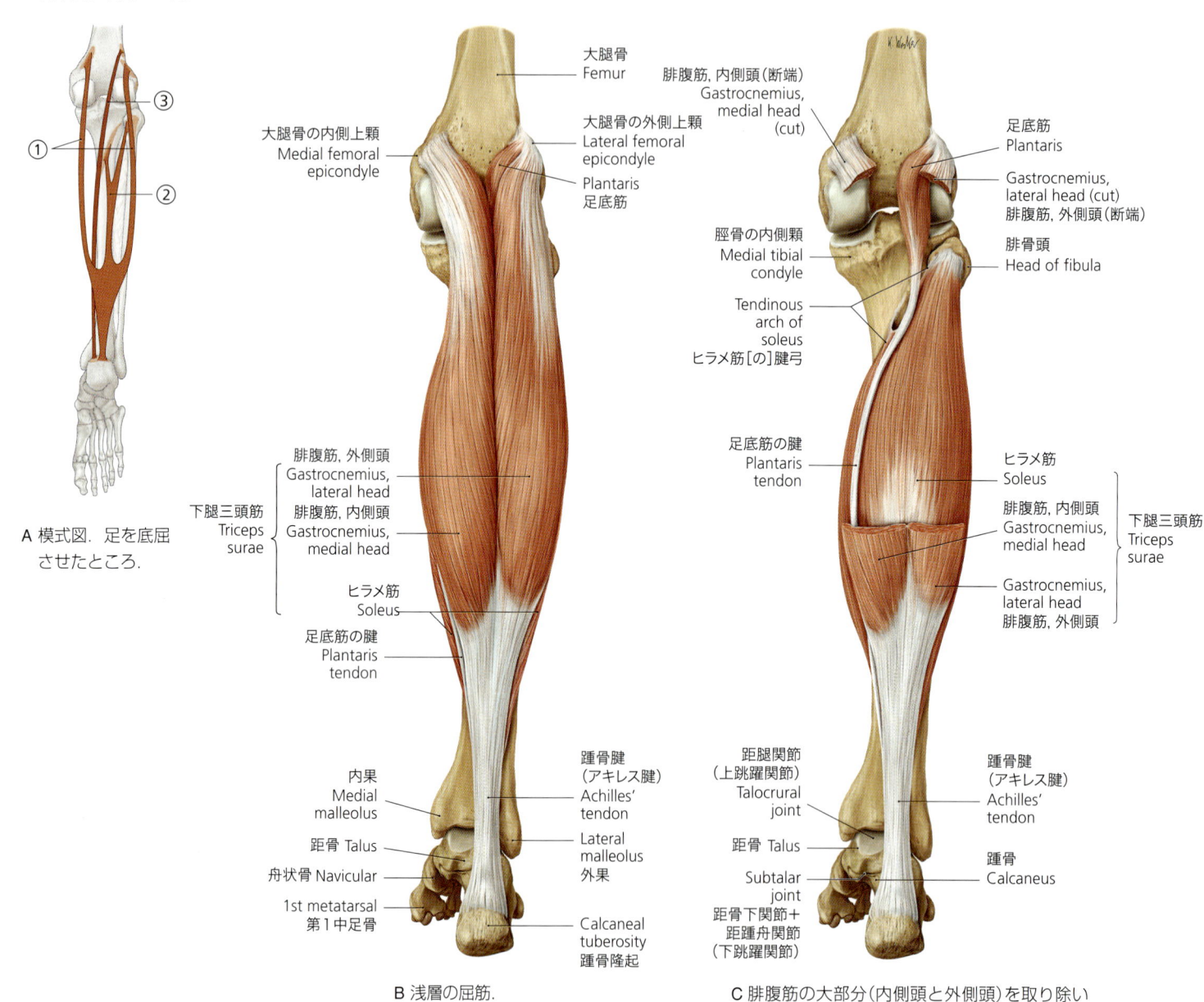

A 模式図．足を底屈させたところ．

ラベル（左図）：
- 大腿骨 Femur
- 大腿骨の内側上顆 Medial femoral epicondyle
- 大腿骨の外側上顆 Lateral femoral epicondyle
- 足底筋 Plantaris
- 腓腹筋, 外側頭 Gastrocnemius, lateral head
- 腓腹筋, 内側頭 Gastrocnemius, medial head
- 下腿三頭筋 Triceps surae
- ヒラメ筋 Soleus
- 足底筋の腱 Plantaris tendon
- 内果 Medial malleolus
- 距骨 Talus
- 舟状骨 Navicular
- 第1中足骨 1st metatarsal
- 踵骨腱（アキレス腱）Achilles' tendon
- 外果 Lateral malleolus
- 踵骨隆起 Calcaneal tuberosity

B 浅層の屈筋．

ラベル（右図）：
- 腓腹筋, 内側頭（断端）Gastrocnemius, medial head (cut)
- 足底筋 Plantaris
- 腓腹筋, 外側頭（断端）Gastrocnemius, lateral head (cut)
- 腓骨頭 Head of fibula
- 脛骨の内側顆 Medial tibial condyle
- ヒラメ筋［の］腱弓 Tendinous arch of soleus
- 足底筋の腱 Plantaris tendon
- ヒラメ筋 Soleus
- 腓腹筋, 内側頭 Gastrocnemius, medial head
- 下腿三頭筋 Triceps surae
- 腓腹筋, 外側頭 Gastrocnemius, lateral head
- 距腿関節（上跳躍関節）Talocrural joint
- 距骨 Talus
- 距骨下関節＋距踵舟関節（下跳躍関節）Subtalar joint
- 踵骨腱（アキレス腱）Achilles' tendon
- 踵骨 Calcaneus

C 腓腹筋の大部分（内側頭と外側頭）を取り除いたところ．

表 25.4　下腿後面の筋（浅層の屈筋）

筋		起始	停止	神経支配	作用
下腿三頭筋	①腓腹筋	大腿骨（内側顆，外側顆）	踵骨腱（アキレス腱）を介して踵骨粗面に停止する	脛骨神経（S1, S2）	・距腿関節：底屈 ・膝関節：屈曲（腓腹筋）
	②ヒラメ筋	腓骨（頭，頸，後面），脛骨（ヒラメ筋腱弓を介してヒラメ筋線から起始する）			
	③足底筋	大腿骨（外側顆，腓腹筋外側頭よりも近位で起始する）			ほとんど無視できるが，膝の屈曲時に膝窩動静脈が圧迫されるのを防いでいる可能性がある

図 25.25 深層の屈筋
右下腿．足を底屈させたところ．後方から見たところ．

A 模式図．

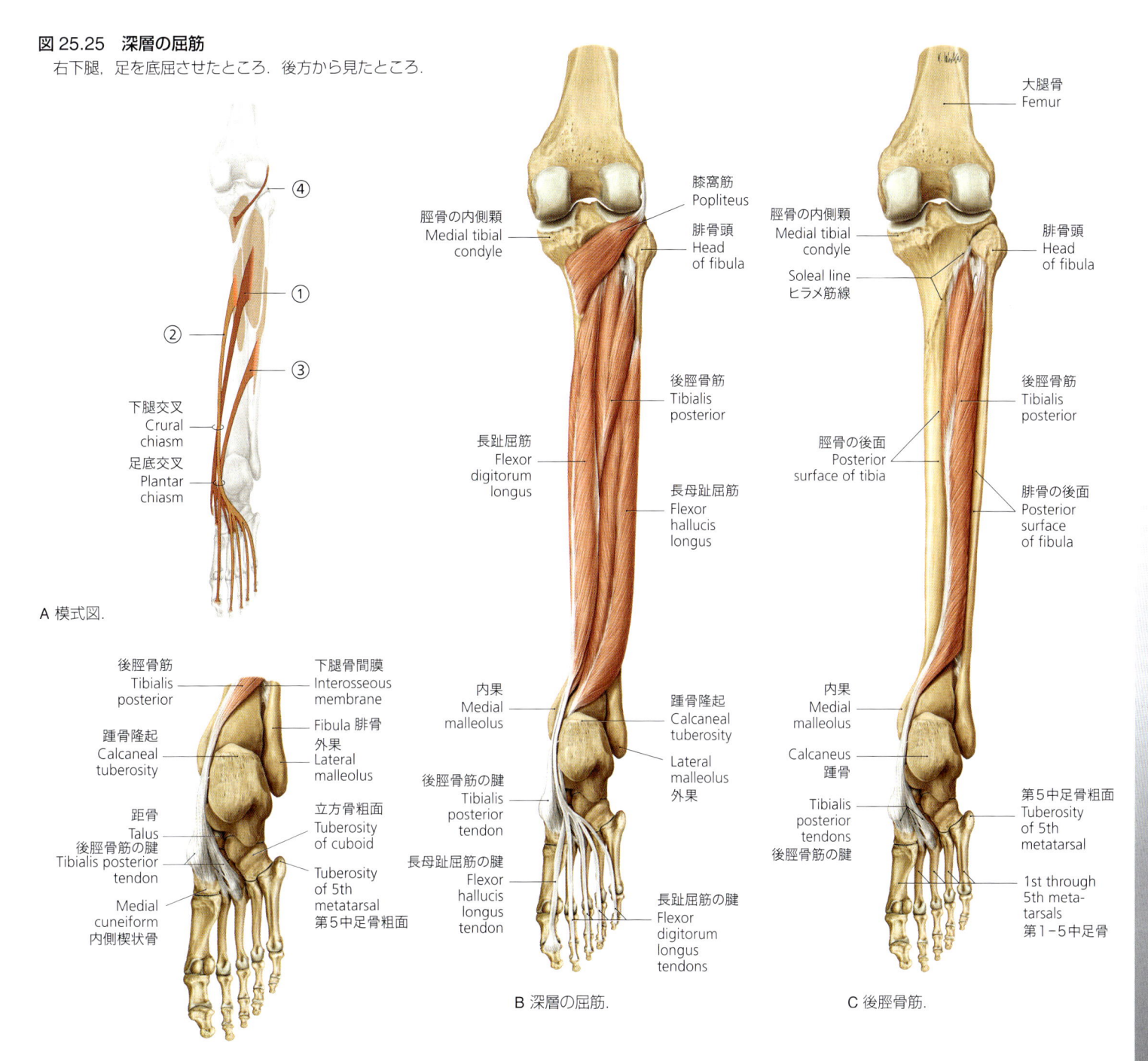

B 深層の屈筋．

C 後脛骨筋．

D 後脛骨筋の停止．

表 25.5	下腿後面の筋（深層の屈筋）			
筋	起始	停止	神経支配	作用
①後脛骨筋	骨間膜，脛骨と腓骨（骨間膜付着部の近傍）	舟状骨粗面，内側・中間・外側楔状骨，第2-4中足骨底	脛骨神経（L4, L5）	・距腿関節：底屈 ・距骨下関節：内反（回外） ・縦足弓と横足弓の保持
②長趾屈筋	脛骨（後面の中間3分の1）	第2-5末節骨底	脛骨神経（L5-S2）	・距腿関節：底屈 ・距骨下関節：内反（回外） ・第2-5趾のMTP関節とIP関節：底屈
③長母趾屈筋	腓骨（後面の遠位3分の2），隣接する骨間膜	第1末節骨底		・距腿関節：底屈 ・距骨下関節：内反 ・第1趾のMTP関節とIP関節：底屈 ・内側縦足弓の保持
④膝窩筋	大腿骨の外側顆，外側半月の後角	脛骨後面（ヒラメ筋の起始部よりも上方）	脛骨神経（L4-S1）	膝関節：屈曲，内旋（関節を安定化する）

IP関節＝趾節間関節，MTP関節＝中足趾節関節．

足の骨
Bones of the Foot

図26.1 足の骨格の区分

右足，足背面（上方から見たところ）．記載解剖学では足の骨格を足根骨，中足骨，前足骨（趾骨）に区分する．一方，機能的あるいは臨床的な観点からは，後足，中足，前足に区分する．

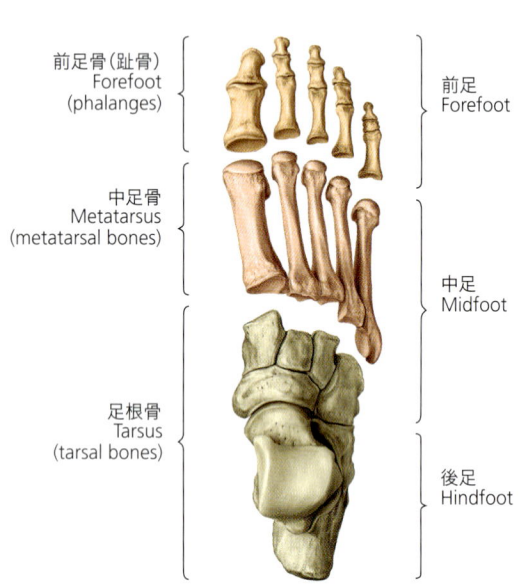

- 前足骨（趾骨） Forefoot (phalanges)
- 中足骨 Metatarsus (metatarsal bones)
- 足根骨 Tarsus (tarsal bones)

- 前足 Forefoot
- 中足 Midfoot
- 後足 Hindfoot

図26.2 右足の骨

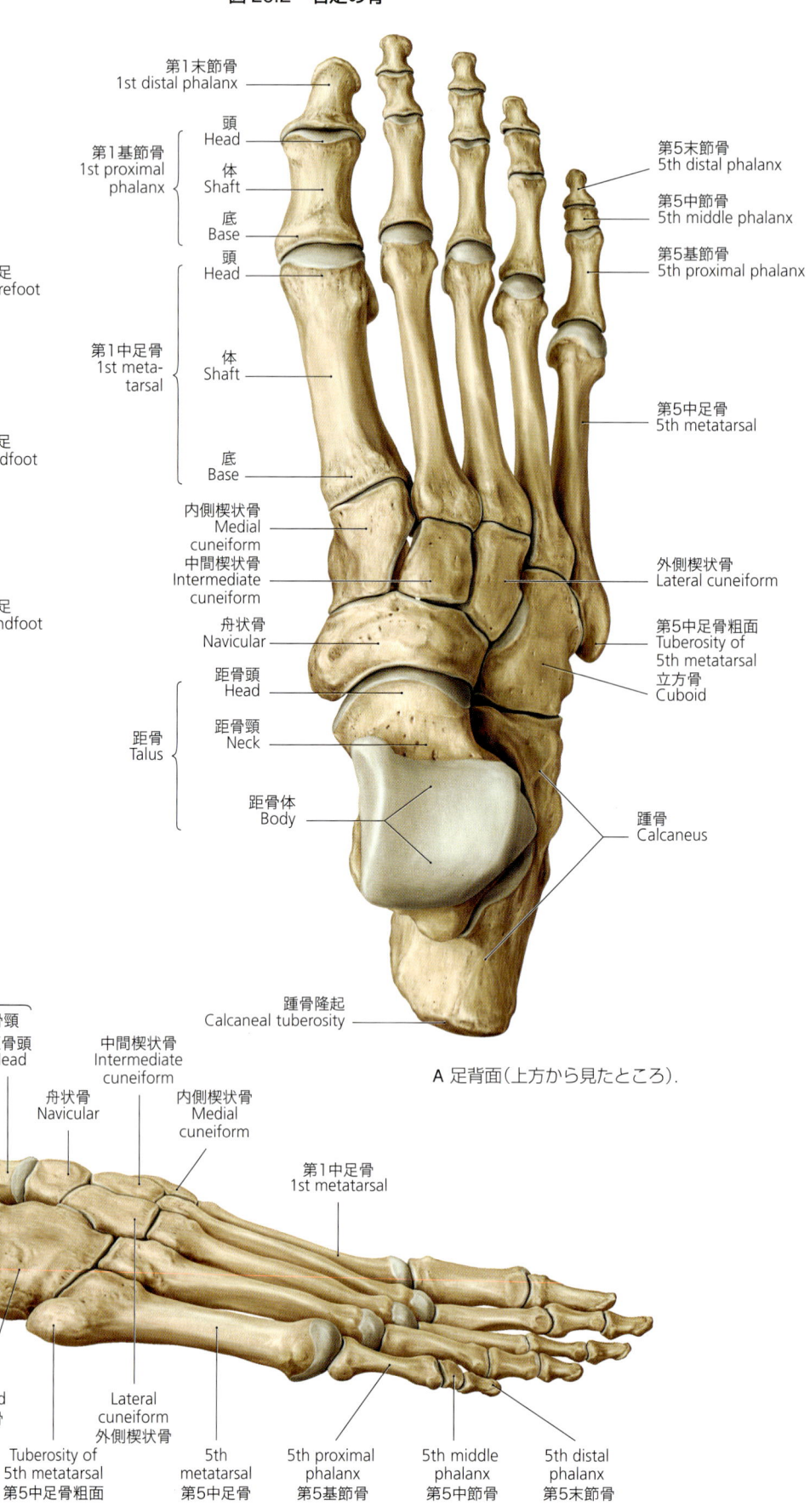

- 第1末節骨 1st distal phalanx
- 第1基節骨 1st proximal phalanx
  - 頭 Head
  - 体 Shaft
  - 底 Base
- 第1中足骨 1st metatarsal
  - 頭 Head
  - 体 Shaft
  - 底 Base
- 内側楔状骨 Medial cuneiform
- 中間楔状骨 Intermediate cuneiform
- 舟状骨 Navicular
- 距骨 Talus
  - 距骨頭 Head
  - 距骨頸 Neck
  - 距骨体 Body
- 第5末節骨 5th distal phalanx
- 第5中節骨 5th middle phalanx
- 第5基節骨 5th proximal phalanx
- 第5中足骨 5th metatarsal
- 外側楔状骨 Lateral cuneiform
- 第5中足骨粗面 Tuberosity of 5th metatarsal
- 立方骨 Cuboid
- 踵骨 Calcaneus
- 踵骨隆起 Calcaneal tuberosity

A 足背面（上方から見たところ）．

- 距骨 Talus
  - 距骨体 Body
  - 距骨頸 Neck
  - 距骨頭 Head
  - 距骨後突起 Posterior process
- 踵骨 Calcaneus
- 踵骨隆起 Calcaneal tuberosity
- 舟状骨 Navicular
- 中間楔状骨 Intermediate cuneiform
- 内側楔状骨 Medial cuneiform
- 第1中足骨 1st metatarsal
- 立方骨 Cuboid
- 外側楔状骨 Lateral cuneiform
- 第5中足骨粗面 Tuberosity of 5th metatarsal
- 第5中足骨 5th metatarsal
- 第5基節骨 5th proximal phalanx
- 第5中節骨 5th middle phalanx
- 第5末節骨 5th distal phalanx
- 踵骨隆起外側突起 Lateral process of calcaneal tuberosity
- 踵骨隆起内側突起 Medial process of calcaneal tuberosity

B 外側方から見たところ．

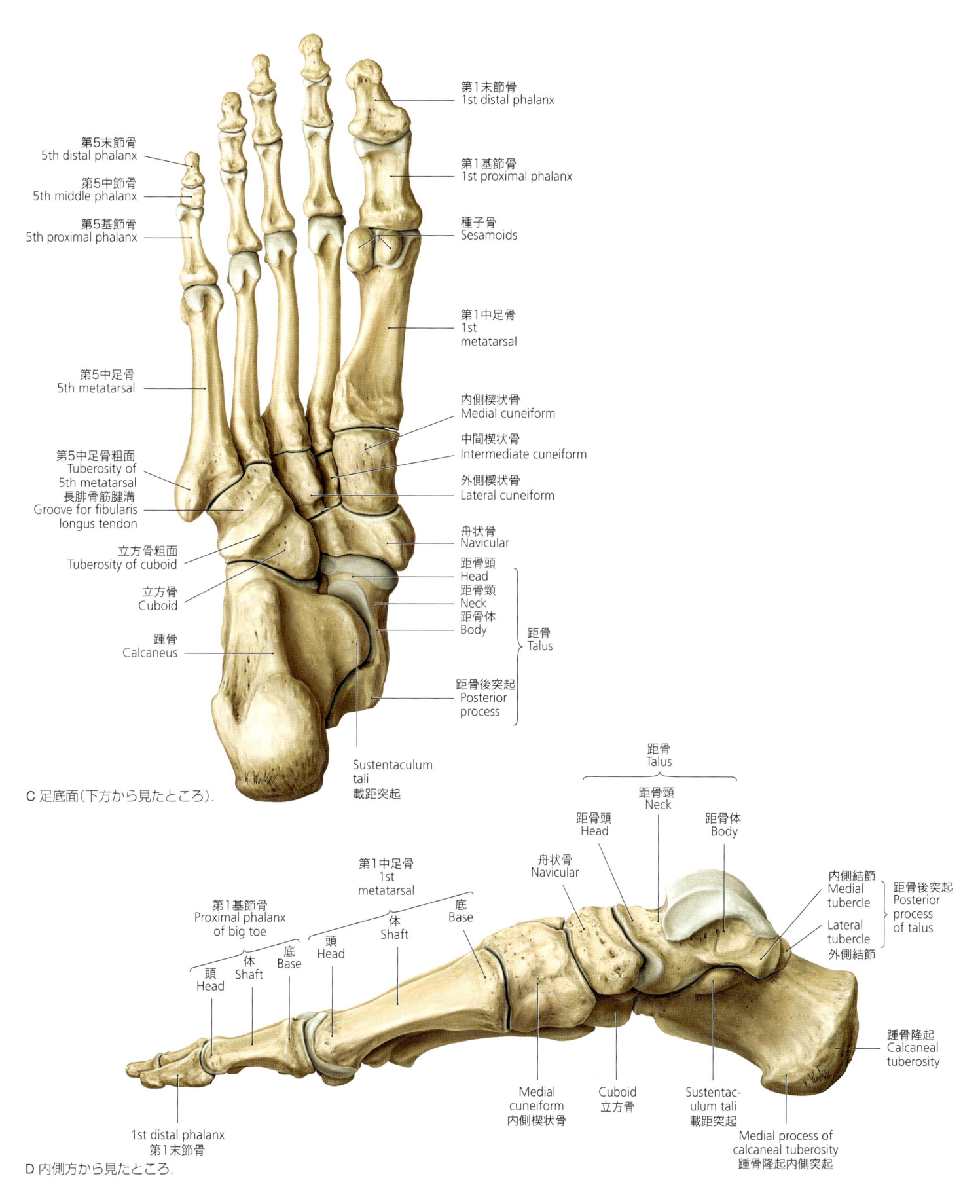

C 足底面（下方から見たところ）．

D 内側方から見たところ．

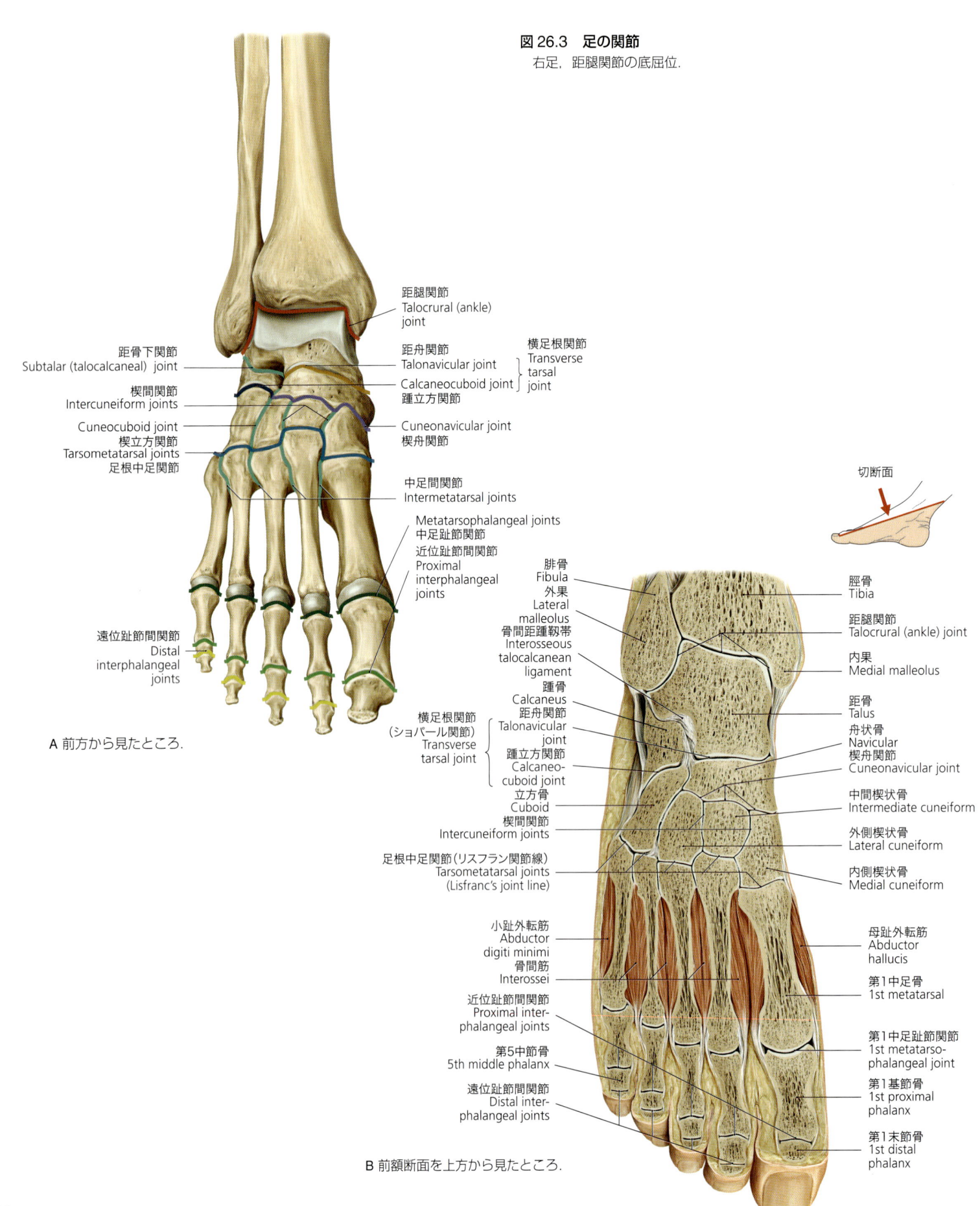

足の関節 (1)
Joints of the Foot (I)

図 26.3　足の関節
右足，距腿関節の底屈位．

距腿関節
Talocrural (ankle) joint

距骨下関節
Subtalar (talocalcaneal) joint

距舟関節
Talonavicular joint

楔間関節
Intercuneiform joints

踵立方関節
Calcaneocuboid joint

横足根関節
Transverse tarsal joint

楔舟関節
Cuneonavicular joint

楔立方関節
Cuneocuboid joint

足根中足関節
Tarsometatarsal joints

中足間関節
Intermetatarsal joints

中足趾節関節
Metatarsophalangeal joints

近位趾節間関節
Proximal interphalangeal joints

遠位趾節間関節
Distal interphalangeal joints

A 前方から見たところ．

切断面

腓骨
Fibula

外果
Lateral malleolus

骨間距踵靱帯
Interosseous talocalcanean ligament

踵骨
Calcaneus

距舟関節
Talonavicular joint

横足根関節（ショパール関節）
Transverse tarsal joint

踵立方関節
Calcaneo-cuboid joint

立方骨
Cuboid

楔間関節
Intercuneiform joints

足根中足関節（リスフラン関節線）
Tarsometatarsal joints (Lisfranc's joint line)

小趾外転筋
Abductor digiti minimi

骨間筋
Interossei

近位趾節間関節
Proximal interphalangeal joints

第5中節骨
5th middle phalanx

遠位趾節間関節
Distal interphalangeal joints

脛骨
Tibia

距腿関節
Talocrural (ankle) joint

内果
Medial malleolus

距骨
Talus

舟状骨
Navicular

楔舟関節
Cuneonavicular joint

中間楔状骨
Intermediate cuneiform

外側楔状骨
Lateral cuneiform

内側楔状骨
Medial cuneiform

母趾外転筋
Abductor hallucis

第1中足骨
1st metatarsal

第1中足趾節関節
1st metatarsophalangeal joint

第1基節骨
1st proximal phalanx

第1末節骨
1st distal phalanx

B 前額断面を上方から見たところ．

図26.4 近位関節面
右足，近位方向から見たところ．

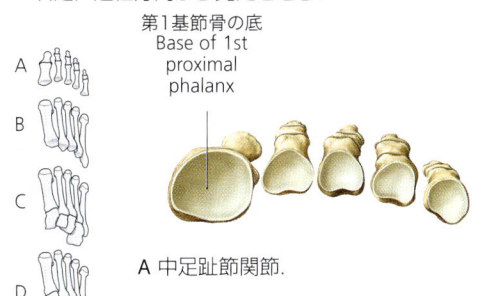

A 中足趾節関節．
- 第1基節骨の底 / Base of 1st proximal phalanx

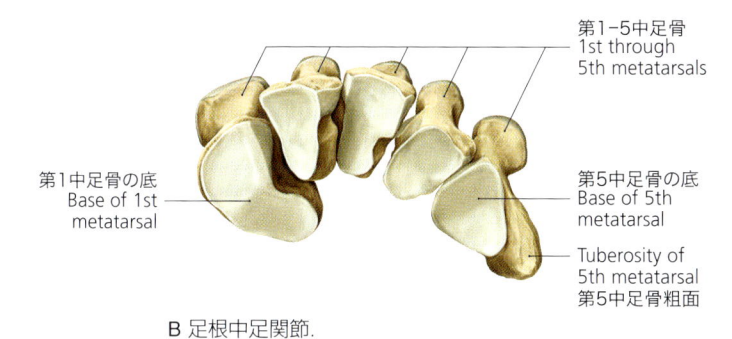

B 足根中足関節．
- 第1中足骨の底 / Base of 1st metatarsal
- 第1–5中足骨 / 1st through 5th metatarsals
- 第5中足骨の底 / Base of 5th metatarsal
- Tuberosity of 5th metatarsal / 第5中足骨粗面

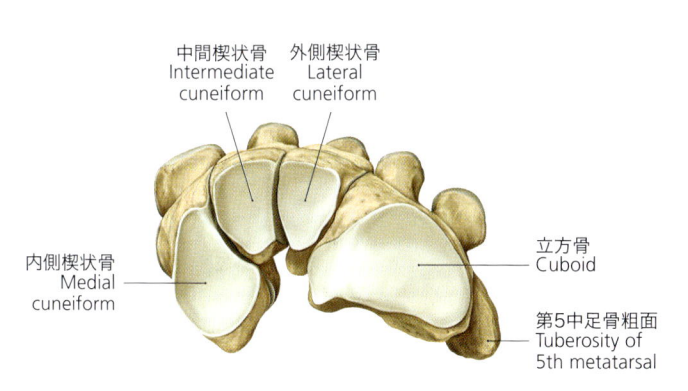

C 楔舟関節と踵立方関節．
- 内側楔状骨 / Medial cuneiform
- 中間楔状骨 / Intermediate cuneiform
- 外側楔状骨 / Lateral cuneiform
- 立方骨 / Cuboid
- 第5中足骨粗面 / Tuberosity of 5th metatarsal

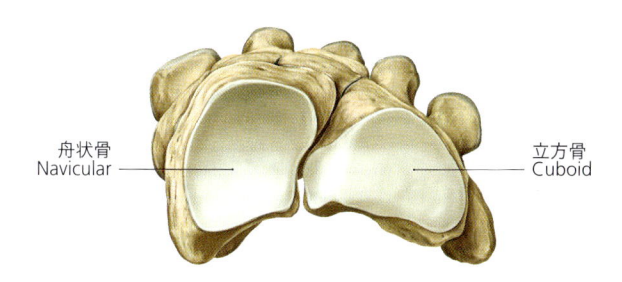

D 距舟関節と踵立方関節．
- 舟状骨 / Navicular
- 立方骨 / Cuboid

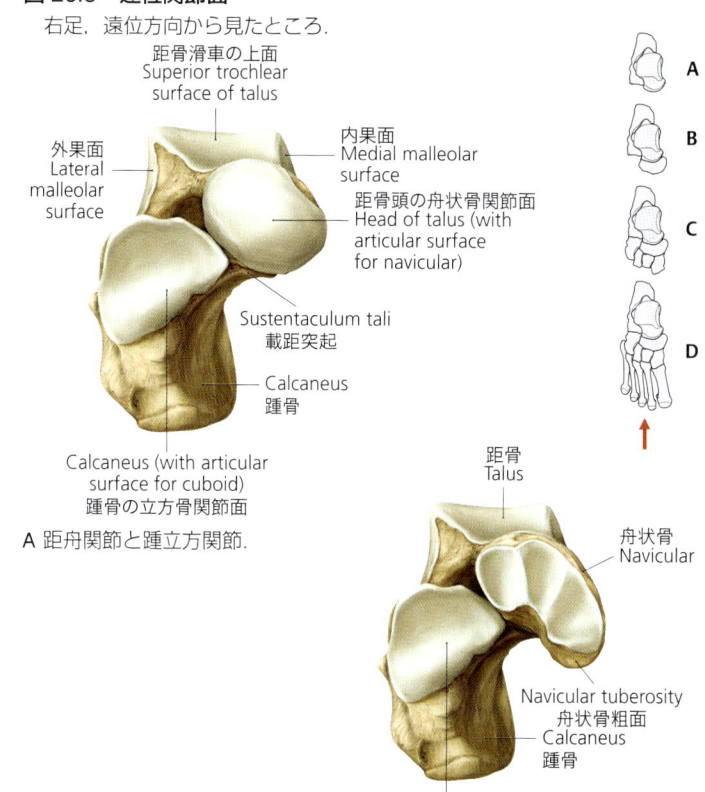

図26.5 遠位関節面
右足，遠位方向から見たところ．

A 距舟関節と踵立方関節．
- 距骨滑車の上面 / Superior trochlear surface of talus
- 外果面 / Lateral malleolar surface
- 内果面 / Medial malleolar surface
- 距骨頭の舟状骨関節面 / Head of talus (with articular surface for navicular)
- Sustentaculum tali / 載距突起
- Calcaneus / 踵骨
- Calcaneus (with articular surface for cuboid) / 踵骨の立方骨関節面

B 楔舟関節と踵立方関節．
- 距骨 / Talus
- 舟状骨 / Navicular
- Navicular tuberosity / 舟状骨粗面
- Calcaneus / 踵骨
- Calcaneus (with articular surface for cuboid) / 踵骨の立方骨関節面

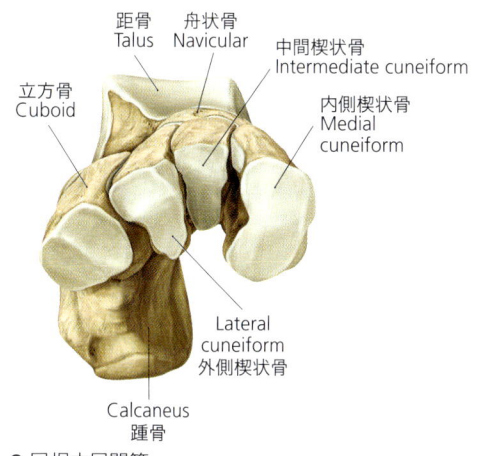

C 足根中足関節．
- 距骨 / Talus
- 舟状骨 / Navicular
- 中間楔状骨 / Intermediate cuneiform
- 内側楔状骨 / Medial cuneiform
- 立方骨 / Cuboid
- Lateral cuneiform / 外側楔状骨
- Calcaneus / 踵骨

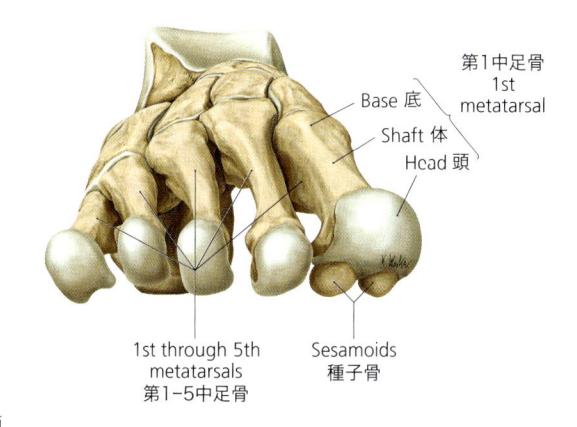

D 中足趾節関節．
- 第1中足骨 / 1st metatarsal
- Base 底
- Shaft 体
- Head 頭
- 1st through 5th metatarsals / 第1–5中足骨
- Sesamoids / 種子骨

足の関節(2)
Joints of the Foot (II)

図 26.6 距腿関節と距骨下関節
右足．距腿関節では，脛骨と腓骨の遠位端が作るくぼみ(足関節窩)に距骨滑車がはまり込んでいる．距骨下関節は骨間距踵靱帯によって，前区(距踵舟関節)と後区(距踵関節)に分けられる(p.409 参照)．

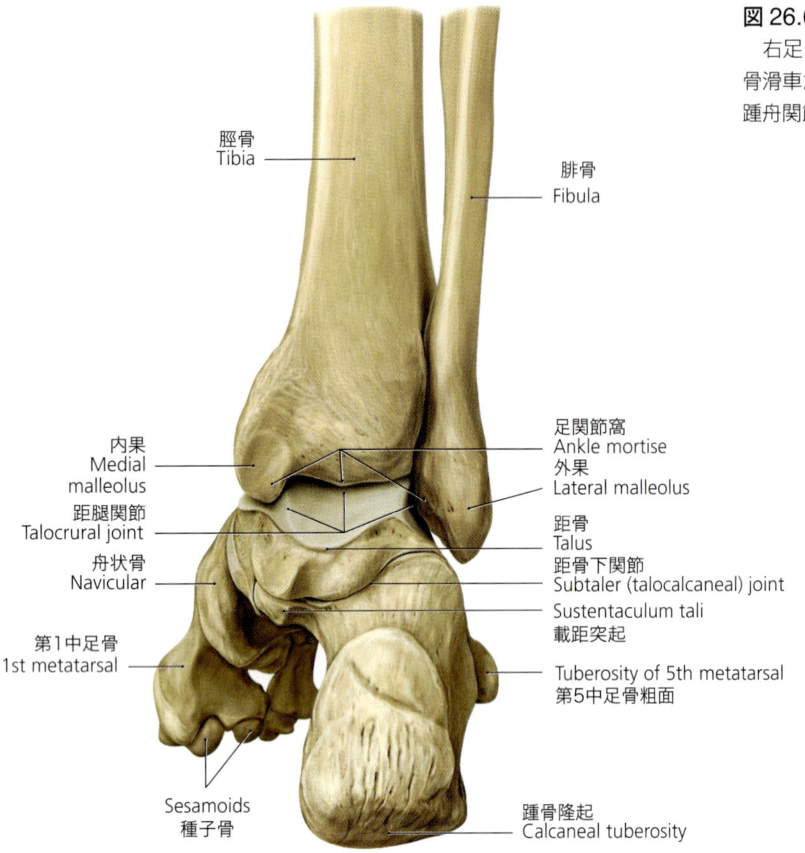

A 後方から見たところ．足は中立位(0°)にある．

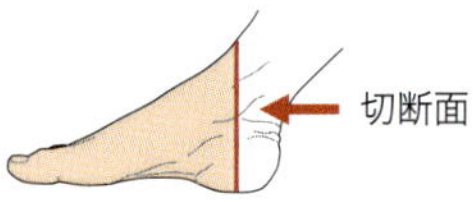

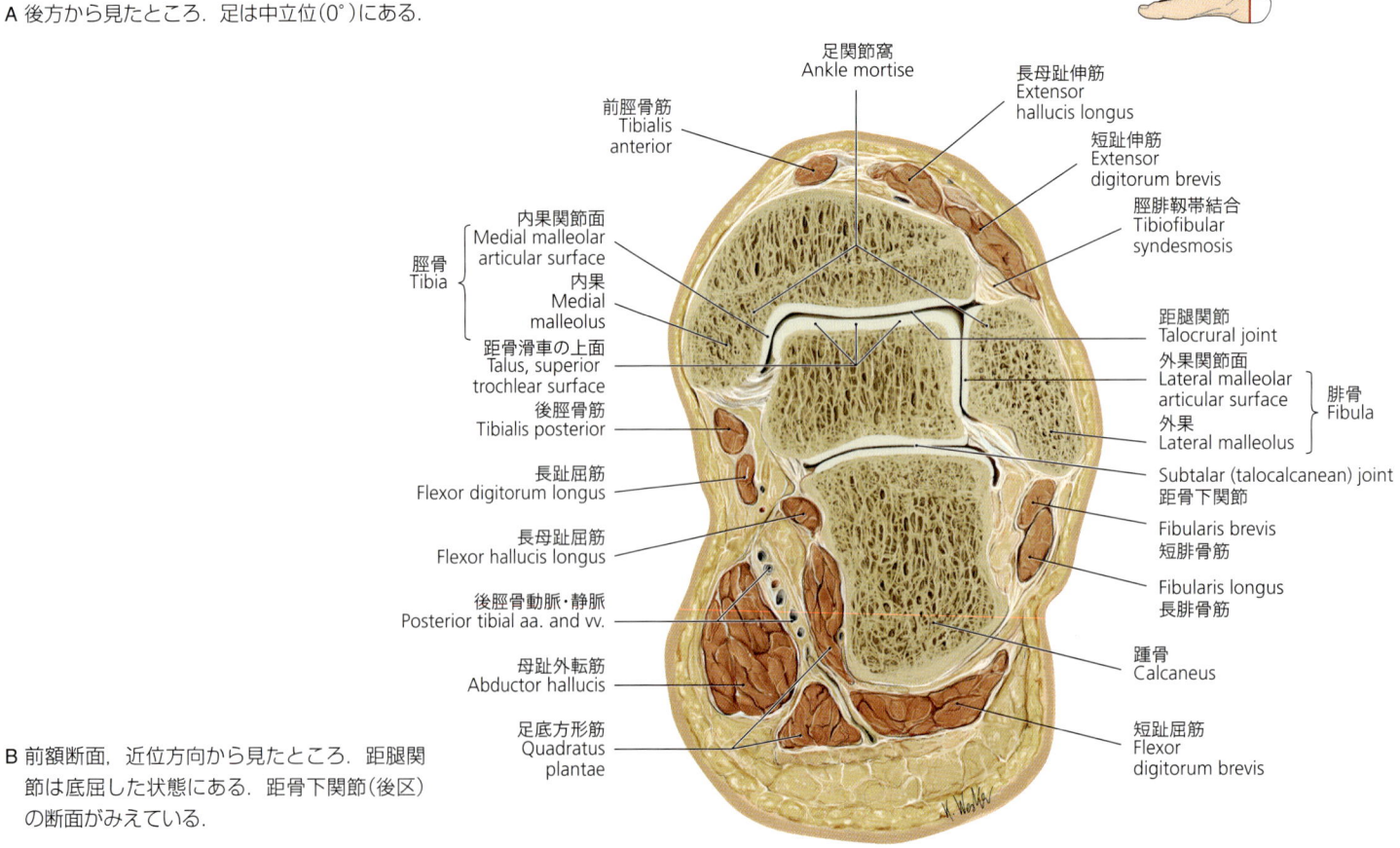

ラベル：
- 脛骨 Tibia
- 腓骨 Fibula
- 内果 Medial malleolus
- 足関節窩 Ankle mortise
- 外果 Lateral malleolus
- 距腿関節 Talocrural joint
- 距骨 Talus
- 舟状骨 Navicular
- 距骨下関節 Subtaler (talocalcaneal) joint
- 載距突起 Sustentaculum tali
- 第1中足骨 1st metatarsal
- 第5中足骨粗面 Tuberosity of 5th metatarsal
- 種子骨 Sesamoids
- 踵骨隆起 Calcaneal tuberosity

B 前額断面，近位方向から見たところ．距腿関節は底屈した状態にある．距骨下関節(後区)の断面がみえている．

ラベル：
- 足関節窩 Ankle mortise
- 長母趾伸筋 Extensor hallucis longus
- 前脛骨筋 Tibialis anterior
- 短趾伸筋 Extensor digitorum brevis
- 内果関節面 Medial malleolar articular surface
- 脛骨 Tibia
- 脛腓靱帯結合 Tibiofibular syndesmosis
- 内果 Medial malleolus
- 距腿関節 Talocrural joint
- 距骨滑車の上面 Talus, superior trochlear surface
- 外果関節面 Lateral malleolar articular surface
- 後脛骨筋 Tibialis posterior
- 外果 Lateral malleolus
- 腓骨 Fibula
- 長趾屈筋 Flexor digitorum longus
- 距骨下関節 Subtalar (talocalcanean) joint
- 長母趾屈筋 Flexor hallucis longus
- 短腓骨筋 Fibularis brevis
- 後脛骨動脈・静脈 Posterior tibial aa. and vv.
- 長腓骨筋 Fibularis longus
- 母趾外転筋 Abductor hallucis
- 踵骨 Calcaneus
- 足底方形筋 Quadratus plantae
- 短趾屈筋 Flexor digitorum brevis

切断面

図 26.7　距腿関節と距骨下関節：矢状断面
右足．内側方から見たところ．

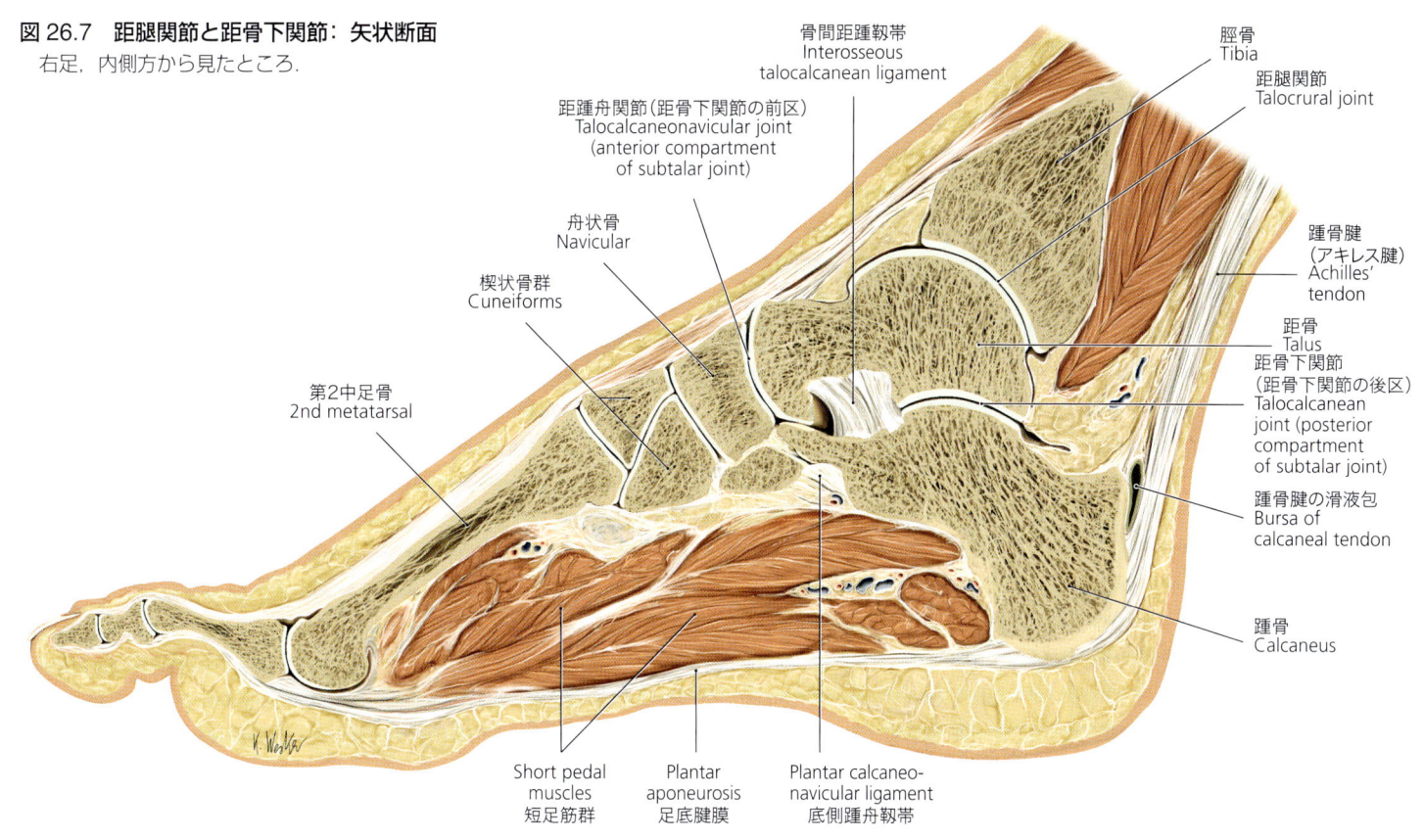

- 骨間距踵靱帯 Interosseous talocalcanean ligament
- 脛骨 Tibia
- 距腿関節 Talocrural joint
- 距踵舟関節（距骨下関節の前区）Talocaneonavicular joint (anterior compartment of subtalar joint)
- 舟状骨 Navicular
- 踵骨腱（アキレス腱）Achilles' tendon
- 楔状骨群 Cuneiforms
- 距骨 Talus
- 距骨下関節（距骨下関節の後区）Talocalcanean joint (posterior compartment of subtalar joint)
- 第2中足骨 2nd metatarsal
- 踵骨腱の滑液包 Bursa of calcaneal tendon
- 踵骨 Calcaneus
- 短足筋群 Short pedal muscles
- 足底腱膜 Plantar aponeurosis
- 底側踵舟靱帯 Plantar calcaneonavicular ligament

図 26.8　距腿関節
右足．

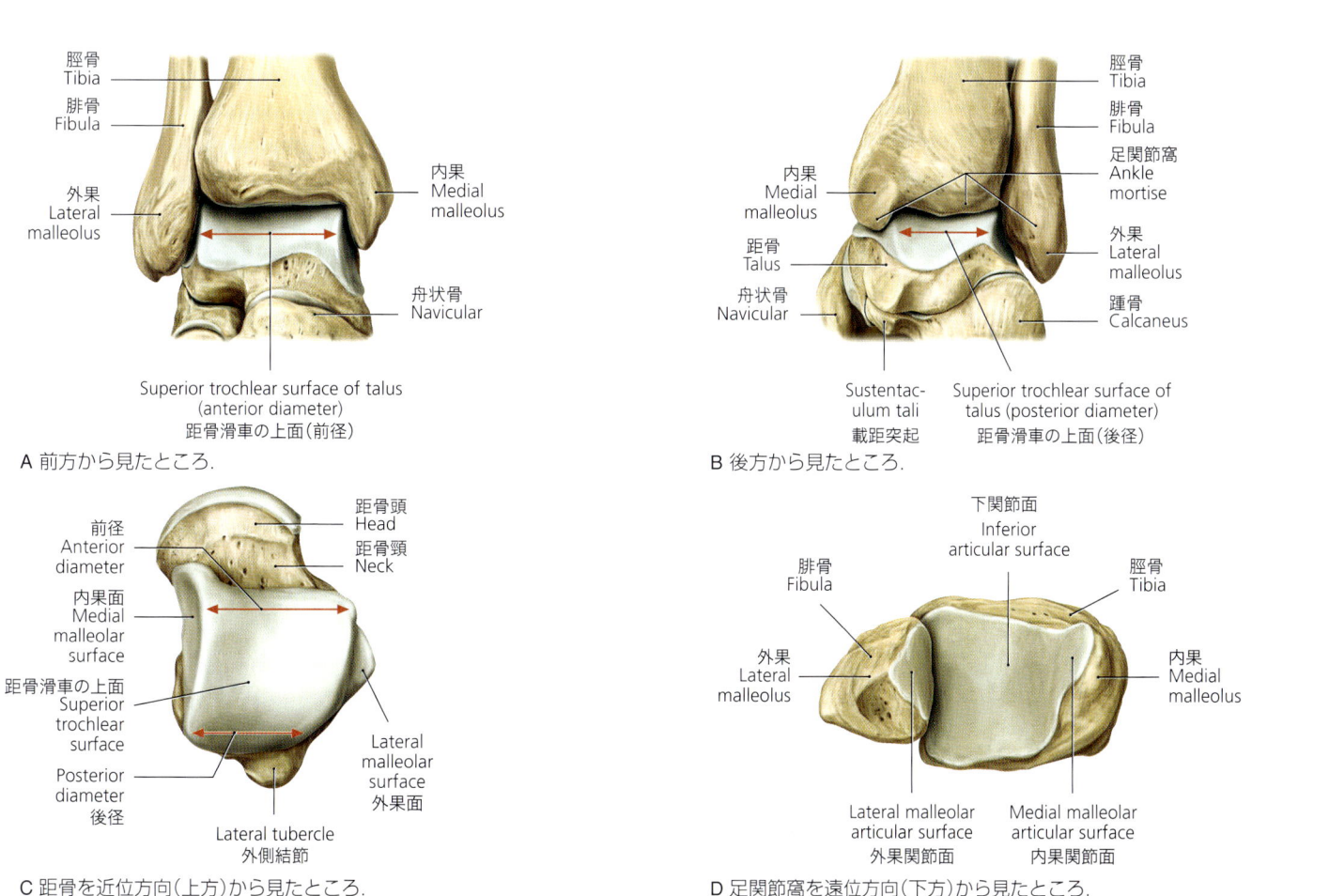

A 前方から見たところ．
- 脛骨 Tibia
- 腓骨 Fibula
- 外果 Lateral malleolus
- 内果 Medial malleolus
- 舟状骨 Navicular
- 距骨滑車の上面（前径）Superior trochlear surface of talus (anterior diameter)

B 後方から見たところ．
- 脛骨 Tibia
- 腓骨 Fibula
- 足関節窩 Ankle mortise
- 内果 Medial malleolus
- 外果 Lateral malleolus
- 距骨 Talus
- 舟状骨 Navicular
- 踵骨 Calcaneus
- 載距突起 Sustentaculum tali
- 距骨滑車の上面（後径）Superior trochlear surface of talus (posterior diameter)

C 距骨を近位方向（上方）から見たところ．
- 距骨頭 Head
- 距骨頸 Neck
- 前径 Anterior diameter
- 内果面 Medial malleolar surface
- 距骨滑車の上面 Superior trochlear surface
- 後径 Posterior diameter
- 外果面 Lateral malleolar surface
- 外側結節 Lateral tubercle

D 足関節窩を遠位方向（下方）から見たところ．
- 下関節面 Inferior articular surface
- 腓骨 Fibula
- 脛骨 Tibia
- 外果 Lateral malleolus
- 内果 Medial malleolus
- 外果関節面 Lateral malleolar articular surface
- 内果関節面 Medial malleolar articular surface

足の関節(3)
Joints of the Foot (III)

図 26.9 距骨下関節とその靱帯
右足．距骨下関節を外してある．距骨下関節は骨間距踵靱帯によって，前区（距踵舟関節）と後区（距踵関節）に分けられる．

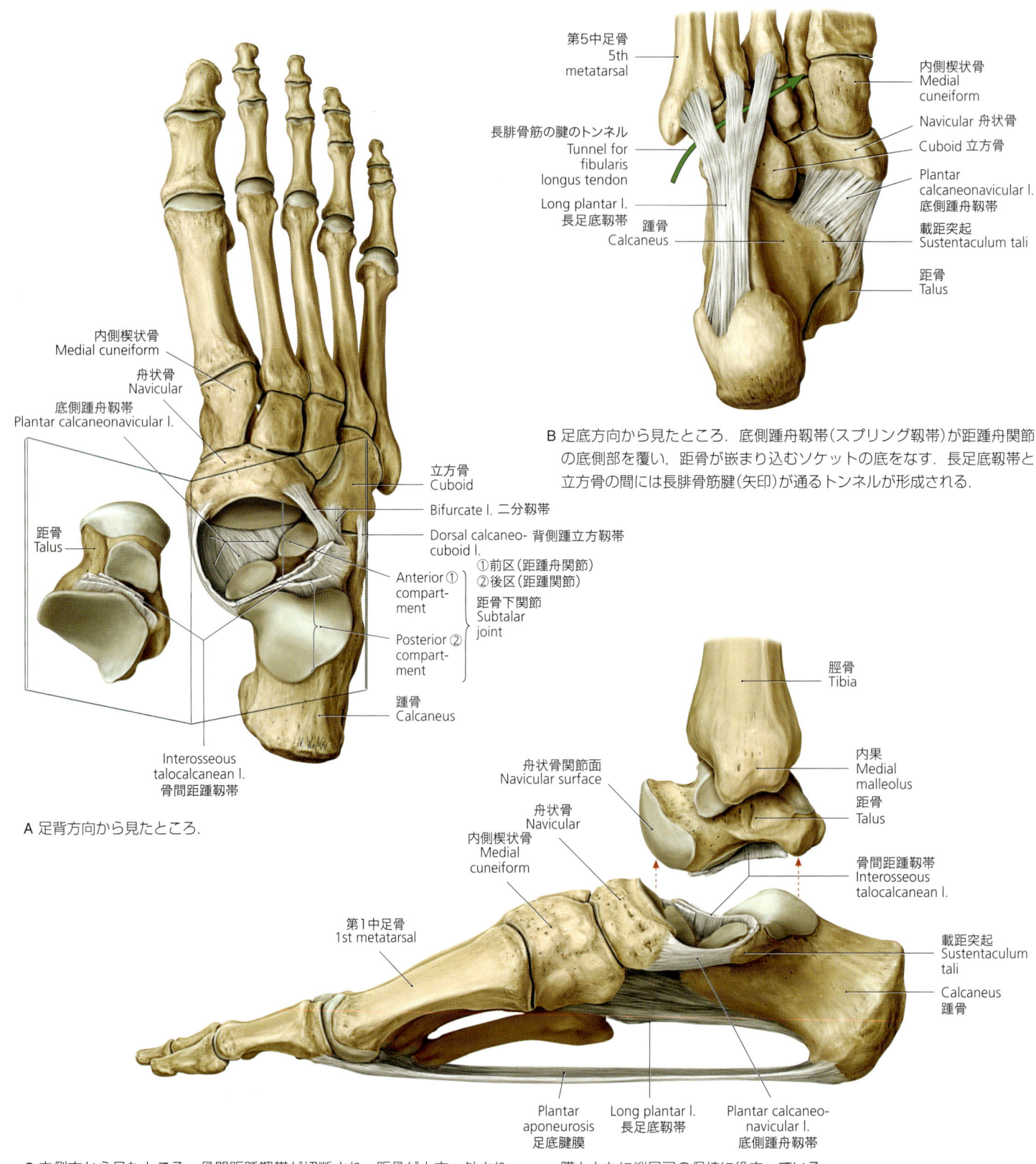

主要ラベル（図A：足背方向から見たところ）
- 内側楔状骨 Medial cuneiform
- 舟状骨 Navicular
- 底側踵舟靱帯 Plantar calcaneonavicular l.
- 距骨 Talus
- 立方骨 Cuboid
- 二分靱帯 Bifurcate l.
- 背側踵立方靱帯 Dorsal calcaneo-cuboid l.
- ①前区（距踵舟関節）Anterior compartment
- ②後区（距踵関節）Posterior compartment
- 距骨下関節 Subtalar joint
- 踵骨 Calcaneus
- 骨間距踵靱帯 Interosseous talocalcanean l.

A 足背方向から見たところ．

図B ラベル
- 第5中足骨 5th metatarsal
- 長腓骨筋の腱のトンネル Tunnel for fibularis longus tendon
- 長足底靱帯 Long plantar l.
- 踵骨 Calcaneus
- 内側楔状骨 Medial cuneiform
- 舟状骨 Navicular
- 立方骨 Cuboid
- 底側踵舟靱帯 Plantar calcaneonavicular l.
- 載距突起 Sustentaculum tali
- 距骨 Talus

B 足底方向から見たところ．底側踵舟靱帯（スプリング靱帯）が距踵舟関節の底側部を覆い，距骨が嵌まり込むソケットの底をなす．長足底靱帯と立方骨の間には長腓骨筋腱（矢印）が通るトンネルが形成される．

図C ラベル
- 舟状骨関節面 Navicular surface
- 舟状骨 Navicular
- 内側楔状骨 Medial cuneiform
- 第1中足骨 1st metatarsal
- 脛骨 Tibia
- 内果 Medial malleolus
- 距骨 Talus
- 骨間距踵靱帯 Interosseous talocalcanean l.
- 載距突起 Sustentaculum tali
- 踵骨 Calcaneus
- 足底腱膜 Plantar aponeurosis
- 長足底靱帯 Long plantar l.
- 底側踵舟靱帯 Plantar calcaneonavicular l.

C 内側方から見たところ．骨間距踵靱帯が切断され，距骨が上方へ外されている．底側踵舟靱帯に注目すること．この靱帯は長足底靱帯や足底腱膜とともに縦足弓の保持に役立っている．

図 26.10 距骨と踵骨

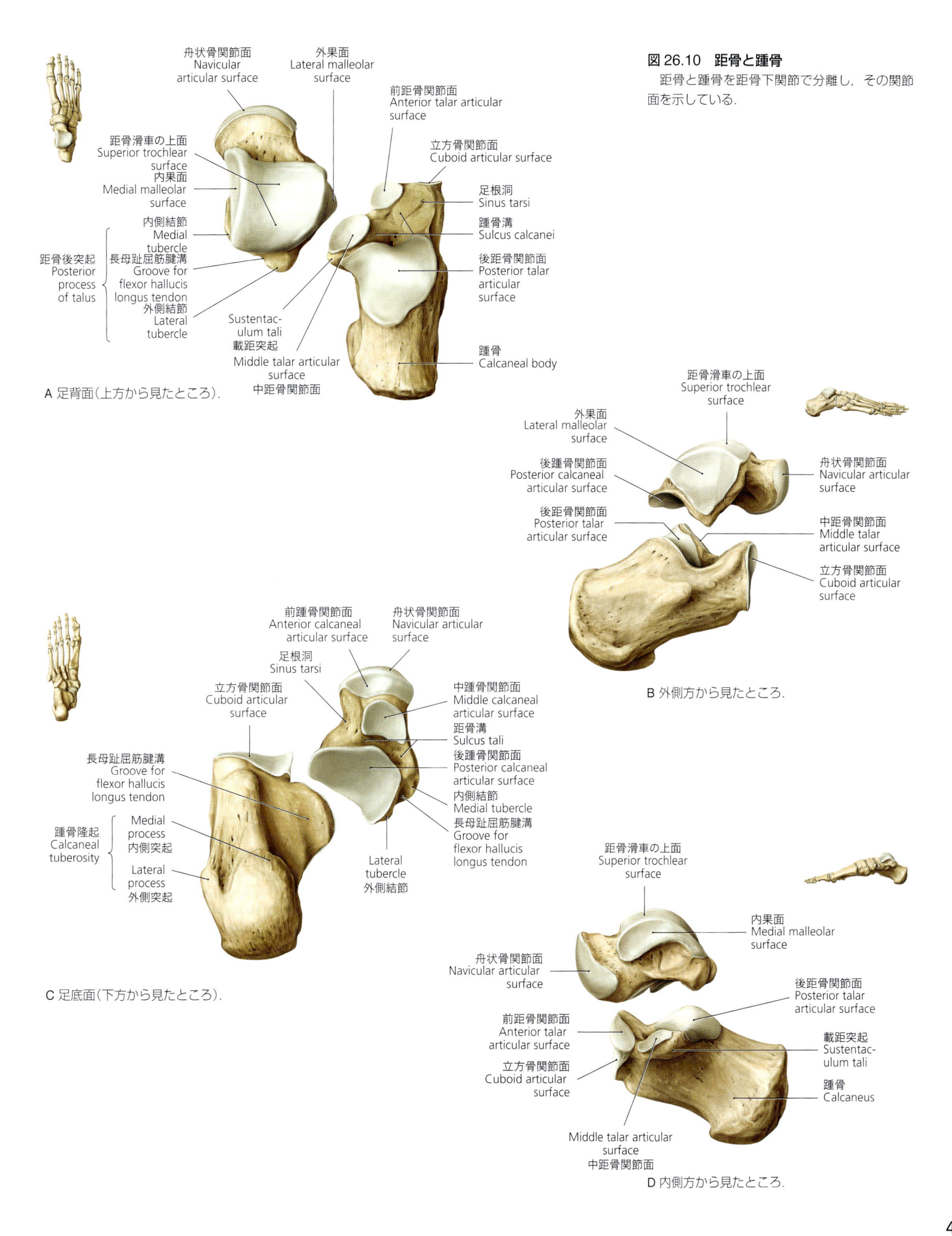

距骨と踵骨を距骨下関節で分離し，その関節面を示している．

A 足背面（上方から見たところ）．

- 舟状骨関節面 Navicular articular surface
- 外果面 Lateral malleolar surface
- 前距骨関節面 Anterior talar articular surface
- 距骨滑車の上面 Superior trochlear surface
- 内果面 Medial malleolar surface
- 立方骨関節面 Cuboid articular surface
- 足根洞 Sinus tarsi
- 踵骨溝 Sulcus calcanei
- 後距骨関節面 Posterior talar articular surface
- 距骨後突起 Posterior process of talus
  - 内側結節 Medial tubercle
  - 長母趾屈筋腱溝 Groove for flexor hallucis longus tendon
  - 外側結節 Lateral tubercle
- 載距突起 Sustentaculum tali
- 中距骨関節面 Middle talar articular surface
- 踵骨 Calcaneal body

B 外側方から見たところ．

- 距骨滑車の上面 Superior trochlear surface
- 外果面 Lateral malleolar surface
- 後踵骨関節面 Posterior calcaneal articular surface
- 後距骨関節面 Posterior talar articular surface
- 舟状骨関節面 Navicular articular surface
- 中距骨関節面 Middle talar articular surface
- 立方骨関節面 Cuboid articular surface

C 足底面（下方から見たところ）．

- 前踵骨関節面 Anterior calcaneal articular surface
- 舟状骨関節面 Navicular articular surface
- 立方骨関節面 Cuboid articular surface
- 足根洞 Sinus tarsi
- 中踵骨関節面 Middle calcaneal articular surface
- 距骨溝 Sulcus tali
- 後踵骨関節面 Posterior calcaneal articular surface
- 内側結節 Medial tubercle
- 長母趾屈筋腱溝 Groove for flexor hallucis longus tendon
- 外側結節 Lateral tubercle
- 長母趾屈筋腱溝 Groove for flexor hallucis longus tendon
- 踵骨隆起 Calcaneal tuberosity
  - 内側突起 Medial process
  - 外側突起 Lateral process

D 内側方から見たところ．

- 距骨滑車の上面 Superior trochlear surface
- 内果面 Medial malleolar surface
- 舟状骨関節面 Navicular articular surface
- 前距骨関節面 Anterior talar articular surface
- 立方骨関節面 Cuboid articular surface
- 後距骨関節面 Posterior talar articular surface
- 載距突起 Sustentaculum tali
- 踵骨 Calcaneus
- 中距骨関節面 Middle talar articular surface

足首と足の靱帯
Ligaments of the Ankle & Foot

足の靱帯は5つに分類できる（距腿関節の靱帯，距骨下関節の靱帯，中足の靱帯，前足の靱帯，足底の靱帯）．内側・外側（側副）靱帯は距骨下関節を安定に保つうえで極めて重要である．

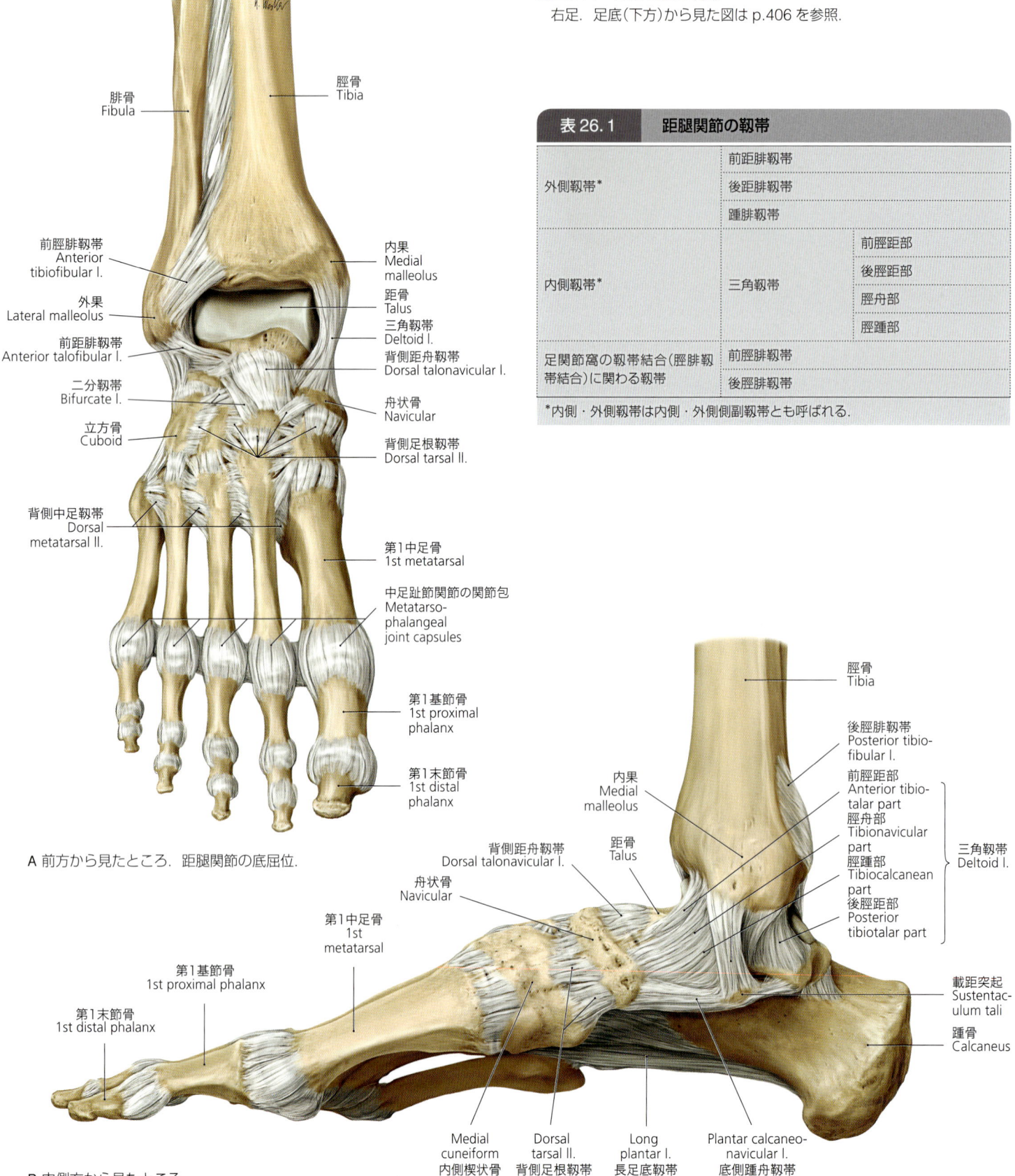

図26.11 足首と足の靱帯
右足．足底（下方）から見た図はp.406を参照．

表26.1	距腿関節の靱帯		
外側靱帯*	前距腓靱帯		
	後距腓靱帯		
	踵腓靱帯		
内側靱帯*	三角靱帯	前脛距部	
		後脛距部	
		脛舟部	
		脛踵部	
足関節窩の靱帯結合（脛腓靱帯結合）に関わる靱帯	前脛腓靱帯		
	後脛腓靱帯		

*内側・外側靱帯は内側・外側側副靱帯とも呼ばれる．

A 前方から見たところ．距腿関節の底屈位．

B 内側方から見たところ．

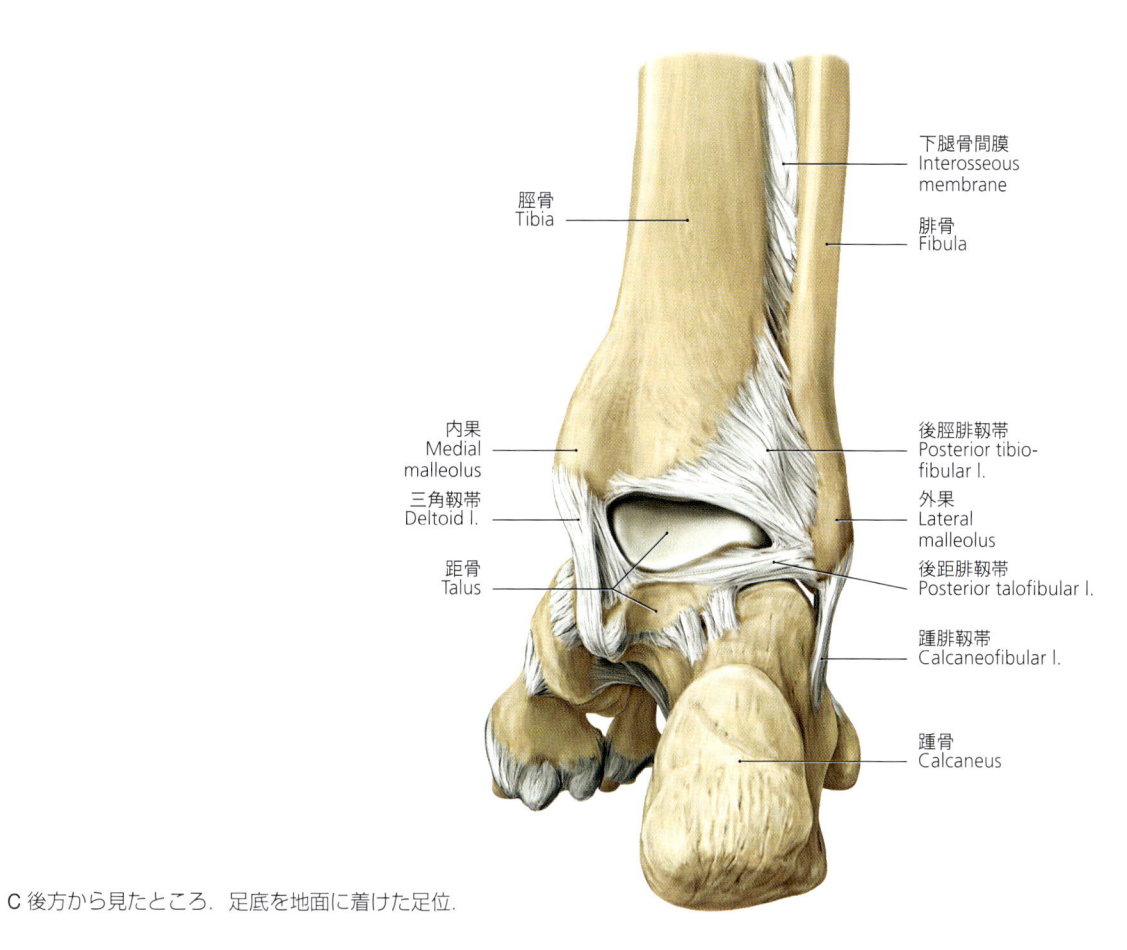

C 後方から見たところ．足底を地面に着けた足位．

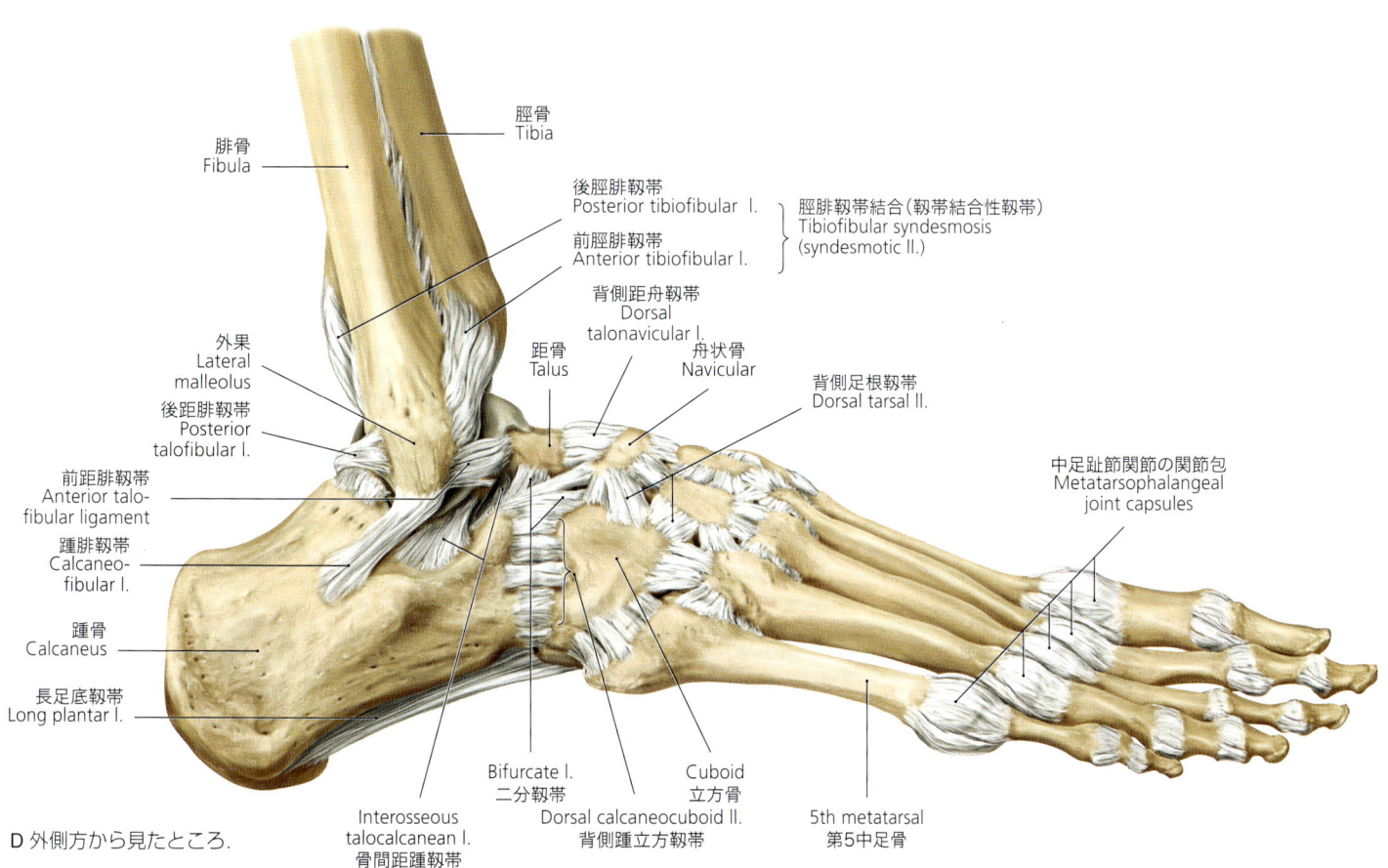

D 外側方から見たところ．

土踏まずと足底弓
Plantar Vault & Arches of the Foot

図 26.12　土踏まず
右足．足で発生した力は2つの外側足放線と3つの内側足放線に伝わる．これらの足放線は，足底に縦足弓と横足弓を形成し，足が垂直負荷を吸収するうえで役立っている．

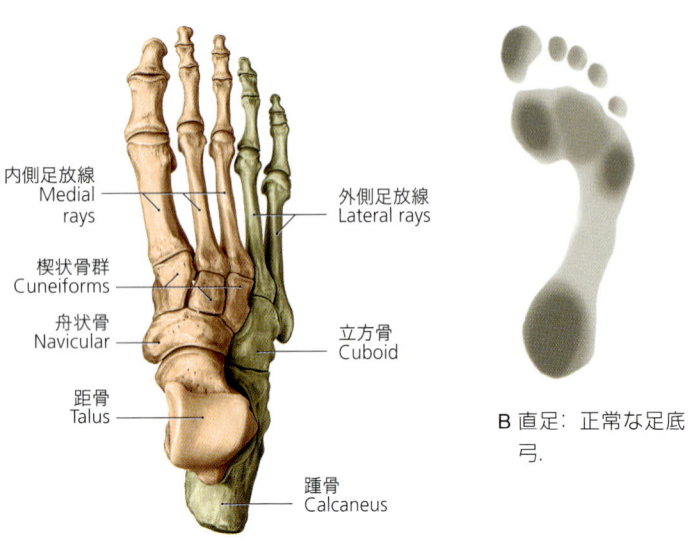

- 内側足放線 Medial rays
- 外側足放線 Lateral rays
- 楔状骨群 Cuneiforms
- 舟状骨 Navicular
- 立方骨 Cuboid
- 距骨 Talus
- 踵骨 Calcaneus

A 上方から見たところ．外側足放線を緑で，内側足放線を赤で示してある．

B 直足：正常な足底弓．

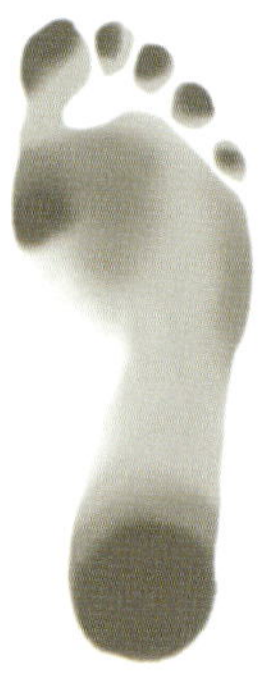

C 扁平足：縦足弓の消失．

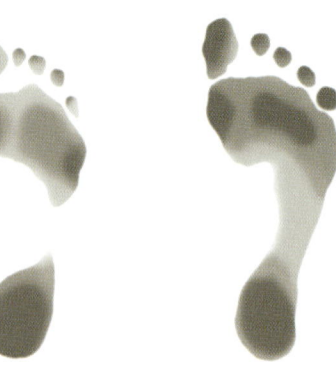

D 凹足：縦足弓の高さの増加．

E 開帳足：横足弓の消失．

図 26.13　横足弓の安定化構造
右足．横足弓を維持する能動的・受動的な安定化構造がある．能動的な安定化構造は筋であり，受動的なのは靱帯である．Note：前足骨にできるアーチには，受動的な安定化構造しか備わっていない．一方，中足骨と足根骨にできるアーチは主として能動的に安定化される．

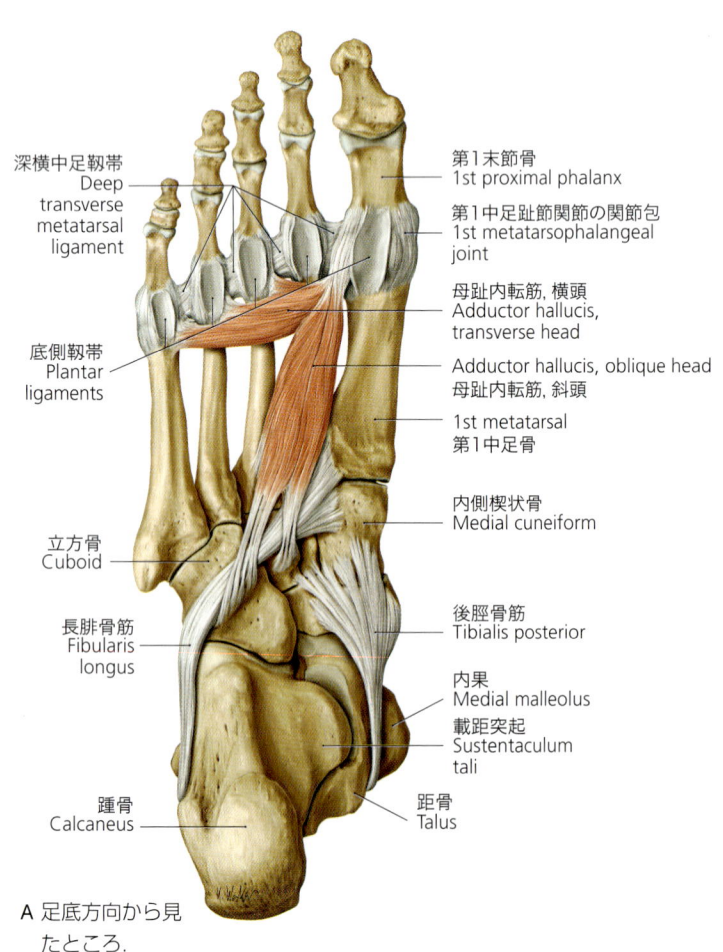

- 深横中足靱帯 Deep transverse metatarsal ligament
- 第1末節骨 1st proximal phalanx
- 第1中足趾節関節の関節包 1st metatarsophalangeal joint
- 母趾内転筋，横頭 Adductor hallucis, transverse head
- 母趾内転筋，斜頭 Adductor hallucis, oblique head
- 第1中足骨 1st metatarsal
- 底側靱帯 Plantar ligaments
- 内側楔状骨 Medial cuneiform
- 立方骨 Cuboid
- 長腓骨筋 Fibularis longus
- 後脛骨筋 Tibialis posterior
- 内果 Medial malleolus
- 載距突起 Sustentaculum tali
- 踵骨 Calcaneus
- 距骨 Talus

A 足底方向から見たところ．

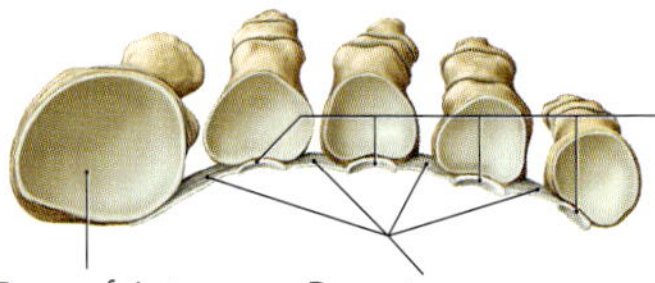

B 前足骨のアーチ，近位方向から見たところ．
- 足底靱帯 Plantar ligaments
- 第1基節骨の底 Base of 1st proximal phalanx
- 深横中足靱帯 Deep transverse metatarsal ligament

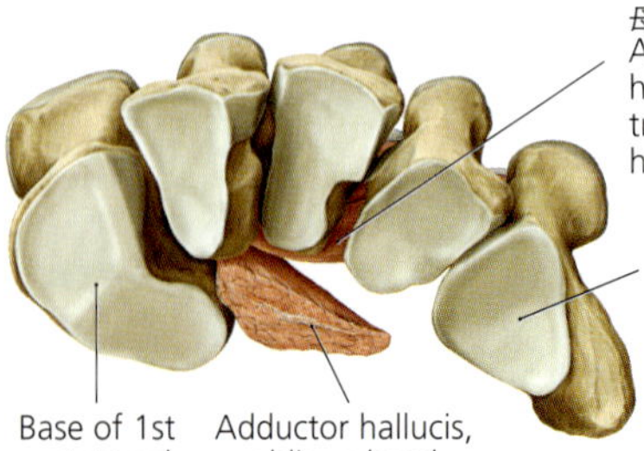

C 中足骨のアーチ，近位方向から見たところ．
- 母趾内転筋，横頭 Adductor hallucis, transverse head
- 第5中足骨の底 Base of 5th metatarsal
- 第1中足骨の底 Base of 1st metatarsal
- 母趾内転筋，斜頭 Adductor hallucis, oblique head
- 中間楔状骨 Intermediate cuneiform
- 外側楔状骨 Lateral cuneiform

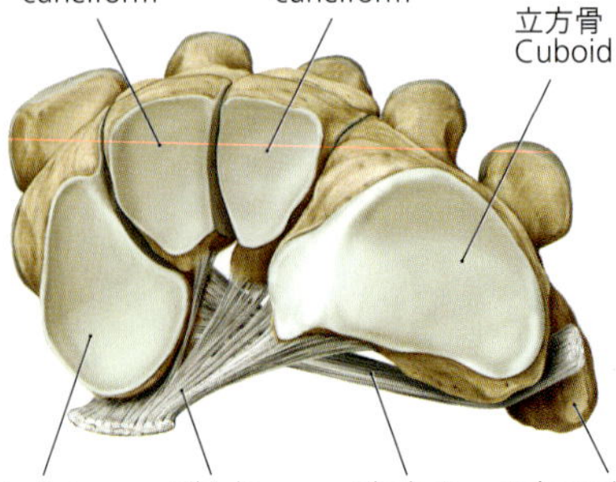

D 足根骨のアーチ，近位方向から見たところ．
- 立方骨 Cuboid
- 内側楔状骨 Medial cuneiform
- 後脛骨筋 Tibialis posterior
- 長腓骨筋 Fibularis longus
- 第5中足骨粗面 Tuberosity of 5th metatarsal

図 26.14　縦足弓の安定化構造
右足，内側方から見たところ．

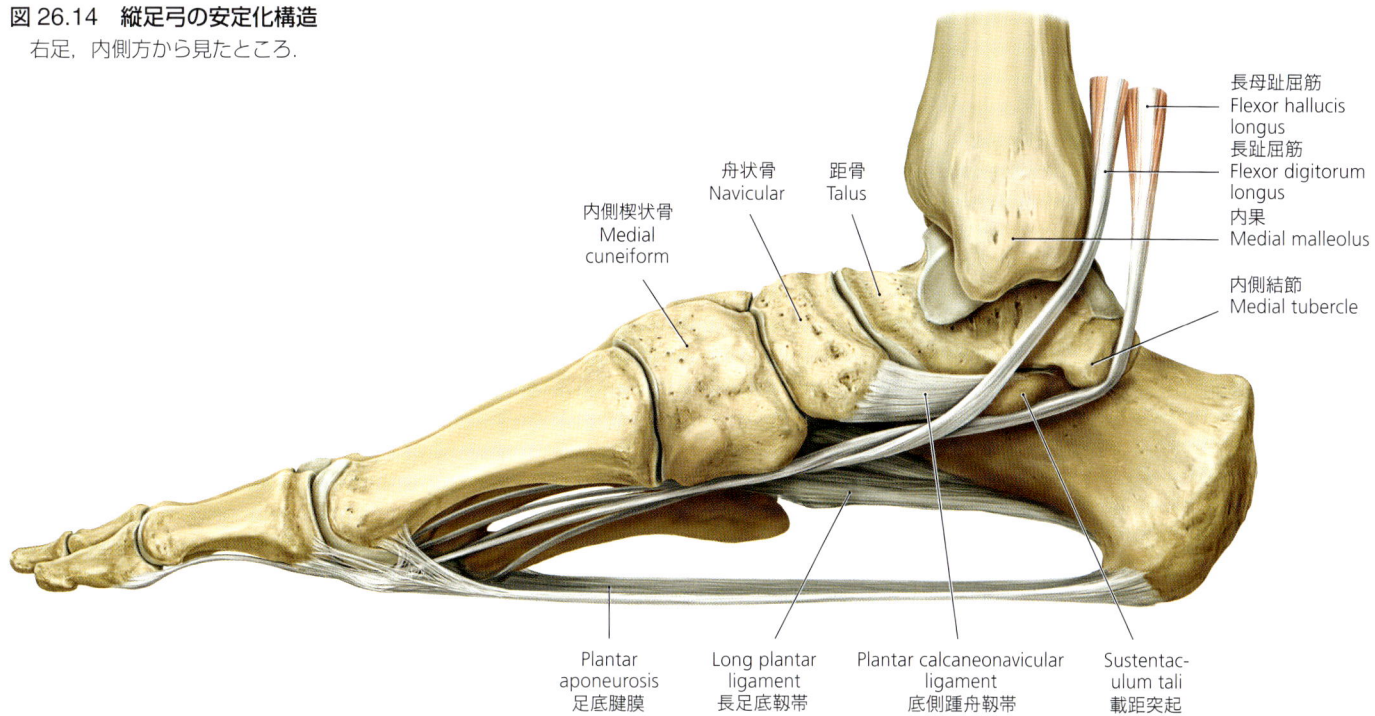

A 縦足弓の受動的安定化構造．

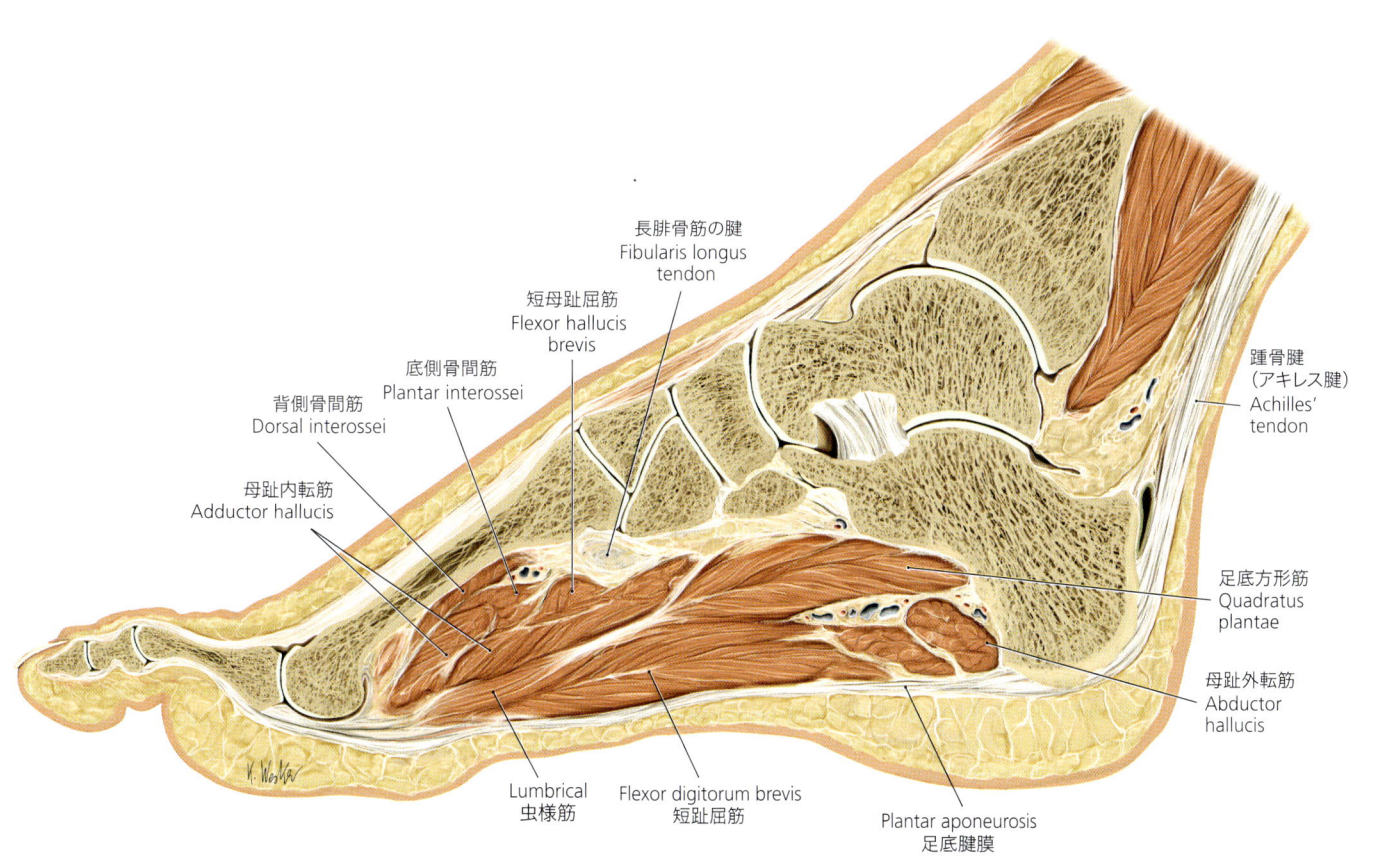

ラベル：
- 内側楔状骨 Medial cuneiform
- 舟状骨 Navicular
- 距骨 Talus
- 長母趾屈筋 Flexor hallucis longus
- 長趾屈筋 Flexor digitorum longus
- 内果 Medial malleolus
- 内側結節 Medial tubercle
- Plantar aponeurosis 足底腱膜
- Long plantar ligament 長足底靱帯
- Plantar calcaneonavicular ligament 底側踵舟靱帯
- Sustentaculum tali 載距突起

B 縦足弓の能動的安定化構造．第2足放線を通る矢状断面．主要な能動的安定化構造は，母趾外転筋，短母趾屈筋，短小趾屈筋，足底方形筋，小趾外転筋である．

ラベル：
- 背側骨間筋 Dorsal interossei
- 底側骨間筋 Plantar interossei
- 短母趾屈筋 Flexor hallucis brevis
- 長腓骨筋の腱 Fibularis longus tendon
- 母趾内転筋 Adductor hallucis
- 踵骨腱（アキレス腱）Achilles' tendon
- 足底方形筋 Quadratus plantae
- 母趾外転筋 Abductor hallucis
- Lumbrical 虫様筋
- Flexor digitorum brevis 短趾屈筋
- Plantar aponeurosis 足底腱膜

足底の筋
Muscles of the Sole of the Foot

図 26.15 足底腱膜
右足，足底方向から見たところ．足底腱膜は強靱であり，中央部が最も厚い．足の辺縁で足背筋膜（示されていない）に移行する．

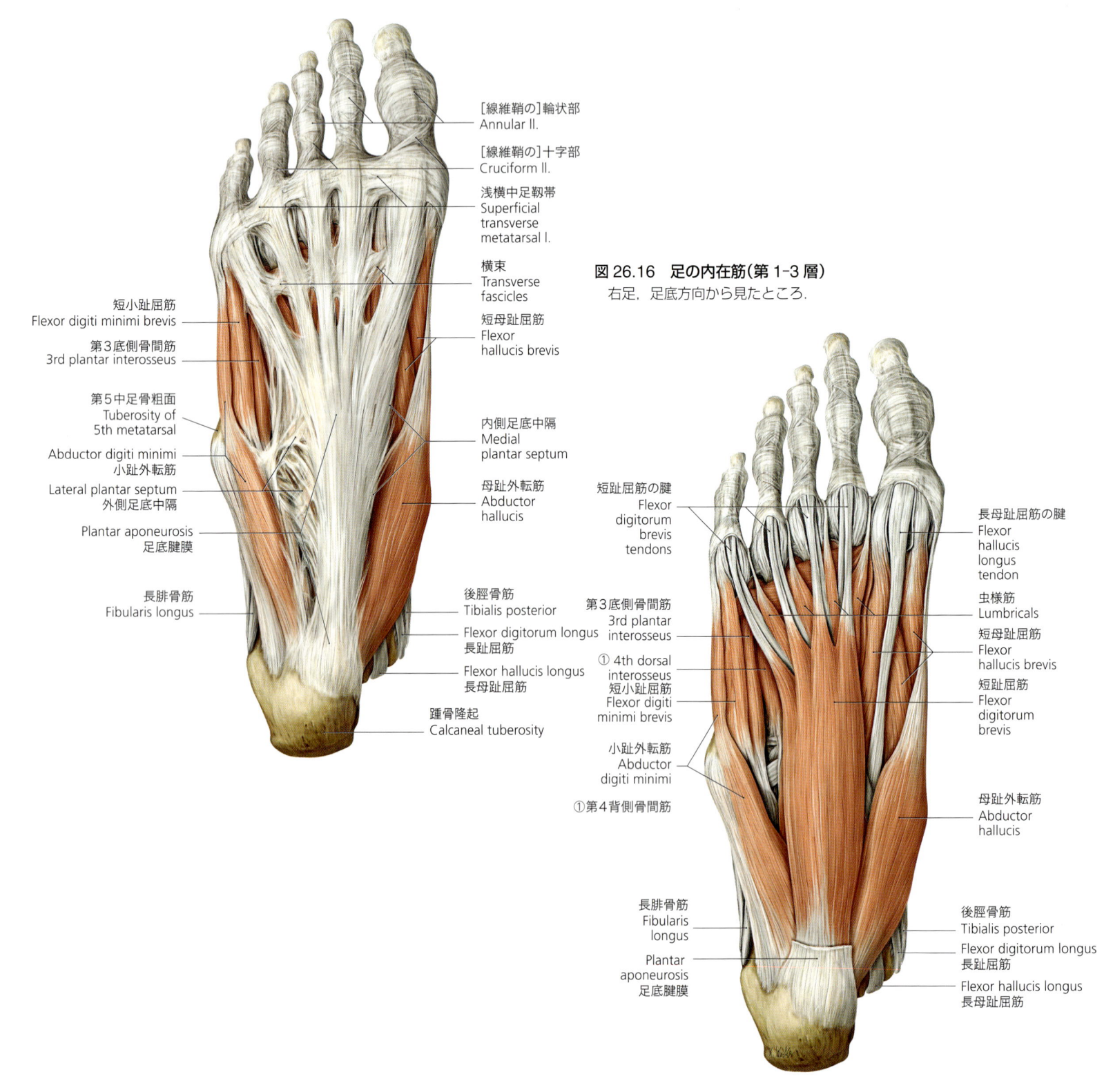

- ［線維鞘の］輪状部 Annular ll.
- ［線維鞘の］十字部 Cruciform ll.
- 浅横中足靱帯 Superficial transverse metatarsal l.
- 横束 Transverse fascicles
- 短母趾屈筋 Flexor hallucis brevis
- 内側足底中隔 Medial plantar septum
- 母趾外転筋 Abductor hallucis
- 後脛骨筋 Tibialis posterior
- 長趾屈筋 Flexor digitorum longus
- 長母趾屈筋 Flexor hallucis longus
- 踵骨隆起 Calcaneal tuberosity
- 短小趾屈筋 Flexor digiti minimi brevis
- 第3底側骨間筋 3rd plantar interosseus
- 第5中足骨粗面 Tuberosity of 5th metatarsal
- 小趾外転筋 Abductor digiti minimi
- 外側足底中隔 Lateral plantar septum
- 足底腱膜 Plantar aponeurosis
- 長腓骨筋 Fibularis longus

図 26.16 足の内在筋（第1-3層）
右足，足底方向から見たところ．

- 短趾屈筋の腱 Flexor digitorum brevis tendons
- 長母趾屈筋の腱 Flexor hallucis longus tendon
- 虫様筋 Lumbricals
- 短母趾屈筋 Flexor hallucis brevis
- 短趾屈筋 Flexor digitorum brevis
- 母趾外転筋 Abductor hallucis
- 後脛骨筋 Tibialis posterior
- 長趾屈筋 Flexor digitorum longus
- 長母趾屈筋 Flexor hallucis longus
- 第3底側骨間筋 3rd plantar interosseus
- ① 第4背側骨間筋 ① 4th dorsal interosseus
- 短小趾屈筋 Flexor digiti minimi brevis
- 小趾外転筋 Abductor digiti minimi
- 長腓骨筋 Fibularis longus
- 足底腱膜 Plantar aponeurosis

A 第1層（最浅層）．足底腱膜は浅横中足靱帯を含めて取り除いてある．

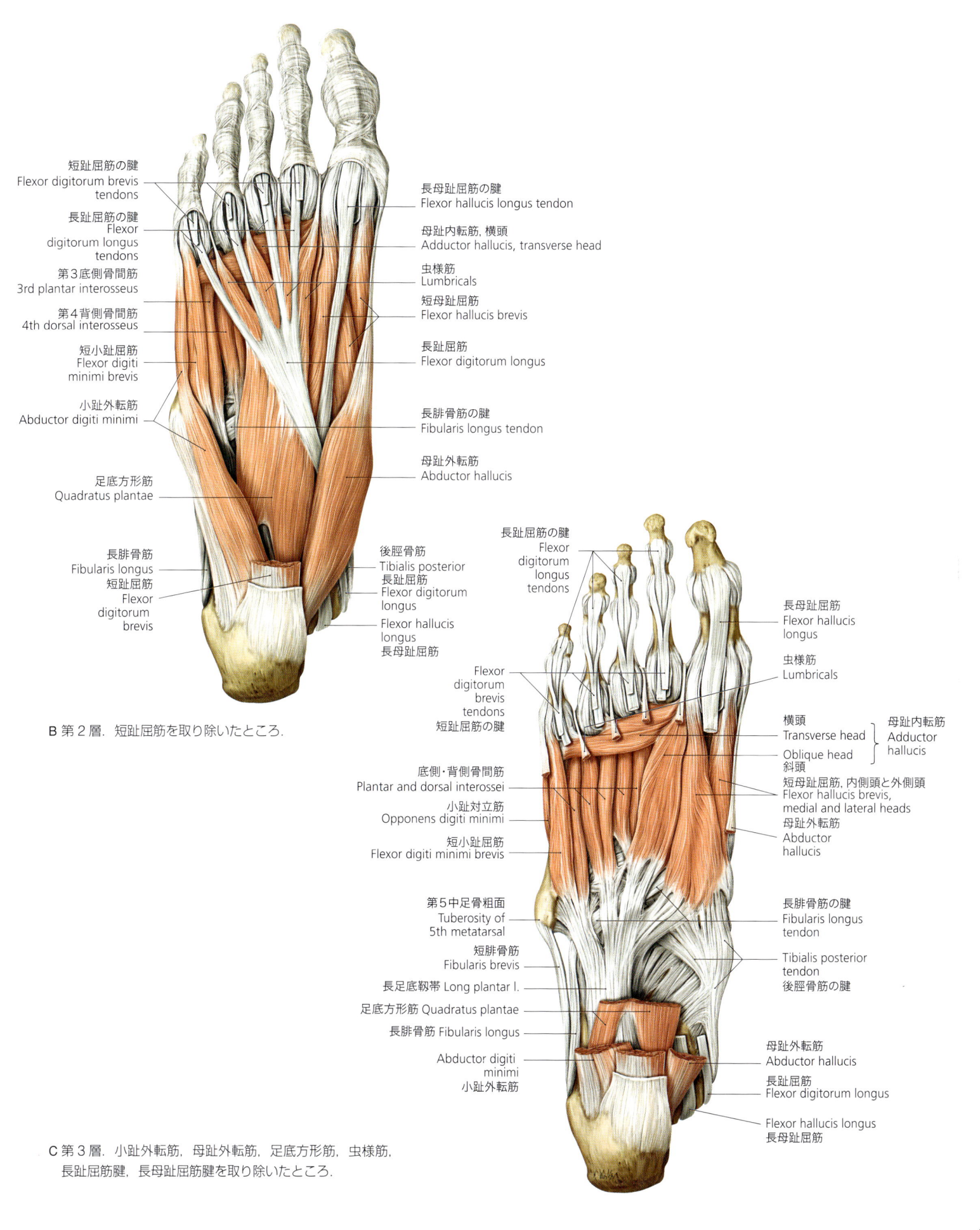

| 短趾屈筋の腱 Flexor digitorum brevis tendons
| 長趾屈筋の腱 Flexor digitorum longus tendons
| 第3底側骨間筋 3rd plantar interosseus
| 第4背側骨間筋 4th dorsal interosseus
| 短小趾屈筋 Flexor digiti minimi brevis
| 小趾外転筋 Abductor digiti minimi
| 足底方形筋 Quadratus plantae
| 長腓骨筋 Fibularis longus
| 短趾屈筋 Flexor digitorum brevis

長母趾屈筋の腱 Flexor hallucis longus tendon
母趾内転筋, 横頭 Adductor hallucis, transverse head
虫様筋 Lumbricals
短母趾屈筋 Flexor hallucis brevis
長趾屈筋 Flexor digitorum longus
長腓骨筋の腱 Fibularis longus tendon
母趾外転筋 Abductor hallucis
後脛骨筋 Tibialis posterior
長趾屈筋 Flexor digitorum longus
長母趾屈筋 Flexor hallucis longus

B 第2層. 短趾屈筋を取り除いたところ.

長趾屈筋の腱 Flexor digitorum longus tendons
短趾屈筋の腱 Flexor digitorum brevis tendons
底側・背側骨間筋 Plantar and dorsal interossei
小趾対立筋 Opponens digiti minimi
短小趾屈筋 Flexor digiti minimi brevis
第5中足骨粗面 Tuberosity of 5th metatarsal
短腓骨筋 Fibularis brevis
長足底靭帯 Long plantar l.
足底方形筋 Quadratus plantae
長腓骨筋 Fibularis longus
小趾外転筋 Abductor digiti minimi

長母趾屈筋 Flexor hallucis longus
虫様筋 Lumbricals
母趾内転筋 Adductor hallucis { 横頭 Transverse head / 斜頭 Oblique head }
短母趾屈筋, 内側頭と外側頭 Flexor hallucis brevis, medial and lateral heads
母趾外転筋 Abductor hallucis
長腓骨筋の腱 Fibularis longus tendon
後脛骨筋の腱 Tibialis posterior tendon
母趾外転筋 Abductor hallucis
長趾屈筋 Flexor digitorum longus
長母趾屈筋 Flexor hallucis longus

C 第3層. 小趾外転筋, 母趾外転筋, 足底方形筋, 虫様筋, 長趾屈筋腱, 長母趾屈筋腱を取り除いたところ.

足の筋と腱鞘
Muscles & Tendon Sheaths of the Foot

下肢

図26.17 足の内在筋(第4層)
右足，足底方向から見たところ．

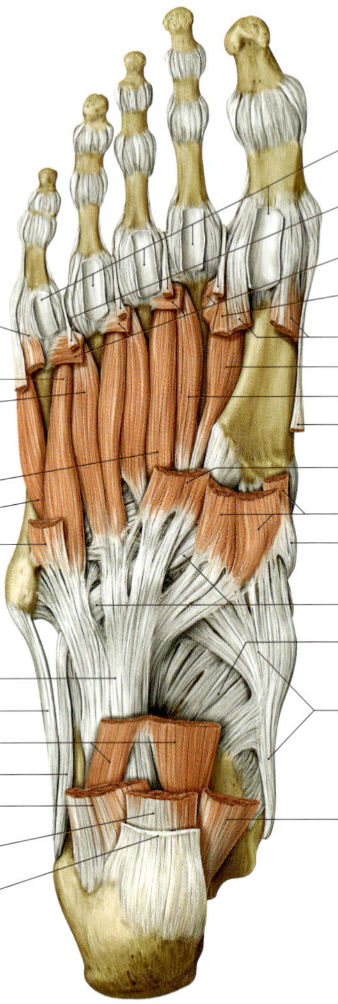

足底靱帯 Plantar ligaments
第1-4虫様筋 1st through 4th lumbricals
横頭 Transverse head ｝母趾内転筋 Adductor hallucis
斜頭 Oblique head
短小趾屈筋 Flexor digiti minimi brevis
第3底側骨間筋 3rd plantar interosseus
第4背側骨間筋 4th dorsal interosseus
第1底側骨間筋 1st plantar interosseus
小趾対立筋 Opponens digiti minimi
Flexor digiti minimi brevis 短小趾屈筋
長足底靱帯 Long plantar l.
短腓骨筋 Fibularis brevis
足底方形筋 Quadratus plantae
長腓骨筋 Fibularis longus
小趾外転筋 Abductor digiti minimi
短趾屈筋 Flexor digitorum brevis
Plantar aponeurosis 足底腱膜

Flexor hallucis brevis 短母趾屈筋
1st dorsal interosseus 第1背側骨間筋
2nd dorsal interosseus 第2背側骨間筋
Abductor hallucis 母趾外転筋
母趾内転筋, 斜頭 Adductor hallucis, oblique head
短母趾屈筋 Flexor hallucis brevis
Tibialis anterior tendon 前脛骨筋の腱
長腓骨筋の腱 Fibularis longus tendon
Plantar calcaneonavicular l. 底側踵舟靱帯
後脛骨筋の腱 Tibialis posterior tendon
母趾外転筋 Abductor hallucis

A 第4層(最深層)．母趾内転筋，短小趾屈筋，短母趾屈筋を取り除いたところ．

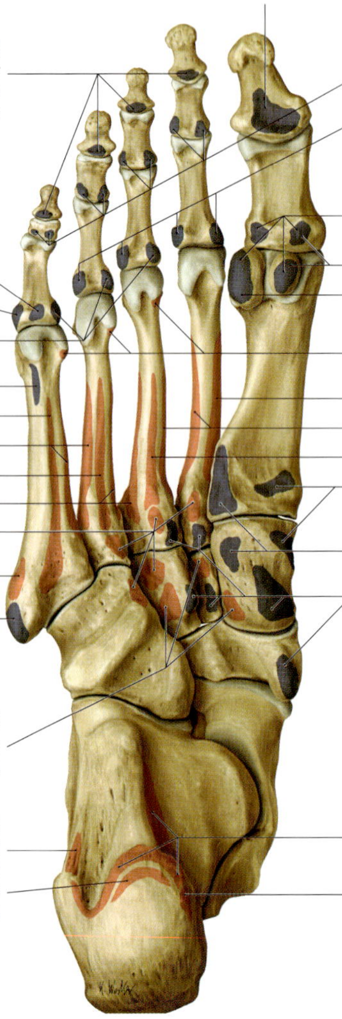

長趾屈筋 Flexor digitorum longus
短小趾屈筋 Flexor digiti minimi brevis
小趾外転筋 Abductor digiti minimi
第1-3底側骨間筋 1st through 3rd plantar interossei
小趾対立筋 Opponens digiti minimi
第3底側骨間筋 3rd plantar interosseus
第4背側骨間筋 4th dorsal interosseus
第2底側骨間筋 2nd plantar interosseus
第3背側骨間筋 3rd dorsal interosseus
母趾内転筋, 斜頭 Adductor hallucis, oblique head
短小趾屈筋 Flexor digiti minimi brevis
小趾外転筋と短腓骨筋 Abductor digiti minimi and fibularis brevis
短母趾屈筋 Flexor hallucis brevis
小趾外転筋 Abductor digiti minimi
短趾屈筋 Flexor digitorum brevis

長母趾屈筋 Flexor hallucis longus
短趾屈筋 Flexor digitorum brevis
第1-4背側骨間筋 1st through 4th dorsal interossei
短母趾屈筋 Flexor hallucis brevis
母趾外転筋 Abductor hallucis
Adductor hallucis 母趾内転筋 母趾内転筋, 横頭 Adductor hallucis, transverse head
1st dorsal interosseus ①
2nd dorsal interosseus ②
1st plantar interosseus ③
Tibialis anterior 前脛骨筋
長腓骨筋 Fibularis longus
後脛骨筋 Tibialis posterior
①第1背側骨間筋
②第2背側骨間筋
③第1底側骨間筋
足底方形筋 Quadratus plantae
母趾外転筋 Abductor hallucis

B 足における筋の起始(赤)と停止(青)．

図 26.18 足首の腱鞘と支帯

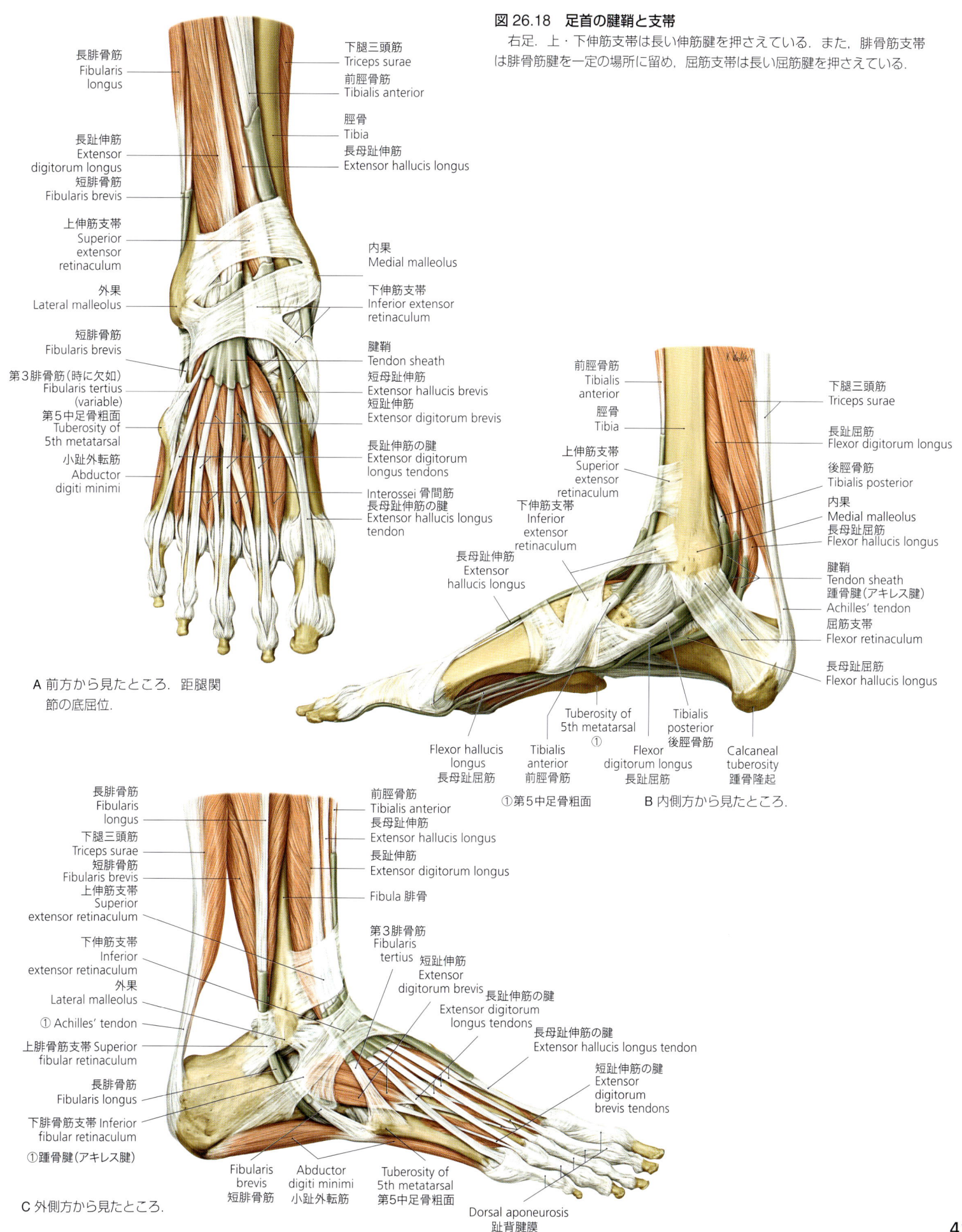

右足．上・下伸筋支帯は長い伸筋腱を押さえている．また，腓骨筋支帯は腓骨筋腱を一定の場所に留め，屈筋支帯は長い屈筋腱を押さえている．

A 前方から見たところ．距腿関節の底屈位．

B 内側方から見たところ．
① 第5中足骨粗面

C 外側方から見たところ．
① 踵骨腱（アキレス腱）

個々の筋(1)
Muscle Facts (I)

足背にある筋は2種類のみ(短趾屈筋,短母趾屈筋)である.しかし,足底にある筋は4つの複雑な層からなり,足底弓を支えている.

図 26.19　足背の内在筋
右足,足背方向から見たところ.

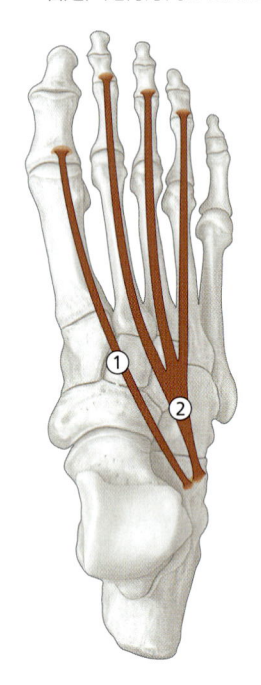

A 模式図.

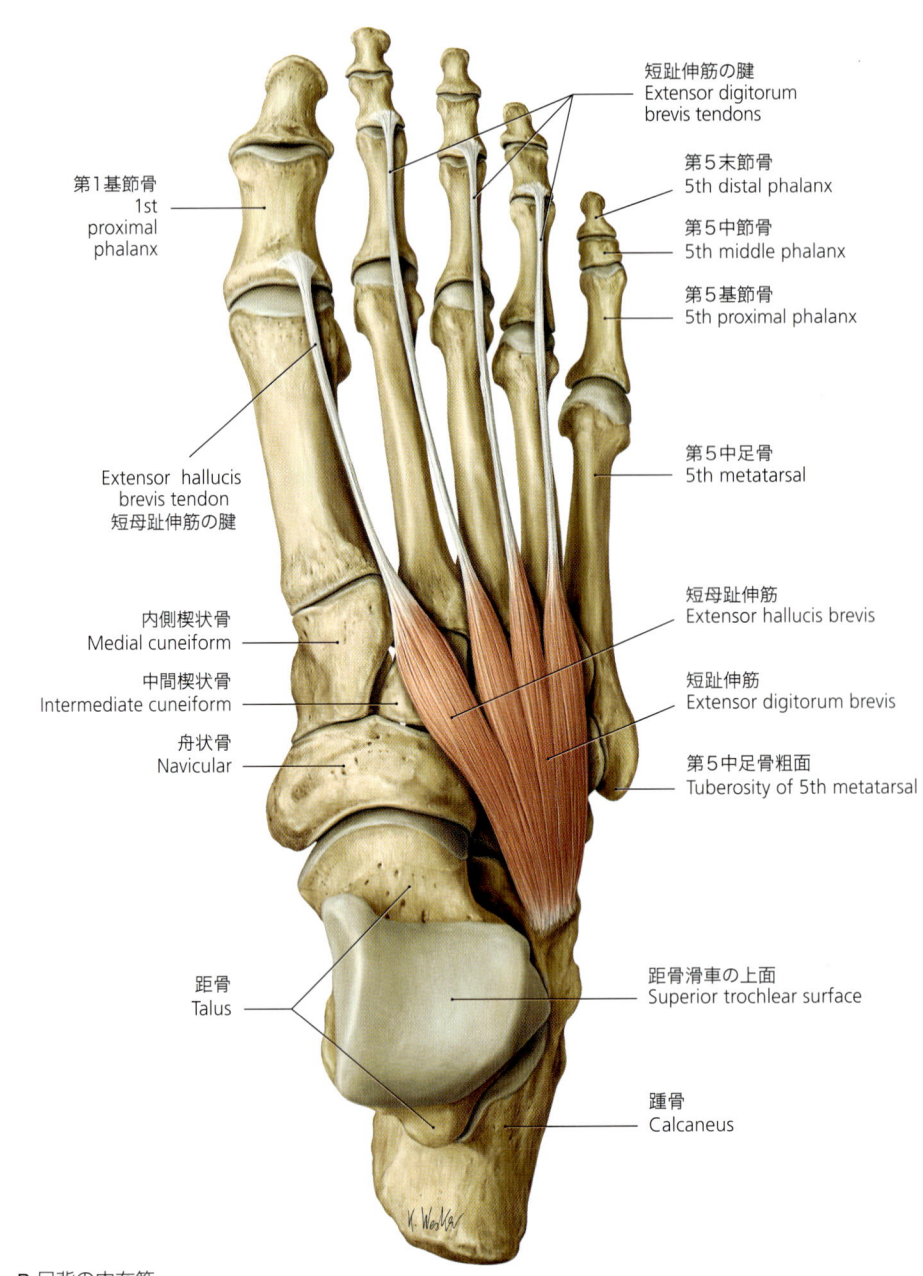

- 短趾伸筋の腱 / Extensor digitorum brevis tendons
- 第1基節骨 / 1st proximal phalanx
- 第5末節骨 / 5th distal phalanx
- 第5中節骨 / 5th middle phalanx
- 第5基節骨 / 5th proximal phalanx
- 第5中足骨 / 5th metatarsal
- Extensor hallucis brevis tendon / 短母趾伸筋の腱
- 内側楔状骨 / Medial cuneiform
- 中間楔状骨 / Intermediate cuneiform
- 舟状骨 / Navicular
- 短母趾伸筋 / Extensor hallucis brevis
- 短趾伸筋 / Extensor digitorum brevis
- 第5中足骨粗面 / Tuberosity of 5th metatarsal
- 距骨滑車の上面 / Superior trochlear surface
- 距骨 / Talus
- 踵骨 / Calcaneus

B 足背の内在筋.

表 26.2　足背の内在筋

筋	起始	停止	神経支配	作用
①短母趾伸筋	踵骨(足背面)	第1趾(趾背腱膜と基節骨底)	深腓骨神経(L5, S1)	第1趾のMTP関節を伸展する
②短趾伸筋		第2-4趾(趾背腱膜,中節骨底)		第2-4趾のMTP関節とPIP関節を伸展する

MTP関節=中足趾節関節,PIP関節=近位趾節間関節.

図 26.20　足底の内在筋（表層：第1層）
右足．足底方向から見たところ．

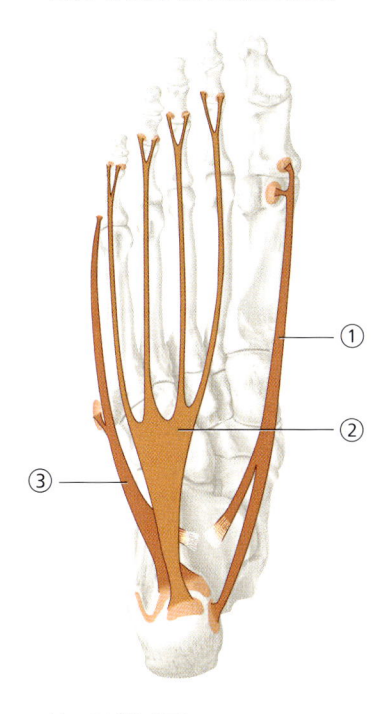

A 第1層（模式図）．

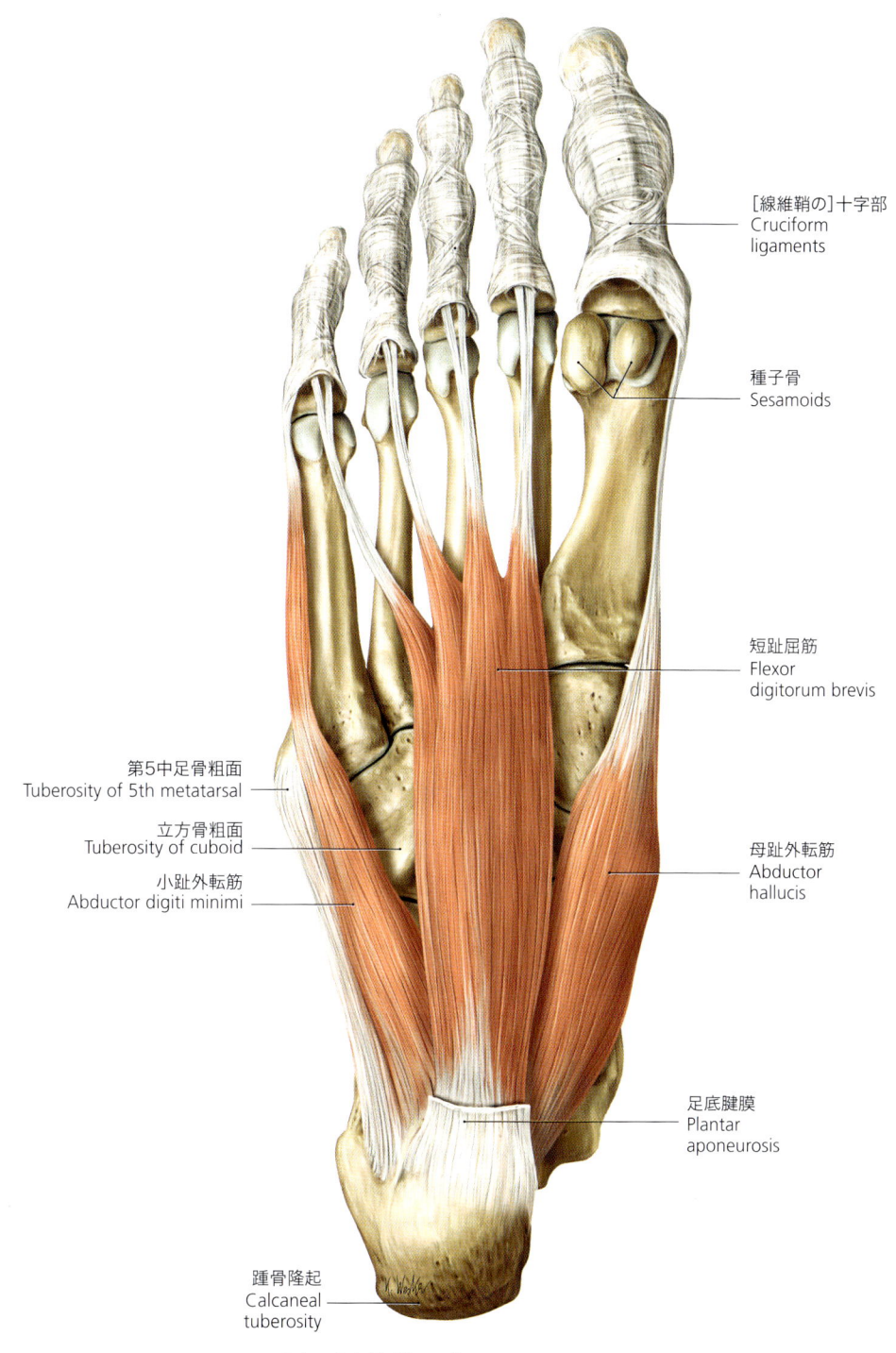

[線維鞘の]十字部
Cruciform ligaments

種子骨
Sesamoids

短趾屈筋
Flexor digitorum brevis

第5中足骨粗面
Tuberosity of 5th metatarsal

立方骨粗面
Tuberosity of cuboid

小趾外転筋
Abductor digiti minimi

母趾外転筋
Abductor hallucis

足底腱膜
Plantar aponeurosis

踵骨隆起
Calcaneal tuberosity

B 足底の内在筋（第1層）．

表 26.3　足底の内在筋（深層：第1層）

筋	起始	停止	神経支配	作用
①母趾外転筋	踵骨隆起（内側突起）	第1趾（内側種子骨を介して基節骨底に停止）	内側足底神経 (S1, S2)	・第1趾のMTP関節：第1趾の屈曲と外転 ・縦足弓の保持
②短趾屈筋	踵骨隆起（内側結節），足底腱膜	第2-5趾（中節骨の側面）		・第2-5趾のMTP関節とPIP関節：屈曲 ・縦足弓の保持
③小趾外転筋		第5趾（基節骨底），第5中足骨（粗面）	外側足底神経（S1-S3）	・第5趾のMTP関節：屈曲 ・第5趾の外転 ・縦足弓の保持

MTP関節＝中足趾節関節，PIP関節＝近位趾節間関節．

個々の筋（2）
Muscle Facts (II)

図 26.21　足底の内在筋（深層：第2-4層）
右足，足底方向から見たところ．

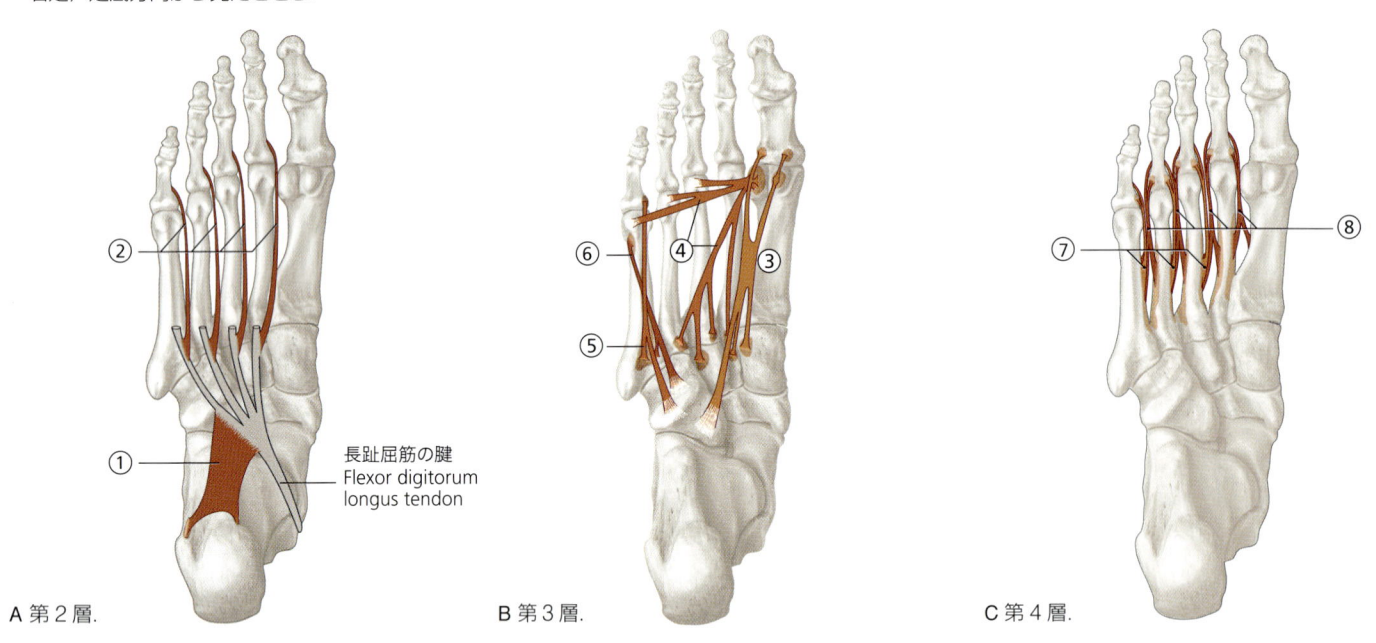

A 第2層．
B 第3層．
C 第4層．

長趾屈筋の腱
Flexor digitorum longus tendon

表 26.4　足底の内在筋（深層：第2-4層）

筋	起始	停止	神経支配	作用
①足底方形筋	踵骨隆起の足底面（内側縁と底側縁）	長趾屈筋腱（外側縁）	外側足底神経（S1-S3）	・長趾屈筋腱の方向を変える，またこの筋の作用を補助する
②虫様筋（4つの筋）	長趾屈筋腱（内側縁）	第2-5趾（趾背腱膜）	第1虫様筋：内側足底神経（S2, S3） 第2-4虫様筋：外側足底神経（S2, S3）	・第2-5趾のMTP関節：屈曲 ・第2-5趾のIP関節：伸展 ・第2-5趾を第1趾に近づける
③短母趾屈筋	立方骨，外側楔状骨，底側踵立方靱帯	第1基節骨底（内側・外側種子骨を介して停止する）	内側頭：内側足底神経（S1, S2） 外側頭：外側足底神経（S1, S2）	・第1趾のMTP関節：屈曲 ・縦足弓の保持
④母趾内転筋	斜頭：第2-4中足骨底 横頭：第3-5趾のMTP関節，深横中足靱帯	第1基節骨底（共通腱が外側種子骨を介して停止する）	外側足底神経，深枝（S2, S3）	・第1趾のMTP関節：屈曲 ・第1趾の内転 ・横頭：横足弓の保持 ・斜頭：縦足弓の保持
⑤短小趾屈筋	第5中足骨底，長足底靱帯	第5基節骨底	外側足底神経，浅枝（S2, S3）	・第5趾のMTP関節：屈曲
⑥小趾対立筋*	長足底靱帯，長腓骨筋腱の足底腱鞘	第5中足骨		・第5趾を下内方に引く
⑦底側骨間筋（3つの筋）	第3-5中足骨（内側縁）	第3-5基節骨底の内側面	外側足底神経（S2, S3）	・第3-5趾のMTP関節：屈曲 ・第3-5趾のIP関節：伸展 ・第3-5趾を第2趾に近づける（内転）
⑧背側骨間筋（4つの筋）	第1-5中足骨（2頭が隣接する中足骨の側面から起始する）	第1背側骨間筋：第2基節骨底の内側面 第2-4背側骨間筋：第2-4基節骨底の外側面，第2-4趾の趾背腱膜		・第2-4趾のMTP関節：屈曲 ・第2-4趾のIP関節：伸展 ・第3・4趾を第2趾から離す（外転）

IP関節＝趾節間関節，MTP関節＝中足趾節関節．*欠損する場合もある．

図 26.22 足底の内在筋（深層：第2-4層）
右足．足底方向から見たところ．

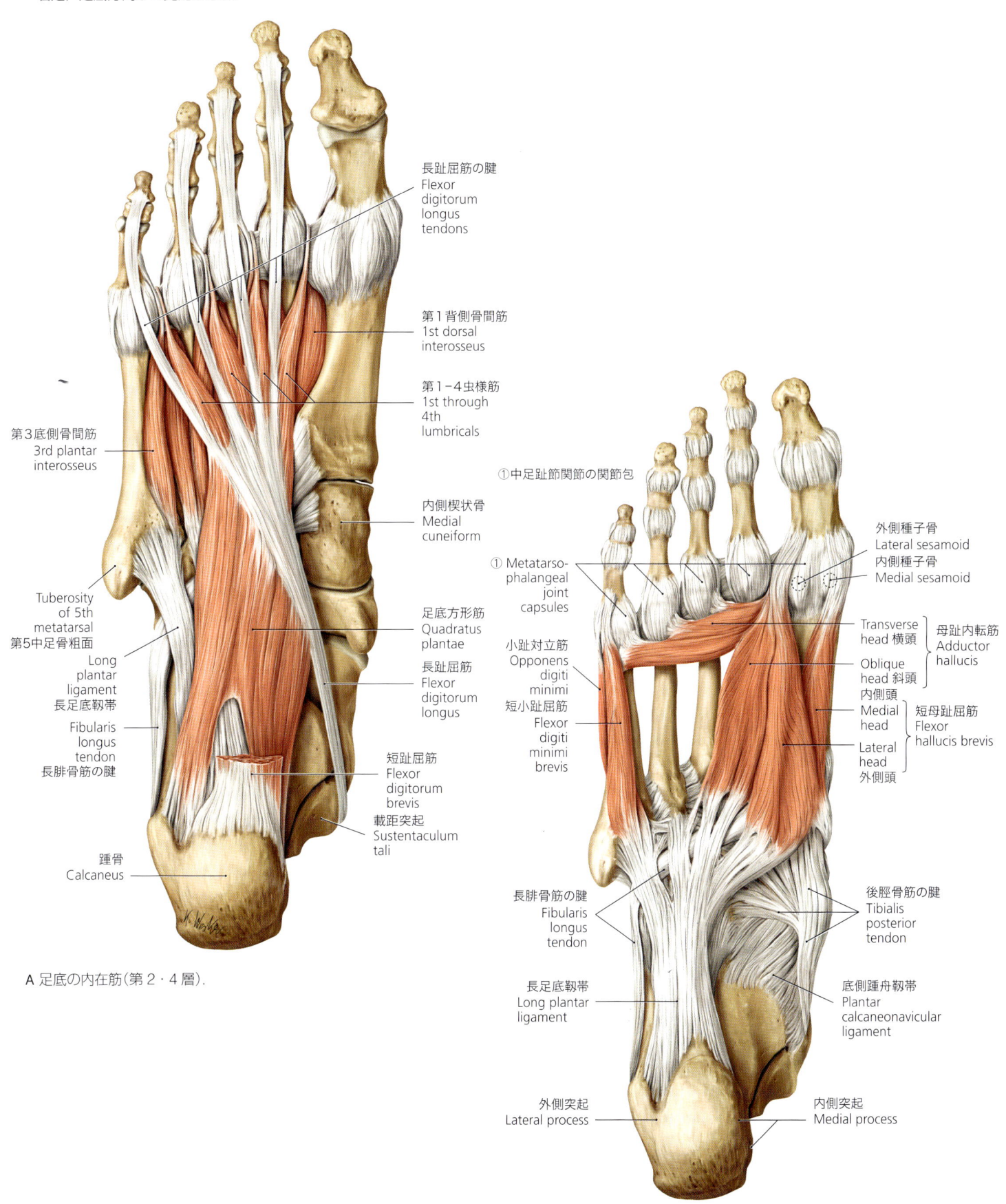

- 長趾屈筋の腱 Flexor digitorum longus tendons
- 第1背側骨間筋 1st dorsal interosseus
- 第1-4虫様筋 1st through 4th lumbricals
- 内側楔状骨 Medial cuneiform
- 足底方形筋 Quadratus plantae
- 長趾屈筋 Flexor digitorum longus
- 短趾屈筋 Flexor digitorum brevis
- 載距突起 Sustentaculum tali
- 第3底側骨間筋 3rd plantar interosseus
- 第5中足骨粗面 Tuberosity of 5th metatarsal
- 長足底靱帯 Long plantar ligament
- 長腓骨筋の腱 Fibularis longus tendon
- 踵骨 Calcaneus

A 足底の内在筋（第2・4層）．

- ①中足趾節関節の関節包 Metatarsophalangeal joint capsules
- 外側種子骨 Lateral sesamoid
- 内側種子骨 Medial sesamoid
- 母趾内転筋 Adductor hallucis ｛横頭 Transverse head／斜頭 Oblique head｝
- 短母趾屈筋 Flexor hallucis brevis ｛内側頭 Medial head／外側頭 Lateral head｝
- 小趾対立筋 Opponens digiti minimi
- 短小趾屈筋 Flexor digiti minimi brevis
- 長腓骨筋の腱 Fibularis longus tendon
- 後脛骨筋の腱 Tibialis posterior tendon
- 長足底靱帯 Long plantar ligament
- 底側踵舟靱帯 Plantar calcaneonavicular ligament
- 外側突起 Lateral process
- 内側突起 Medial process

B 足底の内在筋（第3層）．

下肢の動脈
Arteries of the Lower Limb

図 27.1　下肢の動脈
右下肢.

- 総腸骨動脈 Common iliac a.
- 外腸骨動脈 External iliac a.
- 大腿深動脈 Profunda femoris a.
- 内転筋管 Adductor canal
- 腹大動脈 Abdominal aorta
- 内腸骨動脈 Internal iliac a.
- 鼠径靭帯 Inguinal ligament
- 大腿動脈 Femoral a.
- [内転筋] 腱裂孔 Adductor hiatus
- 膝窩動脈 Popliteal a.
- 前脛骨動脈 Anterior tibial a.
- 下腿骨間膜 Interosseous membrane
- 後脛骨動脈 Posterior tibial a.
- 腓骨動脈 Fibular a.
- 足背動脈 Dorsal pedal a.
- 内側足底動脈 Medial plantar a.

A 前方から見たところ.

B 後方から見たところ.

図 27.2　足底の動脈
右足, 足底方向から見たところ.

- 固有底側趾動脈 Proper plantar digital aa.
- 総底側趾動脈 Common plantar digital aa.
- 底側中足動脈 Plantar metatarsal aa.
- 深足底動脈弓 Deep plantar arch
- 浅枝 Superficial branch
- 深枝 Deep branch
- 内側足底動脈 Medial plantar a.
- 外側足底動脈 Lateral plantar a.
- 母趾外転筋 Abductor hallucis
- 内側足底動脈 Medial plantar a.
- 後脛骨動脈 Posterior tibial a.

- 腹大動脈 Abdominal aorta
- 総腸骨動脈 Common iliac a.
- 内腸骨動脈 Internal iliac a.
- 深腸骨回旋動脈 Deep circumflex iliac a.
- 浅腹壁動脈 Superficial epigastric a.
- 浅腸骨回旋動脈 Superficial circumflex iliac a.
- 梨状筋 Piriformis
- 外側大腿回旋動脈 Lateral circumflex femoral a.
- 大腿深動脈 Profunda femoris a.
- 第1-3貫通動脈 1st through 3rd perforating aa.
- Superior and inferior gluteal aa. 上・下殿動脈
- 外腸骨動脈 External iliac a.
- 下腹壁動脈 Inferior epigastric a.
- 外陰部動脈 External pudendal aa.
- 内側大腿回旋動脈 Medial circumflex femoral a.
- 大腿動脈 Femoral a.
- 内転筋管と大内転筋 Adductor canal (with adductor magnus)
- [内転筋] 腱裂孔 Adductor hiatus
- 膝窩動脈 Popliteal a.
- 下行膝動脈 Descending genicular a.
- 外側上・下膝動脈 Lateral superior and inferior genicular aa.
- 前脛骨反回動脈 Anterior tibial recurrent a.
- 内側上・下膝動脈 Medial superior and inferior genicular aa.
- 下腿骨間膜 Interosseous membrane
- 前脛骨動脈 Anterior tibial a.
- 前外果動脈 Anterior lateral malleolar a.
- 外側足根動脈 Lateral tarsal a.
- 弓状動脈 Arcuate a.
- 前内果動脈 Anterior medial malleolar a.
- 足背動脈 Dorsal pedal a.
- 背側中足動脈 Dorsal metatarsal aa.

C 動脈の走行, 前方から見たところ.

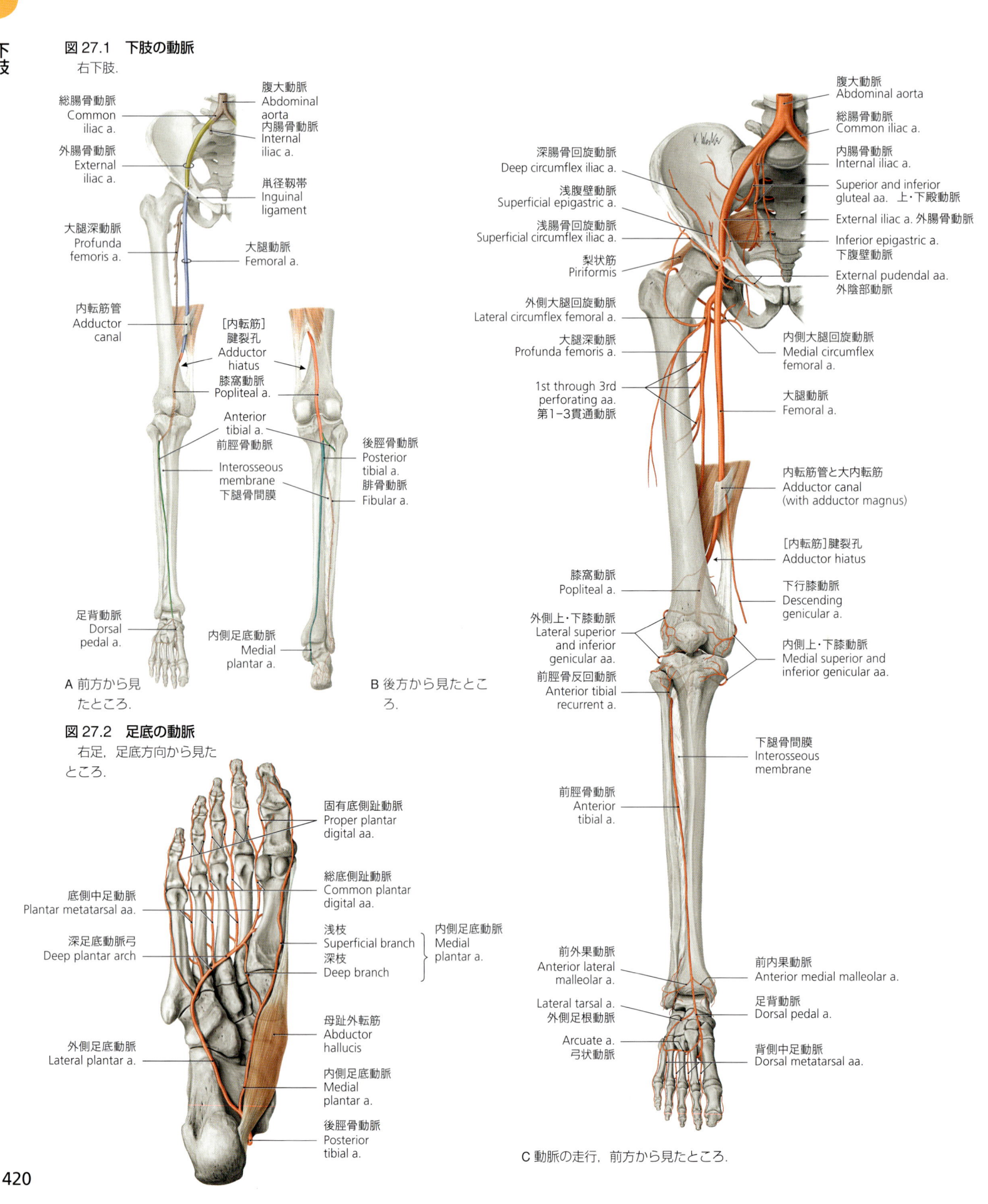

臨床

大腿骨頭壊死

大腿骨頭の骨折（骨粗鬆症患者でよくみられる）や脱臼によって，大腿骨頸の動脈や大腿骨頭窩動脈が損傷されると大腿骨頭は壊死する．

図 27.3 大腿骨頭の動脈
右股関節，前方から見たところ．

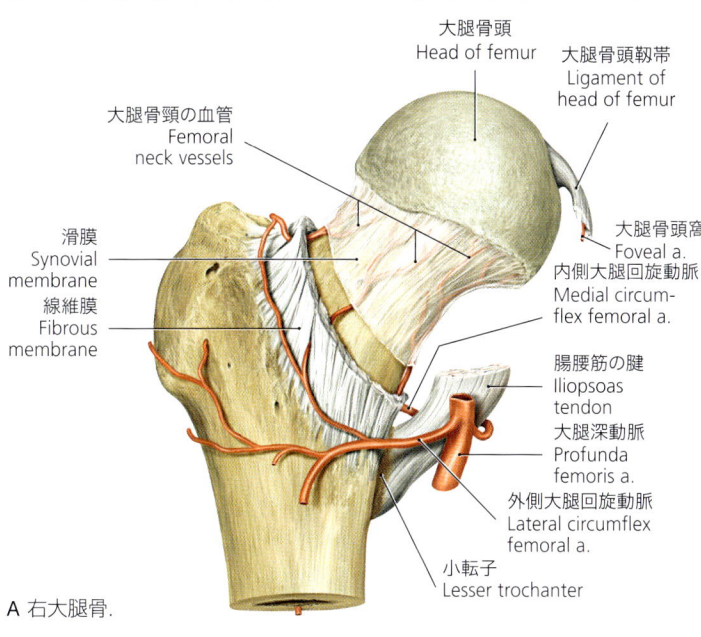

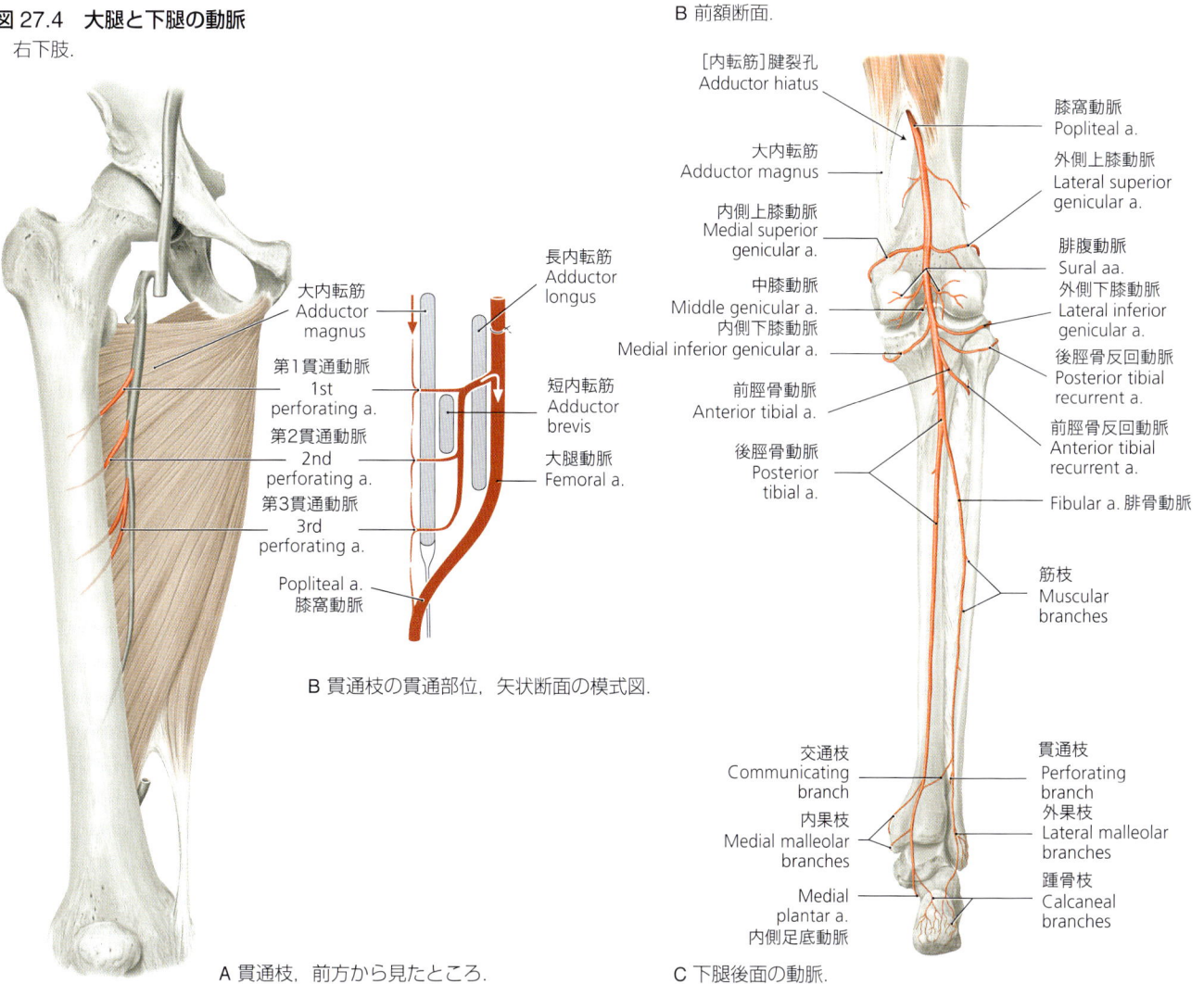

A 右大腿骨．

- 大腿骨頭 Head of femur
- 大腿骨頭靱帯 Ligament of head of femur
- 大腿骨頭の血管 Femoral neck vessels
- 滑膜 Synovial membrane
- 線維膜 Fibrous membrane
- 大腿骨頭窩動脈 Foveal a.
- 内側大腿回旋動脈 Medial circumflex femoral a.
- 腸腰筋の腱 Iliopsoas tendon
- 大腿深動脈 Profunda femoris a.
- 外側大腿回旋動脈 Lateral circumflex femoral a.
- 小転子 Lesser trochanter

B 前額断面．

- 寛骨臼蓋 Acetabular roof
- 寛骨臼の関節唇 Acetabular labrum
- 線維膜 Fibrous membrane
- 滑膜 Synovial membrane
- 寛骨臼窩 Acetabular fossa
- 大腿骨頭靱帯 Ligament of head of femur
- 閉鎖動脈 Obturator a.
- 輪帯 Zona orbicularis
- 内側大腿回旋動脈 Medial circumflex femoral a.

図 27.4 大腿と下腿の動脈
右下肢．

A 貫通枝，前方から見たところ．

- 大内転筋 Adductor magnus
- 第1貫通動脈 1st perforating a.
- 第2貫通動脈 2nd perforating a.
- 第3貫通動脈 3rd perforating a.
- 膝窩動脈 Popliteal a.

B 貫通枝の貫通部位，矢状断面の模式図．

- 長内転筋 Adductor longus
- 短内転筋 Adductor brevis
- 大腿動脈 Femoral a.

C 下腿後面の動脈．

- ［内転筋］腱裂孔 Adductor hiatus
- 大内転筋 Adductor magnus
- 内側上膝動脈 Medial superior genicular a.
- 中膝動脈 Middle genicular a.
- 内側下膝動脈 Medial inferior genicular a.
- 前脛骨動脈 Anterior tibial a.
- 後脛骨動脈 Posterior tibial a.
- 膝窩動脈 Popliteal a.
- 外側上膝動脈 Lateral superior genicular a.
- 腓腹動脈 Sural aa.
- 外側下膝動脈 Lateral inferior genicular a.
- 後脛骨反回動脈 Posterior tibial recurrent a.
- 前脛骨反回動脈 Anterior tibial recurrent a.
- 腓骨動脈 Fibular a.
- 筋枝 Muscular branches
- 交通枝 Communicating branch
- 内果枝 Medial malleolar branches
- 内側足底動脈 Medial plantar a.
- 貫通枝 Perforating branch
- 外果枝 Lateral malleolar branches
- 踵骨枝 Calcaneal branches

下肢の静脈とリンパ管
Veins & Lymphatics of the Lower Limb

図 27.5 下肢の静脈
右下肢，前方から見たところ．

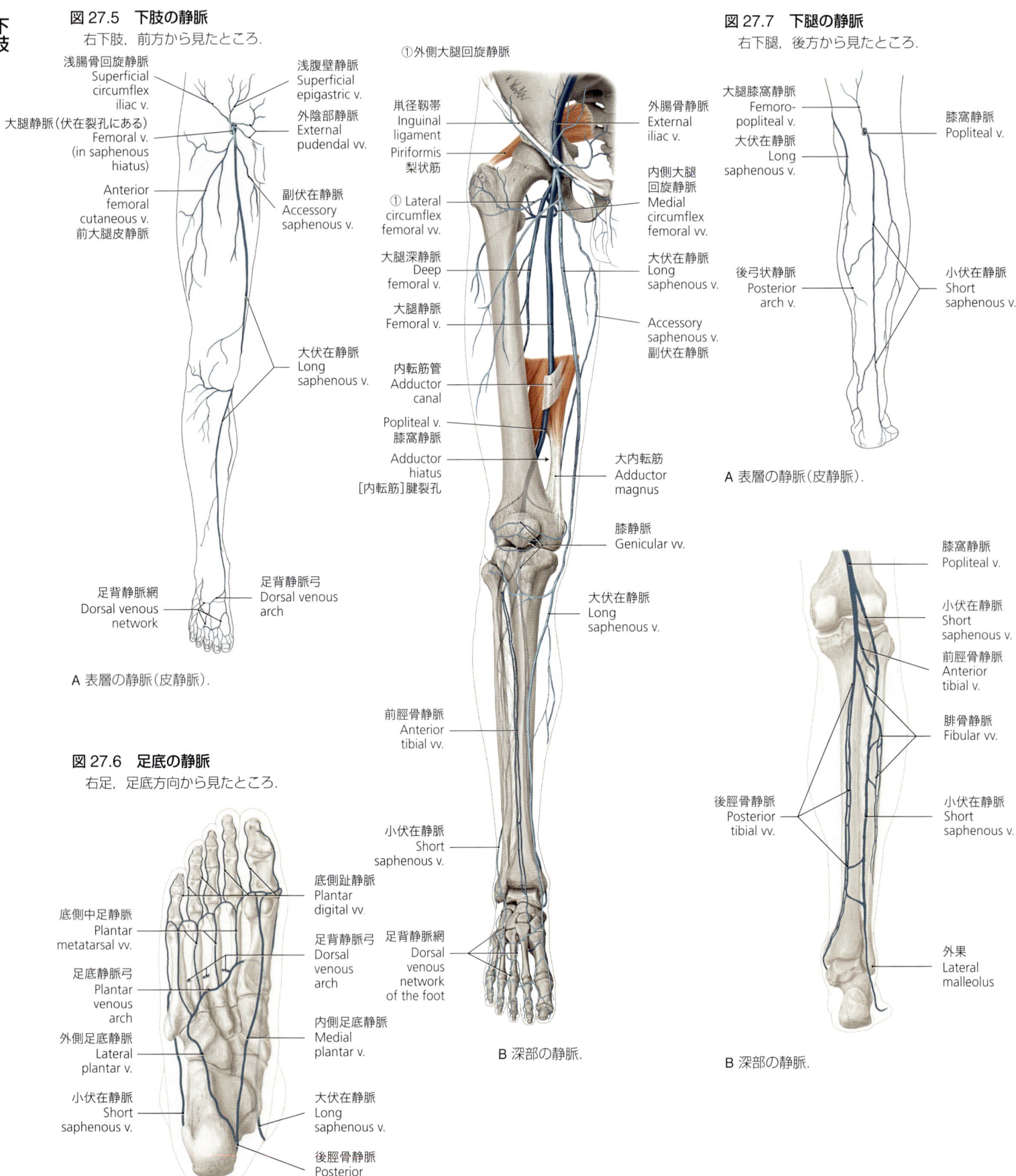

- 浅腸骨回旋静脈 Superficial circumflex iliac v.
- 大腿静脈（伏在裂孔にある）Femoral v. (in saphenous hiatus)
- 前大腿皮静脈 Anterior femoral cutaneous v.
- 浅腹壁静脈 Superficial epigastric v.
- 外陰部静脈 External pudendal vv.
- 副伏在静脈 Accessory saphenous v.
- 大伏在静脈 Long saphenous v.
- 足背静脈網 Dorsal venous network
- 足背静脈弓 Dorsal venous arch

A 表層の静脈（皮静脈）．

図 27.6 足底の静脈
右足，足底方向から見たところ．

- 底側中足静脈 Plantar metatarsal vv.
- 足底静脈弓 Plantar venous arch
- 外側足底静脈 Lateral plantar v.
- 小伏在静脈 Short saphenous v.
- 底側趾静脈 Plantar digital vv.
- 足背静脈弓 Dorsal venous arch
- 内側足底静脈 Medial plantar v.
- 大伏在静脈 Long saphenous v.
- 後脛骨静脈 Posterior tibial vv.

- ①外側大腿回旋静脈
- 鼠径靱帯 Inguinal ligament
- 梨状筋 Piriformis
- ① Lateral circumflex femoral vv.
- 大腿深静脈 Deep femoral v.
- 大腿静脈 Femoral v.
- 内転筋管 Adductor canal
- 膝窩静脈 Popliteal v.
- 内転筋腱裂孔 Adductor hiatus
- 前脛骨静脈 Anterior tibial vv.
- 小伏在静脈 Short saphenous v.
- 足背静脈網 Dorsal venous network of the foot
- 外腸骨静脈 External iliac v.
- 内側大腿回旋静脈 Medial circumflex femoral vv.
- 大伏在静脈 Long saphenous v.
- 副伏在静脈 Accessory saphenous v.
- 大内転筋 Adductor magnus
- 膝静脈 Genicular vv.
- 大伏在静脈 Long saphenous v.

B 深部の静脈．

図 27.7 下腿の静脈
右下腿，後方から見たところ．

- 大腿膝窩静脈 Femoro-popliteal v.
- 大伏在静脈 Long saphenous v.
- 後弓状静脈 Posterior arch v.
- 膝窩静脈 Popliteal v.
- 小伏在静脈 Short saphenous v.

A 表層の静脈（皮静脈）．

- 膝窩静脈 Popliteal v.
- 小伏在静脈 Short saphenous v.
- 前脛骨静脈 Anterior tibial v.
- 腓骨静脈 Fibular vv.
- 後脛骨静脈 Posterior tibial vv.
- 小伏在静脈 Short saphenous v.
- 外果 Lateral malleolus

B 深部の静脈．

図 27.8　臨床的に重要な穿通静脈
右下肢，内側方から見たところ．

- 外腸骨静脈 External iliac v.
- 大伏在静脈 Long saphenous v.
- ドッドの静脈群 Dodd's vv.
- 大腿静脈 Femoral v.
- 大腿静脈 Femoral v.
- 大伏在静脈 Long saphenous v.
- ボイドの静脈群 Boyd's vv.
- 後脛骨静脈 Posterior tibial vv.
- 後弓状静脈 Posterior arch v.
- コケットの静脈群 Cockett's vv.

図 27.9　表層のリンパ管
右下肢．矢印はリンパの主な流れを示している．

- 浅鼠径リンパ節 Superficial inguinal l.n.
- 前内側束 Anteromedial bundle
- 大伏在静脈 Long saphenous v.

A 前方から見たところ．

- 肛門 Anus
- 陰嚢 Scrotum
- 浅膝窩リンパ節 Superficial popliteal l.n.
- 小伏在静脈 Short saphenous v.
- 後外側束 Posterolateral bundle

B 後方から見たところ．

図 27.10　リンパ節とリンパ流路
右下肢，前方から見たところ．

- 総腸骨リンパ節
- 腰リンパ節
  - 下大静脈 Inferior vena cava
  - 総腸骨静脈 Common iliac v.
- 外腸骨リンパ節
  - 外腸骨静脈 External iliac v.
  - ・リンパ流入
    - －深鼠径リンパ節から
    - －膀胱，陰茎と亀頭，子宮から
- 内腸骨リンパ節
  - ・リンパ流入
    - －骨盤臓器
    - －骨盤壁
    - －殿筋
    - －勃起器官
    - －深部会陰領域
  - Internal ① iliac v.
  - ①内腸骨静脈
- 上外側浅鼠径リンパ節 Superolateral l.n.
- 上内側浅鼠径リンパ節 Superomedial l.n.
- 下浅鼠径リンパ節 Inferior l.n.
- 深鼠径リンパ節
  - ・リンパ流入
    - －下肢の深部領域
- 浅鼠径リンパ節
  - ・リンパ流入
    - －下肢の皮膚
      （ふくらはぎと足の外側縁を除く）
    - －臍下部の腹壁
    - －腰部
    - －殿部，腸管，肛門領域
    - －外陰部
      （女性では，子宮円索に沿った子宮底部）
- Inguinal ligament 鼠径靱帯
- Long saphenous v. 大伏在静脈
- 大腿静脈 Femoral v.
- 深膝窩リンパ節
  - ・リンパ流入
    - －下腿
    - －足
- 膝窩静脈 Popliteal v.
- 小伏在静脈 Short saphenous v.
- 浅膝窩リンパ節
  - ・リンパ流入
    - －足の外側縁
    - －ふくらはぎ

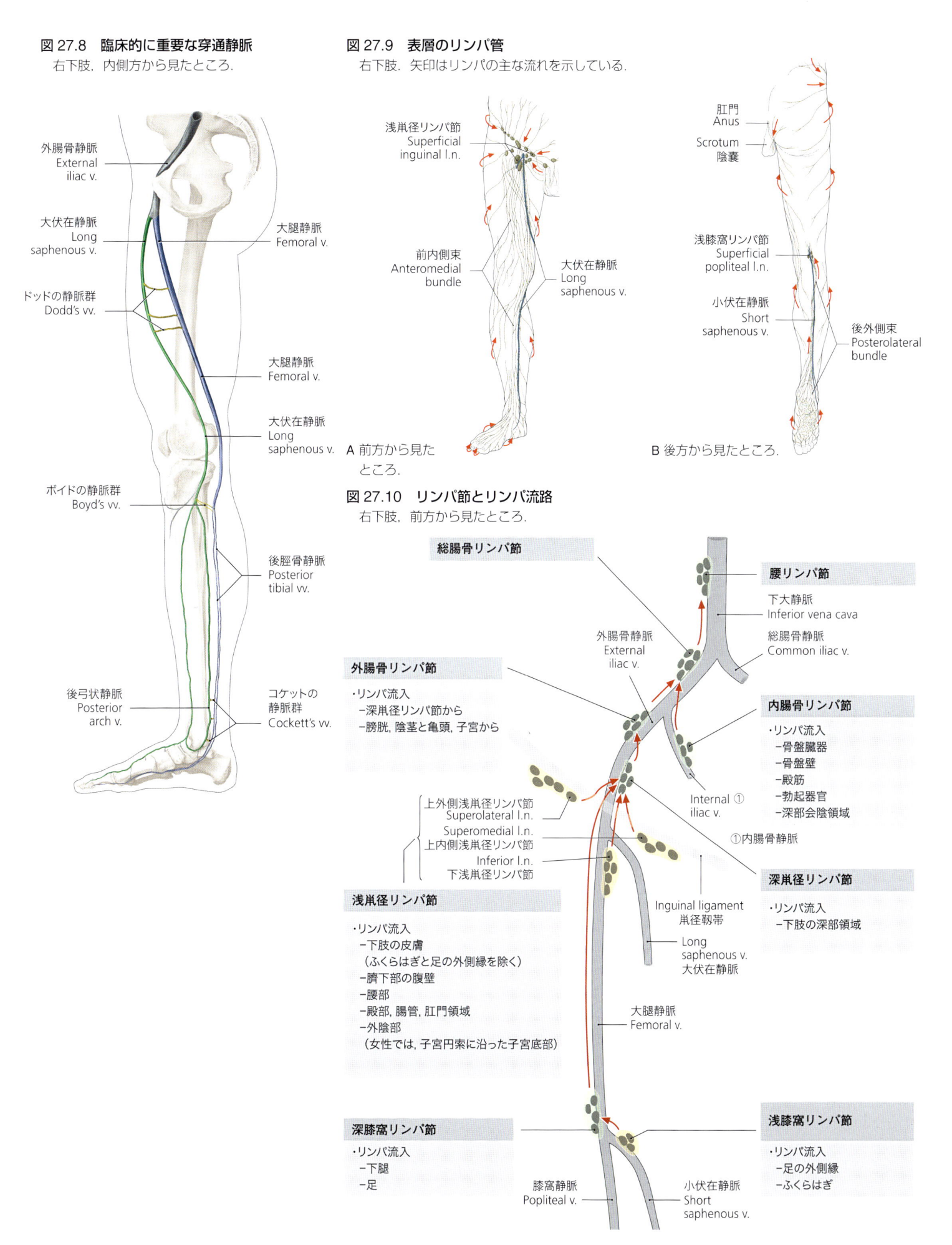

腰仙骨神経叢
Lumbosacral Plexus

腰仙骨神経叢から出る神経は，下肢の知覚と運動に関与する．この神経叢は，腰神経と仙骨神経の前枝によって形成されるが，肋下神経（T12）や尾骨神経（Co1）からの枝も参加する．

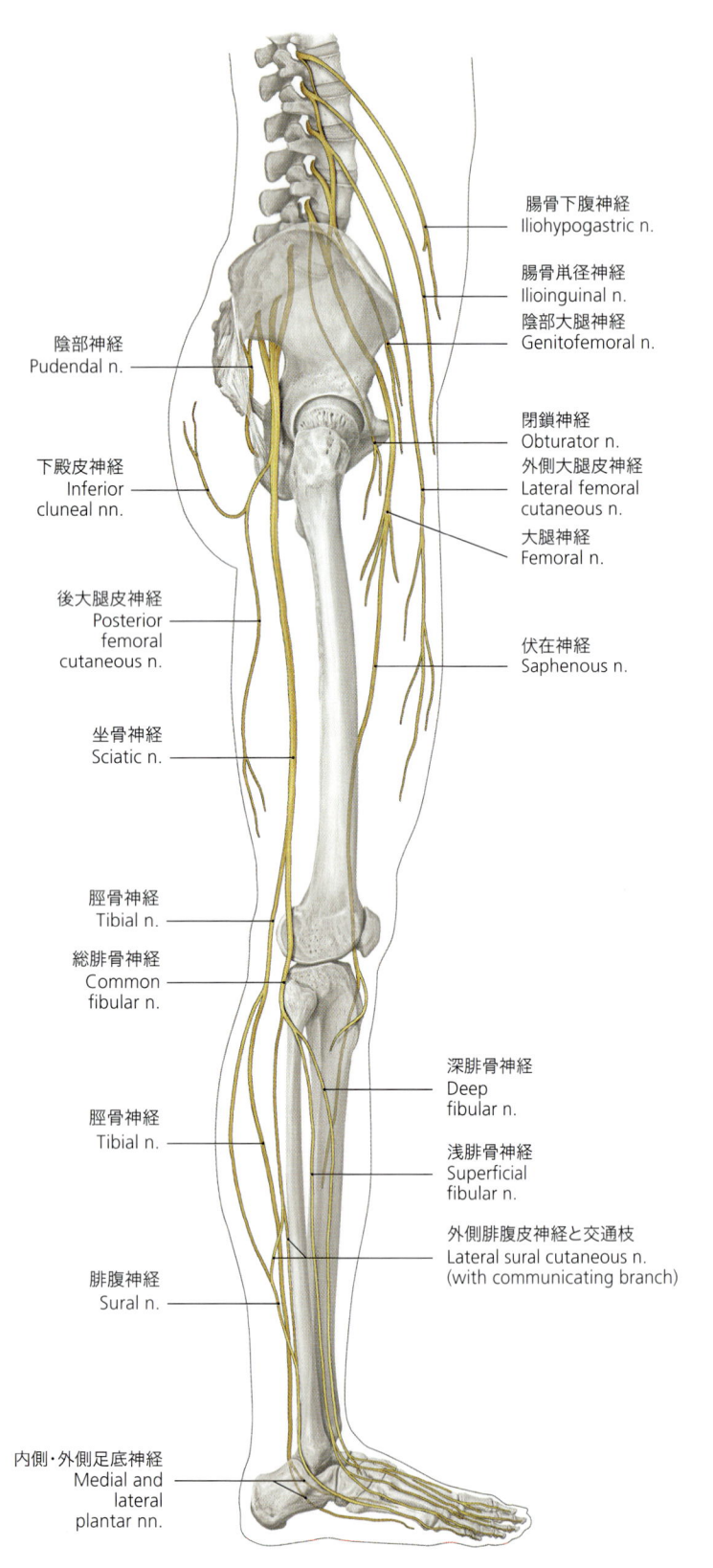

図の主要ラベル：
- 腸骨下腹神経 Iliohypogastric n.
- 腸骨鼠径神経 Ilioinguinal n.
- 陰部大腿神経 Genitofemoral n.
- 陰部神経 Pudendal n.
- 閉鎖神経 Obturator n.
- 下殿皮神経 Inferior cluneal nn.
- 外側大腿皮神経 Lateral femoral cutaneous n.
- 大腿神経 Femoral n.
- 後大腿皮神経 Posterior femoral cutaneous n.
- 伏在神経 Saphenous n.
- 坐骨神経 Sciatic n.
- 脛骨神経 Tibial n.
- 総腓骨神経 Common fibular n.
- 深腓骨神経 Deep fibular n.
- 浅腓骨神経 Superficial fibular n.
- 外側腓腹皮神経と交通枝 Lateral sural cutaneous n. (with communicating branch)
- 腓腹神経 Sural n.
- 内側・外側足底神経 Medial and lateral plantar nn.

表 27.1　腰仙骨神経叢から出る神経

腰神経叢			
腸骨下腹神経		T12–L1	p. 427
腸骨鼠径神経		L1	p. 427
陰部大腿神経		L1–L2	p. 427
外側大腿皮神経		L2–L3	p. 427
閉鎖神経		L2–L4	p. 428
大腿神経		L2–L4	p. 429
仙骨神経叢			
上殿神経		L4–S1	p. 431
下殿神経		L5–S1	p. 431
後大腿皮神経		S1–S3	p. 430
坐骨神経	総腓骨神経	L4–S2	p. 432
坐骨神経	脛骨神経	L4–S3	p. 433
陰部神経		S2–S4	pp. 194, 202

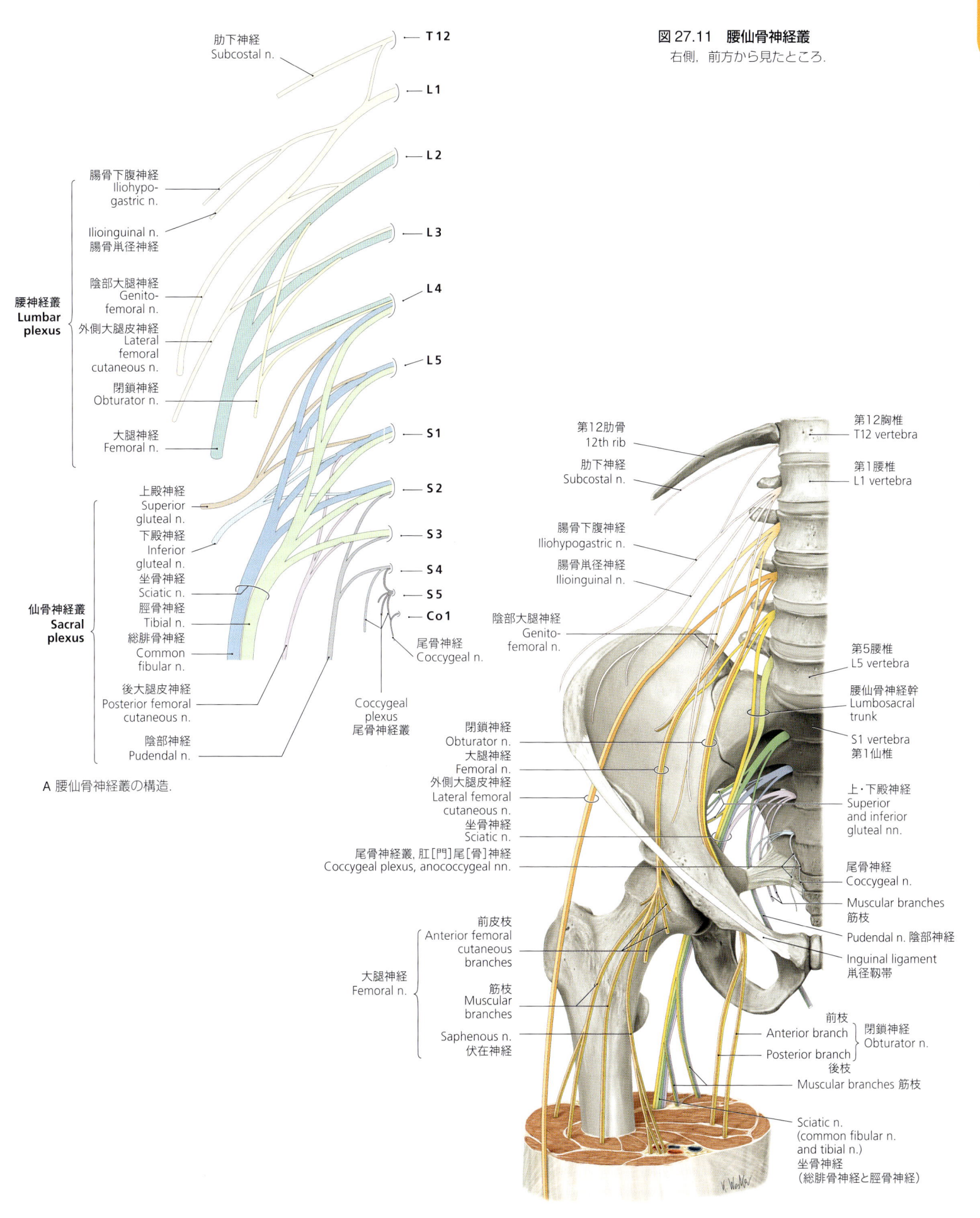

図 27.11 腰仙骨神経叢
右側．前方から見たところ．

腰神経叢
Lumbar plexus
- 腸骨下腹神経 Iliohypogastric n.
- Ilioinguinal n. 腸骨鼡径神経
- 陰部大腿神経 Genitofemoral n.
- 外側大腿皮神経 Lateral femoral cutaneous n.
- 閉鎖神経 Obturator n.
- 大腿神経 Femoral n.

仙骨神経叢
Sacral plexus
- 上殿神経 Superior gluteal n.
- 下殿神経 Inferior gluteal n.
- 坐骨神経 Sciatic n.
- 脛骨神経 Tibial n.
- 総腓骨神経 Common fibular n.
- 後大腿皮神経 Posterior femoral cutaneous n.
- 陰部神経 Pudendal n.

肋下神経 Subcostal n. — T12
L1
L2
L3
L4
L5
S1
S2
S3
S4
S5
Co1
尾骨神経 Coccygeal n.
Coccygeal plexus 尾骨神経叢

A 腰仙骨神経叢の構造．

第12肋骨 12th rib
肋下神経 Subcostal n.
腸骨下腹神経 Iliohypogastric n.
腸骨鼡径神経 Ilioinguinal n.
陰部大腿神経 Genitofemoral n.
閉鎖神経 Obturator n.
大腿神経 Femoral n.
外側大腿皮神経 Lateral femoral cutaneous n.
坐骨神経 Sciatic n.
尾骨神経叢，肛[門]尾[骨]神経 Coccygeal plexus, anococcygeal nn.
前皮枝 Anterior femoral cutaneous branches
大腿神経 Femoral n.
筋枝 Muscular branches
Saphenous n. 伏在神経

第12胸椎 T12 vertebra
第1腰椎 L1 vertebra
第5腰椎 L5 vertebra
腰仙骨神経幹 Lumbosacral trunk
S1 vertebra 第1仙椎
上・下殿神経 Superior and inferior gluteal nn.
尾骨神経 Coccygeal n.
Muscular branches 筋枝
Pudendal n. 陰部神経
Inguinal ligament 鼡径靱帯
前枝 Anterior branch / 閉鎖神経 Obturator n.
Posterior branch 後枝
Muscular branches 筋枝
Sciatic n. (common fibular n. and tibial n.)
坐骨神経（総腓骨神経と脛骨神経）

B 腰仙骨神経叢の走行．

腰神経叢の枝
Nerves of the Lumbar Plexus

表27.2 腰神経から出る神経

神経	脊髄分節	支配筋	皮枝
腸骨下腹神経	T12-L1	腹横筋, 内腹斜筋（下部）	前皮枝, 外側皮枝
腸骨鼡径神経	L1		男性：前陰嚢神経 女性：前陰唇神経
陰部大腿神経	L1-L2	男性：精巣挙筋（陰部枝）	陰部枝, 大腿枝
外側大腿皮神経	L2-L3	—	外側大腿皮神経
閉鎖神経	L2-L4	p. 428 参照	
大腿神経		p. 429 参照	
短い筋枝, 神経叢から直接出る	T12-L4	大腰筋 腰方形筋 腸骨筋 腰横突間筋	—

図 27.12 鼡径部における皮神経の分布
男性の右鼡径部，前方から見たところ．

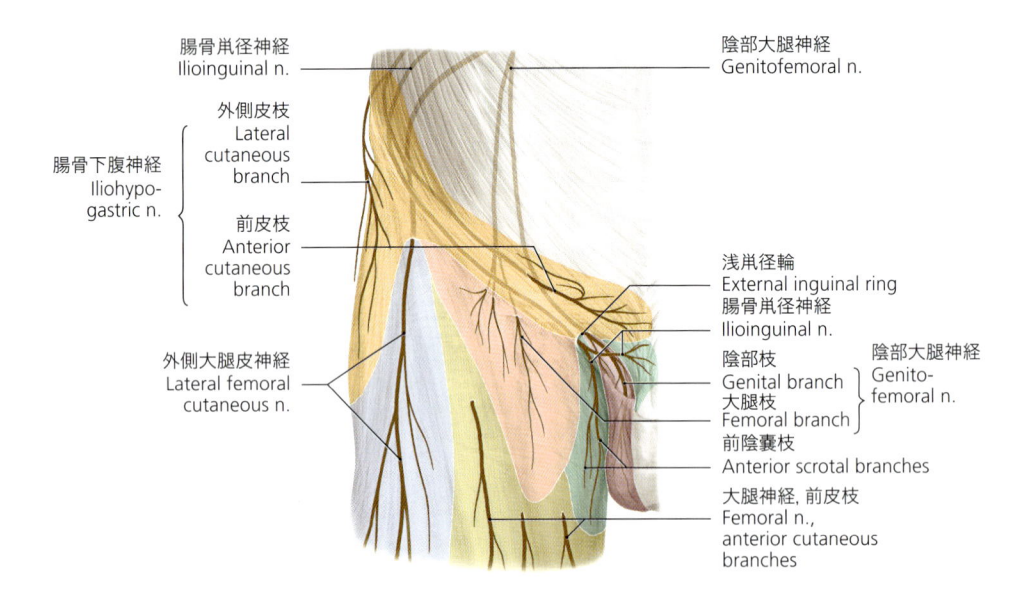

図 27.13 腰神経叢から出る神経
右側，前方から見たところ．前腹壁を取り除いてある．

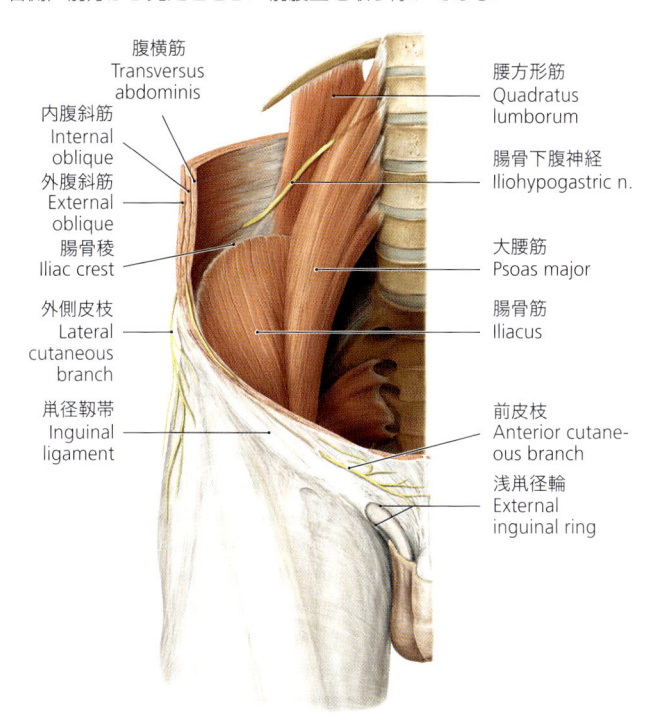

A 腸骨下腹神経.

B 腸骨鼡径神経.

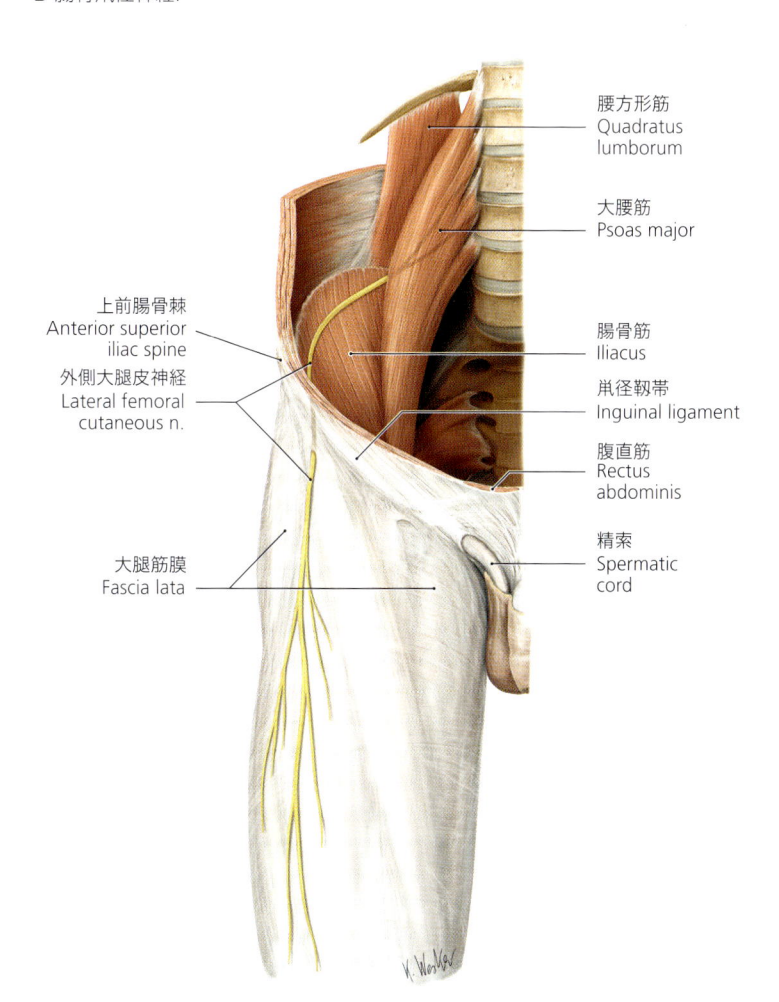

C 陰部大腿神経.

D 外側大腿皮神経.

腰神経叢の枝：閉鎖神経と大腿神経
Nerves of the Lumbar Plexus: Obturator & Femoral Nerves

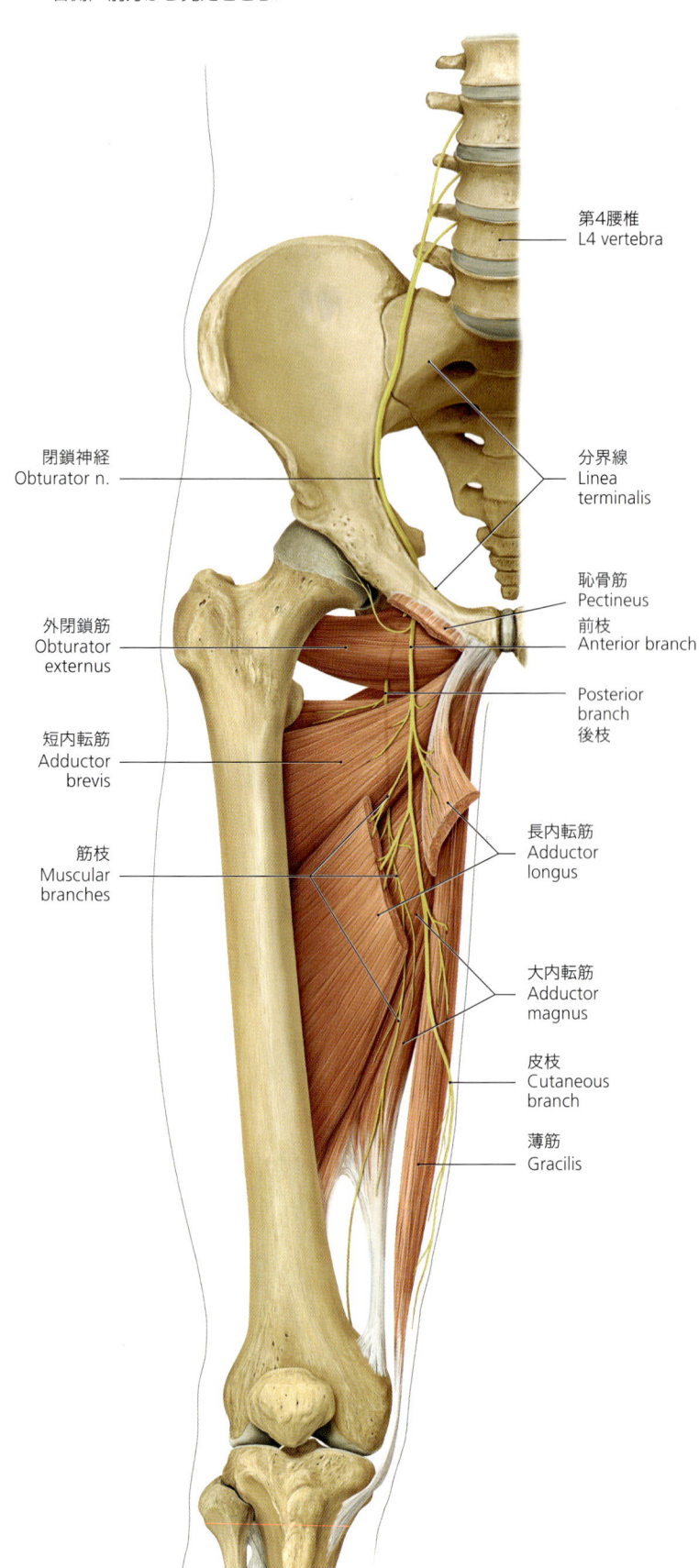

図 27.14　閉鎖神経：皮枝の分布
右下肢．内側方から見たところ．

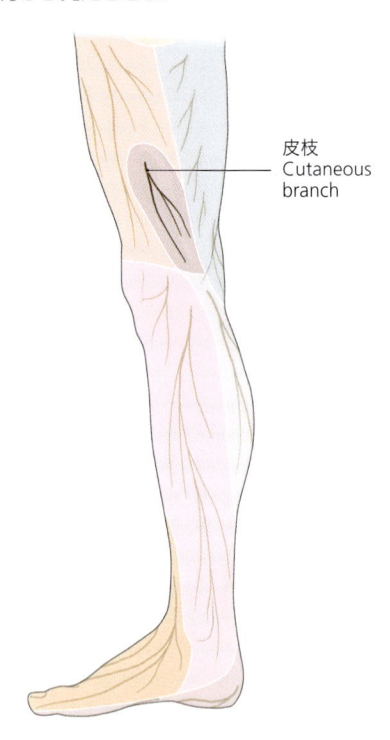

皮枝
Cutaneous branch

図 27.15　閉鎖神経
右側，前方から見たところ．

- 第4腰椎 L4 vertebra
- 分界線 Linea terminalis
- 閉鎖神経 Obturator n.
- 恥骨筋 Pectineus
- 外閉鎖筋 Obturator externus
- 前枝 Anterior branch
- 短内転筋 Adductor brevis
- Posterior branch 後枝
- 長内転筋 Adductor longus
- 筋枝 Muscular branches
- 大内転筋 Adductor magnus
- 皮枝 Cutaneous branch
- 薄筋 Gracilis

表 27.3　閉鎖神経(L2-L4)

運動枝		支配筋
直接枝		外閉鎖筋
前枝		長内転筋
		短内転筋
		薄筋
		恥骨筋
後枝		大内転筋
感覚枝		
		皮枝

図 27.16 大腿神経
右側，前方から見たところ．

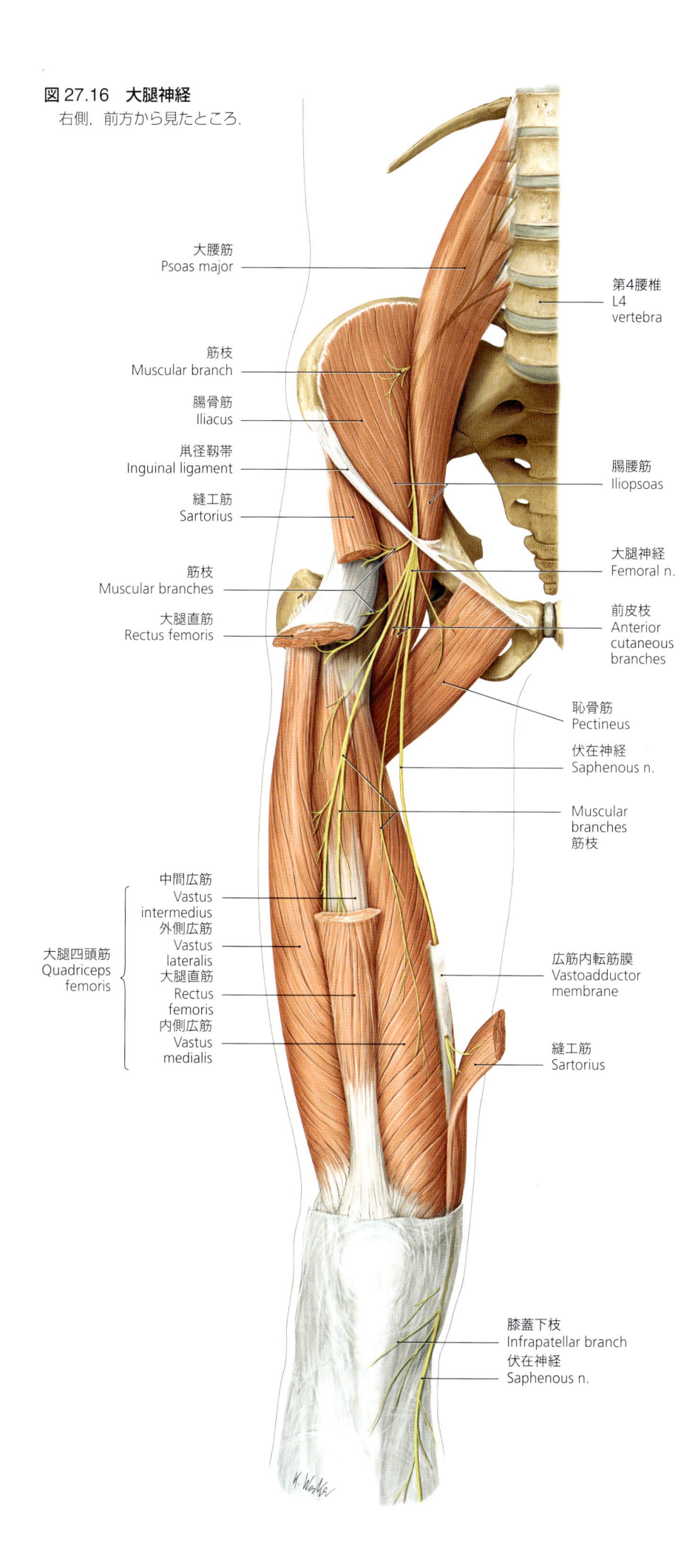

- 大腰筋 Psoas major
- 筋枝 Muscular branch
- 腸骨筋 Iliacus
- 鼠径靱帯 Inguinal ligament
- 縫工筋 Sartorius
- 筋枝 Muscular branches
- 大腿直筋 Rectus femoris
- 第4腰椎 L4 vertebra
- 腸腰筋 Iliopsoas
- 大腿神経 Femoral n.
- 前皮枝 Anterior cutaneous branches
- 恥骨筋 Pectineus
- 伏在神経 Saphenous n.
- Muscular branches 筋枝
- 大腿四頭筋 Quadriceps femoris
  - 中間広筋 Vastus intermedius
  - 外側広筋 Vastus lateralis
  - 大腿直筋 Rectus femoris
  - 内側広筋 Vastus medialis
- 広筋内転筋膜 Vastoadductor membrane
- 縫工筋 Sartorius
- 膝蓋下枝 Infrapatellar branch
- 伏在神経 Saphenous n.

図 27.17 大腿神経：皮枝の分布
右下肢，前方から見たところ．

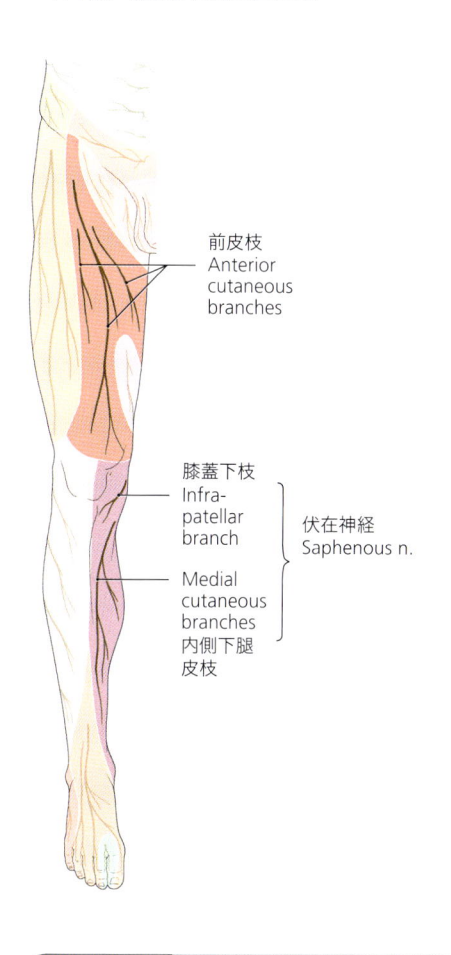

- 前皮枝 Anterior cutaneous branches
- 膝蓋下枝 Infra-patellar branch
- Medial cutaneous branches 内側下腿皮枝
- 伏在神経 Saphenous n.

表 27.4 大腿神経（L2-L4）

運動枝	支配筋
筋枝	腸腰筋
	恥骨筋
	縫工筋
	大腿四頭筋
感覚枝	
前皮枝	
伏在神経	

仙骨神経叢の枝
Nerves of the Sacral Plexus

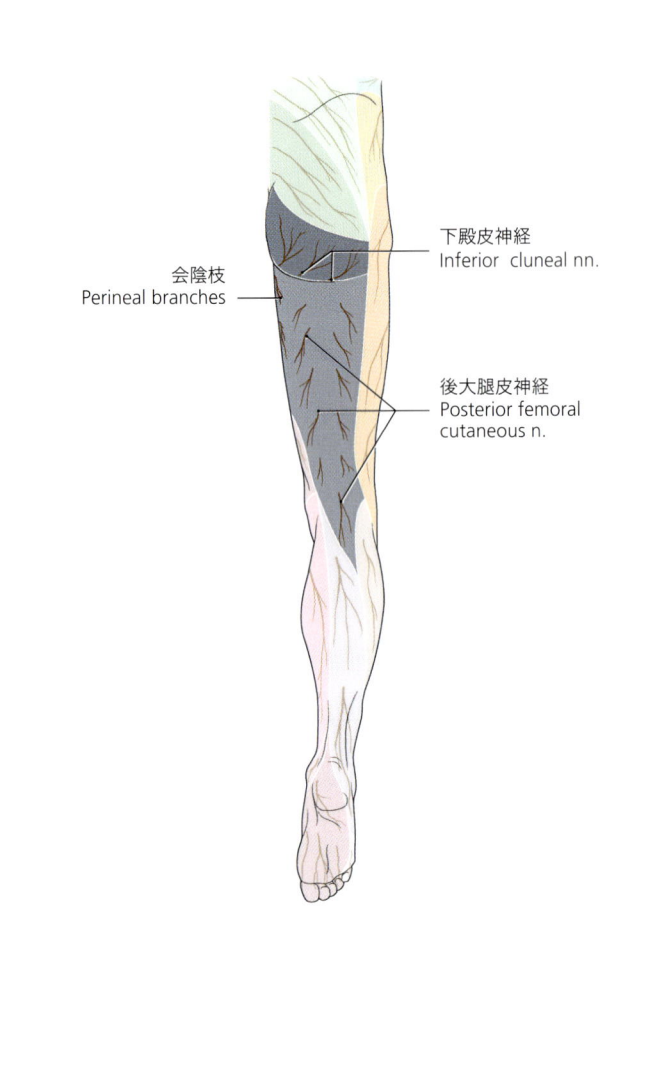

表 27.5　仙骨神経叢から出る神経

神経		脊髄分節	支配筋	皮枝	
上殿神経		L4-S1	中殿筋，小殿筋，大腿筋膜張筋	―	
下殿神経		L5-S2	大殿筋	―	
後大腿皮神経		S1-S3	―	後大腿皮神経	下殿皮神経
					会陰枝
直接枝	梨状筋枝	S1-S2	梨状筋	―	
	内閉鎖筋枝	L5-S1	内閉鎖筋	―	
	大腿方形筋枝		大腿方形筋	―	
坐骨神経	総腓骨神経	L4-S2	p. 432 参照	―	
	脛骨神経	L4-S3	p. 433 参照	―	
陰部神経		S2-S4	骨盤底筋群	下直腸神経，会陰神経	
尾骨神経		S5-Co1	尾骨筋	肛門尾骨神経	

図 27.18　殿部に分布する皮神経
右側，後方から見たところ．

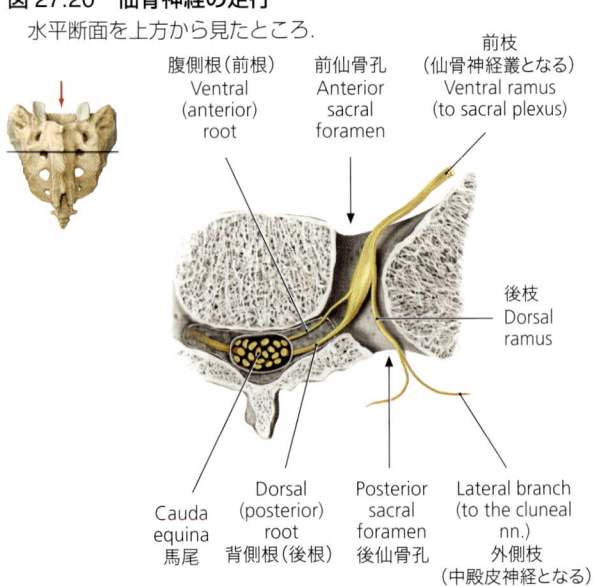

図 27.19　後大腿皮神経の分布
右下肢，後方から見たところ．

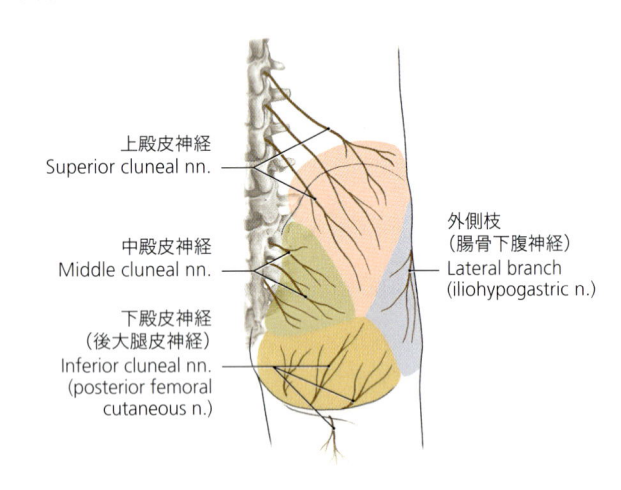

図 27.20　仙骨神経の走行
水平断面を上方から見たところ．

図 27.21 仙骨神経叢から出る神経
右下肢.

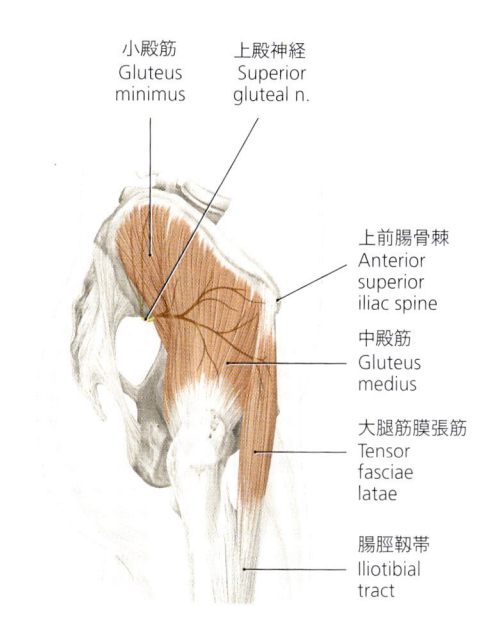

A 上殿神経, 外側方から見たところ.

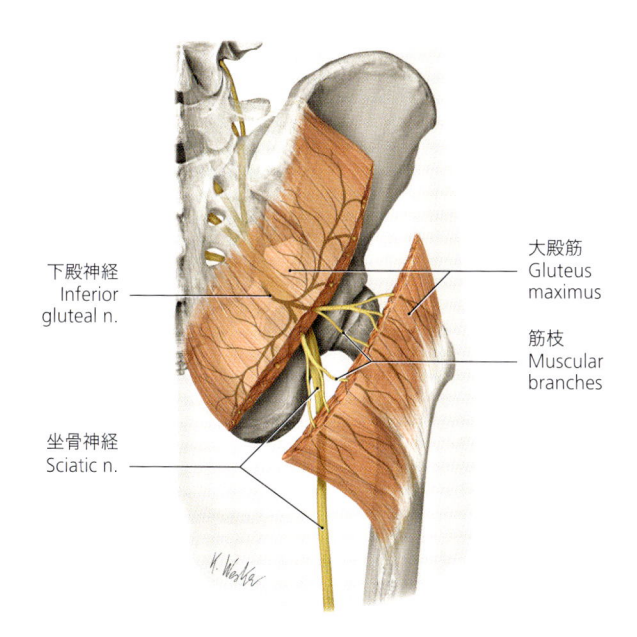

B 下殿神経, 後方から見たところ.

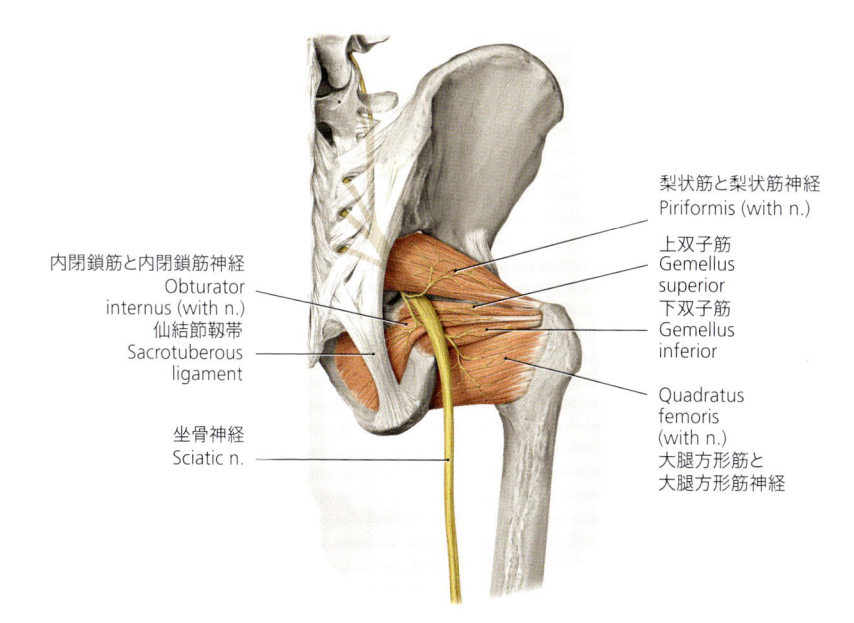

C 仙骨神経叢から直接出る筋枝, 後方から見たところ.

臨床

中・小殿筋の筋力低下

立脚側の中・小殿筋は骨盤を前額面内で安定に保つ働きがある. また, 中・小殿筋に筋力低下や麻痺がみられる場合には, 股関節を外転する力が弱まる. 中・小殿筋の麻痺は, 上殿神経の損傷(例えば, 不適切な筋肉内注射が原因となる)によって生じる. 中・小殿筋麻痺の患者は患側で片脚立ちすると, 骨盤が正常側(遊脚側)に傾く. これをトレンデレンブルグ試験が陽性であるという. このような患者が歩行する際には, 平衡を保とうとして上体を患側側に振り出す. これにより, 重心は患側(立脚側)の下肢に移動し, 遊脚側の骨盤が挙上する(デュシェンヌ跛行). 両側の中・小殿筋が麻痺すると, 患者は典型的な動揺歩行を示すようになる.

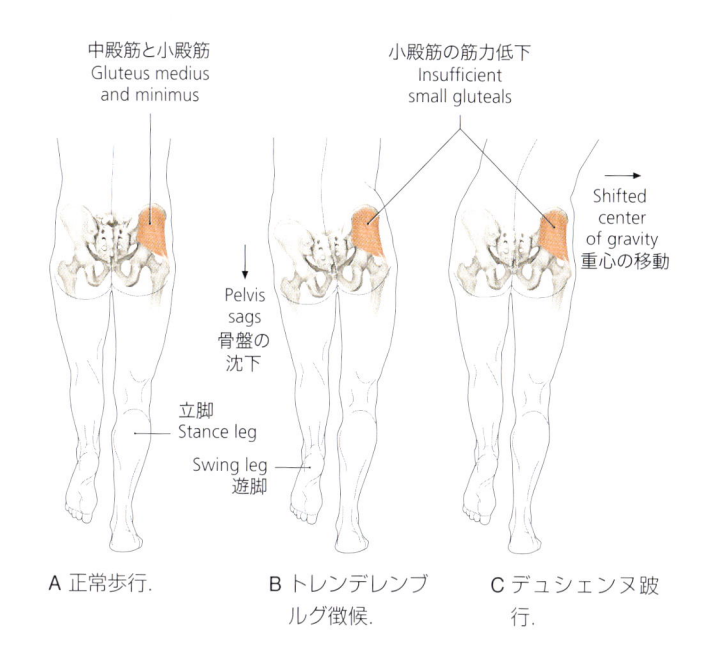

A 正常歩行.

B トレンデレンブルグ徴候.

C デュシェンヌ跛行.

仙骨神経叢の枝：坐骨神経
Nerves of the Sacral Plexus: Sciatic Nerve

> 坐骨神経からは数種類の筋枝が直接分かれる．通常，これらの筋枝が出た後に，坐骨神経は膝窩よりも近位で脛骨神経と総腓骨神経に分かれる．

図27.22 総腓骨神経：皮枝の分布

- 外側腓腹皮神経 Lateral sural cutaneous n.
- 腓腹神経との交通枝 Fibular communicating branch
- 中間足背皮神経 Intermediate dorsal cutaneous n.
- 内側足背皮神経 Medial dorsal cutaneous n.
- 母趾外側の背側趾神経 Lateral cutaneous n. of big toe
- 第2趾内側の背側趾神経 Medial cutaneous n. of 2nd toe
- 深腓骨神経 Deep fibular n.
- 内側足背皮神経 Medial dorsal cutaneous n.
- 中間足背皮神経 Intermediate dorsal cutaneous n.
- 浅腓骨神経 Superficial fibular n.

A 右の下腿と足，前方から見たところ．
B 右の下腿と足，外側方から見たところ．

図27.23 総腓骨神経
右下肢，外側方から見たところ．

- 上前腸骨棘 Anterior superior iliac spine
- 坐骨神経 Sciatic n.
- 脛骨神経 Tibial n.
- 総腓骨神経 Common fibular n.
- 大腿二頭筋，短頭 Biceps femoris, short head
- 大腿二頭筋，長頭 Biceps femoris, long head
- 腓骨頸 Neck of fibula
- 腓骨頭 Head of fibula
- 深腓骨神経 Deep fibular n.
- 浅腓骨神経 Superficial fibular n.
- 前脛骨筋 Tibialis anterior
- 長腓骨筋 Fibularis longus
- 長趾伸筋 Extensor digitorum longus
- 短腓骨筋 Fibularis brevis
- 浅腓骨神経 Superficial fibular n.
- 長母趾伸筋 Extensor hallucis longus
- 内側足背皮神経 Medial dorsal cutaneous n.
- 外果 Lateral malleolus
- 中間足背皮神経 Intermediate dorsal cutaneous n.

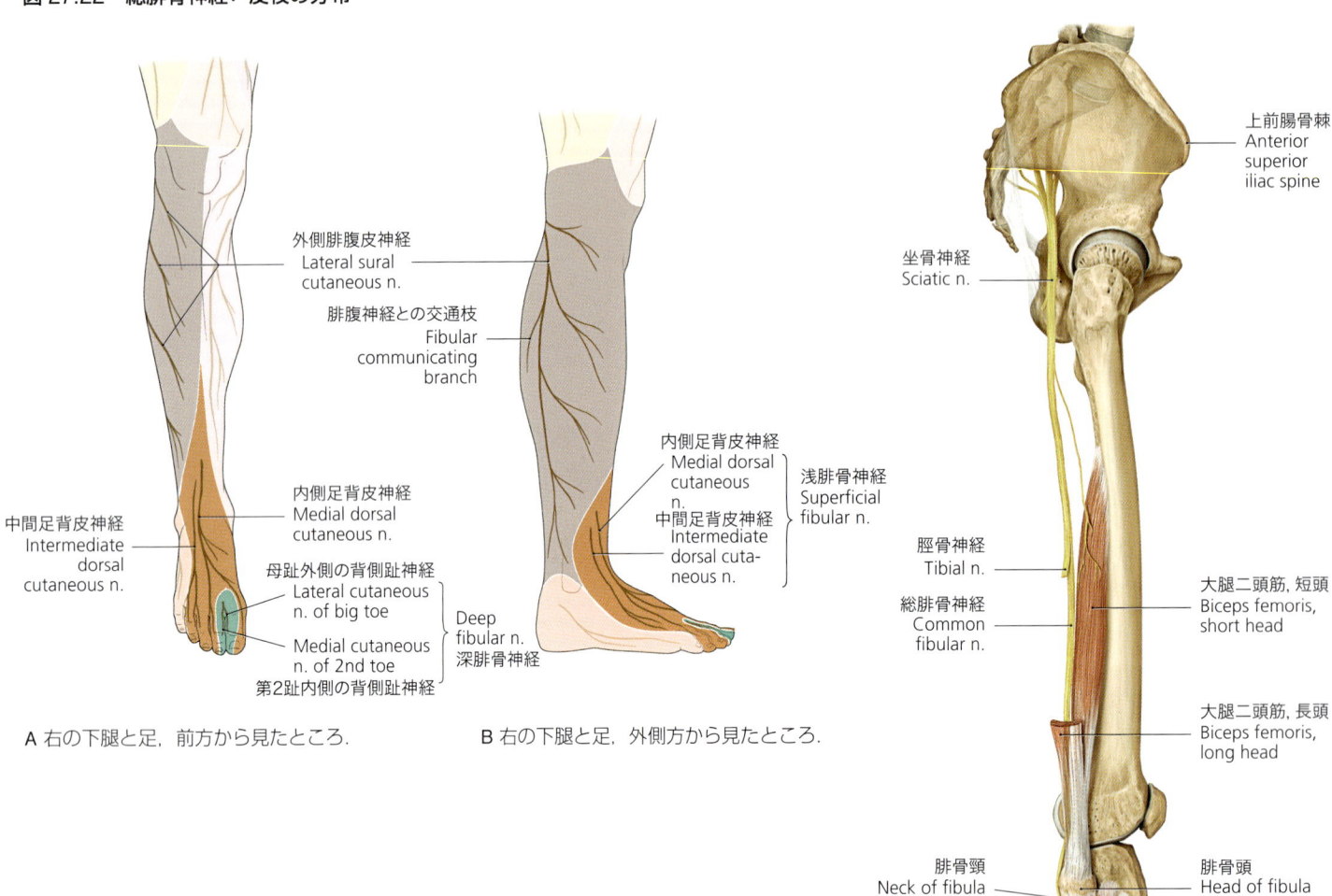

表27.6　総腓骨神経（L4-S2）

神経	支配筋	感覚枝
坐骨神経（総腓骨神経部）から直接出る筋枝	大腿二頭筋（短頭）	―
浅腓骨神経	長・短腓骨筋	内側足背神経 中間足背神経
深腓骨神経	前脛骨筋 長・短趾伸筋 長・短母趾伸筋 第三腓骨筋	背側趾神経（第1趾の外側縁と第2趾の内側縁に分布する）

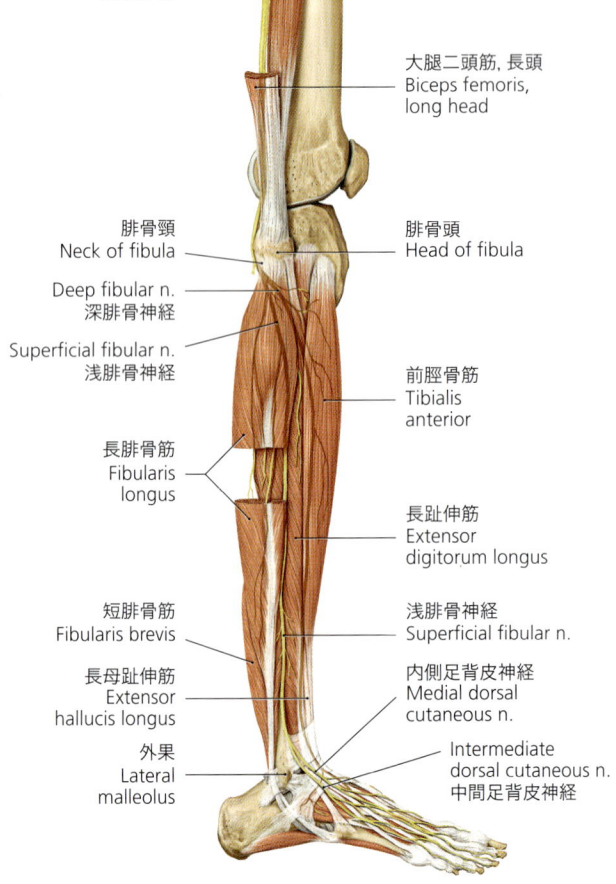

図 27.24　脛骨神経
右下肢．

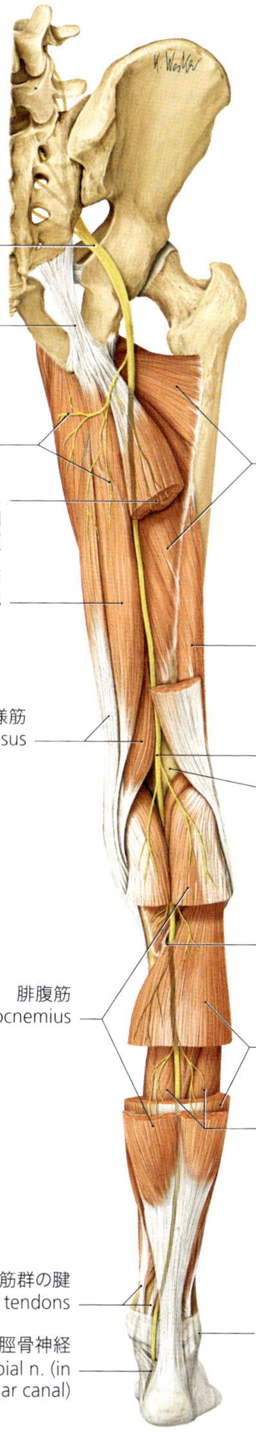

A 後方から見たところ．

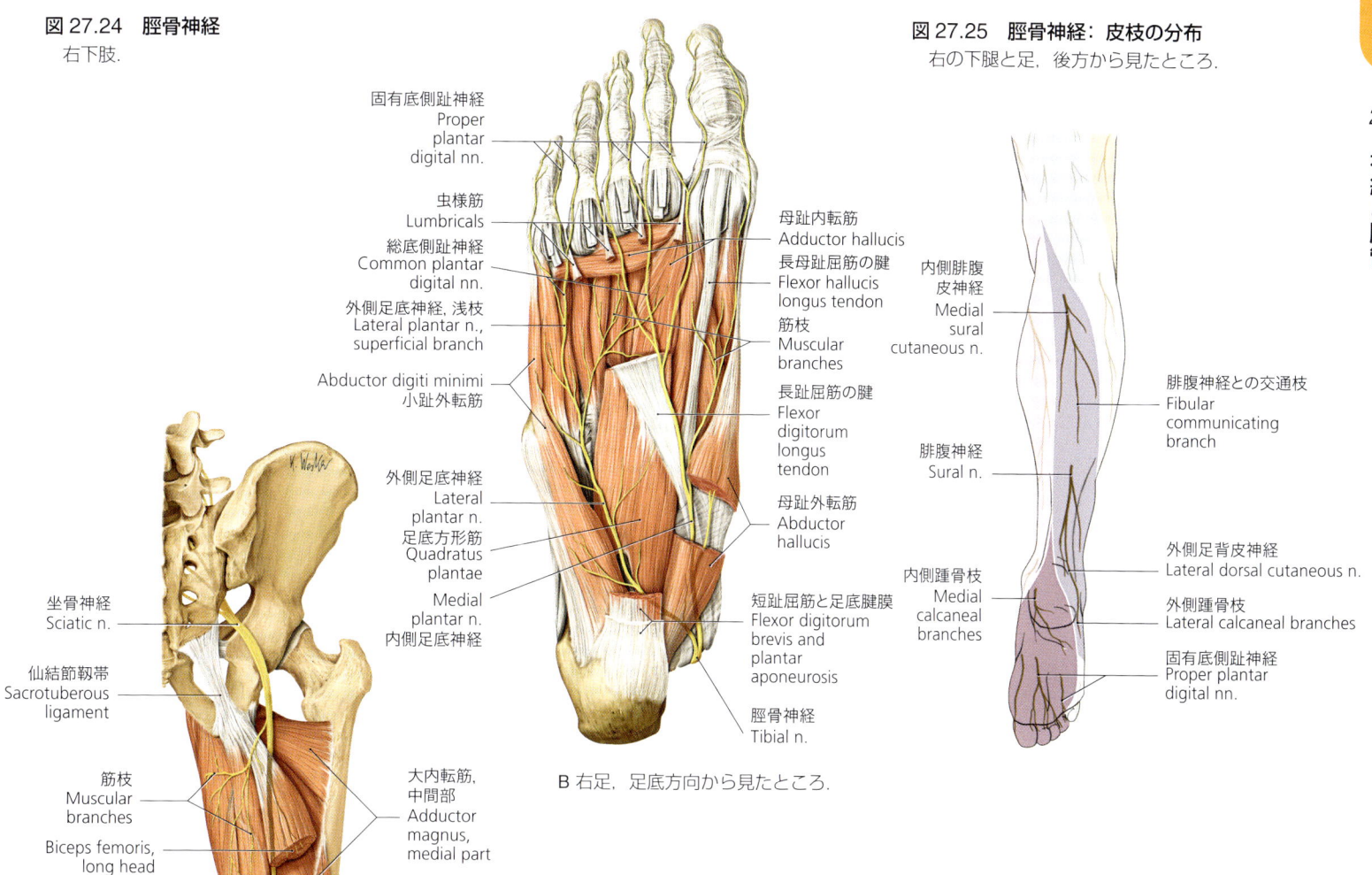

- 坐骨神経 Sciatic n.
- 仙結節靱帯 Sacrotuberous ligament
- 筋枝 Muscular branches
- 大腿二頭筋, 長頭 Biceps femoris, long head
- 半腱様筋 Semitendinosus
- 半膜様筋 Semimembranosus
- 腓腹筋 Gastrocnemius
- 深層の屈筋群の腱 Deep flexor tendons
- (内果管内の)脛骨神経 Tibial n. (in malleolar canal)
- 大内転筋, 中間部 Adductor magnus, medial part
- 大腿二頭筋, 短頭 Biceps femoris, short head
- 脛骨神経 Tibial n.
- 膝窩 Popliteal fossa
- ヒラメ筋[の]腱弓 Tendinous arch of soleus
- ヒラメ筋 Soleus
- 深層の屈筋群 Deep flexors
- 外果 Lateral malleolus

B 右足．足底方向から見たところ．

- 固有底側趾神経 Proper plantar digital nn.
- 虫様筋 Lumbricals
- 総底側趾神経 Common plantar digital nn.
- 外側足底神経, 浅枝 Lateral plantar n., superficial branch
- 小趾外転筋 Abductor digiti minimi
- 外側足底神経 Lateral plantar n.
- 足底方形筋 Quadratus plantae
- 内側足底神経 Medial plantar n.
- 母趾内転筋 Adductor hallucis
- 長母趾屈筋の腱 Flexor hallucis longus tendon
- 筋枝 Muscular branches
- 長趾屈筋の腱 Flexor digitorum longus tendon
- 母趾外転筋 Abductor hallucis
- 短趾屈筋と足底腱膜 Flexor digitorum brevis and plantar aponeurosis
- 脛骨神経 Tibial n.

図 27.25　脛骨神経：皮枝の分布
右の下腿と足, 後方から見たところ．

- 内側腓腹皮神経 Medial sural cutaneous n.
- 腓腹神経との交通枝 Fibular communicating branch
- 腓腹神経 Sural n.
- 外側足背皮神経 Lateral dorsal cutaneous n.
- 内側踵骨枝 Medial calcaneal branches
- 外側踵骨枝 Lateral calcaneal branches
- 固有底側趾神経 Proper plantar digital nn.

表27.7	脛骨神経(L4-S3)	
神経	支配筋	感覚枝
坐骨神経(脛骨神経部)から直接出る筋枝	半腱様筋 半膜様筋 大腿二頭筋(長頭) 大内転筋(内側部)	—
脛骨神経	下腿三頭筋 足底筋 膝窩筋 後脛骨筋 長趾屈筋 長母趾屈筋	内側腓腹皮神経 内側・外側踵骨枝 外側足背皮神経
内側足底神経	母趾外転筋 短趾屈筋 短母趾屈筋(内側頭) 第1・2虫様筋	固有底側趾神経
外側足底神経	短母趾屈筋(外側頭) 足底方形筋 小趾外転筋 短小趾屈筋 小趾対立筋 第3・4虫様筋 第1-3底側骨間筋 第1-4背側骨間筋 母趾内転筋	固有底側趾神経

下肢の皮神経と皮静脈
Superficial Nerves & Vessels of the Lower Limb

図 27.26　皮膚の神経分布：前方から見たところ
右下肢.

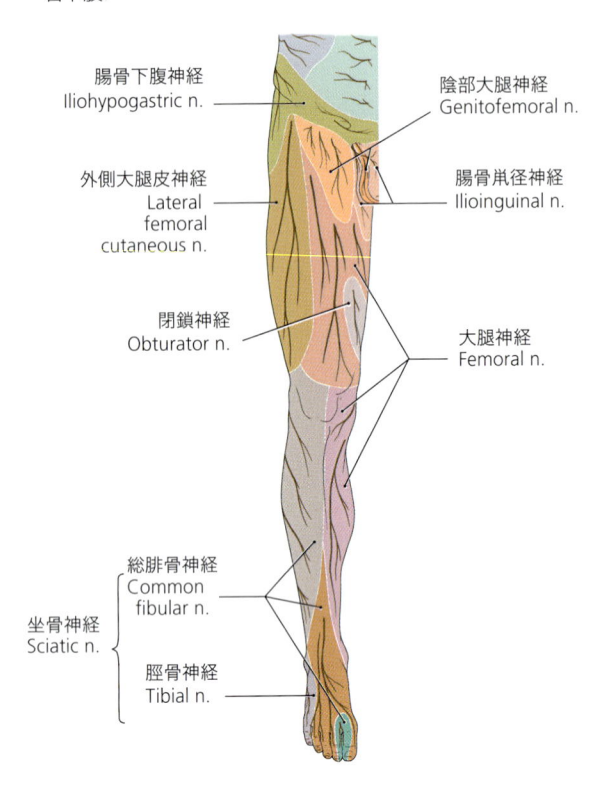

- 腸骨下腹神経 Iliohypogastric n.
- 陰部大腿神経 Genitofemoral n.
- 外側大腿皮神経 Lateral femoral cutaneous n.
- 腸骨鼠径神経 Ilioinguinal n.
- 閉鎖神経 Obturator n.
- 大腿神経 Femoral n.
- 総腓骨神経 Common fibular n.
- 坐骨神経 Sciatic n.
- 脛骨神経 Tibial n.

A 皮神経の分布.

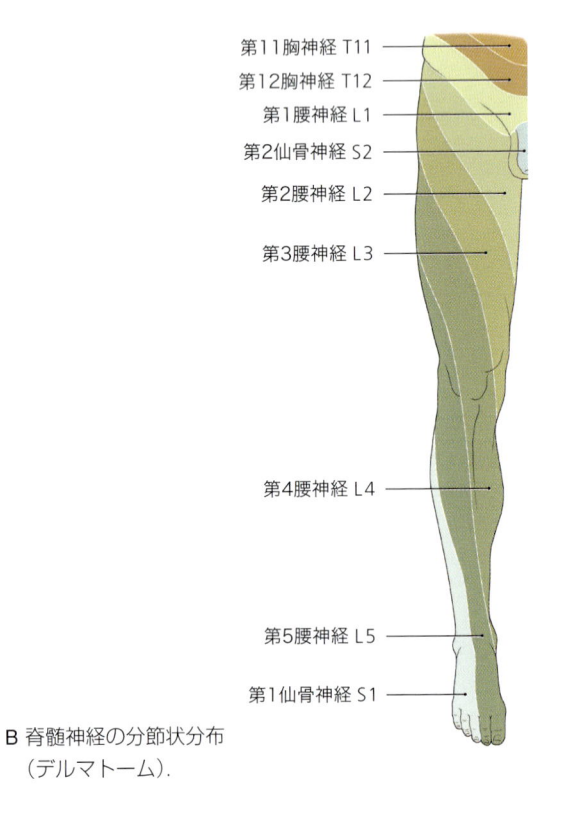

- 第11胸神経 T11
- 第12胸神経 T12
- 第1腰神経 L1
- 第2仙骨神経 S2
- 第2腰神経 L2
- 第3腰神経 L3
- 第4腰神経 L4
- 第5腰神経 L5
- 第1仙骨神経 S1

B 脊髄神経の分節状分布（デルマトーム）.

図 27.27　皮静脈と皮神経
右下肢.

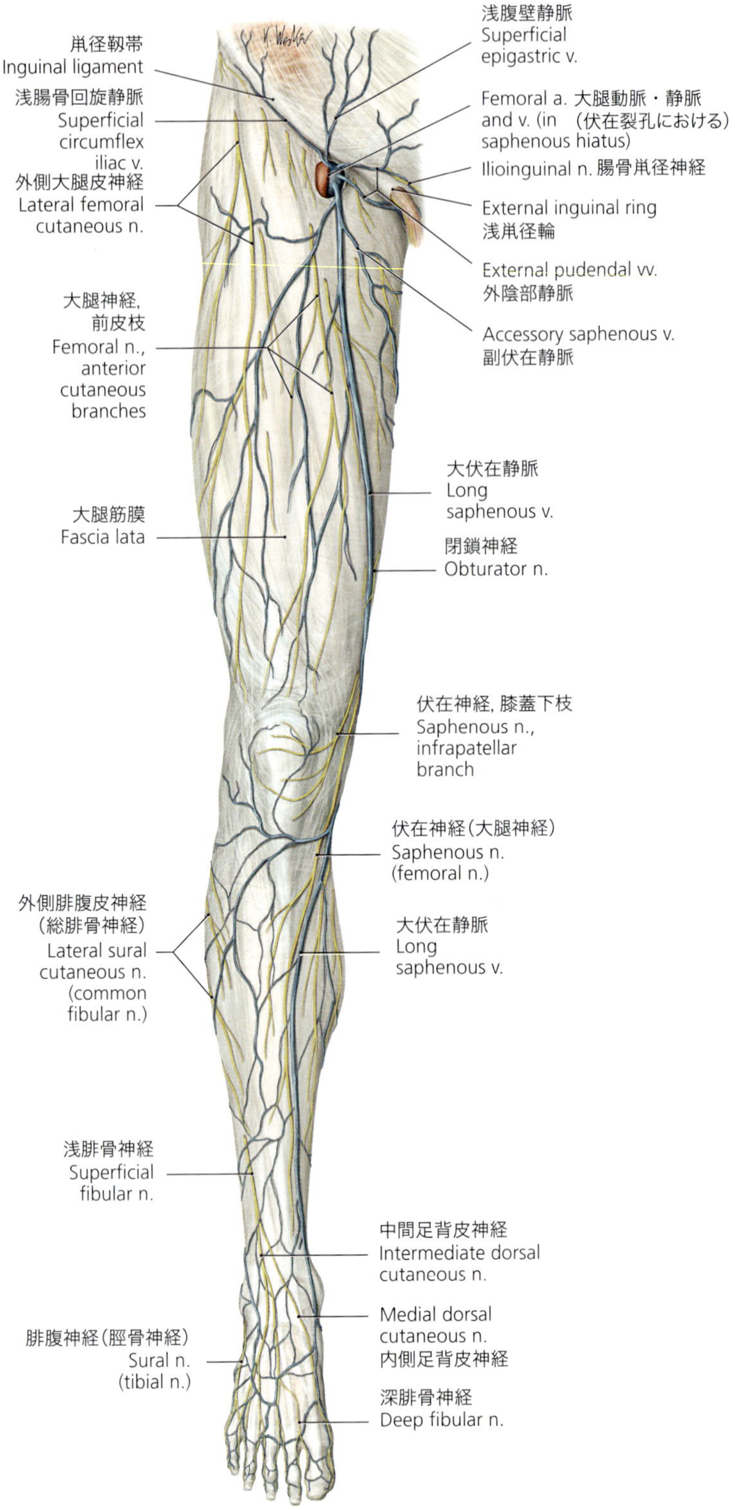

- 鼠径靱帯 Inguinal ligament
- 浅腸骨回旋静脈 Superficial circumflex iliac v.
- 外側大腿皮神経 Lateral femoral cutaneous n.
- 大腿神経, 前皮枝 Femoral n., anterior cutaneous branches
- 大腿筋膜 Fascia lata
- 浅腹壁静脈 Superficial epigastric v.
- 大腿動脈・静脈（伏在裂孔における）Femoral a. and v. (in saphenous hiatus)
- 腸骨鼠径神経 Ilioinguinal n.
- 浅鼠径輪 External inguinal ring
- 外陰部静脈 External pudendal vv.
- 副伏在静脈 Accessory saphenous v.
- 大伏在静脈 Long saphenous v.
- 閉鎖神経 Obturator n.
- 伏在神経, 膝蓋下枝 Saphenous n., infrapatellar branch
- 伏在神経（大腿神経）Saphenous n. (femoral n.)
- 外側腓腹皮神経（総腓骨神経）Lateral sural cutaneous n. (common fibular n.)
- 大伏在静脈 Long saphenous v.
- 浅腓骨神経 Superficial fibular n.
- 中間足背皮神経 Intermediate dorsal cutaneous n.
- 腓腹神経（脛骨神経）Sural n. (tibial n.)
- 内側足背皮神経 Medial dorsal cutaneous n.
- 深腓骨神経 Deep fibular n.

A 前方から見たところ.

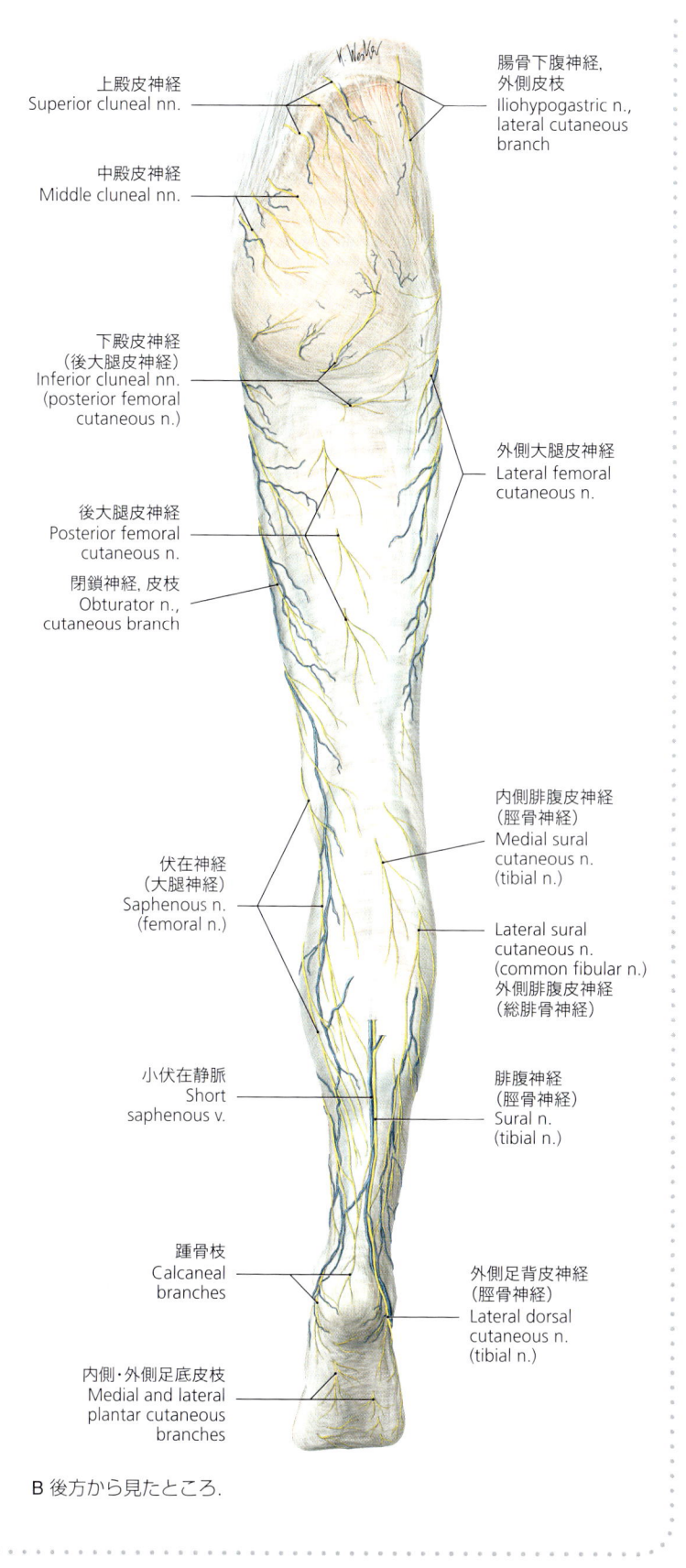

図 27.28 皮膚の神経分布：後方から見たところ
右下肢.

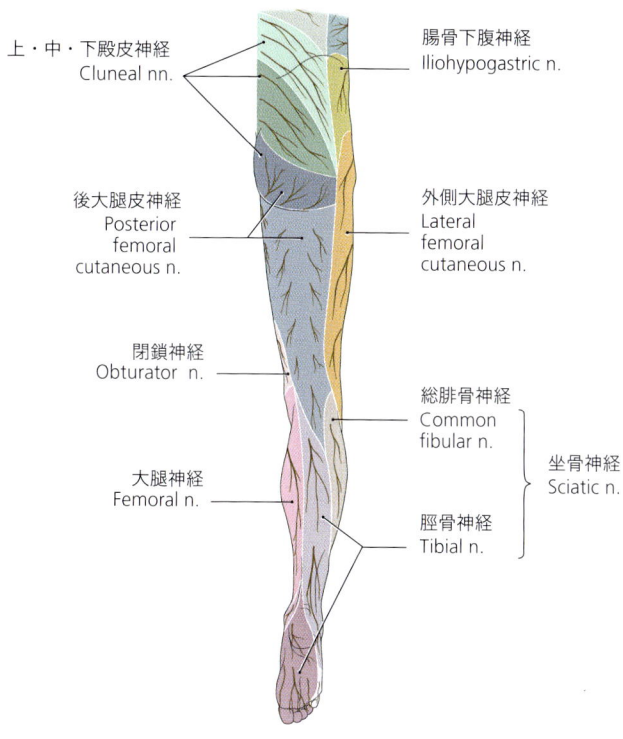

左図（下肢後面、皮神経の走行）:
- 上殿皮神経 Superior cluneal nn.
- 腸骨下腹神経, 外側皮枝 Iliohypogastric n., lateral cutaneous branch
- 中殿皮神経 Middle cluneal nn.
- 下殿皮神経（後大腿皮神経）Inferior cluneal nn. (posterior femoral cutaneous n.)
- 外側大腿皮神経 Lateral femoral cutaneous n.
- 後大腿皮神経 Posterior femoral cutaneous n.
- 閉鎖神経, 皮枝 Obturator n., cutaneous branch
- 内側腓腹皮神経（脛骨神経）Medial sural cutaneous n. (tibial n.)
- 伏在神経（大腿神経）Saphenous n. (femoral n.)
- Lateral sural cutaneous n. (common fibular n.) 外側腓腹皮神経（総腓骨神経）
- 小伏在静脈 Short saphenous v.
- 腓腹神経（脛骨神経）Sural n. (tibial n.)
- 踵骨枝 Calcaneal branches
- 外側足背皮神経（脛骨神経）Lateral dorsal cutaneous n. (tibial n.)
- 内側・外側足底皮枝 Medial and lateral plantar cutaneous branches

B 後方から見たところ.

右上図（皮神経の分布）:
- 上・中・下殿皮神経 Cluneal nn.
- 腸骨下腹神経 Iliohypogastric n.
- 後大腿皮神経 Posterior femoral cutaneous n.
- 外側大腿皮神経 Lateral femoral cutaneous n.
- 閉鎖神経 Obturator n.
- 総腓骨神経 Common fibular n.
- 大腿神経 Femoral n.
- 脛骨神経 Tibial n.
- 坐骨神経 Sciatic n.

A 皮神経の分布.

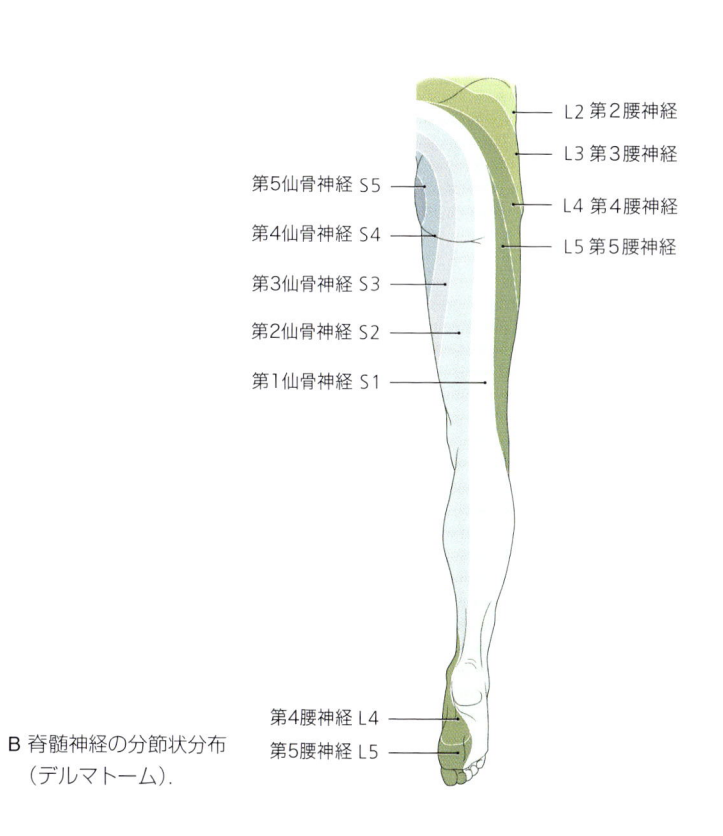

右下図（脊髄神経の分節状分布、デルマトーム）:
- L2 第2腰神経
- L3 第3腰神経
- L4 第4腰神経
- L5 第5腰神経
- 第5仙骨神経 S5
- 第4仙骨神経 S4
- 第3仙骨神経 S3
- 第2仙骨神経 S2
- 第1仙骨神経 S1
- 第4腰神経 L4
- 第5腰神経 L5

B 脊髄神経の分節状分布（デルマトーム）.

鼡径部の局所解剖
Topography of the Inguinal Region

図 27.29 浅層にある静脈とリンパ節
男性の右鼡径部，前方から見たところ．
伏在裂孔を覆う篩状筋膜を取り除いてある．

- 浅鼡径リンパ節と上外側浅鼡径リンパ節 / Superficial and superolateral inguinal l.n.
- 鼡径靭帯 / Inguinal ligament
- 外腸骨静脈 / External iliac v.
- 浅腸骨回旋静脈 / Superficial circumflex iliac v.
- 浅腹壁静脈 / Superficial epigastric v.
- 伏在裂孔 / Saphenous hiatus
- 大腿動脈・静脈 / Femoral a. and v.
- 前大腿皮静脈 / Anterior femoral cutaneous v.
- 外腸骨リンパ節 / External iliac l.n.
- ローゼンミュラーのリンパ節 / Rosenmüller's l.n.
- 外陰部静脈 / External pudendal v.
- 浅鼡径リンパ節と上内側浅鼡径リンパ節 / Superficial and superomedial inguinal l.n.
- 深鼡径リンパ節 / Deep inguinal l.n.
- 浅鼡径リンパ節と下浅鼡径リンパ節 / Superficial and inferior inguinal l.n.
- 大伏在静脈 / Long saphenous v.

図 27.30 鼡径部
男性の右鼡径部，前方から見たところ．

- 外腹斜筋 / External oblique
- 内腹斜筋 / Internal oblique
- 腹横筋 / Transversus abdominis
- 外側大腿皮神経 / Lateral femoral cutaneous n.
- 浅腸骨回旋動脈・静脈 / Superficial circumflex iliac a. and v.
- 鼡径靭帯 / Inguinal ligament
- 陰部大腿神経，大腿枝 / Genitofemoral n., femoral branch
- 浅鼡径輪 / Superficial inguinal ring
- 大腿動脈・静脈（伏在裂孔にある）/ Femoral a. and v. (in saphenous hiatus)
- 白線 / Linea alba
- 腹直筋 / Rectus abdominis
- 腹直筋鞘，前葉 / Anterior rectus sheath
- 浅腹筋膜 / Superficial abdominal fascia
- 外腹斜筋腱膜 / External oblique aponeurosis
- 腸骨鼡径神経 / Ilioinguinal n.
- 陰部大腿神経，陰部枝 / Genitofemoral n., genital branch
- 反転靭帯 / Reflex ligament
- 精索（断端）/ Spermatic cord (cut)
- 裂孔靭帯 / Lacunar ligament
- 外陰部動脈・静脈 / External pudendal a. and v.
- 前大腿皮静脈 / Anterior femoral cutaneous v.
- 大伏在静脈 / Long saphenous v.
- 恥骨筋 / Pectineus

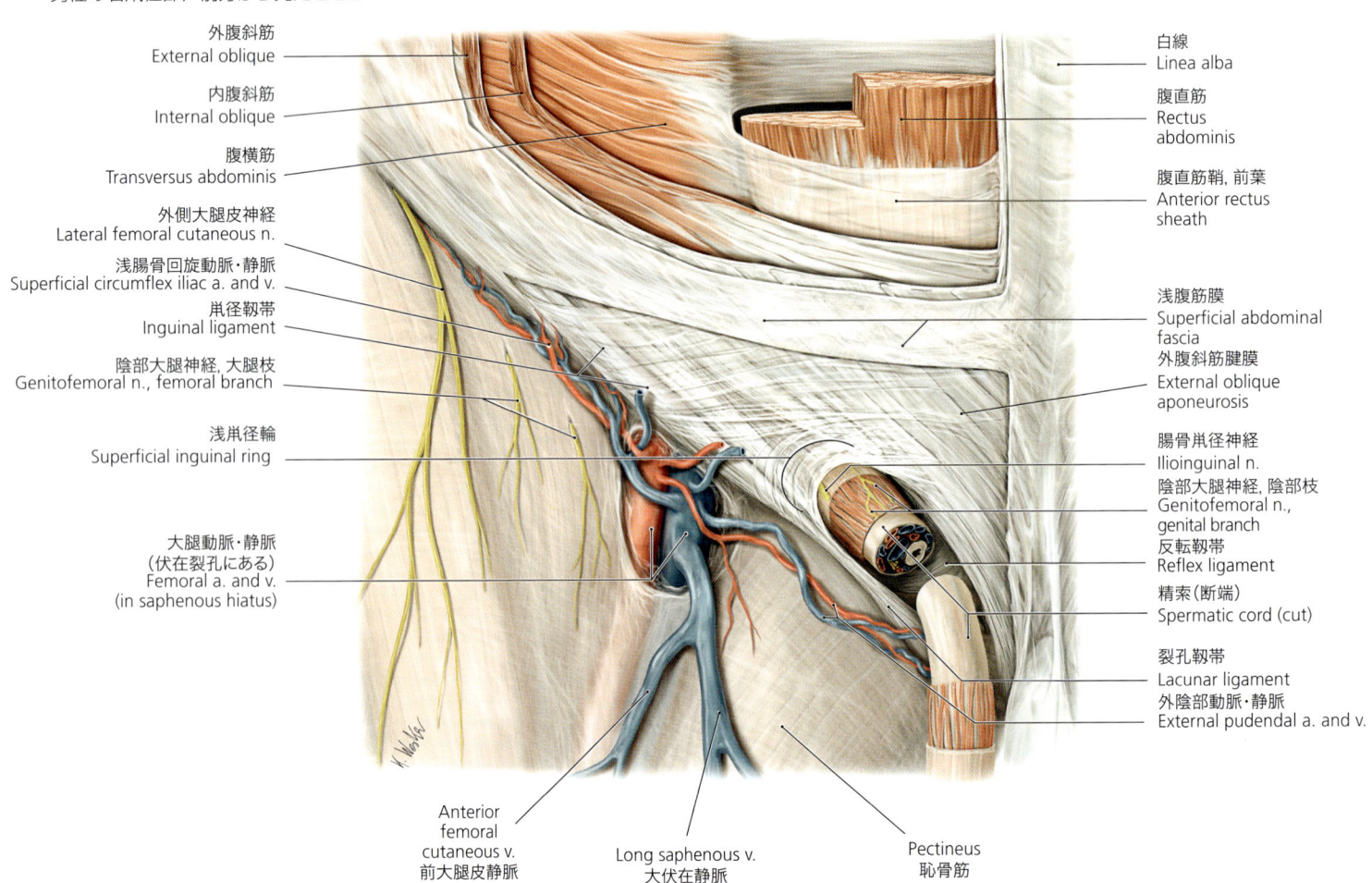

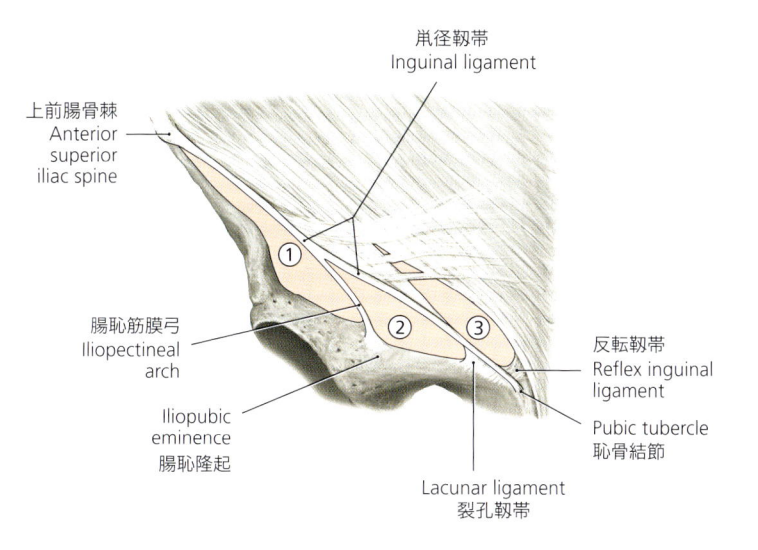

表27.8	鼠径部の構造	
部位	境界	内容
①筋裂孔	上前腸骨棘 鼠径靱帯 腸恥筋膜弓	大腿神経 外側大腿皮神経 腸骨筋 大腰筋
②血管裂孔	鼠径靱帯 腸恥筋膜弓 裂孔靱帯	大腿動脈・静脈 陰部大腿神経（大腿枝） ローゼンミュラーのリンパ節
③外鼠径輪	内側脚 外側脚 反転靱帯	腸骨鼠径神経 陰部大腿神経（陰部枝） 精索 子宮円索

図27.31 筋裂孔と血管裂孔
右鼠径部，前方から見たところ．

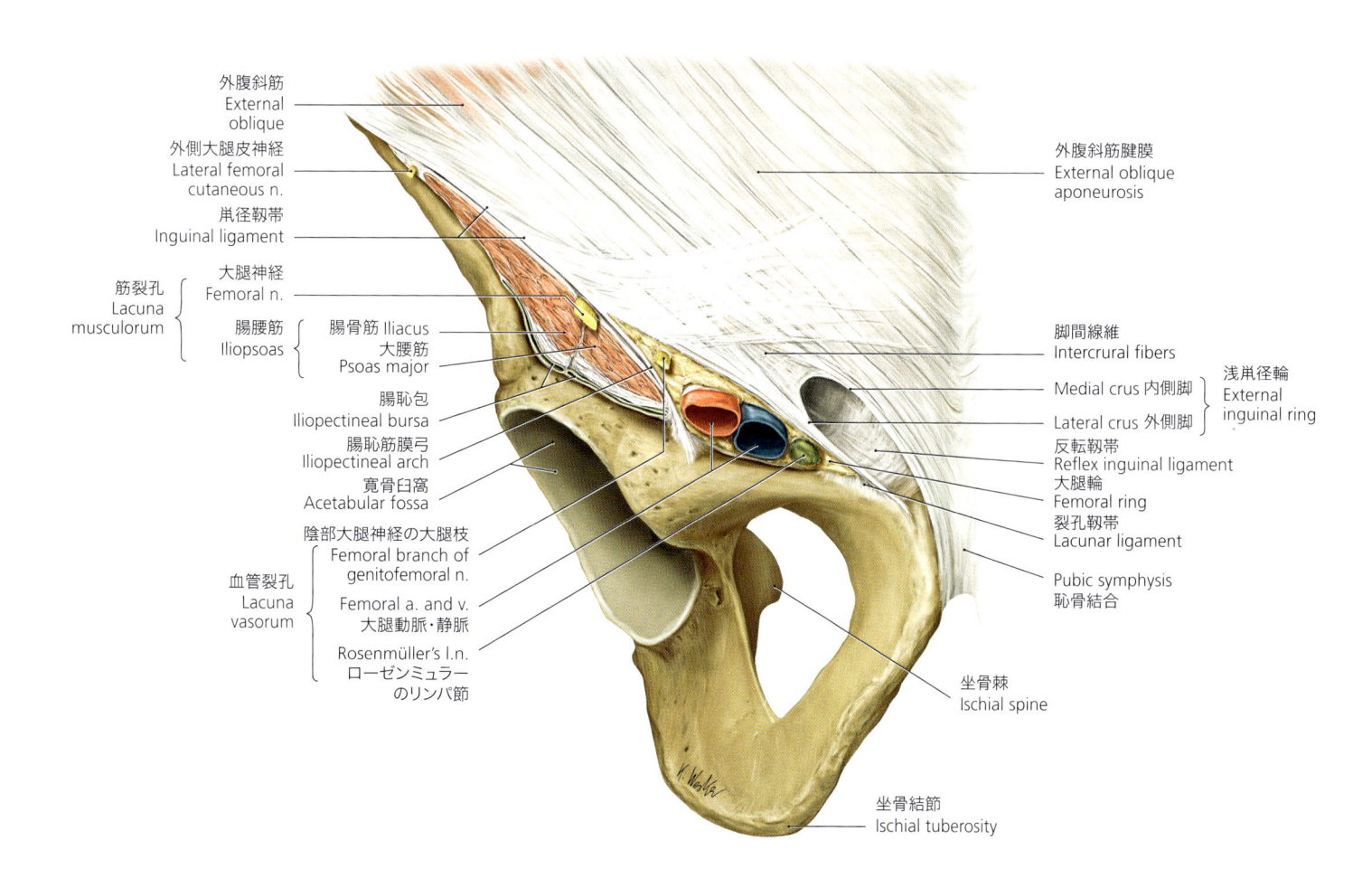

殿部の局所解剖
Topography of the Gluteal Region

図 27.32 殿部
右殿部，後方から見たところ．

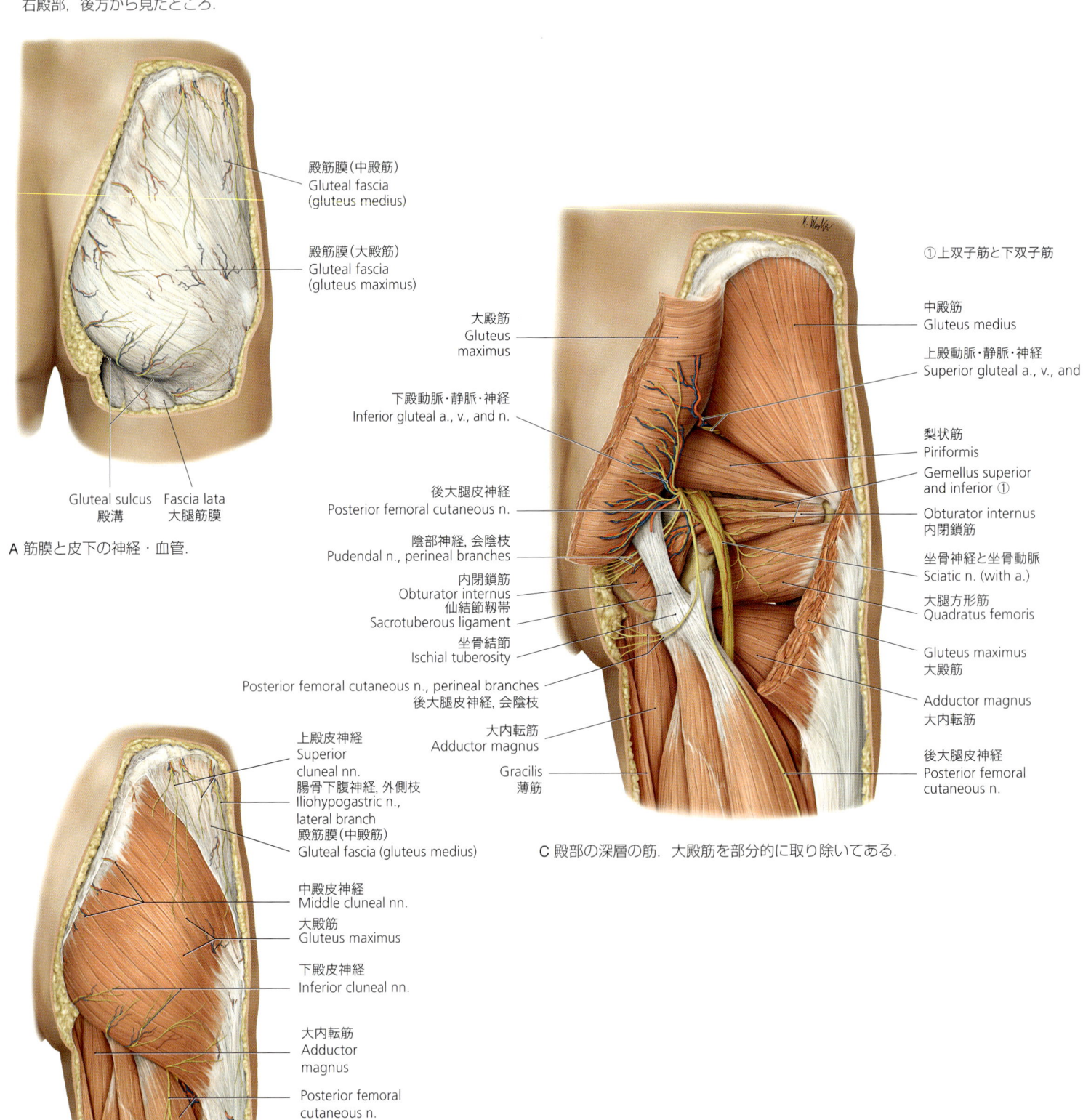

A 筋膜と皮下の神経・血管．

- 殿筋膜（中殿筋） Gluteal fascia (gluteus medius)
- 殿筋膜（大殿筋） Gluteal fascia (gluteus maximus)
- Gluteal sulcus 殿溝
- Fascia lata 大腿筋膜

B 殿部の表層の筋．大腿筋膜を取り除いてある．

- 上殿皮神経 Superior cluneal nn.
- 腸骨下腹神経，外側枝 Iliohypogastric n., lateral branch
- 殿筋膜（中殿筋） Gluteal fascia (gluteus medius)
- 中殿皮神経 Middle cluneal nn.
- 大殿筋 Gluteus maximus
- 下殿皮神経 Inferior cluneal nn.
- 大内転筋 Adductor magnus
- 後大腿皮神経 Posterior femoral cutaneous n. (with biceps femoris, long head) 後大腿皮神経と大腿二頭筋，長頭
- Semimembranosus 半膜様筋
- Semitendinosus 半腱様筋

C 殿部の深層の筋．大殿筋を部分的に取り除いてある．

- 大殿筋 Gluteus maximus
- 下殿動脈・静脈・神経 Inferior gluteal a., v., and n.
- 後大腿皮神経 Posterior femoral cutaneous n.
- 陰部神経，会陰枝 Pudendal n., perineal branches
- 内閉鎖筋 Obturator internus
- 仙結節靱帯 Sacrotuberous ligament
- 坐骨結節 Ischial tuberosity
- 後大腿皮神経，会陰枝 Posterior femoral cutaneous n., perineal branches
- 大内転筋 Adductor magnus
- Gracilis 薄筋
- ①上双子筋と下双子筋
- 中殿筋 Gluteus medius
- 上殿動脈・静脈・神経 Superior gluteal a., v., and n.
- 梨状筋 Piriformis
- Gemellus superior and inferior ①
- 内閉鎖筋 Obturator internus
- 坐骨神経と坐骨動脈 Sciatic n. (with a.)
- 大腿方形筋 Quadratus femoris
- Gluteus maximus 大殿筋
- Adductor magnus 大内転筋
- 後大腿皮神経 Posterior femoral cutaneous n.

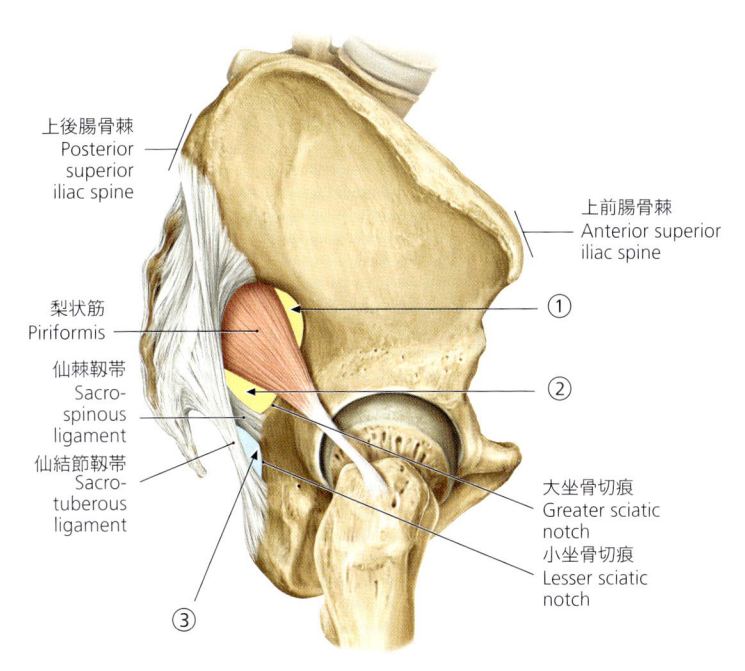

表27.9	坐骨孔		
孔		通過する構造	境界
大坐骨孔	①梨状筋上孔	上殿動脈・静脈・神経	大坐骨切痕 仙棘靱帯 仙骨
	②梨状筋下孔	下殿動脈・静脈・神経 内陰部動脈・静脈 陰部神経 坐骨神経 後大腿皮神経	
③小坐骨孔		内陰部動脈・静脈 陰部神経 内閉鎖筋腱	小坐骨切痕 仙棘靱帯 仙結節靱帯

図 27.33 殿部と坐骨直腸窩
右殿部，後方から見たところ．大殿筋と中殿筋を取り除いてある．

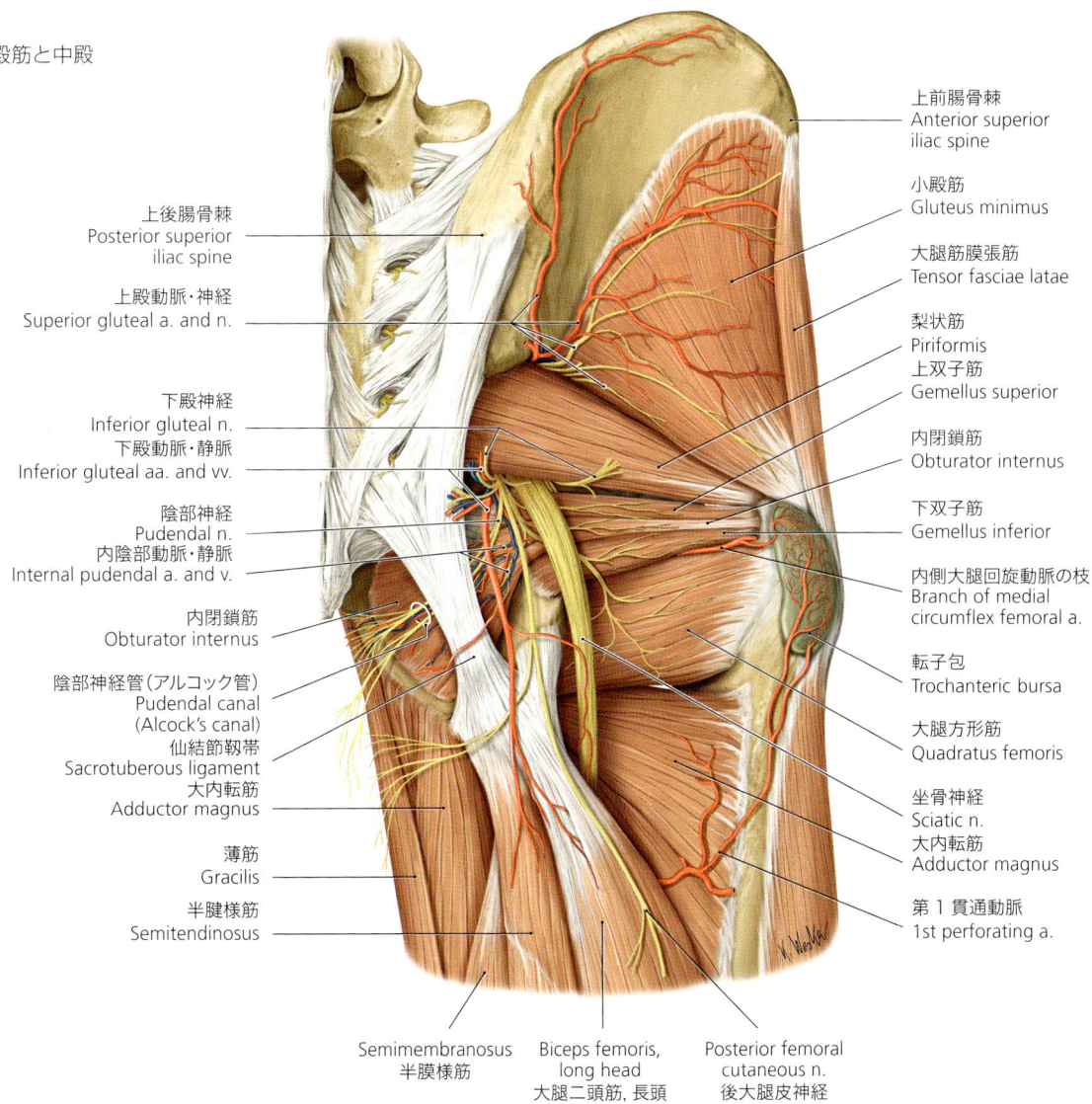

大腿の前面と後面の局所解剖
Topography of the Anterior & Posterior Thigh

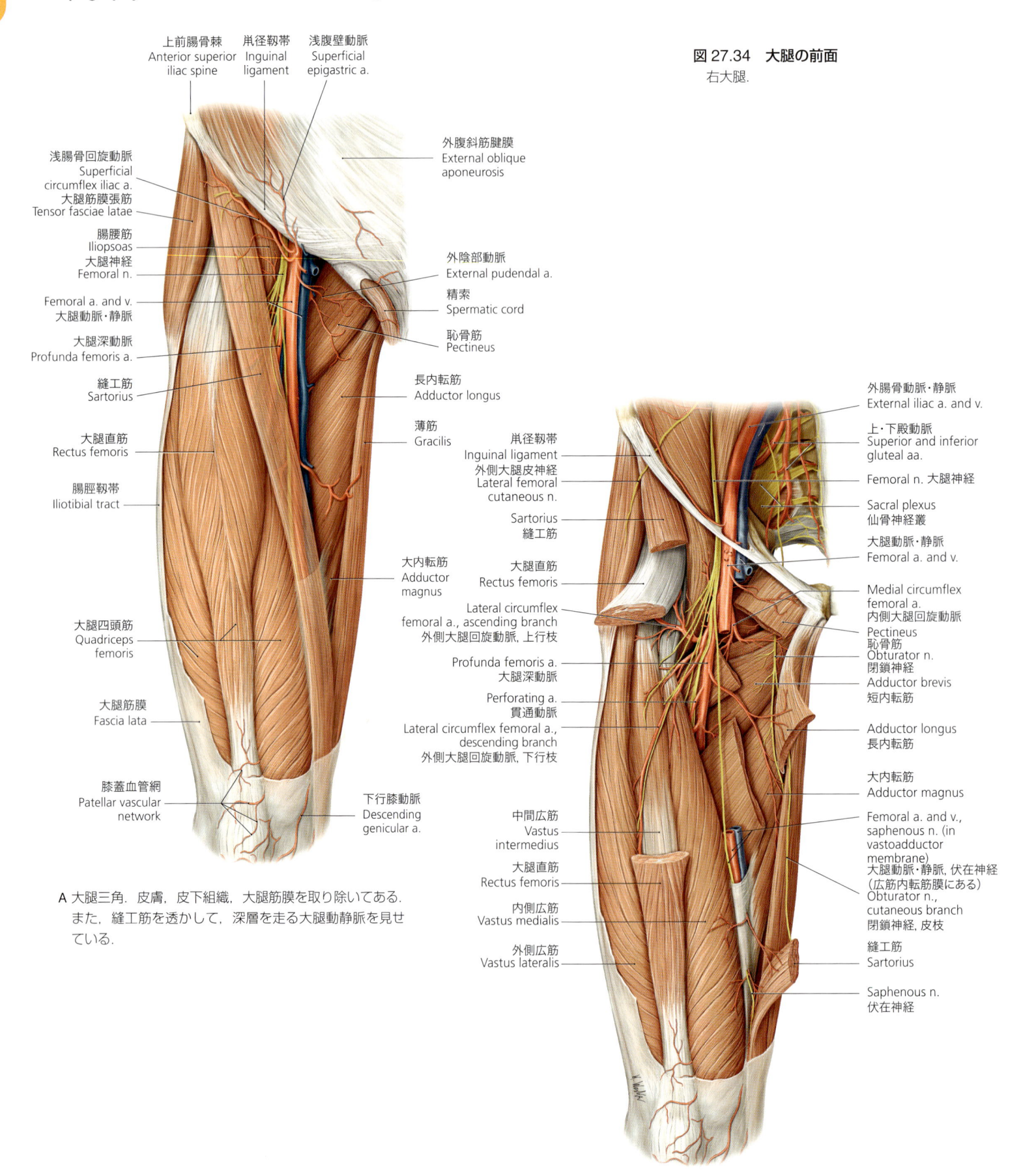

図 27.34　大腿の前面
右大腿.

A 大腿三角．皮膚，皮下組織，大腿筋膜を取り除いてある．また，縫工筋を透かして，深層を走る大腿動静脈を見せている．

B 大腿前面の神経と動静脈．前腹壁を取り除いてある．また，縫工筋，大腿直筋，長内転筋，恥骨筋を部分的に取り除いてある．

図 27.35　大腿の後面
右大腿.

A 殿部と大腿．大腿筋膜を取り除いてある．

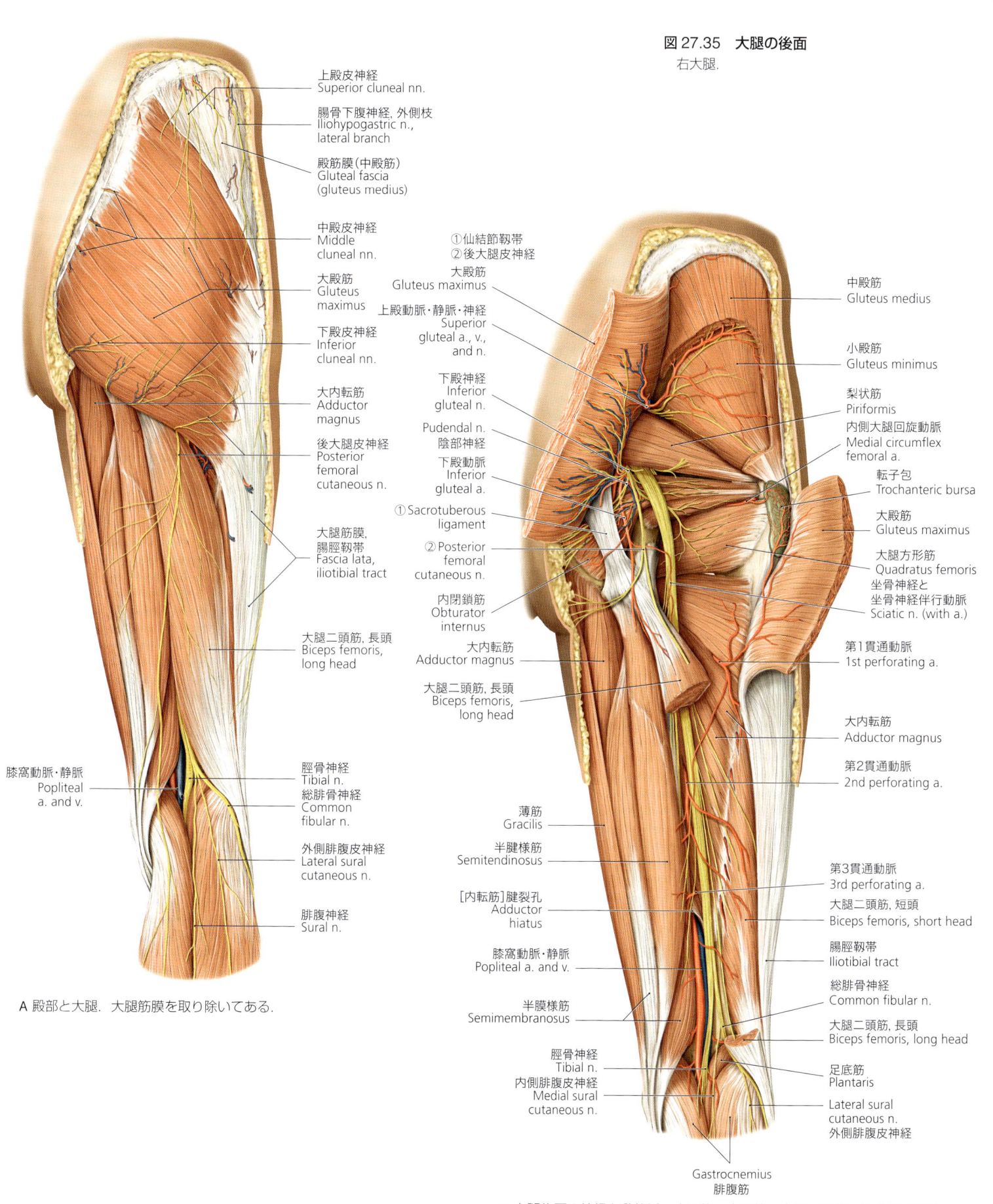

B 大腿後面の神経と動静脈．大殿筋，中殿筋，大腿二頭筋を部分的に取り除いてある．

下腿の後面と内側面の局所解剖
Topography of the Posterior & Medial Leg

図 27.36 下腿の後面
右下腿，後方から見たところ．

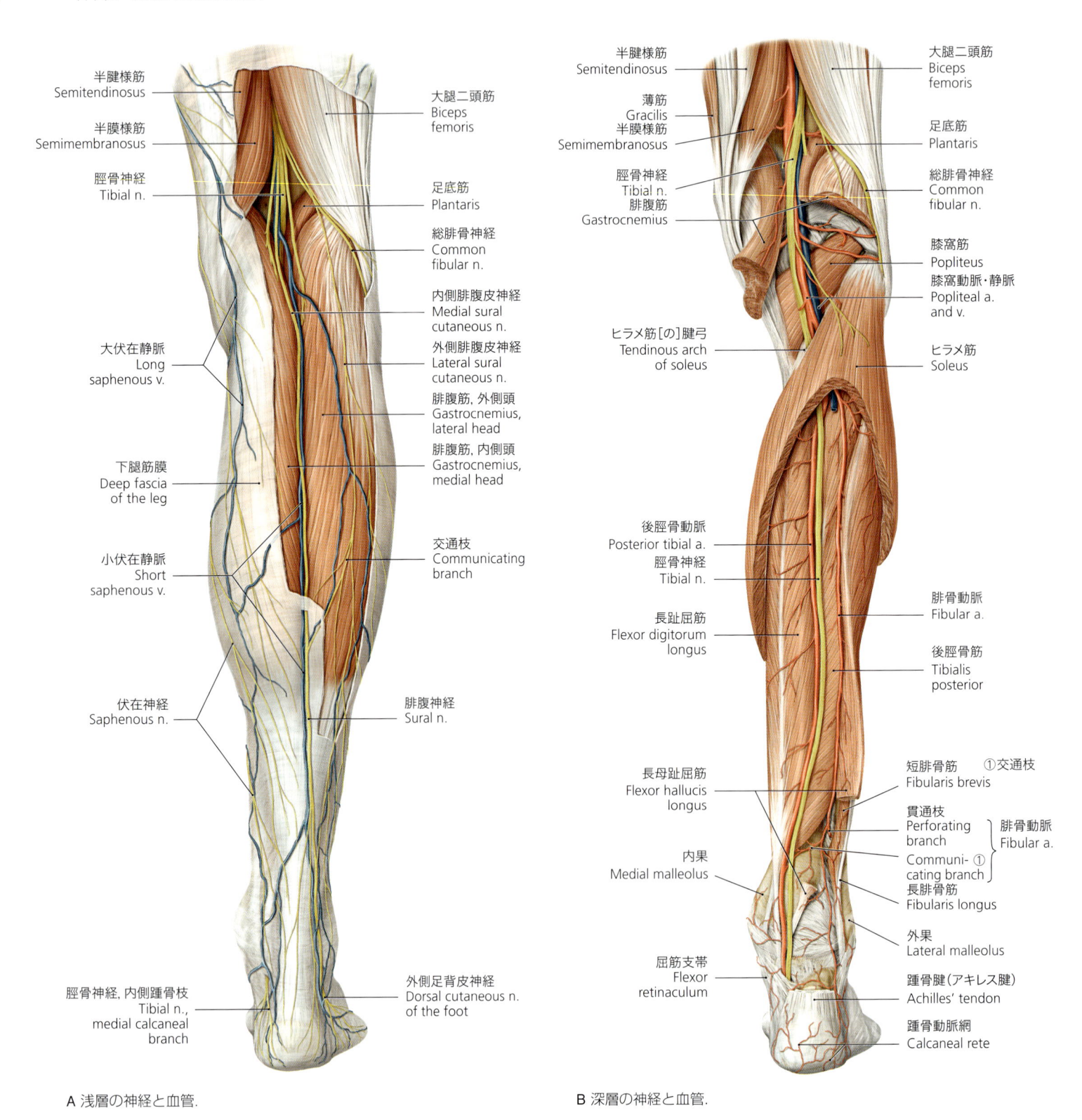

A 浅層の神経と血管．

B 深層の神経と血管．

図 27.37 膝窩
右下肢，後方から見たところ．

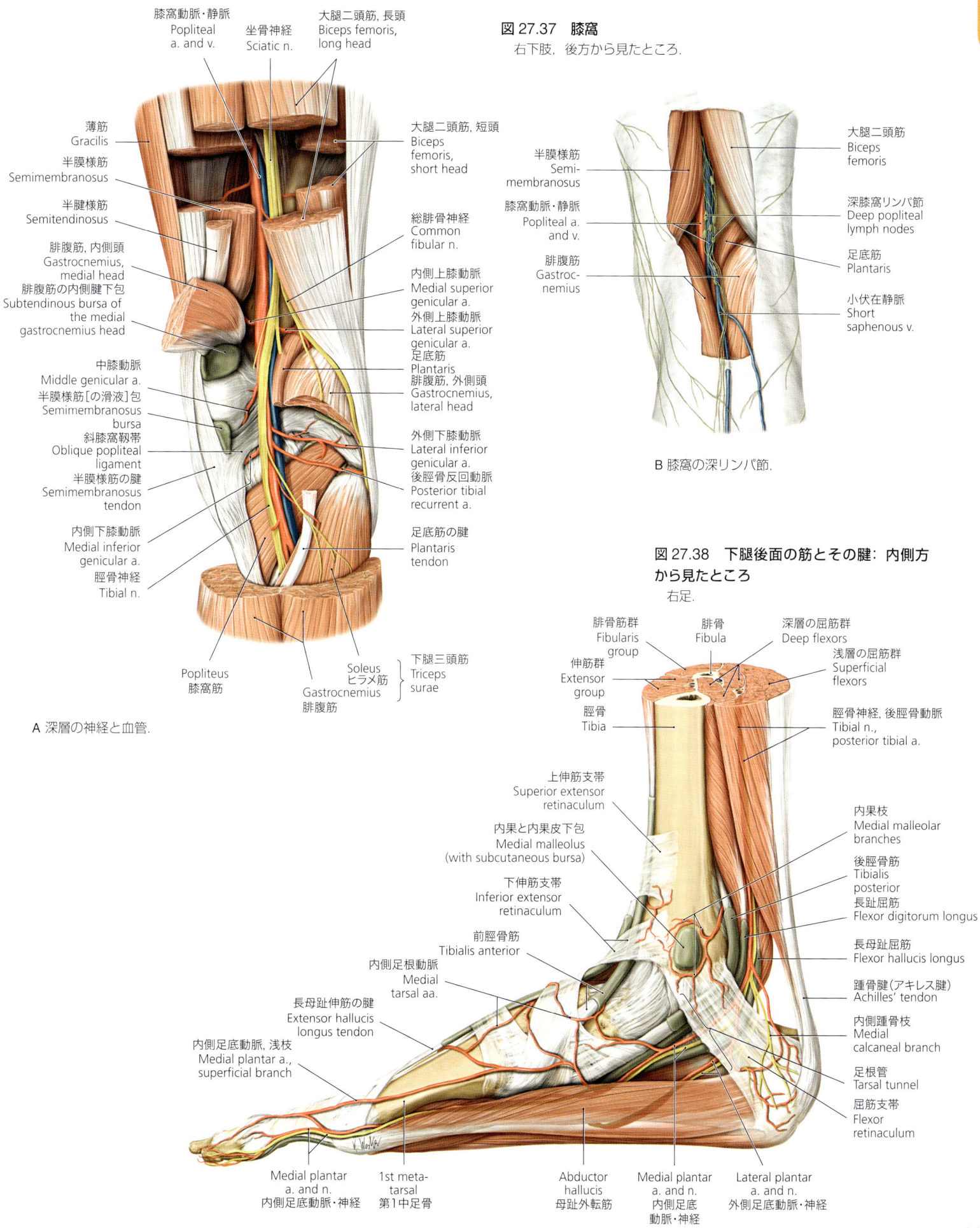

A 深層の神経と血管．

- 膝窩動脈・静脈 Popliteal a. and v.
- 坐骨神経 Sciatic n.
- 大腿二頭筋，長頭 Biceps femoris, long head
- 薄筋 Gracilis
- 半膜様筋 Semimembranosus
- 半腱様筋 Semitendinosus
- 腓腹筋，内側頭 Gastrocnemius, medial head
- 腓腹筋の内側腱下包 Subtendinous bursa of the medial gastrocnemius head
- 中膝動脈 Middle genicular a.
- 半膜様筋[の滑液]包 Semimembranosus bursa
- 斜膝窩靱帯 Oblique popliteal ligament
- 半膜様筋の腱 Semimembranosus tendon
- 内側下膝動脈 Medial inferior genicular a.
- 脛骨神経 Tibial n.
- 大腿二頭筋，短頭 Biceps femoris, short head
- 総腓骨神経 Common fibular n.
- 内側上膝動脈 Medial superior genicular a.
- 外側上膝動脈 Lateral superior genicular a.
- 足底筋 Plantaris
- 腓腹筋，外側頭 Gastrocnemius, lateral head
- 外側下膝動脈 Lateral inferior genicular a.
- 後脛骨反回動脈 Posterior tibial recurrent a.
- 足底筋の腱 Plantaris tendon
- Popliteus 膝窩筋
- Soleus ヒラメ筋
- Gastrocnemius 腓腹筋
- 下腿三頭筋 Triceps surae

B 膝窩の深リンパ節．

- 半膜様筋 Semimembranosus
- 膝窩動脈・静脈 Popliteal a. and v.
- 腓腹筋 Gastrocnemius
- 大腿二頭筋 Biceps femoris
- 深膝窩リンパ節 Deep popliteal lymph nodes
- 足底筋 Plantaris
- 小伏在静脈 Short saphenous v.

図 27.38 下腿後面の筋とその腱：内側方から見たところ
右足．

- 腓骨筋群 Fibularis group
- 腓骨 Fibula
- 深層の屈筋群 Deep flexors
- 伸筋群 Extensor group
- 浅層の屈筋群 Superficial flexors
- 脛骨 Tibia
- 脛骨神経，後脛骨動脈 Tibial n., posterior tibial a.
- 上伸筋支帯 Superior extensor retinaculum
- 内果枝 Medial malleolar branches
- 内果と内果皮下包 Medial malleolus (with subcutaneous bursa)
- 後脛骨筋 Tibialis posterior
- 長趾屈筋 Flexor digitorum longus
- 下伸筋支帯 Inferior extensor retinaculum
- 長母趾屈筋 Flexor hallucis longus
- 前脛骨筋 Tibialis anterior
- 踵骨腱（アキレス腱）Achilles' tendon
- 内側足根動脈 Medial tarsal aa.
- 内側踵骨枝 Medial calcaneal branch
- 長母趾伸筋の腱 Extensor hallucis longus tendon
- 足根管 Tarsal tunnel
- 内側足底動脈，浅枝 Medial plantar a., superficial branch
- 屈筋支帯 Flexor retinaculum
- Medial plantar a. and n. 内側足底動脈・神経
- 1st metatarsal 第1中足骨
- Abductor hallucis 母趾外転筋
- Medial plantar a. and n. 内側足底動脈・神経
- Lateral plantar a. and n. 外側足底動脈・神経

下腿の外側面と前面の局所解剖
Topography of the Lateral & Anterior Leg

図 27.39　下腿と足の神経と血管：外側方から見たところ
右の下腿と足．長腓骨筋と長趾伸筋の起始部を取り除いてある．

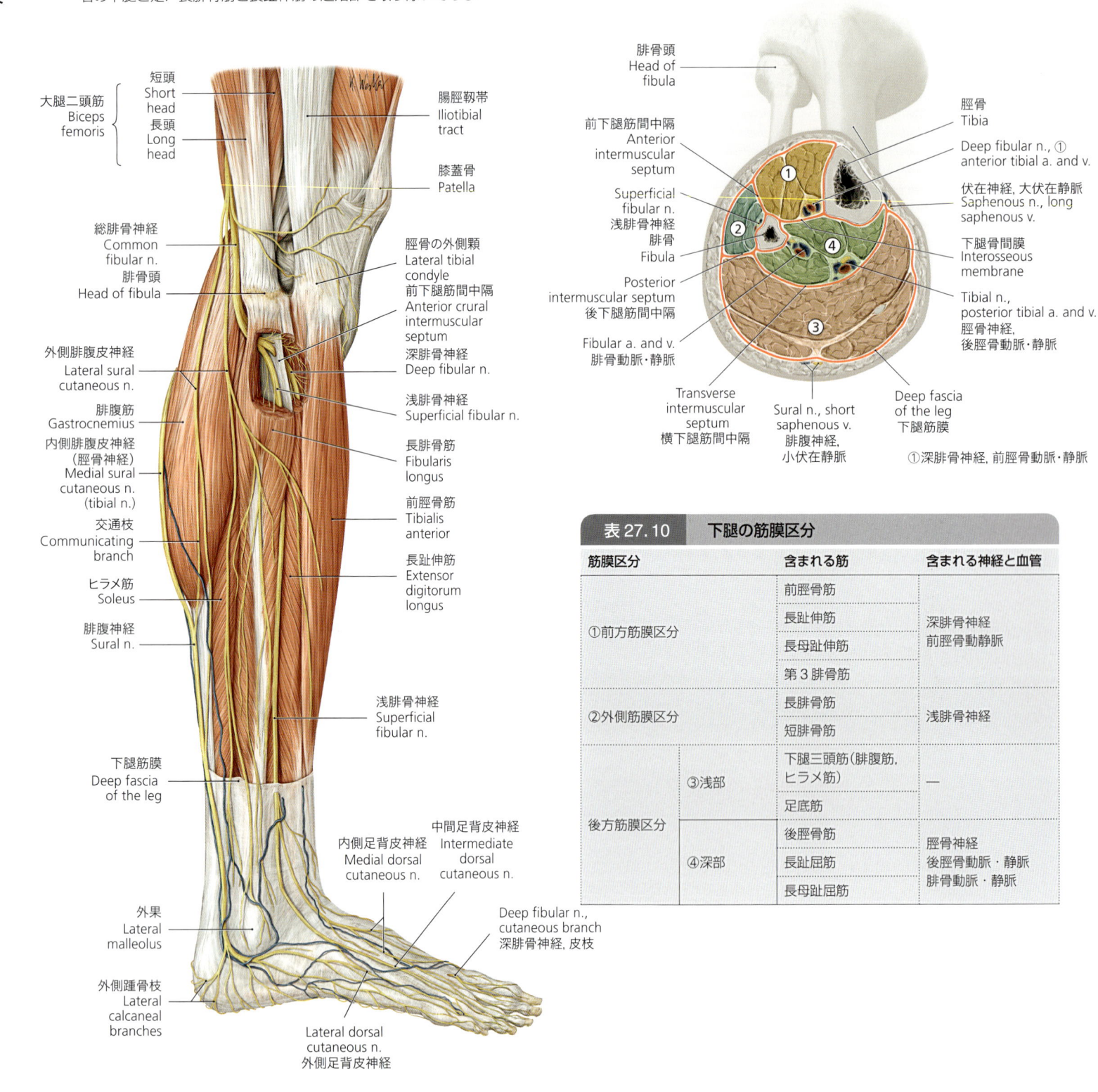

Labels (left leg image):
- 大腿二頭筋 Biceps femoris — 短頭 Short head, 長頭 Long head
- 腸脛靱帯 Iliotibial tract
- 膝蓋骨 Patella
- 総腓骨神経 Common fibular n.
- 腓骨頭 Head of fibula
- 脛骨の外側顆 Lateral tibial condyle
- 前下腿筋間中隔 Anterior crural intermuscular septum
- 深腓骨神経 Deep fibular n.
- 外側腓腹皮神経 Lateral sural cutaneous n.
- 浅腓骨神経 Superficial fibular n.
- 腓腹筋 Gastrocnemius
- 内側腓腹皮神経（脛骨神経）Medial sural cutaneous n. (tibial n.)
- 長腓骨筋 Fibularis longus
- 前脛骨筋 Tibialis anterior
- 交通枝 Communicating branch
- 長趾伸筋 Extensor digitorum longus
- ヒラメ筋 Soleus
- 腓腹神経 Sural n.
- 浅腓骨神経 Superficial fibular n.
- 下腿筋膜 Deep fascia of the leg
- 内側足背皮神経 Medial dorsal cutaneous n.
- 中間足背皮神経 Intermediate dorsal cutaneous n.
- 外果 Lateral malleolus
- 深腓骨神経, 皮枝 Deep fibular n., cutaneous branch
- 外側踵骨枝 Lateral calcaneal branches
- 外側足背皮神経 Lateral dorsal cutaneous n.

Labels (cross-section):
- 腓骨頭 Head of fibula
- 前下腿筋間中隔 Anterior intermuscular septum
- 浅腓骨神経 Superficial fibular n.
- 腓骨 Fibula
- 後下腿筋間中隔 Posterior intermuscular septum
- 腓骨動脈・静脈 Fibular a. and v.
- 横下腿筋間中隔 Transverse intermuscular septum
- 腓腹神経, 小伏在静脈 Sural n., short saphenous v.
- 下腿筋膜 Deep fascia of the leg
- 脛骨神経, 後脛骨動脈・静脈 Tibial n., posterior tibial a. and v.
- 下腿骨間膜 Interosseous membrane
- 伏在神経, 大伏在静脈 Saphenous n., long saphenous v.
- 深腓骨神経, 前脛骨動脈・静脈 Deep fibular n., ① anterior tibial a. and v.
- 脛骨 Tibia
- ①深腓骨神経, 前脛骨動脈・静脈

表 27.10　下腿の筋膜区分

筋膜区分		含まれる筋	含まれる神経と血管
①前方筋膜区分		前脛骨筋	深腓骨神経 前脛骨動静脈
		長趾伸筋	
		長母趾伸筋	
		第3腓骨筋	
②外側筋膜区分		長腓骨筋	浅腓骨神経
		短腓骨筋	
後方筋膜区分	③浅部	下腿三頭筋（腓腹筋, ヒラメ筋）	—
		足底筋	
	④深部	後脛骨筋	脛骨神経 後脛骨動脈・静脈 腓骨動脈・静脈
		長趾屈筋	
		長母趾屈筋	

臨床

コンパートメント症候群

筋の浮腫や血腫により，筋区画内における組織圧が高くなる．高まった組織圧により神経や血管が圧迫を受け，これにより区画内の構造が虚血に陥り，筋や神経に不可逆的な障害を残すことがある．下腿の前コンパートメント症候群は最もよくみられ，患者はひどい痛みに見舞われ，趾を背屈させることができない．このような場合，緊急的に下腿筋膜を切開し，筋区画内の組織圧を下げ，神経と血管を圧迫から解放しなければならない．

図 27.40 下腿と足の神経と血管：前方から見たところ

右の下腿と足，底屈位．

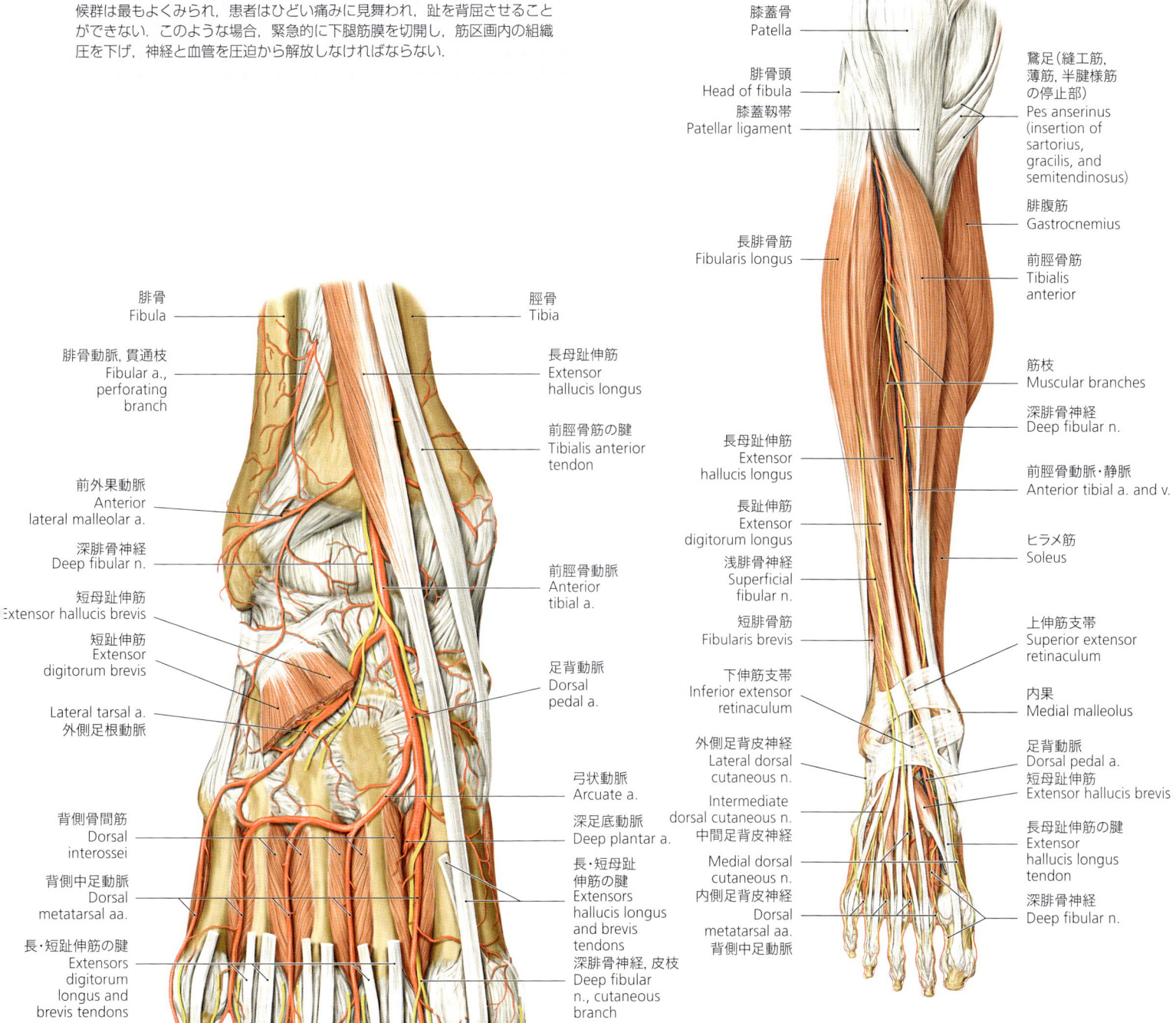

A 足背の神経と血管．

B 下腿の神経と血管．皮膚，皮下組織，筋膜を取り除いてある．前脛骨筋と長母趾伸筋を内側へ引いてある．

足底の局所解剖
Topography of the Sole of the Foot

図 27.41 足の神経と血管：足底
右足，足底方向から見たところ．

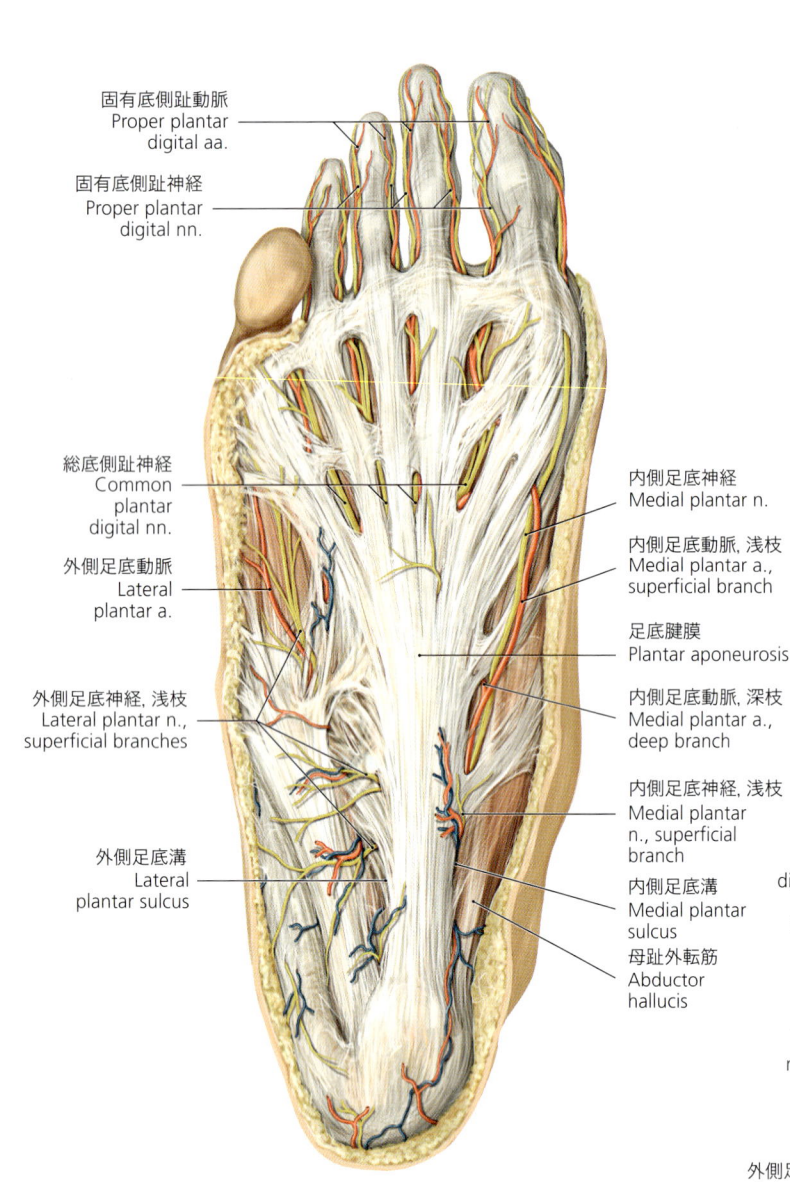

- 固有底側趾動脈 Proper plantar digital aa.
- 固有底側趾神経 Proper plantar digital nn.
- 総底側趾神経 Common plantar digital nn.
- 外側足底動脈 Lateral plantar a.
- 外側足底神経, 浅枝 Lateral plantar n., superficial branches
- 外側足底溝 Lateral plantar sulcus
- 内側足底神経 Medial plantar n.
- 内側足底動脈, 浅枝 Medial plantar a., superficial branch
- 足底腱膜 Plantar aponeurosis
- 内側足底動脈, 深枝 Medial plantar a., deep branch
- 内側足底神経, 浅枝 Medial plantar n., superficial branch
- 内側足底溝 Medial plantar sulcus
- 母趾外転筋 Abductor hallucis

A 浅層．皮膚，皮下組織，筋膜を取り除いてある．

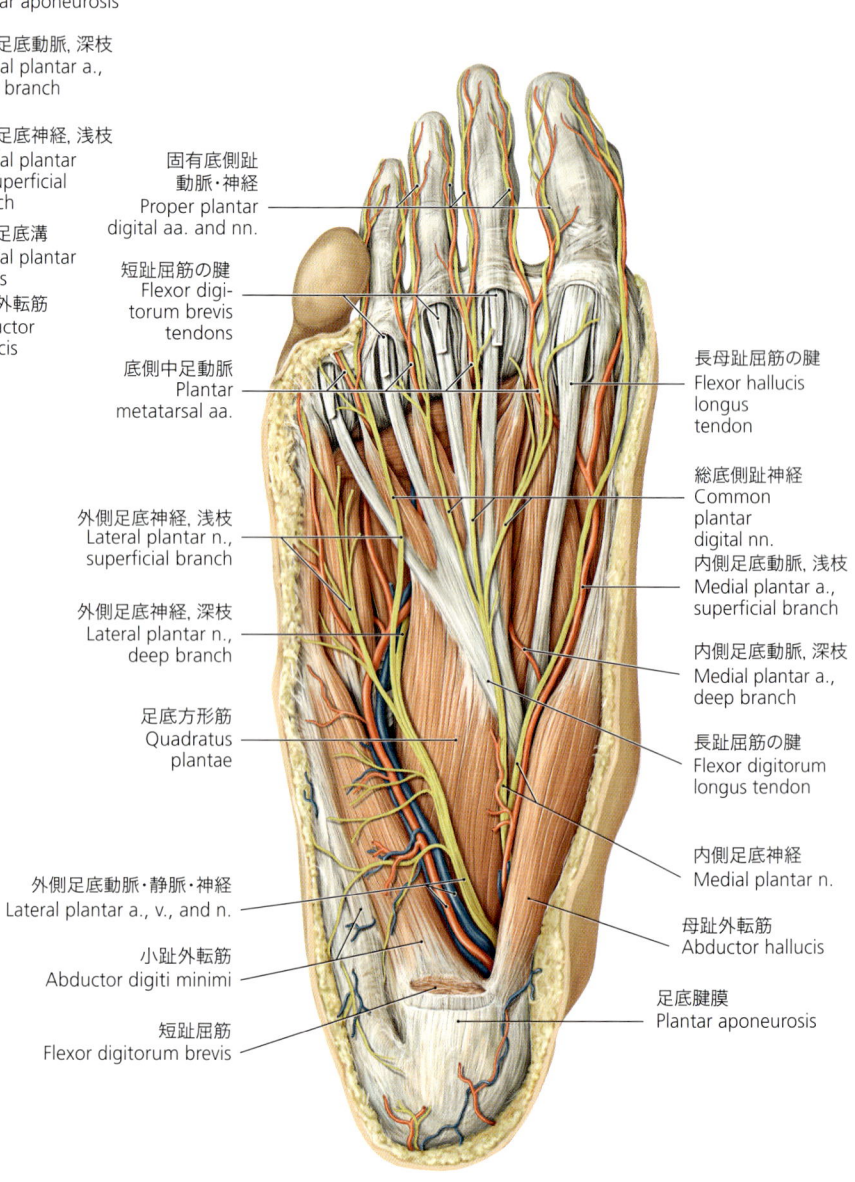

- 固有底側趾動脈・神経 Proper plantar digital aa. and nn.
- 短趾屈筋の腱 Flexor digitorum brevis tendons
- 底側中足動脈 Plantar metatarsal aa.
- 外側足底神経, 浅枝 Lateral plantar n., superficial branch
- 外側足底神経, 深枝 Lateral plantar n., deep branch
- 足底方形筋 Quadratus plantae
- 外側足底動脈・静脈・神経 Lateral plantar a., v., and n.
- 小趾外転筋 Abductor digiti minimi
- 短趾屈筋 Flexor digitorum brevis
- 長母趾屈筋の腱 Flexor hallucis longus tendon
- 総底側趾神経 Common plantar digital nn.
- 内側足底動脈, 浅枝 Medial plantar a., superficial branch
- 内側足底動脈, 深枝 Medial plantar a., deep branch
- 長趾屈筋の腱 Flexor digitorum longus tendon
- 内側足底神経 Medial plantar n.
- 母趾外転筋 Abductor hallucis
- 足底腱膜 Plantar aponeurosis

B 中間層．足底腱膜，短趾伸筋を取り除いたところ．

27 神経と脈管

固有底側趾動脈・神経
Proper plantar digital aa. and nn.

短趾屈筋の腱
Flexor digitorum brevis tendons

底側骨間筋
Plantar interossei

底側中足動脈
Plantar metatarsal aa.

深足底動脈弓
Deep plantar arch

外側足底神経, 深枝
Lateral plantar n., deep branch

足底方形筋
Quadratus plantae

外側足底動脈・静脈・神経
Lateral plantar a., v., and n.

短趾屈筋
Flexor digitorum brevis

長趾屈筋の腱
Flexor digitorum longus tendons

虫様筋
Lumbricals

横頭
Transverse head
斜頭
Oblique head
母趾内転筋
Adductor hallucis

短母趾屈筋
Flexor hallucis brevis

内側足底動脈, 深枝
Medial plantar a., deep branch

長母趾屈筋の腱
Flexor hallucis longus tendon

内側足底動脈
Medial plantar a.

内側足底神経
Medial plantar n.

母趾外転筋
Abductor hallucis

足底腱膜
Plantar aponeurosis

C 深層. 長趾伸筋の腱と虫様筋を取り除いたところ. また, 母趾内転筋の斜頭を部分的に取り除いてある.

図 27.42　足の神経と血管：前額断面
遠位方向（前方）から見たところ.

長趾伸筋
Extensor digitorum longus

第3中足骨
3rd metatarsal

長趾伸筋
Extensor digitorum longus

外側足背皮神経
Lateral dorsal cutaneous n.

背側中足動脈
Dorsal metatarsal a.

小趾外転筋
Abductor digiti minimi

小趾対立筋
Opponens digiti minimi

短小趾屈筋
Flexor digiti minimi brevis

外側足底動脈・静脈
Lateral plantar a. and v.

外側足底中隔
Lateral plantar septum

外側足底神経, 浅枝
Lateral plantar n., superficial branch

足底方形筋
Quadratus plantae

長腓骨筋
Fibularis longus

長趾屈筋腱膜
Aponeurosis of flexor digitorum longus

短趾屈筋
Flexor digitorum brevis

中間足背皮神経
Intermediate dorsal cutaneous n.

骨間筋
Interossei

長趾伸筋
Extensor digitorum longus

深腓骨神経, 足背動脈
Deep fibular n., dorsal pedal a.

短母趾伸筋
Extensor hallucis brevis

長母趾伸筋
Extensor hallucis longus

内側足背皮神経
Medial dorsal cutaneous n.

第2中足骨
2nd metatarsal

内側楔状骨
Medial cuneiform

前脛骨筋
Tibialis anterior

足底筋膜の深層
Deep layer of plantar fascia

伏在神経, 皮枝
Saphenous n., cutaneous branch

母趾外転筋
Abductor hallucis

外側足底神経, 深枝
Lateral plantar n., deep branch

短母趾屈筋
Flexor hallucis brevis

長母趾屈筋
Flexor hallucis longus

内側足底中隔
Medial plantar septum

内側足底動脈・神経
Medial plantar a. and n.

足底腱膜
Plantar aponeurosis

深足底動脈弓
Deep plantar arch

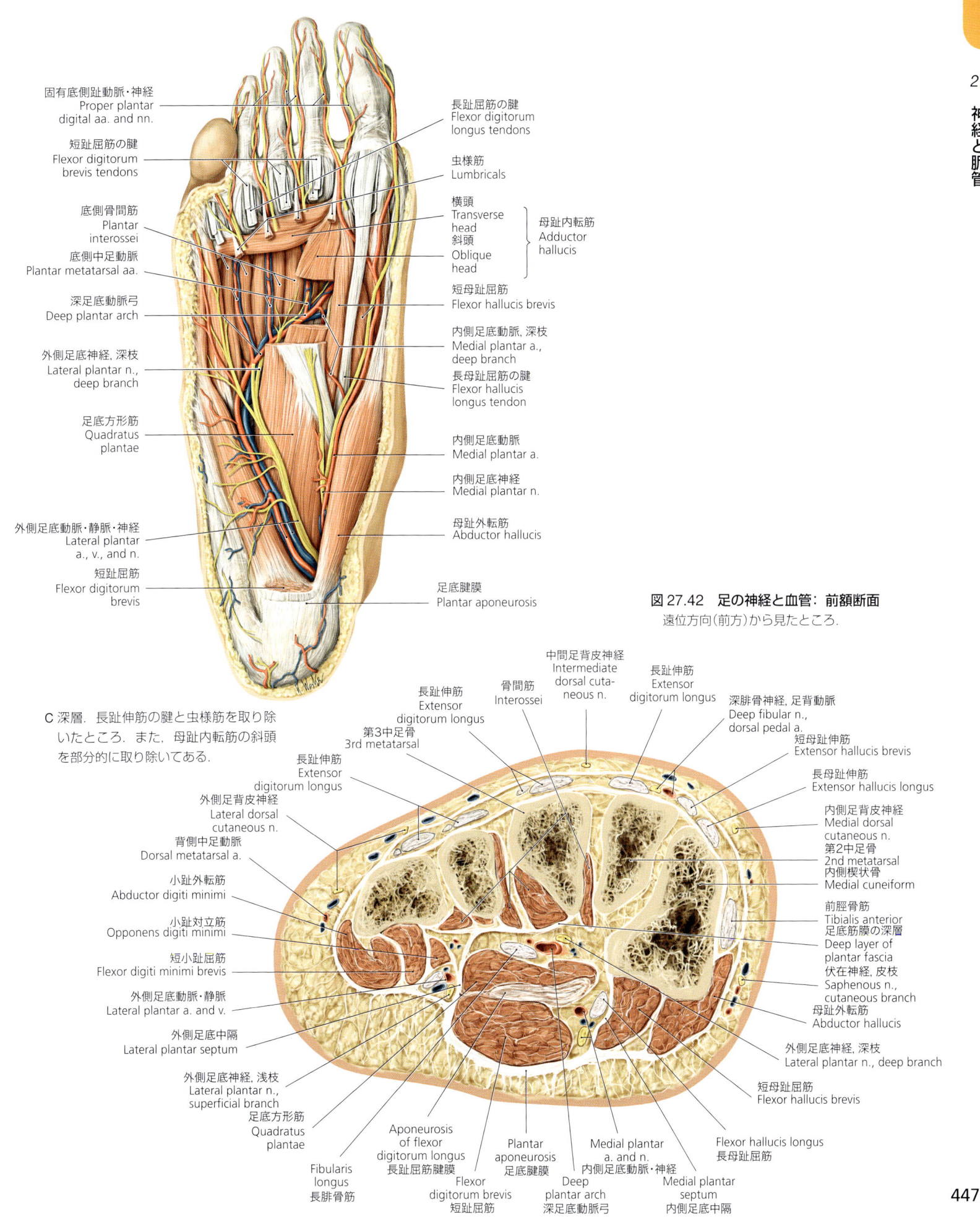

大腿と下腿の断面解剖
Transverse Sections of the Thigh & Leg

下肢

図 27.43 立体断面
右下肢，後方から見たところ．

大殿筋	Gluteus maximus
梨状筋	Piriformis
上双子筋と下双子筋	Gemellus superior and inferior
内閉鎖筋	Obturator internus
薄筋	Gracilis
大内転筋	Adductor magnus
半腱様筋	Semitendinosus
大腿二頭筋, 長頭	Biceps femoris, long head
内側広筋	Vastus medialis
縫工筋	Sartorius
薄筋	Gracilis
長内転筋と短内転筋	Adductors brevis and longus
坐骨神経	Sciatic n.
大内転筋	Adductor magnus
半腱様筋	Semitendinosus
半膜様筋	Semimembranosus
腓腹筋	Gastrocnemius
脛骨	Tibia
ヒラメ筋	Soleus
下腿三頭筋	Triceps surae
腓腹筋	Gastrocnemius
踵骨腱（アキレス腱）	Achilles' tendon
腸骨稜	Iliac crest
中殿筋	Gluteus medius
小殿筋	Gluteus minimus
大腿筋膜張筋	Tensor fasciae latae
大殿筋	Gluteus maximus
大腿方形筋	Quadratus femoris
大内転筋	Adductor magnus
腸脛靱帯	Iliotibial tract
大腿骨	Femur
大腿直筋	Rectus femoris
中間広筋	Vastus intermedius
外側広筋	Vastus lateralis
大腿二頭筋, 短頭	Biceps femoris, short head
腸脛靱帯	Iliotibial tract
大腿二頭筋, 長頭	Biceps femoris, long head
足底筋	Plantaris
腓骨	Fibula
下腿骨間膜	Interosseous membrane

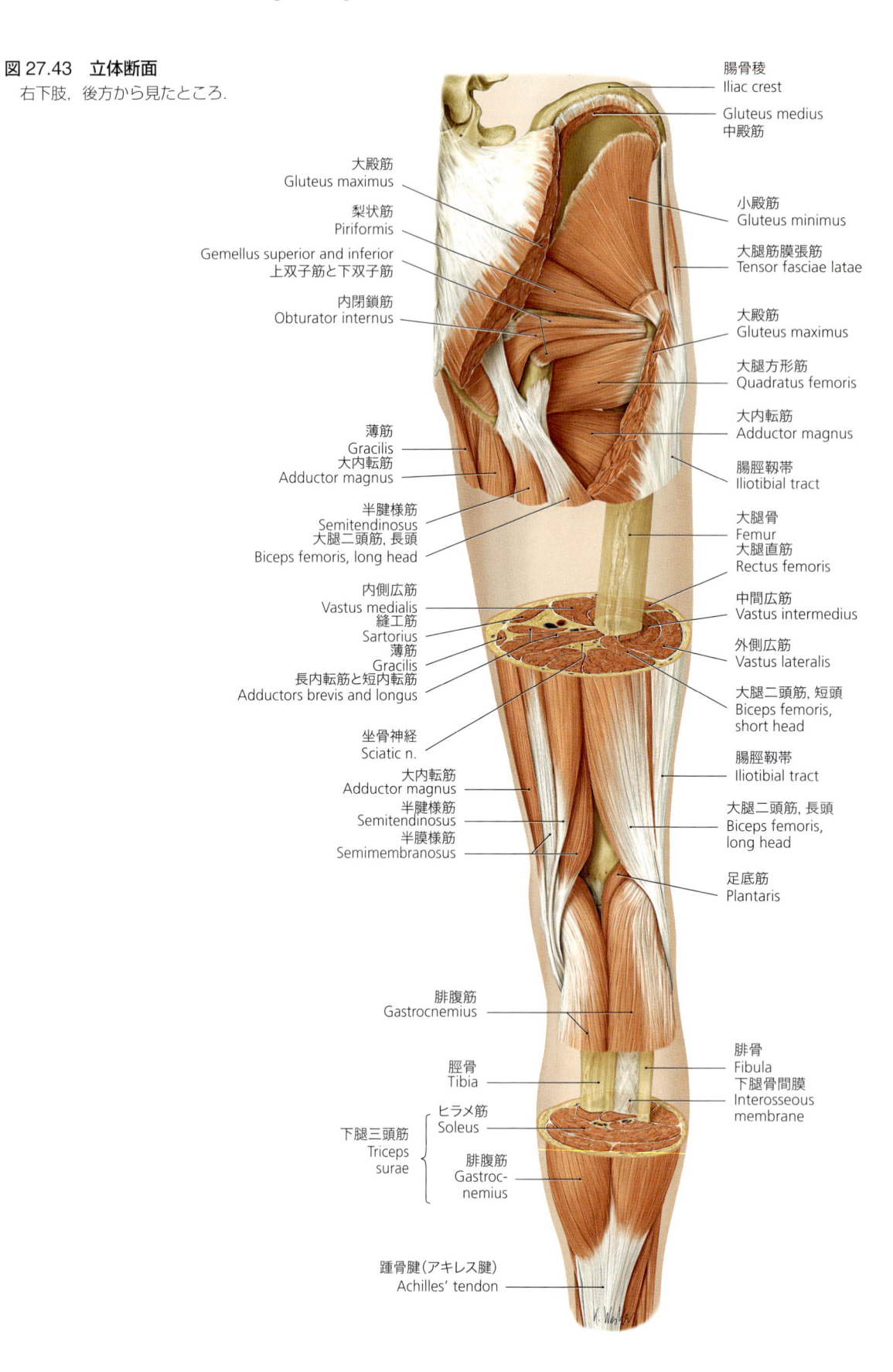

図 27.44 横断面
右下肢, 後面. 近位方向（上方）から見たところ.

大腿四頭筋 Quadriceps femoris
- 内側広筋 Vastus medialis
- 中間広筋 Vastus intermedius
- 大腿直筋 Rectus femoris
- 外側広筋 Vastus lateralis

前面（腹側） ↑

- Medial intermuscular septum 内側大腿筋間中隔
- 縫工筋 Sartorius
- 大腿動脈・静脈 Femoral a. and v.
- 深大腿動脈・静脈 Profunda femoris a., deep femoral v.
- 短内転筋 Adductor brevis
- 長内転筋 Adductor longus
- 薄筋 Gracilis
- 大内転筋 Adductor magnus
- Semimembranosus 半膜様筋
- Semitendinosus 半腱様筋
- 大腿骨 Femur
- 腸脛靱帯 Iliotibial tract
- 坐骨神経 Sciatic n.
- 外側大腿筋間中隔 Lateral intermuscular septum
- Short head 短頭
- Long head 長頭
- 大腿二頭筋 Biceps femoris

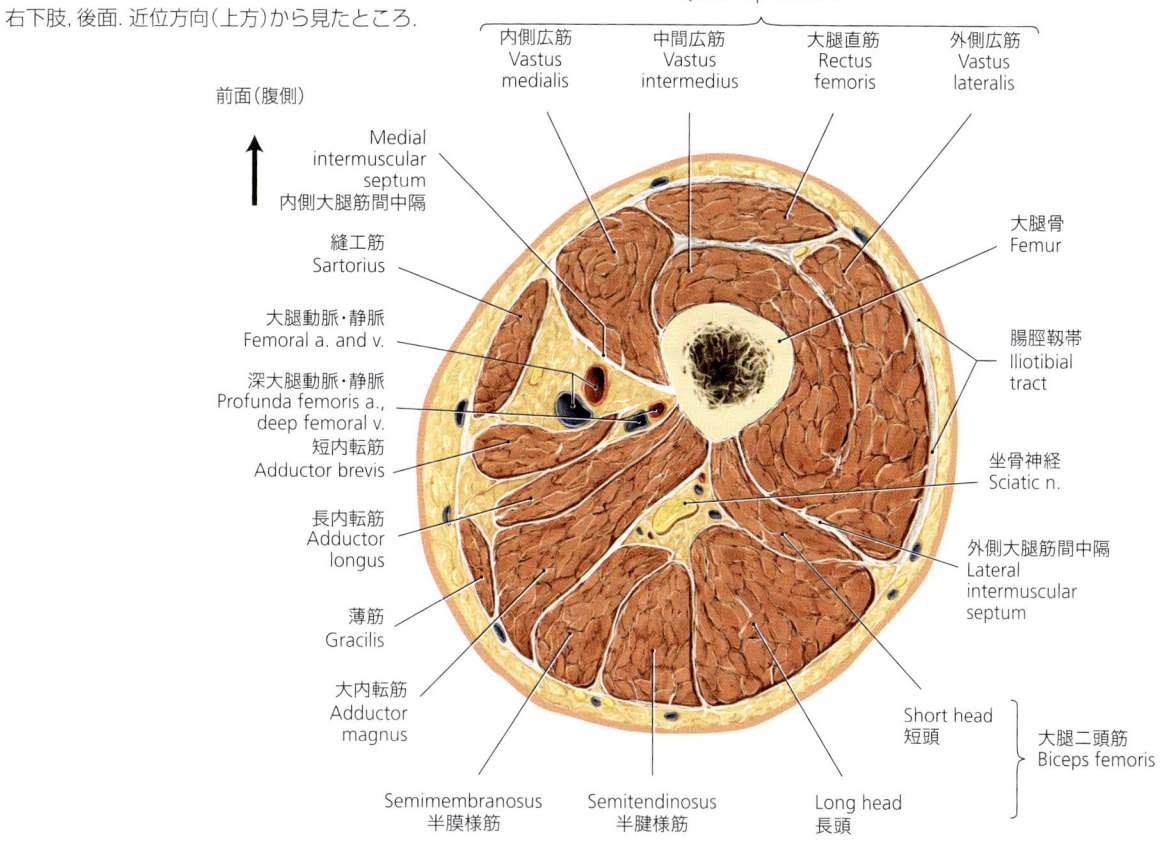

A 大腿（図 27.43 における断面）.

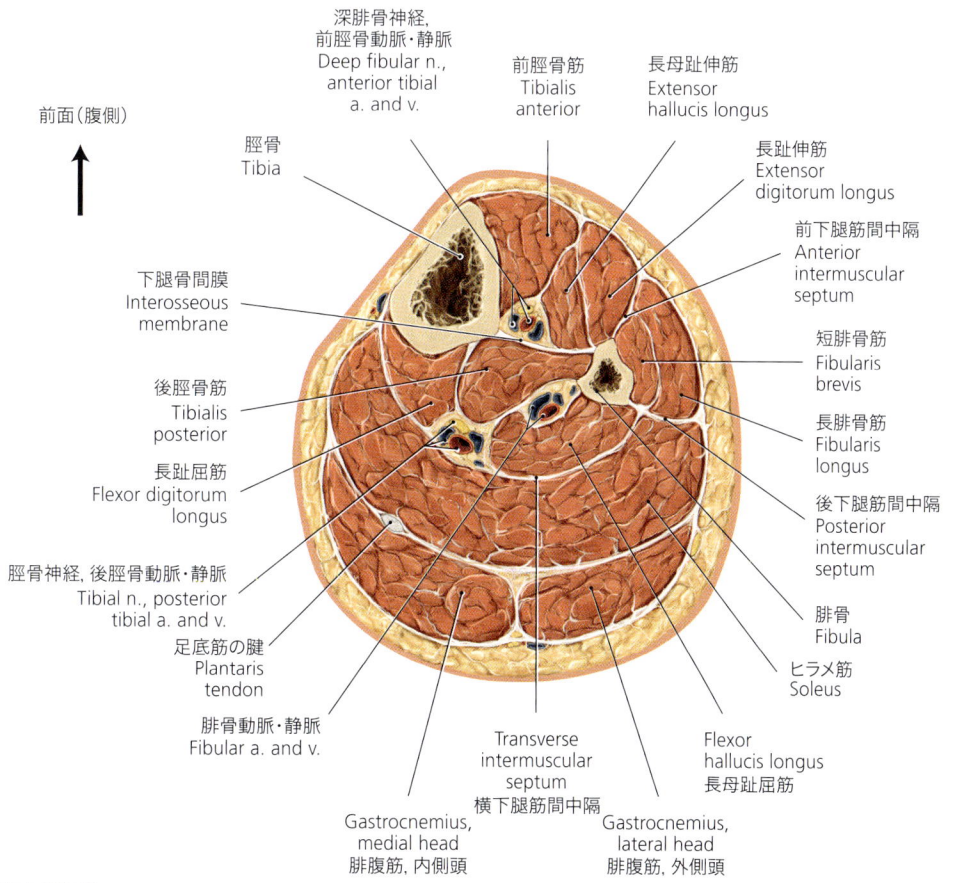

前面（腹側） ↑

- 深腓骨神経, 前脛骨動脈・静脈 Deep fibular n., anterior tibial a. and v.
- 前脛骨筋 Tibialis anterior
- 長母趾伸筋 Extensor hallucis longus
- 脛骨 Tibia
- 長趾伸筋 Extensor digitorum longus
- 下腿骨間膜 Interosseous membrane
- 前下腿筋間中隔 Anterior intermuscular septum
- 後脛骨筋 Tibialis posterior
- 短腓骨筋 Fibularis brevis
- 長趾屈筋 Flexor digitorum longus
- 長腓骨筋 Fibularis longus
- 脛骨神経, 後脛骨動脈・静脈 Tibial n., posterior tibial a. and v.
- 後下腿筋間中隔 Posterior intermuscular septum
- 足底筋の腱 Plantaris tendon
- 腓骨 Fibula
- ヒラメ筋 Soleus
- 腓骨動脈・静脈 Fibular a. and v.
- Transverse intermuscular septum 横下腿筋間中隔
- Flexor hallucis longus 長母趾屈筋
- Gastrocnemius, medial head 腓腹筋, 内側頭
- Gastrocnemius, lateral head 腓腹筋, 外側頭

B 下腿（図 27.43 における断面）.

下肢

体表解剖
Surface Anatomy

図28.1 下肢：前方から見たところ

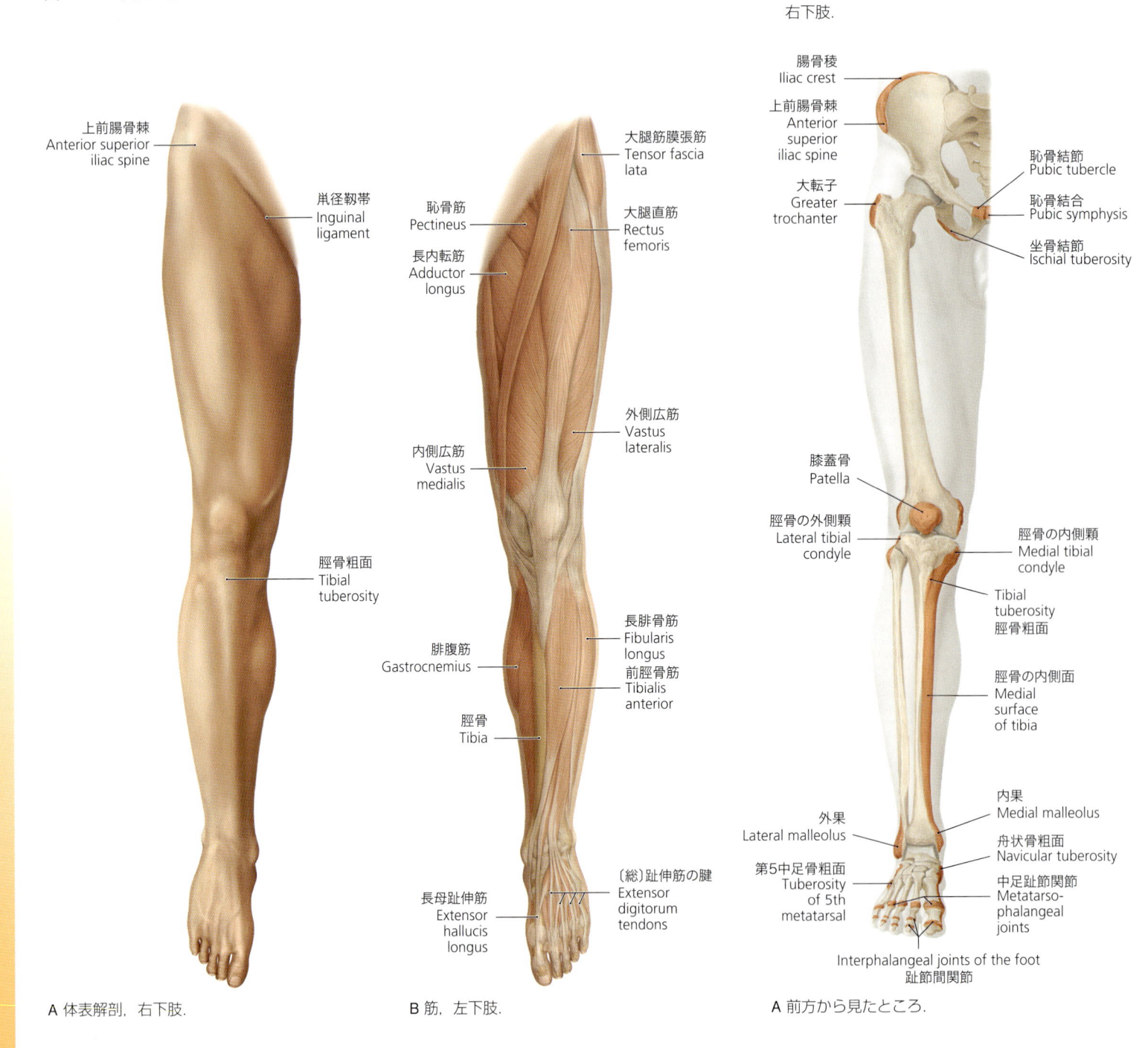

- 上前腸骨棘 Anterior superior iliac spine
- 鼠径靱帯 Inguinal ligament
- 脛骨粗面 Tibial tuberosity

A 体表解剖，右下肢.

- 大腿筋膜張筋 Tensor fascia lata
- 恥骨筋 Pectineus
- 大腿直筋 Rectus femoris
- 長内転筋 Adductor longus
- 外側広筋 Vastus lateralis
- 内側広筋 Vastus medialis
- 長腓骨筋 Fibularis longus
- 腓腹筋 Gastrocnemius
- 前脛骨筋 Tibialis anterior
- 脛骨 Tibia
- 長母趾伸筋 Extensor hallucis longus
- （総）趾伸筋の腱 Extensor digitorum tendons

B 筋，左下肢.

図28.2 体表から触知できる骨の隆起

右下肢.

- 腸骨稜 Iliac crest
- 上前腸骨棘 Anterior superior iliac spine
- 大転子 Greater trochanter
- 恥骨結節 Pubic tubercle
- 恥骨結合 Pubic symphysis
- 坐骨結節 Ischial tuberosity
- 膝蓋骨 Patella
- 脛骨の外側顆 Lateral tibial condyle
- 脛骨の内側顆 Medial tibial condyle
- 脛骨粗面 Tibial tuberosity
- 脛骨の内側面 Medial surface of tibia
- 外果 Lateral malleolus
- 内果 Medial malleolus
- 第5中足骨粗面 Tuberosity of 5th metatarsal
- 舟状骨粗面 Navicular tuberosity
- 中足趾節関節 Metatarso-phalangeal joints
- Interphalangeal joints of the foot 趾節間関節

A 前方から見たところ.

Q1：体表から股関節を触知することはできない．体表の構造をもとに，大腿骨頭の位置を正確に把握するにはどのようにすればよいか？

図 28.3 下肢：後方から見たところ

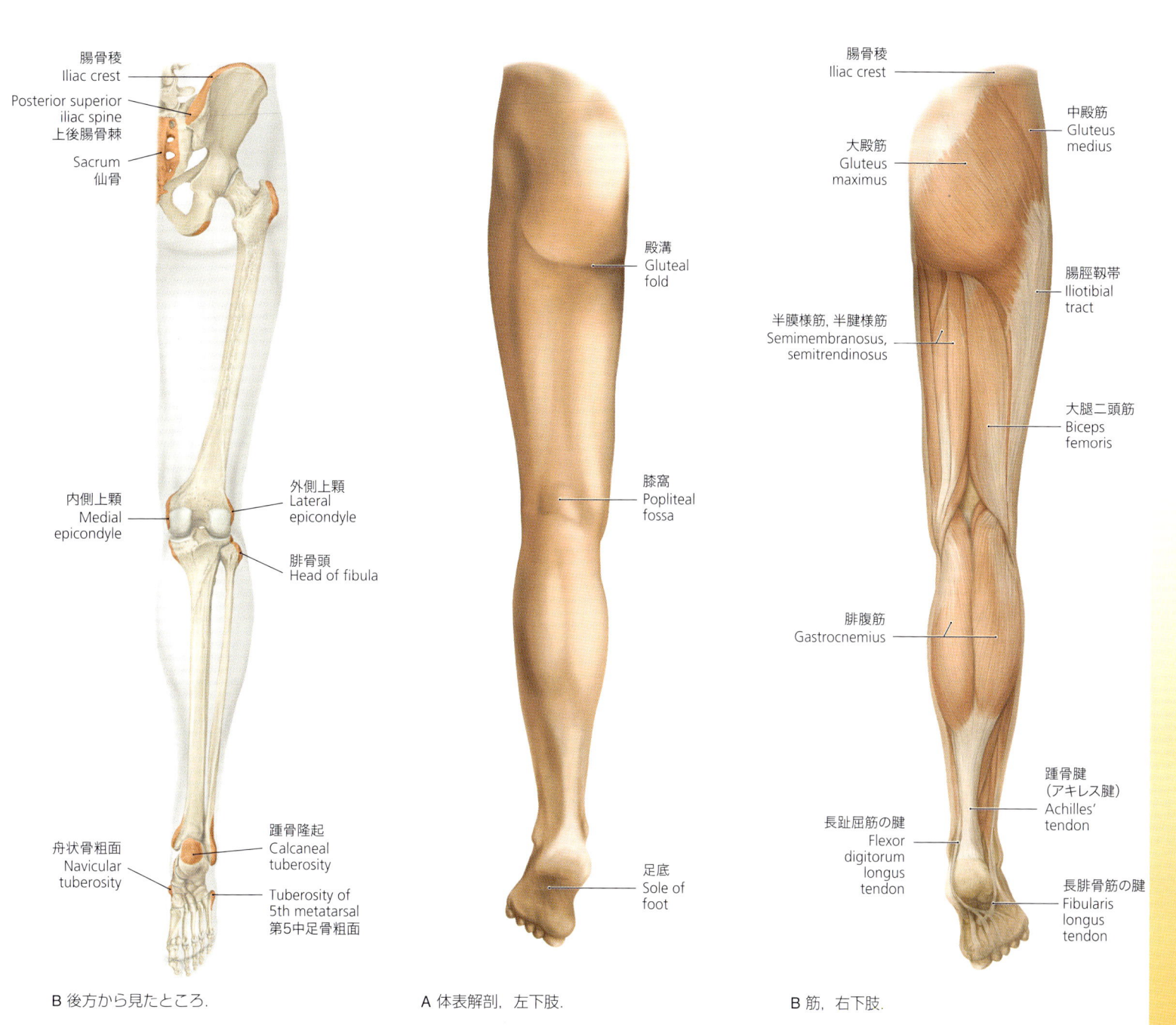

- 腸骨稜 Iliac crest
- Posterior superior iliac spine 上後腸骨棘
- Sacrum 仙骨
- 内側上顆 Medial epicondyle
- 外側上顆 Lateral epicondyle
- 腓骨頭 Head of fibula
- 舟状骨粗面 Navicular tuberosity
- 踵骨隆起 Calcaneal tuberosity
- Tuberosity of 5th metatarsal 第5中足骨粗面

B 後方から見たところ．

- 殿溝 Gluteal fold
- 膝窩 Popliteal fossa
- 足底 Sole of foot

A 体表解剖，左下肢．

- 腸骨稜 Iliac crest
- 中殿筋 Gluteus medius
- 大殿筋 Gluteus maximus
- 腸脛靱帯 Iliotibial tract
- 半膜様筋，半腱様筋 Semimembranosus, semitrendinosus
- 大腿二頭筋 Biceps femoris
- 腓腹筋 Gastrocnemius
- 踵骨腱（アキレス腱）Achilles' tendon
- 長趾屈筋の腱 Flexor digitorum longus tendon
- 長腓骨筋の腱 Fibularis longus tendon

B 筋，右下肢．

Q2: 次の神経の位置を把握するには，触知できる構造のうちどれを利用すればよいか？ ①殿部における坐骨神経，②膝における総腓骨神経，③足首における脛骨神経

答えは p. 627 を参照．

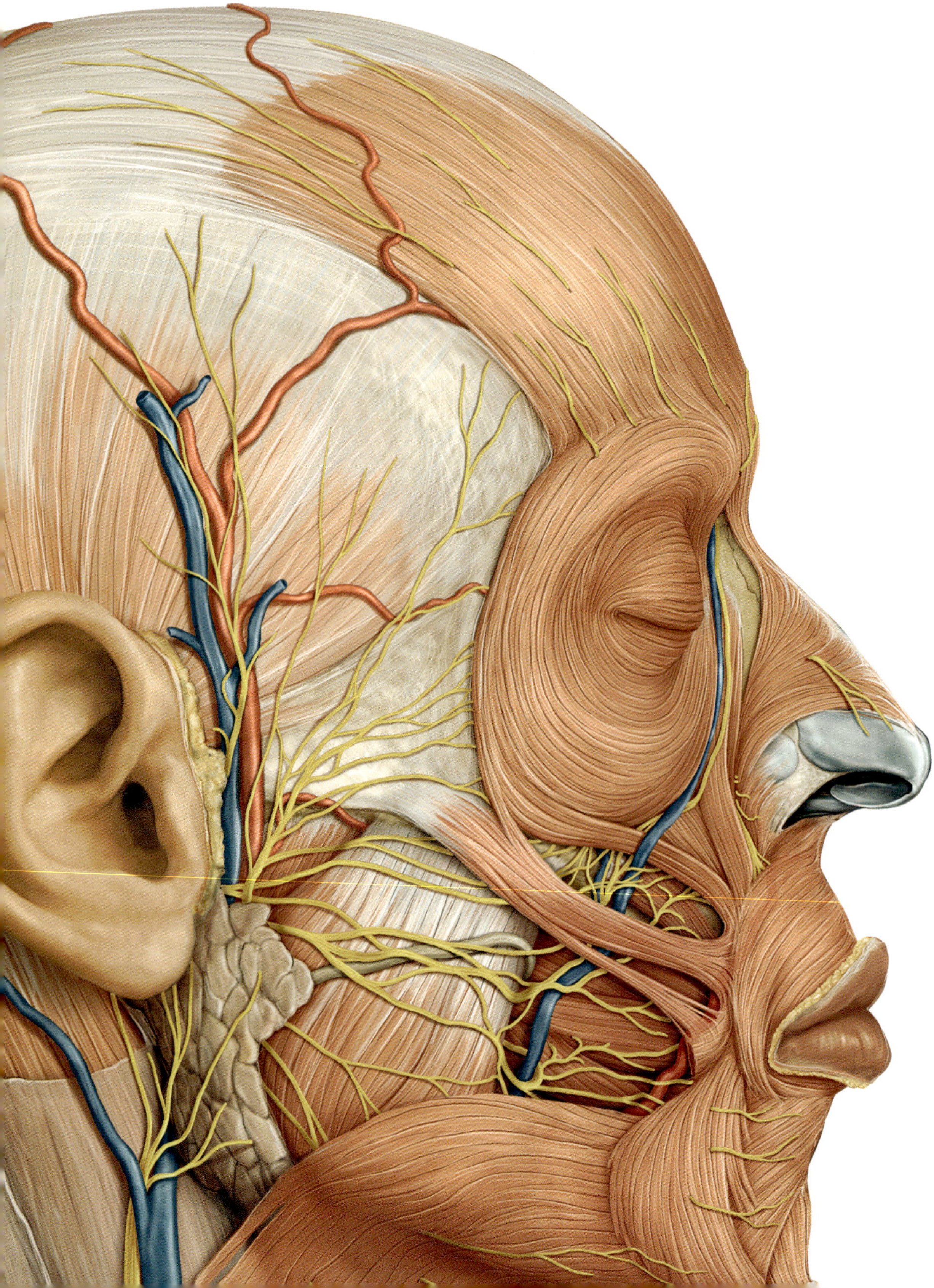

頭頸部
Head & Neck

29. 頭部の骨
- 頭蓋：側面と前面 ……………………………… 454
- 頭蓋：後面と頭蓋冠 …………………………… 456
- 頭蓋底 …………………………………………… 458
- 篩骨と蝶形骨 …………………………………… 460

30. 頭部・顔面の筋
- 表情筋と咀嚼筋 ………………………………… 462
- 頭部の筋，起始と停止 ………………………… 464
- 頭部の筋（1） …………………………………… 466
- 頭部の筋（2） …………………………………… 468

31. 脳神経
- 脳神経の概観 …………………………………… 470
- 脳神経：嗅神経（CN I）と視神経（CN II） …… 472
- 脳神経：動眼神経（CN III），滑車神経（CN IV），外転神経（CN VI） ……………………… 474
- 脳神経：三叉神経（CN V） …………………… 476
- 脳神経：顔面神経（CN VII） ………………… 478
- 脳神経：内耳神経（CN VIII） ………………… 480
- 脳神経：舌咽神経（CN IX） …………………… 482
- 脳神経：迷走神経（CN X） …………………… 484
- 脳神経：副神経（CN XI）と舌下神経（CN XII） … 486

32. 頭部・顔面の神経と血管
- 顔面の神経支配 ………………………………… 488
- 頭頸部の動脈 …………………………………… 490
- 外頸動脈：前枝，内側枝，後枝 ……………… 492
- 外頸動脈：終枝 ………………………………… 494
- 頭頸部の静脈 …………………………………… 496
- 顔面浅層の局所解剖 …………………………… 498
- 耳下腺咬筋部と側頭窩の局所解剖 …………… 500
- 側頭下窩の局所解剖 …………………………… 502
- 翼口蓋窩の局所解剖 …………………………… 504

33. 眼窩と眼
- 眼窩の骨 ………………………………………… 506
- 眼窩の筋 ………………………………………… 508
- 眼窩の神経と血管 ……………………………… 510
- 眼窩の局所解剖 ………………………………… 512
- 眼窩と眼瞼 ……………………………………… 514
- 眼球 ……………………………………………… 516
- 角膜，虹彩，水晶体 …………………………… 518

34. 鼻腔と鼻
- 鼻腔の骨 ………………………………………… 520
- 副鼻腔 …………………………………………… 522
- 鼻腔の神経と血管 ……………………………… 524

35. 側頭骨と耳
- 側頭骨 …………………………………………… 526
- 外耳と外耳道 …………………………………… 528
- 中耳：鼓室 ……………………………………… 530
- 中耳：耳小骨連鎖と鼓膜 ……………………… 532
- 中耳：中耳の動脈 ……………………………… 534
- 内耳 ……………………………………………… 536

36. 口腔・咽頭
- 口腔の骨 ………………………………………… 538
- 顎関節 …………………………………………… 540
- 歯 ………………………………………………… 542
- 口腔の筋 ………………………………………… 544
- 口腔の神経支配 ………………………………… 546
- 舌 ………………………………………………… 548
- 口腔と唾液腺の局所解剖 ……………………… 550
- 扁桃と咽頭 ……………………………………… 552
- 咽頭筋 …………………………………………… 554
- 咽頭の神経と血管 ……………………………… 556

37. 頸部
- 頸部の骨と靱帯 ………………………………… 558
- 頸部の筋肉（1） ………………………………… 560
- 頸部の筋肉（2） ………………………………… 562
- 頸部の筋肉（3） ………………………………… 564
- 頸部の動脈と静脈 ……………………………… 566
- 頸部の神経支配 ………………………………… 568
- 喉頭：軟骨と構造 ……………………………… 570
- 喉頭：筋と区分 ………………………………… 572
- 喉頭の神経と血管，甲状腺と副甲状腺（上皮小体） … 574
- 頸部の局所解剖：部位と筋膜 ………………… 576
- 前頸部の局所解剖 ……………………………… 578
- 前頸部と外側頸三角部の局所解剖 …………… 580
- 外側頸三角部の局所解剖 ……………………… 582
- 後頸部の局所解剖 ……………………………… 584
- 頸部のリンパ管 ………………………………… 586

38. 体表解剖
- 体表解剖 ………………………………………… 588

頭蓋：側面と前面
Anterior & Lateral Skull

図 29.1　頭蓋の側面
左外側方から見たところ．

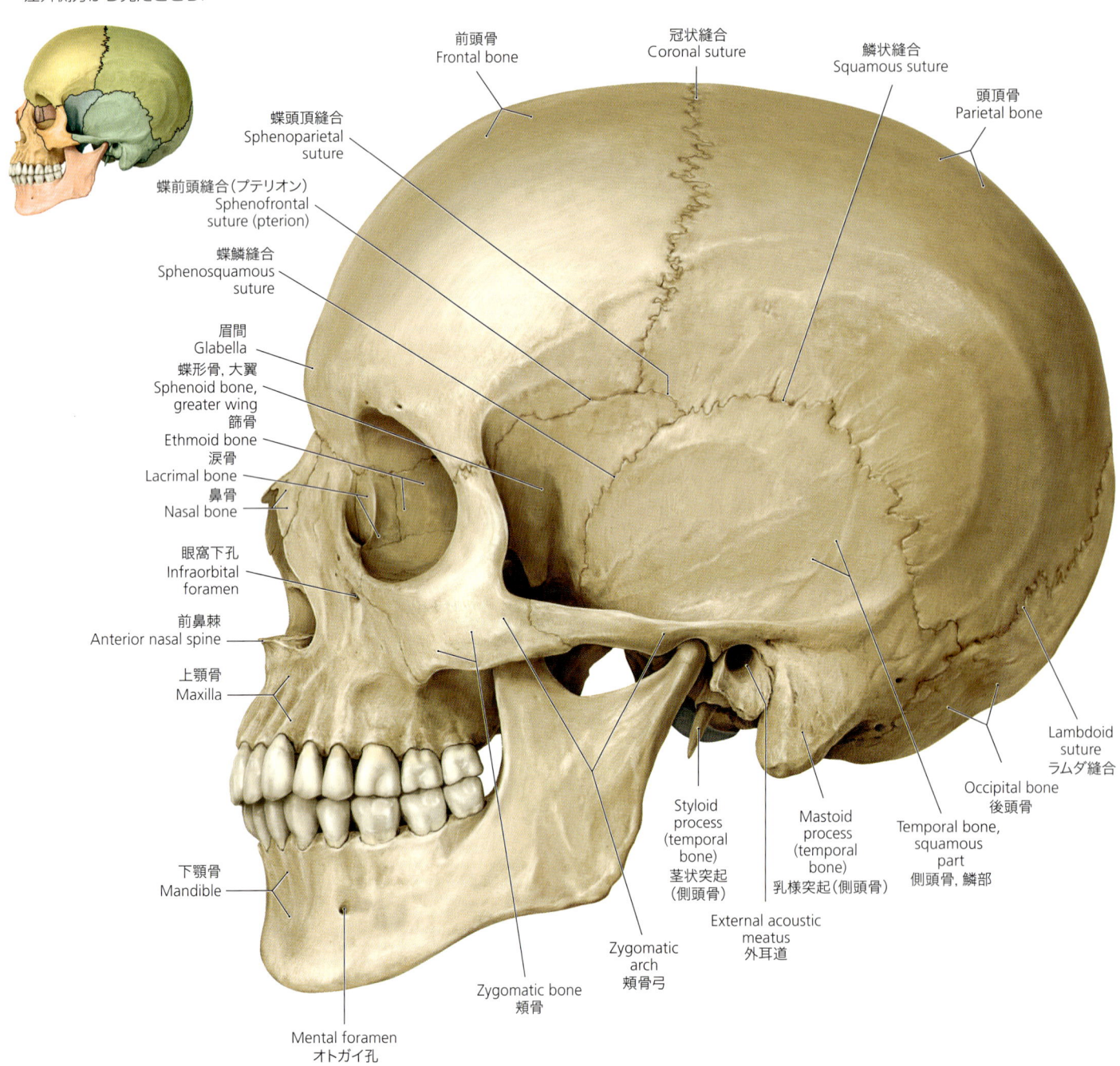

ラベル（図中）：
- 前頭骨　Frontal bone
- 冠状縫合　Coronal suture
- 鱗状縫合　Squamous suture
- 頭頂骨　Parietal bone
- 蝶頭頂縫合　Sphenoparietal suture
- 蝶前頭縫合（プテリオン）　Sphenofrontal suture (pterion)
- 蝶鱗縫合　Sphenosquamous suture
- 眉間　Glabella
- 蝶形骨，大翼　Sphenoid bone, greater wing
- 篩骨　Ethmoid bone
- 涙骨　Lacrimal bone
- 鼻骨　Nasal bone
- 眼窩下孔　Infraorbital foramen
- 前鼻棘　Anterior nasal spine
- 上顎骨　Maxilla
- 下顎骨　Mandible
- Mental foramen　オトガイ孔
- Zygomatic bone　頬骨
- Styloid process (temporal bone)　茎状突起（側頭骨）
- Zygomatic arch　頬骨弓
- Mastoid process (temporal bone)　乳様突起（側頭骨）
- External acoustic meatus　外耳道
- Temporal bone, squamous part　側頭骨，鱗部
- Occipital bone　後頭骨
- Lambdoid suture　ラムダ縫合

表 29.1　頭蓋の骨

頭蓋は脳頭蓋（灰色）と顔面頭蓋（オレンジ色）に分けられる．脳頭蓋は脳を保護し，顔面頭蓋は顔面の諸部分を収容して，保護する．

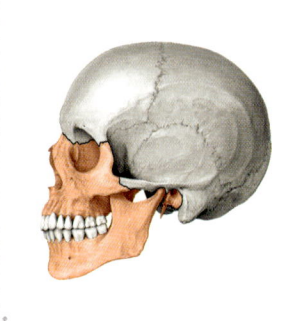

脳頭蓋	顔面頭蓋	
・篩骨（篩板）*	・篩骨	・鋤骨
・前頭骨	・舌骨	・上顎骨
・後頭骨	・下鼻甲介	・下顎骨
・頭頂骨	・涙骨	・鼻骨
・蝶形骨	・蝶形骨（翼状突起）	・口蓋骨
・側頭骨（岩様部と鱗部）	・側頭骨	・頬骨

*篩骨の大部分は顔面頭蓋にある．蝶形骨の大部分は脳頭蓋にある．側頭骨は二部に分けられる．

図29.2 頭蓋の前面
前方から見たところ.

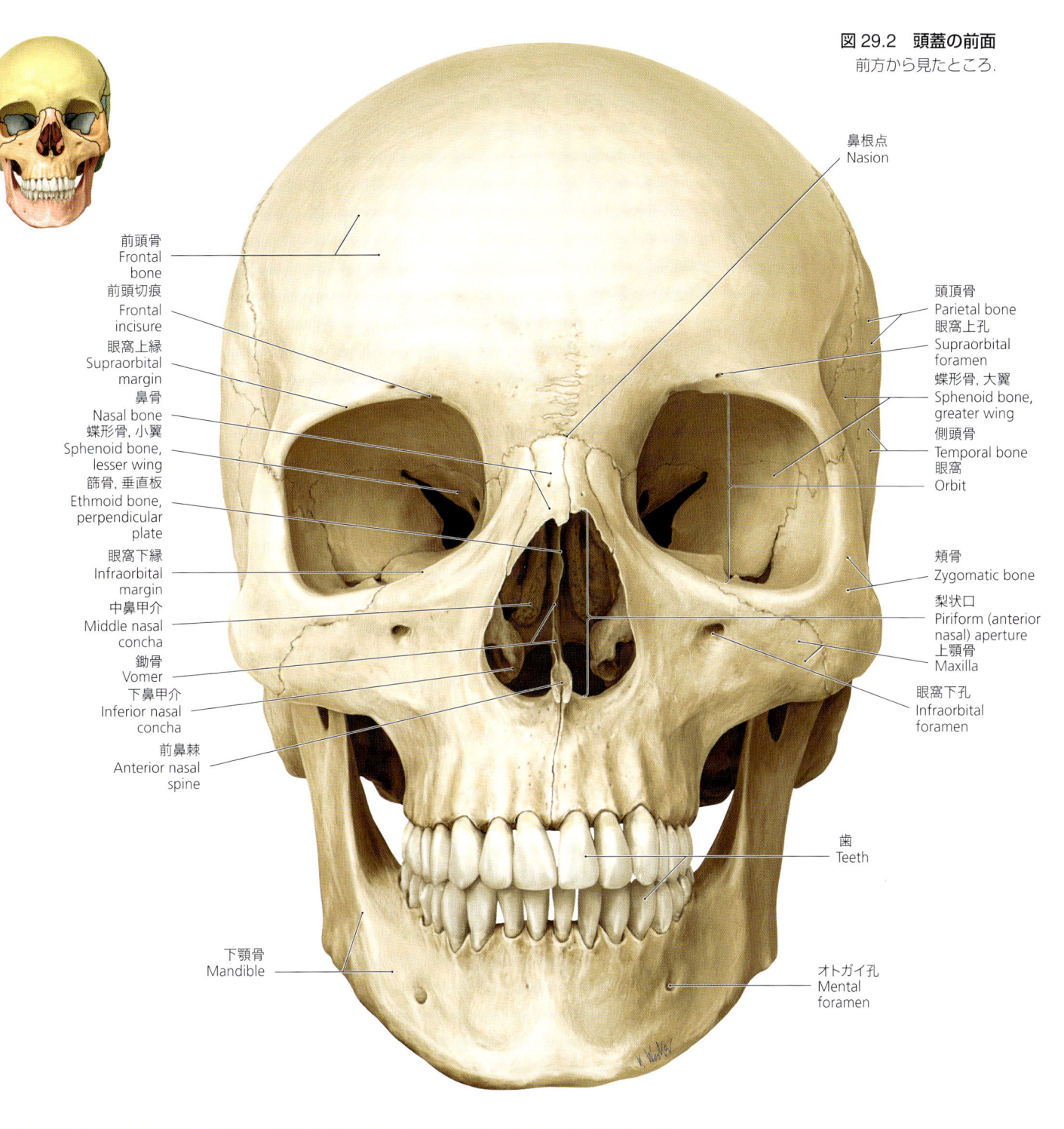

ラベル:
- 前頭骨 Frontal bone
- 前頭切痕 Frontal incisure
- 眼窩上縁 Supraorbital margin
- 鼻骨 Nasal bone
- 蝶形骨, 小翼 Sphenoid bone, lesser wing
- 篩骨, 垂直板 Ethmoid bone, perpendicular plate
- 眼窩下縁 Infraorbital margin
- 中鼻甲介 Middle nasal concha
- 鋤骨 Vomer
- 下鼻甲介 Inferior nasal concha
- 前鼻棘 Anterior nasal spine
- 下顎骨 Mandible
- 鼻根点 Nasion
- 頭頂骨 Parietal bone
- 眼窩上孔 Supraorbital foramen
- 蝶形骨, 大翼 Sphenoid bone, greater wing
- 側頭骨 Temporal bone
- 眼窩 Orbit
- 頬骨 Zygomatic bone
- 梨状口 Piriform (anterior nasal) aperture
- 上顎骨 Maxilla
- 眼窩下孔 Infraorbital foramen
- 歯 Teeth
- オトガイ孔 Mental foramen

臨床

顔面骨折
顔面骨格は枠状の構造であるために骨折線は特徴的なパターンを示し，ル・フォールⅠ型，ル・フォールⅡ型，ル・フォールⅢ型と分類される．

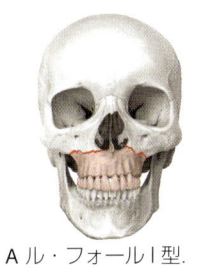

A ル・フォールⅠ型. 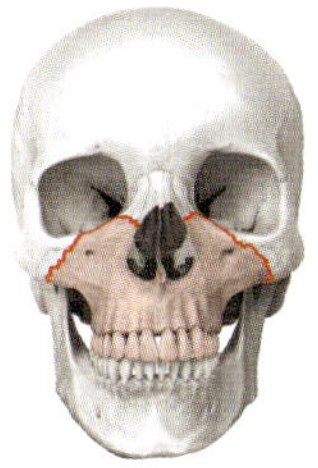　B ル・フォールⅡ型. 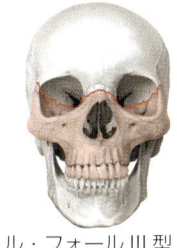　C ル・フォールⅢ型.

29 頭部の骨

頭蓋：後面と頭蓋冠
Posterior Skull & Calvaria

図 29.3　頭蓋
後方から見たところ．

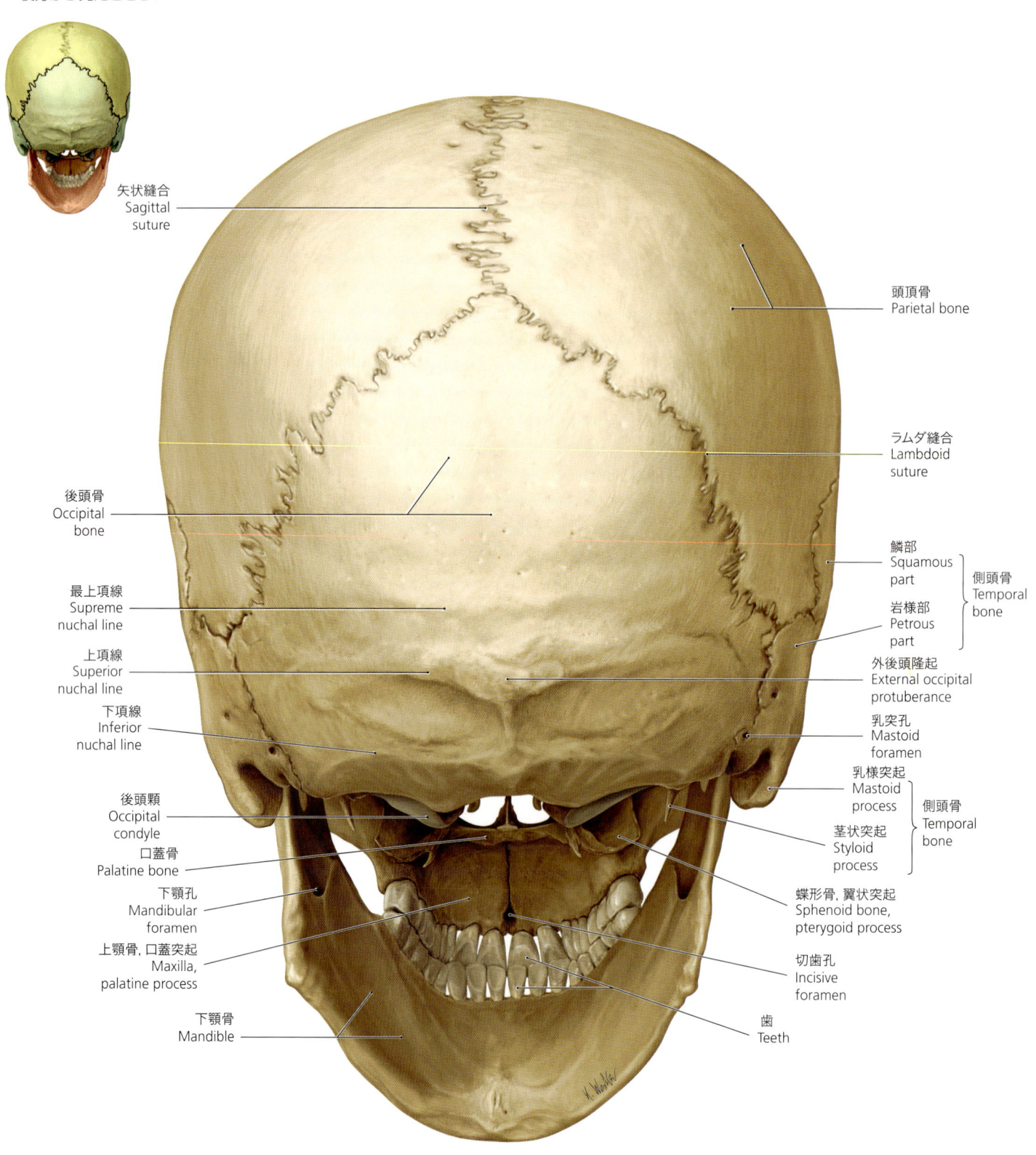

- 矢状縫合　Sagittal suture
- 頭頂骨　Parietal bone
- ラムダ縫合　Lambdoid suture
- 後頭骨　Occipital bone
- 鱗部　Squamous part ｝側頭骨 Temporal bone
- 岩様部　Petrous part
- 最上項線　Supreme nuchal line
- 外後頭隆起　External occipital protuberance
- 上項線　Superior nuchal line
- 乳突孔　Mastoid foramen
- 下項線　Inferior nuchal line
- 乳様突起　Mastoid process ｝側頭骨 Temporal bone
- 後頭顆　Occipital condyle
- 茎状突起　Styloid process
- 口蓋骨　Palatine bone
- 蝶形骨，翼状突起　Sphenoid bone, pterygoid process
- 下顎孔　Mandibular foramen
- 切歯孔　Incisive foramen
- 上顎骨，口蓋突起　Maxilla, palatine process
- 歯　Teeth
- 下顎骨　Mandible

図 29.4 頭蓋冠

図 29.5 頭蓋冠の構造
断面.

板間静脈 Diploic vv.
導出静脈 Emissary v.
頭皮 Scalp
硬膜静脈洞 Dural sinus
外板 Outer table
板間層 Diploë
内板 Inner table
硬膜 Dura mater
頭蓋冠 Calvaria

前頭骨 Frontal bone
冠状縫合 Coronal suture
頭頂骨 Parietal bone
矢状縫合 Sagittal suture
Parietal foramen 頭頂孔
Occipital bone 後頭骨
Lambdoid suture ラムダ縫合

A 頭蓋冠の外面，上方から見たところ．

前頭骨 Frontal bone
前頭稜 Frontal crest
前頭洞 Frontal sinus
動脈溝 Arterial grooves
頭頂骨 Parietal bone
クモ膜顆粒小窩 Granular foveolae (for arachnoid granulations)
上矢状洞溝 Groove for superior sagittal sinus
Parietal foramen 頭頂孔

B 頭蓋冠の内面，下方から見たところ．頭蓋冠の内面には硬膜の動脈，硬膜静脈洞，クモ膜顆粒の溝がある (pp.606-610 参照).

29 頭部の骨

457

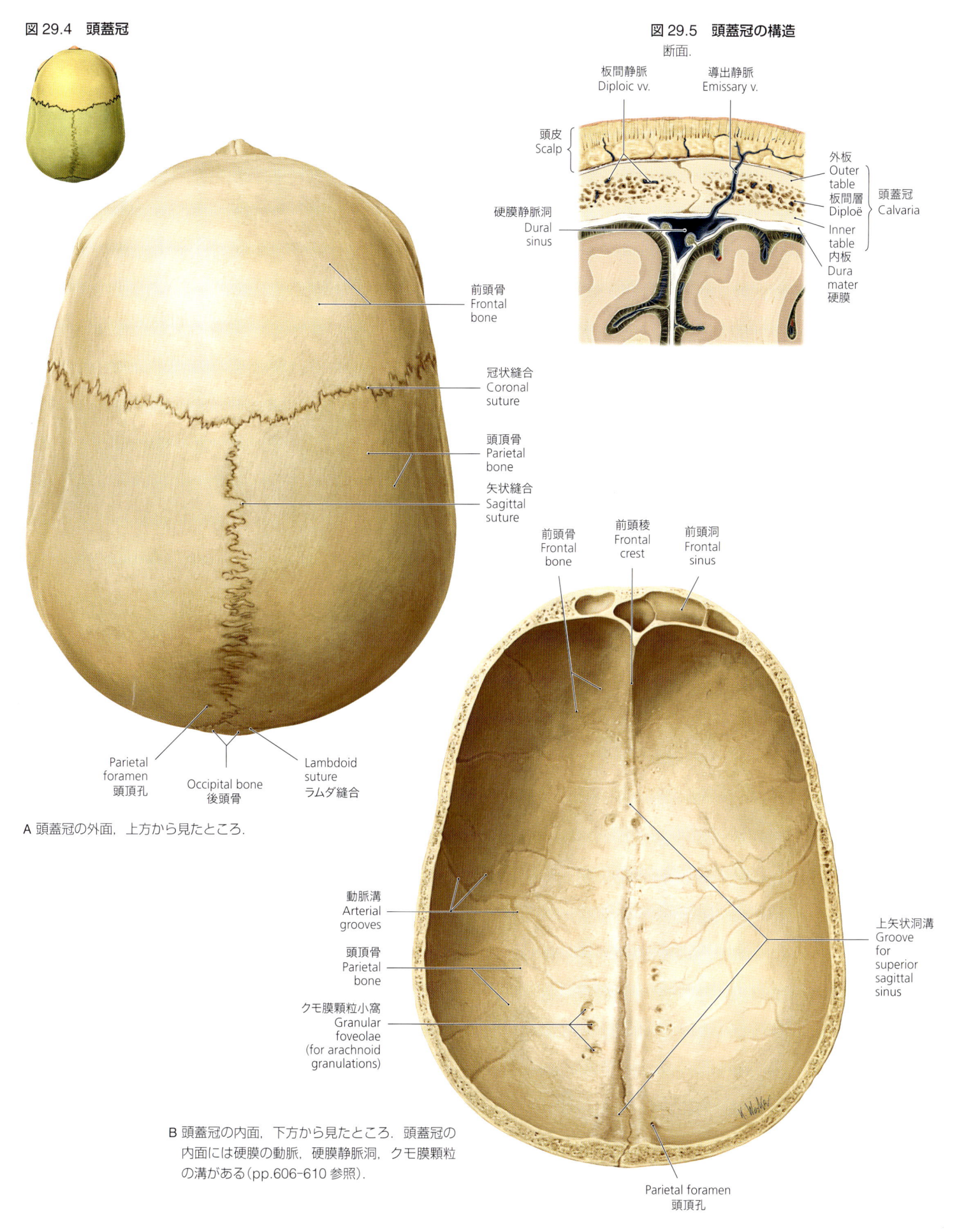

頭蓋底
Base of the Skull

図 29.6　頭蓋底，外面
下方から見たところ．神経や血管（p.490 参照）を通す開口部と管に注目．
Note: この方向からは鼻腔の後方部も見ることができる．

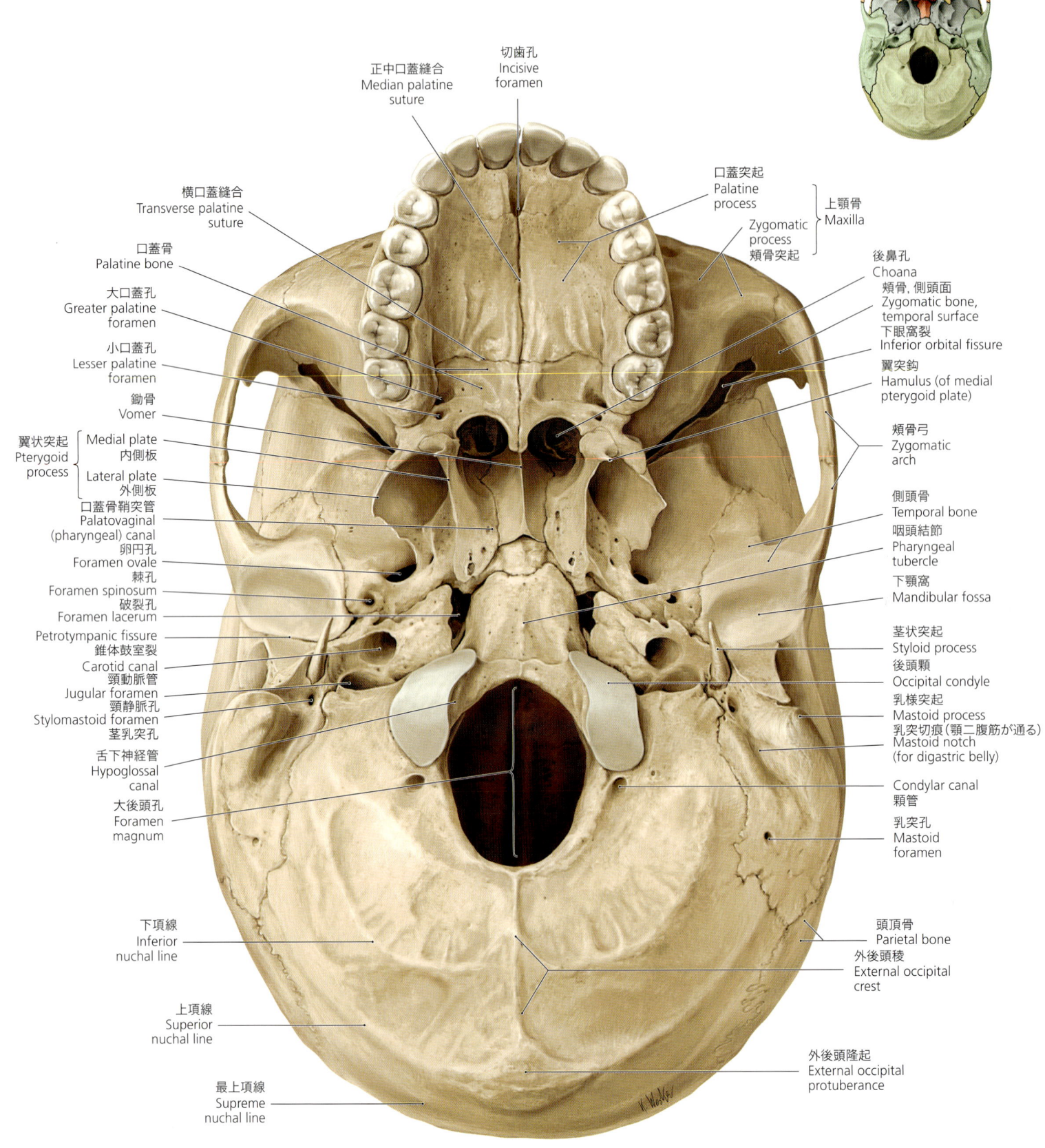

- 正中口蓋縫合 / Median palatine suture
- 切歯孔 / Incisive foramen
- 横口蓋縫合 / Transverse palatine suture
- 口蓋骨 / Palatine bone
- 大口蓋孔 / Greater palatine foramen
- 小口蓋孔 / Lesser palatine foramen
- 鋤骨 / Vomer
- 翼状突起 / Pterygoid process
  - Medial plate 内側板
  - Lateral plate 外側板
- 口蓋骨鞘突管 / Palatovaginal (pharyngeal) canal
- 卵円孔 / Foramen ovale
- 棘孔 / Foramen spinosum
- 破裂孔 / Foramen lacerum
- 錐体鼓室裂 / Petrotympanic fissure
- 頸動脈管 / Carotid canal
- 頸静脈孔 / Jugular foramen
- 茎乳突孔 / Stylomastoid foramen
- 舌下神経管 / Hypoglossal canal
- 大後頭孔 / Foramen magnum
- 下項線 / Inferior nuchal line
- 上項線 / Superior nuchal line
- 最上項線 / Supreme nuchal line
- 口蓋突起 / Palatine process
- 頬骨突起 / Zygomatic process
- 上顎骨 / Maxilla
- 後鼻孔 / Choana
- 頬骨，側頭面 / Zygomatic bone, temporal surface
- 下眼窩裂 / Inferior orbital fissure
- 翼突鉤 / Hamulus (of medial pterygoid plate)
- 頬骨弓 / Zygomatic arch
- 側頭骨 / Temporal bone
- 咽頭結節 / Pharyngeal tubercle
- 下顎窩 / Mandibular fossa
- 茎状突起 / Styloid process
- 後頭顆 / Occipital condyle
- 乳様突起 / Mastoid process
- 乳突切痕（顎二腹筋が通る）/ Mastoid notch (for digastric belly)
- 顆管 / Condylar canal
- 乳突孔 / Mastoid foramen
- 頭頂骨 / Parietal bone
- 外後頭稜 / External occipital crest
- 外後頭隆起 / External occipital protuberance

図 29.7 頭蓋窩

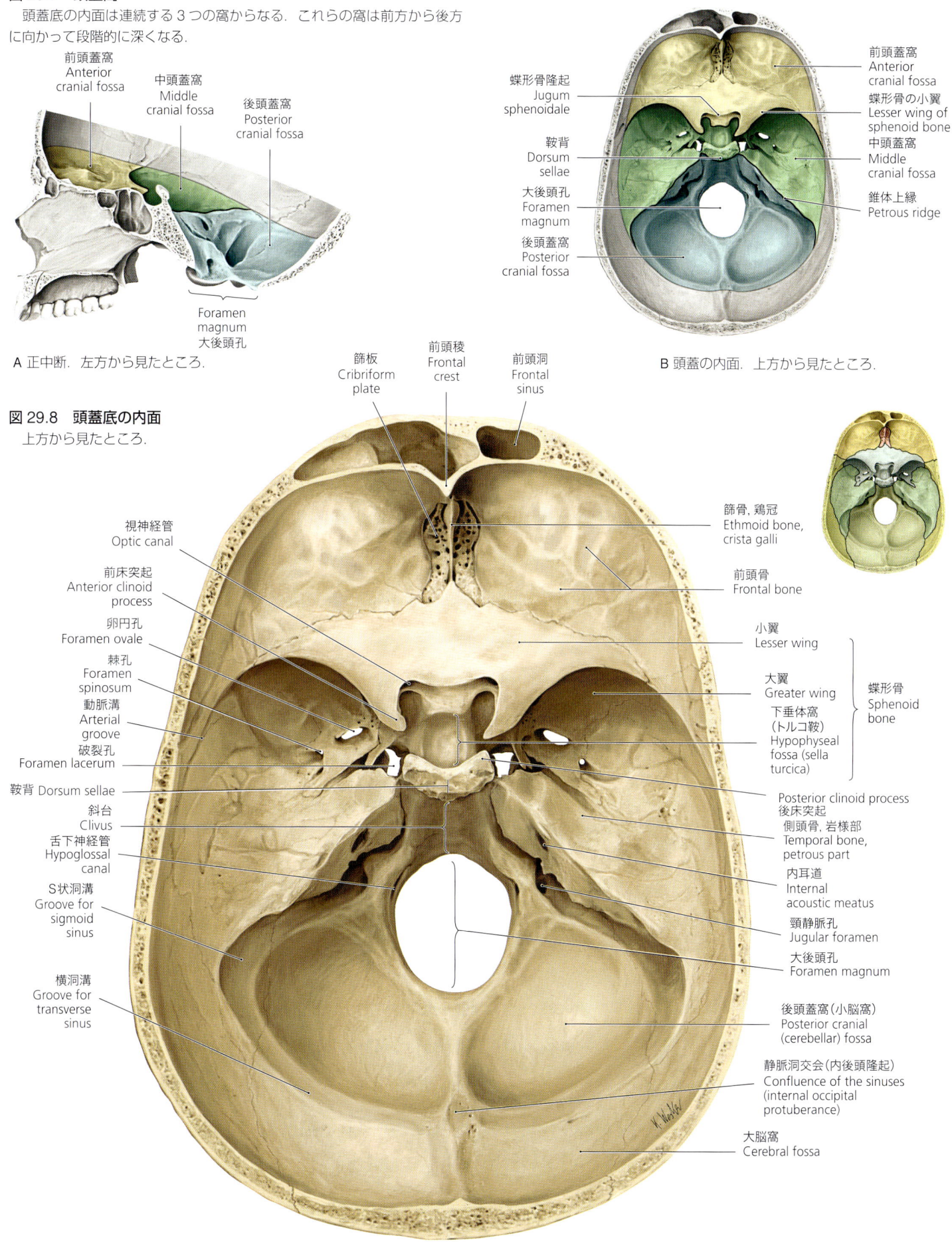

頭蓋底の内面は連続する3つの窩からなる．これらの窩は前方から後方に向かって段階的に深くなる．

- 前頭蓋窩 Anterior cranial fossa
- 中頭蓋窩 Middle cranial fossa
- 後頭蓋窩 Posterior cranial fossa
- 大後頭孔 Foramen magnum

A 正中断．左方から見たところ．

- 蝶形骨隆起 Jugum sphenoidale
- 鞍背 Dorsum sellae
- 大後頭孔 Foramen magnum
- 後頭蓋窩 Posterior cranial fossa
- 前頭蓋窩 Anterior cranial fossa
- 蝶形骨の小翼 Lesser wing of sphenoid bone
- 中頭蓋窩 Middle cranial fossa
- 錐体上縁 Petrous ridge

B 頭蓋の内面．上方から見たところ．

図 29.8 頭蓋底の内面

上方から見たところ．

- 篩板 Cribriform plate
- 前頭稜 Frontal crest
- 前頭洞 Frontal sinus
- 視神経管 Optic canal
- 前床突起 Anterior clinoid process
- 卵円孔 Foramen ovale
- 棘孔 Foramen spinosum
- 動脈溝 Arterial groove
- 破裂孔 Foramen lacerum
- 鞍背 Dorsum sellae
- 斜台 Clivus
- 舌下神経管 Hypoglossal canal
- S状洞溝 Groove for sigmoid sinus
- 横洞溝 Groove for transverse sinus
- 篩骨，鶏冠 Ethmoid bone, crista galli
- 前頭骨 Frontal bone
- 小翼 Lesser wing
- 大翼 Greater wing
- 下垂体窩（トルコ鞍）Hypophyseal fossa (sella turcica)
- 蝶形骨 Sphenoid bone
- 後床突起 Posterior clinoid process
- 側頭骨，岩様部 Temporal bone, petrous part
- 内耳道 Internal acoustic meatus
- 頸静脈孔 Jugular foramen
- 大後頭孔 Foramen magnum
- 後頭蓋窩（小脳窩）Posterior cranial (cerebellar) fossa
- 静脈洞交会（内後頭隆起）Confluence of the sinuses (internal occipital protuberance)
- 大脳窩 Cerebral fossa

篩骨と蝶形骨
Ethmoid & Sphenoid Bones

構造の複雑な篩骨と蝶形骨を分離して示す．頭蓋の他の骨は個々の領域ごとに示す：眼窩（pp.506-507 参照），鼻腔（pp.520-521 参照），口腔（pp.538-539 参照），耳（pp.526-527 参照）．

図 29.9　篩骨
篩骨は鼻腔や副鼻腔の中心となる骨である（pp.520-523 参照）．

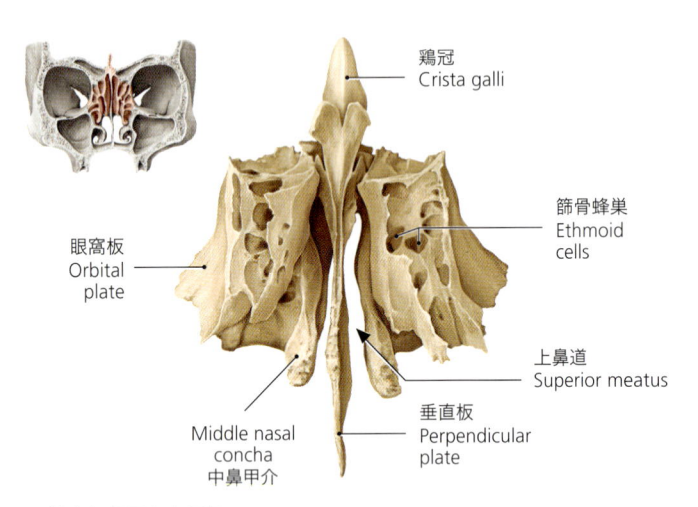

A 前方から見たところ．

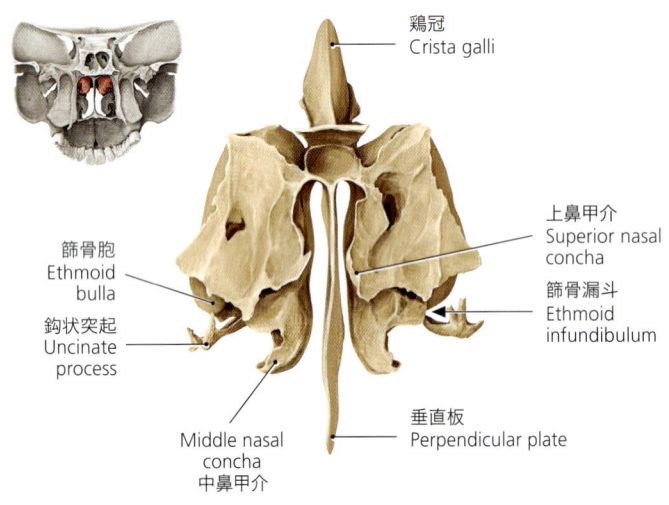

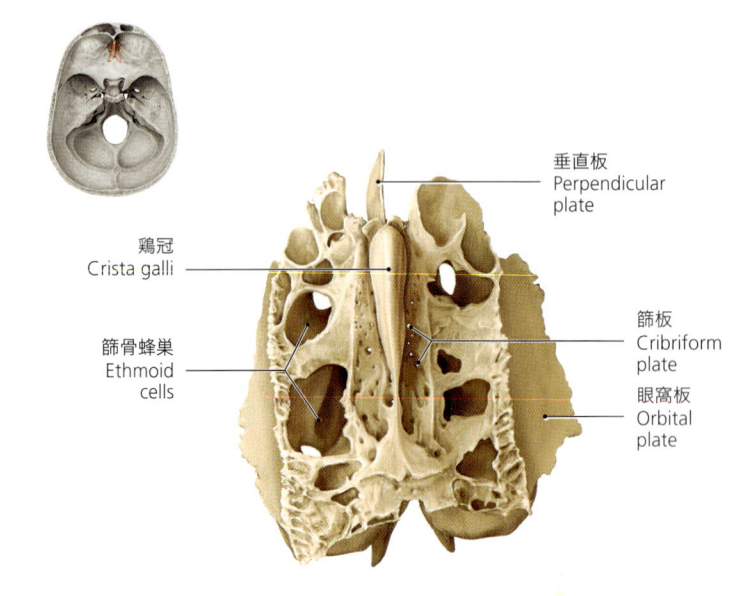

ラベル：鶏冠 Crista galli／篩骨蜂巣 Ethmoid cells／上鼻道 Superior meatus／垂直板 Perpendicular plate／Middle nasal concha 中鼻甲介／眼窩板 Orbital plate

B 上方から見たところ．

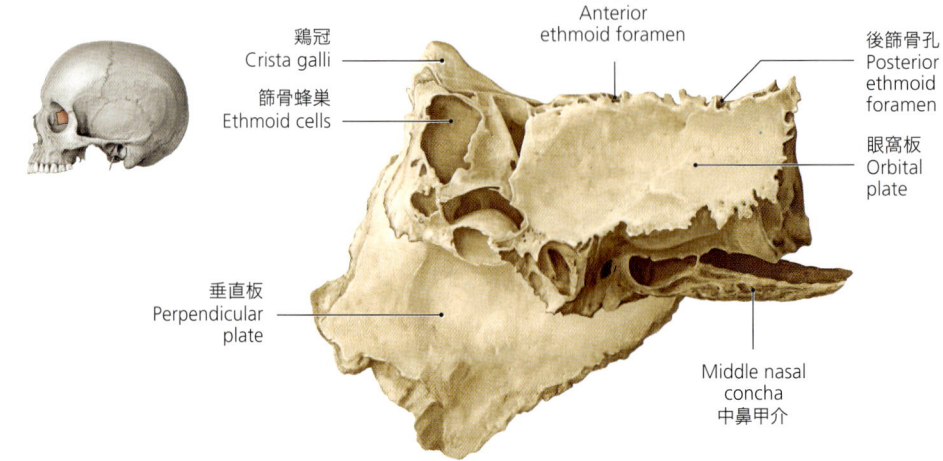

ラベル：垂直板 Perpendicular plate／篩板 Cribriform plate／眼窩板 Orbital plate／鶏冠 Crista galli／篩骨蜂巣 Ethmoid cells

C 後方から見たところ．

ラベル：鶏冠 Crista galli／上鼻甲介 Superior nasal concha／篩骨漏斗 Ethmoid infundibulum／垂直板 Perpendicular plate／Middle nasal concha 中鼻甲介／鈎状突起 Uncinate process／篩骨胞 Ethmoid bulla

D 左外側方から見たところ．

ラベル：鶏冠 Crista galli／篩骨蜂巣 Ethmoid cells／前篩骨孔 Anterior ethmoid foramen／後篩骨孔 Posterior ethmoid foramen／眼窩板 Orbital plate／垂直板 Perpendicular plate／Middle nasal concha 中鼻甲介

図 29.10 蝶形骨

蝶形骨は人体において最も複雑な構造の骨である.

A 前方から見たところ.

- 小翼 Lesser wing
- 蝶形骨稜 Sphenoid crest
- 蝶形骨洞口 Aperture of sphenoid sinus
- 眼窩面 Orbital surface
- 側頭面 Temporal surface
- 正円孔 Foramen rotundum
- 上眼窩裂 Superior orbital fissure
- 翼突管 Pterygoid canal
- 翼突鈎 Pterygoid hamulus
- Pterygoid fossa 翼突窩
- 内側板 Medial plate
- 外側板 Lateral plate
- 翼状突起 Pterygoid process

B 上方から見たところ.

- 小翼 Lesser wing
- 視神経管 Optic canal
- 蝶形骨隆起 Jugum sphenoidale
- 上眼窩裂 Superior orbital fissure
- 大翼 Greater wing
- 卵円孔 Foramen ovale
- Foramen spinosum 棘孔
- Tuberculum sellae 鞍結節
- Hypophyseal fossa 下垂体窩
- Posterior clinoid process 後床突起
- 正円孔 Foramen rotundum
- 前床突起 Anterior clinoid process

C 後方から見たところ.

- 小翼 Lesser wing
- 視神経管 Optic canal
- 後床突起 Posterior clinoid process
- 前床突起 Anterior clinoid process
- 翼突管 Pterygoid canal
- Dorsum sellae 鞍背
- Pterygoid fossa 翼突窩
- 上眼窩裂 Superior orbital fissure
- 大翼, 大脳面 Greater wing, cerebral surface
- 正円孔 Foramen rotundum
- 海綿質の骨梁 Cancellous trabeculae
- 内側板 Medial plate
- 外側板 Lateral plate
- 翼状突起 Pterygoid process

D 下方から見たところ. Note: 蝶形骨稜の下には鋤骨がある(p.538参照).

- 小翼 Lesser wing
- 蝶形骨稜 Sphenoid crest
- 蝶形骨洞口 Aperture of sphenoid sinus
- 大翼 Greater wing
- 正円孔 Foramen rotundum
- 内側板 Medial plate
- 外側板 Lateral plate
- 翼状突起 Pterygoid process
- Foramen ovale 卵円孔
- Foramen spinosum 棘孔
- 大翼 Greater wing
- Temporal surface 側頭面
- Pterygoid hamulus 翼突鈎
- Superior orbital fissure 上眼窩裂
- Body 体
- Pterygoid fossa 翼突窩

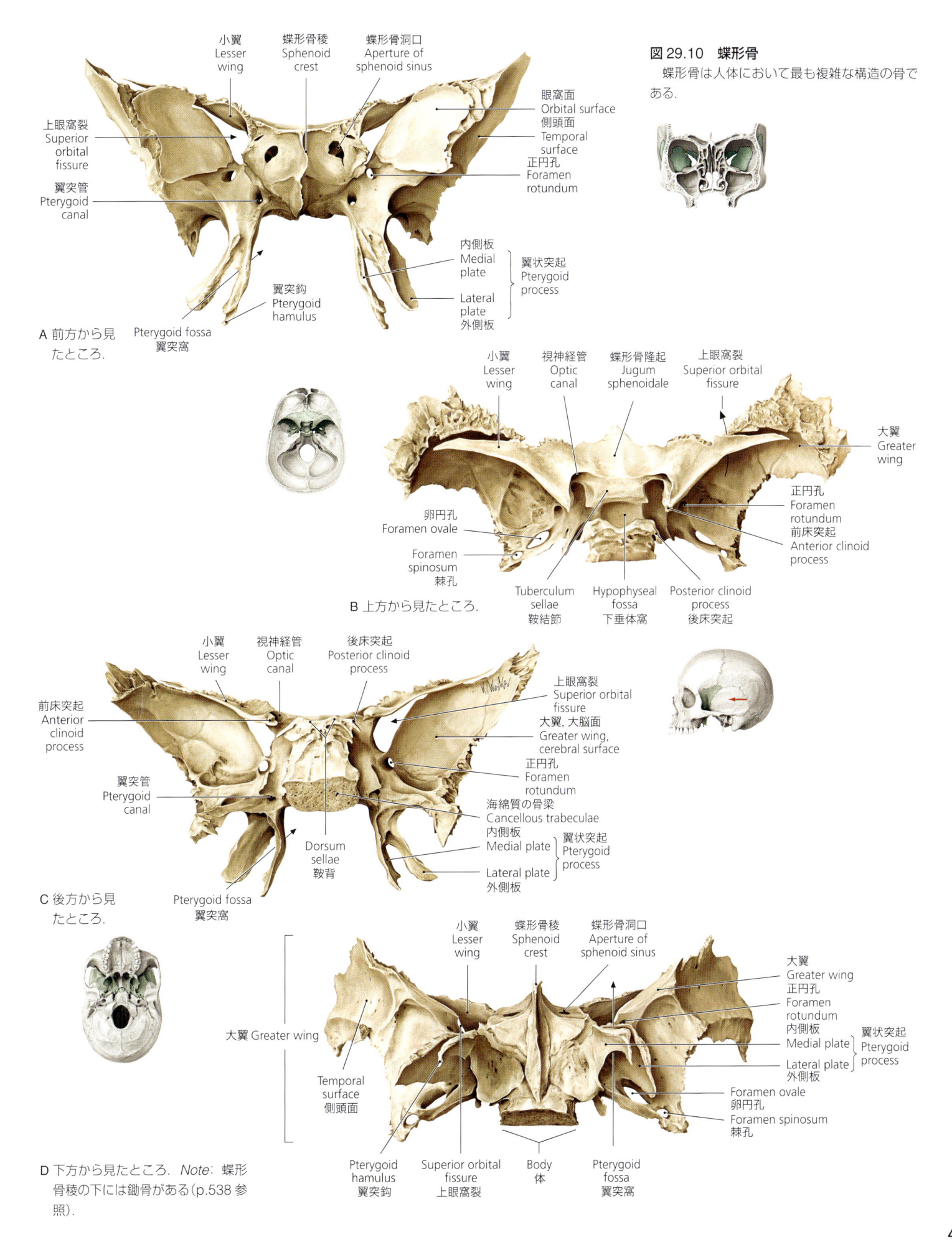

表情筋と咀嚼筋
Muscles of Facial Expression & of Mastication

頭蓋と顔面の筋肉は2つのグループに分類される．顔面の表情筋は顔面浅層の筋からなる．咀嚼筋は咀嚼時の下顎の運動を行う．

図30.1　表情筋

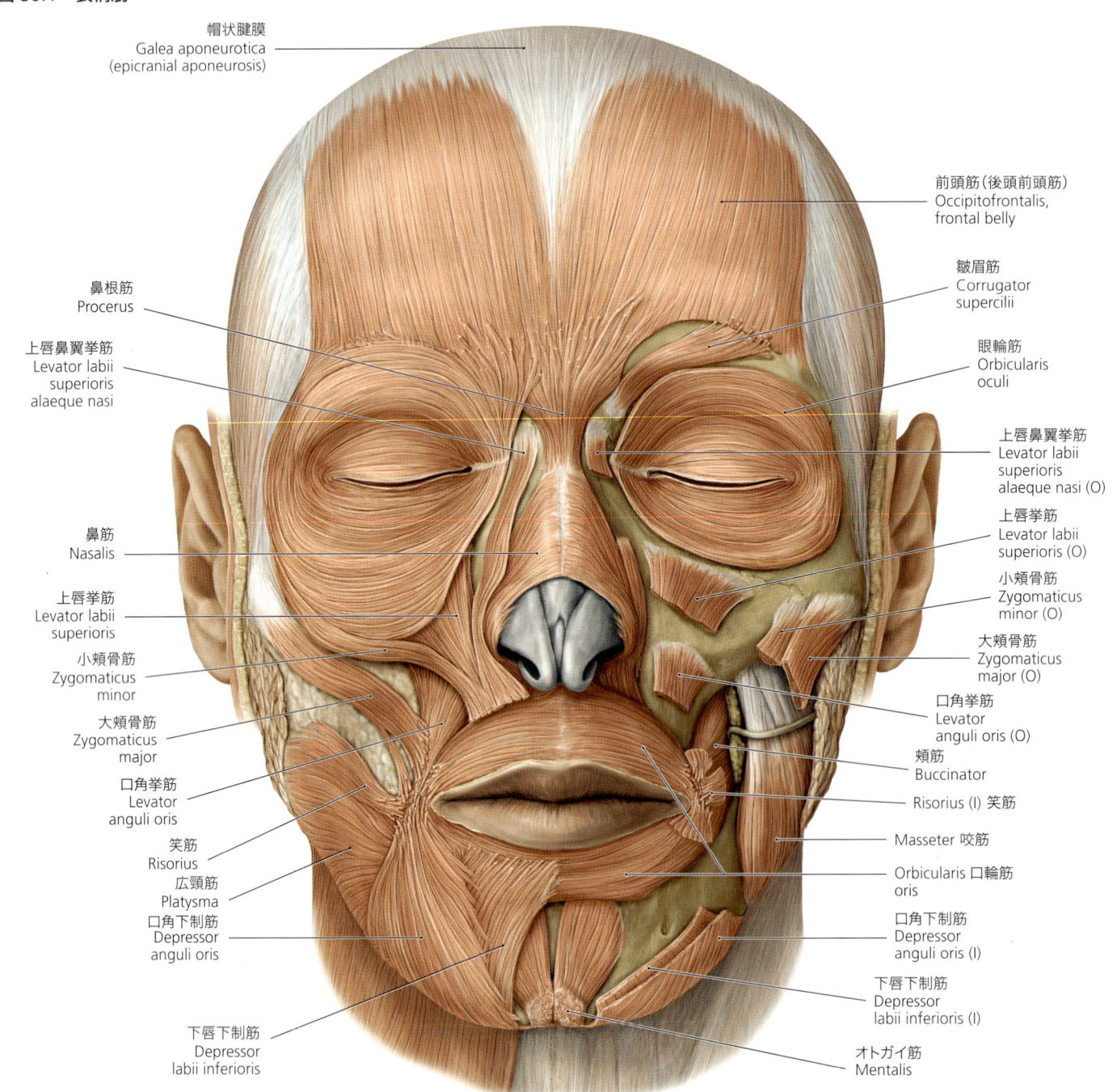

- 帽状腱膜 Galea aponeurotica (epicranial aponeurosis)
- 前頭筋（後頭前頭筋） Occipitofrontalis, frontal belly
- 皺眉筋 Corrugator supercilii
- 眼輪筋 Orbicularis oculi
- 鼻根筋 Procerus
- 上唇鼻翼挙筋 Levator labii superioris alaeque nasi
- 上唇鼻翼挙筋 Levator labii superioris alaeque nasi (O)
- 上唇挙筋 Levator labii superioris (O)
- 鼻筋 Nasalis
- 小頬骨筋 Zygomaticus minor (O)
- 上唇挙筋 Levator labii superioris
- 大頬骨筋 Zygomaticus major (O)
- 小頬骨筋 Zygomaticus minor
- 口角挙筋 Levator anguli oris (O)
- 大頬骨筋 Zygomaticus major
- 頬筋 Buccinator
- 口角挙筋 Levator anguli oris
- Risorius (I) 笑筋
- 笑筋 Risorius
- Masseter 咬筋
- 広頚筋 Platysma
- Orbicularis 口輪筋 oris
- 口角下制筋 Depressor anguli oris
- 口角下制筋 Depressor anguli oris (I)
- 下唇下制筋 Depressor labii inferioris (I)
- 下唇下制筋 Depressor labii inferioris
- オトガイ筋 Mentalis

A 前方から見たところ．左半分では筋の起始をO，停止をIで示している．

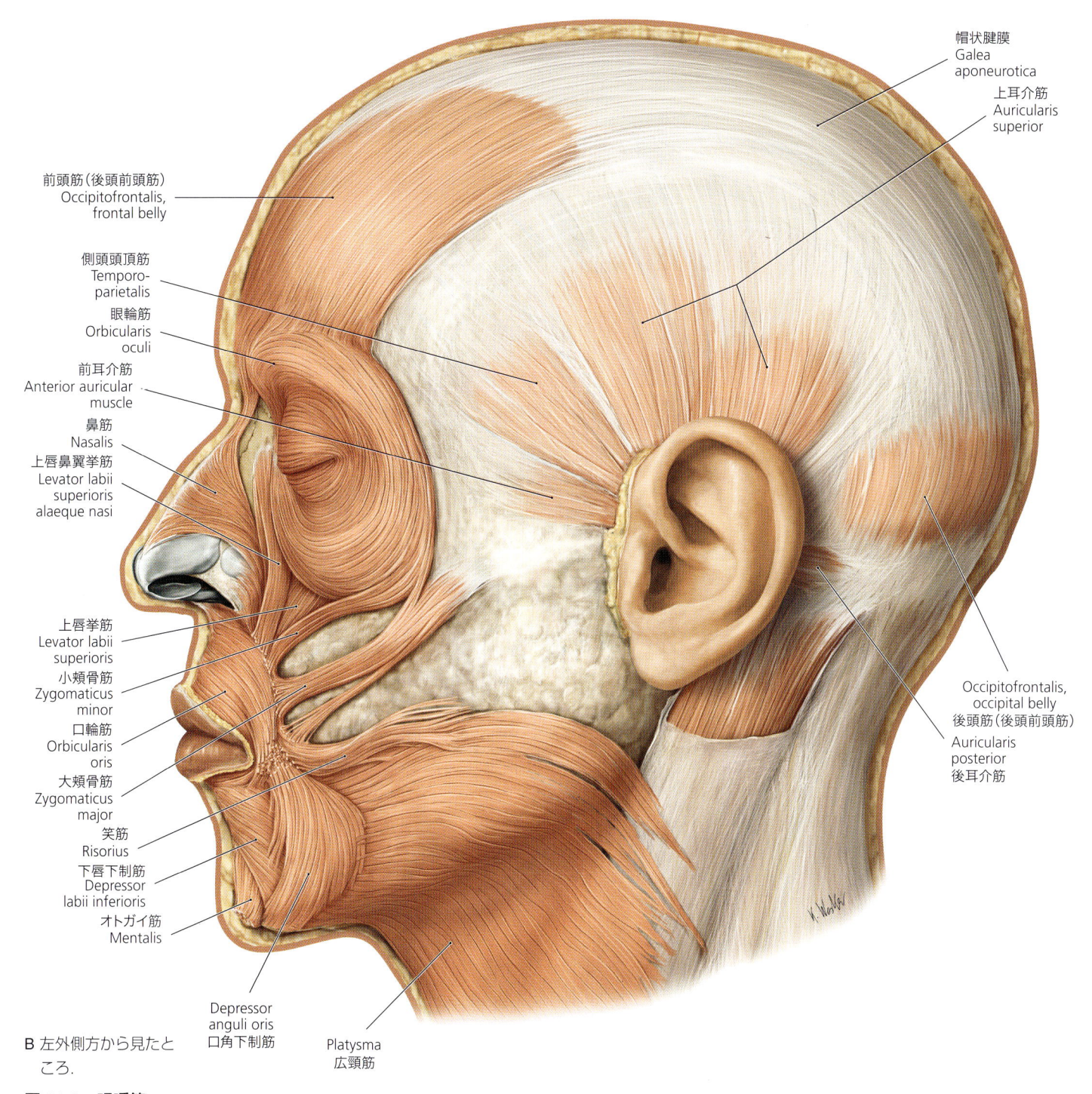

30 頭部・顔面の筋

帽状腱膜
Galea aponeurotica

上耳介筋
Auricularis superior

前頭筋(後頭前頭筋)
Occipitofrontalis, frontal belly

側頭頭頂筋
Temporo-parietalis

眼輪筋
Orbicularis oculi

前耳介筋
Anterior auricular muscle

鼻筋
Nasalis

上唇鼻翼挙筋
Levator labii superioris alaeque nasi

上唇挙筋
Levator labii superioris

小頬骨筋
Zygomaticus minor

口輪筋
Orbicularis oris

大頬骨筋
Zygomaticus major

笑筋
Risorius

下唇下制筋
Depressor labii inferioris

オトガイ筋
Mentalis

Occipitofrontalis, occipital belly
後頭筋(後頭前頭筋)

Auricularis posterior
後耳介筋

Depressor anguli oris
口角下制筋

Platysma
広頸筋

B 左外側方から見たところ.

図30.2 咀嚼筋
左外側方から見たところ.

側頭筋
Temporalis

顎関節の関節包
Capsule of temporo-mandibular joint

茎状突起
Styloid process

咬筋
Masseter
{ Deep part 深部
  Superficial part 浅部 }

A 浅層.

側頭筋
Temporalis

外側翼突筋
Lateral pterygoid

外側靱帯
Lateral ligament

内側翼突筋
Medial pterygoid

Masseter 咬筋

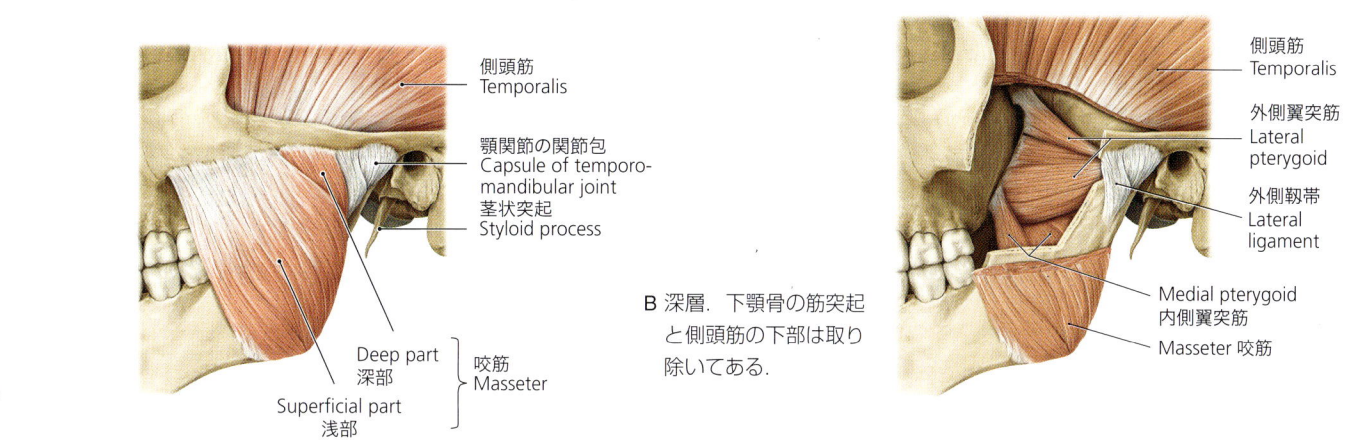

B 深層. 下顎骨の筋突起と側頭筋の下部は取り除いてある.

463

頭部の筋，起始と停止
Muscle Origins & Insertions on the Skull

図 30.3　頭蓋の側面：起始と停止
左外側方から見たところ．赤色が筋の起始，青色が停止．*Note*：一般に表情筋は骨に停止せず，皮膚やほかの表情筋に停止する．

表情筋 Facial muscles
神経支配：顔面神経（CN VII）

- 後頭筋 Occipitofrontalis, （後頭前頭筋） occipital belly
- 皺眉筋 Corrugator supercilii
- 眼輪筋 Orbicularis oculi
  - 眼窩部 Orbital part
  - 涙嚢部 Lacrimal part
- 上唇鼻翼挙筋 Levator labii superioris alaeque nasi
- 大頬骨筋 Zygomaticus major
- 小頬骨筋 Zygomaticus minor
- 口角挙筋 Levator anguli oris
- 鼻筋 Nasalis
  - 横部 Transverse part
  - 翼部 Alar part
- 鼻中隔下制筋 Depressor septi nasi
- 口輪筋 Orbicularis oris
- 頬筋 Buccinator
- オトガイ筋 Mentalis
- 口輪筋 Orbicularis oris
- 下唇下制筋 Depressor labii inferioris
- 口角下制筋 Depressor anguli oris
- 広頸筋 Platysma

胸鎖乳突筋と僧帽筋 Sternocleidomastoid and trapezius
神経支配：副神経（CN XI）

- Sternocleidomastoid 胸鎖乳突筋
- Trapezius 僧帽筋

項部の筋，固有背筋 Nuchal muscles, intrinsic back muscles
神経支配：頸神経の後枝

- Semispinalis capitis 頭半棘筋
- Obliquus capitis superior 上頭斜筋
- 大後頭直筋 Rectus capitis posterior major
- 小後頭直筋 Rectus capitis posterior minor
- 頭板状筋 Splenius capitis
- 頭最長筋 Longissimus capitis

咀嚼筋 Muscles of mastication
神経支配：下顎神経（CN V$_3$）

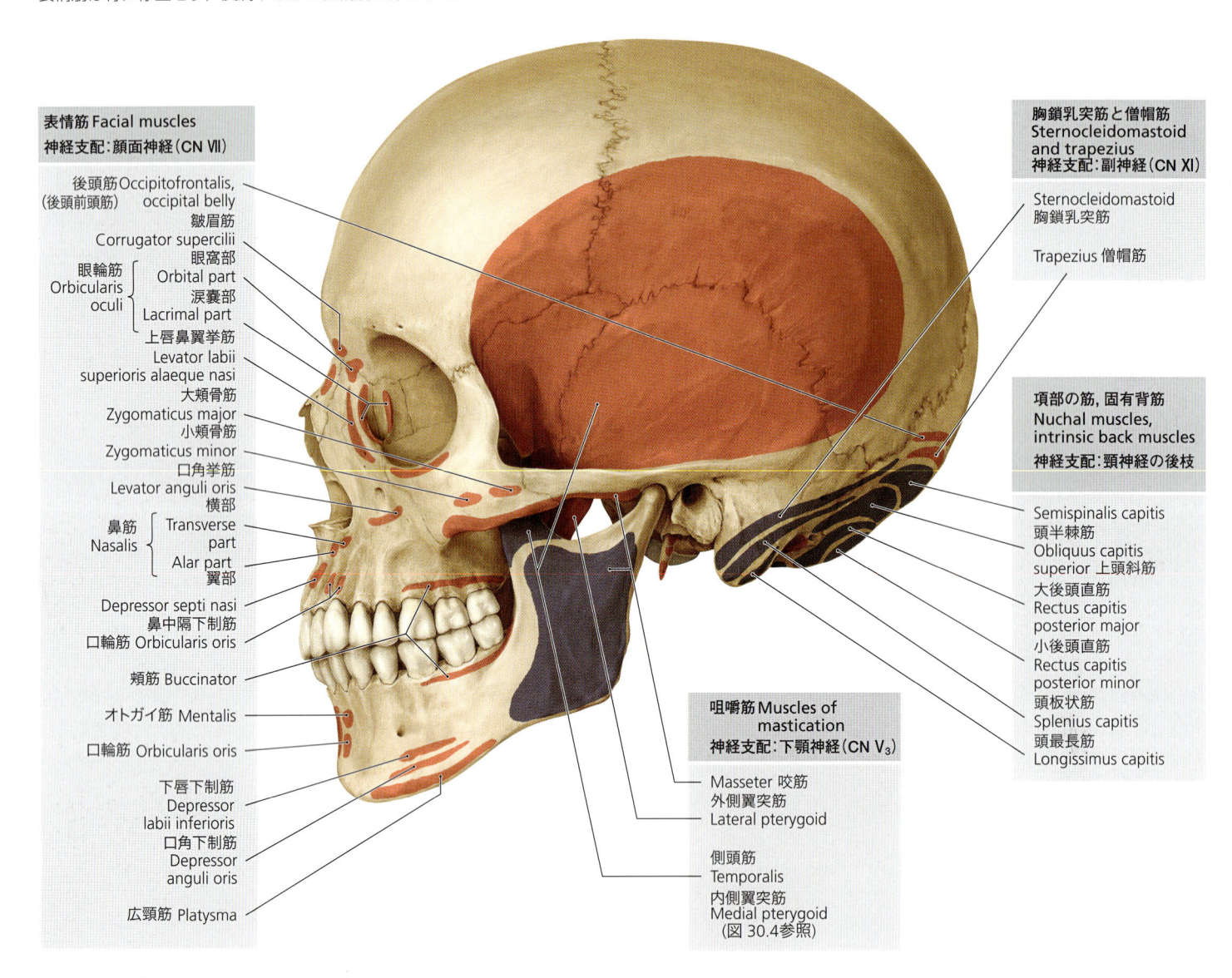

- Masseter 咬筋
- 外側翼突筋 Lateral pterygoid
- 側頭筋 Temporalis
- 内側翼突筋 Medial pterygoid（図 30.4 参照）

図 30.4　下顎骨：起始と停止
下顎骨右半分を内側方から見たところ．

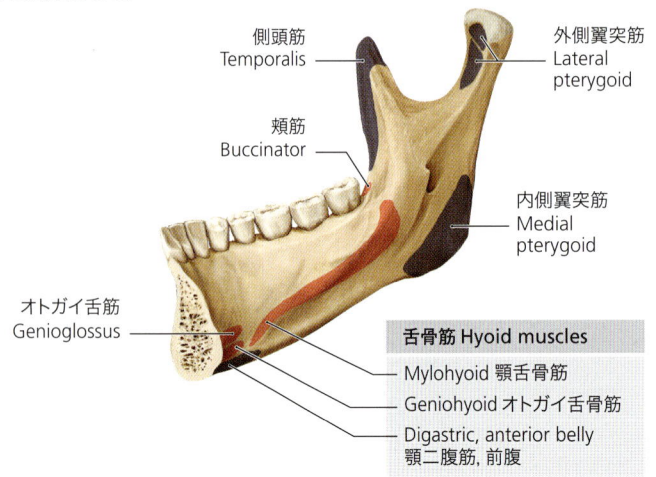

- 側頭筋 Temporalis
- 外側翼突筋 Lateral pterygoid
- 頬筋 Buccinator
- 内側翼突筋 Medial pterygoid
- オトガイ舌筋 Genioglossus

舌骨筋 Hyoid muscles

- Mylohyoid 顎舌骨筋
- Geniohyoid オトガイ舌骨筋
- Digastric, anterior belly 顎二腹筋，前腹

図 30.5　頭蓋底：起始と停止
頭蓋の外面を下方から見たところ．

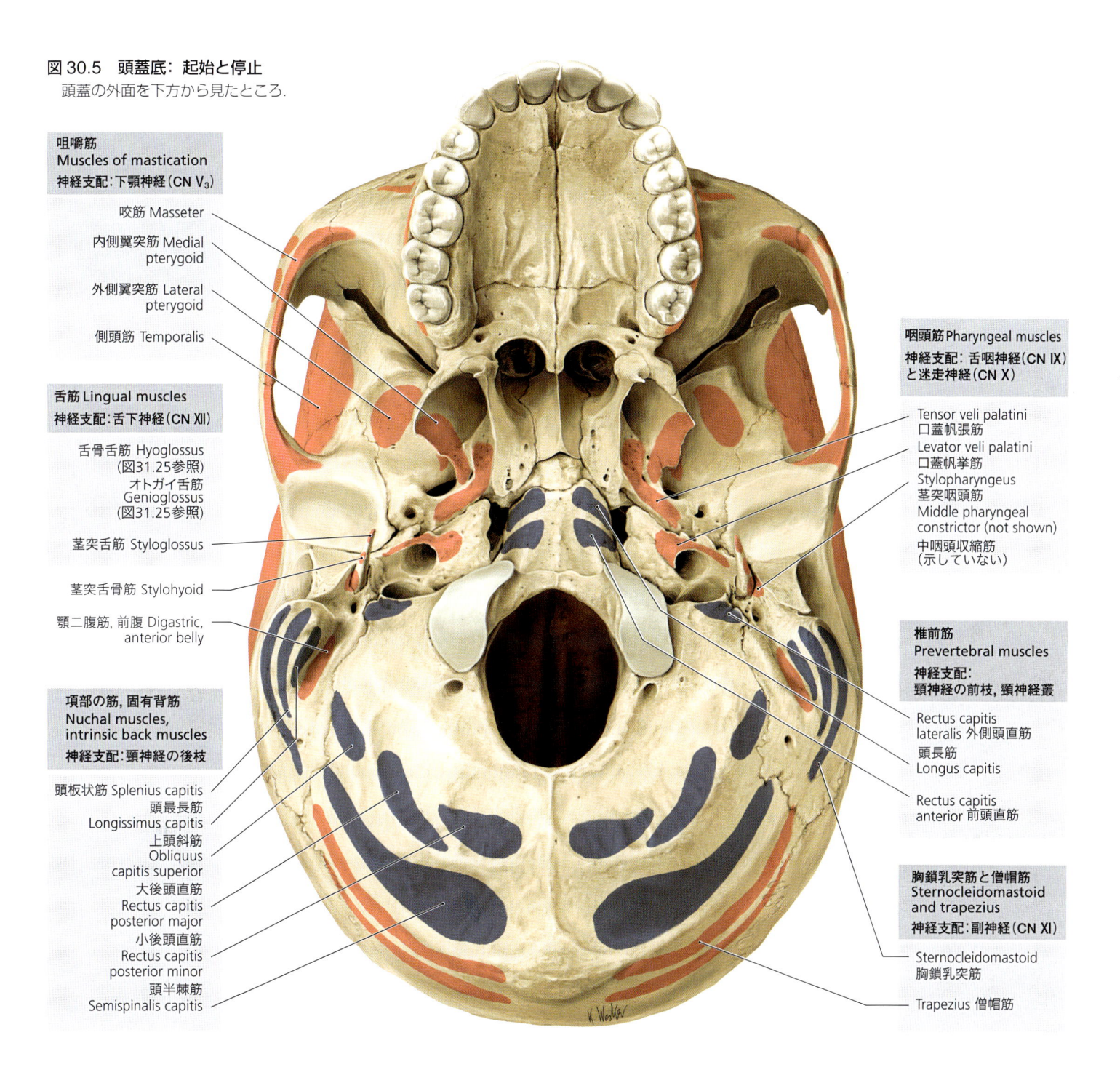

咀嚼筋 Muscles of mastication
神経支配：下顎神経（CN V₃）
- 咬筋 Masseter
- 内側翼突筋 Medial pterygoid
- 外側翼突筋 Lateral pterygoid
- 側頭筋 Temporalis

舌筋 Lingual muscles
神経支配：舌下神経（CN XII）
- 舌骨舌筋 Hyoglossus（図31.25参照）
- オトガイ舌筋 Genioglossus（図31.25参照）
- 茎突舌筋 Styloglossus
- 茎突舌骨筋 Stylohyoid
- 顎二腹筋, 前腹 Digastric, anterior belly

項部の筋, 固有背筋 Nuchal muscles, intrinsic back muscles
神経支配：頸神経の後枝
- 頭板状筋 Splenius capitis
- 頭最長筋 Longissimus capitis
- 上頭斜筋 Obliquus capitis superior
- 大後頭直筋 Rectus capitis posterior major
- 小後頭直筋 Rectus capitis posterior minor
- 頭半棘筋 Semispinalis capitis

咽頭筋 Pharyngeal muscles
神経支配：舌咽神経（CN IX）と迷走神経（CN X）
- Tensor veli palatini 口蓋帆張筋
- Levator veli palatini 口蓋帆挙筋
- Stylopharyngeus 茎突咽頭筋
- Middle pharyngeal constrictor (not shown) 中咽頭収縮筋（示していない）

椎前筋 Prevertebral muscles
神経支配：頸神経の前枝, 頸神経叢
- Rectus capitis lateralis 外側頭直筋
- Longus capitis 頭長筋
- Rectus capitis anterior 前頭直筋

胸鎖乳突筋と僧帽筋 Sternocleidomastoid and trapezius
神経支配：副神経（CN XI）
- Sternocleidomastoid 胸鎖乳突筋
- Trapezius 僧帽筋

図 30.6　舌骨：起始と停止

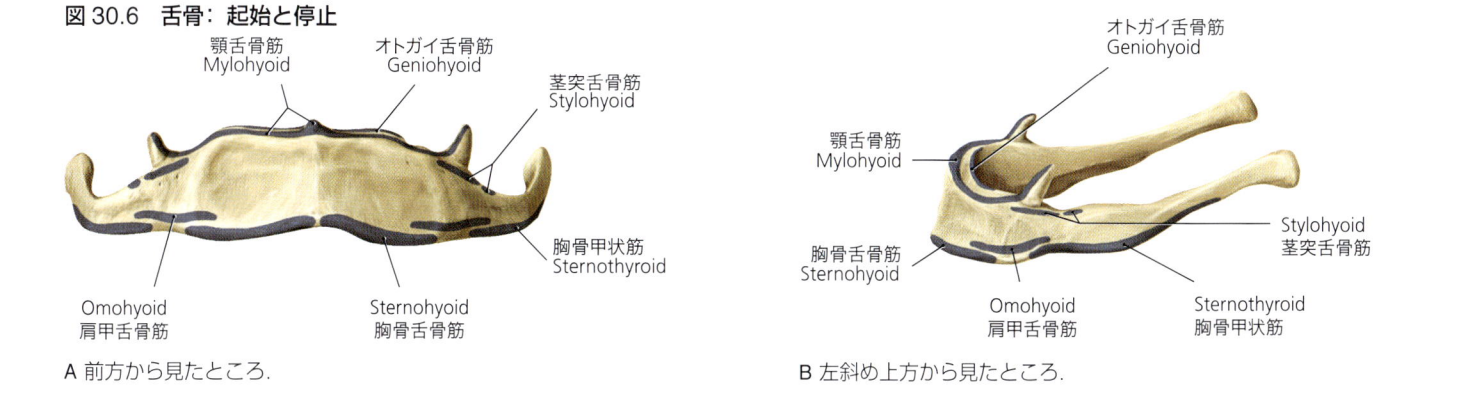

A 前方から見たところ．
- 顎舌骨筋 Mylohyoid
- オトガイ舌骨筋 Geniohyoid
- 茎突舌骨筋 Stylohyoid
- 胸骨甲状筋 Sternothyroid
- Omohyoid 肩甲舌骨筋
- Sternohyoid 胸骨舌骨筋

B 左斜め上方から見たところ．
- オトガイ舌骨筋 Geniohyoid
- 顎舌骨筋 Mylohyoid
- 胸骨舌骨筋 Sternohyoid
- Stylohyoid 茎突舌骨筋
- Omohyoid 肩甲舌骨筋
- Sternothyroid 胸骨甲状筋

頭部の筋 (1)
Muscle Facts (I)

> 表情筋は骨や筋膜から起始し，顔面の皮下組織に停止しているので，皮膚を引っ張ることで表情に影響を及ぼすことができる．

図 30.7　前頭筋
前方から見たところ．

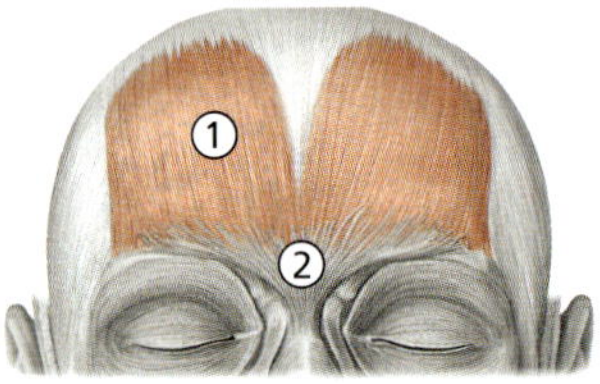

図 30.8　眼瞼裂と鼻
前方から見たところ．

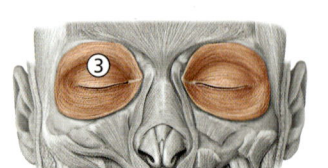

A　眼輪筋．

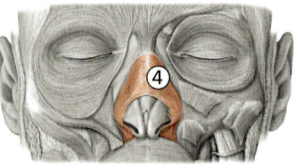

B　鼻筋．

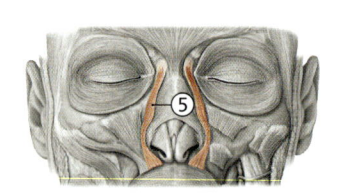

C　上唇鼻翼挙筋．

図 30.9　耳の筋
左外側方から見たところ．

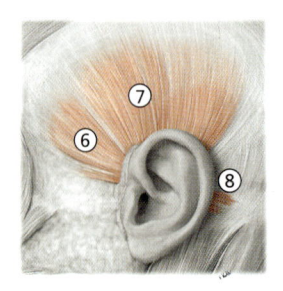

表 30.1　表情筋（顔面筋）：額，鼻，耳

筋	起始	停止*	主な作用**
頭蓋冠			
①前頭筋	帽状腱膜	眉と額の皮膚と皮下組織	眉を挙上，額の皮膚にヒダを作る
眼瞼裂と鼻			
②鼻根筋	鼻骨，外側鼻軟骨（上部）	額下部の眉間の皮膚	眉の内側角を引下げ，鼻背に横方向のヒダを作る
③眼輪筋	眼窩内側縁，内側眼瞼靱帯，涙骨	眼窩縁の皮膚，上瞼板，下瞼板	眼裂の括約筋として働く（眼瞼を閉じる） ・眼瞼部は軽く閉ざす ・眼窩部は強く閉ざす（まばたき）
④鼻筋	上顎骨（犬歯上部）	鼻軟骨	鼻中隔に向かって鼻翼を引くことで鼻孔をせばめる
⑤上唇鼻翼挙筋	上顎骨（前頭突起）	鼻翼軟骨と上唇	上唇を引上げ，鼻孔を開く
耳			
⑥前耳介筋	側頭筋膜（前部）	耳輪	耳を上方と前方に引く
⑦上耳介筋	頭部側方の帽状腱膜	耳介上部	耳を持ち上げる
⑧後耳介筋	乳様突起	耳甲介腔	耳を上方と後方に引く

*表情筋は骨に停止しない．
**表情筋はすべて耳下腺神経叢（p.478 参照）から起こる側頭枝，頬骨枝，頬筋枝，下顎縁枝，頸枝を通して顔面神経（CN VII）によって支配される．

図 30.10　口の筋肉
左外側方から見たところ.

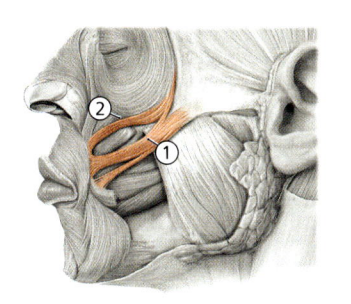

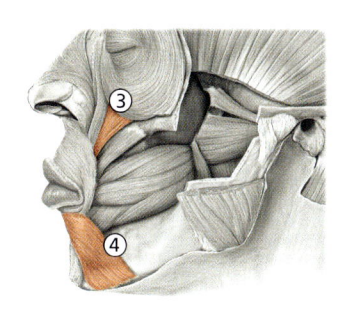

A 大頰骨筋と小頰骨筋.　　B 上唇挙筋と下唇下制筋.　　C 口角挙筋と口角下制筋.　　D 頰筋.

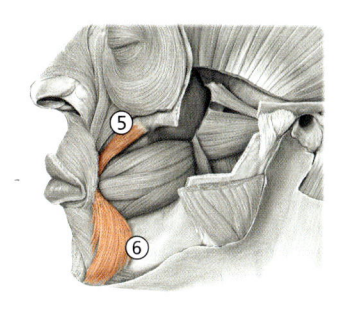

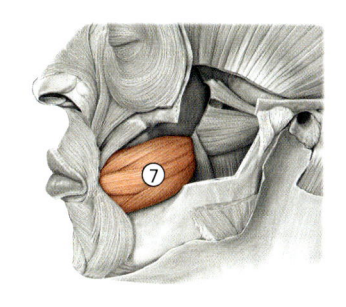

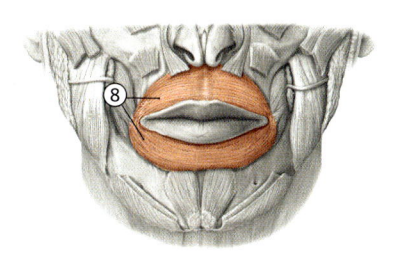

E 口輪筋，前方から見たところ.　　　　F オトガイ筋，前方から見たところ.

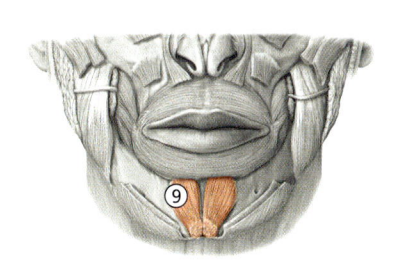

表30.2	表情筋（顔面筋）：口と頸		
筋	起始	停止*	主な作用**
口			
①大頰骨筋	頰骨（外面，後部）	口角の皮膚	口角を外上方に引く
②小頰骨筋		口角のすぐ内側の上唇	上唇を上方に引く
上唇鼻翼挙筋（図 30.8C 参照）	上顎骨（前頭突起）	鼻翼軟骨と上唇	上唇を引上げ，鼻孔を開く
③上唇挙筋	上顎骨（前頭突起）と眼窩下縁	上唇の皮膚，鼻翼軟骨	上唇を引上げ，鼻孔を広げ，口角を上げる
④下唇下制筋	下顎骨（斜線の前部）	下唇の正中線；反対側からの筋肉と混ざる	下唇を外下方に引く
⑤口角挙筋	上顎骨（眼窩下孔の下部）	口角の皮膚	口角を上げ，鼻唇溝の形成を助ける
⑥口角下制筋	下顎骨（犬歯・小臼歯・第一大臼歯下部の斜線）	口角の皮膚；口輪筋と混ざる	口角を外下方に引く
⑦頰筋	下顎骨，上下顎の歯槽突起，翼突下顎縫線	口角，口輪筋	頰を臼歯に押しつけ，舌と協力して食物を咬合面間に留め，また口腔前庭より外に追い出す；口腔から空気を吹き出す／息を強く吹き出すときに拡張を抑える 片側：口を片側に引く
⑧口輪筋	皮膚の深層 上側：上顎骨（正中面） 下側：下顎骨	唇の粘膜	口の括約筋として働く ・唇を引き締め，突き出す（口笛を吹くとき，すうとき，キスをするときなど） ・拡張を抑える（息を強く吹き出すとき）
笑筋（p.462 参照）	咬筋の筋膜	口角の皮膚	顔をしかめるときなどに口角を外に引く
⑨オトガイ筋	下顎骨（切歯窩）	オトガイ部の皮膚	下唇を持ち上げ，突き出す
頸			
広頸筋（p.463 参照）	頸部下部と胸部上部の皮膚	下顎骨（下縁），顔面下部の皮膚，口角	顔面下部の皮膚と口を下げ，ヒダを作る；頸の皮膚を緊張させる；下顎骨の強制下制を助ける

*表情筋は骨に停止しない.
**表情筋はすべて耳下腺神経叢から起こる側頭枝，頰骨枝，頰筋枝，下顎縁枝，頸枝を通して顔面神経（CN VII）によって支配される.

頭部の筋（2）
Muscle Facts (II)

咀嚼筋は顔面の耳下腺部と側頭下部に浅層から深層にかけて位置する．咀嚼筋は下顎骨に付着し下顎神経（CN V₃）から運動性神経支配を受ける．口を開くのを助ける口腔底の筋肉については p.562 を参照．

表30.3　咀嚼筋：咬筋と側頭筋

筋	起始	停止	神経支配	作用
①咬筋	浅部：頬骨弓（前2/3） 深部：頬骨弓（後1/3）	下顎角（咬筋粗面）	下顎神経（CN V₃）の咬筋神経	下顎骨を引き上げ，前に突き出す
②側頭筋	側頭窩（下側頭線）	下顎骨筋突起（先端と内側面）	下顎神経（CN V₃）の深側頭神経	垂直線維：下顎骨を引き上げる 水平線維：下顎骨を後方に引く 片側：下顎骨を外側に動かす（咀嚼時）

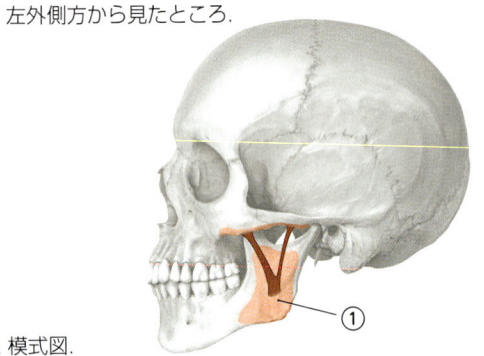

図30.11　咬筋
左外側方から見たところ．

A 模式図．

B 側頭筋と咬筋．

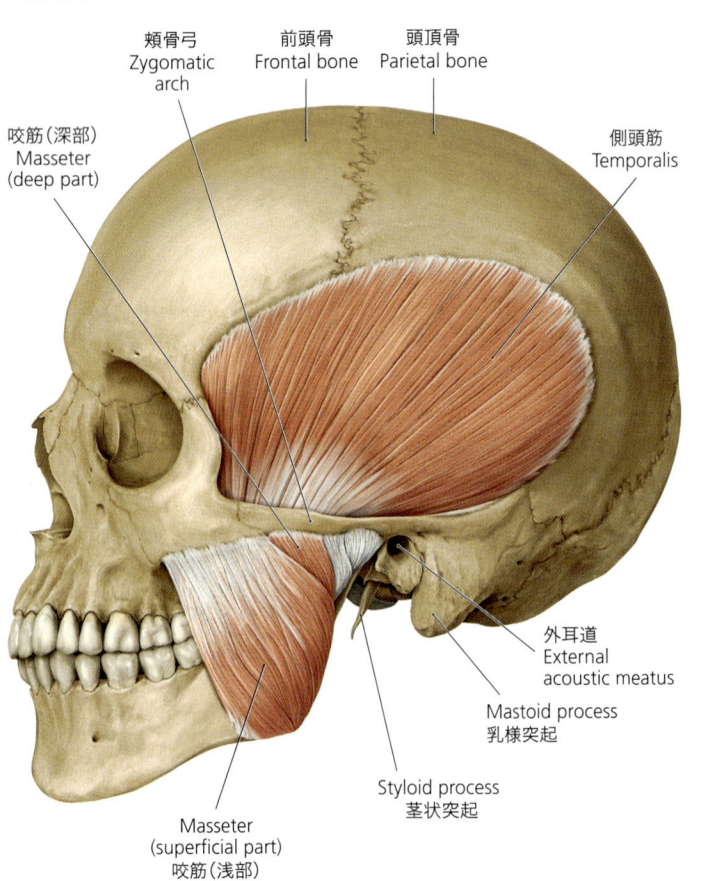

ラベル：頬骨弓 Zygomatic arch／前頭骨 Frontal bone／頭頂骨 Parietal bone／側頭筋 Temporalis／咬筋（深部）Masseter (deep part)／外耳道 External acoustic meatus／乳様突起 Mastoid process／茎状突起 Styloid process／咬筋（浅部）Masseter (superficial part)

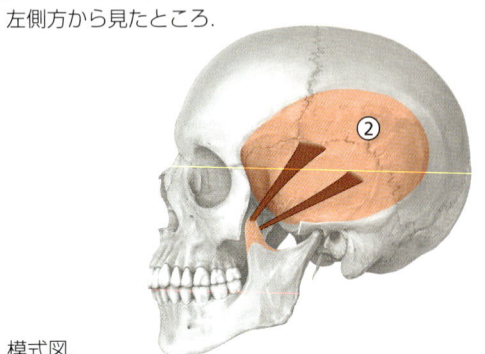

図30.12　側頭筋
左側方から見たところ．

A 模式図．

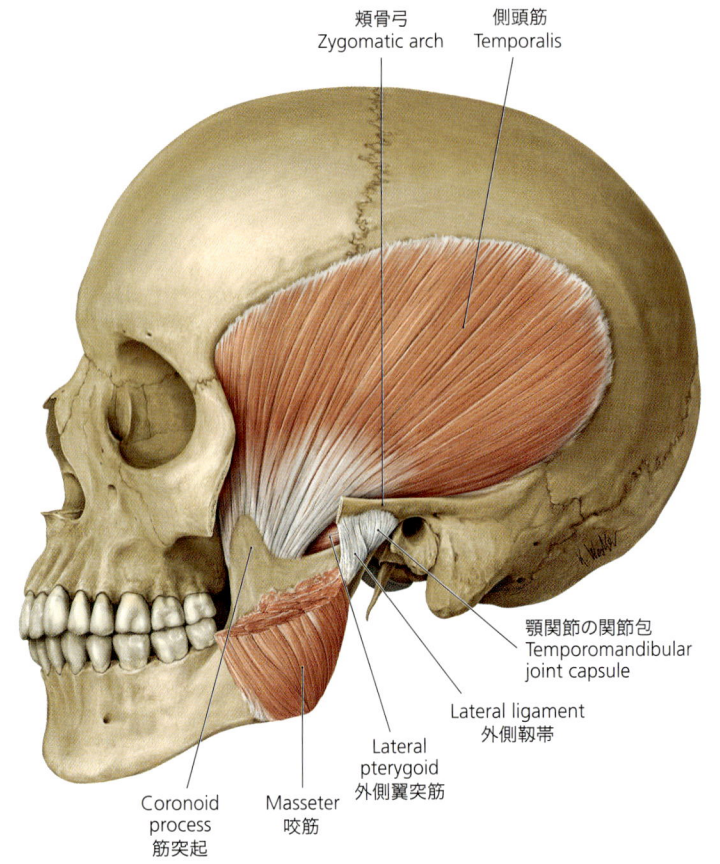

B 側頭筋．咬筋と頬骨弓は取り除いてある．

ラベル：頬骨弓 Zygomatic arch／側頭筋 Temporalis／顎関節の関節包 Temporomandibular joint capsule／外側靱帯 Lateral ligament／外側翼突筋 Lateral pterygoid／咬筋 Masseter／筋突起 Coronoid process

表 30.4　咀嚼筋：翼突筋

筋		起始	停止	神経支配	作用
外側翼突筋	③上頭	蝶形骨の大翼（側頭下稜）	顎関節（関節円板）	下顎神経（CN V$_3$）の外側翼突筋神経	両側：下顎骨を前に突き出す（関節円板を前方に引く） 片側：下顎骨を外側に動かす（咀嚼時）
	④下頭	翼状突起の外側版（外側面）	下顎骨（関節突起）		
内側翼突筋	⑤浅頭	上顎骨（粗面）	下顎角内面の翼突筋粗面	下顎神経（CN V$_3$）の内側翼突筋神経	下顎骨を引き上げる
	⑥深頭	外側翼突板と翼突窩の内側面			

図 30.13　外側翼突筋
左外側方から見たところ.

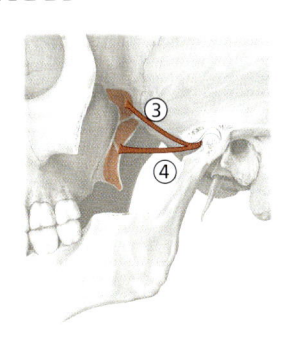

A 模式図.

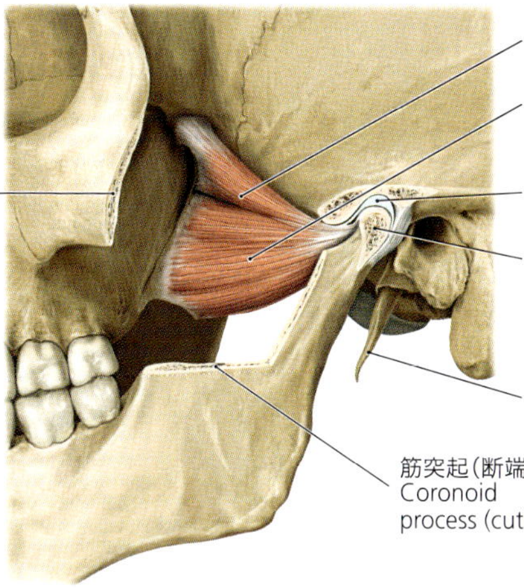

B 外側翼突筋．下顎骨の筋突起は取り除いてある.

図 30.14　内側翼突筋
左外側方から見たところ.

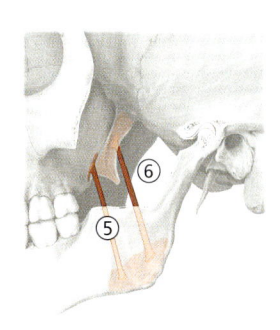

A 模式図.

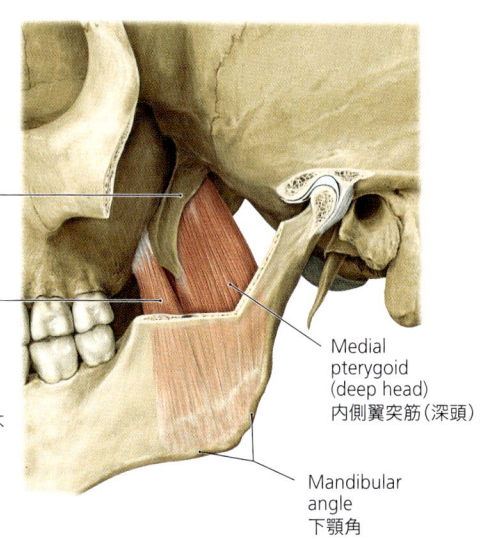

B 内側翼突筋．下顎骨の筋突起は取り除いてある.

図 30.15　咀嚼筋が作る吊り紐
斜め後方から見たところ.

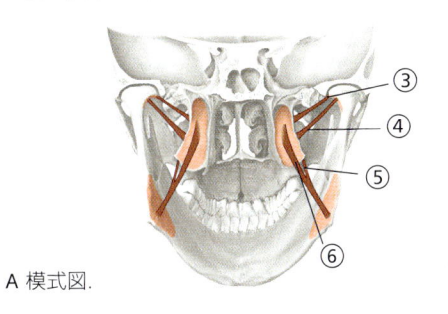

A 模式図.

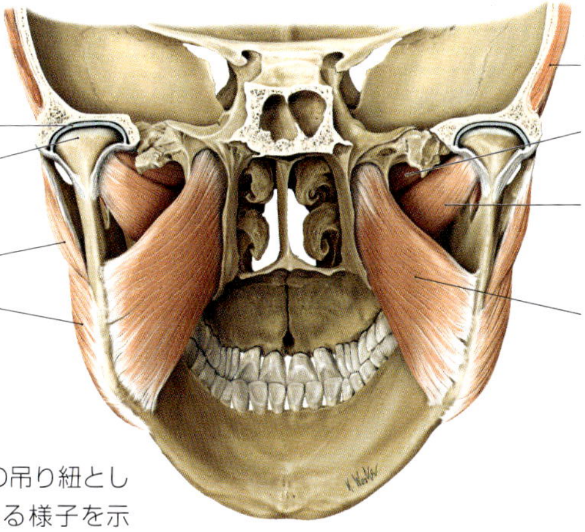

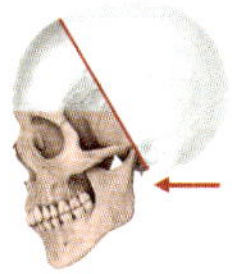

B 咬筋と内側翼突筋が筋性の吊り紐として下顎骨を吊り下げている様子を示す.

脳神経の概観
Cranial Nerves: Overview

図 31.1 脳神経

頭蓋底を内方から見たところ．12 対の脳神経は脳幹からあらわれる順にローマ数字で示される．*Note*：感覚線維と運動線維は脳幹の同じ部位で出入りする．この点が脊髄神経と異なる．脊髄神経では運動線維は前根から出て，感覚線維は後根から入る．

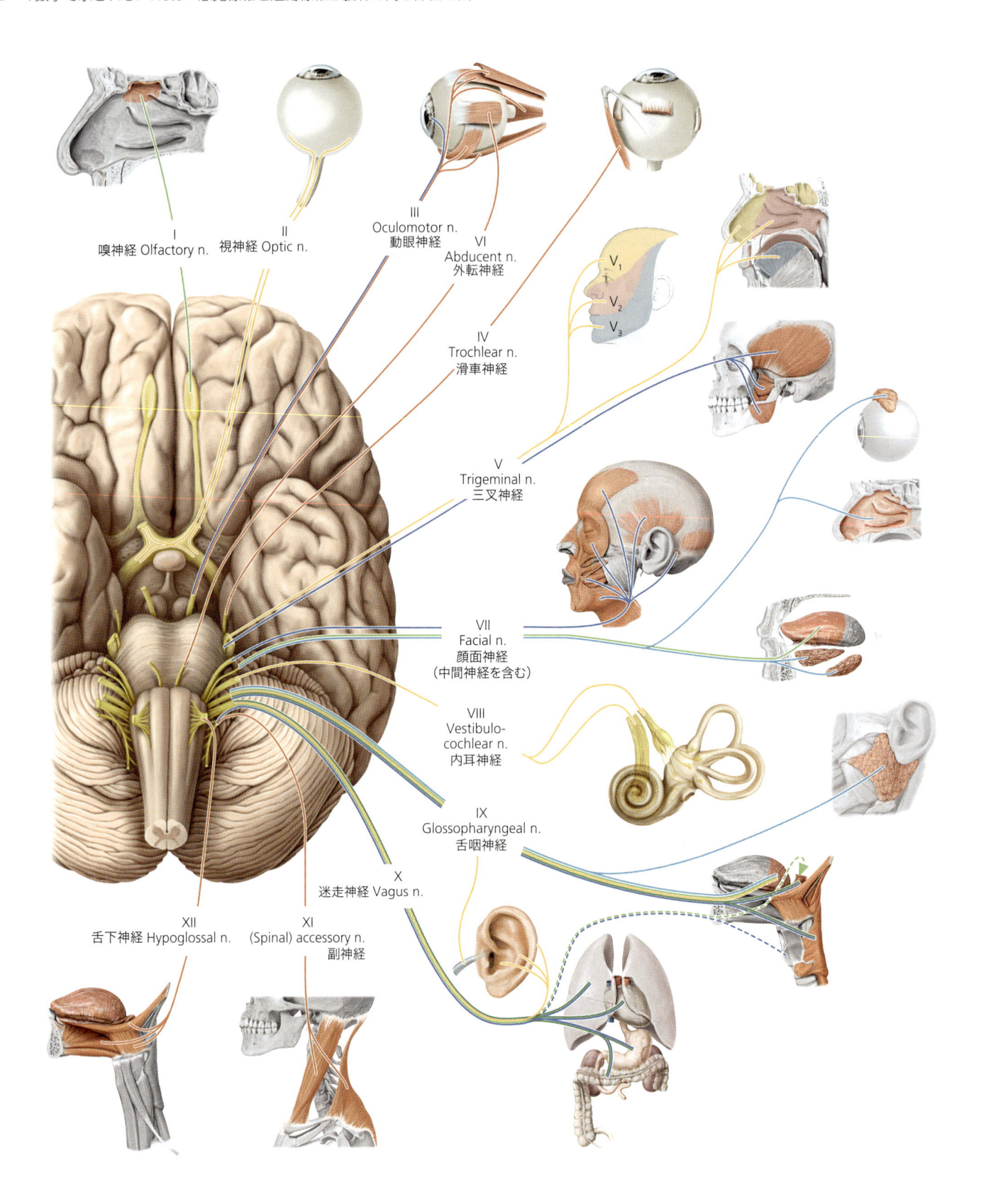

- I 嗅神経 Olfactory n.
- II 視神経 Optic n.
- III 動眼神経 Oculomotor n.
- IV 滑車神経 Trochlear n.
- V 三叉神経 Trigeminal n.
- VI 外転神経 Abducent n.
- VII 顔面神経（中間神経を含む） Facial n.
- VIII 内耳神経 Vestibulocochlear n.
- IX 舌咽神経 Glossopharyngeal n.
- X 迷走神経 Vagus n.
- XI 副神経 (Spinal) accessory n.
- XII 舌下神経 Hypoglossal n.

脳神経には求心性（感覚）線維と遠心性（運動）線維があり，さらに体性あるいは自律（臓性）神経系に分類される（pp. 622-623 参照）．体性神経線維は外部環境との相互作用を可能にし，臓性神経線維は内臓の自律活動を調節する．一般の線維のほかに，脳神経には特定の構造（聴覚器，味蕾など）と結びついた特殊線維も含まれる．脳神経線維は特定の核に起始あるいは停止するが，この核も一般と特殊，体性と臓性，求心性と遠心性に分類される．

表31.1　脳神経線維と脳神経核

この色分けは神経線維と神経核の分類を示すために以下の章でも用いる．

	神経線維	例		神経線維	例
	一般体性遠心性線維（体性運動機能）	骨格筋を支配		一般体性求心性線維（体性感覚）	皮膚と筋紡錘からのインパルスを伝える
	一般臓性遠心性線維（内臓運動機能）	内臓平滑筋，眼筋，心臓，唾液腺などを支配		特殊体性求心性線維	網膜，聴覚器，前庭器からのインパルスを伝える
	特殊臓性遠心性線維	鰓弓由来の骨格筋と心筋を支配		一般臓性求心性線維（臓性感覚）	内臓，血管からのインパルスを伝える
				特殊臓性求心性線維	味蕾，嗅粘膜からのインパルスを伝える

図31.2　脳神経の核

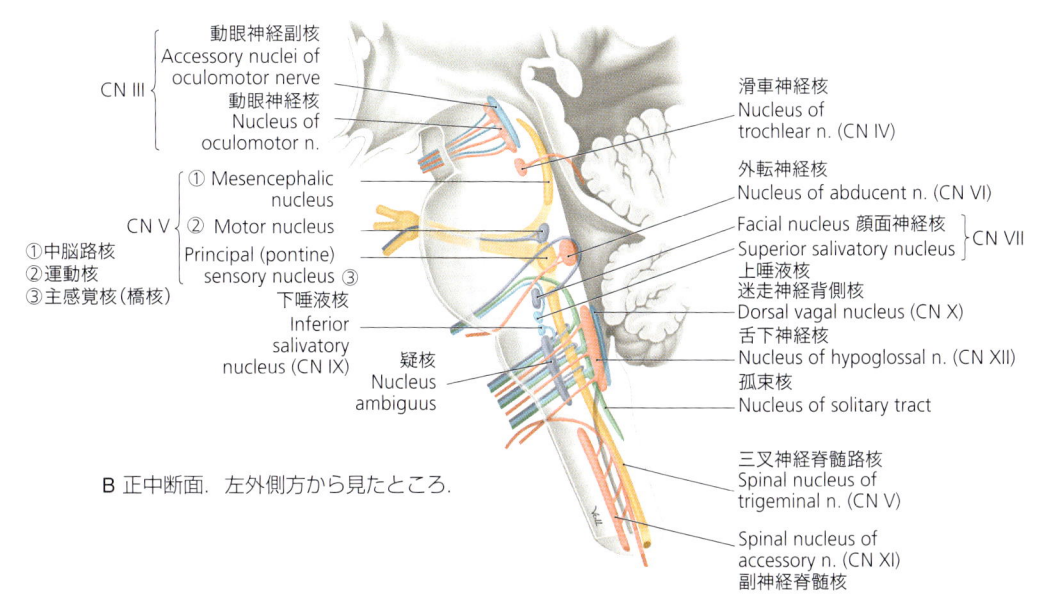

脳神経（CN III-XII）の感覚線維と運動線維は脳幹の特定の核に出入りする．

遠心性（運動）神経核 Efferent (motor) nuclei
- 動眼神経核 Oculomotor n. nuclei (CN III)
- 滑車神経核 Nucleus of trochlear n. (CN IV)
- 外転神経核 Nucleus of abducent n. (CN VI)
- 顔面神経核 Facial nucleus (CN VII)
- 唾液核 Salivatory nuclei
- 疑核 Nucleus ambiguus
- 迷走神経背側核 Dorsal vagal nucleus
- 舌下神経核 Nucleus of hypoglossal n. (CN XII)
- 副神経脊髄核 Spinal nucleus of accessory n. (CN XI)

求心性（感覚）神経核 Afferent (sensory) nuclei
- 三叉神経核群 Trigeminal n. nuclei (CN V)
- CN V
- CN VII
- CN VI
- CN VIII
- CN IX
- CN X
- 三叉神経脊髄路核 Spinal nucleus of trigeminal n. (CN V)
- 孤束核 Nucleus of solitary tract

A 後方から見たところ．小脳を取り除いてある．

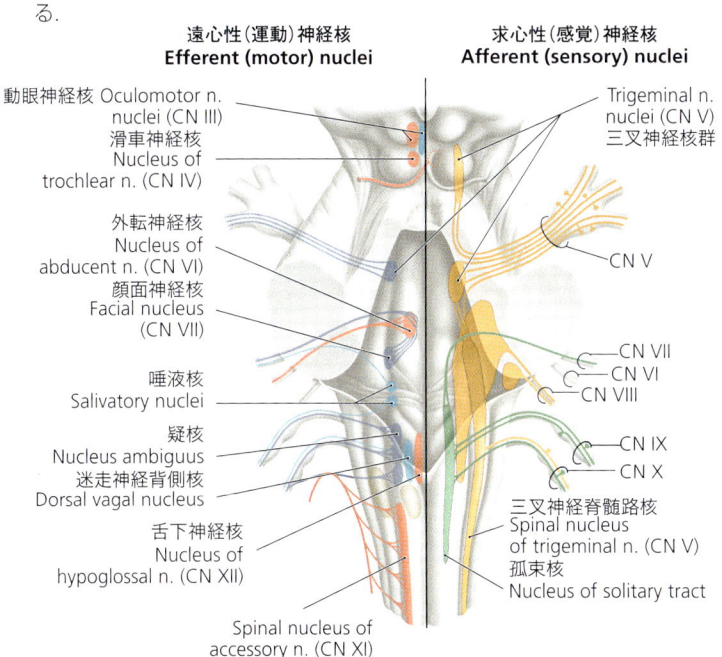

表31.2　脳神経

脳神経	起始部	機能的線維型
CN I: 嗅神経	終脳*	●
CN II: 視神経	間脳*	●
CN III: 動眼神経	中脳	● ●
CN IV: 滑車神経		●
CN V: 三叉神経	橋	● ●
CN VI: 外転神経		●
CN VII: 顔面神経		● ● ● ●
CN VIII: 内耳神経		●
CN IX: 舌咽神経	延髄	● ● ● ● ●
CN X: 迷走神経		● ● ● ●
CN XI: 副神経		● ●
CN XII: 舌下神経		●

*嗅神経と視神経は真の神経というよりは脳の延長である．それゆえ脳幹の核とは関係しない．

CN III
- 動眼神経副核 Accessory nuclei of oculomotor nerve
- 動眼神経核 Nucleus of oculomotor n.

CN V
- ① Mesencephalic nucleus
- ② Motor nucleus
- ③ Principal (pontine) sensory nucleus

①中脳路核
②運動核
③主感覚核（橋核）

- 下唾液核 Inferior salivatory nucleus (CN IX)
- 疑核 Nucleus ambiguus
- 滑車神経核 Nucleus of trochlear n. (CN IV)
- 外転神経核 Nucleus of abducent n. (CN VI)
- 顔面神経核 Facial nucleus / 上唾液核 Superior salivatory nucleus } CN VII
- 迷走神経背側核 Dorsal vagal nucleus (CN X)
- 舌下神経核 Nucleus of hypoglossal n. (CN XII)
- 孤束核 Nucleus of solitary tract
- 三叉神経脊髄路核 Spinal nucleus of trigeminal n. (CN V)
- 副神経脊髄核 Spinal nucleus of accessory n. (CN XI)

B 正中断面．左外側方から見たところ．

脳神経：嗅神経（CN I）と視神経（CN II）
CN I & II: Olfactory & Optic Nerves

> 嗅神経と視神経は真の末梢神経ではなく，それぞれ終脳と間脳の延長（神経路）である．そのため脳幹の脳神経核とは関係しない．

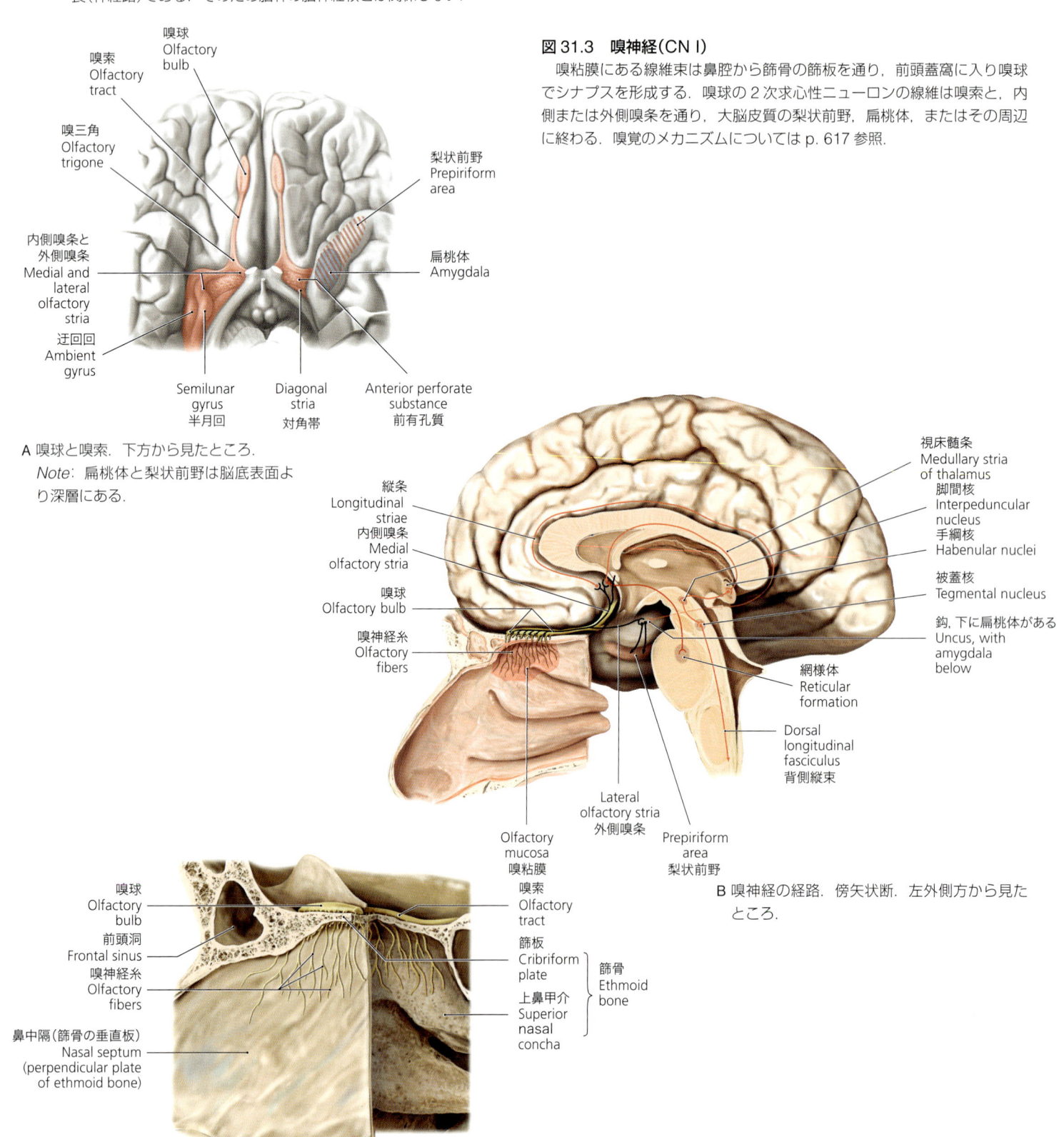

図31.3 嗅神経（CN I）

嗅粘膜にある線維束は鼻腔から篩骨の篩板を通り，前頭蓋窩に入り嗅球でシナプスを形成する．嗅球の2次求心性ニューロンの線維は嗅索と，内側または外側嗅条を通り，大脳皮質の梨状前野，扁桃体，またはその周辺に終わる．嗅覚のメカニズムについては p. 617 参照．

A 嗅球と嗅索．下方から見たところ．
Note：扁桃体と梨状前野は脳底表面より深層にある．

B 嗅神経の経路．傍矢状断．左外側方から見たところ．

C 嗅神経糸．左鼻中隔の一部と右鼻腔の外壁．左外側方から見たところ．

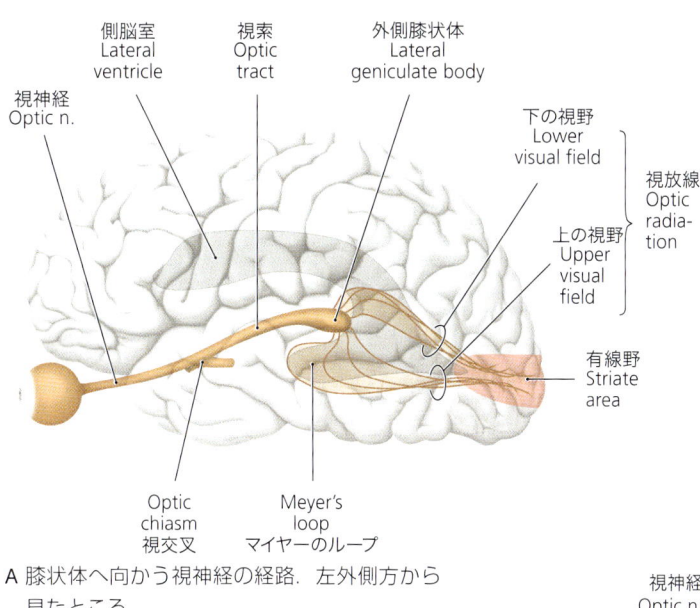

図 31.4 視神経（CN II）

視神経は眼球から視神経管を通り中頭蓋窩に至る．左右の視神経は間脳の下部で視交叉を作り，その後に左右の視索に分かれる．それぞれの視索は外側根と内側根に分かれる．視交叉において多くの網膜神経節細胞からの軸索が，正中線を横切り脳の反対側に向かう．視覚のメカニズムについては p.619 参照．

A 膝状体へ向かう視神経の経路．左外側方から見たところ．

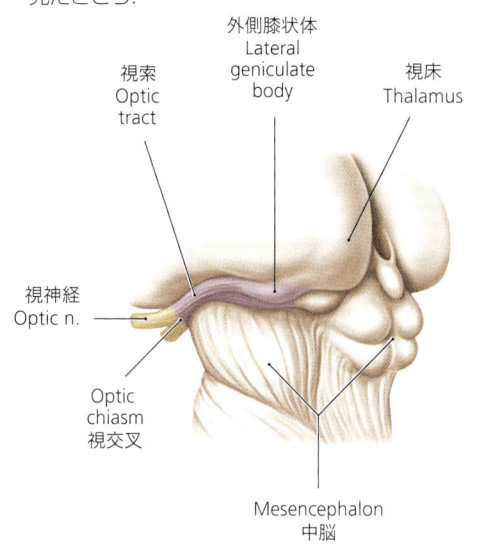

B 視索の終端．脳幹左側を後方から見たところ．視神経は網膜神経節細胞の軸索から構成されている．これらの軸索は主に間脳の外側膝状体と中脳の上丘に終わる．

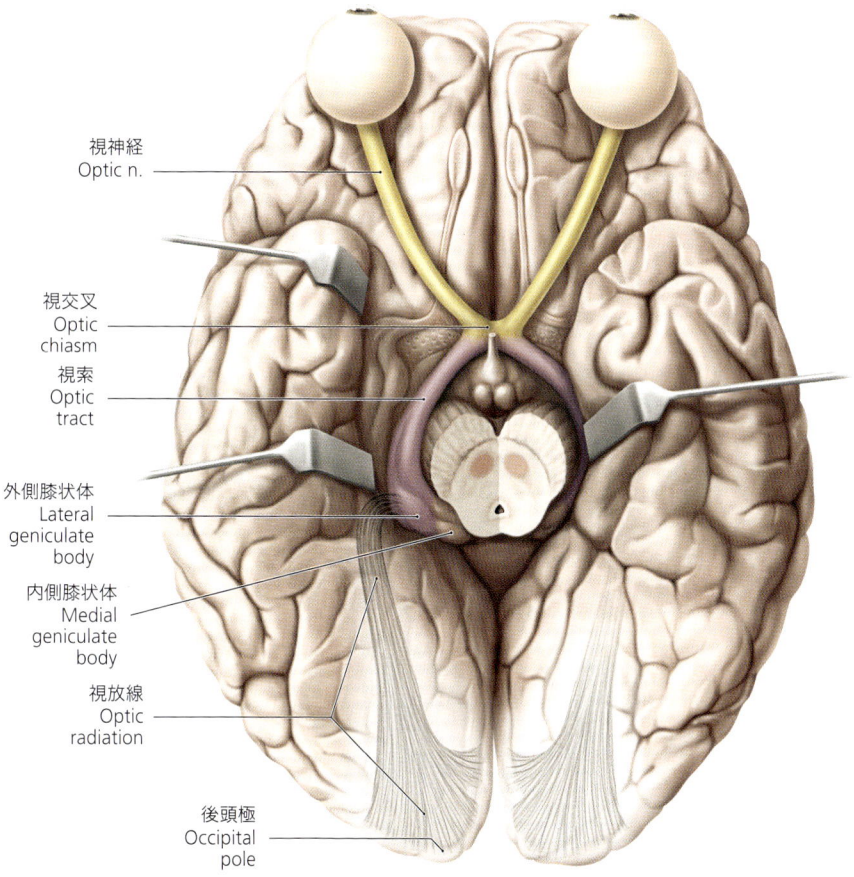

C 視神経の走行．脳の底面．

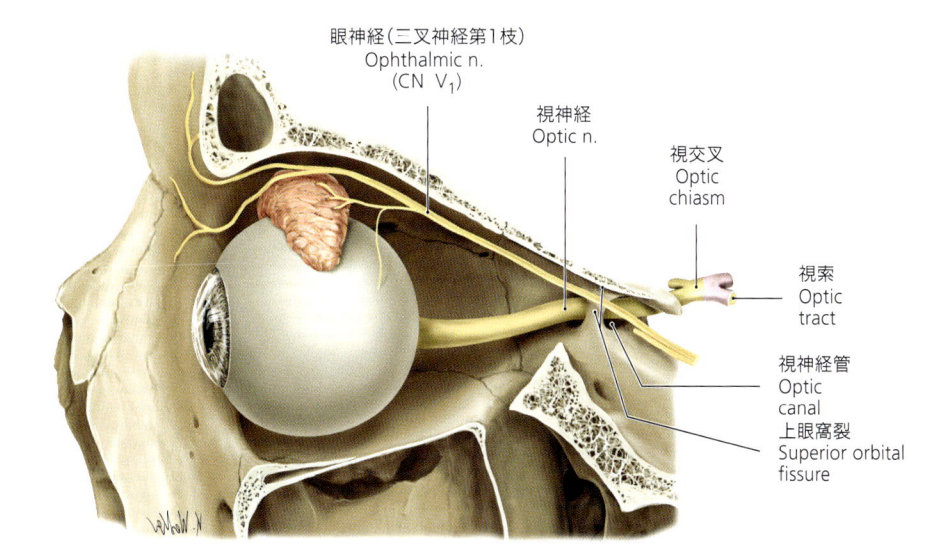

D 左眼窩における視神経．外側方から見たところ．視神経は視神経管を通って眼窩に至る．
Note：ほかの脳神経は上眼窩裂を通って眼窩に入る．

脳神経：動眼神経（CN III），滑車神経（CN IV），外転神経（CN VI）
CN III, IV & VI: Oculomotor, Trochlear & Abducent Nerves

脳神経 III，IV，VI は外眼筋を支配する（p.509 参照）．このうち動眼神経（CN III）だけが体性遠心性線維と臓性遠心性線維を含み，さらに複数の外眼筋と内眼筋を支配する唯一の神経でもある．

図 31.5 動眼神経，滑車神経，外転神経の核
脳神経のうち，すべての線維が対側に向かうのは滑車神経（CN IV）だけである．また滑車神経は脳幹の背側から出る唯一の脳神経であり，従って硬膜内でたどる経路が最も長い．

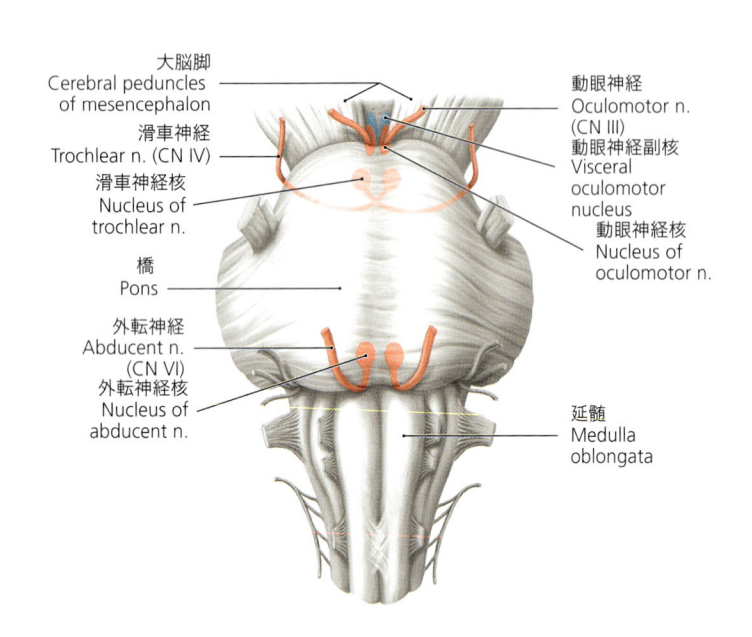

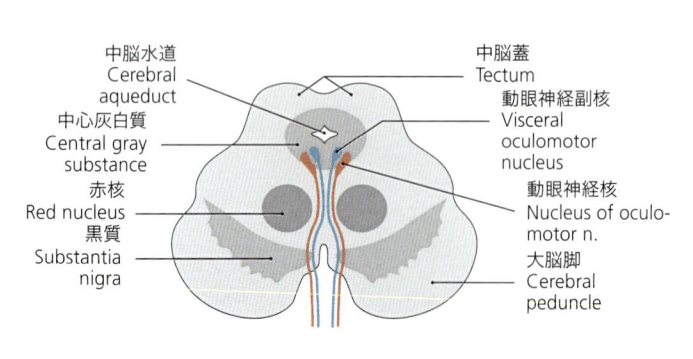

A 外眼筋の脳神経の起始部．脳幹を前方から見たところ．

B 動眼神経核．横断面．上方から見たところ．

表 31.3 外眼筋の脳神経

経路*	線維	核	機能	障害時の影響
動眼神経（CN III）				
中脳から前方に走行	体性遠心性線維	動眼神経核	分布 ・上眼瞼挙筋 ・上直筋，内側直筋，下直筋 ・下斜筋	動眼神経の完全麻痺（外眼筋と内眼筋の麻痺） ・眼瞼下垂（眼瞼が下に垂れる） ・下方および外側への注視の偏り ・複視（二重視） ・散瞳（瞳孔散大） ・遠近調節困難（毛様体麻痺）
	臓性遠心性線維	動眼神経副核（エーディンガー-ウェストファル核）	毛様体神経節のニューロンとシナプスを形成する 分布 ・瞳孔括約筋 ・毛様体筋	
滑車神経（CN IV）				
脳幹後面の正中線近くから起こり，大脳脚の周囲を前方に走行	体性遠心性線維	滑車神経核	分布 ・上斜筋	・複視 ・障害側の眼が上方やや外側に偏る（下斜筋優位）
外転神経（CN VI）				
硬膜外を長く走行**	体性遠心性線維	外転神経核	分布 ・外側直筋	・複視 ・障害側の眼が上方に偏る

*この 3 つの神経はすべて上眼窩裂から眼窩に入る．動眼神経と外転神経は総腱輪を通る．
**外転神経は硬膜外を走行する．そのため外転神経麻痺は髄膜炎やクモ膜下出血に関連して起こりやすい．

Note: 動眼神経は内眼筋を副交感性に支配し，外眼筋の大部分と上眼瞼挙筋には体性運動性に支配する．動眼神経の副交感性線維は毛様体神経節でシナプスを形成する．

Note: 動眼神経麻痺が起こると，その影響が副交感性線維だけにあらわれる場合や体性線維だけにあらわれる場合，さらに両方に同時にあらわれる場合がある．

図 31.6 外眼筋を支配する神経の経路
右眼窩．

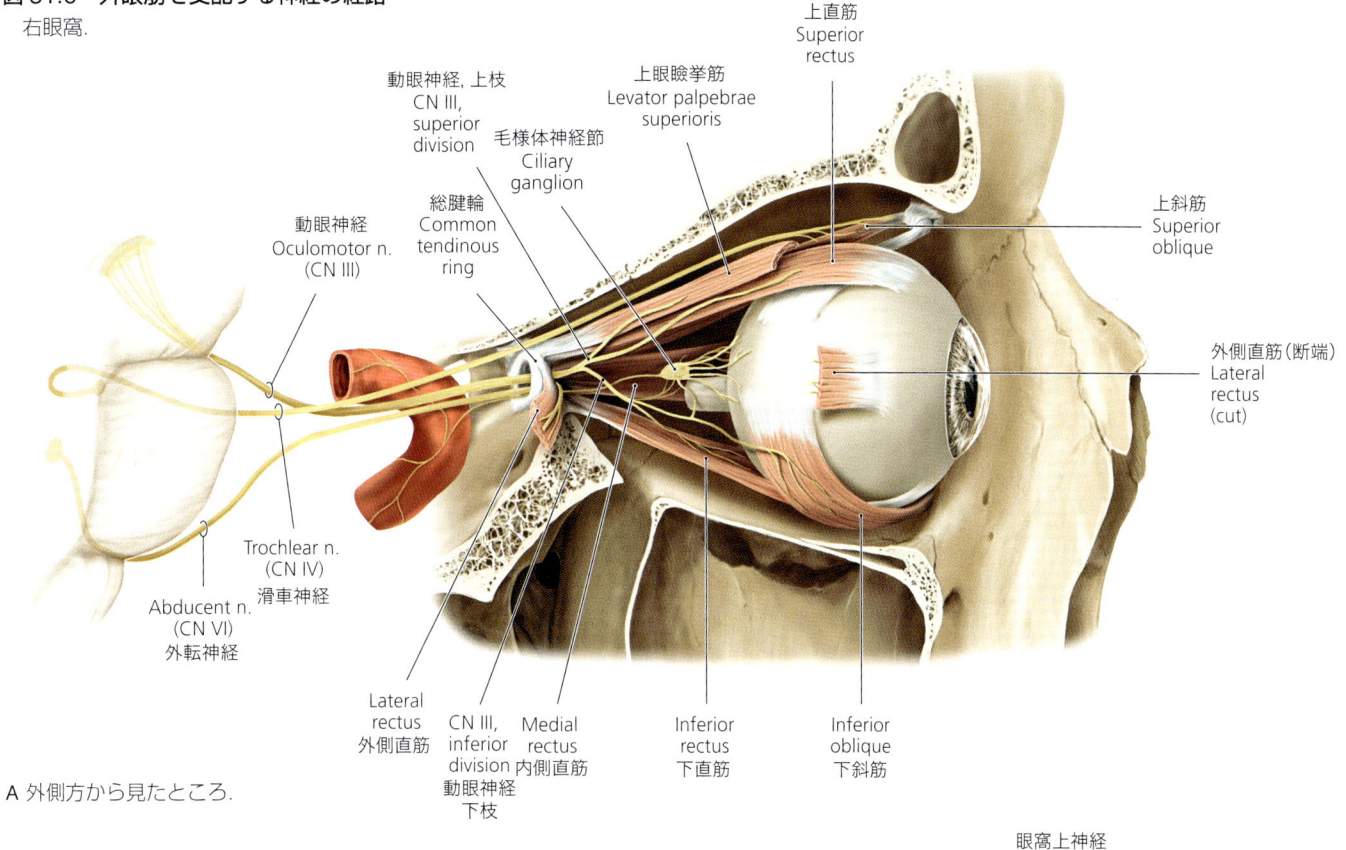

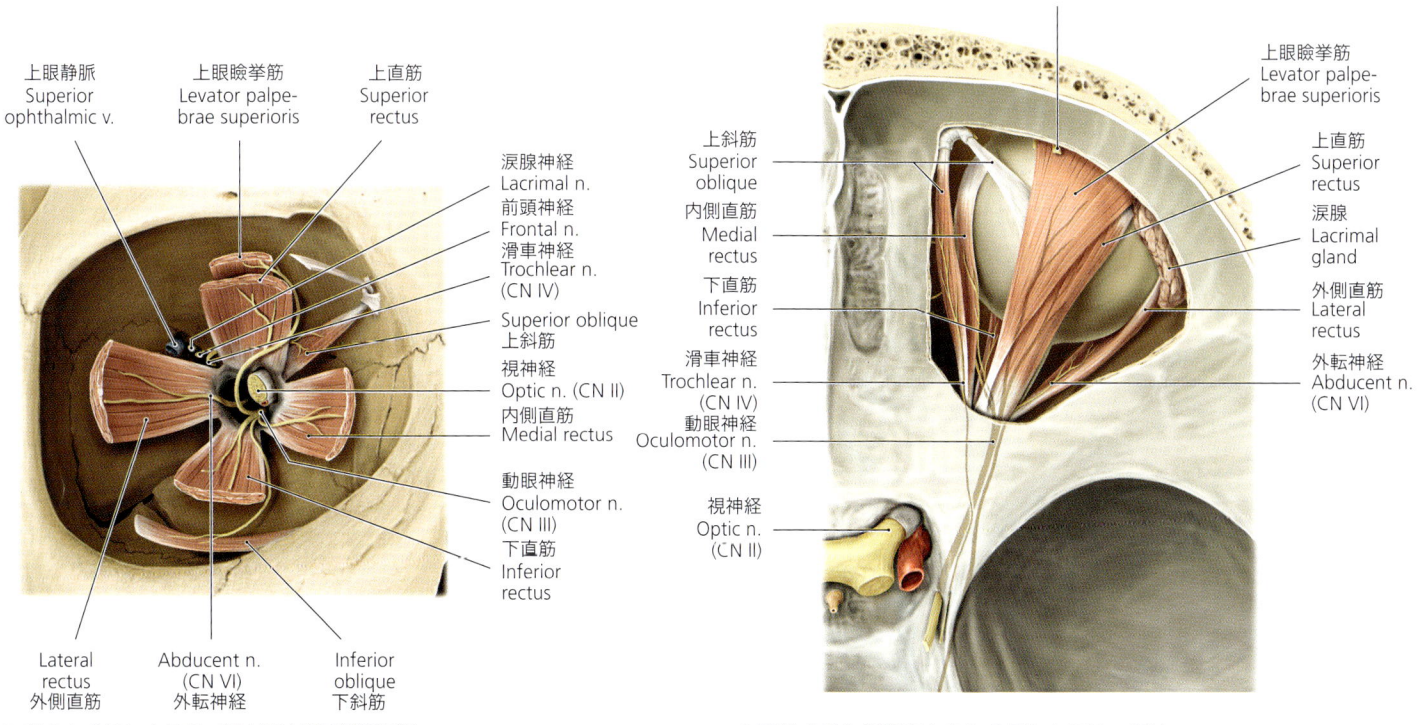

A 外側方から見たところ．

B 前方から見たところ．視神経は視神経管を通って眼窩にあらわれる．視神経管は動眼神経・滑車神経・外転神経があらわれる上眼窩裂より正中側にある．

C 開放された眼窩を上方から見たところ．視神経管と上眼窩裂との関係に注意．

脳神経：三叉神経(CN V)
CN V: Trigeminal Nerve

三叉神経は頭部の感覚神経で，3つの求心性神経核がある．咀嚼筋からの固有感覚線維を受けとる三叉神経中脳路核，触覚を主に伝達する三叉神経主感覚核（橋核），痛覚と温度覚を主に伝達する三叉神経脊髄路核の3つである．三叉神経運動核は咀嚼筋を支配する．

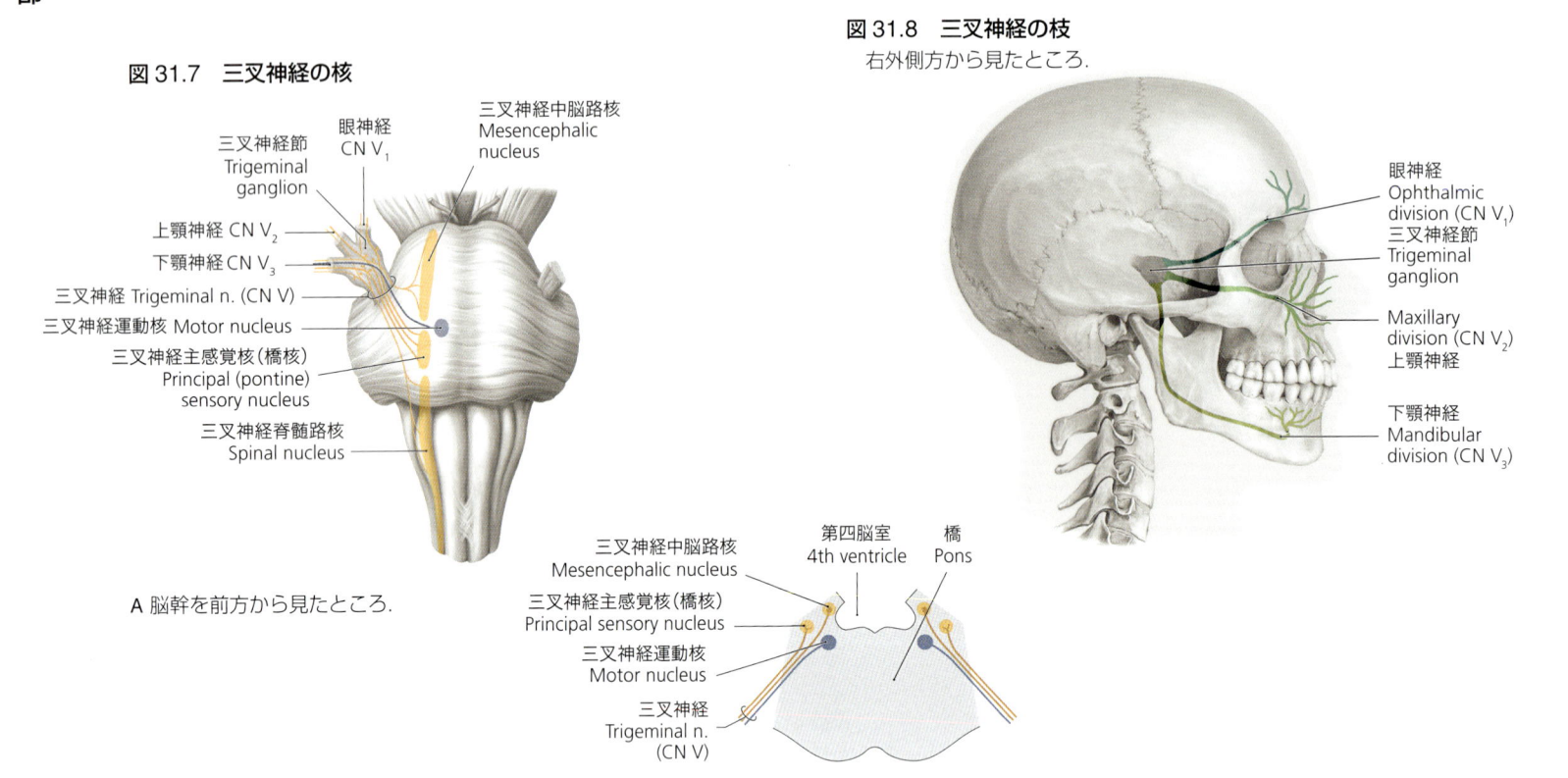

図 31.7 三叉神経の核

- 眼神経 CN V₁
- 三叉神経節 Trigeminal ganglion
- 上顎神経 CN V₂
- 下顎神経 CN V₃
- 三叉神経 Trigeminal n. (CN V)
- 三叉神経運動核 Motor nucleus
- 三叉神経主感覚核（橋核） Principal (pontine) sensory nucleus
- 三叉神経脊髄路核 Spinal nucleus
- 三叉神経中脳路核 Mesencephalic nucleus

A 脳幹を前方から見たところ．

- 三叉神経中脳路核 Mesencephalic nucleus
- 三叉神経主感覚核（橋核） Principal sensory nucleus
- 三叉神経運動核 Motor nucleus
- 三叉神経 Trigeminal n. (CN V)
- 第四脳室 4th ventricle
- 橋 Pons

B 橋の横断面．上方から見たところ．

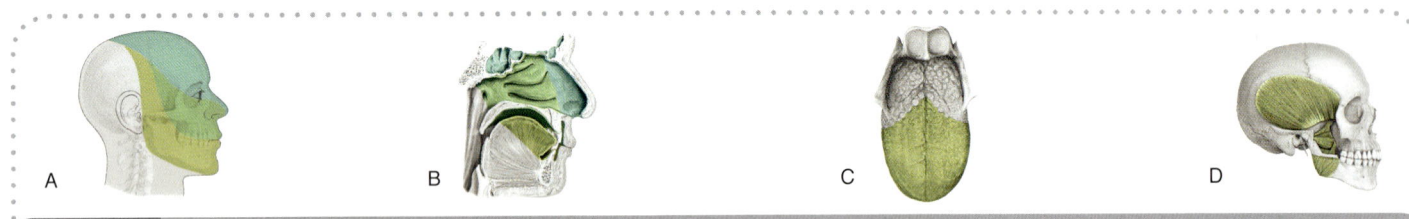

図 31.8 三叉神経の枝
右外側方から見たところ．

- 眼神経 Ophthalmic division (CN V₁)
- 三叉神経節 Trigeminal ganglion
- 上顎神経 Maxillary division (CN V₂)
- 下顎神経 Mandibular division (CN V₃)

A / B / C / D

表 31.4　三叉神経(CN V)

経路	線維	核	機能	障害時の影響
中頭蓋窩から外に出る 眼神経(CN V₁)：上眼窩裂を通り，眼窩に入る 上顎神経(CN V₂)：正円孔を通り，翼口蓋窩に入る 下顎神経(CN V₃)：卵円孔を通り，頭蓋底の下面に出る	体性求心性線維	・三叉神経主感覚核（橋核） ・三叉神経中脳路核 ・三叉神経脊髄路核	分布： ・顔面皮膚(A) ・鼻咽頭粘膜(B) ・舌(前2/3)(C) 角膜反射に関与（眼瞼の反射性閉合）	・感覚の消失（外傷性神経障害） ・眼の帯状疱疹（水痘・帯状疱疹ウイルス），顔面帯状疱疹
	特殊臓性遠心性線維	三叉神経運動核	分布（CN V₃を経由） ・咀嚼筋（側頭筋，咬筋，外側翼突筋，内側翼突筋）(D) ・口腔底筋（顎舌骨筋，顎二腹筋前腹） ・鼓膜張筋 ・口蓋帆張筋	
	臓性遠心性線維の経路*		・涙腺神経(CN V₁の枝)は，顔面神経の副交感性線維を，頬骨神経(CN V₂の枝)と合流して涙腺まで運ぶ ・舌神経(CN V₃の枝)は顔面神経の副交感性線維を鼓索神経と合流して顎下腺および舌下腺に運ぶ ・耳介側頭神経(CN V₃の枝)は舌咽神経の副交感性線維を耳下腺まで運ぶ	
	臓性求心性線維の経路*		顔面神経の味覚線維（鼓索神経）は，舌神経とともに進み，舌の前2/3に分布する	

*一部の脳神経の線維は三叉神経の枝や小枝に合流して，それぞれの支配領域に至る．

図 31.9 三叉神経の枝の経路
右外側方から見たところ．

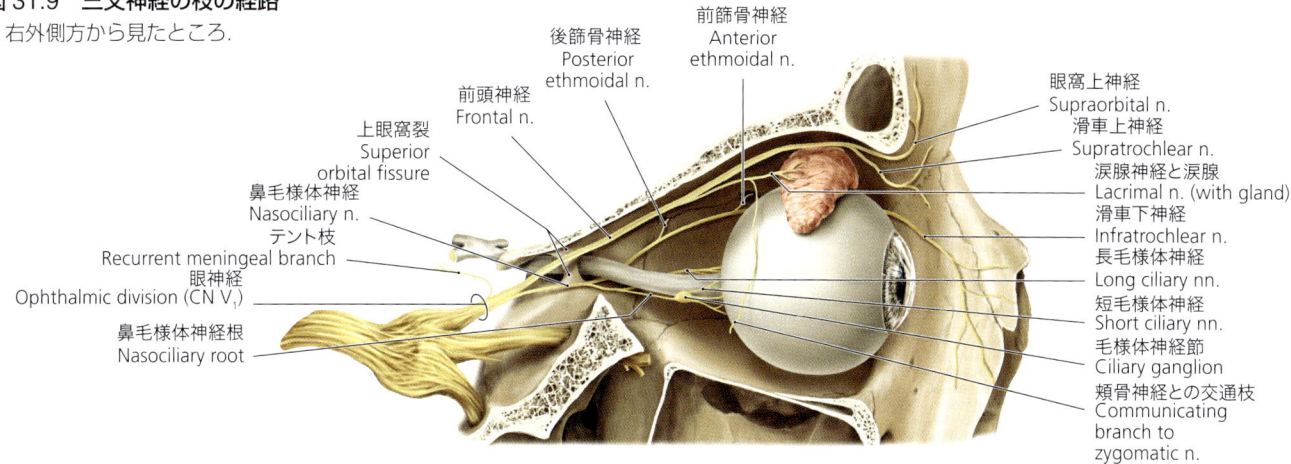

A 眼神経（CN V₁）．右眼窩を部分的に開放してある．

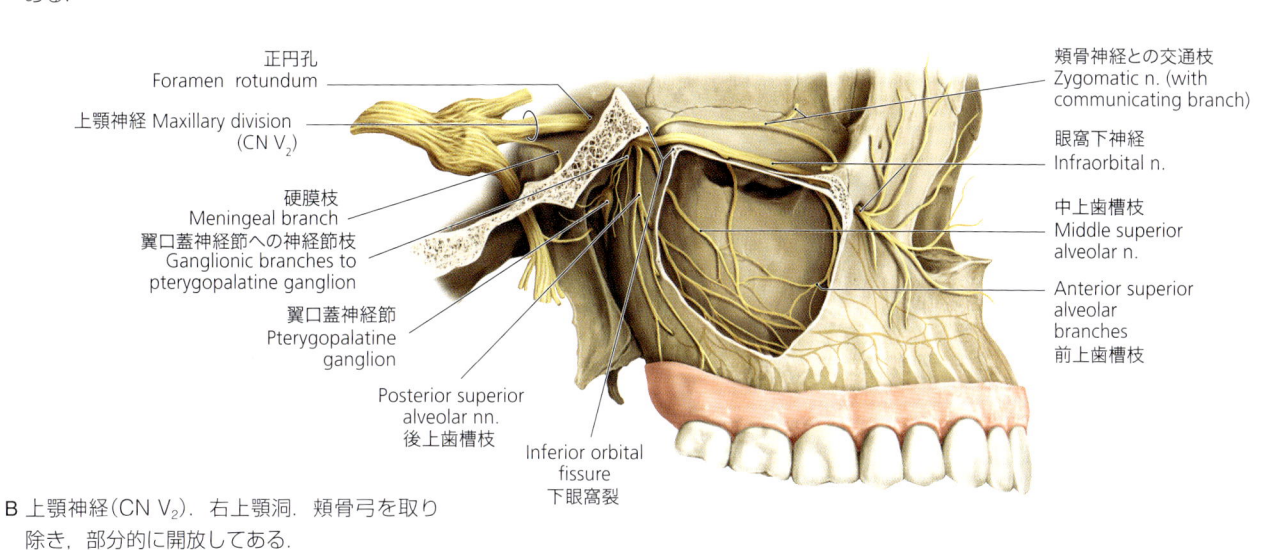

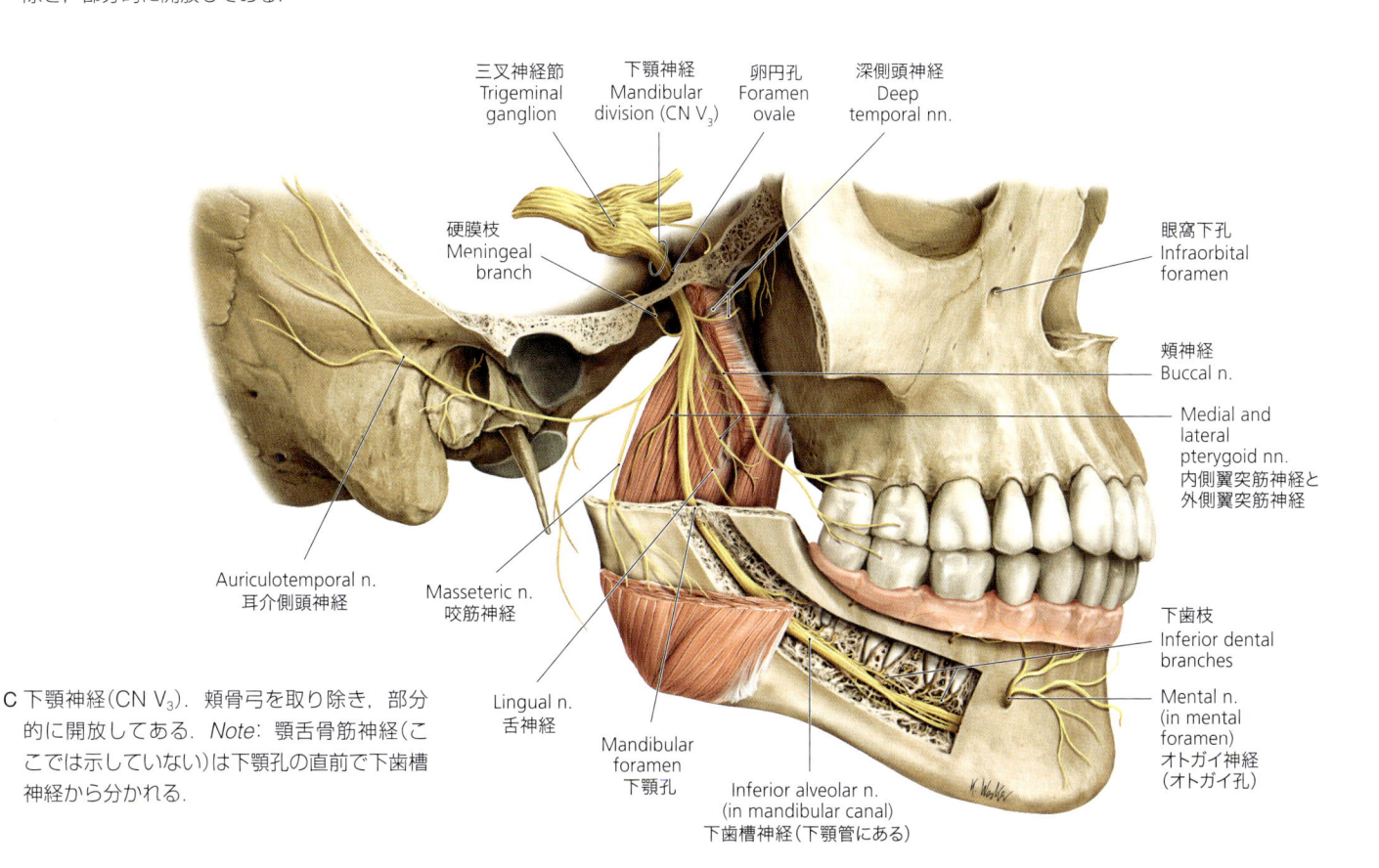

B 上顎神経（CN V₂）．右上顎洞．頬骨弓を取り除き，部分的に開放してある．

C 下顎神経（CN V₃）．頬骨弓を取り除き，部分的に開放してある．*Note*：顎舌骨筋神経（ここでは示していない）は下顎孔の直前で下歯槽神経から分かれる．

脳神経：顔面神経（CN VII）
CN VII: Facial Nerve

顔面神経は，主に顔面神経核からの特殊臓性遠心性（鰓性）線維を表情筋に運ぶ．上唾液核からの臓性遠心性（副交感性）線維は，臓性求心性（の味覚）線維とまとまって中間神経を形成する．

図 31.10 顔面神経の核

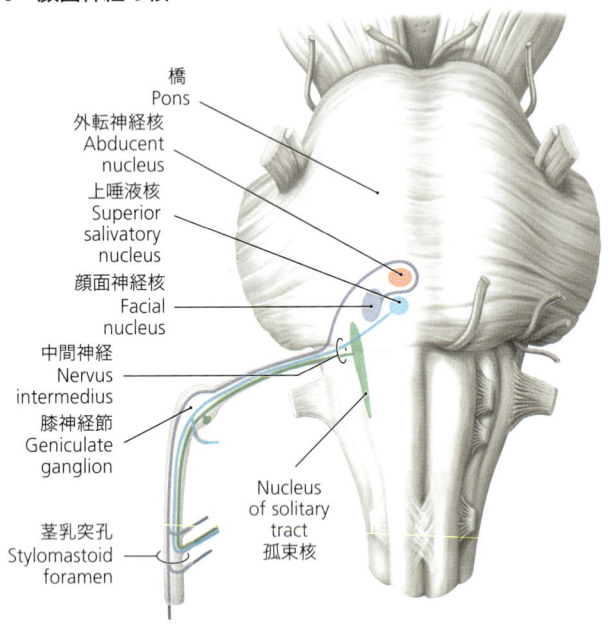

A 脳幹，前方から見たところ．

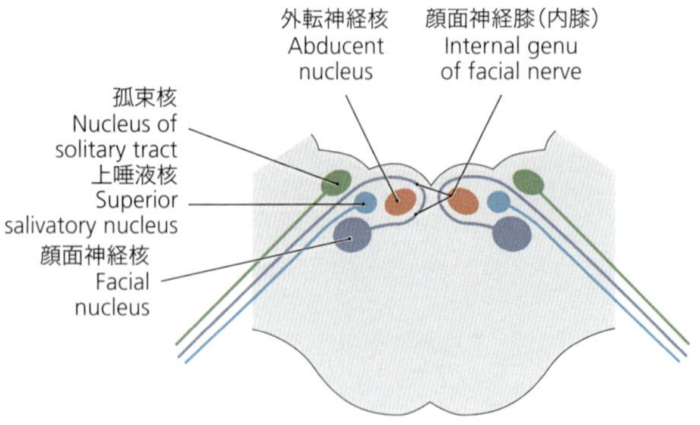

B 橋の横断面，上方から見たところ．

図 31.11 顔面神経の枝
右側方から見たところ．

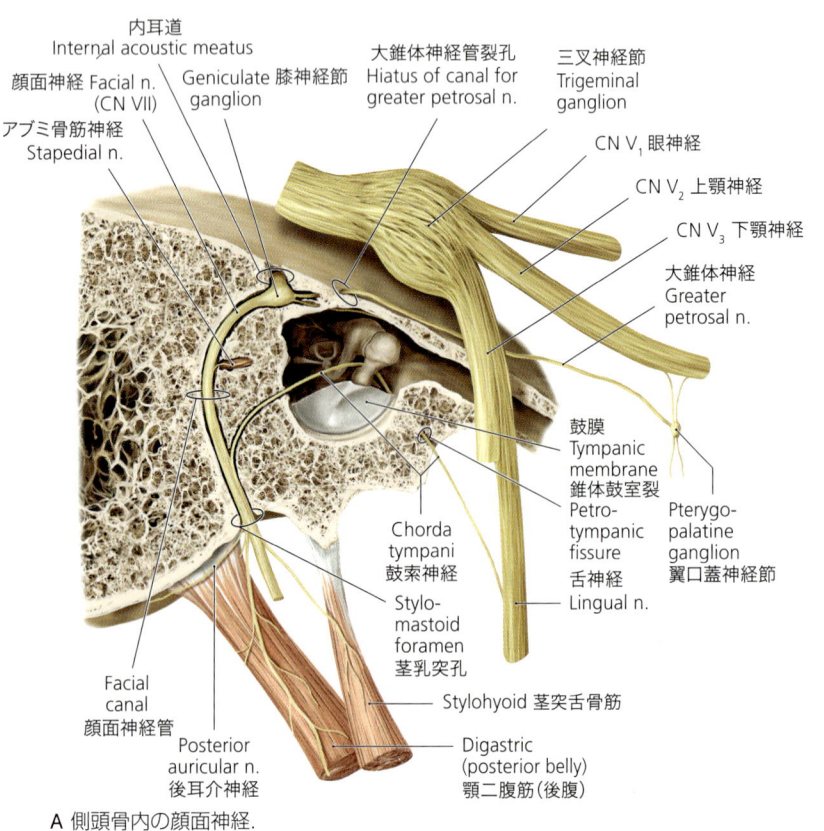

A 側頭骨内の顔面神経．

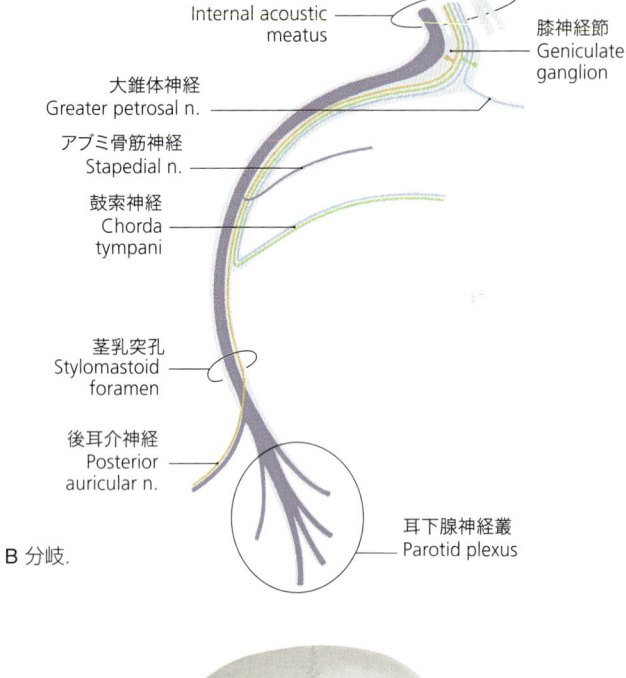

B 分岐．

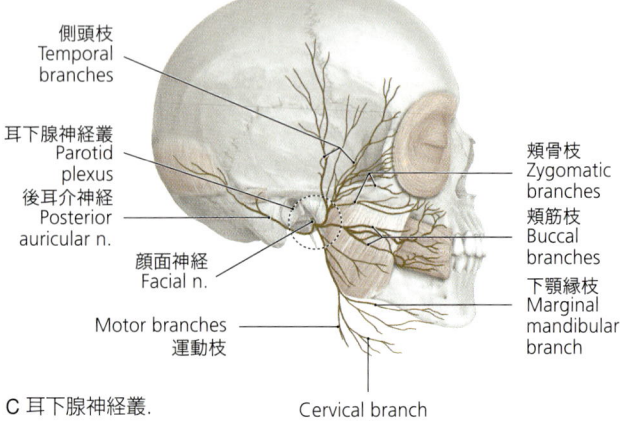

C 耳下腺神経叢．

表31.5　顔面神経（CN VII）

経路	線維	核	機能	障害時の影響
橋とオリーブの間の橋小脳三角から起こり，内耳道から側頭骨の岩様部に入り， ・大錐体神経 ・アブミ骨筋神経 ・鼓索神経 に分かれる 臓性遠心性線維の一部は茎乳突孔を通って頭蓋底に向かい，耳下腺内神経叢を作る	特殊臓性遠心性線維	顔面神経核	分布 ・表情筋 ・茎突舌骨筋 ・顎二腹筋の後腹 ・アブミ骨筋	末梢の顔面神経の障害：障害側の表情筋の麻痺 味覚，涙液分泌，唾液分泌の関連障害など
	臓性遠心性線維（副交感性）*	上唾液核	翼口蓋神経節または顎下神経節のニューロンとシナプスを形成する 分布 ・涙腺 ・鼻粘膜，硬口蓋，軟口蓋の小腺 ・顎下腺 ・舌下腺 ・舌背の小唾液腺	
	特殊臓性求心性線維*	孤束核	膝神経節からの末梢性突起は鼓索神経を作る（舌からの味覚線維）	
	体性求心性線維		耳介，外耳道の皮膚，鼓膜の外面からの感覚性線維は顔面神経経由で三叉神経主感覚核に行く	

*中間神経を形成し，顔面神経核からの臓性遠心性線維と合流する．

図31.12　顔面神経の走行

右外側方から見たところ．臓性遠心性（副交感性）線維と特殊臓性求心性（の味覚）線維は黒線で示してある．

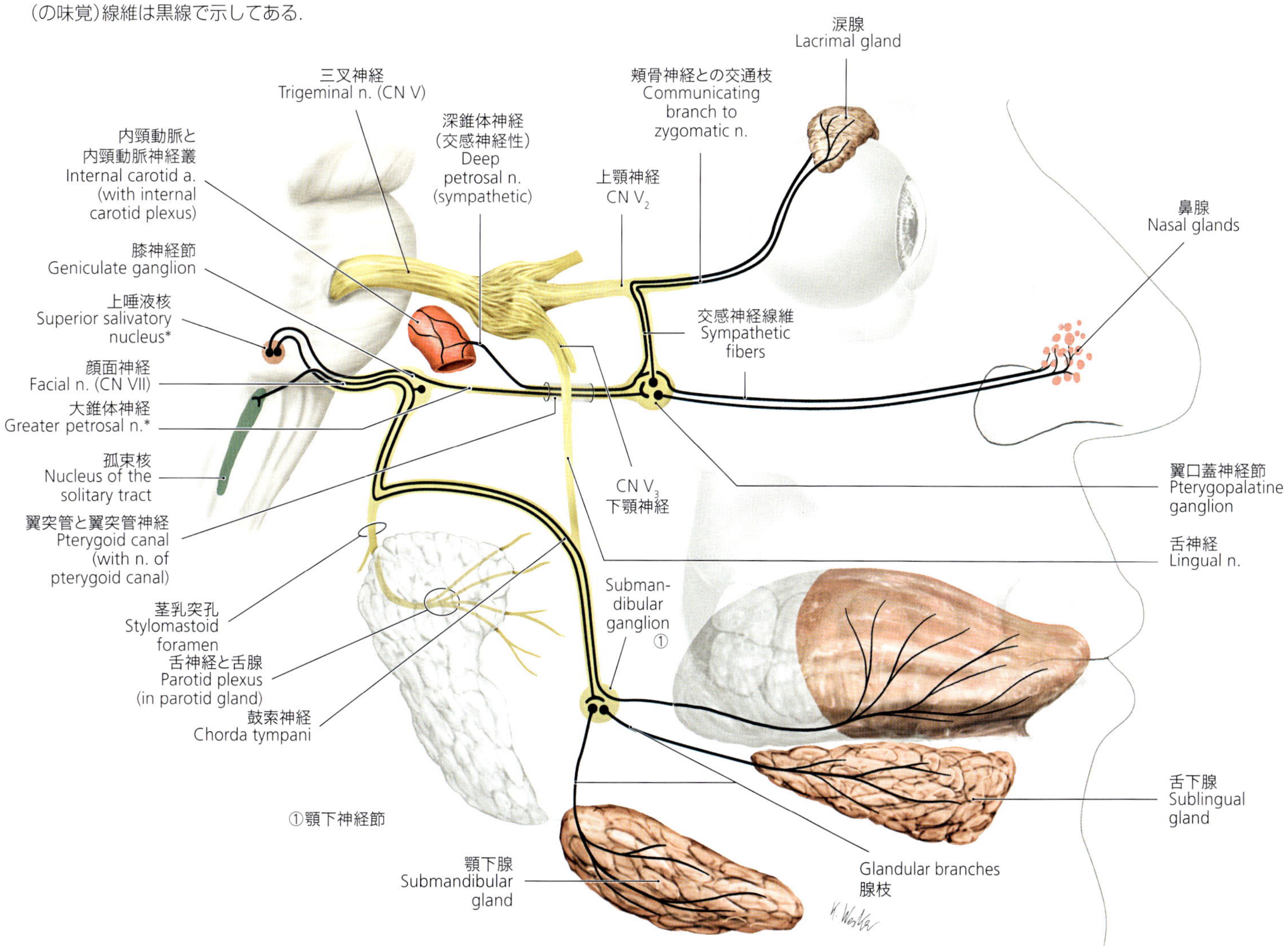

*副交感性．

脳神経：内耳神経（CN VIII）
CN VIII: Vestibulocochlear Nerve

内耳神経は2つの根からなる特殊体性求心性神経である．前庭神経は平衡器（p.618参照）からの興奮を伝え，蝸牛神経は聴覚器（p.616参照）からの興奮を伝える．

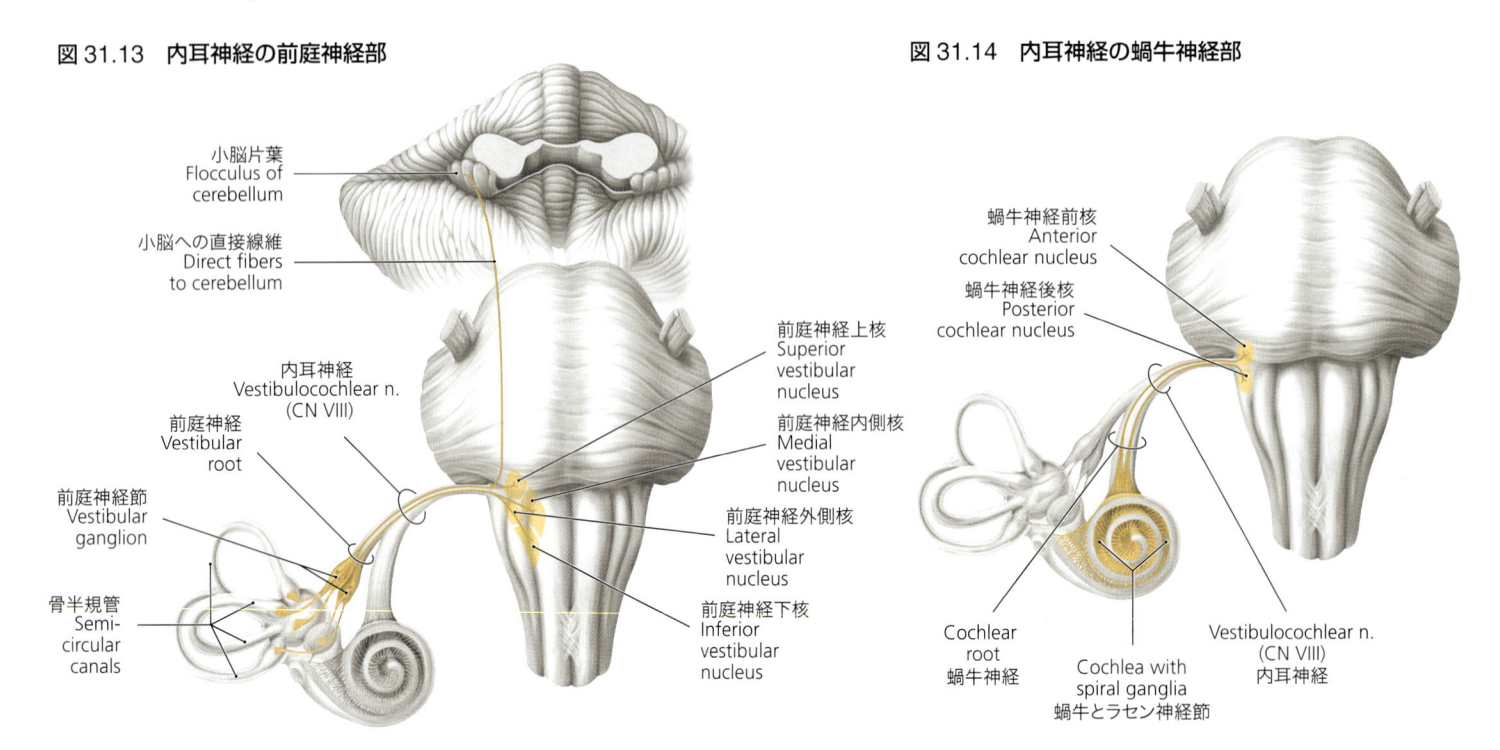

図31.13　内耳神経の前庭神経部

A 延髄と橋，小脳を前方から見たところ．

B 延髄上部の横断面．

図31.14　内耳神経の蝸牛神経部

A 延髄と橋，小脳を前方から見たところ．

B 延髄上部の横断面．

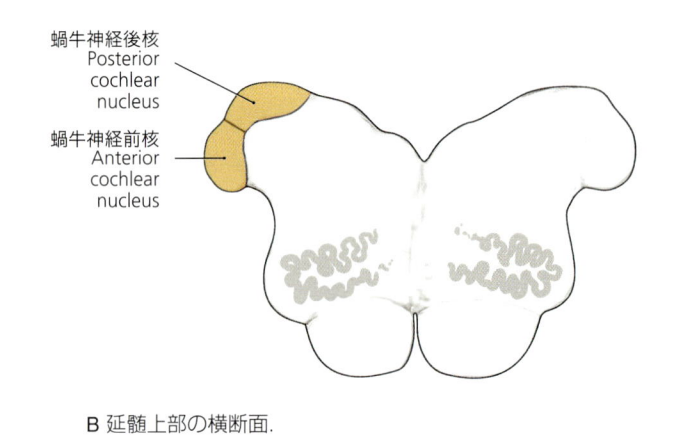

表31.6　内耳神経（CN VIII）

神経	経路	線維	核	機能	障害時の影響
前庭神経	内耳から内耳道を経由して橋小脳三角に至り，そこで脳に入る	特殊体性求心性線維	前庭神経外側核，前庭神経内側核，前庭神経上核，前庭神経下核	骨半規管，球形嚢，卵形嚢からの末梢枝は前庭神経節を経由して，その後4つの前庭神経核に至る．	眩暈
蝸牛神経			蝸牛神経後核と蝸牛神経前核	コルチ器の有毛細胞から始まる末梢枝はラセン神経節を経由して，2つの蝸牛神経核に至る．	聴覚障害

図 31.15 前庭神経節と蝸牛神経節（ラセン神経節）

Note: 前庭神経と蝸牛神経は側頭骨の岩様部において，別個の構造となっている．

図 31.16 側頭骨内の内耳神経

A 鼓室の内側壁．斜め矢状断面．

B 内耳道内の脳神経．右内耳道を斜め後方から見たところ．

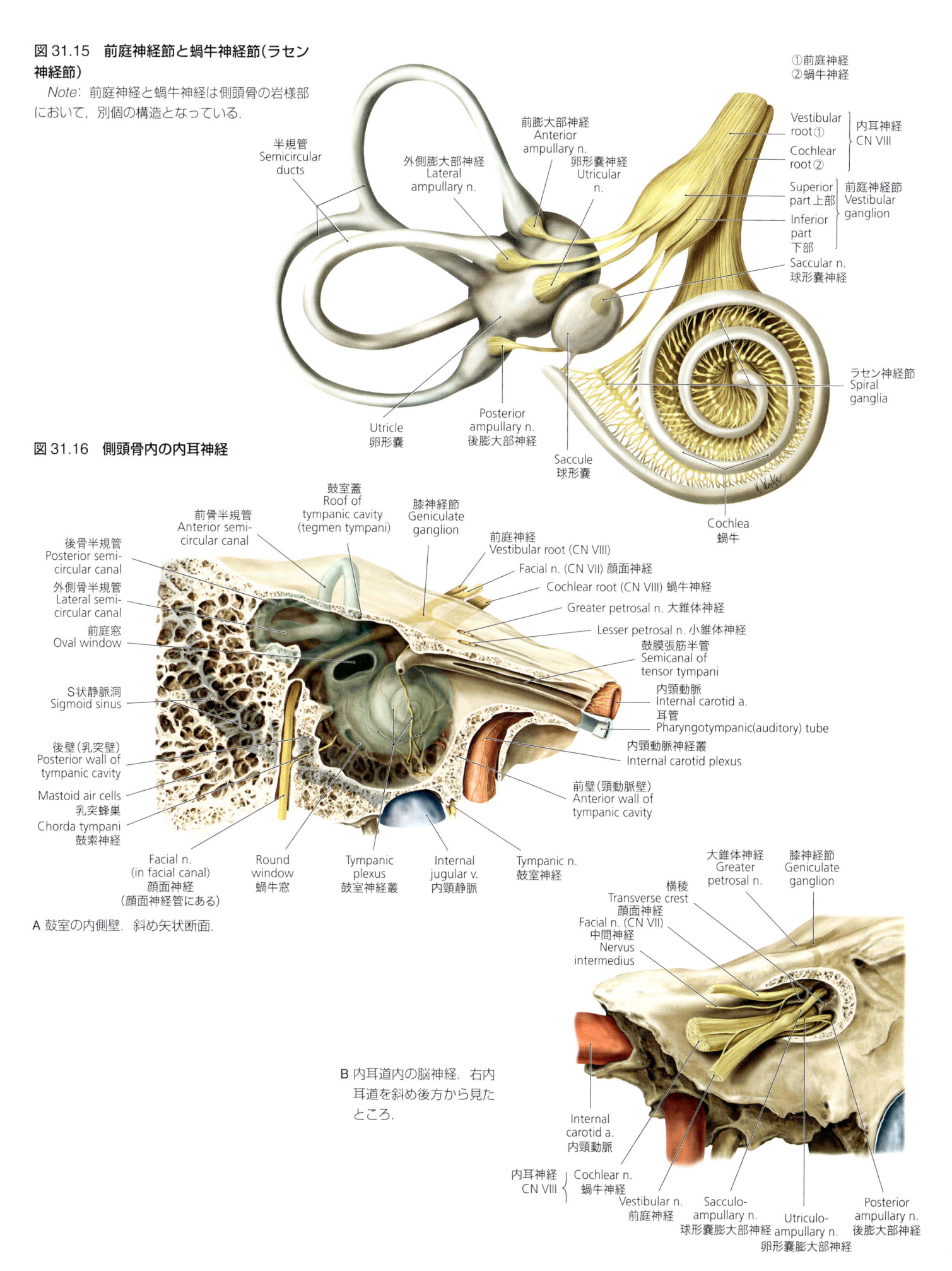

脳神経：舌咽神経（CN IX）
CN IX: Glossopharyngeal Nerve

図 31.17　舌咽神経核

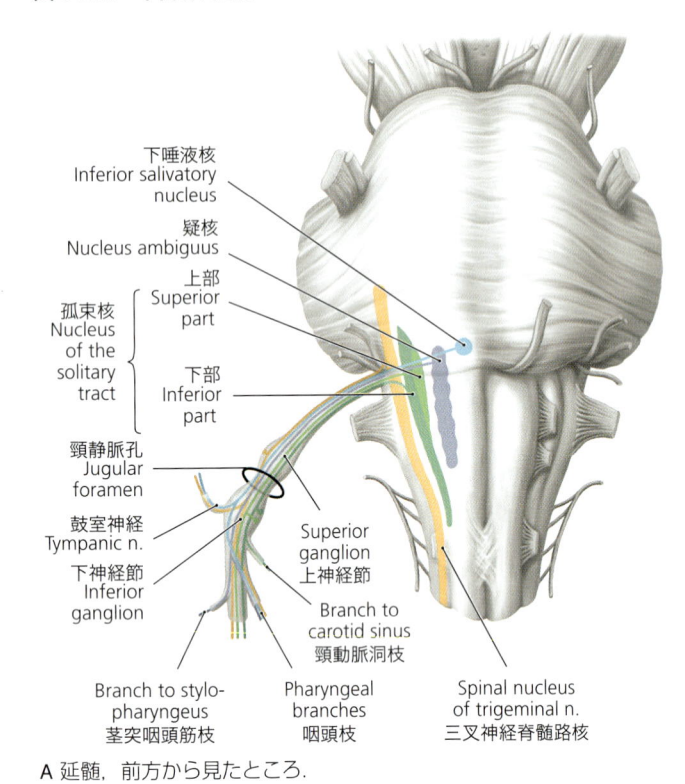

A　延髄，前方から見たところ．

B　延髄の横断面．上方から見たところ．三叉神経の核は示していない．

図 31.18　舌咽神経の走行
左外側方から見たところ．Note：迷走神経（CN X）の線維と舌咽神経（CN IX）の線維は咽頭神経叢を形成して，頸動脈洞に分布する．

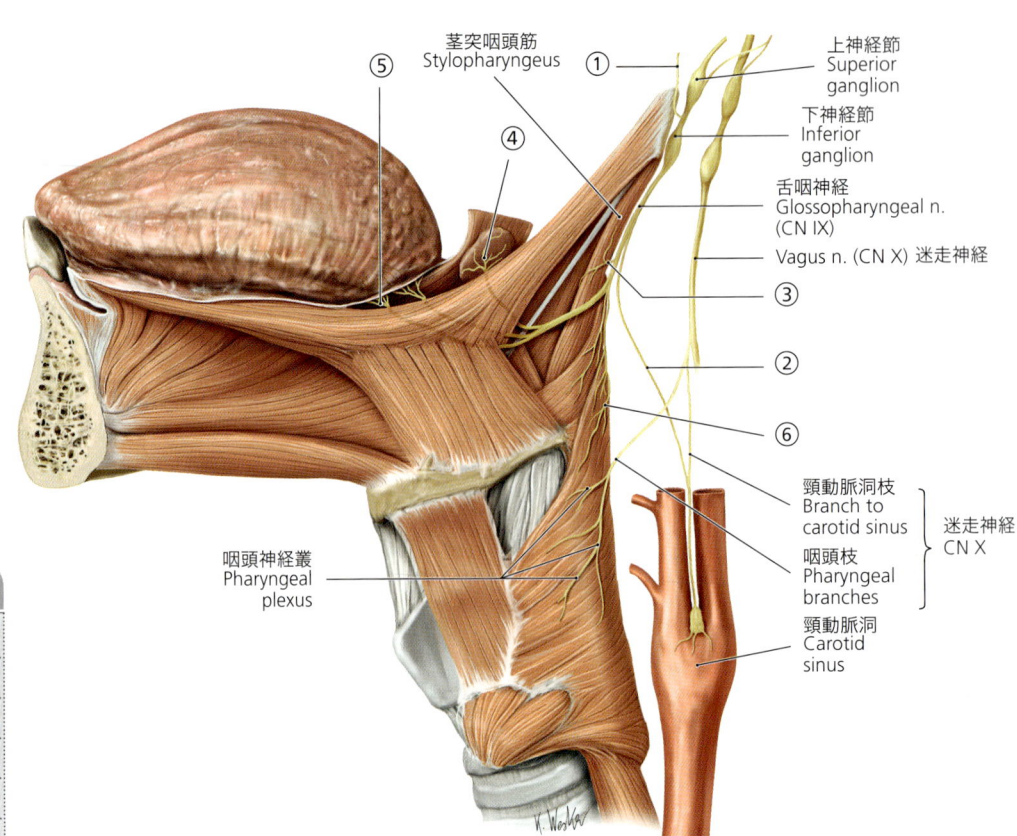

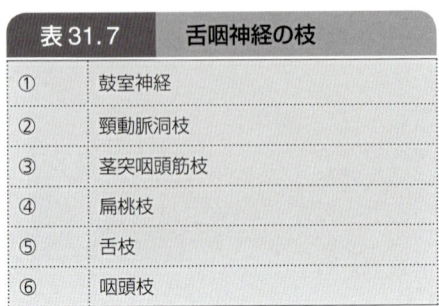

表 31.7	舌咽神経の枝
①	鼓室神経
②	頸動脈洞枝
③	茎突咽頭筋枝
④	扁桃枝
⑤	舌枝
⑥	咽頭枝

| | | | | A | | B | | C | | D | | E | | F | |

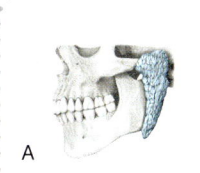

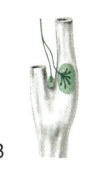

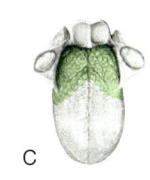

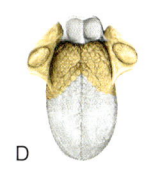

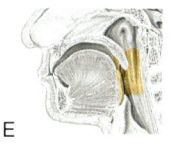

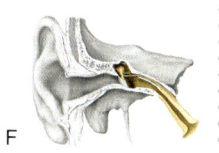

表31.8　舌咽神経（CN IX）

経路	線維	核	機能	障害時の影響
延髄から起こり，頸静脈孔から頭蓋腔を出る	臓性遠心性線維（副交感性）	下唾液核	副交感性節前線維は耳神経節に向かう 節後線維の分布： ・耳下腺(A) ・頬腺 ・口唇腺	舌咽神経の単独の障害は稀である．一般に頸静脈孔を通る迷走神経と副神経延髄根の障害を伴い，頭蓋底骨折時に障害が起こりやすい
	特殊臓性遠心性線維（鰓性）	疑核	分布： ・咽頭収縮筋（咽頭枝は迷走神経とともに咽頭神経叢を作る） ・茎突咽頭筋	
	臓性求心性線維	孤束核下部	頸動脈小体の化学受容器(B)と頸動脈洞の圧受容器から感覚情報を受け取る	
	特殊臓性求心性線維	孤束核上部	舌の後1/3(C)からの感覚情報を舌咽神経下神経節を通して受け取る	
	体性求心性線維	三叉神経脊髄路核	頭蓋内の上神経節と頭蓋外の下神経節からの末梢枝は以下の部位から起こる ・舌，軟口蓋，咽頭粘膜，扁桃(D,E) ・鼓室，鼓膜の内側面，耳管の粘膜（鼓室神経叢）(F) ・外耳と外耳道の皮膚（迷走神経と混ざっている）	

図31.19　鼓室内にある舌咽神経
左前外側方から見たところ．鼓室神経は耳神経節に行く臓性遠心性（副交感性節前）線維と鼓室と耳管に行く体性求心性線維を含み，内頸動脈神経叢から頸鼓神経を経由して来る交感性線維と合流して鼓室神経叢を形成する．

図31.20　舌咽神経の臓性遠心性（副交感性）線維

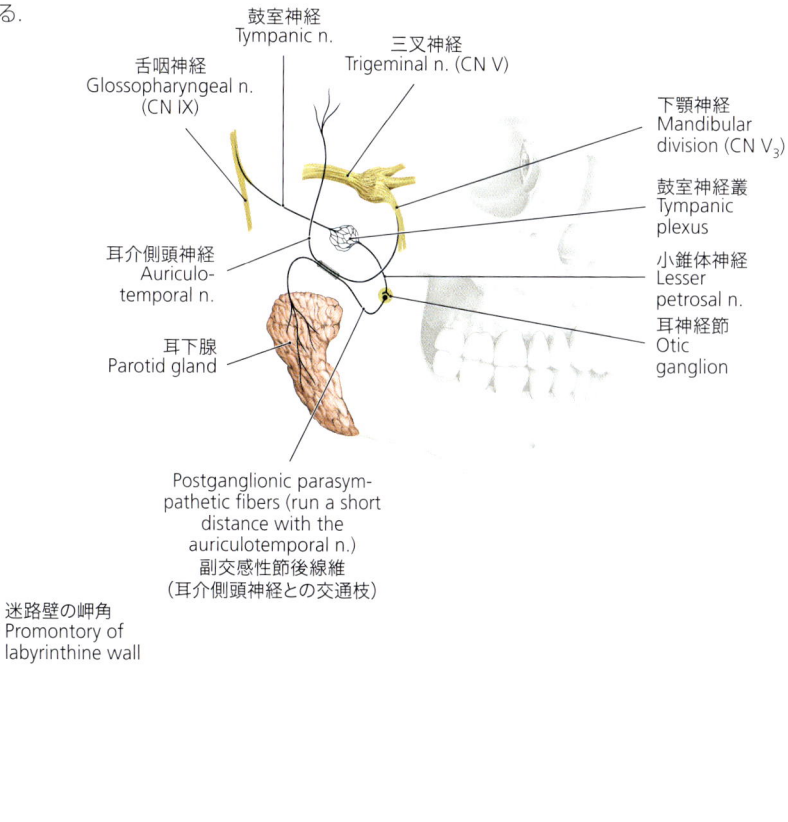

脳神経：迷走神経（CN X）
CN X: Vagus Nerve

図 31.21　迷走神経の核

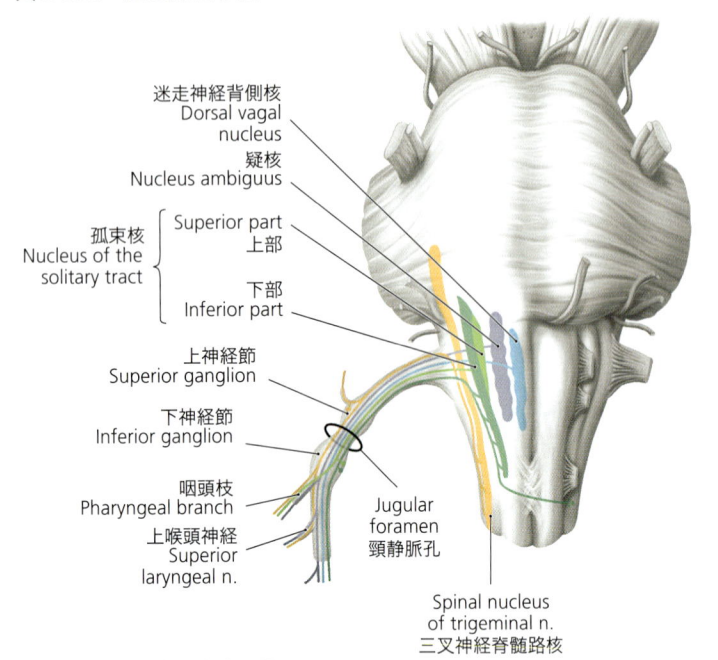

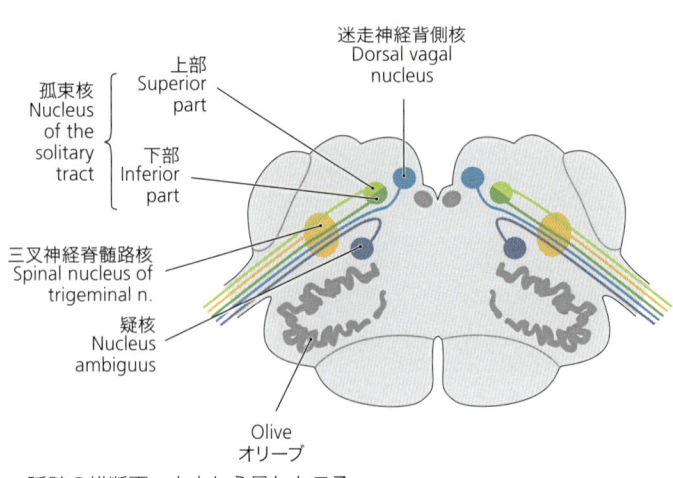

A 延髄を前方から見たところ．

B 延髄の横断面．上方から見たところ．

表 31.9　迷走神経（CN X）

経路	線維	核	機能	障害時の影響
延髄から起こり，頸静脈孔を通って頭蓋腔から出る．迷走神経は脳神経の中で最も広範囲に分布し，頭部・頸部・胸部（p. 91 参照）・腹部（p. 237 参照）の枝に分かれる	特殊臓性遠心性線維（鰓性）	疑核	分布： ・咽頭筋（舌咽神経とともに咽頭神経叢を通して） ・軟口蓋の筋 ・喉頭筋（輪状甲状筋に分布する上喉頭神経，その他の喉頭筋に分布する下喉頭神経）	反回神経は声帯を外転させる唯一の筋である輪状披裂筋の臓性運動性に支配する．片側の損傷は嗄声が引き起こされ，両側の損傷は呼吸困難に陥る
	臓性遠心性線維（副交感性）	迷走神経背側核	椎前神経節または壁内神経節でシナプスを形成する．胸部内臓と腹部内臓の平滑筋と腺に分布（A）	
	体性求心性線維	三叉神経脊髄路核	上神経節（頸静脈神経節）には後頭蓋窩の硬膜（C）と耳の皮膚（D），外耳道（E）からの末梢枝が至る	
	特殊臓性求心性線維	孤束核上部	下神経節（節状神経節）には喉頭蓋の味蕾（F）からの末梢枝が至る．	
	臓性求心性線維	孤束核下部	下神経節には以下から末梢枝が至る ・咽頭下部の食道移行部の粘膜（G） ・声帯ヒダより上（上喉頭神経）・下（下喉頭神経）の喉頭粘膜（G） ・大動脈弓の圧受容器（B） ・大動脈小体の化学受容器（B） ・胸部・腹部の内臓（A）	

図 31.22 迷走神経の走行

迷走神経は頸部で4つの枝を出す．下喉頭神経は，反回神経の終枝である．
Note: 左反回神経は大動脈弓の下を回り，右反回神経は鎖骨下動脈の下を回る．

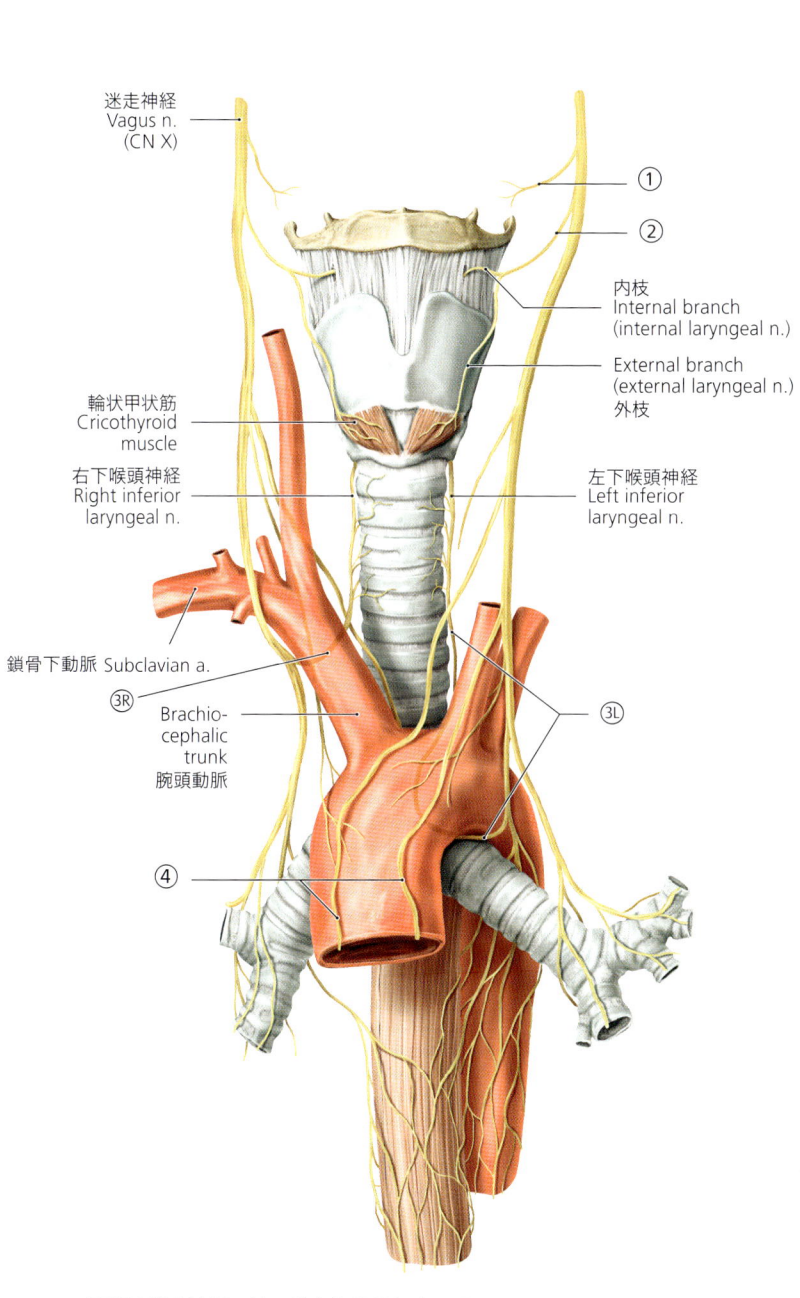

表 31.10	頸部の迷走神経の枝
①	咽頭枝
②	上喉頭神経
③R	右反回神経
③L	左反回神経
④	頸心臓枝

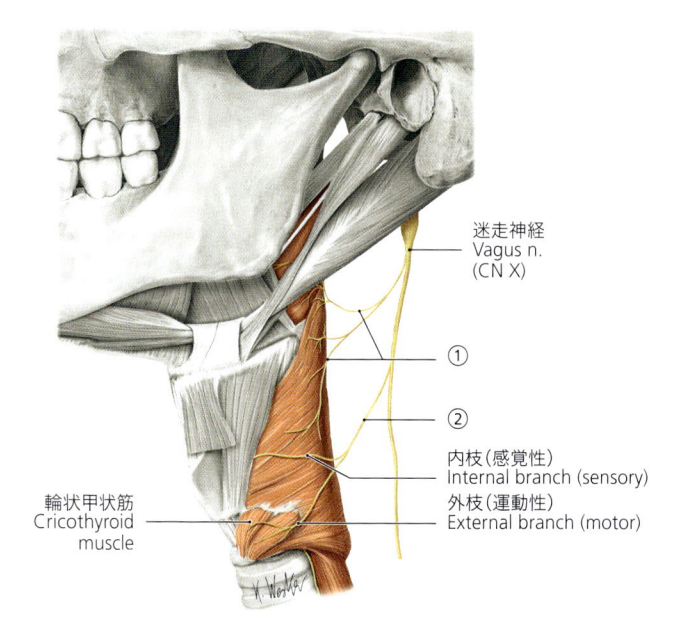

迷走神経 Vagus n. (CN X)
内枝 Internal branch (internal laryngeal n.)
External branch (external laryngeal n.) 外枝
輪状甲状筋 Cricothyroid muscle
右下喉頭神経 Right inferior laryngeal n.
左下喉頭神経 Left inferior laryngeal n.
鎖骨下動脈 Subclavian a.
Brachiocephalic trunk 腕頭動脈

A 頸部の迷走神経の枝．前方から見たところ．

迷走神経 Vagus n. (CN X)
内枝（感覚性） Internal branch (sensory)
外枝（運動性） External branch (motor)
輪状甲状筋 Cricothyroid muscle

B 咽頭と喉頭の筋への分布．左外側方から見たところ．

脳神経：副神経(CN XI)と舌下神経(CN XII)
CN XI & XII: Accessory & Hypoglossal Nerves

> 伝統的に副神経(CN XI)の延髄根とされてきたものは，現在では迷走神経(CN X)の一部として考えられ，脊髄根と短い距離だけ合流しているが，すぐに分離する．延髄根の線維は迷走神経を介して分配されるが，脊髄根の線維は副神経(CN XI)として伸びていく．

図 31.23　副神経
脳幹を後方から見たところ(小脳は取り除いてある)．*Note*：わかりやすくするために右側の筋肉を示す．

図 31.24　副神経の障害
右の副神経の障害．

A　僧帽筋麻痺，後方から見たところ．

B　胸鎖乳突筋麻痺．右前外側方から見たところ．

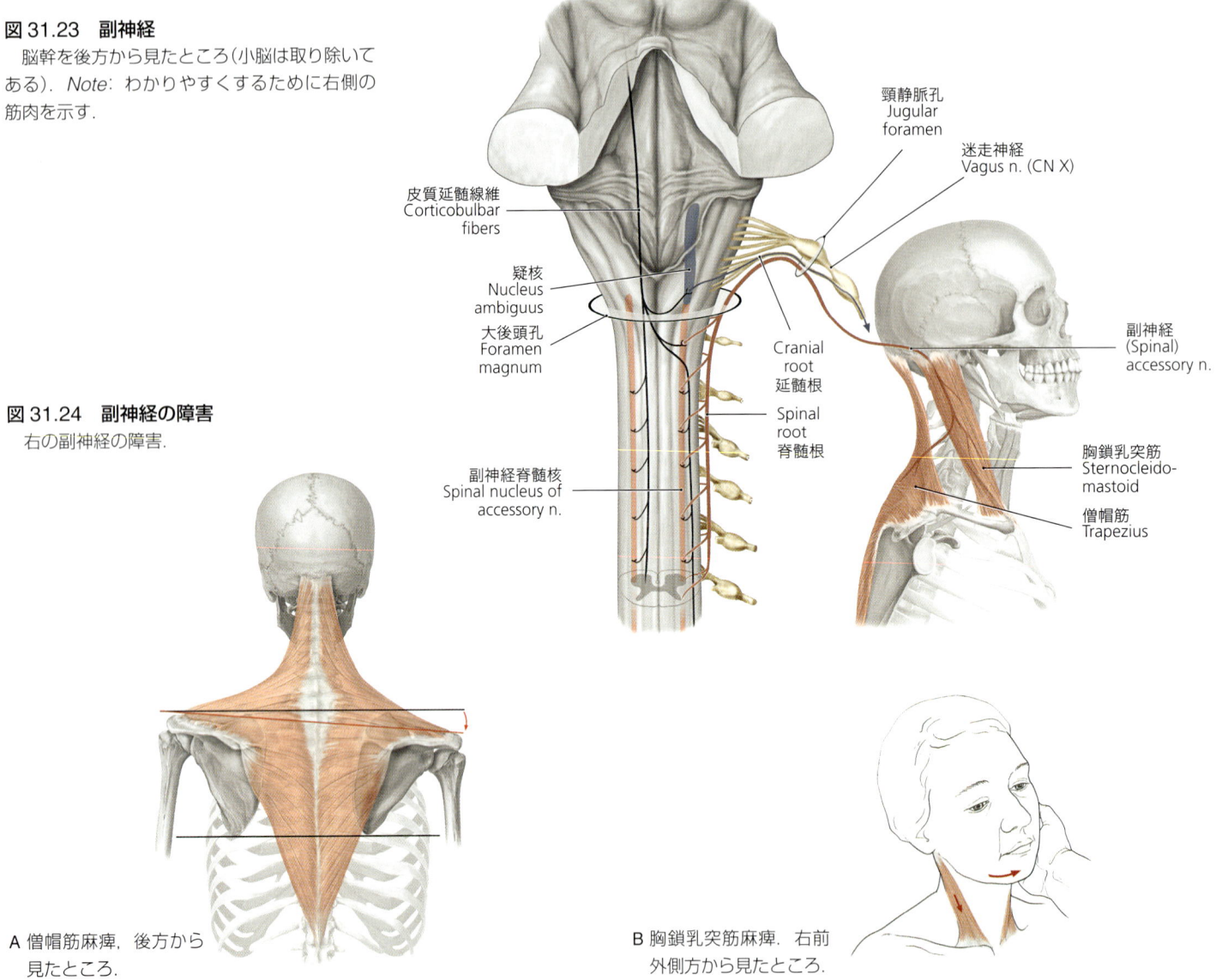

表 31.11	副神経(CN XI)			
経路	線維	核	機能	障害時の影響
脊髄根はC1-C5/6の脊髄から起こって上行し，大後頭孔から頭蓋に入り，延髄からの延髄根と合流する．両根は頸静脈孔で頭蓋から出る．延髄根の線維は頸静脈孔で迷走神経と合流する(内枝)．脊髄根は外枝として項部を下行する	特殊臓性遠心性線維	疑核の尾側部	迷走神経と合流し，反回神経とともに分布する分布・輪状甲状筋以外の喉頭の筋	僧帽筋麻痺：障害側の肩が下がり，腕を水平以上に挙上することが困難になる．この麻痺は頸部の手術(リンパ節の生検など)の際に重要である．僧帽筋は第3-第4/第5頸神経にも支配されているので，副神経が傷害されても僧帽筋は完全には麻痺しない胸鎖乳突筋麻痺：斜頸(ねじれた頸，つまり頸の回転が困難になる)．副神経だけが分布するので片側が障害されると弛緩性の麻痺が起こる．両側が障害されると，頭部を直立させることができない
	体性遠心性線維	副神経脊髄核	副神経外枝を作る分布・僧帽筋・胸鎖乳突筋	

図 31.25 舌下神経
脳幹を後方から見たところ（小脳は取り除いてある）．*Note*：甲状舌骨筋とオトガイ舌骨筋を支配する第1頸神経は短い距離だけ舌下神経とともに進む．

図 31.26 舌下神経核
Note：舌下神経核には反対側の皮質ニューロンが分布している．

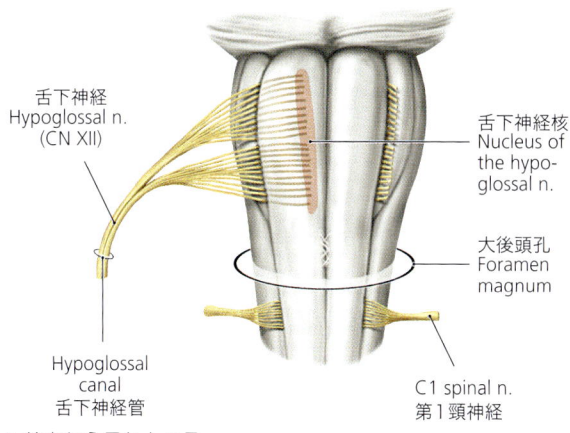

A 前方から見たところ．

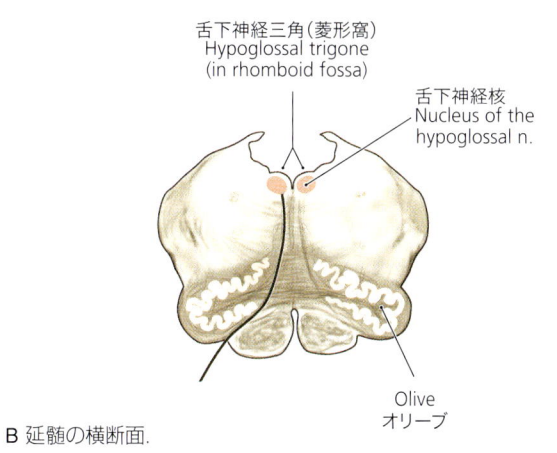

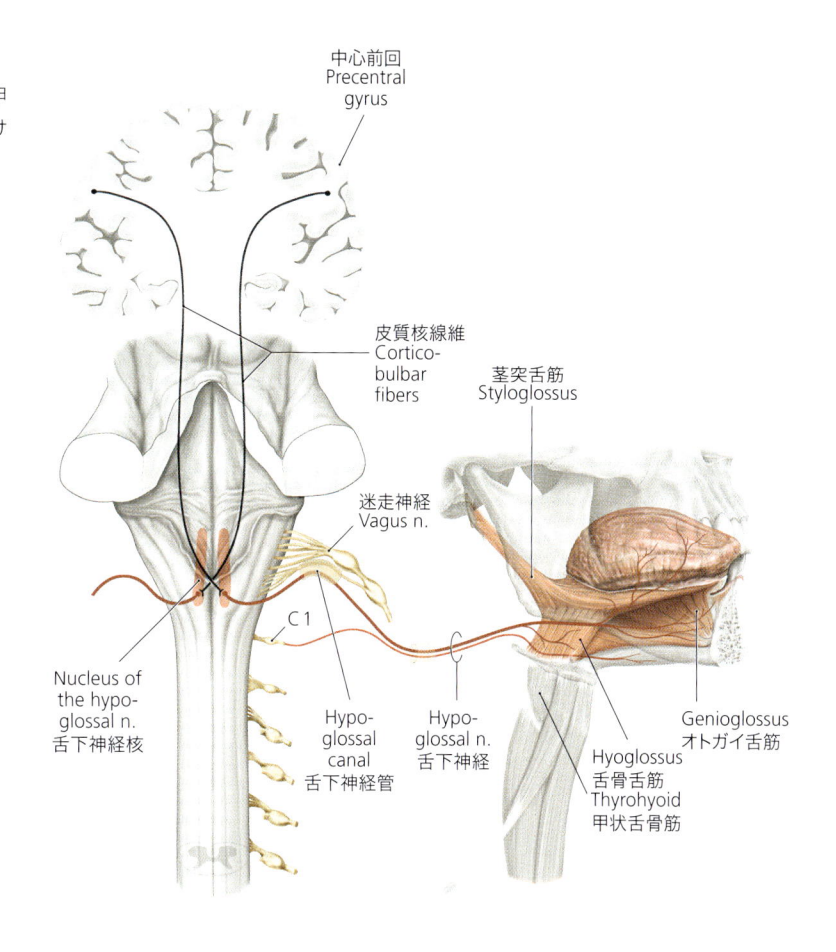

B 延髄の横断面．

図 31.27 舌下神経の障害
上方から見たところ．

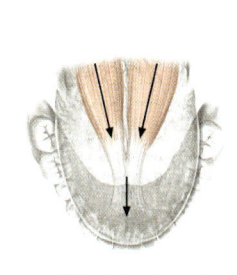

A 正常なオトガイ舌筋．

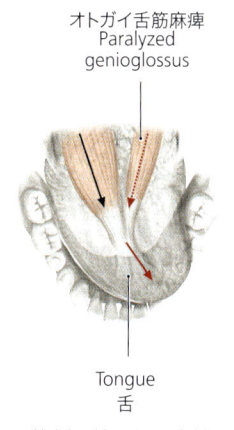

B 片側の核または末梢の障害．

表 31.12　舌下神経（CN XII）

経路	線維	核	機能	障害時の影響
延髄から起こり，舌下神経管を通って頭蓋腔から出て，迷走神経の傍を下行する．舌下神経は舌骨の上で舌根に入る	体性遠心性線維	舌下神経核	分布 ・内舌筋と外舌筋（口蓋舌筋以外．口蓋舌筋は迷走神経の支配を受ける）	中枢の舌下神経麻痺（核上位）：舌は障害された側の反対側へ曲がる 核または末梢の麻痺：舌は，健常な側の筋が優位になるため，障害がある側に曲がる 弛緩麻痺：両核が障害されると，舌を突き出すことができない

顔面の神経支配
Innervation of the Face

図 32.1 顔の運動神経
左外側方から見たところ．表情筋は顔面神経（CN VII）の5つの枝によって運動性に神経支配される．咀嚼筋は三叉神経の下顎神経（CN V_3）によって運動性に神経支配される．

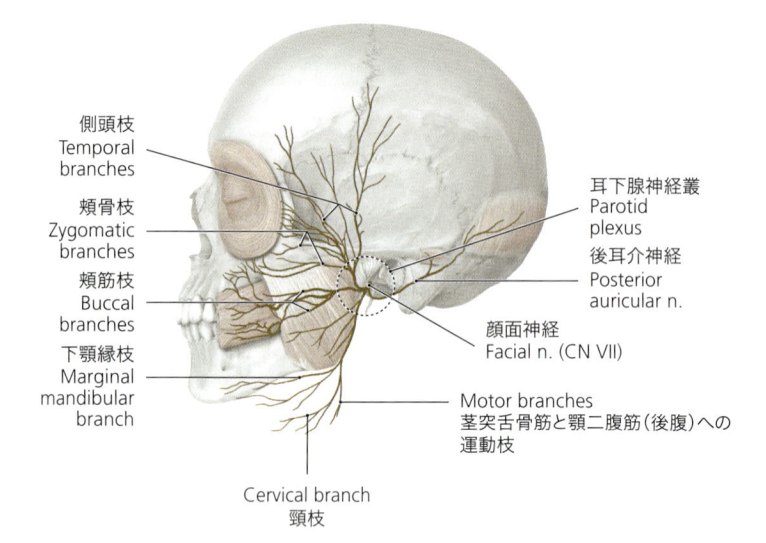

- 側頭枝 Temporal branches
- 頬骨枝 Zygomatic branches
- 頬筋枝 Buccal branches
- 下顎縁枝 Marginal mandibular branch
- 耳下腺神経叢 Parotid plexus
- 後耳介神経 Posterior auricular n.
- 顔面神経 Facial n. (CN VII)
- Motor branches 茎突舌骨筋と顎二腹筋（後腹）への運動枝
- Cervical branch 頸枝

A 表情筋の運動神経支配．

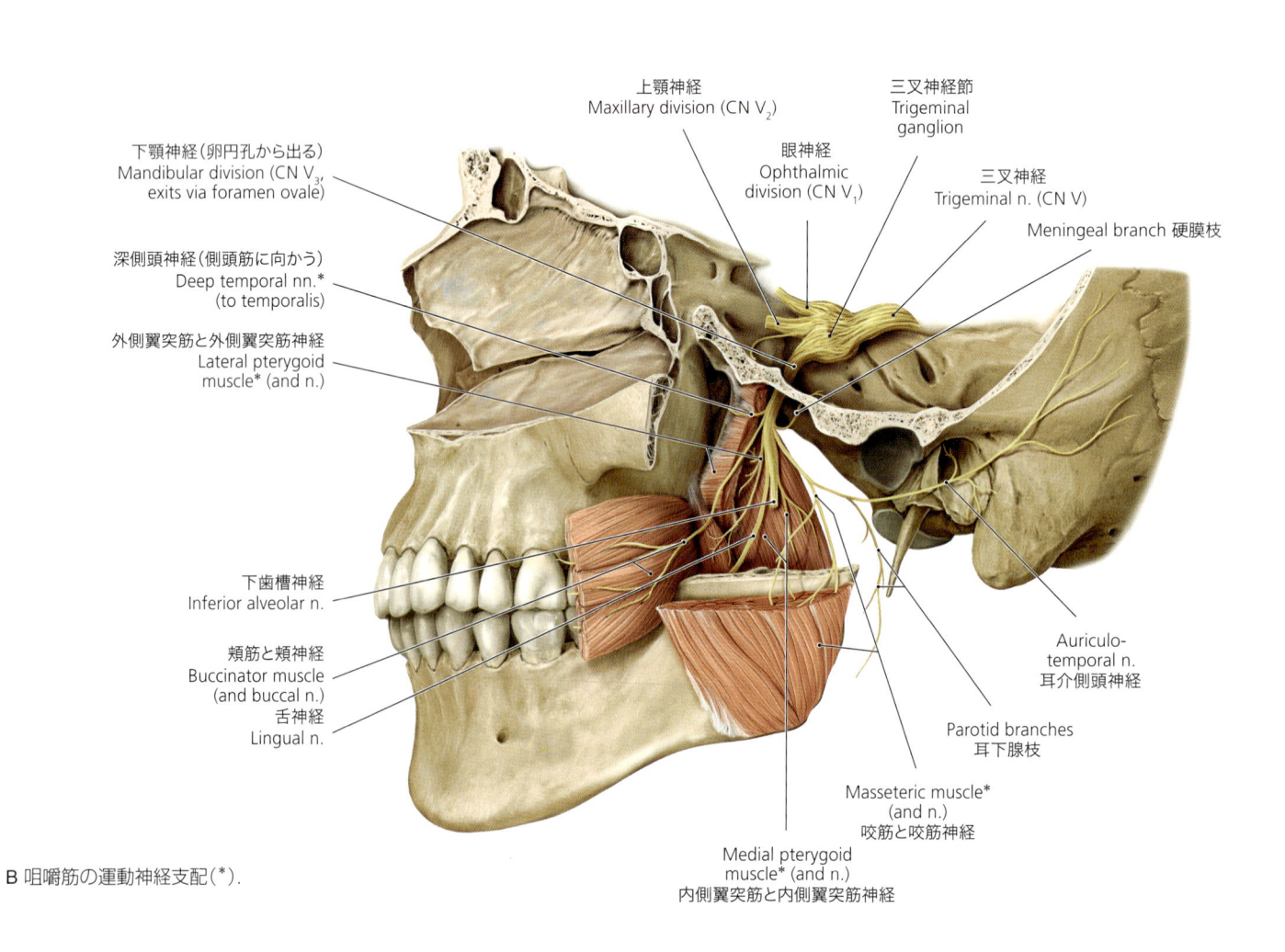

- 上顎神経 Maxillary division (CN V_2)
- 眼神経 Ophthalmic division (CN V_1)
- 三叉神経節 Trigeminal ganglion
- 三叉神経 Trigeminal n. (CN V)
- 下顎神経（卵円孔から出る）Mandibular division (CN V_3, exits via foramen ovale)
- Meningeal branch 硬膜枝
- 深側頭神経（側頭筋に向かう）Deep temporal nn.* (to temporalis)
- 外側翼突筋と外側翼突筋神経 Lateral pterygoid muscle* (and n.)
- 下歯槽神経 Inferior alveolar n.
- 頬筋と頬神経 Buccinator muscle (and buccal n.)
- 舌神経 Lingual n.
- Auriculo-temporal n. 耳介側頭神経
- Parotid branches 耳下腺枝
- Masseteric muscle* (and n.) 咬筋と咬筋神経
- Medial pterygoid muscle* (and n.) 内側翼突筋と内側翼突筋神経

B 咀嚼筋の運動神経支配（*）．

図 32.2 顔面の感覚神経支配

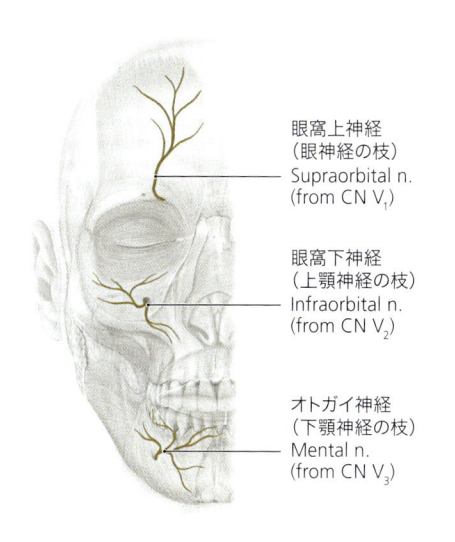

A 三叉神経からの感覚神経，前方から見たところ．眼窩上神経，眼窩下神経，オトガイ神経のそれぞれから感覚枝が出て，それぞれ眼窩の上部，眼窩の下部，オトガイ部に分布する．

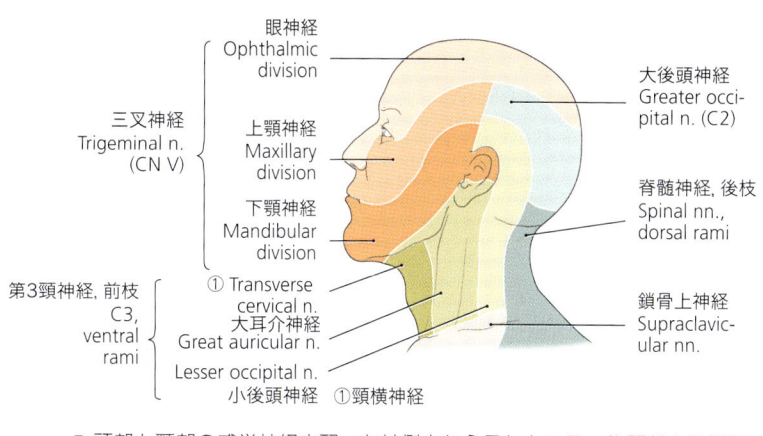

- 眼窩上神経（眼神経の枝） Supraorbital n. (from CN V₁)
- 眼窩下神経（上顎神経の枝） Infraorbital n. (from CN V₂)
- オトガイ神経（下顎神経の枝） Mental n. (from CN V₃)

B 頭部と頸部の感覚神経支配，左外側方から見たところ．後頭部と後頭下部は脊髄神経の後枝（青色）によって支配される．大後頭神経は第2頸神経（C2）の後枝である．

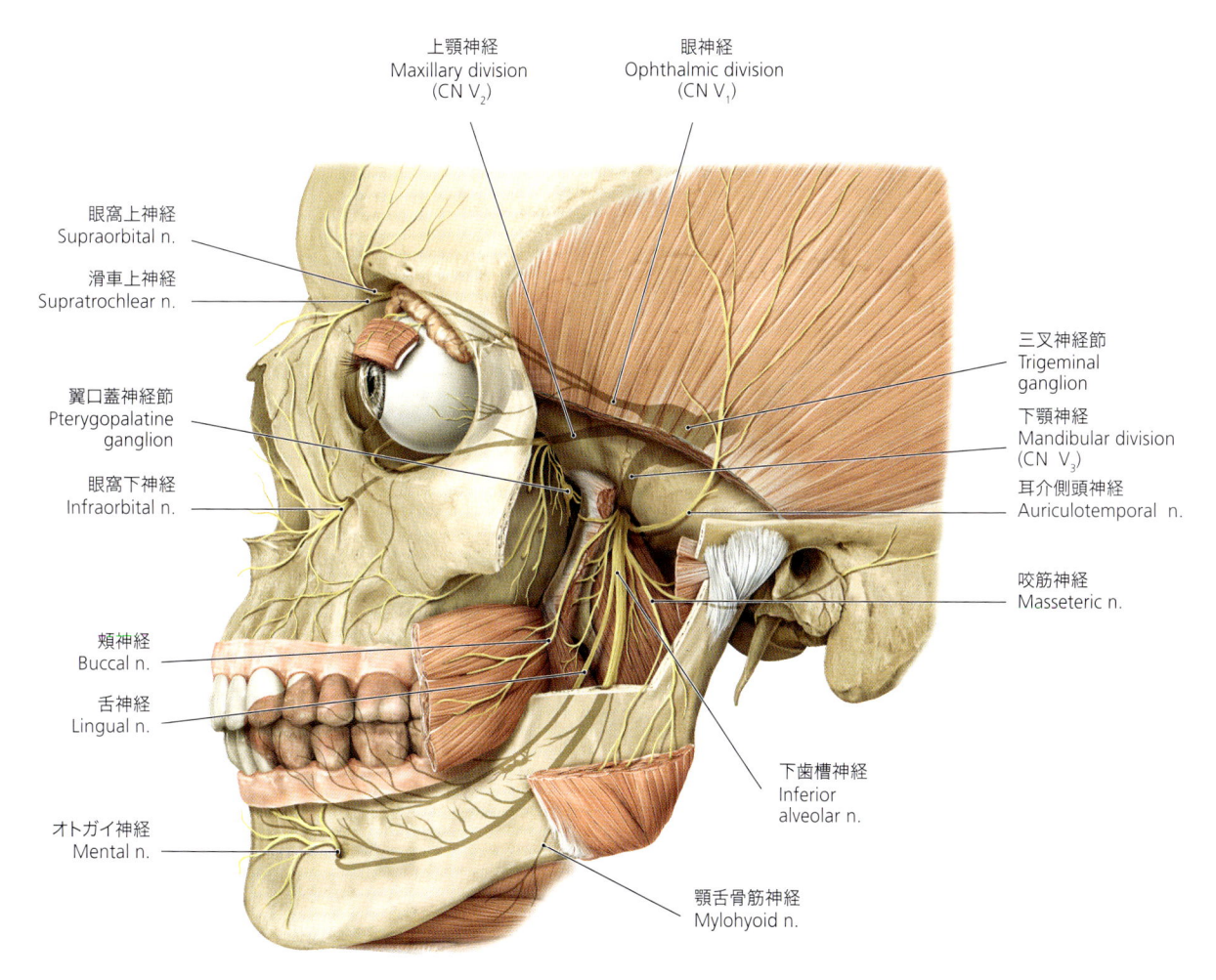

三叉神経 Trigeminal n. (CN V)
- 眼神経 Ophthalmic division
- 上顎神経 Maxillary division
- 下顎神経 Mandibular division

第3頸神経，前枝 C3, ventral rami
- 頸横神経 Transverse cervical n.
- 大耳介神経 Great auricular n.
- 小後頭神経 Lesser occipital n.

- 大後頭神経 Greater occipital n. (C2)
- 脊髄神経，後枝 Spinal nn., dorsal rami
- 鎖骨上神経 Supraclavicular nn.

C 三叉神経の枝，左外側方から見たところ．

- 上顎神経 Maxillary division (CN V₂)
- 眼神経 Ophthalmic division (CN V₁)
- 眼窩上神経 Supraorbital n.
- 滑車上神経 Supratrochlear n.
- 翼口蓋神経節 Pterygopalatine ganglion
- 眼窩下神経 Infraorbital n.
- 頰神経 Buccal n.
- 舌神経 Lingual n.
- オトガイ神経 Mental n.
- 三叉神経節 Trigeminal ganglion
- 下顎神経 Mandibular division (CN V₃)
- 耳介側頭神経 Auriculotemporal n.
- 咬筋神経 Masseteric n.
- 下歯槽神経 Inferior alveolar n.
- 顎舌骨筋神経 Mylohyoid n.

頭頸部の動脈
Arteries of the Head & Neck

頭頸部には総頸動脈の枝が分布する．総頸動脈は頸動脈分岐部で内頸動脈と外頸動脈に分かれる．内頸動脈は脳に主に分布する（p.606）が，その枝は眼窩と鼻中隔で外頸動脈と吻合する．頭部と頸部の構造物に分布するのは主に外頸動脈である．

図 32.3 内頸動脈
左外側方から見たところ．内頸動脈の脳以外への枝の中で最も重要なのは眼動脈である．眼動脈は鼻中隔上部(p.524)と眼窩(p.512)に分布する．脳の動脈についてはpp.608-609参照．

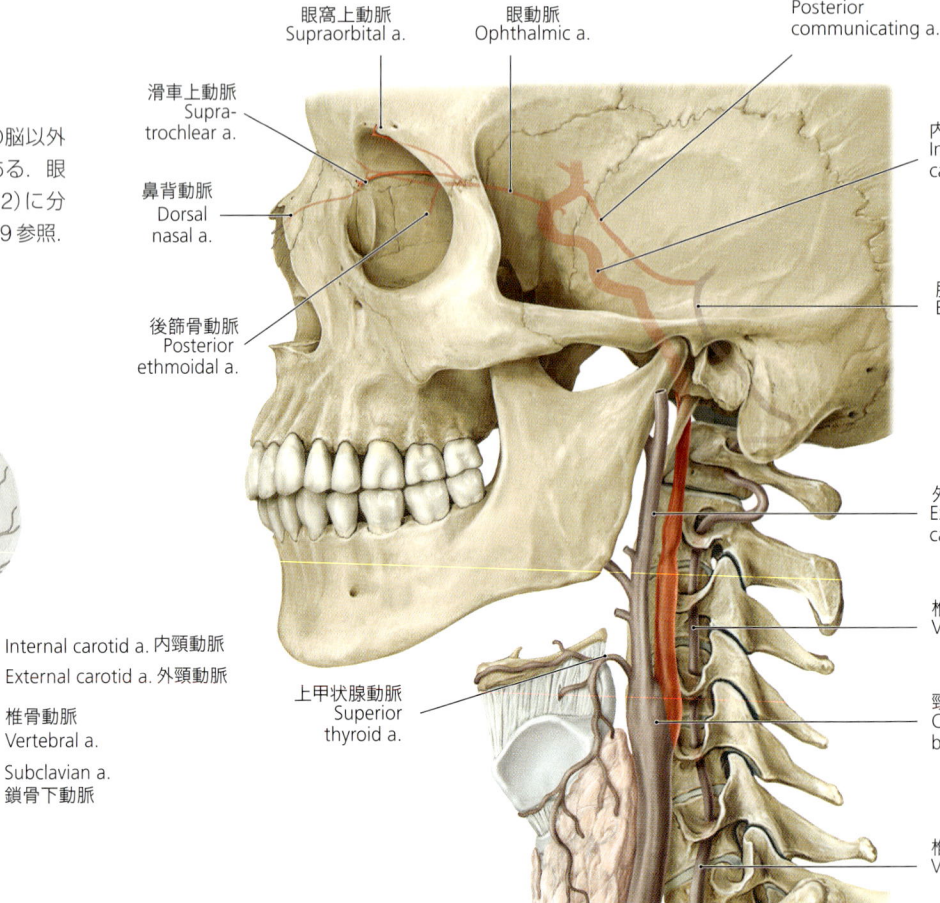

A 模式図．

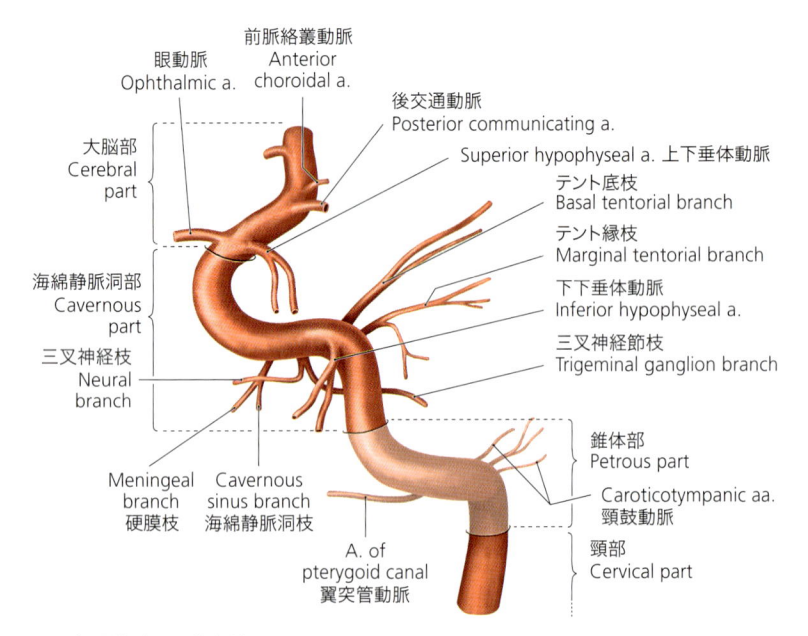

B 内頸動脈の区分と枝．

C 内頸動脈の走行．

眼窩上動脈 Supraorbital a.
眼動脈 Ophthalmic a.
後交通動脈 Posterior communicating a.
滑車上動脈 Supratrochlear a.
内頸動脈 Internal carotid a.
鼻背動脈 Dorsal nasal a.
後篩骨動脈 Posterior ethmoidal a.
脳底動脈 Basilar a.
外頸動脈 External carotid a.
椎骨動脈 Vertebral a.
上甲状腺動脈 Superior thyroid a.
頸動脈分岐部 Carotid bifurcation
椎骨動脈 Vertebral a.
鎖骨下動脈 Subclavian a.

眼動脈 Ophthalmic a.
眼角動脈 Angular a.
顔面動脈 Facial a.
総頸動脈 Common carotid a.
Internal carotid a. 内頸動脈
External carotid a. 外頸動脈
椎骨動脈 Vertebral a.
Subclavian a. 鎖骨下動脈

眼動脈 Ophthalmic a.
前脈絡叢動脈 Anterior choroidal a.
後交通動脈 Posterior communicating a.
Superior hypophyseal a. 上下垂体動脈
大脳部 Cerebral part
テント底枝 Basal tentorial branch
テント縁枝 Marginal tentorial branch
海綿静脈洞部 Cavernous part
下下垂体動脈 Inferior hypophyseal a.
三叉神経枝 Neural branch
三叉神経節枝 Trigeminal ganglion branch
Meningeal branch 硬膜枝
Cavernous sinus branch 海綿静脈洞枝
錐体部 Petrous part
Caroticotympanic aa. 頸鼓動脈
A. of pterygoid canal 翼突管動脈
頸部 Cervical part

臨床

頸動脈アテローム性硬化症

頸動脈はしばしばプラークの形成によって動脈壁が硬化するアテローム性硬化症を起こす．超音波によって動脈の状態を検査することができる．*Note*：頸動脈のアテローム性硬化症がない場合でも，冠性心疾患や他の場所でのアテローム性硬化の疑いを排除することはできない．

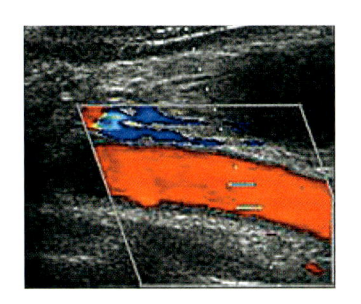

A 正常血液を示す総頸動脈．

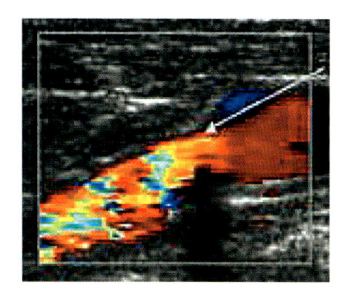

B 頸動脈球における石灰化プラーク．

図 32.4　外頸動脈，概観
左外側方から見たところ．

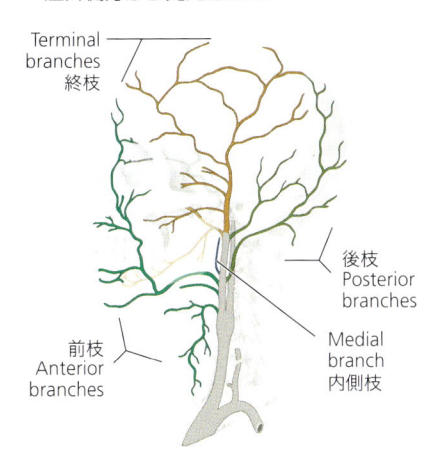

A 外頸動脈の模式図．

表 32.1	外頸動脈の枝
枝のグループ	枝の名称
前枝（p.492）	上甲状腺動脈
	舌動脈
	顔面動脈
内側枝（p.492）	上行咽頭動脈
後枝（p.493）	後頭動脈
	後耳介動脈
終枝（p.494）	顎動脈
	浅側頭動脈

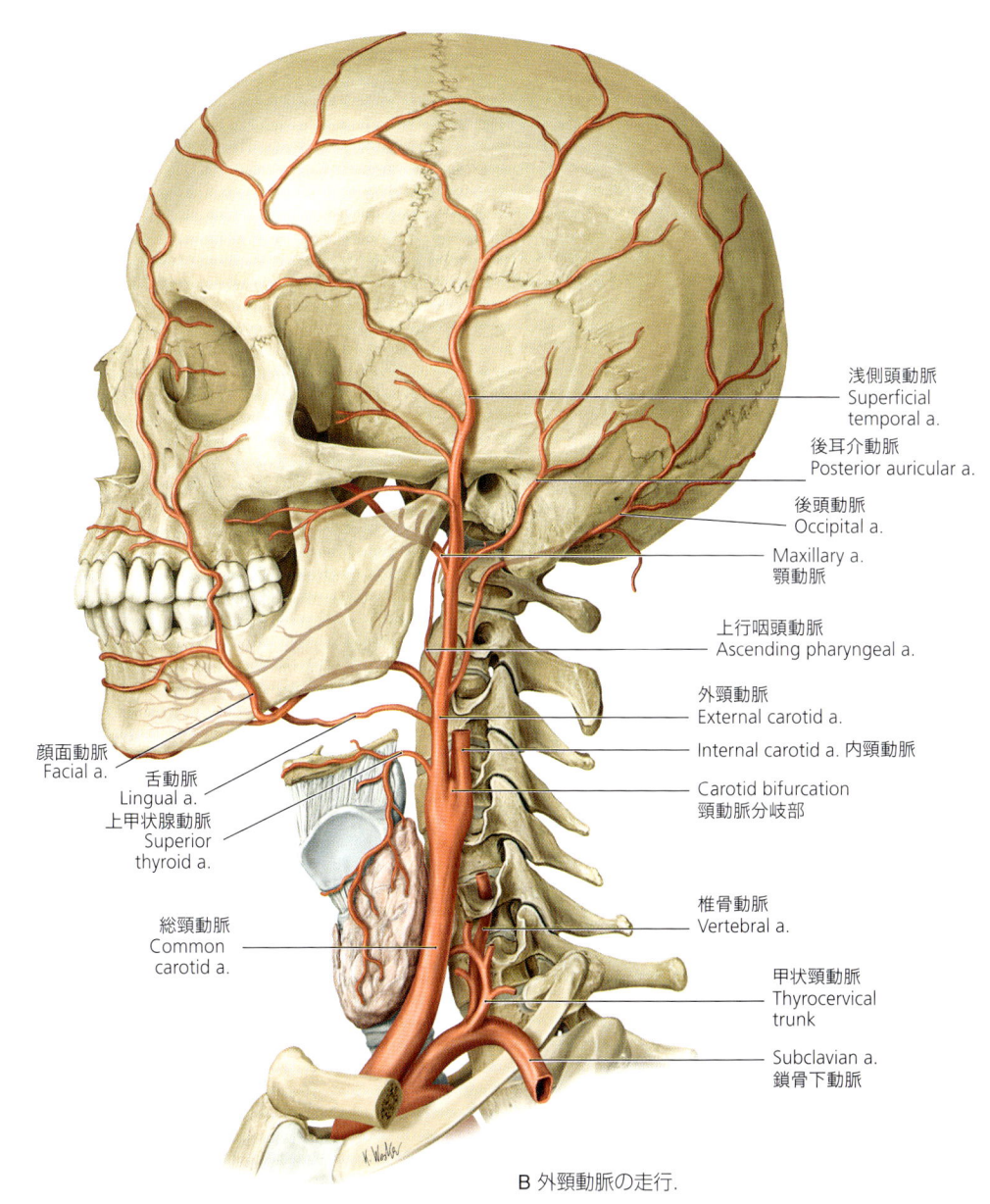

B 外頸動脈の走行．

外頸動脈：前枝，内側枝，後枝
External Carotid Artery: Anterior, Medial & Posterior Branches

図 32.5　前枝と内側枝

左外側方から見たところ．前枝の動脈は，眼窩(p.510)，耳(p.534)，喉頭(p.575)，咽頭(p.556)，口腔などの頭頸部の前側の構造に分布する．*Note*：眼角動脈は，内頸動脈から起こる眼動脈の枝である鼻背動脈と吻合する．

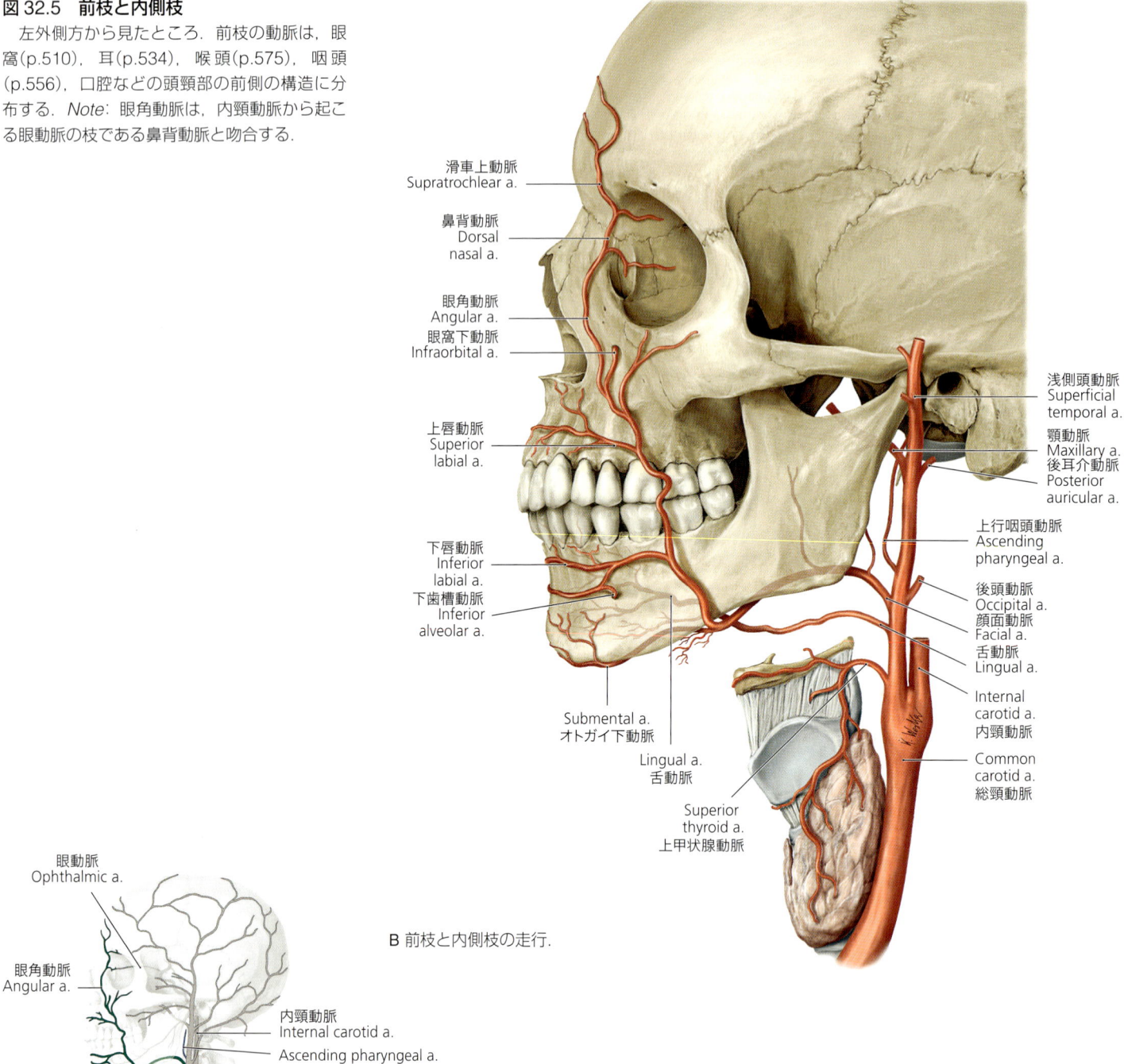

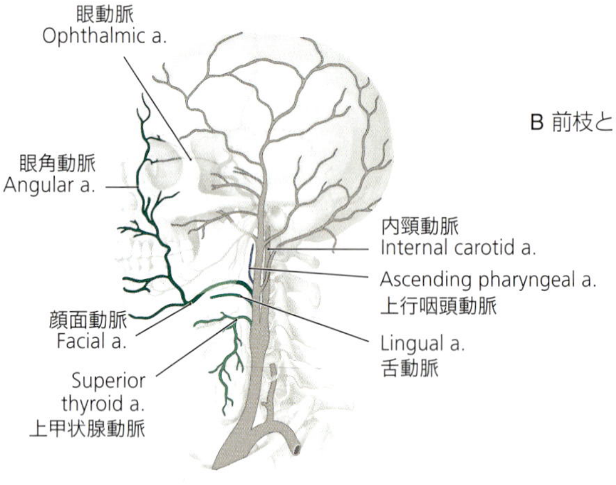

滑車上動脈 Supratrochlear a.
鼻背動脈 Dorsal nasal a.
眼角動脈 Angular a.
眼窩下動脈 Infraorbital a.
上唇動脈 Superior labial a.
下唇動脈 Inferior labial a.
下歯槽動脈 Inferior alveolar a.
Submental a. オトガイ下動脈
Lingual a. 舌動脈
Superior thyroid a. 上甲状腺動脈
浅側頭動脈 Superficial temporal a.
顎動脈 Maxillary a.
後耳介動脈 Posterior auricular a.
上行咽頭動脈 Ascending pharyngeal a.
後頭動脈 Occipital a.
顔面動脈 Facial a.
舌動脈 Lingual a.
Internal carotid a. 内頸動脈
Common carotid a. 総頸動脈

B 前枝と内側枝の走行．

眼動脈 Ophthalmic a.
眼角動脈 Angular a.
内頸動脈 Internal carotid a.
Ascending pharyngeal a. 上行咽頭動脈
顔面動脈 Facial a.
Lingual a. 舌動脈
Superior thyroid a. 上甲状腺動脈

A 前枝と内側枝の動脈．顔面には血液が豊富に供給されているために，顔面が傷害されると大量に出血するが，急速に治癒する．外頸動脈の枝同士の間，また外頸動脈と眼動脈の枝の間には吻合が多数存在する．

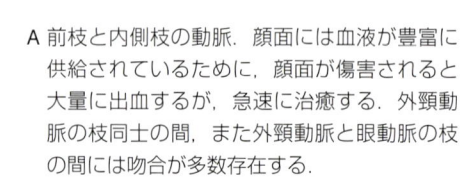

図 32.6 後枝

左側方から見たところ．外頸動脈の後枝は耳（p.534），後頭（p.499），後頸部（p.585）に分布する．

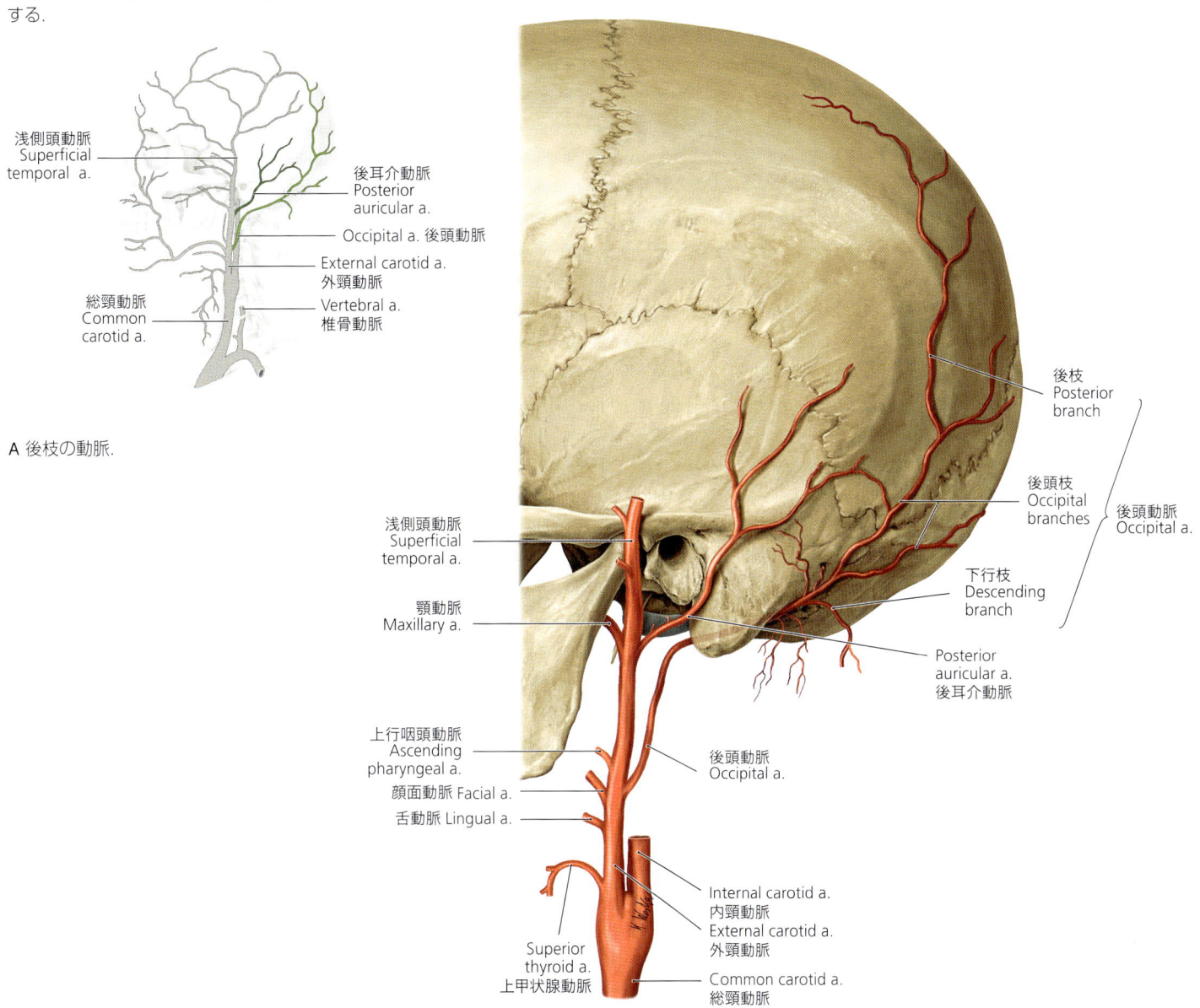

A 後枝の動脈．

B 後枝の走行．

表 32.2	外頸動脈の前枝，内側枝，後枝	
枝	動脈	区分と分布
前枝	上甲状腺動脈	腺枝（甲状腺へ），上喉頭動脈，胸鎖乳突筋枝
	舌動脈	舌背枝（舌根，喉頭蓋へ），舌下動脈（舌下腺，舌，口腔底，口腔へ）
	顔面動脈	上行口蓋動脈（咽頭壁，軟口蓋，耳管へ），扁桃枝（口蓋扁桃へ），オトガイ下動脈（口腔底，顎下腺へ），上唇動脈・下唇動脈，眼角動脈（鼻根へ）
内側枝	上行咽頭動脈	咽頭枝，下鼓室動脈（内耳の粘膜へ），後硬膜動脈
後枝	後頭動脈	後頭枝，下行枝（後頸筋へ）
	後耳介動脈	茎乳突孔動脈（顔面神経管内の顔面神経へ），後鼓室動脈，耳介枝，後頭枝，耳下腺枝

終枝については表 32.3 を参照．

外頸動脈：終枝
External Carotid Artery: Terminal Branches

外頸動脈の終枝は浅側頭動脈と顎動脈の2つの大きな動脈からなる．浅側頭動脈は頭蓋外側部に分布し，顎動脈は顔面の内部構造の主要な動脈である．

図32.7 浅側頭動脈
左外側方から見たところ．浅側頭動脈の炎症は激しい頭痛を引き起こす．浅側頭動脈の前頭枝は高齢者では皮下の浅層に走行をたどることができる．

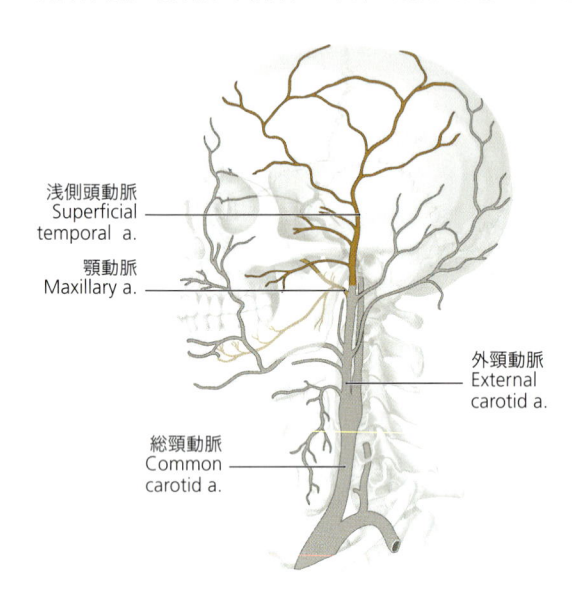

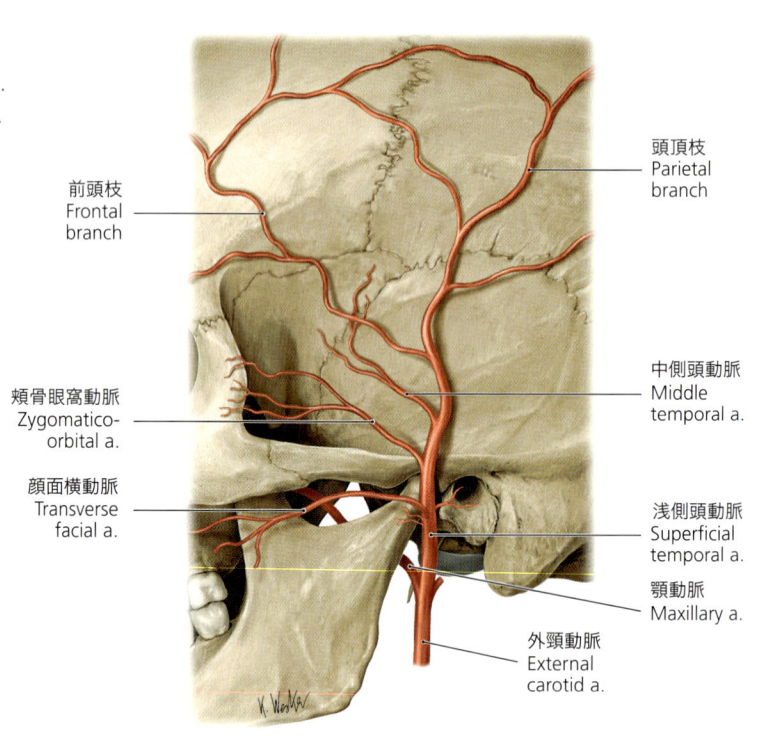

A 終枝の動脈．

B 浅側頭動脈の走行．

表32.3　外頸動脈の末梢枝

枝	動脈		区分と分布	
終枝	浅側頭動脈		顔面横動脈（頬骨弓より下方の軟部組織へ），前頭枝，頭頂枝，頬骨眼窩動脈（眼窩の外側壁へ）	
	顎動脈	下顎部	下歯槽動脈（下顎骨，歯，歯肉へ），中硬膜動脈，深耳介動脈（顎関節，外耳道へ），前鼓室動脈	
		翼突筋部	咬筋動脈，前・後深側頭動脈，翼突筋枝，頬動脈	
		翼口蓋部	後上歯槽動脈（上顎大臼歯，上顎洞，歯肉へ）；眼窩下動脈（上顎歯槽へ）	
			下行口蓋動脈	大口蓋動脈（硬口蓋へ）
				小口蓋動脈（軟口蓋，口蓋扁桃，咽頭壁へ）
			蝶口蓋動脈	外側後鼻枝（鼻腔の側壁，鼻甲介へ）
				中隔後鼻枝（鼻中隔へ）

図 32.8　顎動脈
左外側方から見たところ．顎動脈は下顎部（青）・翼突筋部（緑）・翼口蓋部（黄）の3つの部分からなる．

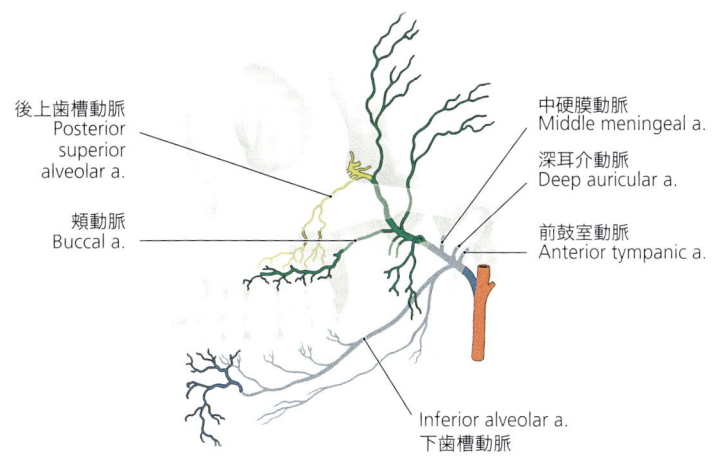

A　顎動脈の枝．

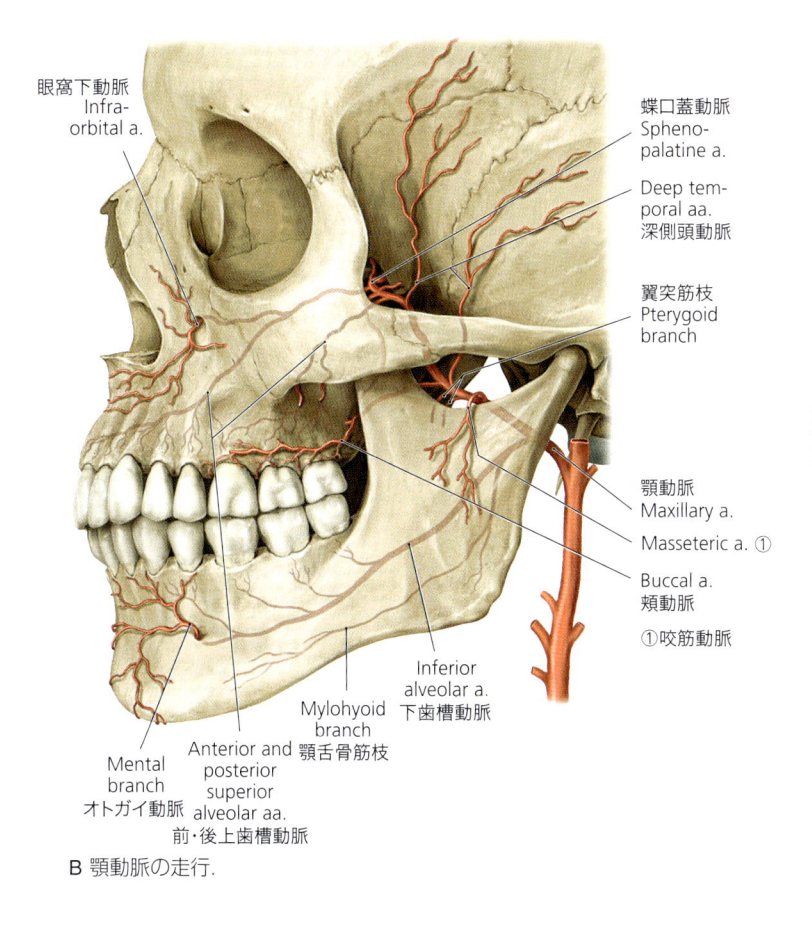

- 後上歯槽動脈 Posterior superior alveolar a.
- 頬動脈 Buccal a.
- 中硬膜動脈 Middle meningeal a.
- 深耳介動脈 Deep auricular a.
- 前鼓室動脈 Anterior tympanic a.
- 下歯槽動脈 Inferior alveolar a.

B　顎動脈の走行．

- 眼窩下動脈 Infra-orbital a.
- 蝶口蓋動脈 Spheno-palatine a.
- 深側頭動脈 Deep temporal aa.
- 翼突筋枝 Pterygoid branch
- 顎動脈 Maxillary a.
- 咬筋動脈① Masseteric a. ①
- 頬動脈 Buccal a.
- 下歯槽動脈 Inferior alveolar a.
- 顎舌骨筋枝 Mylohyoid branch
- 前・後上歯槽動脈 Anterior and posterior superior alveolar aa.
- オトガイ動脈 Mental branch
- ①咬筋動脈

臨床

中硬膜動脈

中硬膜動脈は髄膜とその上にある頭蓋冠に分布する．一般に頭部の外傷によって動脈が破裂すると硬膜外血腫が生じる．

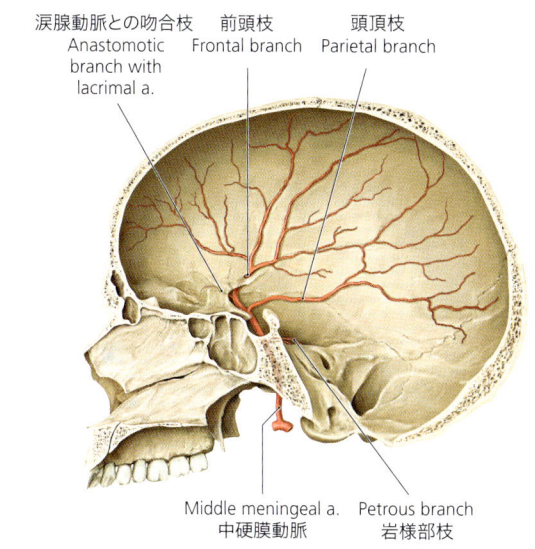

A　右中硬膜動脈．頭蓋を内側方から見たところ．

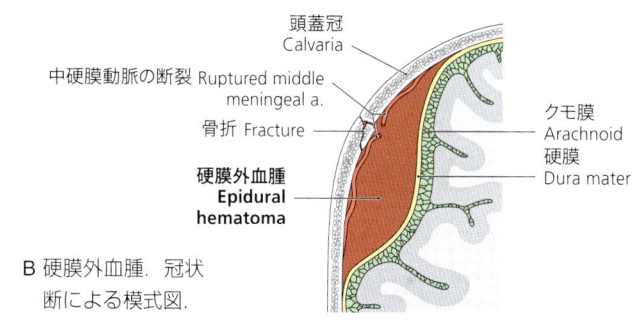

- 涙腺動脈との吻合枝 Anastomotic branch with lacrimal a.
- 前頭枝 Frontal branch
- 頭頂枝 Parietal branch
- 中硬膜動脈 Middle meningeal a.
- 岩様部枝 Petrous branch

B　硬膜外血腫．冠状断による模式図．

- 頭蓋冠 Calvaria
- 中硬膜動脈の断裂 Ruptured middle meningeal a.
- 骨折 Fracture
- 硬膜外血腫 Epidural hematoma
- クモ膜 Arachnoid
- 硬膜 Dura mater

蝶口蓋動脈

蝶口蓋動脈は鼻腔の壁に分布する．蝶口蓋動脈の枝から重篤な咽頭鼻部出血が起こった場合，翼口蓋窩で顎動脈を結紮する必要がある．

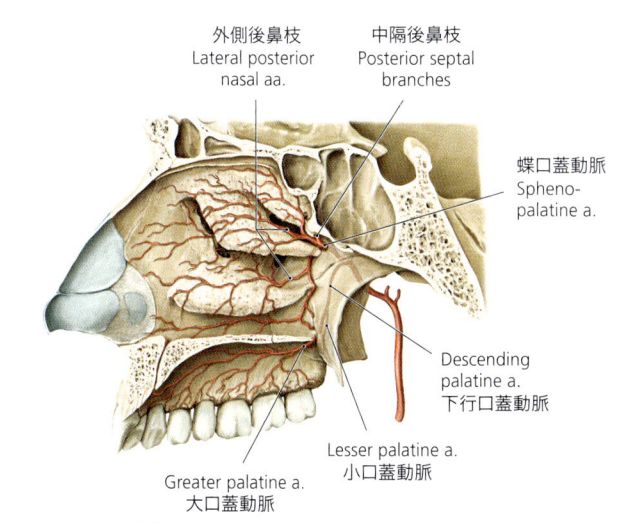

C　鼻腔の外側壁，左外側方から見たところ．

- 外側後鼻枝 Lateral posterior nasal aa.
- 中隔後鼻枝 Posterior septal branches
- 蝶口蓋動脈 Spheno-palatine a.
- 下行口蓋動脈 Descending palatine a.
- 小口蓋動脈 Lesser palatine a.
- 大口蓋動脈 Greater palatine a.

頭頸部の静脈
Veins of the Head & Neck

図 32.9 頭頸部の静脈
左外側方から見たところ．頭頸部の静脈は腕頭静脈に流れ込む．
Note: 左腕頭静脈と右腕頭静脈は対称ではない．

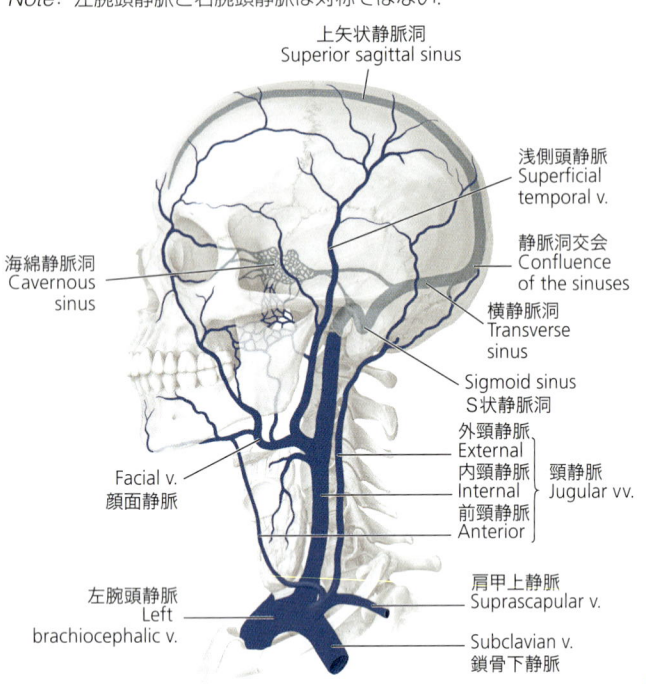

表 32.4	主要な浅静脈	
静脈	排出される領域	位置
内頸静脈	頭蓋内部（脳を含む）	頸動脈鞘内
外頸静脈	頭部（浅層）	頸筋膜の浅葉内
前頸静脈	頸部，頭部の一部	

A 頭頸部の主な静脈．

B 頭頸部の浅静脈．*Note*: 静脈の走行は変異に富む．

図 32.10 頭部の深静脈

左外側方から見たところ．下顎骨の下顎枝，関節突起，筋突起は取り除いてある．翼突筋静脈叢は下顎枝と咀嚼筋の間にある静脈網である．海綿静脈洞は顔面静脈の枝をS状静脈洞に連絡する．

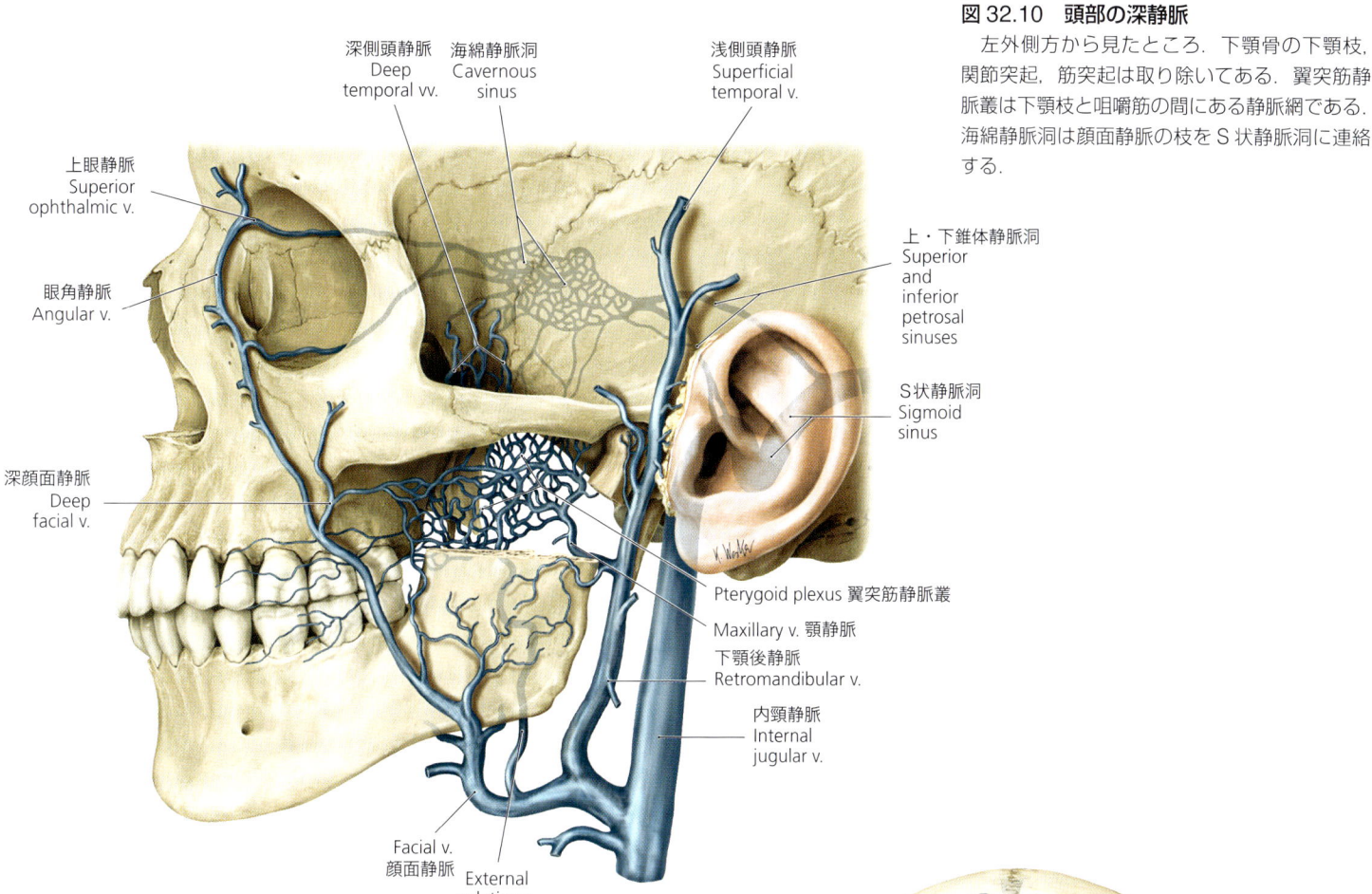

(図：頭蓋骨の左外側面観。以下のラベルが示されている)
- 深側頭静脈 Deep temporal vv.
- 海綿静脈洞 Cavernous sinus
- 浅側頭静脈 Superficial temporal v.
- 上眼静脈 Superior ophthalmic v.
- 眼角静脈 Angular v.
- 上・下錐体静脈洞 Superior and inferior petrosal sinuses
- 深顔面静脈 Deep facial v.
- S状静脈洞 Sigmoid sinus
- Pterygoid plexus 翼突筋静脈叢
- Maxillary v. 顎静脈
- 下顎後静脈 Retromandibular v.
- 内頸静脈 Internal jugular v.
- Facial v. 顔面静脈
- External palatine v. 外口蓋静脈

図 32.11 後頭部の静脈

後方から見たところ．後頭部の浅静脈は板間静脈に流れ込む導出静脈を経由して硬膜静脈洞に連絡する（p.457 の頭蓋冠を参照）．*Note*：外椎骨静脈叢は椎骨全長にわたって存在する．

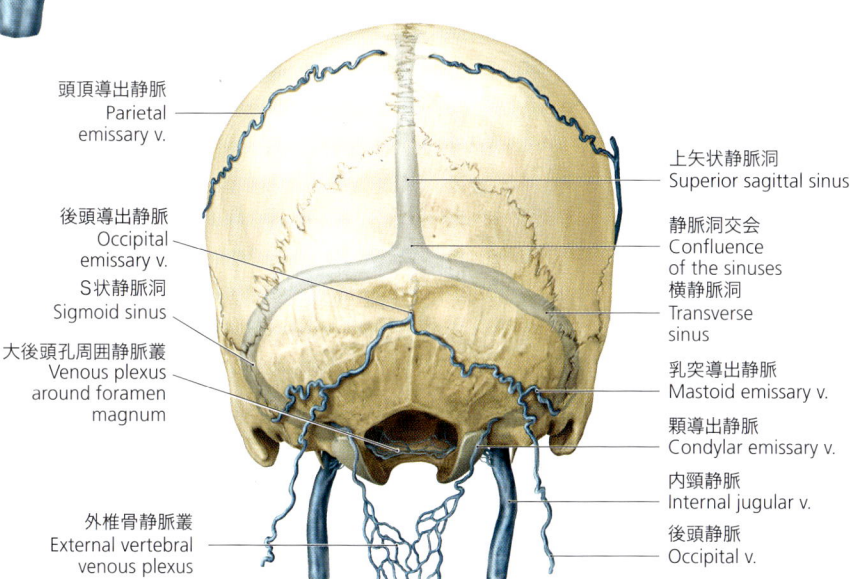

(図：頭蓋骨の後面観。以下のラベルが示されている)
- 頭頂導出静脈 Parietal emissary v.
- 上矢状静脈洞 Superior sagittal sinus
- 後頭導出静脈 Occipital emissary v.
- 静脈洞交会 Confluence of the sinuses
- S状静脈洞 Sigmoid sinus
- 横静脈洞 Transverse sinus
- 大後頭孔周囲静脈叢 Venous plexus around foramen magnum
- 乳突導出静脈 Mastoid emissary v.
- 顆導出静脈 Condylar emissary v.
- 内頸静脈 Internal jugular v.
- 外椎骨静脈叢 External vertebral venous plexus
- 後頭静脈 Occipital v.

表 32.5 静脈吻合

頭頸部の大きな静脈吻合は感染拡大の経路となる．

頭蓋外の静脈	連絡する静脈	静脈洞
眼角静脈	上眼静脈，下眼静脈	海綿静脈洞*
口蓋扁桃静脈	翼突筋静脈叢，下眼静脈	
浅側頭静脈	頭頂導出静脈	上矢状静脈洞
後頭静脈	後頭導出静脈	横静脈洞，静脈洞交会
後耳介静脈	乳突導出静脈	S状静脈洞
外椎骨静脈叢	顆導出静脈	

*顔面領域の細菌感染が深部まで広がると，海綿静脈洞血栓症に至ることがある．

顔面浅層の局所解剖
Topography of the Superficial Face

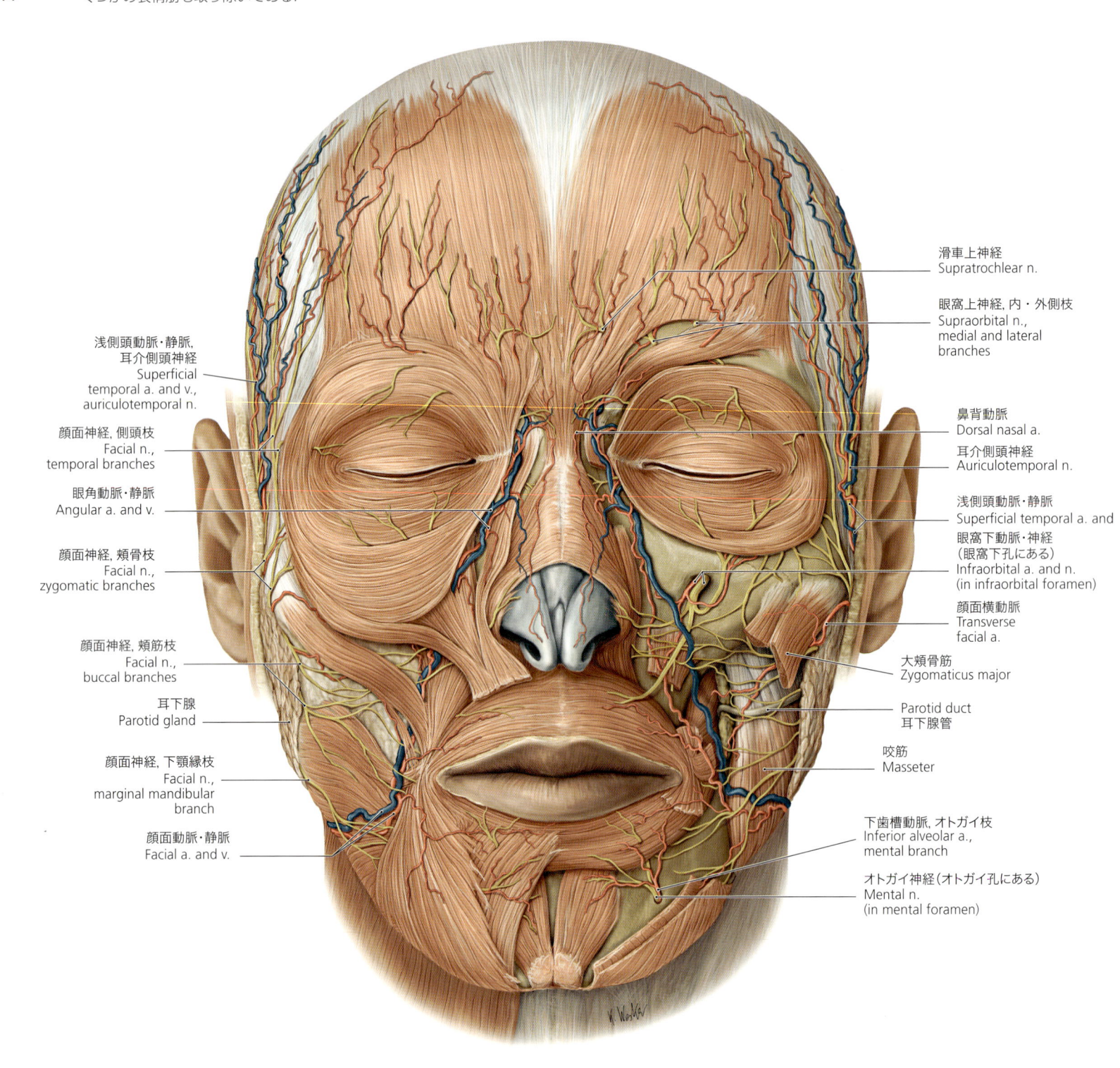

図 32.12　顔面浅層の神経・血管
前方から見たところ．皮膚と脂肪組織は取り除いてある．左半分ではいくつかの表情筋も取り除いてある．

- 浅側頭動脈・静脈, 耳介側頭神経
  Superficial temporal a. and v., auriculotemporal n.
- 顔面神経, 側頭枝
  Facial n., temporal branches
- 眼角動脈・静脈
  Angular a. and v.
- 顔面神経, 頬骨枝
  Facial n., zygomatic branches
- 顔面神経, 頬筋枝
  Facial n., buccal branches
- 耳下腺
  Parotid gland
- 顔面神経, 下顎縁枝
  Facial n., marginal mandibular branch
- 顔面動脈・静脈
  Facial a. and v.

- 滑車上神経
  Supratrochlear n.
- 眼窩上神経, 内・外側枝
  Supraorbital n., medial and lateral branches
- 鼻背動脈
  Dorsal nasal a.
- 耳介側頭神経
  Auriculotemporal n.
- 浅側頭動脈・静脈
  Superficial temporal a. and v.
- 眼窩下動脈・神経（眼窩下孔にある）
  Infraorbital a. and n. (in infraorbital foramen)
- 顔面横動脈
  Transverse facial a.
- 大頬骨筋
  Zygomaticus major
- 耳下腺管
  Parotid duct
- 咬筋
  Masseter
- 下歯槽動脈, オトガイ枝
  Inferior alveolar a., mental branch
- オトガイ神経（オトガイ孔にある）
  Mental n. (in mental foramen)

図 32.13 頭部浅層の神経・血管
左外側方から見たところ.

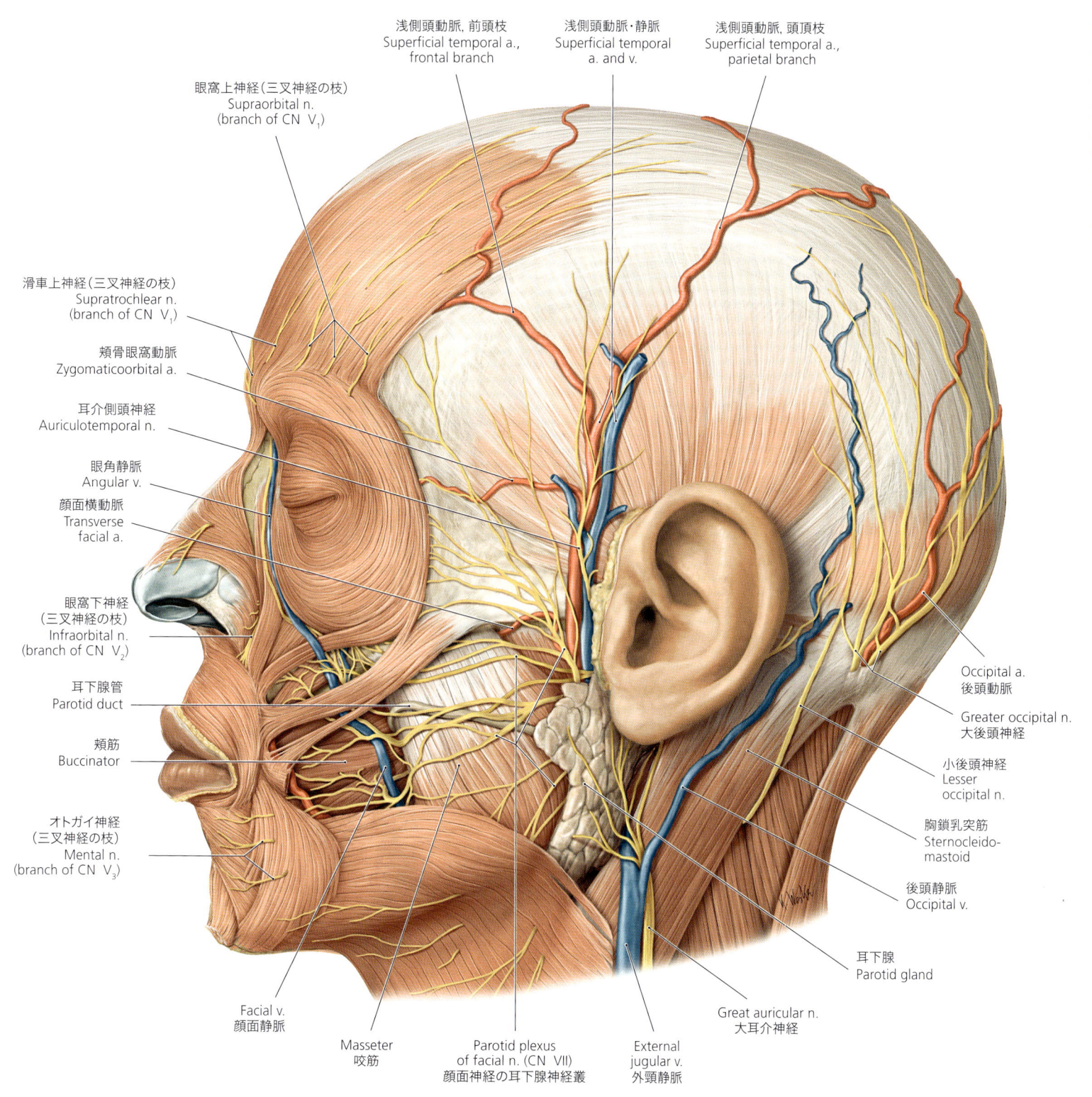

- 眼窩上神経（三叉神経の枝） Supraorbital n. (branch of CN V₁)
- 浅側頭動脈, 前頭枝 Superficial temporal a., frontal branch
- 浅側頭動脈・静脈 Superficial temporal a. and v.
- 浅側頭動脈, 頭頂枝 Superficial temporal a., parietal branch
- 滑車上神経（三叉神経の枝） Supratrochlear n. (branch of CN V₁)
- 頬骨眼窩動脈 Zygomaticoorbital a.
- 耳介側頭神経 Auriculotemporal n.
- 眼角静脈 Angular v.
- 顔面横動脈 Transverse facial a.
- 眼窩下神経（三叉神経の枝） Infraorbital n. (branch of CN V₂)
- 耳下腺管 Parotid duct
- 頬筋 Buccinator
- オトガイ神経（三叉神経の枝） Mental n. (branch of CN V₃)
- 後頭動脈 Occipital a.
- 大後頭神経 Greater occipital n.
- 小後頭神経 Lesser occipital n.
- 胸鎖乳突筋 Sternocleidomastoid
- 後頭静脈 Occipital v.
- 耳下腺 Parotid gland
- 大耳介神経 Great auricular n.
- 外頸静脈 External jugular v.
- 顔面神経の耳下腺神経叢 Parotid plexus of facial n. (CN VII)
- 咬筋 Masseter
- 顔面静脈 Facial v.

耳下腺咬筋部と側頭窩の局所解剖
Topography of the Parotid Region & Temporal Fossa

図 32.14 耳下腺咬筋部
左外側方から見たところ．耳下腺，胸鎖乳突筋，頭部の静脈は取り除いてある．耳下腺床と頸動脈三角を示している．

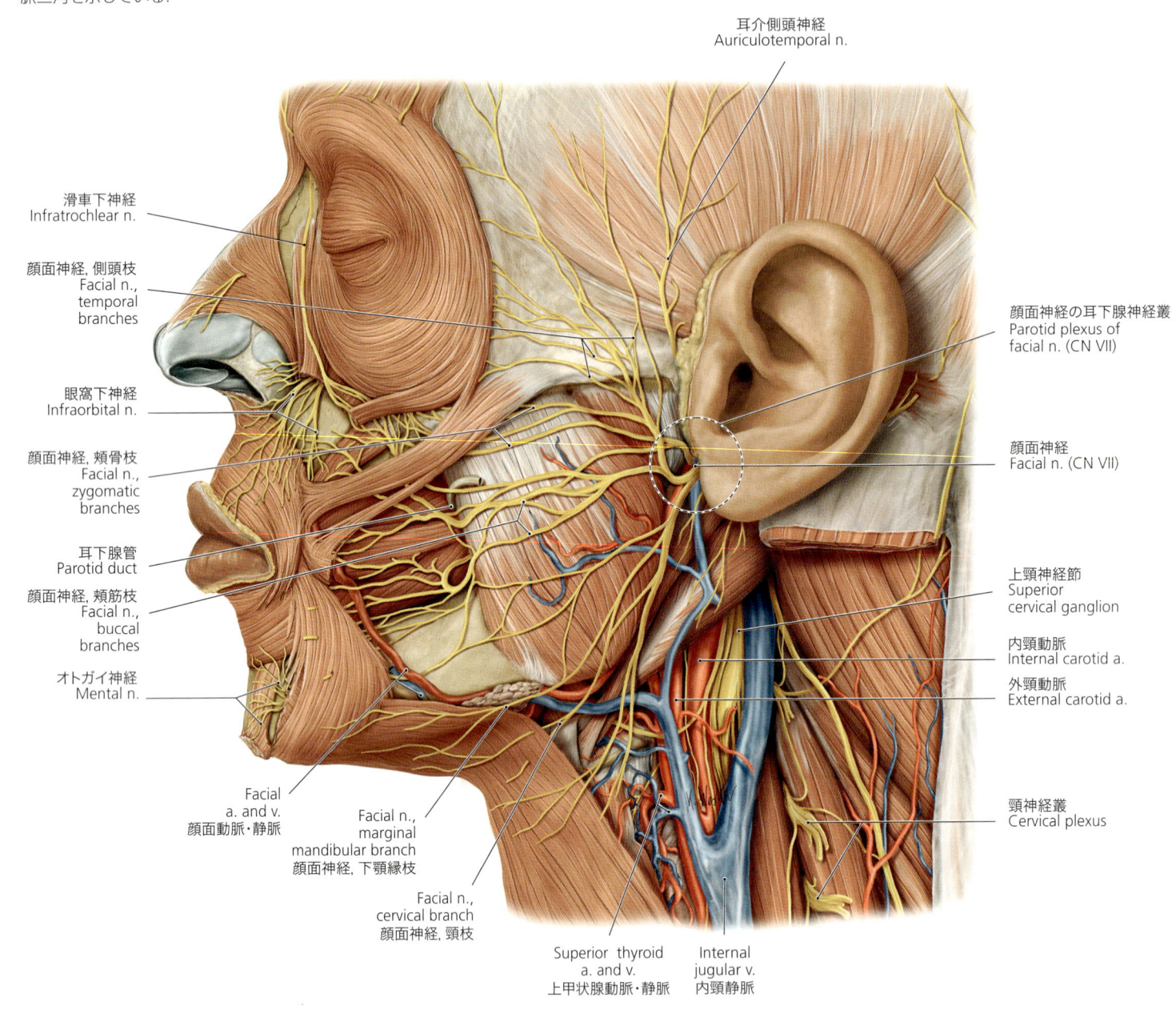

図 32.15 側頭窩

左外側方から見たところ．胸鎖乳突筋と咬筋は取り除いてある．側頭窩と顎関節 (p.540) を示している．

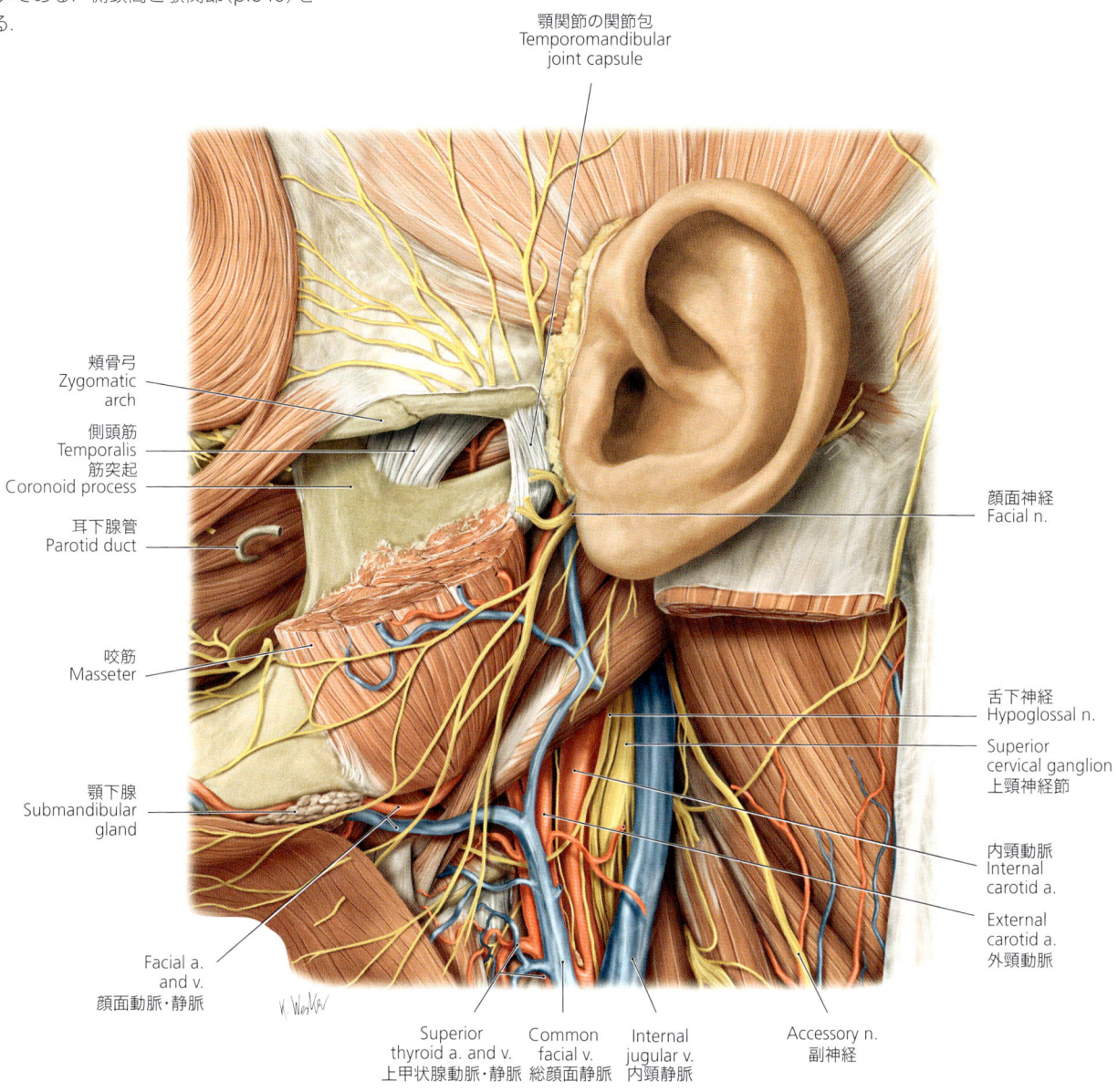

側頭下窩の局所解剖
Topography of the Infratemporal Fossa

図 32.16　側頭下窩：浅層

左外側方から見たところ．下顎枝は取り除いてある．*Note*：顎舌骨筋神経（p.547 参照）は下顎孔の直前で下歯槽神経から出る．

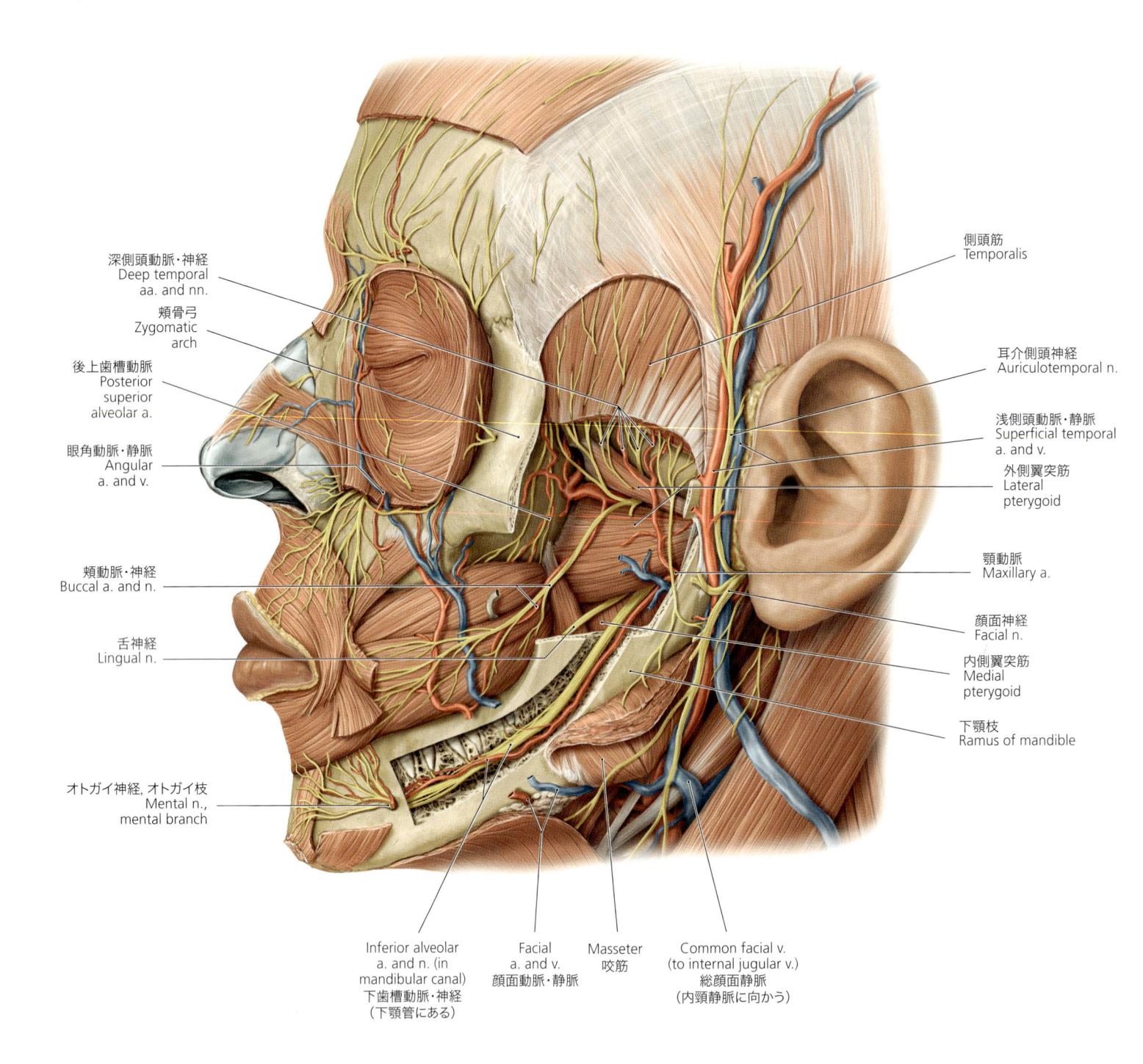

図 32.17　側頭下窩：深層
左外側方から見たところ．外側翼突筋の上頭と下頭は取り除いてある．側頭下窩の深層と下顎神経を示している．下顎神経は卵円孔を通って側頭下窩に入り，下顎管へ至る．

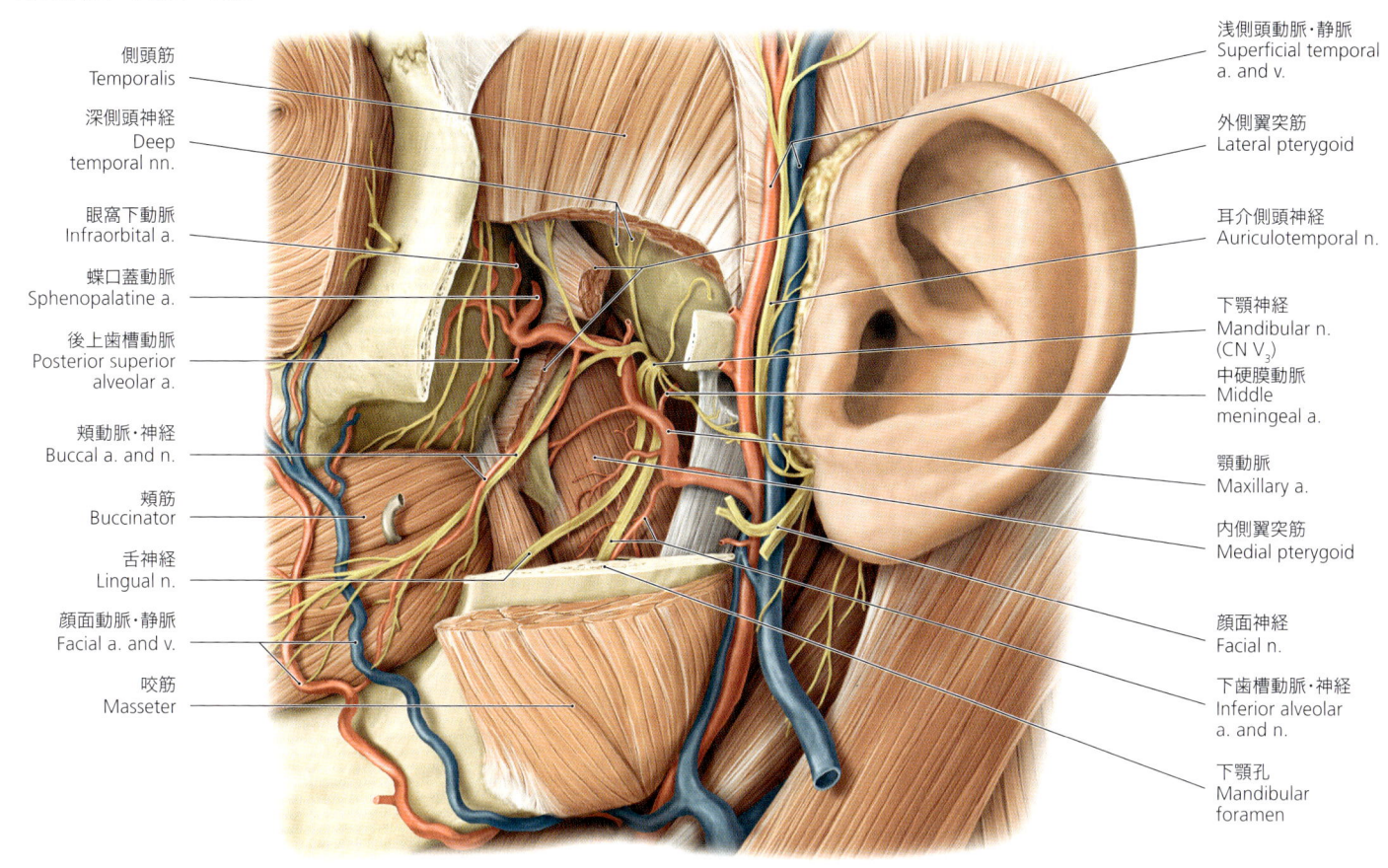

- 側頭筋　Temporalis
- 深側頭神経　Deep temporal nn.
- 眼窩下動脈　Infraorbital a.
- 蝶口蓋動脈　Sphenopalatine a.
- 後上歯槽動脈　Posterior superior alveolar a.
- 頬動脈・神経　Buccal a. and n.
- 頬筋　Buccinator
- 舌神経　Lingual n.
- 顔面動脈・静脈　Facial a. and v.
- 咬筋　Masseter
- 浅側頭動脈・静脈　Superficial temporal a. and v.
- 外側翼突筋　Lateral pterygoid
- 耳介側頭神経　Auriculotemporal n.
- 下顎神経　Mandibular n. (CN V₃)
- 中硬膜動脈　Middle meningeal a.
- 顎動脈　Maxillary a.
- 内側翼突筋　Medial pterygoid
- 顔面神経　Facial n.
- 下歯槽動脈・神経　Inferior alveolar a. and n.
- 下顎孔　Mandibular foramen

図 32.18　側頭下窩の下顎神経（CN V₃）

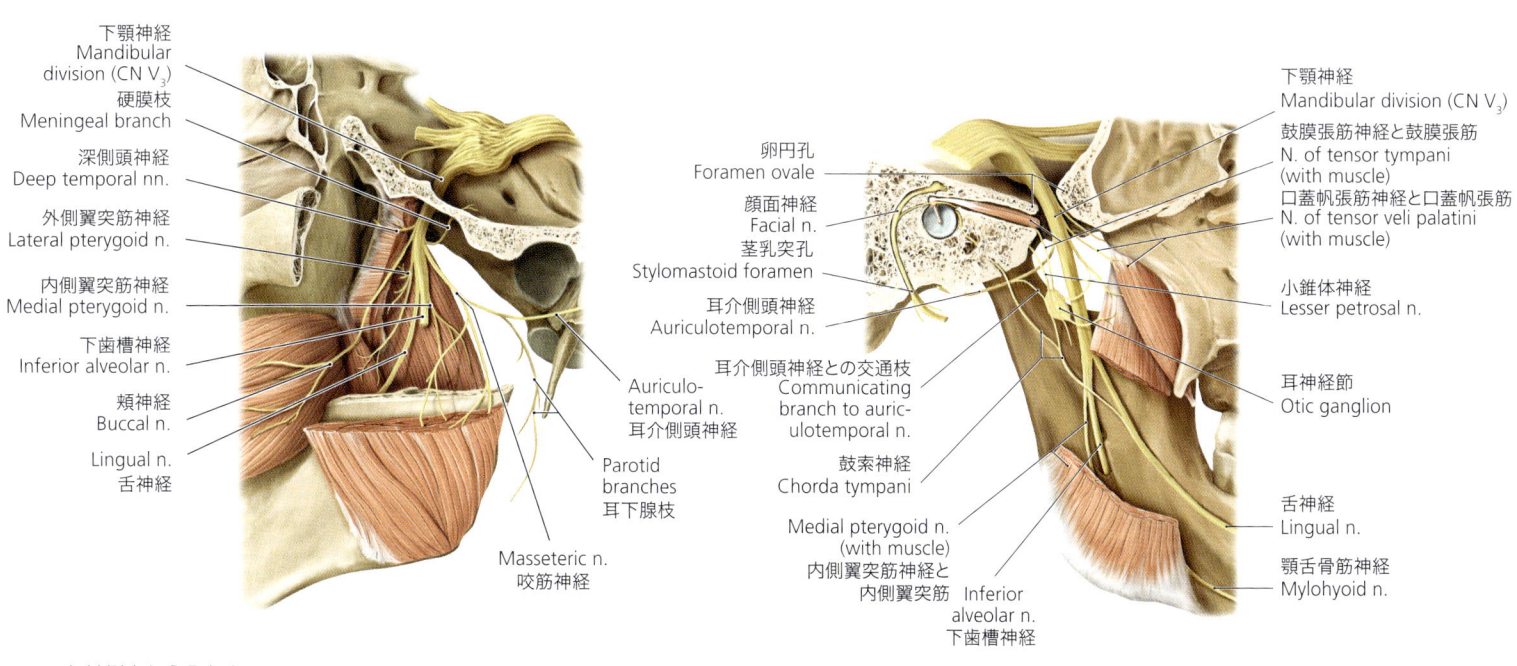

- 下顎神経　Mandibular division (CN V₃)
- 硬膜枝　Meningeal branch
- 深側頭神経　Deep temporal nn.
- 外側翼突筋神経　Lateral pterygoid n.
- 内側翼突筋神経　Medial pterygoid n.
- 下歯槽神経　Inferior alveolar n.
- 頬神経　Buccal n.
- 舌神経　Lingual n.
- 耳介側頭神経　Auriculotemporal n.
- 耳下腺枝　Parotid branches
- 咬筋神経　Masseteric n.
- 下顎神経　Mandibular division (CN V₃)
- 卵円孔　Foramen ovale
- 顔面神経　Facial n.
- 茎乳突孔　Stylomastoid foramen
- 耳介側頭神経　Auriculotemporal n.
- 耳介側頭神経との交通枝　Communicating branch to auriculotemporal n.
- 鼓索神経　Chorda tympani
- 内側翼突筋神経と内側翼突筋　Medial pterygoid n. (with muscle)
- 下歯槽神経　Inferior alveolar n.
- 鼓膜張筋神経と鼓膜張筋　N. of tensor tympani (with muscle)
- 口蓋帆張筋神経と口蓋帆張筋　N. of tensor veli palatini (with muscle)
- 小錐体神経　Lesser petrosal n.
- 耳神経節　Otic ganglion
- 舌神経　Lingual n.
- 顎舌骨筋神経　Mylohyoid n.

A　左外側方から見たところ．　　B　内側方から見たところ．

翼口蓋窩の局所解剖
Topography of the Pterygopalatine Fossa

翼口蓋窩は眼窩尖の下方にあるピラミッド状の小さな空間である．側頭下窩と連続し，両者の間に明確な境界はない．翼口蓋窩は中頭蓋窩，眼窩，鼻腔，口腔を進む神経・血管が交差する場である．

表 32.6　翼口蓋窩の区分

方向	境界構造	方向	境界構造
上方	蝶形骨大翼，下眼窩裂と連絡する	後方	翼状突起（外側板）
前方	上顎結節	外側	翼上顎裂経由で側頭下窩と通じる
内側	口蓋骨垂直板	下方	なし，咽頭後隙に開く

図 32.19　翼口蓋窩の動脈

左外側方から見たところ．顎動脈は側頭下窩の外側翼突筋の上を走り（図 32.16 参照），翼上顎裂から翼口蓋窩に入る．

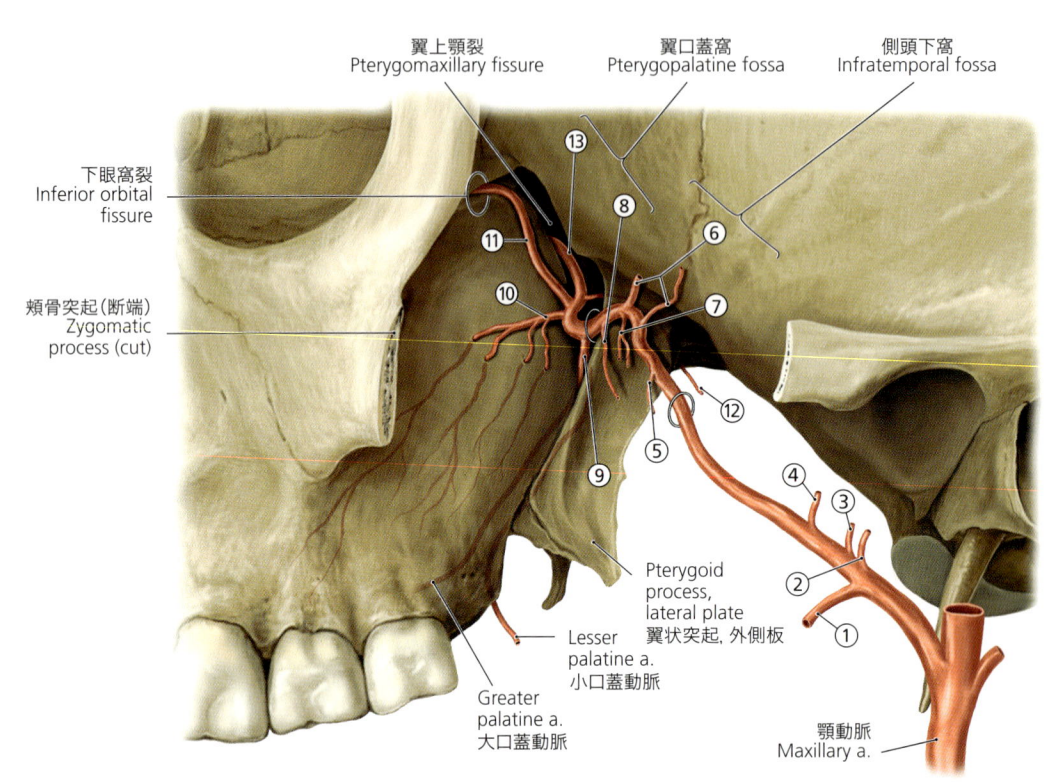

表 32.7　顎動脈の枝

枝	動脈		分布
下顎部	①下歯槽動脈		下顎骨，歯，歯肉
	②前鼓室動脈		鼓室
	③深耳介動脈		顎関節，外耳道
	④中硬膜動脈		頭蓋冠，硬膜，前頭蓋窩・中頭蓋窩
翼突筋部	⑤咬筋動脈		咬筋
	⑥前・後深側頭動脈		側頭筋
	⑦翼突筋枝		翼突筋
	⑧頬動脈		頬粘膜
翼口蓋部	⑨下行口蓋動脈	大口蓋動脈	硬口蓋
		小口蓋動脈	軟口蓋，口蓋扁桃，咽頭壁
	⑩後上歯槽動脈		上顎臼歯，上顎洞，歯肉
	⑪眼窩下動脈		上顎歯槽
	⑫翼突管動脈		
	⑬蝶口蓋動脈	外側後鼻枝	鼻腔側壁，鼻甲介
		中隔後鼻枝	鼻中隔

三叉神経の上顎神経（CN V₂, p.477 参照）は中頭蓋窩から正円孔を通り，翼口蓋窩に入る．副交感性の翼口蓋神経節には大錐体神経（顔面神経の中間神経の副交感神経根）からの節前線維が入る．翼口蓋神経節では，節前線維が涙腺，口蓋腺，鼻腺を支配する神経節細胞とシナプスを形成する．深錐体神経の交感性線維（交感神経根）と上顎神経の感覚線維（感覚根）は，シナプスを形成せずに，翼口蓋神経節を通過する．

図 32.20　翼口蓋窩の神経
左外側方から見たところ．

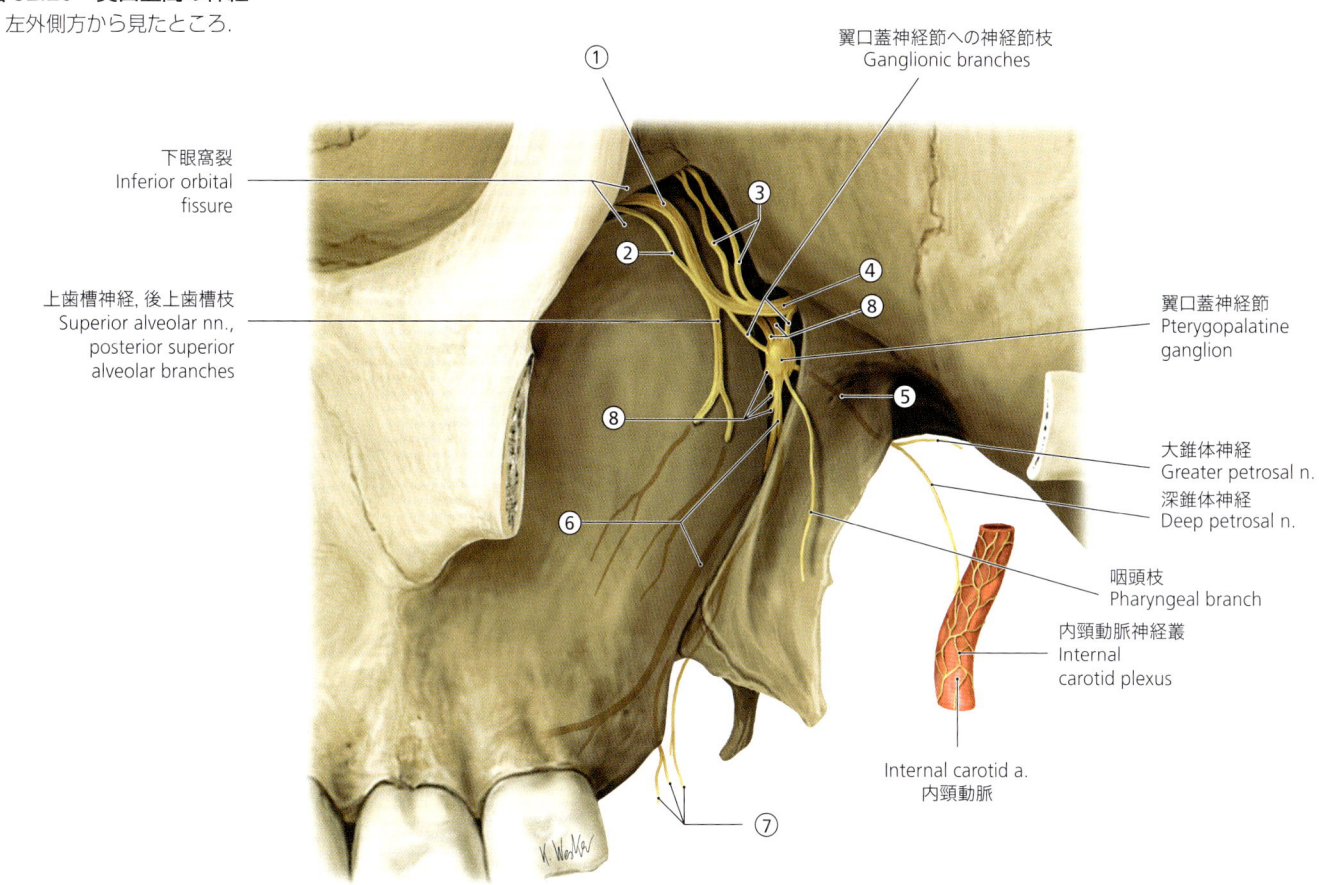

表 32.8　翼口蓋窩への神経・血管の通路

由来	経路	通過する神経	通過する血管
眼窩	下眼窩裂	①眼窩下神経	眼窩下動脈（および伴行静脈）
		②頬骨神経	下眼静脈
		③眼窩枝（上顎神経の枝）	
中頭蓋窩	正円孔	④上顎神経（CN V₂）	
頭蓋底	翼突管	⑤翼突管神経（大錐体神経，深錐体神経）	翼突管動脈（および伴行静脈）
口蓋	大口蓋管	⑥大口蓋神経	下行口蓋動脈
			大口蓋動脈
	小口蓋管	⑦小口蓋神経	小口蓋動脈（下行口蓋動脈の終枝）
鼻腔	蝶口蓋孔	⑧内側上後鼻枝，外側上後鼻枝，下後鼻枝（鼻口蓋神経，上顎神経より）	蝶口蓋動脈（および伴行静脈）

眼窩の骨
Bones of the Orbit

図 33.1 眼窩の骨

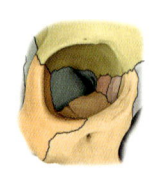

A 前方から見たところ.

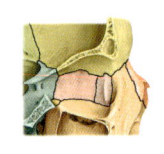

B 右眼窩を右外側方から見たところ.

表 33.1	眼窩の神経・血管の通る開口部		
開口部*	神経		血管
視神経管	視神経(CN II)		眼動脈
上眼窩裂	動眼神経(CN III) 滑車神経(CN IV) 外転神経(CN VI)	三叉神経の眼神経(CN V_1) ・涙腺神経 ・前頭神経 ・鼻毛様体神経	上眼静脈
下眼窩裂	眼窩下神経(CN V_2) 頬骨神経(CN V_2)		眼窩下動脈・静脈, 下眼静脈
眼窩下管	眼窩下神経(CN V_2), 眼窩下動脈・静脈		
眼窩上孔	眼窩上神経(外側枝)		眼窩上動脈
前頭切痕	眼窩上神経(内側枝)		滑車上動脈
前篩骨孔	前篩骨神経, 前篩骨動脈・静脈		
後篩骨孔	後篩骨神経, 後篩骨動脈・静脈		

*涙嚢から続く鼻涙管は骨性の鼻涙管を通る.

眼窩と眼

C 右の眼窩を左外側方から見たところ．

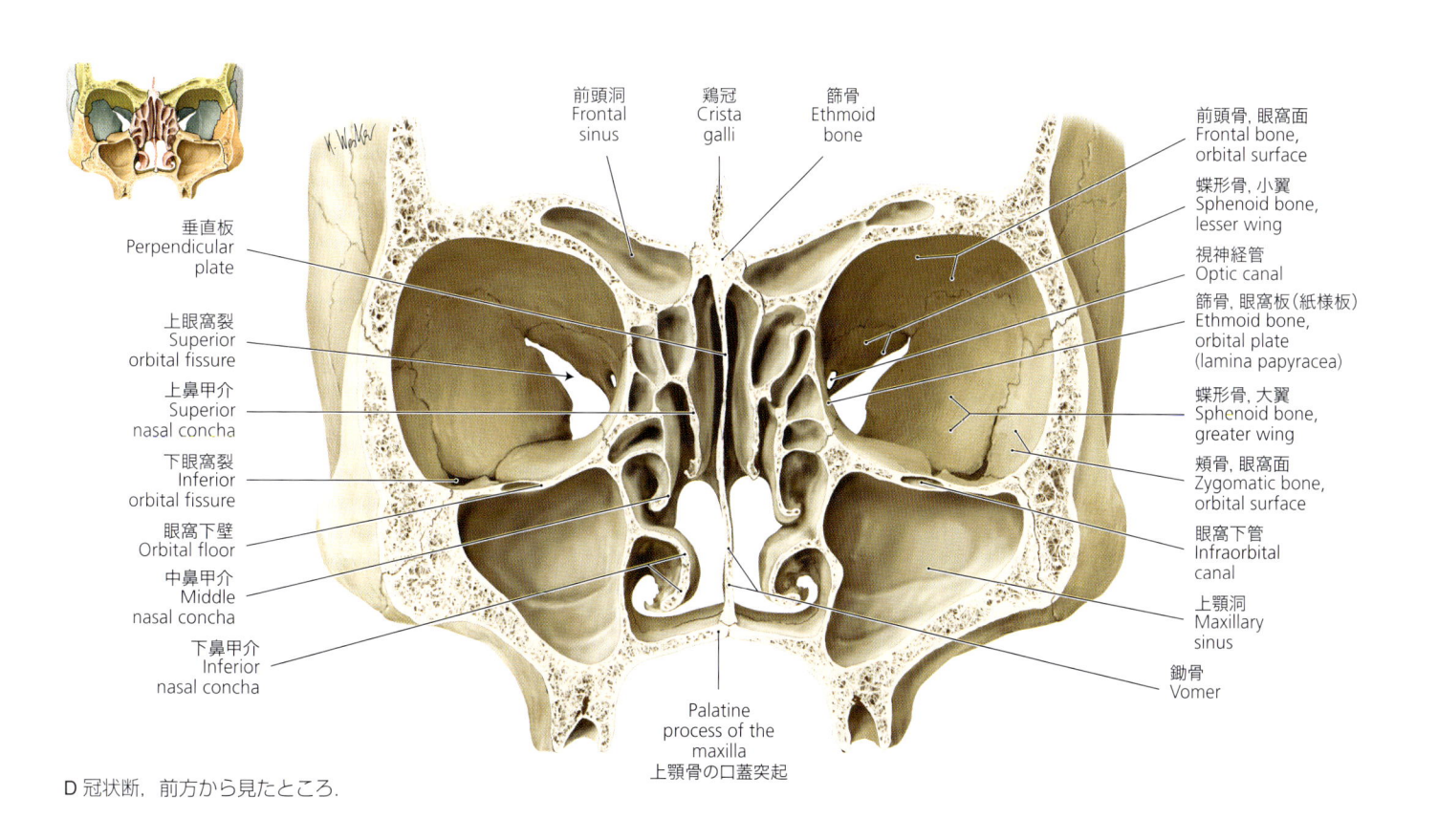

主な構造ラベル：
- 前頭洞 Frontal sinus
- 前頭骨, 眼窩面 Frontal bone, orbital surface
- 上眼窩裂 Superior orbital fissure
- 頬骨, 眼窩面 Zygomatic bone, orbital surface
- 蝶形骨, 小翼 Sphenoid bone, lesser wing
- 頬骨眼窩孔 Zygomatico-orbital foramen
- 蝶形骨, 大翼 Sphenoid bone, greater wing
- 上顎骨, 眼窩面 Maxilla, orbital surface
- 眼窩下管 Infraorbital canal
- 下眼窩裂 Inferior orbital fissure
- 上顎洞 Maxillary sinus
- 口蓋骨, 錐体突起 Palatine bone, pyramidal process

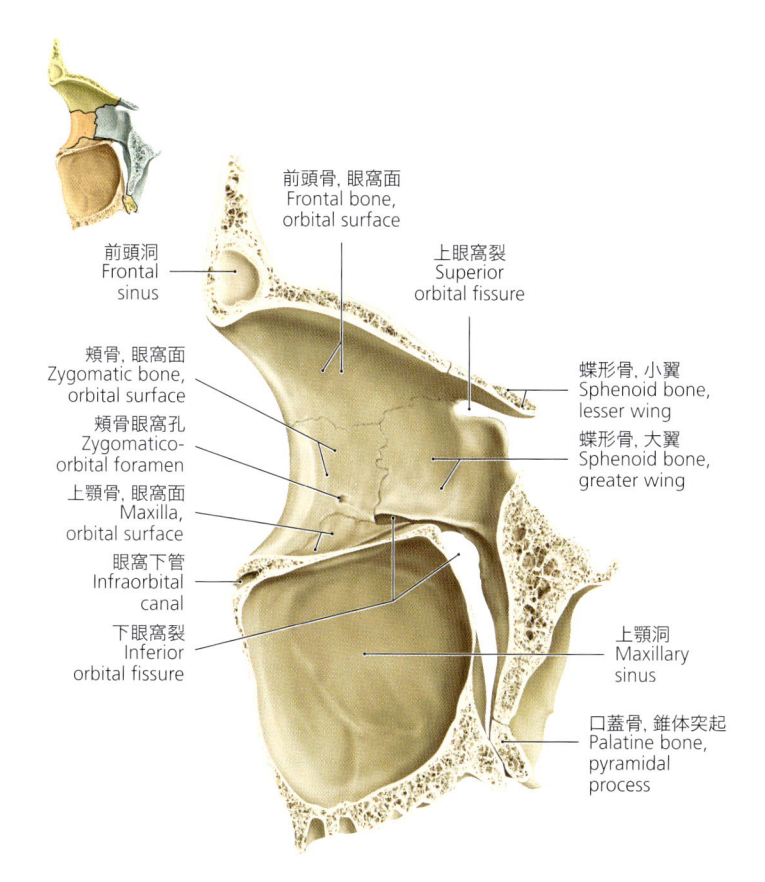

表 33.2　眼窩周囲の構造

方向	境界を成す構造
上方	前頭洞
	前頭蓋窩
内側	篩骨蜂巣
下方	上顎洞

眼窩と臨床的に重要な関係にある深部構造

蝶形骨洞	下垂体
中頭蓋窩	海綿静脈洞
視交叉	翼口蓋窩

D 冠状断，前方から見たところ．

主な構造ラベル：
- 前頭洞 Frontal sinus
- 鶏冠 Crista galli
- 篩骨 Ethmoid bone
- 前頭骨, 眼窩面 Frontal bone, orbital surface
- 蝶形骨, 小翼 Sphenoid bone, lesser wing
- 視神経管 Optic canal
- 篩骨, 眼窩板（紙様板）Ethmoid bone, orbital plate (lamina papyracea)
- 蝶形骨, 大翼 Sphenoid bone, greater wing
- 頬骨, 眼窩面 Zygomatic bone, orbital surface
- 眼窩下管 Infraorbital canal
- 上顎洞 Maxillary sinus
- 鋤骨 Vomer
- 垂直板 Perpendicular plate
- 上眼窩裂 Superior orbital fissure
- 上鼻甲介 Superior nasal concha
- 下眼窩裂 Inferior orbital fissure
- 眼窩下壁 Orbital floor
- 中鼻甲介 Middle nasal concha
- 下鼻甲介 Inferior nasal concha
- 上顎骨の口蓋突起 Palatine process of the maxilla

眼窩の筋
Muscles of the Orbit

図 33.2　外眼筋

右眼球. A以外は上面. 眼球は，4つの直筋(上直筋，下直筋，内側直筋，外側直筋)と2つの斜筋(上斜筋，下斜筋)の6つの外在筋によって動かされる.

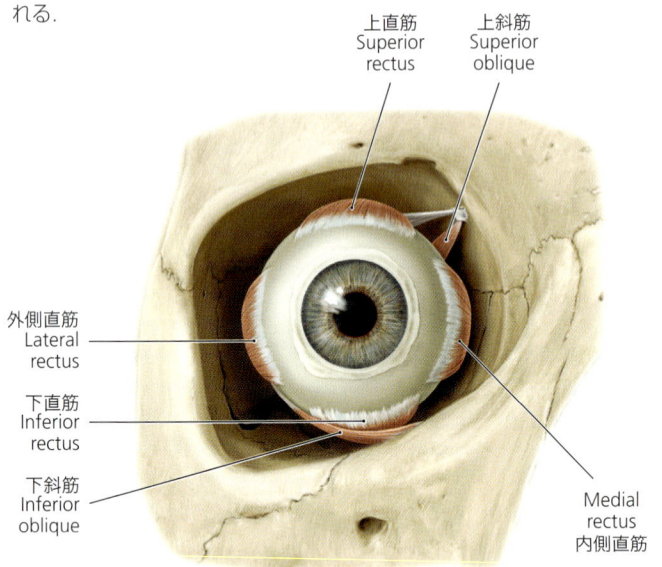

A　前方から見たところ.

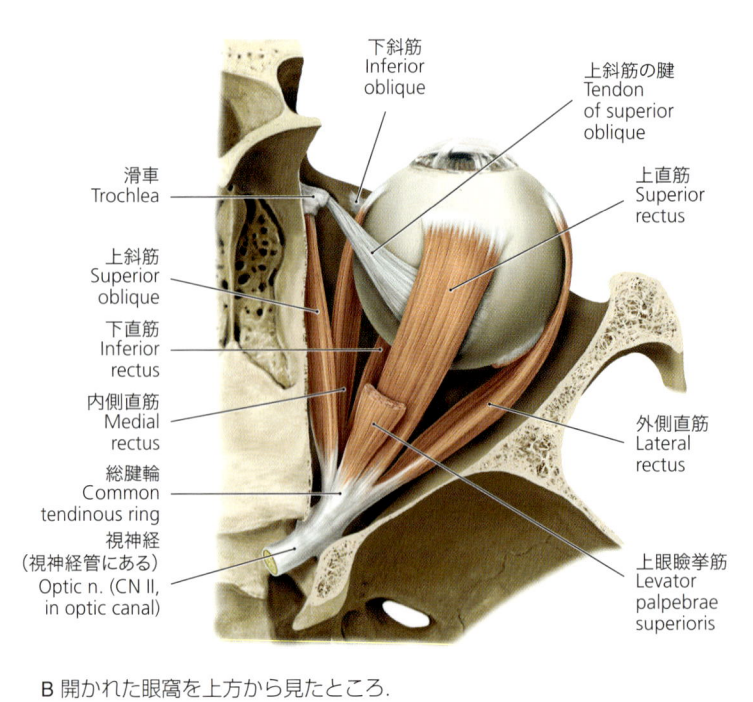

B　開かれた眼窩を上方から見たところ.

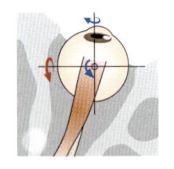

C　上直筋. 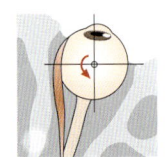　　D　内側直筋. 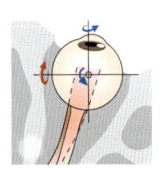　　E　下直筋. 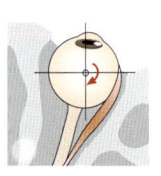　　F　外側直筋. 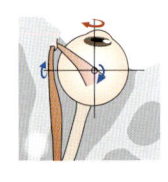　　G　上斜筋. 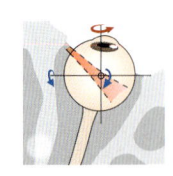　　H　下斜筋.

表 33.3　外眼筋

筋肉	起始	停止	主な作用(赤色)	副次的な作用(青色)	神経支配
上直筋	総腱輪	強膜	上転	内転と内旋	動眼神経(CN III)，上枝
内側直筋			内転	なし	動眼神経(CN III)，下枝
下直筋			下転	内転と外旋	
外側直筋			外転	なし	外転神経(CN VI)
上斜筋	蝶形骨*		下転，外転	内旋	滑車神経(CN IV)
下斜筋	眼窩内側縁		上転，外転	外旋	動眼神経(CN III)，下枝

*上斜筋の停止腱は眼窩上内側縁に付着する腱性のループ(滑車)を通る.

図 33.3　注視の基本的な方向

注視の基本的な方向は6つあり，眼球運動診断ではすべてを検査する.

Note: ある方向への注視では，左右の眼球で同じ筋が使われるのではなく，異なる筋が働く必要がある. そのため，2つの脳神経が必要となる.

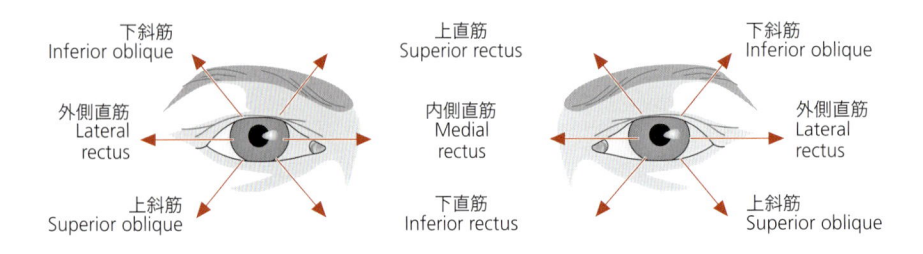

図 33.4 外眼筋の神経支配.
右眼球. 右外側方から見たところ. 眼窩の外側壁は取り除いてある.

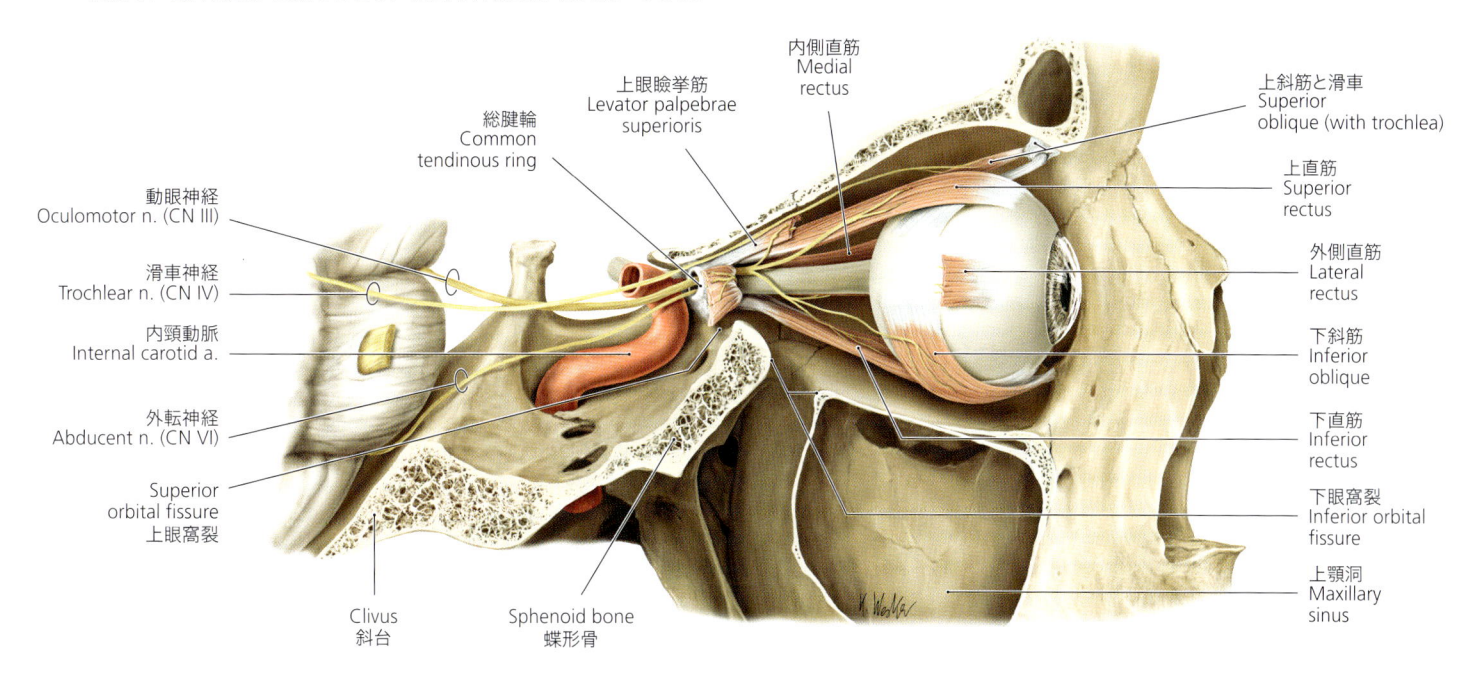

内側直筋 Medial rectus
上眼瞼挙筋 Levator palpebrae superioris
総腱輪 Common tendinous ring
動眼神経 Oculomotor n. (CN III)
滑車神経 Trochlear n. (CN IV)
内頸動脈 Internal carotid a.
外転神経 Abducent n. (CN VI)
Superior orbital fissure 上眼窩裂
Clivus 斜台
Sphenoid bone 蝶形骨
上斜筋と滑車 Superior oblique (with trochlea)
上直筋 Superior rectus
外側直筋 Lateral rectus
下斜筋 Inferior oblique
下直筋 Inferior rectus
下眼窩裂 Inferior orbital fissure
上顎洞 Maxillary sinus

臨床

眼球運動麻痺

眼球運動麻痺は外眼筋や関連する脳神経核や神経路の損傷によって起こる. ある外眼筋の筋力が低下したり麻痺すると, 眼球の偏位が起こる. 外眼筋の協調作用の障害によって片方の眼の視軸が正常からずれる. そのため患者には像が二重に見える複視が生じる.

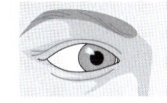

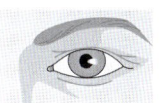

A 外転神経麻痺.
　外側直筋の障害.

B 滑車神経麻痺.
　上斜筋の障害.

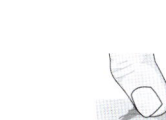

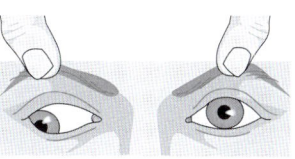

C 動眼神経完全麻痺.
　上直筋, 下直筋, 内側直筋, 下斜筋の障害.

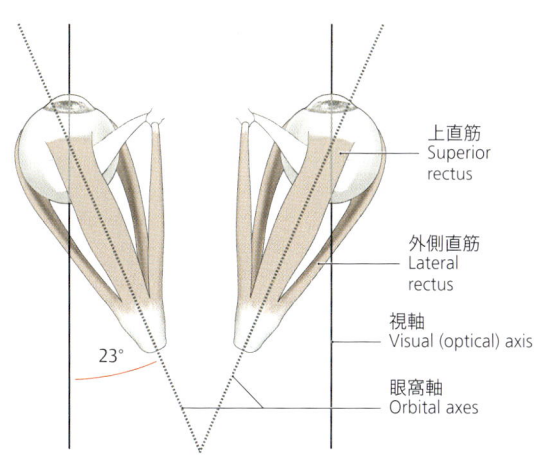

上直筋 Superior rectus
外側直筋 Lateral rectus
視軸 Visual (optical) axis
眼窩軸 Orbital axes

D 正常の視軸と眼窩軸.

眼窩の神経と血管
Neurovasculature of the Orbit

図 33.5　眼窩の静脈
右眼窩．右外側方から見たところ．眼窩の外側壁を取り除き，上顎洞を開いてある．

ラベル:
- 滑車上静脈 Supratrochlear v.
- 鼻背静脈 Dorsal nasal v.
- 上眼静脈 Superior ophthalmic v.
- 涙腺静脈 Lacrimal v.
- 眼角静脈 Angular v.
- 海綿静脈洞 Cavernous sinus
- Ophthalmic v. 眼静脈
- Inferior ophthalmic v. 下眼静脈
- Infraorbital v. 眼窩下静脈
- Facial v. 顔面静脈

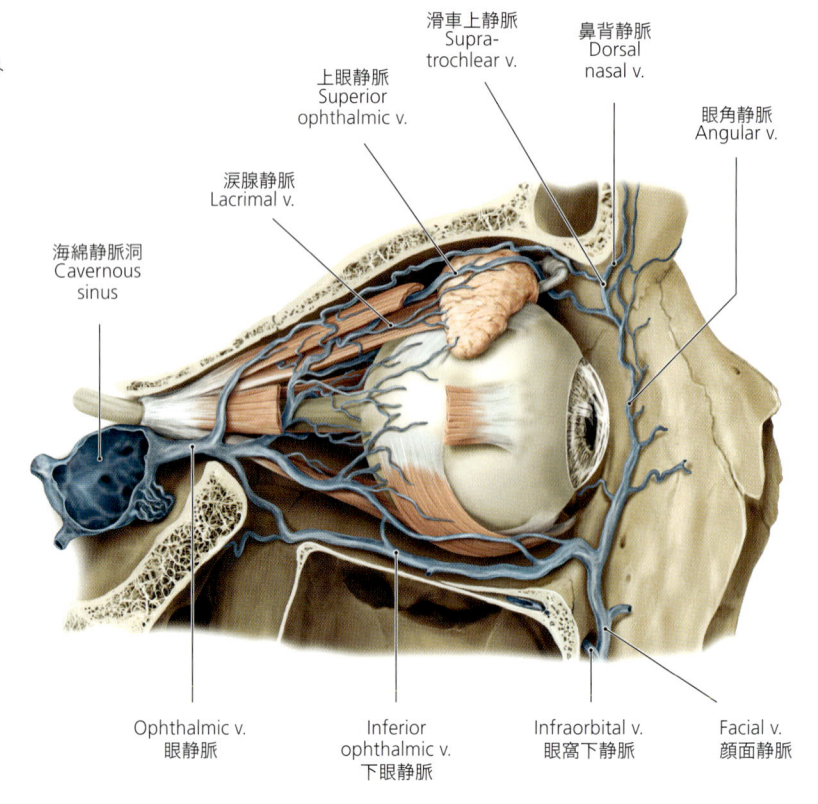

図 33.6　眼窩の動脈
右眼窩，上方から見たところ．視神経管と眼窩の上壁を開いてある．

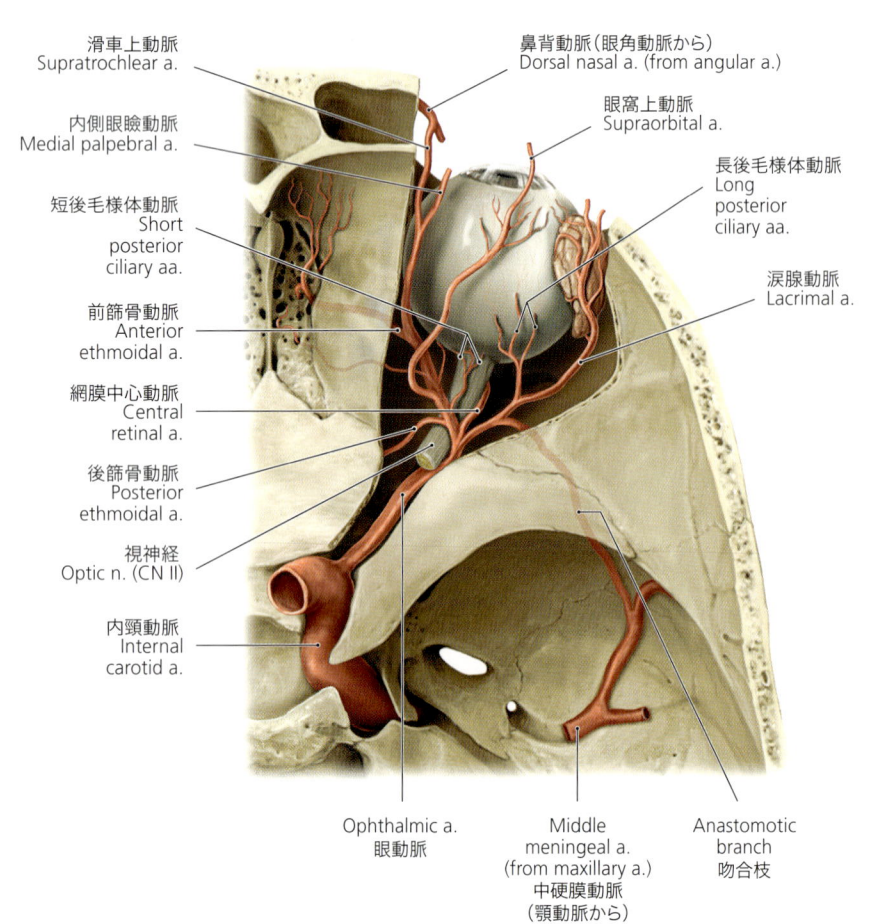

ラベル:
- 滑車上動脈 Supratrochlear a.
- 鼻背動脈（眼角動脈から） Dorsal nasal a. (from angular a.)
- 内側眼瞼動脈 Medial palpebral a.
- 眼窩上動脈 Supraorbital a.
- 短後毛様体動脈 Short posterior ciliary aa.
- 長後毛様体動脈 Long posterior ciliary aa.
- 前篩骨動脈 Anterior ethmoidal a.
- 涙腺動脈 Lacrimal a.
- 網膜中心動脈 Central retinal a.
- 後篩骨動脈 Posterior ethmoidal a.
- 視神経 Optic n. (CN II)
- 内頸動脈 Internal carotid a.
- Ophthalmic a. 眼動脈
- Middle meningeal a. (from maxillary a.) 中硬膜動脈（顎動脈から）
- Anastomotic branch 吻合枝

図 33.7 眼窩の神経支配
右眼窩，右外側方から見たところ．外側壁を取り除いてある．

- 動眼神経 Oculomotor n. (CN III)
- 内頸動脈と内頸動脈神経叢 Internal carotid a. with internal carotid plexus
- 動眼神経，上枝 Oculomotor n., superior branch
- 前頭神経 Frontal n.
- 涙腺神経と涙腺 Lacrimal n. (with gland)
- 眼窩上神経 Supraorbital n.
- 滑車下神経 Infratrochlear n.
- 滑車神経 Trochlear n. (CN IV)
- 長毛様体神経 Long ciliary nn.
- 鼻毛様体神経 Nasociliary n.
- 眼神経 Ophthalmic division (CN V₁)
- 短毛様体神経 Short ciliary nn.
- 三叉神経 Trigeminal n. (CN V)
- 毛様体神経節 Ciliary ganglion
- 三叉神経節 Trigeminal ganglion
- 副交感神経根 Parasympathetic root
- 下顎神経 Mandibular division (CN V₃)
- 外転神経 Abducent n. (CN VI)
- 上顎神経 Maxillary division (CN V₂)
- 視神経 Optic n. (CN II)
- 動眼神経，下枝 Oculomotor n., inferior branch
- 交感神経根 Sympathetic root
- 鼻毛様体神経根 Nasociliary root

図 33.8 眼窩の脳神経
前頭蓋窩と中頭蓋窩．上方から見たところ．海綿静脈洞の外側壁と上壁，眼窩の上壁，眼窩骨膜の一部を取り除いてある．三叉神経節は外側に翻転してある．

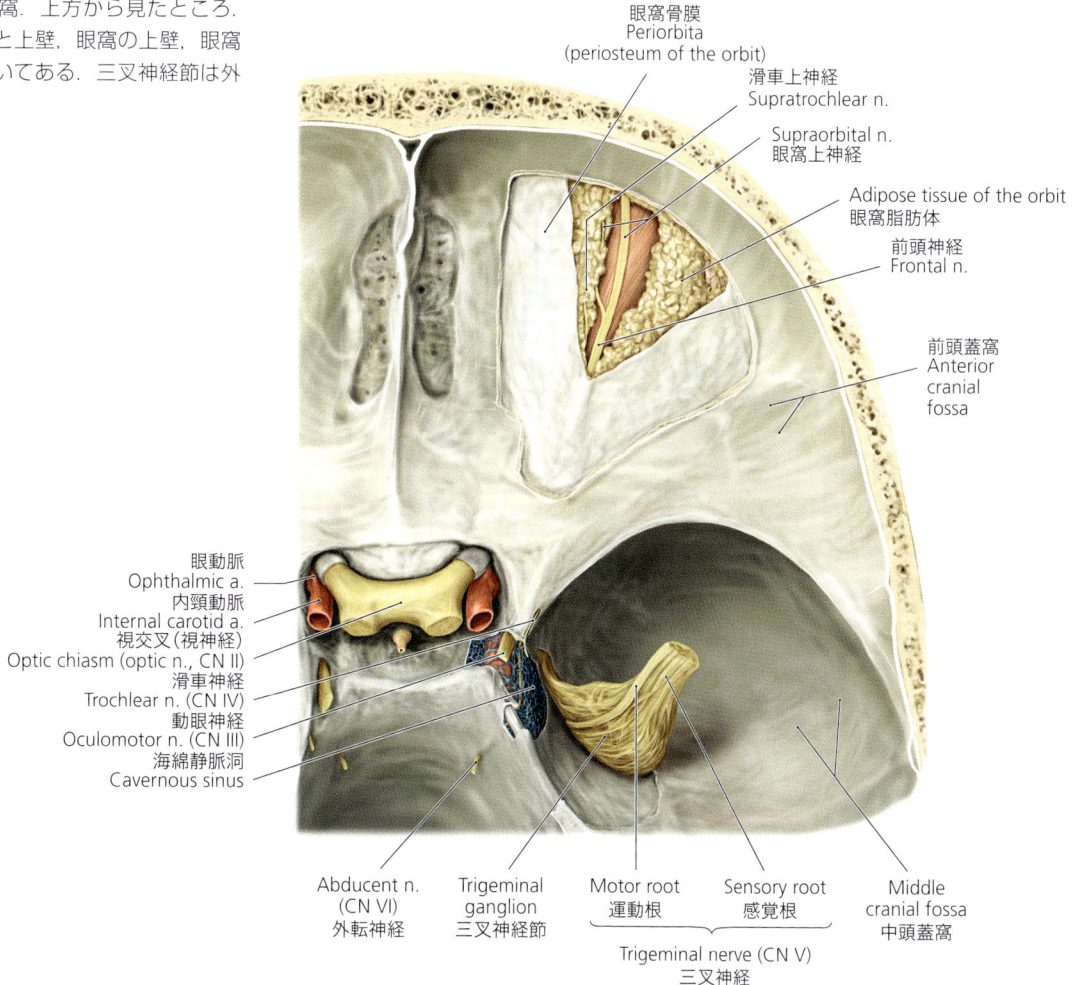

- 眼窩骨膜 Periorbita (periosteum of the orbit)
- 滑車上神経 Supratrochlear n.
- 眼窩上神経 Supraorbital n.
- 眼窩脂肪体 Adipose tissue of the orbit
- 前頭神経 Frontal n.
- 前頭蓋窩 Anterior cranial fossa
- 眼動脈 Ophthalmic a.
- 内頸動脈 Internal carotid a.
- 視交叉 (視神経) Optic chiasm (optic n., CN II)
- 滑車神経 Trochlear n. (CN IV)
- 動眼神経 Oculomotor n. (CN III)
- 海綿静脈洞 Cavernous sinus
- 外転神経 Abducent n. (CN VI)
- 三叉神経節 Trigeminal ganglion
- 運動根 Motor root
- 感覚根 Sensory root
- 中頭蓋窩 Middle cranial fossa
- 三叉神経 Trigeminal nerve (CN V)

眼窩の局所解剖
Topography of the Orbit

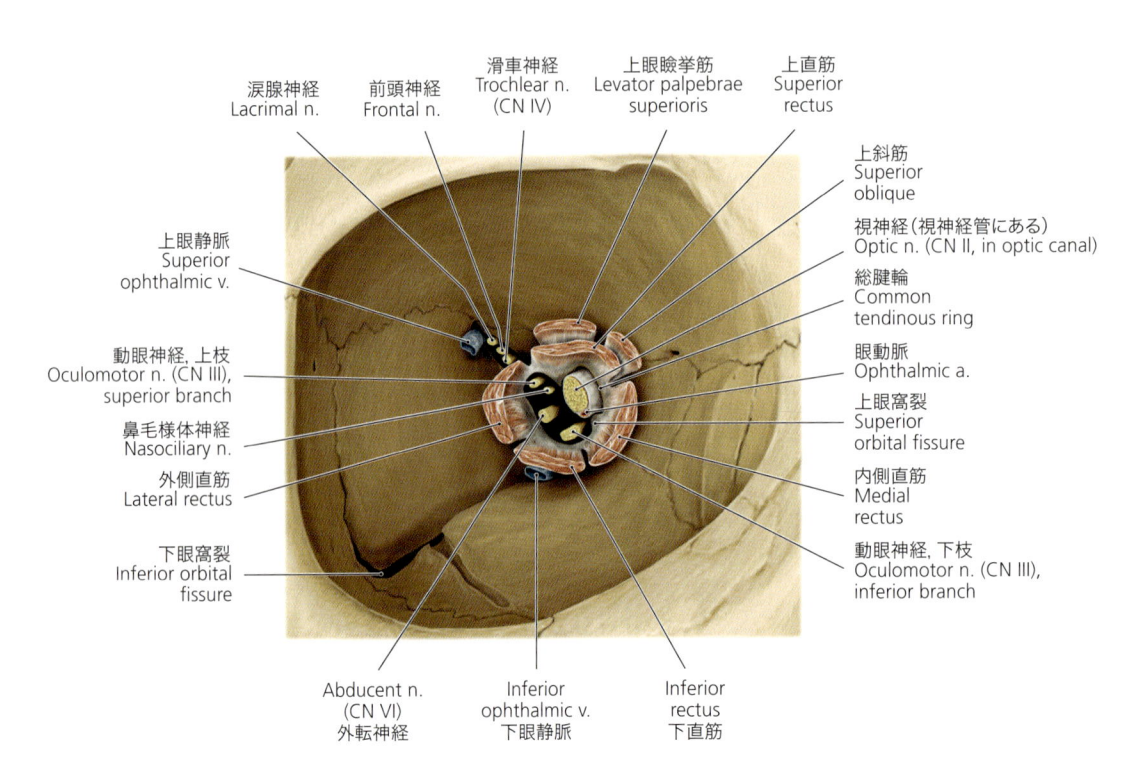

図 33.9 眼窩の神経・血管
前方から見たところ．右側は眼輪筋を，左側は眼窩隔膜を一部取り除いてある．

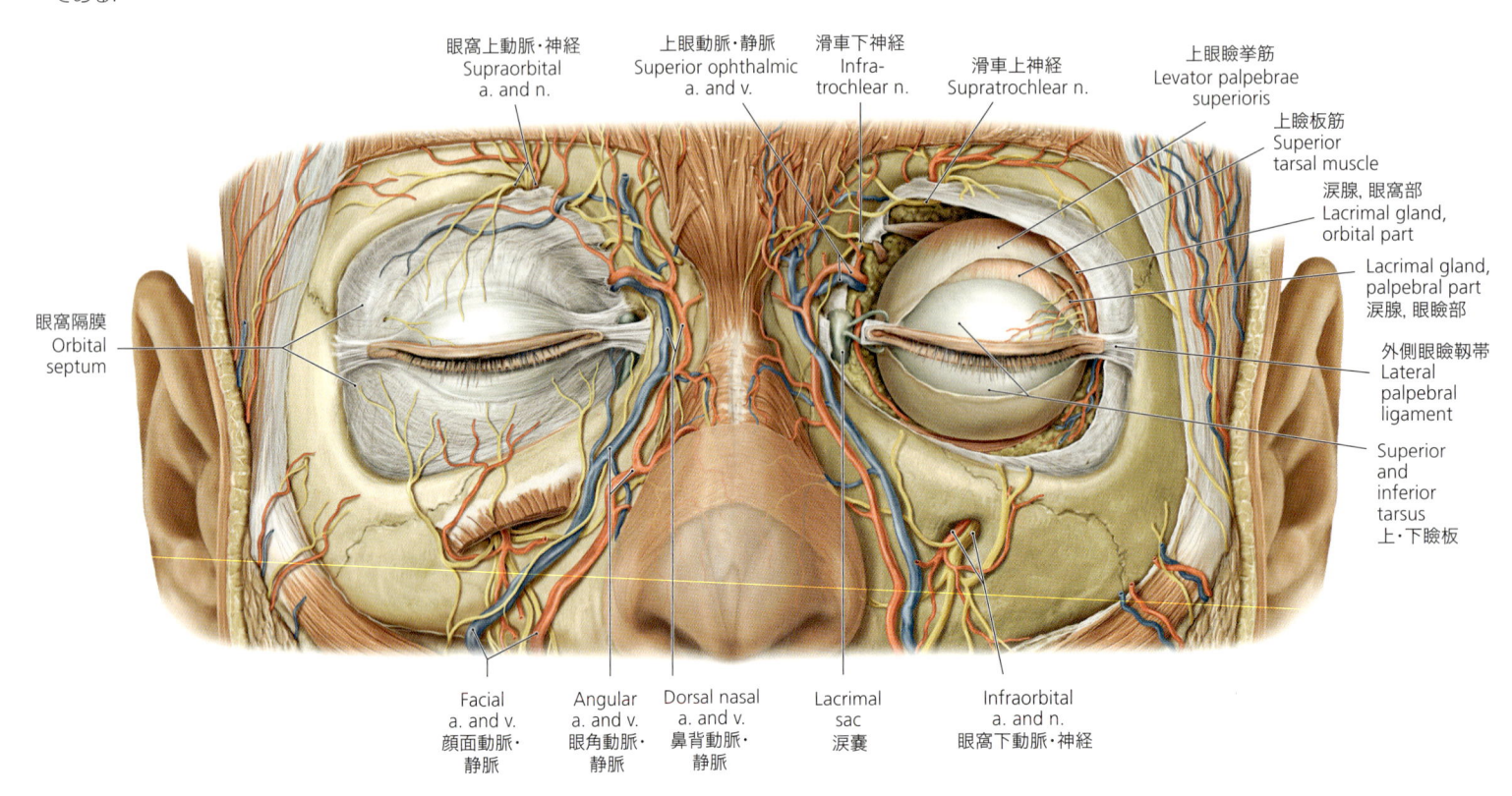

図 33.10 眼窩を通過する神経・血管
前方から見たところ．眼窩内の構造を取り除いてある．*Note*：視神経と眼動脈は視神経管を通る．残りの神経・血管は上眼窩裂を通る．

図 33.11　眼窩の神経・血管

上方から見たところ．眼窩の上壁の骨，眼窩骨膜，眼窩脂肪体を取り除いてある．

A 眼窩上部．

- 滑車下神経 Infratrochlear n.
- 篩板 Cribriform plate
- 前篩骨動脈・神経 Anterior ethmoidal a. and n.
- 滑車上動脈・神経 Supratrochlear a. and n.
- 後篩骨動脈・神経 Posterior ethmoidal a. and n.
- 眼窩上動脈 Supraorbital a.
- 鼻毛様体神経 Nasociliary n.
- 滑車神経 Trochlear n. (CN IV)
- 上眼静脈 Superior ophthalmic v.
- 眼窩上動脈・神経 Supraorbital aa. and nn.
- 上眼瞼挙筋 Levator palpebrae superioris
- 涙腺動脈・神経と涙腺 Lacrimal a. and n. (with gland)
- 上直筋 Superior rectus
- 外転神経 Abducent n. (CN VI)
- 下眼静脈 Inferior ophthalmic v.
- 前頭神経 Frontal n.

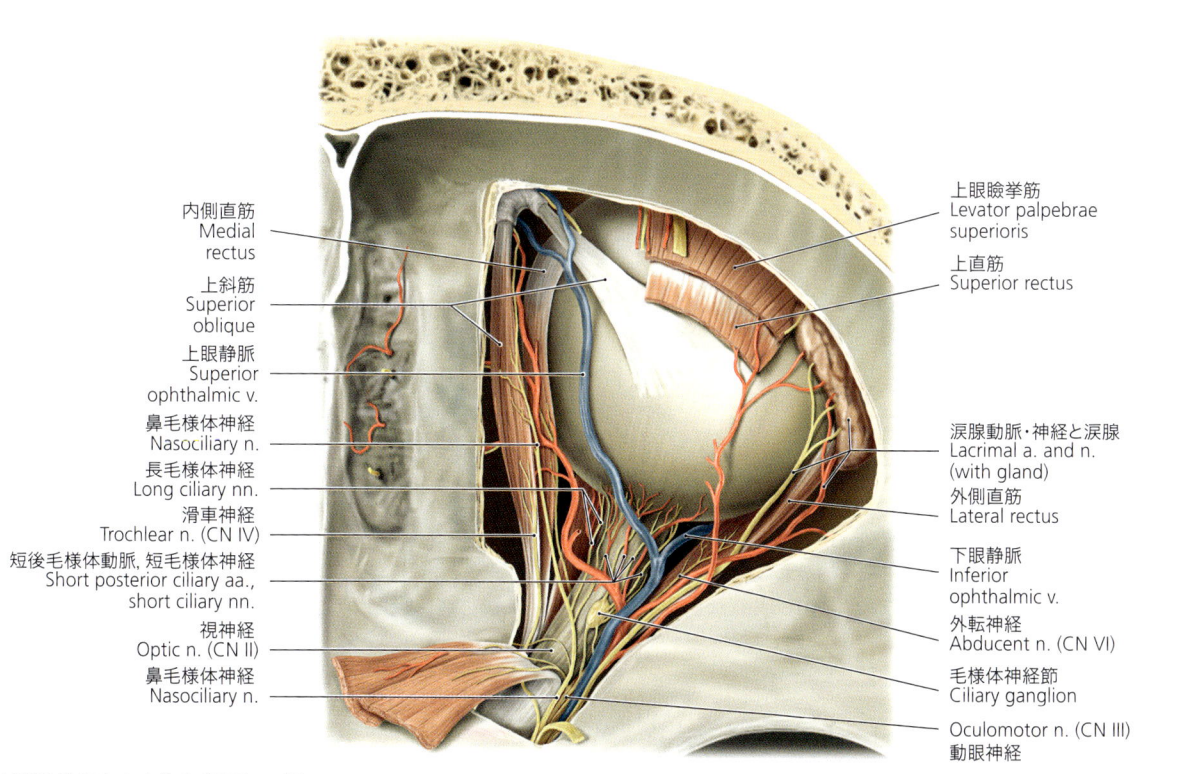

B 眼窩中部．上眼瞼挙筋と上直筋を翻転し，視神経を示す．

- 内側直筋 Medial rectus
- 上斜筋 Superior oblique
- 上眼静脈 Superior ophthalmic v.
- 鼻毛様体神経 Nasociliary n.
- 長毛様体神経 Long ciliary nn.
- 滑車神経 Trochlear n. (CN IV)
- 短後毛様体動脈，短毛様体神経 Short posterior ciliary aa., short ciliary nn.
- 視神経 Optic n. (CN II)
- 鼻毛様体神経 Nasociliary n.
- 上眼瞼挙筋 Levator palpebrae superioris
- 上直筋 Superior rectus
- 涙腺動脈・神経と涙腺 Lacrimal a. and n. (with gland)
- 外側直筋 Lateral rectus
- 下眼静脈 Inferior ophthalmic v.
- 外転神経 Abducent n. (CN VI)
- 毛様体神経節 Ciliary ganglion
- 動眼神経 Oculomotor n. (CN III)

眼窩と眼瞼
Orbit & Eyelid

図33.12 眼窩の局所解剖
右眼窩の矢状断．左外側方から見たところ．

Labels:
- 眼窩の上壁 Orbital roof
- 眼窩骨膜 Periorbita
- 眼窩脂肪体 Adipose tissue of the orbit
- 眼球 Eyeball
- 眼窩隔膜 Orbital septum
- 下斜筋 Inferior oblique
- 眼窩下神経 Infraorbital n.
- 強膜外隙 Episcleral space
- 眼球鞘（テノン嚢） Bulbar fascia (Tenon's capsule)
- Orbital floor 眼窩下壁
- Maxillary sinus 上顎洞
- 強膜 Sclera
- 上眼瞼挙筋 Levator palpebrae superioris
- 上直筋 Superior rectus
- 視神経と視神経外鞘 Optic n. (with dural sheath)
- 下直筋 Inferior rectus

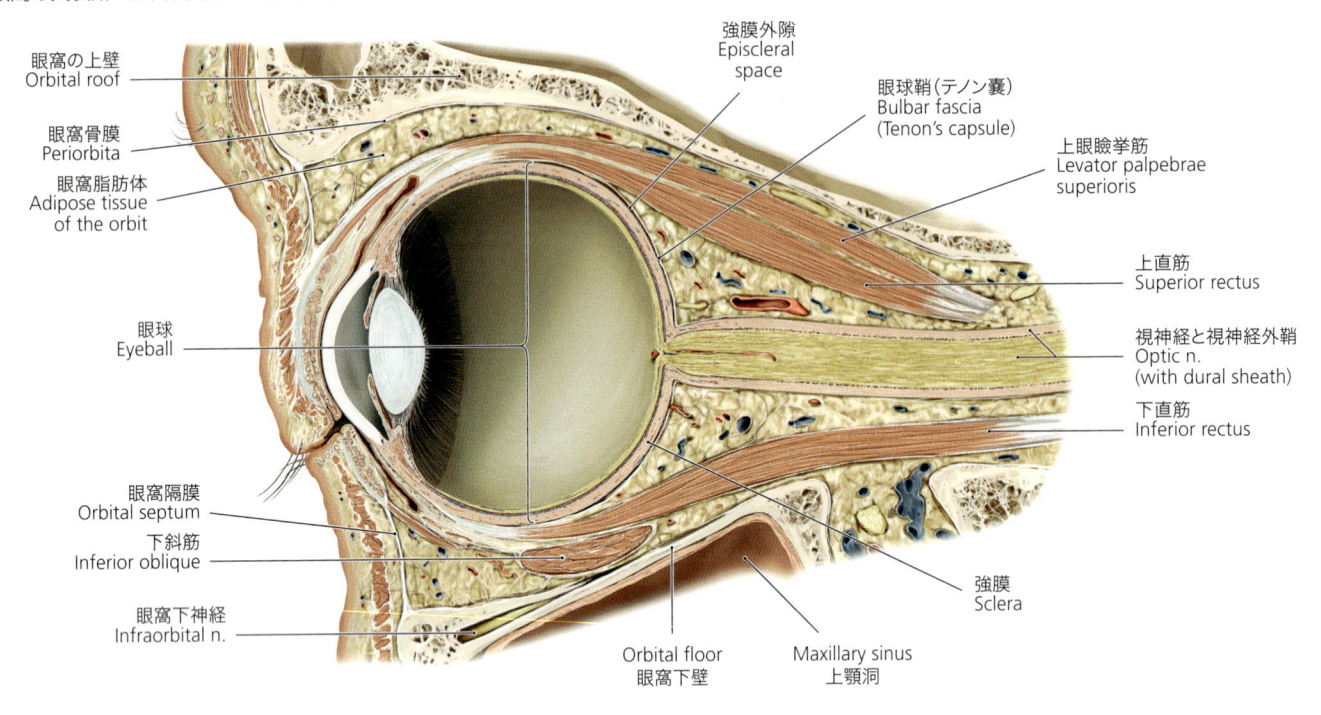

図33.13 眼瞼と結膜
眼窩前方，矢状断．

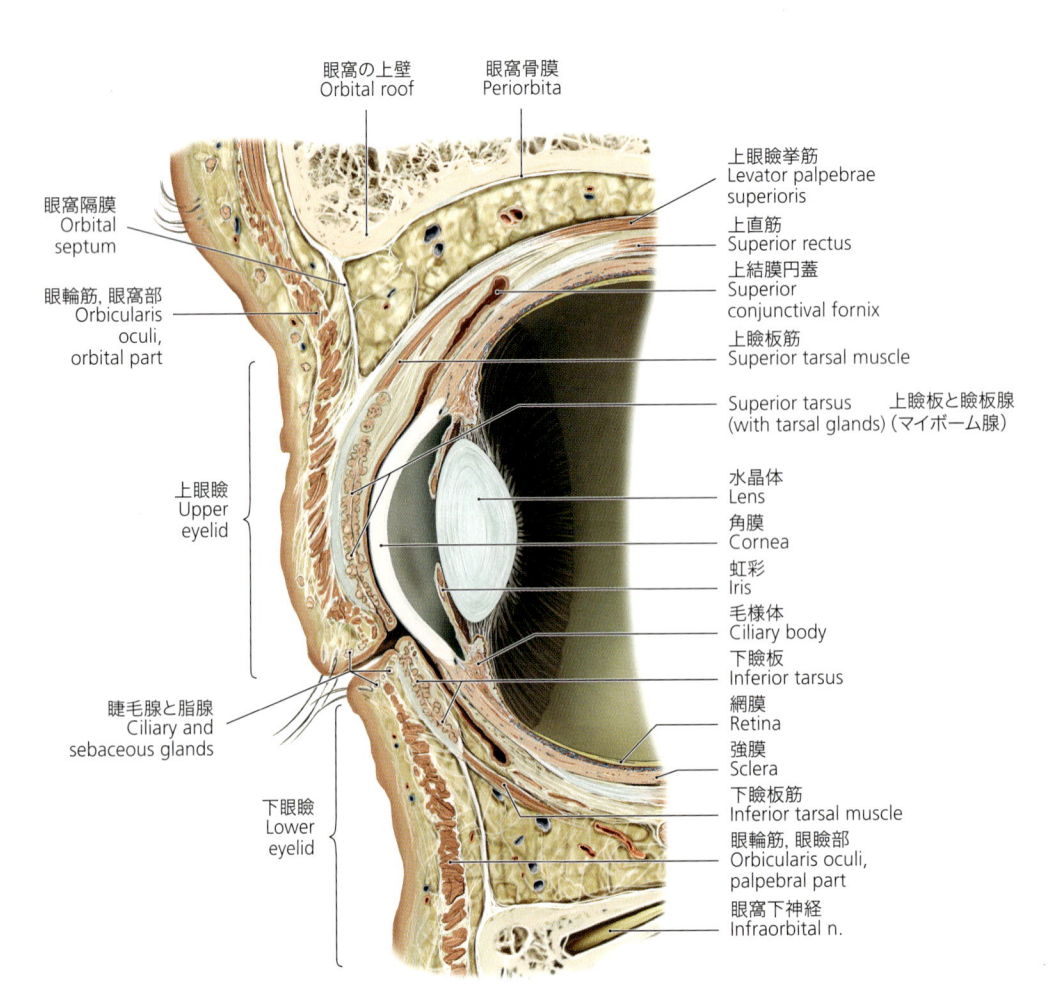

Labels:
- 眼窩の上壁 Orbital roof
- 眼窩骨膜 Periorbita
- 眼窩隔膜 Orbital septum
- 眼輪筋，眼窩部 Orbicularis oculi, orbital part
- 上眼瞼 Upper eyelid
- 睫毛腺と脂腺 Ciliary and sebaceous glands
- 下眼瞼 Lower eyelid
- 上眼瞼挙筋 Levator palpebrae superioris
- 上直筋 Superior rectus
- 上結膜円蓋 Superior conjunctival fornix
- 上瞼板筋 Superior tarsal muscle
- 上瞼板と瞼板腺（マイボーム腺） Superior tarsus (with tarsal glands)
- 水晶体 Lens
- 角膜 Cornea
- 虹彩 Iris
- 毛様体 Ciliary body
- 下瞼板 Inferior tarsus
- 網膜 Retina
- 強膜 Sclera
- 下瞼板筋 Inferior tarsal muscle
- 眼輪筋，眼瞼部 Orbicularis oculi, palpebral part
- 眼窩下神経 Infraorbital n.

図 33.14　涙器
右眼球，前方から見たところ．眼窩隔膜を一部取り除き，上眼瞼挙筋の停止腱を切開してある．

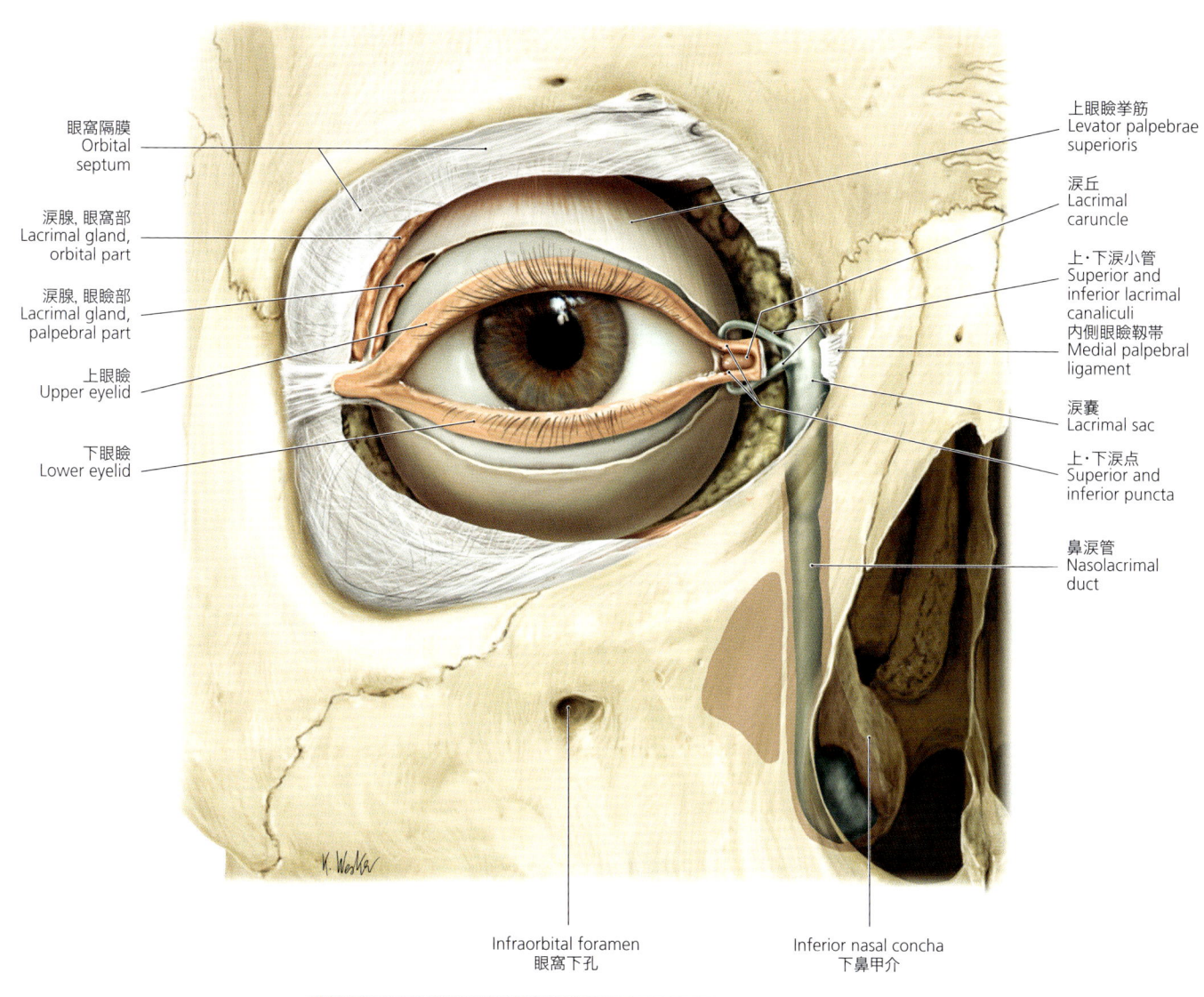

眼窩隔膜
Orbital septum

涙腺，眼窩部
Lacrimal gland, orbital part

涙腺，眼瞼部
Lacrimal gland, palpebral part

上眼瞼
Upper eyelid

下眼瞼
Lower eyelid

上眼瞼挙筋
Levator palpebrae superioris

涙丘
Lacrimal caruncle

上・下涙小管
Superior and inferior lacrimal canaliculi

内側眼瞼靱帯
Medial palpebral ligament

涙嚢
Lacrimal sac

上・下涙点
Superior and inferior puncta

鼻涙管
Nasolacrimal duct

Infraorbital foramen
眼窩下孔

Inferior nasal concha
下鼻甲介

臨床

涙液の排出

閉経後の女性は涙腺での涙液産生不足のためしばしば慢性的にドライアイ（乾性角結膜炎）になる．（細菌による）急性の涙腺炎症は一般的ではないが，激しい炎症を起こし，触診すると極めて軟らかいのが特徴である．上眼瞼は特徴的なS字カーブを描く．

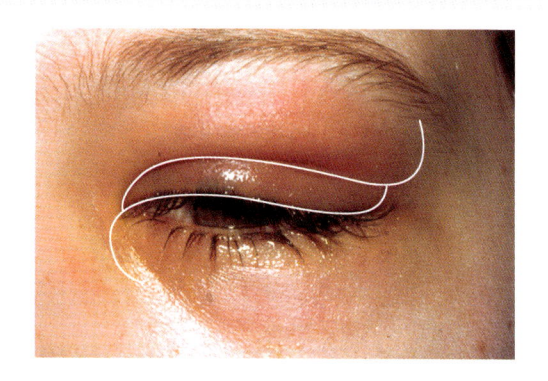

33　眼窩と眼

眼球
Eyeball

図 33.15 眼球の構造
右眼球の横断面．上方から見たところ．
Note：視神経円板を通って視神経に沿う眼窩軸は，眼球の中心から中心窩に向かう視軸から23°ずれている．

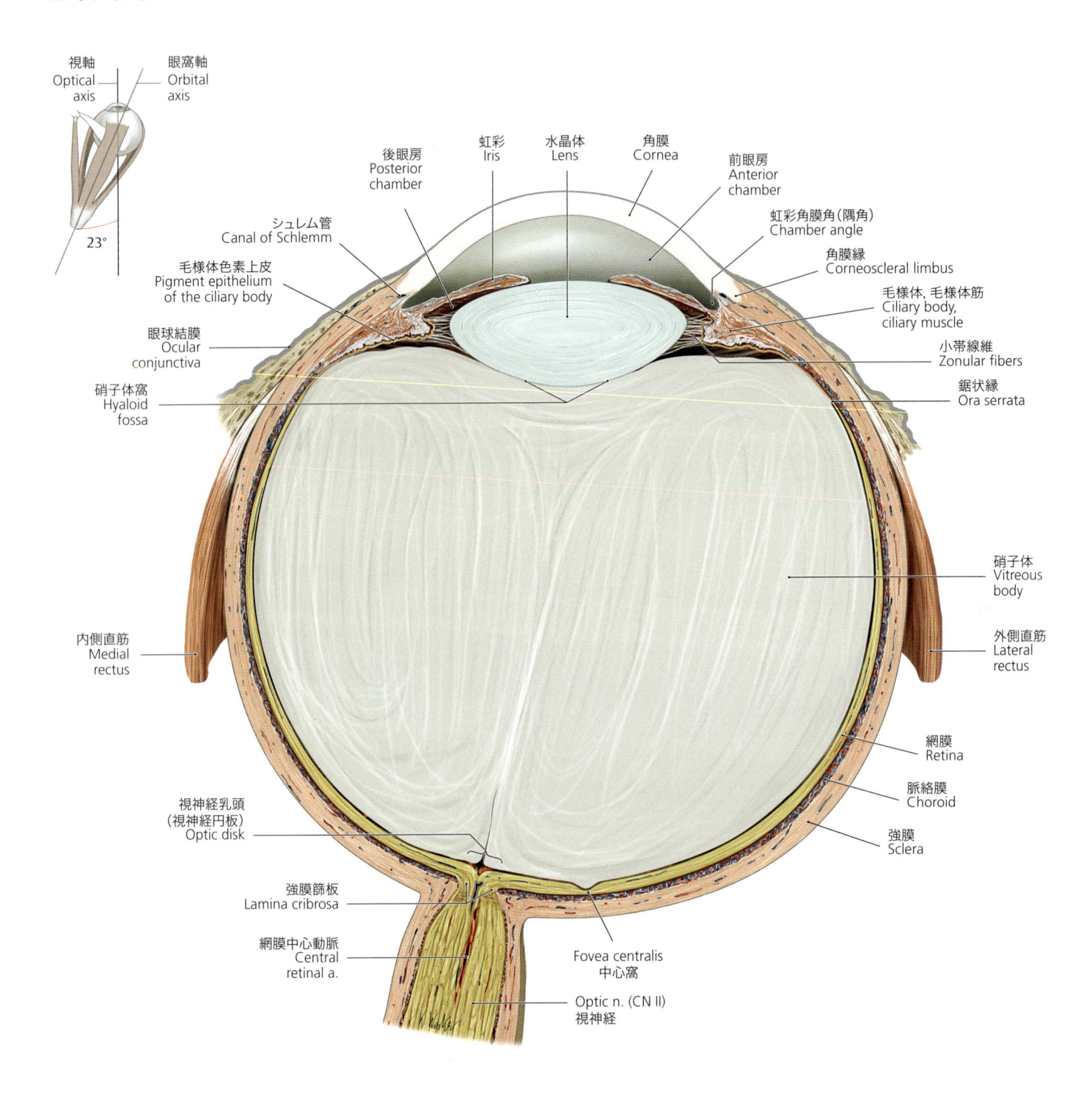

- 視軸 Optical axis
- 眼窩軸 Orbital axis
- 23°
- 後眼房 Posterior chamber
- 虹彩 Iris
- 水晶体 Lens
- 角膜 Cornea
- 前眼房 Anterior chamber
- シュレム管 Canal of Schlemm
- 虹彩角膜角（隅角）Chamber angle
- 毛様体色素上皮 Pigment epithelium of the ciliary body
- 角膜縁 Corneoscleral limbus
- 毛様体，毛様体筋 Ciliary body, ciliary muscle
- 眼球結膜 Ocular conjunctiva
- 小帯線維 Zonular fibers
- 硝子体窩 Hyaloid fossa
- 鋸状縁 Ora serrata
- 硝子体 Vitreous body
- 内側直筋 Medial rectus
- 外側直筋 Lateral rectus
- 網膜 Retina
- 脈絡膜 Choroid
- 視神経乳頭（視神経円板）Optic disk
- 強膜 Sclera
- 強膜篩板 Lamina cribrosa
- 網膜中心動脈 Central retinal a.
- Fovea centralis 中心窩
- Optic n. (CN II) 視神経

図33.16 眼球の血管

視神経を通る高さでの横断面．上方から見たところ．眼球の動脈は眼動脈から起こり，眼動脈は内頸動脈の終枝の1つである．血液は4～8本の渦静脈を介して上・下眼静脈に注ぐ．

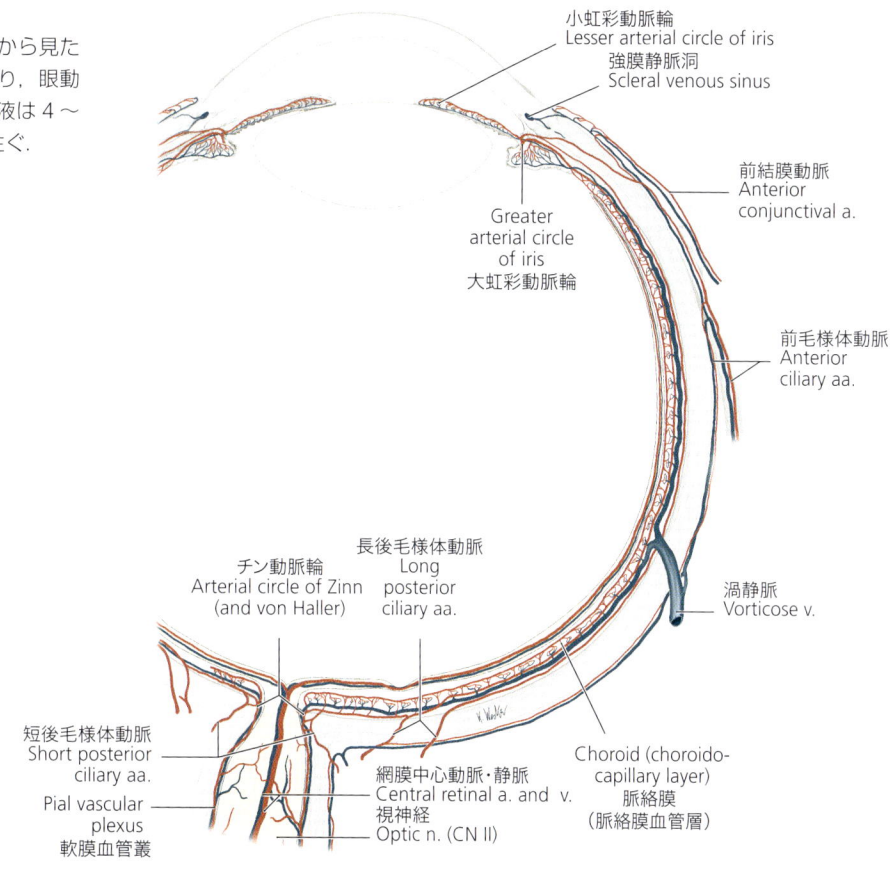

- 小虹彩動脈輪 Lesser arterial circle of iris
- 強膜静脈洞 Scleral venous sinus
- 前結膜動脈 Anterior conjunctival a.
- 大虹彩動脈輪 Greater arterial circle of iris
- 前毛様体動脈 Anterior ciliary aa.
- チン動脈輪 Arterial circle of Zinn (and von Haller)
- 長後毛様体動脈 Long posterior ciliary aa.
- 渦静脈 Vorticose v.
- 短後毛様体動脈 Short posterior ciliary aa.
- 網膜中心動脈・静脈 Central retinal a. and v.
- 視神経 Optic n. (CN II)
- 脈絡膜（脈絡膜血管層）Choroid (choroido-capillary layer)
- 軟膜血管叢 Pial vascular plexus

臨床

眼底

眼底は毛細血管を直接検査できる人体唯一の場所である．眼底の検査により高血圧や糖尿病によって生じる血管の変化を観察できる．視神経乳頭（視神経円板）の検査は，頭蓋内圧を測定して多発性硬化症を診断する際に重要である．

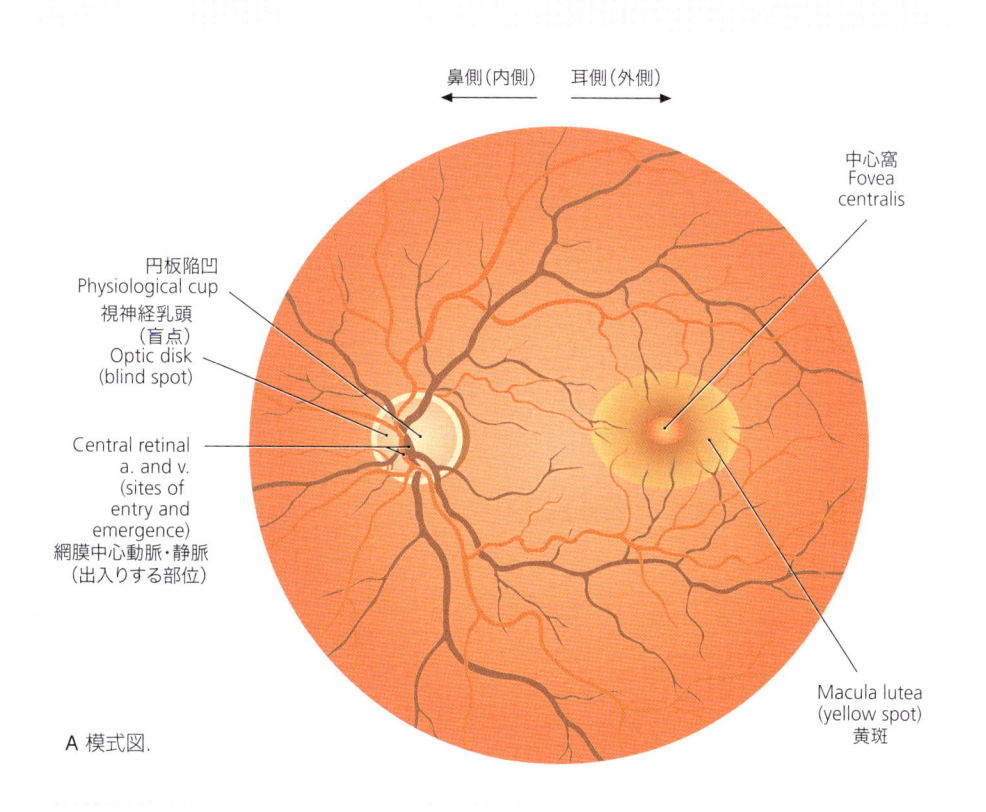

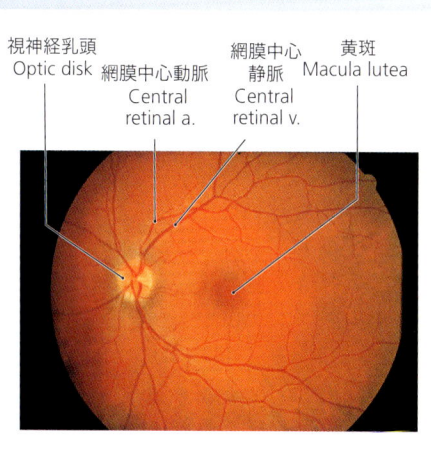

鼻側（内側）← →耳側（外側）

- 円板陥凹 Physiological cup
- 視神経乳頭（盲点）Optic disk (blind spot)
- Central retinal a. and v. (sites of entry and emergence) 網膜中心動脈・静脈（出入りする部位）
- 中心窩 Fovea centralis
- Macula lutea (yellow spot) 黄斑

A 模式図．

- 視神経乳頭 Optic disk
- 網膜中心動脈 Central retinal a.
- 網膜中心静脈 Central retinal v.
- 黄斑 Macula lutea

B 検眼鏡による正常な眼底．

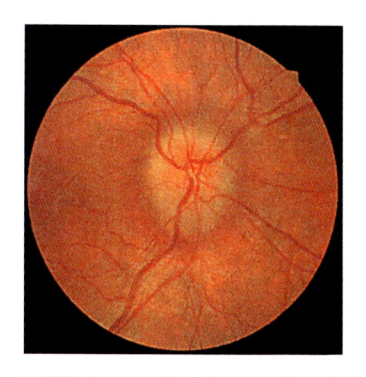

C 頭蓋内圧の亢進；視神経円板の辺縁が不鮮明になる．

角膜，虹彩，水晶体
Cornea, Iris & Lens

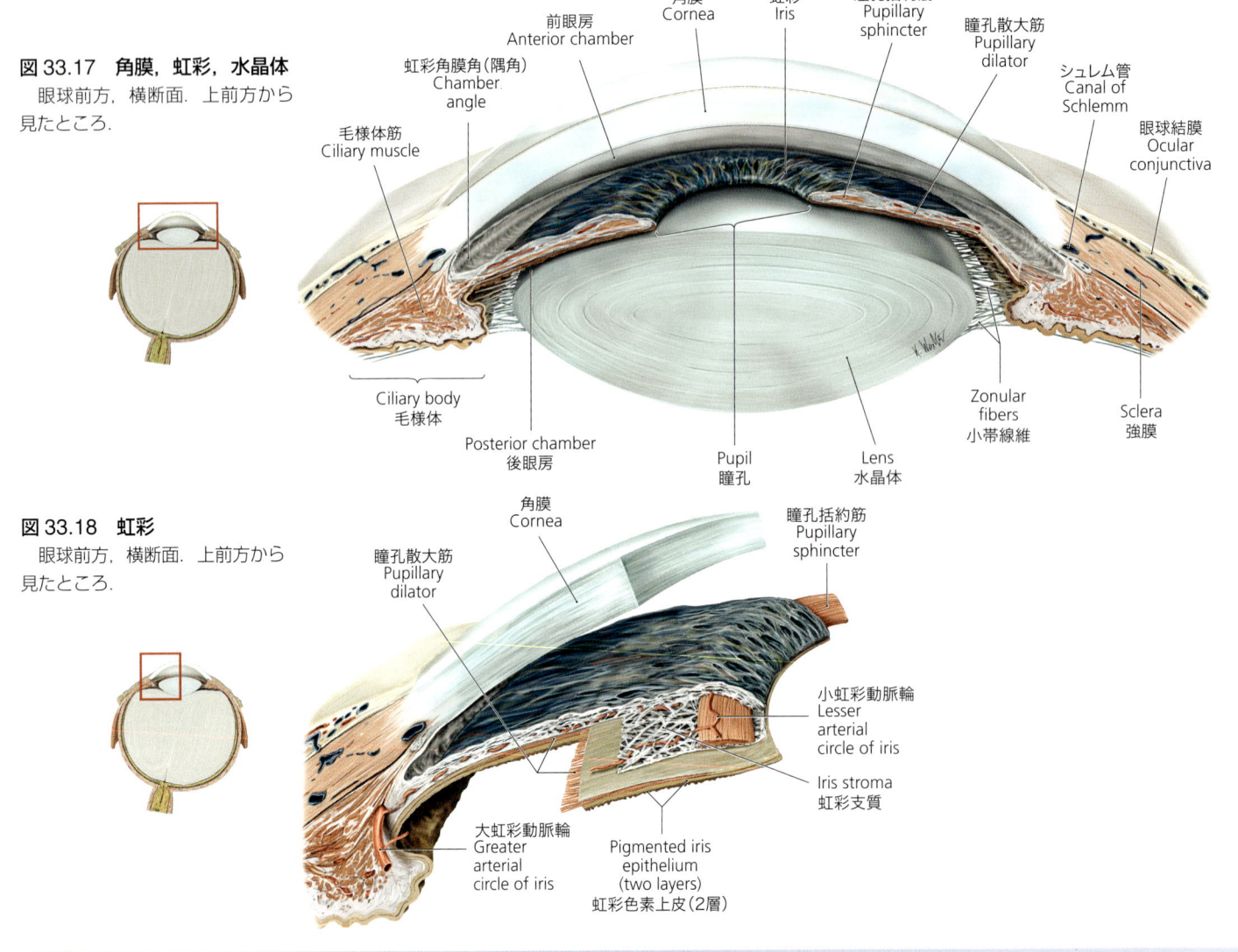

図 33.17 角膜，虹彩，水晶体
眼球前方，横断面．上前方から見たところ．

図 33.18 虹彩
眼球前方，横断面．上前方から見たところ．

臨床

緑内障

後眼房で産生される眼房水は瞳孔を経由して前眼房に入る．眼房水は小柱網の間隙からシュレム管に入り，強膜静脈洞に入って強膜上静脈に至る．眼房水排出路の閉塞によって眼内圧亢進（緑内障）が起こり，篩板で視神経が締め付けられる．この圧迫によって失明することもある．最も一般的な緑内障（症例のほぼ90％）は慢性緑内障（開放隅角緑内障）である．急性緑内障はまれであるが，充血，激しい頭痛，眼痛，悪心，強膜上静脈拡張，角膜浮腫が特徴である．

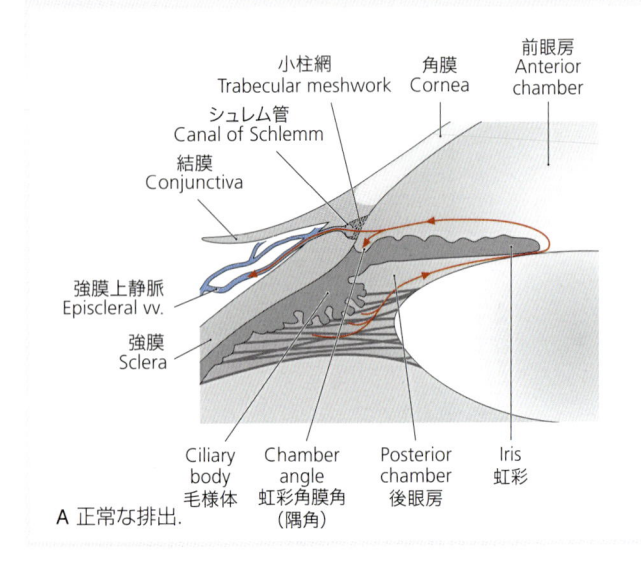

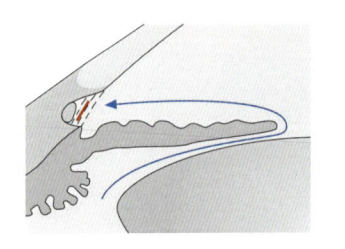

A 正常な排出．

B 慢性緑内障（開放隅角緑内障）．小柱網からの排出が障害される．

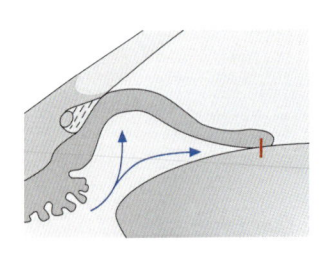

C 急性緑内障（閉塞隅角緑内障）．隅角が虹彩組織によって閉塞される．眼房水は前眼房に流出できず，虹彩の一部が持ち上げられて隅角を閉塞する．

図 33.19　瞳孔
　瞳孔の大きさは，虹彩の2つの内眼筋すなわち瞳孔を収縮させる瞳孔括約筋（副交感神経支配）と瞳孔を拡張させる瞳孔散大筋（交感神経支配）によって調節されている．

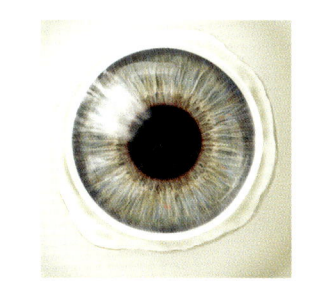

A　正常の大きさ．

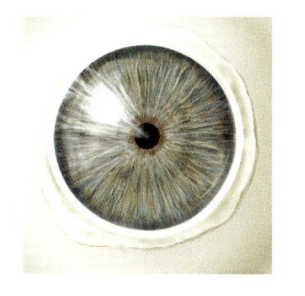

B　極度の縮小（縮瞳）．

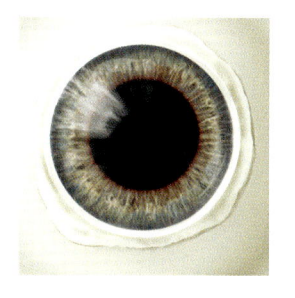

C　極度の拡大（散瞳）．

図 33.20　水晶体と毛様体
　後方から見たところ．水晶体の曲率は輪状の毛様体筋線維によって調節される．

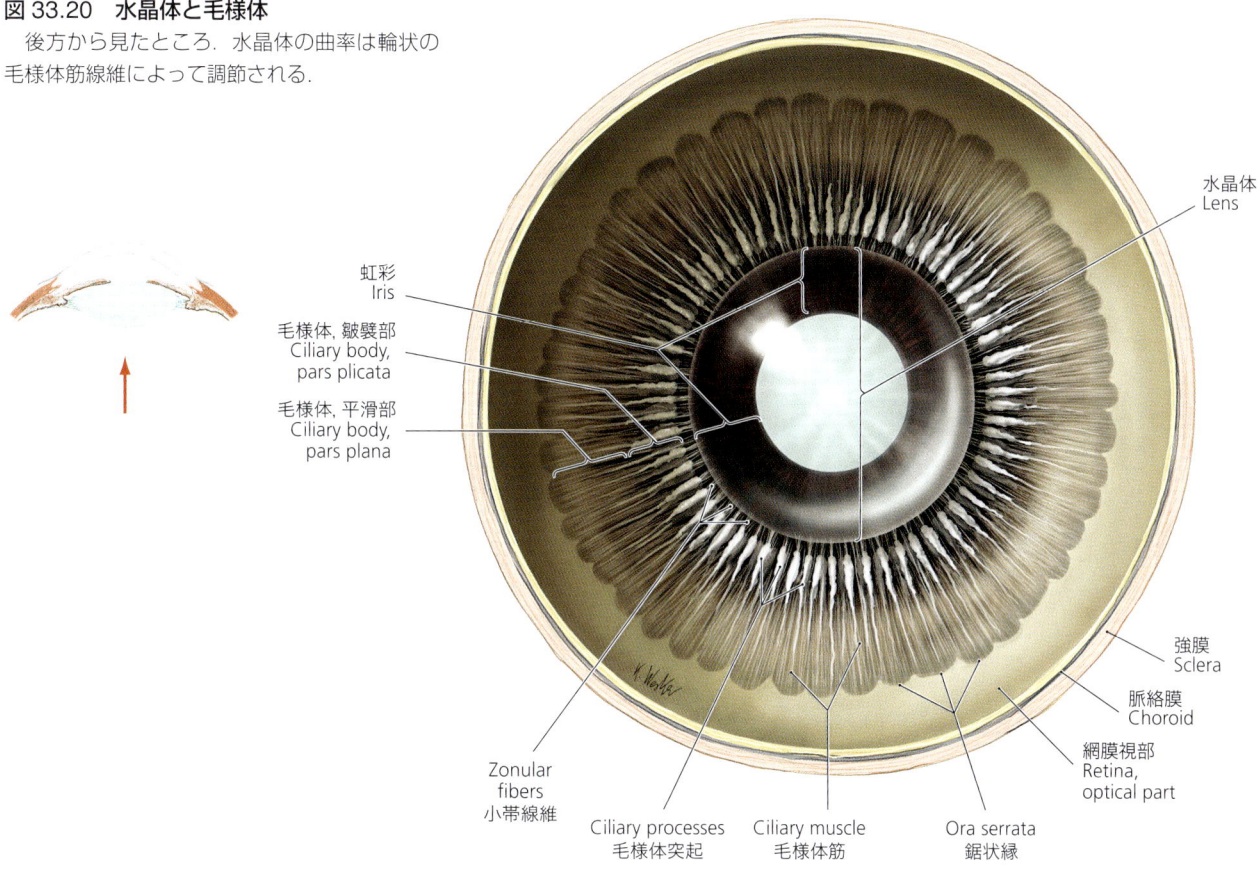

水晶体 Lens
虹彩 Iris
毛様体，皺襞部 Ciliary body, pars plicata
毛様体，平滑部 Ciliary body, pars plana
強膜 Sclera
脈絡膜 Choroid
網膜視部 Retina, optical part
Zonular fibers 小帯線維
Ciliary processes 毛様体突起
Ciliary muscle 毛様体筋
Ora serrata 鋸状縁

図 33.21　水晶体の光屈折
　横断面．上方から見たところ．正常において光線は水晶体と角膜で屈折して網膜表面の焦点（中心窩）に向かう．遠くを見るときは，平行な光線が遠方の光源から入射し，小帯線維が緊張して毛様体筋が弛緩することで，水晶体が平らになる．近くを見るときは，毛様体筋が収縮して小帯線維が弛緩し，水晶体が円形になる．

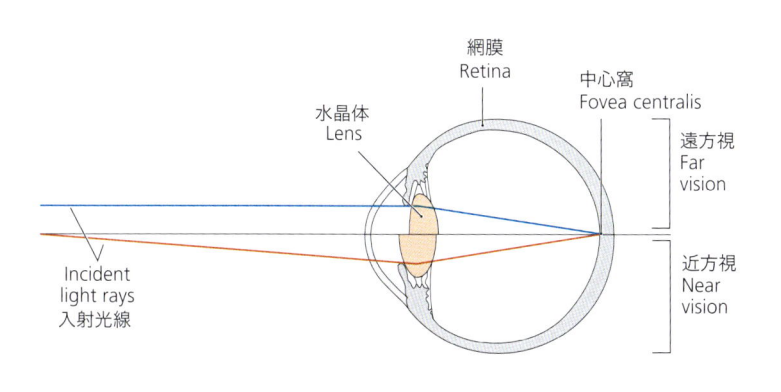

網膜 Retina
水晶体 Lens
中心窩 Fovea centralis
遠方視 Far vision
近方視 Near vision
Incident light rays 入射光線

A　正常な水晶体調節．

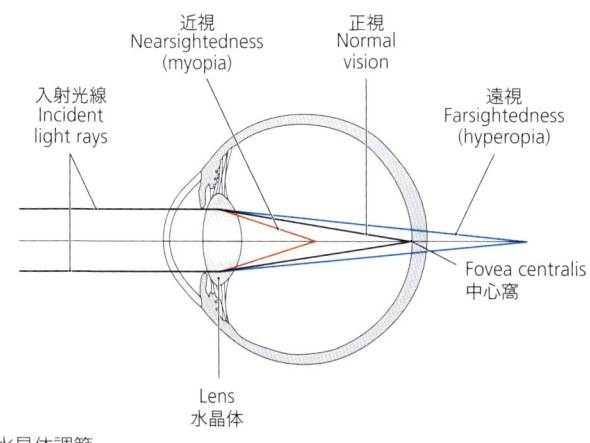

近視 Nearsightedness (myopia)
正視 Normal vision
遠視 Farsightedness (hyperopia)
入射光線 Incident light rays
Fovea centralis 中心窩
Lens 水晶体

B　異常な水晶体調節．

鼻腔の骨
Bones of the Nasal Cavity

図 34.1　鼻の骨格

鼻の骨格は上部は骨，下部は軟骨からなる．外鼻孔（鼻翼）の近位部は結合組織からなり，小片の軟骨が埋もれている．

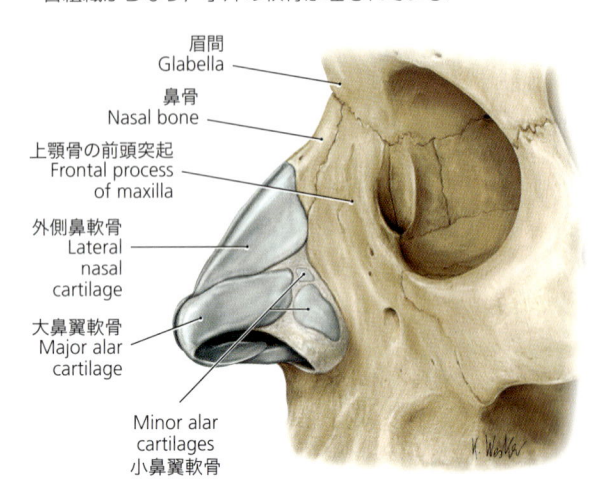

眉間 Glabella
鼻骨 Nasal bone
上顎骨の前頭突起 Frontal process of maxilla
外側鼻軟骨 Lateral nasal cartilage
大鼻翼軟骨 Major alar cartilage
Minor alar cartilages 小鼻翼軟骨

大鼻翼軟骨 Major alar cartilage
外側脚 Lateral crus
内側脚 Medial crus
外鼻孔 Naris
鼻中隔軟骨 Septal cartilage
前鼻棘 Anterior nasal spine
鼻翼 Nasal ala

A 左外側方から見たところ．

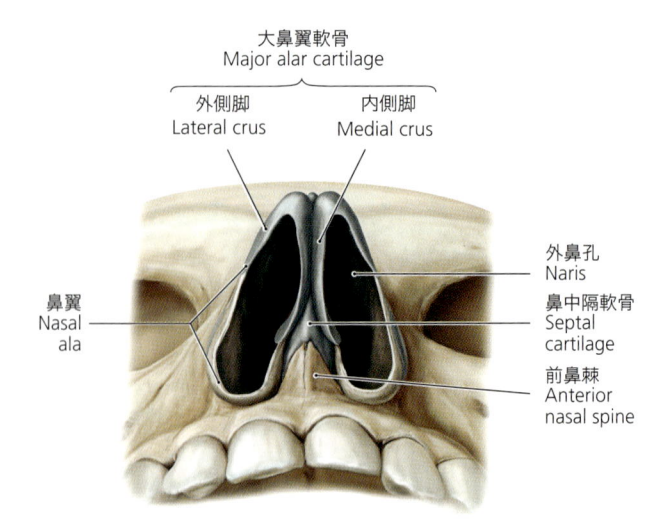

B 下方から見たところ．

図 34.2　鼻腔の骨

左右の鼻腔は外側壁に囲まれ，鼻中隔で隔てられている．空気は梨状口から鼻腔に入り，上鼻道，中鼻道，下鼻道の3つの鼻道（矢印で示す）を通る．3つの鼻道は上鼻甲介，中鼻甲介，下鼻甲介で隔てられる．空気は後鼻孔を経て咽頭鼻部に入る．

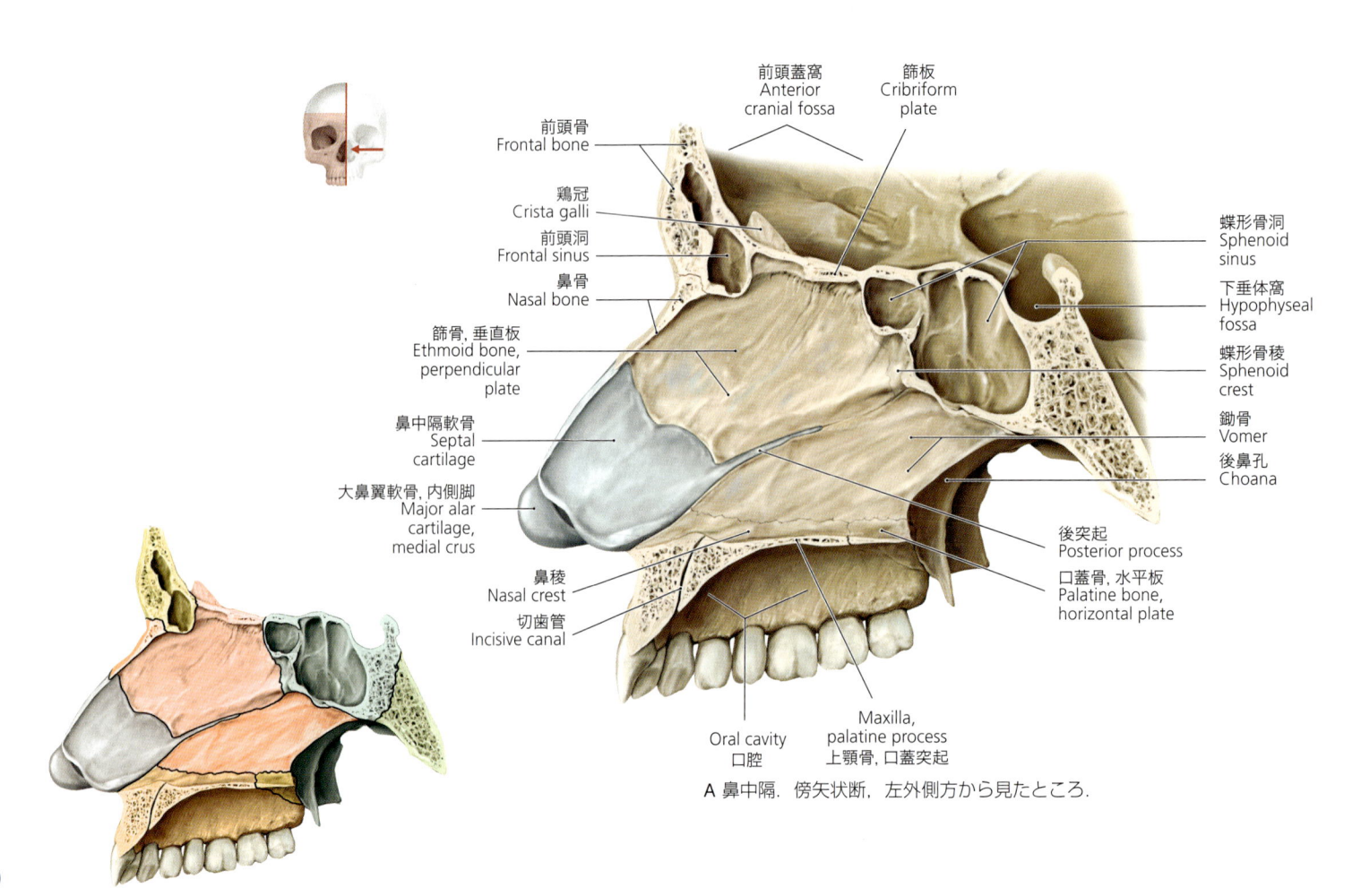

前頭蓋窩 Anterior cranial fossa
篩板 Cribriform plate
前頭骨 Frontal bone
鶏冠 Crista galli
前頭洞 Frontal sinus
鼻骨 Nasal bone
篩骨，垂直板 Ethmoid bone, perpendicular plate
鼻中隔軟骨 Septal cartilage
大鼻翼軟骨，内側脚 Major alar cartilage, medial crus
鼻稜 Nasal crest
切歯管 Incisive canal
蝶形骨洞 Sphenoid sinus
下垂体窩 Hypophyseal fossa
蝶形骨稜 Sphenoid crest
鋤骨 Vomer
後鼻孔 Choana
後突起 Posterior process
口蓋骨，水平板 Palatine bone, horizontal plate
Oral cavity 口腔
Maxilla, palatine process 上顎骨，口蓋突起

A 鼻中隔．傍矢状断，左外側方から見たところ．

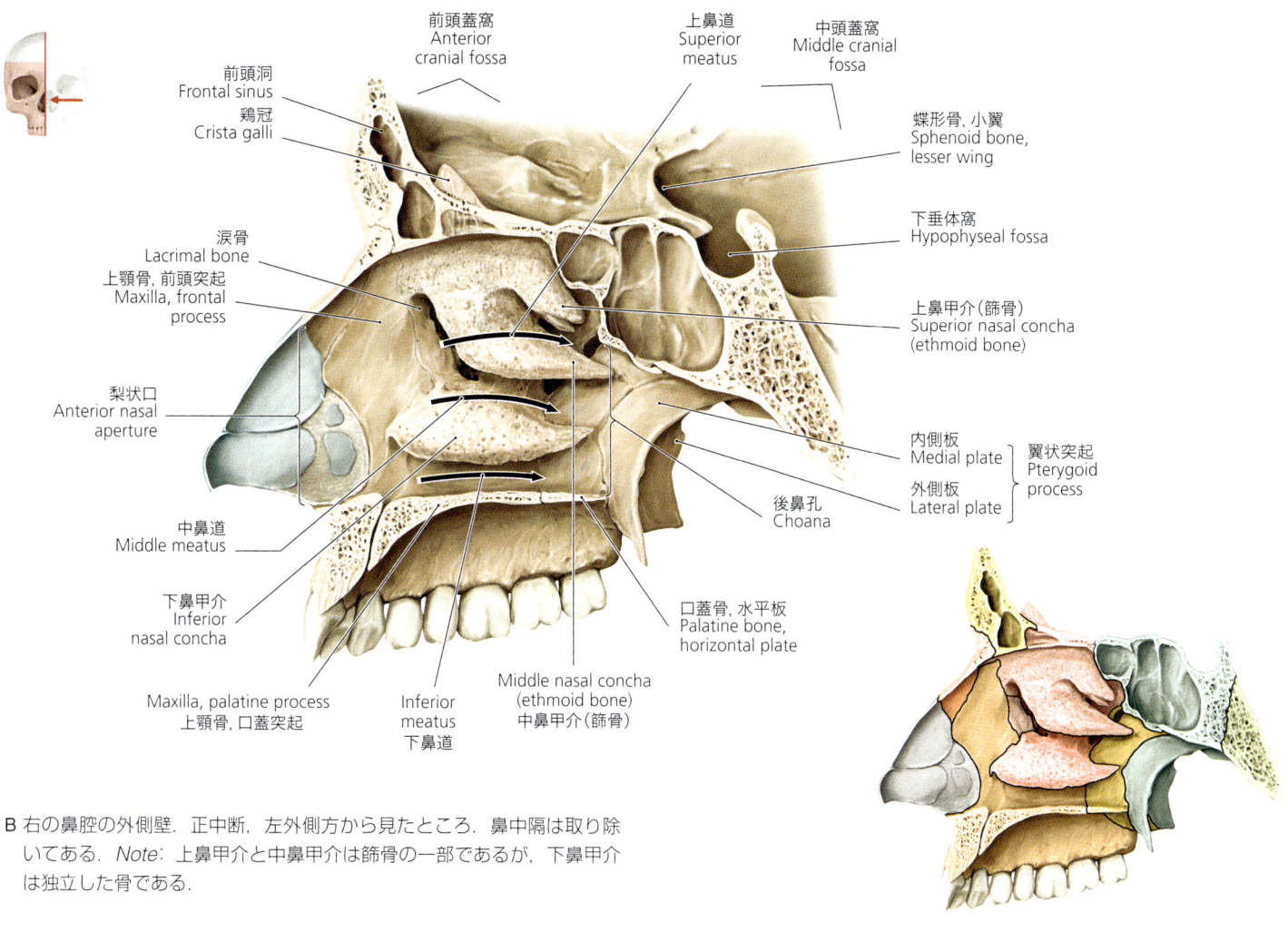

34 鼻腔と鼻

B 右の鼻腔の外側壁．正中断，左外側方から見たところ．鼻中隔は取り除いてある．Note：上鼻甲介と中鼻甲介は篩骨の一部であるが，下鼻甲介は独立した骨である．

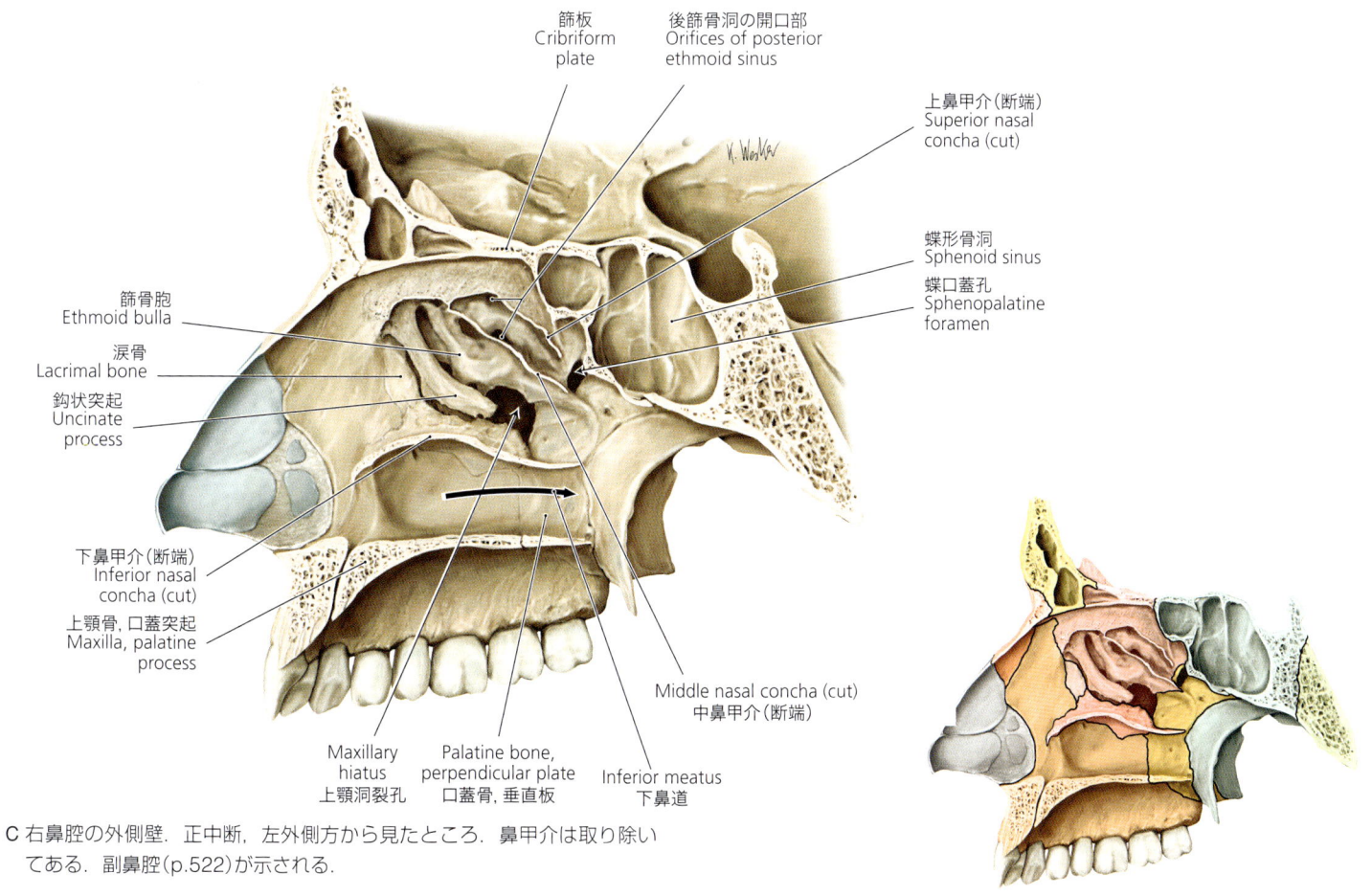

Labels (figure B):
- 前頭洞 Frontal sinus
- 鶏冠 Crista galli
- 前頭蓋窩 Anterior cranial fossa
- 上鼻道 Superior meatus
- 中頭蓋窩 Middle cranial fossa
- 蝶形骨, 小翼 Sphenoid bone, lesser wing
- 下垂体窩 Hypophyseal fossa
- 涙骨 Lacrimal bone
- 上顎骨, 前頭突起 Maxilla, frontal process
- 上鼻甲介（篩骨）Superior nasal concha (ethmoid bone)
- 梨状口 Anterior nasal aperture
- 内側板 Medial plate ／ 外側板 Lateral plate ｝翼状突起 Pterygoid process
- 中鼻道 Middle meatus
- 後鼻孔 Choana
- 下鼻甲介 Inferior nasal concha
- 口蓋骨, 水平板 Palatine bone, horizontal plate
- 上顎骨, 口蓋突起 Maxilla, palatine process
- 下鼻道 Inferior meatus
- 中鼻甲介（篩骨）Middle nasal concha (ethmoid bone)

C 右鼻腔の外側壁．正中断，左外側方から見たところ．鼻甲介は取り除いてある．副鼻腔（p.522）が示される．

Labels (figure C):
- 篩板 Cribriform plate
- 後篩骨洞の開口部 Orifices of posterior ethmoid sinus
- 上鼻甲介（断端）Superior nasal concha (cut)
- 蝶形骨洞 Sphenoid sinus
- 蝶口蓋孔 Sphenopalatine foramen
- 篩骨胞 Ethmoid bulla
- 涙骨 Lacrimal bone
- 鉤状突起 Uncinate process
- 下鼻甲介（断端）Inferior nasal concha (cut)
- 上顎骨, 口蓋突起 Maxilla, palatine process
- 上顎洞裂孔 Maxillary hiatus
- 口蓋骨, 垂直板 Palatine bone, perpendicular plate
- 中鼻甲介（断端）Middle nasal concha (cut)
- 下鼻道 Inferior meatus

副鼻腔
Paranasal Air Sinuses

図 34.3 副鼻腔の位置
前頭洞，篩骨洞，上顎洞，蝶形骨洞からなる副鼻腔は，空気で満たされた空洞で，頭蓋の重さを軽くする．

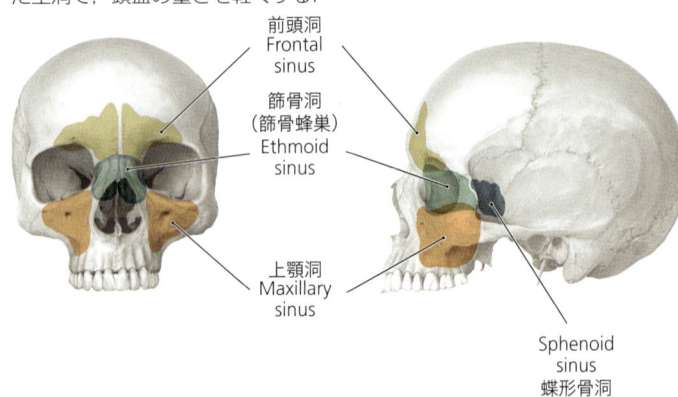

前頭洞 Frontal sinus
篩骨洞（篩骨蜂巣）Ethmoid sinus
上顎洞 Maxillary sinus
Sphenoid sinus 蝶形骨洞

A 前方から見たところ．　　B 左外側方から見たところ．

20歳／12歳／8歳／4歳／1歳
1歳／4歳／8歳／12歳／20歳／60歳〜

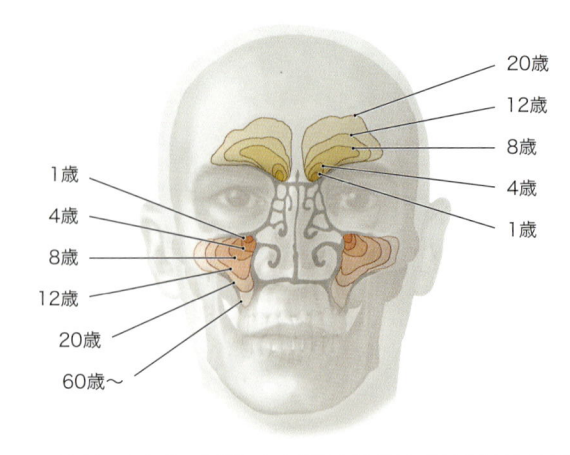

C 副鼻腔の含気化．前頭洞と上顎洞は頭蓋の成長を通じて次第に大きくなっていく．

表 34.1	鼻腔に開口する構造
鼻腔への通路	洞，管
蝶篩陥凹	蝶形骨洞（青）
上鼻道	後篩骨蜂巣（緑）
中鼻道	前篩骨蜂巣・中篩骨蜂巣（緑）
	前頭洞（黄）
	上顎洞（オレンジ）
下鼻道	鼻涙管（赤）

図 34.4 副鼻腔
副鼻腔からの粘膜分泌物の排液路と鼻涙管は鼻腔に開口する．

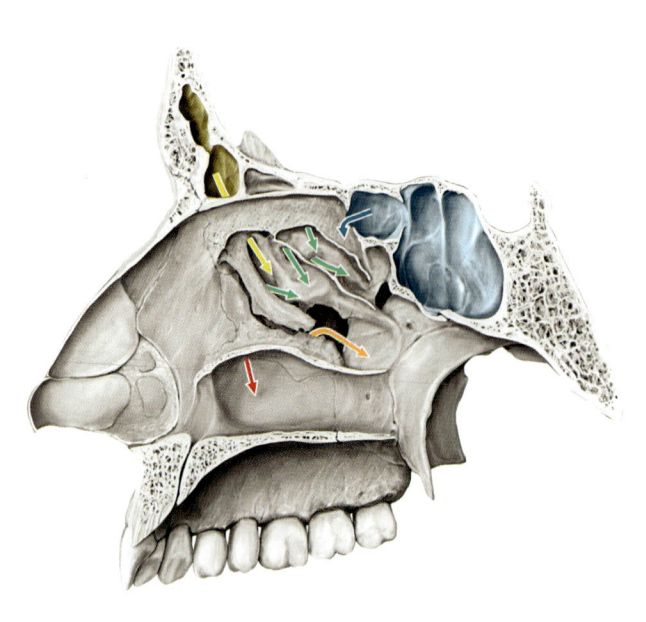

A 副鼻腔と鼻涙管の開口部．矢状断，右鼻腔を左外側方から見たところ．

上鼻甲介 Superior nasal concha
前頭洞 Frontal sinus
鼻腔 Nasal cavity
中鼻甲介 Middle nasal concha
鼻中隔 Nasal septum
下鼻甲介 Inferior nasal concha
眼窩 Orbit
篩骨洞（篩骨蜂巣）Ethmoid sinus
上顎洞 Maxillary sinus

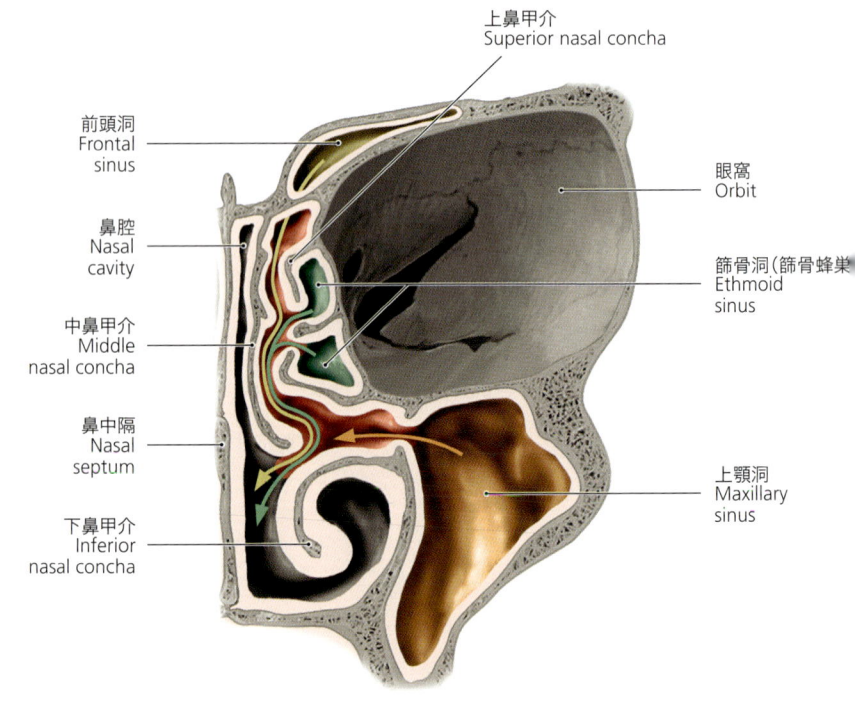

B 左側の鼻腔の副鼻腔と洞口鼻道系（osteomeatal unit）．冠状断，前方から見たところ．

図 34.5　副鼻腔の骨性構造
冠状断，前方から見たところ．

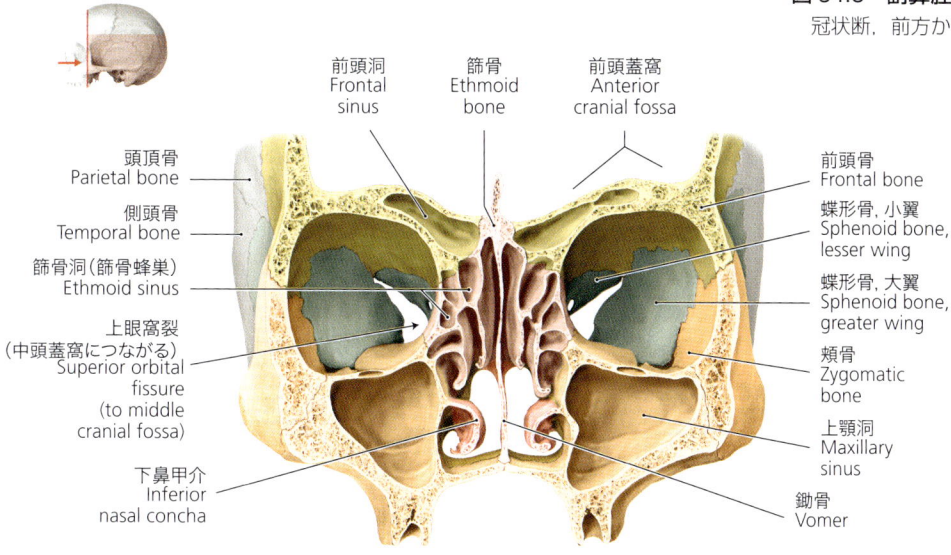

A 副鼻腔の骨．

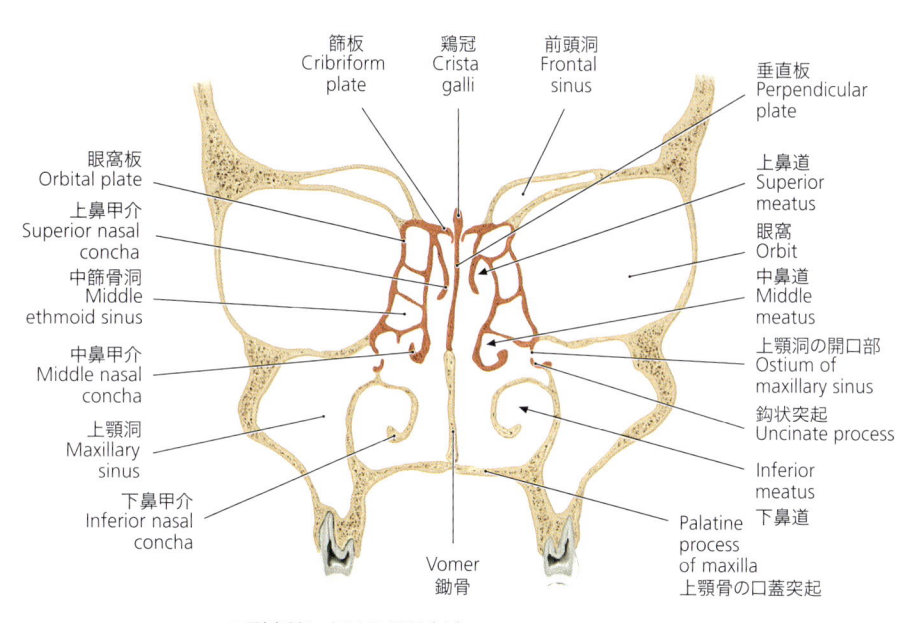

ラベル（左上から時計回り）：
- 頭頂骨 Parietal bone
- 側頭骨 Temporal bone
- 篩骨洞（篩骨蜂巣）Ethmoid sinus
- 上眼窩裂（中頭蓋窩につながる）Superior orbital fissure (to middle cranial fossa)
- 下鼻甲介 Inferior nasal concha
- 前頭洞 Frontal sinus
- 篩骨 Ethmoid bone
- 前頭蓋窩 Anterior cranial fossa
- 前頭骨 Frontal bone
- 蝶形骨，小翼 Sphenoid bone, lesser wing
- 蝶形骨，大翼 Sphenoid bone, greater wing
- 頬骨 Zygomatic bone
- 上顎洞 Maxillary sinus
- 鋤骨 Vomer

B 副鼻腔における篩骨（赤）．

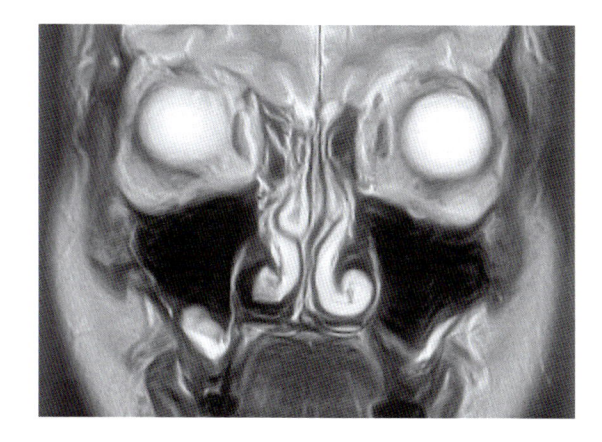

ラベル：
- 篩板 Cribriform plate
- 鶏冠 Crista galli
- 前頭洞 Frontal sinus
- 垂直板 Perpendicular plate
- 眼窩板 Orbital plate
- 上鼻甲介 Superior nasal concha
- 中篩骨洞 Middle ethmoid sinus
- 中鼻甲介 Middle nasal concha
- 上顎洞 Maxillary sinus
- 下鼻甲介 Inferior nasal concha
- 鋤骨 Vomer
- 上鼻道 Superior meatus
- 眼窩 Orbit
- 中鼻道 Middle meatus
- 上顎洞の開口部 Ostium of maxillary sinus
- 鈎状突起 Uncinate process
- 下鼻道 Inferior meatus
- 上顎骨の口蓋突起 Palatine process of maxilla

C 副鼻腔の MR 像．

臨床

鼻中隔弯曲
　正常位の鼻中隔は鼻腔をほぼ対称に隔てている．鼻中隔が極端に外側に偏位すると鼻腔が閉塞されるが，軟骨を除去すること（鼻中隔形成術）で解消される．

副鼻腔炎
　篩骨洞の粘膜が炎症によって腫脹すると，前頭洞と上顎洞から洞口鼻道系（図 34.4 参照）への分泌液の流れが阻害される．この阻害により，分泌液とともに細菌もほかの副鼻腔に移っていき，二次的炎症を起こすことがある．慢性副鼻腔炎の患者には，狭窄した部位を外科的に拡張することで有効な排膿路を確立することができる．

鼻腔の神経と血管
Neurovasculature of the Nasal Cavity

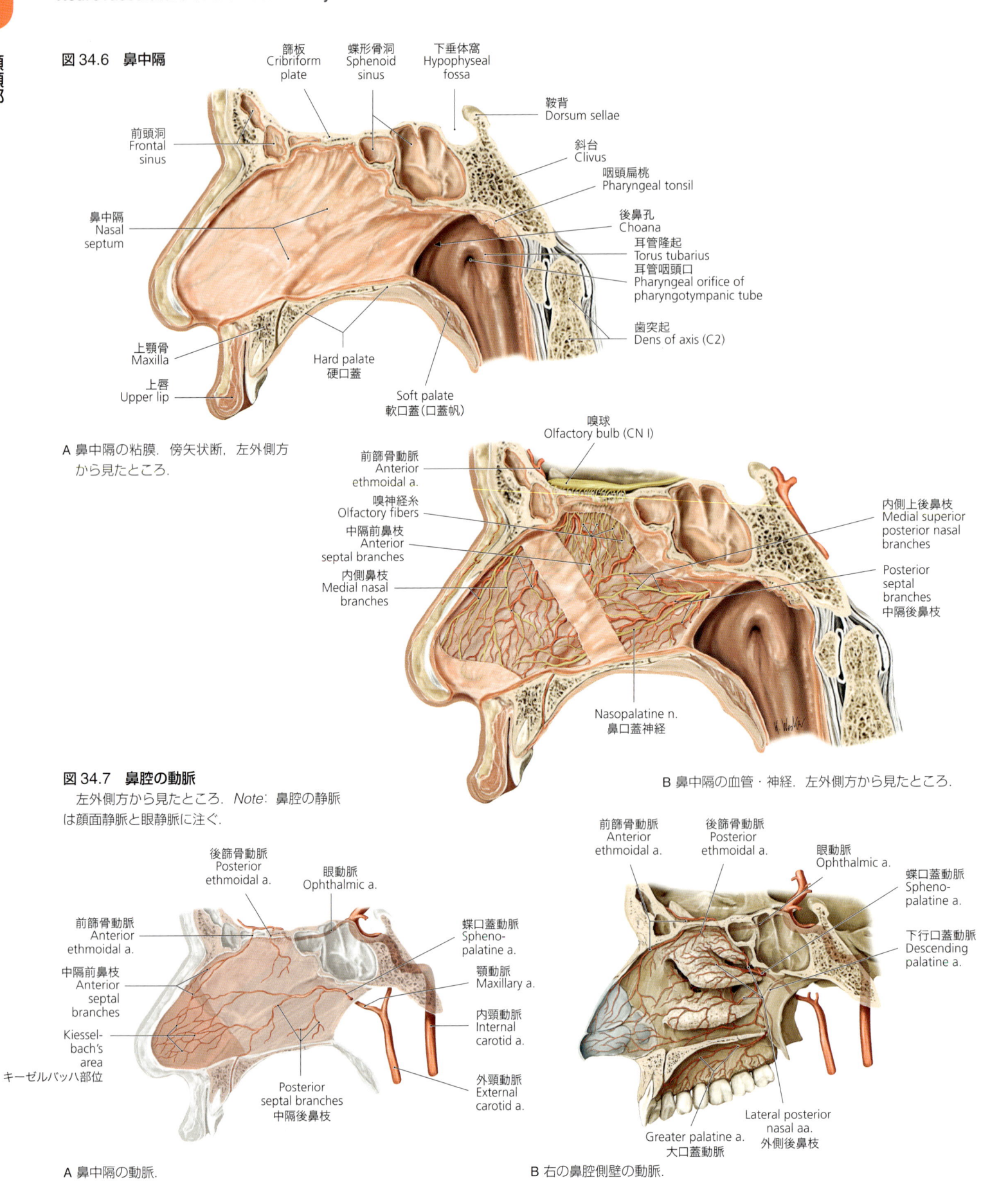

図 34.6 鼻中隔

A 鼻中隔の粘膜．傍矢状断，左外側方から見たところ．

B 鼻中隔の血管・神経．左外側方から見たところ．

図 34.7 鼻腔の動脈

左外側方から見たところ．Note：鼻腔の静脈は顔面静脈と眼静脈に注ぐ．

A 鼻中隔の動脈．

B 右の鼻腔側壁の動脈．

図 34.8 鼻腔の側壁

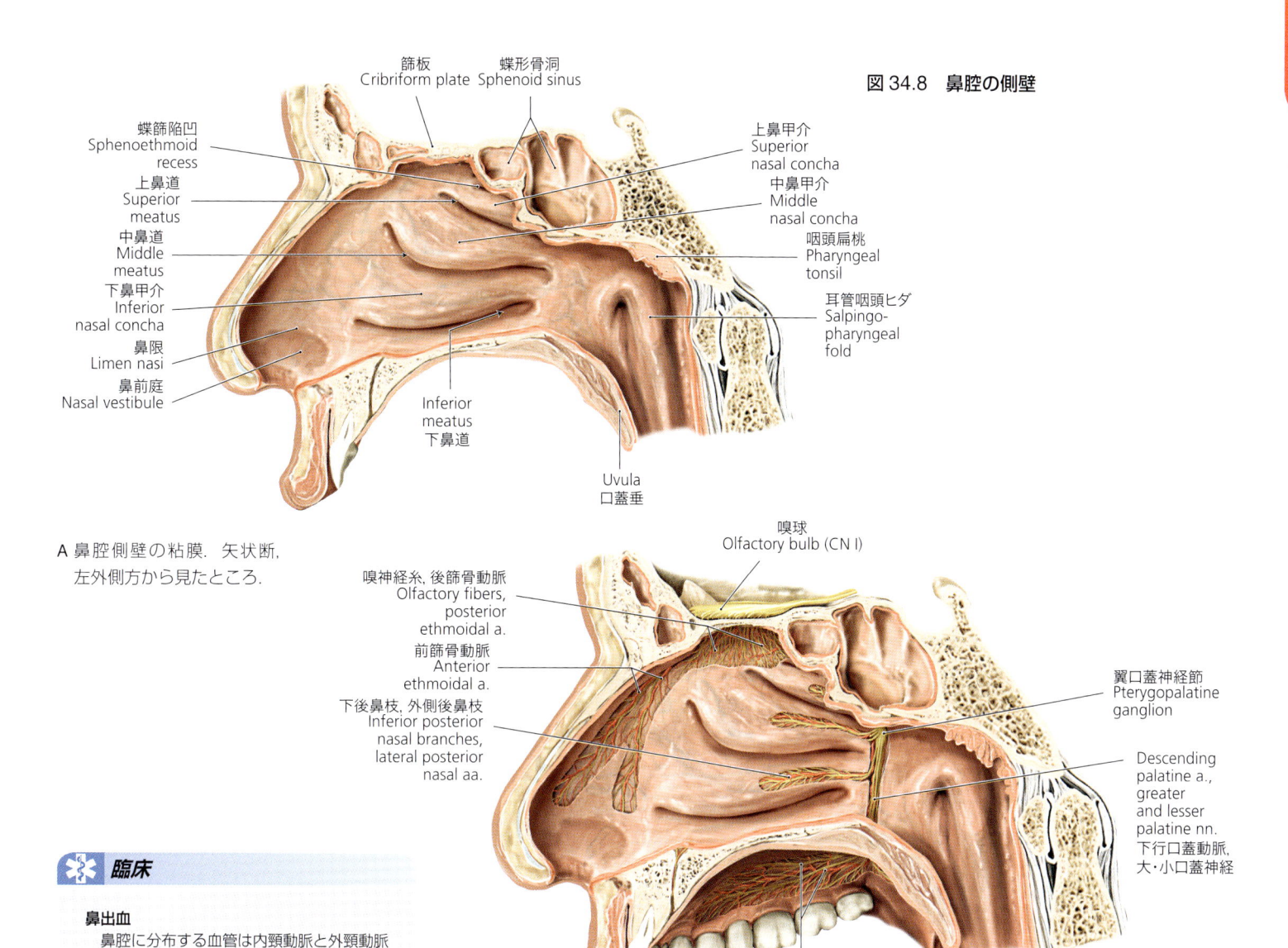

A 鼻腔側壁の粘膜．矢状断，左外側方から見たところ．

B 鼻腔側壁の神経・血管．左外側方から見たところ．

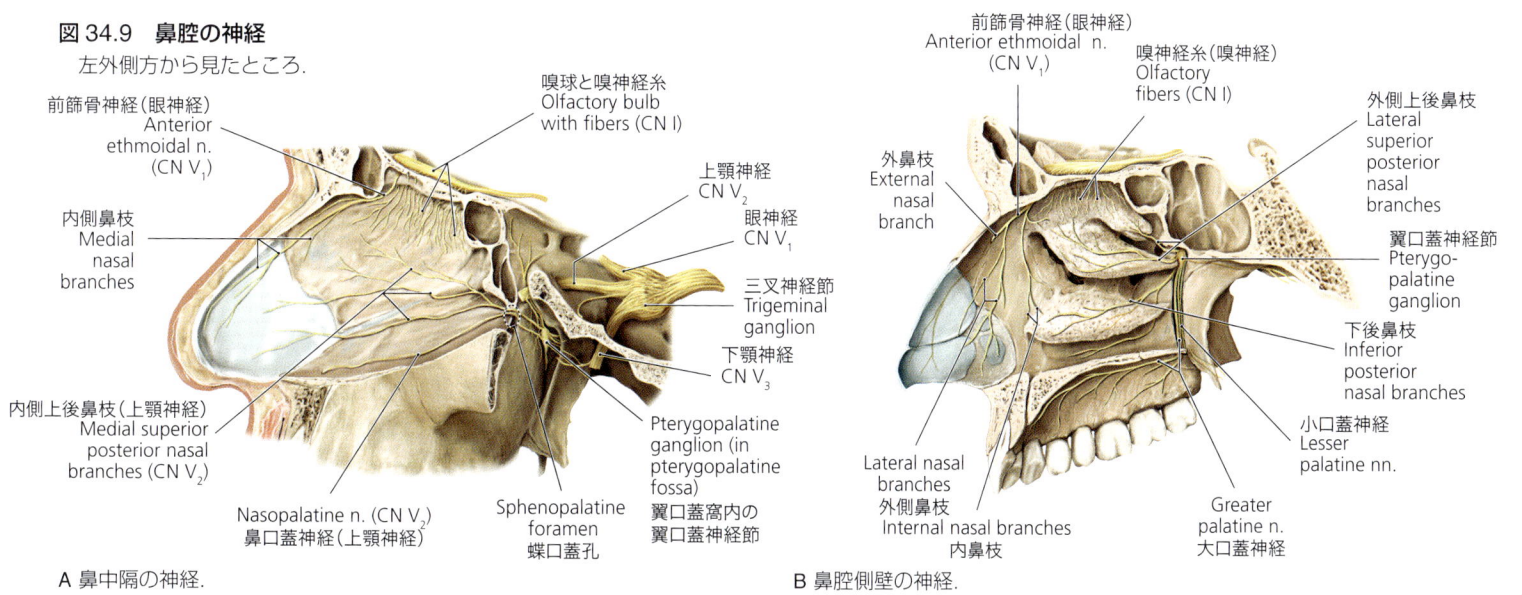

臨床

鼻出血

鼻腔に分布する血管は内頸動脈と外頸動脈の両方から起こる．鼻中隔の前部には，高密度で血管が分布する部位があり，キーゼルバッハ部位と呼ばれる．この部位は激しい鼻出血の最も起こりやすい部位である．

図 34.9 鼻腔の神経

左外側方から見たところ．

A 鼻中隔の神経．

B 鼻腔側壁の神経．

側頭骨
Temporal Bone

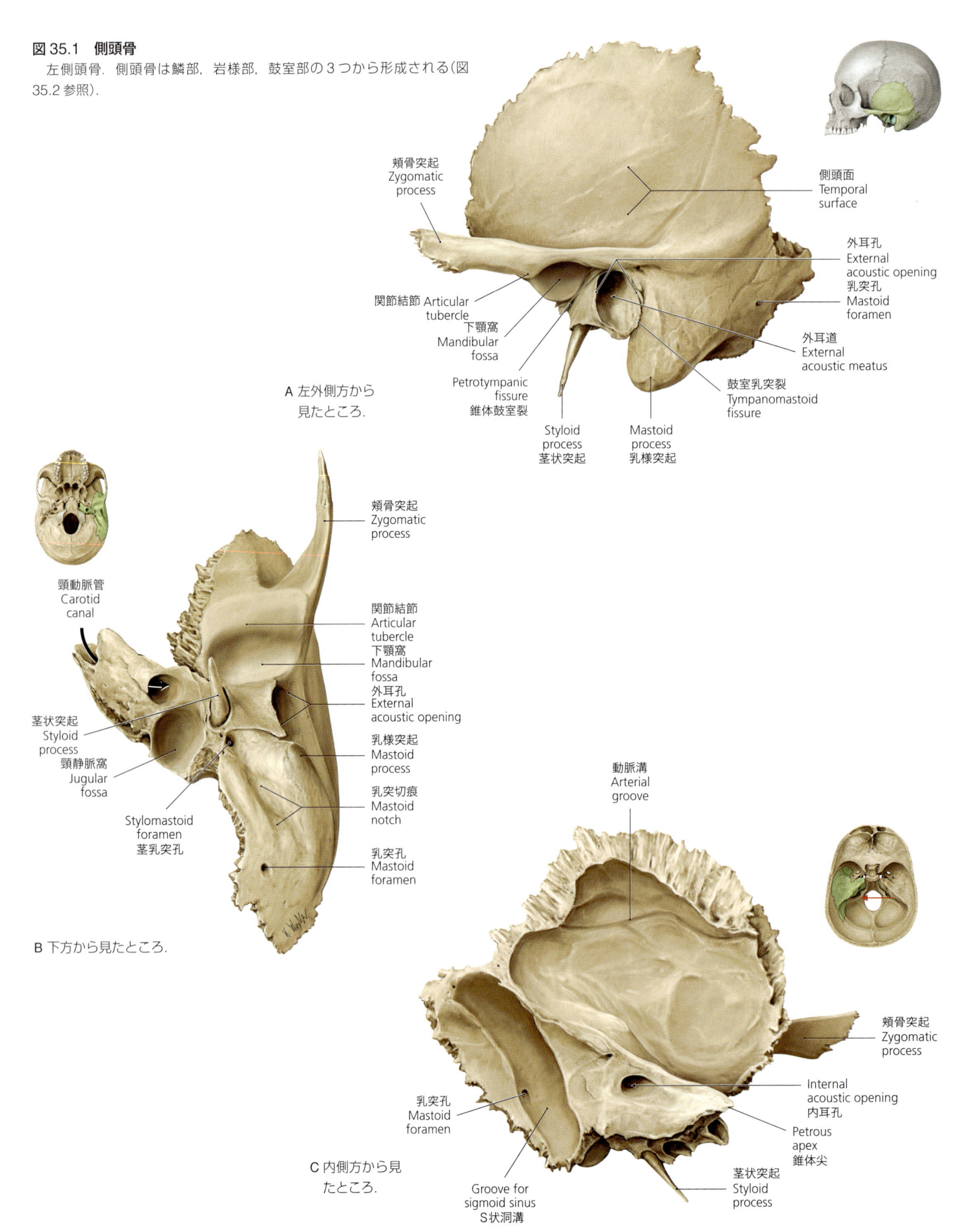

図 35.1　側頭骨
左側頭骨．側頭骨は鱗部，岩様部，鼓室部の3つから形成される（図35.2 参照）．

A 左外側方から見たところ．

- 頬骨突起 Zygomatic process
- 側頭面 Temporal surface
- 外耳孔 External acoustic opening
- 乳突孔 Mastoid foramen
- 関節結節 Articular tubercle
- 下顎窩 Mandibular fossa
- 外耳道 External acoustic meatus
- 錐体鼓室裂 Petrotympanic fissure
- 鼓室乳突裂 Tympanomastoid fissure
- 茎状突起 Styloid process
- 乳様突起 Mastoid process

B 下方から見たところ．

- 頸動脈管 Carotid canal
- 頬骨突起 Zygomatic process
- 関節結節 Articular tubercle
- 下顎窩 Mandibular fossa
- 外耳孔 External acoustic opening
- 乳様突起 Mastoid process
- 茎状突起 Styloid process
- 頸静脈窩 Jugular fossa
- 茎乳突孔 Stylomastoid foramen
- 乳突切痕 Mastoid notch
- 乳突孔 Mastoid foramen

C 内側方から見たところ．

- 動脈溝 Arterial groove
- 頬骨突起 Zygomatic process
- 内耳孔 Internal acoustic opening
- 錐体尖 Petrous apex
- 茎状突起 Styloid process
- 乳突孔 Mastoid foramen
- S状洞溝 Groove for sigmoid sinus

図 35.2 側頭骨の部分

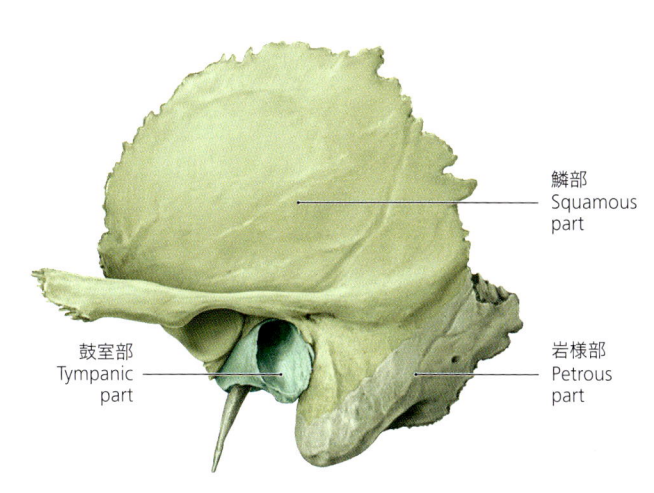

A 左外側方から見たところ．

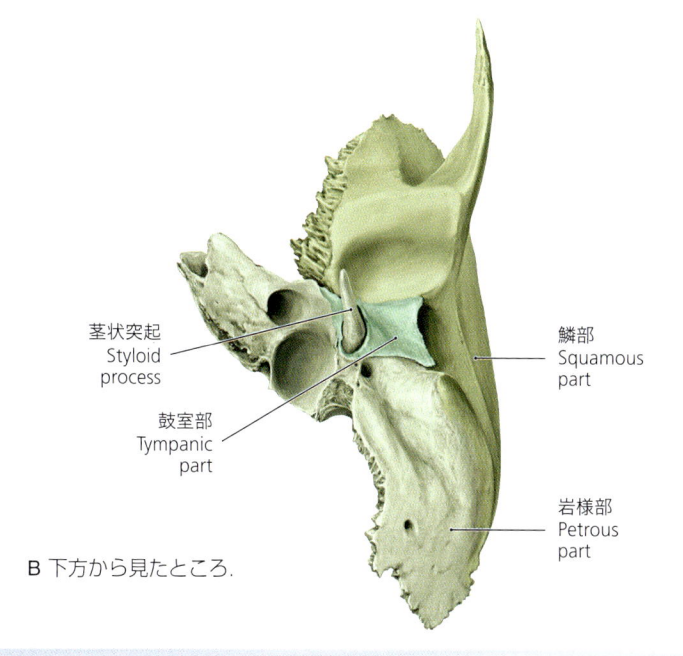

- 鱗部 Squamous part
- 鼓室部 Tympanic part
- 岩様部 Petrous part

B 下方から見たところ．

- 茎状突起 Styloid process
- 鼓室部 Tympanic part
- 鱗部 Squamous part
- 岩様部 Petrous part

臨床

側頭骨内部の構造

乳様突起には中耳と連絡する乳突蜂巣が含まれる．中耳は咽頭鼻部を介して耳管にも連絡する．細菌は耳管を通って咽頭鼻部から中耳へ移動することもある．重篤な場合には細菌が乳突蜂巣から頭蓋腔に入り，髄膜炎を引き起こすこともある．

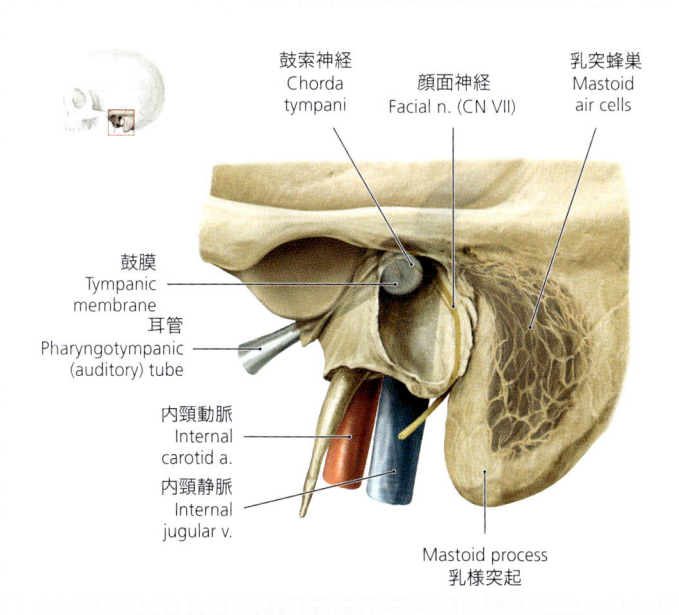

- 鼓索神経 Chorda tympani
- 顔面神経 Facial n. (CN VII)
- 乳突蜂巣 Mastoid air cells
- 鼓膜 Tympanic membrane
- 耳管 Pharyngotympanic (auditory) tube
- 内頸動脈 Internal carotid a.
- 内頸静脈 Internal jugular v.
- Mastoid process 乳様突起

温水（44℃）あるいは冷水（30℃）を外耳道に注ぐと半規管の内リンパに対流が生じ，眼振（律動眼振，前庭動眼反射）を引き起こすことができる．この温度眼振検査は原因不明のめまいの診断に重要である．温度眼振検査では半規管が垂直位になるように患者の向きを変える必要がある．

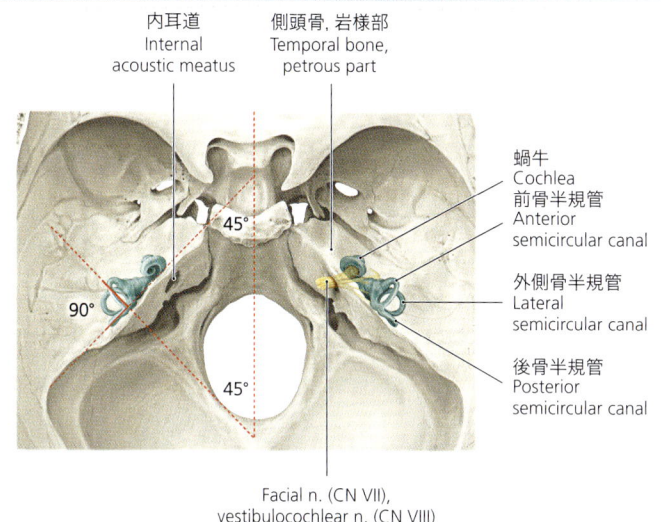

- 内耳道 Internal acoustic meatus
- 側頭骨，岩様部 Temporal bone, petrous part
- 蝸牛 Cochlea
- 前骨半規管 Anterior semicircular canal
- 外側骨半規管 Lateral semicircular canal
- 後骨半規管 Posterior semicircular canal
- Facial n. (CN VII), vestibulocochlear n. (CN VIII) 顔面神経，内耳神経

側頭骨の岩様部には中耳，内耳，鼓膜が含まれる．骨半規管は冠状面，矢状面，横断面に対して約45°を成している．

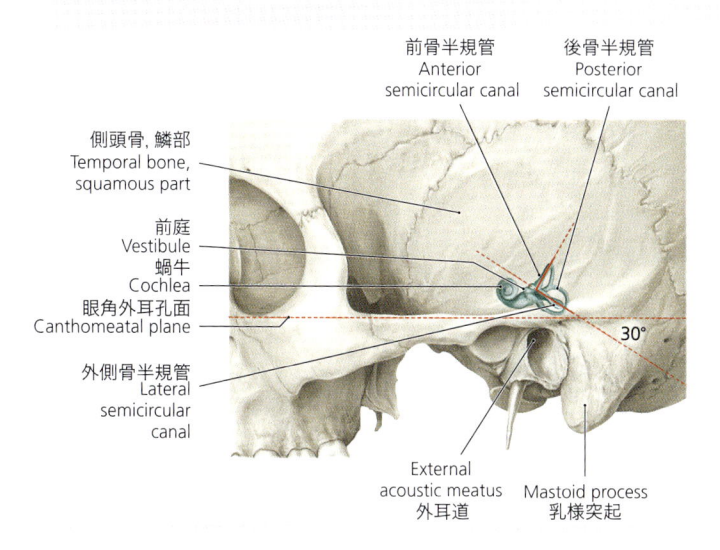

- 前骨半規管 Anterior semicircular canal
- 後骨半規管 Posterior semicircular canal
- 側頭骨，鱗部 Temporal bone, squamous part
- 前庭 Vestibule
- 蝸牛 Cochlea
- 眼角外耳孔面 Canthomeatal plane
- 外側骨半規管 Lateral semicircular canal
- External acoustic meatus 外耳道
- Mastoid process 乳様突起

外耳と外耳道
External Ear & Auditory Canal

聴覚器は大きく外耳，中耳，内耳の3つに分けられる．外耳と中耳は音の伝達器官で，内耳が実際の聴覚器（p.619参照）である．内耳には平衡覚のための器官である前庭器も含まれる（p.618参照）．

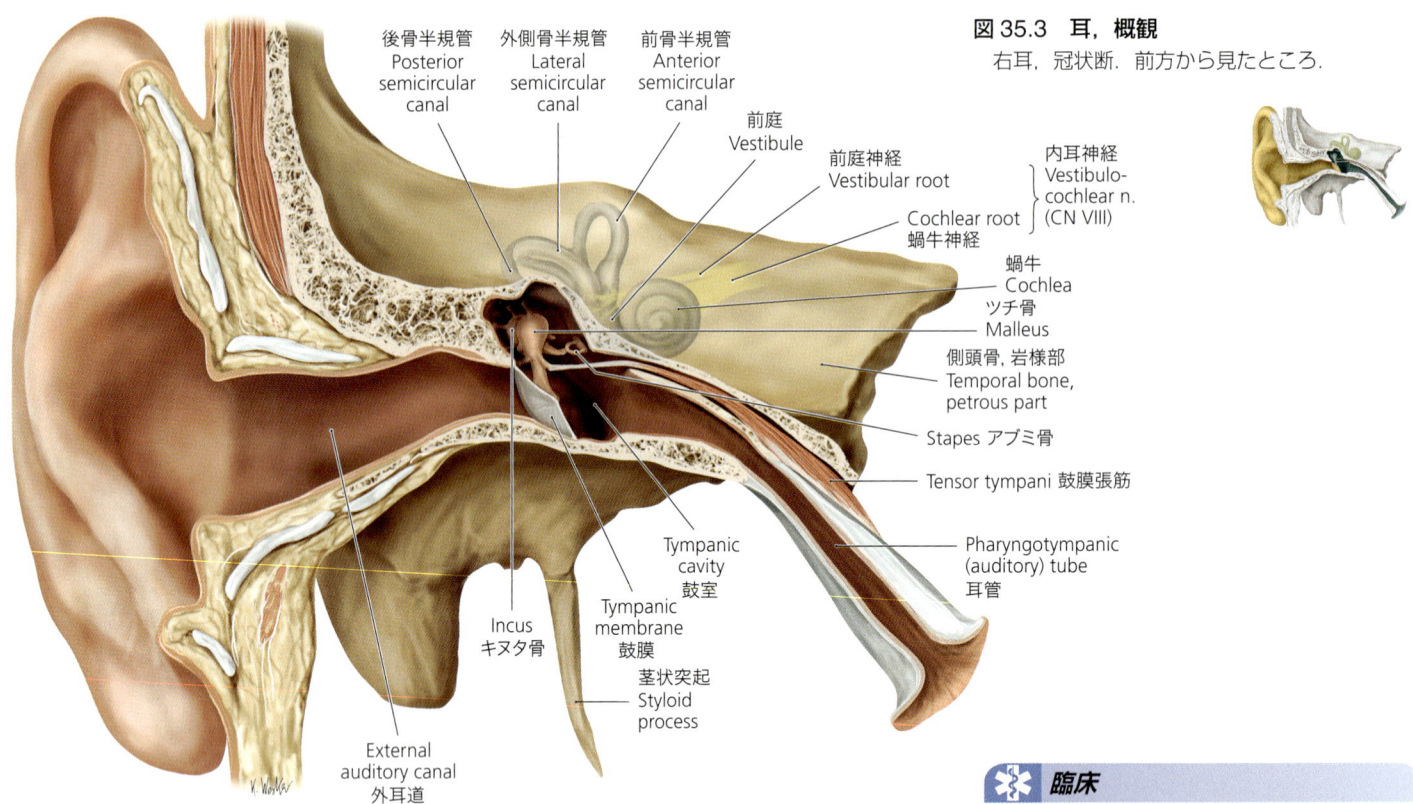

図35.3　耳，概観
右耳，冠状断．前方から見たところ．

ラベル：
- 後骨半規管 Posterior semicircular canal
- 外側骨半規管 Lateral semicircular canal
- 前骨半規管 Anterior semicircular canal
- 前庭 Vestibule
- 前庭神経 Vestibular root
- 蝸牛神経 Cochlear root
- 内耳神経 Vestibulocochlear n. (CN VIII)
- 蝸牛 Cochlea
- ツチ骨 Malleus
- 側頭骨，岩様部 Temporal bone, petrous part
- Stapes アブミ骨
- Tensor tympani 鼓膜張筋
- Pharyngotympanic (auditory) tube 耳管
- Tympanic cavity 鼓室
- Tympanic membrane 鼓膜
- 茎状突起 Styloid process
- Incus キヌタ骨
- External auditory canal 外耳道

図35.4　外耳道
右耳，冠状断．前方から見たところ．鼓膜は外耳道と中耳の鼓室を境界する．外耳道の外側1/3は軟骨性で，内側2/3は骨性（側頭骨の鼓室部）である．

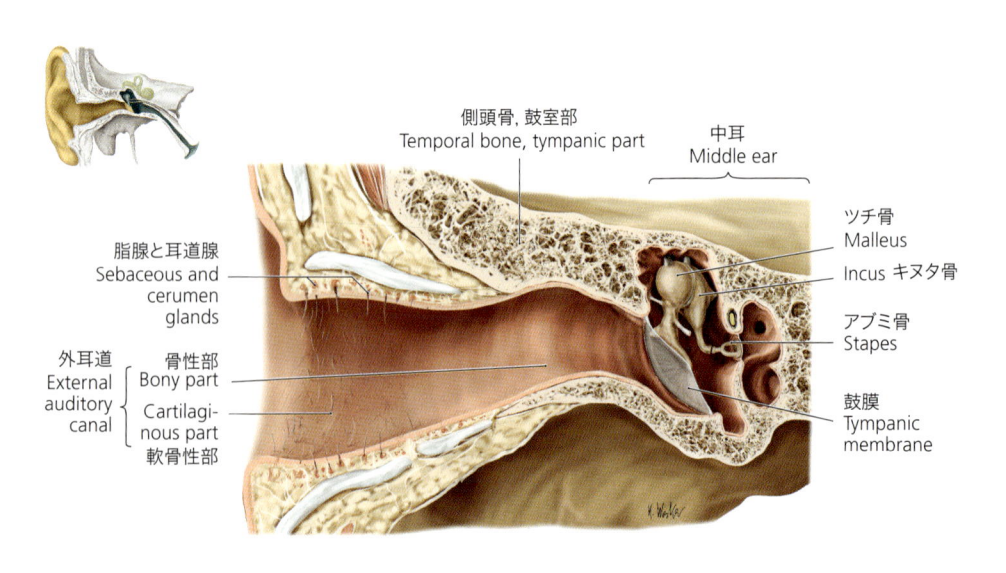

ラベル：
- 側頭骨，鼓室部 Temporal bone, tympanic part
- 中耳 Middle ear
- 脂腺と耳道腺 Sebaceous and cerumen glands
- 外耳道 External auditory canal
  - 骨性部 Bony part
  - 軟骨性部 Cartilaginous part
- ツチ骨 Malleus
- Incus キヌタ骨
- アブミ骨 Stapes
- 鼓膜 Tympanic membrane

臨床

外耳道の弯曲
外耳道は軟骨性部で大きく弯曲している．オトスコープ（耳鏡）を挿入するときは，耳介を後上方に引くと外耳道がまっすぐになり，耳鏡を挿入することができる．

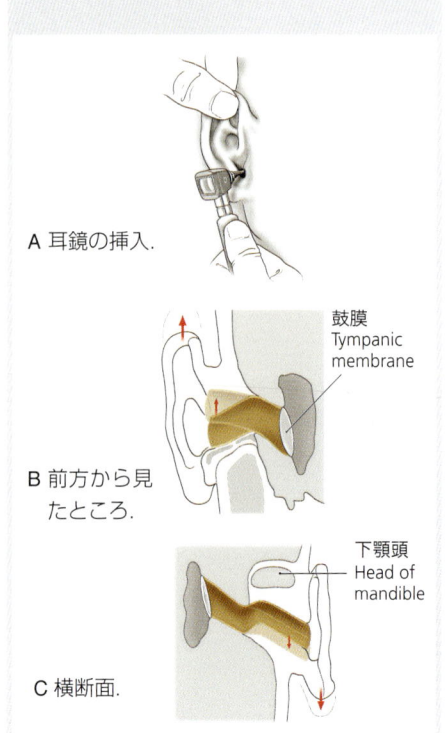

A 耳鏡の挿入．
B 前方から見たところ．（鼓膜 Tympanic membrane）
C 横断面．（下顎頭 Head of mandible）

図 35.5　耳介の構造

耳介には，音を振動させるための漏斗状の音受容器である軟骨のフレームがある．耳介筋は表情筋だと考えられているが，ヒトでは退化している．

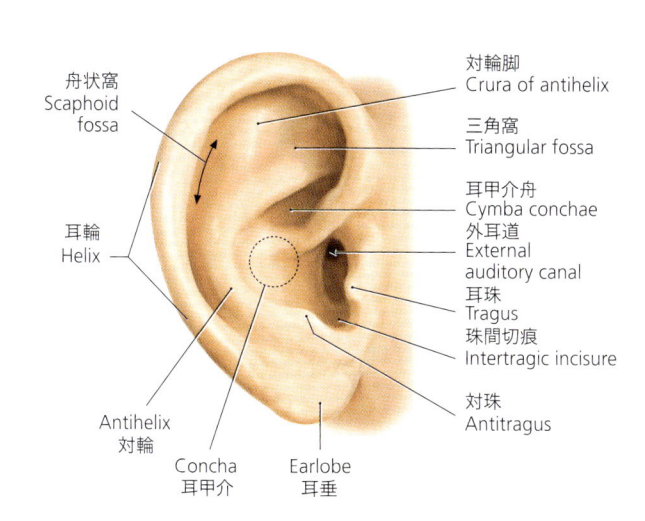

A 右の耳介，外側方から見たところ．

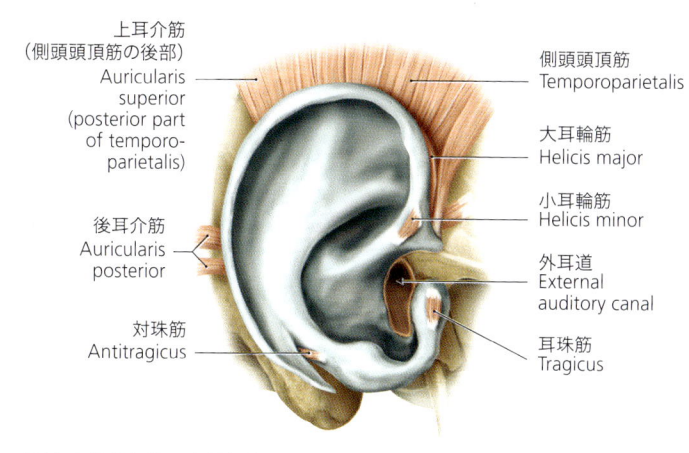

- 舟状窩 Scaphoid fossa
- 対輪脚 Crura of antihelix
- 三角窩 Triangular fossa
- 耳甲介舟 Cymba conchae
- 外耳道 External auditory canal
- 耳珠 Tragus
- 珠間切痕 Intertragic incisure
- 耳輪 Helix
- 対珠 Antitragus
- 対輪 Antihelix
- 耳甲介 Concha
- 耳垂 Earlobe

B 耳介の軟骨と筋．右外側方から見たところ．

- 上耳介筋（側頭頭頂筋の後部）Auricularis superior (posterior part of temporoparietalis)
- 側頭頭頂筋 Temporoparietalis
- 大耳輪筋 Helicis major
- 小耳輪筋 Helicis minor
- 外耳道 External auditory canal
- 耳珠筋 Tragicus
- 後耳介筋 Auricularis posterior
- 対珠筋 Antitragicus

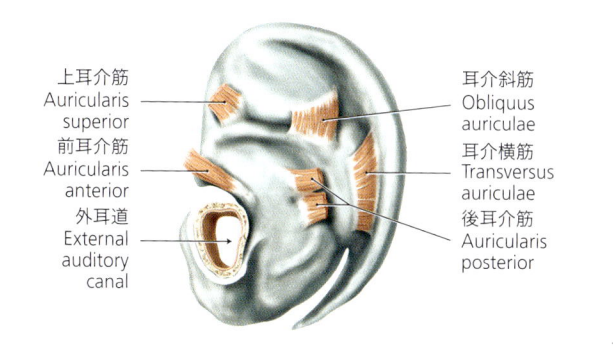

C 耳介の軟骨と筋．後面を内側方から見たところ．

- 上耳介筋 Auricularis superior
- 耳介斜筋 Obliquus auriculae
- 前耳介筋 Auricularis anterior
- 耳介横筋 Transversus auriculae
- 外耳道 External auditory canal
- 後耳介筋 Auricularis posterior

図 35.6　耳介の動脈

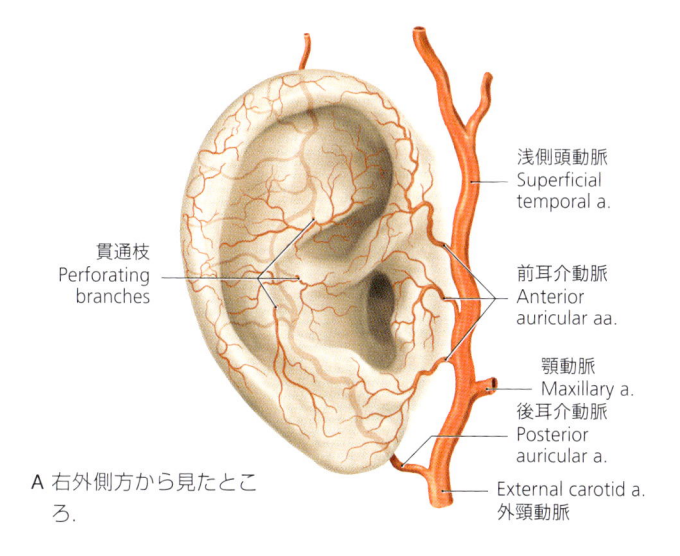

A 右外側方から見たところ．

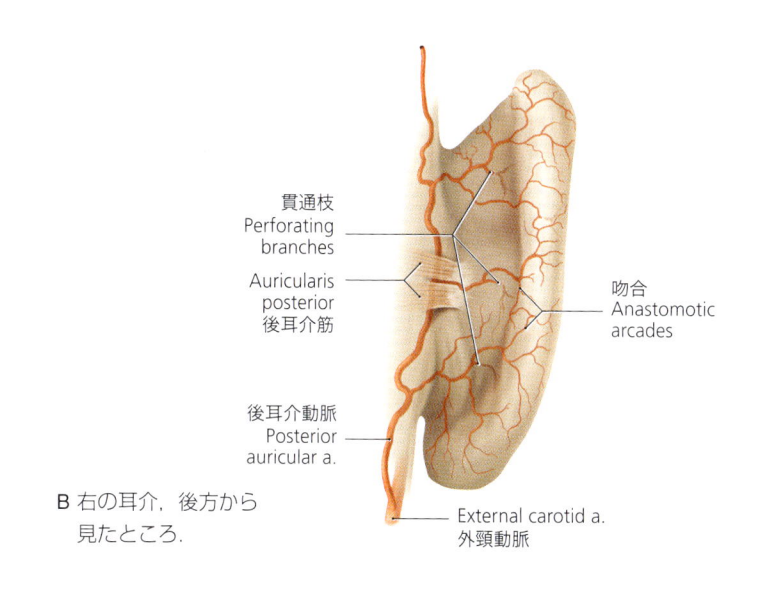

- 貫通枝 Perforating branches
- 浅側頭動脈 Superficial temporal a.
- 前耳介動脈 Anterior auricular aa.
- 顎動脈 Maxillary a.
- 後耳介動脈 Posterior auricular a.
- 外頸動脈 External carotid a.

B 右の耳介，後方から見たところ．

- 貫通枝 Perforating branches
- 後耳介筋 Auricularis posterior
- 吻合 Anastomotic arcades
- 後耳介動脈 Posterior auricular a.
- 外頸動脈 External carotid a.

図 35.7　耳介の神経

A 右外側方から見たところ．

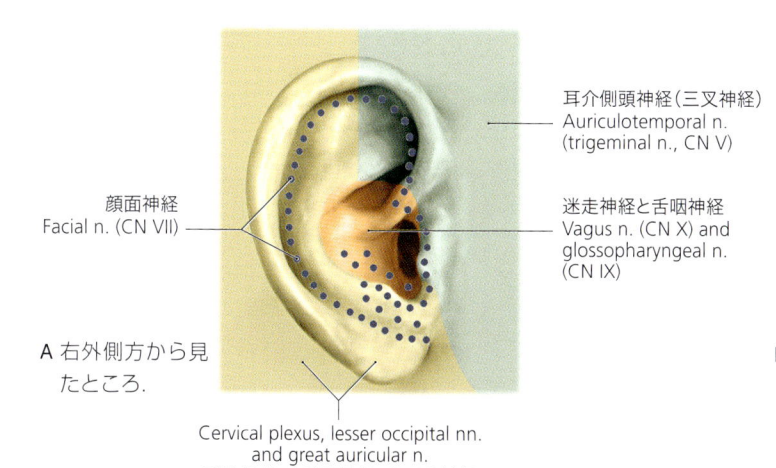

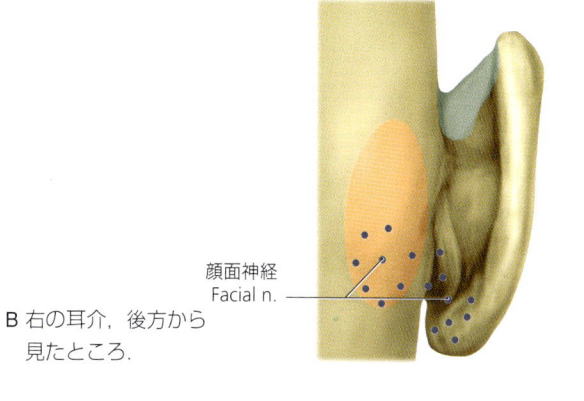

- 顔面神経 Facial n. (CN VII)
- 耳介側頭神経（三叉神経）Auriculotemporal n. (trigeminal n., CN V)
- 迷走神経と舌咽神経 Vagus n. (CN X) and glossopharyngeal n. (CN IX)
- 頸神経叢，小後頭神経，大耳介神経 Cervical plexus, lesser occipital nn. and great auricular n.

B 右の耳介，後方から見たところ．

- 顔面神経 Facial n.

中耳：鼓室
Middle Ear: Tympanic Cavity

図 35.8 中耳
右岩様部．上方から見たところ．中耳の鼓室は前方で耳管によって咽頭につながっており，後方で乳突蜂巣につながっている．

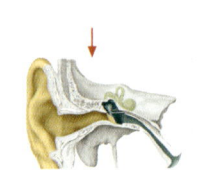

図 35.9 鼓室と耳管
鼓室を開き，内側方から見たところ．

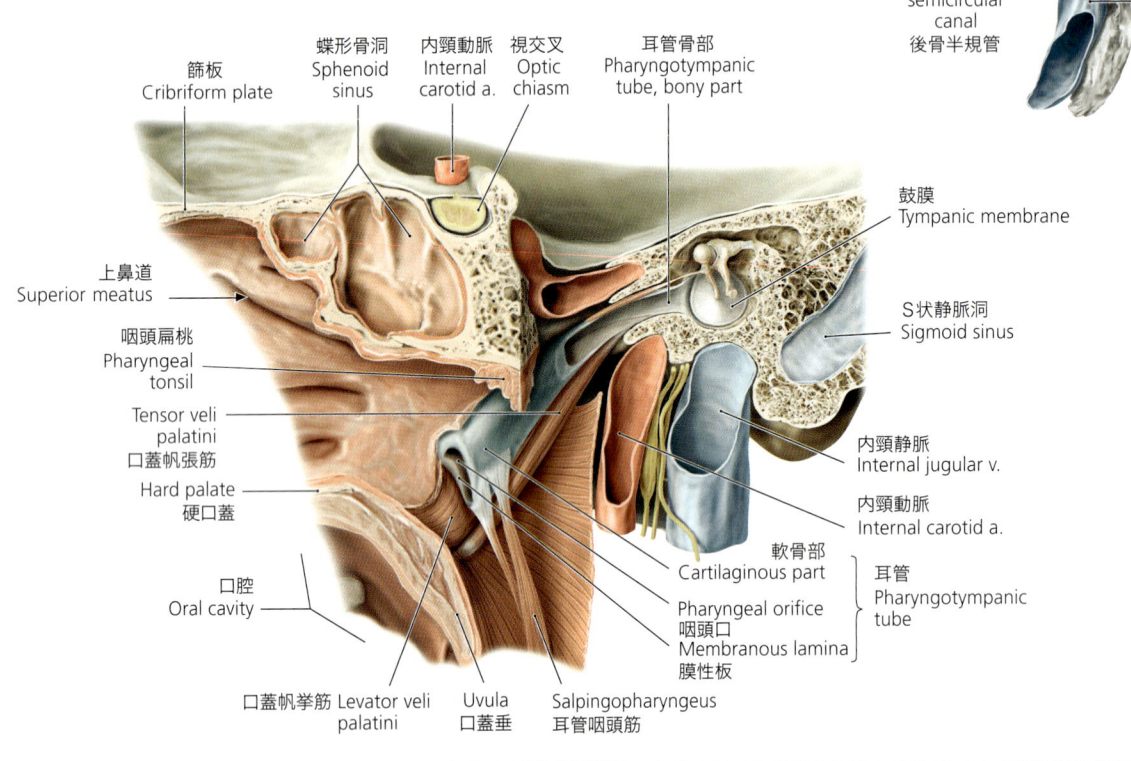

表 35.1	鼓室の境界			
慢性化膿性中耳炎（中耳の炎症）では，病原菌が周囲の領域に広がる可能性がある．				
方向	壁	解剖学的境界	近傍の構造	炎症
前方	頸動脈壁	耳管開口部	頸動脈管	
外側	鼓膜壁	鼓膜	外耳	
上方	室蓋壁	鼓室蓋	中頭蓋窩	髄膜炎，（特に側頭葉の）脳膿瘍
内側	迷路壁	蝸牛基底回転上の岬角	内耳	
			CSF 腔（錐体尖を介して）	外転神経麻痺，三叉神経過敏，視力障害（グラデニーゴ症候群）
下方	頸静脈壁	側頭骨鼓室部	頸静脈球	
			S 状静脈洞	静脈洞血栓症
後方	乳突壁	乳突洞口	乳突蜂巣	乳突炎
			顔面神経管	顔面神経麻痺

図 35.10 鼓室

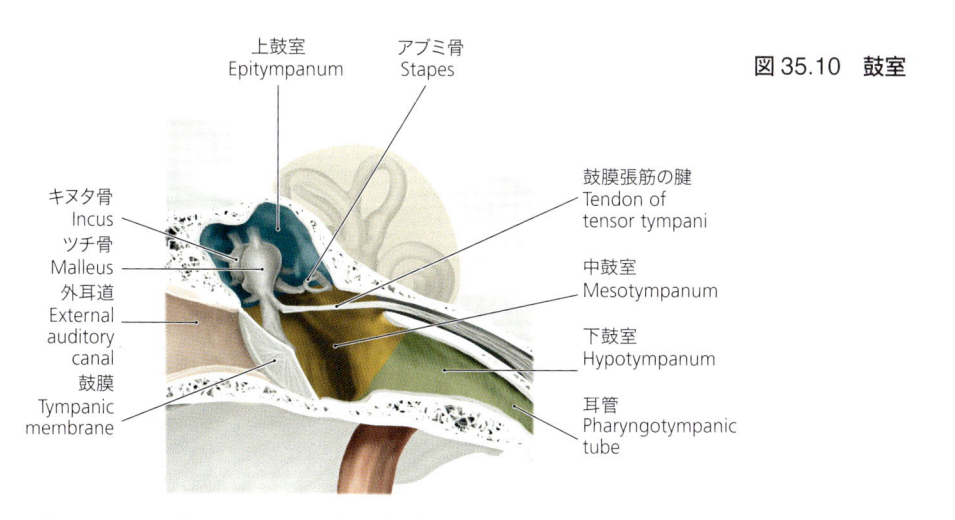

A 鼓室のレベル．前方から見たところ．鼓室は，上鼓室，中鼓室，下鼓室の3つのレベルに分けられる．

- 上鼓室 Epitympanum
- アブミ骨 Stapes
- キヌタ骨 Incus
- ツチ骨 Malleus
- 外耳道 External auditory canal
- 鼓膜 Tympanic membrane
- 鼓膜張筋の腱 Tendon of tensor tympani
- 中鼓室 Mesotympanum
- 下鼓室 Hypotympanum
- 耳管 Pharyngotympanic tube

B 右鼓室，前方から見たところ．前壁は取り除いてある．

- 乳突洞口 Aditus (inlet) to mastoid antrum
- ツチ骨 Malleus
- キヌタ骨 Incus
- 鼓索神経 Chorda tympani
- 鼓膜張筋 Tensor tympani
- アブミ骨筋の腱 Tendon of stapedius
- 鼓膜 Tympanic membrane
- 小錐体神経 Lesser petrosal n.
- 顔面神経管にある顔面神経 Facial n. (CN VII) in facial canal
- 外側半規管隆起 Prominence of lateral semicircular canal
- 顔面神経管隆起 Prominence of facial canal
- アブミ骨 Stapes
- 岬角 Promontory
- 鼓室神経叢 Tympanic plexus
- 鼓室神経 Tympanic n.

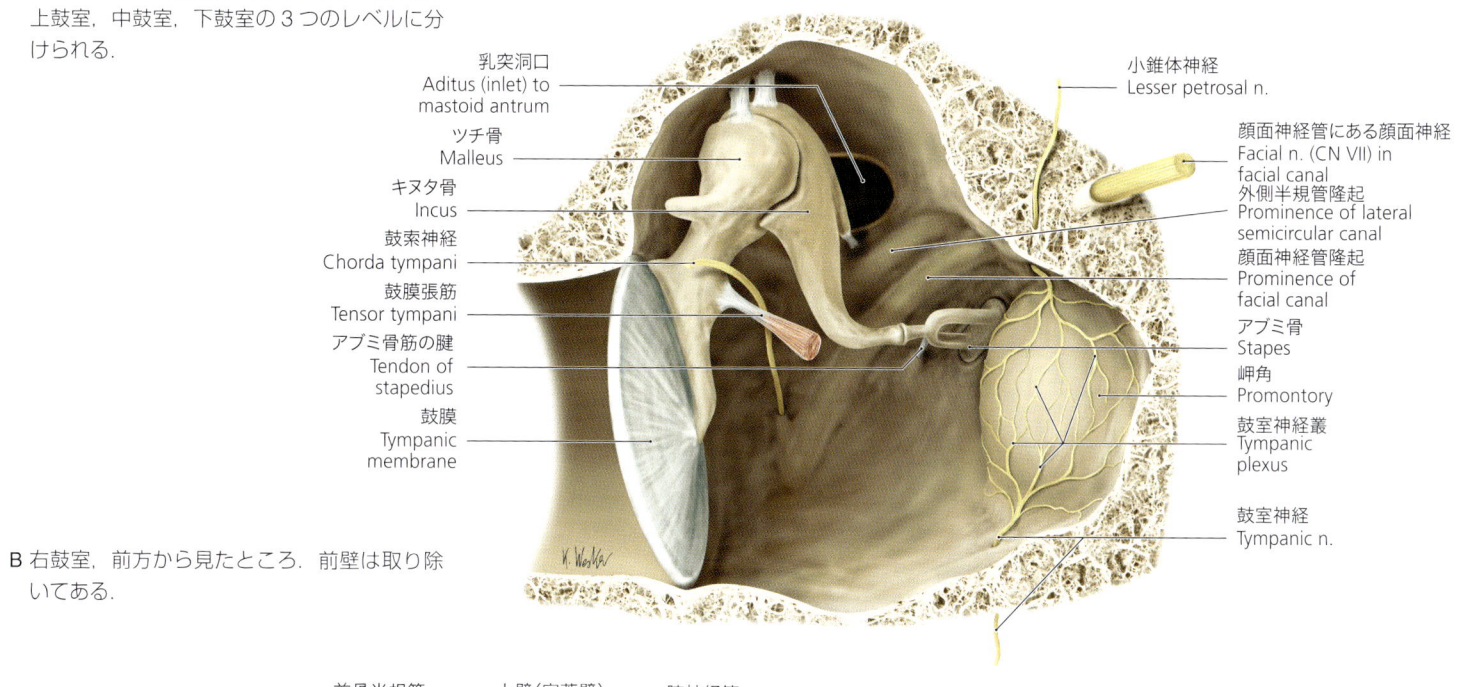

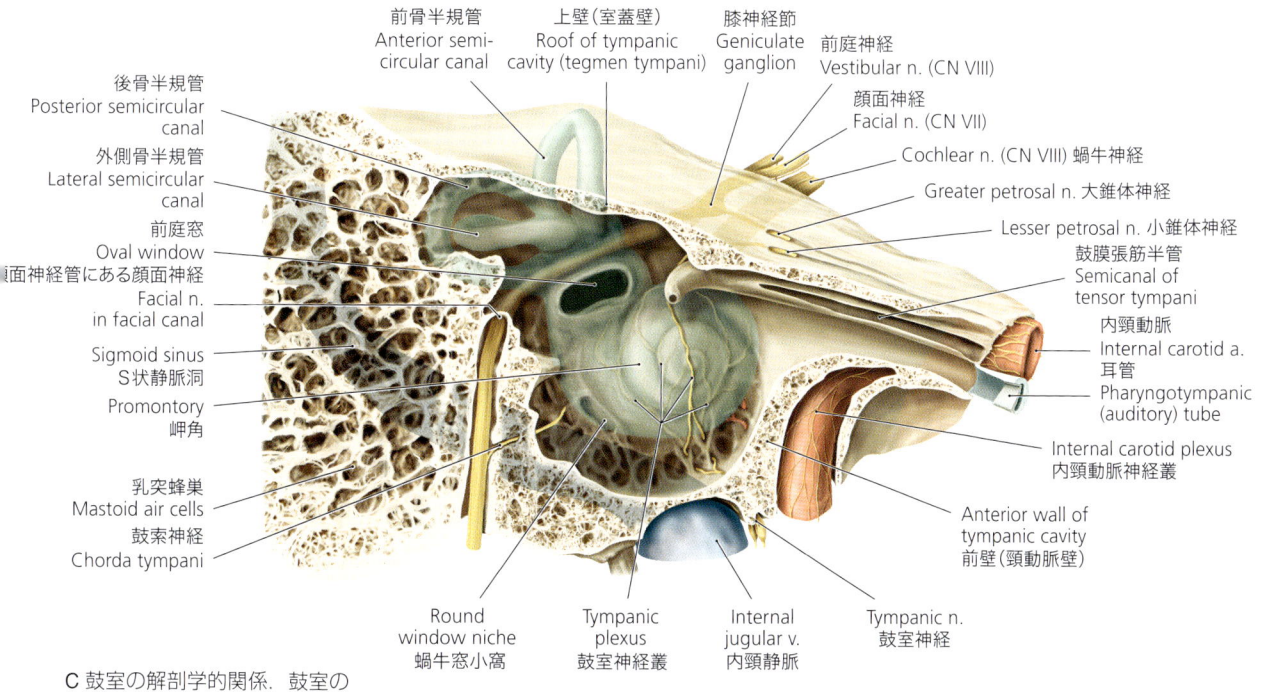

C 鼓室の解剖学的関係．鼓室の内側壁，斜め矢状断．

- 後骨半規管 Posterior semicircular canal
- 外側骨半規管 Lateral semicircular canal
- 前庭窓 Oval window
- 顔面神経管にある顔面神経 Facial n. in facial canal
- S状静脈洞 Sigmoid sinus
- 岬角 Promontory
- 乳突蜂巣 Mastoid air cells
- 鼓索神経 Chorda tympani
- 前骨半規管 Anterior semicircular canal
- 上壁（室蓋壁） Roof of tympanic cavity (tegmen tympani)
- 膝神経節 Geniculate ganglion
- 前庭神経 Vestibular n. (CN VIII)
- 顔面神経 Facial n. (CN VII)
- Cochlear n. (CN VIII) 蝸牛神経
- Greater petrosal n. 大錐体神経
- Lesser petrosal n. 小錐体神経
- 鼓膜張筋半管 Semicanal of tensor tympani
- 内頸動脈 Internal carotid a.
- 耳管 Pharyngotympanic (auditory) tube
- 内頸動脈神経叢 Internal carotid plexus
- 前壁（頸動脈壁） Anterior wall of tympanic cavity
- 鼓室神経 Tympanic n.
- 内頸静脈 Internal jugular v.
- 鼓室神経叢 Tympanic plexus
- 蝸牛窓小窩 Round window niche

中耳：耳小骨連鎖と鼓膜
Middle Ear: Ossicular Chain & Tympanic Membrane

図 35.11　耳小骨
左耳．耳小骨は3つの骨からなり，関節によって鼓膜から前庭窓までつながっている．

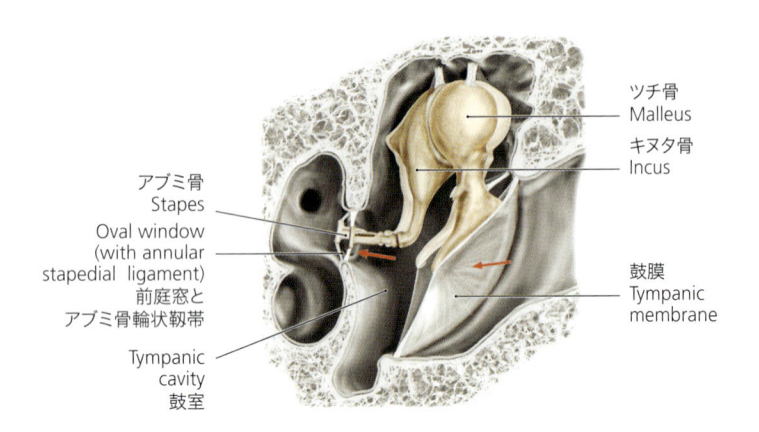

A　中耳の耳小骨．左耳，前方から見たところ．

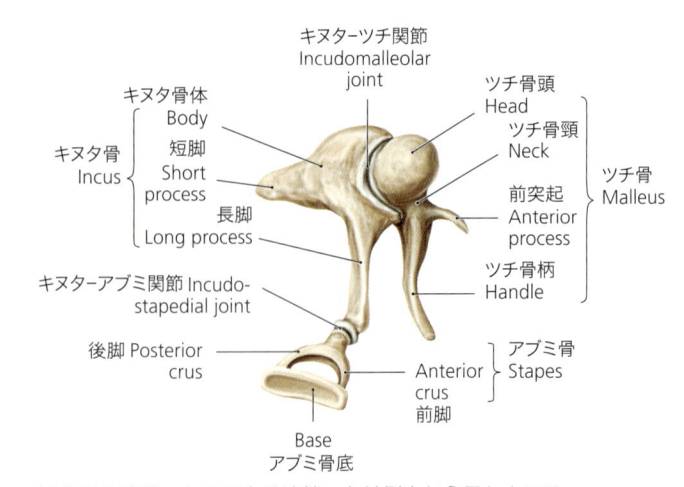

B　耳小骨の連鎖．左の耳小骨連鎖，右外側方から見たところ．

図 35.12　ツチ骨
左耳．

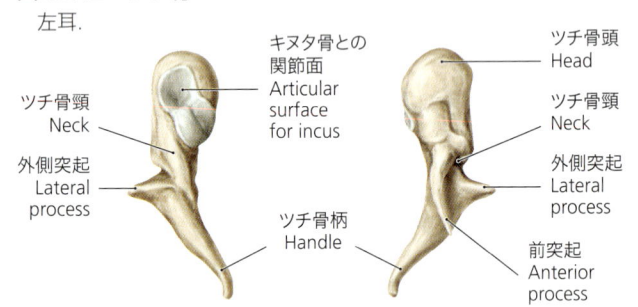

A　後方から見たところ．

B　前方から見たところ．

図 35.13　キヌタ骨
左耳．

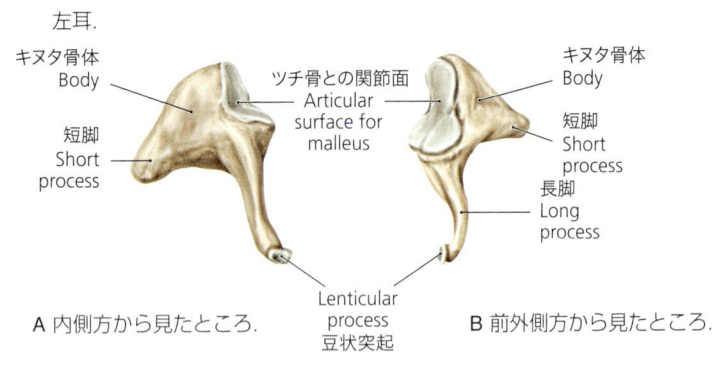

A　内側方から見たところ．

B　前外側方から見たところ．

図 35.14　アブミ骨
左耳．

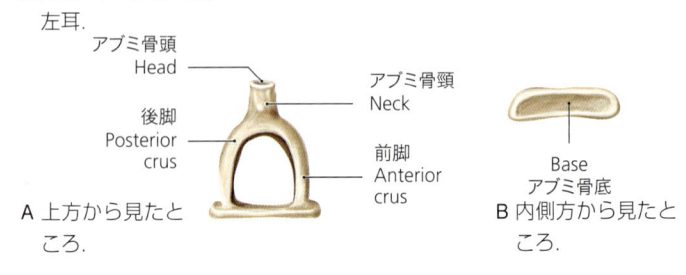

A　上方から見たところ．

B　内側方から見たところ．

図 35.15　鼓膜
右鼓膜．鼓膜は，前上(I)，前下(II)，後下(III)，後上(IV)の4つの部分に分割される．

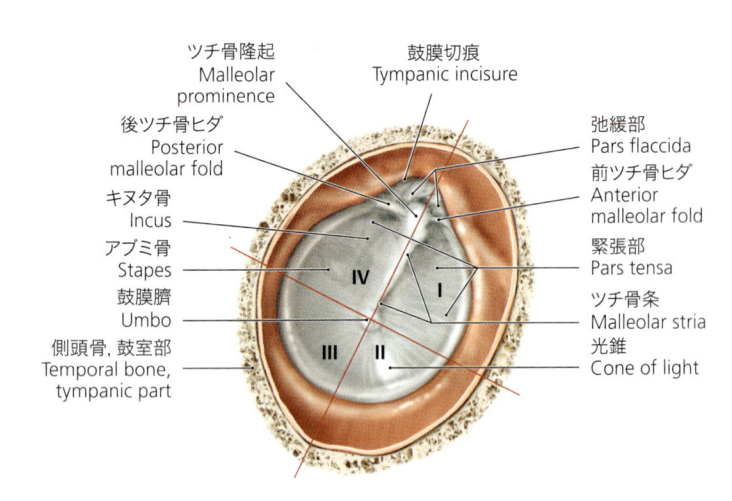

A　右鼓膜，外側方から見たところ．

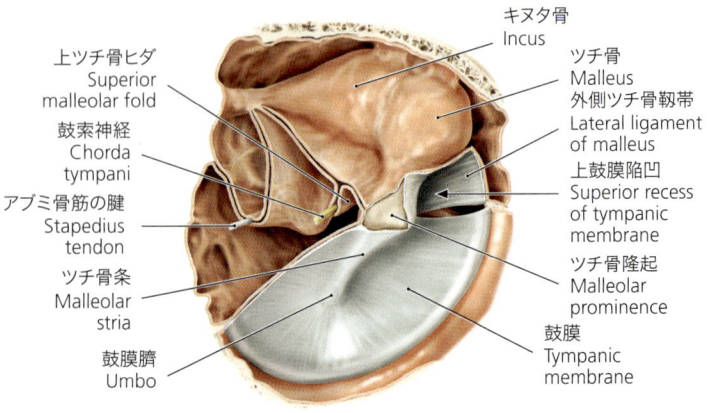

B　鼓膜内の粘膜．後外側方から見たところ．鼓膜を一部取り除いてある．

図 35.16 鼓室の耳小骨連鎖

右耳，外側方から見たところ．耳小骨連鎖の靱帯と中耳の筋（アブミ骨筋と鼓膜張筋）を示す．

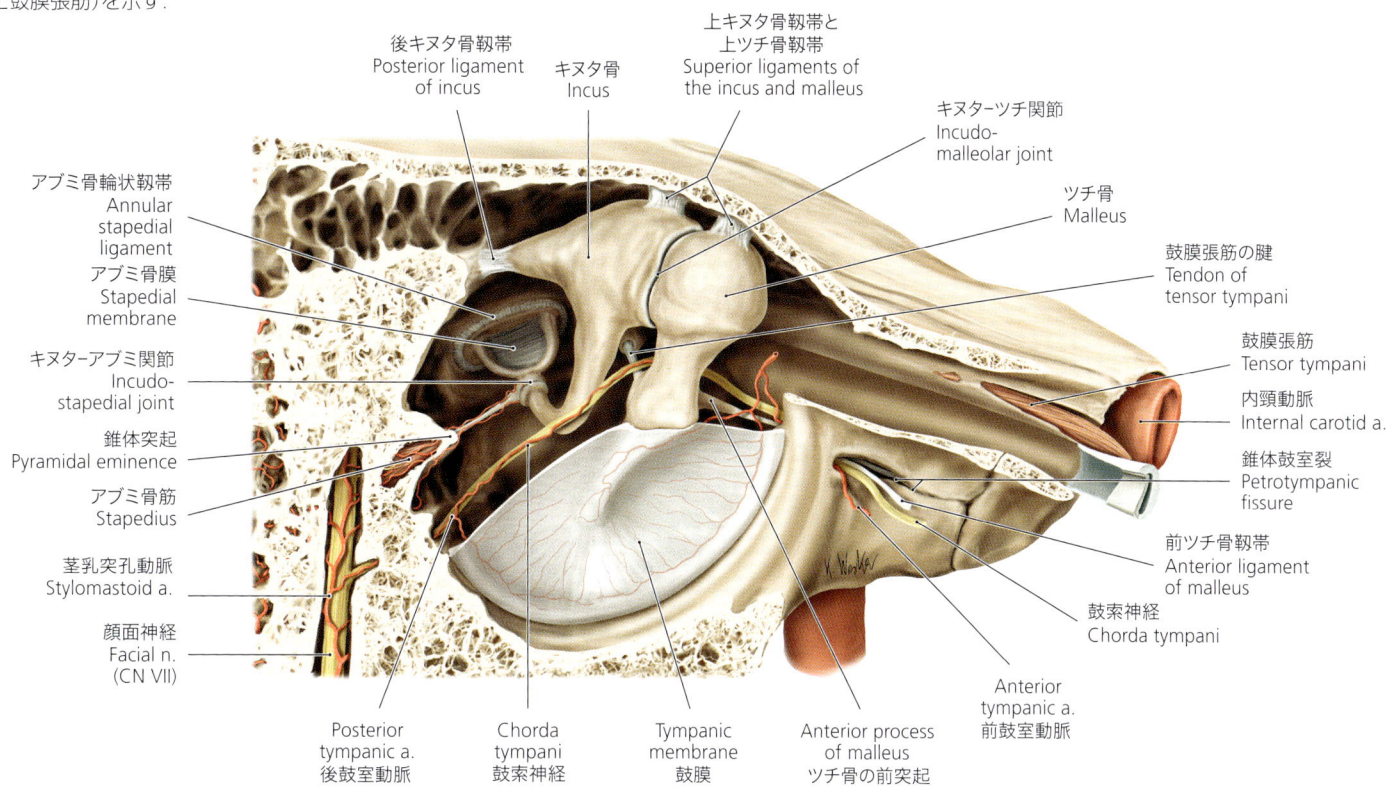

主な標識：
- 後キヌタ骨靱帯 Posterior ligament of incus
- キヌタ骨 Incus
- 上キヌタ骨靱帯と上ツチ骨靱帯 Superior ligaments of the incus and malleus
- キヌターツチ関節 Incudo-malleolar joint
- ツチ骨 Malleus
- アブミ骨輪状靱帯 Annular stapedial ligament
- アブミ骨膜 Stapedial membrane
- 鼓膜張筋の腱 Tendon of tensor tympani
- 鼓膜張筋 Tensor tympani
- 内頸動脈 Internal carotid a.
- キヌターアブミ関節 Incudo-stapedial joint
- 錐体突起 Pyramidal eminence
- アブミ骨筋 Stapedius
- 錐体鼓室裂 Petrotympanic fissure
- 前ツチ骨靱帯 Anterior ligament of malleus
- 茎乳突孔動脈 Stylomastoid a.
- 鼓索神経 Chorda tympani
- 顔面神経 Facial n. (CN VII)
- 後鼓室動脈 Posterior tympanic a.
- 鼓索神経 Chorda tympani
- 鼓膜 Tympanic membrane
- ツチ骨の前突起 Anterior process of malleus
- 前鼓室動脈 Anterior tympanic a.

臨床

聴覚における耳小骨連鎖

音波は外耳道を通り，鼓膜を振動させる．耳小骨連鎖はこの振動を前庭窓に伝え，そこで内耳の液体に振動が伝えられる．液体中の音波は高いインピーダンス（振動に対する抵抗）を受けるために，中耳で増幅する必要がある．鼓膜と前庭窓の表面積の差により音圧は17倍になる．さらに耳小骨連鎖のてこの作用によって全体として22倍に増幅される．耳小骨連鎖が鼓膜とアブミ骨底の間で音圧を変換できないと，20dBの伝音難聴が生じる．聴覚についてはp.619参照．

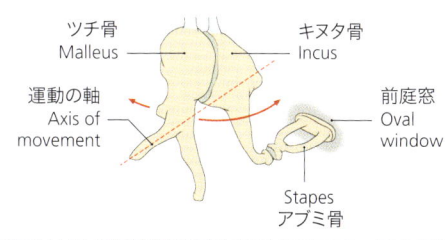

A 鼓膜の振動は耳小骨連鎖の振動を引き起こす．耳小骨連鎖の構造のために，てこの作用によって音波は1.3倍に増強される．

- ツチ骨 Malleus
- キヌタ骨 Incus
- 運動の軸 Axis of movement
- 前庭窓 Oval window
- アブミ骨 Stapes

B アブミ骨の通常の位置は前庭窓と同じ面にある．

- 錐体突起 Pyramidal eminence
- アブミ骨筋の腱 Stapedius tendon
- 前庭窓とアブミ骨輪状靱帯 Oval window with annular stapedial ligament

C 耳小骨連鎖の振動はアブミ骨を傾斜させる．前庭窓のアブミ骨膜に対するアブミ骨底の運動に対応して，波動が内耳の流体柱に引き起こされる．

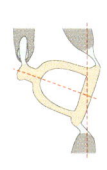

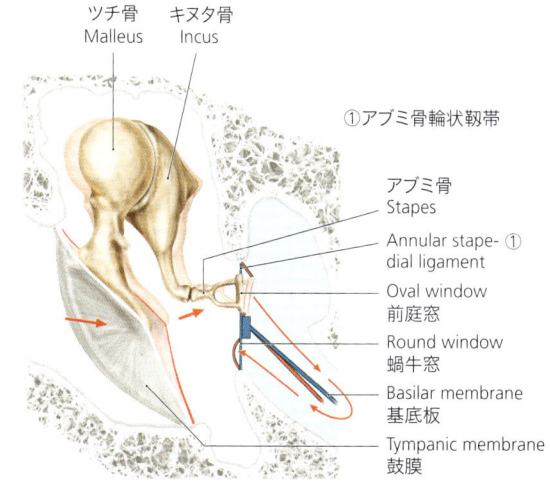

D 耳小骨連鎖による音波の伝導．

- ツチ骨 Malleus
- キヌタ骨 Incus
- ①アブミ骨輪状靱帯
- アブミ骨 Stapes
- Annular stapedial ligament ①
- 前庭窓 Oval window
- 蝸牛窓 Round window
- 基底板 Basilar membrane
- 鼓膜 Tympanic membrane

中耳の動脈
Arteries of the Middle Ear

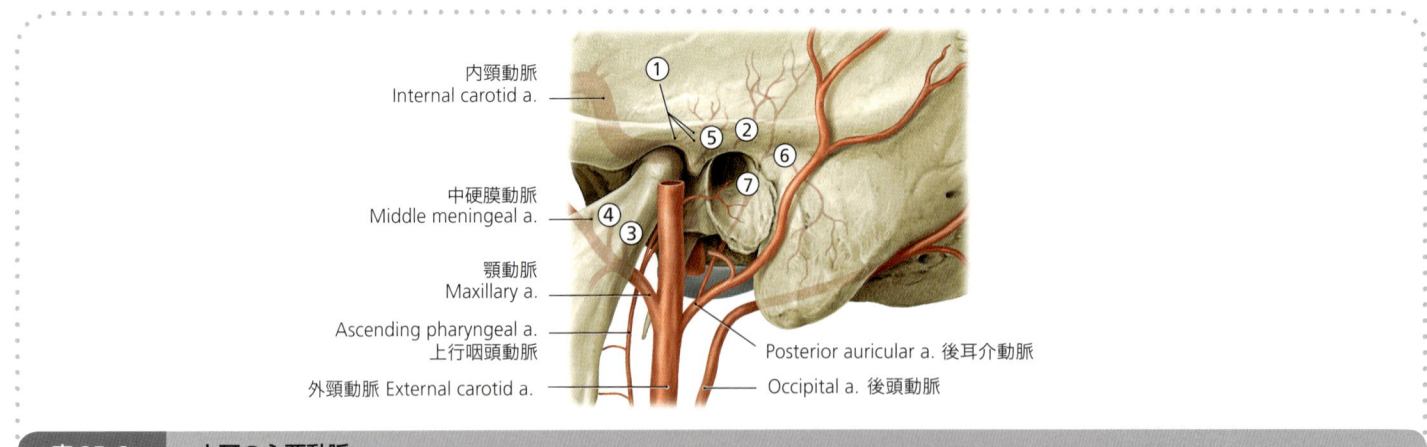

起始	動脈		分布
内頸動脈	①頸鼓動脈		鼓室前壁，耳管
外頸動脈	(内側枝)上行咽頭動脈	②下鼓室動脈	鼓室下壁，岬角
	(終枝)顎動脈	③深耳介動脈	鼓室下壁，鼓膜
		④前鼓室動脈	鼓膜，乳突洞，ツチ骨，キヌタ骨
	中硬膜動脈	⑤上鼓室動脈	室蓋壁，鼓膜張筋，アブミ骨
	(後枝)後耳介動脈	茎乳突孔動脈	
		⑥茎乳突孔動脈	鼓室後壁，乳突蜂巣，アブミ骨筋，アブミ骨
		⑦後鼓室動脈	鼓索神経，鼓膜，ツチ骨

表35.2 中耳の主要動脈

図35.17 中耳の動脈：耳小骨連鎖と鼓膜
右鼓膜，内側方から見たところ．炎症が起こると鼓膜の動脈は拡張し，この図で示したように見えるようになる．

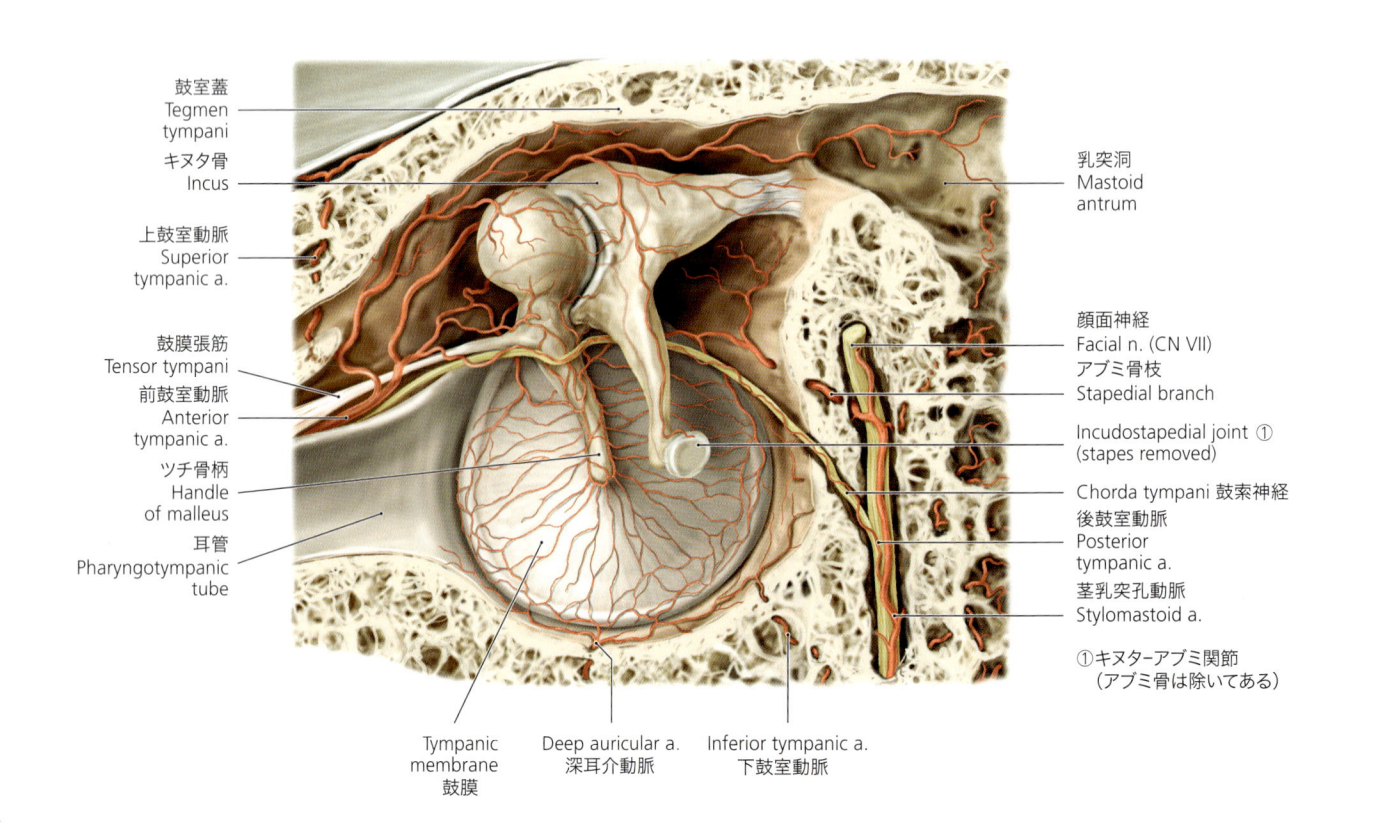

図 35.18 中耳の動脈：鼓室

右側頭骨の岩様部．前面．ツチ骨，キヌタ骨，鼓索神経の一部，前鼓室動脈は取り除いてある．

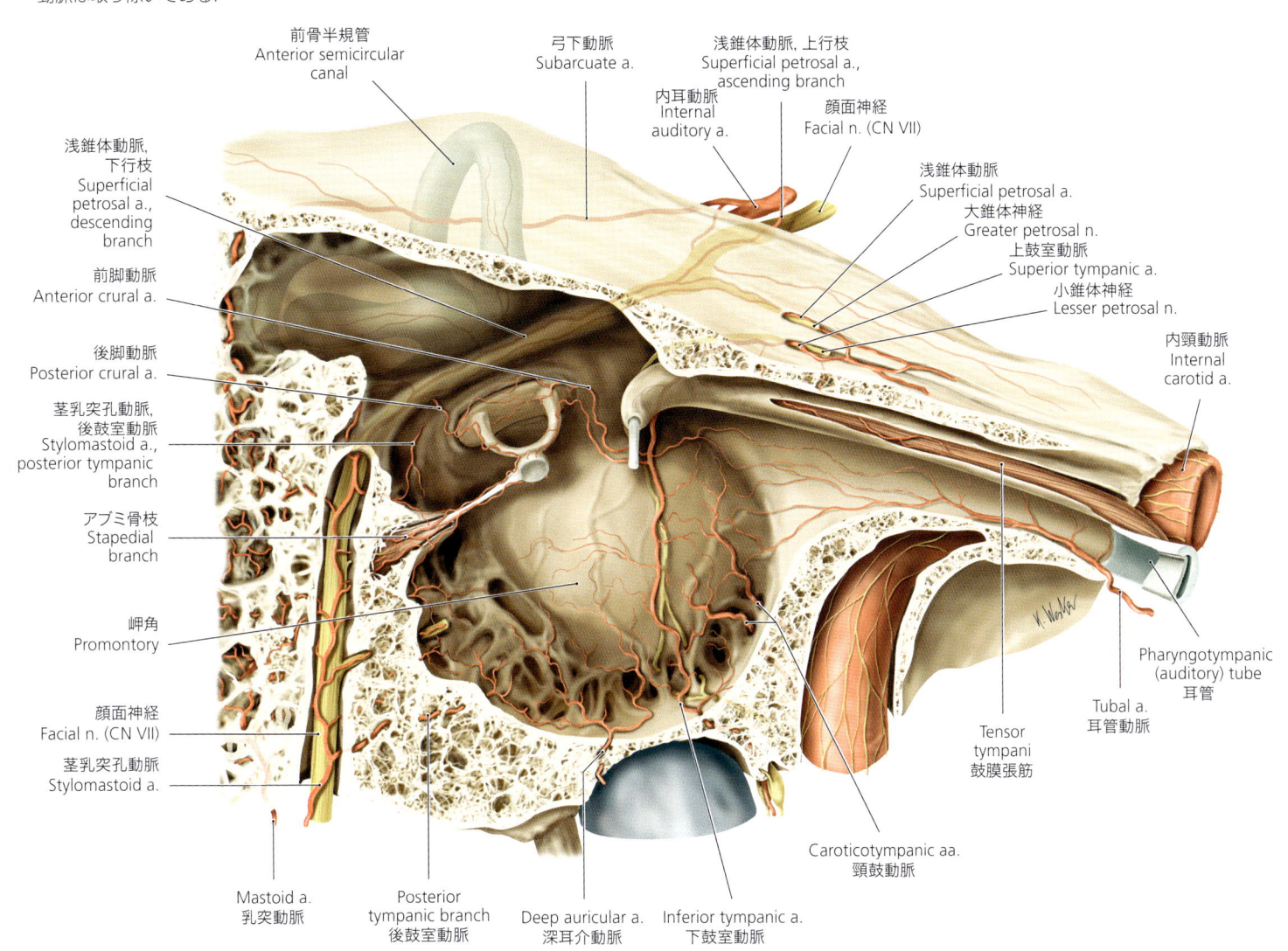

- 前骨半規管 Anterior semicircular canal
- 弓下動脈 Subarcuate a.
- 浅錐体動脈，上行枝 Superficial petrosal a., ascending branch
- 内耳動脈 Internal auditory a.
- 顔面神経 Facial n. (CN VII)
- 浅錐体動脈，下行枝 Superficial petrosal a., descending branch
- 浅錐体動脈 Superficial petrosal a.
- 大錐体神経 Greater petrosal n.
- 上鼓室動脈 Superior tympanic a.
- 小錐体神経 Lesser petrosal n.
- 前脚動脈 Anterior crural a.
- 後脚動脈 Posterior crural a.
- 内頸動脈 Internal carotid a.
- 茎乳突孔動脈，後鼓室動脈 Stylomastoid a., posterior tympanic branch
- アブミ骨枝 Stapedial branch
- 岬角 Promontory
- Pharyngotympanic (auditory) tube 耳管
- 顔面神経 Facial n. (CN VII)
- 茎乳突孔動脈 Stylomastoid a.
- Tubal a. 耳管動脈
- Tensor tympani 鼓膜張筋
- Mastoid a. 乳突動脈
- Posterior tympanic branch 後鼓室動脈
- Deep auricular a. 深耳介動脈
- Inferior tympanic a. 下鼓室動脈
- Caroticotympanic aa. 頸鼓動脈

内耳
Inner Ear

内耳は平衡覚を司る前庭器と聴覚を司る聴覚器からなり，どちらも側頭骨岩様部にある骨迷路内の膜迷路が構成している．骨迷路は外リンパで満たされ，膜迷路は内リンパで満たされている．

図 35.19　前庭器
右外側方から見たところ．

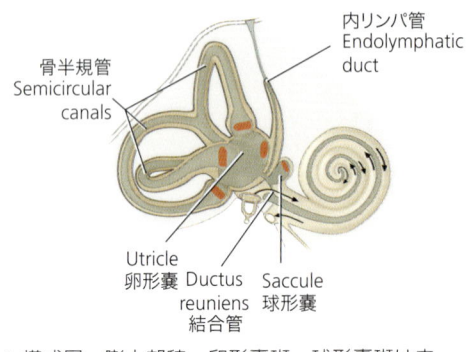

A 模式図．膨大部稜，卵形嚢斑，球形嚢斑は赤で示す．

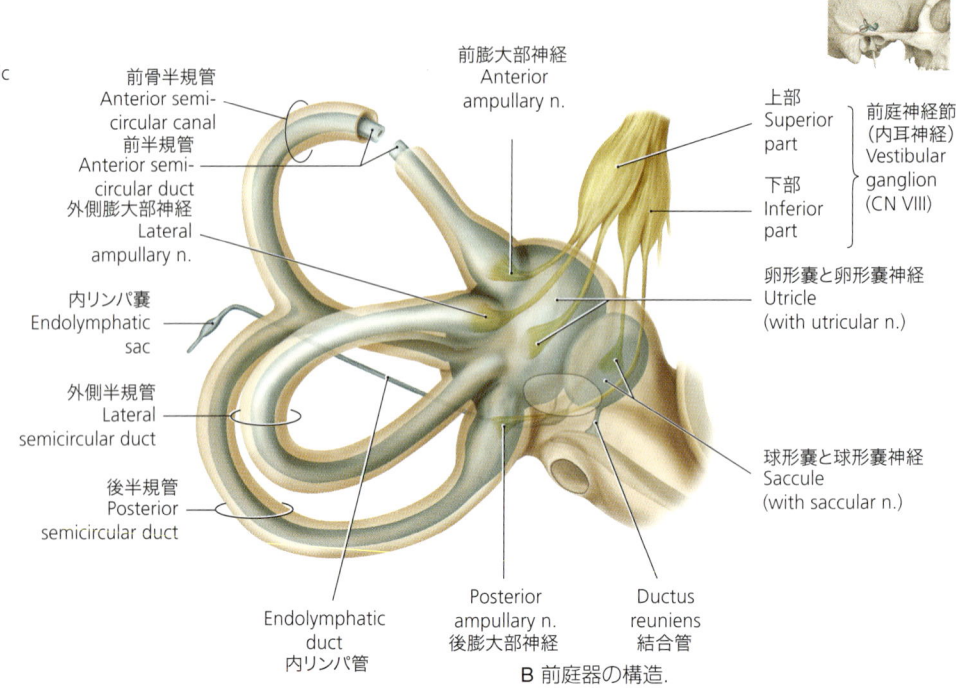

B 前庭器の構造．

図 35.20　聴覚器
蝸牛は，蝸牛迷路と骨性の外殻からなり，聴覚器の感覚上皮（コルチ器）が含まれる．

A 模式図．

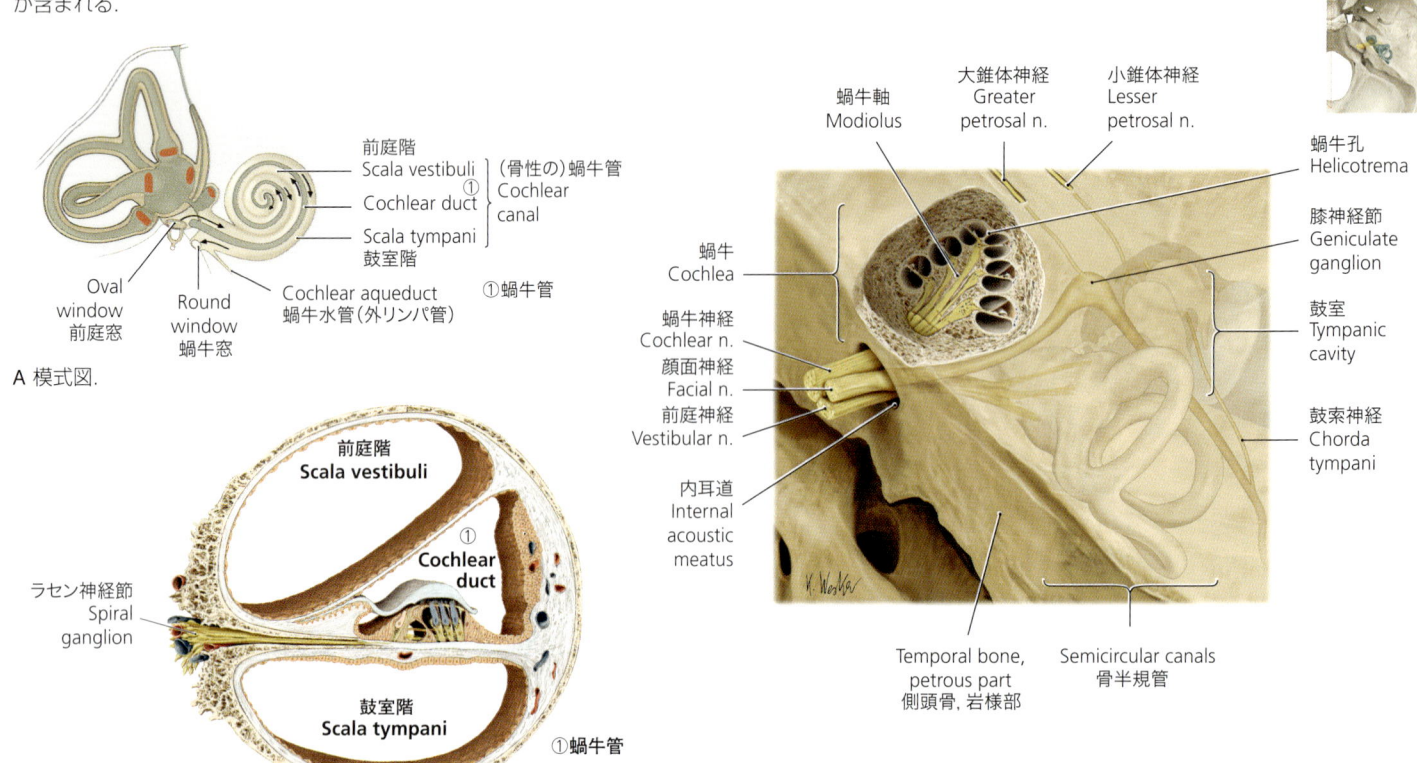

B （骨性の）蝸牛管の領域．横断面．

C 蝸牛の位置．側頭骨岩様部を上方から見たところ．蝸牛は横断してある．蝸牛の骨性の管（ラセン管）は骨性の軸（蝸牛軸）を 2.5 回転する．

図 35.21 膜迷路の神経

右耳，前方から見たところ．内耳神経（CN VIII；p.480 参照）は内耳から内耳道を通って脳幹へ求心性のインパルスを伝える．内耳神経は前庭神経と蝸牛神経に分かれる．*Note*：半規管の感覚器は回転加速度に対応し，球形嚢斑と卵形嚢斑は水平方向と垂直方向の直線加速度に対応する．

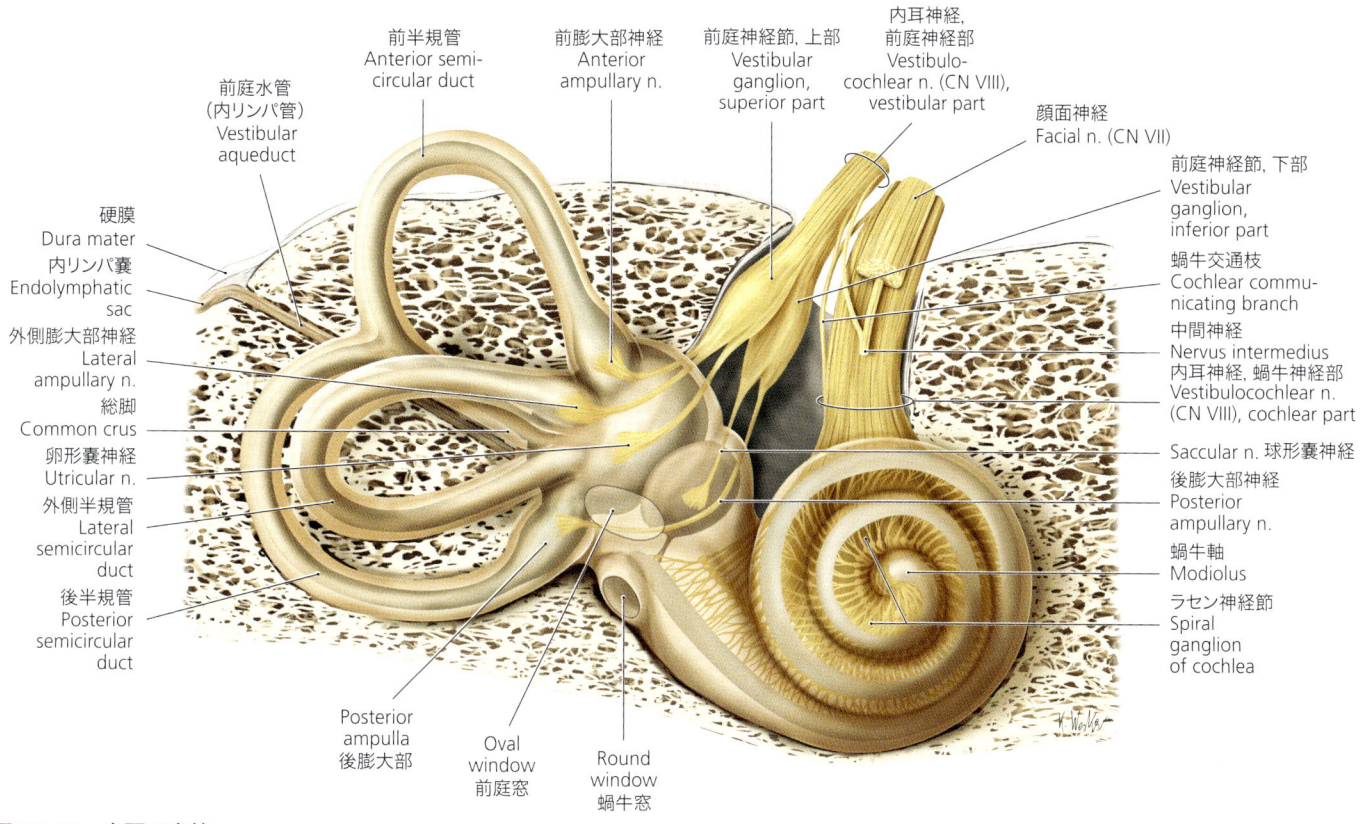

図 35.22 内耳の血管

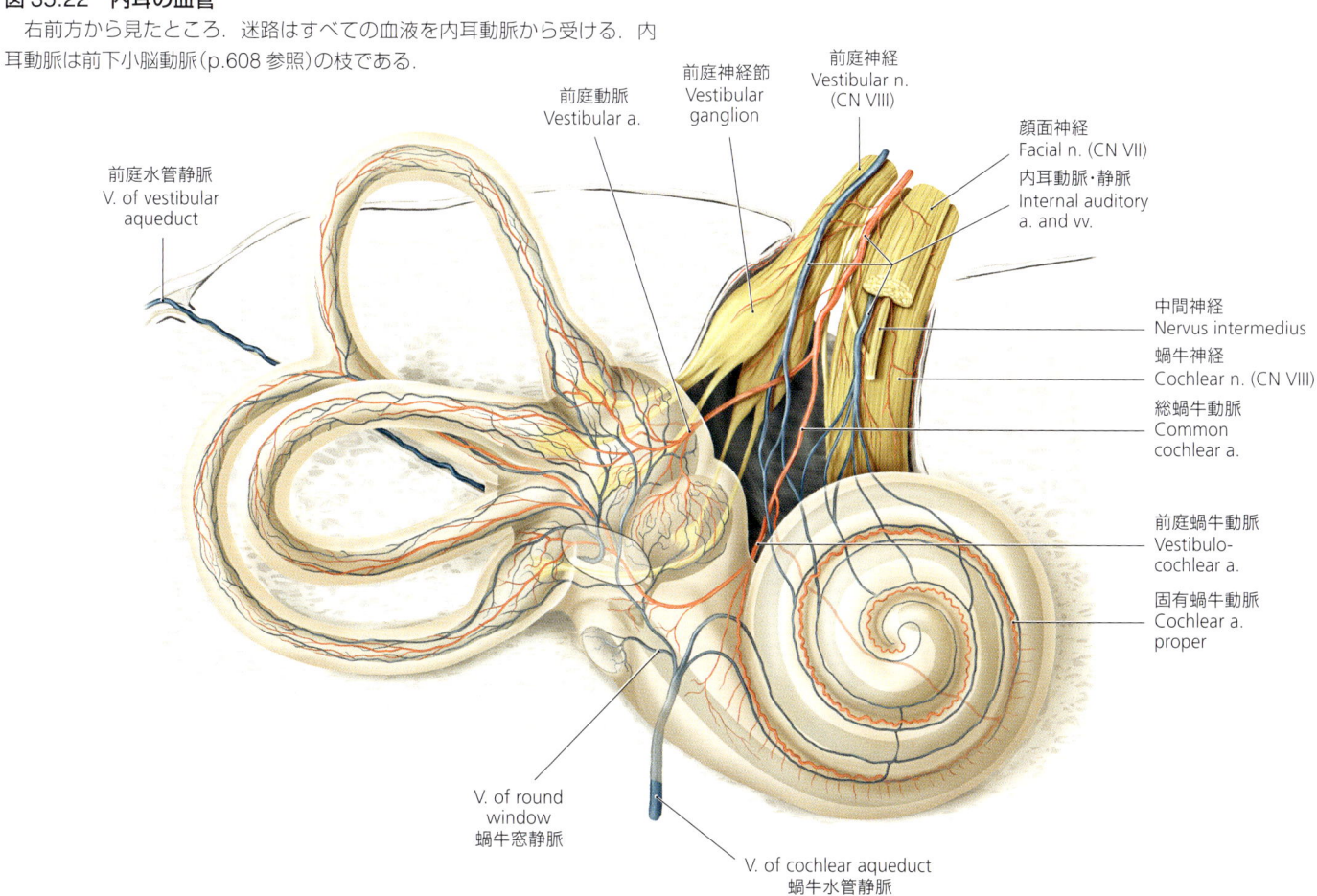

右前方から見たところ．迷路はすべての血液を内耳動脈から受ける．内耳動脈は前下小脳動脈（p.608 参照）の枝である．

口腔の骨
Bones of the Oral Cavity

鼻腔底（上顎骨と口蓋骨）は口蓋の上壁である硬口蓋を作る．上顎骨の水平方向の2つの突起（口蓋突起）が成長し，最終的には正中口蓋縫合で癒合する．癒合が不完全の場合には口蓋裂となる．

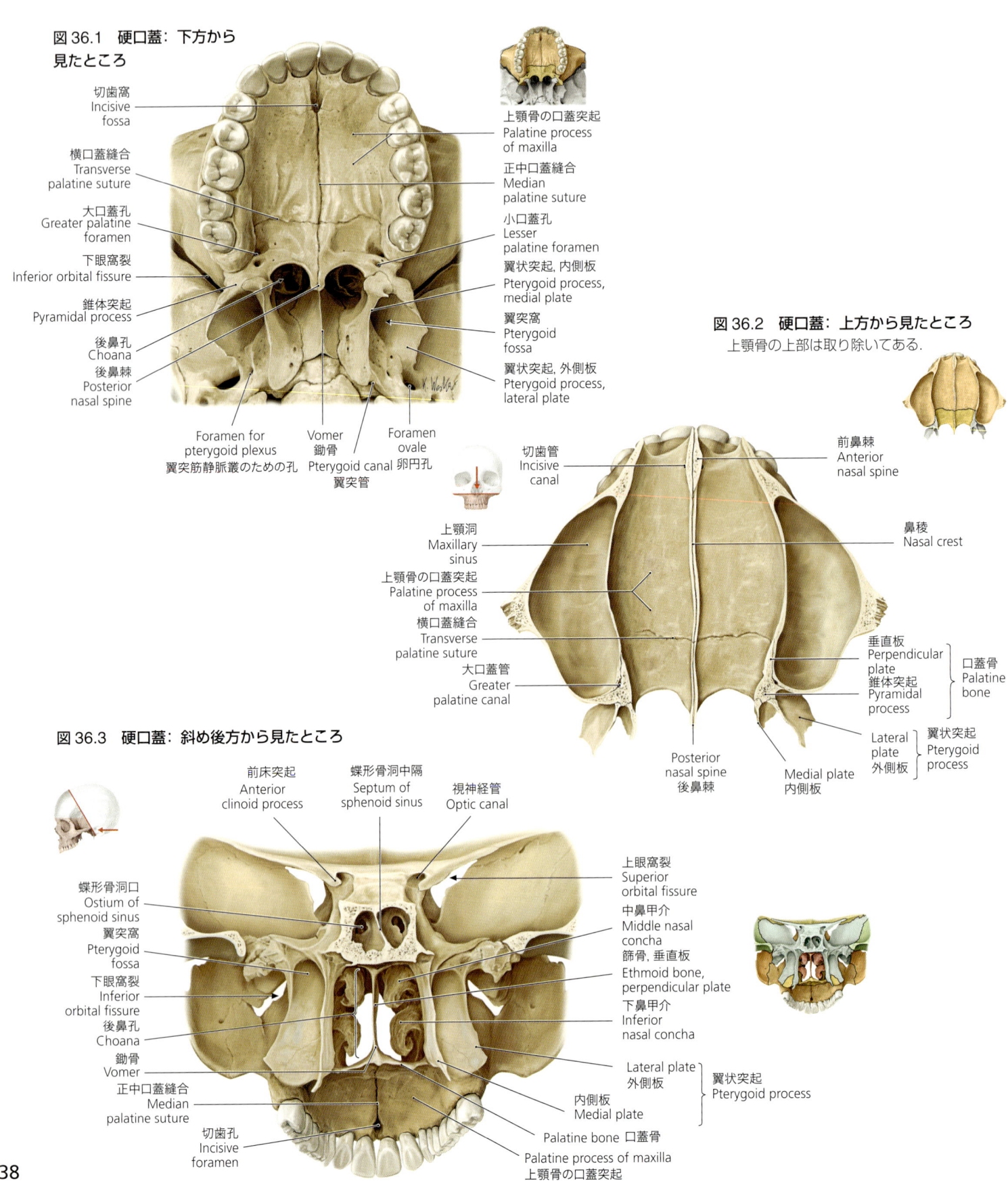

図36.1　硬口蓋：下方から見たところ

- 切歯窩 Incisive fossa
- 横口蓋縫合 Transverse palatine suture
- 大口蓋孔 Greater palatine foramen
- 下眼窩裂 Inferior orbital fissure
- 錐体突起 Pyramidal process
- 後鼻孔 Choana
- 後鼻棘 Posterior nasal spine
- 上顎骨の口蓋突起 Palatine process of maxilla
- 正中口蓋縫合 Median palatine suture
- 小口蓋孔 Lesser palatine foramen
- 翼状突起, 内側板 Pterygoid process, medial plate
- 翼突窩 Pterygoid fossa
- 翼状突起, 外側板 Pterygoid process, lateral plate
- 翼突筋静脈叢のための孔 Foramen for pterygoid plexus
- 鋤骨 Vomer
- 翼突管 Pterygoid canal
- 卵円孔 Foramen ovale

図36.2　硬口蓋：上方から見たところ
上顎骨の上部は取り除いてある．

- 切歯管 Incisive canal
- 前鼻棘 Anterior nasal spine
- 上顎洞 Maxillary sinus
- 鼻稜 Nasal crest
- 上顎骨の口蓋突起 Palatine process of maxilla
- 横口蓋縫合 Transverse palatine suture
- 大口蓋管 Greater palatine canal
- 後鼻棘 Posterior nasal spine
- 垂直板 Perpendicular plate
- 錐体突起 Pyramidal process
- 口蓋骨 Palatine bone
- 内側板 Medial plate
- 外側板 Lateral plate
- 翼状突起 Pterygoid process

図36.3　硬口蓋：斜め後方から見たところ

- 前床突起 Anterior clinoid process
- 蝶形骨洞中隔 Septum of sphenoid sinus
- 視神経管 Optic canal
- 蝶形骨洞口 Ostium of sphenoid sinus
- 翼突窩 Pterygoid fossa
- 下眼窩裂 Inferior orbital fissure
- 後鼻孔 Choana
- 鋤骨 Vomer
- 正中口蓋縫合 Median palatine suture
- 切歯孔 Incisive foramen
- 上眼窩裂 Superior orbital fissure
- 中鼻甲介 Middle nasal concha
- 篩骨, 垂直板 Ethmoid bone, perpendicular plate
- 下鼻甲介 Inferior nasal concha
- 外側板 Lateral plate
- 内側板 Medial plate
- 口蓋骨 Palatine bone
- 上顎骨の口蓋突起 Palatine process of maxilla
- 翼状突起 Pterygoid process

A 前方から見たところ．

図 36.4 下顎骨
下顎骨は顎関節(p.540)によって顔面頭蓋(内臓頭蓋)と連結している．

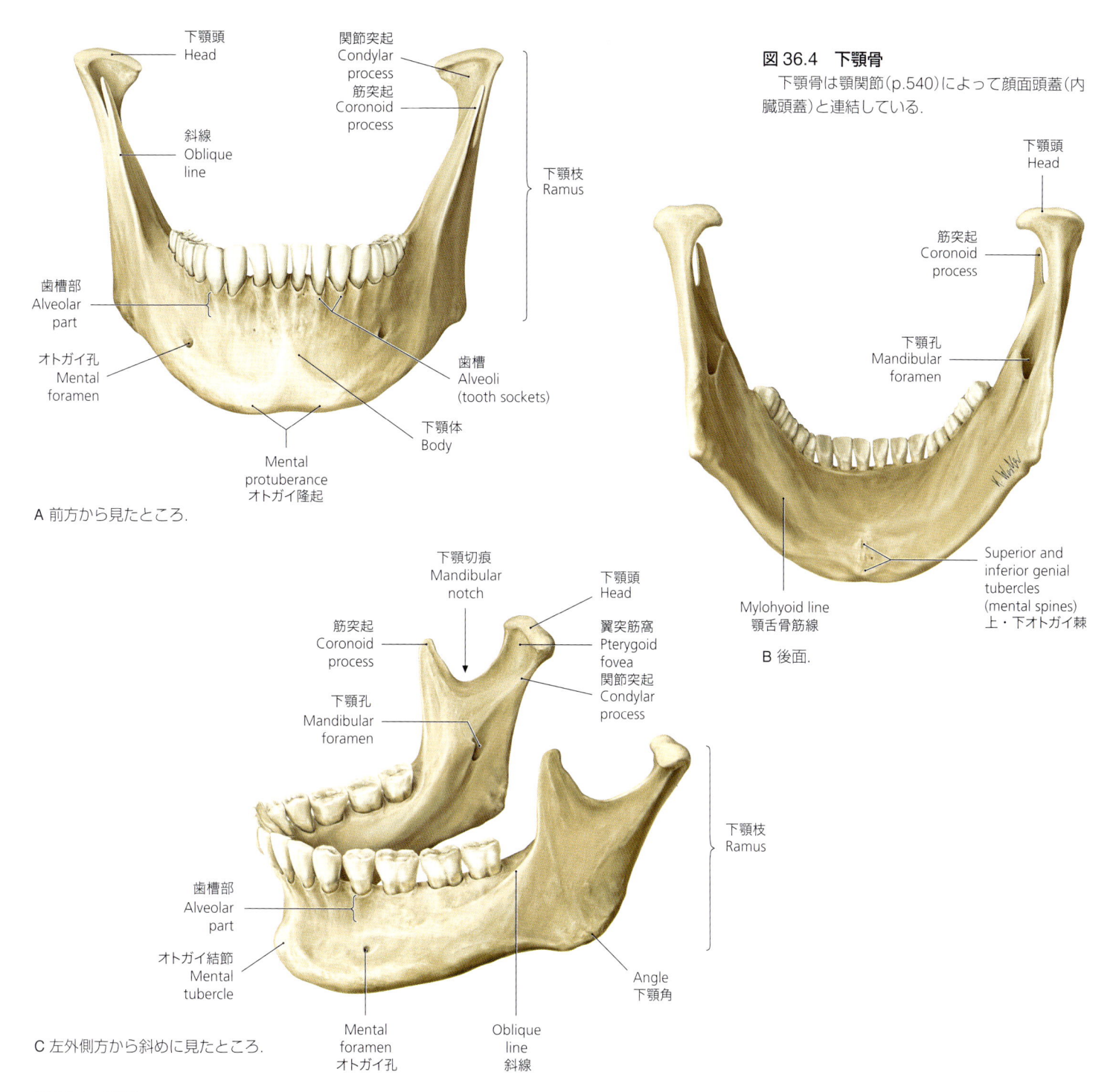

B 後面．

C 左外側方から斜めに見たところ．

図 36.5 舌骨
舌骨は口腔底と喉頭をつなぐ筋によって吊り下げられて頸部にある．頭蓋の骨と見なされない場合もあるが，舌骨は口腔底の筋肉の付着部となっている．大角と体は頸部で触知できる．

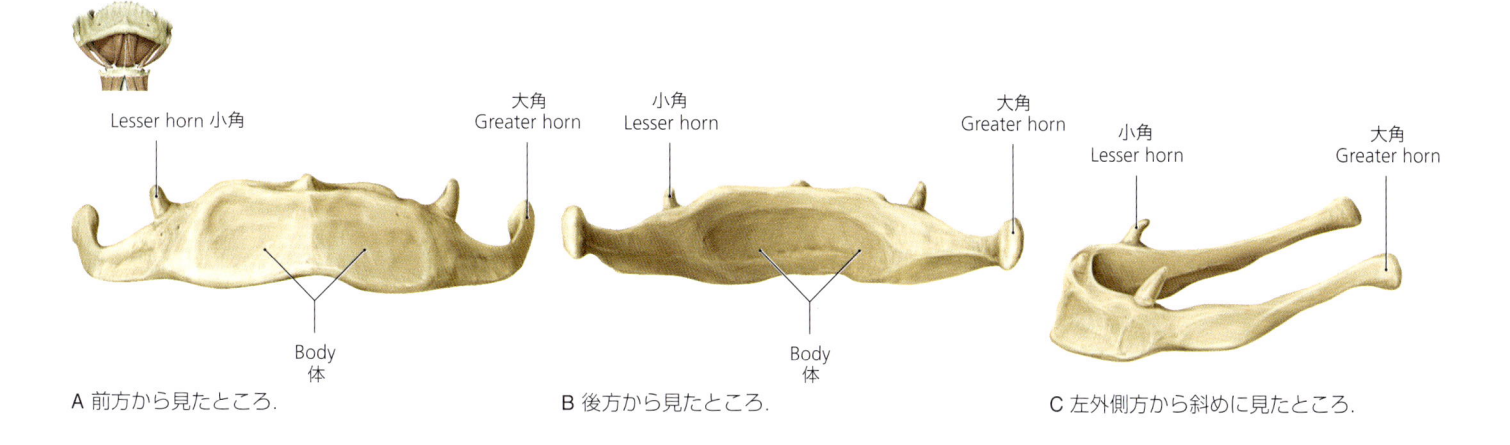

A 前方から見たところ．　　B 後方から見たところ．　　C 左外側方から斜めに見たところ．

顎関節
Temporomandibular joint

図 36.6 顎関節
顎関節では，下顎頭が下顎窩と関節を作る．

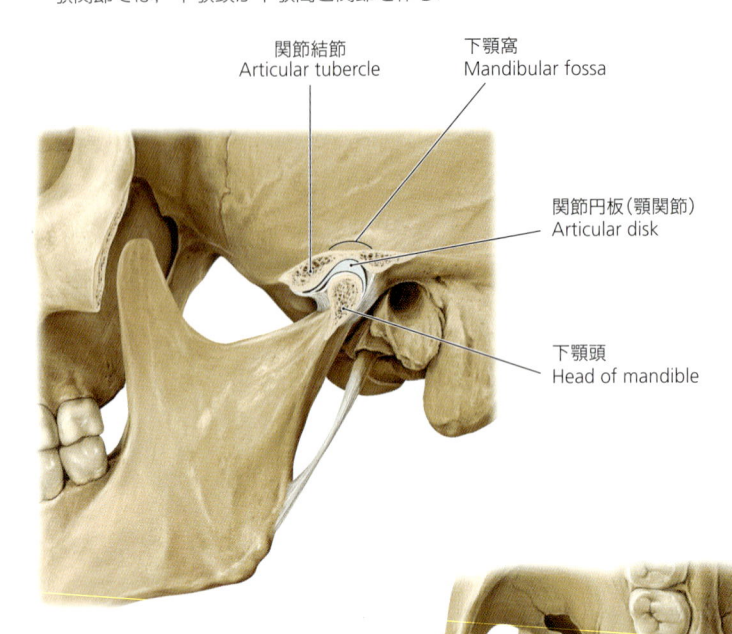

- 関節結節 Articular tubercle
- 下顎窩 Mandibular fossa
- 関節円板（顎関節） Articular disk
- 下顎頭 Head of mandible

A 左外側方から見たところ．顎関節は矢状方向に切開してある．

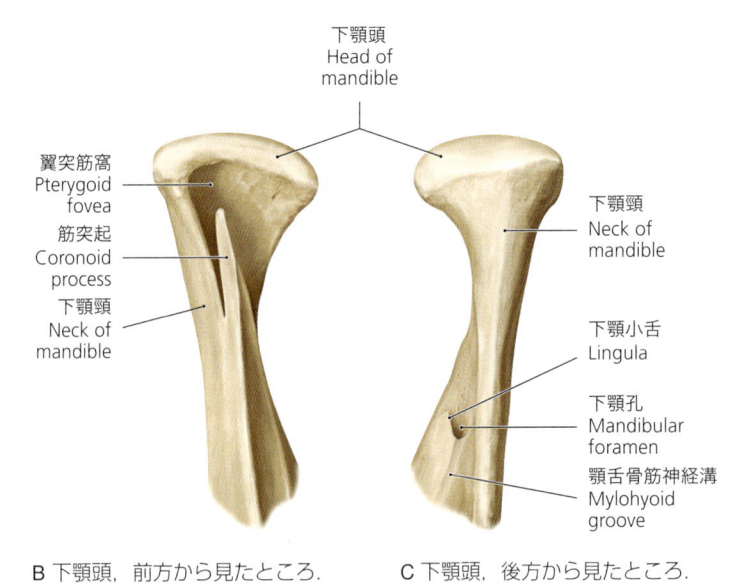

- 下顎頭 Head of mandible
- 翼突筋窩 Pterygoid fovea
- 筋突起 Coronoid process
- 下顎頸 Neck of mandible
- 下顎頸 Neck of mandible
- 下顎小舌 Lingula
- 下顎孔 Mandibular foramen
- 顎舌骨筋神経溝 Mylohyoid groove

B 下顎頭，前方から見たところ．

C 下顎頭，後方から見たところ．

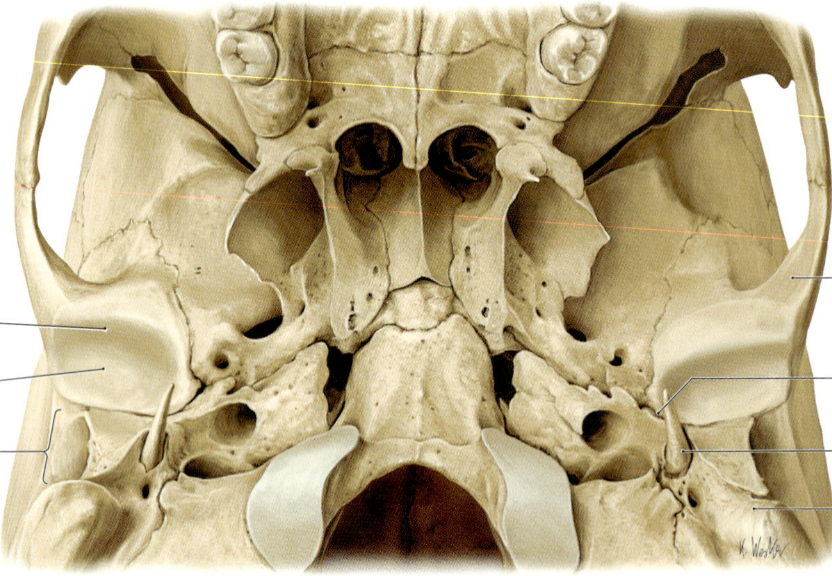

- 関節結節 Articular tubercle
- 下顎窩 Mandibular fossa
- 外耳道 External acoustic meatus (auditory canal)
- 側頭骨の頬骨突起 Zygomatic process of temporal bone
- 錐体鼓室裂 Petrotympanic fissure
- 茎状突起 Styloid process
- 乳様突起 Mastoid process

D 顎関節の下顎窩．下方から見たところ．

図 36.7 顎関節の靱帯

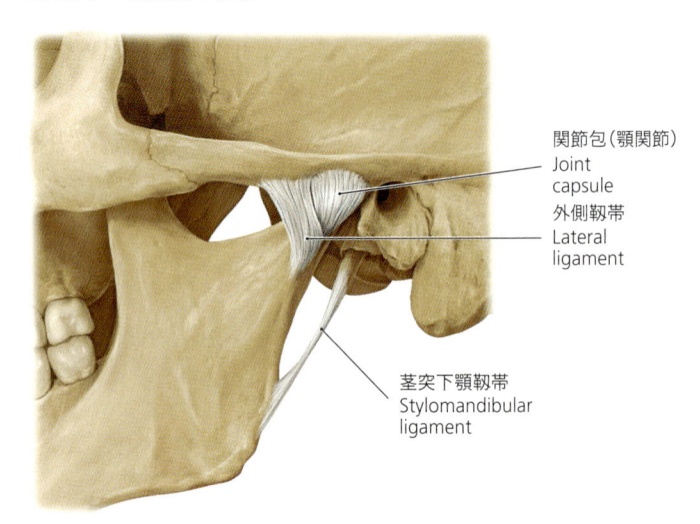

- 関節包（顎関節） Joint capsule
- 外側靱帯 Lateral ligament
- 茎突下顎靱帯 Stylomandibular ligament

A 左の顎関節，外側方から見たところ．

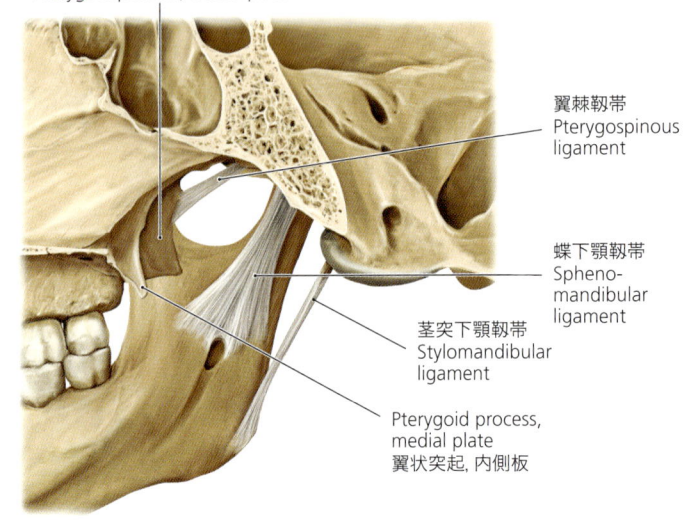

- 翼状突起，外側板 Pterygoid process, lateral plate
- 翼棘靱帯 Pterygospinous ligament
- 蝶下顎靱帯 Sphenomandibular ligament
- 茎突下顎靱帯 Stylomandibular ligament
- 翼状突起，内側板 Pterygoid process, medial plate

B 右の顎関節，内側方から見たところ．

図 36.8　顎関節の運動
左外側方から見たところ．15°までの開口では，下顎頭は下顎窩の中に留まっている．15°以上の開口では，下顎頭は前方に滑走し関節結節上にある．

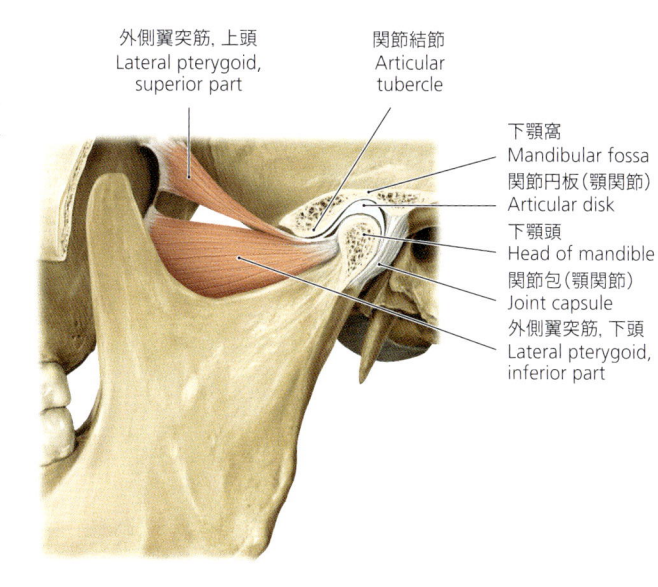

外側翼突筋, 上頭
Lateral pterygoid, superior part

関節結節
Articular tubercle

下顎窩
Mandibular fossa

関節円板（顎関節）
Articular disk

下顎頭
Head of mandible

関節包（顎関節）
Joint capsule

外側翼突筋, 下頭
Lateral pterygoid, inferior part

A 閉口時．

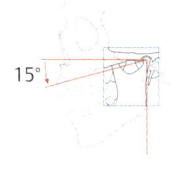

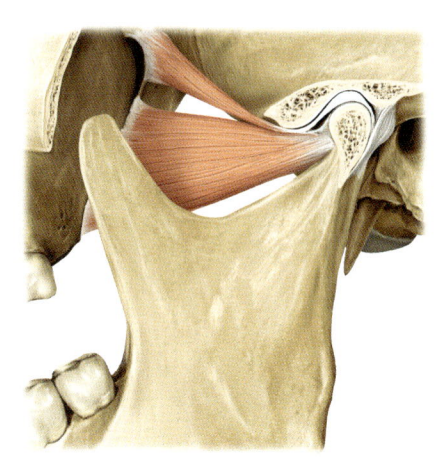

B 15°までの開口時．

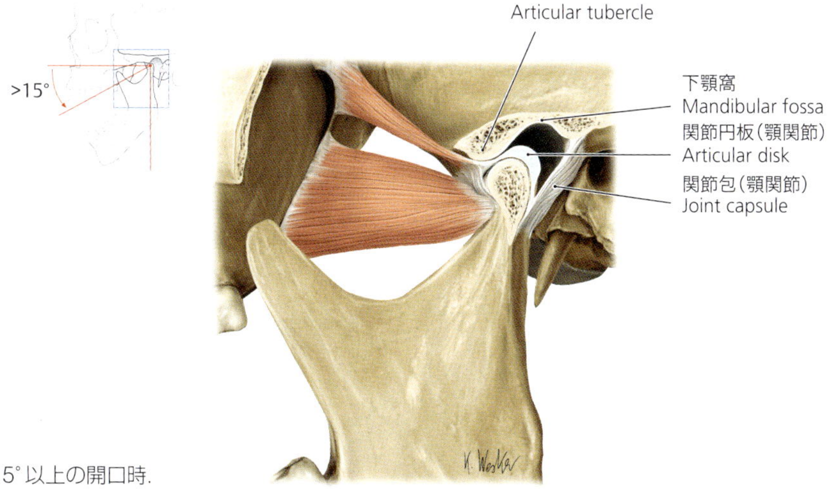

関節結節
Articular tubercle

下顎窩
Mandibular fossa

関節円板（顎関節）
Articular disk

関節包（顎関節）
Joint capsule

C 15°以上の開口時．

臨床

顎関節の脱臼
下顎頭が関節結節を超えて，脱臼が生じることがある．この場合に下顎骨は突出位で固定され，下顎の歯列を押すことで整復される．

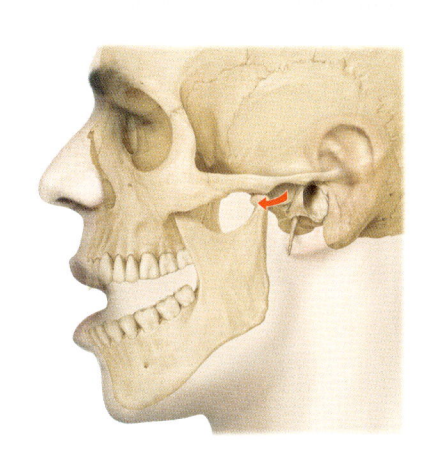

図 36.9　顎関節の関節包の神経支配
上方から見たところ．

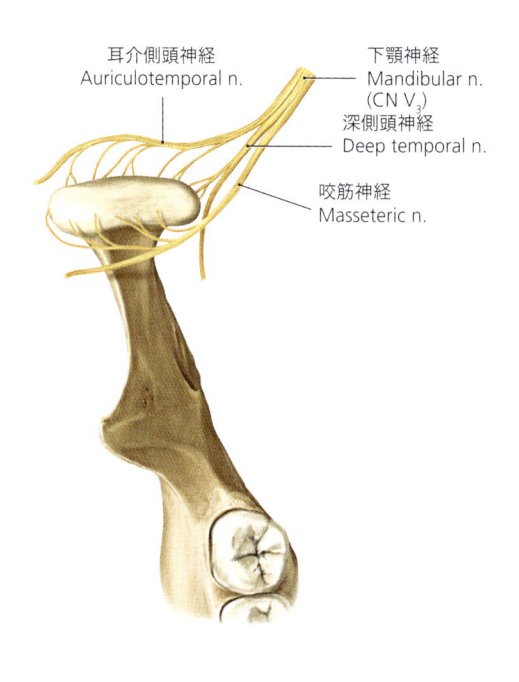

耳介側頭神経
Auriculotemporal n.

下顎神経
Mandibular n. (CN V_3)

深側頭神経
Deep temporal n.

咬筋神経
Masseteric n.

歯
Teeth

図 36.10 歯の構造
歯は，硬組織（エナメル質，象牙質，セメント質）と軟組織（歯髄）からなり，歯冠，歯頸，歯根に分けられる．

歯冠 Crown
歯頸 Neck
歯根 Root

A 歯の主要な部分．

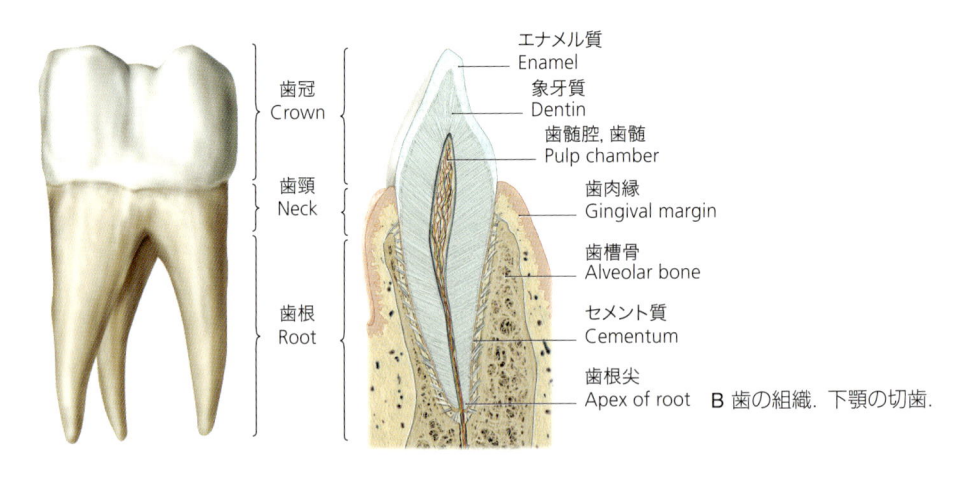

エナメル質 Enamel
象牙質 Dentin
歯髄腔，歯髄 Pulp chamber
歯肉縁 Gingival margin
歯槽骨 Alveolar bone
セメント質 Cementum
歯根尖 Apex of root

B 歯の組織．下顎の切歯．

図 36.11 永久歯
上顎と下顎の左右半側には，3本の前歯（2本の切歯，1本の犬歯）と5本の臼歯（2本の小臼歯，3本の大臼歯）がある．

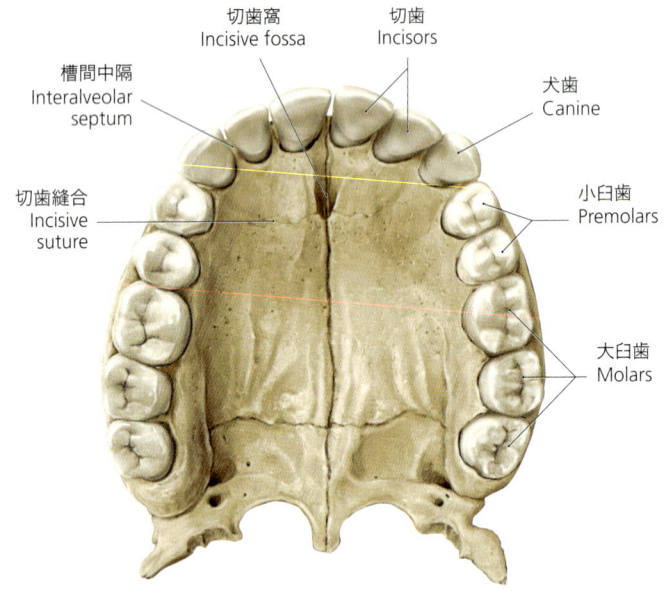

切歯窩 Incisive fossa
切歯 Incisors
槽間中隔 Interalveolar septum
犬歯 Canine
切歯縫合 Incisive suture
小臼歯 Premolars
大臼歯 Molars

A 上顎の歯．下方から見たところ．

大臼歯 Molars
小臼歯 Premolars
犬歯 Canine
Interalveolar septum 槽間中隔
Incisors 切歯

B 下顎の歯．上方から見たところ．

図 36.12 歯の面．
歯の上面は咬合面として知られている．

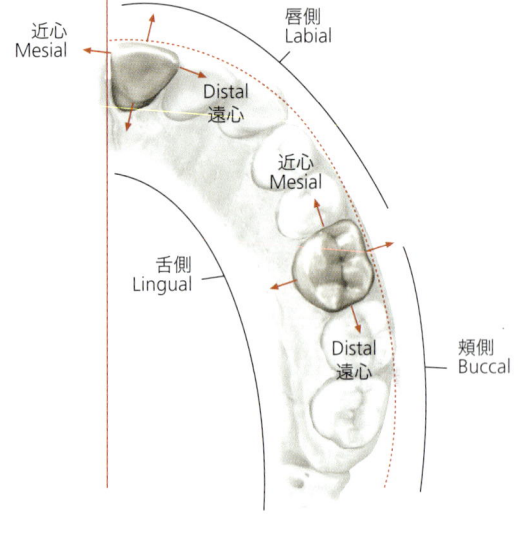

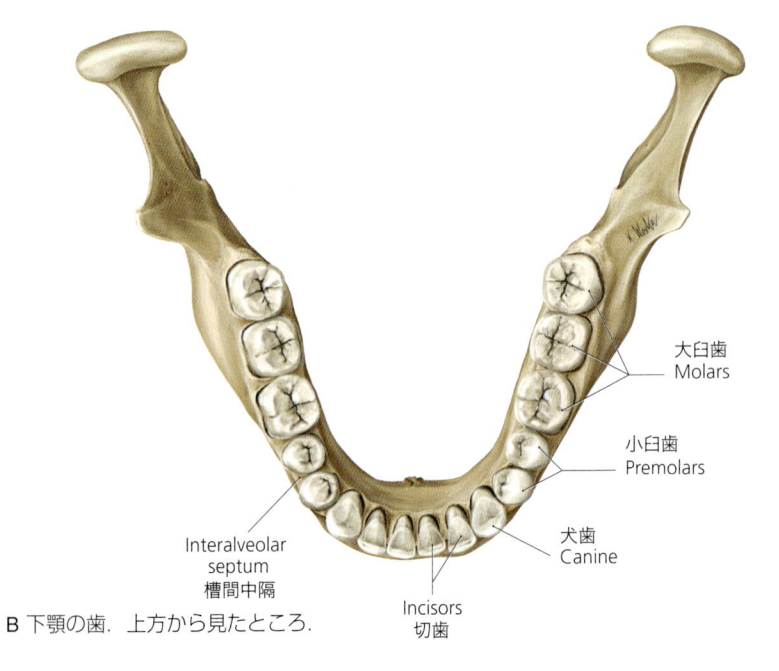

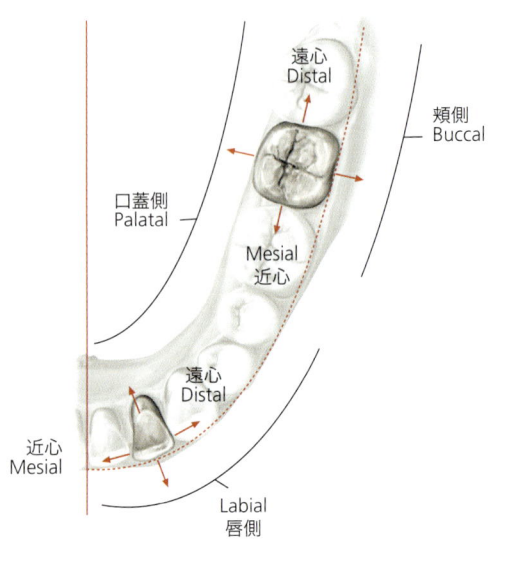

近心 Mesial
唇側 Labial
遠心 Distal
近心 Mesial
舌側 Lingual
遠心 Distal
頬側 Buccal

遠心 Distal
頬側 Buccal
口蓋側 Palatal
近心 Mesial
遠心 Distal
近心 Mesial
唇側 Labial

図 36.13 歯の記号
アメリカでは，32本の永久歯は，上下左右の4域に分けずに数える．

Note: 20本の乳歯は，上顎で右から左にAからJ，下顎で左から右にKからTと表される．上顎の右第2小臼歯はAである．

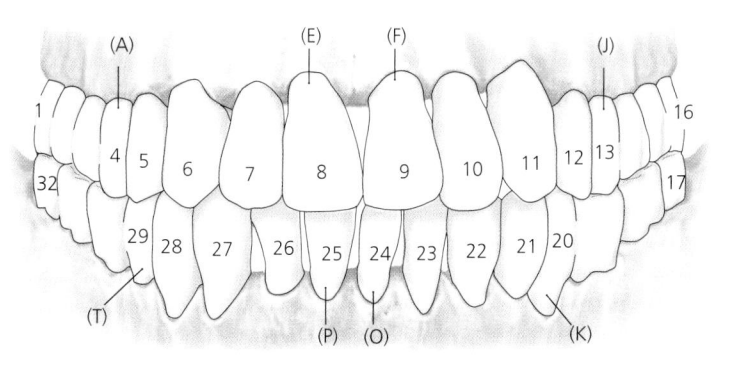

図 36.14 歯のパノラマ断層像
歯のパノラマ断層像(DPT)は，顎関節，上顎洞，上・下顎骨および歯の状態(齲歯の病変や智歯の位置など)を予備的に知ることができる．(断層写真，Dr. U. J. Rother, Director of the Department of Diagnostic Radiology, Center for Dentistry and Oromaxillofacial Surgery, Eppendorf University Medical Center, Hamburg, Germany のご厚意による)

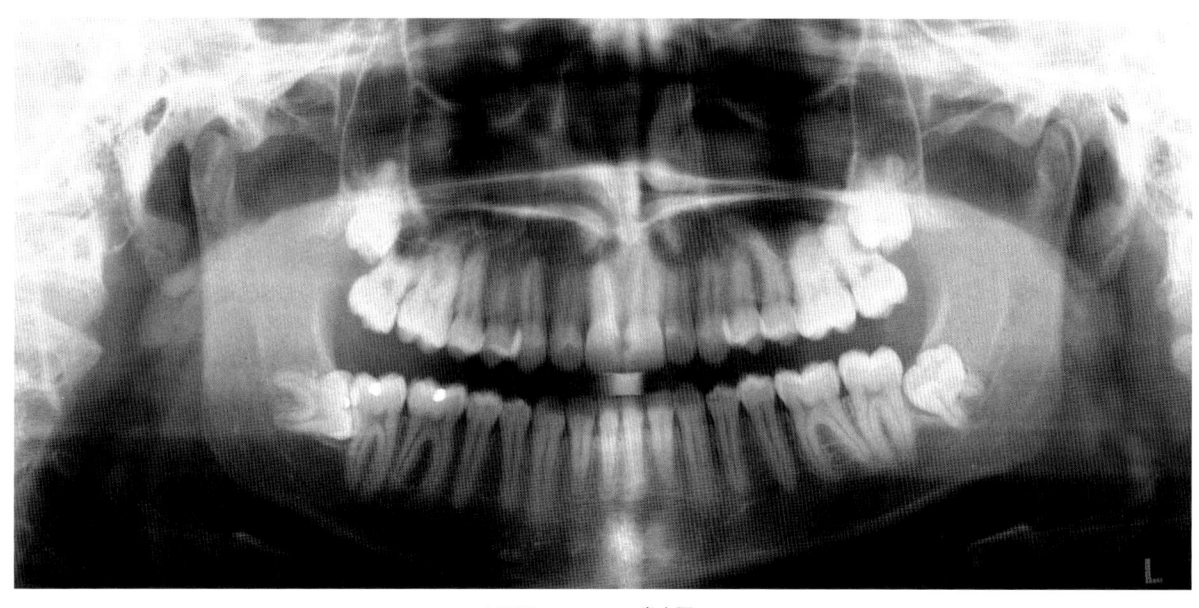

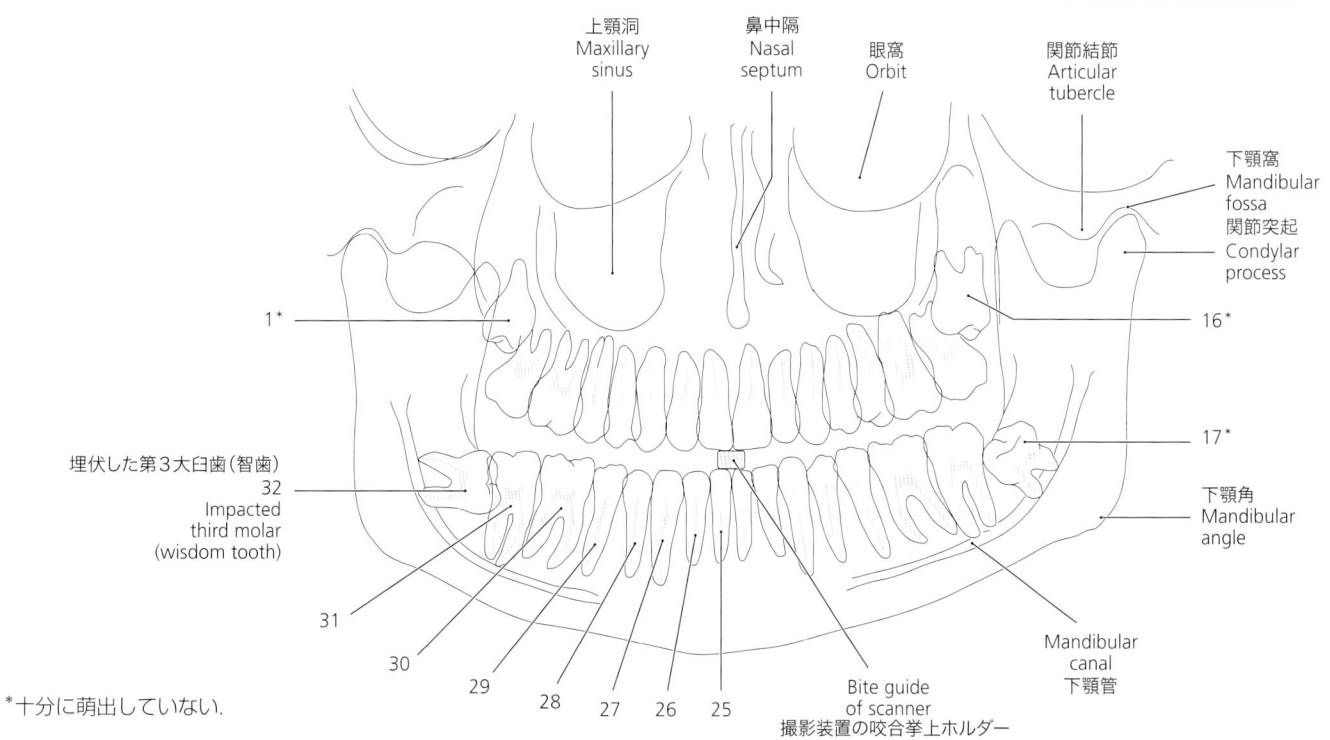

上顎洞 Maxillary sinus
鼻中隔 Nasal septum
眼窩 Orbit
関節結節 Articular tubercle
下顎窩 Mandibular fossa
関節突起 Condylar process
埋伏した第3大臼歯(智歯) Impacted third molar (wisdom tooth)
下顎角 Mandibular angle
下顎管 Mandibular canal
Bite guide of scanner 撮影装置の咬合挙上ホルダー

*十分に萌出していない．

口腔の筋
Oral Cavity Muscle Facts

図 36.15 口腔底の筋
舌骨下筋群は pp.562-563 参照.

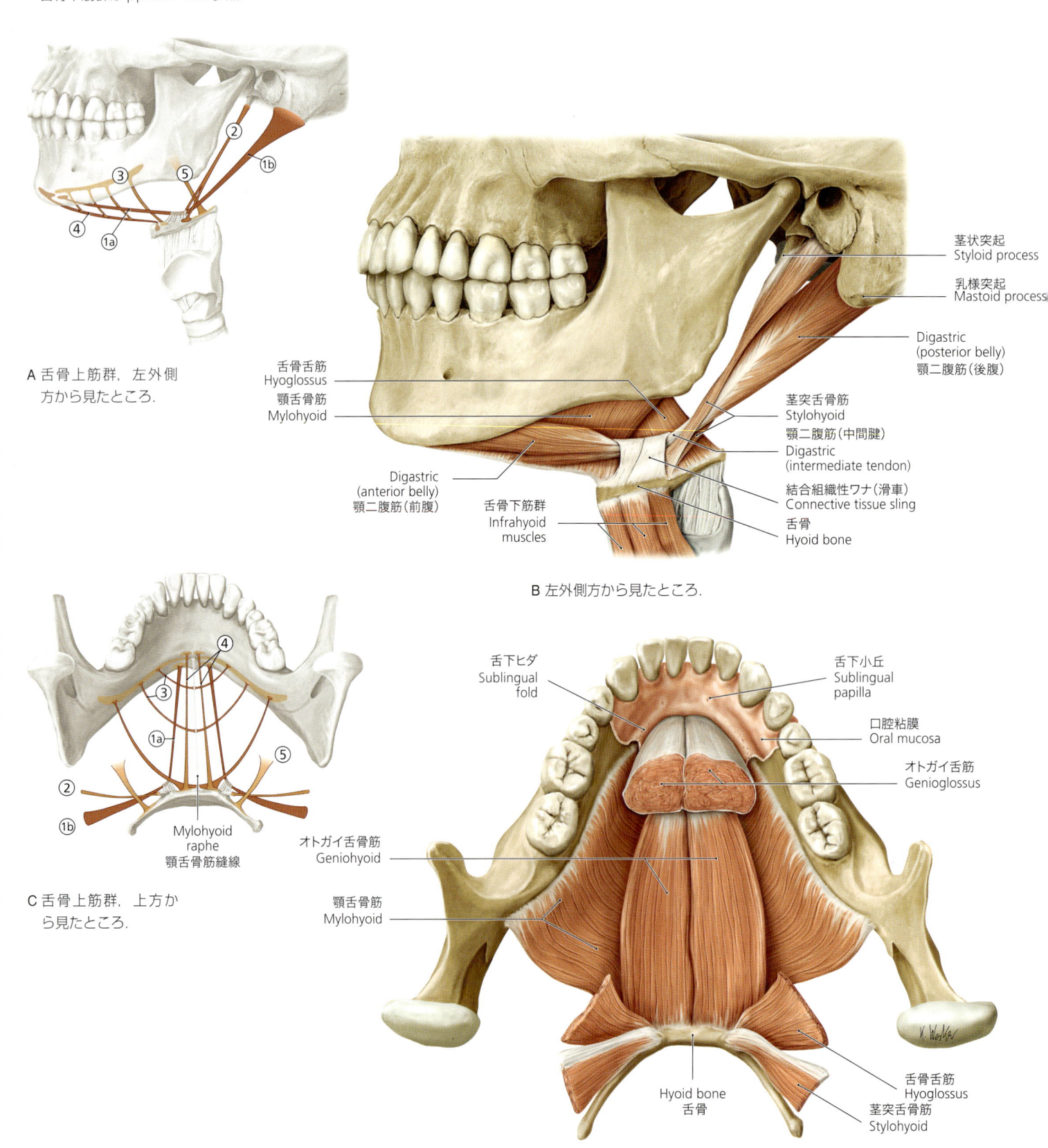

A 舌骨上筋群, 左外側方から見たところ.

C 舌骨上筋群, 上方から見たところ.

Mylohyoid raphe
顎舌骨筋縫線

B 左外側方から見たところ.

- 茎状突起 Styloid process
- 乳様突起 Mastoid process
- 舌骨舌筋 Hyoglossus
- 顎舌骨筋 Mylohyoid
- 顎二腹筋(前腹) Digastric (anterior belly)
- 舌骨下筋群 Infrahyoid muscles
- 顎二腹筋(後腹) Digastric (posterior belly)
- 茎突舌骨筋 Stylohyoid
- 顎二腹筋(中間腱) Digastric (intermediate tendon)
- 結合組織性ワナ(滑車) Connective tissue sling
- 舌骨 Hyoid bone

D 下顎骨と舌骨, 上方から見たところ.

- 舌下ヒダ Sublingual fold
- 舌下小丘 Sublingual papilla
- 口腔粘膜 Oral mucosa
- オトガイ舌筋 Genioglossus
- オトガイ舌骨筋 Geniohyoid
- 顎舌骨筋 Mylohyoid
- 舌骨 Hyoid bone
- 舌骨舌筋 Hyoglossus
- 茎突舌骨筋 Stylohyoid

表36.1　舌骨上筋

筋肉		起始	停止		神経支配	作用
①顎二腹筋	ⓐ前腹	下顎骨の二腹筋窩	線維性の滑車を伴う中間腱を介して停止	舌骨体	下顎神経の枝の顎舌骨筋神経	嚥下時に舌骨を挙上し，下顎の開口を補助する
	ⓑ後腹	側頭骨の乳様突起内側にある乳突切痕			顔面神経	
②茎突舌骨筋		側頭骨の茎状突起	分裂した腱を介して停止			
③顎舌骨筋		下顎骨の顎舌骨筋線	正中腱を介して停止（顎舌骨筋縫線）		下顎神経の枝の顎舌骨筋神経	口腔底を持ち上げ，緊張させる．嚥下時に舌骨を前方に引き，下顎の開口を助ける．咀嚼時に下顎の側方運動を助ける
④オトガイ舌骨筋		下顎骨の下オトガイ棘	舌骨体に停止		舌下神経（CN XII）を経由する第1頸神経（C1）の前枝	嚥下時に舌骨を前方に引き，下顎の開口を助ける
⑤舌骨舌筋		舌骨大角の上縁	舌の側方		舌下神経（CN XII）	舌を押し下げる

図36.16　軟口蓋の筋

下方から見たところ．軟口蓋は口腔の後部の境界を成し，口腔と咽頭を区分している．

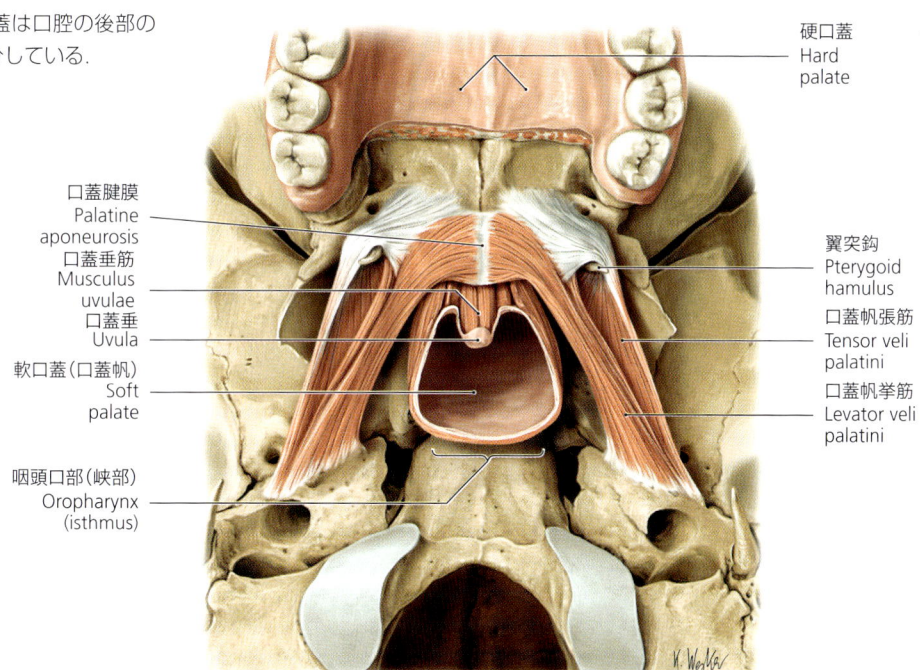

表36.2　軟口蓋の筋肉

筋	起始	停止	神経支配	作用
口蓋帆張筋	翼状突起内側板の舟状窩，蝶形骨棘，耳管軟骨	口蓋腱膜	内側翼突筋神経（下顎神経の枝で耳神経節を経由する）	軟口蓋を緊張させる．嚥下時やあくび時に耳管開口部を開く
口蓋帆挙筋	耳管軟骨，側頭骨岩様部		咽頭神経叢（迷走神経 CN X）を経由する副神経（CN XI）の延髄根	軟口蓋を水平位まで持ち上げる
口蓋垂筋	口蓋垂の粘膜	口蓋腱膜，後鼻棘		口蓋垂を持ち上げ，短くする
口蓋舌筋*	舌の側方	口蓋腱膜		舌後部を持ち上げる．軟口蓋を舌へ牽引する
口蓋咽頭筋*				軟口蓋を緊張させる．嚥下時に咽頭壁を上方・前方・内側に引く

* pp.548，555参照．

口腔の神経支配
Innervation of the Oral Cavity

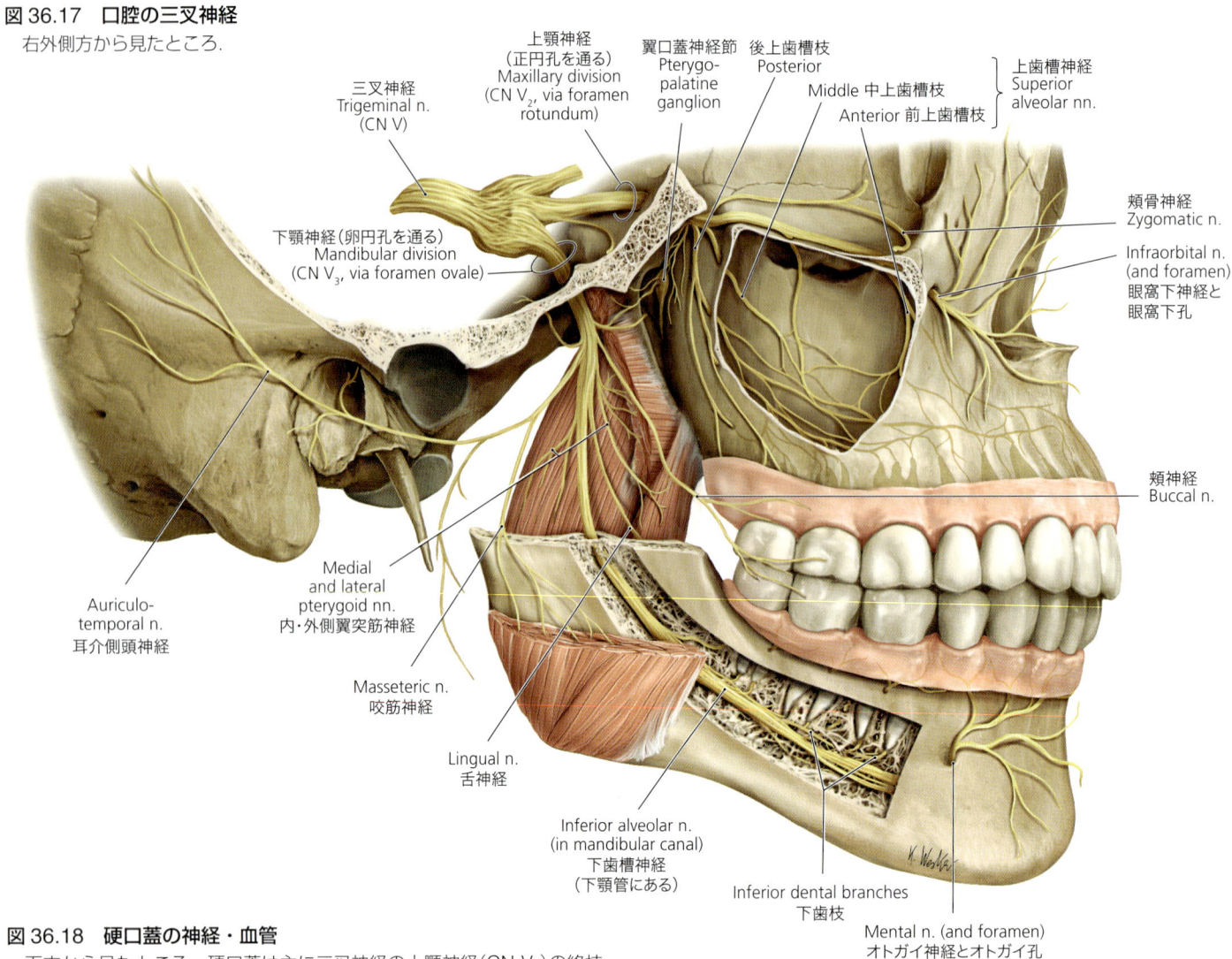

図 36.17　口腔の三叉神経
右外側方から見たところ．

図 36.18　硬口蓋の神経・血管
下方から見たところ．硬口蓋は主に三叉神経の上顎神経（CN V₂）の終枝によって感覚性神経支配を受ける．硬口蓋の動脈は，顎動脈から起こる．

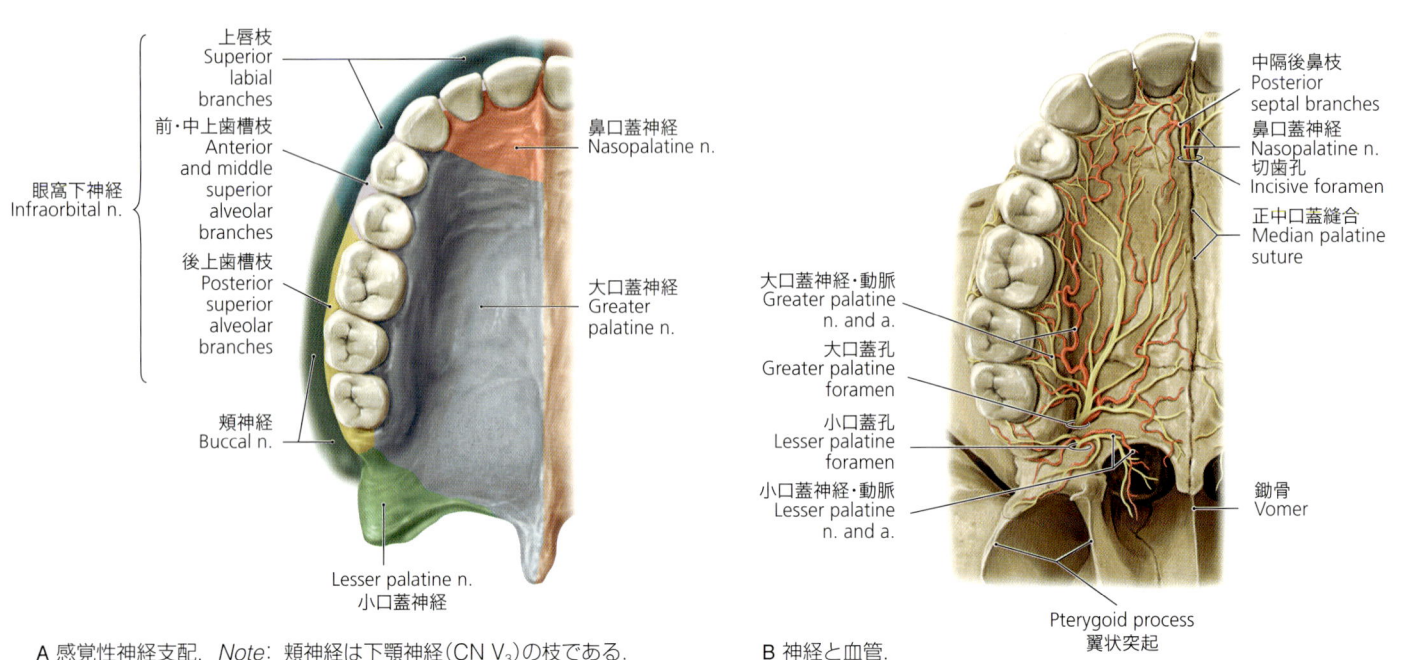

A 感覚性神経支配．*Note*：頬神経は下顎神経（CN V₃）の枝である．　　B 神経と血管．

口腔底の筋肉の神経支配は複雑で，三叉神経（CN V₃），顔面神経（CN VII），舌下神経（CN XII）を経由する第1頸神経によって支配される．

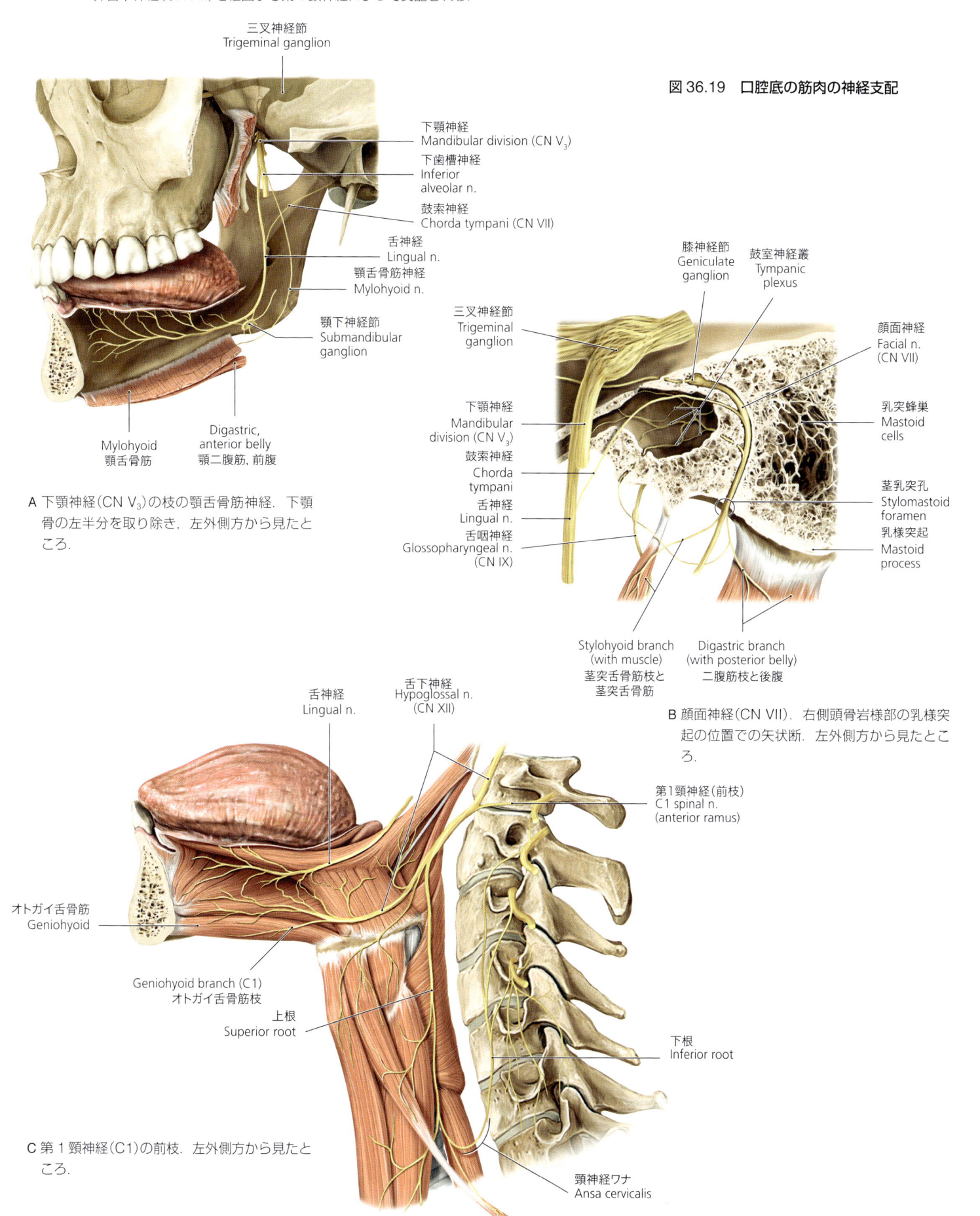

図 36.19　口腔底の筋肉の神経支配

A　下顎神経（CN V₃）の枝の顎舌骨筋神経．下顎骨の左半分を取り除き，左外側方から見たところ．

B　顔面神経（CN VII）．右側頭骨岩様部の乳様突起の位置での矢状断．左外側方から見たところ．

C　第1頸神経（C1）の前枝．左外側方から見たところ．

舌
Tongue

舌背は感覚機能（味覚と微細な触覚識別，p.616参照）を助ける高度に分化した粘膜で覆われている．舌には咀嚼，嚥下，発語において舌の運動機能を助ける非常に強力な筋肉が備わっている．

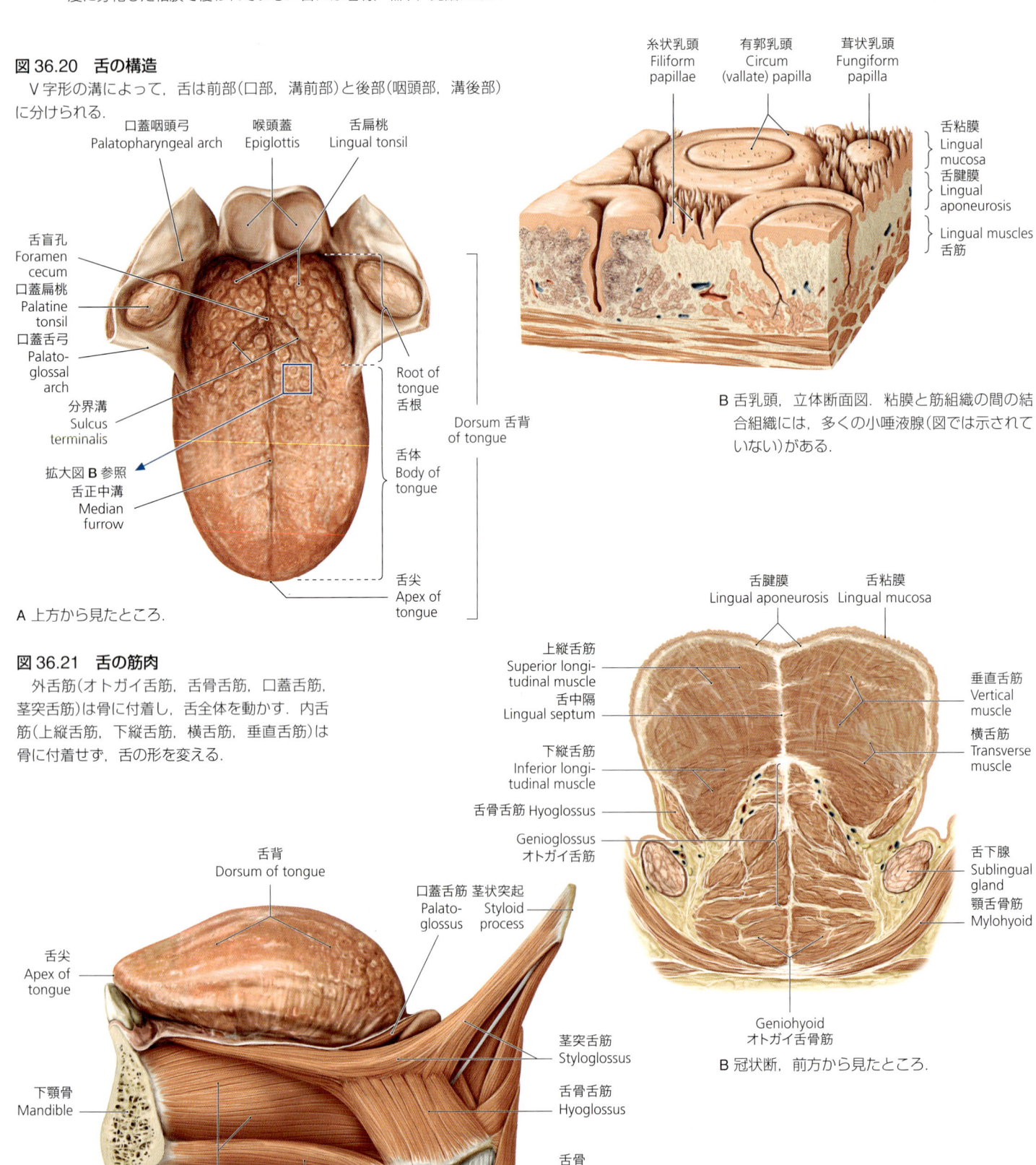

図 36.20 舌の構造
V字形の溝によって，舌は前部（口部，溝前部）と後部（咽頭部，溝後部）に分けられる．

A 上方から見たところ．

B 舌乳頭，立体断面図．粘膜と筋組織の間の結合組織には，多くの小唾液腺（図では示されていない）がある．

図 36.21 舌の筋肉
外舌筋（オトガイ舌筋，舌骨舌筋，口蓋舌筋，茎突舌筋）は骨に付着し，舌全体を動かす．内舌筋（上縦舌筋，下縦舌筋，横舌筋，垂直舌筋）は骨に付着せず，舌の形を変える．

A 左外側方から見たところ．

B 冠状断，前方から見たところ．

図 36.22 舌の体性感覚性神経支配と味覚神経支配
前方から見たところ．

図 36.23 舌の神経・血管
口蓋舌筋は迷走神経（CN X）から体性運動性の神経支配を受ける．他の舌筋は舌下神経（CN XII）に支配される．

味覚 Taste
- 迷走神経 Vagus n. (CN X)
- 舌咽神経 Glossopharyngeal n. (CN IX)
- 顔面神経（鼓索神経経由）Facial n. (CN VII, via chorda tympani)

体性感覚 Somatic sensation
- 迷走神経 Vagus n. (CN X)
- 舌咽神経 Glossopharyngeal n. (CN IX)
- 舌神経（下顎神経）Lingual n. (mandibular n., CN V₃)

- 舌尖 Apex of tongue
- 前舌腺 Anterior lingual glands
- 舌小帯 Frenulum
- 舌下ヒダ Sublingual fold
- 舌下小丘 Sublingual papilla
- 舌深動脈・静脈 Deep lingual a. and v.
- 舌神経 Lingual n.
- 顎下腺管 Submandibular duct

A 舌を下方から見たところ．

- 舌深動脈 Deep lingual a.
- 舌神経 Lingual n. (CN V₃)
- 茎状突起 Styloid process
- 舌咽神経 Glossopharyngeal n. (CN IX)
- 顎下神経節 Submandibular ganglion
- 舌下神経 Hypoglossal n. (CN XII)
- 舌動脈（外頸動脈から）Lingual a. (from external carotid a.)
- 舌静脈（内頸静脈に向かう）Lingual v. (to internal jugular v.)
- 舌骨 Hyoid bone
- 下顎骨 Mandible
- オトガイ下動脈・静脈 Submental a. and v.
- 舌下動脈 Sublingual a.

B 左外側方から見たところ．

臨床

片側性の舌下神経麻痺
舌下神経の障害によって，障害を受けた側のオトガイ舌筋が麻痺し，障害を受けていない側の健常なオトガイ舌筋が優位になる．舌を突出させると，麻痺側へ偏位する．

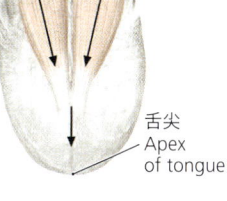

A 正常な舌下神経による舌の能動的突出．
- 舌尖 Apex of tongue

B 片側の舌下神経障害による舌の能動的突出．
- ①患側の麻痺したオトガイ舌筋
- ① Paralyzed genioglossus on affected side

口腔と唾液腺の局所解剖
Topography of the Oral Cavity & Salivary Glands

口腔は鼻腔の下方にあり，咽頭の前方に位置する．口腔は硬口蓋と軟口蓋，舌，口腔底の筋肉，口蓋垂で囲まれる．

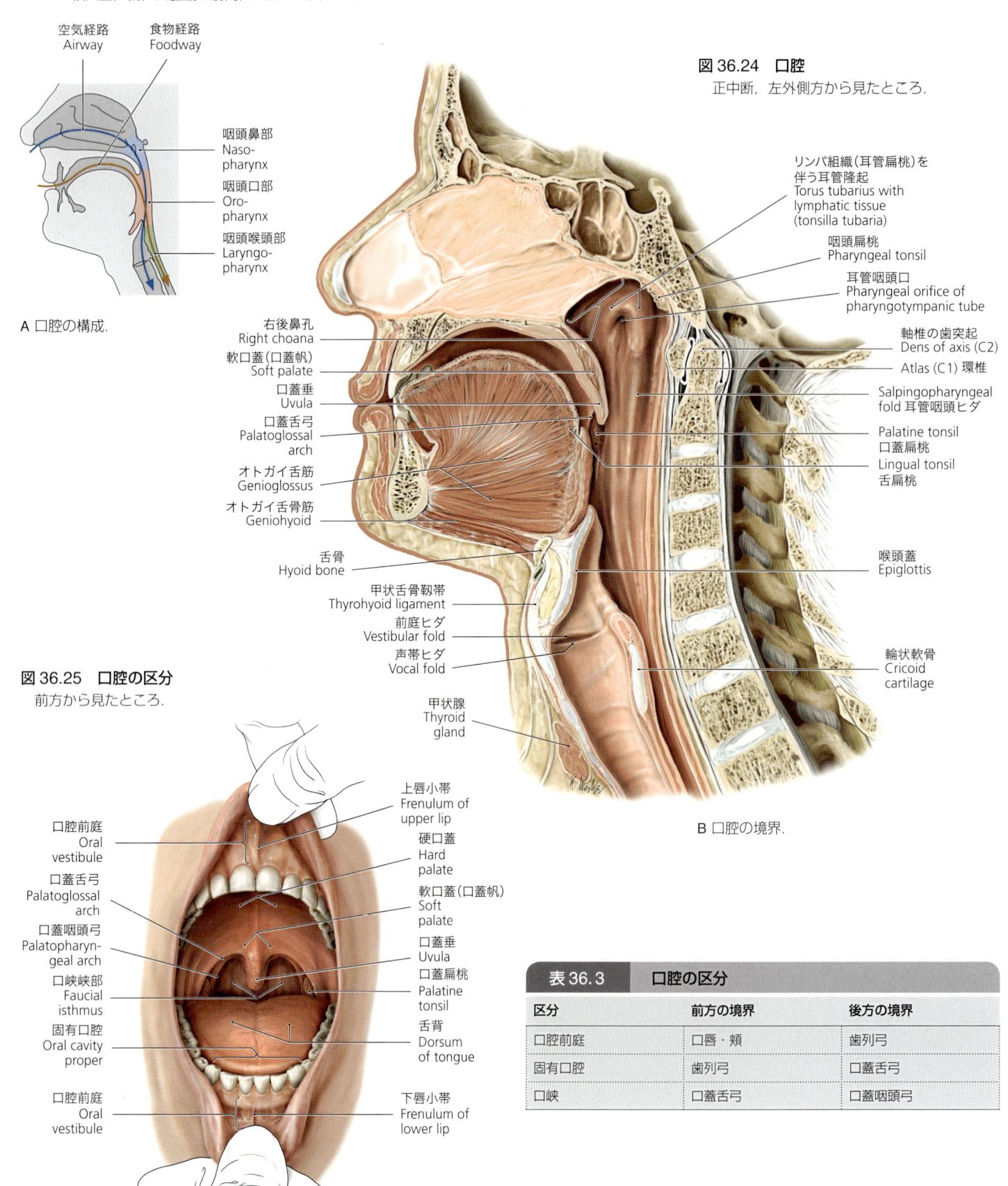

A 口腔の構成．

- 空気経路 Airway
- 食物経路 Foodway
- 咽頭鼻部 Nasopharynx
- 咽頭口部 Oropharynx
- 咽頭喉頭部 Laryngopharynx

図 36.24　口腔
正中断，左外側方から見たところ．

- リンパ組織（耳管扁桃）を伴う耳管隆起 Torus tubarius with lymphatic tissue (tonsilla tubaria)
- 咽頭扁桃 Pharyngeal tonsil
- 耳管咽頭口 Pharyngeal orifice of pharyngotympanic tube
- 右後鼻孔 Right choana
- 軟口蓋（口蓋帆）Soft palate
- 口蓋垂 Uvula
- 口蓋舌弓 Palatoglossal arch
- オトガイ舌筋 Genioglossus
- オトガイ舌骨筋 Geniohyoid
- 舌骨 Hyoid bone
- 甲状舌骨靱帯 Thyrohyoid ligament
- 前庭ヒダ Vestibular fold
- 声帯ヒダ Vocal fold
- 甲状腺 Thyroid gland
- 軸椎の歯突起 Dens of axis (C2)
- 環椎 Atlas (C1)
- 耳管咽頭ヒダ Salpingopharyngeal fold
- 口蓋扁桃 Palatine tonsil
- 舌扁桃 Lingual tonsil
- 喉頭蓋 Epiglottis
- 輪状軟骨 Cricoid cartilage

B 口腔の境界．

図 36.25　口腔の区分
前方から見たところ．

- 口腔前庭 Oral vestibule
- 口蓋舌弓 Palatoglossal arch
- 口蓋咽頭弓 Palatopharyngeal arch
- 口峡峡部 Faucial isthmus
- 固有口腔 Oral cavity proper
- 口腔前庭 Oral vestibule
- 上唇小帯 Frenulum of upper lip
- 硬口蓋 Hard palate
- 軟口蓋（口蓋帆）Soft palate
- 口蓋垂 Uvula
- 口蓋扁桃 Palatine tonsil
- 舌背 Dorsum of tongue
- 下唇小帯 Frenulum of lower lip

表 36.3	口腔の区分	
区分	前方の境界	後方の境界
口腔前庭	口唇・頬	歯列弓
固有口腔	歯列弓	口蓋舌弓
口峡	口蓋舌弓	口蓋咽頭弓

大唾液腺（耳下腺，顎下腺，舌下腺）は左右に3対ある．耳下腺は純粋な（水様の）漿液腺である．舌下腺は主に粘液腺であり，顎下腺は漿粘液性の混合腺である．

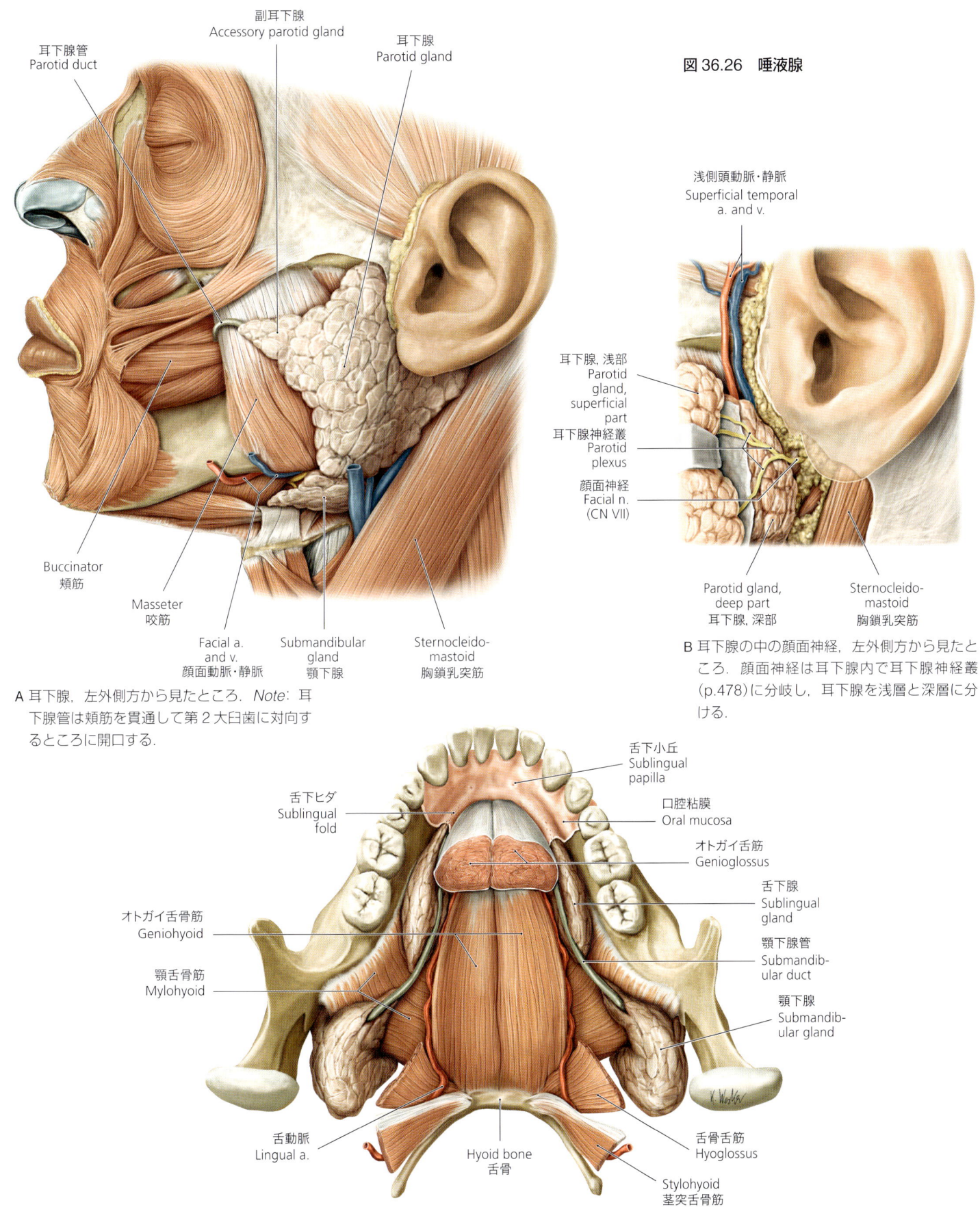

図 36.26　唾液腺

A 耳下腺，左外側方から見たところ．*Note*: 耳下腺管は頬筋を貫通して第2大臼歯に対向するところに開口する．

B 耳下腺の中の顔面神経，左外側方から見たところ．顔面神経は耳下腺内で耳下腺神経叢（p.478）に分岐し，耳下腺を浅層と深層に分ける．

C 顎下腺と舌下腺，上方から見たところ．舌は取り除いてある．

扁桃と咽頭
Tonsils & Pharynx

頭頸部

図 36.27 扁桃

A 口蓋扁桃，前方から見たところ．

- 軟口蓋（口蓋帆） Soft palate
- 扁桃窩 Tonsillar fossa
- 口蓋垂 Uvula
- 口蓋舌弓 Palatoglossal arch
- 口蓋咽頭弓 Palato-pharyngeal arch
- 口蓋扁桃 Palatine tonsil

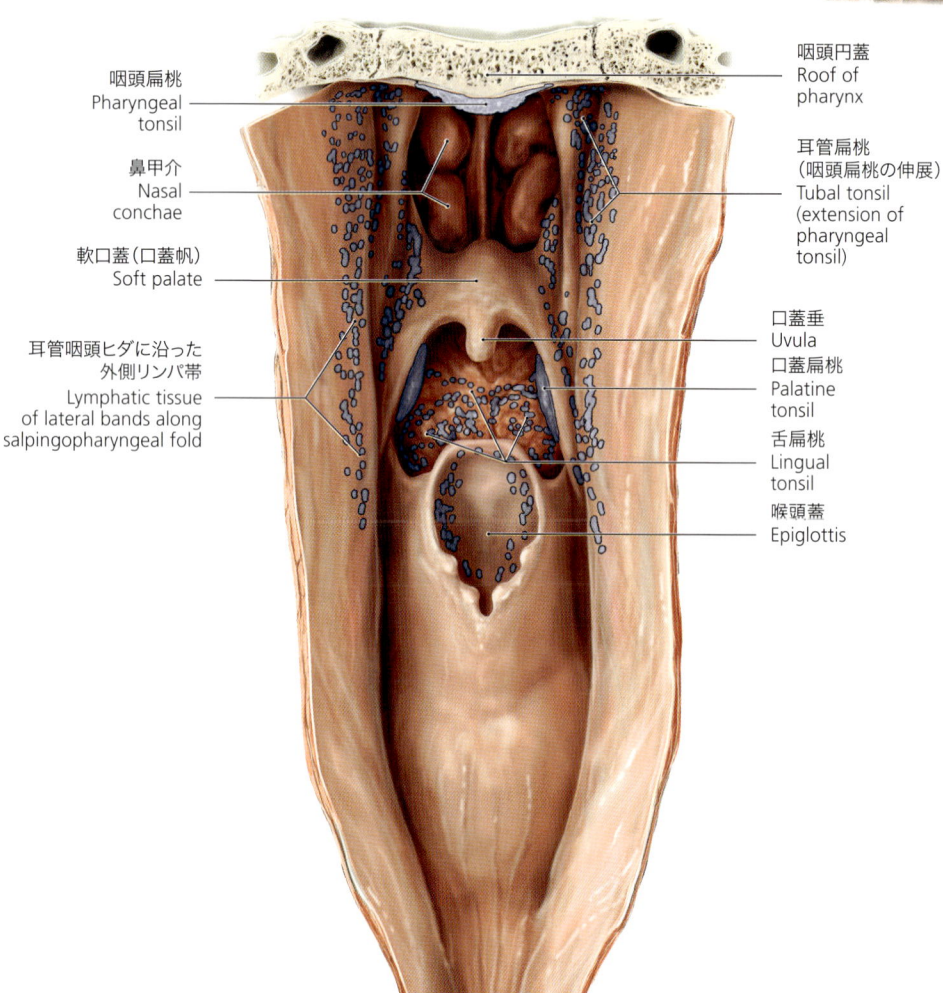

B 咽頭扁桃．咽頭円蓋の矢状断面．

- 後鼻孔 Choana
- 咽頭円蓋 Roof of pharynx
- 鼻中隔 Nasal septum
- 耳管隆起 Torus tubarius
- 軟口蓋（口蓋帆） Soft palate
- 口蓋垂 Uvula
- 咽頭扁桃 Pharyngeal tonsil
- 耳管開口部（耳管咽頭口） Pharyngeal orifice of pharyngo-tympanic tube
- 第2頸椎（軸椎）の歯突起 Dens of axis (C2)
- 耳管咽頭ヒダ Salpingo-pharyngeal fold

C ワルダイエル咽頭輪．咽頭を後方から見たところ．開放してある．

- 咽頭扁桃 Pharyngeal tonsil
- 鼻甲介 Nasal conchae
- 軟口蓋（口蓋帆） Soft palate
- 耳管咽頭ヒダに沿った外側リンパ帯 Lymphatic tissue of lateral bands along salpingopharyngeal fold
- 咽頭円蓋 Roof of pharynx
- 耳管扁桃（咽頭扁桃の伸展） Tubal tonsil (extension of pharyngeal tonsil)
- 口蓋垂 Uvula
- 口蓋扁桃 Palatine tonsil
- 舌扁桃 Lingual tonsil
- 喉頭蓋 Epiglottis

表 36.4 ワルダイエル咽頭輪

扁桃	個数
咽頭扁桃	1
耳管扁桃	2
口蓋扁桃	2
舌扁桃	1
外側リンパ帯	2

臨床

扁桃感染症
重度のウィルス感染や細菌感染による口蓋扁桃の異常肥大によって咽頭口部が閉塞され，嚥下が困難になる．

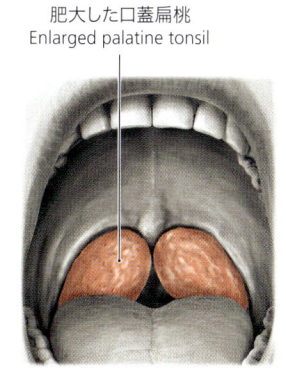

肥大した口蓋扁桃
Enlarged palatine tonsil

幼・小児では咽頭扁桃が特によく発達しているが，6，7歳になると消退し始める．咽頭扁桃の異常肥大はよく見られ，咽頭鼻部にまで膨れ，気道を閉塞するので口呼吸を余儀なくされる．

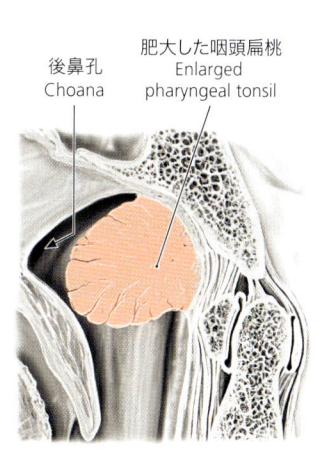

後鼻孔
Choana

肥大した咽頭扁桃
Enlarged pharyngeal tonsil

図 36.28 咽頭粘膜

開放した咽頭，後方から見たところ．咽頭の前部には，後鼻孔（鼻腔へ），口峡峡部（口腔へ），喉頭口（喉頭へ）の3つの開口部がある．

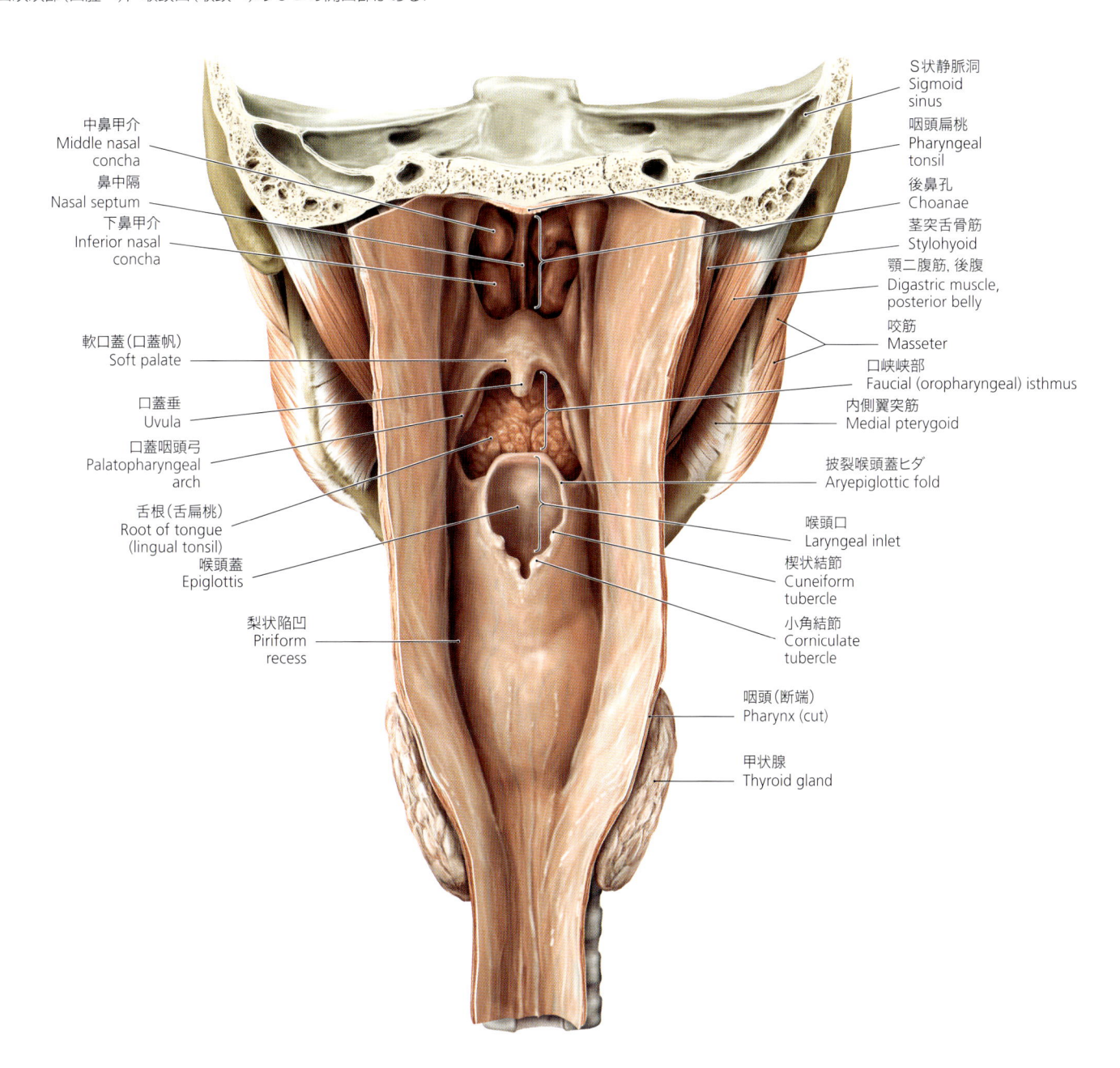

- 中鼻甲介 Middle nasal concha
- 鼻中隔 Nasal septum
- 下鼻甲介 Inferior nasal concha
- 軟口蓋（口蓋帆）Soft palate
- 口蓋垂 Uvula
- 口蓋咽頭弓 Palatopharyngeal arch
- 舌根（舌扁桃）Root of tongue (lingual tonsil)
- 喉頭蓋 Epiglottis
- 梨状陥凹 Piriform recess
- S状静脈洞 Sigmoid sinus
- 咽頭扁桃 Pharyngeal tonsil
- 後鼻孔 Choanae
- 茎突舌骨筋 Stylohyoid
- 顎二腹筋，後腹 Digastric muscle, posterior belly
- 咬筋 Masseter
- 口峡峡部 Faucial (oropharyngeal) isthmus
- 内側翼突筋 Medial pterygoid
- 披裂喉頭蓋ヒダ Aryepiglottic fold
- 喉頭口 Laryngeal inlet
- 楔状結節 Cuneiform tubercle
- 小角結節 Corniculate tubercle
- 咽頭（断端）Pharynx (cut)
- 甲状腺 Thyroid gland

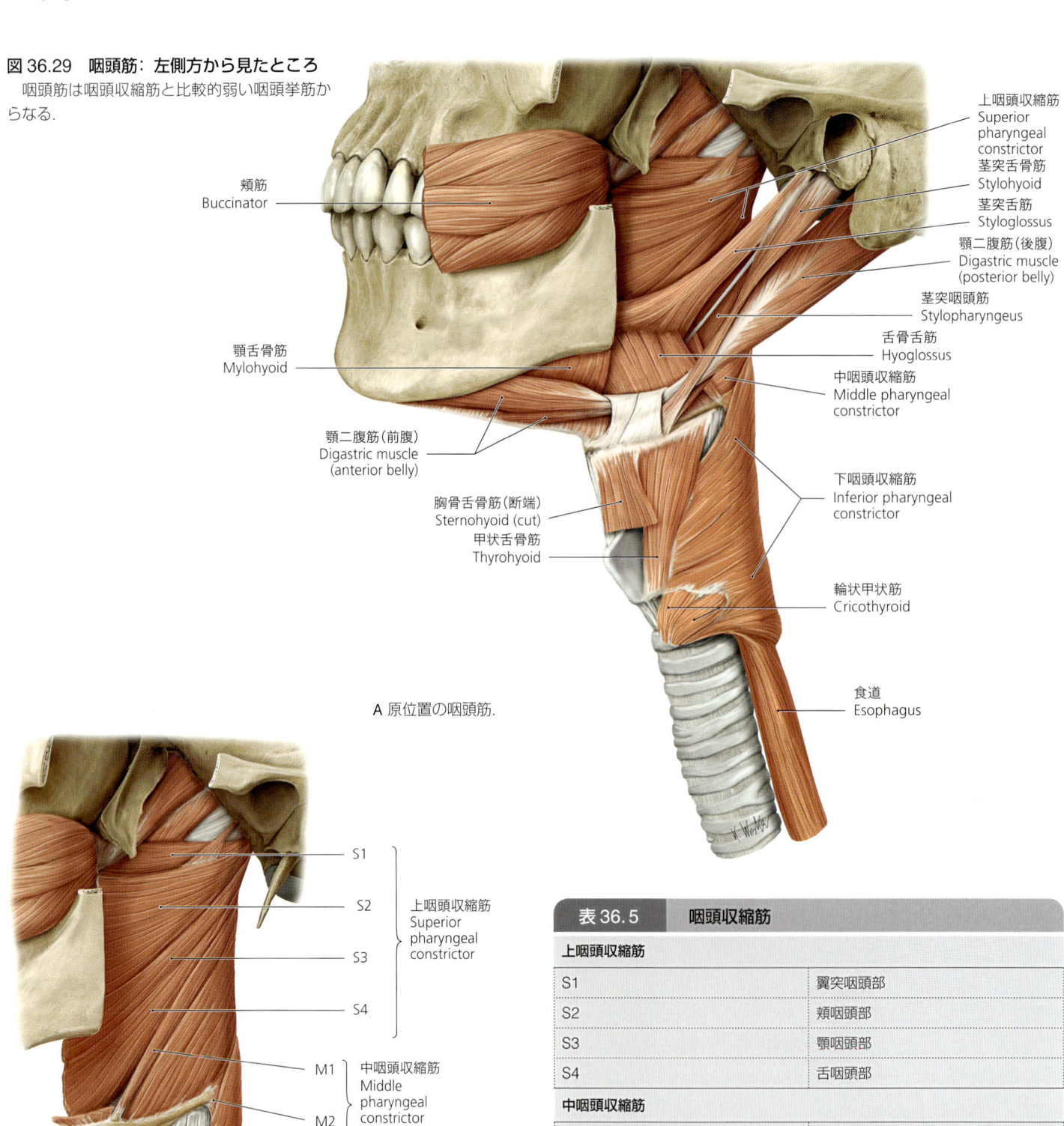

咽頭筋
Pharyngeal Muscles

図 36.29 咽頭筋：左側方から見たところ
咽頭筋は咽頭収縮筋と比較的弱い咽頭挙筋からなる．

- 頬筋 Buccinator
- 顎舌骨筋 Mylohyoid
- 顎二腹筋（前腹） Digastric muscle (anterior belly)
- 胸骨舌骨筋（断端） Sternohyoid (cut)
- 甲状舌骨筋 Thyrohyoid
- 上咽頭収縮筋 Superior pharyngeal constrictor
- 茎突舌骨筋 Stylohyoid
- 茎突舌筋 Styloglossus
- 顎二腹筋（後腹） Digastric muscle (posterior belly)
- 茎突咽頭筋 Stylopharyngeus
- 舌骨舌筋 Hyoglossus
- 中咽頭収縮筋 Middle pharyngeal constrictor
- 下咽頭収縮筋 Inferior pharyngeal constrictor
- 輪状甲状筋 Cricothyroid
- 食道 Esophagus

A 原位置の咽頭筋．

B 咽頭収縮筋の区分．

表 36.5	咽頭収縮筋
上咽頭収縮筋	
S1	翼突咽頭部
S2	頬咽頭部
S3	顎咽頭部
S4	舌咽頭部
中咽頭収縮筋	
M1	小角咽頭部
M2	大角咽頭部
下咽頭収縮筋	
I1	甲状咽頭部
I2	輪状咽頭部

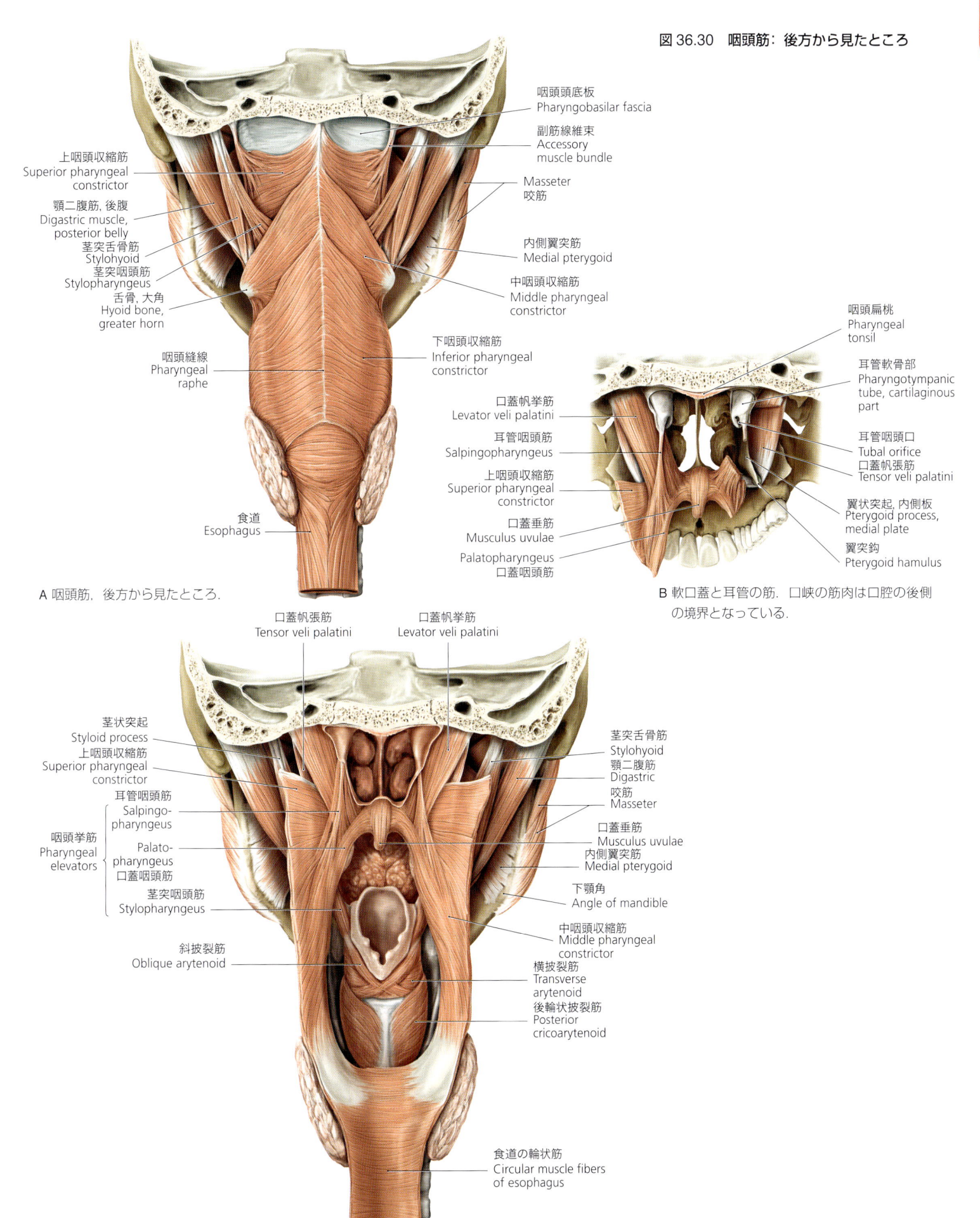

図 36.30 咽頭筋：後方から見たところ

A 咽頭筋，後方から見たところ．

B 軟口蓋と耳管の筋．口峡の筋肉は口腔の後側の境界となっている．

C 開いた咽頭の筋．

咽頭の神経と血管
Neurovasculature of the Pharynx

図 36.31 咽頭周囲隙の神経・血管
後方から見たところ．脊柱と後側にあるすべての構造は取り除いてある．

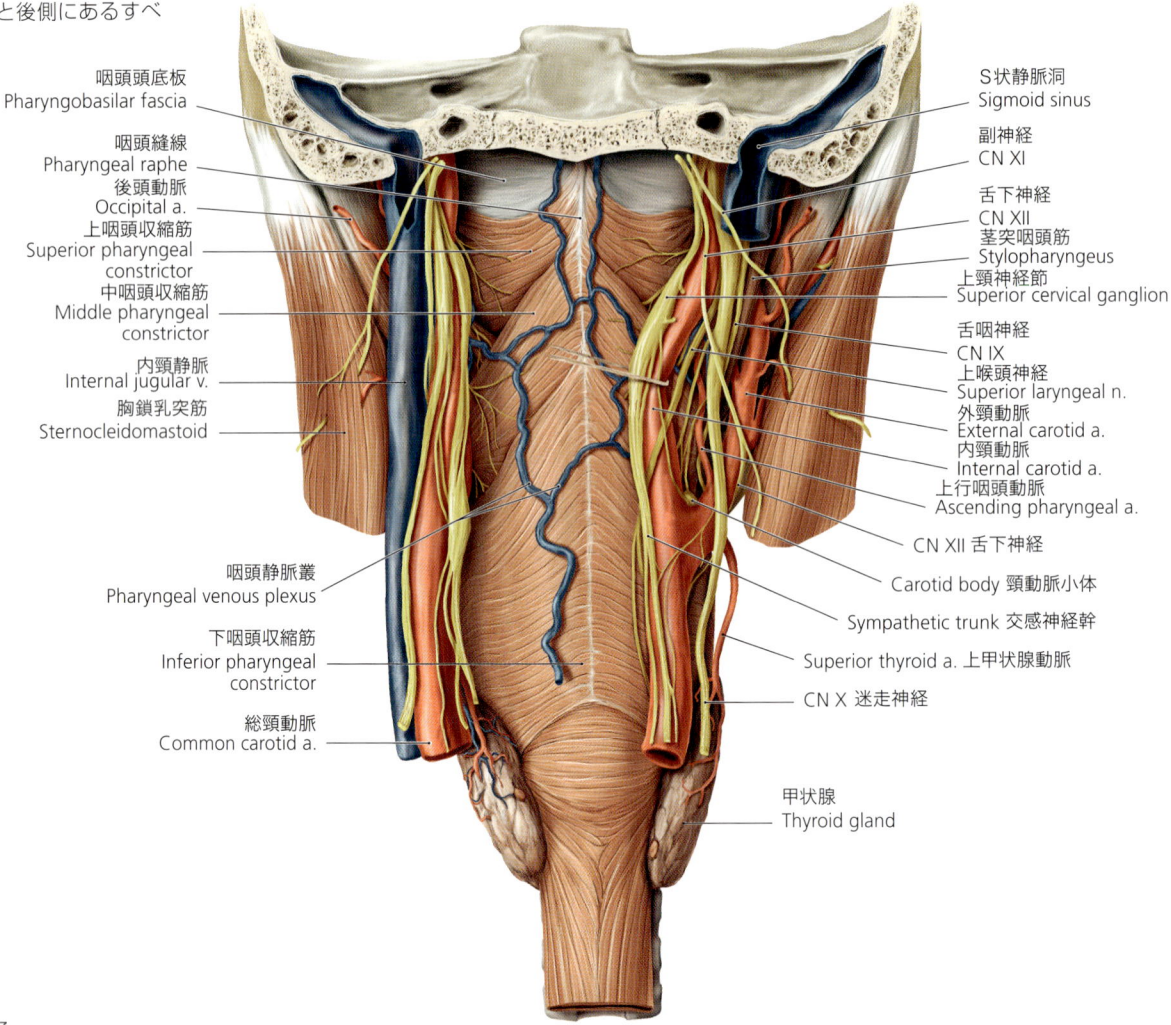

ラベル（左側）:
- 咽頭頭底板 Pharyngobasilar fascia
- 咽頭縫線 Pharyngeal raphe
- 後頭動脈 Occipital a.
- 上咽頭収縮筋 Superior pharyngeal constrictor
- 中咽頭収縮筋 Middle pharyngeal constrictor
- 内頸静脈 Internal jugular v.
- 胸鎖乳突筋 Sternocleidomastoid
- 咽頭静脈叢 Pharyngeal venous plexus
- 下咽頭収縮筋 Inferior pharyngeal constrictor
- 総頸動脈 Common carotid a.

ラベル（右側）:
- S状静脈洞 Sigmoid sinus
- 副神経 CN XI
- 舌下神経 CN XII
- 茎突咽頭筋 Stylopharyngeus
- 上頸神経節 Superior cervical ganglion
- 舌咽神経 CN IX
- 上喉頭神経 Superior laryngeal n.
- 外頸動脈 External carotid a.
- 内頸動脈 Internal carotid a.
- 上行咽頭動脈 Ascending pharyngeal a.
- CN XII 舌下神経
- Carotid body 頸動脈小体
- Sympathetic trunk 交感神経幹
- Superior thyroid a. 上甲状腺動脈
- CN X 迷走神経
- 甲状腺 Thyroid gland

図 36.32 咽頭周囲隙
横断面．上方から見たところ．

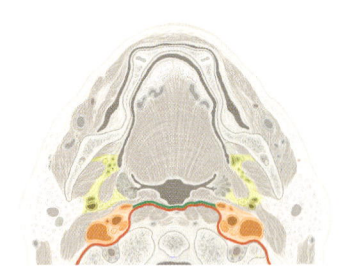

A 咽頭周囲隙．咽頭周囲隙は，咽頭後隙（緑）と咽頭側隙に分けられる．咽頭側隙はさらに前部（黄），後部（オレンジ）に分けられる．頸筋膜（椎前葉，赤）に注意せよ．

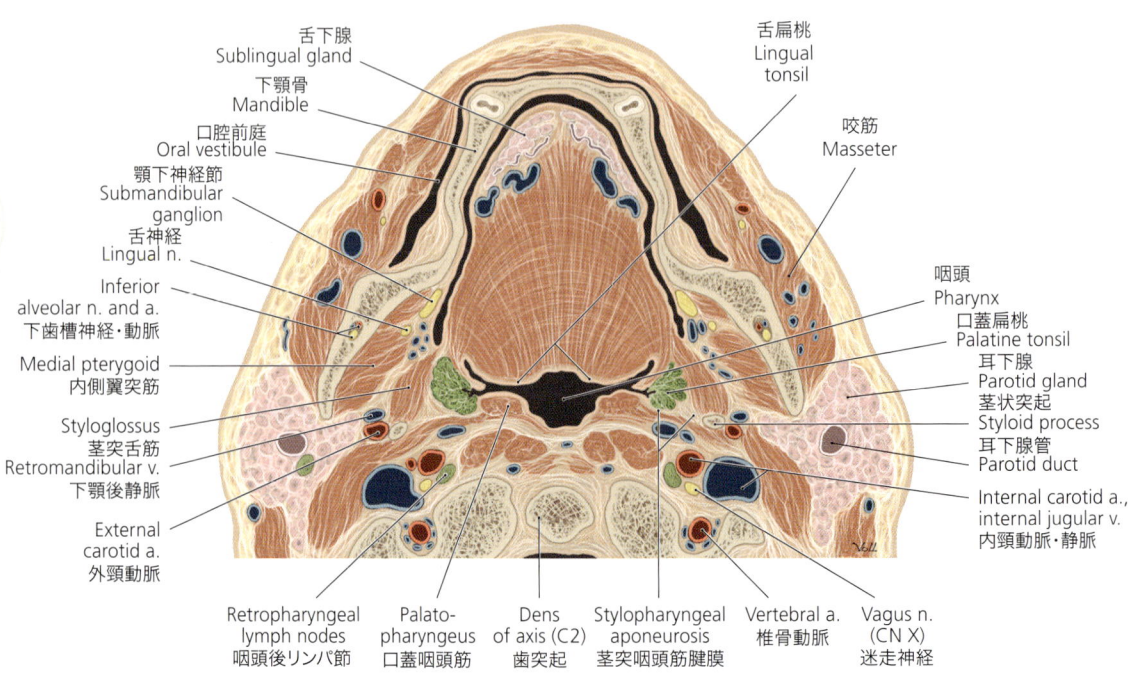

ラベル:
- 舌下腺 Sublingual gland
- 下顎骨 Mandible
- 口腔前庭 Oral vestibule
- 顎下神経節 Submandibular ganglion
- 舌神経 Lingual n.
- Inferior alveolar n. and a. 下歯槽神経・動脈
- Medial pterygoid 内側翼突筋
- Styloglossus 茎突舌筋
- Retromandibular v. 下顎後静脈
- External carotid a. 外頸動脈
- Retropharyngeal lymph nodes 咽頭後リンパ節
- Palato-pharyngeus 口蓋咽頭筋
- Dens of axis (C2) 歯突起
- Stylopharyngeal aponeurosis 茎突咽頭筋腱膜
- Vertebral a. 椎骨動脈
- Vagus n. (CN X) 迷走神経
- 舌扁桃 Lingual tonsil
- 咬筋 Masseter
- 咽頭 Pharynx
- 口蓋扁桃 Palatine tonsil
- 耳下腺 Parotid gland
- 茎状突起 Styloid process
- 耳下腺管 Parotid duct
- Internal carotid a., internal jugular v. 内頸動脈・静脈

B 扁桃窩の高さにおける水平断面．上方から見たところ．

図 36.33 開いた咽頭の神経・血管
後方から見たところ.

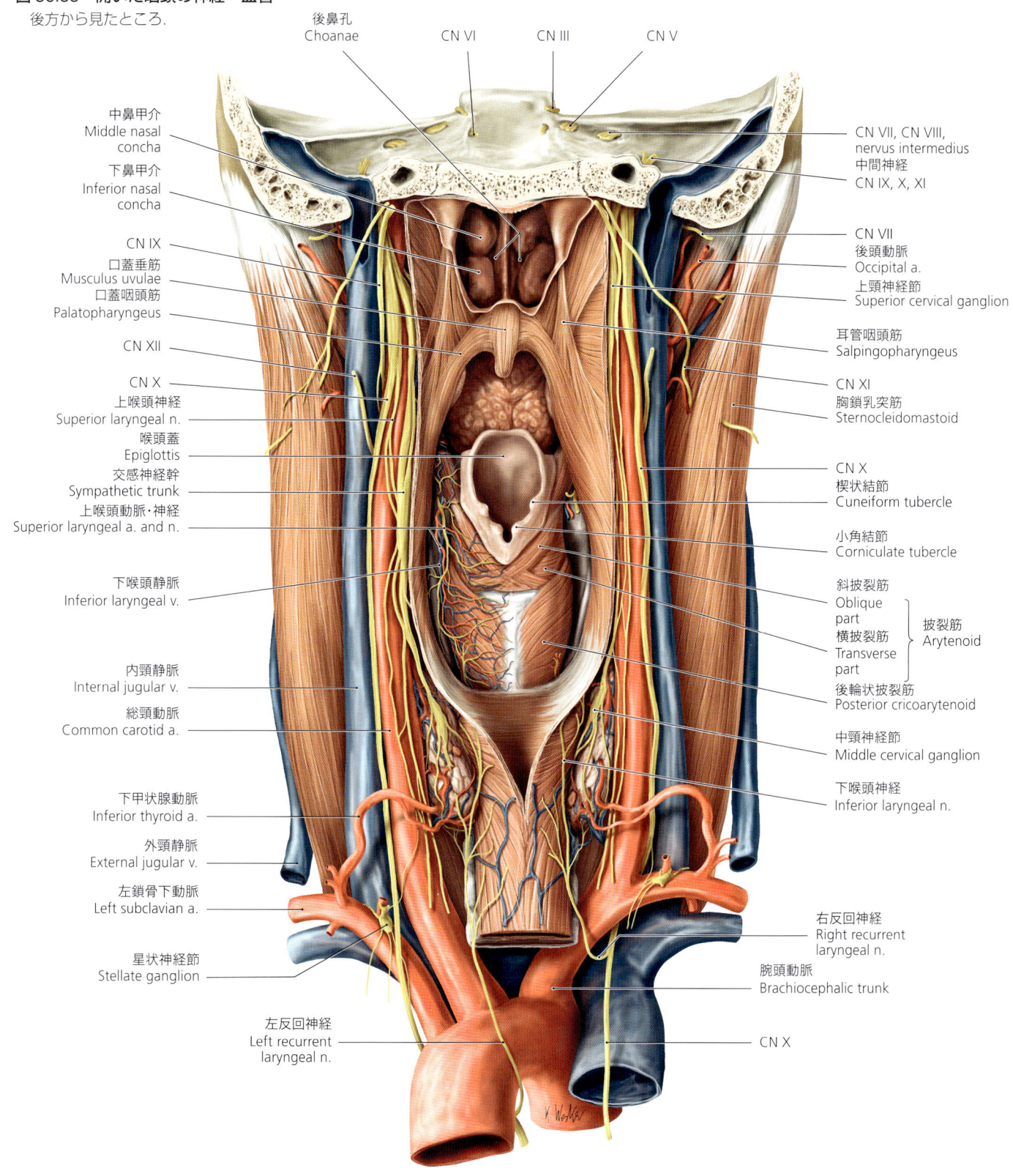

後鼻孔	Choanae
	CN VI
	CN III
	CN V
中鼻甲介	Middle nasal concha
下鼻甲介	Inferior nasal concha
	CN VII, CN VIII, nervus intermedius
中間神経	
	CN IX, X, XI
CN IX	
口蓋垂筋	Musculus uvulae
口蓋咽頭筋	Palatopharyngeus
	CN VII
後頭動脈	Occipital a.
上頚神経節	Superior cervical ganglion
CN XII	
耳管咽頭筋	Salpingopharyngeus
CN X	
上喉頭神経	Superior laryngeal n.
CN XI	
胸鎖乳突筋	Sternocleidomastoid
喉頭蓋	Epiglottis
交感神経幹	Sympathetic trunk
上喉頭動脈・神経	Superior laryngeal a. and n.
CN X	
楔状結節	Cuneiform tubercle
小角結節	Corniculate tubercle
下喉頭静脈	Inferior laryngeal v.
斜披裂筋	Oblique part
横披裂筋	Transverse part
披裂筋	Arytenoid
内頚静脈	Internal jugular v.
後輪状披裂筋	Posterior cricoarytenoid
総頚動脈	Common carotid a.
中頚神経節	Middle cervical ganglion
下喉頭神経	Inferior laryngeal n.
下甲状腺動脈	Inferior thyroid a.
外頚静脈	External jugular v.
左鎖骨下動脈	Left subclavian a.
右反回神経	Right recurrent laryngeal n.
星状神経節	Stellate ganglion
腕頭動脈	Brachiocephalic trunk
左反回神経	Left recurrent laryngeal n.
	CN X

CN III = 動眼神経，CN V = 三叉神経，CN VI = 外転神経，
CN VII = 顔面神経，CN VIII = 内耳神経，CN IX = 舌咽神経，
CN X = 迷走神経，CN XI = 副神経，CN XII = 舌下神経
脳神経は第31章参照.

頸部の骨と靱帯
Bones & Ligaments of the Neck

図 37.1 頸部の境界
左外側方から見たところ.

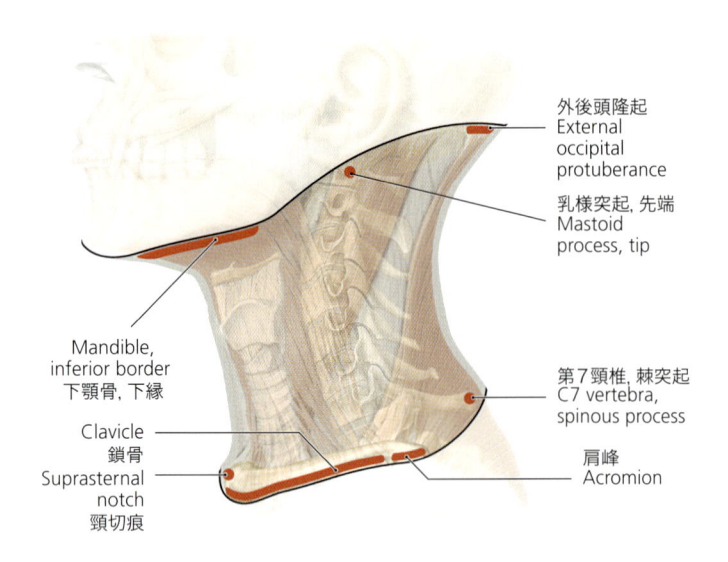

- 外後頭隆起 External occipital protuberance
- 乳様突起, 先端 Mastoid process, tip
- Mandible, inferior border 下顎骨, 下縁
- Clavicle 鎖骨
- Suprasternal notch 頸切痕
- 第7頸椎, 棘突起 C7 vertebra, spinous process
- 肩峰 Acromion

表 37.1	頸の骨と関節	
頸椎		p.6
舌骨		p.539
頭蓋-脊柱の連結	環椎後頭関節	p.16
	環軸関節	
鉤椎関節		p.15
椎間関節		p.14
喉頭		p.571

図 37.2 頸部の骨の構造
左側方から見たところ.

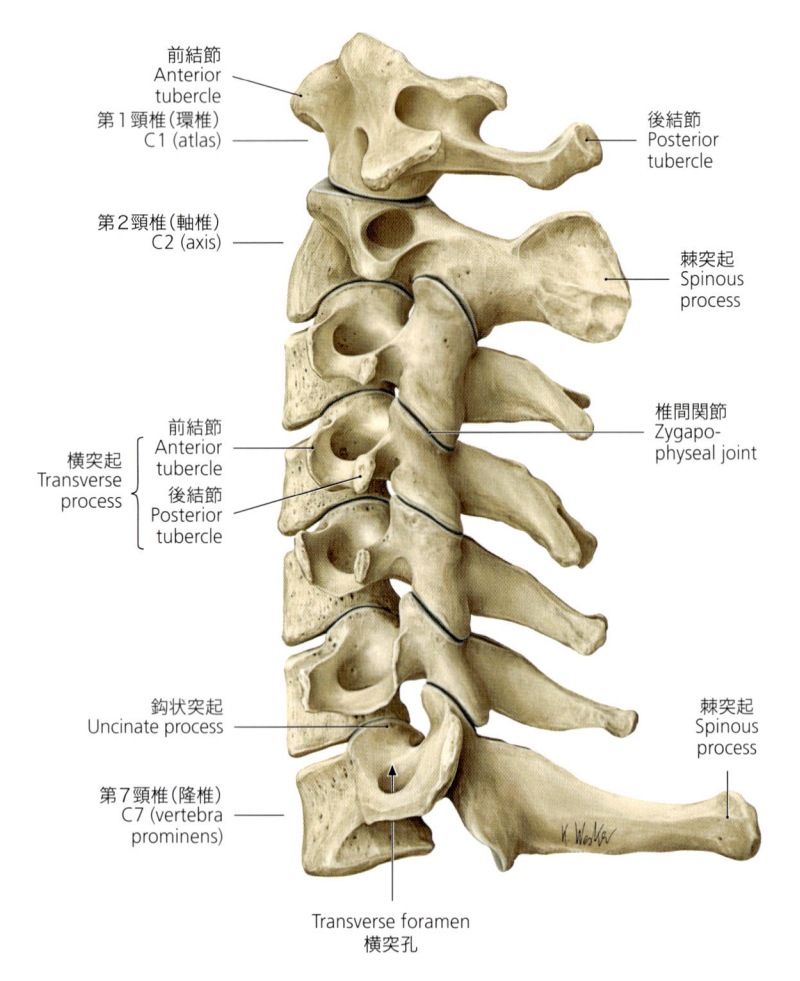

- 前結節 Anterior tubercle
- 第1頸椎(環椎) C1 (atlas)
- 後結節 Posterior tubercle
- 第2頸椎(軸椎) C2 (axis)
- 棘突起 Spinous process
- 椎間関節 Zygapophyseal joint
- 前結節 Anterior tubercle
- 横突起 Transverse process
- 後結節 Posterior tubercle
- 鉤状突起 Uncinate process
- 棘突起 Spinous process
- 第7頸椎(隆椎) C7 (vertebra prominens)
- Transverse foramen 横突孔

A 頸椎. 頸椎の7個の椎骨は頭部の荷重を支えるように特殊化している.

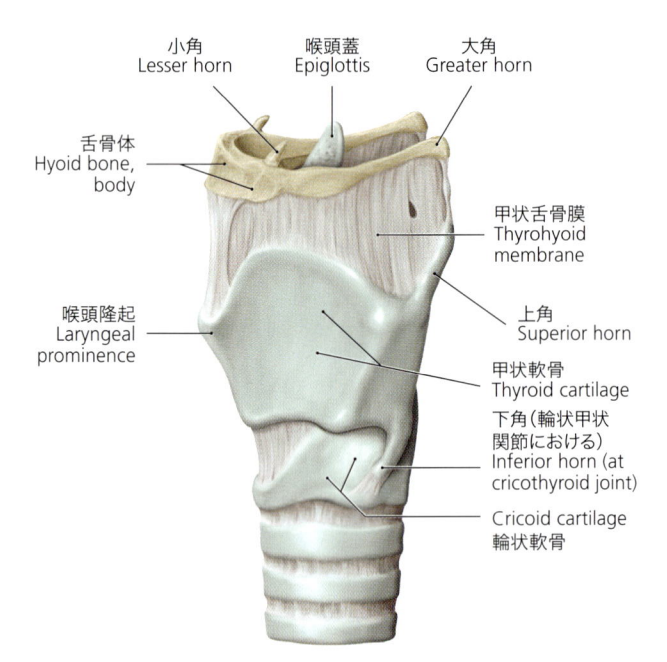

- 小角 Lesser horn
- 喉頭蓋 Epiglottis
- 大角 Greater horn
- 舌骨体 Hyoid bone, body
- 甲状舌骨膜 Thyrohyoid membrane
- 喉頭隆起 Laryngeal prominence
- 上角 Superior horn
- 甲状軟骨 Thyroid cartilage
- 下角(輪状甲状関節における) Inferior horn (at cricothyroid joint)
- Cricoid cartilage 輪状軟骨

B 舌骨と喉頭. 舌骨は舌骨上筋群と舌骨下筋群の付着部となっている. *Note*: 喉頭は, 主に甲状舌骨膜によって舌骨にぶら下がっている.

図 37.3 頸椎の靱帯

正中断，左外側方から見たところ．頭蓋-脊柱連結の靱帯については p.16 参照．

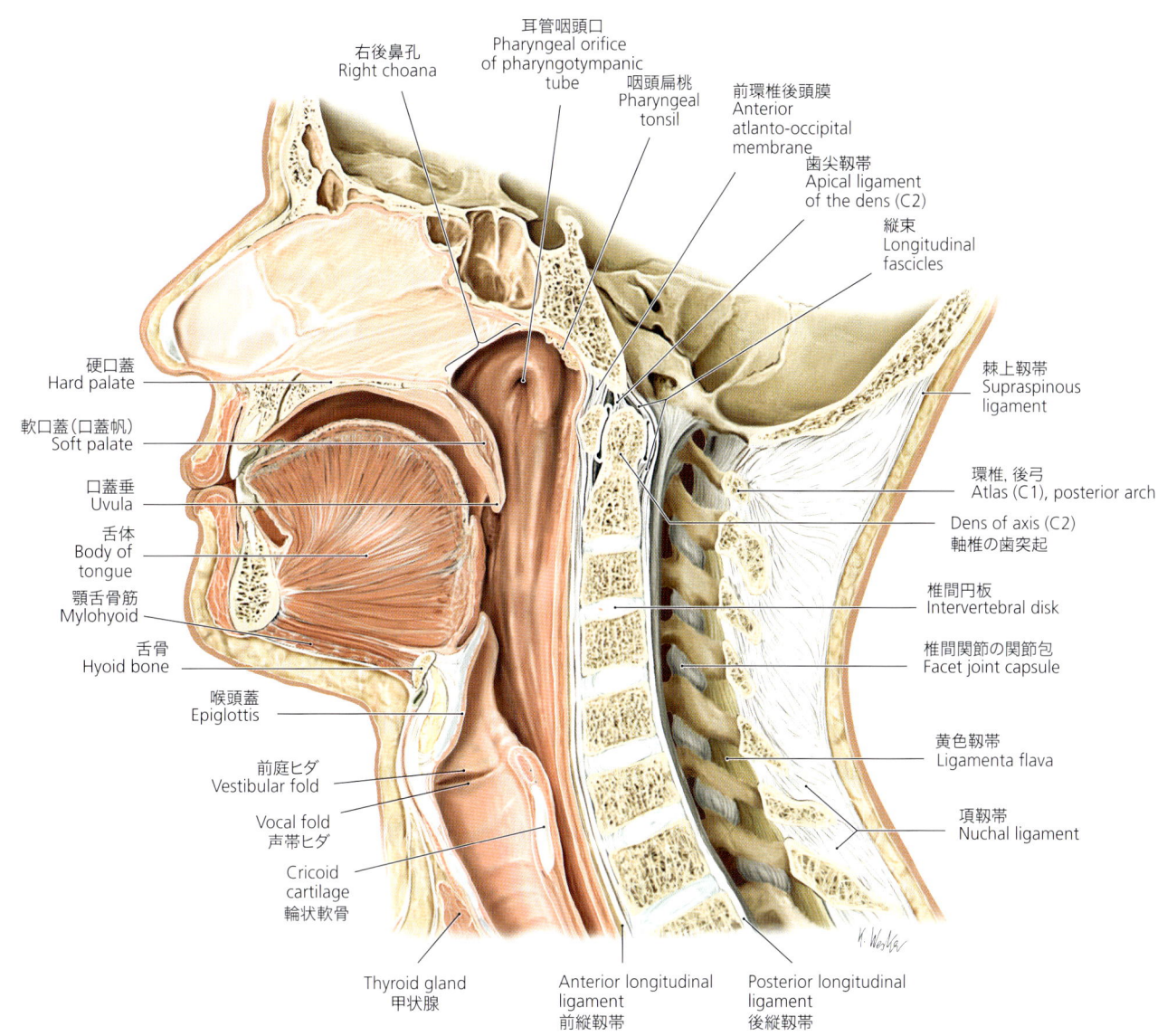

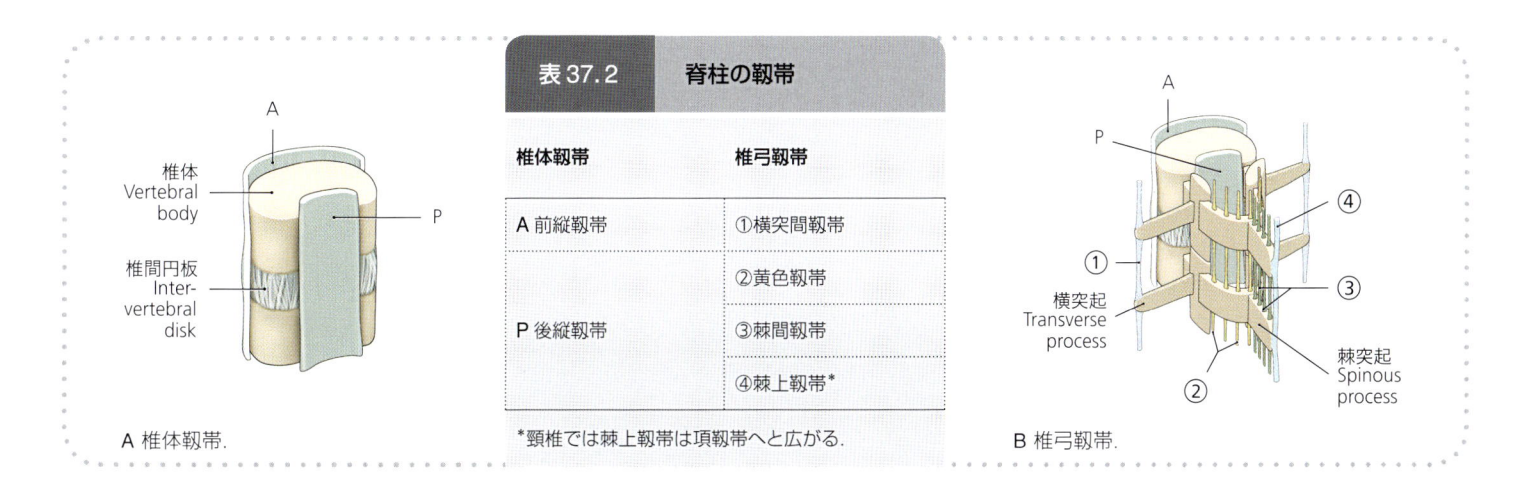

図中ラベル（時計回り・上段から）:
- 右後鼻孔 Right choana
- 耳管咽頭口 Pharyngeal orifice of pharyngotympanic tube
- 咽頭扁桃 Pharyngeal tonsil
- 前環椎後頭膜 Anterior atlanto-occipital membrane
- 歯尖靱帯 Apical ligament of the dens (C2)
- 縦束 Longitudinal fascicles
- 棘上靱帯 Supraspinous ligament
- 環椎，後弓 Atlas (C1), posterior arch
- 軸椎の歯突起 Dens of axis (C2)
- 椎間円板 Intervertebral disk
- 椎間関節の関節包 Facet joint capsule
- 黄色靱帯 Ligamenta flava
- 項靱帯 Nuchal ligament
- 後縦靱帯 Posterior longitudinal ligament
- 前縦靱帯 Anterior longitudinal ligament
- 甲状腺 Thyroid gland
- 輪状軟骨 Cricoid cartilage
- 声帯ヒダ Vocal fold
- 前庭ヒダ Vestibular fold
- 喉頭蓋 Epiglottis
- 舌骨 Hyoid bone
- 顎舌骨筋 Mylohyoid
- 舌体 Body of tongue
- 口蓋垂 Uvula
- 軟口蓋（口蓋帆）Soft palate
- 硬口蓋 Hard palate

A 椎体靱帯
- 椎体 Vertebral body
- 椎間円板 Intervertebral disk
- A 前縦靱帯
- P 後縦靱帯

表 37.2　脊柱の靱帯

椎体靱帯	椎弓靱帯
A 前縦靱帯	①横突間靱帯
	②黄色靱帯
P 後縦靱帯	③棘間靱帯
	④棘上靱帯*

*頸椎では棘上靱帯は項靱帯へと広がる．

B 椎弓靱帯
- ①横突間靱帯 — 横突起 Transverse process
- ②黄色靱帯
- ③棘間靱帯
- ④棘上靱帯 — 棘突起 Spinous process

頸部の筋肉(1)
Muscle Facts (I)

局所解剖学の観点では，頸には6つの主要な筋のグループがある．機能的には，広頸筋は表情筋であり，僧帽筋は上肢帯の筋，後頸の筋は固有背筋である．後頭下の筋(短い項筋と頭蓋-脊柱連結の筋肉)はこの章で頸部深層の筋として扱う．

表37.3　頸の筋肉の分類

I	頸部浅層の筋		III	舌骨上の筋	
	広頸筋，胸鎖乳突筋，僧帽筋	図37.4		顎二腹筋，オトガイ舌骨筋，顎舌骨筋，茎突舌骨筋	図37.7A
II	後頸の筋(固有背筋)		IV	舌骨下の筋	
	⑥頭半棘筋　⑦頸半棘筋	p.32参照		胸骨舌骨筋，胸骨甲状筋，甲状舌骨筋，肩甲舌骨筋	図37.7B
	⑧頭板状筋　⑨頸板状筋		V	椎骨前の筋	
	⑩頭最長筋　⑪頸最長筋	p.30参照		頭長筋，頸長筋，前頭直筋，外側頭直筋	図37.9A
	⑫頸腸肋筋		VI	頸部外側(深層)の筋	
	後頭下の筋(短い項筋と頭蓋-脊柱連結の筋)	図37.9C		前斜角筋，中斜角筋，後斜角筋	図37.9B

図37.4　頸部浅層の筋
詳細については表37.4参照．

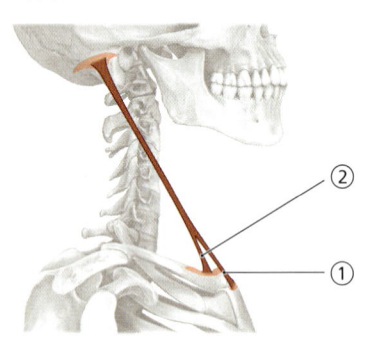

A　胸鎖乳突筋．

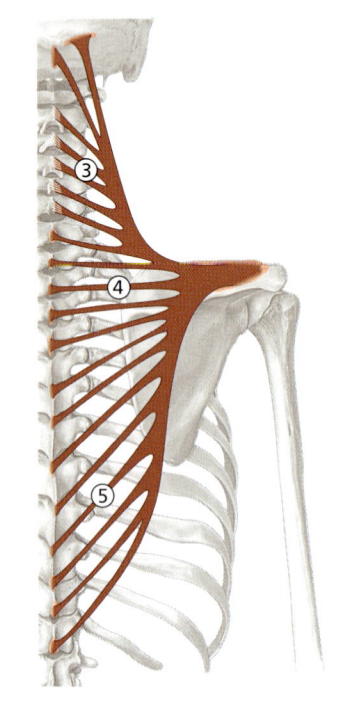

B　僧帽筋．

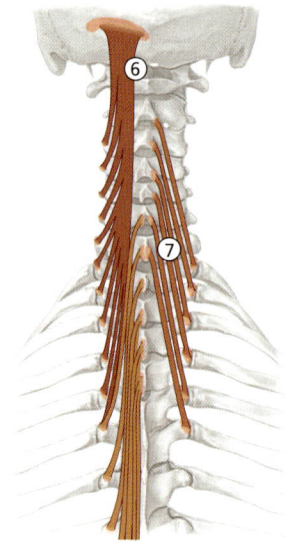

図37.5　後頸の筋

A　半棘筋．

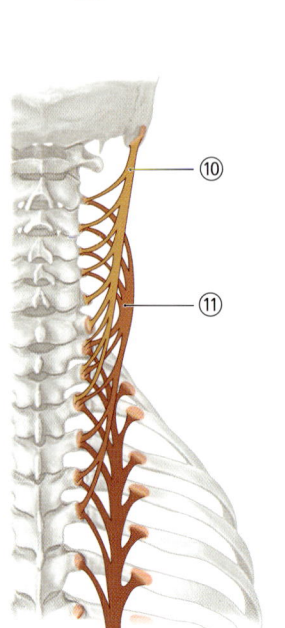

B　板状筋．

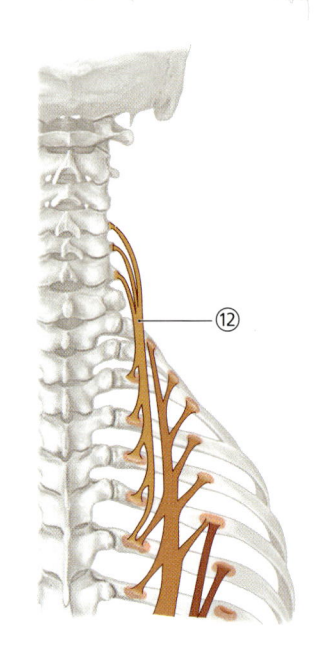

C　最長筋．

D　腸肋筋．

図 37.6　頸部浅層の筋

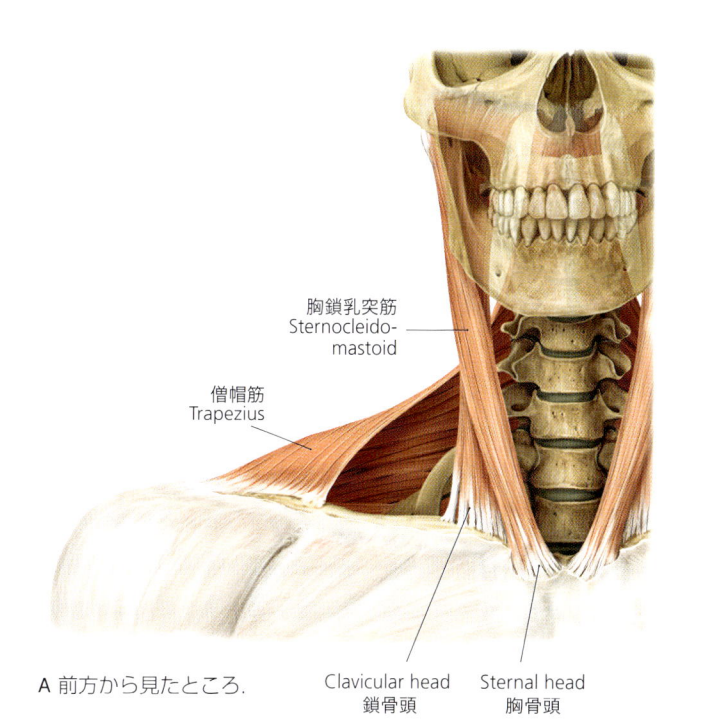

A 前方から見たところ．
B 左外側方から見たところ． 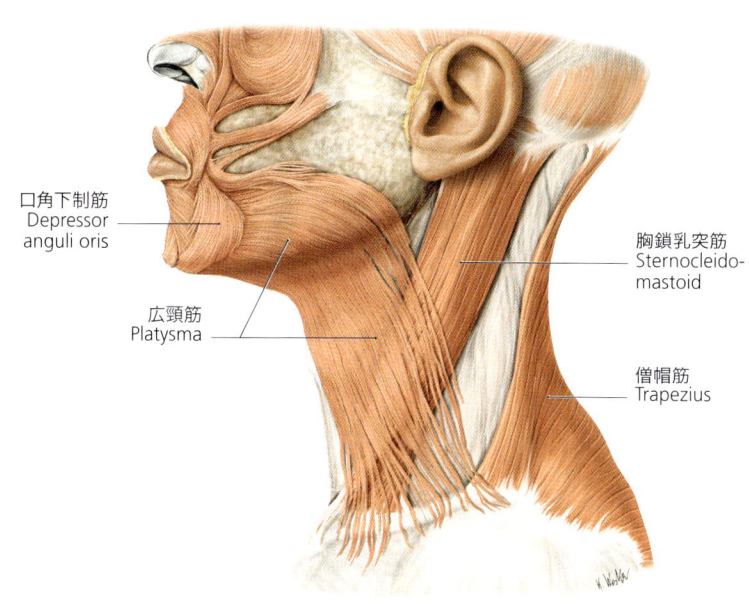
C 後方から見たところ．右側の僧帽筋は取り除いてある． 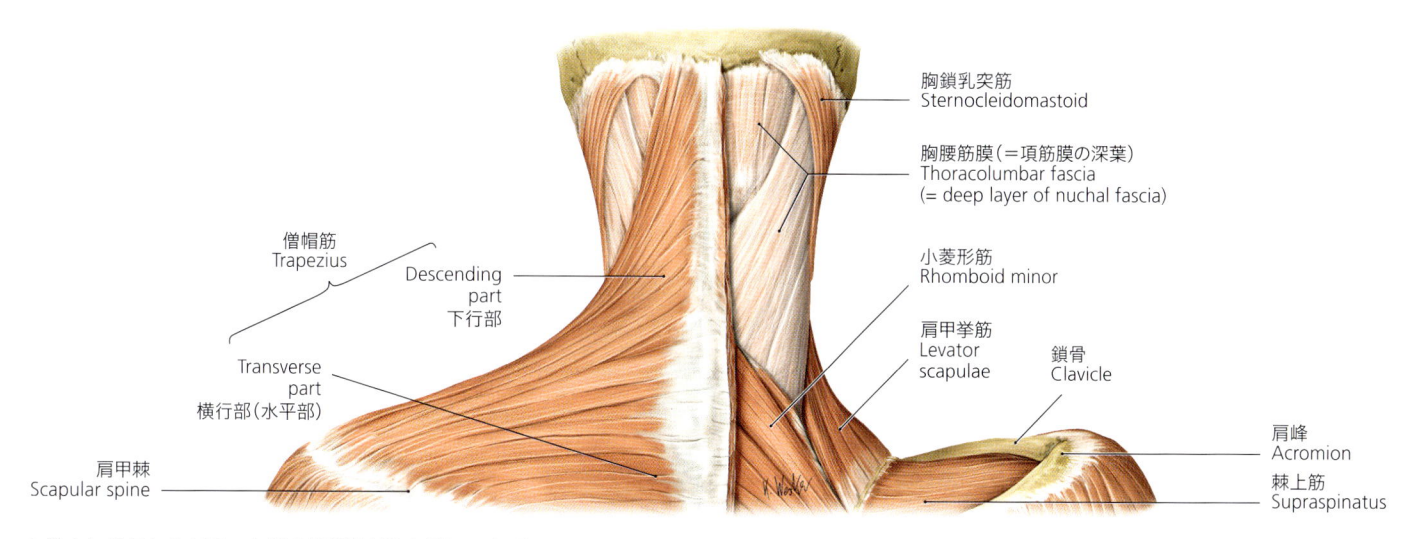

表 37.4	頸部浅層の筋				
筋		起始	停止	神経支配	作用
広頸筋		頸部の下部と胸部上外側の皮膚	下顎骨下縁，顔面下部と口角の皮膚	顔面神経（CN VII）の頸枝	顔面下部と口の皮膚を下に引いてしわを作り，頸の皮膚を緊張させ，下顎の強制下制を助ける
胸鎖乳突筋	①胸骨頭	胸骨柄	側頭骨の乳様突起，後頭骨の上項線	運動神経：副神経（CN XI） 痛覚と固有覚：頸神経叢（C2, C3）	片側：同側に頭部を傾け，対側に回転させる 両側：頭部を上に向け，頭部が固定されている場合には呼吸を助ける
	②鎖骨頭	鎖骨の内側1/3			
僧帽筋	③下行部*	後頭骨，第1-7頸椎棘突起	鎖骨の外側1/3		肩甲骨を上斜めに引いて，関節窩を下方に回す

*④横行部と⑤上行部については p.276 参照．

頸部の筋肉（2）
Muscle Facts (II)

表 37.5　舌骨上の筋

舌骨上の筋は咀嚼の補助筋とも考えられる

筋		起始	停止		神経支配	作用
顎二腹筋	①a 前腹	下顎骨の二腹筋窩	線維性の滑車を伴う中間腱を介して停止	舌骨体	下顎神経(CN V₃)の枝の顎舌骨筋神経	嚥下時に舌骨を挙上し，下顎の開口を補助する
	①b 後腹	側頭骨乳様突起の内側にある乳突切痕			顔面神経(CN VII)	
②茎突舌骨筋		側頭骨の茎状突起	分岐した腱を介して停止		顔面神経(CN VII)	
③顎舌骨筋		下顎骨の顎舌骨筋線	正中腱が縫線（顎舌骨筋縫線）に停止		下顎神経(CN V₃)の枝の顎舌骨筋神経	口腔底を持ち上げ，緊張させる．嚥下時に舌骨を前方に引き，下顎の開口を助ける．咀嚼時に下顎の横方向の運動を助ける
④オトガイ舌骨筋		下顎骨のオトガイ棘（下棘）	直接停止		舌下神経(CN XII)を経由する第1頸神経(C1)の前枝	嚥下時に舌骨を前方に引き，下顎の開口を助ける

図 37.7　舌骨上と舌骨下の筋

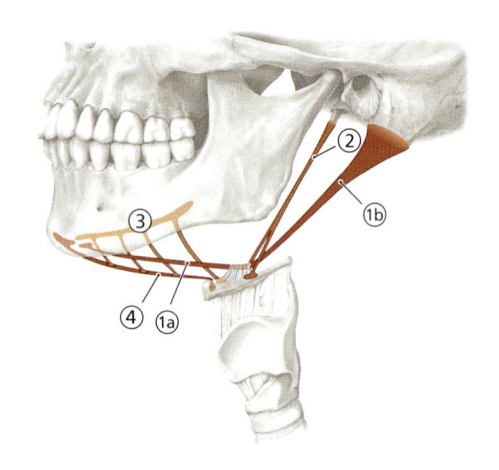

A　舌骨上の筋．左外側方から見たところ．

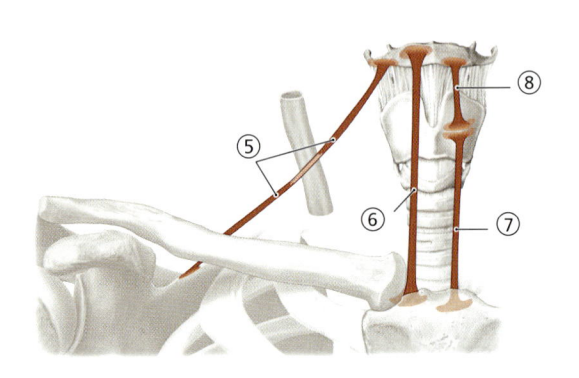

B　舌骨下の筋．左外側方から見たところ．

表 37.6　舌骨下の筋

筋	起始	停止	神経支配	作用
⑤肩甲舌骨筋	肩甲骨の上縁	舌骨体	頸神経叢の頸神経ワナ(C1-C3)	舌骨を押し下げて固定し，発声時と嚥下の最終相において喉頭と舌骨を下げる*
⑥胸骨舌骨筋	胸骨柄と胸鎖関節後面		頸神経ワナ(C2-C3)	
⑦胸骨甲状筋	胸骨柄の後面	甲状軟骨の斜線	頸神経ワナ(C2-C3)	
⑧甲状舌骨筋	甲状軟骨の斜線	舌骨体	舌下神経(CN XII)を経由する第1頸神経(C1)の前枝	舌骨を押し下げて固定し，嚥下時に喉頭を挙上

*肩甲舌骨筋は中間腱で頸筋膜を緊張させる．

図 37.8　舌骨上および舌骨下の筋

茎突舌骨筋
Stylohyoid

顎二腹筋，後腹
Digastric, posterior belly

顎二腹筋，前腹
Digastric, anterior belly

甲状舌骨筋
Thyrohyoid

胸骨甲状筋
Sternothyroid

Mylohyoid
顎舌骨筋

肩甲舌骨筋，上腹と下腹
Omohyoid, superior and inferior belly

胸骨舌骨筋
Sternohyoid

肩甲舌骨筋の中間腱
Intermediate tendon of omohyoid

A　左外側方から見たところ．

筋突起
Coronoid process

オトガイ舌骨筋
Geniohyoid

顎舌骨筋線
Mylohyoid line

下顎頭
Head of mandible

Mandibular ramus
下顎枝

Mylohyoid
顎舌骨筋

Hyoid bone (body)
舌骨(体)

B　口腔底にある顎舌骨筋とオトガイ舌骨筋．後上方から見たところ．

顎舌骨筋
Mylohyoid

顎舌骨筋縫線
Mylohyoid raphe

舌骨
Hyoid bone

甲状舌骨筋
Thyrohyoid

甲状軟骨
Thyroid cartilage

胸骨甲状筋
Sternothyroid

前腹
Anterior belly

後腹
Posterior belly

顎二腹筋
Digastric

茎突舌骨筋
Stylohyoid

胸骨舌骨筋
Sternohyoid

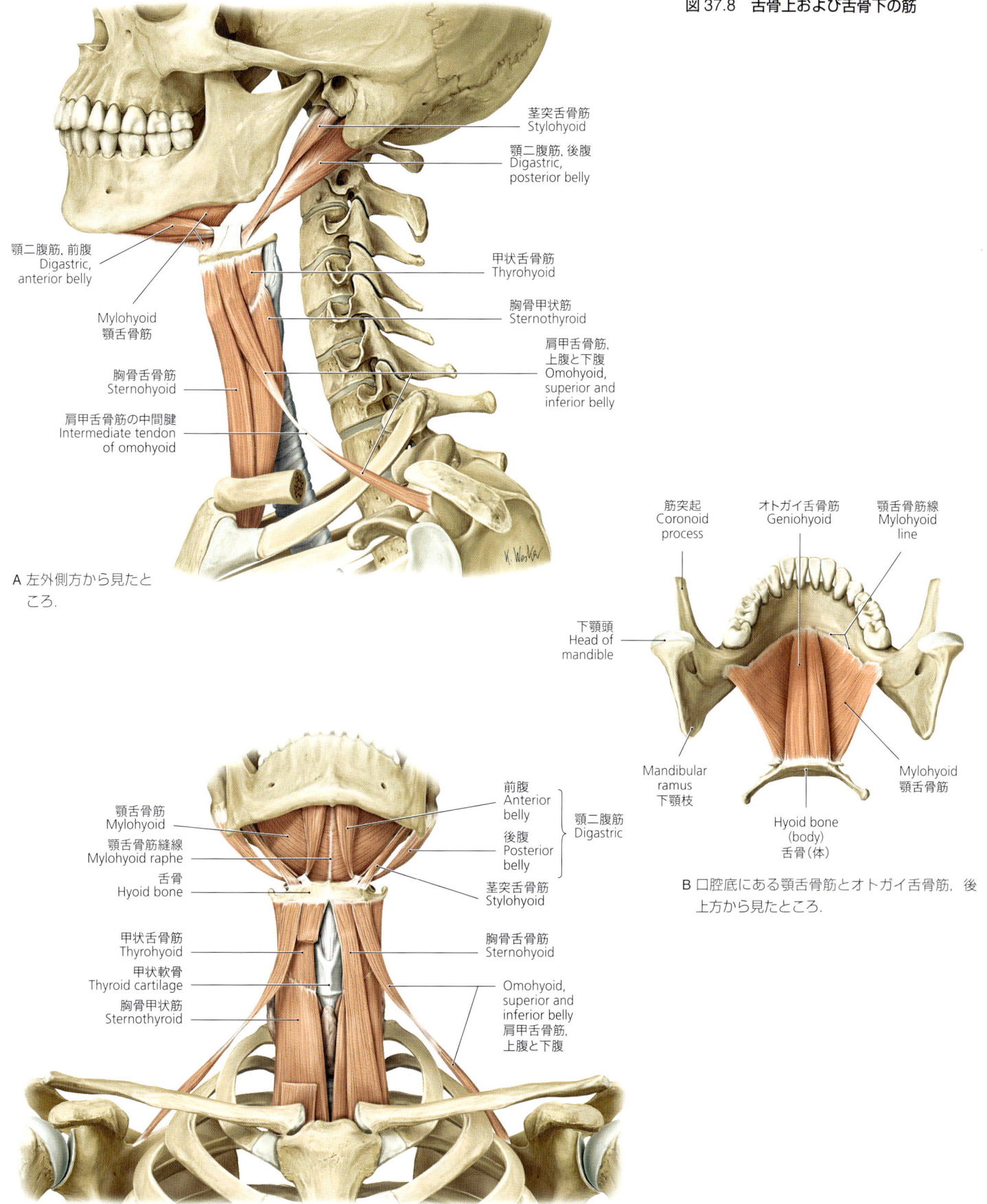

Omohyoid, superior and inferior belly
肩甲舌骨筋，上腹と下腹

C　前方から見たところ．右側では胸骨舌骨筋の一部を取り除いてある．

563

頸部の筋肉(3)
Muscle Facts (III)

図 37.9　頸部深層の筋

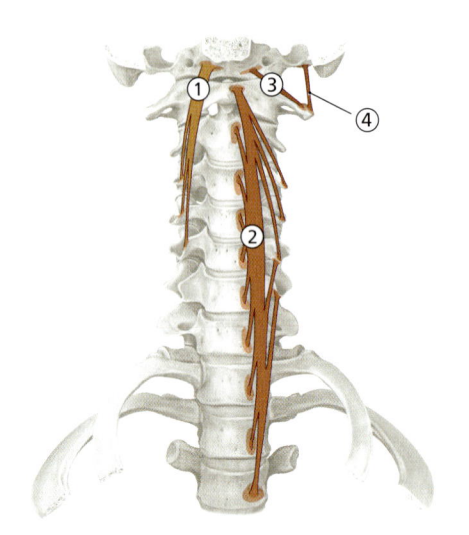

A 椎骨前の筋，前方から見たところ．

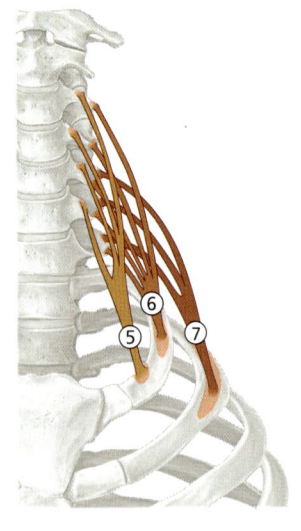

B 斜角筋，前方から見たところ．

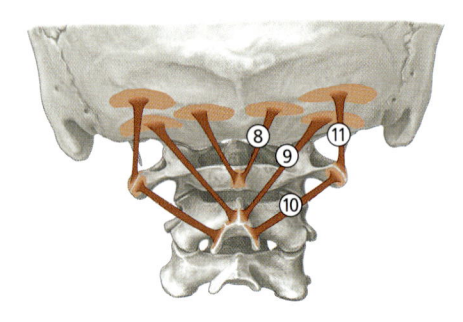

C 後頭下の筋，後方から見たところ．

表 37.7　頸部深層の筋

筋		起始	停止	神経支配	作用
椎骨前の筋					
①頭長筋		第3-6頸椎(C3-C6)の横突起の前結節	後頭骨の基底部	頸神経叢の直接の枝(C1-C3)	環椎後頭関節で頭部の屈曲
②頸長筋	垂直部(中間部)	第5頸椎-第3胸椎(C5-T3)の椎体の前面	第2-4頸椎(C2-C4)の前面	頸神経叢の直接の枝(C2-C6)	片側：頸椎を傾け，反対側に回旋 両側：頸椎の前方への屈曲
	上斜部	第3-5頸椎(C3-C5)の横突起の前結節	環椎(C1)の前結節		
	下斜部	第1-3胸椎(T1-T3)の椎体の前面	第5-6頸椎(C5-C6)の横突起の前結節		
③前頭直筋		環椎(C1)の外側部	後頭骨の基底部	第1・2頸神経(C1-C2)の前枝	片側：環椎後頭関節の外屈 両側：環椎後頭関節の屈曲
④外側頭直筋		環椎(C1)の横突起	後頭骨の基底部(後頭顆より外側)		
斜角筋					
⑤前斜角筋		第3-6頸椎(C3-6)の横突起の前結節	第1肋骨の斜角筋結節		肋骨が動く場合：努力呼吸時に上位肋骨を挙上 肋骨が固定されている場合：(片側)頸椎を同側に曲げる，(両側)頸部の屈曲
⑥中斜角筋		環椎(C1)および軸椎(C2)の横突起，第3-7頸椎(C3-C7)の横突起の後結節	第1肋骨の鎖骨下動脈溝の後側	頸・腕神経叢(C3-C8)からの直接の枝	
⑦後斜角筋		第5-7頸椎(C5-C7)の横突起の後結節	第2肋骨の外側面		
後頭下の筋(短い項筋と頭蓋-脊柱連結の筋)					
⑧小後頭直筋		環椎(C1)の後結節	後頭骨下項線の内側1/3	第1頸神経(C1)の後枝(後頭下神経)	片側：頭を同側に回旋 両側：頭を後屈
⑨大後頭直筋		軸椎(C2)の棘突起	後頭骨下項線の中間1/3		
⑩下頭斜筋			環椎(C1)の横突起		
⑪上頭斜筋		環椎(C1)の横突起	後頭骨の大後頭直筋停止部の上部		片側：頭を同側に傾け，反対側に回旋 両側：頭を後屈

図37.10 頸部深層の筋

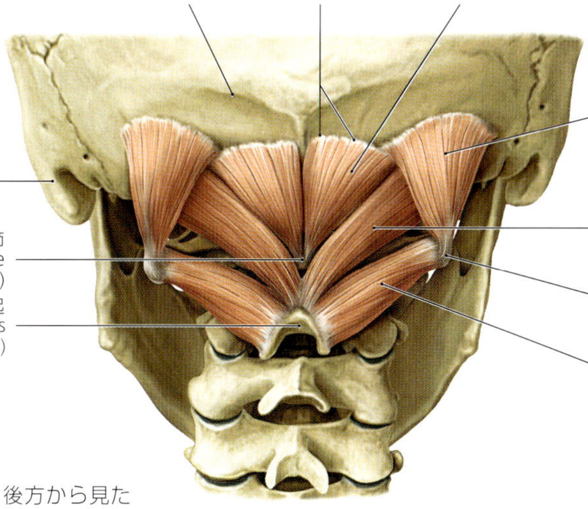

上項線 Superior nuchal line
下項線 Inferior nuchal line
小後頭直筋 Rectus capitis posterior minor
上頭斜筋 Obliquus capitis superior
乳様突起 Mastoid process
大後頭直筋 Rectus capitis posterior major
環椎の後結節 Posterior tubercle of atlas (C1)
環椎の横突起 Transverse process of atlas (C1)
軸椎の棘突起 Spinous process of axis (C2)
下頭斜筋 Obliquus capitis inferior

A 後頭下の筋，後方から見たところ．

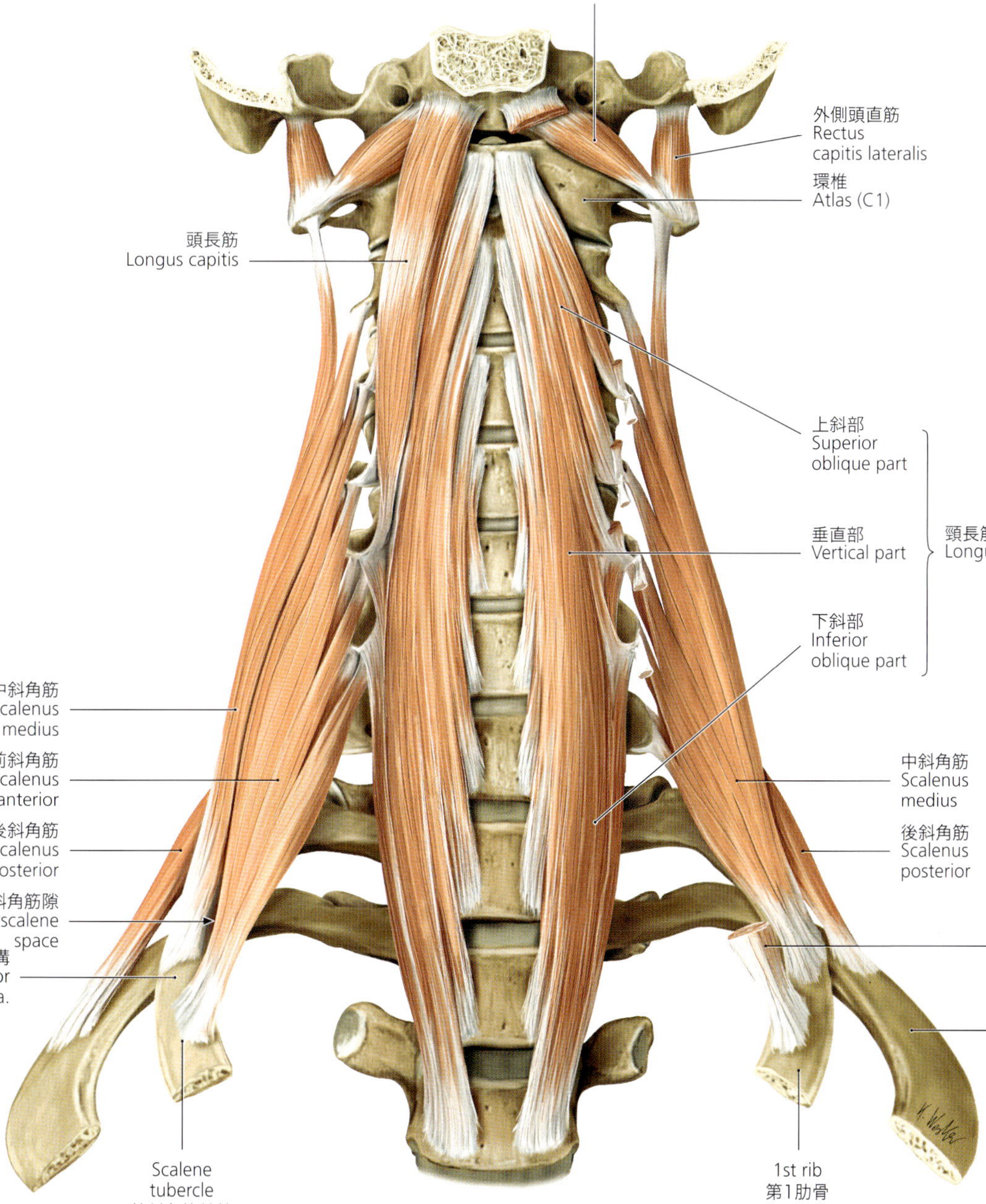

前頭直筋 Rectus capitis anterior
外側頭直筋 Rectus capitis lateralis
環椎 Atlas (C1)
頭長筋 Longus capitis
上斜部 Superior oblique part
垂直部 Vertical part　　頸長筋 Longus colli
下斜部 Inferior oblique part
中斜角筋 Scalenus medius
前斜角筋 Scalenus anterior
後斜角筋 Scalenus posterior
斜角筋隙 Interscalene space
鎖骨下動脈溝 Groove for subclavian a.
中斜角筋 Scalenus medius
後斜角筋 Scalenus posterior
前斜角筋（断端）Scalenus anterior (cut)
第2肋骨 2nd rib
Scalene tubercle 前斜角筋結節
1st rib 第1肋骨

B 椎骨前の筋と斜角筋，前方から見たところ．左側では頭長筋と前斜角筋は取り除いてある．

頸部の動脈と静脈
Arteries & Veins of the Neck

図 37.11　頸部の動脈
左外側方から見たところ．頸部の構造には主に外頸動脈（前枝）と鎖骨下動脈（椎骨動脈，肋頸動脈，甲状頸動脈）が血液を供給する．

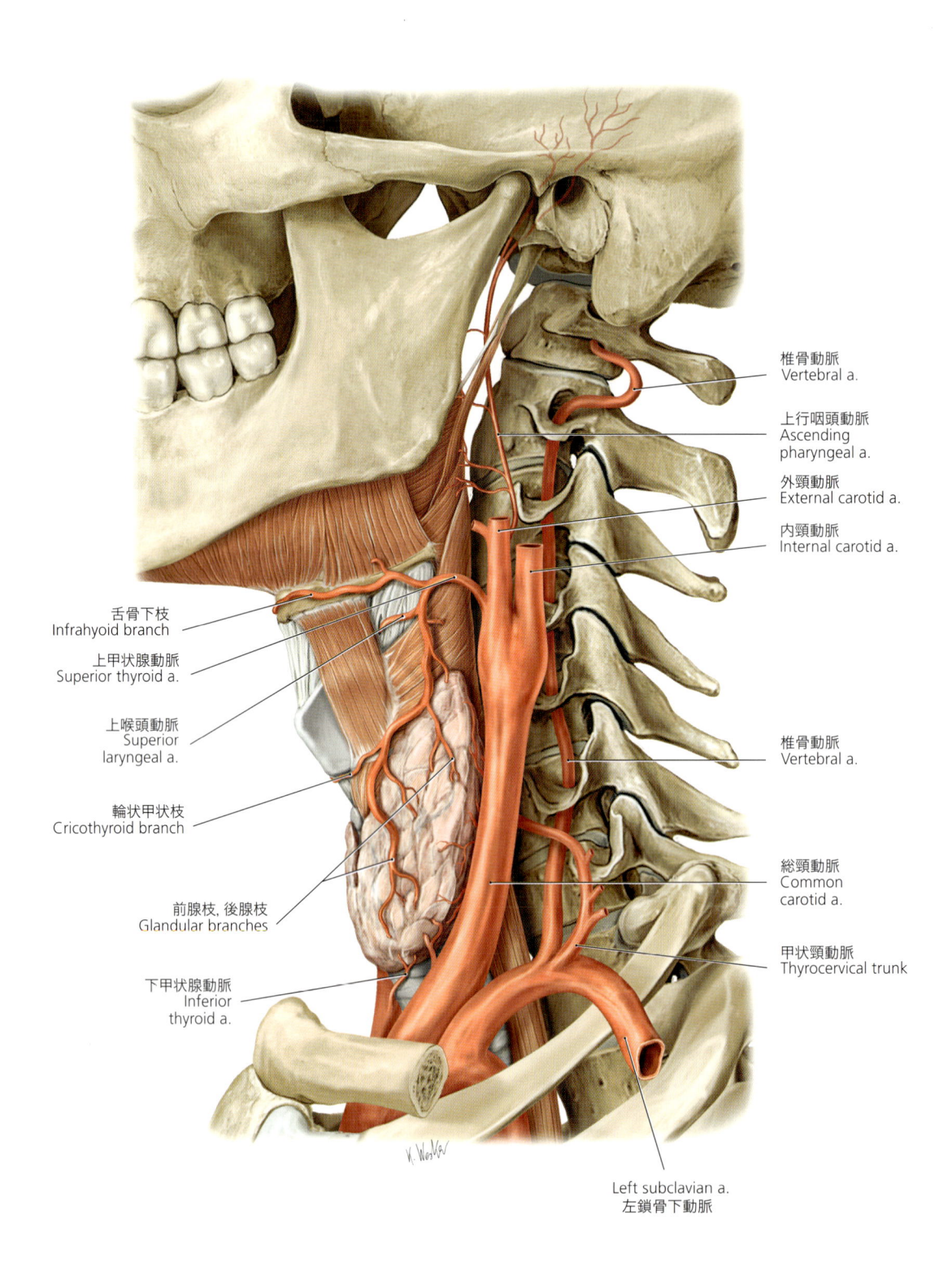

- 椎骨動脈　Vertebral a.
- 上行咽頭動脈　Ascending pharyngeal a.
- 外頸動脈　External carotid a.
- 内頸動脈　Internal carotid a.
- 舌骨下枝　Infrahyoid branch
- 上甲状腺動脈　Superior thyroid a.
- 上喉頭動脈　Superior laryngeal a.
- 輪状甲状枝　Cricothyroid branch
- 前腺枝, 後腺枝　Glandular branches
- 下甲状腺動脈　Inferior thyroid a.
- 椎骨動脈　Vertebral a.
- 総頸動脈　Common carotid a.
- 甲状頸動脈　Thyrocervical trunk
- Left subclavian a. 左鎖骨下動脈

図 37.12 頸部の静脈

左外側方から見たところ．頸部の主要な静脈は，内頸静脈，外頸静脈，前頸静脈である．

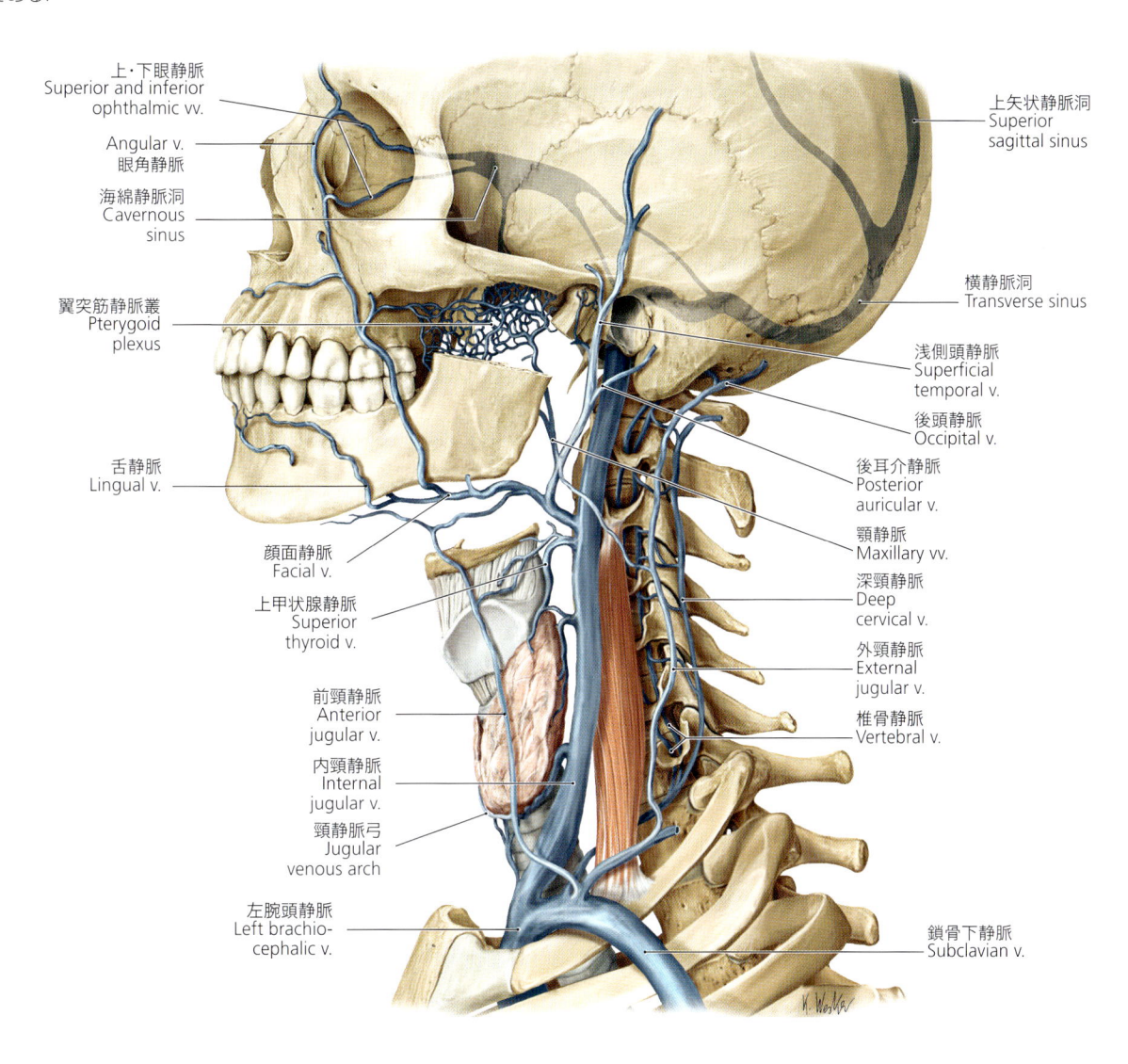

- 上・下眼静脈 Superior and inferior ophthalmic vv.
- 眼角静脈 Angular v.
- 海綿静脈洞 Cavernous sinus
- 翼突筋静脈叢 Pterygoid plexus
- 舌静脈 Lingual v.
- 顔面静脈 Facial v.
- 上甲状腺静脈 Superior thyroid v.
- 前頸静脈 Anterior jugular v.
- 内頸静脈 Internal jugular v.
- 頸静脈弓 Jugular venous arch
- 左腕頭静脈 Left brachiocephalic v.
- 上矢状静脈洞 Superior sagittal sinus
- 横静脈洞 Transverse sinus
- 浅側頭静脈 Superficial temporal v.
- 後頭静脈 Occipital v.
- 後耳介静脈 Posterior auricular v.
- 顎静脈 Maxillary vv.
- 深頸静脈 Deep cervical v.
- 外頸静脈 External jugular v.
- 椎骨静脈 Vertebral v.
- 鎖骨下静脈 Subclavian v.

臨床

頸部の静脈と血流障害

臨床的要因（慢性肺疾患，縦隔腫瘍，感染症など）によって右心への血流が障害されると，血液は上大静脈でせき止められ，後には頸静脈にも血液が貯まる．これにより頸静脈（ときにはさらに細い静脈）に顕著な瘤ができる．

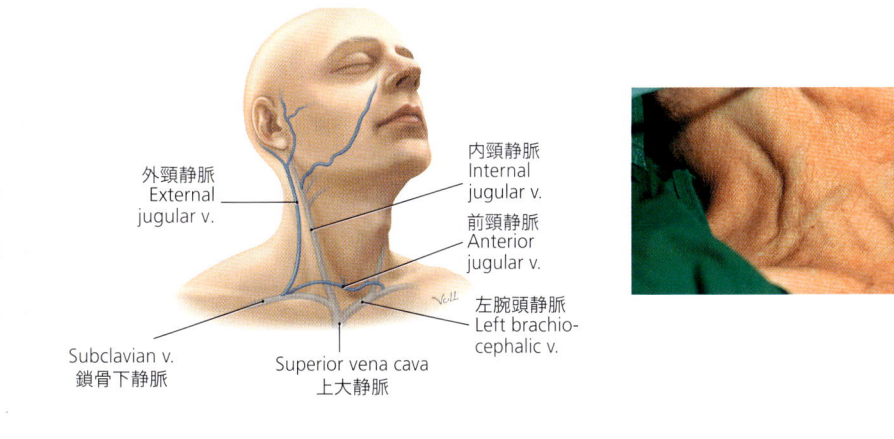

- 外頸静脈 External jugular v.
- 内頸静脈 Internal jugular v.
- 前頸静脈 Anterior jugular v.
- 左腕頭静脈 Left brachiocephalic v.
- 鎖骨下静脈 Subclavian v.
- 上大静脈 Superior vena cava

頸部の神経支配
Innervation of the Neck

表 37.8 頸部の脊髄神経の枝

後枝

	神経	感覚機能	運動機能
C1	後頭下神経	C1 は皮膚分節に与らない	
C2	大後頭神経	C2 皮膚分節	後頸部の固有筋を支配
C3	第3後頭神経	C3 皮膚分節	

前枝

	感覚神経	感覚機能	運動神経	運動機能
C1	—	—		
C2	小後頭神経	頸神経叢の感覚部をなし，前頸部と外頸部を支配	頸神経ワナを作る(頸神経叢の運動部)	甲状舌骨筋以外の舌骨下の筋を支配
C2-C3	大耳介神経			
C2-C3	頸横神経			
C3-C4	鎖骨上神経			
			横隔神経を作る*	横隔膜と心膜を支配

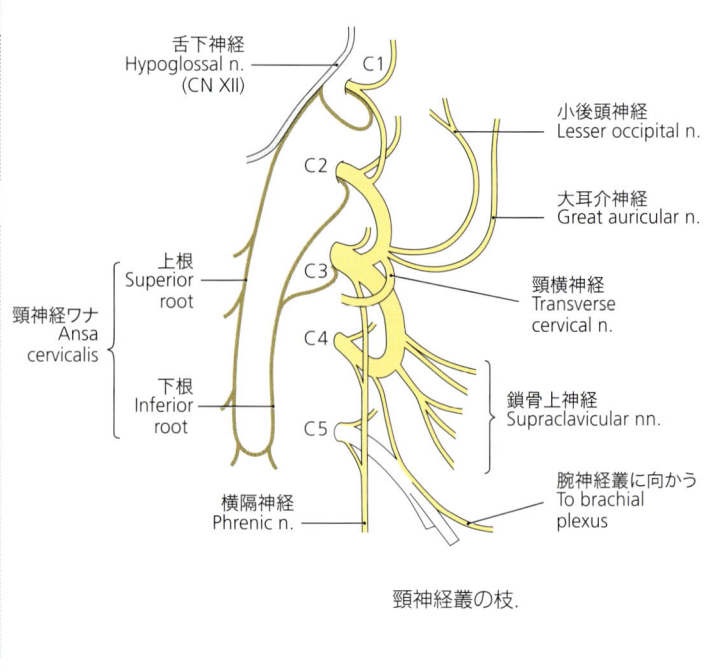

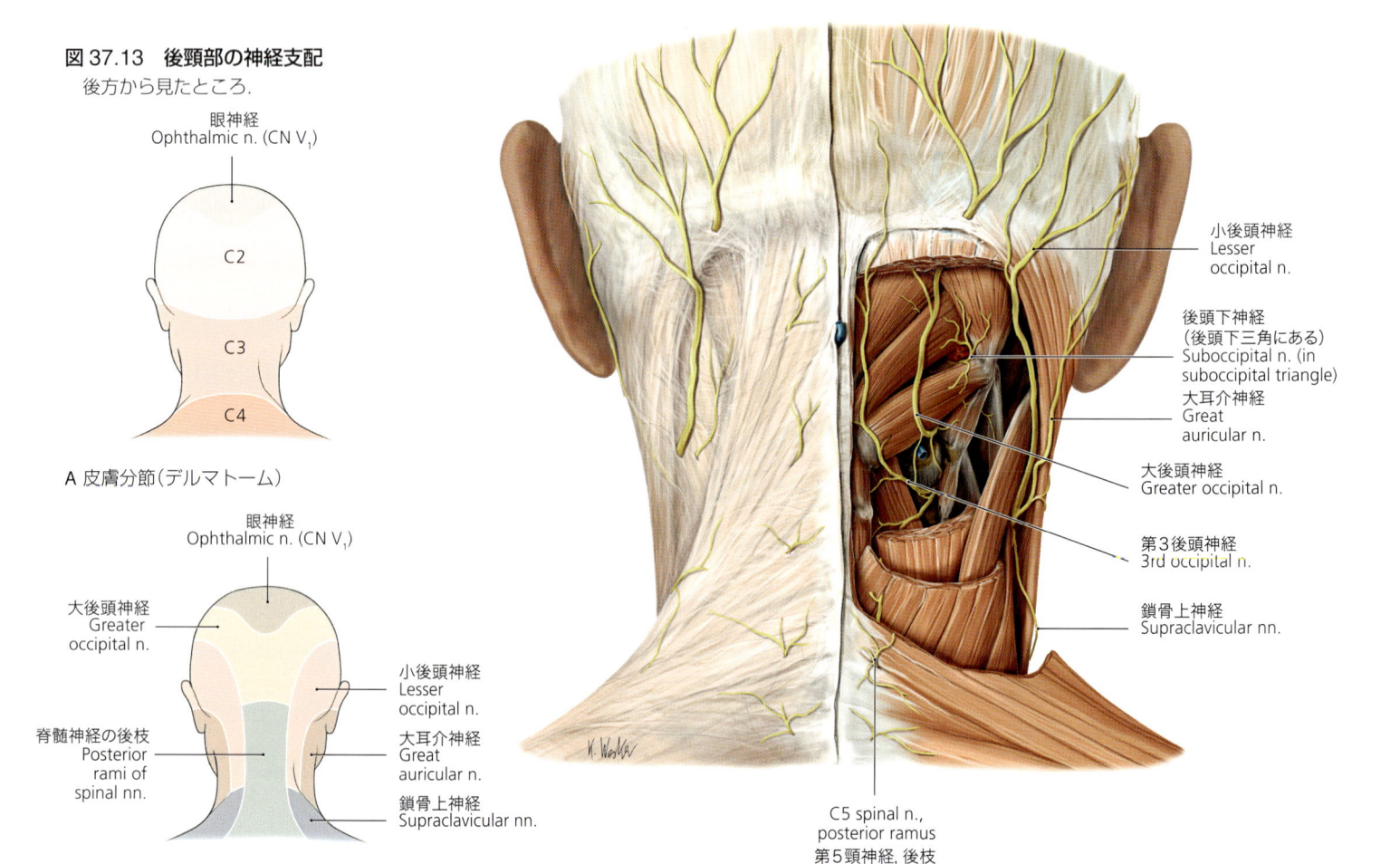

*C3-C5 の前枝が合流して横隔神経を作る(p.54 参照).

頸神経叢の枝.

図 37.13 後頸部の神経支配
後方から見たところ.

A 皮膚分節(デルマトーム)

B 皮神経の領域.

C 脊髄神経の枝.

図 37.14　前・外側頸部の感覚神経支配
左外側方から見たところ.

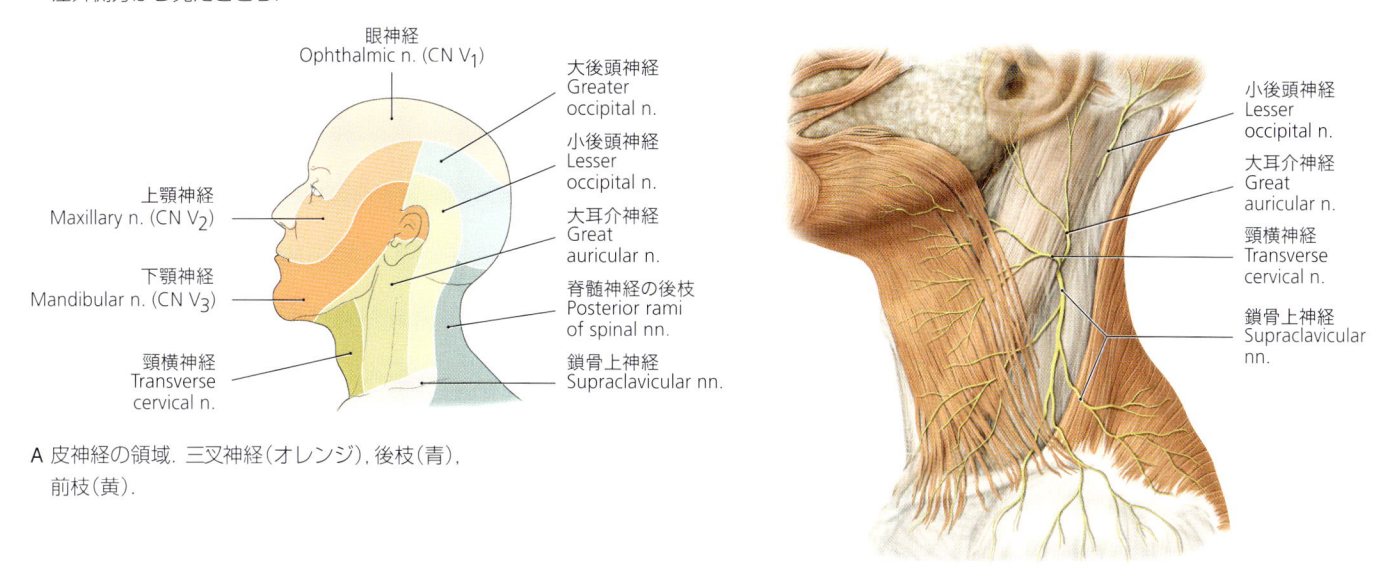

眼神経 Ophthalmic n. (CN V$_1$)
大後頭神経 Greater occipital n.
小後頭神経 Lesser occipital n.
上顎神経 Maxillary n. (CN V$_2$)
大耳介神経 Great auricular n.
下顎神経 Mandibular n. (CN V$_3$)
脊髄神経の後枝 Posterior rami of spinal nn.
頸横神経 Transverse cervical n.
鎖骨上神経 Supraclavicular nn.

A 皮神経の領域. 三叉神経(オレンジ), 後枝(青), 前枝(黄).

小後頭神経 Lesser occipital n.
大耳介神経 Great auricular n.
頸横神経 Transverse cervical n.
鎖骨上神経 Supraclavicular nn.

B 頸神経叢の感覚神経.

図 37.15　前・外側頸部の運動神経支配
左外側方から見たところ.

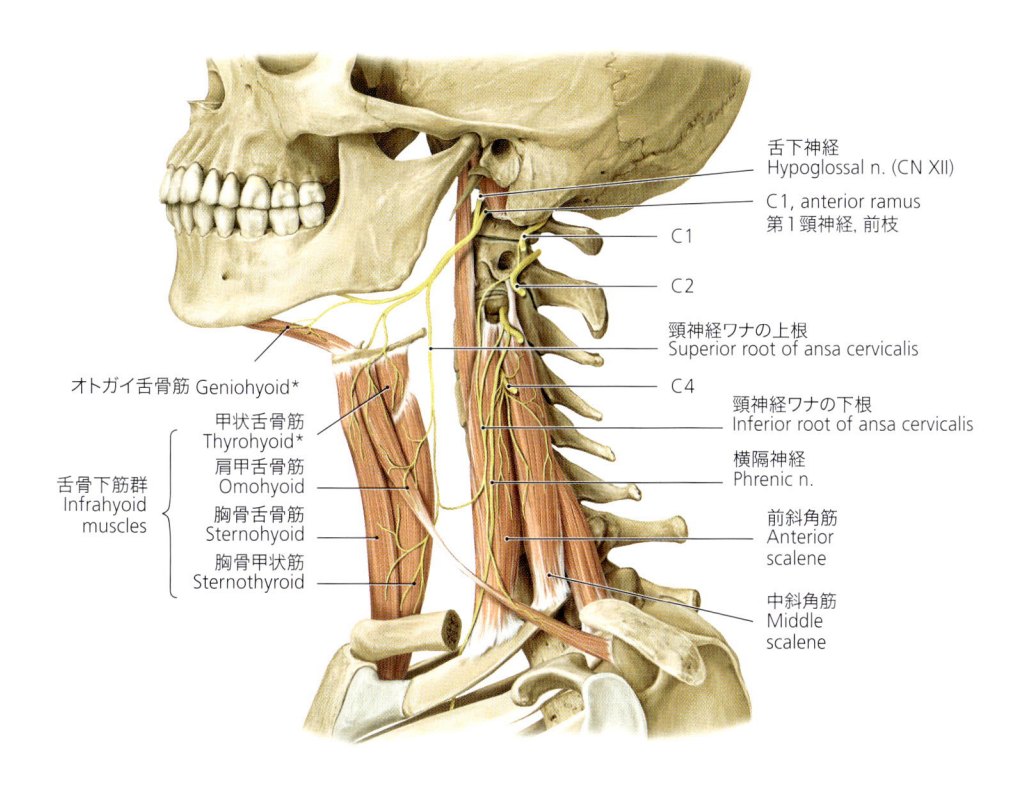

舌下神経 Hypoglossal n. (CN XII)
C1, anterior ramus 第1頸神経, 前枝
C1
C2
頸神経ワナの上根 Superior root of ansa cervicalis
C4
頸神経ワナの下根 Inferior root of ansa cervicalis
横隔神経 Phrenic n.
前斜角筋 Anterior scalene
中斜角筋 Middle scalene

オトガイ舌骨筋 Geniohyoid*
甲状舌骨筋 Thyrohyoid*
肩甲舌骨筋 Omohyoid
胸骨舌骨筋 Sternohyoid
胸骨甲状筋 Sternothyoid
舌骨下筋群 Infrahyoid muscles

*舌下神経と伴行する. 第1頸神経(C1)の前枝によって支配される.

喉頭：軟骨と構造
Larynx: Cartilage & Structure

図 37.16 喉頭軟骨
左外側方から見たところ．喉頭は，喉頭蓋軟骨，甲状軟骨，輪状軟骨，1対の披裂軟骨，1対の小角軟骨の5つの軟骨からなる．これらの軟骨は互いに，また気管や舌骨と弾性のある靱帯でつながっている．

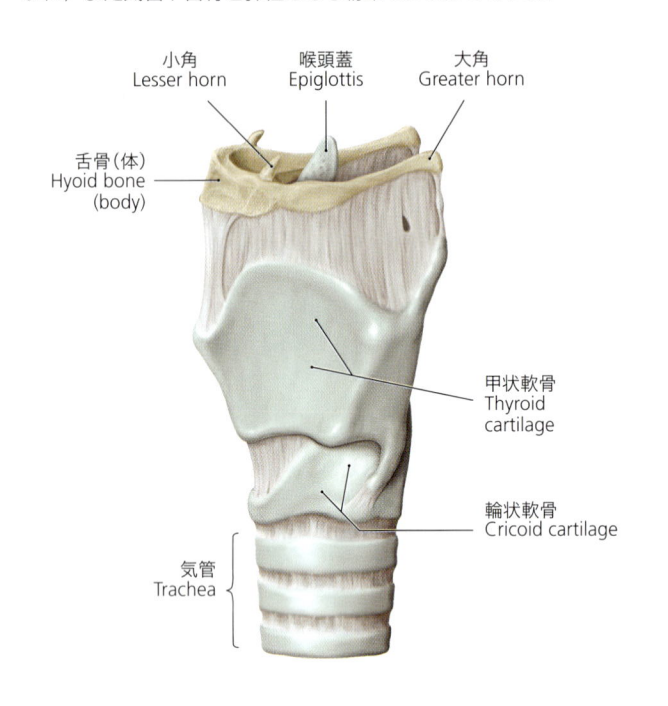

- 小角 Lesser horn
- 喉頭蓋 Epiglottis
- 大角 Greater horn
- 舌骨（体）Hyoid bone (body)
- 甲状軟骨 Thyroid cartilage
- 輪状軟骨 Cricoid cartilage
- 気管 Trachea

図 37.17 喉頭蓋軟骨
喉頭蓋の内部骨格は，弾性軟骨の喉頭蓋軟骨からなり，嚥下終了時に喉頭蓋が自動的に元の位置に戻るようになっている．

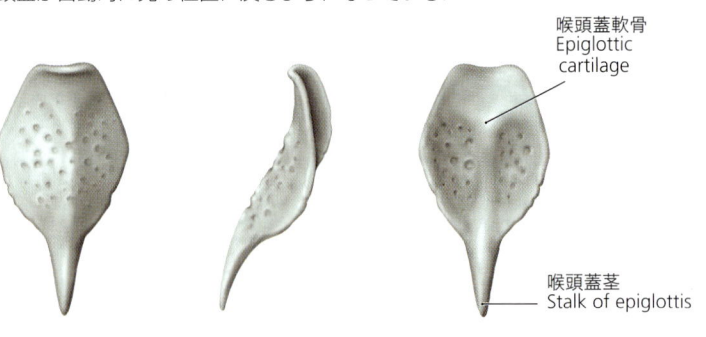

- 喉頭蓋軟骨 Epiglottic cartilage
- 喉頭蓋茎 Stalk of epiglottis

A 舌側面（前方から見たところ）．
B 左外側方から見たところ．
C 喉頭面（後方から見たところ）．

図 37.18 甲状軟骨
左外側面．

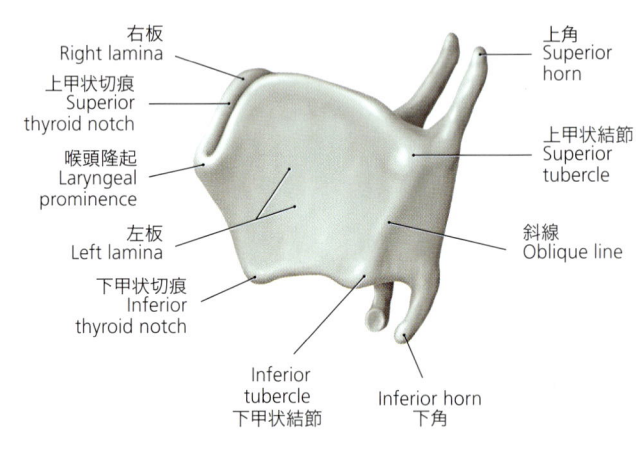

- 右板 Right lamina
- 上甲状切痕 Superior thyroid notch
- 喉頭隆起 Laryngeal prominence
- 左板 Left lamina
- 下甲状切痕 Inferior thyroid notch
- 上角 Superior horn
- 上甲状結節 Superior tubercle
- 斜線 Oblique line
- 下甲状結節 Inferior tubercle
- 下角 Inferior horn

図 37.19 輪状軟骨

- 披裂関節面 Articular facet for arytenoid cartilage
- 甲状関節面 Articular facet for thyroid cartilage
- 輪状軟骨弓 Arch
- 輪状軟骨板 Lamina

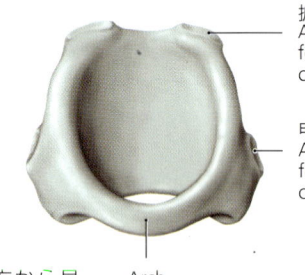

A 前方から見たところ．（Arch 輪状軟骨弓）
B 左外側方から見たところ．
C 後方から見たところ．

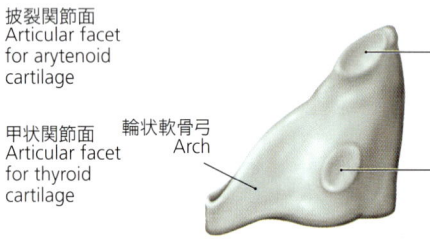

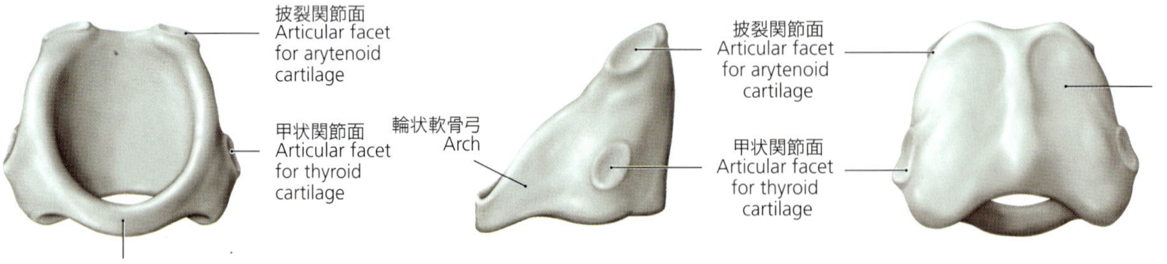

図 37.20 披裂軟骨と小角軟骨
右側の軟骨．

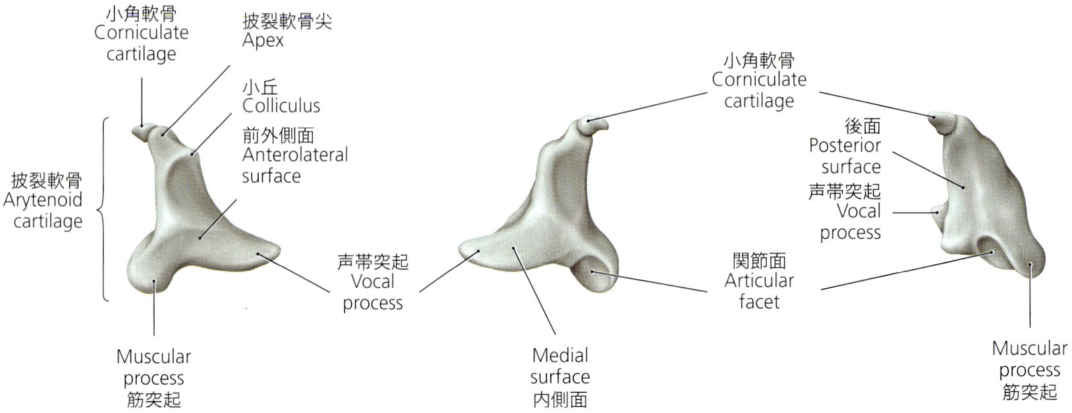

- 小角軟骨 Corniculate cartilage
- 披裂軟骨尖 Apex
- 小丘 Colliculus
- 前外側面 Anterolateral surface
- 披裂軟骨 Arytenoid cartilage
- 声帯突起 Vocal process
- 筋突起 Muscular process
- 内側面 Medial surface
- 後面 Posterior surface
- 関節面 Articular facet

A 右外側方から見たところ．
B 内側方から見たところ．
C 後方から見たところ．

図 37.21　喉頭の構造

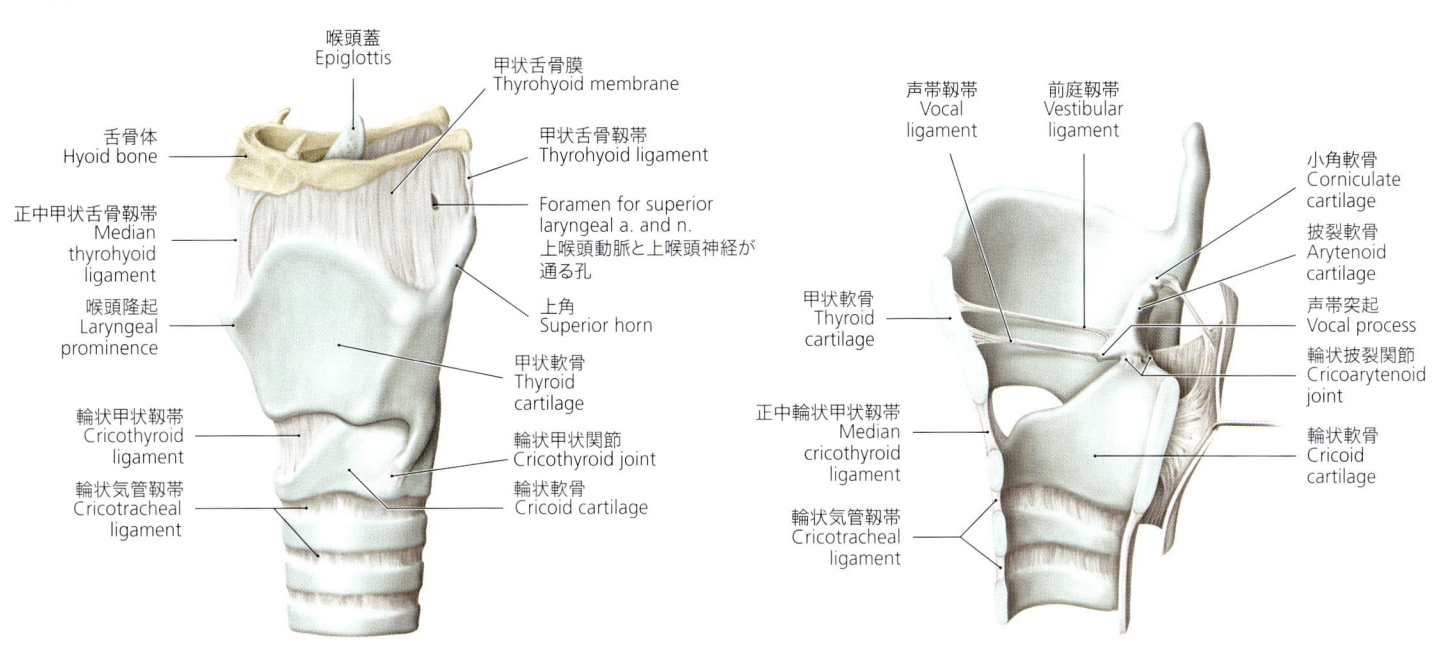

A 左前斜方向から見たところ．

B 矢状断，左内側方から見たところ．披裂軟骨は発声時に声帯ヒダの位置を変化させる．

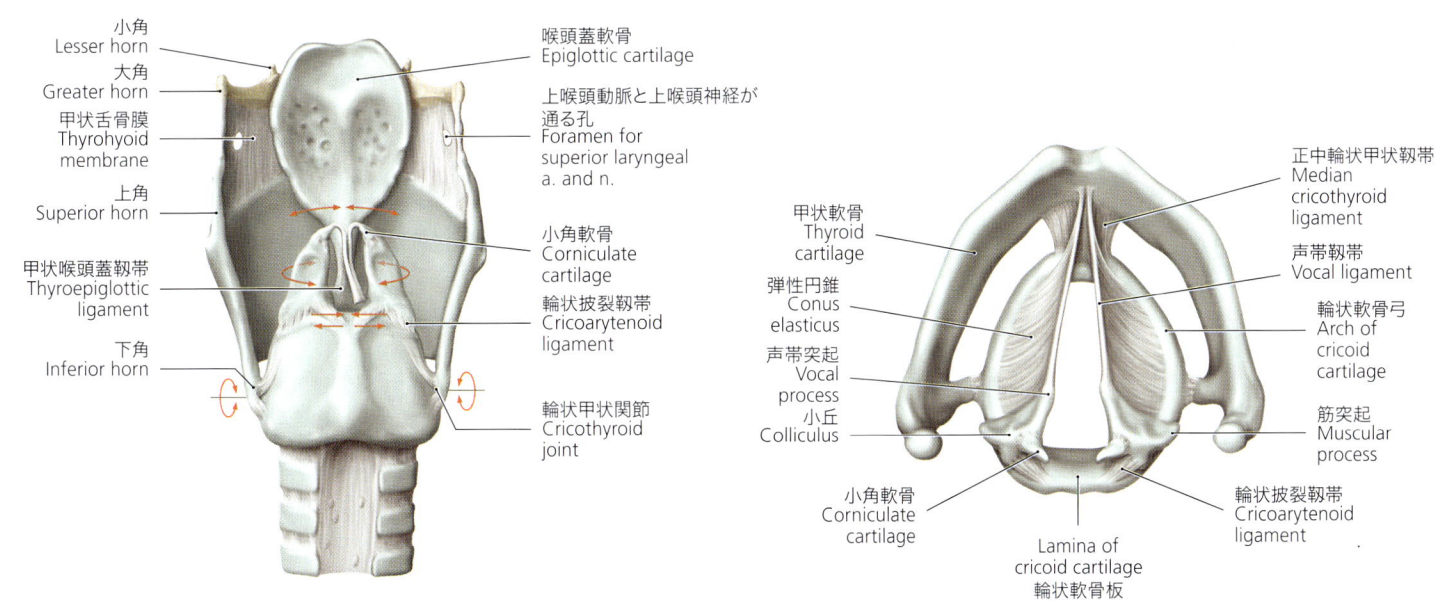

C 後方から見たところ．矢印は喉頭の関節における種々の運動の方向を示す．

D 上方から見たところ．

喉頭：筋と区分
Larynx: Muscles & Levels

図 37.22　喉頭筋

喉頭の筋は喉頭軟骨を動かし，それぞれの相対的な位置を変えて，声帯ヒダの緊張や位置に影響を与える．喉頭全体を動かす筋（舌骨上と舌骨下の筋）は p. 562 に解説している．

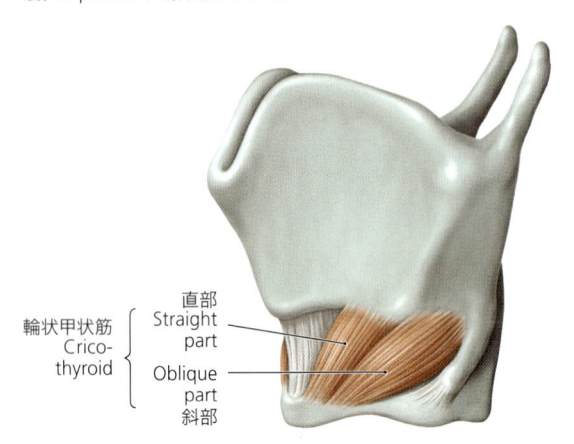

A 外喉頭筋，左外側斜方から見たところ．

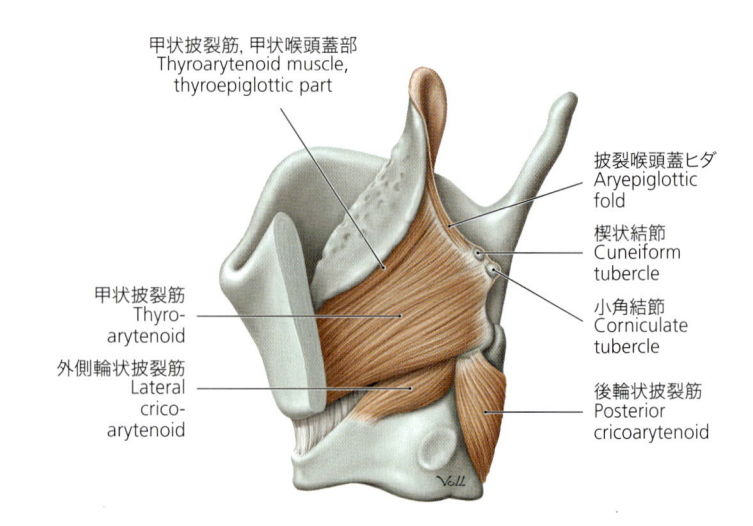

- 輪状甲状筋 Cricothyroid
  - 直部 Straight part
  - 斜部 Oblique part

B 内喉頭筋，左外側方から見たところ．甲状軟骨の左半分は取り除いてある．喉頭蓋と甲状披裂筋が示される．

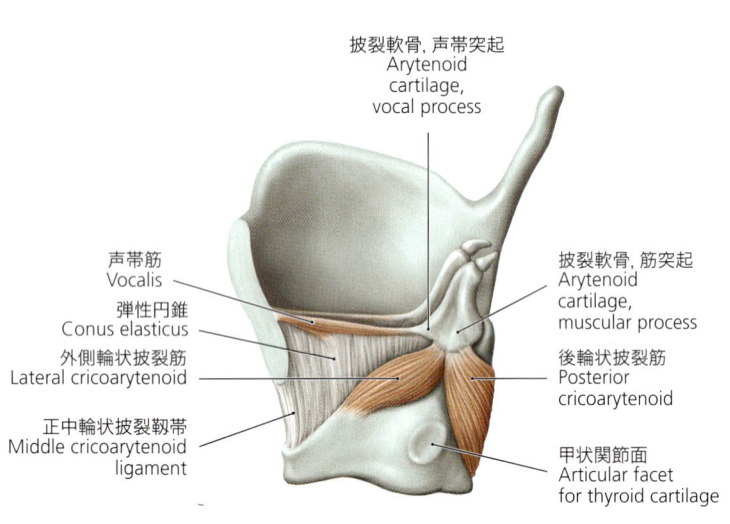

- 甲状披裂筋，甲状喉頭蓋部 Thyroarytenoid muscle, thyroepiglottic part
- 披裂喉頭蓋ヒダ Aryepiglottic fold
- 楔状結節 Cuneiform tubercle
- 甲状披裂筋 Thyro-arytenoid
- 小角結節 Corniculate tubercle
- 外側輪状披裂筋 Lateral cricoarytenoid
- 後輪状披裂筋 Posterior cricoarytenoid

C 左外側方から見たところ．喉頭蓋は取り除いてある．

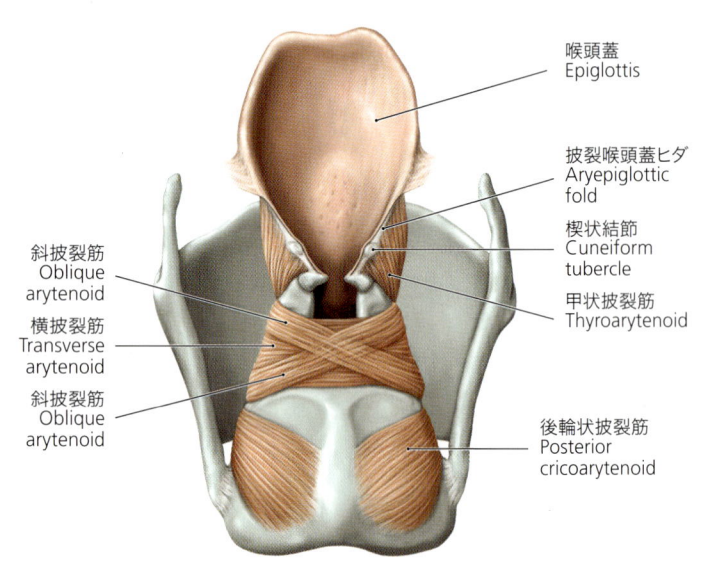

- 披裂軟骨，声帯突起 Arytenoid cartilage, vocal process
- 声帯筋 Vocalis
- 弾性円錐 Conus elasticus
- 外側輪状披裂筋 Lateral cricoarytenoid
- 正中輪状披裂靱帯 Middle cricoarytenoid ligament
- 披裂軟骨，筋突起 Arytenoid cartilage, muscular process
- 後輪状披裂筋 Posterior cricoarytenoid
- 甲状関節面 Articular facet for thyroid cartilage

D 後方から見たところ．

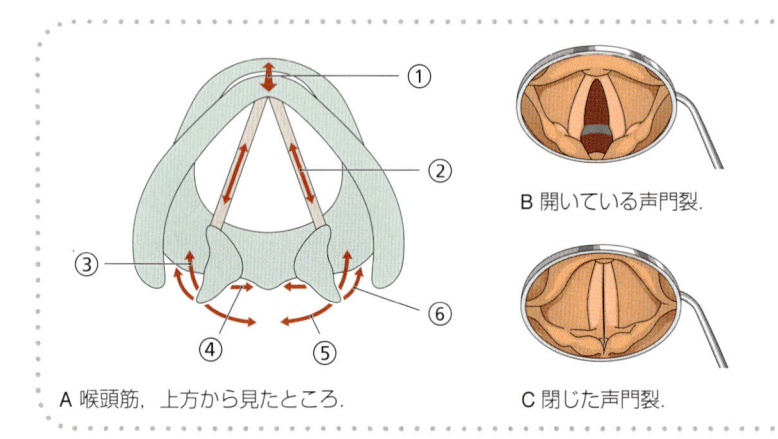

- 喉頭蓋 Epiglottis
- 披裂喉頭蓋ヒダ Aryepiglottic fold
- 楔状結節 Cuneiform tubercle
- 甲状披裂筋 Thyroarytenoid
- 斜披裂筋 Oblique arytenoid
- 横披裂筋 Transverse arytenoid
- 斜披裂筋 Oblique arytenoid
- 後輪状披裂筋 Posterior cricoarytenoid

A 喉頭筋，上方から見たところ．
B 開いている声門裂．
C 閉じた声門裂．

表 37.9　喉頭筋の作用

筋	作用	声門裂への効果
①輪状甲状筋*	声帯ヒダの緊張	なし
②声帯筋		
③甲状披裂筋	声帯ヒダの内転	閉じる
④横披裂筋		
⑤後輪状披裂筋	声帯ヒダの外転	開く
⑥外側輪状披裂筋	声帯ヒダの内転	閉じる

*輪状甲状筋は喉頭の外面にある唯一の筋である．

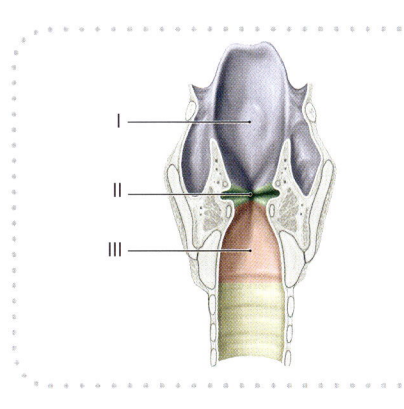

表37.10	喉頭の区分	
区分	領域	範囲
I	声門上腔（喉頭前庭）	喉頭の入口（喉頭口）から前庭ヒダまで
II	声門間腔（喉頭室）	前庭ヒダから喉頭室（粘膜の外側への膨出）を通り，声帯ヒダまで
III	声門下腔	声帯ヒダから輪状軟骨の下縁まで

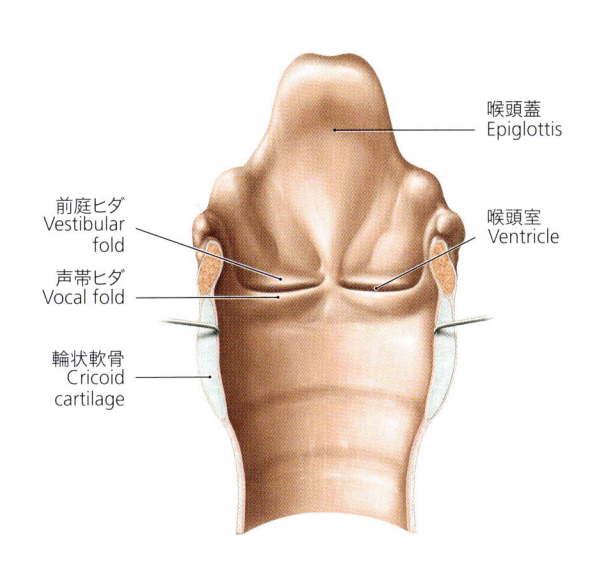

図 37.23　喉頭腔

A 後方から見たところ．喉頭は切り広げられている．

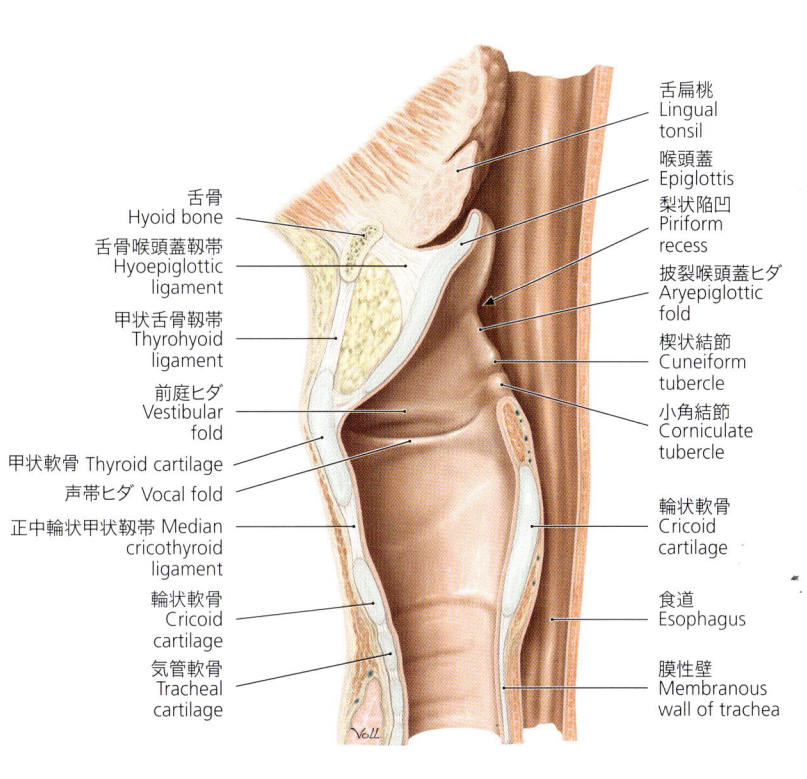

B 正中矢状断，左外側方から見たところ．

図 37.24　前庭ヒダと声帯ヒダ
冠状断，上方から見たところ．

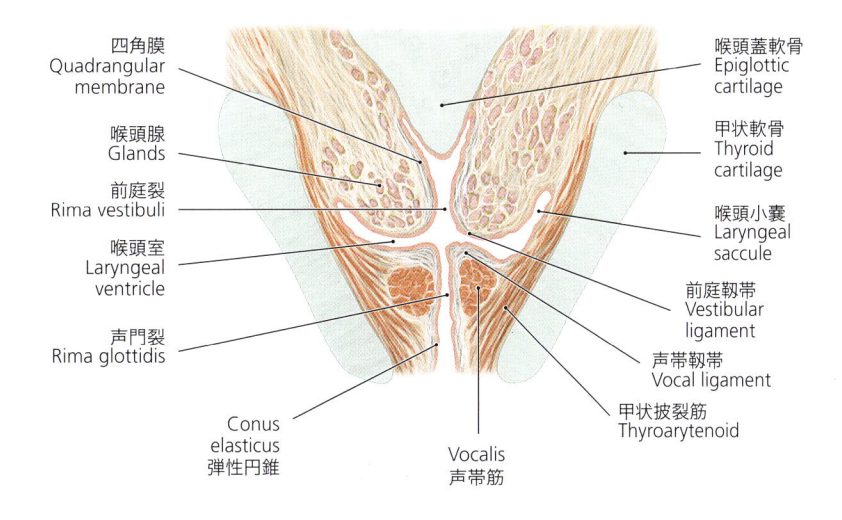

37
頸部

573

喉頭の神経と血管，甲状腺と副甲状腺（上皮小体）
Neurovasculature of the Larynx, Thyroid & Parathyroids

図 37.25　甲状腺と副甲状腺（上皮小体）

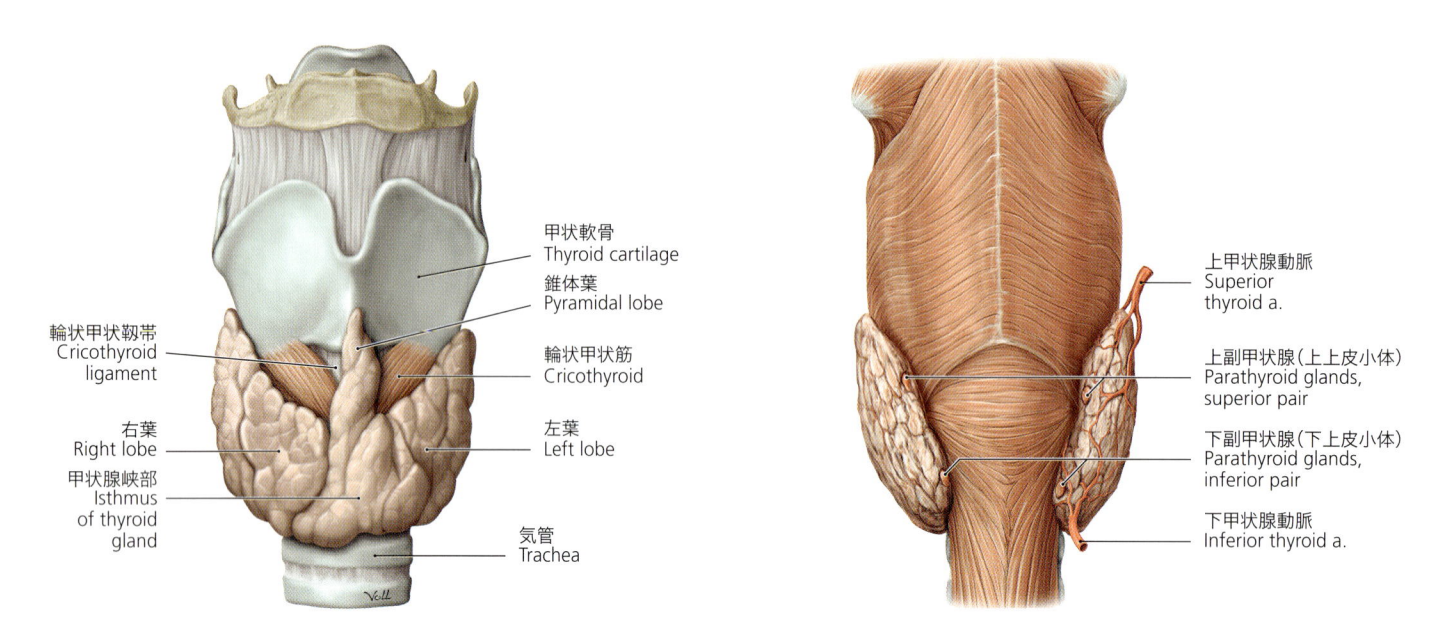

A　甲状腺，前方から見たところ．

B　甲状腺と副甲状腺（上皮小体），後方から見たところ．

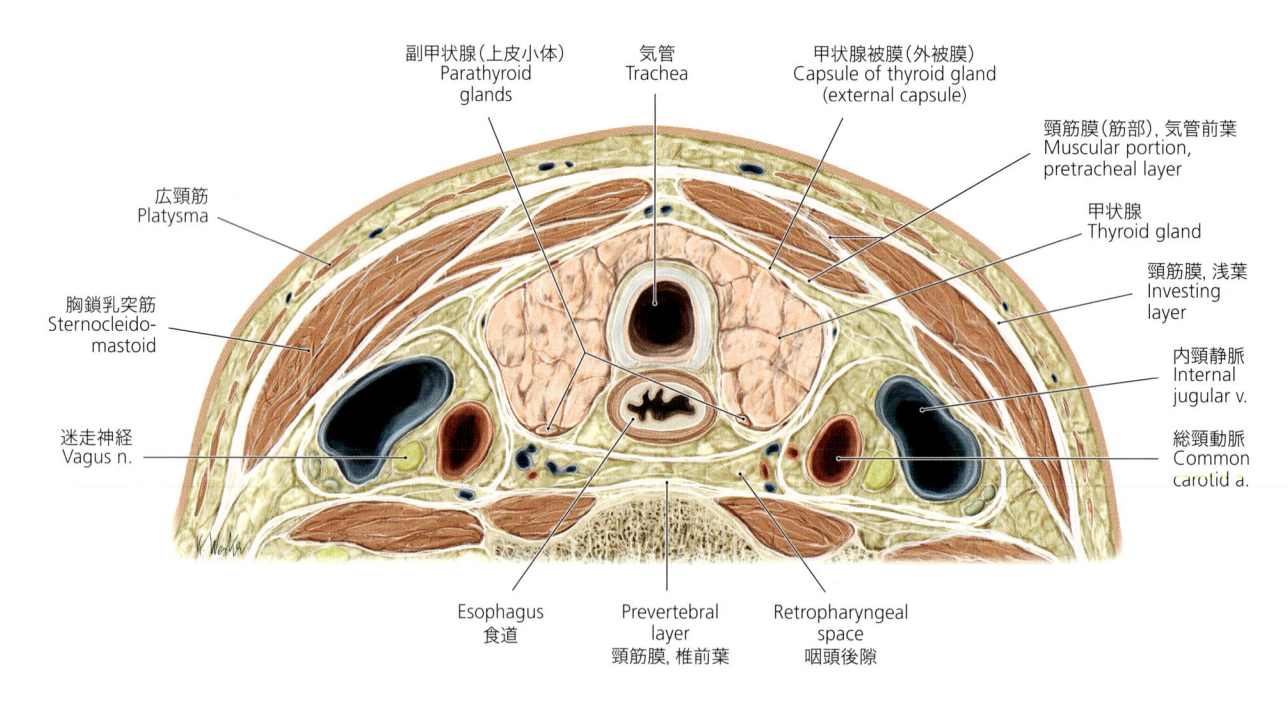

C　甲状腺と副甲状腺の局所解剖的な関係．頸筋膜については p.577 参照．

図 37.26　動脈と神経
前方から見たところ.

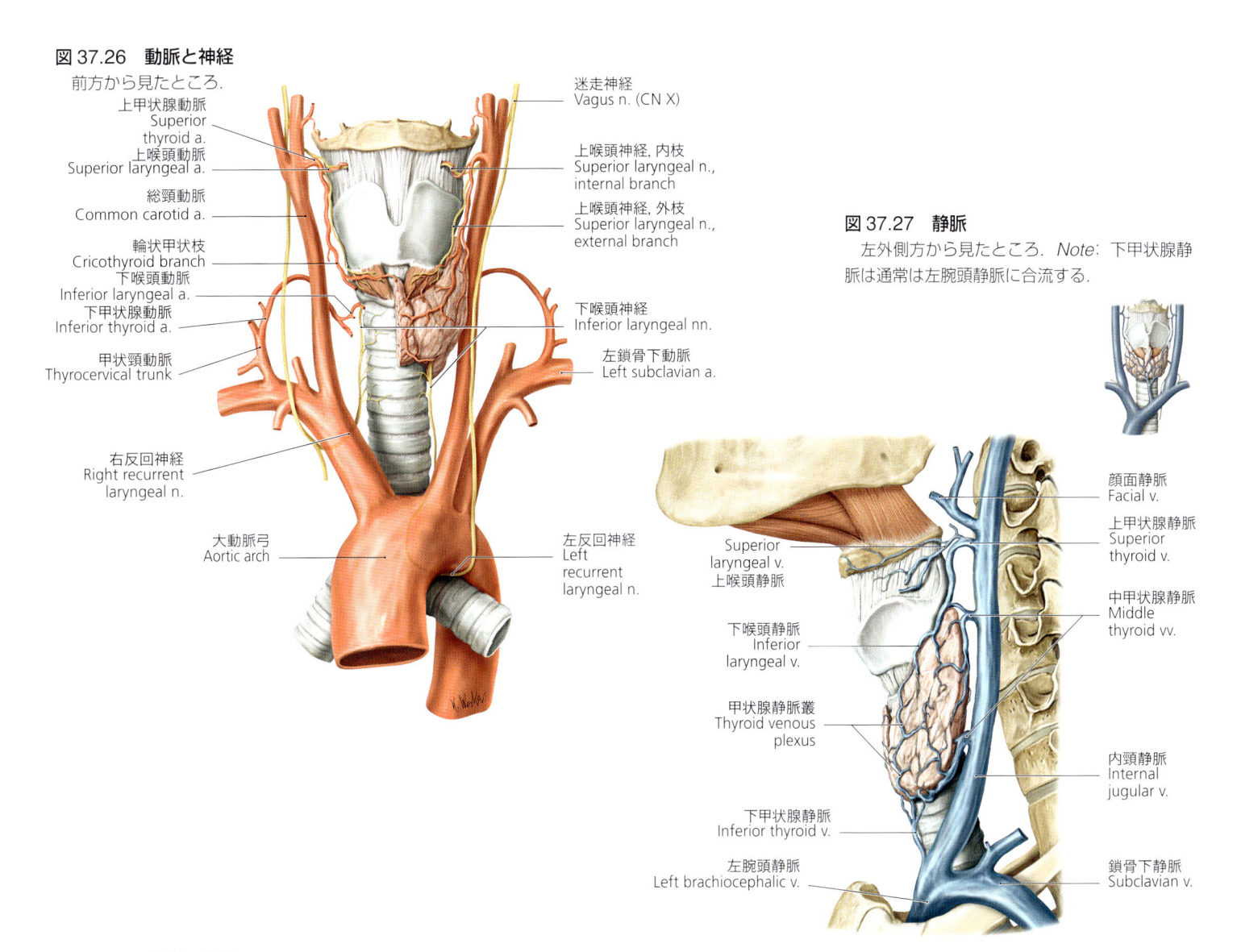

- 上甲状腺動脈 Superior thyroid a.
- 上喉頭動脈 Superior laryngeal a.
- 総頸動脈 Common carotid a.
- 輪状甲状枝 Cricothyroid branch
- 下喉頭動脈 Inferior laryngeal a.
- 下甲状腺動脈 Inferior thyroid a.
- 甲状頸動脈 Thyrocervical trunk
- 右反回神経 Right recurrent laryngeal n.
- 大動脈弓 Aortic arch
- 迷走神経 Vagus n. (CN X)
- 上喉頭神経, 内枝 Superior laryngeal n., internal branch
- 上喉頭神経, 外枝 Superior laryngeal n., external branch
- 下喉頭神経 Inferior laryngeal nn.
- 左鎖骨下動脈 Left subclavian a.
- 左反回神経 Left recurrent laryngeal n.

図 37.27　静脈
左外側方から見たところ. Note: 下甲状腺静脈は通常は左腕頭静脈に合流する.

- 上喉頭静脈 Superior laryngeal v.
- 下喉頭静脈 Inferior laryngeal v.
- 甲状腺静脈叢 Thyroid venous plexus
- 下甲状腺静脈 Inferior thyroid v.
- 左腕頭静脈 Left brachiocephalic v.
- 顔面静脈 Facial v.
- 上甲状腺静脈 Superior thyroid v.
- 中甲状腺静脈 Middle thyroid vv.
- 内頸静脈 Internal jugular v.
- 鎖骨下静脈 Subclavian v.

図 37.28　神経・血管
左外側方から見たところ.

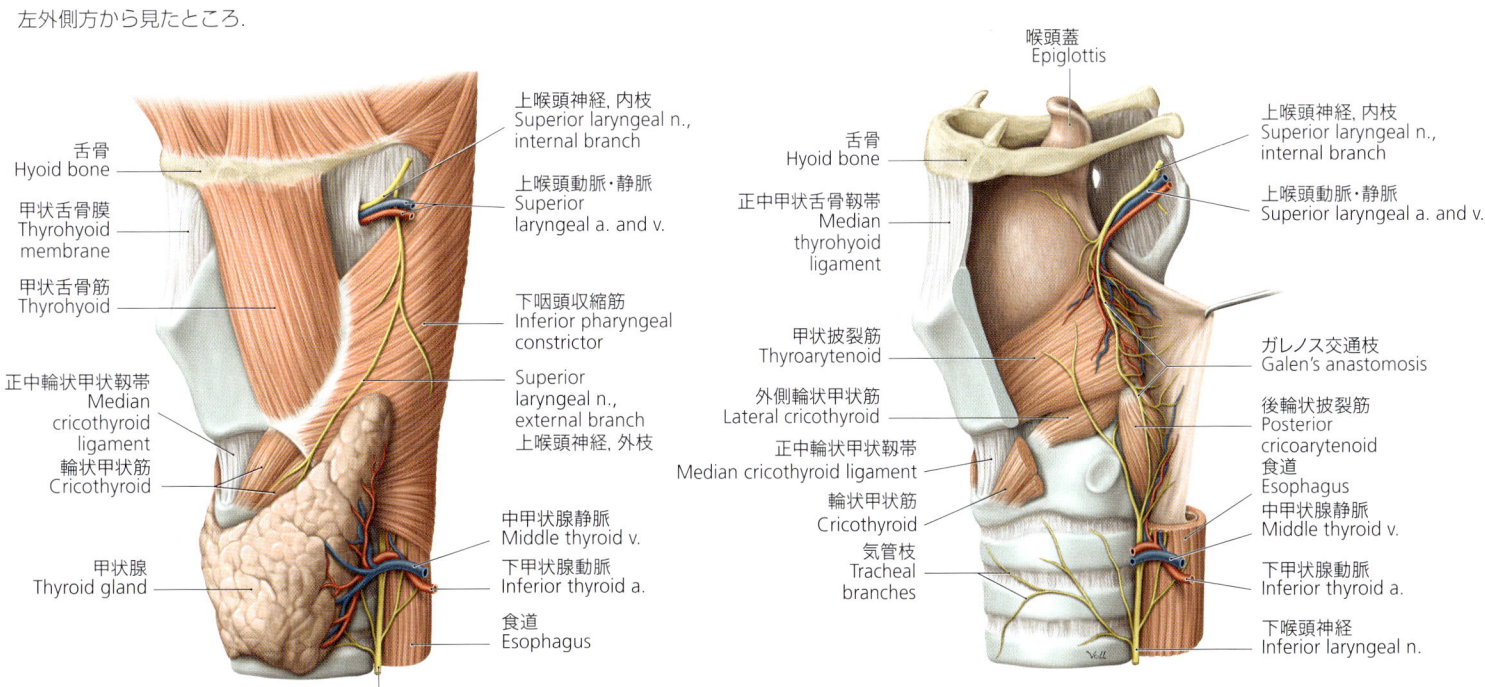

A 浅層.

- 舌骨 Hyoid bone
- 甲状舌骨膜 Thyrohyoid membrane
- 甲状舌骨筋 Thyrohyoid
- 正中輪状甲状靱帯 Median cricothyroid ligament
- 輪状甲状筋 Cricothyroid
- 甲状腺 Thyroid gland
- 上喉頭神経, 内枝 Superior laryngeal n., internal branch
- 上喉頭動脈・静脈 Superior laryngeal a. and v.
- 下咽頭収縮筋 Inferior pharyngeal constrictor
- 上喉頭神経, 外枝 Superior laryngeal n., external branch
- 中甲状腺静脈 Middle thyroid v.
- 下甲状腺動脈 Inferior thyroid a.
- 食道 Esophagus
- 下喉頭神経 Inferior laryngeal n.

B 深層. 輪状甲状筋と甲状軟骨の左板は取り除き, 咽頭粘膜を後ろに引いてある.

- 喉頭蓋 Epiglottis
- 舌骨 Hyoid bone
- 正中甲状舌骨靱帯 Median thyrohyoid ligament
- 甲状披裂筋 Thyroarytenoid
- 外側輪状甲状筋 Lateral cricothyroid
- 正中輪状甲状靱帯 Median cricothyroid ligament
- 輪状甲状筋 Cricothyroid
- 気管枝 Tracheal branches
- 上喉頭神経, 内枝 Superior laryngeal n., internal branch
- 上喉頭動脈・静脈 Superior laryngeal a. and v.
- ガレノス交通枝 Galen's anastomosis
- 後輪状披裂筋 Posterior cricoarytenoid
- 食道 Esophagus
- 中甲状腺静脈 Middle thyroid v.
- 下甲状腺動脈 Inferior thyroid a.
- 下喉頭神経 Inferior laryngeal n.

頸部の局所解剖：部位と筋膜
Topography of the Neck: Regions & Fascia

表37.11　頸の部位

部位	区分	構造物
①前頸部（前頸三角）	顎下三角	顎下腺，顎下リンパ節，舌下神経（CN XII），顔面動脈・顔面静脈
	オトガイ下三角	オトガイ下リンパ節
	筋三角	胸骨甲状筋，胸骨舌骨筋，甲状腺，副甲状腺（上皮小体）
	頸動脈三角	頸動脈分岐部，頸動脈小体，舌下神経（CN XII），迷走神経（CN X）
②胸鎖乳突筋部*		胸鎖乳突筋，頸動脈，内頸静脈，迷走神経（CN X），頸静脈リンパ節
③外側頸三角部（後頸三角）	肩甲鎖骨三角	鎖骨下動脈，肩甲下動脈，鎖骨上リンパ節
	後頭三角	副神経（CN XI），腕神経叢の神経幹，頸横動脈，頸神経叢の後枝
④後頸部		後頭下の筋肉，椎骨動脈，頸神経叢

*胸鎖乳突筋部は小鎖骨上窩も含む．

A 右前方から見たところ．

B 左後方から見たところ．

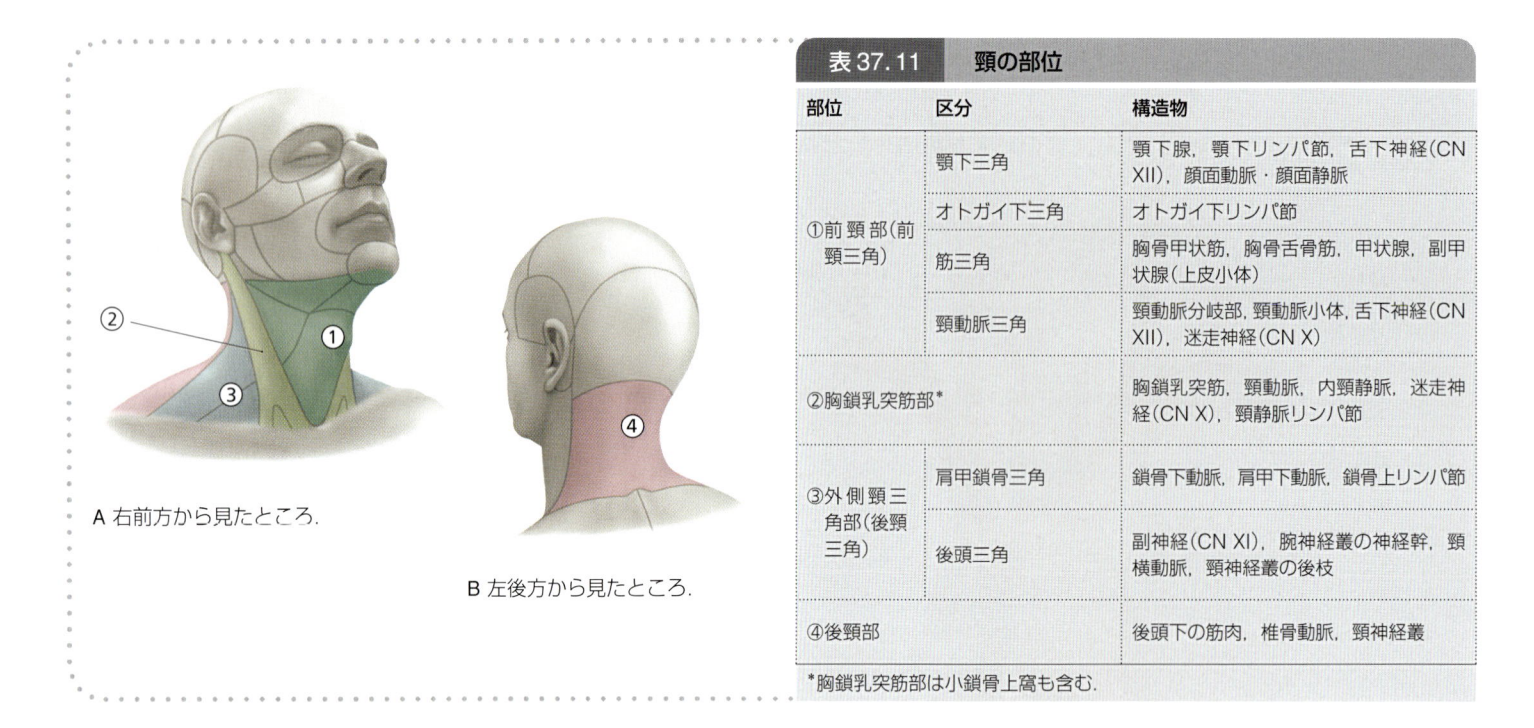

図 37.29　頸部の部位

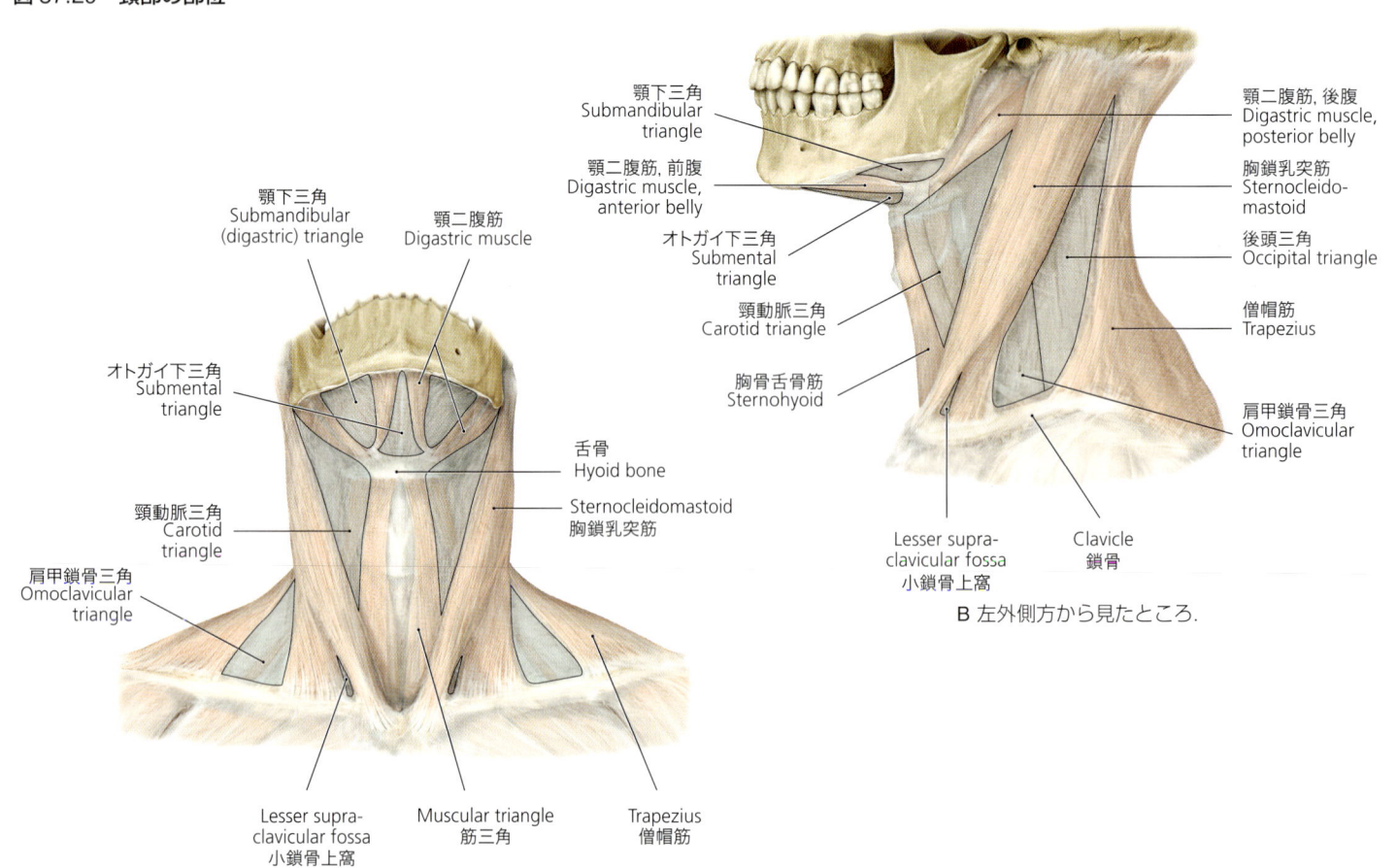

A 前方から見たところ．

B 左外側方から見たところ．

表 37.12　頸筋膜

頸筋膜は頸部の構造を囲む4層に分けられる.

葉	層	種類	特徴
①浅葉	浅筋膜	筋を包む	頸全体を覆う. 2葉に分かれて胸鎖乳突筋と僧帽筋を包む
気管前葉	②気管前筋膜		舌骨下筋を包む
	③内臓筋膜	内臓を包む	甲状腺, 喉頭, 気管, 咽頭, 食道を取り囲む
④椎前葉	椎前筋膜	筋を包む	脊柱の頸部と付着する筋肉を取り囲む
⑤頸動脈鞘		神経・血管を包む	総頸動脈, 内頸静脈, 迷走神経を包む

A 第5頸椎の高さでの水平断面.

B 正中矢状断, 左外側方から見たところ.

項靱帯 Nuchal ligament
脊髄 Spinal cord

図 37.30　頸筋膜
前方から見たところ.

下顎骨 Mandible
耳下腺 Parotid gland
頸筋膜, 浅葉 ① Investing layer
胸鎖乳突筋 Sternocleidomastoid
胸骨舌骨筋 Sternohyoid
頸動脈鞘 Carotid sheath ⑤
気管前葉の内臓部 ③ Visceral portion, pretracheal layer
肩甲舌骨筋 Omohyoid
気管前葉の筋部 ② Muscular portion, pretracheal layer
頸筋膜, 椎前葉 Prevertebral ④ layer
僧帽筋 Trapezius
鎖骨 Clavicle

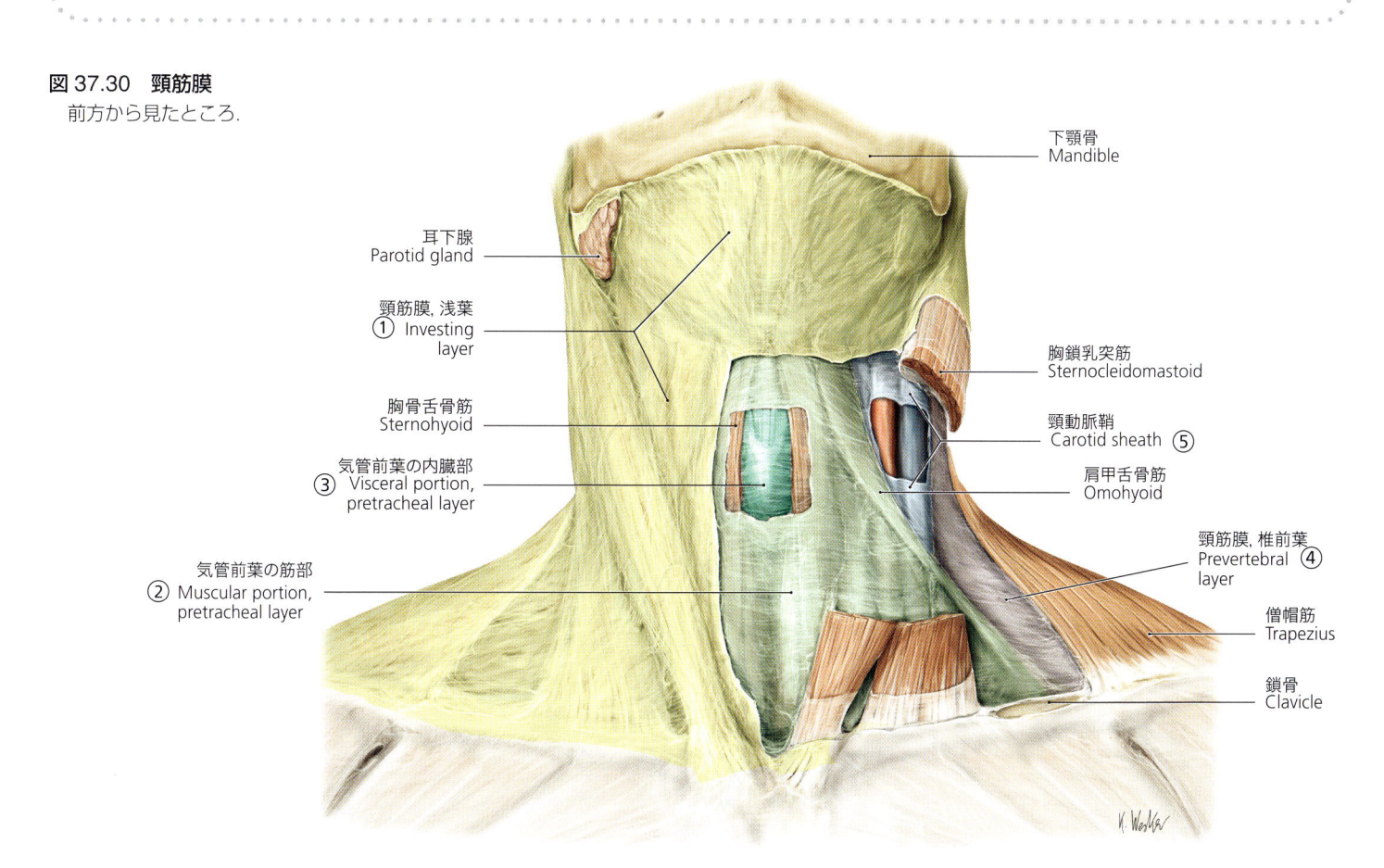

前頸部の局所解剖
Topography of the Anterior Cervical Region

図 37.31　前頸三角
前方から見たところ．

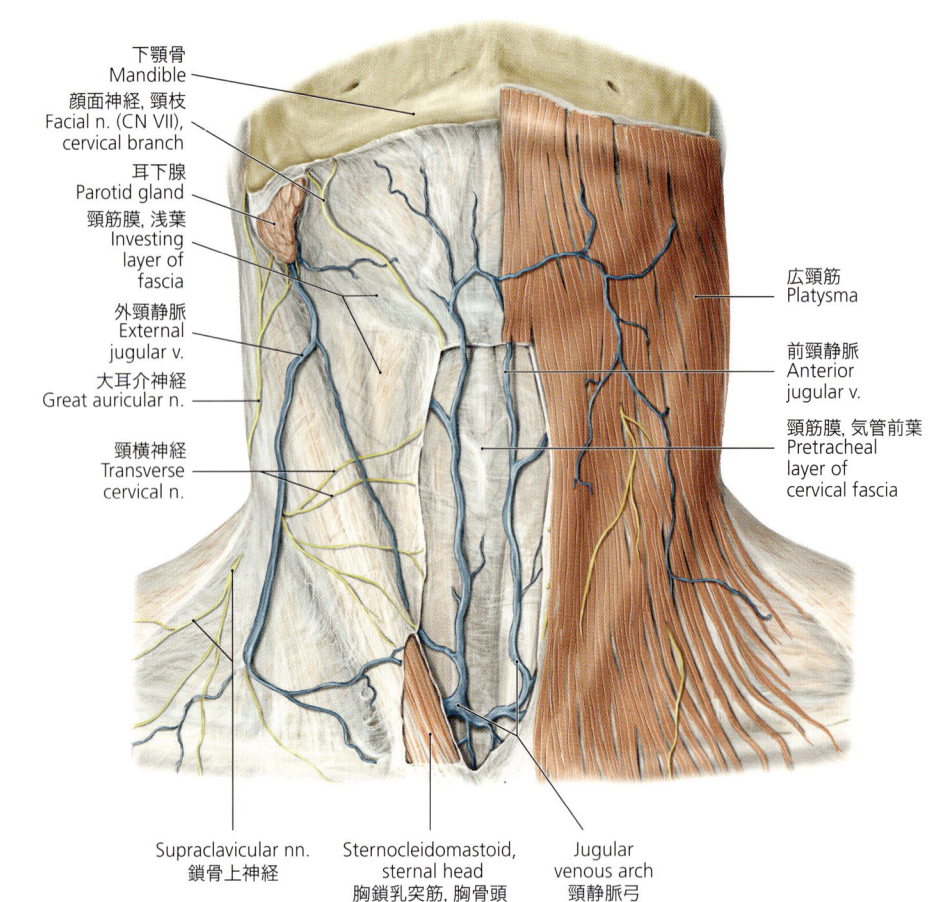

A 浅層．皮下にある広頸筋は右側では剥離してある．中央部では頸筋膜を見えるようにしてある．

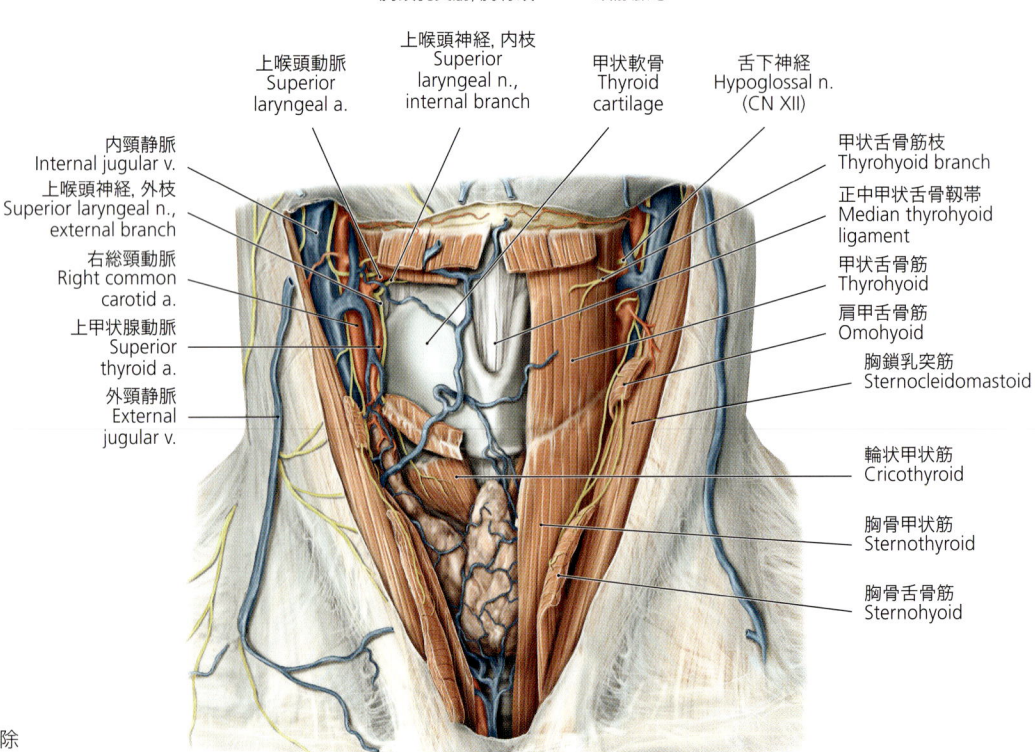

ラベル（上図）：
- 下顎骨 Mandible
- 顔面神経, 頸枝 Facial n. (CN VII), cervical branch
- 耳下腺 Parotid gland
- 頸筋膜, 浅葉 Investing layer of fascia
- 外頸静脈 External jugular v.
- 大耳介神経 Great auricular n.
- 頸横神経 Transverse cervical n.
- 広頸筋 Platysma
- 前頸静脈 Anterior jugular v.
- 頸筋膜, 気管前葉 Pretracheal layer of cervical fascia
- 鎖骨上神経 Supraclavicular nn.
- 胸鎖乳突筋, 胸骨頭 Sternocleidomastoid, sternal head
- 頸静脈弓 Jugular venous arch

B 深層．気管前葉（頸筋膜の中間層）は取り除いてある．

ラベル（下図）：
- 上喉頭動脈 Superior laryngeal a.
- 上喉頭神経, 内枝 Superior laryngeal n., internal branch
- 甲状軟骨 Thyroid cartilage
- 舌下神経 Hypoglossal n. (CN XII)
- 内頸静脈 Internal jugular v.
- 上喉頭神経, 外枝 Superior laryngeal n., external branch
- 右総頸動脈 Right common carotid a.
- 上甲状腺動脈 Superior thyroid a.
- 外頸静脈 External jugular v.
- 甲状舌骨筋枝 Thyrohyoid branch
- 正中甲状舌骨靱帯 Median thyrohyoid ligament
- 甲状舌骨筋 Thyrohyoid
- 肩甲舌骨筋 Omohyoid
- 胸鎖乳突筋 Sternocleidomastoid
- 輪状甲状筋 Cricothyroid
- 胸骨甲状筋 Sternothyroid
- 胸骨舌骨筋 Sternohyoid

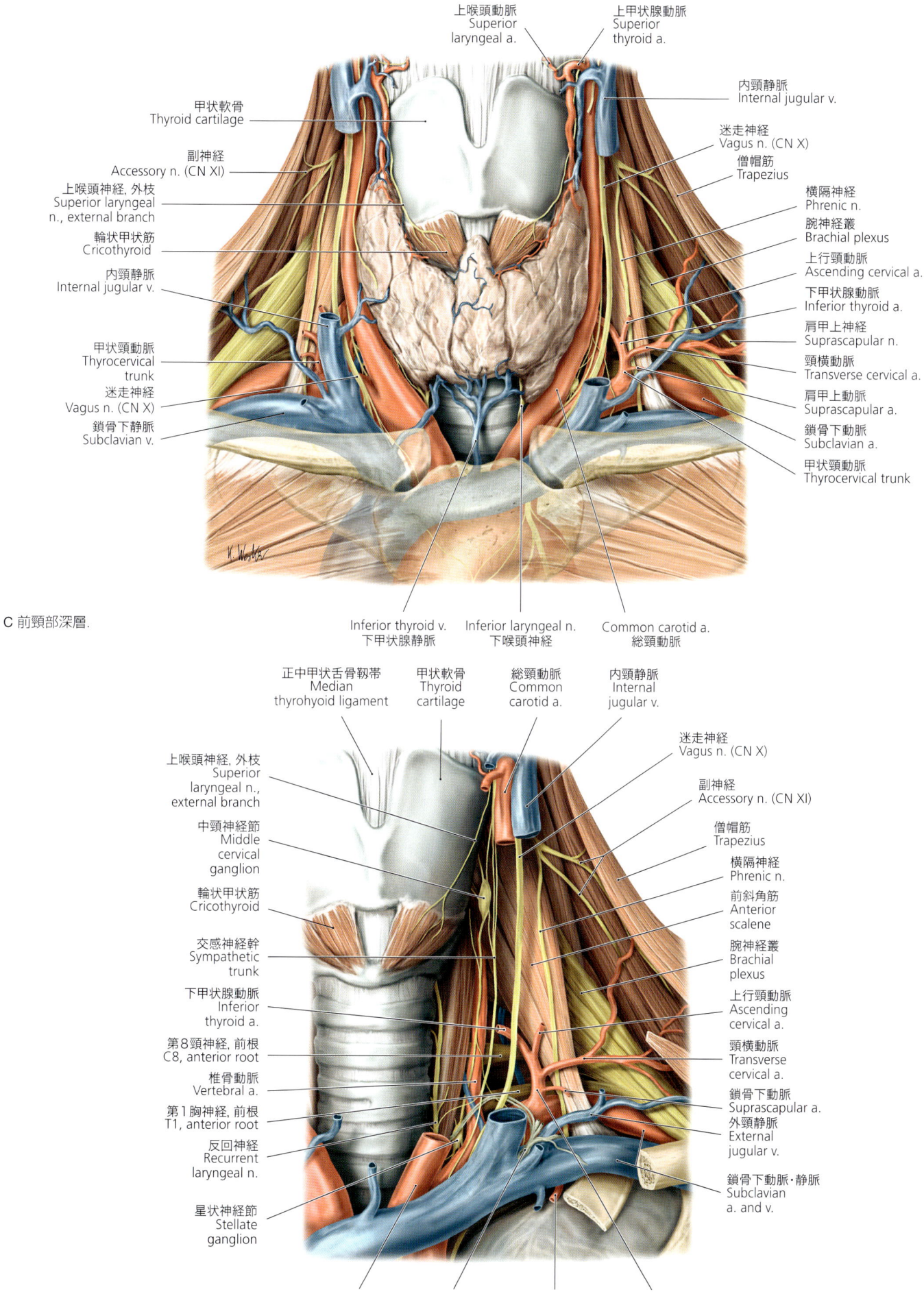

37

頸部

C 前頸部深層.

- 甲状軟骨 Thyroid cartilage
- 副神経 Accessory n. (CN XI)
- 上喉頭神経, 外枝 Superior laryngeal n., external branch
- 輪状甲状筋 Cricothyroid
- 内頸静脈 Internal jugular v.
- 甲状頸動脈 Thyrocervical trunk
- 迷走神経 Vagus n. (CN X)
- 鎖骨下静脈 Subclavian v.
- 上喉頭動脈 Superior laryngeal a.
- 上甲状腺動脈 Superior thyroid a.
- 内頸静脈 Internal jugular v.
- 迷走神経 Vagus n. (CN X)
- 僧帽筋 Trapezius
- 横隔神経 Phrenic n.
- 腕神経叢 Brachial plexus
- 上行頸動脈 Ascending cervical a.
- 下甲状腺動脈 Inferior thyroid a.
- 肩甲上神経 Suprascapular n.
- 頸横動脈 Transverse cervical a.
- 肩甲上動脈 Suprascapular a.
- 鎖骨下動脈 Subclavian a.
- 甲状頸動脈 Thyrocervical trunk
- Inferior thyroid v. 下甲状腺静脈
- Inferior laryngeal n. 下喉頭神経
- Common carotid a. 総頸動脈

D 頸の底部.

- 正中甲状舌骨靱帯 Median thyrohyoid ligament
- 甲状軟骨 Thyroid cartilage
- 総頸動脈 Common carotid a.
- 内頸静脈 Internal jugular v.
- 上喉頭神経, 外枝 Superior laryngeal n., external branch
- 中頸神経節 Middle cervical ganglion
- 輪状甲状筋 Cricothyroid
- 交感神経幹 Sympathetic trunk
- 下甲状腺動脈 Inferior thyroid a.
- 第8頸神経, 前根 C8, anterior root
- 椎骨動脈 Vertebral a.
- 第1胸神経, 前根 T1, anterior root
- 反回神経 Recurrent laryngeal n.
- 星状神経節 Stellate ganglion
- 迷走神経 Vagus n. (CN X)
- 副神経 Accessory n. (CN XI)
- 僧帽筋 Trapezius
- 横隔神経 Phrenic n.
- 前斜角筋 Anterior scalene
- 腕神経叢 Brachial plexus
- 上行頸動脈 Ascending cervical a.
- 頸横動脈 Transverse cervical a.
- 鎖骨下動脈 Suprascapular a.
- 外頸静脈 External jugular v.
- 鎖骨下動脈・静脈 Subclavian a. and v.
- Common carotid a. 総頸動脈
- Thoracic duct 胸管
- Internal thoracic a. 内胸動脈
- Thyrocervical trunk 甲状頸動脈

579

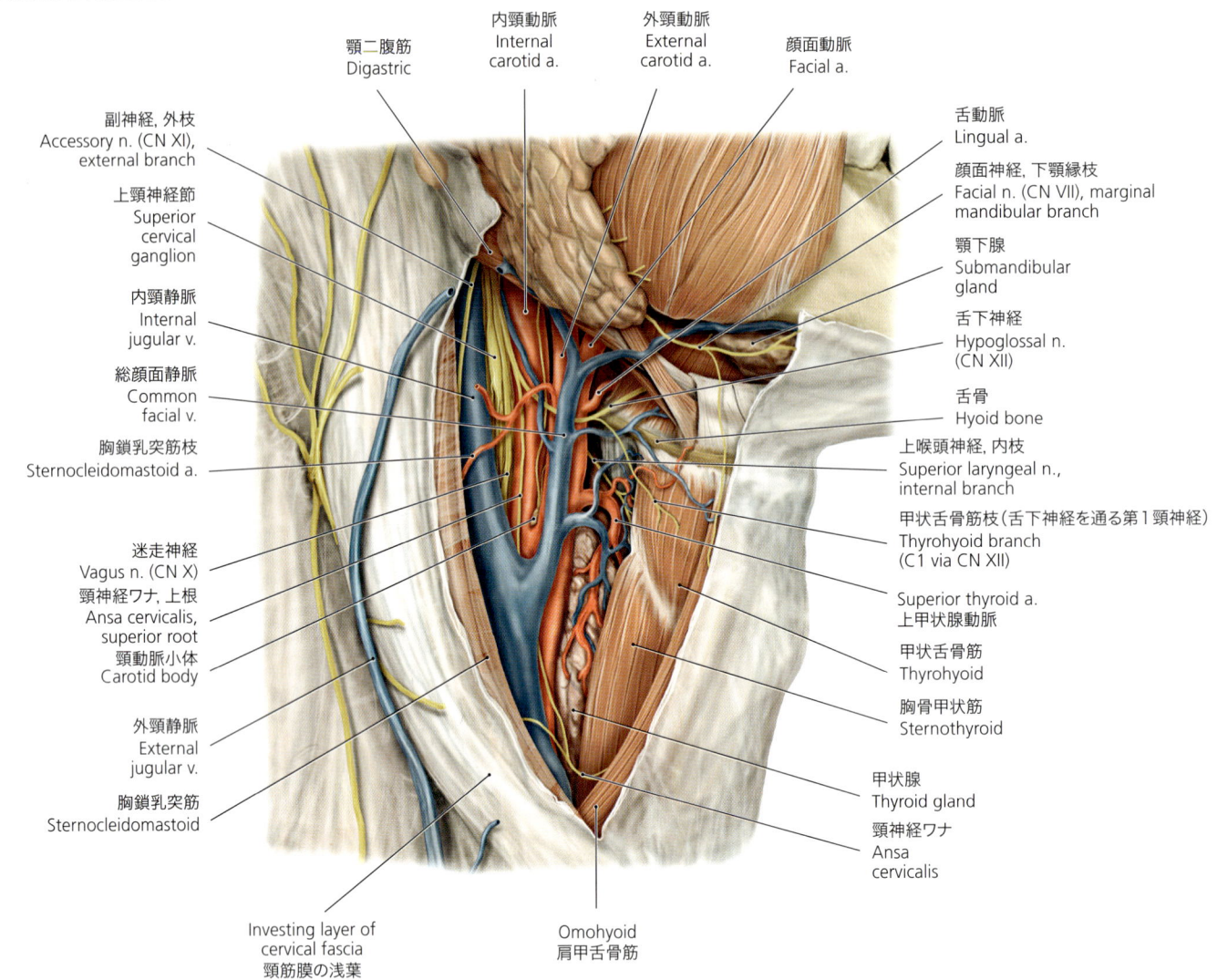

前頸部と外側頸三角部の局所解剖
Topography of the Anterior & Lateral Cervical Regions

図37.32 頸動脈三角
右外側方から見たところ．

図37.33 外側頸三角部の深層
右外側方から見たところ．胸鎖乳突筋の大部分を取り除いてある．

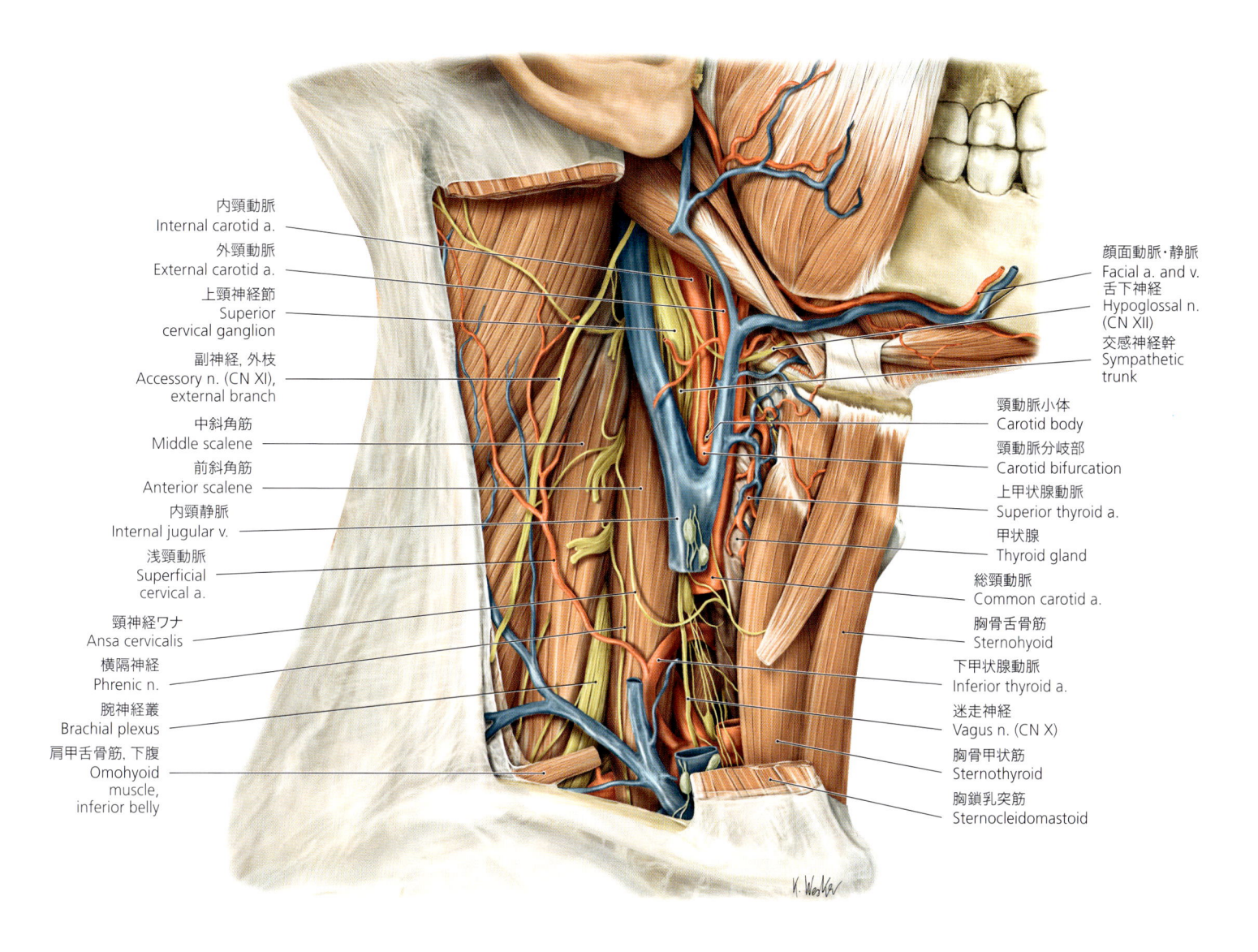

- 内頸動脈 Internal carotid a.
- 外頸動脈 External carotid a.
- 上頸神経節 Superior cervical ganglion
- 副神経，外枝 Accessory n. (CN XI), external branch
- 中斜角筋 Middle scalene
- 前斜角筋 Anterior scalene
- 内頸静脈 Internal jugular v.
- 浅頸動脈 Superficial cervical a.
- 頸神経ワナ Ansa cervicalis
- 横隔神経 Phrenic n.
- 腕神経叢 Brachial plexus
- 肩甲舌骨筋，下腹 Omohyoid muscle, inferior belly
- 顔面動脈・静脈 Facial a. and v.
- 舌下神経 Hypoglossal n. (CN XII)
- 交感神経幹 Sympathetic trunk
- 頸動脈小体 Carotid body
- 頸動脈分岐部 Carotid bifurcation
- 上甲状腺動脈 Superior thyroid a.
- 甲状腺 Thyroid gland
- 総頸動脈 Common carotid a.
- 胸骨舌骨筋 Sternohyoid
- 下甲状腺動脈 Inferior thyroid a.
- 迷走神経 Vagus n. (CN X)
- 胸骨甲状筋 Sternothyroid
- 胸鎖乳突筋 Sternocleidomastoid

外側頸三角部の局所解剖
Topography of the Lateral Cervical Region

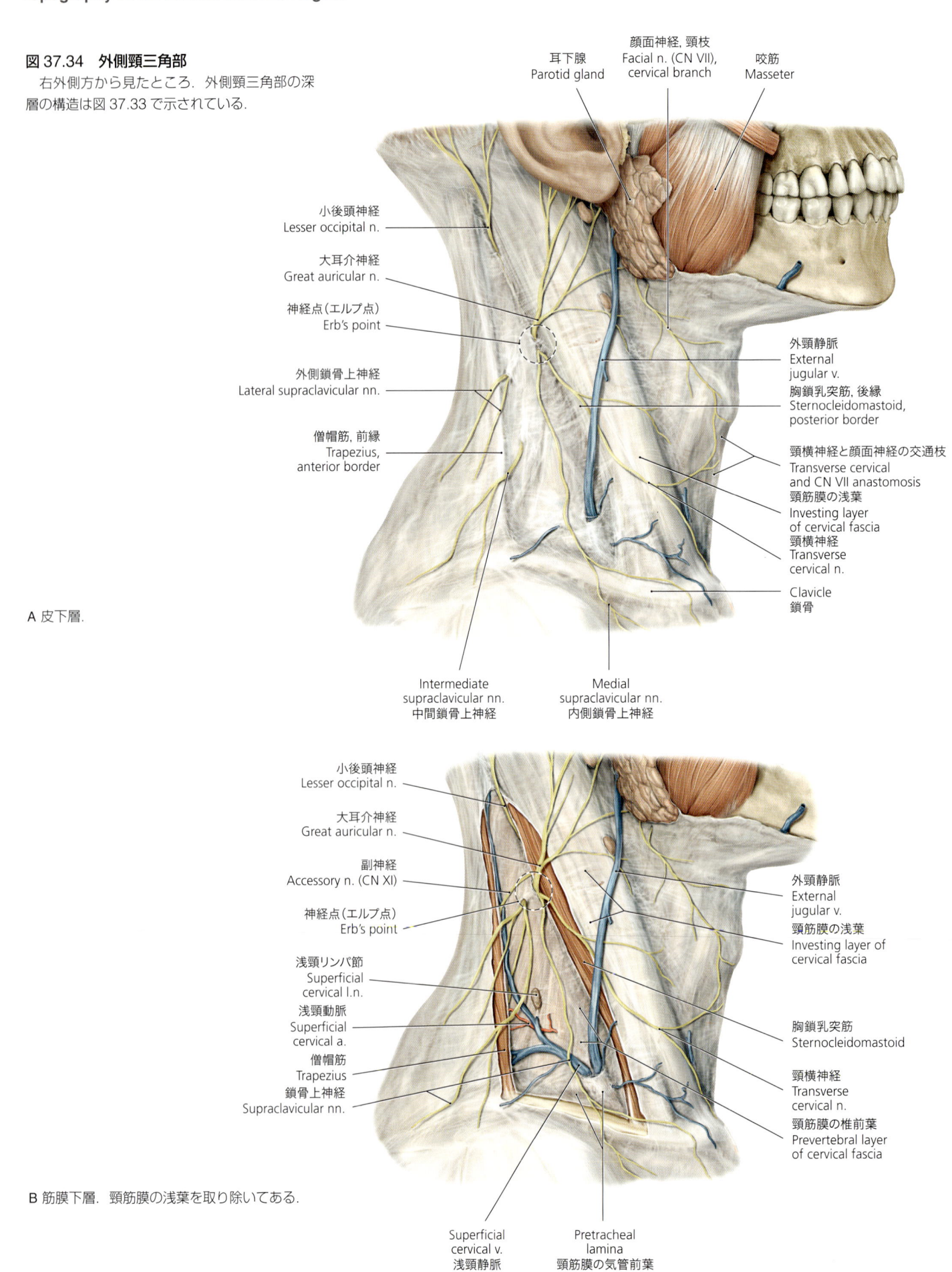

図 37.34 外側頸三角部
右外側方から見たところ．外側頸三角部の深層の構造は図 37.33 で示されている．

A 皮下層．

- 小後頭神経 Lesser occipital n.
- 大耳介神経 Great auricular n.
- 神経点（エルプ点）Erb's point
- 外側鎖骨上神経 Lateral supraclavicular nn.
- 僧帽筋，前縁 Trapezius, anterior border
- 耳下腺 Parotid gland
- 顔面神経，頸枝 Facial n. (CN VII), cervical branch
- 咬筋 Masseter
- 外頸静脈 External jugular v.
- 胸鎖乳突筋，後縁 Sternocleidomastoid, posterior border
- 頸横神経と顔面神経の交通枝 Transverse cervical and CN VII anastomosis
- 頸筋膜の浅葉 Investing layer of cervical fascia
- 頸横神経 Transverse cervical n.
- Clavicle 鎖骨
- Intermediate supraclavicular nn. 中間鎖骨上神経
- Medial supraclavicular nn. 内側鎖骨上神経

B 筋膜下層．頸筋膜の浅葉を取り除いてある．

- 小後頭神経 Lesser occipital n.
- 大耳介神経 Great auricular n.
- 副神経 Accessory n. (CN XI)
- 神経点（エルプ点）Erb's point
- 浅頸リンパ節 Superficial cervical l.n.
- 浅頸動脈 Superficial cervical a.
- 僧帽筋 Trapezius
- 鎖骨上神経 Supraclavicular nn.
- 外頸静脈 External jugular v.
- 頸筋膜の浅葉 Investing layer of cervical fascia
- 胸鎖乳突筋 Sternocleidomastoid
- 頸横神経 Transverse cervical n.
- 頸筋膜の椎前葉 Prevertebral layer of cervical fascia
- Superficial cervical v. 浅頸静脈
- Pretracheal lamina 頸筋膜の気管前葉

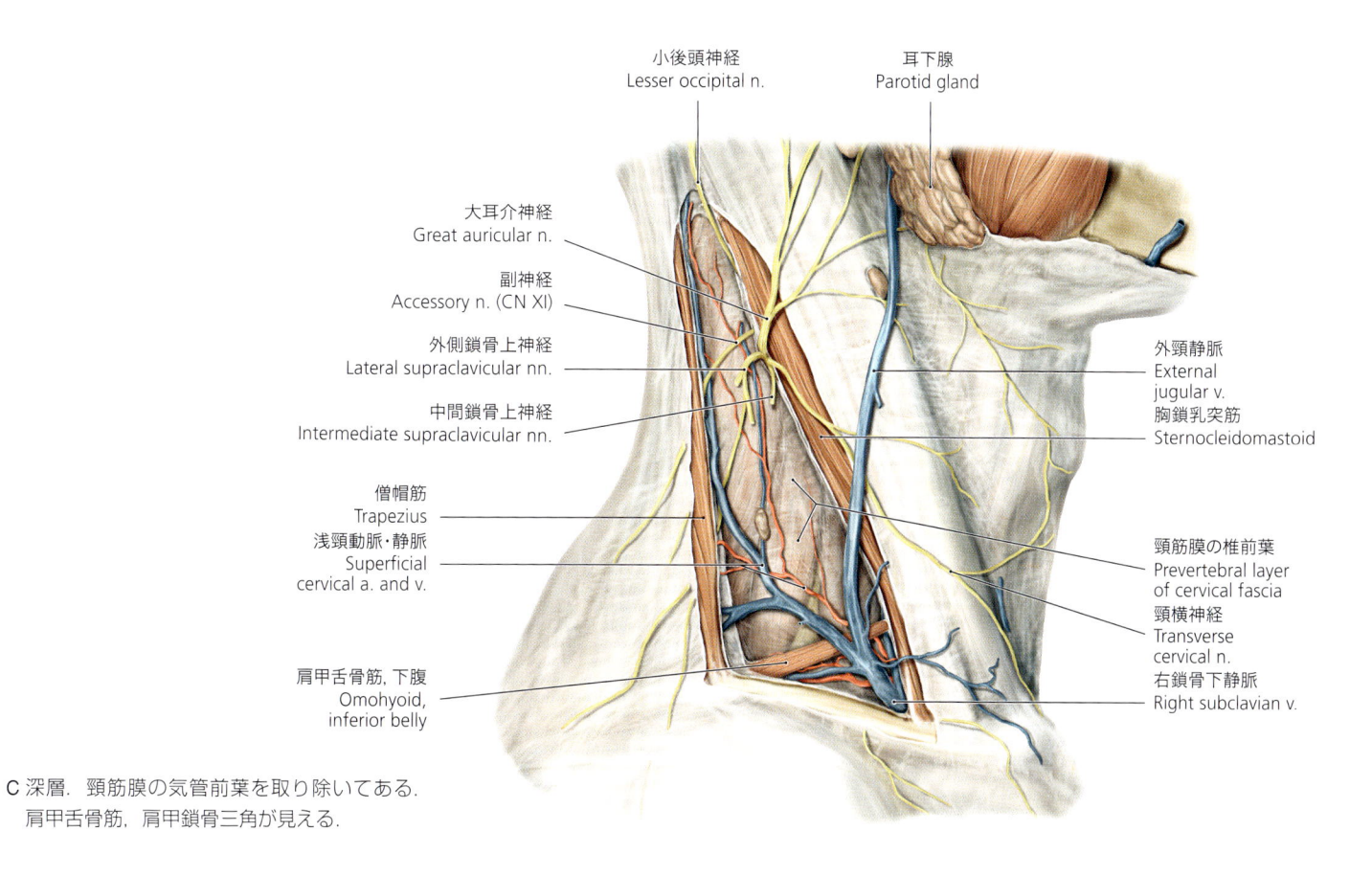

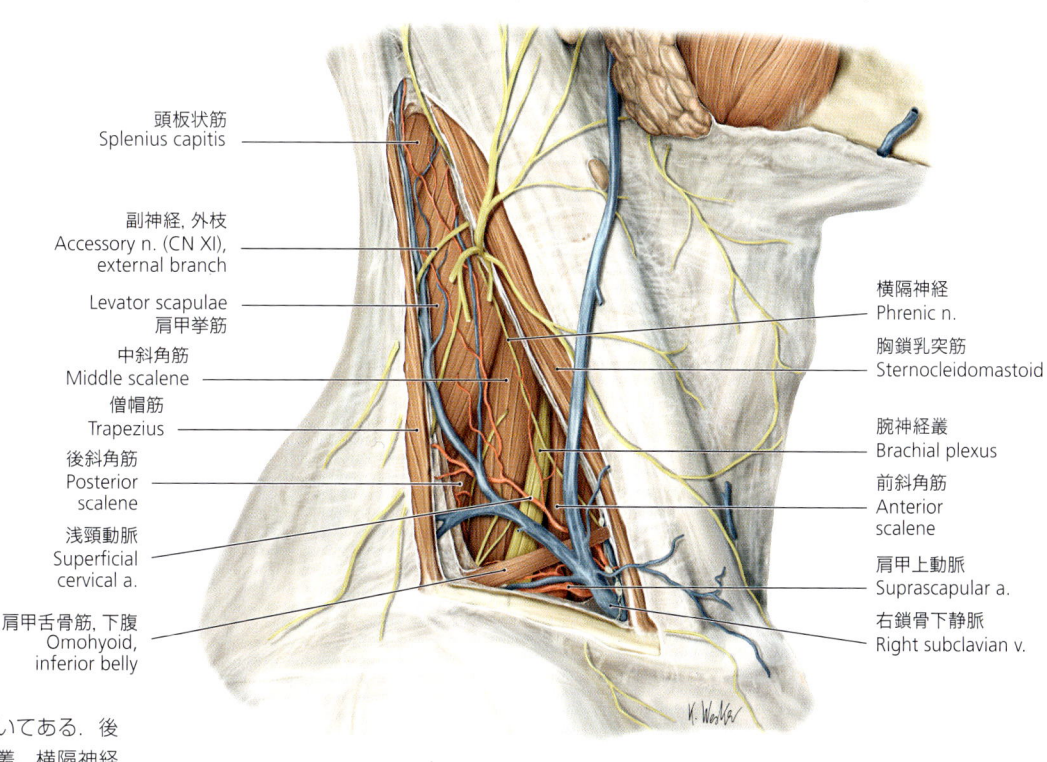

| 小後頭神経 Lesser occipital n.
| 耳下腺 Parotid gland
| 大耳介神経 Great auricular n.
| 副神経 Accessory n. (CN XI)
| 外側鎖骨上神経 Lateral supraclavicular nn.
| 中間鎖骨上神経 Intermediate supraclavicular nn.
| 僧帽筋 Trapezius
| 浅頸動脈・静脈 Superficial cervical a. and v.
| 肩甲舌骨筋, 下腹 Omohyoid, inferior belly
| 外頸静脈 External jugular v.
| 胸鎖乳突筋 Sternocleidomastoid
| 頸筋膜の椎前葉 Prevertebral layer of cervical fascia
| 頸横神経 Transverse cervical n.
| 右鎖骨下静脈 Right subclavian v.

C 深層. 頸筋膜の気管前葉を取り除いてある. 肩甲舌骨筋, 肩甲鎖骨三角が見える.

| 頭板状筋 Splenius capitis
| 副神経, 外枝 Accessory n. (CN XI), external branch
| 肩甲挙筋 Levator scapulae
| 中斜角筋 Middle scalene
| 僧帽筋 Trapezius
| 後斜角筋 Posterior scalene
| 浅頸動脈 Superficial cervical a.
| 肩甲舌骨筋, 下腹 Omohyoid, inferior belly
| 横隔神経 Phrenic n.
| 胸鎖乳突筋 Sternocleidomastoid
| 腕神経叢 Brachial plexus
| 前斜角筋 Anterior scalene
| 肩甲上動脈 Suprascapular a.
| 右鎖骨下静脈 Right subclavian v.

D 深層. 頸筋膜の椎前葉を取り除いてある. 後頸三角の深層にある筋, 腕神経叢, 横隔神経が見える.

後頸部の局所解剖
Topography of the Posterior Cervical Region

図 37.35 後頭部と後頸部
後方から見たところ．左側の皮下層と右側の筋膜下層．後頭部は厳密には頭部の一部であるが，頸部の血管と神経と連続しているために本項で解説する．

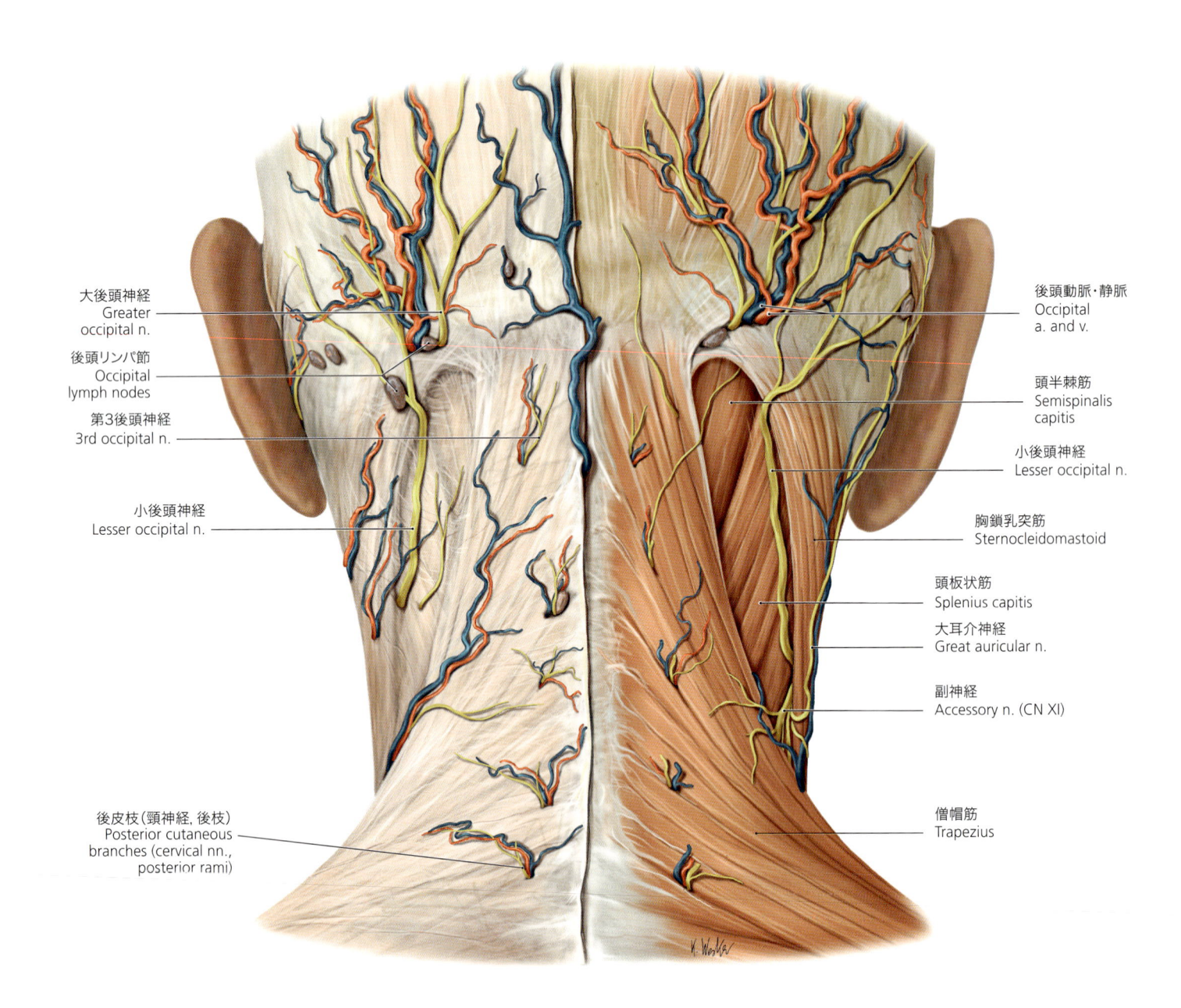

- 大後頭神経 Greater occipital n.
- 後頭リンパ節 Occipital lymph nodes
- 第3後頭神経 3rd occipital n.
- 小後頭神経 Lesser occipital n.
- 後皮枝（頸神経, 後枝） Posterior cutaneous branches (cervical nn., posterior rami)
- 後頭動脈・静脈 Occipital a. and v.
- 頭半棘筋 Semispinalis capitis
- 小後頭神経 Lesser occipital n.
- 胸鎖乳突筋 Sternocleidomastoid
- 頭板状筋 Splenius capitis
- 大耳介神経 Great auricular n.
- 副神経 Accessory n. (CN XI)
- 僧帽筋 Trapezius

図 37.36　後頭下三角
右側，後方から見たところ．後頭下三角の境界は後頭下の筋（大後頭直筋，上頭斜筋，下頭斜筋）であり，椎骨動脈が通っている．左右の椎骨動脈は環椎後頭膜を出た後で合流して脳底動脈を形成する．

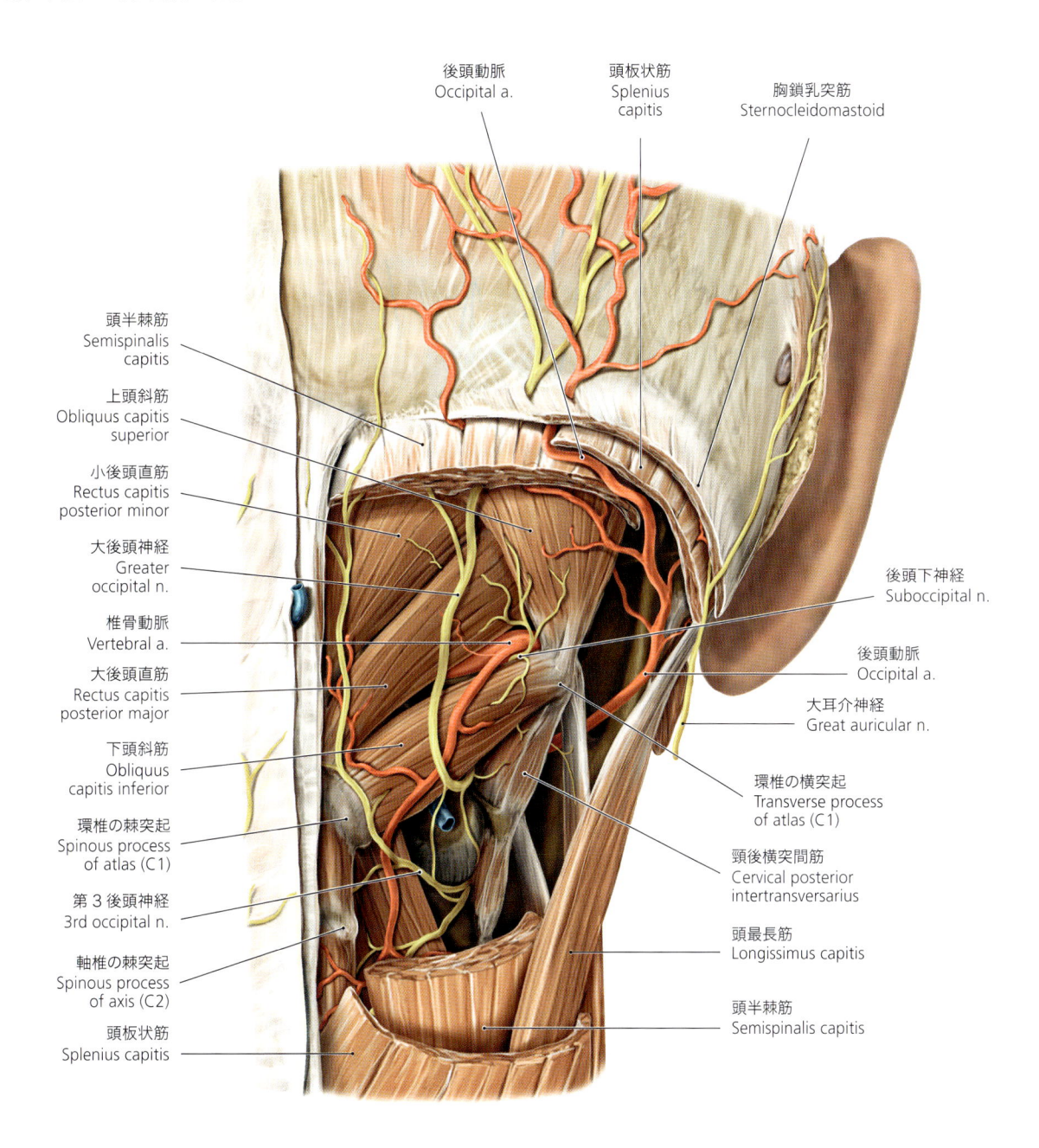

後頭動脈 Occipital a.
頭板状筋 Splenius capitis
胸鎖乳突筋 Sternocleidomastoid
頭半棘筋 Semispinalis capitis
上頭斜筋 Obliquus capitis superior
小後頭直筋 Rectus capitis posterior minor
大後頭神経 Greater occipital n.
椎骨動脈 Vertebral a.
大後頭直筋 Rectus capitis posterior major
下頭斜筋 Obliquus capitis inferior
環椎の棘突起 Spinous process of atlas (C1)
第3後頭神経 3rd occipital n.
軸椎の棘突起 Spinous process of axis (C2)
頭板状筋 Splenius capitis
後頭下神経 Suboccipital n.
後頭動脈 Occipital a.
大耳介神経 Great auricular n.
環椎の横突起 Transverse process of atlas (C1)
頸後横突間筋 Cervical posterior intertransversarius
頭最長筋 Longissimus capitis
頭半棘筋 Semispinalis capitis

頸部のリンパ管
Lymphatics of the Neck

図 37.37　頸部のリンパ流路
右外側方から見たところ．

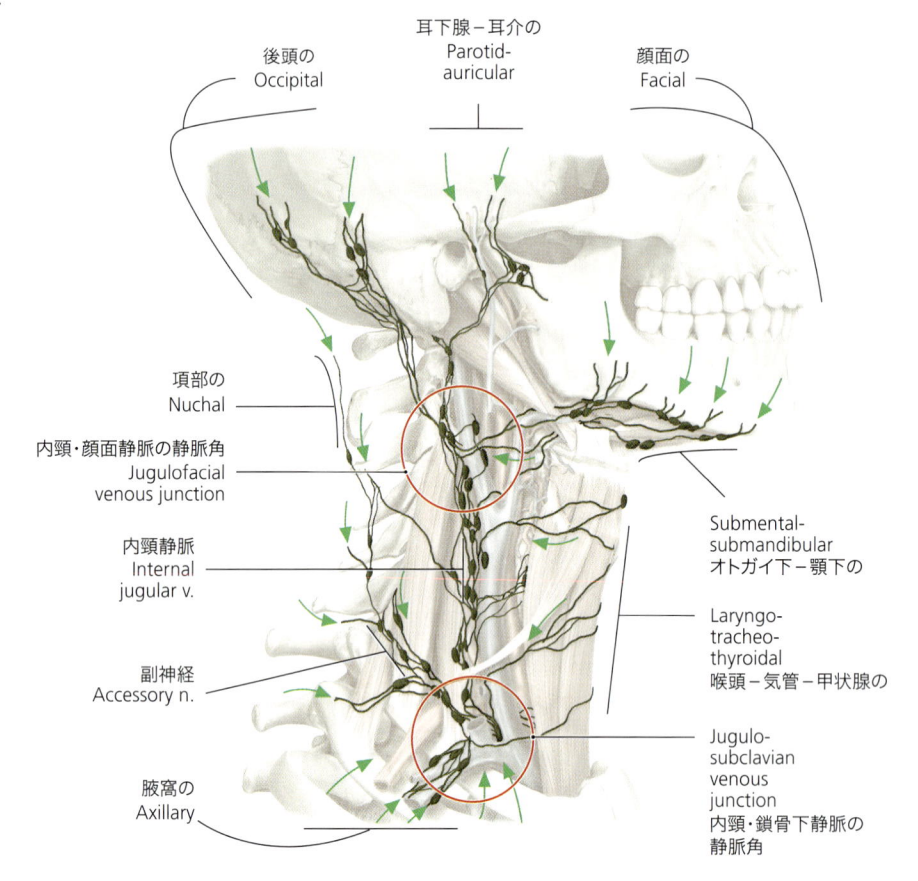

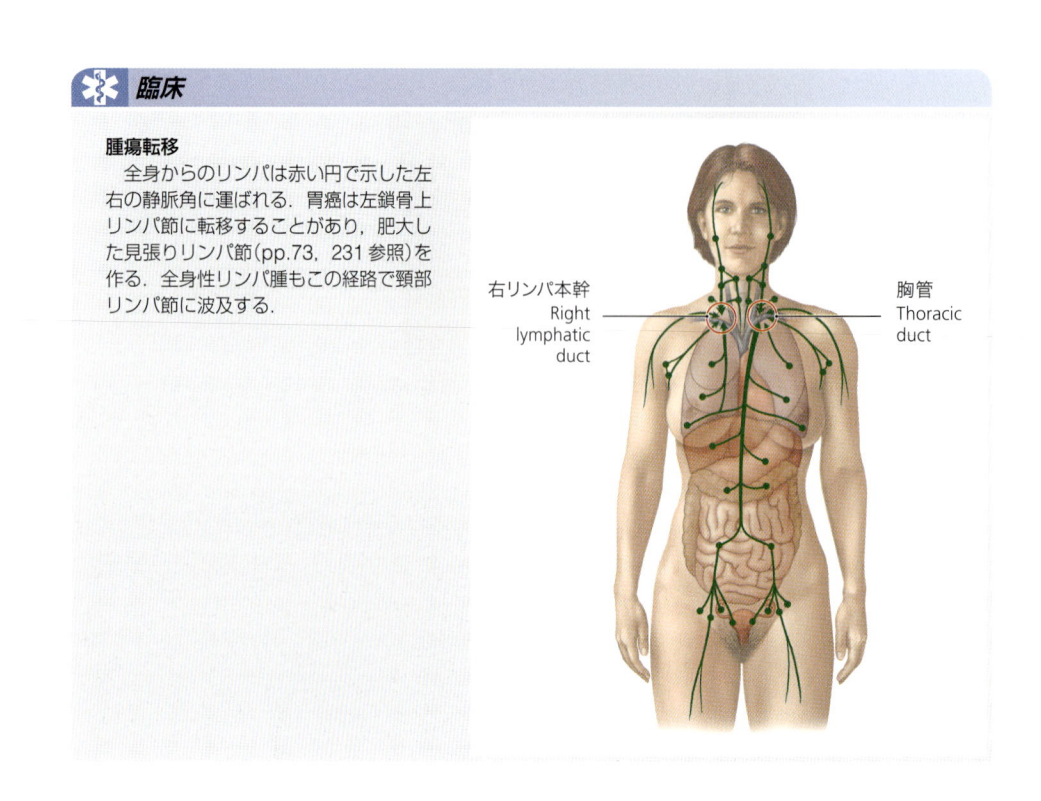

- 後頭の Occipital
- 耳下腺−耳介の Parotid-auricular
- 顔面の Facial
- 項部の Nuchal
- 内頸・顔面静脈の静脈角 Jugulofacial venous junction
- 内頸静脈 Internal jugular v.
- 副神経 Accessory n.
- 腋窩の Axillary
- オトガイ下−顎下の Submental-submandibular
- 喉頭−気管−甲状腺の Laryngo-tracheo-thyroidal
- 内頸・鎖骨下静脈の静脈角 Jugulo-subclavian venous junction

臨床

腫瘍転移

全身からのリンパは赤い円で示した左右の静脈角に運ばれる．胃癌は左鎖骨上リンパ節に転移することがあり，肥大した見張りリンパ節(pp.73, 231 参照)を作る．全身性リンパ腫もこの経路で頸部リンパ節に波及する．

- 右リンパ本幹 Right lymphatic duct
- 胸管 Thoracic duct

図 37.38　浅頸リンパ節
右外側方から見たところ．

耳介後リンパ節 Retroauricular lymph nodes
後頭リンパ節 Occipital lymph node
浅耳下腺リンパ節 Superficial parotid lymph nodes
乳突リンパ節 Mastoid lymph nodes
Deep parotid lymph nodes 深耳下腺リンパ節
浅前頸リンパ節 Anterior superficial cervical lymph nodes
外側頸リンパ節の浅リンパ節 Lateral superficial cervical lymph nodes

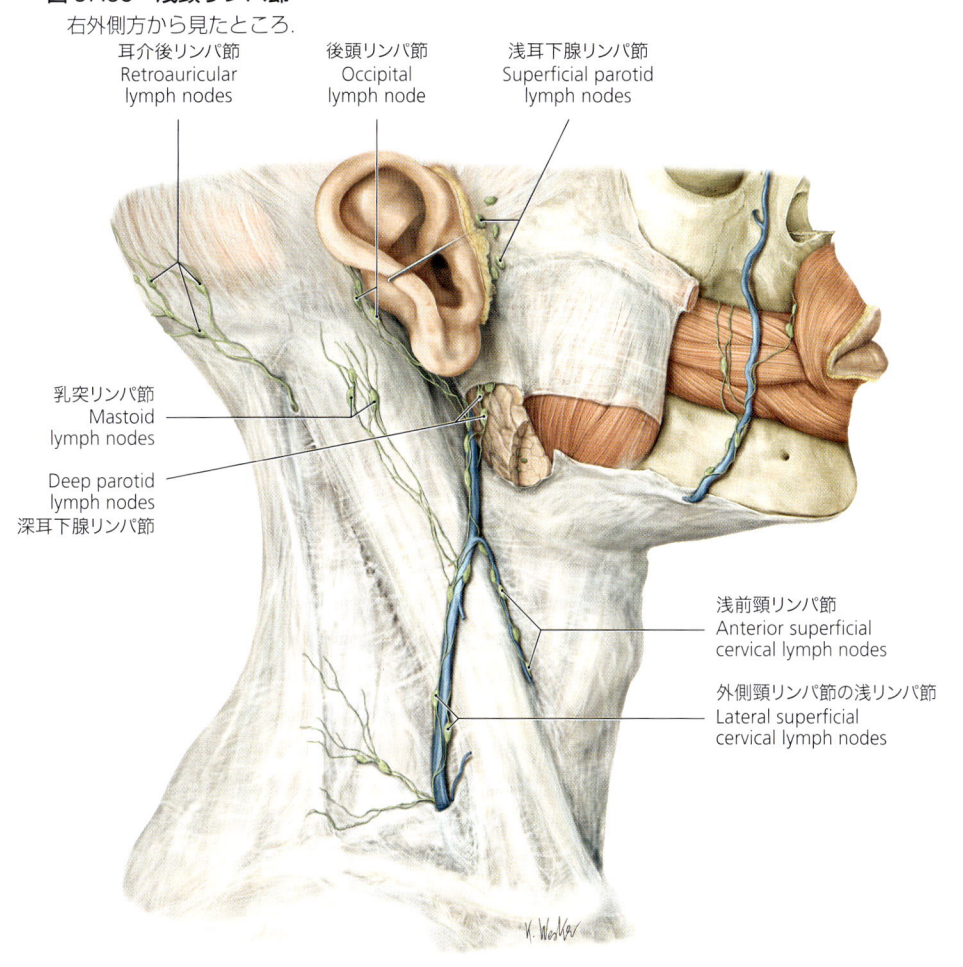

表 37.13	頸部浅層のリンパ節
リンパ節	分布域
耳介後リンパ節	後頭部
後頭リンパ節	
乳突リンパ節	
浅耳下腺リンパ節	耳下腺耳介部
深耳下腺リンパ節	
浅前頸リンパ節	胸鎖乳突筋部
外側頸リンパ節の浅リンパ節	

図 37.39　深頸リンパ節
右外側方から見たところ．

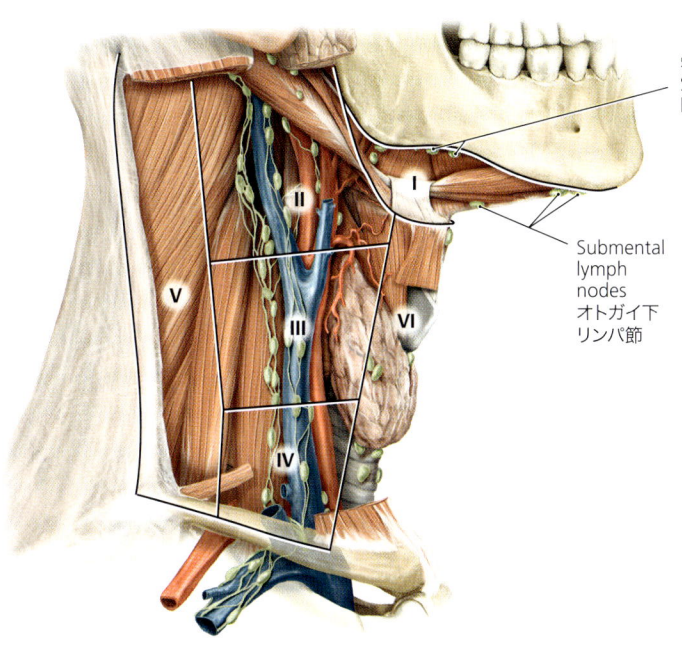

顎下リンパ節 Submandibular lymph nodes
Submental lymph nodes オトガイ下リンパ節

表 37.14	頸部深層のリンパ節		
区分	リンパ節		分布域
I	オトガイ下リンパ節		顔
	顎下リンパ節		
II	外頸リンパ節	上外側グループ	
III		中外側グループ	項部，喉頭-気管-甲状腺部
IV		下外側グループ	
V	後頸三角のリンパ節		項部
VI	前頸リンパ節		喉頭-気管-甲状腺部

体表解剖
Surface Anatomy

図 38.1　頭部と後頭下の体表解剖

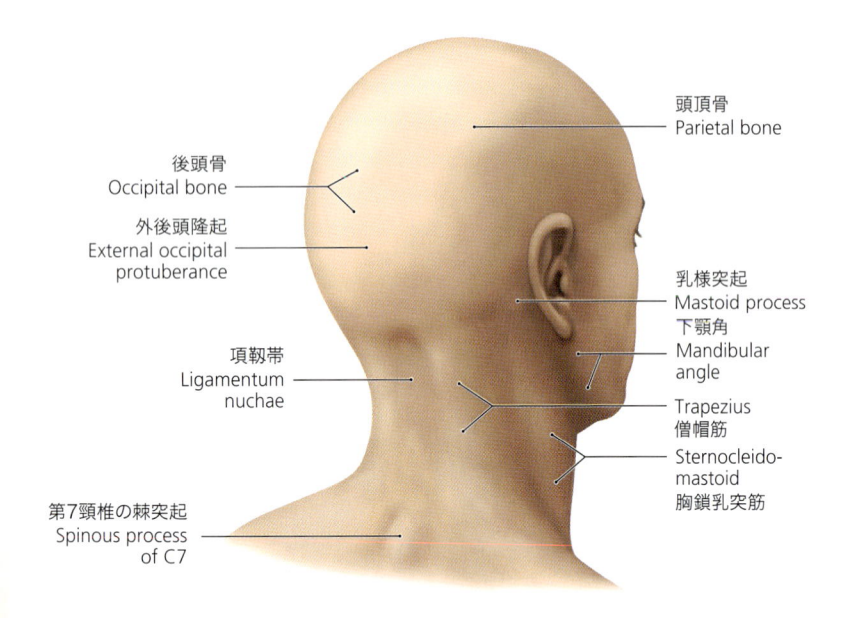

後頭骨
Occipital bone

頭頂骨
Parietal bone

外後頭隆起
External occipital protuberance

乳様突起
Mastoid process

下顎角
Mandibular angle

項靱帯
Ligamentum nuchae

Trapezius
僧帽筋

Sternocleido-mastoid
胸鎖乳突筋

第7頸椎の棘突起
Spinous process of C7

Q1：胸鎖乳突筋後縁の上 2/3 の高さから麻酔剤を注入するのは，何のためか？

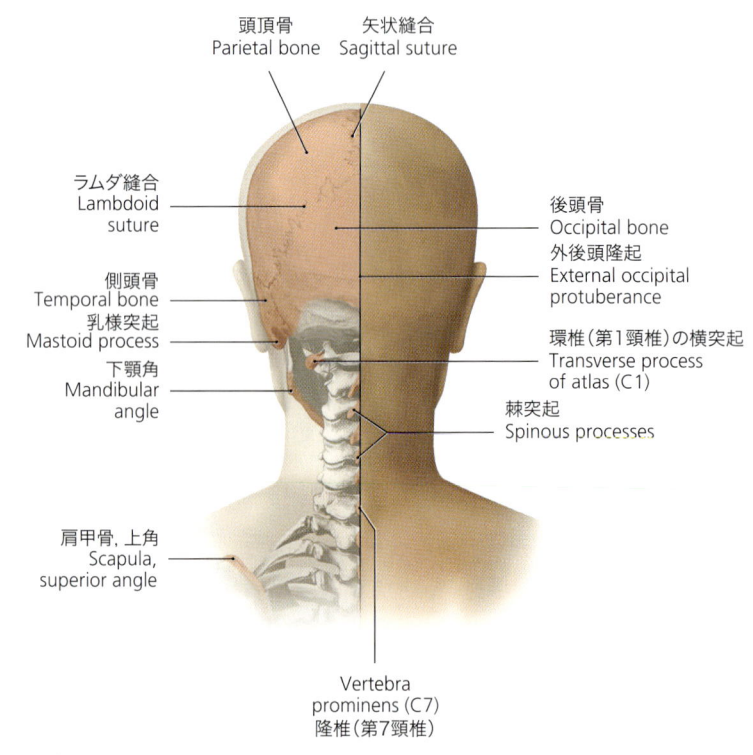

A 体表解剖，右後外側方から見たところ．

Q2：静脈洞交会の静脈血を聴診するには，どの触知可能な部分を目安とすればよいか？

頭頂骨
Parietal bone

矢状縫合
Sagittal suture

ラムダ縫合
Lambdoid suture

側頭骨
Temporal bone

乳様突起
Mastoid process

下顎角
Mandibular angle

後頭骨
Occipital bone

外後頭隆起
External occipital protuberance

環椎（第1頸椎）の横突起
Transverse process of atlas (C1)

棘突起
Spinous processes

肩甲骨，上角
Scapula, superior angle

Vertebra prominens (C7)
隆椎（第7頸椎）

B 触知可能な骨突起，後方から見たところ．

図 38.2 顔と頸部の体表解剖

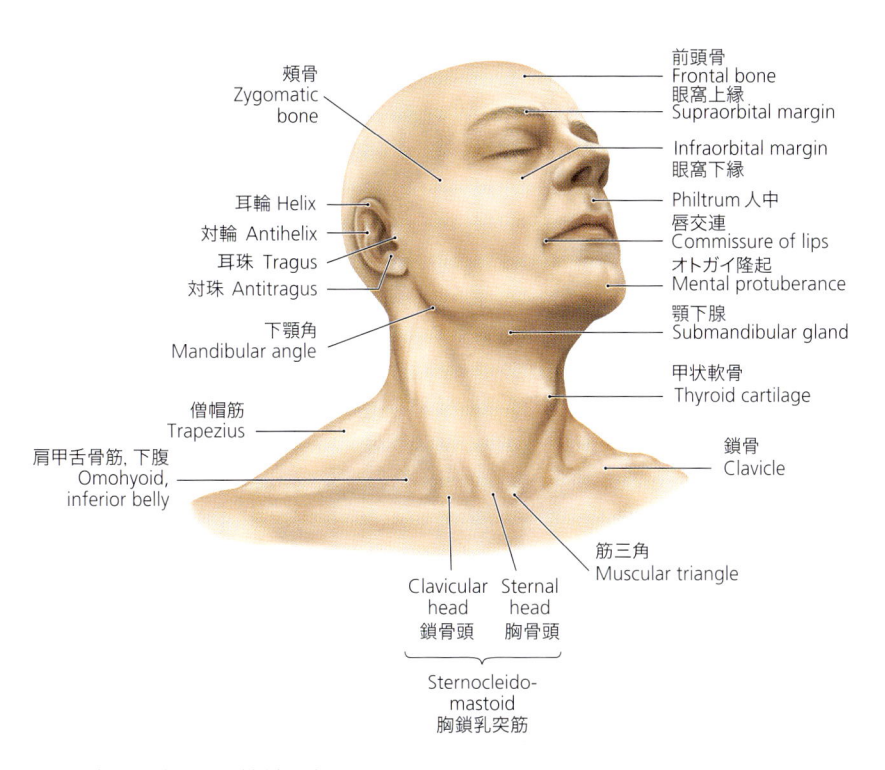

A 体表解剖，右前外側方から見たところ．

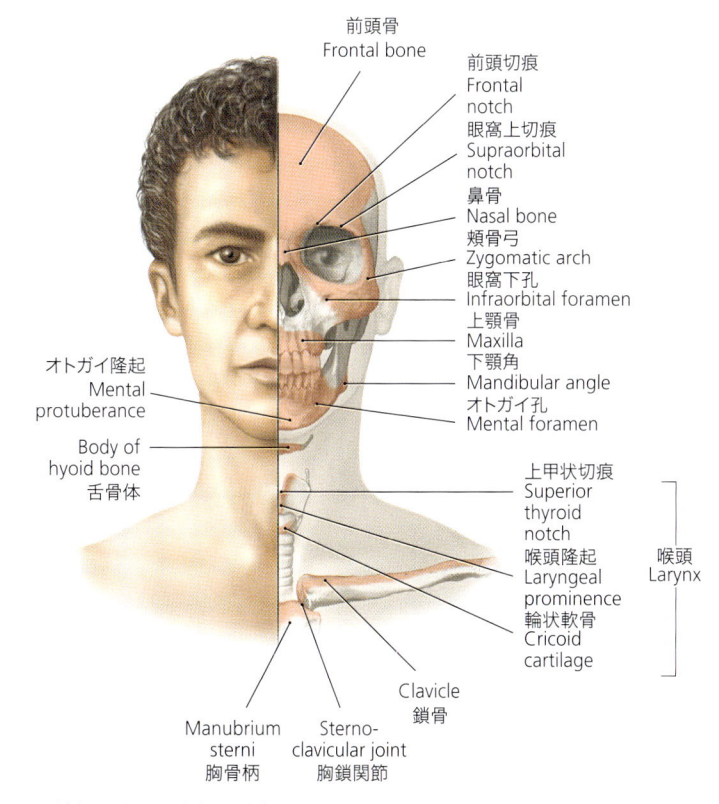

B 触知可能な骨突起，前方から見たところ．

Q3: 外側頸三角部（後頸三角）の境界をなすものは何か？ この領域に含まれ，上肢の筋肉を運動性に支配をする構造を2つ挙げよ．

Q4: 頸動脈三角の境界をなすものは何か？頸動脈三角内の頸動脈鞘に含まれ，垂直方向に走る血管以外の構造を1つ挙げよ．

Q5: 「アダムの林檎」として知られる解剖学的構造は何か？

解答は p. 626 を参照．

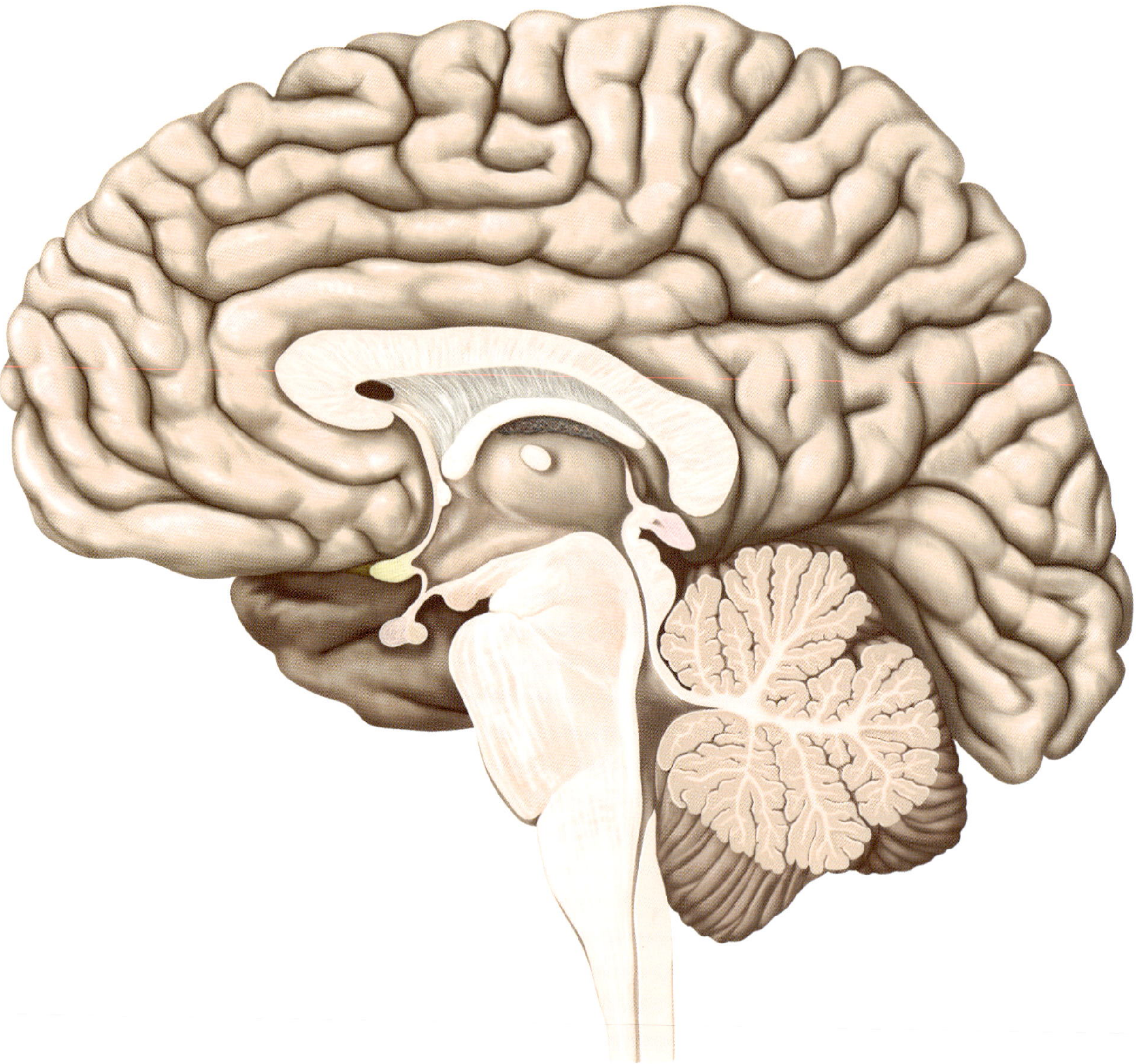

神経解剖
Neuroanatomy

39. 脳と脊髄
- 神経系：概観 … 592
- 大脳 … 594
- 大脳と間脳 … 596
- 間脳，脳幹，小脳 … 598
- 脊髄 … 600
- 髄膜 … 602
- 脳室と脳脊髄液の空間 … 604

40. 脳と脊髄の血管
- 硬膜静脈洞と脳の静脈 … 606
- 脳の動脈 … 608
- 脊髄の動脈と静脈 … 610

41. 機能系
- 神経回路：概観 … 612
- 一般感覚と運動の伝導路 … 614
- 特殊感覚の伝導路(1) … 616
- 特殊感覚の伝導路(2) … 618
- 特殊感覚の伝導路(3) … 620

42. 自律神経系
- 自律神経系 … 622

神経系：概観
Nervous System: Overview

図 39.1　中枢神経系と末梢神経系

神経系は中枢神経系と末梢神経系に区分される．中枢神経系は脳と脊髄からなり，これらはひとつの機能ユニットを形成する．末梢神経系は脳や脊髄から出る神経からなる（脳からは脳神経，脊髄からは脊髄神経が出る）．

図 39.2　ニューロン（神経細胞）

神経系はニューロン（神経細胞）とそれを支持するグリア細胞からなるが，グリア細胞のほうが圧倒的に多い（約 10 倍）．個々のニューロンの細胞体からは，1本の軸索（情報伝達領域）と1本以上の樹状突起（情報受容領域）が伸びている．シナプスにおける神経伝達物質の放出により，標的ニューロンに興奮性もしくは抑制性のシナプス後電位が生じる．シナプス後電位がある閾値を超えると，次に活動電位が発生し，軸索終末部から神経伝達物質が放出される．

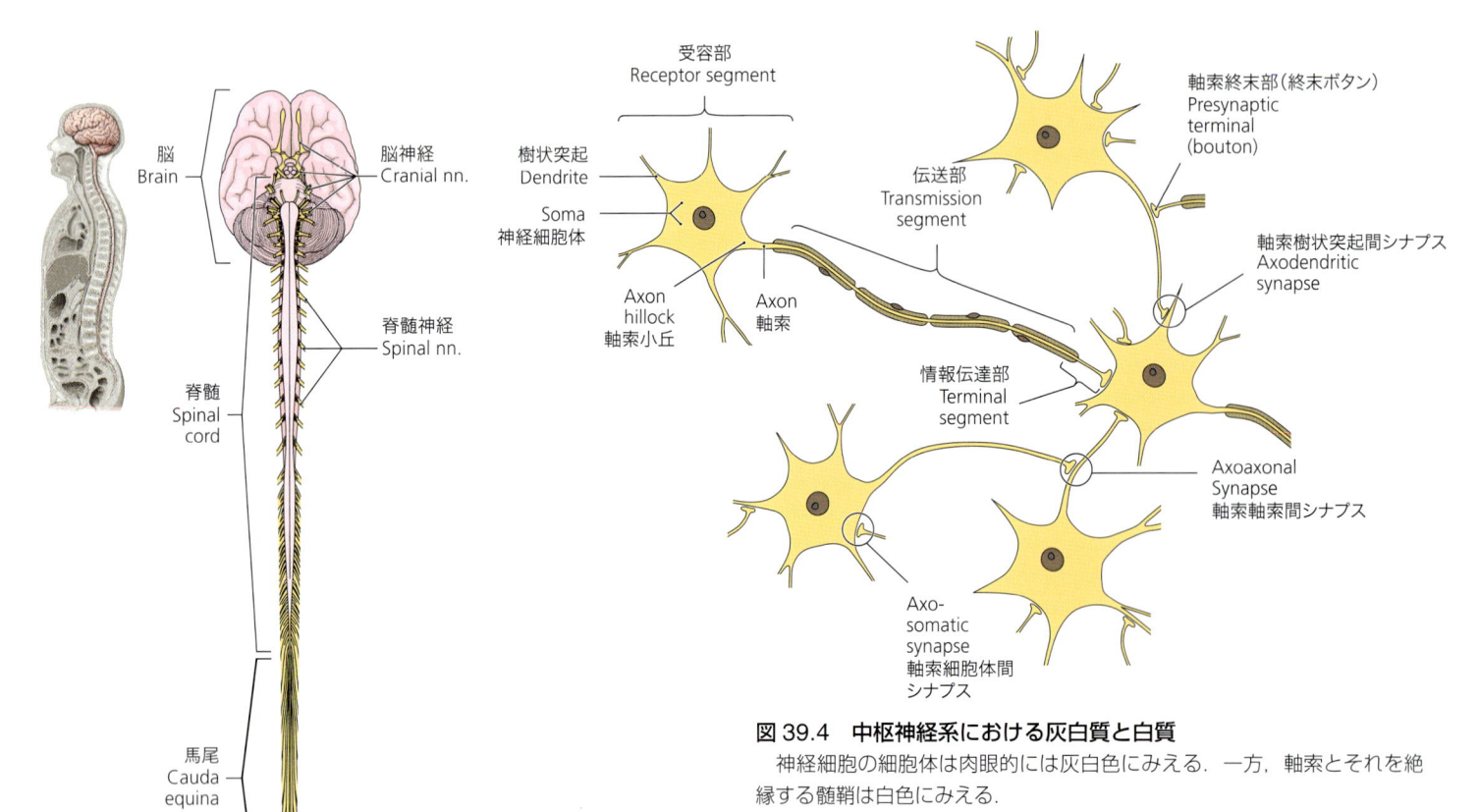

図 39.3　髄鞘形成

ある種のグリア細胞は軸索を層状に包みこんで，髄鞘（ミエリン鞘）を形成する．髄鞘が形成されることにより，軸索は電気的に絶縁され，活動電位の伝導速度が速くなる．中枢神経系では，1つのオリゴデンドロサイト（稀突起神経膠細胞）が複数の軸索を包み込み，軸索を形成する．末梢神経系では，1つのシュワン細胞が1本の軸索だけを包み込み，髄鞘を形成する．

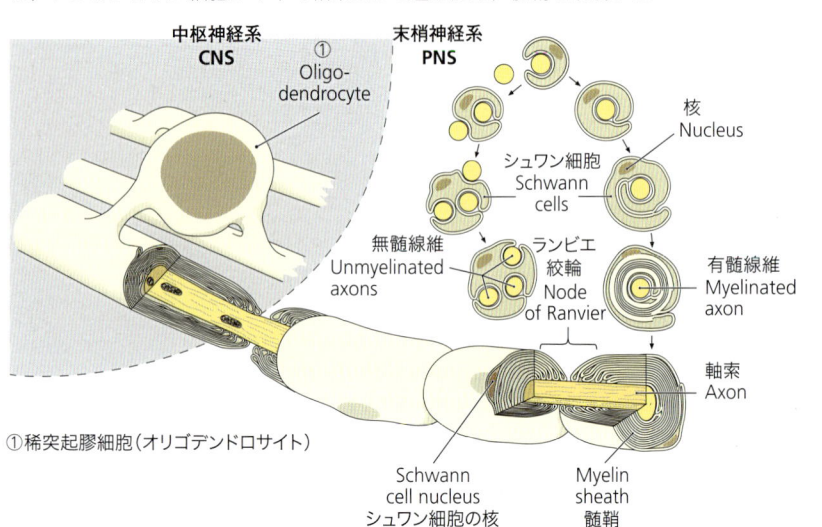

① 稀突起膠細胞（オリゴデンドロサイト）

図 39.4　中枢神経系における灰白質と白質

神経細胞の細胞体は肉眼的には灰白色にみえる．一方，軸索とそれを絶縁する髄鞘は白色にみえる．

A　脳の前額断面．

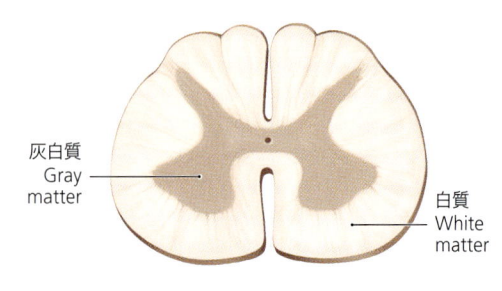

B　脊髄の横断面．

表 39.1　脳の発生

	発生初期の脳	成人の脳		構造
神経管	前脳胞（前脳）	終脳（大脳）		大脳皮質，大脳白質，大脳基底核
		間脳		視床上部（松果体），背側視床，腹側視床，視床下部
	中脳胞（中脳）	中脳*		中脳蓋（上丘と下丘），中脳被蓋，大脳脚
	菱脳胞（後脳）	後脳	小脳	小脳皮質，小脳核，小脳脚
			橋*	神経核，神経路
		髄脳	延髄*	

*中脳，橋，延髄を合わせて脳幹と呼ぶ．

図 39.5　脳の発生
左外側方から見たところ．

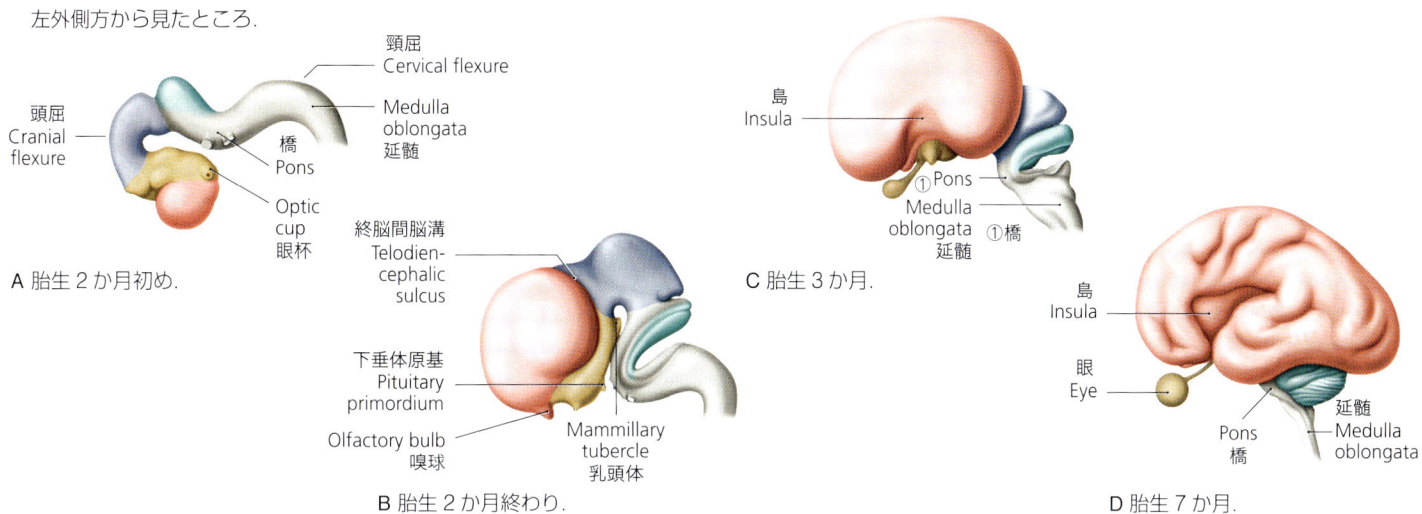

A　胎生 2 か月初め．

B　胎生 2 か月終わり．

C　胎生 3 か月．

D　胎生 7 か月．

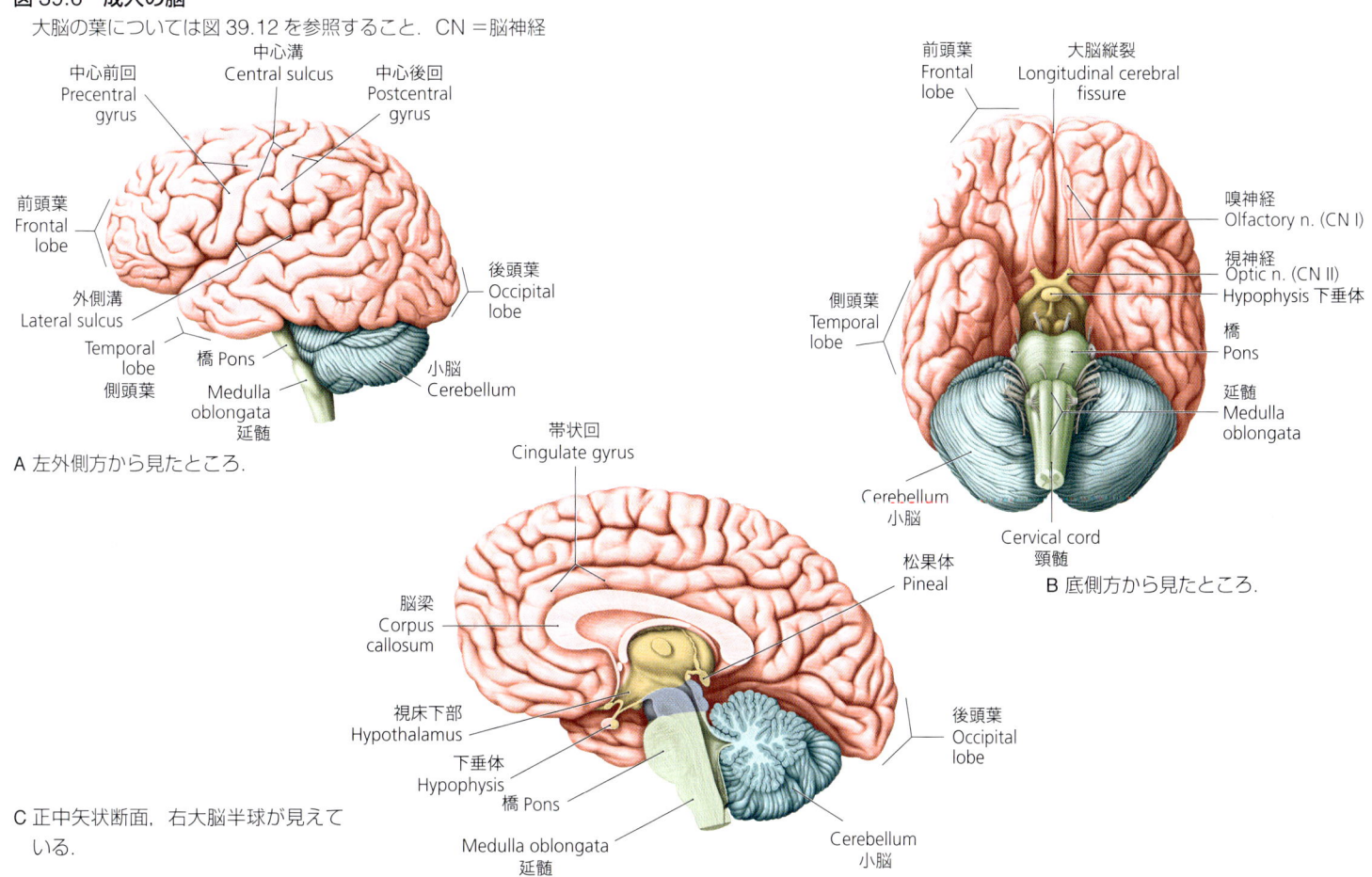

図 39.6　成人の脳
大脳の葉については図 39.12 を参照すること．CN ＝脳神経

A　左外側方から見たところ．

B　底側方から見たところ．

C　正中矢状断面，右大脳半球が見えている．

大脳
Telencephalon

図 39.7 大脳の区分
前額断面を前方から見たところ．大脳は大脳皮質，大脳白質，基底核に区分される．大脳皮質はさらに不等皮質と等皮質（新皮質）に分けられる．

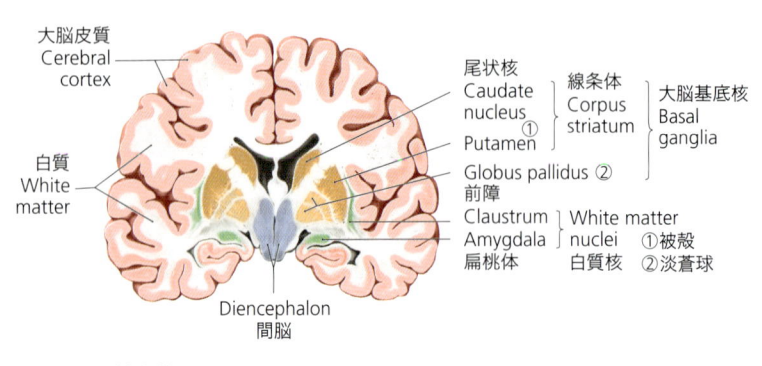

- 大脳皮質 Cerebral cortex
- 白質 White matter
- 尾状核 Caudate nucleus
- 被殻 Putamen ①
- Globus pallidus ② 淡蒼球
- 前障 Claustrum
- 扁桃体 Amygdala
- 線条体 Corpus striatum
- 大脳基底核 Basal ganglia
- White matter nuclei 白質核 ①被殻 ②淡蒼球
- 間脳 Diencephalon

図 39.8 大脳白質
特殊な剖出方法により，大脳白質の表層にある線維構造を示している．

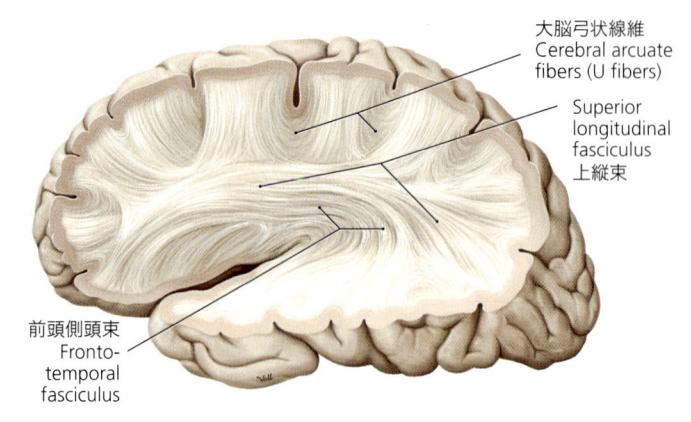

- 大脳弓状線維 Cerebral arcuate fibers (U fibers)
- 上縦束 Superior longitudinal fasciculus
- 前頭側頭束 Fronto-temporal fasciculus

A 左大脳半球を外側方から見たところ．

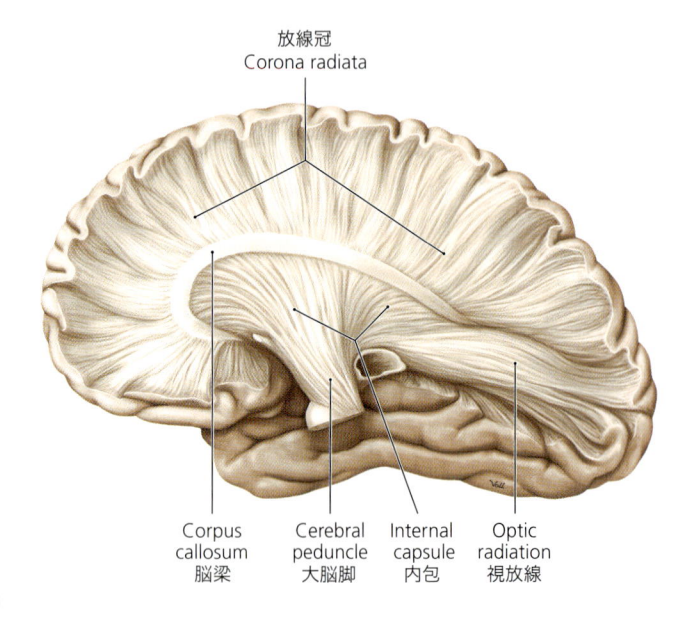

図 39.9 基底核
水平断面を上方から見たところ．基底核は運動系（p.615 参照）にとって必須の要素である．

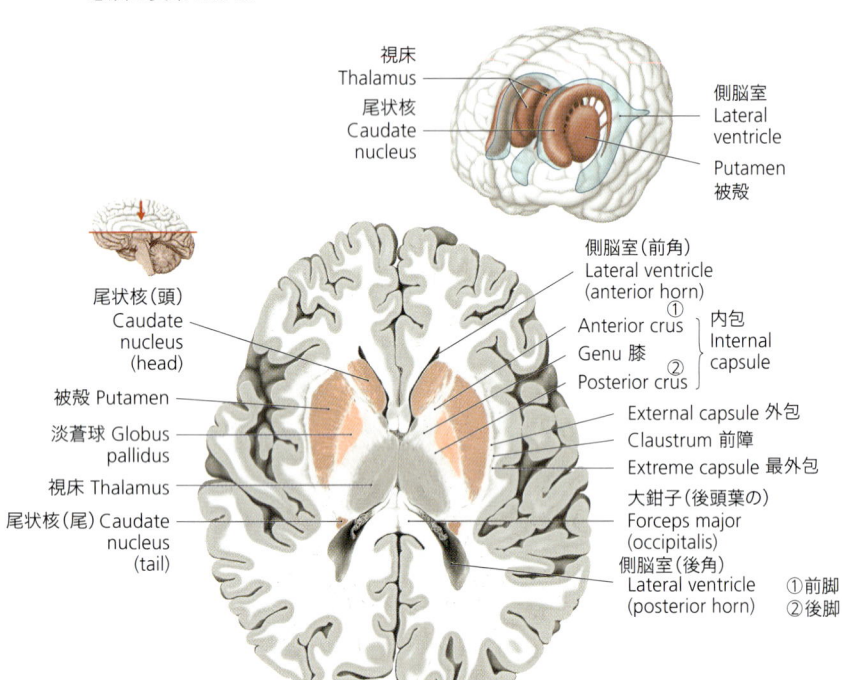

- 視床 Thalamus
- 尾状核 Caudate nucleus
- 側脳室 Lateral ventricle
- 被殻 Putamen
- 尾状核（頭）Caudate nucleus (head)
- 被殻 Putamen
- 淡蒼球 Globus pallidus
- 視床 Thalamus
- 尾状核（尾）Caudate nucleus (tail)
- 側脳室（前角）Lateral ventricle (anterior horn)
- Anterior crus ①
- Genu 膝
- Posterior crus ②
- 内包 Internal capsule
- External capsule 外包
- Claustrum 前障
- Extreme capsule 最外包
- 大鉗子（後頭葉の）Forceps major (occipitalis)
- 側脳室（後角）Lateral ventricle (posterior horn)
- ①前脚 ②後脚

- 放線冠 Corona radiata
- 脳梁 Corpus callosum
- 大脳脚 Cerebral peduncle
- 内包 Internal capsule
- 視放線 Optic radiation

B 右大脳半球の内側方から見たところ．

図 39.10 不等皮質
3層構造の不等皮質は，嗅皮質（青）と海馬（ピンク）に見られる．

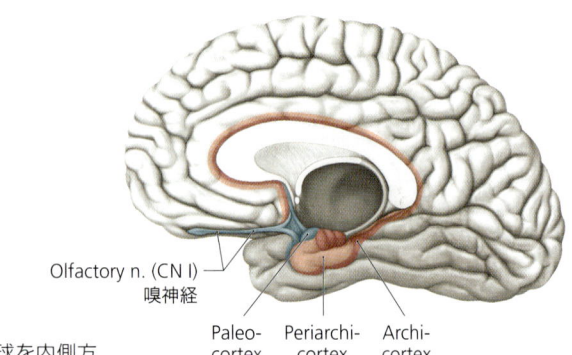

- Olfactory n. (CN I) 嗅神経
- Paleo-cortex 古皮質
- Periarchi-cortex 周原皮質
- Archi-cortex 原皮質

A 右大脳半球を内側方から見たところ．

- 嗅球 Olfactory bulb
- 嗅索 Olfactory tract
- 嗅三角 Olfactory trigone
- 嗅神経 Olfactory n. (CN I)
- 周原皮質 Periarchicortex
- 原皮質 Archicortex

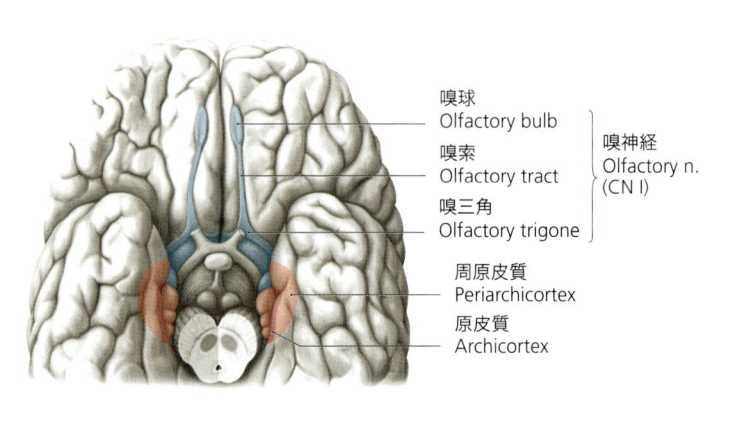

B 底側方から見たところ．

図 39.11 等皮質：円柱状の構成

等皮質は形態学的には6つの水平な層に区分され、機能的には皮質円柱が集合したものとみなせる。

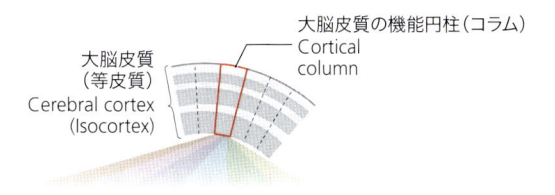

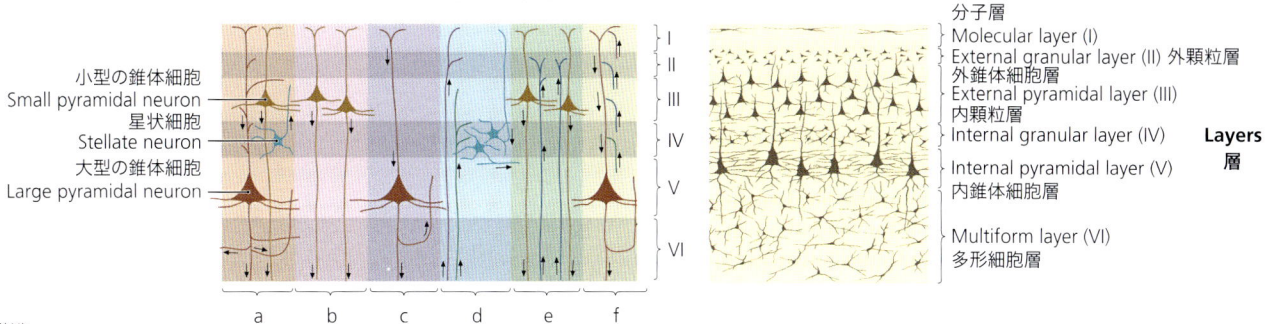

大脳皮質の機能円柱（コラム） Cortical column
大脳皮質（等皮質） Cerebral cortex (Isocortex)

- 小型の錐体細胞 Small pyramidal neuron
- 星状細胞 Stellate neuron
- 大型の錐体細胞 Large pyramidal neuron

Layers 層
- 分子層 Molecular layer (I)
- 外顆粒層 External granular layer (II)
- 外錐体細胞層 External pyramidal layer (III)
- 内顆粒層 Internal granular layer (IV)
- 内錐体細胞層 Internal pyramidal layer (V)
- 多形細胞層 Multiform layer (VI)

Columns 機能円柱（コラム）

A 等皮質の組織構造。

中心溝 Central sulcus
外側溝 Lateral sulcus

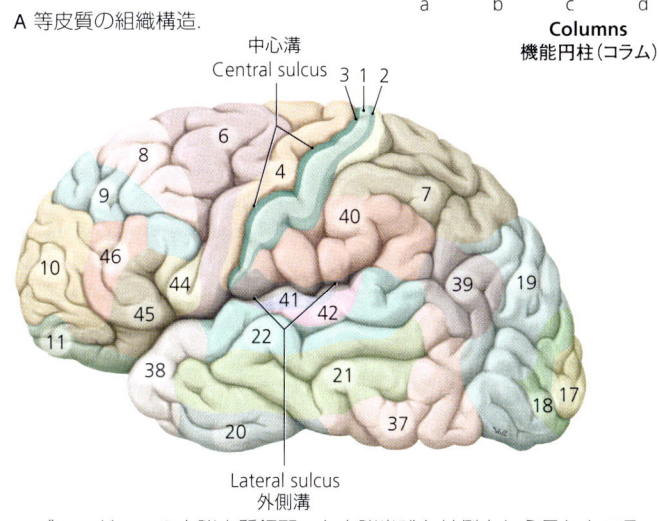

B ブロードマンの大脳皮質領野、左大脳半球を外側方から見たところ。

頭頂後頭溝 Parieto-occipital sulcus
鳥距溝 Calcarine sulcus

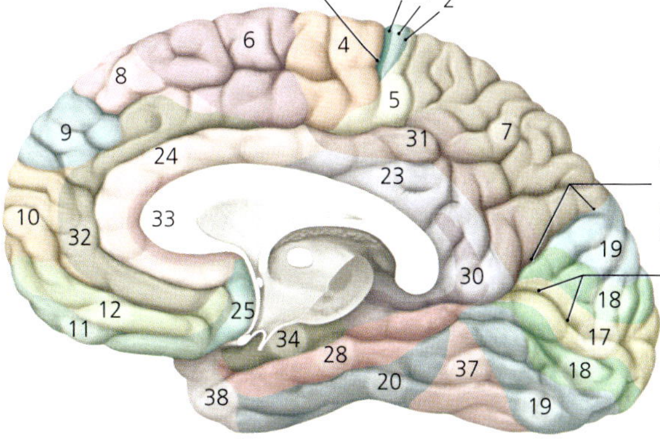

C ブロードマンの大脳皮質領野、右大脳半球を内側方から見たところ。

図 39.12 大脳半球の葉

等皮質は機能的に関連する領域（葉）に区分されることもある。

- Frontal lobe 前頭葉
- Parietal lobe 頭頂葉
- Temporal lobe 側頭葉
- Occipital lobe 後頭葉
- Insular lobe (insula) ①
- Limbic lobe (limbus) ②

①島葉（島）　②辺縁葉（辺縁系）

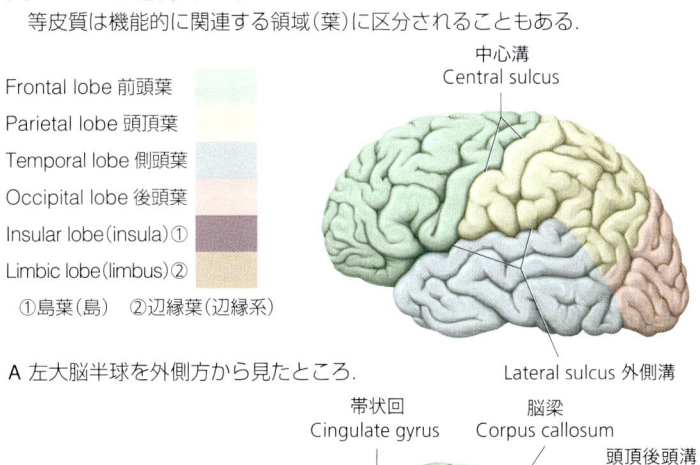

中心溝 Central sulcus
Lateral sulcus 外側溝

A 左大脳半球を外側方から見たところ。

島 Insula

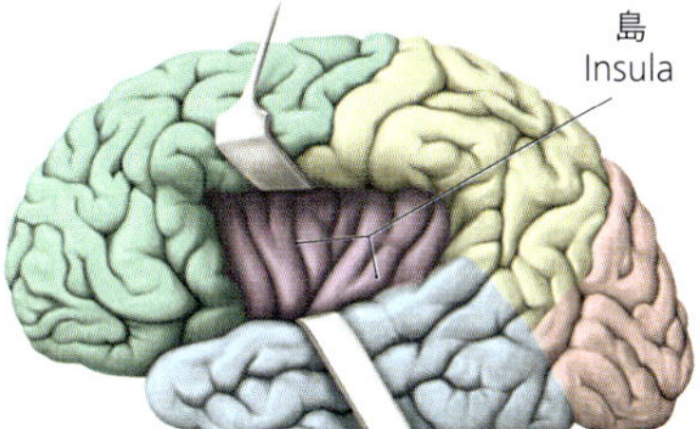

B 左大脳半球を外側方から見たところ。外側溝を開いて島をみせている。

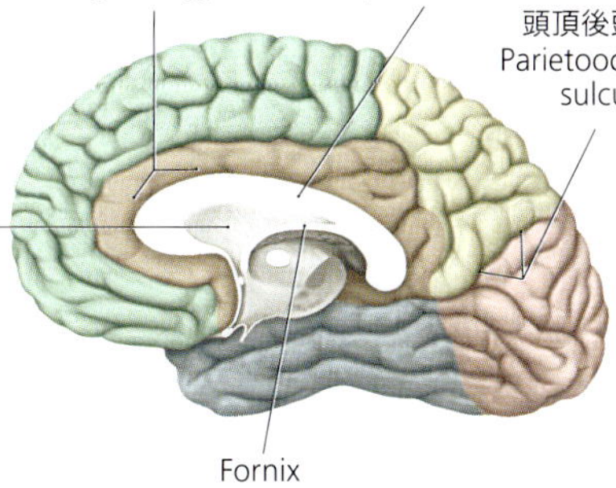

帯状回 Cingulate gyrus
脳梁 Corpus callosum
頭頂後頭溝 Parietooccipital sulcus
透明中隔 Septum pellucidum
脳弓 Fornix

C 右大脳半球を内側方から見たところ。

前頭極 Frontal pole
嗅神経 Olfactory n. (CN I)
視神経 Optic n. (CN II)
下垂体 Hypophysis
乳頭体 Mammillary body
中脳 Mesencephalon
後頭極 Occipital pole
大脳縦裂 Longitudinal cerebral fissure

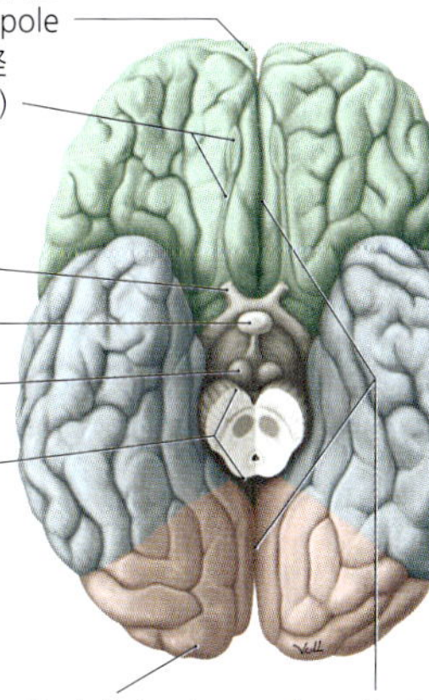

D 底側方から見たところ。脳幹を取り除いてある。

大脳と間脳
Telencephalon & Diencephalon

図 39.13 海馬とその関連構造
海馬, 脳弓, 扁桃体は辺縁系 (p.621 参照) の主要な構造である.

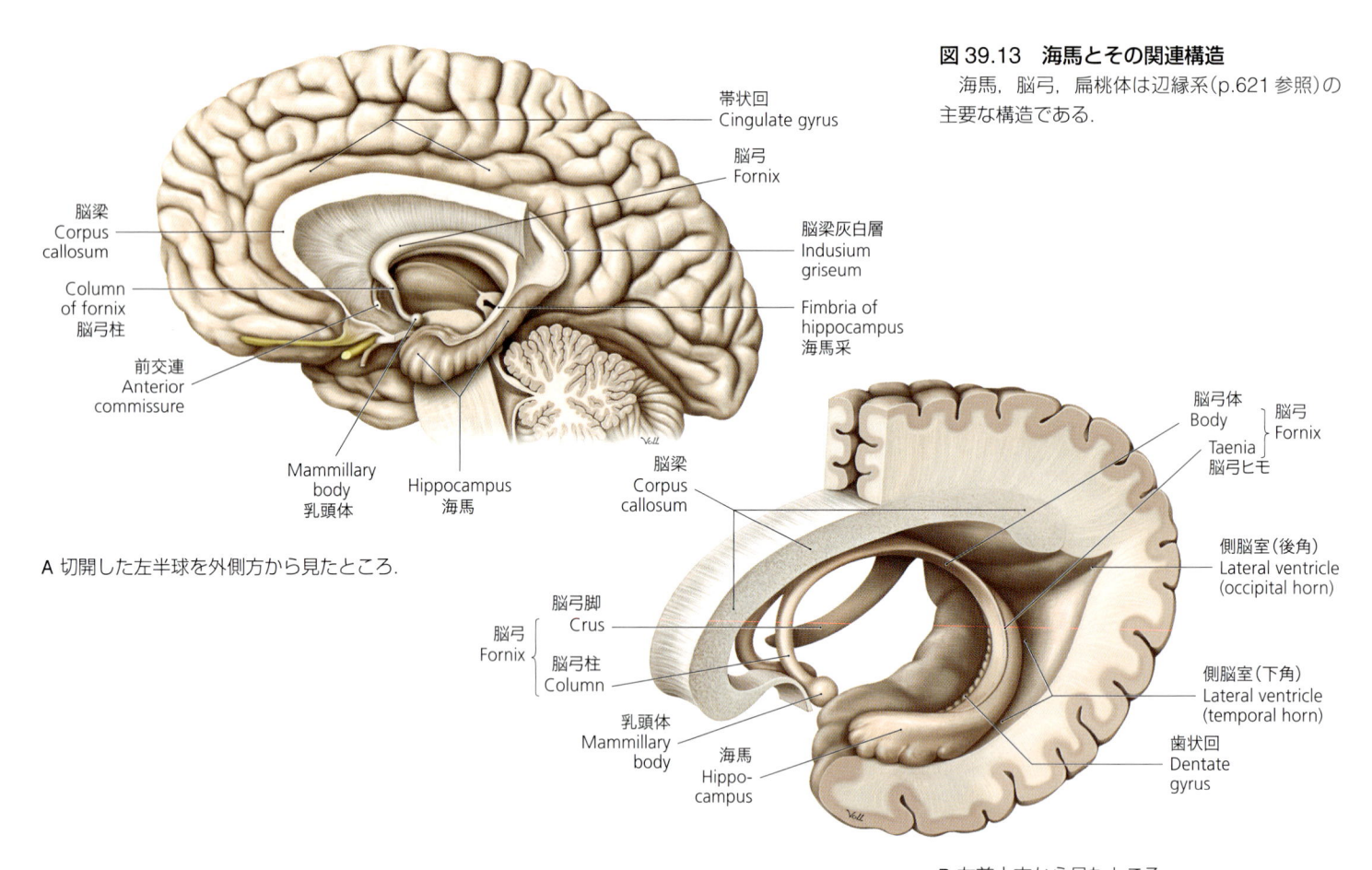

A 切開した左半球を外側方から見たところ.

B 左前上方から見たところ.

図 39.14 間脳
正中矢状断面. 間脳の主要な構造は視床, 視床下部, 脳下垂体の後葉である. 間脳から大脳を取り外した図は p.598 を参照.

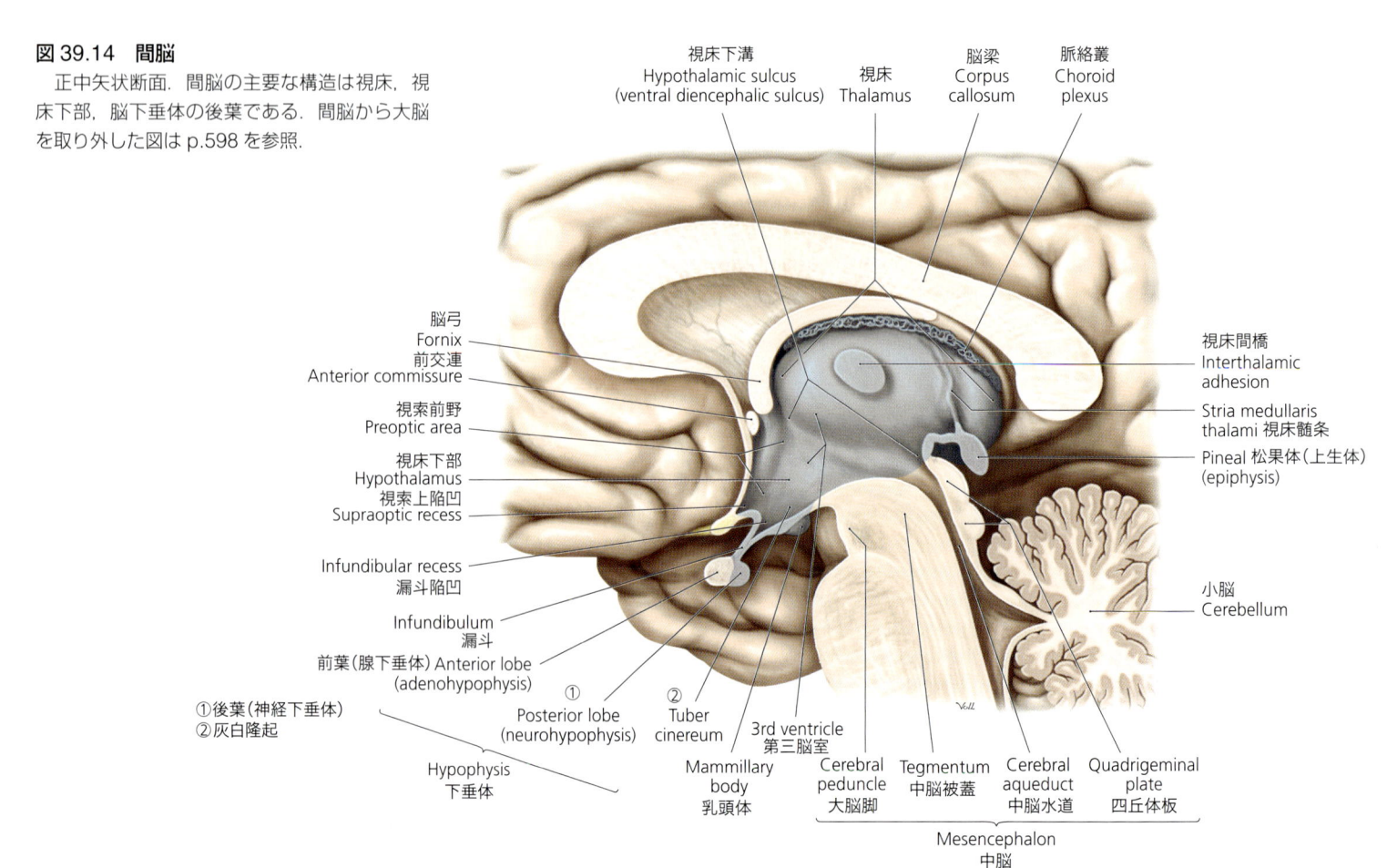

図 39.15 大脳と間脳：内部構造
やや傾いた前額断面．

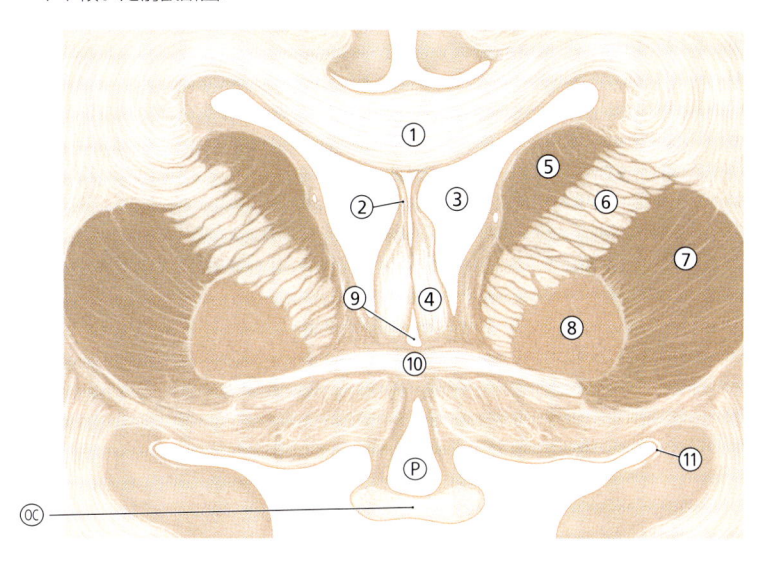

A 視交叉を通る断面．

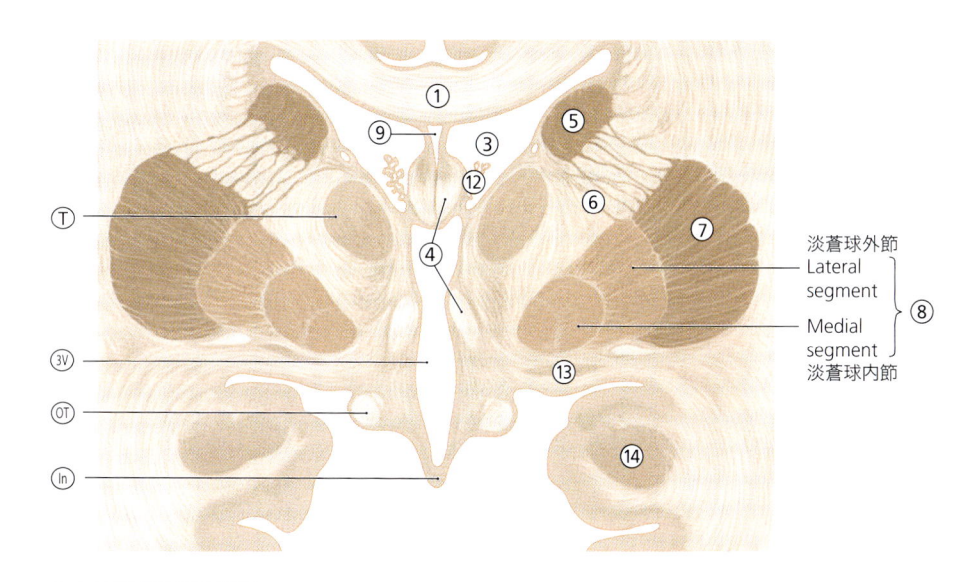

B 灰白隆起を通る断面．

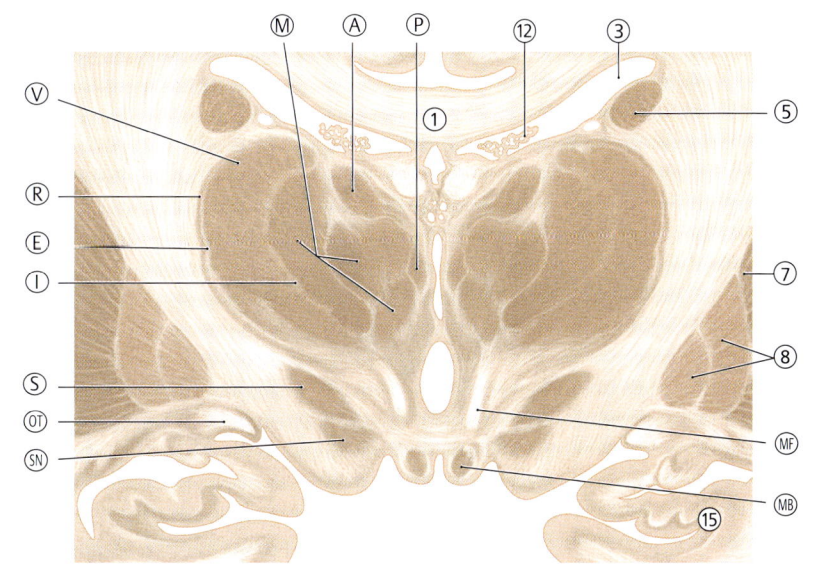

C 乳頭体を通る断面．

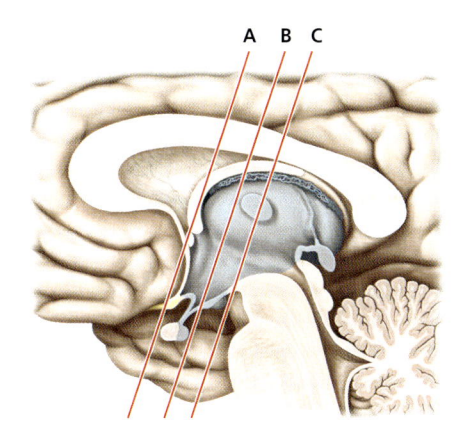

表 39.2		間脳の構造
ⓟ		視索上陥凹
ⓞⓒ		視交叉
③ⓥ		第三脳室
ⓞⓣ		視索
ⓘⓝ		漏斗
		視床（視床核）
Ⓣ	Ⓡ	視床網様核
	Ⓔ	外側髄板
	Ⓥ	視床外側腹側核群
	Ⓘ	内側髄板
	Ⓜ	視床内側核群
	Ⓐ	視床前核群
	Ⓟ	視床室傍核群
Ⓢ		視床下核
ⓈⓃ*		黒質
ⓂⒻ		乳頭体視床束
ⓂⒷ		乳頭体

*本来は中脳に含まれる．

表 39.3	大脳の構造
①	脳梁
②	透明中隔
③	側脳室
④	脳弓
⑤	尾状核
⑥	内包
⑦	被核
⑧	淡蒼球
⑨	透明中隔腔
⑩	前交連
⑪	外側嗅条
⑫	脈絡叢
⑬	基底核（マイネル核）
⑭	扁桃体
⑮	海馬

淡蒼球外節 Lateral segment
淡蒼球内節 Medial segment ⑧

間脳，脳幹，小脳
Diencephalon, Brainstem & Cerebellum

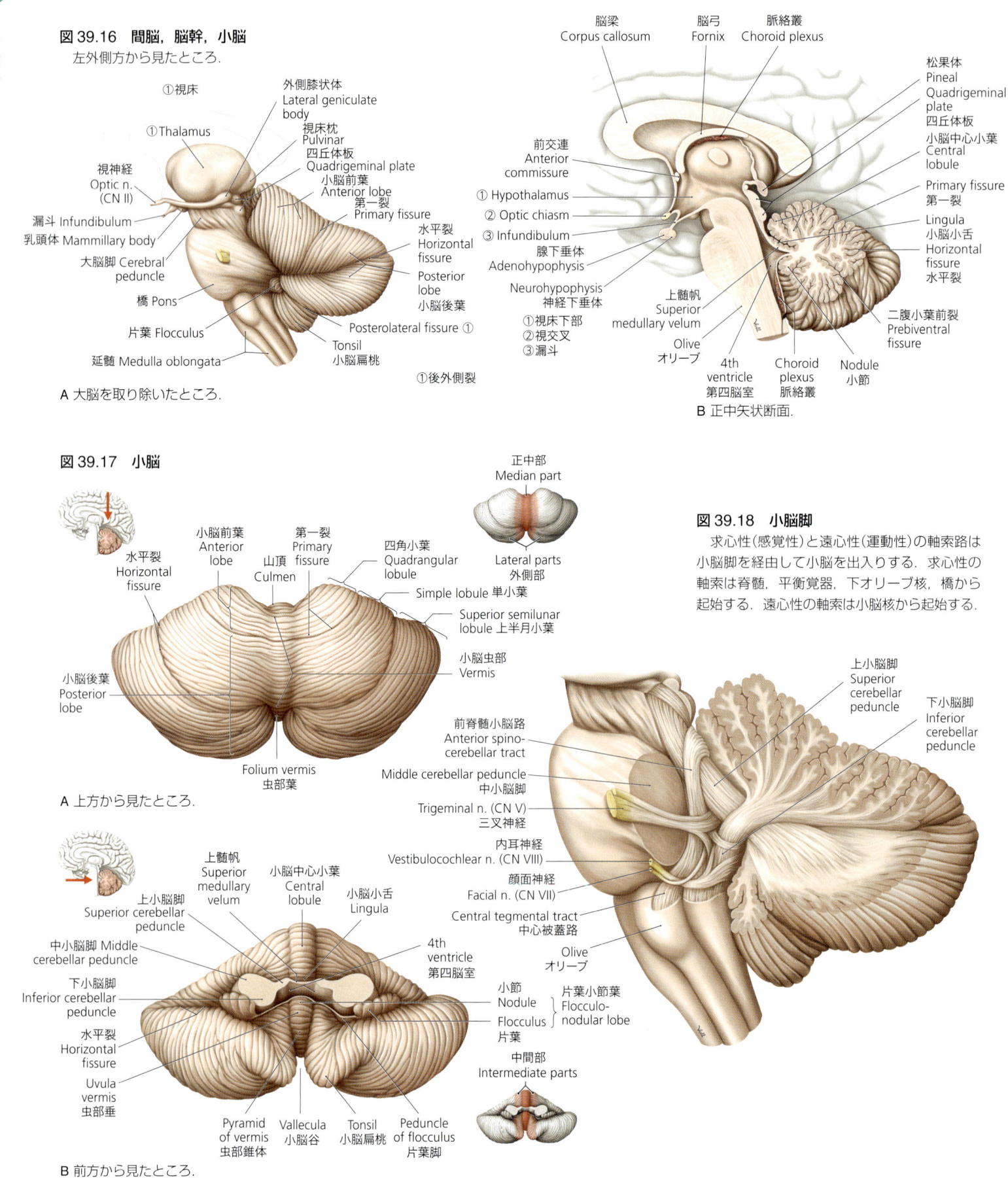

図 39.16　間脳，脳幹，小脳
左外側方から見たところ．

①視床 Thalamus
外側膝状体 Lateral geniculate body
視床枕 Pulvinar
四丘体板 Quadrigeminal plate
小脳前葉 Anterior lobe
第一裂 Primary fissure
視神経 Optic n. (CN II)
漏斗 Infundibulum
乳頭体 Mammillary body
大脳脚 Cerebral peduncle
橋 Pons
片葉 Flocculus
延髄 Medulla oblongata
水平裂 Horizontal fissure
小脳後葉 Posterior lobe
Posterolateral fissure ①
小脳扁桃 Tonsil
①後外側裂

A 大脳を取り除いたところ．

脳梁 Corpus callosum
脳弓 Fornix
脈絡叢 Choroid plexus
前交連 Anterior commissure
①視床下部 Hypothalamus
②視交叉 Optic chiasm
③漏斗 Infundibulum
腺下垂体 Adenohypophysis
神経下垂体 Neurohypophysis
①視床下部
②視交叉
③漏斗
上髄帆 Superior medullary velum
第四脳室 4th ventricle
オリーブ Olive
脈絡叢 Choroid plexus
松果体 Pineal
四丘体板 Quadrigeminal plate
小脳中心小葉 Central lobule
第一裂 Primary fissure
小脳小舌 Lingula
水平裂 Horizontal fissure
二腹小葉前裂 Prebiventral fissure
小節 Nodule

B 正中矢状断面．

図 39.17　小脳

水平裂 Horizontal fissure
小脳前葉 Anterior lobe
山頂 Culmen
第一裂 Primary fissure
四角小葉 Quadrangular lobule
単小葉 Simple lobule
上半月小葉 Superior semilunar lobule
小脳虫部 Vermis
小脳後葉 Posterior lobe
虫部葉 Folium vermis
正中部 Median part
外側部 Lateral parts

A 上方から見たところ．

上髄帆 Superior medullary velum
小脳中心小葉 Central lobule
小脳小舌 Lingula
第四脳室 4th ventricle
小節 Nodule
片葉 Flocculus
片葉小節葉 Flocculo-nodular lobe
上小脳脚 Superior cerebellar peduncle
中小脳脚 Middle cerebellar peduncle
下小脳脚 Inferior cerebellar peduncle
水平裂 Horizontal fissure
虫部垂 Uvula vermis
虫部錐体 Pyramid of vermis
小脳谷 Vallecula
小脳扁桃 Tonsil
片葉脚 Peduncle of flocculus
中間部 Intermediate parts

B 前方から見たところ．

図 39.18　小脳脚

求心性（感覚性）と遠心性（運動性）の軸索路は小脳脚を経由して小脳を出入りする．求心性の軸索は脊髄，平衡覚器，下オリーブ核，橋から起始する．遠心性の軸索は小脳核から起始する．

前脊髄小脳路 Anterior spinocerebellar tract
中小脳脚 Middle cerebellar peduncle
三叉神経 Trigeminal n. (CN V)
内耳神経 Vestibulocochlear n. (CN VIII)
顔面神経 Facial n. (CN VII)
中心被蓋路 Central tegmental tract
オリーブ Olive
上小脳脚 Superior cerebellar peduncle
下小脳脚 Inferior cerebellar peduncle

図 39.19 脳幹

脳幹は生命維持中枢である．また，脳幹には 10 対の脳神経（第 III–XII 脳神経）が出入りする．脳神経とその核については p.470 で概観できる．

A 脳幹の各部位．
- 間脳 Diencephalon
- 中脳 Mesencephalon
- 下垂体 Hypophysis
- 橋 Pons
- 延髄 Medulla oblongata
- 中脳水道 Cerebral aqueduct
- 小脳 Cerebellum
- 第四脳室 4th ventricle
- 菱形窩 Rhomboid fossa

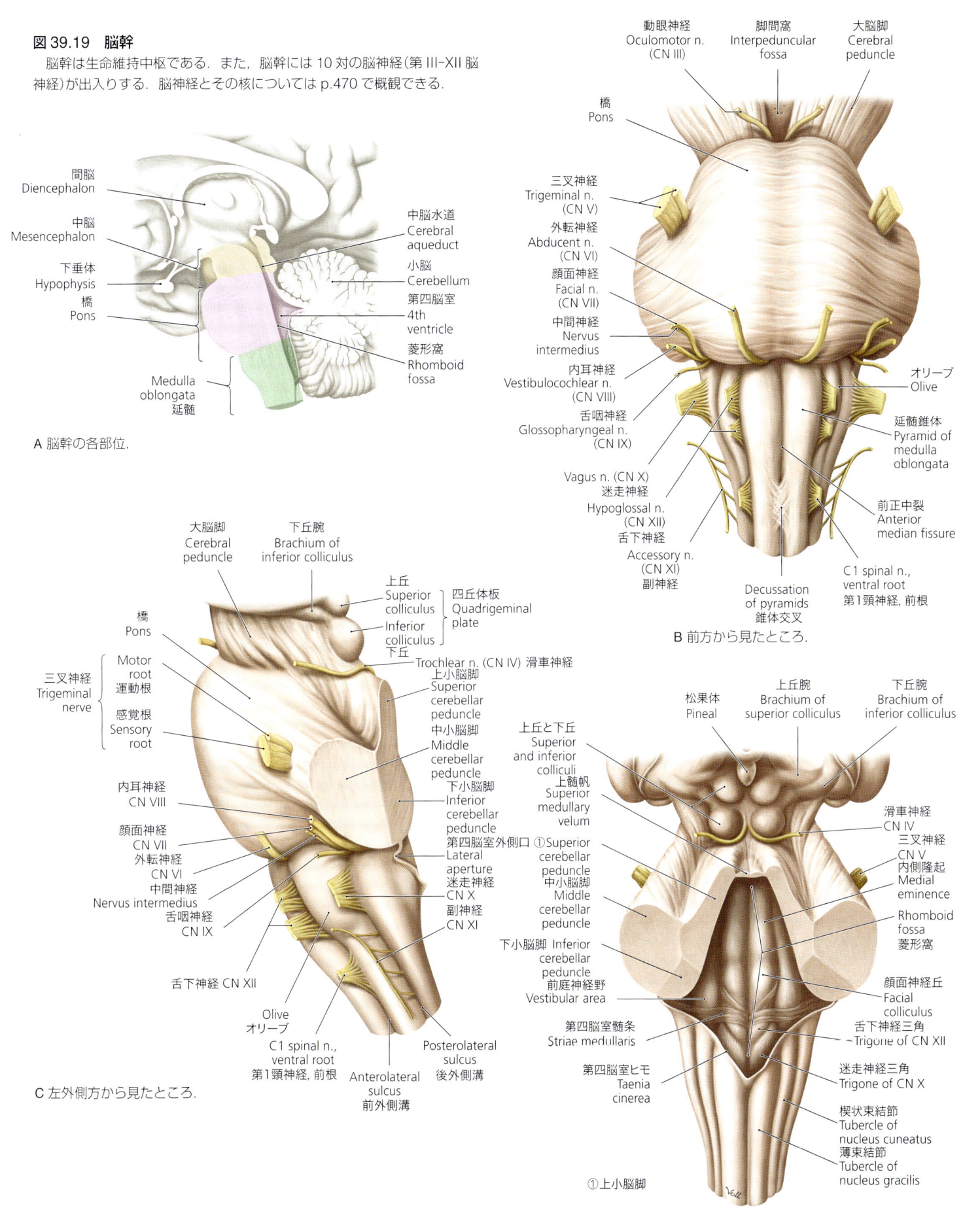

B 前方から見たところ．
- 動眼神経 Oculomotor n. (CN III)
- 脚間窩 Interpeduncular fossa
- 大脳脚 Cerebral peduncle
- 橋 Pons
- 三叉神経 Trigeminal n. (CN V)
- 外転神経 Abducent n. (CN VI)
- 顔面神経 Facial n. (CN VII)
- 中間神経 Nervus intermedius
- 内耳神経 Vestibulocochlear n. (CN VIII)
- 舌咽神経 Glossopharyngeal n. (CN IX)
- 迷走神経 Vagus n. (CN X)
- 舌下神経 Hypoglossal n. (CN XII)
- 副神経 Accessory n. (CN XI)
- 錐体交叉 Decussation of pyramids
- オリーブ Olive
- 延髄錐体 Pyramid of medulla oblongata
- 前正中裂 Anterior median fissure
- 第1頸神経, 前根 C1 spinal n., ventral root

C 左外側方から見たところ．
- 大脳脚 Cerebral peduncle
- 下丘腕 Brachium of inferior colliculus
- 上丘 Superior colliculus
- 下丘 Inferior colliculus
- 四丘体板 Quadrigeminal plate
- 滑車神経 Trochlear n. (CN IV)
- 橋 Pons
- 三叉神経 Trigeminal nerve
  - 運動根 Motor root
  - 感覚根 Sensory root
- 上小脳脚 Superior cerebellar peduncle
- 中小脳脚 Middle cerebellar peduncle
- 下小脳脚 Inferior cerebellar peduncle
- 第四脳室外側口 Lateral aperture
- 内耳神経 CN VIII
- 顔面神経 CN VII
- 外転神経 CN VI
- 中間神経 Nervus intermedius
- 舌咽神経 CN IX
- 迷走神経 CN X
- 副神経 CN XI
- 舌下神経 CN XII
- オリーブ Olive
- 第1頸神経, 前根 C1 spinal n., ventral root
- 前外側溝 Anterolateral sulcus
- 後外側溝 Posterolateral sulcus

D 後方から見たところ．
- 松果体 Pineal
- 上丘腕 Brachium of superior colliculus
- 下丘腕 Brachium of inferior colliculus
- 上丘と下丘 Superior and inferior colliculi
- 上髄帆 Superior medullary velum
- ①上小脳脚 Superior cerebellar peduncle
- 中小脳脚 Middle cerebellar peduncle
- 下小脳脚 Inferior cerebellar peduncle
- 前庭神経野 Vestibular area
- 第四脳室髄条 Striae medullaris
- 第四脳室ヒモ Taenia cinerea
- 滑車神経 CN IV
- 三叉神経 CN V
- 内側隆起 Medial eminence
- 菱形窩 Rhomboid fossa
- 顔面神経丘 Facial colliculus
- 舌下神経三角 Trigone of CN XII
- 迷走神経三角 Trigone of CN X
- 楔状束結節 Tubercle of nucleus cuneatus
- 薄束結節 Tubercle of nucleus gracilis

①上小脳脚

脊髄
Spinal Cord

図 39.20　脊髄と脊髄分節

脊髄は 31 節の脊髄分節からなり，個々の脊髄分節は体幹と四肢のある特定の領域を支配する（図 39.22 参照）．求心性（感覚性）の後根糸と遠心性（運動性）の前根糸はそれぞれ何本かが集まり，後根と前根を形成する．この 2 種類の根はいったん融合したのち，求心性と遠心性の成分が混合した前枝と後枝に再び分かれる．前枝および後枝は様々な枝に分かれる．

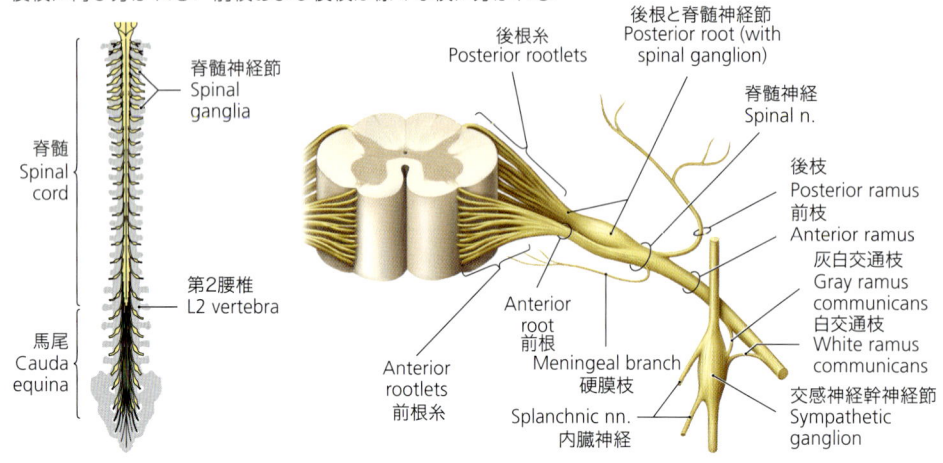

A　脊髄，後方から見たところ．

B　脊髄分節，前方から見たところ．

図 39.21　現位置における脊髄

後方から見たところ．脊柱管を開いたところ．

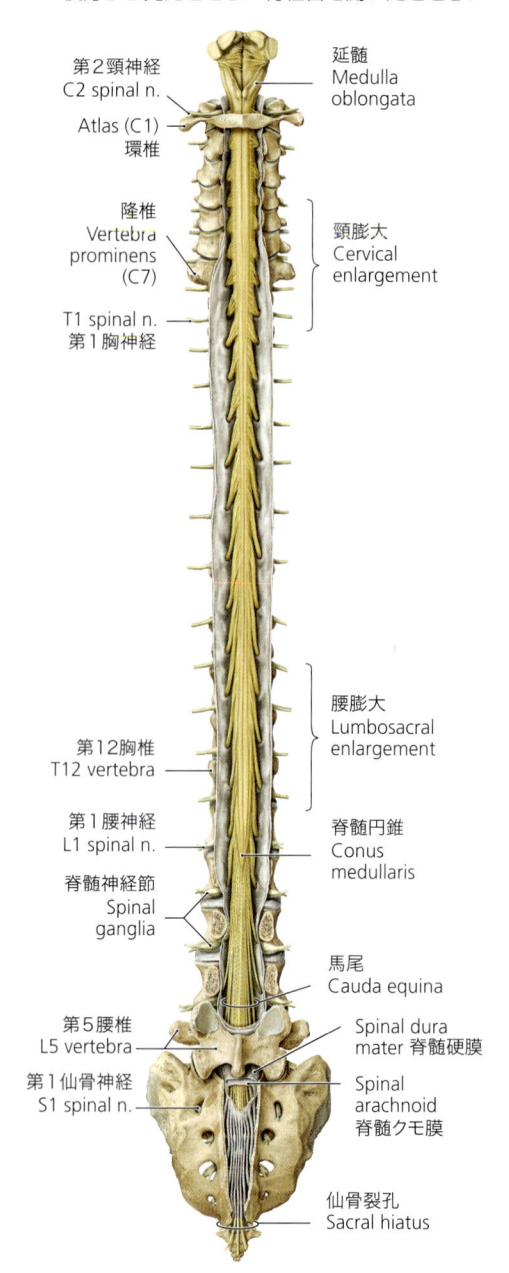

図 39.22　脊髄分節の支配領域と脊髄障害

脊髄は 4 つの主要な領域（頸髄，胸髄，腰髄，仙髄）に区分される．脊髄分節には番号がつけられている．この番号は，脊髄分節から出た脊髄神経が通る椎間孔の高さによって決められる．（Note：番号は脊髄分節の近傍にある椎骨と必ずしも対応しない．）

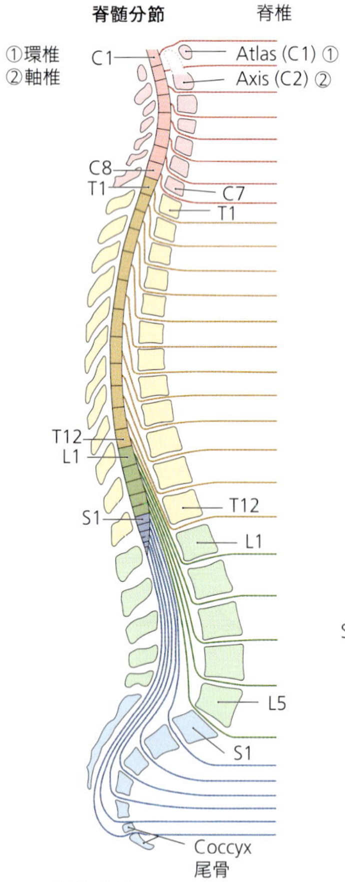

A　脊髄分節．

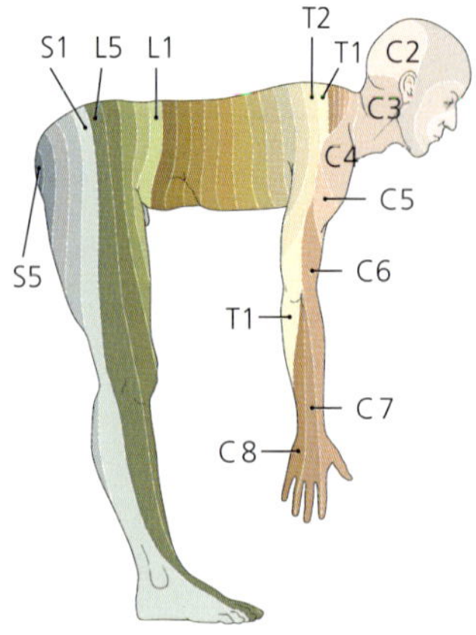

B　デルマトーム（皮膚分節）．それぞれの脊髄分節は特定のデルマトームを支配する．

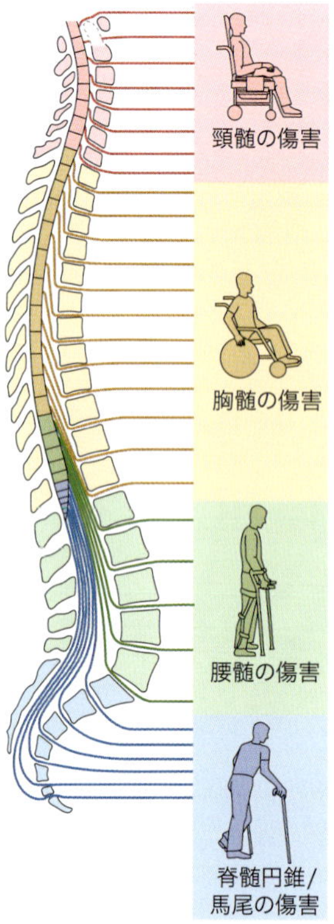

C　脊髄障害．

図 39.23 現位置における脊髄：横断面
上方から見たところ．

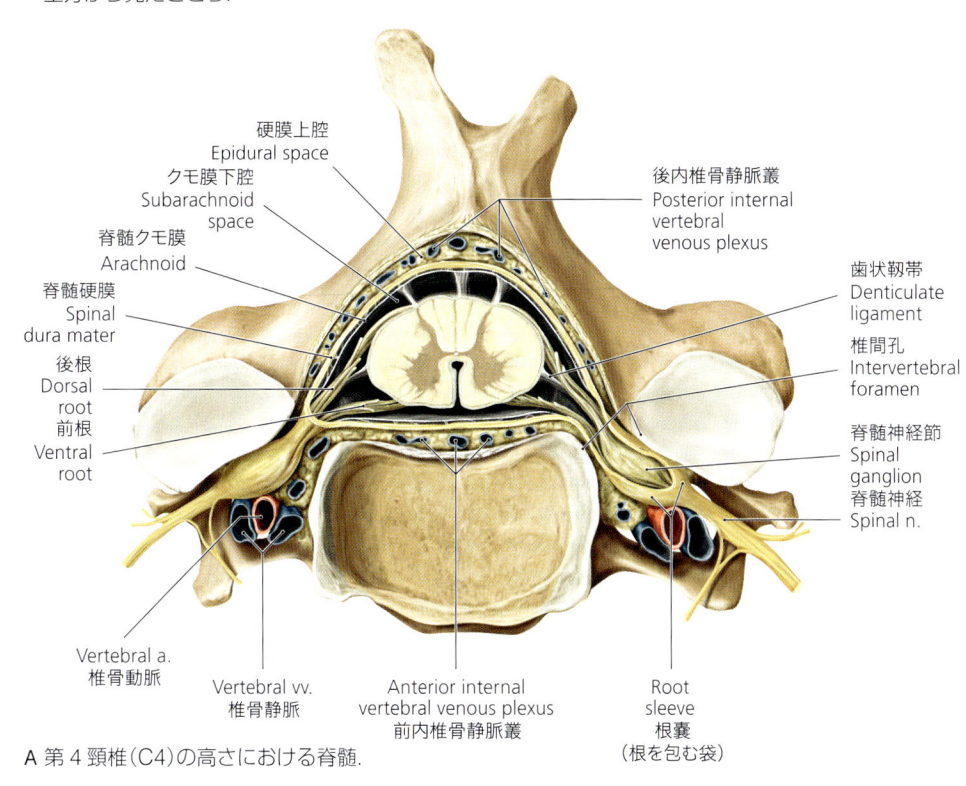

A 第4頸椎（C4）の高さにおける脊髄．

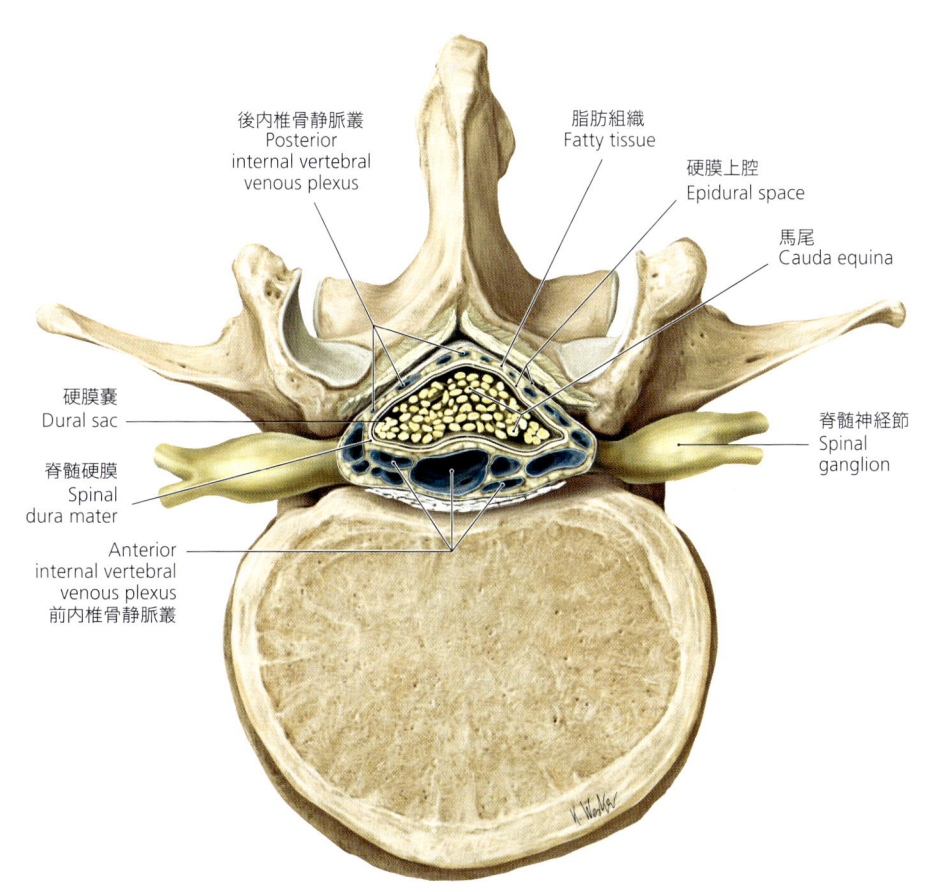

B 第2腰椎（L2）の高さにおける脊髄．

臨床

腰椎穿刺
穿刺針を腰椎の高さで硬膜嚢に刺入すると，針は神経根（馬尾）の間をすり抜けて通り，神経根や脊髄を損傷することはない．したがって，脳脊髄液を採取する場合には，第3・4腰椎間に穿刺針を刺入する(2)．このとき，患者には体を前屈させた体位を取らせ，腰椎の棘突起の間を開いておく．

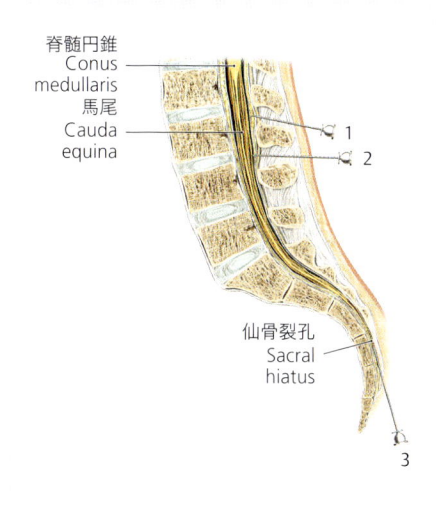

麻酔
腰椎麻酔は腰椎穿刺と同様の方法で行われる(2)．硬膜外麻酔は，カテーテルを硬膜上腔に留置し，硬膜嚢を貫通しない(1)．また，仙骨裂孔を通じて注射針を刺入して，硬膜外麻酔を行う場合もある(3)．

図 39.24 馬尾
成人では，脊髄はほぼ第1腰椎の高さで終わる．これより下の脊柱管内は，前根と後根によって満たされている．この2種類の根は椎間孔において融合し，その後再び前枝と後枝に分かれる（p.36 参照）．

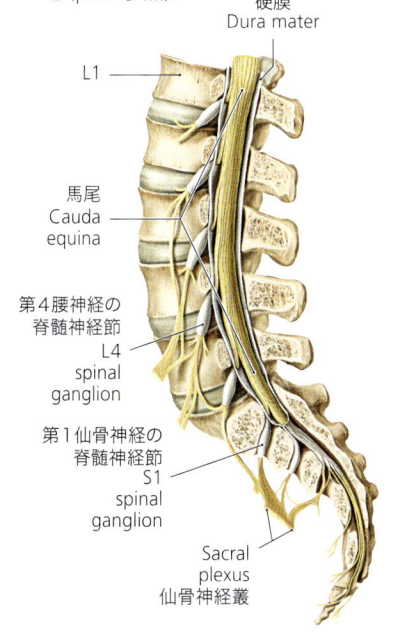

髄膜
Meninges

脳と脊髄は髄膜によって覆われる．髄膜は硬膜，クモ膜，軟膜の3層からなる．クモ膜と軟膜の間にある空間はクモ膜下腔と呼ばれ，脳脊髄液で満たされている（p.604参照）．脊髄の髄膜についてはp.601参照．

図 39.25 髄膜
脳の静脈（硬膜静脈洞）については p.606 参照．

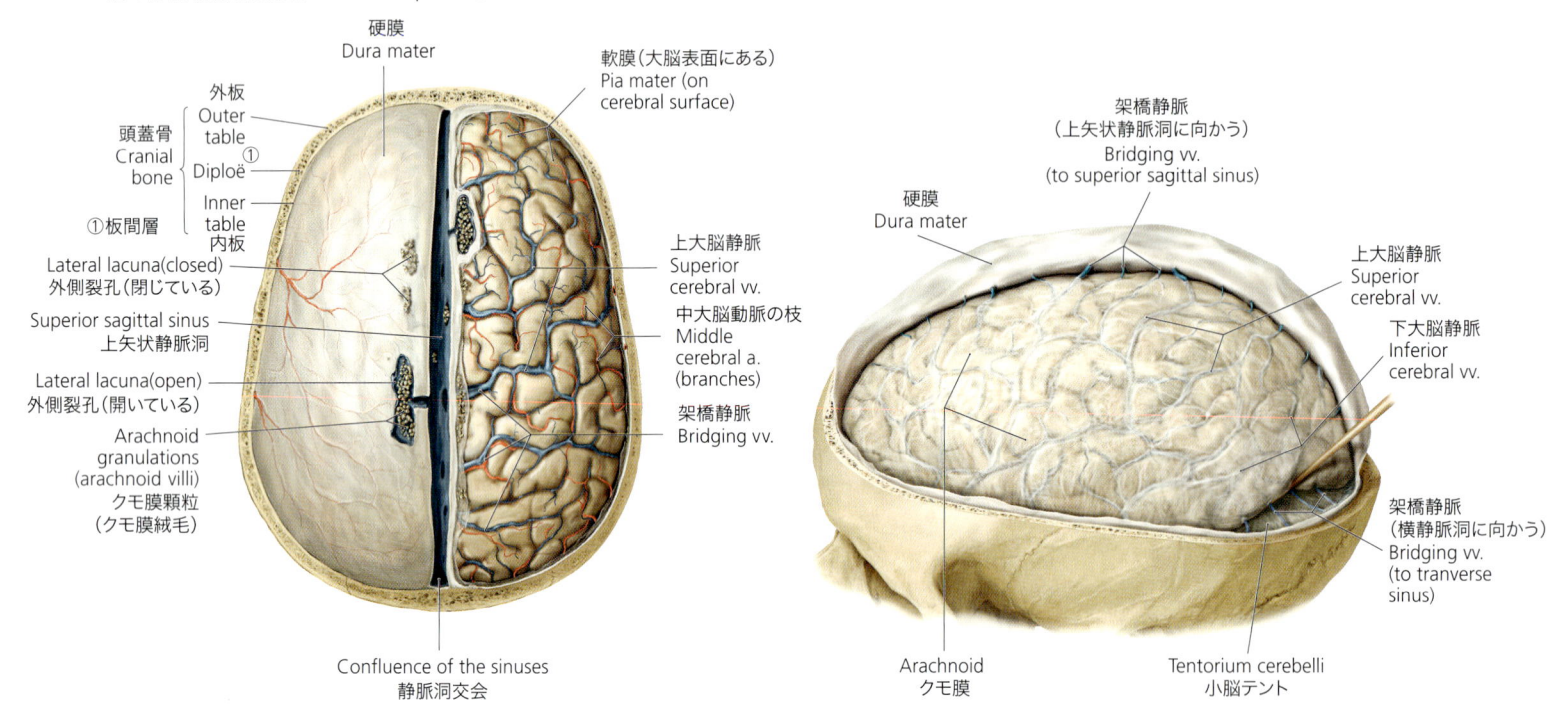

主な名称（図中ラベル）

- 硬膜 Dura mater
- 軟膜（大脳表面にある）Pia mater (on cerebral surface)
- 外板 Outer table
- 頭蓋骨 Cranial bone
- ①板間層 Diploë
- 内板 Inner table
- 外側裂孔（閉じている）Lateral lacuna (closed)
- 上矢状静脈洞 Superior sagittal sinus
- 外側裂孔（開いている）Lateral lacuna (open)
- クモ膜顆粒（クモ膜絨毛）Arachnoid granulations (arachnoid villi)
- 静脈洞交会 Confluence of the sinuses
- 上大脳静脈 Superior cerebral vv.
- 中大脳動脈の枝 Middle cerebral a. (branches)
- 架橋静脈 Bridging vv.
- 架橋静脈（上矢状静脈洞に向かう）Bridging vv. (to superior sagittal sinus)
- 下大脳静脈 Inferior cerebral vv.
- 架橋静脈（横静脈洞に向かう）Bridging vv. (to transverse sinus)
- クモ膜 Arachnoid
- 小脳テント Tentorium cerebelli
- 板間静脈 Diploic vv.
- 硬膜外血腫 Epidural hematoma
- 頭蓋骨 Cranial bone
- 内皮様細胞層 Neurothelium
- クモ膜 Arachnoid
- Subdural hemorrhage 硬膜下出血
- クモ膜小柱 Arachnoid trabeculae
- 大脳皮質 Cerebral cortex
- 軟膜 Pia mater
- 大脳動脈 Cerebral a.
- クモ膜下腔 Subarachnoid space
- 大脳静脈 Cerebral v.
- 髄膜性の内層 Meningeal layer
- 骨膜性の外層 Periosteal layer
- 上矢状静脈洞 Superior sagittal sinus
- 導出静脈 Emissary v.
- 帽状腱膜 Galea aponeurotica
- 頭皮 Scalp
- 外板 Outer table
- 板間層 Diploë
- 内板 Inner table
- 頭皮の静脈 Scalp vv.
- クモ膜顆粒小窩 Granular foveola
- 外側裂孔とクモ膜顆粒 Lateral lacuna with arachnoid granulations
- 大脳鎌 Falx cerebri
- 架橋静脈 Bridging v.
- 上大脳静脈 Superior cerebral vv.

A 上方から見たところ．左側では硬膜（髄膜の外層）が見えている．右側では軟膜（髄膜の内層）を被った脳が見えている．クモ膜顆粒（クモ膜の突出部）は脳脊髄液を吸収する場所である．

B クモ膜（髄膜の中間層），左上方から見たところ．

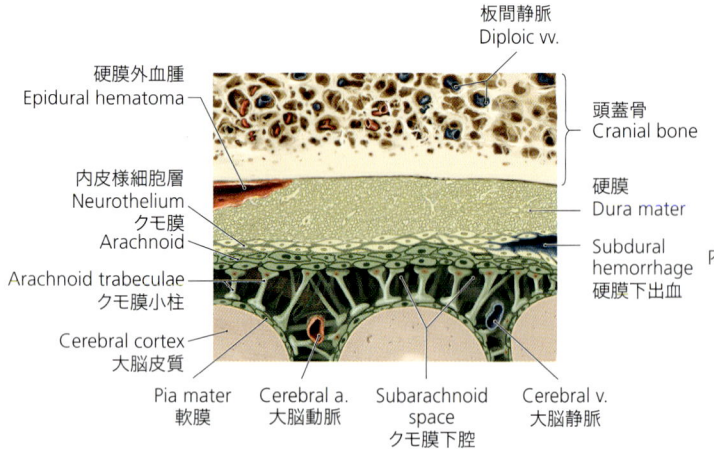

C 髄膜の層，前額断面を前方から見たところ．

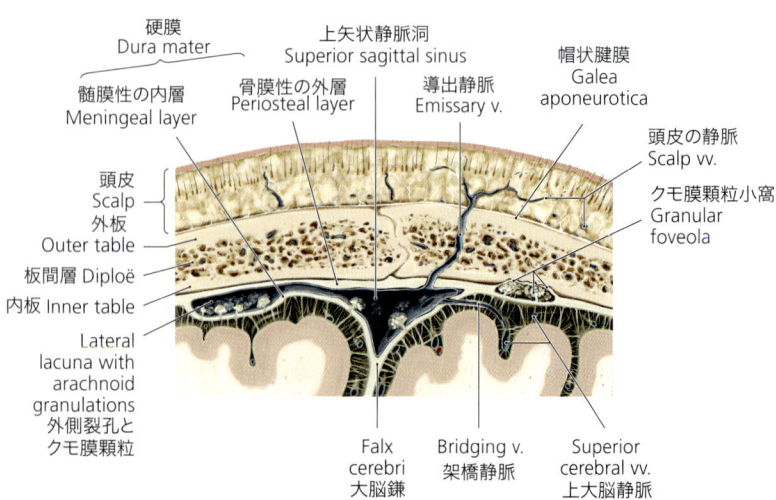

D 硬膜と頭蓋冠，前額断面を前方から見たところ．

臨床

脳外出血

硬い骨である頭蓋冠と柔らかな脳実質の間で生じた出血（脳外出血）により，脳が圧迫され，障害が現れる場合がある．血腫の増大により頭蓋内圧が高まると，直接圧迫されている部位だけでなく，血腫から離れた部位も損傷を受ける．脳外出血は硬膜との位置関係により3つのタイプに分けられる．脳の動脈については p.608 を参照．

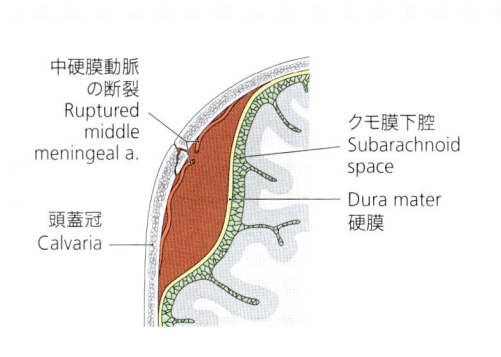

A 硬膜外血腫（硬膜の上にできる）．
- 中硬膜動脈の断裂 Ruptured middle meningeal a.
- 頭蓋冠 Calvaria
- クモ膜下腔 Subarachnoid space
- Dura mater 硬膜

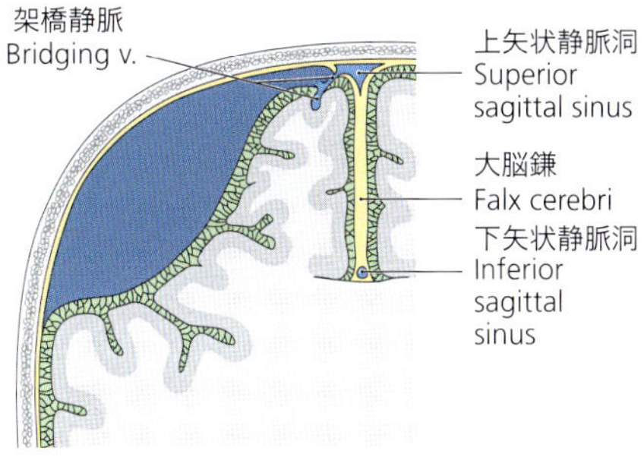

B 硬膜下血腫（硬膜の下にできる）．
- 架橋静脈 Bridging v.
- 上矢状静脈洞 Superior sagittal sinus
- 大脳鎌 Falx cerebri
- 下矢状静脈洞 Inferior sagittal sinus

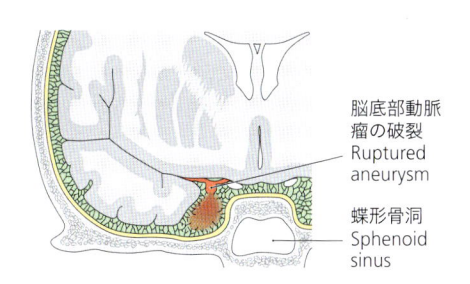

C クモ膜下出血．
- 脳底部動脈瘤の破裂 Ruptured aneurysm
- 蝶形骨洞 Sphenoid sinus

図 39.26　硬膜中隔

左前上方から見たところ．主要な硬膜中隔は大脳鎌，小脳テント，小脳鎌（この図では見えない）である．硬膜中隔は脳の特定の部位に入り込み，各部位を分離する．

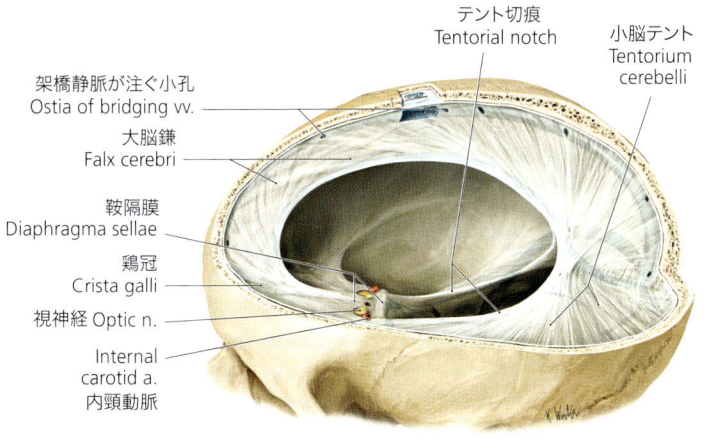

- 架橋静脈が注ぐ小孔 Ostia of bridging vv.
- テント切痕 Tentorial notch
- 小脳テント Tentorium cerebelli
- 大脳鎌 Falx cerebri
- 鞍隔膜 Diaphragma sellae
- 鶏冠 Crista galli
- 視神経 Optic n.
- 内頸動脈 Internal carotid a.

図 39.27　硬膜の支配神経

上方から見たところ．右側の小脳テントを取り除いてある．

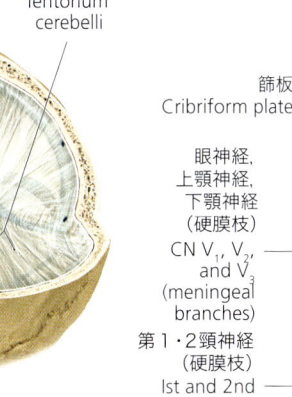

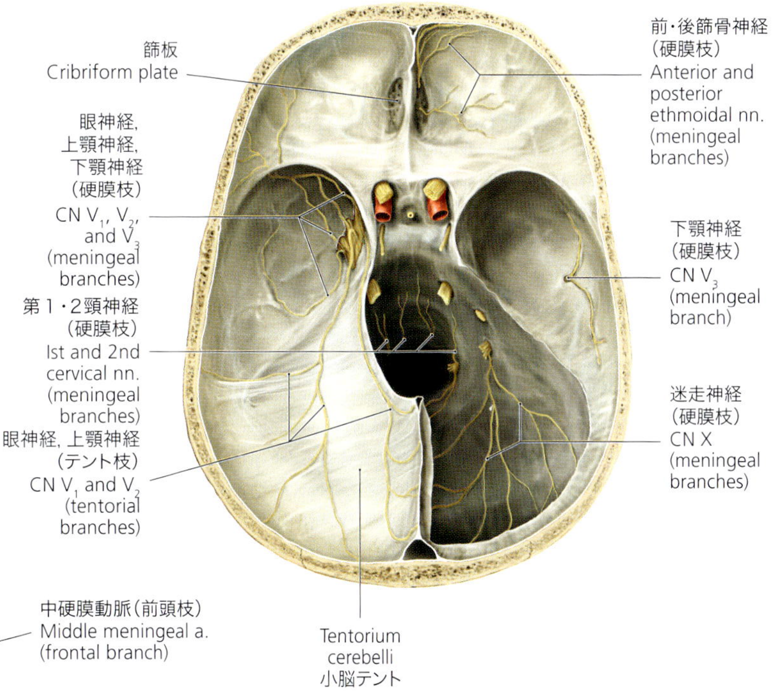

- 篩板 Cribriform plate
- 前・後篩骨神経（硬膜枝）Anterior and posterior ethmoidal nn. (meningeal branches)
- 眼神経，上顎神経，下顎神経（硬膜枝）CN V₁, V₂, and V₃ (meningeal branches)
- 下顎神経（硬膜枝）CN V₃ (meningeal branch)
- 第1・2頸神経（硬膜枝）1st and 2nd cervical nn. (meningeal branches)
- 眼神経，上顎神経（テント枝）CN V₁ and V₂ (tentorial branches)
- 迷走神経（硬膜枝）CN X (meningeal branches)
- 小脳テント Tentorium cerebelli

図 39.28　硬膜の動脈

正中矢状断面．左内側方から見たところ．脳の動脈については p.608 を参照．

- 中硬膜動脈（前頭枝）Middle meningeal a. (frontal branch)
- 中硬膜動脈（頭頂枝）Middle meningeal a. (parietal branch)
- 後頭動脈（乳突枝）Occipital a. (mastoid branch)
- ①中硬膜動脈（頭蓋底の棘孔を通る）Middle meningeal a. ① (via foramen spinosum)
- 椎骨動脈（枝）Vertebral a. (branches)

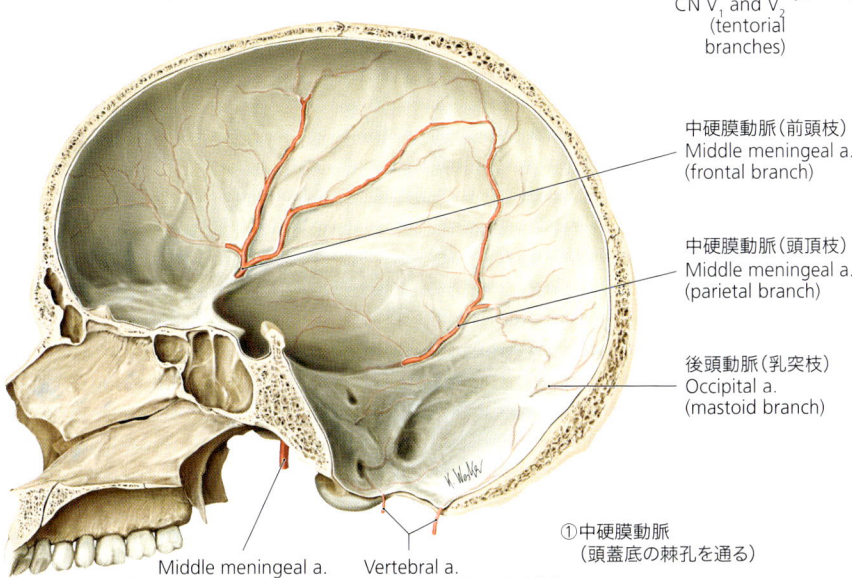

脳室と脳脊髄液の空間
Ventricles & CSF Spaces

図 39.29 脳脊髄液の循環
脳と脊髄は脳脊髄液の中に浮かんでいる．脳脊髄液は脈絡叢で作られ，脳室やクモ膜下腔を満たす．

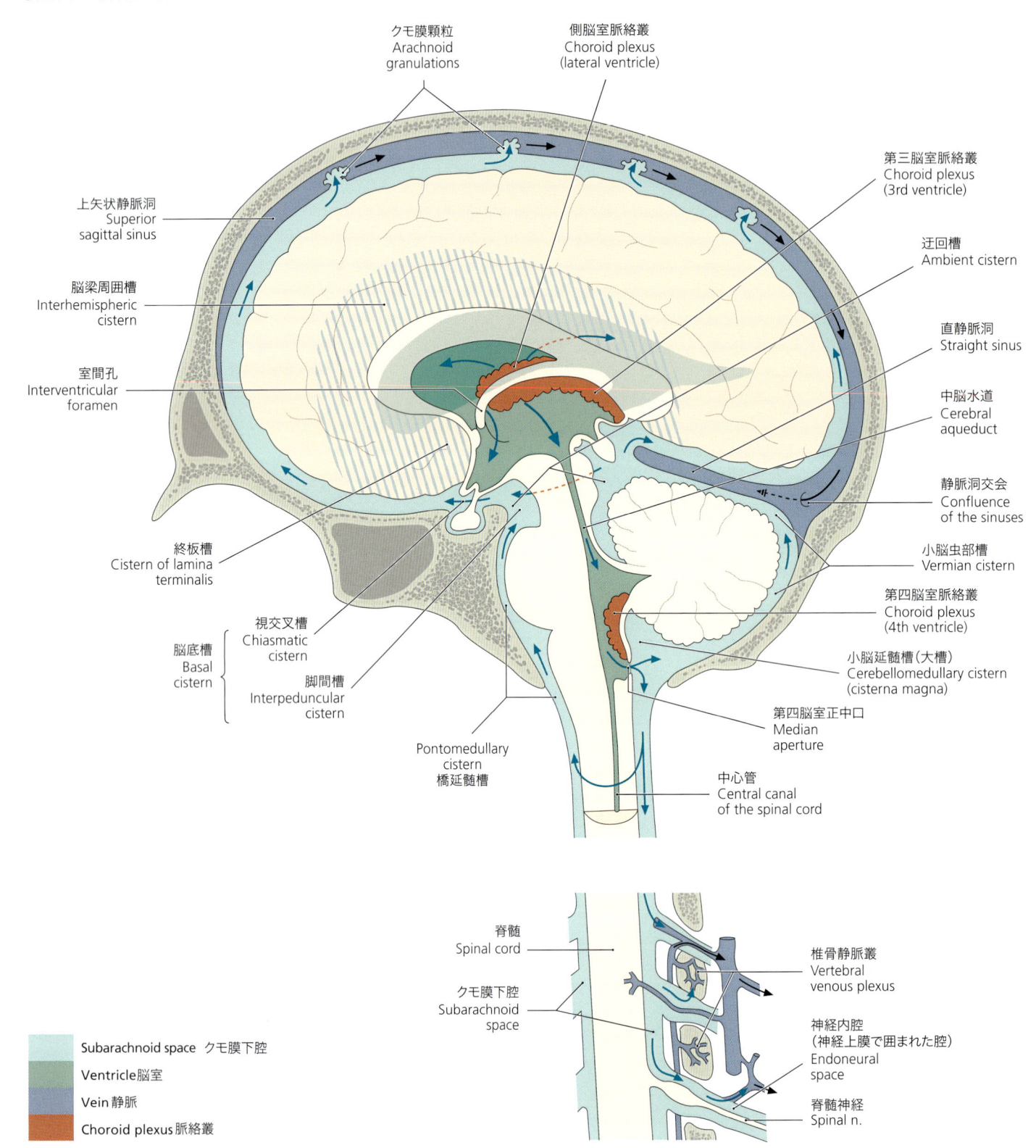

- クモ膜顆粒 Arachnoid granulations
- 側脳室脈絡叢 Choroid plexus (lateral ventricle)
- 第三脳室脈絡叢 Choroid plexus (3rd ventricle)
- 上矢状静脈洞 Superior sagittal sinus
- 迂回槽 Ambient cistern
- 脳梁周囲槽 Interhemispheric cistern
- 直静脈洞 Straight sinus
- 室間孔 Interventricular foramen
- 中脳水道 Cerebral aqueduct
- 静脈洞交会 Confluence of the sinuses
- 終板槽 Cistern of lamina terminalis
- 小脳虫部槽 Vermian cistern
- 視交叉槽 Chiasmatic cistern
- 第四脳室脈絡叢 Choroid plexus (4th ventricle)
- 脳底槽 Basal cistern
- 小脳延髄槽（大槽） Cerebellomedullary cistern (cisterna magna)
- 脚間槽 Interpeduncular cistern
- 第四脳室正中口 Median aperture
- 橋延髄槽 Pontomedullary cistern
- 中心管 Central canal of the spinal cord
- 脊髄 Spinal cord
- 椎骨静脈叢 Vertebral venous plexus
- クモ膜下腔 Subarachnoid space
- 神経内腔（神経上膜で囲まれた腔） Endoneural space
- 脊髄神経 Spinal n.

凡例:
- Subarachnoid space クモ膜下腔
- Ventricle 脳室
- Vein 静脈
- Choroid plexus 脈絡叢

図 39.30　脳室系

脳室系は脊髄にある中心管に連なる．脳室系の鋳型標本をみると4つの脳室が連絡している様子がわかる．

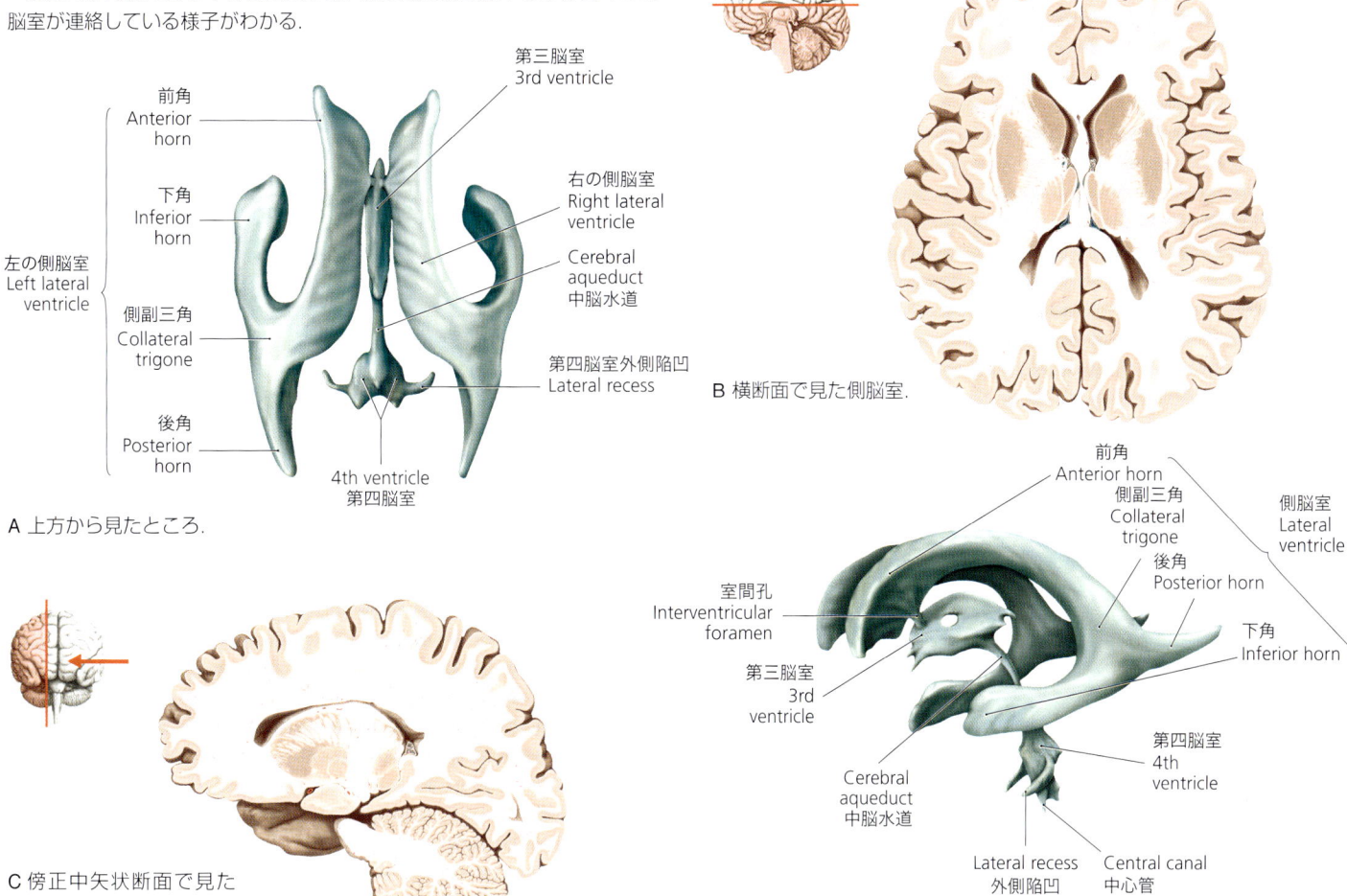

左の側脳室 Left lateral ventricle
- 前角 Anterior horn
- 下角 Inferior horn
- 側副三角 Collateral trigone
- 後角 Posterior horn

第三脳室 3rd ventricle
右の側脳室 Right lateral ventricle
Cerebral aqueduct 中脳水道
第四脳室外側陥凹 Lateral recess
4th ventricle 第四脳室

A　上方から見たところ．

B　横断面で見た側脳室．

前角 Anterior horn
側副三角 Collateral trigone
後角 Posterior horn
側脳室 Lateral ventricle
下角 Inferior horn
室間孔 Interventricular foramen
第三脳室 3rd ventricle
第四脳室 4th ventricle
Cerebral aqueduct 中脳水道
Lateral recess 外側陥凹
Central canal 中心管

C　傍正中矢状断面で見た左側脳室．

D　左外側方から見たところ．

図 39.31　脳室系とその周辺構造

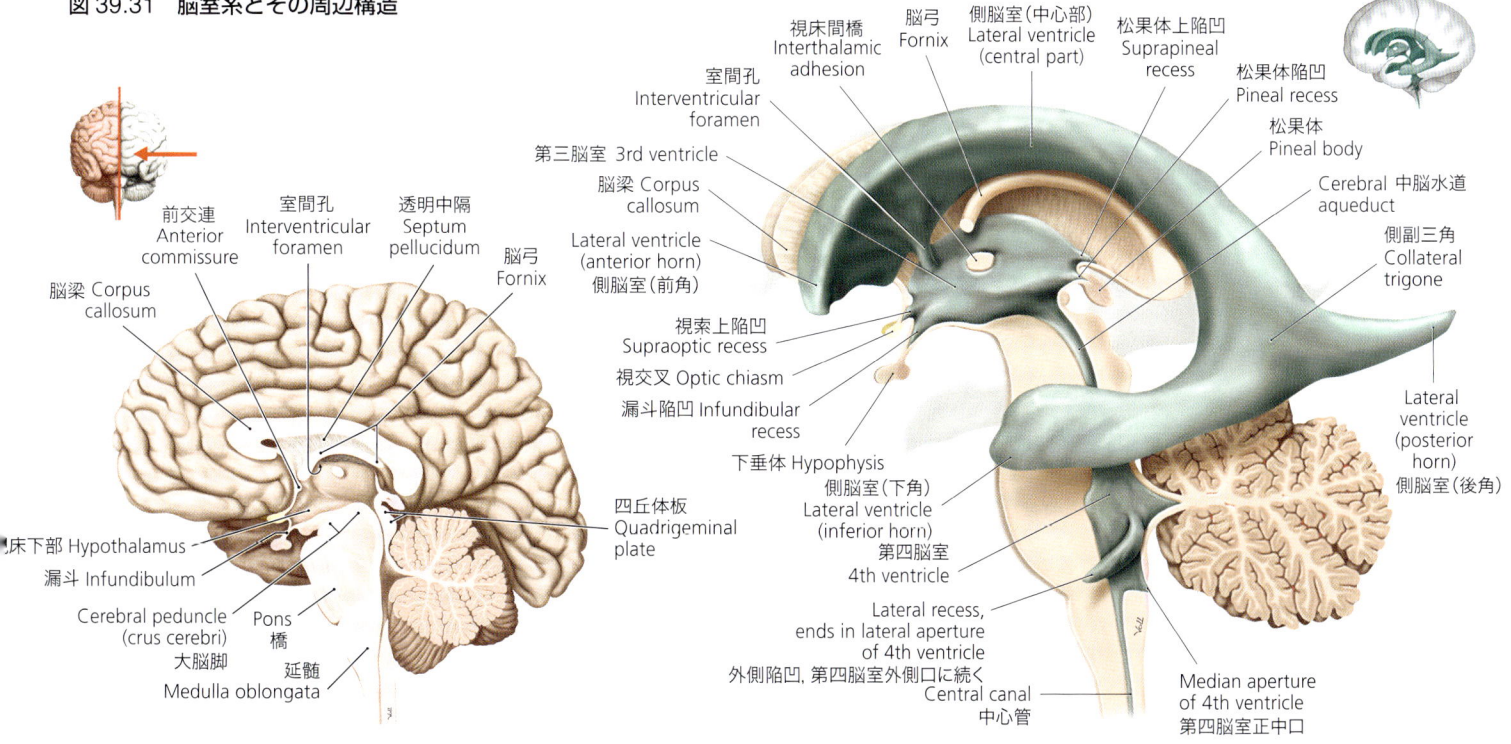

前交連 Anterior commissure
脳梁 Corpus callosum
室間孔 Interventricular foramen
透明中隔 Septum pellucidum
脳弓 Fornix
四丘体板 Quadrigeminal plate
床下部 Hypothalamus
漏斗 Infundibulum
Cerebral peduncle (crus cerebri) 大脳脚
Pons 橋
Medulla oblongata 延髄

視床間橋 Interthalamic adhesion
脳弓 Fornix
側脳室（中心部）Lateral ventricle (central part)
松果体上陥凹 Suprapineal recess
松果体陥凹 Pineal recess
松果体 Pineal body
室間孔 Interventricular foramen
第三脳室 3rd ventricle
脳梁 Corpus callosum
Lateral ventricle (anterior horn) 側脳室（前角）
視索上陥凹 Supraoptic recess
視交叉 Optic chiasm
漏斗陥凹 Infundibular recess
下垂体 Hypophysis
側脳室（下角）Lateral ventricle (inferior horn)
第四脳室 4th ventricle
Lateral recess, ends in lateral aperture of 4th ventricle
外側陥凹, 第四脳室外側口に続く
Central canal 中心管
Cerebral aqueduct 中脳水道
側副三角 Collateral trigone
Lateral ventricle (posterior horn) 側脳室（後角）
Median aperture of 4th ventricle 第四脳室正中口

A　正中矢状断面で見た第三・四脳室．

B　脳室系とその周辺構造．

硬膜静脈洞と脳の静脈
Dural Sinuses & Veins of the Brain

神経解剖

表 40.1	主要な硬膜静脈洞		
上方部		下方部	
①	上矢状静脈洞	⑦	海綿静脈洞
②	下矢状静脈洞	⑧	前海綿間静脈洞
③	直静脈洞	⑨	後海綿間静脈洞
④	静脈洞交会	⑩	蝶形頭頂静脈洞
⑤	横静脈洞	⑪	上錐体静脈洞
⑥	S状静脈洞	⑫	下錐体静脈洞

後頭静脈洞も上方部に含まれる（図40.2参照）．

大脳鎌 Falx cerebri
Tentorium cerebelli 小脳テント

図 40.1　静脈洞交会
後方から見たところ．

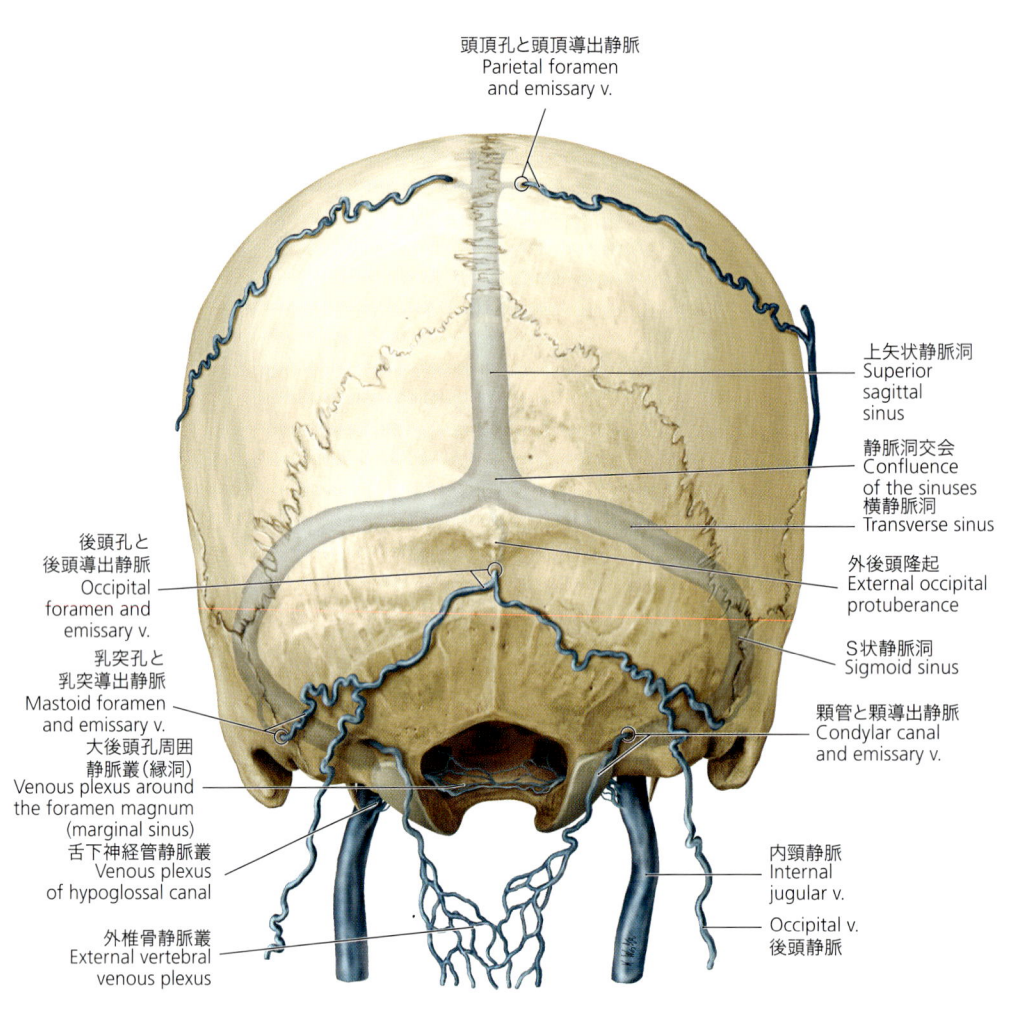

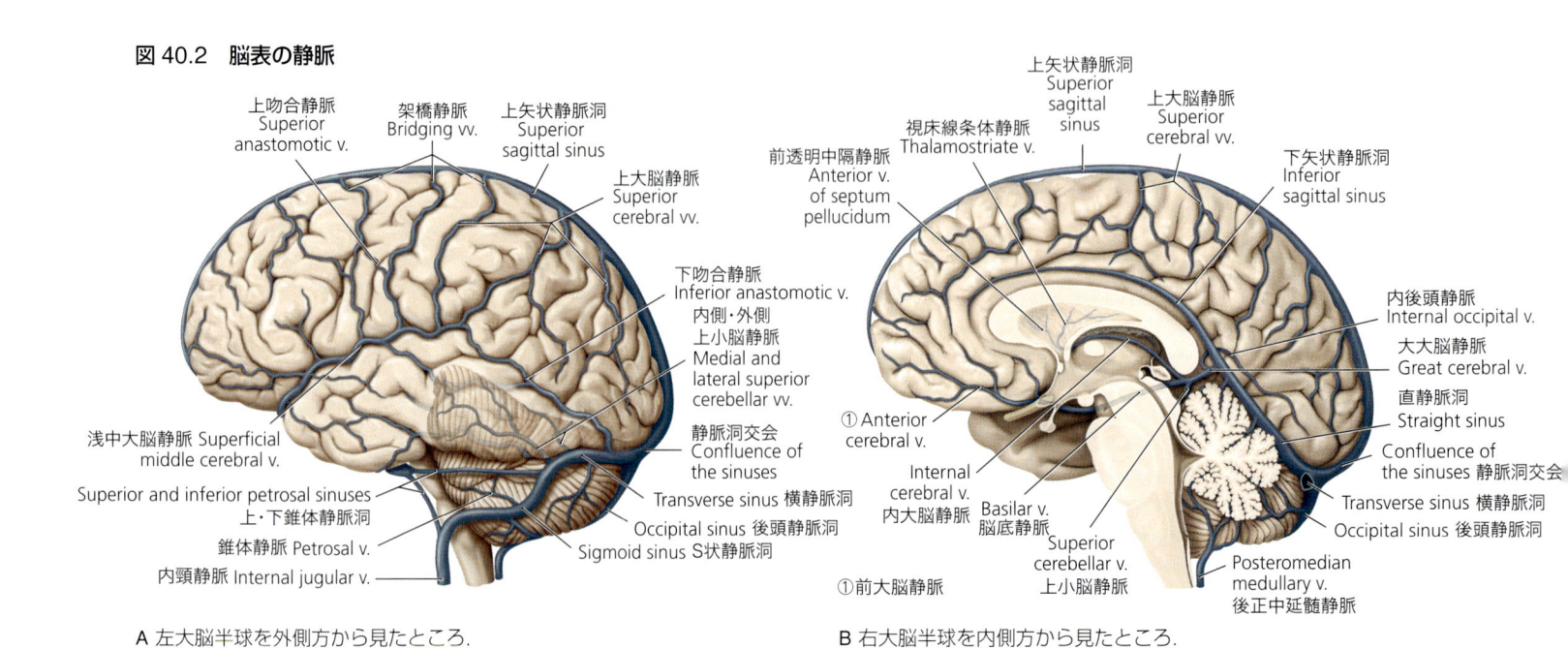

頭頂孔と頭頂導出静脈　Parietal foramen and emissary v.
上矢状静脈洞　Superior sagittal sinus
静脈洞交会　Confluence of the sinuses
横静脈洞　Transverse sinus
後頭孔と後頭導出静脈　Occipital foramen and emissary v.
外後頭隆起　External occipital protuberance
乳突孔と乳突導出静脈　Mastoid foramen and emissary v.
S状静脈洞　Sigmoid sinus
大後頭孔周囲静脈叢（縁洞）　Venous plexus around the foramen magnum (marginal sinus)
顆管と顆導出静脈　Condylar canal and emissary v.
舌下神経管静脈叢　Venous plexus of hypoglossal canal
内頸静脈　Internal jugular v.
外椎骨静脈叢　External vertebral venous plexus
後頭静脈　Occipital v.

図 40.2　脳表の静脈

上吻合静脈　Superior anastomotic v.
架橋静脈　Bridging vv.
上矢状静脈洞　Superior sagittal sinus
上大脳静脈　Superior cerebral vv.
下吻合静脈　Inferior anastomotic v.
内側・外側上小脳静脈　Medial and lateral superior cerebellar vv.
静脈洞交会　Confluence of the sinuses
横静脈洞　Transverse sinus
後頭静脈洞　Occipital sinus
S状静脈洞　Sigmoid sinus
浅中大脳静脈　Superficial middle cerebral v.
上・下錐体静脈洞　Superior and inferior petrosal sinuses
錐体静脈　Petrosal v.
内頸静脈　Internal jugular v.

A　左大脳半球を外側方から見たところ．

視床線条体静脈　Thalamostriate v.
前透明中隔静脈　Anterior v. of septum pellucidum
上矢状静脈洞　Superior sagittal sinus
上大脳静脈　Superior cerebral vv.
下矢状静脈洞　Inferior sagittal sinus
① Anterior cerebral v.　①前大脳静脈
内大脳静脈　Internal cerebral v.
脳底静脈　Basilar v.
上小脳静脈　Superior cerebellar v.
内後頭静脈　Internal occipital v.
大大脳静脈　Great cerebral v.
直静脈洞　Straight sinus
静脈洞交会　Confluence of the sinuses
横静脈洞　Transverse sinus
後頭静脈洞　Occipital sinus
後正中延髄静脈　Posteromedian medullary v.

B　右大脳半球を内側方から見たところ．

図 40.3 脳底の静脈
底側方から見たところ．

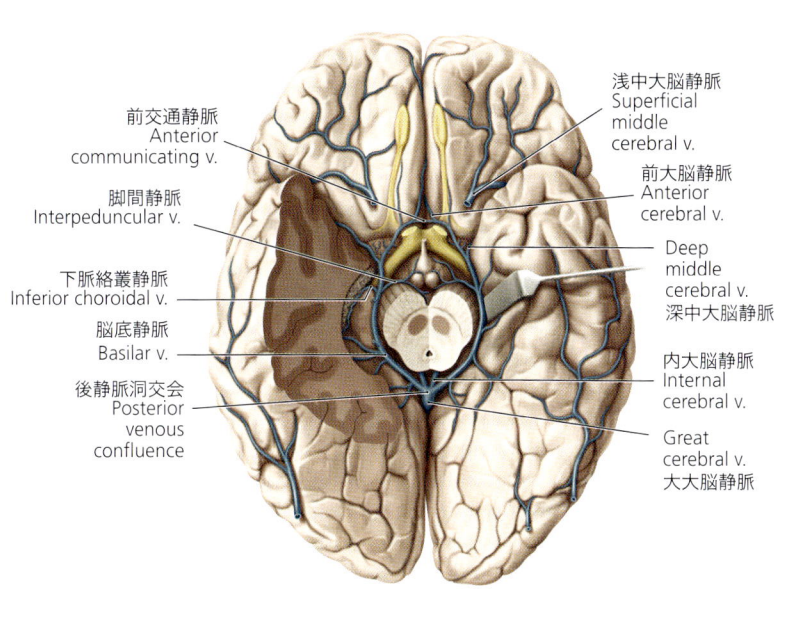

- 前交通静脈 Anterior communicating v.
- 脚間静脈 Interpeduncular v.
- 下脈絡叢静脈 Inferior choroidal v.
- 脳底静脈 Basilar v.
- 後静脈洞交会 Posterior venous confluence
- 浅中大脳静脈 Superficial middle cerebral v.
- 前大脳静脈 Anterior cerebral v.
- 深中大脳静脈 Deep middle cerebral v.
- 内大脳静脈 Internal cerebral v.
- 大大脳静脈 Great cerebral v.

図 40.4 脳幹の静脈
底側方から見たところ．

- 脳底静脈 Basilar v.
- 三叉神経 Trigeminal n. (CN V)
- 横橋静脈 Transverse pontine vv.
- 横延髄静脈 Transverse medullary vv.
- 後正中延髄静脈 Posteromedian medullary v.
- 脚間静脈 Interpeduncular vv.
- 橋中脳静脈 Pontomesencephalic v.
- 上錐体静脈 Superior petrosal v.
- 上小脳静脈 Superior cerebellar vv.
- 前外側・前正中橋静脈 Anterolateral and anteromedian pontine v.

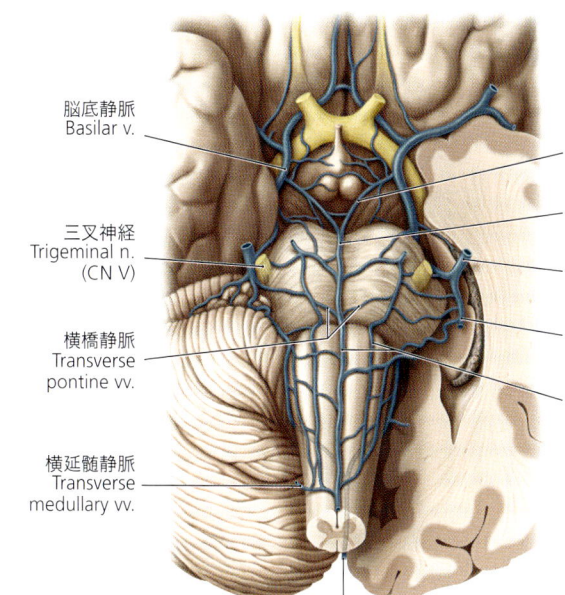

図 40.5 頭蓋底の硬膜静脈洞
頭蓋腔を開き，上方から見たところ．右側の小脳テントを取り除いてある．

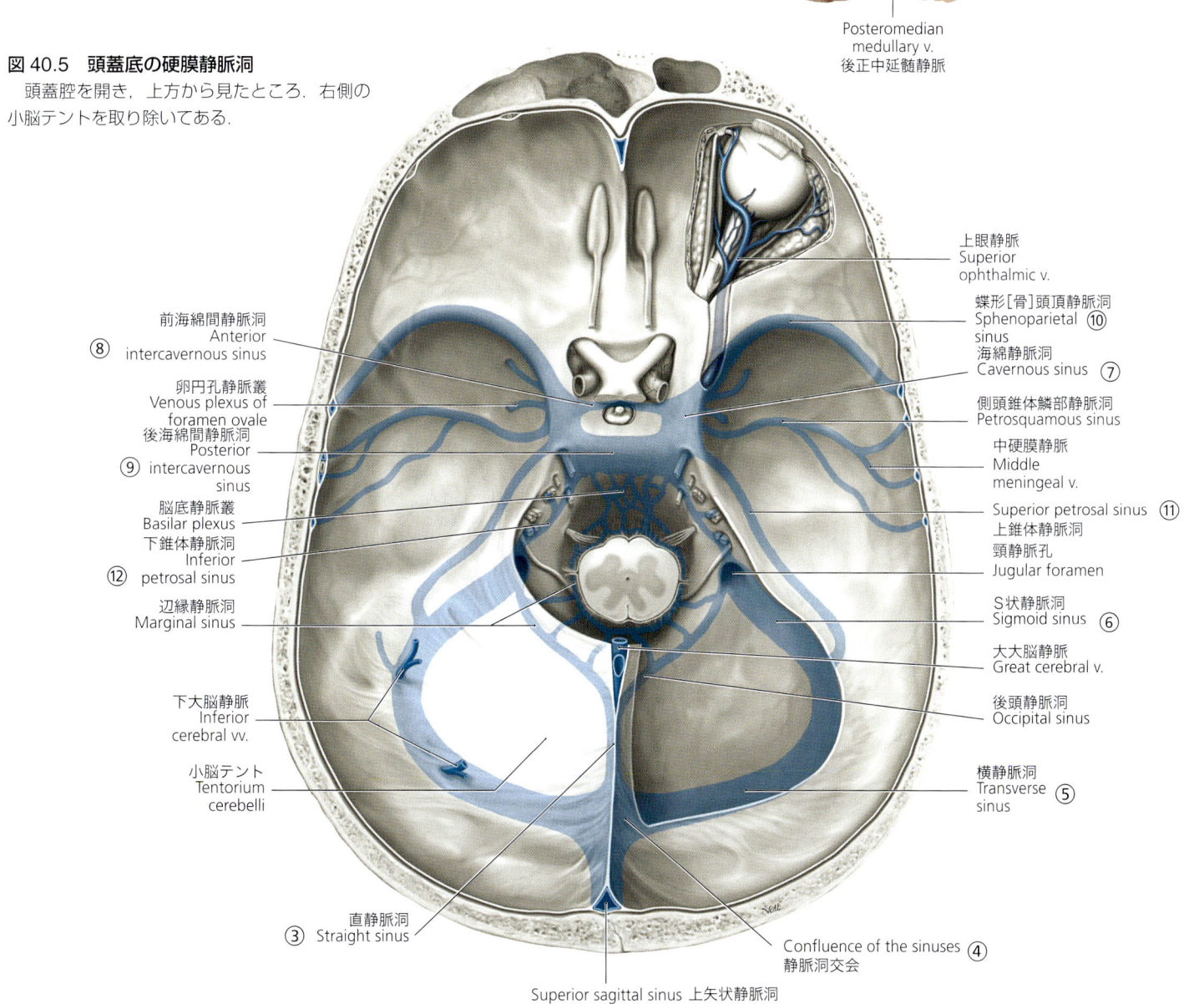

- 前海綿間静脈洞 Anterior intercavernous sinus ⑧
- 卵円孔静脈叢 Venous plexus of foramen ovale
- 後海綿間静脈洞 Posterior intercavernous sinus ⑨
- 脳底静脈叢 Basilar plexus
- 下錐体静脈洞 Inferior petrosal sinus ⑫
- 辺縁静脈洞 Marginal sinus
- 下大脳静脈 Inferior cerebral vv.
- 小脳テント Tentorium cerebelli
- 直静脈洞 Straight sinus ③
- 上眼静脈 Superior ophthalmic v.
- 蝶形[骨]頭頂静脈洞 Sphenoparietal sinus ⑩
- 海綿静脈洞 Cavernous sinus ⑦
- 側頭錐体鱗部静脈洞 Petrosquamous sinus
- 中硬膜静脈 Middle meningeal v.
- 上錐体静脈洞 Superior petrosal sinus ⑪
- 頸静脈孔 Jugular foramen
- S状静脈洞 Sigmoid sinus ⑥
- 大大脳静脈 Great cerebral v.
- 後頭静脈洞 Occipital sinus
- 横静脈洞 Transverse sinus ⑤
- 静脈洞交会 Confluence of the sinuses ④
- 上矢状静脈洞 Superior sagittal sinus ①

脳の動脈
Arteries of the Brain

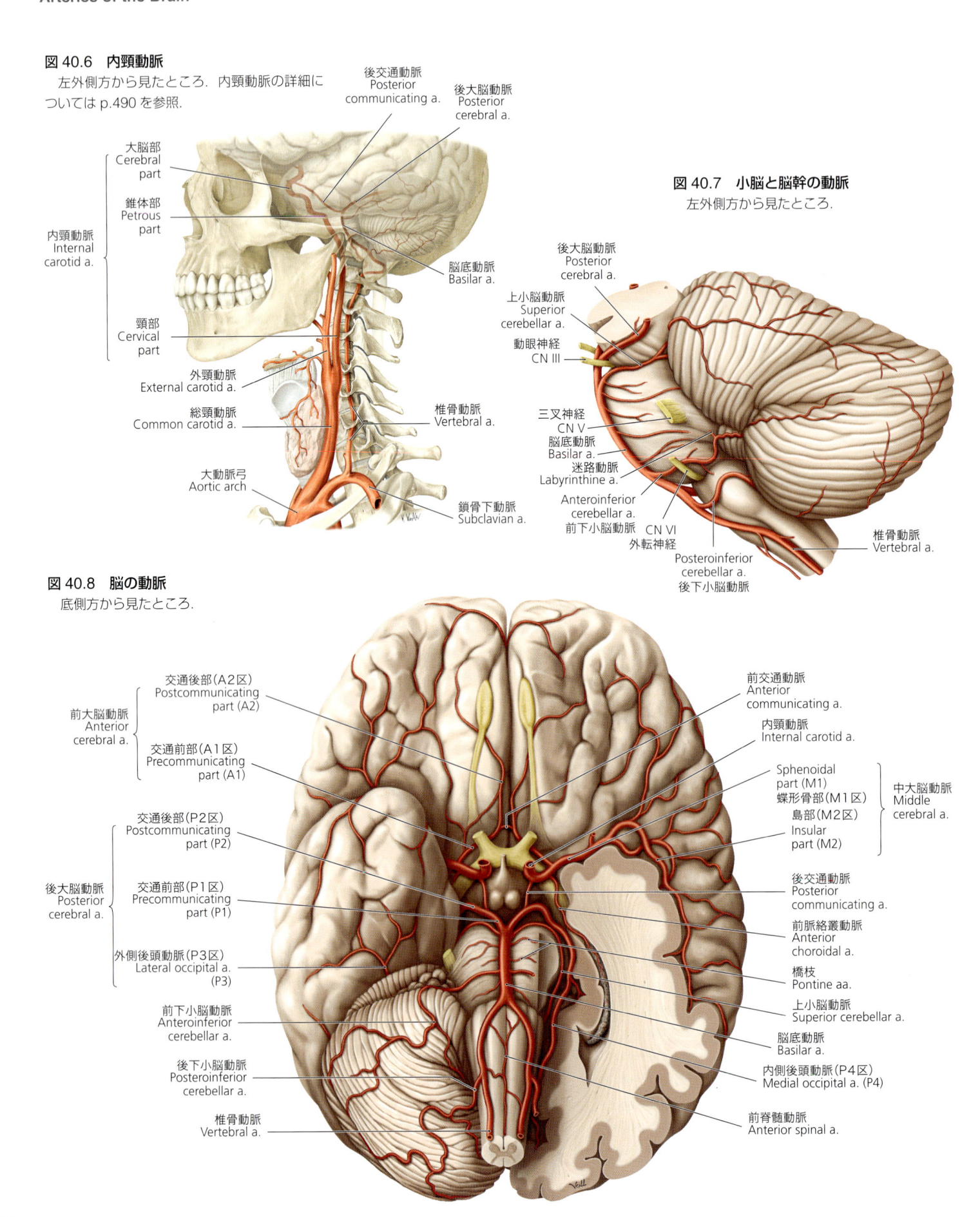

図 40.6 内頸動脈
左外側方から見たところ．内頸動脈の詳細については p.490 を参照．

- 後交通動脈 Posterior communicating a.
- 後大脳動脈 Posterior cerebral a.
- 内頸動脈 Internal carotid a.
  - 大脳部 Cerebral part
  - 錐体部 Petrous part
  - 頸部 Cervical part
- 外頸動脈 External carotid a.
- 総頸動脈 Common carotid a.
- 大動脈弓 Aortic arch
- 脳底動脈 Basilar a.
- 椎骨動脈 Vertebral a.
- 鎖骨下動脈 Subclavian a.

図 40.7 小脳と脳幹の動脈
左外側方から見たところ．

- 後大脳動脈 Posterior cerebral a.
- 上小脳動脈 Superior cerebellar a.
- 動眼神経 CN III
- 三叉神経 CN V
- 脳底動脈 Basilar a.
- 迷路動脈 Labyrinthine a.
- 前下小脳動脈 Anteroinferior cerebellar a.
- 外転神経 CN VI
- 後下小脳動脈 Posteroinferior cerebellar a.
- 椎骨動脈 Vertebral a.

図 40.8 脳の動脈
底側方から見たところ．

- 前大脳動脈 Anterior cerebral a.
  - 交通後部（A2区）Postcommunicating part (A2)
  - 交通前部（A1区）Precommunicating part (A1)
- 後大脳動脈 Posterior cerebral a.
  - 交通後部（P2区）Postcommunicating part (P2)
  - 交通前部（P1区）Precommunicating part (P1)
  - 外側後頭動脈（P3区）Lateral occipital a. (P3)
- 前下小脳動脈 Anteroinferior cerebellar a.
- 後下小脳動脈 Posteroinferior cerebellar a.
- 椎骨動脈 Vertebral a.
- 前交通動脈 Anterior communicating a.
- 内頸動脈 Internal carotid a.
- 中大脳動脈 Middle cerebral a.
  - 蝶形骨部（M1区）Sphenoidal part (M1)
  - 島部（M2区）Insular part (M2)
- 後交通動脈 Posterior communicating a.
- 前脈絡叢動脈 Anterior choroidal a.
- 橋枝 Pontine aa.
- 上小脳動脈 Superior cerebellar a.
- 脳底動脈 Basilar a.
- 内側後頭動脈（P4区）Medial occipital a. (P4)
- 前脊髄動脈 Anterior spinal a.

図 40.9　大脳の動脈

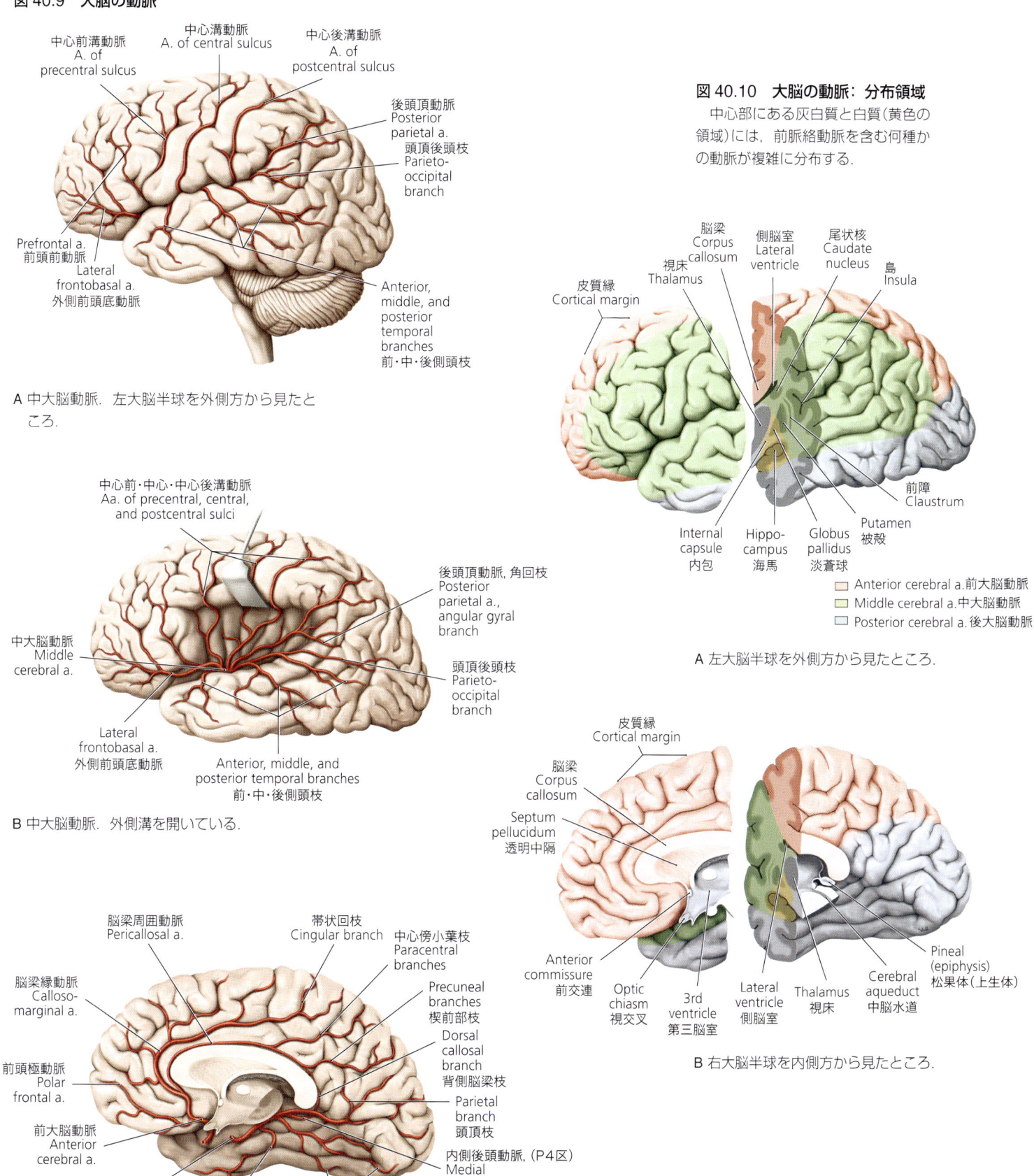

A　中大脳動脈．左大脳半球を外側方から見たところ．

B　中大脳動脈．外側溝を開いている．

C　前・後大脳動脈．右大脳半球を内側方から見たところ．

図 40.10　大脳の動脈：分布領域
中心部にある灰白質と白質（黄色の領域）には，前脈絡動脈を含む何種かの動脈が複雑に分布する．

☐ Anterior cerebral a. 前大脳動脈
☐ Middle cerebral a. 中大脳動脈
☐ Posterior cerebral a. 後大脳動脈

A　左大脳半球を外側方から見たところ．

B　右大脳半球を内側方から見たところ．

脊髄の動脈と静脈
Arteries & Veins of the Spinal Cord

脊髄の動・静脈は，多数の水平系列とこれらを縦に連絡する垂直系列からなる．

図 40.11　脊髄の動脈

不対の前脊髄動脈と1対の後脊髄動脈は通常，椎骨動脈から起始する．これらの3本の動脈は脊髄の表面を下りながら，脊髄に枝を出してゆく．前・後髄節動脈はこの3本の動脈に合流し，血流を補う．脊髄の高さによって，髄節動脈を出す動脈が異なっており，椎骨動脈，上行頸動脈，深頸動脈，肋間動脈，腰動脈，外側仙骨動脈から出る脊髄枝が脊柱管に入り，髄節動脈となる．

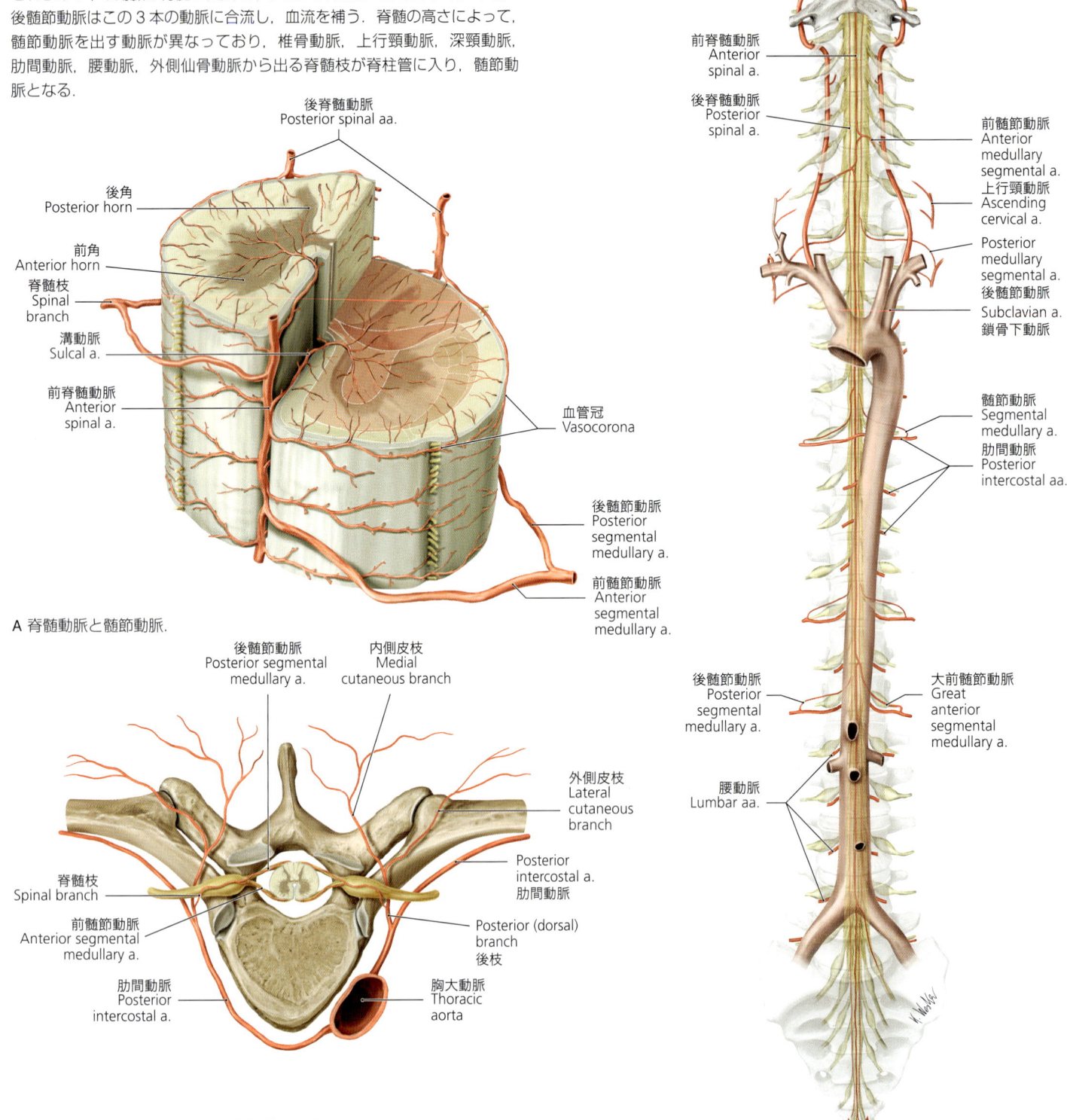

A 脊髄動脈と髄節動脈．

B 髄節動脈の起始．胸部では，髄節動脈は肋間動脈の脊髄枝から起こる（p.34 参照）．

C 脊髄の動脈：全体像．

図40.12 脊髄の静脈

脊髄からの静脈血は脊髄表面の静脈叢を介して，前・後脊髄静脈(各1本)に流れ込む．脊髄静脈と根静脈は，脊髄からの静脈血を内椎骨静脈叢へ導く．椎間静脈と椎体静脈は内・外椎骨静脈叢をつないでおり，これらの静脈叢からの血液は奇静脈系に流れ込む．

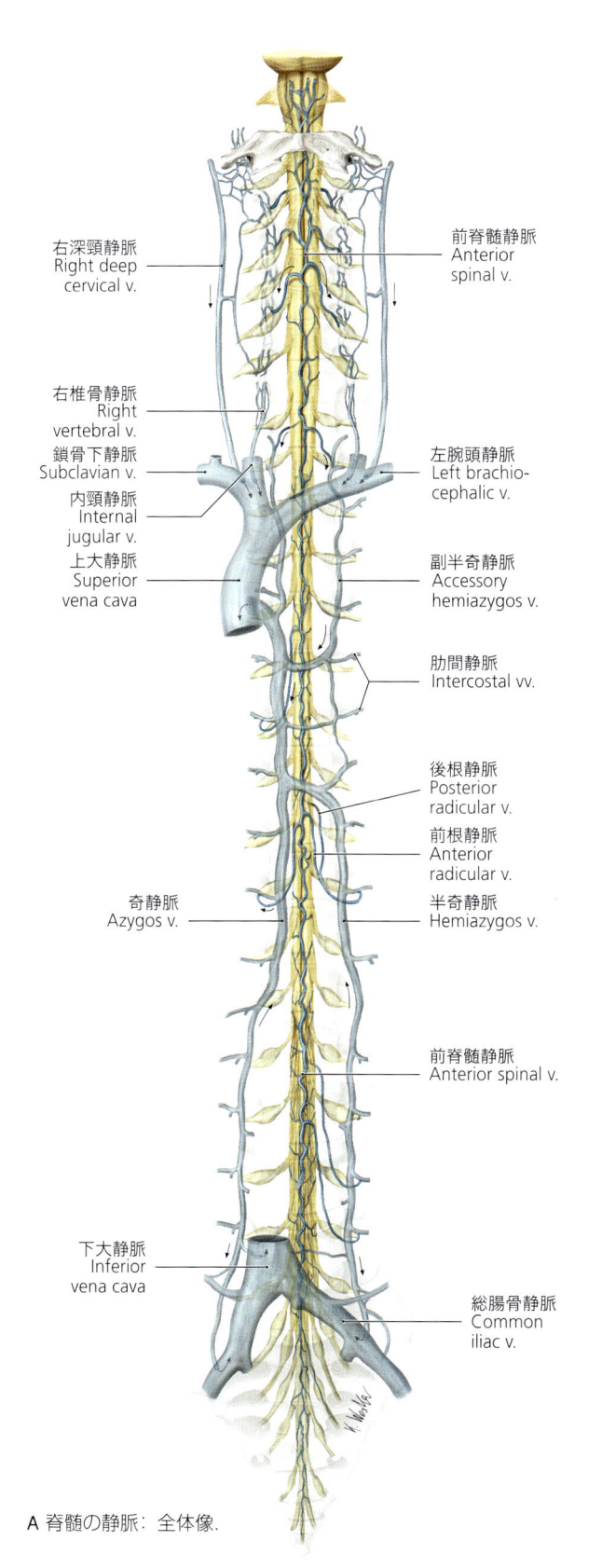

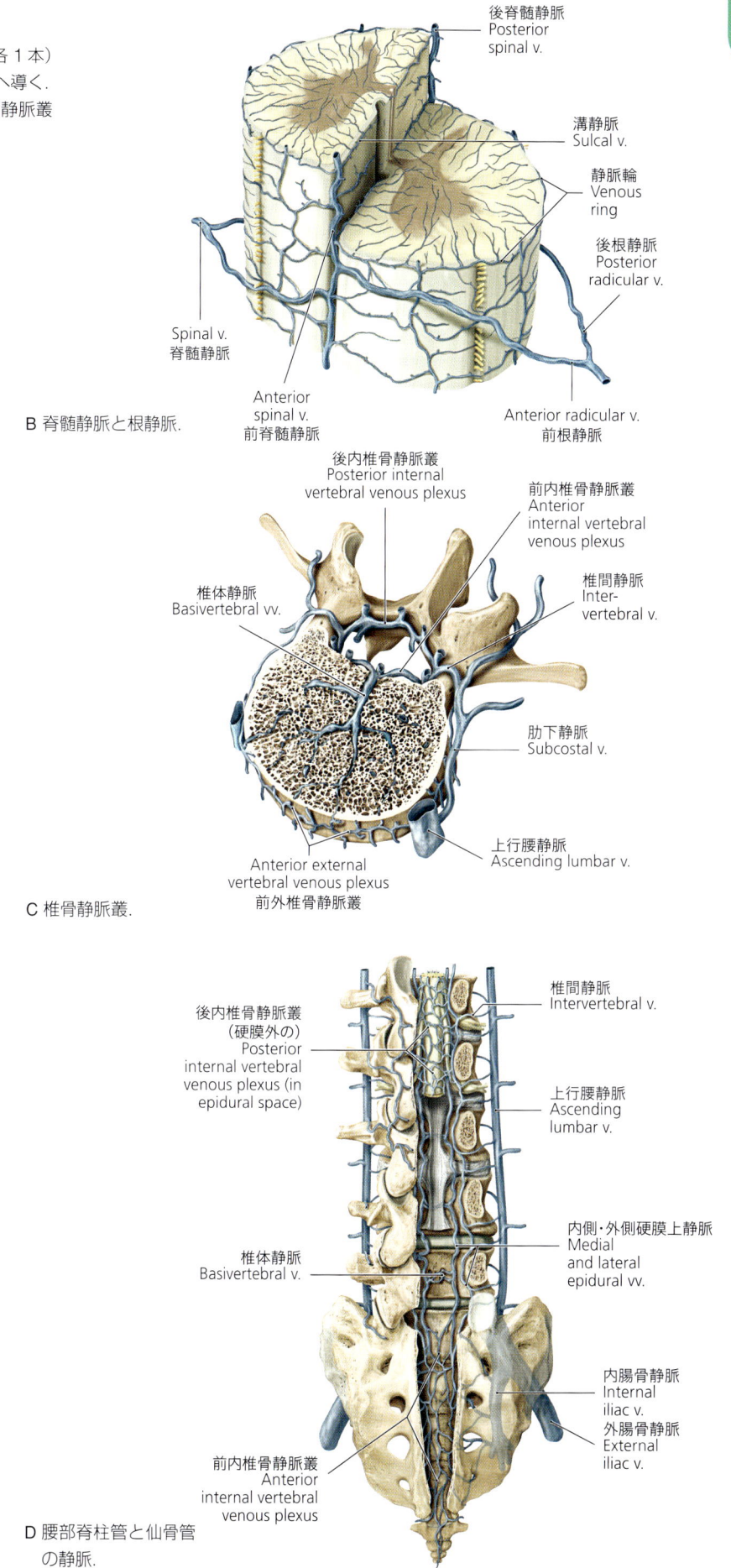

A 脊髄の静脈：全体像．

- 右深頸静脈 Right deep cervical v.
- 前脊髄静脈 Anterior spinal v.
- 右椎骨静脈 Right vertebral v.
- 鎖骨下静脈 Subclavian v.
- 内頸静脈 Internal jugular v.
- 上大静脈 Superior vena cava
- 左腕頭静脈 Left brachio-cephalic v.
- 副半奇静脈 Accessory hemiazygos v.
- 肋間静脈 Intercostal vv.
- 後根静脈 Posterior radicular v.
- 前根静脈 Anterior radicular v.
- 奇静脈 Azygos v.
- 半奇静脈 Hemiazygos v.
- 前脊髄静脈 Anterior spinal v.
- 下大静脈 Inferior vena cava
- 総腸骨静脈 Common iliac v.

B 脊髄静脈と根静脈．

- 後脊髄静脈 Posterior spinal v.
- 溝静脈 Sulcal v.
- 静脈輪 Venous ring
- 後根静脈 Posterior radicular v.
- 脊髄静脈 Spinal v.
- 前脊髄静脈 Anterior spinal v.
- 前根静脈 Anterior radicular v.

C 椎骨静脈叢．

- 後内椎骨静脈叢 Posterior internal vertebral venous plexus
- 前内椎骨静脈叢 Anterior internal vertebral venous plexus
- 椎体静脈 Basivertebral vv.
- 椎間静脈 Intervertebral v.
- 肋下静脈 Subcostal v.
- 上行腰静脈 Ascending lumbar v.
- 前外椎骨静脈叢 Anterior external vertebral venous plexus

D 腰部脊柱管と仙骨管の静脈．

- 椎間静脈 Intervertebral v.
- 後内椎骨静脈叢(硬膜外の) Posterior internal vertebral venous plexus (in epidural space)
- 上行腰静脈 Ascending lumbar v.
- 椎体静脈 Basivertebral v.
- 内側・外側硬膜上静脈 Medial and lateral epidural vv.
- 内腸骨静脈 Internal iliac v.
- 外腸骨静脈 External iliac v.
- 前内椎骨静脈叢 Anterior internal vertebral venous plexus

神経回路：概観
Circuitry

図 41.1 末梢神経系の機能的区分
　末梢神経系の神経線維は情報の流れる方向によって 2 つのタイプ（遠心性線維と求心性線維）に分けられる．遠心性（感覚性）線維は情報を中枢神経に伝え，求心性（運動性）線維は情報を中枢神経の外に送る．これとは別の機能的区分もあり，神経系を体性神経と自律神経の 2 つに分けることもできる．体性神経は外界との相互作用を仲介し，自律（内臓）神経は内臓の機能を調節する．

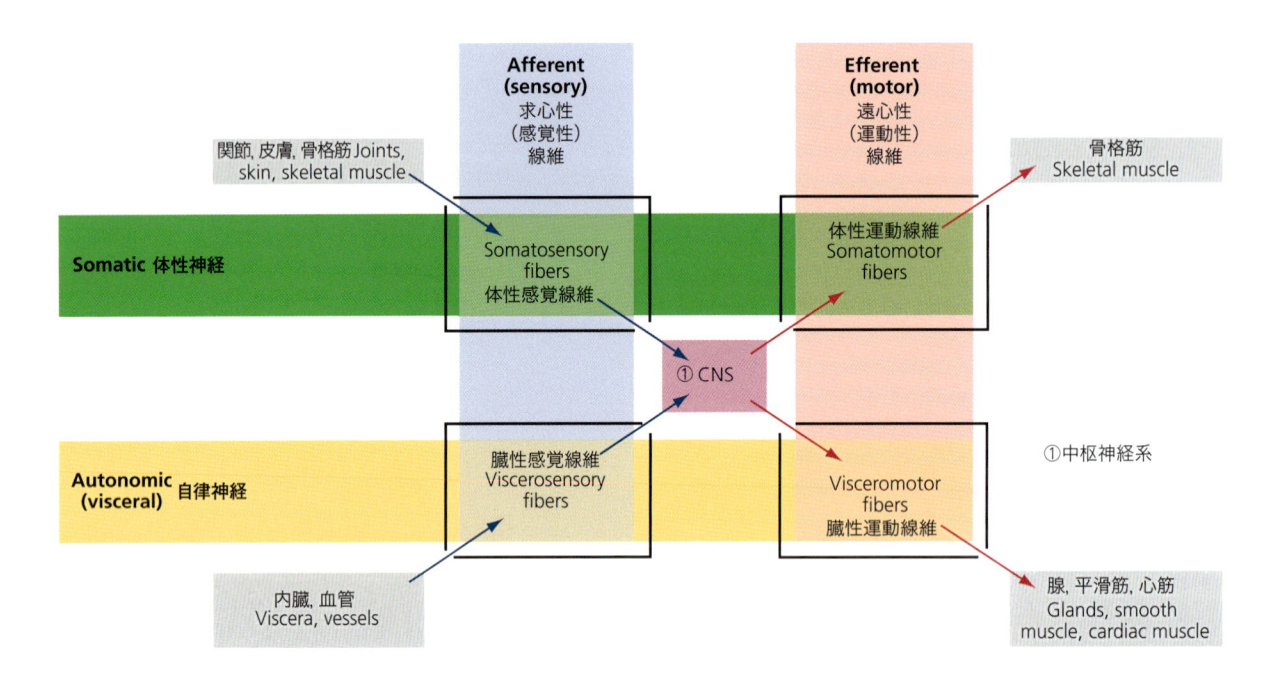

図 41.2 脊髄灰白質の構造
　左前上方から見たところ．脊髄の灰白質は 3 種類の柱（角）に区分される．求心性線維（青）と遠心性線維（赤）の細胞体はこれらの柱の中にあり，同じ機能を持つ細胞どうしが集団を形成する．

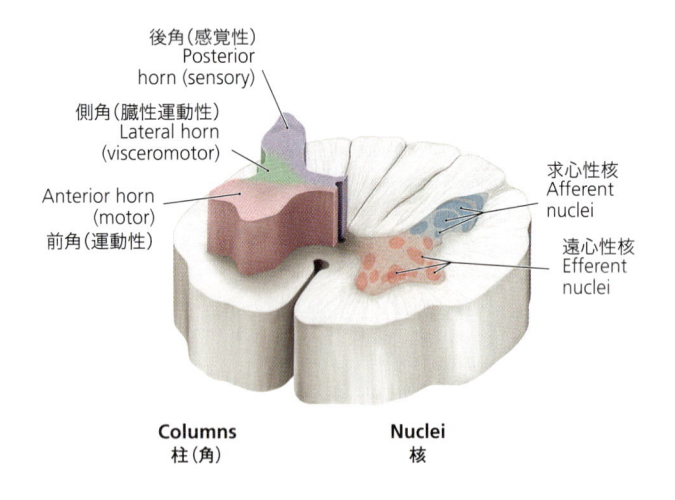

図 41.3 筋の神経支配
　大部分の筋は脊髄前角にある運動柱によって支配される．運動柱は一つの筋を支配する運動ニューロンの細胞体が垂直方向に集まったもので，複数の脊髄分節にまたがって存在する（青，茶）．しかし，指標筋と呼ばれる少数の筋では，支配神経の細胞体は単一の脊髄分節内に存在する．

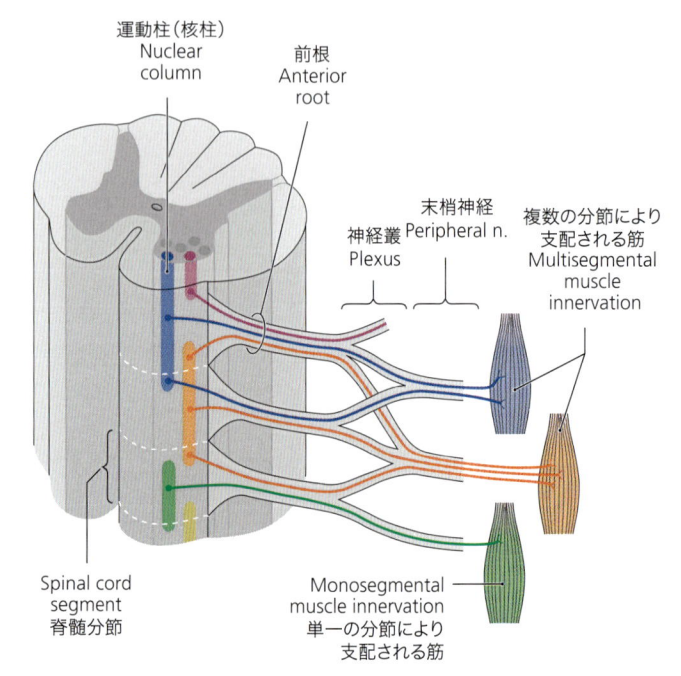

図 41.4 反射

無意識の状態で起こる運動(反射)は脊髄の灰白質によって調節される.

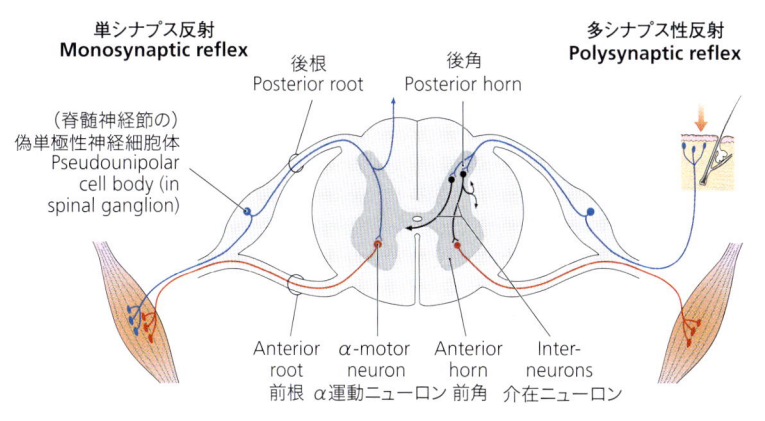

単シナプス反射
Monosynaptic reflex

多シナプス性反射
Polysynaptic reflex

- 後根 Posterior root
- 後角 Posterior horn
- (脊髄神経節の)偽単極性神経細胞体 Pseudounipolar cell body (in spinal ganglion)
- 前根 Anterior root
- α運動ニューロン α-motor neuron
- 前角 Anterior horn
- 介在ニューロン Interneurons

A 多シナプス性反射の反射弓は,筋の内部もしくは筋から離れた部位(例えば皮膚)にある受容器から始まる.これらの受容器からのシグナルは介在ニューロンを介して,筋の収縮を引き起こす.

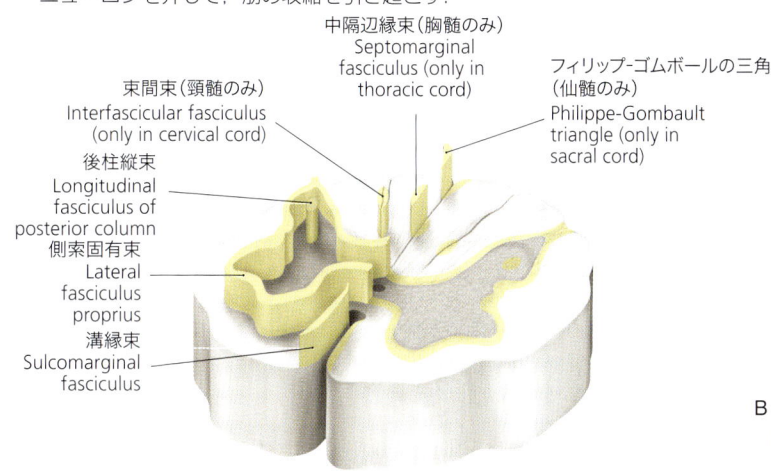

- 中隔辺縁束(胸髄のみ) Septomarginal fasciculus (only in thoracic cord)
- 束間束(頸髄のみ) Interfascicular fasciculus (only in cervical cord)
- フィリップ-ゴムボールの三角(仙髄のみ) Philippe-Gombault triangle (only in sacral cord)
- 後柱縦束 Longitudinal fasciculus of posterior column
- 側索固有束 Lateral fasciculus proprius
- 溝縁束 Sulcomarginal fasciculus

B 脊髄にある主要な固有束.固有束は脊髄に固有の伝導路であり,この中を軸索が上・下行し,脊髄分節の間を連絡する.多分節筋(複数の脊髄分節によって支配される筋)に脊髄反射が起こる場合には,固有束の連絡機能により,個々の分節から出る神経が同調される.

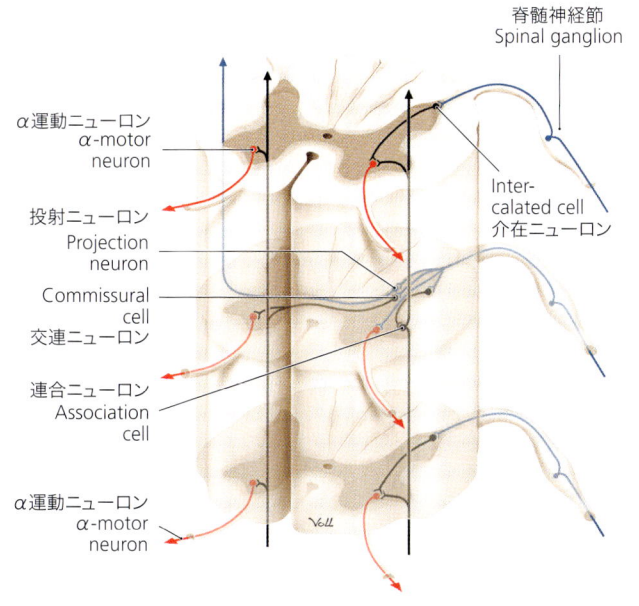

- α運動ニューロン α-motor neuron
- 投射ニューロン Projection neuron
- 交連ニューロン Commissural cell
- 連合ニューロン Association cell
- α運動ニューロン α-motor neuron
- 脊髄神経節 Spinal ganglion
- 介在ニューロン Intercalated cell

C 脊髄の固有路.固有路を黒で示してある.

図 41.5 感覚系と運動系

感覚系(p.614参照)と運動系(p.615参照)は機能的に関連し合っており,ひとつの系(感覚運動系)として記載されることがある.

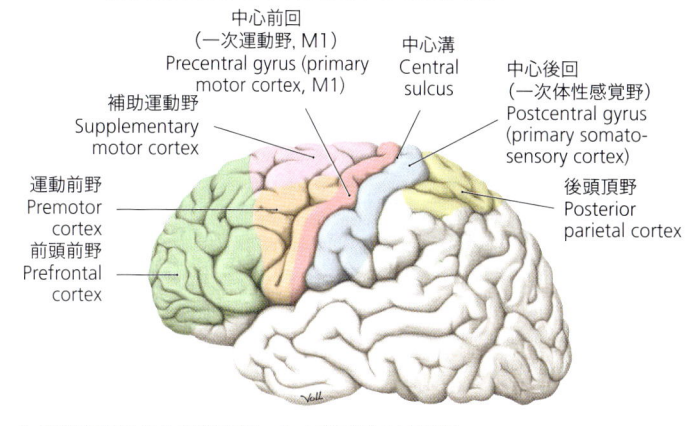

- 中心前回(一次運動野, M1) Precentral gyrus (primary motor cortex, M1)
- 中心溝 Central sulcus
- 中心後回(一次体性感覚野) Postcentral gyrus (primary somatosensory cortex)
- 補助運動野 Supplementary motor cortex
- 運動前野 Premotor cortex
- 前頭前野 Prefrontal cortex
- 後頭頂野 Posterior parietal cortex

A 感覚運動系の大脳皮質野.左大脳半球の外側面.

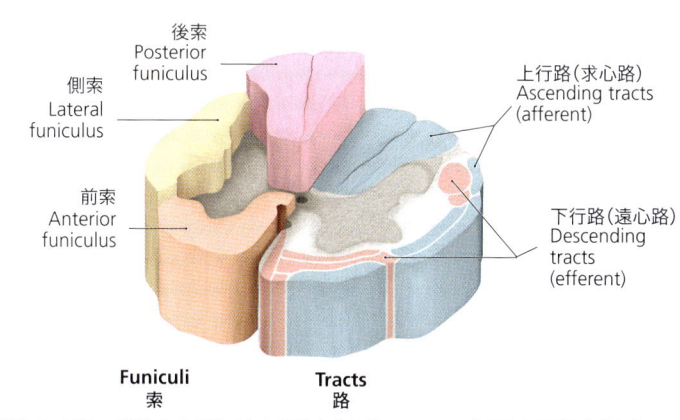

- 後索 Posterior funiculus
- 側索 Lateral funiculus
- 前索 Anterior funiculus
- 上行路(求心路) Ascending tracts (afferent)
- 下行路(遠心路) Descending tracts (efferent)
- Funiculi 索
- Tracts 路

B 脊髄の白質.脊髄の白質には上行路(求心路, p.614参照)と下行路(遠心路, p.615参照)があり,これらの部位には軸索が走り,中枢神経内で情報を伝達する(機能的には末梢神経に相当する).

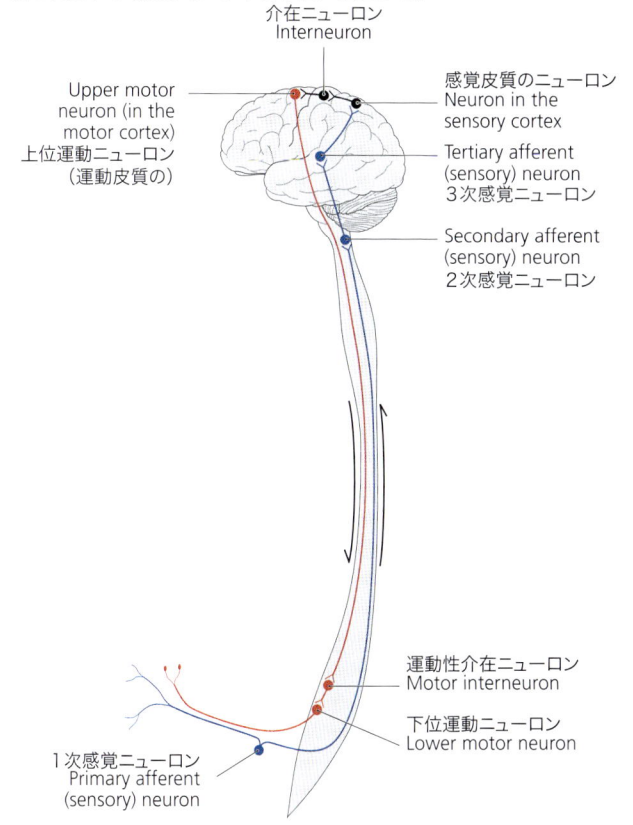

- 介在ニューロン Interneuron
- 上位運動ニューロン(運動皮質の) Upper motor neuron (in the motor cortex)
- 感覚皮質のニューロン Neuron in the sensory cortex
- 3次感覚ニューロン Tertiary afferent (sensory) neuron
- 2次感覚ニューロン Secondary afferent (sensory) neuron
- 運動性介在ニューロン Motor interneuron
- 下位運動ニューロン Lower motor neuron
- 1次感覚ニューロン Primary afferent (sensory) neuron

C 感覚運動系の概観.

一般感覚と運動の伝導路
Sensory & Motor Pathways

図 41.6 感覚情報の経路（上行路）

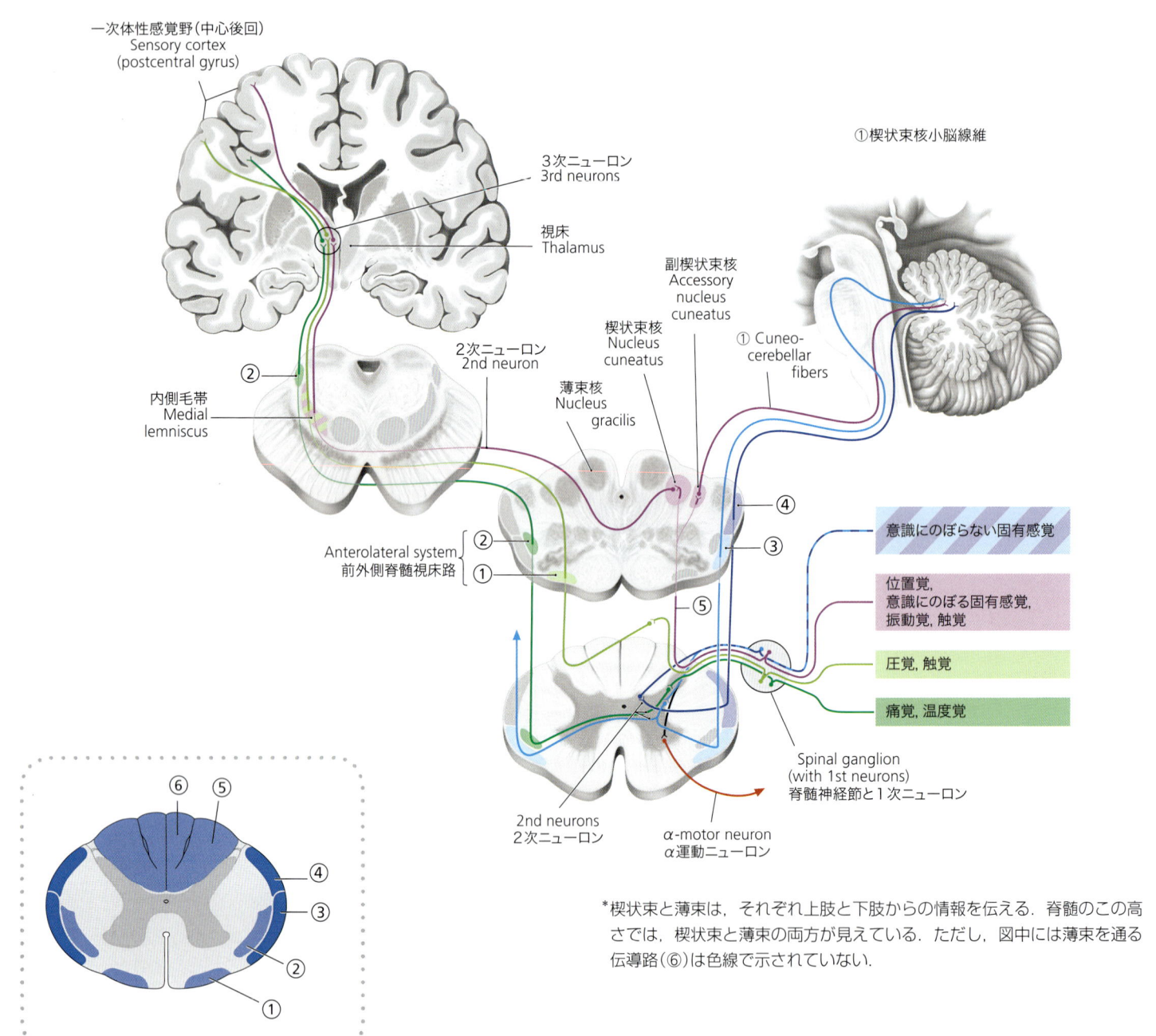

- 一次体性感覚野（中心後回） Sensory cortex (postcentral gyrus)
- 3次ニューロン 3rd neurons
- 視床 Thalamus
- 2次ニューロン 2nd neuron
- 内側毛帯 Medial lemniscus
- 薄束核 Nucleus gracilis
- 楔状束核 Nucleus cuneatus
- 副楔状束核 Accessory nucleus cuneatus
- ①楔状束核小脳線維 Cuneo-cerebellar fibers
- Anterolateral system 前外側脊髄視床路
- 意識にのぼらない固有感覚
- 位置覚，意識にのぼる固有感覚，振動覚，触覚
- 圧覚，触覚
- 痛覚，温度覚
- Spinal ganglion (with 1st neurons) 脊髄神経節と1次ニューロン
- α-motor neuron α運動ニューロン
- 2nd neurons 2次ニューロン

*楔状束と薄束は，それぞれ上肢と下肢からの情報を伝える．脊髄のこの高さでは，楔状束と薄束の両方が見えている．ただし，図中には薄束を通る伝導路（⑥）は色線で示されていない．

表 41.1 脊髄の上行路

伝導路		位置	機能		ニューロン
①	前脊髄視床路	前索	粗大性触圧覚の経路		1次ニューロンの細胞体は脊髄神経節に存在する．2次ニューロンの細胞体は後角に存在し，軸索は前交連を通り，反対側の前索に入る
②	外側脊髄視床路	前索・側索	痛覚，温度覚，くすぐり感，瘙痒感，性感の経路		
③	前脊髄小脳路	側索	意識に上らない固有覚を小脳へ伝える経路（運動の自動的な協調に関与する，たとえばジョギングや自転車に乗ったりするような場合）		1次ニューロンの細胞体は脊髄神経節に存在する．2次ニューロンの細胞体は後角に存在し，軸索は側索を通り，小脳に至る
④	後脊髄小脳路				
⑤	楔状束	後索	意識に上る固有覚（体肢の位置と姿勢についての情報，位置覚）と識別性触圧覚（振動，繊細な圧覚，2点の識別）の経路	上肢からの情報を伝える（楔状束はT3より下には存在しない）	1次ニューロンの細胞体は脊髄神経節に存在し，軸索は同側の後索を上行する．2次ニューロンの細胞体は延髄の後索核（楔状束核・薄束核）に存在し，軸索は反対側の内側毛帯へ入る
⑥	薄束*			下肢からの情報を伝える	

錐体路（皮質脊髄路）
Pyramidal (corticospinal) tract

錐体外路系
Extrapyramidal motor system

図 41.7 運動情報の経路（下行路）

脚 Leg
腕 Arm
顔面 Face

中心前回（一次運動野）
Precentral gyrus (primary motor cortex)

補助運動野
Supplementary motor cortexes

Postcentral gyrus (primary somatosensory cortex)①

錐体外路とともに走る皮質脊髄路
Corticospinal tract (with extrapyramidal fibers)

被蓋核 Tegmental nucleus
赤核 Red nucleus
黒質 Substantia nigra
錐体路 Pyramidal tract

皮質核線維 Corticonuclear fibers
皮質脊髄線維 Corticospinal fibers

①中心後回（一次体性感覚野）

小脳から From cerebellum

外側腹側核 Ventral lateral nucleus
下オリーブ核 Inferior olive
錐体 Pyramid

CN VII
CN XII

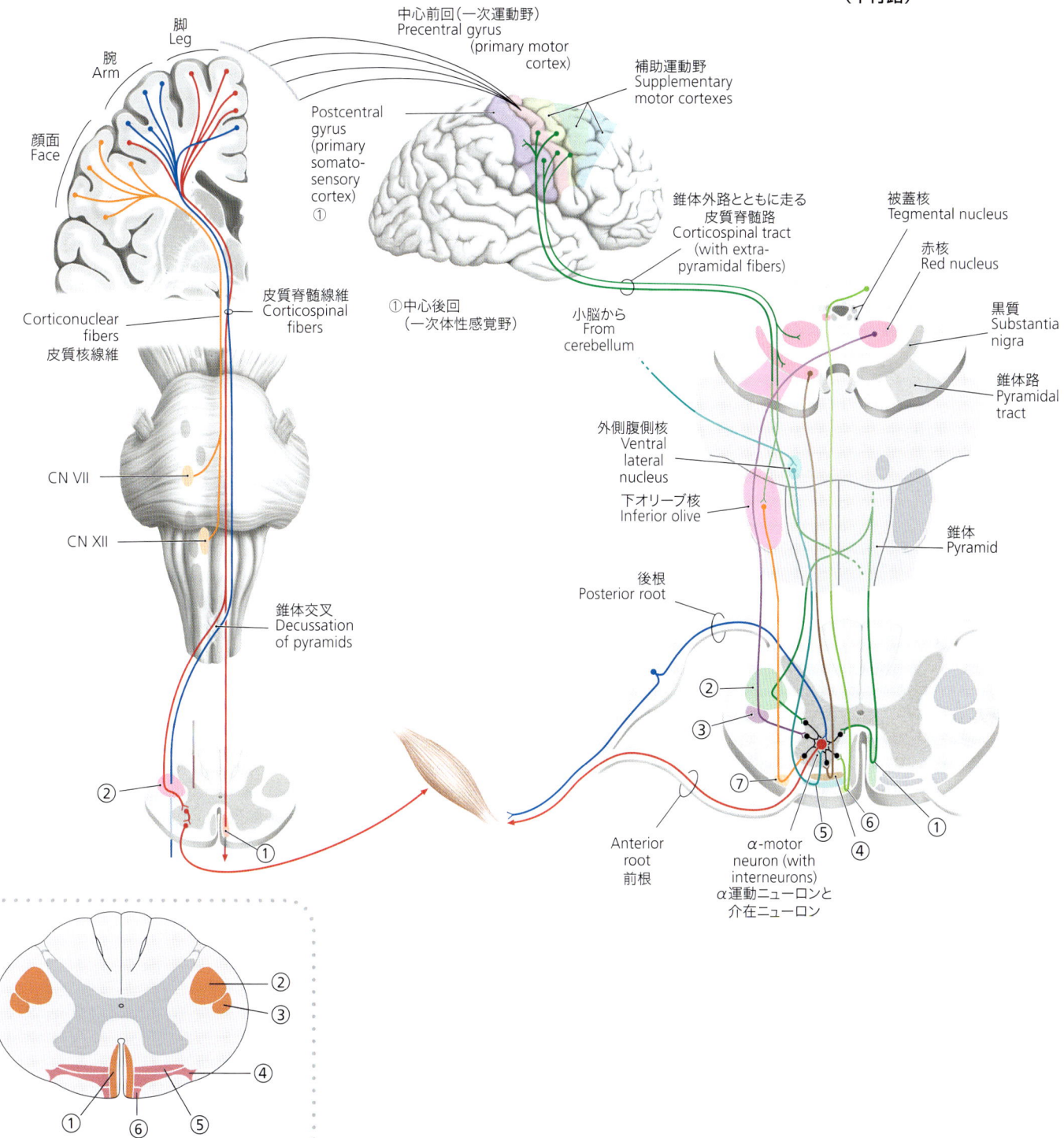

錐体交叉 Decussation of pyramids

後根 Posterior root

前根 Anterior root

α運動ニューロンと介在ニューロン
α-motor neuron (with interneurons)

表 41.2		脊髄の下行路	
伝導路			機能
錐体路	①	前皮質脊髄路	随意運動のための最も重要な経路 1次ニューロンの細胞体は大脳皮質の運動野に存在する 皮質核線維は脳神経の運動核に達する 皮質脊髄線維は脊髄前角の運動神経細胞に達する 皮質網様体線維は網様体核に達する
	②	外側皮質脊髄路	
錐体外路系	③	赤核脊髄路	
	④	網様体脊髄路	
	⑤	前庭脊髄路	自動的な運動（例えば、歩行、ランニング、サイクリング）や習熟した動作のための経路
	⑥	視蓋脊髄路	
	⑦	オリーブ脊髄路	

特殊感覚の伝導路（1）
Sensory Systems (I)

表 41.3　特殊感覚の種類

感覚	脳神経		参照ページ
視覚	視神経（CN II）		p.473
平衡覚	内耳神経（CN VIII）	前庭神経	p.480
聴覚		蝸牛神経	p.481
味覚	顔面神経（CN VII）		p.478
	舌咽神経（CN IX）		p.482
	迷走神経（CN X）		p.484
嗅覚	嗅神経（CN I）		p.472

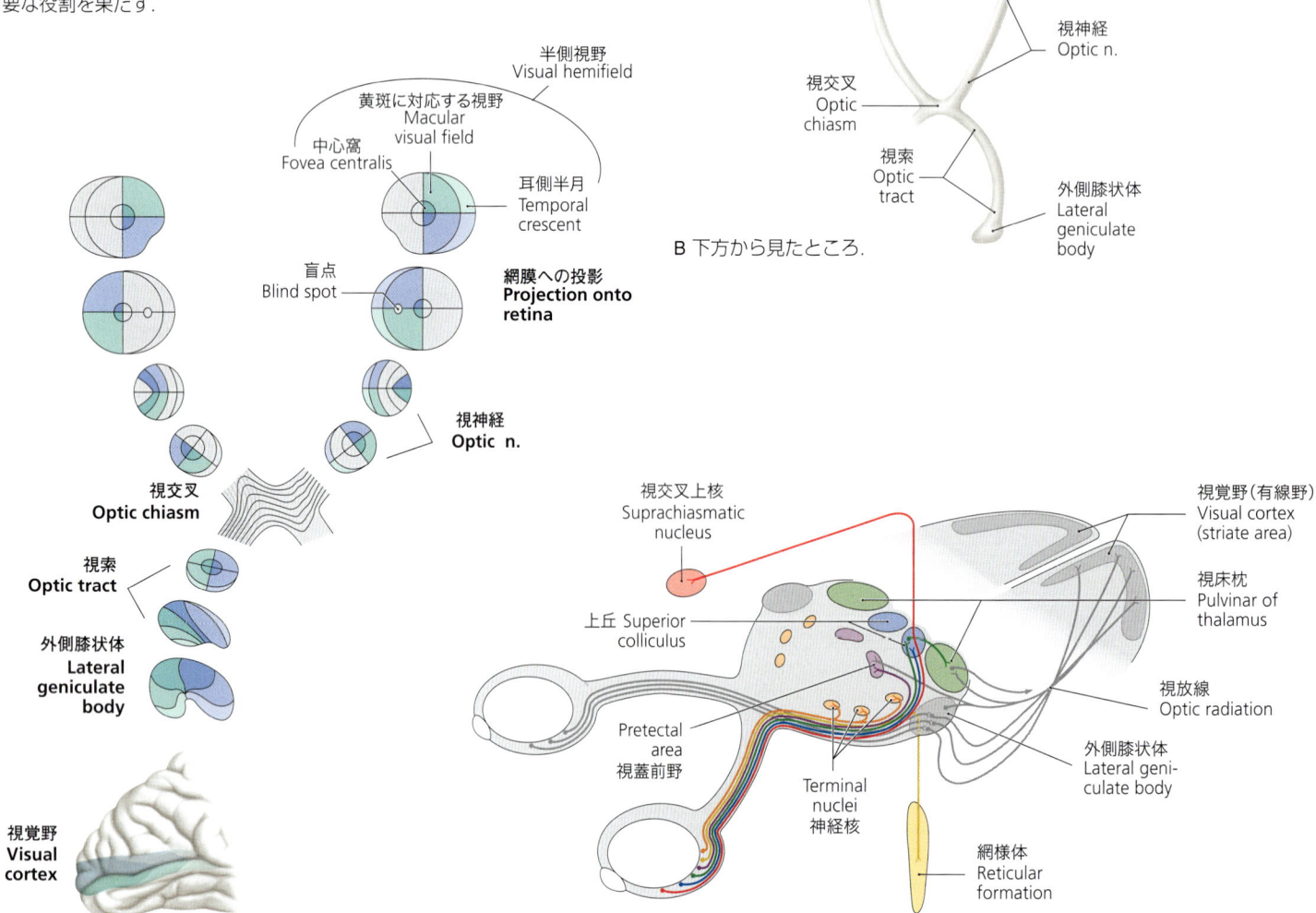

図 41.8　視覚系：概観

A 左外側方から見たところ．

B 下方から見たところ．

図 41.9　視覚情報の経路

　視神経線維の90%が外側膝状体にあるニューロンとシナプスを形成し，さらにこのニューロンは有線野（視覚野）に投射する．この経路は膝状体経路と呼ばれ，意識に上る視覚を生み出す．視神経線維のうち残りの10%は視索の内側根に沿って走り，非膝状体経路を形成する．視覚に関連する情報処理や反射は非随意的に調節されており，この調節に非膝状体経路が重要な役割を果たす．

A 膝状体経路．視野の左半からの情報が伝わる様子．

B 非膝状体経路．

臨床

視覚路の傷害
左の視覚路について，傷害部位とその際に認められる視野欠損を示してある．

1. 視神経の傷害
   患側眼の全盲　●○

2. 視神経交叉（中央部）の傷害
   両耳側半盲（馬に付ける"目隠し革"）　◐◑

3. 視索の傷害
   患側と反対側の同名半盲　◐◐

4. マイヤーのループ（前頭葉）における視放線の傷害
   患側と反対側の上 1/4 盲（"空中に浮ぶ一片のパイ"）

5. 視放線（内側部）の傷害
   患側と反対側の下 1/4 盲

6. 後頭葉の傷害
   患側と反対側の同名半盲，中心視野は保たれる（黄斑回避）

7. 後頭極（皮質領域）の傷害
   中心視野の半分（患側と反対側）が欠ける

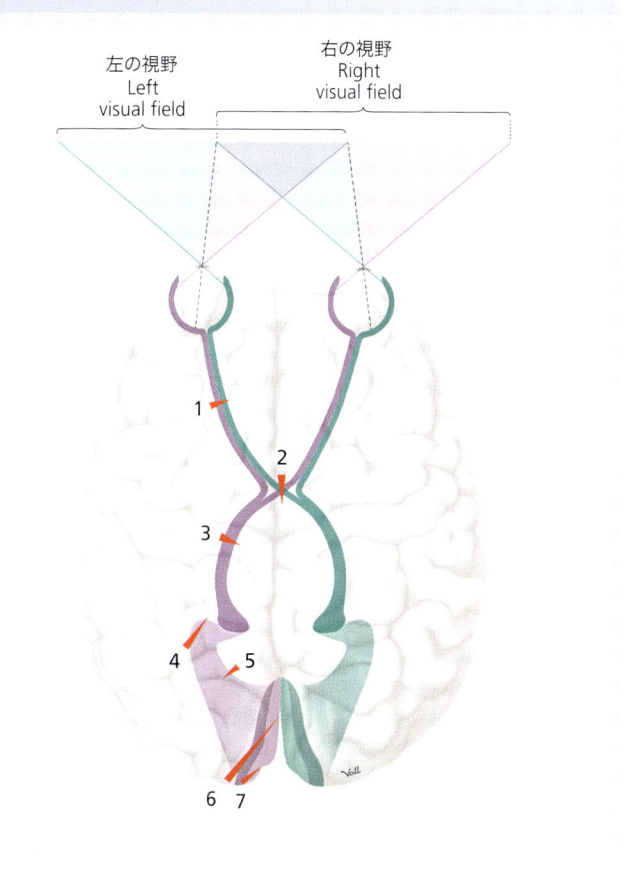

左の視野 Left visual field　右の視野 Right visual field

図 41.10　視覚系における反射

視覚系における反射は，視神経（求心性線維）と外眼筋の支配神経（遠心性線維）によって仲介される．

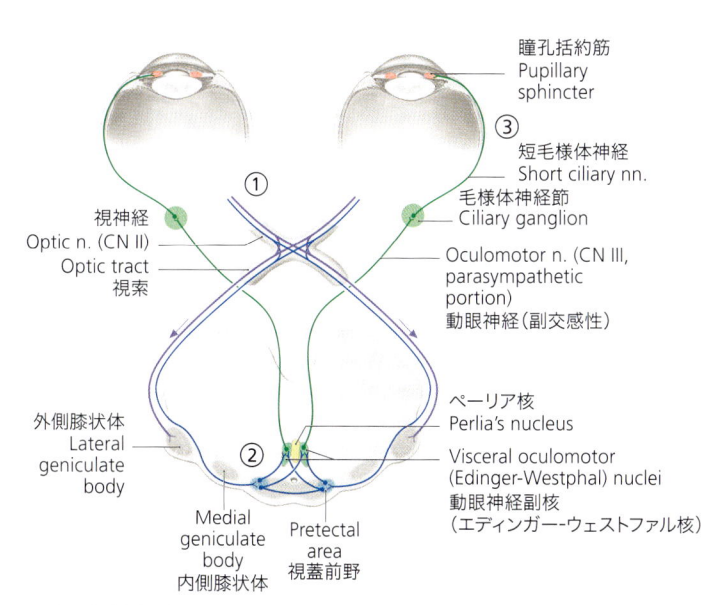

A 瞳孔（対光）反射．
① 網膜からの光情報は視神経を介して伝わる．
② 外側膝状体を素通りし，蓋前野に達する．
③ 動眼神経副核（エディンガー・ウエストファール核）のニューロンが毛様体神経節にある節後線維とシナプスを形成する．この神経節からの信号は，瞳孔括約筋を収縮させる．

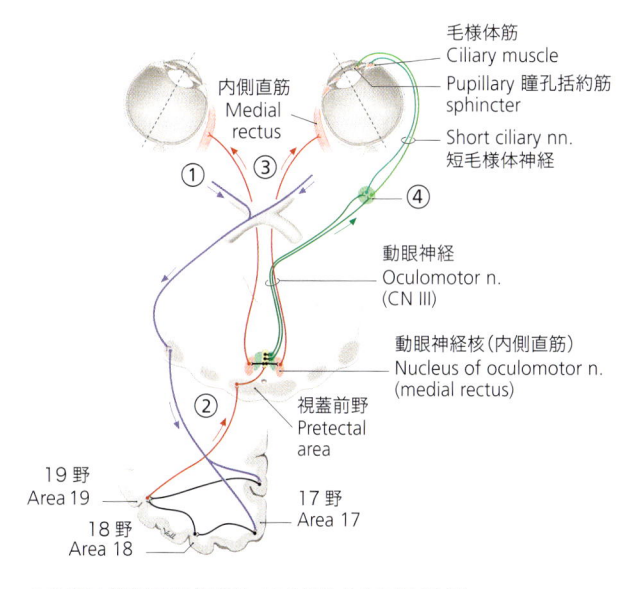

（ラベル：瞳孔括約筋 Pupillary sphincter，短毛様体神経 Short ciliary nn.，毛様体神経節 Ciliary ganglion，動眼神経（副交感性）Oculomotor n. (CN III, parasympathetic portion)，ペーリア核 Perlia's nucleus，動眼神経副核（エディンガー-ウェストファル核）Visceral oculomotor (Edinger-Westphal) nuclei，視神経 Optic n. (CN II)，視索 Optic tract，外側膝状体 Lateral geniculate body，内側膝状体 Medial geniculate body，視蓋前野 Pretectal area）

B 輻輳と遠近調節（接近してくる物体を見る場合）．
① 接近してくる物体からの光を受容する．
② 光情報が 1 次視覚野（17 野）と 2 次視覚野（19 野）を介して，動眼神経核へと送られる．
③ 輻輳：両側の内側直筋が収縮し，眼球の視軸を一点に集める．これにより，接近してくる物体の像は，網膜の中心窩に投影されたまま保たれる．中心窩は網膜の中で最も視力の良い部分である．
④ 遠近調節：水晶体（レンズ）の曲率は毛様体筋の収縮によって増大する．瞳孔括約筋も同時に収縮する．

（ラベル：毛様体筋 Ciliary muscle，瞳孔括約筋 Pupillary sphincter，短毛様体神経 Short ciliary nn.，内側直筋 Medial rectus，動眼神経 Oculomotor n. (CN III)，動眼神経核（内側直筋）Nucleus of oculomotor n. (medial rectus)，視蓋前野 Pretectal area，19 野 Area 19，18 野 Area 18，17 野 Area 17）

特殊感覚の伝導路（2）
Sensory Systems (II)

図 41.11　平衡

体位の平衡は，視覚系，固有覚系，平衡覚系からの情報に基づいて保たれている．これらの3つの系は全てが前庭神経核へ線維を送る．さらに，前庭神経核から出た線維は脊髄や小脳，脳幹に達し，運動の補助や繊細な運動の調節，外眼筋の運動調節にそれぞれ関与する．固有覚（位置覚）とは，空間における体肢の位置についての感覚である．*Note*：前庭神経核から視床や大脳皮質への線維は空間感覚に関与し，視床下部への線維はめまいの際にみられる嘔吐と関係する．

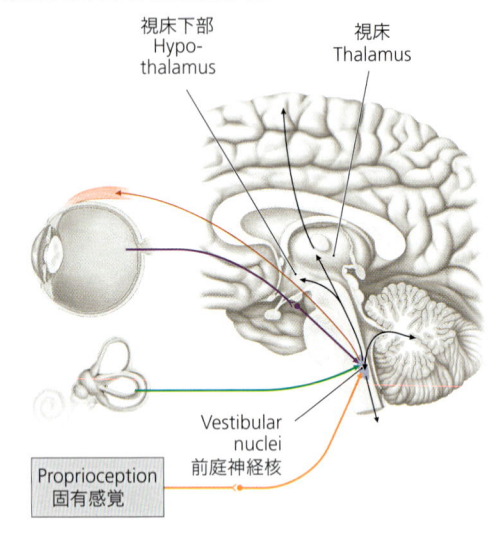

視床下部 Hypothalamus
視床 Thalamus
Vestibular nuclei 前庭神経核
Proprioception 固有感覚

図 41.13　平衡覚系とその神経核

平衡覚系の受容器は内耳の膜迷路に存在する．球形嚢斑と卵形嚢斑は直線加速度を検知するのに対し，半規管の膨大部稜は回転（角）加速度を検知する．

Cortex 皮質
Extraocular muscles 外眼筋
動眼神経核 Nucleus of oculomotor n. (CN III)
滑車神経核 Nucleus of trochlear n. (CN IV)
外転神経核 Nucleus of abducent n. (CN VI)
内側縦束 Medial longitudinal fasciculus (MLF)
Cerebellum 小脳
前庭神経核 Vestibular nuclei
① Superior
② Lateral
③ Medial
④ Inferior
①前庭神経上核
②前庭神経外側核
③前庭神経内側核
④前庭神経下核
前庭小脳線維（下小脳脚を通る）Vestibulocerebellar fibers (via inferior cerebellar peduncle)
前庭神経節 Vestibular ganglion (CN VIII)
Ampullary crests 膨大部稜
Utricle 卵形嚢
Saccule 球形嚢
MLF (to cervical cord) 内側縦束（頚髄へ）
外側前庭脊髄路 Lateral vestibulospinal tract
Reticulospinal tract 網様体脊髄路
To sacral cord 仙髄へ

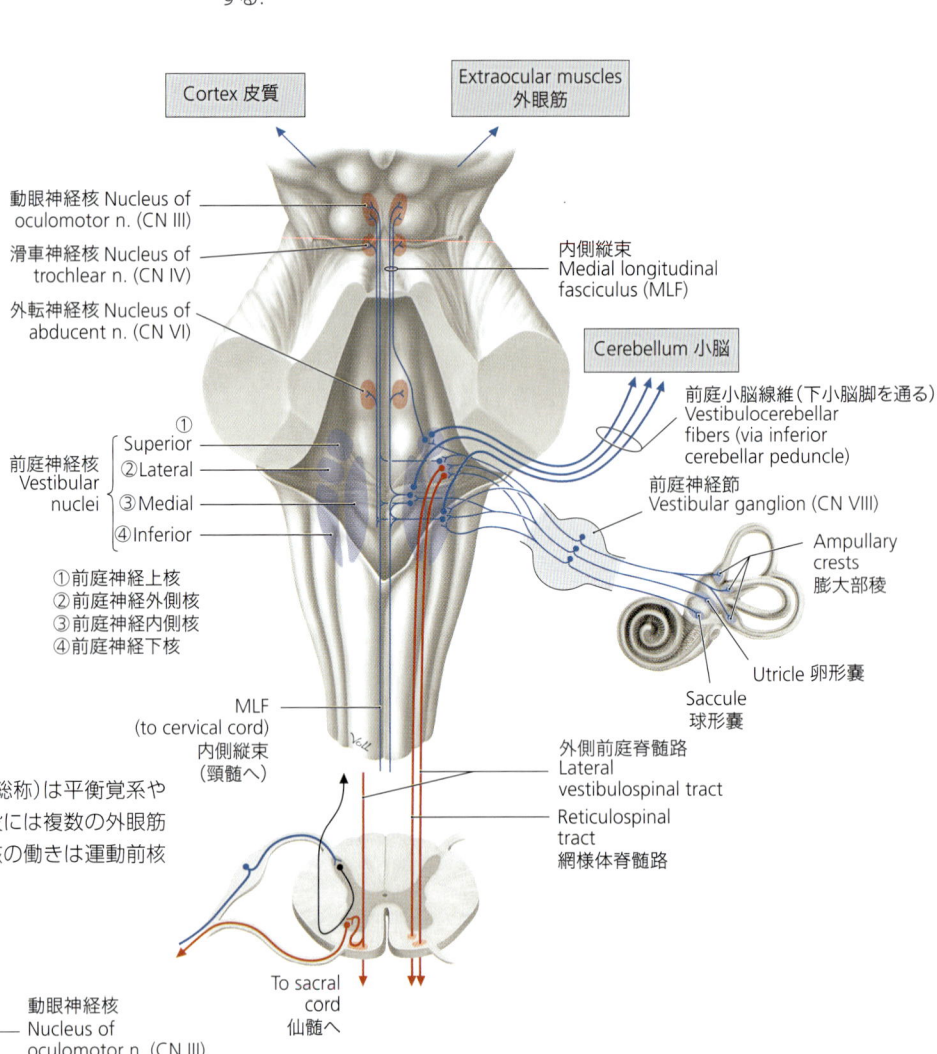

図 41.12　眼球運動核

眼球運動核（滑車神経核，動眼神経核，外転神経核の総称）は平衡覚系や視覚系からの線維を受けている．また，眼球運動の共役には複数の外眼筋とこれらを支配する神経が必要であるため，眼球運動核の働きは運動前核（紫）によって核上性に協調される．

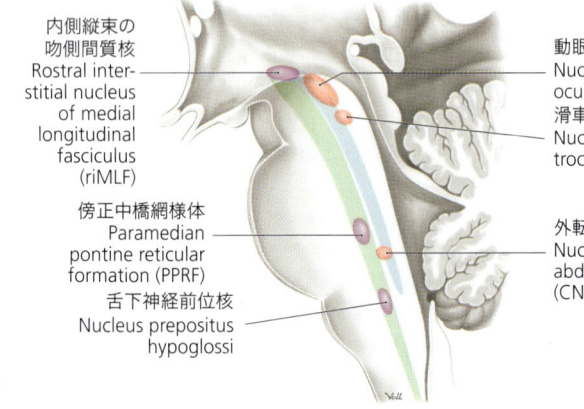

内側縦束の吻側間質核 Rostral interstitial nucleus of medial longitudinal fasciculus (riMLF)
傍正中橋網様体 Paramedian pontine reticular formation (PPRF)
舌下神経前位核 Nucleus prepositus hypoglossi
動眼神経核 Nucleus of oculomotor n. (CN III)
滑車神経核 Nucleus of trochlear n. (CN IV)
外転神経核 Nucleus of abducent n. (CN VI)

- Mesencephalic reticular formation (MRF)　中脳網様体
- Medial longitudinal fasciculus (MLF)　内側縦束
- Oculomotor nuclei　動眼神経核
- Premotor nuclei　運動前核

図 41.14 聴覚系

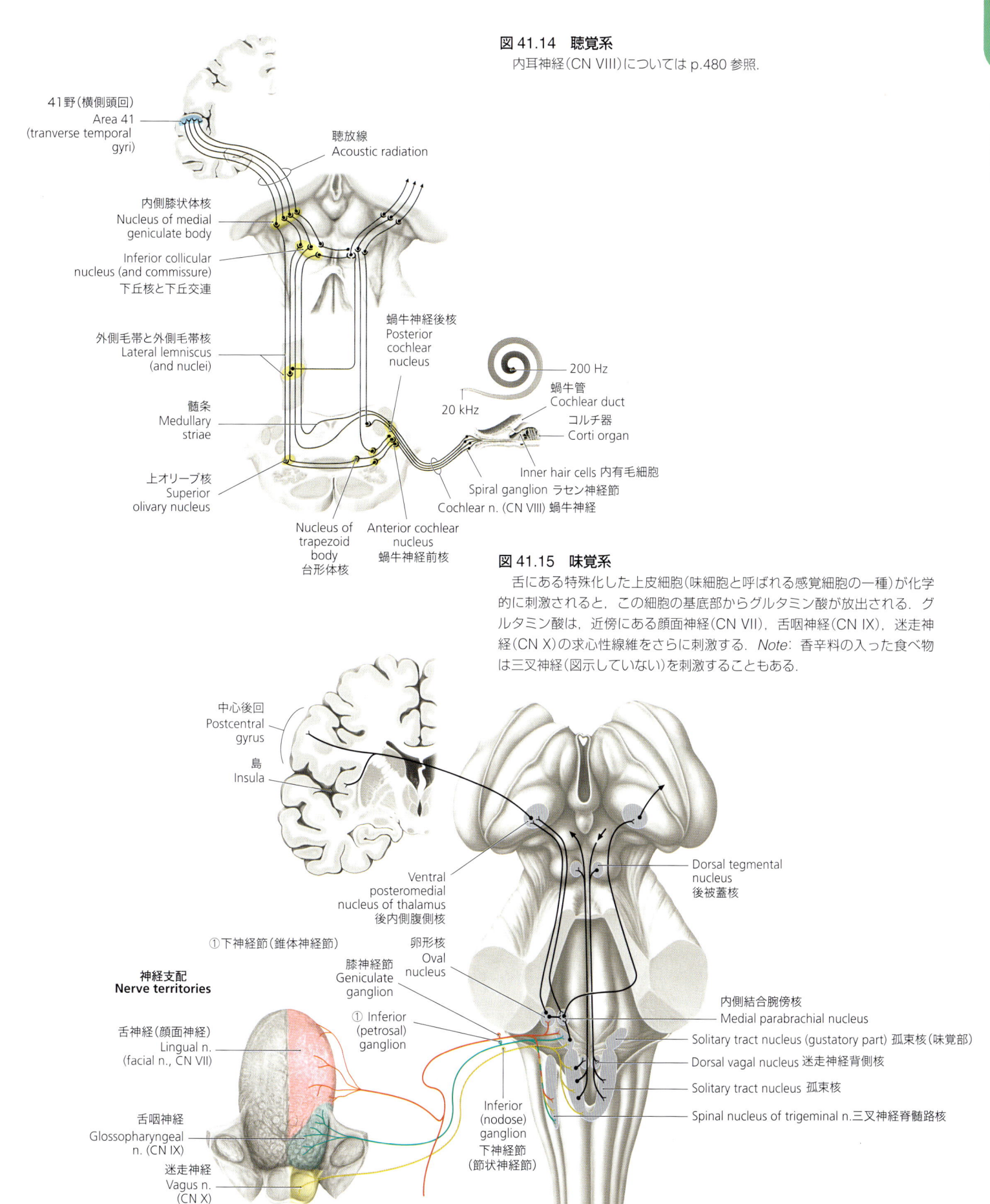

内耳神経（CN VIII）については p.480 参照.

- 41野（横側頭回） Area 41 (tranverse temporal gyri)
- 聴放線 Acoustic radiation
- 内側膝状体核 Nucleus of medial geniculate body
- 下丘核と下丘交連 Inferior collicular nucleus (and commissure)
- 外側毛帯と外側毛帯核 Lateral lemniscus (and nuclei)
- 蝸牛神経後核 Posterior cochlear nucleus
- 髄条 Medullary striae
- 200 Hz
- 20 kHz
- 蝸牛管 Cochlear duct
- コルチ器 Corti organ
- 内有毛細胞 Inner hair cells
- ラセン神経節 Spiral ganglion
- 蝸牛神経 Cochlear n. (CN VIII)
- 上オリーブ核 Superior olivary nucleus
- 台形体核 Nucleus of trapezoid body
- 蝸牛神経前核 Anterior cochlear nucleus

図 41.15 味覚系

舌にある特殊化した上皮細胞（味細胞と呼ばれる感覚細胞の一種）が化学的に刺激されると，この細胞の基底部からグルタミン酸が放出される．グルタミン酸は，近傍にある顔面神経（CN VII），舌咽神経（CN IX），迷走神経（CN X）の求心性線維をさらに刺激する．*Note*：香辛料の入った食べ物は三叉神経（図示していない）を刺激することもある．

- 中心後回 Postcentral gyrus
- 島 Insula
- 後被蓋核 Dorsal tegmental nucleus
- 後内側腹側核 Ventral posteromedial nucleus of thalamus
- ①下神経節（錐体神経節）
- 卵形核 Oval nucleus
- 膝神経節 Geniculate ganglion
- 神経支配 Nerve territories
- 舌神経（顔面神経）Lingual n. (facial n., CN VII)
- ① Inferior (petrosal) ganglion
- 内側結合腕傍核 Medial parabrachial nucleus
- 孤束核（味覚部）Solitary tract nucleus (gustatory part)
- 迷走神経背側核 Dorsal vagal nucleus
- 舌咽神経 Glossopharyngeal n. (CN IX)
- 下神経節（節状神経節）Inferior (nodose) ganglion
- 孤束核 Solitary tract nucleus
- 三叉神経脊髄路核 Spinal nucleus of trigeminal n.
- 迷走神経 Vagus n. (CN X)

特殊感覚の伝導路(3)
Sensory Systems (III)

図 41.16 嗅覚系

嗅覚系は，情報が大脳皮質に至るまでに，視床を介さない唯一の感覚系である(梨状前野が1次嗅覚野だと考えられている)．嗅覚系はその他の大脳皮質ともつながっているため，複雑な感情反応や行動反応を引き起こすことがある(視床下部や視床，辺縁系が関与する)．有害な臭いで吐き気を催したり，食欲をそそる匂いで唾液が分泌されるのはこのためである．

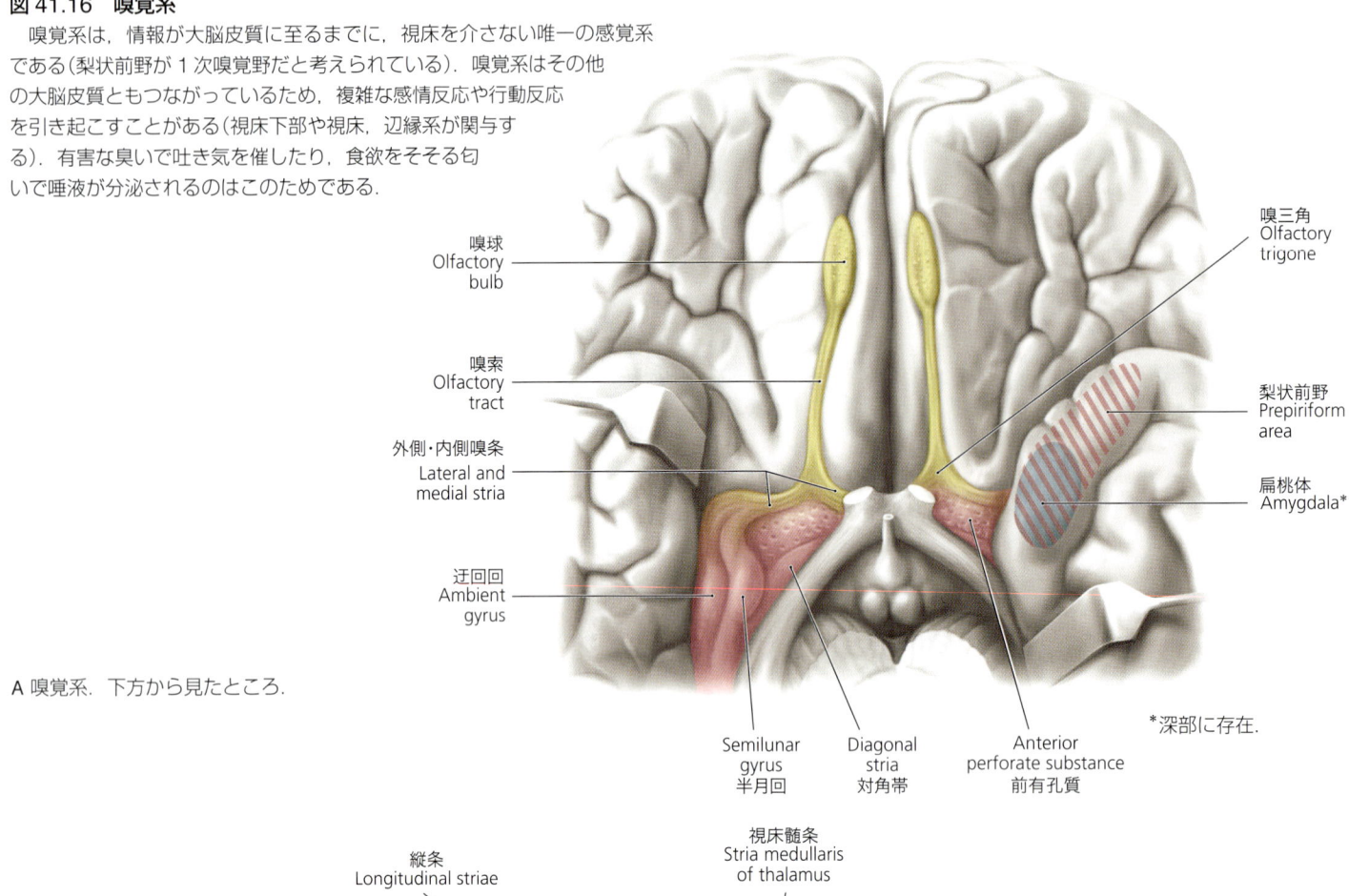

A 嗅覚系．下方から見たところ．

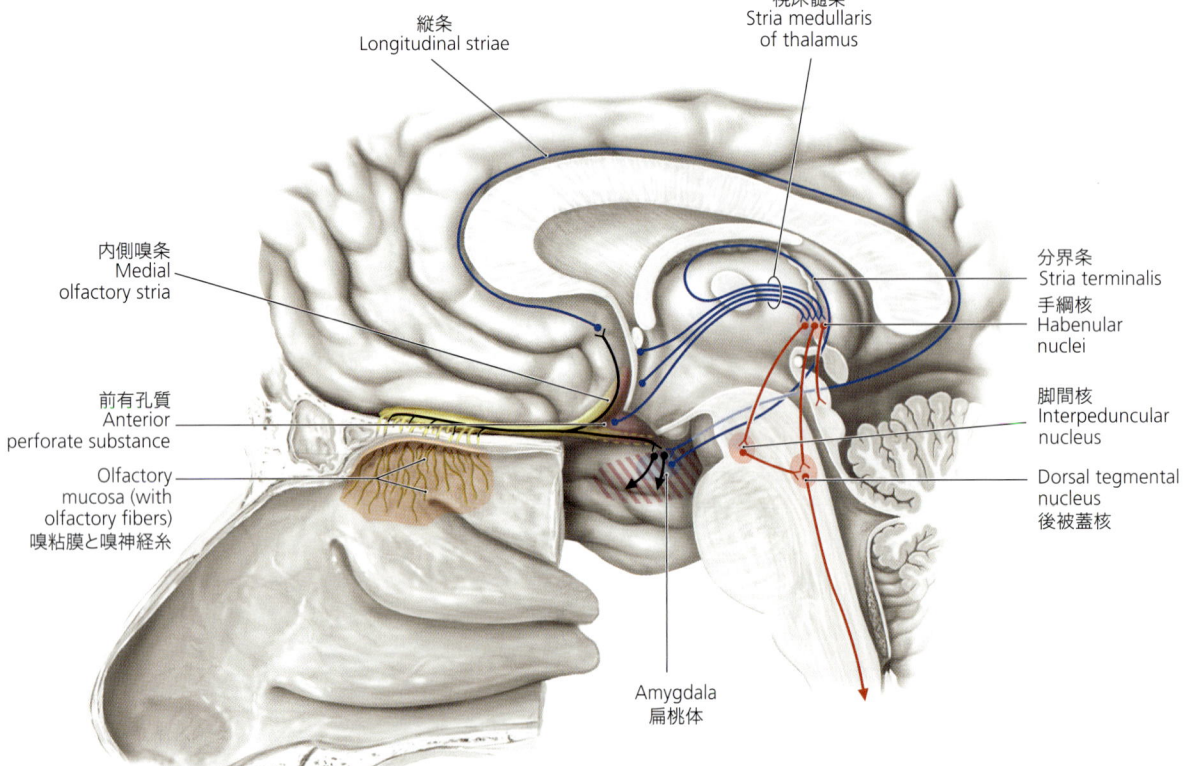

- 嗅球 Olfactory bulb
- 嗅索 Olfactory tract
- 外側・内側嗅条 Lateral and medial stria
- 迂回回 Ambient gyrus
- 嗅三角 Olfactory trigone
- 梨状前野 Prepiriform area
- 扁桃体 Amygdala*
- 半月回 Semilunar gyrus
- 対角帯 Diagonal stria
- 前有孔質 Anterior perforate substance

*深部に存在．

- 縦条 Longitudinal striae
- 視床髄条 Stria medullaris of thalamus
- 内側嗅条 Medial olfactory stria
- 前有孔質 Anterior perforate substance
- 嗅粘膜と嗅神経糸 Olfactory mucosa (with olfactory fibers)
- 分界条 Stria terminalis
- 手綱核 Habenular nuclei
- 脚間核 Interpeduncular nucleus
- 後被蓋核 Dorsal tegmental nucleus
- 扁桃体 Amygdala

B 嗅覚系と関連する核．正中矢状断面で左側の嗅覚系を見たところ．

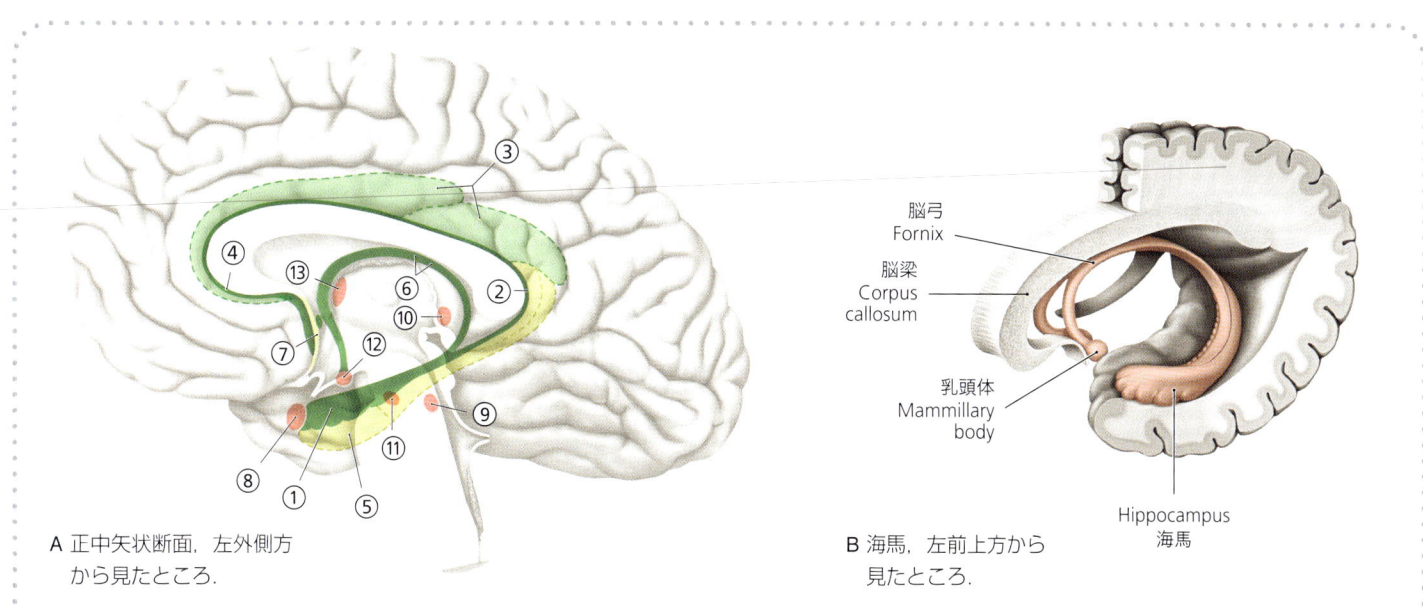

辺縁系は大脳，間脳，中脳の間で情報を交換・統合しており，衝動や感情的行動を調節する．また，辺縁系は記憶や学習においても重要な役割を果たしている．

A 正中矢状断面，左外側方から見たところ．

B 海馬，左前上方から見たところ．

脳弓 Fornix
脳梁 Corpus callosum
乳頭体 Mammillary body
Hippocampus 海馬

表 41.4　辺縁系の構造

外側弓	内側弓*		皮質下核
① 海馬傍回	⑤ 海馬体（海馬，海馬傍回の内側嗅領）		⑧ 扁桃体
② 脳梁灰白層	⑥ 脳弓		⑨ 背側被蓋核
③ 梁下野（嗅傍野）	⑦ 中隔野		⑩ 手綱核
			⑪ 脚間核
④ 帯状回	終傍回		⑫ 乳頭体
			⑬ 視床前核

*内側弓にはブロカ対角帯も含まれる（示されていない）．

図 41.17　辺縁系核

ペーペズ回路は意識的レベルと無意識的レベルに蓄えられた情報を結びつける．

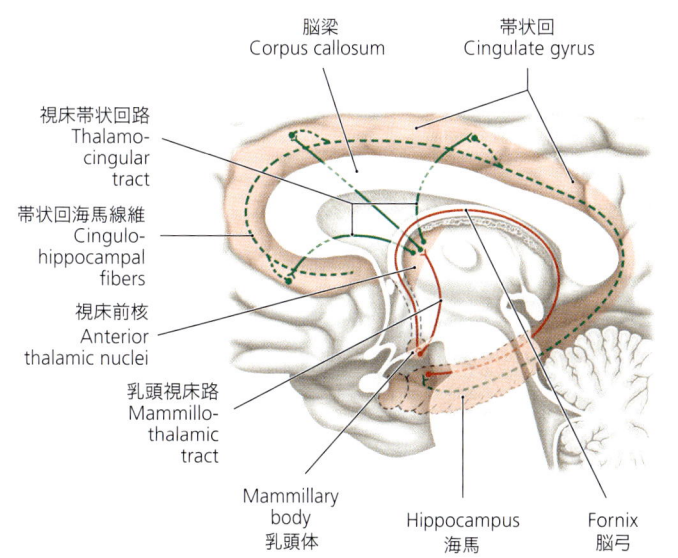

脳梁 Corpus callosum
帯状回 Cingulate gyrus
視床帯状回路 Thalamo-cingular tract
帯状回海馬線維 Cingulo-hippocampal fibers
視床前核 Anterior thalamic nuclei
乳頭視床路 Mammillo-thalamic tract
Mammillary body 乳頭体
Hippocampus 海馬
Fornix 脳弓

図 41.18　辺縁系による末梢自律神経系の調節

辺縁系は自律神経系の標的器官に由来する求心性フィードバック信号を受けている．自律神経系については p. 623 を参照．

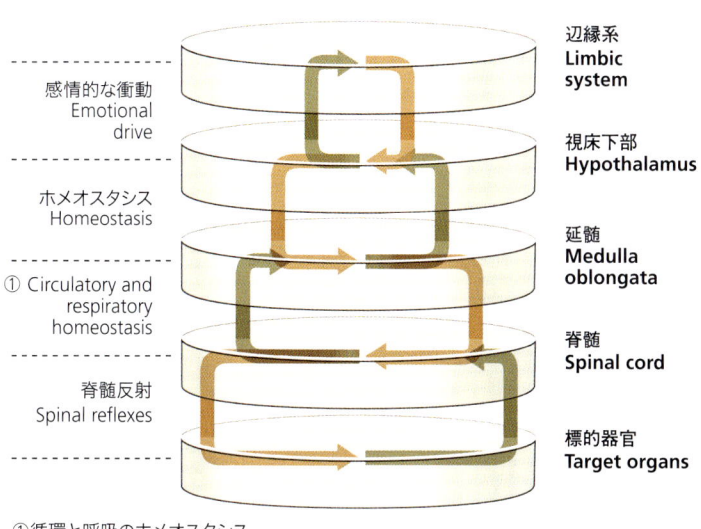

感情的な衝動 Emotional drive — 辺縁系 Limbic system
ホメオスタシス Homeostasis — 視床下部 Hypothalamus
① Circulatory and respiratory homeostasis — 延髄 Medulla oblongata
脊髄反射 Spinal reflexes — 脊髄 Spinal cord
— 標的器官 Target organs

①循環と呼吸のホメオスタシス

自律神経系
Autonomic Nervous System

図 42.1 自律神経系の回路
　自律神経系は平滑筋，心筋，腺に分布し，交感神経系と副交感神経系に区分される．この2つの系は臓器機能(分泌や臓器の血流を含む)をしばしば拮抗的に調節する．緑：求心性線維，紫：遠心性線維．

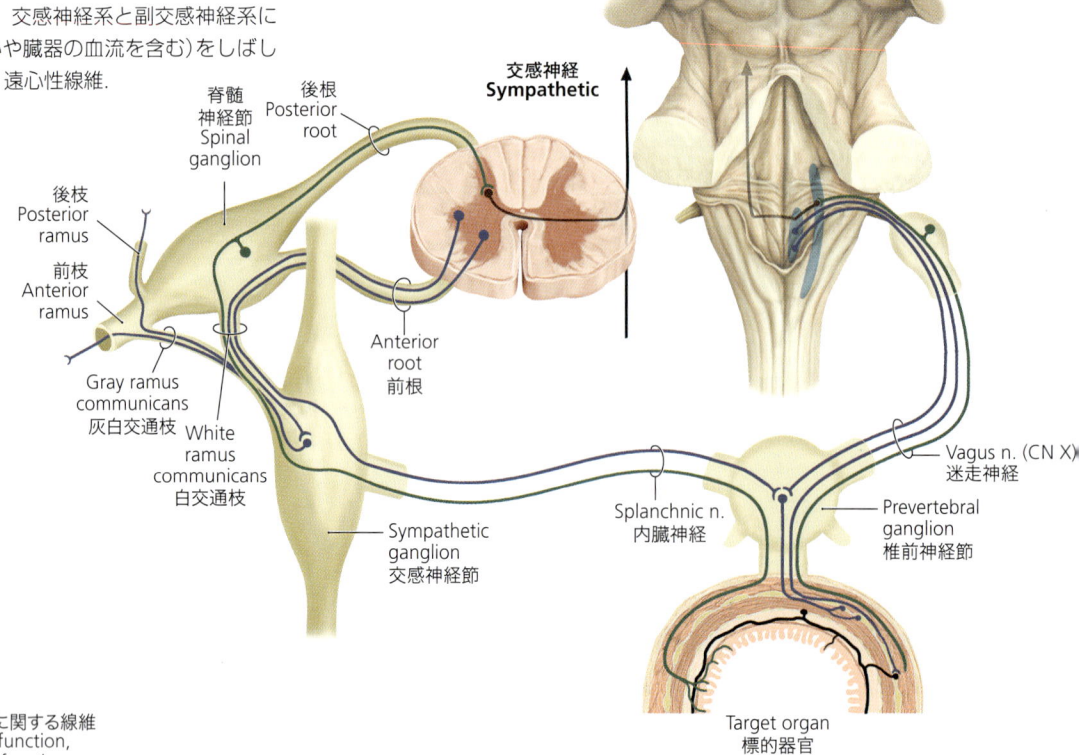

図 42.2 脊髄における自律神経路

図 42.3 自律神経伝達物質の調節作用

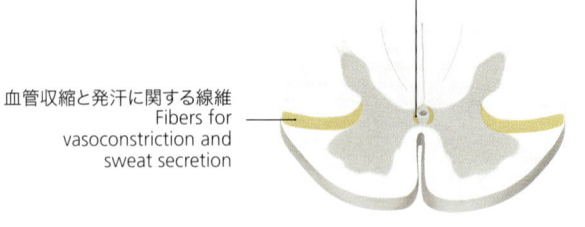

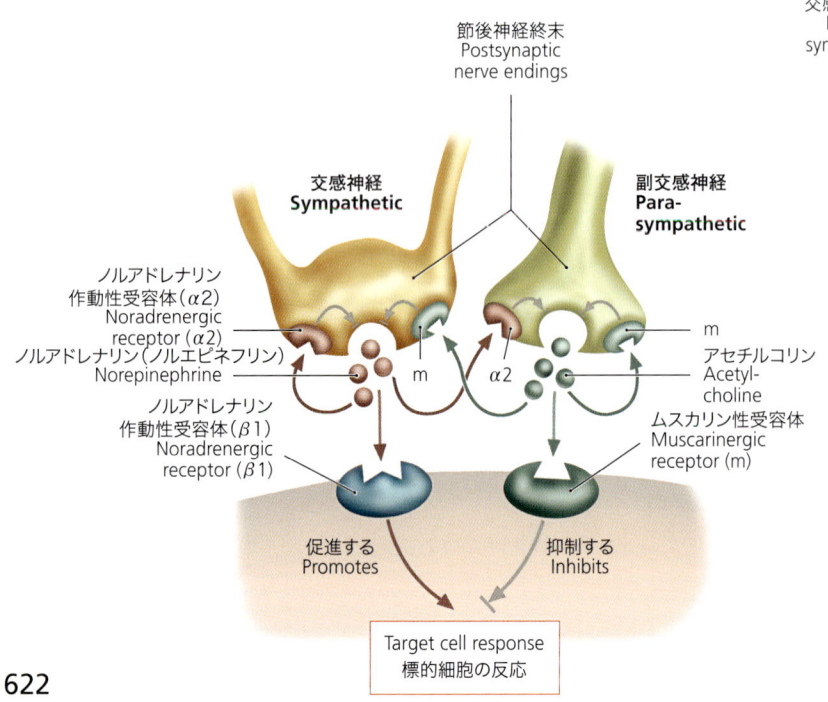

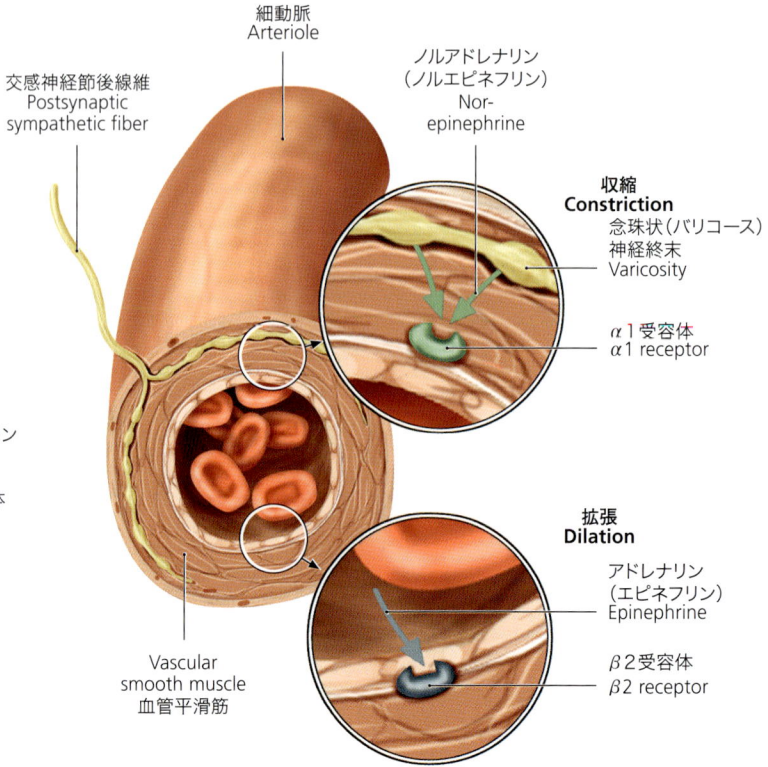

図 42.4 血圧の調節
　交感神経線維はノルアドレナリンを放出し，α1受容体を介して血管平滑筋を収縮させる(結果として血圧が上がる)．循環血液中のアドレナリンはβ2受容体を介して血管の拡張を引き起こす(結果として血圧が下がる)．
Note: 副交感神経線維は血管にほとんど分布しない．

図 42.5 自律神経系

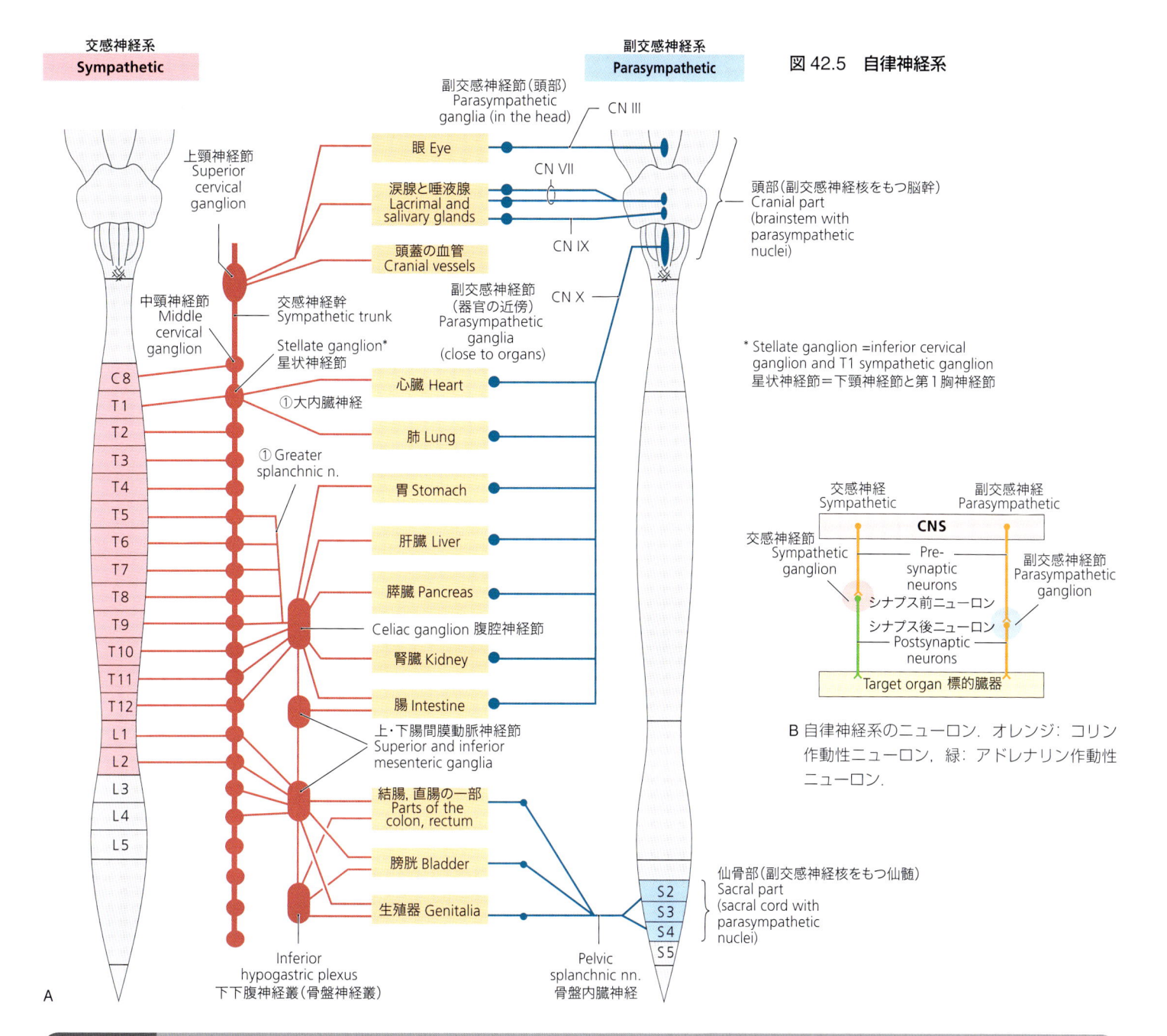

交感神経系 Sympathetic

- 上頸神経節 Superior cervical ganglion
- 中頸神経節 Middle cervical ganglion
- 交感神経幹 Sympathetic trunk
- Stellate ganglion* 星状神経節
- ① 大内臓神経 ① Greater splanchnic n.
- Celiac ganglion 腹腔神経節
- 上・下腸間膜動脈神経節 Superior and inferior mesenteric ganglia
- Inferior hypogastric plexus 下下腹神経叢(骨盤神経叢)

脊髄: C8, T1–T12, L1–L5

副交感神経系 Parasympathetic

- 副交感神経節(頭部) Parasympathetic ganglia (in the head) — CN III, CN VII, CN IX
- 副交感神経節(器官の近傍) Parasympathetic ganglia (close to organs) — CN X
- 頭部(副交感神経核をもつ脳幹) Cranial part (brainstem with parasympathetic nuclei)
- 仙骨部(副交感神経核をもつ仙髄) Sacral part (sacral cord with parasympathetic nuclei) — S2, S3, S4, S5
- Pelvic splanchnic nn. 骨盤内臓神経

標的臓器: 眼 Eye、涙腺と唾液腺 Lacrimal and salivary glands、頭蓋の血管 Cranial vessels、心臓 Heart、肺 Lung、胃 Stomach、肝臓 Liver、膵臓 Pancreas、腎臓 Kidney、腸 Intestine、結腸, 直腸の一部 Parts of the colon, rectum、膀胱 Bladder、生殖器 Genitalia

* Stellate ganglion = inferior cervical ganglion and T1 sympathetic ganglion
星状神経節＝下頸神経節と第1胸神経節

A

B 自律神経系のニューロン．オレンジ：コリン作動性ニューロン，緑：アドレナリン作動性ニューロン．

CNS — シナプス前ニューロン Pre-synaptic neurons、シナプス後ニューロン Postsynaptic neurons、交感神経節 Sympathetic ganglion、副交感神経節 Parasympathetic ganglion、標的臓器 Target organ

表 42.1　交感神経系と副交感神経系の作用

器官(器官系)		交感神経系	副交感神経系
消化管	内輪筋・外縦筋	↓運動性	↑運動性
	括約筋	収縮	弛緩
	腺	↓分泌	↑分泌
脾臓の被膜		収縮	
肝臓		↑グリコーゲンの分解/糖新生	影響を与えない
膵臓	内分泌部	↓インスリンの分泌	
	外分泌部	↓膵液の分泌	↑膵液の分泌
膀胱	排尿筋	弛緩	収縮
	機能的膀胱括約筋	収縮	
精嚢		収縮(射精)	影響を与えない
精管			
子宮		収縮もしくは弛緩(ホルモンの状態に依存)	
動脈		収縮	陰茎と陰核の動脈の弛緩(勃起)

p. 244 も参照すること．

付 録
Appendix

体表解剖に関する問題の解答……………………………626
英文索引……………………………………………………628
和文索引……………………………………………………659

体表解剖に関する問題の解答
Answers to Surface Anatomy Questions

背部 (pp.40-41)

Q1：ミハエリス Michaelis 菱形窩の上縁は L4 の棘突起と左右の後上腸骨棘を結ぶ線からなる．この菱形窩の下縁は腸骨稜のカーブに沿って下り，殿裂に達する．

Q2：肩甲骨の下角の高さには T7 の棘突起がある．また，腸骨稜の高さには L4 の棘突起がある．体表から触知できる骨については p.40 を参照すること．

胸部 (pp.120-121)

Q1：注意深く視診した後に，左右の乳房を触診する．その際には下外側，下内側，上内側，上外側の順に乳房の組織を触診し，その後腋窩を触診して腋窩突起を調べる．乳房からのリンパの大半は腋窩リンパ節に集まる．乳房内側部のリンパは内胸動静脈の傍にある胸骨傍リンパ節に集まる．腋窩リンパ節については p.64 参照．

Q2：大動脈弁は右第 2 肋間隙，肺動脈弁は左第 2 肋間隙で最も聴診しやすい．第 2 肋間隙を確定する際には，触診によって胸骨柄と胸骨体の間の胸骨角を見つければよい．三尖弁（右房室弁）と二尖弁（左房室弁）は左第 5 肋間隙で最も聴診しやすい．肋骨が視認・触知できる場合には鎖骨中線最下部の第 10 肋骨から数えて第 5 肋間隙を確定する．聴診部位については p.87 参照．胸部の基準線については p.120 参照．

腹部・骨盤部 (pp.248-249)

Q1：ほぼ第 4 腰椎の高さにある臍を通る鉛直線と水平線を用いて胸部と腹部を上下左右に 4 つに分ける (p.142 参照)．

LUQ（左上腹部）	肝臓，胃，横行結腸，小腸，脾臓，膵臓，十二指腸，下行結腸，左腎，左副腎，左尿管
RUQ（右上腹部）	肝臓，胃，横行結腸，小腸，胆嚢，膵臓，十二指腸，上行結腸，右腎，右副腎，右尿管
LLQ（左下腹部）	小腸，下行結腸，左尿管，膀胱，生殖器
RLQ（右下腹部）	小腸，上行結腸（盲腸，虫垂），右尿管，膀胱，生殖器

Q2：直接鼠径ヘルニアは中高年の男性によく見られ，損耗によって生じると考えられている．典型的な症状ではヘルニアが鼠径管の中間部分を占め，鼠径三角を通って腹腔から外に出て，さらに浅鼠径輪を通って脱出する．まれに陰嚢に入ることもある．間接鼠径ヘルニアは男児や若年の男性に見られ，先天的な要因によって生じると考えられている．一般にはヘルニアが深鼠径輪から外に出て，鼠径管全体を占め，さらに浅鼠径輪を通って脱出する．まれに陰嚢に入ることもある．鼠径ヘルニアについては p.133 を参照．

上肢 (pp.350-353)

Q1：内側・外側前腕皮神経の両者は，肘窩における静脈穿刺の際に損傷されることがある．内側前腕皮神経は腕神経叢の内側神経束から出る枝であり，外側前腕皮神経は筋皮神経（外側神経束に由来する）の皮神経成分である．

Q2：内側側副靱帯は，肘を屈曲位にして，肘頭，内側・外側上顆，鉤状突起を手がかりにすると触知できる．外側側副靱帯は外側上顆を手がかりにして触知できる．肘の側副靱帯については p.248 を参照すること．

Q3：手首では，尺骨動脈・神経は尺側手根屈筋腱の外側に接して走行する（これらの動脈・神経が尺骨神経管に入るまで）．正中神経は長掌筋と橈側手根屈筋の触知できる腱の間に位置する．橈骨動脈は橈側手根屈筋腱のやや外側に存在する．

Q4：解剖学的嗅ぎタバコ入れの底における圧痛は舟状骨の骨折を示唆する．解剖学的嗅ぎタバコ入れについては p.347，舟状骨骨折については p.299 を参照すること．

下肢 (pp.450-451)

Q1：大腿骨頭は大腿動脈の直ぐ後ろに位置する．大腿動脈は鼡径靱帯の中点から下方に向かって走る．鼡径部の構造については p.436 を参照．

Q2：坐骨神経は大坐骨孔を通り，殿部に現れる．この孔は後上腸骨棘と坐骨結節を結ぶ線の中点に位置する．坐骨神経はさらに殿部において，大腿骨の大転子と坐骨結節を結ぶ線の中点のすぐ内側を通過する（pp.438-439 ページ参照）．総腓骨神経は，大腿二頭筋腱の内側に沿って下行しており，膝窩の外側縁で触知できる（p.442 参照）．脛骨神経は足首において内果と踵骨腱（アキレス腱）の間に位置する（p.442 参照）．

頭頸部 (pp.588-589)

Q1：麻酔剤を胸鎖乳突筋後縁の上 2/3 の高さで注入すると，頸神経叢をブロックすることができる．

Q2：静脈洞交会は外後頭隆起の深部にある．硬膜静脈洞については p.606 を参照．

Q3：外側頸三角部（後頸三角）は，胸鎖乳突筋，僧帽筋，鎖骨によって囲まれる領域で，副神経（CN XI）と腕神経叢が含まれる．頸の部位については p.576 を参照．外側頸三角部（後頸三角）に含まれるものについては p.582 を参照．

Q4：頸動脈三角は，胸骨舌骨筋，顎二腹筋後腹，胸鎖乳突筋によって囲まれる領域で，迷走神経（CN X）が含まれる．頸の部位については p.576 を参照．頸動脈三角に含まれるものについては p.580 を参照．

Q5：甲状軟骨（p.570 参照）は一般に「アダムの林檎」と呼ばれている．

英文索引
Index of English Term

・項目の主要掲載ページは太字で示す.

A

α1 receptor α1受容体 622
α-motor neuron α運動ニューロン 614, 615
Abdominal
- aorta 腹大動脈 23, 34, 55, 56, 143, 146, 149, 156, 175, 180, 206, 207, **208**, 210, 213
- part
-- of esophagus 腹部《食道の》 96
-- of pectoralis major 腹部《大胸筋の》 130, 264, 274
-- of ureter 腹部《尿管の》 180
Abducent nerve(CN Ⅵ) 外転神経 470, 475, **509**, 511-513, 599, 608
Abductor
- digiti minimi
-- 小指外転筋 301, 306-310, 312, **313**
-- 小趾外転筋 402, 412, 413, 415, **417**, 433, 446
- hallucis 母趾外転筋 402, 404, 411-414, **417**, 420, 443, 446, 447
- pollicis
-- brevis 短母指外転筋 306-309, 312, **313**, 353
-- longus 長母指外転筋 288, 290, 291, 296, **297**, 307, 309, 310
--- tendon 長母指外転筋の腱 307, 308
Accessory
- cephalic vein 副橈側皮静脈 318, 331
- collateral ligament 副側副靱帯 304
- hemiazygos vein 副半奇静脈 35, 57, **70**, 71, 79, 99, 117, 611
- nerve(CN Ⅺ) 副神経 470, **486**, 501, 556, 579-584, 599
- nucleus cuneatus 副楔状束核 614
- pancreatic duct 副膵管 160, 172, 174
- parotid gland 副耳下腺 551
- process 副突起 5, 9
- saphenous vein 副伏在静脈 422, 434
- sex glands 付属生殖腺 200
Acetabular
- fossa 寛骨臼窩 125, **359**, 363, 364, 421
- labrum 関節唇《寛骨臼の》 361, 363, 364, 421
- notch 寛骨臼切痕 125, 359
- rim 寛骨臼縁 124-126, 358, **359**, 362
- roof 寛骨臼蓋 364, 421
Acetabulum 寛骨臼 124-126, 129, **358**, 361, 363
Achilles' tendon 踵骨腱(アキレス腱) 393, 394, 398, 405, 411, **415**, 442, 443, 448, 451
Acinus 腺房 111
Acoustic radiation 聴放線 619
Acromial
- angle of scapula 肩峰角《肩甲骨の》 255
- articular surface 肩峰関節面 254, 262
- branch
-- of suprascapular artery 肩峰枝《肩甲上動脈の》 317
-- of thoracoacromial artery 肩峰枝《胸肩峰動脈の》 316
- end of clavicle 肩峰端《鎖骨の》 253, 254, 259
- part of deltoid 肩峰部《三角筋の》 265, 272
Acromioclavicular
- joint 肩鎖関節 47, 252, 258, **259**
- ligament 肩鎖靱帯 259, 261
Acromion 肩峰 22, 40, 253, **255**, 258-262

Adductor
- brevis 短内転筋 367, 372, **376**, 440, 448
- canal 内転筋管 420, 422
- hallucis 母趾内転筋 411, 413, 418, **419**, 447
- hiatus [内転筋]腱裂孔 367, 377, 420-422, 441
- longus 長内転筋 366, 367, 369, 372, **376**, 440, 448, 450
- magnus 大内転筋 194, 203, 366-372, **377**, 421, 439-441, 448
- minimus 小内転筋 377
- muscles 内転筋群 155
- pollicis 母指内転筋 306, 308, 309, 312, **313**
- tubercle of femur 内転筋結節《大腿骨の》 360
Adenohypophysis 腺下垂体 598
Adipose tissue of orbit 眼窩脂肪体 511, **514**
Aditus(inlet) to mastoid antrum 乳突洞口 531
Adventitia of urinary bladder 外膜《膀胱の》 185
Afferent
- (ascending) tracts of spinal cord 求心路(上行路)《脊髄の》 613
- fibers 求心性線維 54
- nuclei 求心性核 612
Alar
- folds 翼状ヒダ 390
- ligaments 翼状靱帯 17
- part of nasalis 翼部《鼻筋の》 464
Alcock's canal(pudendal canal) アルコック管(陰部神経管) 155, 439
Alveolar
- bone 歯槽骨 542
- duct 肺胞管 111
- macrophage 肺胞大食細胞 111
- part of mandible 歯槽部《下顎骨の》 539
- sac 肺胞嚢 111
Alveoli(tooth sockets) 歯槽 539
Alveolus(pulmonary alveolus) 肺胞 111, 116
Ambient
- cistern 迂回槽 604
- gyrus 迂回回 472, 620
Ampulla
- of ductus deferens 精管膨大部 143, 150, 187, 200
- of uterine tube 卵管膨大部 189
Ampullary crests 膨大部稜 618
Amygdala 扁桃体 472, 594, **620**
Anal
- canal 肛門管 166, 167
- cleft 殿裂 41, 136
- columns 肛門柱 167
- pecten 肛門櫛 167
- sinuses 肛門洞 167
- triangle 肛門三角 136
- valves 肛門弁 167
Anastomotic branch with lacrimal artery 涙腺動脈との吻合枝《中硬膜動脈の》 495
Anatomical
- (anatomic) snuffbox 解剖学的嗅ぎタバコ入れ(橈骨窩) **346**, 351-353
- neck of humerus 解剖頸《上腕骨の》 **256**, 257, 260
Anconeus 肘筋 268, 270, **279**, 290
Angular
- artery 眼角動脈 492, 498, 502, **512**
- gyral branch of middle cerebral artery 角回枝《中大脳動脈の》 609
- notch of stomach 角切痕《胃の》 158
- vein 眼角静脈 496-499, 502, **510**, 512, 567

Ankle mortise 足関節窩 356, 380, **404**, 405
Annular
- ligament/s
-- [線維鞘の]輪状部 305, 306, 311, 412
-- 輪状靱帯 110
-- of radius 橈骨輪状靱帯 284-287
- stapedial ligament アブミ骨輪状靱帯 532
Anococcygeal
- ligament 肛門尾骨靱帯 136, 137, 140, 141
- nerves 肛門尾骨神経 203
- raphe 肛門尾骨縫線 141
Anocutaneous line 肛門皮膚線 167
Ansa cervicalis 頸神経ワナ 547, **568**, 569, 578, 580, 581
Antebrachial fascia 前腕筋膜 306
Anterior
-(ventral)
-- rami
--- of intercostal nerves 前枝《肋間神経の》 61
--- of spinal nerve 前枝《脊髄神経の》 **36**, 59, 321
-- root of spinal nerve 前根《脊髄神経の》 59, 321, 430, **600**, 601, 615
- ampullary nerve 前膨大部神経 481, 536, **537**
- antebrachial interosseous nerve 前[前腕]骨間神経 320, 328
- arch of atlas 前弓《環椎の》 7
- articular facet of vertebra 前関節面《椎骨の》 7
- atlantooccipital membrane 前環椎後頭膜 18, 19, **559**
- auricular arteries 前耳介動脈 529
- basal
-- segment of lung 前肺底区 108
-- segmental artery of lung 前肺底動脈 115
-- vein of lung 前肺底静脈 115
- belly of digastric muscle 前腹《顎二腹筋の》 464, 544, 554, **563**
- border
-- of lung 前縁《肺の》 105
-- of radius 前縁《橈骨の》 280, 281
-- of tibia 前縁《脛骨の》 380
- branch/es
-- of external carotid artery 前枝《外頸動脈の》 491, 492
-- of inferior pancreaticoduodenal artery 前下膵十二指腸動脈 211, 212, 219
-- of obturator nerve 前枝《閉鎖神経の》 425, 428
-- of renal artery 前枝《腎動脈の》 209
- calcaneal articular surface of talus 前踵骨関節面《距骨の》 407
- cecal artery 前盲腸動脈 212, 213, **220**, 221
- cerebral
-- artery 前大脳動脈 608, 609
-- vein 前大脳静脈 606, 607
- cervical triangle(region) 前頸三角(前頸部) 576, 578
- chamber of eyeball 前眼房 516, 518
- choroidal artery 前脈絡叢動脈 490, 608
- ciliary arteries 前毛様体動脈 517
- circumflex humeral artery 前上腕回旋動脈 316, 317
- clinoid process 前床突起 459, 461, 538
- cochlear nucleus 蝸牛神経前核 480, 619
- commissure 前交連 596, 598, 605, 609
- communicating
-- artery 前交通動脈 608
-- vein 前交通静脈 607
- conjunctival artery 前結膜動脈 517
- cranial fossa 前頭蓋窩 459, 523

628

Anterolateral surface of humerus

- cruciate ligament 前十字靱帯 387, **388**, 389, 391
- crural
- – artery 前脚動脈 535
- – intermuscular septum 前下腿筋間中隔 444
- crus
- – of internal capsule 前脚《内包の》 594
- – of stapes 前脚《アブミ骨の》 532
- cusp
- – of left atrioventricular valve 前尖《左房室弁の》 86, 87
- – of pulmonary valve 前半月弁《肺動脈弁の》 86, 87
- – of right atrioventricular valve 前尖《右房室弁の》 85-87
- cutaneous
- – branch
- – – of 2nd intercostal nerves 前皮枝《第2肋間神経の》 326
- – – of femoral nerve 前皮枝《大腿神経の》 425, 426, 429, 434
- – – of iliohypogastric nerve 前皮枝《腸骨下腹神経の》 133, 426, 427
- – – of intercostal nerves 前皮枝《肋間神経の》 58, 61, 330
- – – of spinal nerve 前皮枝《脊髄神経の》 **36**, 59
- deep temporal artery 前深側頭動脈 504
- diameter of trochlea of talus 前径《距骨滑車の》 405
- ethmoidal
- – artery 前篩骨動脈 510, 513, **524**, 525
- – foramen 前篩骨孔 460, 506
- – nerve 前篩骨神経 477, 513, **525**
- external vertebral venous plexus 前外椎骨静脈叢 35, 57, 611
- extremity of spleen 前端《脾臓の》 174
- femoral cutaneous vein 前大腿皮静脈 422, 436
- funiculus of spinal cord 前索《脊髄》 613
- gastric plexus 前胃神経叢 74, 98, 238, 245
- glandular branches of superior thyroid artery 前腺枝《上甲状腺動脈の》 566
- gluteal line of ilium 前殿筋線《腸骨の》 125, 359
- horn
- – of lateral ventricle 前角《側脳室の》 594, 605
- – of spinal cord 前角《脊髄の》 612
- inferior
- – iliac spine 下前腸骨棘 124-126, 128, 136, 137, **358**, 359
- – segmental artery of kidney 下前区動脈《腎臓の》 209
- intercavernous sinus 前海綿間静脈洞 607
- intercondylar area of tibia 前顆間区《脛骨の》 381, 391
- intercostal
- – branches of internal thoracic artery 前肋間枝《内胸動脈の》 34, 56
- – veins 前肋間静脈 35, 57
- internal vertebral venous plexus 前内椎骨静脈叢 35, **57**, 601, 611
- internodal bundles 前結節間束 90
- interosseous
- – artery 前骨間動脈 316, **317**, 340, 345
- – veins 前骨間静脈 318
- interventricular
- – (left anterior descending) branch of left coronary artery 前室間枝（前下行枝）《左冠状動脈の》 83, 88

- – sulcus 前室間溝 84
- jugular vein 前頸静脈 **496**, 567, 578
- ligament of malleus 前ツチ骨靱帯 532
- labial
- – branches 前陰唇枝 195
- – commissure 前陰唇交連 192
- lacrimal crest 前涙嚢稜 506
- lateral
- – malleolar artery 前外果動脈 420, 445
- – segment (Segment Ⅵ) of right liver 右外側前区域（区域Ⅵ）《右肝部の》 170
- layer
- – of rectus sheath 前葉《腹直筋鞘の》 134
- – of renal fascia 前葉《腎筋膜の》 176
- ligament of fibular head 前腓骨頭靱帯 388
- lingual glands 前舌腺 549
- lip of uterine os 前唇《外子宮口の》 190
- lobe
- – of adenohypophysis 前葉《腺下垂体の》 596
- – of cerebellum 小脳前葉 598
- longitudinal ligament 前縦靱帯 **18**, 19, 20, 51, 128, 365, 366, 559
- malleolar fold 前ツチ骨ヒダ 532
- medial
- – malleolar artery 前内果動脈 420
- – segment (Segment Ⅴ) of right liver 右内側前区域（区域Ⅴ）《右肝部の》 170
- median fissure 前正中裂 599
- mediastinum 前縦隔 67, 76
- nasal
- – (piriform) aperture 梨状口 455, 521
- – spine 前鼻棘 454, 455, 538
- nuclei of thalamus (anterior thalamic nuclei) 視床前核 597, 621
- papillary muscle 前乳頭筋 85, 87, 90
- part
- – of vagina 前部《腟》 190
- – of ulnar collateral ligament 前部《肘関節の内側側副靱帯》 284
- perforate substance 前有孔質 472, 620
- process of malleus 前突起《ツチ骨の》 532
- radicular
- – artery 前根動脈 56
- – vein 前根静脈 611
- ramus/i
- – of 1st sacral nerve 前枝《第1仙骨神経の》 237, 239, 242
- – of cervical nerve 前枝《頸神経の》 547, 569
- – of lumbar nerves 前枝《腰神経の》 242, 243
- – of sacral nerve 前枝《仙骨神経の》 36
- – of thoracic aorta 前枝《胸大動脈の》 34
- root
- – of C8 前根《第8頸神経の》 579
- – of sacral nerve 前根《仙骨神経の》 36
- rootlets 前根糸 600
- sacral foramina 前仙骨孔 10, 11, 126, 129
- sacrococcygeal ligament 前仙尾靱帯 129
- sacroiliac ligaments 前仙腸靱帯 **128**, 129, 141, 365
- scalene (scalenus anterior) 前斜角筋 51, 77, 317, 321, 564, **565**, 579, 581
- scrotal
- – artery 前陰嚢動脈 202
- – branches of genitofemoral nerve 前陰嚢枝《陰部大腿神経の》 426
- – vein 前陰嚢静脈 202
- segmental
- – artery of lung 前上葉動脈《肺の》 115
- – medullary artery 前髄節動脈 610

- semicircular
- – canal 前骨半規管 528, 530, 531, **536**
- – duct 前半規管 536, 537
- septal branches of anterior ethmoidal artery 中隔前鼻枝《前篩骨動脈の》 524
- spinal
- – artery 前脊髄動脈 608, 610
- – vein 前脊髄静脈 611
- spinocerebellar tract 前脊髄小脳路 598
- sternoclavicular ligament 前胸鎖靱帯 258, 259
- superficial cervical lymph nodes 浅前頸リンパ節 587
- superior
- – alveolar
- – – arteries 前上歯槽動脈 495
- – – branches of superior alveolar nerves 前上歯槽枝《上歯槽神経の》 477, 546
- – iliac spine 上前腸骨棘 40, 120, **124**, 125, 126, 129, 136, 137, 248, 356-359, 362
- – pancreaticoduodenal artery 前上膵十二指腸動脈 207, **211**, 212, 218, 219
- – segmental artery of kidney 上前区動脈《腎臓の》 209
- surface
- – of kidney 前面《腎臓の》 178
- – of patella 前面《膝蓋骨の》 383
- – of suprarenal gland 前面《副腎の》 176
- talar articular surface of calcaneus 前距骨関節面《踵骨》 407
- talofibular ligament 前距腓靱帯 408
- temporal branch of middle cerebral artery 前側頭枝《中大脳動脈の》 609
- tibial
- – artery 前脛骨動脈 **420**, 421, 445
- – recurrent artery 前脛骨反回動脈 420, 421
- – veins 前脛骨静脈 422, 445
- tibiofibular ligament 前脛腓靱帯 408, 409
- tibiotalar part of deltoid ligament 前脛距部《三角靱帯の》 408
- trunk of internal iliac
- – artery 前枝《内腸骨動脈の》 180
- – vein 前枝《内腸骨静脈の》 180
- tubercle
- – of atlas 前結節《環椎の》 7, 558
- – of cervical vertebrae 前結節《頸椎の》 6
- – of transvers process 前結節《横突起の》 7
- – of vertebra 前結節《椎骨の》 5, 7, 18
- tympanic artery 前鼓室動脈 495, 504, 534
- vagal trunk 前迷走神経幹 74, **98**, 237-240, 245
- vaginal
- – column 前腟柱《腟の》 190
- – fornix 前部《腟円蓋の》 151, 184, 188
- vein/s
- – of right ventricle 前右心室静脈 88
- – of septum pellucidum 前透明中隔静脈 606
- wall
- – of stomach 前壁《胃の》 156, 175
- – of tympanic cavity 前壁《頸動脈壁》《鼓室の》 481
- – of upper lobe of lung 前上葉静脈《肺の》 115
- – of vagina 前壁《腟の》 189, 190
Anteroinferior cerebellar artery 前下小脳動脈 608
Anterolateral
- pontine vein 前外側橋静脈 607
- sulcus 前外側溝 599
- surface
- – of arytenoid cartilage 前外側面《披裂軟骨の》 570
- – of humerus 前外側面《上腕骨の》 256

――system（spinothalamic tract） 前外側脊髄視床路 614
Anteromedial
― bundle of lymphatics of lower limb 前内側束《下肢リンパ管の》 423
― surface of humerus 前内側面《上腕骨の》 256
Anteromedian pontine vein 前正中橋静脈 607
Antihelix 対輪 529, 589
Antitragicus 対珠筋 529
Antitragus 対珠 529, 589
Anulus fibrosus 線維輪 12, 20
Anus 肛門 136, 137, 167, 192, 194, 203
Aorta 大動脈 77, 82
Aortic
― arch 大動脈弓 34, **68**, 77, 79, 83, 84, 90, 95, 99, 114
― bifurcation 大動脈分岐部 56, 206, 213
― hiatus（aperture）of diaphragm 大動脈裂孔《横隔膜の》 **52**, 53, 68, 70
― sinus 大動脈洞 87
― valve 大動脈弁 **86**, 87
Aorticorenal ganglia 大動脈腎動脈神経節 236, 237, 239
Aperture of sphenoid sinus 蝶形骨洞口 461
Apex
― of arytenoid cartilage 披裂軟骨尖 570
― of bladder 膀胱尖 181, 201
― of lung 肺尖 105
― of patella 膝蓋骨尖 383
― of prostate 前立腺尖 200
― of root 歯根尖 542
― of sacrum 仙骨尖 10
― of tongue 舌尖 548
Apical
― axillary lymph node 上腋窩リンパ節 64
― ligament of dens 歯尖靱帯 17, 559
― segment of right lung 肺尖区 108
― segmental artery of lung 肺尖動脈 115
― vein of upper lobe of right lung 肺尖静脈 115
Apicoposterior vein of upper lobe of right lung 肺尖後静脈 115
Aponeurosis of transversus abdominis（transversus abdominis aponeurosis） 腹横筋腱膜 131, **134**, 139
Appendicular vein 虫垂静脈 215, 220
Appendix
― of epididymis 精巣上体垂 198
― of testis 精巣垂 198, 205
Aqueous humor 眼房水 518
Arachnoid クモ膜 602
― granulations クモ膜顆粒 602, 604
― trabeculae クモ膜小柱 602
― villi クモ膜絨毛 602
Arch
― of cricoid cartilage 輪状軟骨弓 570, 571
― of the foot 足底弓 410
Archicortex 原皮質 594
Arcuate
― artery of kidney 弓状動脈《腎臓の》 179, **209**, 420, 445
― line
―― of ilium 弓状線《腸骨の》 **124**, 127, 129, 358
―― of pubis 弓状線《恥骨の》 129
―― of rectus sheath 弓状線《腹直筋鞘の》 131, 134, 135, 139
― popliteal ligament 弓状膝窩靱帯 385
― vein of kidney 弓状静脈《腎臓の》 179
Areola 乳輪 62, 121

Areolar
― glands 乳輪腺 62
― venous plexus 乳輪静脈叢 57
Arm 上腕 252
Arterial
― circle of Zinn チン動脈輪 517
― groove 動脈溝 457, 459, 526
Artery
― of central sulcus 中心溝動脈 609
― of ductus deferens 精管動脈 196, 199, **222**, 223
― of pancreatic tail 膵尾動脈 211
― of postcentral sulcus 中心後溝動脈 609
― of precentral sulcus 中心前溝動脈 609
― of pterygoid canal 翼突管動脈 490, 504
― of vestibular bulb 腟前庭球動脈 191, 195
Articular
― branch
―― of median nerve 関節枝《正中神経の》 328
―― of spinal nerve 関節枝《脊髄神経の》 36
― circumference
―― of head of radius 関節環状面《橈骨頭の》 280-282
―― of radius 関節環状面《橈骨の》 281, 287
―― of ulna 関節環状面《尺骨の》 280, 287
― disk
―― of sternoclavicular joint 関節円板《胸鎖関節の》 259
―― of temporomandibular joint 関節円板《顎関節の》 540, 541
― facet
―― for arytenoid cartilage 披裂関節面 570
―― for thyroid cartilage 甲状関節面 570
―― of arytenoid cartilage 関節面《披裂軟骨の》 570
― fovea of radius 関節窩《橈骨の》 280, 281, 286
― surface
―― for navicular（navicular articular surface）of talus 舟状骨関節面《距骨の》 403, 407
―― of lateral malleolus of fibula 外果関節面《腓骨の》 381
―― of medial malleolus（medial malleolar articular surface）of tibia 内果関節面《脛骨の》 381, 404, 405
―― of patella 関節面《膝蓋骨の》 383, 390
― tubercle of temporomandibular joint 関節結節《顎関節の》 526, 540, 541
Articularis genus 膝関節筋 367
Aryepiglottic fold 披裂喉頭蓋ヒダ 553, 572, **573**
Arytenoid 披裂筋 557
― cartilage 披裂軟骨 570, 571
Ascending
― (afferent) tracts of spinal cord 上行路（求心路）《脊髄》 613
― aorta 上行大動脈 **68**, 82-84, 87, 114
― branch
―― of lateral circumflex femoral artery 上行枝《外側大腿回旋動脈の》 440
―― of superficial petrosal artery 上行枝《浅錐体動脈の》 535
― cervical artery 上行頸動脈 317, 579, 610
― colon 上行結腸 142, 145, 147-149, 162, **164**, 165
― lumbar vein 上行腰静脈 35, **215**, 216, 219, 611
― part
―― of duodenum 上部《十二指腸の》 149, **160**, 161, 174

―― of trapezius 上行部《僧帽筋の》 22, 268, 276, 332
― pharyngeal artery 上行咽頭動脈 491, 492, **493**, 534, 556, 566
Atlanto-occipital
― joint 環椎後頭関節 **14**, 16, 18
― ligament 環椎後頭靱帯 17
Atlas（C1） 環椎（第1頸椎, C1） 4, 6, 7, 47, 600
Atrial branch of right coronary artery 心房枝《右冠状動脈の》 88
Atrioventricular（AV）
― node 房室結節 90
― bundle 房室束 90
Auditory
― (pharyngotympanic) tube 耳管 528, **530**, 531
― apparatus 聴覚器 536
― ossicles 耳小骨 532
Auricle 耳介 529
Auricular surface
― of ilium 耳状面《腸骨の》 124, 358
― of sacrum 耳状面《仙骨の》 10, 11
Auricularis
― anterior 前耳介筋 463, 466, **529**
― posterior（posterior auricular muscles） 後耳介筋 463, 466, **529**
― superior（superior auricular muscles） 上耳介筋 463, **466**, 529
Auriculotemporal nerve 耳介側頭神経 477, 488, 489, 499, 500, **502**, 503, 529, 541
Axilla 腋窩 333, 336
Axillary
― artery 腋窩動脈 56, 60, 62, **316**, 317, 320, 335-338
― lymph nodes 腋窩リンパ節 64, 319
― lymphatic plexus 腋窩リンパ叢 64
― nerve 腋窩神経 37, 320, 321, **324**, 330, 331, 333, 337
― recess 腋窩陥凹 261, 262
― vein 腋窩静脈 57, 60, 62, **318**, 335-338
Axis（C2） 軸椎（第2頸椎） 4, 6, 7
Azygos vein 奇静脈 35, 54, 55, 57, 61, **70**, 71, 78, 99, 611

B

Bare area of liver 無漿膜野《肝臓の》 170, 171
Bartholin's gland バルトリン腺 186, 192
Basal
― cistern 脳底槽 604
― ganglia 大脳基底核 592, 594
― tentorial branch of internal carotid artery テント底枝《内頸動脈の》 490
Base
― of lung 肺底 105
― of metacarpals 底《中手骨の》 299, 300
― of middle phalanx 底《中節骨の》 299
― of phalanges ［指（節）骨］底 300
― of prostate 前立腺底 200
― of proximal phalanx 基節骨の底《足の》 400
― of sacrum 仙骨底 5, 11
― of stapes アブミ骨底 532
Basilar
― artery 脳底動脈 490, **608**, 610
― plexus 脳底静脈叢 607
― vein 脳底静脈 606, 607
Basilic
― hiatus 尺側皮静脈の裂孔 **318**, 330
― vein 尺側皮静脈 **318**, 330, 339, 350, 351

Basivertebral vein　椎体静脈　611
Biceps
－brachii　上腕二頭筋　262，264，266，267，**278**，288，289，341，350
－femoris　大腿二頭筋　373，**379**，394，441，442，448，451
Bicipital aponeurosis　上腕二頭筋腱膜　266，288
Bifurcate ligament　二分靱帯　406，**408**，409
Bile
－duct　総胆管　171，**172**，173，175，179，210
－ducts　胆管　172
Bladder trigone　膀胱三角　185
Blind spot　盲点　616
Bochdalek's triangle (lumbocostal triangle)　ボクダレク三角（腰肋三角）　52，53
Body
－（shaft）of rib　肋骨体　45，47
－of（urinary）bladder　膀胱体　181，185，201
－of clitoris　陰核体　193
－of epididymis　精巣上体体　198
－of fornix　脳弓体　596
－of gallbladder　胆嚢体　172
－of hyoid bone　舌骨体　539，558
－of ilium　腸骨体　**124**，125，358，359
－of incus　キヌタ骨体　532
－of ischium　坐骨体　**124**，125，358，359
－of mandible　下顎体　539
－of pancreas　膵体　174，175
－of penis　陰茎体　197
－of pubis　恥骨体　124，125，359
－of sphenoid bone　蝶形骨体　461
－of sternum　胸骨体　44，**46**
－of stomach　胃体　158，159
－of talus　距骨体　**400**，401
－of tongue　舌体　548
Bony part of external auditory canal　骨性部《外耳道の》　528
Boyd's veins　ボイドの静脈群　423
Brachial
－artery　上腕動脈　**316**，317，336-339，341
－lymph node　上腕リンパ節　64
－plexus　腕神経叢　23，66，77，91，320，**321**，326，335，579，581，583
－vein　上腕静脈　**318**，336，337，339
Brachialis　上腕筋　264，267，**278**，288，289
Brachiocephalic
－lymph node　腕頭リンパ節　78，100
－trunk　腕頭動脈　34，68，78，83，84，**316**，557
－vein　腕頭静脈　35，57，**70**，71，77，78，83，99，114
Brachioradialis　腕橈骨筋　270，288，290，291，294，**295**，310，350
Brachium
－of inferior colliculus　下丘腕　599
－of superior colliculus　上丘腕　599
Brain　脳　592
Brainstem　脳幹　599
Breast　乳房　**62**，63，121
Bridging veins　架橋静脈　602，606
Broad ligament of uterus　子宮広間膜　152，**181**，183
Bronchial
－artery　気管支動脈　68，116
－tree　気管支樹　108，**111**
－veins　気管支静脈　117
Bronchiole　細気管支　111
Bronchomediastinal trunk　気管支縦隔リンパ本幹　72

Bronchopulmonary
－lymph node　気管支肺リンパ節　73，100，101，118，**119**
－segments　肺区域　108
Buccal
－artery　頬動脈　495，502，503，**504**
－branches of facial nerve　頬筋枝《顔面神経の》　478，488，498，500
－nerve　頬神経　**477**，488，489，502，503，546
Buccinator　頬筋　462，464，**467**，554
Buccopharyngeal part of superior pharyngeal constrictor　頬咽頭部《上咽頭収縮筋の》　554
Bulb of penis　尿道球　155，**185**，187，197
Bulbar
－fascia (Tenon's capsule)　眼球鞘（テノン嚢）　514
－penile
－－artery　尿道球動脈　202
－－veins　尿道球静脈　202，222
Bulbospongiosus　球海綿体筋　136，137，155，184，185，191，193，197
Bulbourethral gland　尿道球腺　150，184，185，187，197，**200**，201，203，205
Bundle of His　ヒス束　90

[C]

C1
－spinal nerve　第1頸神経　487，547，569
－vertebra　→ Atlas（C1）　第1頸椎（環椎）
C2
－spinal nerve　第2頸神経　569，600
－vertebra　→ Axis（C2）　第2頸椎（軸椎）
C4
－spinal nerve　第4頸神経　322
－vertebra　第4頸椎　601
C5 spinal nerve　第5頸神経　321
C8 spinal nerve　第8頸神経　321
Calcaneal
－branches of fibular artery　踵骨枝《腓骨動脈の》　421
－rete　踵骨動脈網　442
－tuberosity　踵骨隆起　357，**400**，401，404，407，412，415
Calcaneocuboid joint　踵立方関節　402，403
Calcaneofibular ligament　踵腓靱帯　409
Calcaneus　踵骨　356，**400**，401-407，410
Calcarine sulcus　鳥距溝　595
Callosomarginal artery　脳梁縁動脈　609
Calvaria　頭蓋冠　457
Canal of Schlemm　シュレム管　516，518
Canine　犬歯　542
Capitate　有頭骨　253，**298**，299-301，351，352
Capitelum of humerus　上腕骨小頭　**256**，257，282，285
Capitulotrochlear groove of humerus　小頭滑車溝《上腕骨の》　257
Capsular branches of renal artery　被膜枝《腎動脈の》　209
Capsule
－（external capsule）of thyroid gland　甲状腺被膜（外被膜）　574
－of zygapophyseal joint　関節包《椎間関節の》　16，18
Cardia　噴門　158，159
Cardiac
－apex　心尖　83-85，87
－branches of cardiac plexus　心臓枝《心臓神経叢の》　75

－impression　心圧痕　105
－lymphatic ring　噴門リンパ輪　101，230
－notch　心切痕　105
－orifice　噴門口　146，148，149
－plexus　心臓神経叢　75，91
－surface　心外膜　80
Caroticotympanic
－arteries　頸鼓動脈　534，535
－nerve　頸鼓神経　483
Carotid
－bifurcation　頸動脈分岐部　490，491，581
－body　頸動脈小体　556，**580**，581
－branch of glossopharyngeal nerve　頸動脈枝《舌咽神経の》　482
－canal　頸動脈管　458，526
－sheath　頸動脈鞘　23，577
－sinus　頸動脈洞　482
－triangle　頸動脈三角　**576**，580
Carpal
－articular surface of radius　手根関節面《橈骨の》　280，281
－bones　手根骨　252，**298**
－region　手根　342
－tunnel　手根管　303，342
Carpometacarpal joint　手根中手関節　300，301
Cartilaginous part
－of external auditory canal　軟骨性部《外耳道の》　528
－of pharyngotympanic tube　軟骨部《耳管の》　530，555
Cauda equina　馬尾　3，430，592，600，**601**
Caudal gonadal ligament (gubernaculum)　尾側性腺靱帯（導帯）　205
Caudate
－lobe of liver　尾状葉《肝臓の》　146，170，171
－nucleus　尾状核　594，609
－process of liver　尾状突起《肝臓の》　171
Caval hiatus (aperture) of diaphragm　大静脈孔《横隔膜の》　**52**，53，55，70，77
Cavernous
－nerves of penis　陰茎海綿体神経　243
－part of internal carotid artery　海綿静脈洞部《内頸動脈の》　490
－sinus　海綿静脈洞　496，497，510，567，**607**
－－branch of internal carotid artery　海綿静脈洞枝《内頸動脈の》　490
Cecal veins　盲腸静脈　220，221
Cecum　盲腸　142，145，148，152，153，162，**164**，165，182，183
Celiac
－branch of posterior vagal trunk　腹腔枝《後迷走神経幹の》　237，238，240
－ganglia　腹腔神経節　240，245
－lymph node　腹腔リンパ節　100，**226**，228，230-232
－plexus　腹腔神経叢　236
－trunk　腹腔動脈　54，55，143，147，178，206-208，**210**，211，216-219
Cementum　セメント質　542
Central
－axillary lymph node　中心腋窩リンパ節　64
－canal of spinal cord　中心管《脊髄の》　604，605
－gray substance　中心灰白質　474
－lobule of cerebellum　小脳中心小葉　598
－part of lateral ventricle　中心部《側脳室の》　605
－retinal
－－artery　網膜中心動脈　**510**，516，517
－－vein　網膜中心静脈　517
－slip　中間帯　311
－sulcus　中心溝　593，595，613

– tegmental tract　中心被蓋路　598
– tendon of diaphragm　腱中心《横隔膜の》　**52**, 53, 55, 61, 134
– vein of suprarenal gland　中心静脈《副腎の》　176
Cephalic vein　橈側皮静脈　57, 60, **318**, 330, 331, 334-336, 339, 350, 351
Ceratopharyngeal part of middle pharyngeal constrictor　大角咽頭部《中咽頭収縮筋の》　554
Cerebellar
– (posterior cranial) fossa　小脳窩（後頭蓋窩）　459
– peduncles　小脳脚　598
Cerebellomedullary cistern (cisterna magna)　小脳延髄槽（大槽）　604
Cerebellum　小脳　593, **598**, 599
Cerebral
– artery　大脳動脈　602
– aqueduct　中脳水道　474, 599, **604**, 605, 609
– arcuate fibers (U fibers)　大脳弓状線維　594
– cortex　大脳皮質　592, **594**, 595, 602
– fossa　大脳窩　459
– part of internal carotid artery　大脳部《内頸動脈の》　490, **608**
– peduncle　大脳脚　**594**, 598, 599, 605
– surface of sphenoid bone　大脳面《蝶形骨の》　461
Cerumen glands　耳道腺　528
Cervical
– branch of facial nerve　頸枝《顔面神経の》　478, 488, 500, 578, 582
– canal　子宮頸管　188, 189
– cardiac
– – branches of vagus nerve　頸心臓枝《迷走神経の》　485
– – nerves　頸心臓神経　75
– cord　頸髄　593
– enlargement　頸膨大　600
– fascia　頸筋膜　23, 556, 574, **577**, 578
– lymph node　頸リンパ節　64
– nerves　頸神経　584
– part　頸部
– – of esophagus　頸部《食道の》　77, 96
– – of internal carotid artery　頸部《内頸動脈の》　490, **608**
– – of parietal pleura　頸部《壁側胸膜の》　77
– – of trachea　頸部《気管の》　110
– plexus　頸神経叢　500
– posterior intertransversarius　頸後横突間筋　585
– vertebrae [C1–C7]　頸椎　**2**, 4, 6
Cervicothoracic junction　頸胸椎境界　2
Chamber (iridocorneal) angle　虹彩角膜角（隅角）　516, 518
Chiasmatic cistern　視交叉槽　604
Choana　後鼻孔　458, **520**, 521, 524, 538
Chondro-osseous junction　骨軟骨性接合部　51
Chondropharyngeal part of middle pharyngeal constrictor　小角咽頭部《中咽頭収縮筋の》　554
Chorda tympani　鼓索神経　478, 479, **481**, 503, 531, 532, 534, 536, 547
Chordae tendineae　腱索　85, 87
Choroid　脈絡膜　516, 519
– plexus　脈絡叢　596, 598
– – of 3rd ventricle　第三脳室脈絡叢　604
– – of 4th ventricle　第四脳室脈絡叢　604
– – of lateral ventricle　側脳室脈絡叢　604
Ciliary　睫毛腺　514
– body　毛様体　514, 516, 518, **519**

– ganglion　毛様体神経節　475, 477, **511**, 513, 617
– muscle　毛様体筋　516, 518, **519**, 617
– processes　毛様体突起　519
Cingular branch of callosomarginal artery　帯状回枝《脳梁縁動脈の》　609
Cingulate gyrus　帯状回　593, 595, 596, **621**
Cingulo-hippocampal fibers　帯状回海馬線維　621
Circular
– folds　輪状ヒダ　160, 162
– layer　輪筋層
– – of duodenum　輪筋層《十二指腸の》　**160**, 172
– – of esophagus　輪筋層《食道の》　97
– – of rectum　輪筋層《直腸の》　167
Circum (vallate) papilla　有郭乳頭　548
Circumflex
– artery of left coronary artery　回旋枝《左冠状動脈の》　88
– scapular artery　肩甲回旋動脈　316, **317**, 333, 336, 337
Cistern of lamina terminalis　終板槽　604
Cisterna
– chyli　乳ビ槽　72, **226**, 228
– magna (cerebellomedullary cistern)　大槽（小脳延髄槽）　604
Claustrum　前障　594, 609
Clavicle　鎖骨　47, 120, 252, 253, **254**, 258-260, 350
Clavicular
– head of sternocleidomastoid　鎖骨頭《胸鎖乳突筋の》　561
– notch　鎖骨切痕　44, **46**, 49
– part　鎖骨部
– – of deltoid　鎖骨部《三角筋の》　272
– – of pectoralis major　鎖骨部《大胸筋の》　264, 274, 334
Clitoral prepuce (prepuce of clitoris)　陰核包皮　136, 192, 193
Clitoris　陰核　186, 190, **192**, 193
Clivus　斜台　459, 509, 524
Coccygeal
– cornu　尾骨角　10
– nerve　尾骨神経　425
– plexus　尾骨神経叢　425
Coccygeus　尾骨筋　140, 141
Coccyx　尾骨　2-4, **10**, 11, 126, 127, 129, 136, 137, 141, 157, 166
Cochlea　蝸牛　481, 528, **536**
Cochlear
– aqueduct　蝸牛水管　530, 536
– communicating branch　蝸牛交通枝　537
– duct　蝸牛管　**536**, 617
– root (nerve) (CN Ⅷ)　蝸牛神経　480, 481, 528, 536, **537**, 619
Cockett's veins　コケットの静脈群　423
Colic
– branch of ileocolic artery　結腸枝《回結腸動脈の》　212, 213, 220
– impression of liver　結腸圧痕《肝臓の》　170
– surface of pancreas　結腸面《膵臓の》　174
– veins　結腸静脈　215
Collateral
– branch
– – of intercostal nerves　側副枝《肋間神経の》　61
– – of posterior intercostal arteries　側副枝《肋間動脈の》　56
– ligaments
– – of distal interphalangeal joint　側副靭帯《遠位指節間 (DIP) 関節の》　**302**, 304, 305, 308

– – of metacarpophalangeal joint　側副靭帯《中手指節 (MCP) 関節の》　301, **302**, 304, 305
– – of proximal interphalangeal joint　側副靭帯《近位指節間 (PIP) 関節の》　**302**, 304, 305
– trigone of lateral ventricle　側副三角《側脳室の》　605
Colles' fascia → superficial perineal fascia　コリース筋膜（浅会陰筋膜）
Colliculus of arytenoid cartilage　小丘《披裂軟骨の》　570, 571
Colon　結腸　164
Column of fornix　脳弓柱　596
Commissural cusp　交連尖　87
Commissure
– of inferior colliculus　下丘交連　619
– of lips　唇交連　589
Common
– basal vein of lower lobe of lung　総肺底静脈　115
– carotid
– – artery　総頸動脈　34, 68, 317, 335, 491-494, 556, 557, **566**, 575, 578, 579, 581, 608
– – plexus　総頸動脈神経叢　75
– cochlear artery　総蝸牛動脈　537
– crus of semicircular ducts　総脚《半規管の》　537
– facial vein　総顔面静脈　501, 502, 580
– fibular nerve　総腓骨神経　424, 425, **432**, 434, 435, 441-444
– flexor tendon sheath　指屈筋の総腱鞘　306
– hepatic
– – artery　総肝動脈　55, 147, 173, 207, **210**, 211, 212, 218
– – duct　総肝管　172, 173
– iliac
– – artery　総腸骨動脈　206, **208**, 213, 221-225, 420
– – lymph node　総腸骨リンパ節　**226**, 227-229, 234, 235
– – vein　総腸骨静脈　57, **214**, 215, 216, 221, 224, 225, 611
– interosseous artery　総骨間動脈　**316**, 317, 340
– palmar digital
– – arteries　総掌側指動脈　316, 317, **344**, 345
– – nerves　総掌側指神経　328-330
– plantar digital
– – arteries　総底側趾動脈　420
– – nerves　総底側趾神経　433, 446
– tendinous ring　総腱輪　475, **508**, 509
Communicating branch
– of fibular artery　交通枝《腓骨動脈の》　421
– to zygomatic nerve　頬骨神経との交通枝　477
Concha　耳甲介　529
Conducting system of heart　心臓刺激伝導系　90
Condylar
– canal　顆管　458, 606
– emissary vein　顆導出静脈　497, 606
– process of mandible　関節突起《下顎骨の》　539
Condyle of humerus　上腕骨顆　256
Cone of light　光錐　532
Confluence of sinuses　静脈洞交会　496, 497, 602, 604, **606**, 607
Conjunctiva　結膜　514
Conoid
– ligament　円錐靭帯　259
– tubercle　円錐靭帯結節　254
Conus
– arteriosus　動脈円錐　85

- branch of right coronary artery　円錐枝《右冠状動脈の》　88
- elasticus　弾性円錐　571, 572
- medullaris of spinal cord　脊髄円錐　3, 600
Convoluted seminiferous tubules　曲精細管　199
Cooper's (suspensory) ligaments of breast　クーパー靱帯（乳房提靱帯）　63
Coracoacromial
- arch　烏口肩峰弓　259, 261, 262
- ligament　烏口肩峰靱帯　258, 259, **261**, 262
Coracobrachialis　烏口腕筋　264, 265, 267, **274**
Coracoclavicular ligament　烏口鎖骨靱帯　**259**, 261, 332
Coracohumeral ligament　烏口上腕靱帯　261
Coracoid process　烏口突起　47, 120, 253, **255**, 258, 260, 262, 350
Cornea　角膜　514, 516, **518**
Corneoscleral limbus　角膜縁　516
Corniculate
- cartilage　小角軟骨　570, 571
- tubercle　小角結節　553, 573
Corona
- of glans　亀頭冠　197, 202
- radiata　放線冠　594
Coronal suture　冠状縫合　454, 457
Coronary
- ligament of liver　肝冠状間膜　170, 171
- sinus　冠状静脈洞　84, 86, 88
- sulcus　冠状溝　84, 85
Coronoid
- fossa of humerus　鈎突窩《上腕骨の》　256, 283, 285
- process
- - of mandible　筋突起《下顎骨の》　539, 540
- - of ulna　鈎状突起《尺骨の》　280-283, 285, 286
Corpus
- callosum　脳梁　593-595, **596**, 598, 605, 609, 621
- cavernosum of penis　陰茎海綿体　150, 184, 187, **197**, 201, 203
- spongiosum　尿道海綿体　184, 185, 187, **197**, 201, 203
- striatum　線条体　594
Corrugator
- cutis ani　肛門皺皮筋　167
- supercilii　皺眉筋　462, 464
Cortex of suprarenal gland　皮質《副腎の》　176
Corti organ　コルチ器　619
Cortical margin　皮質縁　609
Corticobulbar fibers　皮質延髄線維　486
Corticonuclear fibers　皮質核線維　615
Corticospinal
- (pyramidal) tract　皮質脊髄路（錐体路）　615
- fibers　皮質脊髄線維　615
Costal
- angle　肋骨角　44, 45, 47
- cartilage　肋軟骨　**44**, 45, 49, 130, 259, 265
- facet　肋骨窩　2, 5
- - on transverse process　横突肋骨窩　8
- groove　肋骨溝　61
- margin (arch)　肋骨弓　44, 265
- notch　肋骨切痕　46
- part
- - of diaphragm　肋骨部《横隔膜の》　**52**, 53, 55, 134
- - of parietal pleura　壁側胸膜の肋骨部（肋骨胸膜）　55, 61, 66, 78, 79, **103**, 104
- process　肋骨突起　5, 9

- surface
- - of lung　肋骨面《肺の》　105
- - of scapula　肋骨面《肩甲骨の》　255, 259
- - tubercle　肋骨結節　44, 45, 47, 49
Costocervical trunk　肋頸動脈　34, 317
Costoclavicular ligament　肋鎖靱帯　259
Costodiaphragmatic recess　肋骨横隔洞　103, 104
Costomediastinal recess　肋骨縦隔洞　93
Costotransverse
- joint　肋横突関節　44, 49
- ligament　肋横突靱帯　49
Costovertebral joints　肋椎関節　49
Costoxiphoid ligament　肋剣靱帯　49
Cranial
- fossa　頭蓋窩　459
- nerves　脳神経　470, 592
- root　延髄根　486
Craniocervical junction　頸椎後頭境界　2
Cremaster muscle　精巣挙筋　130, 131, **132**, 133, 196
Cremasteric
- (cremaster) fascia　精巣挙筋膜　132, 133, 196, 198
- artery　精巣挙筋動脈　196, 199
- vein　精巣挙筋静脈　196, 199
Crest
- of greater tuberosity of humerus　大結節稜《上腕骨の》　256
- of lesser tuberosity of humerus　小結節稜《上腕骨の》　256, 257
- of neck of rib　肋骨頸稜　47
Cribriform plate　篩板　459, **460**, 520-525, 603
Cricoarytenoid
- joint　輪状披裂関節　571
- ligament　輪状披裂靱帯　571
Cricoid cartilage　輪状軟骨　96, 110, 550, 558, **570**, 571
Cricopharyngeal part of inferior pharyngeal constrictor　輪状咽頭部《下咽頭収縮筋の》　554
Cricothyroid　輪状甲状筋　485, 554, **572**, 574, 578, 579
- branch of superior thyroid artery　輪状甲状枝《上甲状腺動脈の》　566, 575
- joint　輪状甲状関節　571
- ligament　輪状甲状靱帯　571, 574
Cricotracheal ligament　輪状気管靱帯　571
Crista
- galli　鶏冠　460, 507, 520
- terminalis　分界稜　85
Crown of tooth　歯冠　542
Cruciform ligaments　［線維鞘の］十字部　304-306, 412, 417
Crura of antihelix　対輪脚　529
Crural chiasm　下腿交叉　395, 399
Crus
- of clitoris　陰核脚　151, 155, 184, 186, 191, 193
- of fornix　脳弓脚　596
- of penis　陰茎脚　153, 155, 185, 197
Cubital
- fossa　肘窩　339
- lymph node　肘リンパ節　64, **319**
Cuboid　立方骨　**400**, 402, 403, 406, 410
- articular surface of calaneus　立方骨関節面《踵骨の》　407
Culmen　山頂　598
Cuneiform tubercle　楔状結節　553, **572**, 573
Cuneiforms　楔状骨群　405
Cuneocerebellar fibers　楔状束核小脳線維　614

Cuneocuboid joint　楔立方関節　402
Cuneonavicular joint　楔舟関節　402
Cutaneous
- branch
- - of deep fibular nerve　皮枝《深腓骨神経の》　444, 445
- - of obturator nerve　皮枝《閉鎖神経の》　428, 435, 440
- vein　皮静脈　57
Cymba conchae　耳甲介舟　529
Cystic
- artery　胆嚢動脈　171, **210**, 211
- duct　胆嚢管　171-173
- lymph node　胆嚢リンパ節　231
- vein　胆嚢静脈　215

D

Decussation of pyramids　錐体交叉　599, 615
Deep
- auricular artery　深耳介動脈　495, 504, **534**, 535
- branch
- - of lateral plantar nerve　深枝《外側足底神経の》　446, 447
- - of medial plantar artery　深枝《内側足底動脈の》　420, 446, 447
- - of radial nerve　深枝《橈骨神経の》　320, 339, 341
- - of ulnar artery　深枝《尺骨動脈の》　342, 343, 345
- - of ulnar nerve　深枝《尺骨神経の》　329, 342, 343, 345
- cervical
- - artery　深頸動脈　317
- - lymph node　深頸リンパ節　119
- - vein　深頸静脈　567, 611
- circumflex
- - iliac artery　深腸骨回旋動脈　**208**, 216, 225, 420
- - iliac vein　深腸骨回旋静脈　216, 225
- clitoral
- - artery　陰核深動脈　195
- - veins　陰核深静脈　195
- dorsal
- - clitoral vein　深陰核背静脈　191, 195
- - penile vein　深陰茎背静脈　181, 197, **202**, 203, 222, 223, 225
- facial vein　深顔面静脈　497
- fascia of the leg　下腿筋膜　442, 444
- femoral vein　大腿深静脈　422
- fibular nerve　深腓骨神経　424, **432**, 434, 444, 445
- head
- - of flexor pollicis brevis　深頭《短母指屈筋の》　308
- - of medial pterygoid　深頭《内側翼突筋の》　468
- inguinal
- - lymph node　深鼠径リンパ節　227-229, **234**, 235, 436
- - ring　深鼠径輪　131, **133**, 152, 183
- layer
- - of nuchal fascia　深葉《項筋膜の》　23, 26
- - of thoracolumbar fascia　深葉《胸腰筋膜の》　23, 27
- lingual
- - artery　舌深動脈　549
- - vein　舌深静脈　549
- median cubital vein　深肘正中皮静脈　318, 339
- middle cerebral vein　深中大脳静脈　607

Deep palmar
- palmar
 -- arch　深掌動脈弓　316, 317, 343, **345**
 -- venous arch　深掌静脈弓　318
- parotid lymph nodes　深耳下腺リンパ節　587
- part
 -- of external anal sphincter　深部《外肛門括約筋の》　167
 -- of masseter　深部《咬筋の》　463, 467, 468
 -- of parotid gland　深部《耳下腺の》　551
- penile
 -- artery　陰茎深動脈　197, 202
 -- fascia　深陰茎筋膜　197, 201, 202
 -- veins　陰茎深静脈　202, 222
- petrosal nerve　深錐体神経　479, 505
- plantar
 -- artery　深足底動脈　445
 -- arch　深足底動脈弓　420, 447
- popliteal lymph nodes　深膝窩リンパ節　443
- temporal
 -- arteries　深側頭動脈　495, 502, **504**
 -- nerves　深側頭神経　477, 488, 502, **503**, 541
 -- veins　深側頭静脈　497
- transverse
 -- metacarpal ligament　深横中手靱帯　**302**, 304-307, 311
 -- metatarsal ligament　深横中足靱帯　410
- perineal　深会陰横筋　151, **155**, 184, 190, 191, 193-195, 197, 200, 201
Deferential plexus　精管神経叢　243, 247
Deltoid　三角筋　22, 40, 120, 264-266, 268, 270, **272**, 332, 350, 351
- branch of thoracoacromial artery　三角筋枝《胸肩峰動脈の》　316
- ligament　三角靱帯　**408**, 409
- tuberosity of humerus　三角筋粗面《上腕骨の》　**256**, 272
Deltopectoral groove　三角筋胸筋溝　120, 318
Dens of axis (C2)　歯突起《第2頸椎の》　3, 4, 7, 47, 524, 556
Dentate gyrus　歯状回　596
Denticulate ligament　歯状靱帯　601
Dentin　象牙質　542
Depressor
- anguli oris　口角下制筋　462-464, **467**, 561
- labii inferioris　下唇下制筋　**462**, 463, 464, 467
- septi nasi　鼻中隔下制筋　464
Descending
- aorta　下行大動脈　66, **68**, 79, 93
- branch
 -- of lateral circumflex femoral artery　下行枝《外側大腿回旋動脈の》　440
 -- of occipital artery　下行枝《後頭動脈の》　493
 -- of superficial petrosal artery　下行枝《浅錐体動脈の》　535
- colon　下行結腸　145, 147, 148, 156, 159, 161, **164**, 165, 175, 213
- genicular artery　下行膝動脈　**420**, 440
- palatine artery　下行口蓋動脈　495, **504**, 524, 525
- part
 -- of duodenum　下行部《十二指腸の》　147, 149, **160**, 161, 172, 174, 176
 -- of trapezius　下行部《僧帽筋の》　22, 268, 276, 332, 561
Detrusor vesicae　排尿筋　185
Diagonal conjugate　対角結合線　129
Diagonal stria　対角帯　472, 620

Diaphragm　横隔膜　48, **52**, 53-55, 66, 77, 81, 112
Diaphragma sellae　鞍隔膜　603
Diaphragmatic
- fascia　横隔膜筋膜　81
- part of parietal pleura　壁側胸膜の横隔部（横隔胸膜）　54, 55, 66, 77, 97, **103**, 104, 134
- surface
 -- of lung　横隔面《肺の》　105
 -- of pancreas　横隔面《膵臓の》　174
Diencephalon　間脳　594, **596**, 599
Digastric
- branch of facial nerve　二腹筋枝《顔面神経の》　547
- muscle　顎二腹筋　464, 465, 544, 554, 555, 562, **563**, 580
Diploë of calvaria　板間層《頭蓋冠の》　457, 602
Diploic veins　板間静脈　457, 602
Distal
- extension creases　遠位伸筋線　353
- interphalangeal joint
 -- 遠位指節間（DIP）関節　300, 301, **302**, 304, 305, 311, 352
 -- 遠位趾節間（DIP）関節　402
 -- capsule　関節包《遠位指節間（DIP）関節》　302
 -- crease　遠位指節間（DIP）関節線　353
- phalanges of foot　末節骨《足の》　397, 400, **401**, 402
- phalanx of hand　末節骨《手の》　252, 253, **298**, 300, 301, 305, 311
- radioulnar joint　下橈尺関節　**281**, 286, 287, 301
- transverse crease　遠位横手掌線　353
- wrist crease　遠位手根線　353
Dodd's veins　ドッドの静脈群　423
Dorsal
- (posterior)
 -- branch (ramus) of thoracic aorta　後枝《胸大動脈の》　34, 610
 -- ramus
 --- of posterior intercostal artery　後枝《肋間動脈の》　56, 61
 --- of sacral nerve　後枝《仙骨神経の》　36, 430
 --- of spinal nerve　後枝《脊髄神経の》　**36**, 39, 58, 59, 321, 332, 600
 -- root
 --- of sacral nerve　背側根（後根）《仙骨神経の》　36, 430
 --- of spinal nerve　後根《脊髄神経の》　59, 321, **600**, 601, 615
- aponeurosis　趾背腱膜　415
- branch/es
 -- of palmar digital nerves　背側枝《掌側指神経の》　344, 346
 -- of ulnar nerve　背側枝《尺骨神経の》　329, 331, 346
- calcaneocuboid ligaments　背側踵立方靱帯　406, 409
- callosal branch of posterior cerebral artery　背側脳梁枝《後大脳動脈の》　609
- carpal
 -- artery　背側手根動脈　317, 347
 -- branch
 --- of radial artery　背側手根枝《橈骨動脈の》　347
 --- of ulnar artery　背側手根枝《尺骨動脈の》　317, 341, 347
 -- network　背側手根動脈網　317, 347
 -- tendon sheaths　背側手根腱鞘　310

- carpometacarpal ligaments　背側手根中手靱帯　302
- clitoral
 -- artery　陰核背動脈　191, 195
 -- nerve　陰核背神経　191, 194, 195
- digital
 -- arteries
 --- 背側指動脈　**317**, 344, 347
 --- 背側趾動脈　445
 -- expansion　指背腱膜　297, **311**, 353
 -- nerves
 --- 背側指神経　329, 331, 344, **346**
 --- 背側趾神経　445
 -- veins　背側指静脈　318, 331
- intercarpal ligaments　背側手根間靱帯　302
- interossei
 -- of foot　背側骨間筋《足の》　411-414, 419
 -- of hand　背側骨間筋《手の》　301, 307-311, 314, 315, 352
- longitudinal fasciculus　背側縦束　472
- metacarpal arteries　背側中手動脈　317, 347
- metatarsal
 -- arteries　背側中足動脈　420, 445
 -- ligaments　背側中足靱帯　408
- nerve of penis (dorsal penile nerve)　陰茎背神経　197, 202, 203, **243**
- nasal
 -- artery　鼻背動脈　490, 492, 498, **510**, 512
 -- vein　鼻背静脈　510, 512
- pancreatic artery　後膵動脈　211
- pedal artery　足背動脈　420, 445
- penile
 -- artery　陰茎背動脈　197, **202**, 203, 225
 -- nerve (dorsal nerve of penis)　陰茎背神経　197, 202, 203, **243**
- radiocarpal ligament　背側橈骨手根靱帯　302
- radioulnar ligament　背側橈骨尺靱帯　286, 287, **302**
- root of spinal nerve　後根《脊髄神経の》　59
- scapular
 -- artery　肩甲背動脈　317
 -- nerve　肩甲背神経　320, 321, **322**
- talonavicular ligament　背側距舟靱帯　408, 409
- tarsal ligaments　背側足根靱帯　408, 409
- tegmental nucleus　後被蓋核　619, 620
- tubercle of radius　背側結節《橈骨の》　**280**, 281, 290, 291, 310
- vagal nucleus　迷走神経背核　471, **484**, 619
- venous
 -- arch of foot　足背静脈弓　422
 -- network
 --- of foot　足背静脈網　422
 --- of hand　手背静脈網　**318**, 331, 351, 353
Dorsolateral arm territory　上腕背外側領域　319
Dorsomedial arm territory　上腕背内側領域　319
Dorsum
- of penis　陰茎背　225
- of tongue　舌背　548, 550
- sellae　鞍背　459, 461, 524
Ductus
- deferens　精管　157, 180-182, 187, **196**, 198, 199, 205, 225
- reuniens　結合管　536
Duodenal
- branch of anterior superior pancreaticoduodenal artery　十二指腸枝《前上膵十二指腸動脈の》　211
- bulb　［十二指腸］球部　160
- diverticula　十二指腸憩室　161
- impression of liver　十二指腸圧痕《肝臓の》　170

Duodenojejunal flexure 十二指腸空腸曲 148, 160, 162
Duodenum 十二指腸 142, 143, 146, 148, 149, 156, 159, **160**, 172-175, 210, 213
Dura mater of calvaria 硬膜《頭蓋冠の》 457, 537, 601, **602**
Dural
－sac 硬膜嚢 601
－sheath 視神経外鞘 514
－sinus 硬膜静脈洞 457

E

Earlobe 耳垂 529
Edinger-Westphal（visceral oculomotor）nuclei エディンガー－ウェストファル核（動眼神経副核） 471, **474**, 617
Efferent
－ductules 精巣輸出管 198, 199
－fibers 遠心性線維 54
－nuclei 遠心性核 612
Ejaculatory duct 射精管 187, **200**, 201
Elbow joint 肘関節 252, **282**, 284, 285
Emissary vein 導出静脈 457, 602
Enamel エナメル質 542
Endolymphatic
－duct 内リンパ管 536
－sac 内リンパ嚢 530, 536, 537
Endometrium 子宮内膜 188
Endoneural space 神経内腔 604
Endothoracic fascia 胸内筋膜 53, 61, **103**
Epicolic lymph node 結腸壁リンパ節 233
Epididymal duct 曲精巣上体管 199
Epididymis 精巣上体 187, 196, **198**, 205, 225, 234
Epidural space 硬膜上腔 601
Epiglottic cartilage 喉頭蓋軟骨 570, 571
Epiglottis 喉頭蓋 550, 552, 553, 558, **573**
Epiphyseal
－line 骨端線《大腿骨の》 363
－ring 輪状骨端 12
Epiploic appendices 腹膜垂 144, **145**, 162, 164
Episcleral space 強膜外腔 514
Epitympanum 上鼓室 531
Epoöphoron 卵巣上体 189, 205
Erb's point 神経点（エルブ点） 582
Erector spinae 脊柱起立筋 **31**, 41, 53, 269
Esophageal
－branches 食道動脈 68, 99
－－of recurrent laryngeal nerve 食道枝《反回神経の》 98, 99
－hiatus (aperture) of diaphragm 食道裂孔 52, 55, 70, 77, **97**
－inlet 食道入口 96
－plexus 食道神経叢 74, 75, **98**
－veins 食道静脈 **99**, 215, 218
Esophagus 食道 23, 77-79, **96**, 97, 104, 158, 159
Ethmoid
－bone 篩骨 454, 455, **460**, 506, 507, 520, 523, 538
－bulla 篩骨胞 460, 521
－infundibulum 篩骨漏斗 460
－sinus 篩骨洞（篩骨蜂巣） 522, 523
Excretory duct 排出管 187
Extensor
－carpi
－－radialis
－－－brevis 短橈側手根伸筋 268, 270, 288, 290, 291, 294, **295**, 309, 310
－－－longus 長橈側手根伸筋 268, 270, 288, 290, 291, 294, **295**, 309, 310, 350, 351
－－－－tendon 長橈側手根伸筋の腱 290
－－ulnaris 尺側手根伸筋 268, 270, **290**, 297, 309, 310, 351
－digiti minimi 小指伸筋 290, 296, **297**, 309, 310, 353
－digitorum ［総］指伸筋 268, 270, 290, 296, **297**, 309, 310, 347, 351, 353
－－brevis 短趾伸筋 392, 393, 415, **416**
－－－tendons 短趾伸筋の腱 415, 416
－－longus 長趾伸筋 392, **397**, 404, 415
－－－tendon 長趾伸筋の腱 397, 415
－－tendon
－－－［総］指伸筋の腱 290, 305, 311, 351
－－－［総］趾伸筋の腱 450
－－hallucis
－－－brevis 短母趾伸筋 392, 415, **416**
－－－longus 長母趾伸筋 392, 393, **397**, 404, 415, 450
－－－tendon 長母趾伸筋の腱 397, 415, 443
－indicis 示指伸筋 290, 291, **297**, 309, 310, 353
－－tendon 示指伸筋の腱 352
－pollicis
－－brevis 短母指伸筋 290, 291, 297, 307-309, **310**, 353
－－longus 長母指伸筋 290, 291, 296, **297**, 309, 310, 352, 353
－－－tendon 長母指伸筋の腱 290
－retinaculum
－－of foot 伸筋支帯《足の》 353
－－of hand 伸筋支帯《手の》 310
External
－acoustic opening 外耳孔 526
－anal sphincter 外肛門括約筋 136, 137, 150, 151, 166, **167**, 182-184, 194, 203
－auditory canal (external acoustic meatus) 外耳道 454, 526, **528**, 529, 530
－branch
－－of accessory nerve 外枝《副神経の》 580, 581, 583
－－of superior laryngeal nerve 外枝《上喉頭神経の》 485, **575**, 578, 579
－capsule 外包 594
－(capsule) of thyroid gland 甲状腺被膜（外被膜） 574
－carotid
－－artery 外頸動脈 490, **491**, 492-494, 556, 566, 580, 581, 608
－－plexus 外頸動脈神経叢 75
－ear 外耳 528
－genitalia 外生殖器 186, 192
－granular layer (Ⅱ) 外顆粒層 595
－iliac
－－artery 外腸骨動脈 149, 151, 152, 155, 184, 208, 222, **223**, 224, 225, 420, 440
－－lymph node 外腸骨リンパ節 227-229, **234**, 235, 436
－－vein 外腸骨静脈 151, 155, 184, 216, 222, **223**, 224, 225, 436, 440
－intercostal
－－membrane 外肋間膜 51
－－muscles 外肋間筋 26, 27, 50, **51**, 61, 130
－jugular vein 外頸静脈 496, 499, 557, **567**, 578-580, 582, 583
－medullary lamina 外側髄版 597
－nasal branch of maxillary nerve 外鼻枝《上顎神経の》 525
－oblique 外腹斜筋 22, 26, 40, 53, 61, 130-134, 138, **139**, 248, 264, 268, 269
－－aponeurosis 外腹斜筋腱膜 **130**, 132-134, 139, 436, 440
－occipital
－－crest 外後頭稜 458
－－protuberance 外後頭隆起 24, 25, **456**, 458, 588
－os of uterus 外子宮口 189, **190**, 191
－palatine vein 外口蓋静脈 497
－pudendal
－－arteries 外陰部動脈 202, **225**, 420, 436, 440
－－veins 外陰部静脈 57, 202, **225**, 422, 434, 436
－pyramidal layer (Ⅲ) 外錐体細胞層 595
－spermatic fascia 外精筋膜 132, 196, 198, **199**, 202
－urethral orifice 外尿道口 136, **185**, 190, 192, 194, 197
－vertebral venous plexus 外椎骨静脈叢 **35**, 497, 606
Extraocular muscle 外眼筋 508
Extrapyramidal motor system 錐体外路系 615
Extreme capsule 最外包 594
Eyeball 眼球 514, **516**
Eyelid 眼瞼 514

F

Facial
－artery 顔面動脈 **298**, 491-493, 498, 500, 501, 512
－canal 顔面神経管 478
－colliculus 顔面神経丘 599
－nerve (CN Ⅶ) 顔面神経 **478**, 479, 488, 498, 500, 501, 547, 551, 599
－nucleus 顔面神経核 471, 478
－vein 顔面静脈 **496**, 497-501, 512, 567
Falciform ligament of liver 肝鎌状間膜 144, 159, **171**
Fallopian tube ファロービウス管 151
False ribs 仮肋 45
Falx cerebri 大脳鎌 602, 603
Fascia lata 大腿筋膜 133, **438**, 440, 441
Faucial isthmus 口峡部 550, 553
Female
－pelvis 女性骨盤 126
－urethra 女性尿道 185
Femoral
－artery 大腿動脈 157, 196, 208, 225, **420**, 434, 436, 440
－branch of genitofemoral nerve 大腿枝《陰部大腿神経の》 426, 427, 436
－nerve 大腿神経 135, 157, 424-426, **429**, 434, 435, 440
－ring 大腿輪 135, 437
－vein 大腿静脈 57, 157, 196, 208, 225, **422**, 423, 434, 436, 440
Femoropatellar joint 膝蓋大腿関節 386
Femoropopliteal vein 大腿膝窩静脈 422
Femur 大腿骨 356, **360**, 361, 362, 364, 365, 448
Fibrous
－appendix of liver 線維付着《肝臓の》 171
－capsule
－－of kidney 線維被膜《腎臓の》 23, 178, 179, 209
－－of suprarenal gland 線維被膜《副腎の》 176

Fibrous lumbar triangle

- lumbar triangle (of Grynfeltt) 上腰三角（グランフェルト三角） 39
- membrane 線維膜 365
- pericardium 線維性心膜 77-79, **80**, 81, 83
- stroma 線維性間質 196

Fibula 腓骨 356, **380**, 381, 404, 405, 415, 448

Fibular
- artery 腓骨動脈 **420**, 421, 442, 445
- veins 腓骨静脈 422

Fibularis
- brevis 短腓骨筋 392-394, **396**, 404, 413-415, 442, 445
- longus 長腓骨筋 373, 392-394, **396**, 404, 410, 412, 413, 415, 442, 450
- - tendon 長腓骨筋の腱 **396**, 411, 413, 414, 419, 451
- tertius 第3腓骨筋 392, 393, 396, **397**, 415

Filiform papillae 糸状乳頭 548
Fimbria of hippocampus 海馬采 596

Flexor
- carpi
- - radialis 橈側手根屈筋 288, **292**, 293, 306, 309, 350
- - - tendon 橈側手根屈筋の腱 307, 308, 352
- - ulnaris 尺側手根屈筋 268, 270, 288, 290, **293**, 306, 309, 350, 351
- - - tendon 尺側手根屈筋の腱 302, 307, 308, 352
- digiti
- - minimi
- - - brevis
- - - - 短小指屈筋 306-309, **312**, 313
- - - - 短小趾屈筋 412-414, **418**, 419
- digitorum
- - brevis 短趾屈筋 404, 411, 412, **417**, 446, 447
- - - tendons 短趾屈筋の腱 412, 413, 446, 447
- - longus 長趾屈筋 394, 395, **399**, 411-413, 415, 419, 442, 443
- - - tendon 長趾屈筋の腱 **413**, 418, 419, 446, 447, 451
- - profundus 深指屈筋 289-291, **293**, 307, 309, 311
- - - tendons 深指屈筋の腱 288, 289, 304, 305, **306**, 307, 308, 311, 315
- - superficialis 浅指屈筋 288, 289, 292, **293**, 306, 309, 311, 342
- - - tendon 浅指屈筋の腱 288, 304-308, 311
- hallucis
- - brevis 短母趾屈筋 411-414, 418, **419**, 447
- - longus 長母趾屈筋 394, 395, **399**, 404, 411, 413, 415, 442, 443
- - - tendon 長母趾屈筋の腱 399, **412**, 413, 446, 447
- pollicis
- - brevis 短母指屈筋 306, 308, 309, 312, **313**, 353
- - longus 長母指屈筋 288, 289, 292, **293**, 306, 307, 309
- - - tendon 長母指屈筋の腱 288, **289**, 306, 308
- retinaculum
- - of foot 屈筋支帯《足の》 **415**, 442, 443
- - of hand 屈筋支帯《手の》 303, **306**, 307, 308, 328, 329, 344

Flexors of forearm 前腕屈筋 289

Floating ribs 浮遊肋 45
Flocculonodular lobe 片葉小節葉 598
Flocculus 片葉 598
Folium vermis 虫部葉 598
Follicular stigm 卵胞口 188
Foot 足 356

Foramen
- cecum 舌盲孔 548
- lacerum 破裂孔 458, 459
- magnum 大後頭孔 **458**, 459, 486
- ovale 卵円孔 **458**, 459, 461, 477, 503, 538
- rotundum 正円孔 461, **477**, 506
- spinosum 棘孔 458, 459, **461**

Forceps major 大鉗子 594
Forearm 前腕 252
Forefoot 前足（前足骨） 400
Fornix 脳弓 595, **596**, 598, 605, 621

Fossa
- of lacrimal sac 涙嚢窩 506
- ovalis 卵円窩 85

Fourth ventricle 第四脳室 598, 599, **605**

Fovea
- centralis 中心窩 516, 616
- of femoral head 大腿骨頭窩 360, 361, 364

Free margin of ovary 自由縁《卵巣の》 188

Frenulum
- of ileal orifice 回腸口小帯 164
- of lower lip 下唇小帯 550
- of tongue 舌小帯 549
- of upper lip 上唇小帯 550

Frontal
- belly of occipitofrontalis 前頭《後頭前頭筋の》 462, 463
- bone 前頭骨 454, **455**, 457, 459, 506, 507, 520, 523
- branch
- - of middle meningeal artery 前頭枝《中硬膜動脈の》 495, 603
- - of superficial temporal artery 前頭枝《浅側頭動脈の》 494, 499
- crest 前頭稜 457, 459
- incisure 前頭切痕 455, 506
- lobe 前頭葉 593
- nerve 前頭神経 475, 477, **511**, 512, 513
- pole 前頭極 595
- process of maxilla 前頭突起《上顎骨の》 506, 520, 521
- sinus 前頭洞 457, 459, 472, **507**, 520-524

Frontotemporal fasciculus 前頭側頭束 594

Fundus
- of bladder 膀胱底 201
- of gallbladder 胆嚢底 172
- of stomach 胃底 158, 159

Fungiform papilla 茸状乳頭 548

G

Galea aponeurotica 帽状腱膜 462, 463, 602
Galen's anastomosis ガレノス交通枝 575
Gallbladder 胆嚢 142, 144, 146-148, 156, 159, 163, 168, 171, **172**, 173, 175, 210
Ganglion impar 不対神経節 236, 237
Gartner's duct ガルトナー管 205

Gastric
- artery 胃動脈 210
- impression of liver 胃圧痕《肝臓の》 170
- plexus 胃神経叢 91, 238
- surface
- - of pancreas 胃面《膵臓の》 174

- - of spleen 胃面《脾臓の》 148, 175
Gastrocnemius 腓腹筋 392, 394, **398**, 442, 448, 450, 451
Gastrocolic ligament 胃結腸間膜 146, 147
Gastroduodenal artery 胃十二指腸動脈 207, 210, **211**, 212, 218-221
Gastrosplenic ligament 胃脾間膜 147, **148**, 149, 163, 168

Gemellus
- inferior 下双子筋 370-372, **375**, 438, 439, 448
- superior 上双子筋 370-372, 374, **375**, 438, 439, 448

General
- somatic efferent fiber (somatomotor function) 一般体性遠心性線維（体性運動機能） 471
- visceral efferent fiber (visceromotor function) 一般臓性遠心性線維（内臓運動機能） 471

Genicular veins 膝静脈 422
Geniculate ganglion 膝神経節 **478**, 479, 536, 547, 619
Genioglossus オトガイ舌筋 464, 465, **544**, 548, 550
Geniohyoid オトガイ舌骨筋 465, 544, 548, 550, 562, **563**
- branch of C1 オトガイ舌骨筋枝《第1頸神経の》 547

Genital
- branch of genitofemoral nerve 陰部枝《陰部大腿神経の》 133, 196, 203, 426, **427**, 436
- organs
- - of female 生殖器《女性の》 186
- - of male 生殖器《男性の》 187

Genitofemoral nerve 陰部大腿神経 132, 133, 179, 194, 196, 424-426, **427**, 434, 436

Genu of internal capsule 内包膝 594
Gingival margin 歯肉縁 542
Glabella 眉間 454, 520

Glans
- of clitoris 陰核亀頭 136, 186, 193, 194
- penis 陰茎亀頭 137, 185, 187, **197**, 198, 201, 202, 225

Glenohumeral
- joint 肩甲上腕関節 258, 260
- ligaments 関節上腕靱帯 261

Glenoid
- cavity of scapula 関節窩《肩甲骨の》 **255**, 259, 260, 262
- labrum of scapula 関節唇《肩甲骨の》 262

Globus pallidus 淡蒼球 594, 609

Glossopharyngeal
- nerve (CN IX) 舌咽神経 470, **482**, 483, 547, 599, 619
- part of superior pharyngeal constrictor 舌咽頭部《上咽頭収縮筋の》 554

Gluteal
- aponeurosis 殿筋腱膜 22
- fascia 殿筋膜 438, 441
- fold (sulcus) 殿溝 41, 438, 451
- region 殿部 438
- surface of ilium 殿筋面《腸骨の》 125, 126, 359
- tuberosity of femur 殿筋粗面《大腿骨の》 360, 362

Gluteus
- maximus 大殿筋 40, 136, 137, 157, 194, 203, 369-374, **375**, 438, 441, 451
- medius 中殿筋 40, 367, 370-374, **375**, 438, 441, 448, 451

– minimus 小殿筋 367, 370-372, 374, **375**, 439, 441, 448
Gonad primordium 性腺原基 205
Graafian follicle グラーフ卵胞 188
Gracilis 薄筋 194, 203, 366, 367, 369-371, **376**, 438-442, 448
Granular foveolae クモ膜顆粒小窩 457, 602
Gray
– matter
––（substance）of spinal cord 灰白質《脊髄の》 592, 612
–– of brain 灰白質《脳の》 592
– ramus communicans 灰白交通枝 59, **237**, 242, 243, 600, 622
Great
– anterior segmental medullary artery 大前髄節動脈 610
– auricular nerve 大耳介神経 37, 38, 334, 499, **568**, 569, 578, 582-585
– cardiac vein 大心臓静脈 88
– cerebral vein 大大脳静脈 606, 607
– pancreatic artery 大膵動脈 211
Greater
– arterial circle of iris 大虹彩動脈輪 517, 518
– curvature of stomach 大弯《胃の》 158, 159
– horn of hyoid bone 大角《舌骨の》 539, 558, 570
– occipital nerve 大後頭神経 37, 38, 499, **568**, 584, 585
– omentum 大網 143, **144**, 146-148, 156, 159, 175
– palatine
–– artery 大口蓋動脈 495, **504**, 524, 525, 546
–– canal 大口蓋管 538
–– foramen 大口蓋孔 458, 538
–– nerve 大口蓋神経 **505**, 525, 546
– petrosal nerve 大錐体神経 **478**, 479, 481, 505
– sciatic
–– foramen 大坐骨孔 129, 439
–– notch 大坐骨切痕 **125**, 126, 359, 439
– splanchnic nerve 大内臓神経 55, 74, 78, 98, 72, 237, 238-240, 245, 623
– trochanter 大転子 40, 356, 357, **360**, 361-365, 370, 450
– tubercle（tuberosity）of humerus 大結節《上腕骨の》 253, 256, 257, 259, **260**, 350, 351
– vestibular gland 大前庭腺 186, 205
– wing of sphenoid bone 大翼《蝶形骨の》 454, 455, 459, **461**, 507, 523
Groove
– for fibularis longus tendon 長腓骨筋腱溝 401
– for flexor hallucis longus tendon 長母趾屈筋腱溝 407
– for sigmoid sinus S状洞溝 459, 526
– for subclavian artery 鎖骨下動脈溝 47, 565
– for subclavian vein 鎖骨下静脈溝 47
– for subclavius muscle 鎖骨下筋溝 254
– for superior sagittal sinus 上矢状洞溝 457
– for transverse sinus 横洞溝 459
– for vena cava 大静脈溝 171
– for vertebral artery 椎骨動脈溝 **6**, 7, 16, 17

[H]

Habenular nuclei 手綱核 472, 620
Hamate 有鈎骨 298, 301
Hand 手 252
Handle of malleus ツチ骨柄 532, 534

Hard palate 硬口蓋 **524**, 530, 538, 550
Haustra of colon 結腸膨起 164, 165
Head
– of caudate nucleus 尾状核頭 594
– of epididymis 精巣上体頭 198
– of femur 大腿骨頭 155, 157, **360**, 361-363, 421
– of fibula 腓骨頭 356, 357, **380**, 381, 393, 451
– of humerus 上腕骨頭 **256**, 257-260
– of malleus ツチ骨頭 532
– of mandible 下顎頭 539-541, 563
– of metacarpals 中手骨の頭 299, 300, 353
– of middle phalanx of hand 中節骨の頭《手の》 299
– of pancreas 膵頭 174, 175
– of phalanges ［指（節）骨］頭 300
– of proximal phalanx of foot 基節骨の頭《足の》 400
– of radius 橈骨頭 252, 253, **281**, 282, 285, 351
– of rib 肋骨頭 45, 47
– of stapes アブミ骨頭 532
– of talus 距骨頭 **400**, 401, 405
– of tibia 脛骨頭 380
– of ulna 尺骨頭 280, 281, 286
Heart 心臓 82, **84**
Helicis
– major 大耳輪筋 529
– minor 小耳輪筋 529
Helicotrema 蝸牛孔 536
Helix 耳輪 529, 589
Hemiazygos vein 半奇静脈 35, 54, 55, 57, **70**, 71, 79, 99, 117, 214, 215, 611
Hepatic
– branch
–– of anterior vagal trunk 肝枝《前迷走神経幹の》 238, 240
–– of posterior vagal trunk 肝枝《後迷走神経幹の》 238
– duct 肝管 177
– lymph node 肝リンパ節 230, 231
– plexus 肝神経叢 238, 240, 245
– surface of diaphragm 肝臓の付着部《横隔膜の》 146
– veins 肝静脈 82, 216, 218, 219
Hepatoduodenal ligament 肝十二指腸間膜 146, 148, 149, **159**, 163, 168, 177
Hepato-esophageal ligament 肝食道間膜 159
Hepatogastric ligament 肝胃間膜 143, 148, **159**, 163, 168
Hepatopancreatic
– ampulla 胆膵管膨大部 172
– duct 胆膵管 173
Hesselbach's triangle ヘッセルバッハ三角 133
Hiatus of canal for greater petrosal nerve 大錐体神経管裂孔 478
Hilum
– of lung 肺門 105
– of spleen 脾門 174
Hindfoot 後足 400
Hip
– bone 寛骨 124, 125, 356, **358**
– joint 股関節 356, **362**, 363, 364
Hippocampus 海馬 596, 609, **621**
Hook of hamate 有鈎骨鈎 299, 350, 352
Horizontal
– fissure
–– of cerebellum 水平裂《小脳の》 598
–– of lung 水平裂《肺の》 93, 104, 105, 109

– part of duodenum 水平部《十二指腸の》 143, 148, 149, **160**, 161, 172, 174
– plate of palatine bone 水平板《口蓋骨の》 521
Humeral
– axillary lymph node 上腕腋窩リンパ節 64
– head
–– of flexor digitorum superficialis 上腕頭《浅指屈筋の》 292
–– of pronator teres 上腕頭《円回内筋の》 289
Humeroradial joint 腕橈関節 282
Humeroulnar joint 腕尺関節 282, 283
Humerus 上腕骨 252, 253, **256**, 257, 259, 260
Hyaline cartilage end plate 硝子軟骨性関節面 12
Hyaloid fossa 硝子体窩 516
Hyoepiglottic ligament 舌骨喉頭蓋靭帯 573
Hyoglossus 舌骨舌筋 465, **544**, 545, 548, 554
Hyoid
– bone 舌骨 465, **539**, 544, 558
– muscles 舌骨筋 464
Hypogastric nerve 下腹神経 **237**, 239, 241-243, 247
Hypoglossal
– canal 舌下神経管 458, 459, 487
– nerve（CN XII）舌下神経 470, **487**, 501, 547, 549, 580, 581, 599
– trigone 舌下神経三角 487
Hypophyseal fossa（sella turcica）of sphenoid bone 下垂体窩《蝶形骨の》 459, **461**, 520, 521, 524
Hypophysis 下垂体 593, 595, **596**, 599, 605
Hypothalamic sulcus（ventral diencephalic sulcus）視床下溝 596
Hypothalamus 視床下部 593, **596**, 598, 618
Hypothenar eminence 小指球 350, 352, 353
Hypotympanum 下鼓室 531

[I]

Ileal
– arteries 回腸動脈 212, 220, **221**
– branch of ileocolic artery 回腸枝《回結腸動脈の》 212, 213, 220
– veins 回腸静脈 215, 220, **221**
Ileocecal orifice 回腸口 164
Ileocolic
– artery 回結腸動脈 207, **212**, 213, 220, 221, 241
– lymph node 回結腸リンパ節 232, 233
– labrum（superior lip）回結腸唇（上唇） 164
– vein 回結腸静脈 215, **220**, 221
Ileum 回腸 142-145, 148, 153, **162**, 165, 182
Iliac
– crest 腸骨稜 4, 22, 40, 120, **124**, 125-127, 268, 356-359, 362, 364, 365, 450, 451
– fossa 腸骨窩 124, 126, 127
– part of latissimus dorsi 腸骨部《広背筋の》 277
– plexus 腸骨動脈神経叢 239, 243
– tubercle 腸骨結節 126, 127
– tuberosity 腸骨粗面 **124**, 126, 127, 129, 358
– wing 腸骨翼 125, 126, 359
Iliacus 腸骨筋 134, 135, 139, 180, 225, 366, 367, 369, 374, **375**, 376
Iliococcygeus 腸骨尾骨筋 140, 141
Iliocostalis 腸肋筋 26, 30, 560
– cervicis 頚腸肋筋 27, **30**, 31
– lumborum 腰腸肋筋 27, 30, **31**

‒ thoracis 胸腸肋筋 27，**31**
Iliofemoral ligament 腸骨大腿靱帯 364，365，367
Iliohypogastric nerve 腸骨下腹神経 37，58，133，176，178，179，424-426，**427**，434，435，438，441
Ilioinguinal nerve 腸骨鼡径神経 132，176，178，179，194，196，202，203，424-426，**427**，434，436
Iliolumbar
‒ artery 腸腰動脈 208，222，223
‒ ligament 腸腰靱帯 **128**，365
‒ triangle 下腰三角（プチ三角）39
Iliopectineal
‒ arch 腸恥筋膜弓 135，437
‒ bursa 腸恥包 437
Iliopsoas 腸腰筋 135，138，**139**，157，366，367，429，440
Iliopubic eminence 腸恥隆起 127，437
Iliotibial tract 腸脛靱帯 366，367，370，**373**，440，441，448，451
Ilium 腸骨 **124**，125-127，129，181，359
Impression for costoclavicular ligament 肋鎖靱帯圧痕 254
Incisive
‒ canal 切歯管 520，538
‒ foramen 切歯孔 456，458，538
‒ fossa 切歯窩 538，542
‒ suture 切歯縫合 542
Incisors 切歯 542
Incudo-malleolar joint キヌタ-ツチ関節 532
Incudo-stapedial joint キヌタ-アブミ関節 532
Incus キヌタ骨 528，530，531，**532**
Indusium griseum 脳梁灰白層 596
Inferior
‒ (temporal) horn of lateral ventricle 下角《側脳室の》596，605
‒ alveolar
‒‒ artery 下歯槽動脈 492，**495**，502-504，556
‒‒ nerve 下歯槽神経 477，488，498，502，503，**546**，547，556
‒ anastomotic vein 下吻合静脈 606
‒ angle of scapula (inferior scapular angle) 下角《肩甲骨の》4，40，253，**255**，351
‒ articular
‒‒ facet of vertebra 下関節面《椎骨の》6-9
‒‒ process 下関節突起 5-9
‒‒ surface of tibia 下関節面《脛骨の》381，405
‒ basal vein of lower lobe of lung 下肺底静脈 115
 belly of omohyoid 下腹《肩甲舌骨筋の》563
‒ border
‒‒ of liver 下縁《肝臓の》171
‒‒ of lung 下縁《肺の》105
‒‒ of pancreas 下縁《膵臓の》174
‒ branch of oculomotor nerve 下枝《動眼神経の》475，511，512
‒ cerebellar peduncle 下小脳脚 598，599
‒ cerebral veins 下大脳静脈 602，607
‒ cervical ganglion 下頸神経節 91
‒ choroidal vein 下脈絡叢静脈 607
‒ cluneal nerves 下殿皮神経 39，194，203，424，430，435，**438**，441
‒ collicular nucleus 下丘核 619
‒ colliculus of quadrigeminal plate 下丘《四丘体板の》599
‒ costal facet 下肋骨窩 5，8，49
‒ dental branches of inferior alveolar nerve 下歯枝《下歯槽神経の》477，546

‒ duodenal
‒‒ flexure 下十二指腸曲 160
‒‒ recess 下十二指腸陥凹 161
‒ epigastric
‒‒ artery 下腹壁動脈 133，135，180，208，222，**225**，420
‒‒ vein 下腹壁静脈 133，135，180，215，216，**225**
‒ extensor retinaculum 下伸筋支帯 415，443
‒ fascia of pelvic diaphragm (inferior pelvic diaphragmatic fascia) 下骨盤隔膜筋膜 136，137，152，153，**154**，167，191
‒ fibular retinaculum 下腓骨筋支帯 415
‒ ganglion 下神経節 482，483，**484**，619
‒ gluteal
‒‒ artery 下殿動脈 **222**，224，420，438-441
‒‒ line of ilium 下殿筋線《腸骨の》125，359
‒‒ nerve 下殿神経 425，**431**，438，439，441
‒‒ veins 下殿静脈 216，**222**，223，224，438，439
‒ head (part) of lateral pterygoid 下頭《外側翼突筋の》469，541
‒ horn
‒‒ of lateral ventricle 下角《側脳室の》596，605
‒‒ of thyroid cartilage 下角《甲状軟骨の》558，570，571
‒ hypogastric plexus 下下腹神経叢（骨盤神経叢）236，**239**，244-247，623
‒ hypophyseal artery 下下垂体動脈 490
‒ inguinal lymph node 下浅鼡径リンパ節 423，436
‒ labial artery 下唇動脈 492
‒ lacrimal canaliculi 下涙小管 515
‒ laryngeal
‒‒ artery 下喉頭動脈 575
‒‒ nerve 下喉頭神経 485，557，**575**，579
‒‒ vein 下喉頭静脈 557，**575**
‒ lateral brachial cutaneous nerve 下外側上腕皮神経 **325**，330-332
‒ lip 回盲唇（下唇）164
‒ lobar bronchi 下葉気管支 77，104
‒ lobe of lung 下葉《肺の》93，104，105
‒ longitudinal muscle 下縦舌筋 548
‒ meatus 下鼻道 **521**，525
‒ mediastinum 下縦隔 66
‒ mesenteric
‒‒ artery 下腸間膜動脈 149，180，206-208，**213**，216，217，221，223-225
‒‒ ganglion 下腸間膜動脈神経節 **237**，239，241，244-247
‒‒ lymph node 下腸間膜リンパ節 226-228，**233**，234，235
‒‒ plexus 下腸間膜神経叢 236，**237**，239，241-245
‒‒ vein 下腸間膜静脈 215，219，220，**221**，224
‒ nasal concha 下鼻甲介 455，507，515，**521**，522，523，525，538，553
‒ nuchal line 下項線 25，28，**456**，458
‒ oblique 下斜筋 475，**508**，509，514
‒‒ part of longus colli 下斜部《頸長筋の》29，565
‒ olive 下オリーブ核 615
‒ ophthalmic vein 下眼静脈 496，**510**，512，513，567
‒ orbital fissure 下眼窩裂 458，477，**506**，507，509，538
‒ pair of parathyroid glands 下副甲状腺（下上皮小体）574

‒ pancreatic
‒‒ artery 下膵動脈 211，219
‒‒ lymph node 下膵リンパ節 231
‒ pancreaticoduodenal
‒‒ artery 下膵十二指腸動脈 207，**211**，212，218
‒‒ vein 下膵十二指腸静脈 215
‒ part
‒‒ of nucleus of solitary tract 下部《孤束核の》482，484
‒‒ of vestibular ganglion 下部《前庭神経節の》481，536，537
‒ pelvic diaphragmatic fascia (inferior fascia of pelvic diaphragm) 下骨盤隔膜筋膜 136，137，152，153，**154**，167，191
‒ petrosal sinus 下錐体静脈洞 497，**607**
‒ pharyngeal constrictor 下咽頭収縮筋 77，97，**554**，555
‒ phrenic
‒‒ artery 下横隔動脈 **54**，68，178，179，208，217
‒‒ lymph node 下横隔リンパ節 **101**，118，226，228，229
‒‒ vein 下横隔静脈 178，214，216，217
‒ pole of kidney 下端《腎臓の》178
‒ posterior nasal branches of greater palatine nerve 下後鼻枝《大口蓋神経の》525
‒ pubic ramus 恥骨下枝 124-126，136，137，150-153，155，191，358，359
‒ puncta 下涙点 515
‒ recess of omental bursa 下陥凹《網嚢の》146
‒ rectal
‒‒ artery 下直腸動脈 195，202，203，222，223，**224**
‒‒ nerves 下直腸神経 194，195，202，203，243
‒‒ plexus 下直腸動脈神経叢 243，245
‒‒ veins 下直腸静脈 195，202，203，215，222，223，**224**
‒ rectus 下直筋 475，**508**，509，514
‒ root of ansa cervicalis 下根《頸神経ワナの》547，568，569
‒ sagittal sinus 下矢状静脈洞 606
‒ salivatory nucleus 下唾液核 471，482
‒ segmental artery of renal artery 下区動脈《腎動脈の》209
‒ suprarenal artery 下副腎動脈 177-179，208，**209**，217
‒ tarsal muscle 下瞼板筋 514
‒ tarsus 下瞼板 514
‒ thoracic aperture 胸郭下口 44
‒ thyroid
‒‒ artery 下甲状腺動脈 99，317，557，566，574，**575**，579，581
‒‒ notch 下甲状切痕 570
‒‒ tubercle 下甲状結節 570
‒‒ vein 下甲状腺静脈 54，66，70，77，99，**575**，579
‒ tracheobronchial lymph node 下気管気管支リンパ節 100，101，118，**119**
‒ transverse rectal fold 下直腸横ヒダ 167
‒ tympanic artery 下鼓室動脈 534，535
‒ ulnar collateral artery 下尺側側副動脈 **316**，338-340
‒ vena cava 下大静脈 35，55，57，70，71，82，88，208，210-215，**216**，217-220
‒ vertebral notch 下椎切痕 8，9
‒ vesical
‒‒ artery 下膀胱動脈 157，208，222，**223**，225

– – vein 下膀胱静脈 216, **223**
– vestibular nucleus 前庭神経下核 480, 618
Inflection points 内弯点 3
Infraclavicular fossa 鎖骨下窩 334
Infraglenoid tubercle of scapula 関節下結節《肩甲骨の》 **255**, 260
Infraglottic cavity (subglottic space) 声門下腔 573
Infrahyoid
– branch of superior thyroid artery 舌骨下枝《上甲状腺動脈の》 566
– muscles 舌骨下筋群 544, 569
Infraorbital
– artery 眼窩下動脈 492, 495, 498, 503, **504**, 512
– canal 眼窩下管 **506**, 507
– foramen 眼窩下孔 454, 455, 477, **506**, 515
– groove 眼窩下溝 506
– margin 眼窩下縁 455, 589
– nerve 眼窩下神経 477, 498-500, **505**, 512
– vein 眼窩下静脈 510
Infrapatellar
– branch of saphenous nerve 膝蓋下枝《伏在神経の》 429, 434
– bursa 深膝蓋下包 390, 391
– fat pad 膝蓋下脂肪体 390, 391
Infraspinatus 棘下筋 22, 262, 269, 270, **273**, 351
Infraspinous
– fascia 棘下筋膜 332
– fossa of scapula 棘下窩《肩甲骨の》 **255**, 260, 261
Infrasternal angle 胸骨下角 48
Infratemporal fossa 側頭下窩 502, 503
Infratrochlear nerve 滑車下神経 477, 500, **511**, 512, 513
Infundibular recess 漏斗陥凹 596, 605
Infundibulum
– of gallbladder 胆嚢漏斗 172
– of hypophysis 漏斗《下垂体の》 596, 598, 605
– of uterine tube 卵管漏斗 189
Inguinal
– canal 鼠径管 **133**, 187
– ligament 鼠径靱帯 **128**, 130, 131, 133, 135, 139, 225, 248, 364-366, 436, 437, 440, 450
– region 鼠径部 **132**, 436
Inlet (aditus) to mastoid antrum 乳突洞口 531
Inner
– hair cells 内有毛細胞 619
– lip of iliac crest 内唇《腸骨稜の》 127
– oblique fibers of stomach 斜線維《胃の》 158
– table of clavaria 内板《頭蓋冠の》 457, 602
Innermost intercostals 最内肋間筋 50, **51**, 61
Insula 島 595, 609, 619
Insular part (M2) of middle cerebral artery 島部 (M2区)《中大脳動脈の》 608
Interalveolar septum
– 槽間中隔 542
– 肺胞中隔 111
Interatrial
– bundle 心房間束 90
– septum 心房中隔 85, 87
Intercapitular veins 中手骨頭間静脈 318, 331
Interclavicular ligament 鎖骨間靱帯 259
Intercondylar
– eminence of tibia 顆間隆起《脛骨の》 380-382
– line of femur 顆間線《大腿骨の》 360
– notch of femur 顆間窩《大腿骨の》 360, 382
Intercostal
– lymph node 肋間リンパ節 73, 118

– lymphatics 肋間リンパ管 72, 100
– muscles 肋間筋 50
– nerves 肋間神経 36, 37, 39, 55, **58**, 60-62, 74, 78, 79, 98, 156, 330
– vein 肋間静脈 60, 78, 79, 156, 611
Intercostobrachial nerves 肋間上腕神経 **36**, 58, 321, 326, 330, 331
Intercrural fibers 脚間線維 133, 437
Intercuneiform joints 楔間関節 402
Interfoveolar ligament 窩間靱帯 133, 135
Interganglionic trunk of sympathetic trunk 節間枝《交感神経幹の》 237
Interhemispheric cistern 脳梁周囲槽 604
Interlobar
– artery 葉間動脈 179, 209
– vein 葉間静脈 179
Interlobular artery 小葉間動脈 209
Intermediate
– cuneiform 中間楔状骨 **400**, 401-403, 410
– dorsal cutaneous nerve 中間足背皮神経 432, 434, 444, 445
– hepatic veins 中間肝静脈 171
– lacunar lymph node 中間裂孔リンパ節 228, 229, 235
– laryngeal cavity (transglottic space) 喉頭室（声門間腔）573
– line of iliac crest 中間線《腸骨稜の》 127
– lumbar lymph node 中間腰リンパ節 156, **228**, 229, 234, 235
– mesenteric lymph node 中間腸間膜リンパ節 232
– supraclavicular nerves 中間鎖骨上神経 582, 583
– tendon
– – of digastric muscle 中間腱《顎二腹筋の》 544
– – of omohyoid 中間腱《肩甲舌骨筋の》 563
Intermesenteric plexus 腸間膜動脈間神経叢 236, **237**, 239, 241-244, 247
Intermetatarsal joints 中足間関節 402
Internal
– acoustic
– – meatus 内耳道 459
– – opening 内耳孔 526
– anal sphincter 内肛門括約筋 167
– auditory artery 内耳動脈 535
– branch of superior laryngeal nerve 内枝《上喉頭神経の》 485, **575**, 578, 580
– capsule 内包 594, 609
– carotid
– – artery 内頸動脈 34, 481, **490**, 491-493, 500, 501, 510, 524, 532, 556, 566, 580, 581, 608
– – plexus 内頸動脈神経叢 75, 481, **483**, 505
– cerebral vein 内大脳静脈 606, 607
– genitalia 内生殖器 186
– genu of facial nerve 顔面神経膝（内膝）478
– granular layer (Ⅳ) 内顆粒層 595
– iliac
– – artery 内腸骨動脈 **34**, 202, 208, 222-225, 420
– – lymph node 内腸骨リンパ節 **227**, 228, 229, 235
– – vein 内腸骨静脈 35, 202, 216, 222-225, 611
– intercostals 内肋間筋 50, **51**, 61, 130
– jugular vein 内頸静脈 23, 35, 57, 70, 71, 114, 335, **496**, 497, 500, 501, 556, 557, 567, 575, 578, 580, 581, 606, 611
– medullary lamina 内側髄板 597

– nasal branches of maxillary nerve 内鼻枝《上顎神経の》 525
– oblique 内腹斜筋 22, 26, 27, 130, 131, 133, 138, **139**, 268, 269, 525
– – aponeurosis 内腹斜筋腱膜 **130**, 134, 139
– occipital
– – protuberance 内後頭隆起 18
– – vein 内後頭静脈 606
– os 内子宮口 189
– pudendal
– – artery 内陰部動脈 195, 202, 203, 208, 222, 223, **224**, 439
– – vein 内陰部静脈 195, 202, 203, 216, 222, 223, **224**, 439
– pyramidal layer (Ⅴ) 内錐体細胞層 595
– spermatic fascia 内精筋膜 133, 196, 198, **199**, 225
– thoracic
– – artery 内胸動脈 34, 54, 55, **56**, 60-62, 66, 68, 77, 99, 156, 316, 317
– – veins 内胸静脈 35, 55, **57**, 60-62, 66, 70, 77, 155, 156, 185, 215
– urethral orifice 内尿道口 155, 185
interneurons 介在ニューロン 615
Interossei
– of foot 骨間筋《足の》 392, 402, 415
– of hand 骨間筋《手の》 307-309
Interosseous
– border
– – of radius 骨間縁《橈骨の》 280, **281**
– – of ulna 骨間縁《尺骨の》 280, **281**
– membrane
– – of forearm 前腕骨間膜 281, **286**, 292, 293, 295, 301, 317
– – of leg 下腿骨間膜 380, 420, 448
– recurrent artery 反回骨間動脈 317, 341
– sacroiliac ligaments 骨間仙腸靱帯 128, 129
– slip 骨間筋腱線維 311
– talocalcanean ligament 骨間距踵靱帯 402, 405, 406, **409**
Interpectoral axillary lymph node 胸筋間腋窩リンパ節 64
Interpeduncular
– cistern 脚間槽 604
– fossa 脚間窩 599
– nucleus 脚間核 472, 620
– veins 脚間静脈 607
Interphalangeal (IP) joint
– of hand 指節間関節 253, 301, 350
– of foot 趾節間関節 357, 450
Interscalene space 斜角筋隙 321, 565
Interspinales 棘間筋 32, **33**
– cervicis 頸棘間筋 25, 27
– lumborum 腰棘間筋 27, 32, **33**
Interspinous
– distance of anterior iliac spines 上前腸骨棘間径 127
– ligaments 棘間靱帯 12, 18, 19, **20**
Intertendinous connections of extensor digitorum 腱間結合《[総]指伸筋の》 290, 310
Interthalamic adhesion 視床間橋 596, 605
Intertragic incisure 珠間切痕 529
Intertransversarii cervicis 頸横突間筋 25
Intertransversarii 横突間筋 32
– laterales lumborum 腰外側横突間筋 27, 32, **33**
– mediales lumborum 腰内側横突間筋 27, 32, **33**
Intertransverse ligaments 横突間靱帯 17, 18, **20**, 21

Intertrochanteric
- crest 転子間稜《大腿骨の》 360, 362, 365
- line 転子間線《大腿骨の》 360, 362, 365

Intertubercular
- groove of humerus 結節間溝《上腕骨の》 **256**, 257, 259-262
- synovial sheath 結節間滑液鞘 261

Interureteral fold 尿管間ヒダ 185

Interventricular
- foramen 室間孔 604, 605
- septum 心室中隔 **85**, 87, 90, 93

Intervertebral
- disk 椎間円板 2-4, **12**, 20, 21, 44, 49, 129
- foramen 椎間孔 2, **8**, 9, 12, 601
- surface 椎間面 12
- vein 椎間静脈 35, 611

Intestinal trunk 腸リンパ本幹 226, 228

Intra-articular ligament of head of rib 関節内肋骨頭靱帯 49

Intrapulmonary lymph node 肺内リンパ節 73, 118, **119**

Intrinsic back muscles 固有背筋 23, 53, 61

Investing layer (superficial layer) of cervical fascia 浅葉《頸筋膜の》 23, 574, 577, 578, 580

IP joint crease 指節間関節線 353

iridocorneal (chamber) angle 虹彩角膜角（隅角） 516, 518

Iris 虹彩 514, 516, **518**, 519

Iris stroma 虹彩支質 518

Ischial
- ramus 坐骨枝 124-126, 136, 137, 359
- spine 坐骨棘 **124**, 125-127, 129, 136, 141, 157, 356, 358, 359, 362, 364, 365
- tuberosity 坐骨結節 40, **124**, 125, 126, 129, 136, 137, 141, 194, 203, 356-359, 362, 365, 450

Ischioanal fossa 坐骨肛門窩（坐骨直腸窩） 154, 155

Ischiocavernosus 坐骨海綿体筋 136, 137, **140**, 155, 191, 193, 194, 197, 203

Ischiofemoral ligament 坐骨大腿靱帯 364, 365

Ischiopubic ramus of hip bone 坐骨恥骨枝《寛骨の》 197

Ischium 坐骨 **124**, 125, 126, 359

Isocortex 等皮質 595

Isthmus
- of thyroid gland 甲状腺峡部 574
- of uterine tube 卵管峡部 189

J・K

Jejunal
- arteries 空腸動脈 **212**, 220, 221
- veins 空腸静脈 215, **220**, 221

Jejunum 空腸 142-145, 160, 161, **162**, 165, 173, 174

Joint
- capsule
- - of elbow joint 関節包《肘関節の》 285
- - of glenohumeral joint 関節包《肩関節の》 261, 262
- - of knee joint 関節包《膝関節の》 390
- - of temporomandibular joint 関節包《顎関節の》 463, 540, 541
- of head of rib 肋骨頭関節 49
- space of sternocostal joint 関節隙《胸肋関節の》 49

Jugular
- foramen 頸静脈孔 **458**, 459, 486, 607
- fossa 頸静脈窩 526
- notch 頸切痕 44, **46**, 120
- trunk 頸リンパ本幹 72
- venous arch 頸静脈弓 567, 578
- veins 頸静脈 496

Jugum sphenoidale 蝶形骨隆起 459, 461

Junction of esophageal and gastric mucosae (Z line) 食道と胃粘膜との境界（Z 線） 97

Juxtaintestinal lymph node 小腸傍リンパ節 232

Kidney 腎臓 23, 142, 147, 149, 156, 159, 161, 175, **176**, 177-180, 186, 187, 209, 218

Kiesselbach's area キーゼルバッハ部位 524

Knee joint 膝関節 356, 382

L

L1 vertebra 第 1 腰椎 4
L2 vertebra 第 2 腰椎 600, 601
L4 vertebra 第 4 腰椎 9
L5 vertebra 第 5 腰椎 150, 151, 364, 365, 600

Labium
- majus 大陰唇 136, 185, 186, 191, **192**
- minus (minor) 小陰唇 136, 185, 186, 190, 191, **192**, 194

Labyrinthine artery 迷路動脈 608

Lacrimal
- artery 涙腺動脈 510, 513
- apparatus 涙器 515
- bone 涙骨 454, 506, 521
- caruncle 涙丘 515
- gland 涙腺 475, **515**
- nerve 涙腺神経 475, 477, **511**, 512, 513
- part of orbicularis oculi 涙嚢部《眼輪筋の》 464
- punetum 涙点 515
- sac 涙嚢 515
- vein 涙腺静脈 510

Lactiferous
- duct 乳管 63
- sinus 乳管洞 63

Lacuna
- musculorum 筋裂孔 437
- vasorum 血管裂孔 437

Lacunar ligament 裂孔靱帯 132, 133, **436**, 437

Lambdoid suture ラムダ縫合 454, **456**, 457

Lamina
- cribrosa of sclera 強膜篩板 516
- of cricoid cartilage 輪状軟骨板 570, 571
- of vertebral arch 椎弓板 5, 7, 8

Large intestine 大腸 164

Laryngeal
- glands 喉頭腺 573
- inlet 喉頭口 553
- prominence 喉頭隆起 558, **570**, 571
- saccule 喉頭小嚢 573

Laryngopharyngeal branch of superior cervical ganglion 喉頭咽頭枝《上頸神経節の》 117

Laryngopharynx 咽頭喉頭部 550

Lateral
- abdominal wall muscles 側腹筋 23
- ampullary nerve 外側膨大部神経 **481**, 536, 537
- angle of scapula 外側角《肩甲骨の》 255
- antebrachial cutaneous nerve 外側前腕皮神経 327, **330**, 331, 339
- aortic lymph node 外側大動脈リンパ節 226, 227, **228**, 229
- aperture of 4th ventricle 第四脳室外側口 599
- arcuate ligament 外側弓状靱帯 52, 53
- bands of hand 外側帯《手の》 311
- basal
- - segment of lung 外側肺底区 108
- - segmental artery of lung 外側肺底動脈 115
- border
- - of humerus 外側縁《上腕骨の》 256
- - of kidney 外側縁《腎臓の》 178
- - of scapula 外側縁《肩甲骨の》 **255**, 260, 262
- branch
- - of iliohypogastric nerve 外側枝《腸骨下腹神経の》 430, 438, 441
- - of left coronary artery 外側枝《左冠状動脈の》 88
- - of sacral nerve 外側枝《仙骨神経の》 36
- - of supraorbital nerve 外側枝《眼窩上神経の》 498
- calcaneal branches of sural nerve 外側踵骨枝《腓腹神経の》 433, 444
- caval lymph node 外側大静脈リンパ節 228
- cervical region (posterior triangle) 外側頸三角部（後頸三角） 576, 582
- circumflex femoral
- - artery 外側大腿回旋動脈 **420**, 440
- - veins 外側大腿回旋静脈 422
- collateral ligament of knee joint 外側側副靱帯《膝関節の》 384-386, 388-390
- condyle
- - of femur 外側顆《大腿骨の》 356, 360, 361, 382
- - of tibia 外側顆《脛骨の》 356, 357, **380**, 381, 382, 393, 450
- cord 外側神経束 320, 321, **326**, 327, 328, 336-338
- costotransverse ligament 外側肋横突靱帯 49
- cricoarytenoid 外側輪状披裂筋 572
- crus
- - of major alar cartilage 外側脚《大鼻翼軟骨の》 520
- - of superficial inguinal ring 外側脚《浅鼠径輪の》 132, 133, 437
- cuneiform 外側楔状骨 **400**, 401-403, 410
- cutaneous branch
- - of 4th intercostal nerves 外側皮枝《第4肋間神経の》 326
- - of iliohypogastric nerve 外側皮枝《腸骨下腹神経の》 58, 426, 427, 435
- - of intercostal nerves 外側皮枝《肋間神経の》 37, 58, 61, 330
- - of posterior intercostal
- - - arteries 外側皮枝《肋間動脈の》 39, **56**, 610
- - - veins 外側皮枝《肋間静脈の》 39
- - of spinal nerve 外側皮枝《脊髄神経の》 **36**, 37, 58, 59
- - of thoracic aorta 外側皮枝《胸大動脈の》 34
- dorsal cutaneous nerve 外側足背神経 433, **435**, 444, 445
- epicondyle
- - of femur 外側上顆《大腿骨の》 357, 360, 382, **451**
- - of humerus 外側上顆《上腕骨の》 253, **256**, 257, 285, 350
- femoral cutaneous nerve 外側大腿皮神経 424-426, **427**, 434-436, 440
- frontobasal artery 外側前頭底動脈 609
- funiculus of spinal cord 側索《脊髄の》 613
- geniculate body 外側膝状体 **473**, 598, 616, 617

- head
  - - of flexor hallucis brevis 外側頭《短母趾屈筋の》 413, 419
  - - of gastrocnemius 外側頭《腓腹筋の》 370, 371, 393, 394, **398**, 442
  - - of triceps brachii 外側頭《上腕三頭筋の》 268, 270, **279**, 333, 350, 351
- horn of spinal cord 側角《脊髄の》 612
- inferior genicular artery 外側下膝動脈 420, 421, **443**
- inguinal fossa 外側鼠径窩 **135**, 153, 182
- intermuscular septum of arm 外側上腕筋間中隔 333
- ligament of malleus 外側ツチ骨靱帯 532
- lacuna 外側裂孔 602
- lacunar lymph node 外側裂孔リンパ節 229
- lemniscus 外側毛帯 619
- ligament of temporomandibular joint 外側靱帯《顎関節の》 463, 468, 540
- lip of femur 外側唇《大腿骨の》 360
- longitudinal patellar retinaculum 外側縦膝蓋支帯 384
- lumbar lymph node 外側腰リンパ節 156
- malleolar
  - - articular surface 外果関節面 404, 405
  - - branches of fibular artery 外果枝《腓骨動脈の》 421
  - - fossa of fibula 外果窩《腓骨の》 380, 381
  - - surface of talus 外果面《距骨の》 403, 405, 407
- malleolus 外果 356, 357, **380**, 381, 394, 404, 405, 442, 444, 450
- mammary branches
  - - of intercostal nerves 外側乳腺枝《肋間神経の》 62
  - - of lateral thoracic artery 外側乳腺枝《外側胸動脈の》 62
- masses of atlas 外側塊《環椎の》 7
- meniscus 外側半月 386, **387**, 388-390
- nasal
  - - branches of maxillary nerve 外側鼻枝《上顎神経の》 525
  - - cartilage 外側鼻軟骨 520
- occipital artery (P3) 外側後頭動脈 (P3区) 608, 609
- olfactory stria 外側嗅条 472, 620
- part
  - - of sacrum 外側部《仙骨の》 5, 10, 11
  - - of vaginal fornix 外側部《腟円蓋の》 189
  - - parts of cerebellum 外側部《小脳の》 598
- pectoral nerve 外側胸筋神経 320, 321, **326**, 334-336
- pericardial lymph node 心膜外側リンパ節 79
- pharyngeal space 咽頭側隙 556
- plantar
  - - artery 外側足底動脈 **420**, 443, 446, 447
  - - nerve 外側足底神経 424, **433**, 443, 446, 447
  - - septum 外側足底中隔 412
  - - sulcus 外側足底溝 446
  - - vein 外側足底静脈 **422**, 446, 447
- plate
  - - of pterygoid process 外側板《翼状突起の》 458, 461, 538
  - - of sphenoid bone 外側板《蝶形骨の》 521
- posterior nasal arteries of sphenopalatine artery 外側後鼻枝《蝶口蓋動脈の》 525
- process
  - - of calcaneal tuberosity 外側突起《踵骨隆起の》 400, 407

- - of malleus 外側突起《ツチ骨の》 532
- pterygoid 外側翼突筋 463-465, 467, **468**, 469, 541
- - nerve 外側翼突筋神経 477, 488, 503, **546**
- rays of foot 外側足放線 410
- recess of 4th ventricle 第四脳室外側陥凹 605
- rectus 外側直筋 475, **508**, 509, 513, 516
- root of median nerve 外側根《正中神経の》 328
- sacral
  - - arteries 外側仙骨動脈 34, 208, **222**
  - - crest 外側仙骨稜 10, 11
  - - veins 外側仙骨静脈 216, **222**, 223
- segment
  - - of globus pallidus 外節《淡蒼球の》 597
  - - of lung 外側中葉区 108
- segmental artery of right lung 外側中葉動脈《右肺の》 115
- semicircular
  - - canal 外側骨半規管 **481**, 528, 530, 531
  - - duct 外側半規管 536, 537
- subtendinous bursa of gastrocnemius 外側腱下包《腓腹筋の》 385
- sulcus 外側溝 593, 595
- superficial cervical lymph nodes 外側頸リンパ節の浅リンパ節 587
- superior
  - - genicular artery 外側上膝動脈 **420**, 421, 443
  - - posterior nasal branches (posterior superior lateral nasal branches) of maxillary nerve 外側上後鼻枝《上顎神経の》 505, 525
  - - supraclavicular nerves 外側鎖骨上神経 582, 583
- supracondylar
  - - line of femur 外側顆上線《大腿骨の》 360
  - - ridge of humerus 外側顆上稜《上腕骨の》 256
- sural cutaneous nerve 外側腓腹皮神経 **432**, 434, 435, 442, 444
- surface
  - - of fibula 外側面《腓骨の》 380
  - - of radius 外側面《橈骨の》 280
  - - of tibia 外側面《脛骨の》 380
- tarsal artery 外側足根動脈 420, 445
- thoracic
  - - artery 外側胸動脈 56, **60**, 62, 316, 335-337
  - - vein 外側胸静脈 **60**, 62
- transverse patellar retinaculum 外側横膝蓋支帯 384
- tubercle of posterior process of talus 外側結節《距骨後突起の》 401, 405, 407
- umbilical fold 外側臍ヒダ **135**, 144, 145, 148, 149, 152, 153, 182, 183
- ventricle 側脳室 473, 594, **605**, 609, 616
- vestibular nucleus 前庭神経外側核 480, 618
- vestibulospinal tract 外側前庭脊髄路 618
Latissimus dorsi 広背筋 22, 26, 40, 268, **277**, 332, 351
- aponeurosis 広背筋腱膜 26
Layngeal vestibule (supraglottic space) 喉頭前庭（声門上腔） 573
Least splanchnic nerve 最下内臓神経 245-247
Left
- anterior lateral segment (Segment Ⅲ) of left liver 左外側前区域（区域Ⅲ）《左肝部の》 170
- ascending lumbar vein 左上行腰静脈 55, 70, 71
- atrioventricular valve 左房室弁 85, **86**, 87
- atrium 左心房 82, 84, **85**, 87, 88, 93
- auricle 左心耳 83, **84**, 85, 88

- brachiocephalic vein 左腕頭静脈 35, 54
- branch of proper hepatic artery 左枝《固有肝動脈の》 171, 210
- broncho-mediastinal trunk 左気管支縦隔リンパ本幹 119
- bundle branch of atrioventricular bundle 左脚《房室束の》 90
- colic
  - - artery 左結腸動脈 149, **207**, 221
  - - flexure 左結腸曲 144, 145, 148, 156, 161, **164**, 165, 175
  - - lymph node 左結腸リンパ節 233
  - - vein 左結腸静脈 149, **215**
- common
  - - carotid artery 左総頸動脈 68, 77, 84, 99
  - - iliac artery 左総腸骨動脈 143, 151, 206, 221, 223, 225
  - - iliac lymph node 左総腸骨リンパ節 226
  - - iliac vein 左総腸骨静脈 71, 143, 151, 216, 221, 223, 225
- coronary
  - - artery 左冠状動脈 83, **88**
  - - trunk 左冠状リンパ本幹 100
- crus of diaphragm 左脚《横隔膜の》 **52**, 53
- cusp
  - - of aortic valve 左半月弁《大動脈弁の》 87
  - - of pulmonary valve 左半月弁《肺動脈弁の》 86
- dome of diaphragm 左天蓋《横隔膜の》 52
- duct of caudate lobe 左尾状葉胆管 172
- fibrous
  - - anulus 左線維輪 86
  - - trigone 左線維三角 86
- gastric
  - - artery 左胃動脈 147, 207, 210-212, **218**, 219, 221
  - - lymph node 左胃リンパ節 **230**, 231
  - - vein 左胃静脈 99, 215, **218**, 219-221
- gastro-omental
  - - artery 左胃大網動脈 207, 210, 211, **218**, 219
  - - lymph node 左胃大網リンパ節 230
  - - vein 左胃大網静脈 215, **218**, 219
- hepatic duct 左肝管 171-173
- hepatic veins 左肝静脈 171
- hypogastric nerve 左下腹神経 237, 239, 242, 243
- inferior
  - - epigastric artery 左下腹壁動脈 208
  - - gluteal artery 左下殿動脈 224
  - - lobar bronchi 左下葉気管支 110
  - - phrenic
    - - - artery 左下横隔動脈 55, 180, 208, 217
    - - - vein 左下横隔静脈 214, 216, 217
  - - pulmonary vein 左下肺静脈 114, 115
  - - rectal
    - - - artery 左下直腸動脈 223, 224
    - - - vein 左下直腸静脈 223
  - - suprarenal artery 左下副腎動脈 180, 208, 217
- internal
  - - iliac
    - - - artery 左内腸骨動脈 180, 225
    - - - vein 左内腸骨静脈 180, 225
  - - jugular vein 左内頸静脈 54, 70, 77, 114
  - - pudendal
    - - - artery 左内陰部動脈 223, 224
    - - - vein 左内陰部静脈 223
- jugular trunk 左頸リンパ本幹 100

- lamina of thyroid cartilage 左板《甲状軟骨の》 570
- lateral
  - - aortic lymph node 左外側大動脈リンパ節 226-229
  - division of left liver 左外側区《左肝部の》 170
  - liver 左肝部 170
- lobe
  - - of liver 左葉《肝臓の》 146, 168, 171
  - - of prostate 左葉《前立腺の》 200
  - - of thymus 左葉《胸腺の》 80
  - - of thyroid gland 左葉《甲状腺の》 574
- lumbar
  - - lymph node 左腰リンパ節 229, 234
  - - trunk 左腰リンパ本幹 72, **226**, 228
- lung 左肺 66, 93, 104, **105**
- main bronchus 左主気管支 68, 79, **110**
- marginal
  - - artery 左辺縁動脈 88
  - - vein 左辺縁静脈 88
- medial
  - - division of left liver 左内側区《左肝部の》 170
  - - segment (Segment Ⅳ) of left liver 左内側区域 (区域Ⅳ)《左肝部の》 170
- middle suprarenal artery 左中副腎動脈 177, 180, 208
- ovarian
  - - artery 左卵巣動脈 179, 216, 217, 219, **225**
  - - vein 左卵巣静脈 214, 216, 217, 219, **225**
- phrenic nerve 左横隔神経 54, 55, 74, 79, 91
- posterior lateral segment (Segment Ⅱ) of left liver 左外側後区域(区域Ⅱ)《左肝部の》 170
- pulmonary
  - - artery 左肺動脈 66, 68, 77, 79, 83, 84, 104, **114**, 115
  - - veins 左肺静脈 70, 77, 79, 84, 88, **114**
- recurrent laryngeal nerve 左反回神経 557, 575
- renal
  - - artery 左腎動脈 143, 177, 179, 180, 208, **209**, 212, 217, 220, 221
  - - vein 左腎静脈 71, 143, 160, 177-180, 212, **214**, 216, 217
- subclavian
  - - artery 左鎖骨下動脈 54, 68, 77, 79, 84, 99, 557, 566, 575
  - - trunk 左鎖骨下リンパ本幹 119
  - - vein 左鎖骨下静脈 54, 70, 77, 79, 114
- superior
  - - gluteal
    - - - artery 左上殿動脈 208
    - - - vein 左上殿静脈 180, 216
  - - intercostal vein 左上肋間静脈 79
  - - lobar bronchus 左上葉気管支 110
  - - pulmonary vein 左上肺静脈 85, 114, 115
  - - suprarenal artery 左上副腎動脈 55, 177, 180
- suprarenal vein 左副腎静脈 176, 179, 180, 214, 216, **217**, 219
- sympathetic trunk 左交感神経幹 98
- testicular
  - - artery 左精巣動脈 179, 180, **217**, 219
  - - vein 左精巣静脈 179, 180, 214, **217**, 219
- triangular ligament 左三角間膜 170, 171
- ventricle 左心室 82-84, **85**, 93

Lens 水晶体 514, 516, **518**, 519
Lenticular process of incus 豆状突起《キヌタ骨の》 532

Lesser
- arterial circle of iris 小虹彩動脈輪 517, 518
- curvature of stomach 小弯《胃の》 158, 159
- horn of hyoid bone 小角《舌骨の》 539, 558, 570
- occipital nerve 小後頭神経 37, 38, 499, 568, **569**, 582-584
- omentum 小網 146, 148, **159**, 163, 168, 210
- palatine
  - - artery 小口蓋動脈 495, **504**, 546
  - - foramen 小口蓋孔 458, 538
  - - nerves 小口蓋神経 **505**, 525, 546
- petrosal nerve 小錐体神経 483, 503
- sac (omental bursa) 網嚢 **146**, 156, 175
- sciatic
  - - foramen 小坐骨孔 129, 439
  - - notch 小坐骨切痕 125, 126, 359, 439
- splanchnic nerve 小内臓神経 **237**, 238-240, 245-247
- supraclavicular fossa 小鎖骨上窩 120, 576
- trochanter 小転子 356, **360**, 362, 364, 365
- tubercle (tuberosity) of humerus 小結節《上腕骨の》 253, **256**, 257, 259, 260, 262, 350
- wing of sphenoid bone 小翼《蝶形骨の》 455, 459, **461**, 507, 521, 523

Levator
- anguli oris 口角挙筋 462, 464, **467**
- ani 肛門挙筋 136, 137, **140**, 141, 150-153, 155, 167, 182-184, 191, 193-195, 203
- hiatus 挙筋門 141
- labii
  - - superioris 上唇挙筋 462, 463, **467**
  - - - alaeque nasi 上唇鼻翼挙筋 462-464, **466**
- palpebrae superioris 上眼瞼挙筋 475, **508**, 509, 514
- scapulae 肩甲挙筋 22, 23, 269, **276**, 561
- veli palatini 口蓋帆挙筋 465, 530, **545**, 555

Levatores
- costarum 肋骨挙筋 27, 32
- - breves 短肋骨挙筋 27, 32, **33**
- - longi 長肋骨挙筋 27, 32, **33**

Ligament
- of head of femur 大腿骨頭靱帯 157, 363, **364**, 421
- of vena cava 大静脈靱帯 171

Ligamenta flava 黄色靱帯 12, 16, 18, 19, **20**, 21, 559

Ligamentum
- arteriosum 動脈管索 77, 79, **83**, 84, 95, 115
- teres of liver 肝円索 163, 168, **170**, 171
- venosum 静脈管索 95, 171

Limbus of fossa ovalis 卵円窩縁 85
Limen nasi 鼻限 525
Line of gravity 重心線 3, 357

Linea
- alba 白線 120, **130**, 131, 134, 139, 248, 436
- aspera 粗線《大腿骨の》 360, 362
- terminalis 分界線 127, 129

Lingual
- artery 舌動脈 491, **492**, 549, 580
- aponeurosis 舌腱膜 548
- branch of glossopharyngeal nerve 舌枝《舌咽神経の》 482
- mucosa 舌粘膜 548
- muscles 舌筋 465, 548

- nerve (CN V₃) 舌神経 477-479, 488, 489, 503, 546, **547**, 549, 619
- papilae 舌乳頭 548
- septum 舌中隔 548
- tonsil 舌扁桃 **548**, 550, 552, 556, 573
- vein 舌静脈 549, 567

Lingula
- of cerebellum 小脳小舌 598
- of lung 小舌《肺の》 105
- of mandible 下顎小舌 540

Lingular
- artery 肺舌動脈 115
- vein 肺舌静脈 115

Lisfranc's joint line リスフラン関節線 402
Liver 肝臓 146, 156, **168**, 170
Lobes of liver 肝葉 170
Lobule of epididymis 精巣小葉《精巣上体の》 198, 199
Lobules of mammary gland 乳腺小葉 63

Long
- ciliary nerves 長毛様体神経 477, **511**, 513
- head
  - - of biceps brachii 長頭《上腕二頭筋の》 262, 264, 266, **278**
  - - of biceps femoris 長頭《大腿二頭筋の》 370, 371, 373, **379**, 441, 448
  - - of triceps brachii 長頭《上腕三頭筋の》 268, 270, **279**, 351
- plantar ligament 長足底靱帯 406, **408**, 409, 411, 413, 414, 419
- posterior ciliary arteries 長後毛様体動脈 510, 517
- process of incus 長脚《キヌタ骨の》 532
- saphenous vein 大伏在静脈 57, **422**, 423, 434, 436, 442
- thoracic nerve 長胸神経 320, 321, **322**, 335-337

Longissimus 最長筋 26, **30**, 560
- capitis 頭最長筋 24, 25, 27, 30, **31**, 464, 465, 585
- cervicis 頸最長筋 30, 31
- thoracis 胸最長筋 27, 30, **31**

Longitudinal
- axis in vagina 膣軸 188
- cerebral fissure 大脳縦裂 593, 595
- cervical axis 子宮頸軸 188
- fascicles 縦束 17, 19, 306, 559
- folds
  - - of esophagus 縦走ヒダ《食道の》 97
  - - of urethra 縦走ヒダ《尿道の》 185
- layer
  - - of duodenum 縦筋層《十二指腸の》 160, 172
  - - of esophagus 縦筋層《食道の》 97
  - - of rectum 縦筋層《直腸の》 167
- striae 縦条 472, 620
- uterine axis 子宮体軸 188

Longus
- capitis 頭長筋 **29**, 465, 565
- colli 頸長筋 23, **29**, 565

Lower
- esophageal (phrenic) constriction 下食道狭窄(横隔膜狭窄) 96
- eyelid 下眼瞼 514, 515
- leg 下腿 356
- subscapular nerve 下肩甲下神経 323, 336, 337
- trunk 下神経幹 321

Lumbar
- arteries 腰動脈 56, 208, 610
- ganglia 腰神経節 **237**, 239, 242, 243

- lymph node 腸リンパ節 226
- nerves 腰神経 242, 243
- part of diaphragm 腰椎部《横隔膜の》 **52**, 55
- plexus 腰神経叢 425
- splanchnic nerves 腰内臓神経 **242**, 243-247
- triangle 腰三角 22
- vein 腰静脈 35, 57, 71, 214, 216
- vertebrae [L1-L5] 腰椎 2, 4, **9**

Lumbocostal triangle (Bochdalek's triangle) 腰肋三角（ボクダレク三角） 52, 53

Lumbosacral
- enlargement 腰膨大 600
- junction 腰仙椎境界 2
- trunk 腰仙骨神経幹 **242**, 243, 425

Lumbrical slip 虫様筋腱線維 311

Lumbricals
- of foot 虫様筋《足の》 411-413, 418, **419**, 447
- of hand 虫様筋《手の》 307, 308, 311, 314, **315**

Lunate 月状骨 **298**, 299-301
- surface of acetabulum 月状面《寛骨臼の》 125, 359, 364

Lungs 肺 104, **105**

Lunules
- of semilunar cusps of aortic valve 半月弁半月《大動脈弁の》 87
- of semilunar cusps of pulmonary valve 半月弁半月《肺動脈弁の》 87

Lymph node リンパ節 73

Lymphatic
- follicles リンパ小節 162
- vessel リンパ管 72

M

Main pancreatic duct (pancreatic duct) 膵管 160, 172, 173, **174**

Major
- alar cartilage 大鼻翼軟骨 520
- calix 大腎杯 179, 209
- duodenal papilla 大十二指腸乳頭 160, 172
- salivary glands 大唾液腺 551

Male
- pelvis 男性骨盤 126
- urethra 男性尿道 185

Malleolar
- groove of tibia 内果溝《脛骨の》 380
- prominence ツチ骨隆起 532
- stria ツチ骨条 532

Malleus ツチ骨 528, 530, 531, **532**

Mammary
- gland 乳腺 63
- lobes 乳腺葉 63

Mammillary
- body 乳頭体 595, **596**, 598, 621
- process of lumber vertebrae 乳頭突起《腰椎の》 9

Mammillothalamic
- fasciculus 乳頭体視床束 597
- tract 乳頭視床路 621

Mandible 下顎骨 454-456, 464, **539**, 540, 556

Mandibular
- angle 下顎角 588, 589
- division (CN V₃) 下顎神経 476, **477**, 483, 488, 489, 503, 511, 541, 546, 547
- foramen 下顎孔 456, **477**, 539, 540
- fossa 下顎窩 458, 526, **540**, 541
- notch 下顎切痕 539

Manubrium of sternum 胸骨柄 44, **46**, 47

Marginal
- artery 結腸辺縁動脈 212
- mandibular branch of facial nerve 下顎縁枝《顔面神経の》 478, **488**, 498, 500, 580
- sinus 辺縁静脈洞 607
- tentorial branch of internal carotid artery テント縁枝《内頸動脈の》 490

Masseter 咬筋 462-465, 467, **468**, 555, 556, 582

Masseteric
- artery 咬筋動脈 495, 504
- nerve 咬筋神経 477, 488, 489, 503, 541, **546**

Mastoid
- antrum 乳突洞 534
- branch of occipital artery 乳突枝《後頭動脈の》 603
- cells (mastoid air cells) 乳突蜂巣 481, 530, **531**, 547
- emissary vein 乳突導出静脈 497, 606
- foramen 乳突孔 456, 458, **526**, 606
- lymph nodes 乳突リンパ節 587
- notch of temporal bone 乳突切痕《側頭骨の》 458, 526
- process of temporal bone 乳様突起《側頭骨の》 16, 24, 454, 456, 458, **526**, 588

Maxilla 上顎骨 454, 455, 456, 458, 507, 521, 524, 538

Maxillary
- artery 顎動脈 491-494, **495**, 502-504, 524, 534
- division (nerve) (CN V₂) 上顎神経 476, **477**, 489, 511, 525, 546
- hiatus 上顎洞裂孔 506, 521
- sinus 上顎洞 506, 507, 514, **522**, 523, 538
- veins 顎静脈 **496**, 497, 567

MCP joint crease 中手指節関節線 353

Medial
- antebrachial
-- cutaneous nerve 内側前腕皮神経 **326**, 330, 331, 338, 339
-- vein 内側前腕静脈 339
- arcuate ligament 内側弓状靱帯 52, 53
- basal
-- segment of lung 内側肺底区 108
-- segmental artery of lung 内側肺底動脈 115
- border
-- of humerus 内側縁《上腕骨の》 257
-- of kidney 内側縁《腎臓の》 178
-- of scapula 内側縁《肩甲骨の》 22, 40, 253, **255**, 259, 269
-- of suprarenal gland 内側縁《副腎の》 176
- brachial cutaneous nerve 内側上腕皮神経 320, 321, **326**, 330, 331, 338
- branch/es
-- of external carotid artery 内側枝《外頸動脈の》 491, 492
-- of spinal nerve 内側枝《脊髄神経の》 36
-- of supraorbital nerve 内側枝《眼窩上神経の》 498
- calcaneal branch of tibial nerve 内側踵骨枝《脛骨神経の》 433, 442, 443
- circumflex femoral
-- artery 内側大腿回旋動脈 **420**, 421, 440, 441
-- veins 内側大腿回旋静脈 422
- collateral ligament of knee joint 内側側副靱帯《膝関節の》 384-386, **388**
- condyle
-- of femur 内側顆《大腿骨の》 356, **360**, 361, 382, 389
-- of tibia 内側顆《脛骨の》 356, 357, **380**, 381, 382, 450
- cord 内側神経束 320, 321, **326**, 328, 329, 337, 338
- crus
-- of major alar cartilage 内側脚《大鼻翼軟骨の》 520
-- of superficial inguinal ring 内側脚《浅鼠径輪の》 132, 133, 437
- cuneiform 内側楔状骨 **400**, 401-403, 406, 410
- cutaneous
-- branch/es
--- of posterior intercostal arteries 内側皮枝《肋間動脈の》 56, 610
--- of saphenous nerve 内側下腿皮枝《伏在神経の》 429
--- of spinal nerve 内側皮枝《脊髄神経の》 37, 58
--- of thoracic aorta 内側皮枝《胸大動脈の》 34
-- dorsal cutaneous nerve 内側足背皮神経 432, **434**, 444, 445
- eminence of floor of 4th ventricle 内側隆起《第四脳室底の》 599
- epicondyle
-- of femur 内側上顆《大腿骨の》 356, 357, **360**, 382, 451
-- of humerus 内側上顆《上腕骨の》 253, **256**, 257, 264, 339, 350
- geniculate body 内側膝状体 473, 617
- head
-- of clavicle 内側頭《鎖骨の》 120
-- of flexor hallucis brevis 内側頭《短母趾屈筋の》 413, 419
-- of gastrocnemius 内側頭《腓腹筋の》 370, 371, 392, 394, **398**, 442
-- of triceps brachii 内側頭《上腕三頭筋の》 270, 279
- inferior genicular artery 内側下膝動脈 420, 421, **443**
- inguinal fossa 内側鼠径窩 135
- intermuscular septum of arm 内側上腕筋間中隔 338
- lacunar lymph node 内側裂孔リンパ節 229
- lemniscus 内側毛帯 614
- lip of femur 内側唇《大腿骨の》 360
- longitudinal
-- fasciculus (MLF) 内側縦束 618
-- patellar retinaculum 内側縦膝蓋支帯 384
- malleolar
-- articular surface (articular surface of medial malleolus) of tibia 内果関節面《脛骨の》 381, 404, 405
-- branches of posterior tibial artery 内果枝《後脛骨動脈の》 421, 443
-- surface of talus 内側面《距骨の》 403, 405, 407
- malleolus of tibia 内果《脛骨の》 380, 381
- mammary
-- branches
--- of intercostal nerves 内側乳腺枝《肋間神経の》 62
--- of internal thoracic artery 内側乳腺枝《内胸動脈の》 56, 62
- meniscus 内側半月 386, **387**, 388-390
- nasal branches of anterior ethmoidal nerve 内側鼻枝《前篩骨神経の》 524, 525

Medial nuclei of thalamus

- nuclei of thalamus　視床内側核群　597
- occipital artery (P4)　内側後頭動脈 (P4区)　608, 609
- olfactory stria　内側嗅条　472, 620
- palpebral
-- artery　内側眼瞼動脈　510
-- ligament　内側眼瞼靱帯　515
- parabrachial nucleus　内側結合腕傍核　619
- pectoral nerve　内側胸筋神経　320, 321, **326**, 334-336
- plantar
-- artery　内側足底動脈　420, 421, 443, 446, **447**
-- nerve　内側足底神経　424, 443, **446**, 447
-- septum　内側足底中隔　412
-- sulcus　内側足底溝　446
-- vein　内側足底静脈　422
- plate
-- of pterygoid process　内側板《翼状突起の》　458, 461, 538
-- of sphenoid bone　内側板《蝶形骨の》　521
- process of calcaneal tuberosity　内側突起《踵骨隆起の》　400, 401, 407
- pterygoid　内側翼突筋　463-465, **469**, 502, 553, 555, 556
-- nerve　内側翼突筋神経　477, 488, 503, **546**
- rays　内側足放線　410
- rectus　内側直筋　475, **508**, 509, 516, 617
- root of median nerve　内側根《正中神経の》　328
- sacral crest　内側仙骨稜　10
- segment
-- of globus pallidus　内節《淡蒼球の》　597
-- of lung　内側中葉区　108
- segmental artery of right lung　内側中葉動脈《右肺の》　115
- subtendinous bursa of gastrocnemius　内側腱下包《腓腹筋の》　385
- superior
-- genicular artery　内側上膝動脈　420, 421, **443**
-- posterior nasal branches (posterior superior medial nasal branches) of maxillary nerve　内側上後鼻枝《上顎神経の》　505, **524**, 525
- supraclavicular nerves　内側鎖骨上神経　582
- supracondylar
-- line of femur　内側顆上線《大腿骨の》　360
-- ridge of humerus　内側顆上稜《上腕骨の》　256, 257
- sural cutaneous nerve　内側腓腹皮神経　**433**, 435, 442, 444
- surface
-- of arytenoid cartilage　内側面《披裂軟骨の》　570
-- of fibula　内側面《腓骨の》　380
-- of ovary　内側面《卵巣の》　188
-- of tibia　内側面《脛骨の》　357, 380, 450
-- of ulna　内側面《尺骨の》　280
- tarsal arteries　内側足根動脈　443
- transverse patellar retinaculum　内側横膝蓋支帯　384
- tubercle of posterior process of talus　内側結節《距骨後突起の》　**401**, 407
- umbilical
-- (umbilicus) fold　内側臍ヒダ　**135**, 145, 148, 149, 152, 153
-- ligaments　内側臍索　95
- vestibular nucleus　前庭神経内側核　480, 618
Median
- antebrachial
-- cutaneous nerve　前腕正中皮神経　321

-- vein　前腕正中皮静脈　**318**, 330, 339
- aperture of 4th ventricle　第四脳室正中口　604, 605
- arcuate ligament　正中弓状靱帯　52, 53
- atlantoaxial joint　正中環軸関節　16, 17
- basilic vein　尺側正中皮静脈　318, 339
- cephalic vein　橈側正中皮静脈　318
- cricoarytenoid ligament　正中輪状披裂靱帯　572
- cricothyroid ligament　正中輪状甲状靱帯　110, 571
- cubital vein　肘正中皮静脈　**318**, 330, 339, 350
- furrow　舌正中溝　548
- nerve　正中神経　60, 320, **328**, 330, 331, 335-342, 345, 346
-- roots　正中神経根　336
- palatine suture　正中口蓋縫合　458, 538
- part of crebellum　正中部《小脳の》　598
- sacral
-- artery　正中仙骨動脈　**34**, 180, 208, 216, 222-225
-- crest　正中仙骨稜　5, **10**, 11, 126, 127
-- vein　正中仙骨静脈　180, 216, 224, 225
- thyrohyoid ligament　正中甲状舌骨靱帯　**571**, 578, 579
- umbilical
-- fold　正中臍ヒダ　**135**, 144, 145, 148, 149, 152, 153, 182, 183
-- ligament　正中臍索　180, **181**, 186, 187
Mediastinal
- part of parietal pleura　壁側胸膜の縦隔部（縦隔胸膜）　54, 55, 66, 77, 80, 83, 97, **103**
- surface of lung　縦隔面《肺の》　105
Mediastinum　縦隔　77
- testis (testicular mediastinum)　精巣縦隔　198, 199
Medulla
- oblongata　延髄　474, 593, 598, **599**, 600, 605
- of suprarenal gland　髄質《副腎の》　176
Medullary
- rays of kidney　髄放線《腎臓の》　179
- striae　髄条　619
Membranous
- labyrinth　膜迷路　537
- lamina of pharyngotympanic tube　膜性板《耳管の》　530
- layer of superficial abdominal fascia　膜様層《浅腹筋膜の》　134
- part
-- of interventricular septum　膜性部《心室中隔の》　87
-- of urethra　隔膜部《尿道の》　155, 185, 197, 200
- wall of trachea　膜性壁《気管の》　573
Meningeal
- branch/es
-- (ramus) of spinal nerves　硬膜枝《脊髄神経の》　**36**, 600
-- of anterior ethmoidal nerve　硬膜枝《前篩骨神経の》　603
-- of cervical nerve　硬膜枝《頸神経の》　603
-- of internal carotid artery　硬膜枝《内頸動脈の》　490
-- of mandibular division　硬膜枝《下顎神経の》　503, 603
-- of maxillary nerve　硬膜枝《上顎神経の》　477, 603
-- of vagus nerve　硬膜枝《迷走神経の》　603
Meninges　髄膜　602

Mental
- branch　オトガイ動脈　495
-- of inferior alveolar artery　オトガイ枝《下歯槽動脈の》　498
-- of mental nerve　オトガイ枝《オトガイ神経の》　502
- foramen　オトガイ孔　454, 455, 539
- nerve　オトガイ神経　477, **489**, 499, 500, 546
- protuberance　オトガイ隆起　539, 589
- tubercle　オトガイ結節　539
Mentalis　オトガイ筋　462-464, **467**
Mesencephalic nucleus of trigeminal nerve　三叉神経中脳路核　471, 619
Mesencephalon　中脳　595, 599
Mesenteric root (root of mesentery)　腸間膜根　149, 161
Mesentery　腸間膜　142, 143, 145, 146, **148**, 163, 165, 175
Mesoappendix　虫垂間膜　149, 164
Mesometrium　子宮間膜　**188**, 189, 235
Mesonephric (wolffian) duct　中腎管（ウォルフ管）　205
Mesosalpinx　卵管間膜　188, 189
Mesotympanum　中鼓室　531
Mesovarial margin　間膜縁　188, 189
Mesovarium　卵巣間膜　188
Metacarpals　中手骨　252, 253, **298**, 300, 301, 304, 305, 311, 315, 351, 352
Metacarpophalangeal (MCP) joint　中手指節 (MCP) 関節　253, 300, 301, **302**, 304, 311, 344, 350, 352
Metatarsal (metatarsus)　中足骨　356, 400, **401**, 402-406, 410
Metatarsophalangeal joint　中足趾節関節　357, 402, 450
- capsules　関節包《中足趾節関節の》　408, 409, 419
Meyer's loop　マイヤーのループ　473, 616
Michaelis' rhomboid　ミハエリス菱形窩　41
Midcarpal joint　手根中央関節　300, 301
Midclavicular line (MCL)　鎖骨中線　120
Middle
- arm territory　上腕中間領域　319
- calcaneal articular surface of talus　中踵骨関節面《距骨の》　407
- cerebellar peduncle　中小脳脚　598, 599
- cerebral artery　中大脳動脈　**608**, 609
- cervical ganglion　中頸神経節　74, 75, 91, 98, 557, **579**, 623
- circular layer of stomach　輪筋層《胃の》　158
- cluneal nerves　中殿皮神経　37, 39, 203, 430, **435**, 438, 441
- colic
-- artery　中結腸動脈　143, 162, **207**, 212, 213, 220, 221
-- lymph node　中結腸リンパ節　233
-- vein　中結腸静脈　162, **215**, 218-221
- collateral artery　中側副動脈　316
- cranial fossa　中頭蓋窩　459
- crease　中位手掌線　353
- ear　中耳　528, 530
- esophageal (thoracic) constriction　中食道狭窄（胸部狭窄）　96
- ethmoid sinus　中篩骨洞　523
- forearm territory　前腕中間領域　319
- genicular artery　中膝動脈　421, 443
- internodal bundles　中結節間束　90
- lobe
-- artery of right lung　中葉動脈《右肺の》　115

644

– – of lung　中葉《肺の》　93, 104, 105
– – vein of right lung　中葉静脈《右肺の》　115
– meatus　中鼻道　**521**, 523, 525
– mediastinum　中縦隔　67, 76
– meningeal
– – artery　中硬膜動脈　**495**, 503, 504, 510, 534, 603
– – vein　中硬膜静脈　607
– nasal concha　中鼻甲介　455, 460, 507, **521**, 522, 523, 525, 538, 553
– phalanx
– – of foot　中節骨《足の》　400-402
– – of hand　中節骨《手の》　252, 298, **299**, 300, 301, 305
– pharyngeal constrictor　中咽頭収縮筋　554, 555
– rectal
– – artery　中直腸動脈　202, 208, **222**, 223-225
– – plexus　中直腸動脈神経叢　239, **242**, 243, 245
– – veins　中直腸静脈　215, 216, **222**, 223, 224
– scalene (scalenus medius)　中斜角筋　51, 317, **564**, 565
– superior alveolar branches of superior alveolar nerves　中上歯槽枝《上歯槽神経の》　477, 546
– suprarenal artery　中副腎動脈　**178**, 179, 217
– talar articular surface of calaneus　中距骨関節面《踵骨の》　407
– temporal
– – artery　中側頭動脈　494
– – branch of middle cerebral artery　中側頭枝《中大脳動脈の》　609
– thyroid veins　中甲状腺静脈　575
– transverse rectal fold　中直腸横ヒダ　167
– trunk (C7)　中神経幹《第7頸神経》　321
Midfoot　中足　400
Minor
– alar cartilages　小鼻翼軟骨　520
– calix　小腎杯　179
– duodenal papilla　小十二指腸乳頭　160, 172
Mitral valve　僧帽弁　→左房室弁
Modiolus　蝸牛軸　535, 537
Molars　大臼歯　542
Molecular layer (Ⅰ)　分子層　595
Mons pubis　恥丘　136, 192
Motor branches
– – of facial nerve　運動枝《顔面神経の》　478
– – of radial nerve　運動枝《橈骨神経の》　337
– nucleus of trigeminal nerve　三叉神経運動核　471, 476
– root
– – of trigeminal nerve　運動根《三叉神経の》　511, 599
Müllerian (paramesonephric) duct　ミュラー管　205
Mucosa
– of esophagus　粘膜《食道の》　97
– of urinary bladder　粘膜《膀胱の》　185
Multifidus　多裂筋　27, 32, **33**
Multiform layer (Ⅵ)　多形細胞層　595
Muscles
– of facial expression　表情筋　462
– of mastication　咀嚼筋　463
Muscular
– branch/es
– – of coccygeal nerve　筋枝《尾骨神経の》　425
– – of femoral nerve　筋枝《大腿神経の》　425, 429
– – of fibular artery　筋枝《腓骨動脈の》　421

– – of inferior gluteal nerve　筋枝《下殿神経の》　431
– – of lateral plantar nerve　筋枝《外側足底神経の》　433
– – of obturator nerve　筋枝《閉鎖神経の》　428
– – of perineal nerves　筋枝《会陰神経の》　203
– – of radial nerve　筋枝《橈骨神経の》　333, 339, 341
– coat (muscularis) of esophagus　筋層《食道の》　97
– part of interventricular septum　筋性部《心室中隔の》　87
– process of arytenoid cartilage　筋突起《披裂軟骨の》　570, 571
– triangle　筋三角　120, 576, 589
Muscularis
– externa
– – of duodenum　外筋層《十二指腸の》　160, 172
– – of rectum　外筋層《直腸の》　167
– – of stomach　外筋層《胃の》　158
– – of urinary bladder　筋層《膀胱の》　185
Musculocutaneous nerve　筋皮神経　320, 321, **327**, 330, 331, 336, 338, 339, 341
Musculophrenic artery　筋横隔動脈　**54**, 55, 56, 61
Musculus uvulae　口蓋垂筋　**545**, 555
Myelin sheath　髄鞘（ミエリン鞘）　592
Mylohyoid　顎舌骨筋　465, 544, 548, 554, 562, **563**
– branch of inferior alveolar artery　顎舌骨筋枝《下歯槽動脈の》　495
– groove　顎舌骨筋神経溝　540
– line　顎舌骨筋線　539, 563
– nerve　顎舌骨筋神経　489, 503, **547**
– raphe　顎舌骨筋縫線　544, 563
Mylopharyngeal part of superior pharyngeal constrictor　顎咽頭部《上咽頭収縮筋の》　554
Myometrium　子宮筋層　188, 189

N

Nail　爪　305
Nasal
– bone　鼻骨　454, 455, 506, **520**
– cavity　鼻腔　520, 522
– conchae　鼻甲介　552
– crest　鼻稜　520, 538
– septum　鼻中隔　522, **524**, 553
– vestibule　鼻前庭　525
Nasalis　鼻筋　462-464, **466**
Nasion　鼻根点　455
Nasociliary
– nerve　鼻毛様体神経　477, **511**, 513
– root　鼻毛様体神経根　477, 511
Nasolacrimal duct　鼻涙管　**515**, 522
Nasopalatine nerve　鼻口蓋神経　**524**, 525, 546
Nasopharynx　咽頭鼻部　550
Navicular　舟状骨　**400**, 401-406
– articular surface (articular surface for navicular) of talus　舟状骨関節面《距骨の》　403, 407
– fossa of urethra　尿道舟状窩　185, 197, 201
– tuberosity　舟状骨粗面　357, 403, 450, 451
Neck
– of bladder　膀胱頸　185, 200, 201
– of femur　大腿骨頸　356, 360-363, 365
– of fibula　腓骨頸　380, 382
– of gallbladder　胆嚢頸　172
– of malleus　ツチ骨頸　532
– of mandible　下顎頸　540
– of radius　橈骨頸　280, 286

– of rib　肋骨頸　45, 47
– of scapula　肩甲頸　255, 261
– of stapes　アブミ骨頸　532
– of talus　距骨頸　**400**, 401, 405
– of tooth　歯頸　542
Nerve
– fiber　神経線維　471
– of pterygoid canal　翼突管神経　479, 505
– of tensor
– – tympani　鼓膜張筋神経　503
– – veli palatini　口蓋帆張筋神経　503
– to subclavius　鎖骨下筋神経　320, 321, **322**
Nervus intermedius　中間神経　478, **481**, 537, 557, 599
Neural branch of internal carotid artery　三叉神経枝《内頸動脈の》　490
Neurocranium　脳頭蓋　454
Neurohypophysis　神経下垂体　598
Neurons　ニューロン　592
Neurothelium　内皮様細胞層　602
Nipple　乳頭　62, 63, 121
Nodose ganglion　節状神経節　619
Nodule　小節　598
– of semilunar cusps　半月弁結節　87
Nuchal
– fascia　項筋膜　23, 26
– ligament　項靱帯　16, 17, 19, 276, **559**, 588
Nucleus/i
– ambiguus　疑核　471, 482, **484**, 486
– cuneatus　楔状束核　614
– gracilis　薄束核　614
– of abducent nerve　外転神経核　**471**, 474, 618
– of cranial nerve　脳神経核　471
– of hypoglossal nerve　舌下神経核　471, 487
– of lateral lemniscus　外側毛帯核　619
– of medial geniculate body　内側膝状体核　619
– of oculomotor nerve　動眼神経核　471, **474**, 617, 618
– of solitary tract　孤束核　471, 478, 479, **482**, 484
– of trapezoid body　台形体核　619
– of trochlear nerve　滑車神経核　471, **474**, 618
– prepositus hypoglossi　舌下神経前位核　618
– pulposus　髄核　12
Nutrient foramina　栄養孔　21

O

Oblique
– arytenoid　斜披裂筋　555, 557, **572**
– cord　斜索　286
– diameter　斜径　127
– fissure of lung　斜裂《肺の》　93, 104, **105**, 109
– head
– – of adductor hallucis　斜頭《母趾内転筋の》　410, 413, 414, **419**, 447
– – of adductor pollicis　斜頭《母指内転筋の》　307, 308, **313**
– line of mandible　斜線《下顎骨の》　539
– line of thyroid cartilage　斜線《甲状軟骨の》　570
– part of cricothyroid　斜部《輪状甲状筋の》　572
– popliteal ligament　斜膝窩靱帯　385
– vein of left atrium　左心房斜静脈　88
Obliquus
– auriculae　耳介斜筋　529
– capitis
– – inferior　下頭斜筋　24, 25, 27, 28, 564, **565**, 585

Obliquus capitis superior

– – superior 上頭斜筋 24, 25, 27, 28, 464, 465, 564, **565**
Obturator
– artery 閉鎖動脈 135, 157, 208, **222**, 223-225, 421
– canal 閉鎖管 141, 157
– externus 外閉鎖筋 155, 367, 372, **377**
– fascia 閉鎖筋膜 136, 137, 141, 152
– foramen 閉鎖孔 **124**, 125, 126, 141, 358, 359
– internus 内閉鎖筋 136, 137, 140, 141, 152, 153, 155, 157, 369-372, 374, **375**, 438, 439, 448
– – fascia 内閉鎖筋筋膜 141
– – nerve 内閉鎖筋神経 431
– lymph node 閉鎖リンパ節 235
– membrane 閉鎖膜 128, 129, 364
– nerve 閉鎖神経 135, 157, 242, 243, 424, 425, **428**, 434, 435, 440
– veins 閉鎖静脈 135, 157, 216, **222**, 223-225
Occipital
– artery 後頭動脈 38, 491-493, 499, 534, 556, 557, **584**, 585
– belly of occipitofrontalis 後頭筋《後頭前頭筋の》 463, 464
– bone 後頭骨 454, **456**, 457
– branches of occipital artery 後頭枝《後頭動脈の》 493
– condyle 後頭顆 16, 456, **458**
– emissary vein 後頭導出静脈 497
– foramen 後頭孔 606
– horn (posterior horn) of lateral ventricle 後角《側脳室の》 594, 596, 605
– lobe 後頭葉 593
– lymph node 後頭リンパ節 **584**, 587
– nerve 後頭神経 37-39, **568**, 584, 585
– pole 後頭極 473, 595
– sinus 後頭静脈洞 607
– triangle 後頭三角 576
– vein 後頭静脈 496, 497, 499, 567, **584**, 606
Occipitofrontalis 後頭前頭筋 462, 463
Occluded part of umbilical artery 閉塞部《臍動脈の》 225
Ocular conjunctiva 眼球結膜 516, 518
Oculomotor nerve (CN III) 動眼神経 470, **474**, 475, 509, 511-513, 599, 608, 617
Olecranon 肘頭 22, 252, 253, **268**, 280, 281, 283, 290, 351
– bursa 肘頭皮下包 283
– fossa of humerus 肘頭窩《上腕骨の》 **256**, 257, 283
Olfactory
– bulb 嗅球 **472**, 524, 525, 594, 620
– fibers 嗅神経糸 472, 524, 525
– mucosa 嗅粘膜 472, 620
– nerve 嗅神経 470, **472**, 593-595
– tract 嗅索 472, 594, **620**
– trigone 嗅三角 472, 594, 620
Olive オリーブ 484, 487, **598**, 599
Omental
– bursa (lesser sac) 網嚢 **146**, 156, 175
– foramen 網嚢孔 143, 148, 168
Omoclavicular triangle 肩甲鎖骨三角 576
Omohyoid 肩甲舌骨筋 332, 465, **563**, 578
Opening of greater vestibular glands 大前庭腺開口部 192
Ophthalmic
– artery 眼動脈 490, 492, **510**, 512, 524

– division (CN V₁) 眼神経 476, **477**, 489, 525
– vein 眼静脈 510
Opponens
– digiti minimi
– – 小指対立筋 307-309, 312, **313**
– – 小趾対立筋 413, 414, 418, **419**
– pollicis 母指対立筋 301, 306-309, **312**, 313
Optic
– canal 視神経管 459, 461, 473, **506**, 507, 538
– chiasm 視交叉 **473**, 511, 598, 605, 609, 616
– disk 視神経円板（視神経乳頭）516
– nerve (CN II) 視神経 470, **473**, 475, 511, 513, 616, 617
– radiation 視放線 473, **594**, 616
– tract 視索 **473**, 616, 617
Optical part of retina 網膜視部 519
Ora serrata 鋸状縁 519
Oral
– cavity 口腔 550
– – proper 固有口腔 550
– mucosa 口腔粘膜 544
– vestibule 口腔前庭 550, 556
Orbicularis
– oculi 眼輪筋 **462**, 463, 464, 466
– oris 口輪筋 462-464, **467**
Orbit 眼窩 455, **506**, 522
Orbital
– branches of maxillary nerve 眼窩枝《上顎神経の》 505
– floor 眼窩下壁 507, 514
– part
– – of lacrimal gland 眼窩部《涙腺の》 515
– – of orbicularis oculi 眼窩部《眼輪筋の》 464
– plate of ethmoid bone 眼窩板《篩骨の》 460, 506, 507, 523
– septum 眼窩隔膜 512, 514, 515
– surface
– – of frontal bone 眼窩面《前頭骨の》 506, 507
– – of maxilla 眼窩面《上顎骨の》 506, 507
– – of sphenoid bone 眼窩面《蝶形骨の》 461
– – of zygomatic bone 眼窩面《頬骨の》 507
Orifice of vermiform appendix 虫垂口 164
Oropharynx 咽頭口部 550
Ossicular chain 耳小骨連鎖 533
Otic ganglion 耳神経節 483, 503
Outer
– lip of iliac crest 外唇《腸骨稜の》 127
– longitudinal layer of stomach 縦筋層《胃の》 158
– table of clavaria 外板《頭蓋冠の》 457, 602
Oval
– nucleus 卵形核 619
– window 前庭窓 **481**, 531, 532, 536
Ovarian
– artery 卵巣動脈 188, 189, 208, **223**
– plexus 卵巣動脈神経叢 **236**, 237, 240, 242, 247
– suspensory ligament 卵巣提索 151, 152, **183**, 184, 186, 205
– vein 卵巣静脈 179, 188, 189, **223**
Ovary 卵巣 151, 152, 155, 181, 183, 186, **188**, 189, 191, 205, 225, 235

P

Palatine
– aponeurosis 口蓋腱膜 545
– bone 口蓋骨 458, 521, **538**

– process of maxilla 口蓋突起《上顎骨の》 456, 458, 507, 521, **538**
– tonsil 口蓋扁桃 548, 550, **552**, 556
Palatoglossal arch 口蓋舌弓 548, 550, **552**
Palatoglossus 口蓋舌筋 548
Palatopharyngeal arch 口蓋咽頭弓 548, 550, **552**, 553
Palatopharyngeus 口蓋咽頭筋 555, 556
Palatovaginal (pharyngeal) canal 口蓋骨鞘突管 458
Paleocortex 古皮質 594
Palm 手掌 350
Palmar
– aponeurosis 手掌腱膜 293, 306, 330
– branch
– – of median nerve 掌枝《正中神経の》 328, 330
– – of ulnar nerve 掌枝《尺骨神経の》 329, 330
– carpal network 掌側手根動脈網 317
– carpometacarpal ligaments 掌側手根中手靱帯 302
– digital
– – arteries 掌側指動脈 316, 317, 344, **345**
– – nerves 掌側指神経 344, 345
– – veins 掌側指静脈 318
– intercarpal ligaments 掌側手根間靱帯 302
– interossei 掌側骨間筋 308, 309, 314, 315
– ligaments 掌側靱帯 **302**, 305, 308, 311
– metacarpal
– – arteries 掌側中手動脈 317, 345
– – ligaments 掌側中手靱帯 302
– – veins 掌側中手静脈 318
– radiocarpal ligament 掌側橈骨手根靱帯 302
– radioulnar ligament 掌側橈骨尺骨靱帯 286, 287, 302
– ulnocarpal ligament 掌側尺骨手根靱帯 302
– venous network 手掌静脈網 350, 353
Palmaris
– brevis 短掌筋 306, 353
– longus 長掌筋 288, **292**, 293
– – tendon 長掌筋の腱 306, 350, 352, 353
Palpebral part of lacrimal gland 眼瞼部《涙腺の》 515
Pampiniform plexus 蔓状静脈叢 196, 198, 199, **225**
Pancreas 膵臓 142, 143, 146-149, 156, 160, 161, 173, **174**, 177, 210
Pancreatic
– branches of splenic artery 膵枝《脾動脈の》 207
– duct (main pancreatic duct) 膵管 160, 172, 173, **174**
– lymph node 膵リンパ節 230
– plexus 膵神経叢 238, 245
– veins 膵静脈 215
Pancreaticoduodenal
– artery 膵十二指腸動脈 220
– lymph node 膵十二指腸リンパ節 231
– vein 膵十二指腸静脈 218, 219
Paracentral branches of anterior cerebral artery 中心傍小葉枝《前大脳動脈の》 609
Paracolic
– gutter 結腸傍溝 149
– lymph node 結腸傍リンパ節 233
Paraesophageal lymph node 食道傍リンパ節 73, 101
Paramedian pontine reticular formation (PPRF) 傍正中橋網様体 618
Paramesonephric (müllerian) duct ミュラー管 205
Paranasal air sinuses 副鼻腔 522

Pararenal fat pad (perirenal fat capsule) of kidney　脂肪被膜《腎臓の》　176-178
Parasternal lymph node　胸骨傍リンパ節　**64**, 73, 118
Parasympathetic
– ganglia　副交感神経節　623
– nervous system　副交感神経系　75, 244
– root　副交感神経根　511
Parathyroid glands　副甲状腺（上皮小体）　574
Paratracheal lymph node　気管傍リンパ節　73, 100, 101, 118, **119**
Paraumbilical (periumbilical) veins　臍傍静脈　57, 215
Paraurethral gland　尿道傍腺　205
Paravaginal tissue　腟傍組織　155
Paraventricular nuclei of thalamus　視床室傍核群　597
Paravertebral ganglia　椎傍神経節　244
Paravesical fossa　膀胱傍陥凹　152, 155, 183
Paravesicular fascia　膀胱傍結合組織　153
Parietal
– bone　頭頂骨　454-456, **457**, 458, 523
– branch
– – of middle meningeal artery　頭頂枝《中硬膜動脈の》　495, 603
– – of superficial temporal artery　頭頂枝《浅側頭動脈の》　494, 499
– emissary vein　頭頂導出静脈　497, 606
– foramen　頭頂孔　457, 606
– layer
– – of serous pericardium　壁側板《漿膜性心膜の》　80, 81
– – of tunica vaginalis　壁側板《精巣鞘膜の》　196, 198
– pelvic fascia　壁側骨盤筋膜　154
– peritoneum　壁側腹膜　23, 103, **134**, 135, 143-145, 149-153, 159, 161, 166, 167, 176, 181-184
– pleura　壁側胸膜　103
Parieto-occipital
– branch of middle cerebral artery　頭頂後頭枝《中大脳動脈の》　609
– sulcus　頭頂後頭溝　595
Parotid
– branches of auriculotemporal nerve　耳下腺枝《耳介側頭神経の》　503
– duct　耳下腺管　499, 501, **551**, 556
– gland　耳下腺　499, **551**, 556, 582, 583
– plexus　耳下腺神経叢　478, 488, 499, 500, **551**
Pars
– flaccida of tympanic membrane　弛緩部《鼓膜の》　532
– plana of ciliary body　平滑部《毛様体の》　519
– plicata of ciliary body　皺襞部《毛様体の》　519
– tensa of tympanic membrane　緊張部《鼓膜の》　532
Patella　膝蓋骨　356, 357, 361, 366, 382, **383**, 390, 391, 450
Patellar
– ligament　膝蓋靱帯　366, 367, 369, 373, **384**, 386, 390, 392, 393
– surface of femur　膝蓋面《大腿骨の》　360, 361, 389
– vascular network　膝蓋血管網　440
Patent part of umbilical artery　開存部《臍動脈の》　225
Pecten pubis　恥骨櫛　**127**, 358
Pectinate muscles　櫛状筋　85

Pectineal
– ligament　恥骨櫛靱帯　133
– line　恥骨筋線　362
Pectineus　恥骨筋　133, 157, 366, 367, **376**, 436, 440, 450
Pectoral
– axillary lymph node　胸筋腋窩リンパ節　64
– branch of thoracoacromial artery　胸筋枝《胸肩峰動脈の》　316
Pectoralis
– major　大胸筋　120, 130, 264-266, **274**, 334, 350
– minor　小胸筋　265, 266, **275**
Pedicle of vertebral arch　椎弓根　5, 7, 8
Peduncle of flocculus　片葉脚　598
Pelvic
– diaphragm　骨盤隔膜　167
– floor　骨盤底　136, **141**
– – muscles　骨盤底の筋　140
– girdle　下肢帯　124, 356, **358**
– inlet　骨盤上口　127
– outlet　骨盤下口　129
– part of ureter　骨盤部《尿管の》　180
– splanchnic nerves　骨盤内臓神経　237, 239, 242, **243**, 244-247, 623
– surface of sacrum　前面《仙骨の》　126
Pelvis　骨盤　154
Penile
– fascia　陰茎筋膜　150, 184
– septum　陰茎中隔　197
– skin　陰茎皮膚　197
– suspensory ligament (suspensory ligament of penis)　陰茎提靱帯　150, 184, 202, 225
Penis　陰茎　137, 187, 196, **197**, 234
Perforating
– arteries　貫通動脈　420, 421, 440, 441, 445
– branch/es
– – of deep palmar arch　貫通枝《深掌動脈弓の》　317
– – of fibular artery　貫通枝《腓骨動脈の》　421, 442
– – of internal thoracic artery　貫通枝《内胸動脈の》　62
– – of median antebrachial vein　貫通枝《前腕正中皮静脈の》　330
Perforator veins　貫通静脈　**318**, 339
Periarchicortex　周原皮質　594
Peribronchial network　気管支周囲リンパ管叢　118
Pericallosal artery　脳梁周囲動脈　609
Pericardiacophrenic
– artery　心膜横隔動脈　**54**, 55, 66, 77, 80
– vein　心膜横隔静脈　**55**, 66, 77, 80
Pericardial
– branches of phrenic nerve　心膜枝《横隔神経の》　54
– cavity　心膜腔　81
Pericardium　心膜　55, 66, **80**, 84
Perimetrium (serosa)　子宮外膜（漿膜）　188, 190
Perineal
– artery　会陰動脈　191, **195**, 202
– body　会陰体（会陰腱中心）　136, **150**, 151-153, 182, 183
– branches
– – of posterior femoral cutaneous nerve　会陰枝《後大腿皮神経の》　194, 430, 438
– – of pudendal nerve　会陰枝《陰部神経の》　438
– flexure　会陰曲　166
– membrane　会陰膜（下尿生殖隔膜筋膜）　136, 137, 152, 153, **191**, 197
– nerves　会陰神経　**194**, 195, 202, 203

– raphe　会陰縫線　136, 137, 192
– region　会陰部（域）　136
Perineum　会陰　**154**, 194, 203
Periorbita　眼窩骨膜　514
Peripharyngeal space　咽頭周囲隙　556
Perirenal fat capsule　脂肪被膜　156
– (pararenal fat pad) of kidney　脂肪被膜《腎臓の》　176-178
Peritoneal cavity　腹膜腔　142, 143, **144**, 148, 154, 176
– of scrotum　精巣鞘膜腔　199
Peritoneum　腹膜　**142**, 143, 154
Periumbilical (paraumbilical) veins　臍傍静脈　57, 215
Perlia's nucleus　ペルリア核　617
Permanent teeth　永久歯　542
Perpendicular plate
– of ethmoid bone　垂直板《篩骨の》　455, **460**, 507, 520, 523, 538
– of palatine bone　垂直板《口蓋骨の》　521, 538
Pes anserinus　鵞足　366, 367, 369, 370, **392**
Petrosal
– ganglion　錐体神経節　619
– vein　錐体静脈　606
Petrosquamous sinus　側頭錐体鱗部静脈洞　607
Petrotympanic fissure　錐体鼓室裂　458, 478, 526, **533**
Petrous
– apex　錐体尖　526
– branch of middle meningeal artery　岩様部枝《中硬膜動脈の》　495
– part
– – of internal carotid artery　錐体部《内頸動脈の》　490, **608**
– – of temporal bone　岩様部《側頭骨の》　456, 459, **527**
– ridge　錐体上縁　459
Peyer's patches　パイエル板　162
Phalangoglenoid ligament　指節関節靱帯　304
Phalanx (phalanges)
– 指（節）骨　252, 253, **298**, 300, 351, 352
– 趾（節）骨　356
Pharyngeal
– branch/es
– – of glossopharyngeal nerve　咽頭枝《舌咽神経の》　482
– – of vagus nerve　咽頭枝《迷走神経の》　482, 484, 485
– constrictors　咽頭収縮筋　554
– elevators　咽頭挙筋　555
– muscles　咽頭筋　554
– orifice of pharyngotympanic tube　耳管咽頭口　524, 530, 550, 552
– plexus　咽頭神経叢　75, **482**
– tonsil　咽頭扁桃　**552**, 553, 555
– tubercle　咽頭結節　458
– venous plexus　咽頭静脈叢　556
Pharyngobasilar fascia　咽頭頭底板　555
Pharyngo-esophageal constriction　咽頭食道狭窄　96
Pharyngotympanic (auditory) tube　耳管　528, **530**, 531
Pharynx　咽頭　553, 556
Philtrum　人中　589
Phrenic
– (lower esophageal) constriction　横隔膜狭窄（下食道狭窄）　96
– nerve　横隔神経　**54**, 55, 66, 77, 93, 321, 568, 569, 579, 581, 583
Phrenicocolic ligament　横隔結腸間膜　147

Phrenicosplenic ligament　横隔脾間膜　161
Pia mater　軟膜　602
Pial vascular plexus　軟膜血管叢　517
Pigment epithelium of ciliary body　毛様体色素上皮　516
Pigmented iris epithelium　虹彩色素上皮　518
Pineal
－ body　松果体　593, 598, 599, **605**
－ recess　松果体陥凹　605
PIP joint crease　近位指節間関節線　353
Piriform
－（anterior nasal）aperture　梨状口　455, 521
－ recess　梨状陥凹　553, 573
Piriformis　梨状筋　140, **141**, 222, 366, 367, 369-371, 375, 420, 438, 439, 441, 448
－ nerve　梨状筋神経　431
Pisiform　豆状骨　253, 299, 301, 350, 352, 353
Placenta　胎盤　94
Plantar
－ aponeurosis　足底腱膜　406, 411, **412**, 446, 447
－ calcaneonavicular ligament　底側踵舟靱帯　406, **408**, 411, 414, 419
－ chiasm　足底交叉　395, 399
－ digital veins　底側趾静脈　422
－ interosseus　底側骨間筋　412-414, 419
－ ligaments　足底靱帯　410
－ metatarsal
－－ arteries　底側中足動脈　**420**, 446, 447
－－ veins　底側中足静脈　422
－ vault　土踏まず　410
－ venous arch　足底静脈弓　422
Plantaris　足底筋　370, 371, 394, **398**, 442, 448
－ tendon　足底筋の腱　394, 398
Platysma　広頸筋　462-464, **561**, 578
Pleural cavity　胸膜腔　**66**, 77, 102, 176
Polar frontal artery　前頭極動脈　609
Pons　橋　474, 478, **598**, 599, 605
Pontine
－ arteries　橋枝　608
－ nucleus（principal sensory nucleus）橋核（三叉神経主感覚核）　471, 476
Pontomedullary cistern　橋延髄槽　604
Pontomesencephalic vein　橋中脳静脈　607
Popliteal
－ artery　膝窩動脈　420-442, **443**
－ fossa　膝窩　370, 451
－ surface of femur　膝窩面《大腿骨の》　360, 382
－ vein　膝窩静脈　422, 441, **443**
Popliteus　膝窩筋　379, 385, 394, **399**, 442
Portal vein　［肝］門脈（肝静脈）　82, 171, 210-212, 215, **218**, 219-221
Postcentral gyrus　中心後回　593, 613-615, 619
Posterior
－（dorsal）
－－ ramus
－－－（branch）of thoracic aorta　後枝《胸大動脈の》　34, 610
－－－ of posterior intercostal arteries　後枝《肋間動脈の》　56, 61
－－－ of sacral nerve　後枝《仙骨神経の》　36, 430
－－－ of spinal nerve　後枝《脊髄神経の》　36, 39, 58, 59, 321, 332, **600**
－－ root
－－－ of sacral nerve　背側根（後根）《仙骨神経の》　36, 430
－－－ of spinal nerve　後根《脊髄神経の》　59, 321, **600**, 601, 615

－ ampullary nerve　後膨大部神経　481, **536**, 537
－ antebrachial cutaneous nerve　後前腕皮神経　325, **331**, 346
－ arch
－－ of atlas　後弓《環椎の》　6, 7
－－ vein　後弓状静脈　422, 423
－ articular facet of vertebra　後関節面《椎骨の》　6
－ atlanto-occipital membrane　後環椎後頭膜　**16**, 17-19, 25
－ auricular
－－ artery　後耳介動脈　491-493, 529, **534**
－－ muscles（auricularis posterior）後耳介筋　463, 466, **529**
－－ nerve　後耳介神経　478, 488
－－ vein　後耳介静脈　496, 567
－ basal
－－ segment of lung　後肺底区　108
－－ segmental artery of lung　後肺底動脈　115
－ belly of digastric muscle　後腹《顎二腹筋》　544, 554, 555, 563
－ border
－－ of radius　後縁《橈骨の》　280
－－ of ulna　後縁《尺骨の》　280
－ brachial cutaneous nerve　後上腕皮神経　325, **331**, 332, 337, 338
－ branch/es
－－ of anterior interosseous artery　後枝《前骨間動脈の》　317
－－ of external carotid artery　後枝《外頸動脈の》　491, 493
－－ of inferior pancreaticoduodenal artery　後下膵十二指腸動脈　211, 212, **219**
－－ of obturator nerve　後枝《閉鎖神経の》　425, 428
－－ of occipital artery　後枝《後頭動脈の》　493
－－ of renal artery　後枝《腎動脈の》　209
－ calcaneal articular surface of talus　後踵骨関節面《距骨の》　407
－ cecal artery　後盲腸動脈　212, 213, 220, **221**
－ cerebral artery　後大脳動脈　608, 609
－ cervical region　後頸部　576, 584
－ chamber of eyeball　後眼房　516, 518
－ circumflex humeral artery　後上腕回旋動脈　316, 317, **333**
－ clinoid process　後床突起　459, 461
－ cochlear nucleus　蝸牛神経後核　480, 619
－ communicating artery　後交通動脈　490, 608
－ cord　後神経束　320, 321, 337
－ cranial（cerebellar）fossa　後頭蓋窩（小脳窩）　459
－ cricoarytenoid　後輪状披裂筋　555, 557, **572**
－ cruciate ligament　後十字靱帯　387, **388**, 389
－ crural artery　後脛動脈　535
－ crus
－－ of internal capsule　後脚《内包の》　594
－－ of stapes　後脚《アブミ骨の》　532
－ cusp
－－ of aortic valve　後半月弁《大動脈弁の》　86
－－ of left atrioventricular valve　後尖《左房室弁の》　86, 87
－－ of right atrioventricular valve　後尖《右房室弁の》　86, 87
－ cutaneous branches of cervical nerves　後皮枝《頸神経の》　584
－ deep temporal artery　後深側頭動脈　504
－ descending（interventricular）artery　後下行枝（後室間枝）　88
－ diameter of trochlea of talus　後径《距骨滑車の》　405
－ ethmoid sinus　後篩骨洞　521

－ ethmoidal
－－ artery　後篩骨動脈　490, 510, 513, **524**, 525
－－ foramen　後篩骨孔　460, **506**
－－ nerve　後篩骨神経　**477**, 513, 603
－ extremity of pancreas　後端《膵臓の》　174
－ femoral cutaneous nerve　後大腿皮神経　194, 203, 424, 425, **430**, 435, 438, 441
－ funiculus of spinal cord　後索《脊髄の》　613
－ gastric
－－ artery　後胃動脈　211
－－ plexus　後胃神経叢　98, 245
－ glandular branches of superior thyroid artery　後腺枝《上甲状腺動脈の》　566
－ gluteal line of ilium　後殿筋線《腸骨の》　125, 375
－ horn
－－（occipital horn）of lateral rentricle　後角《側脳室の》　594, 596, 605
－－ of spinal nerve　後角《脊髄の》　610, 612
－ inferior iliac spine　下後腸骨棘　124-126, **359**, 362
－ intercavernous sinus　後海綿間静脈洞　607
－ intercondylar area of tibia　後顆間区《脛骨の》　381
－ intercostal
－－ arteries　肋間動脈　34, 39, **56**, 61, 68, 77, 98, 99, 610
－－ veins　肋間静脈　35, 54, **57**, 60, 61, 70, 71, 99, 156, 611
－ internal vertebral venous plexus　後内椎骨静脈叢　35, **57**, 601, 611
－ internodal bundles　後結節間束　90
－ interosseous
－－ artery　後骨間動脈　316, 317, **340**, 341
－－ nerve　後［前腕］骨間神経　325, 341
－ interventricular
－－（descending）artery　後室間枝（後下行枝）　88
－－ sulcus　後室間溝　84
－－ vein　後室間静脈（中心臓静脈）　88
－ ligament of fibular head　後腓骨頭靱帯　386, 388
－ labial
－－ branches of perineal artery　後陰唇枝《会陰動脈の》　195
－－ commissure　後陰唇交連　136, **192**, 193
－－ nerves　後陰唇神経　194
－－ veins　後陰唇静脈　195
－ lateral segment（Segment Ⅶ）of right liver　右外側後区域（区域Ⅶ）《右肝部の》　170
－ layer of rectus sheath　後葉《腹直筋鞘の》　134
－ left ventricular branch　左心室後枝　88
－ ligament of incus　後キヌタ骨靱帯　532
－ lip of uterine os　後唇《外子宮口の》　190
－ lobe
－－ of cerebellum　小脳後葉　598
－－ of neurohypophysis　後葉《神経下垂体の》　596
－ longitudinal ligament　後縦靱帯　16, 17, **18**, 19, 21, 559
－ malleolar fold　後ツチ骨ヒダ　532
－ medial segment（Segment Ⅷ）of right liver　右内側後区域（区域Ⅷ）《右肝部の》　170
－ mediastinum　後縦隔　67, **76**
－ meniscofemoral ligament　後半月大腿靱帯　387, 388
－ nasal spine　後鼻棘　538
－ papillary muscle　後乳頭筋　85, 87
－ parietal
－－ artery　後頭頂動脈　609
－－ cortex　後頭頂野　613

- part
- – of vagina 後部《腟の》 190
- – of ulnar collateral ligament 後部《肘関節の内側側副靱帯の》 284
- process
- – of nasal cartilage 後突起《鼻軟骨の》 520
- – of talus 距骨後突起 400, 401, 407
- radicular
- – artery 後根動脈 56
- – vein 後根静脈 611
- ramus
- – of C5 spinal nerve 後枝《第5頸神経の》 37
- – of intercostal nerves 後枝《肋間神経の》 61, 326
- – of spinal nerve 後枝《脊髄神経の》 **36**, 39, 58, 59, 321, 332, **600**
- root of spinal nerve 後根《脊髄神経の》 59, 321, **600**, 601, 615
- rootlets 後根糸 600
- sacral foramen 後仙骨孔 4, **10**, 11, 126, 430
- sacroiliac ligaments 後仙腸靱帯 128, 129, **364**, 365
- scalene(scalenus posterior) 後斜角筋 51, 317, 564, **565**
- scrotal
- – branches of perineal artery 後陰嚢枝《会陰動脈の》 202, 223
- – nerves 後陰嚢神経 202, 203, **243**
- – vein 後陰嚢静脈 202, **222**, 223
- segment of right lung 後上葉区《右肺の》 108
- segmental
- – artery of lung 後上葉動脈《肺の》 115
- – – of kidney 後区動脈《腎臓の》 209
- – medullary artery 後髄節動脈 610
- semicircular
- – canal 骨半規管 481, 528, **530**, 531
- – duct 後半規管 **536**, 537
- septal branches of sphenopalatine artery 中隔後鼻枝《蝶口蓋動脈の》 495, 504, 524, 546
- serratus 後鋸筋 30
- spinal artery 後脊髄動脈 610
- spinal vein 後脊髄静脈 611
- sternoclavicular ligament 後胸鎖靱帯 258
- superior
- – alveolar
- – – artery 後上歯槽動脈 495, 502, 503, **504**
- – – branches of superior alveolar nerves 後上歯槽枝《上歯槽神経の》 505, 546
- – iliac spine 上後腸骨棘 40, 124-126, 129, **357**, 358, 359, 362, 439, 451
- – lateral nasal branches(lateral superior posterior nasal branches) of maxillary nerve 外側上後鼻枝《上顎神経の》 505, 525
- – pancreaticoduodenal artery 後上膵十二指腸動脈 207, 210, 211, 218, **219**
- – pancreaticoduodenal vein 後上膵十二指腸静脈 215
- surface
- – of arytenoid cartilage 後面《披裂軟骨の》 570
- – of fibula 後面《腓骨の》 380
- – of kidney 後面《腎臓の》 178
- – of radius 後面《橈骨の》 280
- – of scapula 後面《肩甲骨の》 255
- – of tibia 後面《脛骨の》 380
- – of ulna 後面《尺骨の》 280
- – of uterus 後面《子宮の》 181
- – talar articular surface of calaneus 後距骨関節面《踵骨の》 407
- – talofibular ligament 後距腓靱帯 409
- – temporal branch of middle cerebral artery 後側頭枝《中大脳動脈の》 609
- – tibial
- – – artery 後脛骨動脈 404, 420, **421**, 442
- – – recurrent artery 後脛骨反回動脈 421, 443
- – – veins 後脛骨静脈 404, **422**, 423
- – tibiofibular ligament 後脛腓靱帯 408, 409
- – tibiotalar part of deltoid ligament 後脛距部《三角靱帯の》 408
- – triangle(lateral cervical region) 後頸三角(外側頸三角部) 576, 582
- – tubercle
- – – of atlas 後結節《環椎の》 7, 17, 558
- – – of cervical vertebrae 後結節《頸椎の》 6
- – – of transvers process 後結節《横突起の》 7
- – tympanic artery 後鼓室動脈 532, **534**, 535
- – vein of upper lobe of right lung 後上葉静脈《右肺の》 115
- – vagal trunk 後迷走神経幹 98, 237, **238**, 239, 240, 245-247
- – vaginal fornix 後部《腟円蓋の》 151, 184, 188
- – vein of left ventricle 左心室後静脈 88
- – venous confluence 後静脈洞交会 607
- – wall
- – – (surface) of stomach 後壁《胃の》 147, 156
- – – of tympanic cavity 後壁《乳突壁》《鼓室の》 481
- – – of vagina 後壁《腟の》 190
- Posteroinferior cerebellar artery 後下小脳動脈 608
- Posterolateral
- – bundle 後外側束 423
- – fissure of cerebellum 後外側裂《小脳の》 598
- – sulcus 後外側溝 599
- Posteromedian medullary vein 後正中延髄静脈 606, 607
- Postsynaptic sympathetic fiber 交感神経節後線維 622
- Preaortic lymph node 大動脈前リンパ節 226, 229
- Prebiventral fissure 二腹小葉前裂 598
- Prececal lymph node 盲腸前リンパ節 233
- Precentral gyrus 中心前回 593, 613, 615
- Precuneal branches of anterior cerebral artery 楔前部枝《前大脳動脈の》 609
- Prefrontal
- – artery 前頭前動脈 609
- – cortex 前頭前野 613
- Premolars 小臼歯 542
- Premotor cortex 運動前野 613
- Preoptic area 視索前野 596
- Prepatellar bursa 膝蓋前皮下包 391
- Prepiriform area 梨状前野 472, 620
- Preprostatic part(prostatic part) of urethra 前立腺部《尿道の》 185, 197, 200
- Prepuce 包皮 201
- – of clitoris(clitoral prepuce) 陰核包皮 136, 192, 193
- – of penis 陰茎包皮 184
- Prerectal fibers 直腸前線維 141
- Pretectal area 視蓋前野 616, 617
- Pretracheal
- – lamina of cervical fascia 気管前筋膜《頸筋膜の》 577
- – layer of cervical fascia 気管前葉《頸筋膜の》 23, 574, 577, 578
- Prevertebral
- – ganglion 椎前神経節 622
- – lymph node 椎前リンパ節 100
- – layer of cervical fascia 椎前葉《頸筋膜の》 23, 577
- Primary fissure 第一裂 598
- Primordium of prostate duct 前立腺原基 205
- Principal sensory(pontine) nucleus 三叉神経主感覚核(橋核) 471, 476
- Procerus 鼻根筋 462, 466
- Processus vaginalis 鞘状突起 196
- Profunda
- – brachii artery 上腕深動脈 **316**, 317, 333
- – femoris artery 大腿深動脈 420, 440
- Prominence of lateral semicircular canal 外側半規管隆起 531
- Promontory
- – lymph node 岬角リンパ節 229, 234, 235
- – of ilium 岬角《腸骨の》 127
- – of sacrum(sacral promontory) 岬角《仙骨の》 **2**, 3, 5, 10, 11, 126, 365, 366, 531
- Pronator
- – quadratus 方形回内筋 288, 289, 292, **293**, 306
- – teres 円回内筋 266, 288, 289, 291, 292, **293**
- Proper
- – cochlear artery 固有蝸牛動脈 537
- – hepatic artery 固有肝動脈 171, 207, **210**, 211, 212, 220, 221
- – ovarian ligament 固有卵巣索 151, 152, 183, 184, **188**, 189, 205
- – palmar digital
- – – artery 固有掌側指動脈 317, 344
- – – nerves 固有掌側指神経 328-331, **344**
- – plantar digital
- – – arteries 固有底側趾動脈 420, **446**, 447
- – – nerves 固有底側趾神経 433, 445, **446**, 447
- Prostate 前立腺 150, 153, 155, 182, 184, 185, 187, 197, **200**, 201, 205, 223
- Prostatic
- – capsule 前立腺被膜 200
- – ductules 前立腺管 185, 197
- – isthmus 前立腺峡部 200
- – part(preprostatic part) of urethra 前立腺部《尿道の》 185, 197, 200
- – plexus 前立腺神経叢 239, **243**, 247
- – utricle 前立腺小室 205
- – venous plexus 前立腺静脈叢 202, 222
- Proximal
- – extension creases 近位伸筋線 353
- – interphalangeal joint
- – – 近位指節間(PIP)関節 300, 301, **302**, 304, 311, 352
- – – 近位趾節間(PIP)関節 402
- – – capsule 関節包《近位指節間(PIP)関節の》 302
- – phalanx
- – – of foot 基節骨《足の》 400-402, 410
- – – of hand 基節骨《手の》 252, 298, 300, 301, 304
- – radioulnar joint 上橈尺関節 281, **282**, 286, 287
- – transverse crease 近位横手掌線 353
- – wrist crease 近位手根線 353
- Psoas
- – fascia 腰筋筋膜 23
- – major 大腰筋 23, 52, 135, 139, 180, 225, 366, 367, 369, 374, **375**
- – minor 小腰筋 52, 369, 374, **375**
- Pterion(sphenofrontal suture) プテリオン(蝶前頭縫合) 454
- Pterygoid
- – branches of posterior deep temporal artery 翼突筋枝《後深側頭動脈の》 495, 504

Pterygoid canal

- canal　翼突管　538
- fossa　翼突窩　461，538
- fovea　翼突筋窩　539，540
- hamulus　翼突筋鈎　461，545
- plexus　翼突筋静脈叢　496，**497**，567
- process of sphenoid bone　翼状突起《蝶形骨の》　456，458，**461**，521，538

Pterygopalatine
- fossa　翼口蓋窩　504，506
- ganglion　翼口蓋神経節　477-479，489，**505**，525，546

Pterygopharyngeal part of superior pharyngeal constrictor　翼突咽頭部《上咽頭収縮筋の》　554

Pterygospinous ligament　翼棘靱帯　540

Pubic
- arcuate ligament　恥骨弓靱帯　141
- symphysis　恥骨結合　124，126，127，**128**，129，141，150，151，191，201，248，357，358，365，366，369，450
- tubercle　恥骨結節　124，126，127，**128**，141，248，356-359，362，364，450

Pubis　恥骨　**124**，125，126，157，166，181，359

Pubococcygeus　恥骨尾骨筋　141，166

Pubofemoral ligament　恥骨大腿靱帯　364，365

Puborectalis　恥骨直腸筋　141，166

Pudendal
- canal（Alcock's canal）　陰部神経管（アルコック管）　155，439
- nerve　陰部神経　**194**，195，202，203，242，243，424，425，438，439，441

Pulmonary
- arteries　肺動脈　114
- alveolus（alveolus）　肺胞　111，116
- ligament　肺間膜　105
- outflow tract of right ventricle　肺動脈口《右心室の》　93
- plexus　肺神経叢　75，91，117
- trunk　肺動脈幹　68，77，83，84，87，90，91，104，**114**，115
- valve　肺動脈弁　**86**，87，88
- veins　肺静脈　82，114

Pulp chamber　歯髄腔　542

Pulvinar of thalamus　視床枕　598，616

Pupil　瞳孔　519

Pupillary
- dilator　瞳孔散大筋　518
- sphincter　瞳孔括約筋　518，617

Purkinje's fibers　プルキンエ線維　90

Putamen　被殻　594，609

Pyloric
- antrum　幽門洞　158，159
- branch of anterior vagal trunk　幽門枝《前迷走神経幹の》　238，240，245
- canal　幽門管　158，159
- orifice　幽門口　158，160
- part of stomach　幽門部《胃の》　156，175
- sphincter　幽門括約筋　160

Pyramid　錐体　615
- of medulla oblongata　延髄錐体　599
- of vermis　虫部錐体　598

Pyramidal
- lobe of thyroid gland　錐体葉《甲状腺の》　574
- process of palatine bone　錐体突起《口蓋骨の》　538
- tract（corticospinal tract）　錐体路（皮質脊髄路）　615

Pyramidalis　錐体筋　131，139

Q

Quadrangular
- lobule of cerebellum　四角小葉《小脳の》　598
- membrane of laryngeal cavity　四角膜《喉頭腔の》　573

Quadrate lobe of liver　方形葉《肝臓の》　171

Quadratus
- femoris　大腿方形筋　155，370，371，374，**375**，438，439，441，448
- femoris nerve　大腿方形筋神経　431
- lumborum　腰方形筋　23，27，52，138，**139**
- plantae　足底方形筋　404，411，413，418，**419**，446，447

Quadriceps femoris　大腿四頭筋　248，**378**，429，440

Quadrigeminal plate　四丘体板　598，599，605

R

Radial
- artery　橈骨動脈　**316**，317，339-342，344，345，347
- bundle territory　橈側リンパ管束領域　319
- carpal
- - collateral ligament　外側手根側副靱帯　302
- - eminence　橈側手根隆起　303
- collateral
- - artery　橈側側副動脈　316，341
- - ligament of proximal radio-ulnar joint　外側側副靱帯《上橈尺関節の》　284-286，301
- group of lymphatics　橈側リンパ管群　**319**
- head of flexor digitorum superficialis　橈骨頭《浅指屈筋の》　289
- nerve　橈骨神経　320，**325**，330，331，333，337，339-341，346
- notch of ulna　橈側切痕《尺骨の》　280，281，287
- recurrent artery　橈側反回動脈　316，339
- tuberosity　橈骨粗面　278，280，**281**
- tunnel　橈骨神経管　325，339
- veins　橈骨静脈　318

Radiate
- ligament of head of rib　放線状肋骨靱帯　49
- sternocostal ligaments　放線状胸肋靱帯　49，51

Radiocarpal joint　橈骨手根関節　300，301

Radioulnar Joints　橈尺関節　286

Radius　橈骨　252，253，**280**，309

Ramus of mandible　下顎枝　539

Rectal
- ampulla　直腸膨大部　167
- venous plexus　直腸静脈叢　216

Rectoprostatic fascia　直腸前立腺筋膜　150，182，201

Rectouterine pouch　直腸子宮窩（ダグラス窩）　151，152，157，**181**，183，184，188，190

Rectovaginal septum　直腸膣中隔　152，190

Rectovesical
- pouch　直腸膀胱窩　143，150，153，182，**184**，201
- septum　直腸膀胱中隔　150，**153**，157，184

Rectum　直腸　143，150-153，157，**166**，167，180-183，201

Rectus
- abdominis　腹直筋　55，120，130，131，133，134，138，**139**，143，150-153，157，182，183，248
- capitis
- - anterior　前頭直筋　29，465
- - lateralis　外側頭直筋　29，465，**565**
- - posterior major　大後頭直筋　24，25，27，28，464，465，**565**，585
- - posterior minor　小後頭直筋　24，25，27，28，464，465，564，**565**，585
- femoris　大腿直筋　366，367，369，373，**378**，429，440，448，450
- sheath　腹直筋鞘　**134**，139，264

Recurrent
- laryngeal nerve　反回神経　66，74，75，77，79，91，98，117，**485**，557，575，579
- meningeal branch of ophthalmic division　テント枝《眼神経の》　477

Red nucleus　赤核　474，615

Reflex［inguinal］ligament　反転靱帯　436，437

Renal
- artery　腎動脈　179，206，208，**209**，217，220，221
- column　腎柱　179
- cortex　腎皮質　178，179
- fascia　腎筋膜　176
- ganglia　腎神経節　247
- hilum　腎門　176，178
- impression of liver　腎圧痕《肝臓の》　170
- medulla　腎髄質　179
- papilla　腎乳頭　179
- pelvis　腎盂（腎盤）　178，179
- plexus　腎神経叢　236，**237**，239，240，246
- pyramid　腎錐体　179
- surface of suprarenal gland　腎面《副腎の》　176
- vein　腎静脈　179，214，216，**217**

Respiratory bronchiole　呼吸細気管支　111，116

Rete testis　精巣網　198，199

Reticular
- formation　網様体　472，616
- nucleus of thalamus　視床網様核　597

Reticulospinal tract　網様体脊髄路　618

Retina　網膜　514，516

Retroaortic lymph node　大動脈後リンパ節　226，228

Retroauricular lymph nodes　耳介後リンパ節　587

Retrocaval lymph node　大静脈後リンパ節　228，229

Retromandibular vein　下顎後静脈　496，497，556

Retroperitoneal space　腹膜後隙　152，153

Retroperitoneum　腹膜後域　176

Retropharyngeal
- lymph nodes　咽頭後リンパ節　556
- space　咽頭後隙　556

Retropubic space　恥骨後隙　150，152，153，201

Retropyloric lymph node　幽門後リンパ節　231

Retrorenal layer of renal fascia　後葉《腎筋膜の》　176

Rhomboid
- （romboideus）major　大菱形筋　22，26，269，**276**
- fossa　菱形窩　599
- minor　小菱形筋　22，26，269，**276**，561

Rib　肋骨　44，45，**47**，263

Right
- ascending lumbar vein　右上行腰静脈　70，71
- atrioventricular
- - orifice　右房室口　85
- - valve　右房室弁　85，**86**，87
- atrium　右心房　82，84，**85**，90，93
- auricle　右心耳　83，**84**，85，88
- branch of proper hepatic artery　右枝《固有肝動脈の》　171，210

−− bronchomediastinal trunk　右気管支縦隔リンパ本幹　119
− bundle branch of atrioventricular bundle　右脚《房室束の》　90
− choana　右後鼻孔　550
− colic
−− artery　右結腸動脈　207, 212, **220**
−− flexure　右結腸曲　145, 147, 148, 159, 161, **164**, 165
−− lymph node　右結腸リンパ節　233
−− vein　右結腸静脈　215, **220**
− common
−− iliac
−−− artery　右総腸骨動脈　149-151, 180, 182, 208, 213, 224, 227
−−− lymph node　右総腸骨リンパ節　226
−−− vein　右総腸骨静脈　149-151, 182, 216, 224
− coronary artery　右冠状動脈　86, 87, **88**
− crus of diaphragm　右脚《横隔膜の》　52, 53
− cusp
−− of aortic valve　右半月弁《大動脈弁の》　87
−− of pulmonary valve　右半月弁《肺動脈弁の》　86
− dome of diaphragm　右天蓋《横隔膜の》　52
− duct of caudate lobe　右尾状葉胆管　172
− fibrous
−− anulus　右線維輪　86
−− trigone　右線維三角　86
− gastric
−− artery　右胃動脈　207, **210**, 211, 212, 218-221
−− vein　右胃静脈　215, 218, 220
− gastro-omental
−− artery　右胃大網動脈　207, 210, 212, **218**, 219-221
−− lymph node　右胃大網リンパ節　**230**
−− vein　右胃大網静脈　215, **218**, 219-221
− hepatic
−− duct　右肝管　171-173
−− vein　右肝静脈　171
− hypogastric nerve　右下腹神経　239, 241-243
− inferior
−− epigastric
−−− artery　右下腹壁動脈　216
−−− vein　右下腹壁静脈　216
−− gluteal
−−− artery　右下殿動脈　208
−−− vein　右下殿静脈　216, 224
−− lobar bronchi　右下葉気管支　110
−− phrenic
−−− artery　右下横隔動脈　55, 217
−−− vein　右下横隔静脈　214, 217
−− pulmonary vein　右下肺静脈　114, 115
−− rectal vein　右下直腸静脈　224
−− suprarenal artery　右下副腎動脈　217
− internal
−− iliac artery　右内腸骨動脈　208, 216, 223, 224
−− jugular vein　右内頸静脈　70, 119
−− pudendal
−−− artery　右内陰部動脈　208
−−− vein　右内陰部静脈　216, 224
− jugular trunk　右頸リンパ本幹　119
− lamina of thyroid cartilage　右板《甲状軟骨の》　570
− lateral aortic lymph node　右外側大動脈リンパ節　226, 229, 227
− liver　右肝部　170

− lobe
−− of liver　右葉《肝臓の》　146, 156, 168, 171
−− of prostate　右葉《前立腺の》　200
−− of thymus　右葉《胸腺の》　80
−− of thyroid gland　右葉《甲状腺の》　574
− lumbar
−− lymph node　右腰リンパ節　229, 234
−− trunk　右腰リンパ本幹　72, 226, 228
− lung　右肺　66, 93, 104, **105**, 176
− lymphatic duct　右リンパ本幹　72
− main bronchus　右主気管支　77, 110
− marginal
−− artery　右縁枝（鋭角縁枝）　88
−− vein　右辺縁静脈　88
− medial division of right liver　右内側区《右肝部の》　170
− middle lobar bronchus　右中葉気管支　110
− ovarian
−− artery　右卵巣動脈　178, 216, **217**
−− vein　右卵巣静脈　178, 214, 216, **217**
− phrenic nerve　右横隔神経　55, 74, 91
− pulmonary
−− artery　右肺動脈　77, 78, 84, 87, 104, **114**, 115
−− veins　右肺静脈　70, 77, 78, 84, 88, 104, **114**
− recurrent laryngeal nerve　右反回神経　575
− renal
−− artery　右腎動脈　156, 175, 177, 178, 217
−− vein　右腎静脈　177, 178, **214**, 216, 217
− subclavian
−− artery　右鎖骨下動脈　34, 68, 78
−− trunk　右鎖骨下リンパ本幹　119
−− vein　右鎖骨下静脈　70, 71, 78, 114, 583
− superior
−− gluteal
−−− artery　右上殿動脈　223, 224
−−− vein　右上殿静脈　223, 224
−− lobar bronchus　右上葉気管支　110
−− pulmonary vein　右上肺静脈　114, 115
−− suprarenal artery　右上副腎動脈　55, 177
−− suprarenal vein　右副腎静脈　176, 178, 180, 214, 216, **217**
−− supreme intercostal vein　右最上肋間静脈　70
− testicular
−− artery　右精巣動脈　178, 180, **217**
−− vein　右精巣静脈　178, 180, 214, **217**
− triangular ligament　右三角間膜　170, 171
− ventricle　右心室　82-84, **85**, 90, 93
Rima
− glottidis　声門裂　573
− vestibuli　前庭裂　573
Risorius　笑筋　462, 463
Roof of tympanic cavity (tegmen tympani)　鼓室蓋　481
Root
− of mesentery (mesenteric root)　腸間膜根　149, 161
− of penis　陰茎根　197
− of tongue　舌根　548, 553
− of tooth　歯根　542
− sleeve　根嚢　601
Rosenmüller's lymph node　ローゼンミュラーのリンパ節　436
Rotatores
− breves　短回旋筋　33
− longi　長回旋筋　32, 33
− muscles　回旋筋　32
− thoracis breves　胸短回旋筋　27
− thoracis longi　胸長回旋筋　27

Round
− ligament of uterus　子宮円索　151, 152, **181**, 183, 184, 186, 191, 205, 223, 225
− window　蝸牛窓　481, 536, **537**
−− niche　蝸牛窓小窩　531
Rugal folds　胃粘膜ヒダ　158

S

Sacciform recess of elbow joint　嚢状陥凹《肘関節の》　284-286, 301
Saccular nerve　球形嚢神経　**481**, 536, 537
Saccule　球形嚢　**481**, 536, 618
Sacculoampullary nerve　球形嚢膨大部神経　481
Sacral
− canal　仙骨管　5, 10, 11, 126, 129
− cornua　仙骨角　10
− ganglia　仙骨神経節　236, 237, 239
− hiatus　仙骨裂孔　10, 126, 129, 600
− lymph node　仙骨リンパ節　227, 228, 234, 235
− nerve　仙骨神経　36, 237, 239, 242, **430**, 600
− plexus　仙骨神経叢　194, 202, 237, 242, **425**, 440, 601
− promontory (promontory of sacrum)　岬角《仙骨の》　2, 3, 5, 10, 11, 126, 365, 366, 531
− splanchnic nerve　仙骨内臓神経　244-246
− triangle　仙骨三角　41
− tuberosity　仙骨粗面　10, 11, 129
Sacrococcygeal joint　仙尾関節　10
Sacroiliac joint　仙腸関節　124, 126, 127, 129, 358
Sacrospinous ligament　仙棘靱帯　**128**, 129, 141, 157, 364, 365, 439
Sacrotuberous ligament　仙結節靱帯　**128**, 129, 141, 364, 365, 370, 371, 375, 438, 439, 441
Sacrum　仙骨　2, 4, 5, **10**, 40, 126, 129, 136, 137, 141, 357, 358, 364, 451
Sagittal
− suture　矢状縫合　456, 457
− thoracic diameter　胸郭矢状径　48
Salivatory nuclei　唾液核　471
Salpingopharyngeal fold　耳管咽頭ヒダ　525, 550, 552
Salpingopharyngeus　耳管咽頭筋　530
Saphenous
− hiatus　伏在裂孔　225, 436
− nerve　伏在神経　424, 425, **429**, 434, 435, 440, 442
Sartorius　縫工筋　248, 366, 367, 369, 373, **378**, 440, 448
Scala
− tympani　鼓室階　536
− vestibuli　前庭階　536
Scalene　斜角筋　23, **50**, 565
− tubercle　前斜角筋結節　565
Scalenus
− anterior (anterior scalene)　前斜角筋　51, 77, 317, 321, 564, **565**, 579, 581
− medius (middle scalene)　中斜角筋　51, 317, **564**, 565
− posterior (posterior scalene)　後斜角筋　51, 317, 564, **565**
Scalp　頭皮　457, 602
Scaphoid　舟状骨　298, **300**, 301
− fossa　舟状窩　529
Scapula　肩甲骨　40, 52, 252, 253, **255**, 262, 269, 272

Scapular
- foramen 肩甲孔 254
- notch 肩甲切痕 47, 255, 259, **260**, 261
- part of latissimus dorsi 肩甲骨部《広背筋の》 277
- spine 肩甲棘 4, 22, 40, 252, 253, **255**, 260, 261, 268, 269, 332, 351, 561

Scapulothoracic joint 肩甲胸郭関節 258
Sciatic nerve 坐骨神経 157, 424, 425, 431, **432**, 434, 435, 438, 439, 441, 448
Sclera 強膜 514, 516, **518**, 519
Scleral venous sinus 強膜静脈洞 517
Scrotal septum 陰嚢中隔 143, 150, 184, **199**, 201
Scrotum 陰嚢 137, 143, 187, **196**, 198, 201, 203, 234
Sebaceous glands 脂腺《眼瞼の》 514
Segmental
- arteries 区域動脈 179
- bronchus 区域気管支 111
- medullary artery of posterlor intercostal artery 髄節動脈《肋間動脈の》 610
- veins 区域静脈 179

Segments of liver 肝区域 170
Semicanal of tensor tympani 鼓膜張筋半管 481, 531
Semicircular
- canals 骨半規管 480, 536
- ducts 半規管 481, 537

Semilunar
- folds 半月ヒダ 164
- gyrus 半月回 472, 620
- line 半月線 120, **131**, 248

Semimembranosus 半膜様筋 369-371, **379**, 394, 438, 441, 442, 448, 451
Seminal
- colliculus 精丘 155, 185, **197**, 200
- vesicle 精嚢 150, 157, 182, 187, 201, 205, **223**, 243

Seminiferous tubules 精細管 199
Semispinalis 半棘筋 **32**, 560
- capitis 頭半棘筋 24-27, 32, **33**, 268, 269, 464, 465
- cervicis 頸半棘筋 24, **32**, 33, 269
- thoracis 胸半棘筋 33

Semitendinosus 半腱様筋 369, 370, **379**, 438, 439, 441, 442, 448, 451
Sensory
- cortex (postcentral gyrus) 一次体性感覚野(中心後回) 614
- root of trigeminal nerve 感覚根《三叉神経の》 511, 599

Septal
- cusp of right atrioventricular valve 中隔尖《右房室弁の》 86, 87
- papillary muscle 中隔乳頭筋 85, 87

Septomarginal trabecula 中隔縁柱 85, 87, 90
Septum 精巣中隔 198, 199
- of sphenoid sinus 蝶形骨洞中隔 538
- pellucidum 透明中隔 595, 605, 609

Serosa (perimetrium) 漿膜(子宮外膜) 188, 190
Serous pericardium 漿膜性心膜 80, 81
Serratus
- anterior 前鋸筋 22, 61, 120, 130, 258, 264, 266, 269, **275**
- posterior inferior 下後鋸筋 22, 23, 26, 30, **31**, 269
- posterior superior 上後鋸筋 26, 31

Sesamoids 種子骨 299, **401**, 403, 404

Shaft
- (body) of rib 肋骨体 45, 47
- of clavicle 鎖骨体 254
- of femur 大腿骨体 360, 363
- of fibula 腓骨体 380
- of humerus 上腕骨体 256, 257
- of metacarpals 中手骨の体 299, 300
- of middle phalanx of hand 中節骨の体《手の》 299
- of phalanges ［指(節)骨］体 **300**
- of proximal phalanx 基節骨の体《足の》 400
- of radius 橈骨体 280
- of tibia 脛骨体 380, 397
- of ulna 尺骨体 280, 351

Short
- ciliary nerves 短毛様体神経 477, **511**, 513, 617
- gastric arteries 短胃動脈 211
- gastric veins 短胃静脈 215, 218, 219
- head
- - of biceps brachii 短頭《上腕二頭筋の》 262, 264, 266, **267**, 278
- - of biceps femoris 短頭《大腿二頭筋の》 371, 373, **379**, 441, 448
- posterior ciliary arteries 短後毛様体動脈 **510**, 513, 517
- process of incus 短脚《キヌタ骨の》 532
- saphenous vein 小伏在静脈 **422**, 423, 435, 442, 443

Shoulder
- girdle 上肢帯 252
- joint 肩関節 252, **258**, 263

Sigmoid
- arteries S状結腸動脈 207, **213**, 221, 224
- colon S状結腸 145, 150-153, **164**, 166, 182, 213
- lymph node S状結腸リンパ節 233
- mesocolon S状結腸間膜 145, **148**, 150, 153, 163, 164, 166, 182
- sinus S状静脈洞 35, 481, 496, 530, 556, **606**, 607
- veins S状結腸静脈 215, **221**, 224

Simple lobule 単小葉 598
Sinoatrial (SA) node 洞房結節 90
Sinus tarsi of calcaneum 足根洞《踵骨の》 407
Skull 頭蓋 454
Small
- cardiac vein 小心臓静脈 88
- intestine 小腸 142, 160

Soft palate 軟口蓋(口蓋帆) 524, 545, 550, **552**, 553
Sole of foot 足底 451
Soleal line of tibia ヒラメ筋線《脛骨の》 380, 382
Soleus ヒラメ筋 392, 394, **398**, 442, 445, 448
Special visceral efferent fibers 特殊臓性遠心性線維 471
Spermatic cord 精索 130-133, **196**, 203, 205, 223, 436, 440
Sphenoethmoid recess 蝶篩陥凹 525
Sphenofrontal suture (pterion) 蝶前頭縫合(プテリオン) 454
Sphenoid
- bone 蝶形骨 454-456, 459, **461**, 507, 521, 523
- crest 蝶形骨稜 461
- sinus 蝶形骨洞 **520**, 521, 522, 524, 525

Sphenoidal part (M1) of middle cerebral artery 蝶形骨部(M1区)《中大脳動脈の》 608
Sphenomandibular ligament 蝶下顎靱帯 540

Sphenopalatine
- artery 蝶口蓋動脈 **495**, 503, 504, 524, 546
- foramen 蝶口蓋孔 525

Sphenoparietal sinus 蝶形[骨]頭頂静脈洞 607
Sphenosquamous suture 蝶鱗縫合 454
Sphincter
- of bile duct 総胆管括約筋 172
- of hepatopancreatic ampulla 胆膵管膨大部括約筋 172
- of pancreatic duct 膵管括約筋 172
- urethrae 尿道括約筋 150, 152, 153

Spinal
- arachnoid 脊髄クモ膜 600, 601
- branch
- - of posterior intercostal arteries 脊髄枝《肋間動脈の》 56, 610
- - of thoracic aorta 脊髄枝《胸大動脈の》 34
- cord 脊髄 3, 23, 36, 61, 592, **600**, 604
- dura mater 脊髄硬膜 600, 601
- furrow 脊柱溝 41
- ganglion 脊髄神経節 36, 59, **600**, 601, 622
- nerve 脊髄神経 36, 37, 39, 58, 59, 592, **600**, 601, 604
- nucleus
- - of accessory nerve 副神経脊髄核 471, 486
- - of trigeminal nerve 三叉神経脊髄路核 471, **476**, 482, 484, 619
- part of deltoid 肩甲棘部《三角筋の》 272
- root 脊髄根 486
- vein 脊髄静脈 611

Spinalis 棘筋 26, 27, **30**
- cervicis 頸棘筋 27, 30, **31**
- thoracis 胸棘筋 27, 30, **31**

Spinous process 棘突起 2, 4, **5**, 6-9, 12, 18, 44, 45, 49
Spiral ganglion ラセン神経節 **480**, 481, 536, 537, 619
Splanchnic nerves 内臓神経 600, 622
Spleen 脾臓 142, 146-148, 156, 159, 161, 168, 173, **174**, 210, 218
Splenic
- artery 脾動脈 55, 143, 147, 173, **174**, 175, 177, 179, 207, 210-212, 218-221
- lymph node 脾リンパ節 230, 231
- plexus 脾神経叢 238, 240, 245
- recess of omental bursa 脾陥凹《網嚢の》 146
- vein 脾静脈 143, **174**, 175, 179, 211, 215, 218-221

Splenius
- capitis 頭板状筋 24-27, 30, **31**, 268, 269, 464, 465
- cervicis 頸板状筋 24, 26, 27, **30**, 31
- muscles 板状筋 30, 31, **560**

Spongy part of urethra 海綿体部《尿道の》 185, 187, **197**, 200, 201
Squamous
- part of temporal bone 鱗部《側頭骨の》 454, 456, **527**
- suture 鱗状縫合 454

Stalk of epiglottis 喉頭蓋茎 570
Stapedial
- membrane アブミ骨膜 532
- nerve アブミ骨筋神経 478

Stapes アブミ骨 528, **532**
Stellate ganglion 星状神経節 75, **557**, 579, 623
Sternal
- angle 胸骨角 44, **46**, 120
- articular surface 胸骨関節面 254

– branches
– – of intercostal nerves　胸骨枝《肋間神経の》　58
– – of internal thoracic artery　胸骨枝《内胸動脈の》　34
– end of clavicle　胸骨端《鎖骨の》　254，259
– head of sternocleidomastoid　胸骨頭《胸鎖乳突筋の》　561
– part of diaphragm　胸骨部《横隔膜の》　**52**，53
Sternoclavicular joint　胸鎖関節　47，258，**259**
Sternocleidomastoid　胸鎖乳突筋　24，120，264，464，560，**561**，578，583
– region　胸鎖乳突筋部　576
Sternocostal joints　胸肋関節　**49**，259
Sternocostal part of pectoralis major　胸肋部《大胸筋の》　130，264，274，334
Sternocostal triangle　胸肋三角　53
Sternohyoid　胸骨舌骨筋　465，562，**563**，578，581
Sternothyroid　胸骨甲状筋　465，562，**563**，578，580
Sternum　胸骨　44，45，**46**，49，61，130，131
Stomach　胃　102，142，144，146，156，**158**，159，175，210
Straight
– part of cricothyroid　直部《輪状甲状筋の》　572
– seminiferous tubules　直精細管　199
– sinus　直静脈洞　604，**606**，607
Stria
– medullaris of thalamus　視床髄条　596，620
– terminalis　分界条　620
Striae medullaris of 4th ventricle　第四脳室髄条　599
Striate area (visual cortex)　有線野（視覚野）　473，616
Styloglossus　茎突舌筋　465，**548**，554，556
Stylohyoid　茎突舌骨筋　465，**544**，554，555，563
– branch of facial nerve　茎突舌骨筋枝《顔面神経の》　547
Styloid process
– of radius　茎状突起《橈骨の》　253，**280**，281，286，287，351，352
– of temporal bone　茎状突起《側頭骨の》　16，454，456，458，**526**，527，528，556
– of ulna　茎状突起《尺骨の》　253，**281**，286，287，351-353
Stylomandibular ligament　茎突下顎靱帯　540
Stylomastoid
– artery　茎乳突孔動脈　534，535
– foramen　茎乳突孔　458，478，479，503，**526**，547
Stylopharyngeal
– aponeurosis　茎突咽頭筋腱膜　556
– branch of glossopharyngeal nerve　茎突咽頭筋枝《舌咽神経の》　482
Stylopharyngeus　茎突咽頭筋　465，482，**554**，555，556
Subacromial
– bursa　肩峰下包　262，263
– space　肩峰下腔　258
Subarachnoid space　クモ膜下腔　601，**602**，604
Subarcuate artery　弓下動脈　535
Subclavian
– artery　鎖骨下動脈　34，56，62，66，316，**317**，335，490，491
– plexus　鎖骨下動脈神経叢　75
– trunk　鎖骨下リンパ本幹　72
– vein　鎖骨下静脈　35，62，66，215，**318**，334，335，567，575，579
Subclavius　鎖骨下筋　265，266，**275**

Subcoracoid bursa　烏口腕筋包　261
Subcostal
– artery　肋下動脈　34
– muscles　肋下筋　51
– nerve　肋下神経　36，**58**，176，179，425
– plane　肋骨下平面　120
– vein　肋下静脈　35，57，611
Subcutaneous
– acromial bursa　肩峰皮下包　263
– bursa of medial malleolus　内果皮下包　443
– part of external anal sphincter　皮下部《外肛門括約筋》　167
– perineal space　会陰皮下隙　155
– venous plexus　皮下静脈叢　167
Subdeltoid bursa　三角筋下包　262，263
Subglottic space (infraglottic cavity)　声門下腔　573
Sublingual
– artery　舌下動脈　549
– fold　舌下ヒダ　544，549
– gland　舌下腺　548，**551**，556
– papilla　舌下小丘　544，549
Submandibular
– (digastric) triangle　顎下三角　576
– duct　顎下腺管　549，551
– ganglion　顎下神経節　479，**547**，549
– gland　顎下腺　501，**551**，580
– lymph nodes　顎下リンパ節　587
Submental
– artery　オトガイ下動脈　492
– lymph nodes　オトガイ下リンパ節　587
– triangle　オトガイ下三角　576
– vein　オトガイ下静脈　496
Submucosa
– of esophagus　粘膜下組織《食道の》　97
– of urinary bladder　粘膜下組織《膀胱の》　185
Suboccipital
– muscles　後頭下筋　28
– nerve　後頭下神経　37，38，**568**，585
Subperitoneal space　腹膜下隙　154
Subpleural
– connective tissue　胸膜下結合組織　116
– network　胸膜下リンパ管叢　118
Subpopliteal recess　膝窩筋下陥凹　385，390
Subpubic angle　恥骨下角　127
Subpyloric lymph node　幽門下リンパ節　230，231
Subscapular
– artery　肩甲下動脈　**316**，317，335，337
– axillary lymph node　肩甲下腋窩リンパ節　64
– fossa　肩甲下窩　255
– nerve　肩甲下神経　320，321
Subscapularis　肩甲下筋　258，262，265，266，**273**
Subserosa　漿膜下組織　133
Substantia nigra　黒質　474，615
Subtaler (talocalcaneal) joint　距骨下関節　402，**404**，406
Subtendinous bursa of subscapularis　腱下包《肩甲下筋の》　262，263
Subthalamic nucleus　視床下核　597
Sulcal
– artery　溝動脈　610
– vein　溝静脈　611
Sulcus
– calcanei　踵骨溝　407
– for spinal nerve　脊髄神経溝　6，7
– tali　距骨溝　407
– terminalis　分界溝　548
Superficial
– abdominal fascia　浅腹筋膜　132，133，**134**，201，436

– branch/es
– – of lateral plantar nerve　浅枝《外側足底神経の》　433，446
– – of medial plantar artery　浅枝《内側足底動脈の》　420，443，446
– – of medial plantar nerve　浅枝《内側足底神経の》　446
– – of radial nerve　浅枝《橈骨神経の》　320，**325**，330，331，339-341，346
– – of ulnar artery　浅枝《尺骨動脈の》　343
– – of ulnar nerve　浅枝《尺骨神経の》　329，342，345
– cervical
– – artery　浅頸動脈　**317**，581-583
– – lymph node　浅頸リンパ節　582
– – vein　浅頸静脈　582，583
– circumflex
– – iliac
– – – artery　浅腸骨回旋動脈　**420**，436，440
– – – vein　浅腸骨回旋静脈　57，**422**，434，436
– dorsal penile veins　浅陰茎背静脈　197，201，202
– epigastric
– – artery　浅腹壁動脈　420，440
– – vein　浅腹壁静脈　57，422，434，**436**
– fascia　浅筋膜　198
– fibular nerve　浅腓骨神経　424，**432**，434，444，445
– head
– – of flexor pollicis brevis　浅頭《短母指屈筋の》　307
– – of medial pterygoid　浅頭《内側翼突筋の》　468
– inguinal
– – lymph node　浅鼠径リンパ節　**227**，228，229，234，235，423，436
– – ring　浅鼠径輪　130，**132**，133，139，196，202，248，436
– layer
– – (investing layer) of cervical fascia　浅葉《頸筋膜の》　23，574，**577**，578，580
– – of nuchal fascia　浅葉《項筋膜の》　23
– – of thoracolumbar fascia　浅葉《胸腰筋膜の》　22，23，26
– middle cerebral vein　浅中大脳静脈　606，607
– palmar
– – arch　浅掌動脈弓　316，317，342，343，**345**
– – branch of radial artery　浅掌枝《橈骨動脈の》　**316**，342，344，345
– – venous arch　浅掌静脈弓　318
– parotid lymph nodes　浅耳下腺リンパ節　587
– part
– – of external anal sphincter　浅部《外肛門括約筋の》　167
– – of masseter　浅部《咬筋の》　463，467，468
– – of parotid gland　浅部《耳下腺の》　551
– pelvic diaphragmatic fascia　浅骨盤隔膜筋膜　154
– penile fascia　浅陰茎筋膜　197，201，202
– perineal fascia　浅会陰筋膜　**136**，137，152，155，191
– petrosal artery　浅錐体動脈　535
– popliteal lymph node　浅膝窩リンパ節　423
– temporal
– – artery　浅側頭動脈　491-493，**494**，499，502，503，529
– – vein　浅側頭静脈　496，**497**，498，502，503，567
– transverse
– – metacarpal ligament　浅横中手靱帯　306
– – metatarsal ligament　浅横中足靱帯　412

Superficial transverse perineal
――perineal　浅会陰横筋　**136**, 137, 193-195, 203
Superior
― alveolar nerves　上歯槽神経　505, 546
― anastomotic vein　上吻合静脈　606
― angle of scapula　上角《肩甲骨の》　253, 255, 259, 351
― articular
―― facet
――― of sacrum　上関節面《仙骨の》　10
――― of vertebra　上関節面《椎骨の》　**5**, 6-9
―― process　上関節突起　**5**, 6-11, 126, 127
― auricular muscles（auricularis superior）　上耳介筋　463, **466**, 529
― basal vein of lower lobe of lung　上肺底静脈　115
― belly of omohyoid　上腹《肩甲舌骨筋の》　563
― border
―― of scapula　上縁《肩甲骨の》　255
―― of spleen　上縁《脾臓の》　148, 174, 175
―― of suprarenal gland　上縁《副腎の》　176
― branch of oculomotor nerve　上枝《動眼神経の》　475, 511, 512
― cerebellar
―― artery　上小脳動脈　608
―― peduncle　上小脳脚　598, 599
―― vein　上小脳静脈　602, 606, 607
― cervical ganglion　上頸神経節　75, 500, 501, **556**, 557, 580, 581, 623
― cluneal nerves　上殿皮神経　37, 39, 58, 203, 430, **435**, 438, 441
― colliculus of quadrigeminal plate　上丘《四丘体板の》　599, 616
― conjunctival fornix　上結膜円蓋　514
― costal facet　上肋骨窩　5, 8, **49**
― costotransverse ligament　上肋横突靱帯　49
― duodenal
―― flexure　上十二指腸曲　160
―― recess　上十二指腸陥凹　161
― epigastric
―― artery　上腹壁動脈　56
―― vein　上腹壁静脈　215
― extensor retinaculum　上伸筋支帯　415, 443, 445
― fascia of pelvic diaphragm　上骨盤隔膜筋膜　152, 153, **167**
― fibular retinaculum　上腓骨筋支帯　415
― ganglion　上神経節　482-484
― gluteal
―― artery　上殿動脈　208, 222, 223, **224**, 420, 438-441
―― nerve　上殿神経　425, **431**, 438, 439, 441
―― vein　上殿静脈　216, 222, **224**, 438, 441
― head（part）of lateral pterygoid　上頭《外側翼突筋の》　469, 541
― horn of thyroid cartilage　上角《甲状軟骨の》　558, **570**, 571
― hypogastric plexus　上下腹神経叢　236, **237**, 239, 241-243, 246, 247
― hypophyseal artery　上下垂体動脈　490
― labial
―― artery　上唇動脈　492
―― branches of infraorbital nerve　上唇枝《眼窩下神経の》　546
― lacrimal canaliculi　上涙小管　515
― laryngeal
―― artery　上喉頭動脈　557, **566**, 575, 578, 579
―― nerve　上喉頭神経　117, 484, **485**, 556, 557, 575, 578-580
―― vein　上喉頭静脈　575
― lateral brachial cutaneous nerve　上外側上腕皮神経　324, 330-332
― ligaments
―― of incus　上キヌタ骨靱帯　532
―― of malleus　上ツチ骨靱帯　532
― lip（ileocolic labrum）　回結腸唇（上唇）　164
― lobar bronchi　上葉気管支　77, 78, 104
― lobe of lung　上葉《肺の》　93, 104, 105
― longitudinal
―― fasciculus　上縦束　594
―― muscle of tongue　上縦舌筋　548
― malleolar fold　上ツチ骨ヒダ　532
― meatus　上鼻道　460, **521**, 523, 525
― mediastinum　上縦隔　**66**, 76
― medullary velum　上髄帆　598, 599
― mesenteric
―― artery　上腸間膜動脈　143, 149, 156, 160, 174, 175, 180, 206-208, 211, **212**, 219-221
―― ganglion　上腸間膜動脈神経節　**237**, 239, 240, 245, 247
―― lymph node　上腸間膜リンパ節　**226**, 227, 228, 231-233
―― plexus　上腸間膜動脈神経叢　**236**, 238, 240, 244, 245
―― vein　上腸間膜静脈　149, 156, 160, 211, 215, **220**, 221
― nasal concha　上鼻甲介　460, 507, **521**, 522, 523, 525
― nuchal line　上項線　16, 24, 25, 28, 269, **456**, 458
― oblique　上斜筋　475, 508
―― part of longus colli　上斜部《頸長筋の》　29, 565
― olivary nucleus　上オリーブ核　619
― ophthalmic
―― artery　上眼動脈　512
―― vein　上眼静脈　496, 497, **510**, 512, 513, 567, 607
― orbital fissure　上眼窩裂　461, 477, **506**, 507, 509, 523, 538
― pair of parathyroid glands　上副甲状腺（上上皮小体）　574
― pancreatic lymph node　上膵リンパ節　231
― part
―― of duodenum　上部《十二指腸の》　148, 149, **160**, 161, 172, 174
―― of nucleus of solitary tract　上部《孤束核の》　482, 484
―― of vestibular ganglion　上部《前庭神経節の》　481, 536, 537
― petrosal
―― sinus　上錐体静脈洞　497, 607
―― vein　上錐体静脈　607
― pharyngeal constrictor　上咽頭収縮筋　**554**, 555
― phrenic
―― arteries　上横隔動脈　54, 55, 61
―― lymph node　上横隔リンパ節　79, 100
― pole of kidney　上端《腎臓の》　178
― pubic ramus　恥骨上枝　124-126, 133, 137, 150, 151, 197, 358, 359
― puncta　上涙点　515
― recess of tympanic membrane　上鼓膜陥凹　532
― rectal
―― artery　上直腸動脈　**207**, 213, 221, 224
―― lymph node　上直腸リンパ節　233
―― plexus　上直腸動脈神経叢　245
―― vein　上直腸静脈　215, **221**, 224
― rectus　上直筋　475, **508**, 509, 514
― root of ansa cervicalis　上根《頸神経ワナの》　547, **568**, 569, 580
― sagittal sinus　上矢状静脈洞　35, 496, 497, 567, 602, 604, **606**, 607
― salivatory nucleus　上唾液核　471, 478, 479
― segment［S Ⅵ］of lung　上-下葉区《肺の》　108
― segmental artery
―― of kidney　上区動脈《腎臓の》　209
―― of lung　上-下葉動脈《肺の》　115
― semilunar lobule　上半月小葉　598
― suprarenal arteries　上副腎動脈　178, 179, 208, **217**
― tarsal muscle　上瞼板筋　514
― tarsus　上瞼板　514
― thoracic
―― artery　最上胸動脈　56, 316, **335**, 336, 337
―― aperture　胸郭上口　44
― thyroid
―― artery　上甲状腺動脈　490, 492, **493**, 500, 501, 556, 566, 574, 578-581
―― notch　上甲状切痕　570
―― tubercle　上甲状結節　570
―― vein　上甲状腺静脈　496, 567, 575
― tracheobronchial lymph node　上気管気管支リンパ節　118, 119
― transverse
―― rectal fold　上直腸横ヒダ　167
―― scapular ligament　上肩甲横靱帯　259, 261, 262
― ulnar collateral artery　上尺側側副動脈　**316**, 338-340
― vein of lower lobe of lung　上-下葉静脈《肺の》　115
― vena cava　上大静脈　35, 54, 57, 66, **70**, 77, 78, 83, 88, 114, 611
― vertebral notch　上椎切痕　**5**, 8, 9, 12
― vesical
―― artery　上膀胱動脈　222, 223, 225
―― vein　上膀胱静脈　223
― vestibular nucleus　前庭神経上核　480, 618
Superipr tympanic artery　上鼓室動脈　534
Superolateral lymph node of superficial inguinal nodes　上外側浅鼠径リンパ節　423, 436
Superomedial lymph node of superficial inguinal nodes　上内側浅鼠径リンパ節　423
Supinator　回外筋　288-291, 296, **297**
Supplementary motor cortex　補助運動野　613, 615
Suprachiasmatic nucleus　視交叉上核　616
Supraclavicular
― lymph node　鎖骨上リンパ節　64
― nerves　鎖骨上神経　37, 58, 62, 330-332, 334, **568**, 569, 578, 582
Supraduodenal artery　十二指腸上動脈　211
Supraglenoid tubercle of scapula　関節上結節《肩甲骨の》　**255**, 260
Supraglottic space（layngeal vestibule）　声門上腔（喉頭前庭）　573
Suprahyoid muscles　舌骨上筋群　544
Supraoptic recess　視索上陥凹　596, 605
Supraorbital
― artery　眼窩上動脈　490, **510**, 512, 513
― foramen　眼窩上孔　455, **506**
― margin　眼窩上縁　455, 589
― nerve　眼窩上神経　475, 477, 489, **498**, 499, 511-513
Suprapatellar pouch　膝蓋上陥凹　390, 391
Suprapineal recess　松果体上陥凹　605

Suprapyloric lymph node　幽門上リンパ節　230, 231
Suprarenal
- gland　副腎　142, 147, 149, 156, 161, 175, **176**, 177-180
- impression of liver　副腎圧痕《肝臓の》　170
- plexus　副腎神経叢　236, **237**, 239
- vein　副腎静脈　178
Suprascapular
- artery　肩甲上動脈　316, **317**, 332, 333, 335
- nerve　肩甲上神経　320, 321, **322**, 332, 333, 579
- vein　肩甲上静脈　496
Supraspinatus　棘上筋　22, 262, 265, 266, 269, 270, **273**, 332
Supraspinous
- fossa of scapula　棘上窩《肩甲骨の》　47, 255
- ligament　棘上靱帯　18, 19, **20**, 559
Supratrochlear
- artery　滑車上動脈　490, 492, **510**, 513
- lymph node　滑車上リンパ節　64
- nerve　滑車上神経　477, 489, 498, 499, **511**, 512, 513
- vein　滑車上静脈　510
Supravaginal part of uterine cervix　腟上部《子宮頸の》　188, 189
Supraventricular crest　室上稜　85
Supravesical fossa　膀胱上窩　135, 152, 183
Supreme
- intercostal
-- artery　最上肋間動脈　317
-- vein　最上肋間静脈　70
- nuchal line　最上項線　456, 458
Sural
- arteries　腓腹動脈　421
- nerve　腓腹神経　424, 433, 434, 435, **442**, 444
Surfactant　サーファクタント（表面活性物質）　111
Surgical neck of humerus　外科頸《上腕骨の》　256
Suspensory
- ligament/s
-- of breast (Cooper's ligaments)　乳房提靱帯（クーパー靱帯）　63
-- of duodenum　十二指腸提筋　160
-- of penis (Penile suspensory ligament)　陰茎提靱帯　150, 184, 202, 225
-- of the ovary　卵巣提索　155
Sustentaculum tali　載距突起　**401**, 403, 404-407, 410
Sympathetic
- ganglion　交感神経幹神経節　36, 600
- nerve　交感神経　622
- nervous system　交感神経系　75, 244
- root　交感神経根　511
- trunk　交感神経幹　**74**, 75, 78, 79, 91, 98, 237, 239, 243, 245-247, 556, 557, 579, 581, 623
Symphyseal surface　恥骨結合面　124, 129, 358
Synovial membrane　滑膜　365

T

T1 spinal nerve　第1胸神経　321, 600
Taenia
- cinerea of 4th ventricle　第四脳室ヒモ　599
- mesocolica　間膜ヒモ　164
- of fornix　脳弓ヒモ　596
- omentalis　大網ヒモ　164

Taeniae coli　自由ヒモ　144, 145, 148, 150, 151, 162-164, 166, 182
Tail
- of caudate nucleus　尾状核尾　594
- of epididymis　精巣上体尾　198
- of pancreas　膵尾　174, 175
Talocalcaneal (subtaler) joint　距骨下関節　402, **404**, 406
Talocalcaneonavicular joint　距踵舟関節　405
Talocrural joint　距腿関節　356, 402, 404, **405**
Talonavicular joint　距舟関節　402
Talus　距骨　400-406, **407**
Tarsal
- glands　瞼板腺　514
- tunnel　足根管　443
Tarsals　足根　356
Tarsometatarsal joints　足根中足関節　402-403
Tarsus (tarsal bones)　足根骨　400
Tectorial membrane of lateral atlanto-axial joint　蓋膜《外側環軸関節の》　16-18
Tectum of midbrain　中脳蓋　474
Teeth　歯　455, 456, **542**
Tegmen tympani (roof of tympanic cavity)　鼓室蓋　481
Tegmental nucleus　被蓋核　472, 615
Telencephalon　大脳　594
Temporal
- bone　側頭骨　16, 454, 456, 458, 459, 523, **526**, 527
- branches of facial nerve　側頭枝《顔面神経の》　478, 488, 498, 500
- crescent　耳側半月　616
- fossa　側頭窩　501
- horn (inferior horn) of lateral ventricle　下角《側脳室の》　596, 605
- lobe　側頭葉　593
- surface
-- of sphenoid bone　側頭面《蝶形骨の》　461
-- of zygomatic bone　側頭面《頬骨の》　458
Temporalis　側頭筋　463-465, **468**, 501
Temporomandibular joint　顎関節　540, 541
Temporoparietalis　側頭頭頂筋　463
Tendinous arch
-- of levator ani　肛門挙筋腱弓　141
-- of soleus　ヒラメ筋［の］腱弓　398, 442
- intersections　腱画　131, 139
Tendon
- of conus　動脈円錐腱　86
- of insertion
-- of biceps brachii　停止腱《上腕二頭筋の》　266, 288
-- of brachioradialis　停止腱《腕橈骨筋の》　295
- of tensor tympani　鼓膜張筋の腱　531
- sheath　腱鞘　415
Tenon's capsule (bulbar fascia)　テノン嚢（眼球鞘）　514
Tensor
- fasciae latae　大腿筋膜張筋　366, 367, 370, 371, 373, 374, **375**, 439, 440, 448, 450
- tympani　鼓膜張筋　**528**, 531, 534
- veli palatini　口蓋帆張筋　530, **545**, 555
Tentorial
- branches of maxillary nerve　テント枝《上顎神経の》　603
- notch　テント切痕　603
Tentorium cerebelli　小脳テント　602, **603**, 607
Teres
- major　大円筋　22, 40, 264-270, **277**, 332, 351
- minor　小円筋　40, 262, 269, 270, **273**

Terminal
- branches of external carotid artery　終枝《外頸動脈の》　491, 494
- bronchiole　終末細気管支　111
- nuclei　神経核　616
- of ileum　終末部《回腸の》　164
Testicular
- artery　精巣動脈　196, 198, 199, **225**
- mediastinum (mediastinum testis)　精巣縦隔　198, 199
- plexus　精巣動脈神経叢　196, 198, 236, **237**, 239, 240, 247
- vein　精巣静脈　196, 198, 199, **225**
Testis　精巣　187, **198**, 205, 225, 234
Thalamocingular tract　視床帯状回路　621
Thalamostriate vein　視床線条体静脈　606
Thalamus　視床　473, 594, **596**, 598, 609, 614, 618
Thenar
- branch of median nerve　母指球枝《正中神経の》　342
- crease　母指線　353
- eminence　母指球　350, 352, 353
Thigh　大腿　356
Third ventricle　第三脳室　596, **605**, 609
Thoracic
- aorta　胸大動脈　55, 56, 61, **68**, 77, 79, 93, 98, 99, 104, 316, 610
- aortic plexus　胸大動脈神経叢　75, 91
- cavity　胸腔　66
- constriction (middle esophageal constriction)　胸部狭窄（中食道狭窄）　96
- duct　胸管　72, 79, **100**, 119, 226, 579
- ganglion　胸神経節　74, 78, 91
- nerve　胸神経　321
- part
-- of esophagus　胸部《食道の》　77, 96, 104
-- of trachea　胸部《気管の》　110
- splanchnic nerves　胸内臓神経　244, 245
- vertebrae [T1-T12]　胸椎　2, 4, **8**
Thoracoacromial artery　胸肩峰動脈　56, **316**, 334-337
Thoracodorsal
- artery　胸背動脈　316, 336, **337**
- nerve　胸背神経　320, 321, **323**, 337
- vein　胸背静脈　**318**, 336
Thoracoepigastric vein　胸腹壁静脈　57, 60, **318**
Thoracolumbar
- fascia　胸腰筋膜　22, **23**, 26, 27, 40, 268, 269, 277
- junction　胸腰椎境界　2
Thorax　胸部　44, 77
Thymus　胸腺　66, 77, 78, **80**
Thyroarytenoid　甲状披裂筋　572
Thyrocervical trunk　甲状頸動脈　34, 56, 68, 316, 317, 335, 491, 566, **575**, 579
Thyroepiglottic
- ligament　甲状喉頭蓋靱帯　571
- part of thyroarytenoid　甲状喉頭蓋部《甲状披裂筋の》　572
Thyrohyoid　甲状舌骨筋　554, 562, **563**, 578, 580
- branch of ansa cervicalis　甲状舌骨筋枝《頸神経ワナの》　578, 580
- ligament　甲状舌骨靱帯　550, **571**, 573
- membrane　甲状舌骨膜　558, **571**
Thyroid
- cartilage　甲状軟骨　110, 120, 558, 563, **570**, 571, 574, 578, 579

Thyroid
– gland 甲状腺 66, 77, 550, 553, **574**, 580, 581
– venous plexus 甲状腺静脈叢 575
Thyropharyngeal part of inferior pharyngeal constrictor 甲状咽頭部《下咽頭収縮筋の》 554
Tibia 脛骨 356, **380**, 381, 382, 404, 405, 448, 450
Tibial
– nerve 脛骨神経 424, 425, **433**, 434, 435, 442, 443
– plateau of tibia 上関節面《脛骨の》 356, 380, 382
– tuberosity 脛骨粗面 356, 357, 373, **380**, 381, 392, 450
Tibialis
– anterior 前脛骨筋 369, 373, 392, 393, **397**, 404, 415, 443, 450
– posterior 後脛骨筋 394, 395, **399**, 404, 410-413, 415, 442, 443
– – tendon 後脛骨筋の腱 399, **413**, 419
Tibiocalcanean part of deltoid ligament 脛踵部《三角靱帯の》 408
Tibiofibular
– joint 脛腓関節 380, 382
– syndesmosis 脛腓靱帯結合 380, 404, 409
Tibionavicular part of deltoid ligament 脛舟部《三角靱帯の》 408
Tongue 舌 548
Tonsil of cerebellum 小脳扁桃 598
Tonsillar
– branch of glossopharyngeal nerve 扁桃枝《舌咽神経の》 482
– fossa 扁桃窩 552
Tonsils 扁桃 552
Torus tubarius 耳管隆起 524, 550, 552
Trabeculae carneae of interventricular septum 肉柱《心室中隔の》 85
Trachea 気管 23, 108, **110**, 570
Tracheal
– bifurcation 気管分岐部 110
– cartilages 気管軟骨 110
Tracheobronchial lymph node 気管気管支リンパ節 73, 100, 101, **118**
Tragicus 耳珠筋 529
Tragus 耳珠 529, 589
Transglottic space (intermediate laryngeal cavity) 声門間腔（喉頭室） 573
Transumbilical plane 臍平面 248
Transversalis fascia 横筋筋膜 23, **131**, 133-135
Transverse
– arytenoid 横披裂筋 555, **572**
– carpal ligament 横手根靱帯 303, 344
– cervical
– – artery 頸横動脈 39, 317, **579**
– – ligament 子宮頸横靱帯（基靱帯） 152, 155
– – nerve 頸横神経 568, 569, 578, 582, 583
– – vein 頸横静脈 334
– colon 横行結腸 102, 142-148, 156, 161, 162, **164**, 165, 175, 176
– facial artery 顔面横動脈 494, **498**, 499
– fascicles
– – of foot 横束（横線維束）《足の》 412
– – of hand 横束（横線維束）《手の》 306
– foramen 横突孔 5, 6, 7, 558
– head
– – of adductor hallucis 横頭《母趾内転筋の》 410, 413, 419, 447
– – of adductor pollicis 横頭《母指内転筋の》 307, 308, 313

– ligament
– – of acetabulum 寛骨臼横靱帯 364
– – of humerus 上腕横靱帯 261, 262
– – of knee 膝横靱帯 387, 388
– ligament of atlas 環椎横靱帯 17, 19
– lines of sacrum 横線《仙骨の》 10
– medullary veins 横延髄静脈 607
– mesocolon 横行結腸間膜 143, **145**, 146-148, 162-165, 175, 177
– muscle of tongue 横舌筋 548
– palatine suture 横口蓋縫合 458, 538
– part
– – of nasalis 横部《鼻筋の》 464
– – of trapezius 横行部（水平部）《僧帽筋の》 22, 268, 276, 332, 561
– – of ulnar collateral ligament 横部《内側側副靱帯の》 284
– pericardial sinus 心膜横洞 81
– perineal ligament 会陰横靱帯 181, **191**, 203
– pontine veins 横橋静脈 607
– process 横突起 4, **5**, 6-9, 18, 20, 44, 45, 49
– – of atlas 横突起《環椎の》 29
– rectal fold 直腸横ヒダ 166
– sinus 横静脈洞 35, 496, 497, 567, **606**, 607
– tarsal joint 横足根関節（ショパール関節） 402
– thoracic diameter 胸郭横径 48
– vesical fold 横膀胱ヒダ 152, 153, 181, **182**, 183
Transversospinales 横突棘筋 33
Transversus
– abdominis 腹横筋 27, 52, 131, 133-135, **138**, 139
– – aponeurosis (aponeurosis of transversus abdominis) 腹横筋腱膜 131, **134**, 139
– auriculae 耳介横筋
– thoracis 胸横筋 50, **51**
Trapezium 大菱形骨 **298**, 300, 301
Trapezius 僧帽筋 23-26, 40, 264, 266, 268, **276**, 332, 464, 465, 560, 561
Trapezoid 小菱形骨 **298**, 299-301, 315
– ligament 菱形靱帯 259
Triangle
– of Grynfeltt (fibrous lumbar triangle) グランフェルト三角（上腰三角） 39
– of Petit プチ三角（下腰三角） 39
Triangular fossa 三角窩 529
Triceps
– brachii 上腕三頭筋 22, 40, 268, 270, **279**, 288, 290, 333, 350, 351
– surae 下腿三頭筋 393, **398**, 415, 448
Tricuspid valve 三尖弁 →右房室弁
Trigeminal
– ganglion 三叉神経節 **476**, 477, 478, 488, 489, 525, 547
– – branch of internal carotid artery 三叉神経節枝《内頸動脈の》 490
– nerve (CN Ⅴ) 三叉神経 470, **476**, 483, 546, 598, 599, 607
– nuclei 三叉神経核群 471
Trigone of CN Ⅹ 迷走神経三角 599
Triquetrum 三角骨 253, **298**, 299, 301, 351, 352
Triradiate cartilage Y軟骨 125, 359
Trochanteric
– bursa 転子包 363, 439, 441
– fossa 転子窩 360
Trochlea 滑車 508

– of humerus 上腕骨滑車 **256**, 257, 282, 283, 285
– of talus 距骨滑車 403-405, 407
Trochlear
– nerve (CN Ⅳ) 滑車神経 470, **474**, 475, 509, 512, 513, 599
– notch of ulna 滑車切痕《尺骨の》 280, 281, 283
True
– conjugate 産科的真結合線 129
– ribs 真肋 45
Tubal
– artery 耳管動脈 535
– branch of uterine artery 卵管枝《子宮動脈の》 225
– tonsil 耳管扁桃 552
Tubarian branch of tympanic plexus 耳管枝《鼓室神経叢の》 483
Tuber cinereum 灰白隆起 596
Tubercle
– of nucleus cuneatus 楔状束結節 599
– of nucleus gracilis 薄束結節 599
– of scaphoid 舟状骨結節 253, 299, 350, 352
– of trapezium 大菱形骨結節 253, **299**, 350, 352, 353
Tuberculum sellae 鞍結節 461
Tuberosity
– for serratus anterior 前鋸筋結節 47
– of 5th metatarsal 第5中足骨粗面 400, **401**, 403, 404, 410, 412, 413, 415, 417, 450, 451
– of cuboid 立方骨粗面 **401**, 417
– of distal phalanx of hand 末節骨粗面《手の》 299, 300, 305
Tunica
– albuginea 白膜 198, 199
– – of corpus cavernosum 陰茎海綿体白膜 197, 202
– – of corpus spongiosum 尿道海綿体白膜 197
– dartos 肉様膜 196, 198, **199**
– vaginalis 精巣鞘膜 196, 198
Tympanic
– canaliculus 鼓室神経小管 483
– cavity 鼓室 481, 528, **530**, 531
– incisure 鼓膜切痕 532
– membrane 鼓膜 478, 528, 531, **532**, 534
– nerve 鼓室神経 481, 482, **483**, 531
– part of temporal bone 鼓室部《側頭骨の》 527
– plexus 鼓室神経叢 481, **483**, 531, 547
Tympanomastoid fissure 鼓室乳突裂 526
Type
– Ⅰ pneumocyte Ⅰ型肺胞上皮細胞 111
– Ⅱ pneumocyte Ⅱ型肺胞上皮細胞 111

U

Ulna 尺骨 252, 253, **280**, 309, 352
Ulnar
– artery 尺骨動脈 316, 317, 339-341, **342**, 343-345, 347
– bundle territory 尺側リンパ管束領域 319
– carpal
– – collateral ligament 内側手根側副靱帯 302
– – eminence 尺側手根隆起 303
– collateral ligament of elbow joint 内側側副靱帯《肘関節の》 **284**, 285, 286, 301
– groove of humerus 尺骨神経溝《上腕骨の》 256, 257
– group of lymphatics 尺側リンパ管群 319

- head of flexor digitorum superficialis 尺骨頭《浅指屈筋の》 289, 292
- nerve 尺骨神経 60, 321, **329**, 330, 331, 335-346
- notch of radius 尺骨切痕《橈骨の》 287
- recurrent artery 尺側反回動脈 316
- tuberosity 尺骨粗面 278, 280, **281**
- tunnel 尺骨神経管(ギヨン管) 342-344
- veins 尺骨静脈 318

Umbilical
- artery 臍動脈 **94**, 95, 208, 222, 223, 225
- cord 臍帯 95
- folds 臍ヒダ 135
- ring 臍輪 139
- vein 臍静脈 94

Umbilicus 臍 **94**, 95, 120, 121, 130, 131, 134

Umbo 鼓膜臍 532

Uncinate
- process
-- of cervical vertebrae 鉤状突起《頸椎の》 6, 7
-- of ethmoid bone 鉤状突起《篩骨の》 420, 521, 523
-- of pancreas 鉤状突起《膵臓の》 143, 174, 175

Uncus of limbic lobe 鉤《辺縁葉の》 472

Unicovertebral joint 鉤椎関節 15

Upper
- esophageal constriction 上食道狭窄 96
- eyelid 上眼瞼 514, 515
- limb 上肢 252
- lip 上唇 524
- subscapular nerve 上肩甲下神経 323, 337
- trunk(C5-C6) 上神経幹(第5・6頸神経) 321

Ureter 尿管 142, 149-151, 157, 166, 177, 178, **180**, 181, 183-187, 216, 225

Ureteral
- branches of renal artery 尿管枝《腎動脈の》 209
- orifice 尿管口 185-187
- plexus 尿管神経叢 **237**, 239, 242, 243, 246

Urethra 尿道 155, **184**, 185, 186, 190, 197, 200

Urethral
- artery 尿道動脈 197, 202
- ampulla 膨大部《尿道の》 185
- carina 尿道隆起《腟の》 190
- crest 尿道稜 197
- glands 尿道腺 185, 197

Urinary bladder 膀胱 142, 143, 150-153, 155, 157, 180, 182, 183, **184**, 185-187, 190, 197, 225, 235

Urogenital
- sinus 尿生殖洞 205
- triangle 尿生殖三角 136

Uterine
- artery 子宮動脈 208, 222, **223**, 225
- body(corpus) 子宮体 151, 184, 188-190
- cavity 子宮腔 188, 189
- cervix 子宮頸 151, 155, 157, 184, 186, **188**
- fundus 子宮底 151, 152, 155, 181, 184, **188**, 189, 191, 225
- isthmus 子宮峡部 188
- ostium of uterine tube 卵管子宮口 189
- part of uterine tube 子宮部《卵管の》 189
- pole 子宮端 188
- tube 卵管 152, 155, 181, 183, 184, 186, 188, **189**, 191, 205, 225, 235
- venous plexus 子宮静脈叢 216, 222, **223**
- veins 子宮静脈 216, 222, **223**, 225

Uterosacral
- fold 子宮仙骨ヒダ(直腸子宮ヒダ) 152, **166**, 181, 183
- ligament 子宮仙骨靱帯(直腸子宮靱帯) 157, **181**, 189, 190

Uterovaginal
- plexus 子宮腟神経叢 242, 247
- venous plexus 子宮腟静脈叢 157, 190

Uterus 子宮 151, 152, 181, 183, 184, 186, **188**, 189-191, 205, 235

Utricle 卵形嚢 536, 618

Utricular nerve 卵形嚢神経 536, 537

Utriculoampullary nerve 卵形嚢膨大部神経 481

Uvula 口蓋垂 525, **545**, 550, 552, 553
- of bladder 膀胱垂 185
- vermis 虫部垂 598

V

Vagina 腟 151, 152, 155, 183, 184, 186, 189, **190**, 191, 205

Vaginal
- artery 腟動脈 **222**, 223, 225
- branch of uterine artery 腟枝《子宮動脈の》 222
- fornix 腟円蓋 151, 188-190
- orifice 腟口 136, 190-192, 194
- part of uterine cervix 腟部《子宮頸の》 188, 189
- rugae 腟粘膜ヒダ 190, 191
- venous plexus 腟静脈叢 222, 223
- vestibule(vestibule of vagina) 腟前庭 155, 186, **190**, 191, 192

Vagus nerve(CN Ⅹ) 迷走神経 23, 66, 74, 75, 77-79, 91, 98, 244, 470, 482, **484**, 485, 549, 556, 579-581, 599, 619, 622

Vallate(circum) papilla 有郭乳頭 548

Vallecula of cerebellum 小脳谷 598

Valve
- of coronary sinus 冠状静脈弁 85
- of foramen ovale 卵円孔弁 85
- of inferior vena cava 下大静脈弁 85

Valved orifice
- of coronary sinus 冠状静脈口 85
- of inferior vena cava 下大静脈口 85

Valves of Kerckring ケルクリングヒダ 160

Vasa recta 直細動脈 212

Vascular pole of ovary 血管極《卵巣の》 188, 189

Vasocorona 血管冠 610

Vastoadductor membrane 広筋内転筋膜 429

Vastus
- intermedius 中間広筋 366, 367, 371, **378**, 429, 440, 448
- lateralis 外側広筋 366, 367, 371, 373, **378**, 429, 440, 448, 450
- medialis 内側広筋 366, 367, 369, **378**, 429, 440, 448, 450

Vein
- of cochlear aqueduct 蝸牛水管静脈 537
- of ductus deferens 精管静脈 196, 199
- of round window 蝸牛窓静脈 537
- of vestibular
-- aqueduct 前庭水管静脈 537
-- bulb 前庭球静脈 195

Venous
- plexus
-- around foramen magnum 大後頭孔周囲静脈叢 497, 606
-- of foramen ovale 卵円孔静脈叢 607
-- of hypoglossal canal 舌下神経管静脈叢 606
- ring 静脈輪 611

Ventral
- (anterior)
-- rami
--- of intercostal nerves 前枝《肋間神経の》 61
--- of spinal nerve 前枝《脊髄神経の》 **36**, 59, 321
-- root of spinal nerve 前根《脊髄神経の》 59, 321, 430, **600**, 601, 615
- diencephalic sulcus(hypothalamic sulcus) 視床下溝 596
- lateral nucleus 外側腹側核 615
- posteromedial nucleus of thalamus 後内側腹側核《視床の》 619
- root of cervical nerve 前根《頸神経の》 599

Ventricle
- 喉頭室 573
- 脳室 605

Ventrolateral thalamic nuclei 視床外側腹側核群 597

Vermian cistern of cerebellum 小脳虫部槽 604

Vermiform appendix 虫垂 142, 153, **164**, 182

Vermis of cerebellum 小脳虫部 598

Vertebra 椎骨 5
- prominens(C7) 隆椎(第7頸椎) 4, 6, 40, 558, 600

Vertebral
- artery 椎骨動脈 34, 38, 56, 68, 316, 317, 490, 491, 556, **566**, 579, 601, 608, 610
- arch 椎弓 **5**, 6, 7, 9, 12
- body 椎体 4-6, 8, 12, 45
- canal 脊柱管(椎管) 3, 12, 20
- column 脊柱 2
- foramen 椎孔 **5**, 7, 9, 12, 45
- part of latissimus dorsi 椎骨部《広背筋の》 277
- plexus 椎骨動脈神経叢 75
- vein 椎骨静脈 567, 601, 611
- venous plexus 椎骨静脈叢 35, 156, 604

Vertical
- muscle of tongue 垂直舌筋 548
- part of longus colli 垂直部《頸長筋の》 29, 565

Vesical
- plexus 膀胱神経叢 239, **242**, 243, 246, 247
- veins 膀胱静脈 222, 225
- venous plexus 膀胱静脈叢 **202**, 216, 222

Vesicoprostatic venous plexus 膀胱前立腺静脈叢 157

Vesicouterine pouch 膀胱子宮窩 151, 152, **181**, 183, 184, 188, 190

Vesicovaginal septum 膀胱腟中隔 190

Vesicular appendices of epoöphoron 胞状垂《卵巣上体の》 189

Vestibular
- artery 前庭動脈 537
- apparatus 前庭器 536
- aqueduct 前庭水管 537
- area 前庭神経野 599
- bulb 前庭球 155, 185, 186, 191, **192**, 193
- fold 前庭ヒダ 550, 573
- ganglion 前庭神経節 480, **481**, 536, 537, 618
- ligament 前庭靱帯 571
- nuclei 前庭神経核 618
- root(CN Ⅷ) 前庭神経 480, **481**, 528

Vestibule 前庭 528, 530
- of omental bursa 網嚢前庭 146, 147
- of vagina(vaginal vestibule) 腟前庭 155, 186, **190**, 191, 192

Vestibulocerebellar fibers 前庭小脳線維 618

Vestibulocochlear
- artery　前庭蝸牛動脈　537
- nerve（CN Ⅷ）　内耳神経　470, **480**, 481, 528, 598, 599

Visceral
- layer
- – of serous pericardium　臓側板《漿膜性心膜の》　80, 81
- – of tunica vaginalis　臓側板《精巣鞘膜の》　196, 198
- oculomotor（Edinger-Westphal）nuclei　動眼神経副核（エディンガー－ウェストファル核）　471, **474**, 617
- pelvic fascia　臓側骨盤筋膜　150, 151, **154**, 182, 183, 185
- peritoneum　臓側腹膜　103, **142**, 143, 167, 182-184, 201
- pleura　臓側胸膜　66
- surface of liver　臓側面《肝臓の》　170

Viscerocranium　顔面頭蓋　454

Visual
- cortex（striate area）　視覚野（有線野）　616
- hemifield　半側視野　616

Vitreous body　硝子体　516

Vocal
- fold　声帯ヒダ　550, 573
- ligament　声帯靱帯　571
- process of arytenoid cartilage　声帯突起《披裂軟骨の》　570, 571

Vocalis　声帯筋　572
Vomer　鋤骨　455, 507, **520**, 523, 538
Vorticose vein　渦静脈　517
Vulva　陰門　154

W・X

White
- matter　白質　592, 594, 613
- –（substance）of spinal cord　白質《脊髄の》　613
- ramus communicans of spinal nerve　白交通枝《脊髄神経の》　59, 600, 622

Wing of sacrum　仙骨翼　5, 10, 11
Wolffian（mesonephric）duct　ウォルフ管（中腎管）　205

Xiphoid process of sternum　剣状突起《胸骨の》　44, 46, 120

Z

Zonular fibers　小帯線維　516, **518**, 519
Zygapophyseal joint　椎間関節　6, 8, 9, **14**, 558

Zygomatic
- arch　頬骨弓　458
- bone　頬骨　**454**, 455, 458, 506, 507, 523
- branches of facial nerve　頬骨枝《顔面神経の》　478, 488, 498, 500
- nerve　頬骨神経　505, 546
- process of temporal bone　頬骨突起《側頭骨の》　458, 526

Zygomatico-orbital
- artery　頬骨眼窩動脈　494, 499
- foramen　頬骨眼窩孔　506, 507

Zygomaticus
- major　大頬骨筋　462-464, **467**, 498
- minor　小頬骨筋　462-464, **467**

和文索引
Index of Japanese Term

- 五十音電話帳方式で配列している．項目の主要掲載ページは太字で示す．
- 派生語や関連語は — をつけて上位の用語の下にまとめている．
- 「右」は「う」，「左」は「さ」，「肩」は「けん」，「膝」は「しつ」に配列している．
- 英文中の a., aa. は artery, arteries を，l., ll. は ligament, ligaments を，n., nn. は nerve, nerves を，v., vv. は vein, veins を表す．

あ

α1受容体　α1 receptor　622
α運動ニューロン　α-motor neuron　614, 615
アキレス腱→踵骨腱　Achilles' tendon
アブミ骨　Stapes　528, **532**
— アブミ骨頸　Neck of stapes　532
— アブミ骨底　Base of stapes　532
— アブミ骨頭　Head of stapes　532
— 後脚　Posterior crus of stapes　532
— 前脚　Anterior crus of stapes　532
アブミ骨筋神経　Stapedial n.　478
アブミ骨膜　Stapedial membrane　532
アブミ骨輪状靱帯　Annular stapedial l.　532
アルコック管（陰部神経管）　Alcock's canal（pudendal canal）　155, 439
鞍隔膜　Diaphragma sellae　603
鞍結節　Tuberculum sellae　461
鞍背　Dorsum sellae　459, 461, 524

い

胃　Stomach　102, 142, 144, 146, 156, **158**, 159, 175, 210
— 胃体　Body of stomach　158, 159
— 胃底　Fundus of stomach　158, 159
— 外筋層　Muscularis externa of stomach　158
— 角切痕　Angular notch of stomach　158
— 後壁　Posterior wall（surface）of stomach　147, 156
— 斜線維　Inner oblique fibers of stomach　158
— 縦筋層　Outer longitudinal layer of stomach　158
— 小弯　Lesser curvature of stomach　158, 159
— 前壁　Anterior wall of stomach　156, 175
— 大弯　Greater curvature of stomach　158, 159
— 幽門部　Pyloric part of stomach　156, 175
— 輪筋層　Middle circular layer of stomach　158
胃圧痕《肝臓の》　Gastric impression of liver　170
胃結腸間膜　Gastrocolic l.　146, 147
胃十二指腸動脈　Gastroduodenal a.　207, 210, **211**, 212, 218-221
胃神経叢　Gastric plexus　91, 238
— 前胃神経叢　Anterior gastric plexus　74, 98, 238, 245
胃動脈　Gastric a.　210
胃粘膜ヒダ　Rugal folds　158
胃脾間膜　Gastrosplenic l.　147, **148**, 149, 163, 168
Ⅰ型肺胞上皮細胞　Type Ⅰ pneumocyte　111
一次体性感覚野（中心後回）　Sensory cortex（postcentral gyrus）　614
一般臓性遠心性線維（内臓運動機能）　General visceral efferent fiber（visceromotor function）　471
一般体性遠心性線維（体性運動機能）　General somatic efferent fiber（somatomotor function）　471
咽頭　Pharynx　553, 556
— 咽頭口部　Oropharynx　550
— 咽頭喉頭部　Laryngopharynx　550
— 咽頭鼻部　Nasopharynx　550
咽頭挙筋　Pharyngeal elevators　555
咽頭筋　Pharyngeal muscles　554
咽頭結節　Pharyngeal tubercle　458
咽頭後隙　Retropharyngeal space　556
咽頭後リンパ節　Retropharyngeal lymph nodes　556
咽頭収縮筋　Pharyngeal constrictors　554
咽頭周囲隙　Peripharyngeal space　556
咽頭静脈叢　Pharyngeal venous plexus　556
咽頭食道狭窄　Pharyngo-esophageal constriction　96
咽頭神経叢　Pharyngeal plexus　75, **482**
咽頭側隙　Lateral pharyngeal space　556
咽頭頭底板　Pharyngobasilar fascia　555
咽頭扁桃　Pharyngeal tonsil　**552**, 553, 555
陰核　Clitoris　186, 190, **192**, 193
— 陰核亀頭　Glans of clitoris　136, 186, 193, 194
— 陰核脚　Crus of clitoris　151, 155, 184, 186, 191, 193
— 陰核体　Body of clitoris　193
陰核深静脈　Deep clitoral vv.　195
陰核深動脈　Deep clitoral a.　195
陰核背神経　Dorsal clitoral n.　191, 194, 195
陰核背動脈　Dorsal clitoral a.　191, 195
陰核包皮　Prepuce of clitoris（clitoral prepuce）　136, 192, 193
陰茎　Penis　137, 187, 196, **197**, 234
— 陰茎亀頭　Glans penis　185, 187, **197**, 198, 201, 202, 225
— 陰茎脚　Crus of penis　153, 155, 185, 197
— 陰茎根　Root of penis　197
— 陰茎体　Body of penis　197
— 陰茎背　Dorsum of penis　225
陰茎海綿体　Corpus cavernosum of penis　150, 184, 187, **197**, 201, 203
陰茎海綿体神経　Cavernous nn. of penis　243
陰茎海綿体白膜　Tunica albuginea of corpus cavernosum　197, 202
陰茎筋膜　Penile fascia　150, 184
陰茎深静脈　Deep penile vv.　202, 222
陰茎深動脈　Deep penile a.　197, 202
陰茎中隔　Penile septum　197
陰茎提靱帯　Suspensory l. of penis（penile suspensory l.）　150, 184, 202, 225
陰茎背神経　Dorsal penile n.（dorsal n. of penis）　197, 202, 203, **243**
陰茎背動脈　Dorsal penile a.　197, **202**, 203, 225
陰茎皮膚　Penile skin　197
陰茎包皮　Prepuce of penis　184
陰嚢　Scrotum　137, 143, 187, **196**, 198, 201, 203, 234
陰嚢中隔　Scrotal septum　143, 150, 184, **199**, 201
陰部神経　Pudendal n.　**194**, 195, 202, 203, 242, 243, 424, 425, 438, 439, 441
— 会陰枝　perineal branches of pudendal n.,　438
陰部神経管（アルコック管）　Pudendal canal（Alcock's canal）　155, 439
陰部大腿神経　Genitofemoral n.　133, 179, 194, 196, 424-426, **427**, 434, 436
— 陰部枝　Genital branch of genitofemoral n.　133, 196, 203, 426, **427**, 436
— 前陰嚢枝　Anterior scrotal branches of genitofemoral n.　426
— 大腿枝　Femoral branch of genitofemoral n.　426, 427, 436
陰門　Vulva　154

う

ウォルフ管（中腎管）　Wolffian（mesonephric）duct　205
右胃静脈　Right gastric v.　215, 218, 220
右胃大網静脈　Right gastro-omental v.　215, **218**, 219-221
右胃大網動脈　Right gastro-omental a.　207, 210, 212, **218**, 219-221
右胃大網リンパ節　Right gastro-omental lymph node　230
右胃動脈　Right gastric a.　207, **210**, 211, 212, 218-221
右縁枝（鋭角縁枝）　Right marginal a.　88
右下肺静脈　Right inferior pulmonary v.　114, 115
右下葉気管支　Right inferior lobar bronchi　110
右肝管　Right hepatic duct　171-173
右肝静脈　Right hepatic v.　171
右肝部　Right liver　170
— 右外側後区域（区域Ⅶ）　Posterior lateral segment（Segment Ⅶ）of right liver　170
— 右外側前区域（区域Ⅵ）　Anterior lateral segment（Segment Ⅵ）of right liver　170
— 右内側区　Right medial division of right liver　170
— 右内側後区域（区域Ⅷ）　Posterior medial segment（Segment Ⅷ）of right liver　170
— 右内側前区域（区域Ⅴ）　Anterior medial segment（Segment Ⅴ）of right liver　170
右冠状動脈　Right coronary a.　86, 87, **88**
— 円錐枝　Conus branch of right coronary a.　88
— 心房枝　Atrial branch of right coronary a.　88
右気管支縦隔リンパ本幹　Right bronchomediastinal trunk　119
右頸リンパ本幹　Right jugular trunk　119
右結腸曲　Right colic flexure　145, 147, 148, 159, 161, **164**, 165
右結腸静脈　Right colic v.　215, **220**
右結腸動脈　Right colic a.　207, 212, **220**
右結腸リンパ節　Right colic lymph node　233
右後鼻孔　Right choana　550
右鎖骨下リンパ本幹　Right subclavian trunk　119
右三角間膜　Right triangular l.　170, 171
右主気管支　Right main bronchus　77, 110
右上肺静脈　Right superior pulmonary v.　114, 115
右上葉気管支　Right superior lobar bronchus　110
右心耳　Right auricle　83, **84**, 85, 88
右心室　Right ventricle　82-84, **85**, 90, 93
— 肺動脈口　Pulmonary outflow tract of right ventricle　93
右心房　Right atrium　82, 84, **85**, 90, 93
右精巣静脈　Right testicular v.　178, 180, 214, **217**
右精巣動脈　Right testicular a.　178, 180, **217**
右線維三角　Right fibrous trigone　86
右線維輪　Right fibrous anulus　86
右中葉気管支　Right middle lobar bronchus　110
右肺　Right lung　66, 93, 104, **105**, 176
— 下葉　Inferior lobe of right lung　93, 104
— 斜裂　Oblique fissure of right lung　93, 104, 105, 109
— 上葉　Superior lobe of right lung　93, 104
— 水平裂　Horizontal fissure of right lung　93, 104, 109
— 中葉　Middle lobe of right lung　93, 104
右肺静脈　Right pulmonary vv.　70, 77, 78, 84, 88, 104, **114**
右肺動脈　Right pulmonary a.　77, 78, 84, 87, 104, **114**, 115
右半月弁《大動脈弁の》　Right cusp of aortic valve　87
右半月弁《肺動脈弁の》　Right cusp of pulmonary valve　86
右尾状葉胆管　Right duct of caudate lobe　172
右副腎静脈　Right suprarenal v.　176, 178, 180, 214, 216, **217**

659

（うへんえんじょうみゃく）

右辺縁静脈　Right marginal v.　88
右房室口　Right atrioventricular orifice　85
右房室弁　Right atrioventricular valve　85, **86**, 87
　— 後尖　Posterior cusp of right atrioventricular valve　86, 87
　— 前尖　Anterior cusp of right atrioventricular valve　85-87
　— 中隔尖　Septal cusp of right atrioventricular valve　86, 87
右腰リンパ節　Right lumbar lymph node　229, 234
右腰リンパ本幹　Right lumbar trunk　72, 226, 228
右卵巣静脈　Right ovarian v.　178, 214, 216, **217**
右卵巣動脈　Right ovarian a.　178, 216, **217**
右リンパ本幹　Right lymphatic duct　72
迂回回　Ambient gyrus　472, 620
迂回槽　Ambient cistern　604
烏口肩峰弓　Coracoacromial arch　259, 261, 262
烏口肩峰靱帯　Coracoacromial l.　258, 259, **261**, 262
烏口鎖骨靱帯　Coracoclavicular l.　**259**, 261, 332
烏口上腕靱帯　Coracohumeral l.　261
烏口突起　Coracoid process　47, 120, 253, **255**, 258, 260, 262, 350
烏口腕筋　Coracobrachialis　264, 265, 267, **274**
烏口腕筋包　Subcoracoid bursa　261
運動前野　Premotor cortex　613

え

エディンガー—ウェストファル核（動眼神経副核）　Edinger–Westphal (visceral oculomotor) nuclei　471, **474**, 617
エナメル質　Enamel　542
エルプ点（神経点）　Erb's point　582
会陰　Perineum　154, 194, 203
　— 会陰体（会陰腱中心）　Perineal body　136, **150**, 151-153, 182, 183
会陰横靱帯　Transverse perineal l.　181, **191**, 203
会陰曲　Perineal flexure　166
会陰神経　Perineal nn.　**194**, 195, 202, 203
　— 筋枝　Muscular branches of perineal nn.　203
会陰動脈　Perineal a.　191, **195**, 202
　— 後陰唇枝　Posterior labial branches of perineal a.　195
　— 後陰嚢枝　Posterior scrotal branches of perineal a.　202, 223
会陰皮下隙　Subcutaneous perineal space　155
会陰部（域）　Perineal region　136
会陰縫線　Perineal raphe　136, 137, 192
会陰膜（下尿生殖隔膜筋膜）　Perineal membrane　136, 137, 152, 153, **191**, 197
永久歯　Permanent teeth　542
栄養孔　Nutrient foramina　21
鋭角縁枝（右縁枝）　Right marginal a.　88
腋窩　Axilla　333, 336
腋窩陥凹　Axillary recess　261, 262
腋窩静脈　Axillary v.　57, 60, 62, **318**, 335-338
腋窩神経　Axillary n.　37, 320, 321, **324**, 330, 331, 333, 337
腋窩動脈　Axillary a.　56, 60, 62, **316**, 317, 320, 335-338
腋窩リンパ節　Axillary lymph nodes　64, 319
腋窩リンパ叢　Axillary lymphatic plexus　64
S状結腸　Sigmoid colon　145, 150-153, **164**, 166, 182, 213
S状結腸間膜　Sigmoid mesocolon　145, **148**, 150, 153, 163, 164, 166, 182

S状結腸静脈　Sigmoid vv.　215, **221**, 224
S状結腸動脈　Sigmoid aa.　207, **213**, 221, 224
S状結腸リンパ節　Sigmoid lymph node　233
S状静脈洞　Sigmoid sinus　35, 481, 496, 530, 556, **606**, 607
S状洞溝　Groove for sigmoid sinus　459, 526
円回内筋　Pronator teres　266, 288, 289, 291, 292, **293**
　— 上腕頭　Humeral head of pronator teres　289
円錐靱帯　Conoid l.　259
円錐靱帯結節　Conoid tubercle　254
延髄　Medulla oblongata　474, 593, 598, **599**, 600, 605
延髄根　Cranial root　486
延髄錐体　Pyramid of medulla oblongata　599
遠位横手掌線　Distal transverse crease　353
遠位指節間（DIP）関節　Distal interphalangeal joint　300, 301, **302**, 304, 305, 311, 352
　— 関節包　Distal interphalangeal joint capsule　302
　— 側副靱帯　Collateral ll. of distal interphalangeal joint　**302**, 304, 305, 308
遠位指節間（DIP）関節線　Distal interphalangeal joint crease　353
遠位趾節間（DIP）関節　Distal interphalangeal joint　402
遠位手根線　Distal wrist crease　353
遠位伸筋線　Distal extension creases　353
遠心性核　Efferent nuclei　612
遠心性線維　Efferent fibers　54

お

オトガイ下三角　Submental triangle　576
オトガイ下静脈　Submental v.　496
オトガイ下動脈　Submental a.　492
オトガイ下リンパ節　Submental lymph nodes　587
オトガイ筋　Mentalis　462-464, **467**
オトガイ結節　Mental tubercle　539
オトガイ孔　Mental foramen　454, 455, 539
オトガイ神経　Mental n.　477, **489**, 499, 500, 546
　— オトガイ枝　Mental branch of mental n.　502
オトガイ舌筋　Genioglossus　464, 465, **544**, 548, 550
オトガイ舌骨筋　Geniohyoid　465, 544, 548, 550, 562, **563**
オトガイ舌骨筋枝《第1頸神経の》　Geniohyoid branch of C1　547
オトガイ動脈　Mental branch　495
オトガイ隆起　Mental protuberance　539, 589
オリーブ　Olive　484, 487, **598**, 599
黄色靱帯　Ligamenta flava　12, 16, 18, 19, **20**, 21, 559
横延髄静脈　Transverse medullary vv.　607
横隔胸膜（壁側胸膜の横隔部）　Diaphragmatic part of parietal pleura　54, 55, 66, 77, 97, **103**, 104, 134
横隔結腸間膜　Phrenicocolic l.　147
横隔神経　Phrenic n.　**54**, 55, 66, 77, 93, 321, 568, 569, 579, 581, 583
　— 右横隔神経　Right phrenic n.　55, 74, 91
　— 左横隔神経　Left phrenic n.　54, 55, 74, 79, 91
　— 心膜枝　Pericardial branches of phrenic n.　54
横隔膜　Diaphragm　48, **52**, 53-55, 66, 77, 81, 112
　— 右脚　Right crus of diaphragm　52, 53
　— 右天蓋　Right dome of diaphragm　52

　— 肝臓の付着部　Hepatic surface of diaphragm　146
　— 胸骨部　Sternal part of diaphragm　**52**, 53
　— 腱中心　Central tendon of diaphragm　**52**, 53, 55, 61, 134
　— 左脚　Left crus of diaphragm　**52**, 53
　— 左天蓋　Left dome of diaphragm　52
　— 腰椎部　Lumbar part of diaphragm　**52**, 55
　— 肋骨部　Costal part of diaphragm　**52**, 53, 55, 134
横隔膜狭窄（下食道狭窄）　Phrenic (lower esophageal) constriction　96
横隔膜筋膜　Diaphragmatic fascia　81
横隔脾間膜　Phrenicosplenic l.　161
横橋静脈　Transverse pontine vv.　607
横筋筋膜　Transversalis fascia　23, **131**, 133-135
横口蓋縫合　Transverse palatine suture　458, 538
横行結腸　Transverse colon　102, 142-148, 156, 161, 162, **164**, 165, 175, 176
横行結腸間膜　Transverse mesocolon　143, **145**, 146-148, 162-165, 175, 177
横手根靱帯　Transverse carpal l.　303, 344
横静脈洞　Transverse sinus　35, 496, 497, 567, **606**, 607
横舌筋　Transverse muscle of tongue　548
横束（横線維束）《足の》　Transverse fascicles of foot　412
横束（横線維束）《手の》　Transverse fascicles of hand　306
横足根関節（ショパール関節）　Transverse tarsal joint　402
横洞溝　Groove for transverse sinus　459
横突間筋　Intertratnsversarii　32
横突間靱帯　Intertransverse ll.　17, 18, **20**, 21
横突起　Transverse process　4, **5**, 6, 7, 18, 20, 44, 45, 49
　— 後結節　Posterior tubercle of transvers process　7
　— 前結節　Anterior tubercle of transvers process　7
横突棘筋　Transversospinales　33
横突孔　Transverse foramen　5-7, 558
横突肋骨窩　Costal facet on transverse process　8
横披裂筋　Transverse arytenoid　555, **572**
横膀胱ヒダ　Transverse vesical fold　152, 153, 181, **182**, 183

か

ガルトナー管　Gartner's duct　205
ガレノス交通枝　Galen's anastomosis　575
下咽頭収縮筋　Inferior pharyngeal constrictor　77, 97, **554**, 555
　— 甲状咽頭部　Thyropharyngeal part of inferior pharyngeal constrictor　554
　— 輪状咽頭部　Cricopharyngeal part of inferior pharyngeal constrictor　554
下オリーブ核　Inferior olive　615
下横隔静脈　Inferior phrenic v.　178, 214, 216, 217
　— 右下横隔静脈　Right inferior phrenic v.　214, 217
　— 左下横隔静脈　Left inferior phrenic v.　214, 216, 217
下横隔動脈　Inferior phrenic a.　**54**, 68, 178, 179, 208, 217
　— 右下横隔動脈　Right inferior phrenic a.　55, 217
　— 左下横隔動脈　Left inferior phrenic a.　55, 180, 208, 217

下横隔リンパ節　Inferior phrenic lymph node　101，118，226，228，229
下下垂体動脈　Inferior hypophyseal a.　490
下下腹神経叢（骨盤神経叢）　Inferior hypogastric plexus　236，**239**，244-247，623
下外側上腕皮神経　Inferior lateral brachial cutaneous n.　**325**，330-332
下角《側脳室の》　Temporal horn of lateral ventricle　596
下顎角　Mandibular angle　588，589
下顎孔　Mandibular foramen　456，**477**，539，540
下顎後静脈　Retromandibular v.　496，497，556
下顎骨　Mandible　454-456，464，**539**，540，556
－下顎窩　Mandibular fossa　458，526，**540**，541
－下顎頸　Neck of mandible　540
－下顎枝　Ramus of mandible　539
－下顎小舌　Lingula of mandible　540
－下顎体　Body of mandible　539
－下顎頭　Head of mandible　539-541，563
－関節突起　Condylar process of mandible　539
－筋突起　Coronoid process of mandible　539，540
－歯槽部　Alveolar part of mandible　539
－斜線　Oblique line of mandible　539
下顎神経　Mandibular division（CN V₃）　476，**477**，483，488，489，503，511，541，546，547
－硬膜枝　Meningeal branch of mandibular division　503，603
下顎切痕　Mandibular notch　539
下関節突起　Inferior articular process　5-9
下眼窩裂　Inferior orbital fissure　458，477，**506**，507，509，538
下眼瞼　Lower eyelid　514，515
下眼静脈　Inferior ophthalmic v.　496，**510**，512，513，567
下気管気管支リンパ節　Inferior tracheobronchial lymph node　100，101，118，**119**
下丘《四丘体板の》　Inferior colliculus of quadrigeminal plate　599
下丘核　Inferior collicular nucleus　619
下丘交連　Commissure of inferior colliculus　619
下丘腕　Brachium of inferior colliculus　599
下区動脈《腎動脈の》　Inferior segmental a. of renal a.　209
下頚神経節　Inferior cervical ganglion　91
下肩甲下神経　Lower subscapular n.　323，336，337
下瞼板　Inferior tarsus　514
下瞼板筋　Inferior tarsal muscle　514
下鼓室　Hypotympanum　531
下鼓室動脈　Inferior tympanic a.　534，535
下甲状結節　Inferior thyroid tubercle　570
下甲状切痕　Inferior thyroid notch　570
下甲状腺静脈　Inferior thyroid v.　54，66，70，77，99，**575**，579
下甲状腺動脈　Inferior thyroid a.　99，317，557，566，574，**575**，579，581
下行結腸　Descending colon　145，147，148，156，159，161，**164**，165，175，213
下行口蓋動脈　Descending palatine a.　495，**504**，524，525
下行膝動脈　Descending genicular a.　**420**，440
下行大動脈　Descending aorta　66，**68**，79，93
下後鋸筋　Serratus posterior inferior　22，23，26，30，**31**，269

下後腸骨棘　Posterior inferior iliac spine　124-126，359，362
下喉頭静脈　Inferior laryngeal v.　557，**575**
下喉頭神経　Inferior laryngeal n.　485，557，**575**，579
下喉頭動脈　Inferior laryngeal a.　575
下項線　Inferior nuchal line　25，28，**456**，458
下骨盤隔膜筋膜　Inferior fascia of pelvic diaphragm（inferior pelvic diaphragmatic fascia）　136，137，152，153，**154**，167，191
下根《頚神経ワナの》　Inferior root of ansa cervicalis　547，568，569
下矢状静脈洞　Inferior sagittal sinus　606
下肢帯　Pelvic girdle　124，356，**358**
下歯槽神経　Inferior alveolar n.　477，488，498，502，503，**546**，547，556
－下歯枝　Inferior dental branches of inferior alveolar n.　477，546
下歯槽動脈　Inferior alveolar a.　492，**495**，502-504，556
－オトガイ枝　Mental branch of inferior alveolar a.　498
－顎舌骨筋枝　Mylohyoid branch of inferior alveolar a.　495
下斜筋　Inferior oblique　475，**508**，509，514
下尺側側副動脈　Inferior ulnar collateral a.　**316**，338-340
下十二指腸陥凹　Inferior duodenal recess　161
下十二指腸曲　Inferior duodenal flexure　160
下縦隔　Inferior mediastinum　66
下縦舌筋　Inferior longitudinal muscle　548
下小脳脚　Inferior cerebellar peduncle　598，599
下上皮小体（下副甲状腺）　Inferior pair of parathyroid glands　574
下食道狭窄（横隔膜狭窄）　Lower esophageal（phrenic）constriction　96
下伸筋支帯　Inferior extensor retinaculum　415，443
下神経幹　Lower trunk　321
下神経節　Inferior ganglion　482，483，**484**，619
下唇（回盲唇）　Inferior lip　164
下唇下制筋　Depressor labii inferioris　**462**，463，464，467
下唇小帯　Frenulum of lower lip　550
下唇動脈　Inferior labial a.　492
下垂体　Hypophysis　593，595，**596**，599，605
－漏斗　Infundibulum of hypophysis　596，598，605
下垂体窩《蝶形骨の》　Hypophyseal fossa（sella turcica）of sphenoid bone　459，**461**，520，521，524
下膵十二指腸静脈　Inferior pancreaticoduodenal v.　215
下膵十二指腸動脈　Inferior pancreaticoduodenal a.　207，**211**，212，218
下膵動脈　Inferior pancreatic a.　211，219
下膵リンパ節　Inferior pancreatic lymph node　231
下錐体静脈洞　Inferior petrosal sinus　497，**607**
下浅鼠径リンパ節　Inferior inguinal lymph node　423，436
下前区動脈　Anterior inferior segmental a. of kidney《腎臓の》　209
下前腸骨棘　Anterior inferior iliac spine　124-126，128，136，137，**358**，359
下双子筋　Gemellus inferior　370-372，**375**，438，439，448
下唾液核　Inferior salivatory nucleus　471，482
下腿　Lower leg　356
下腿筋膜　Deep fascia of the leg　442，444
下腿交叉　Crural chiasm　395，399

下腿骨間膜　Interosseous membrane of leg　380，420，448
下腿三頭筋　Triceps surae　393，**398**，415，448
下大静脈　Inferior vena cava　35，55，57，70，71，82，88，208，210-215，**216**，217-220
下大静脈口　Valved orifice of inferior vena cava　85
下大静脈弁　Valve of inferior vena cava　85
下大脳静脈　Inferior cerebral vv.　602，607
下腸間膜静脈　Inferior mesenteric v.　215，219，220，**221**，224
下腸間膜動脈　Inferior mesenteric a.　149，180，206-208，**213**，216，217，221，223-225
下腸間膜動脈神経節　Inferior mesenteric ganglion　**237**，239，241，244-247
下腸間膜動脈神経叢　Inferior mesenteric plexus　236，**237**，239，241-245
下腸間膜リンパ節　Inferior mesenteric lymph node　226-228，**233**，234，235
下直筋　Inferior rectus　475，**508**，509，514
下直腸横ヒダ　Inferior transverse rectal fold　167
下直腸静脈　Inferior rectal vv.　195，202，203，215，222，223，**224**
－右下直腸静脈　Right inferior rectal v.　224
－左下直腸静脈　Left inferior rectal v.　223
下直腸神経　Inferior rectal nn.　194，195，202，203，**243**
下直腸動脈　Inferior rectal a.　195，202，203，222，223，**224**
－左下直腸動脈　Left inferior rectal a.　223，224
下直腸動脈神経叢　Inferior rectal plexus　243，245
下椎切痕　Inferior vertebral notch　8，9
下殿筋線《腸骨の》　Inferior gluteal line of ilium　125，359
下殿静脈　Inferior gluteal vv.　216，**222**，223，224，438，439
－右下殿静脈　Right inferior gluteal v.　216，224
下殿神経　Inferior gluteal n.　425，**431**，438，439，441
－筋枝　Muscular branches of inferior gluteal n.　431
下殿動脈　Inferior gluteal a.　**222**，224，420，438-441
－右下殿動脈　Right inferior gluteal a.　208
－左下殿動脈　Left inferior gluteal a.　224
下殿皮神経　Inferior cluneal nn.　39，194，203，424，430，435，**438**，441
下頭斜筋　Obliquus capitis inferior　24，25，27，28，564，**565**，585
下橈尺関節　Distal radioulnar joint　281，286，287，301
下尿生殖隔膜筋膜（会陰膜）　Perineal membrane　136，137，152，153，**191**，197
下肺底静脈　Inferior basal v. of lower lobe of lung　115
下腓骨筋支帯　Inferior fibular retinaculum　415
下鼻甲介　Inferior nasal concha　455，507，515，**521**，522，523，525，538，553
下鼻道　Inferior meatus　**521**，525
下副甲状腺（下上皮小体）　Inferior pair of parathyroid glands　574
下副腎動脈　Inferior suprarenal a.　177-179，208，**209**，217
－右下副腎動脈　Right inferior suprarenal a.　217
－左下副腎動脈　Left inferior suprarenal a.　180，208，217
下腹神経　Hypogastric n.　**237**，239，241-243，247

下腹神経（つづき）
— 右下腹神経　Right hypogastric n.　239, 241-243
— 左下腹神経　Left hypogastric n.　237, 239, 242, 243
下腹壁静脈　Inferior epigastric v.　133, 135, 180, 215, 216, **225**
— 右下腹壁静脈　Right inferior epigastric v.　216
下腹壁動脈　Inferior epigastric a.　133, 135, 180, 208, 222, **225**, 420
— 右下腹壁動脈　Right inferior epigastric a.　216
— 左下腹壁動脈　Left inferior epigastric a.　208
下吻合静脈　Inferior anastomotic v.　606
下膀胱静脈　Inferior vesical v.　216, **223**
下膀胱動脈　Inferior vesical a.　157, 208, 222, **223**, 225
下脈絡叢静脈　Inferior choroidal v.　607
下葉気管支　Inferior lobar bronchi　77, 104
下腰三角（プチ三角）　Iliolumbar triangle (of Petit)　39
下涙小管　Inferior lacrimal canaliculi　515
下涙点　Inferior puncta　515
下肋骨窩　Inferior costal facet　5, 8, 49
仮肋　False ribs　45
架橋静脈　Bridging vv.　602, 606
渦静脈　Vorticose v.　517
窩間靱帯　Interfoveolar l.　133, 135
蝸牛　Cochlea　481, 528, **536**
蝸牛管　Cochlear duct　**536**, 619
蝸牛孔　Helicotrema　536
蝸牛交通枝　Cochlear communicating branch　537
蝸牛軸　Modiolus　535, 537
蝸牛神経　Cochlear root (n.) (CN Ⅷ)　480, 481, 528, 536, **537**, 619
蝸牛神経後核　Posterior cochlear nucleus　480, 619
蝸牛神経前核　Anterior cochlear nucleus　480, 619
蝸牛水管　Cochlear aqueduct　530, 536
蝸牛水管静脈　V. of cochlear aqueduct　537
蝸牛窓　Round window　481, 536, **537**
蝸牛窓小窩　Round window niche　531
蝸牛窓静脈　V. of round window　537
顆間窩《大腿骨の》　Intercondylar notch of femur　360, 382
顆間線《大腿骨の》　Intercondylar line of femur　360
顆間隆起《脛骨の》　Intercondylar eminence of tibia　380-382
顆管　Condylar canal　458, 606
顆導出静脈　Condylar emissary v.　497, 606
鵞足　Pes anserinus　366, 367, 369, 370, **392**
介在ニューロン　interneurons　615
灰白交通枝　Gray ramus communicans　59, **237**, 242, 243, 600, 622
灰白質《脊髄の》　Gray matter (substance) of spinal cord　592, 612
灰白質《脳の》　Gray matter of brain　592
灰白隆起　Tuber cinereum　596
回外筋　Supinator　288-291, 296, **297**
回結腸唇（上唇）　Ileocolic labrum (superior lip)　164
回結腸静脈　Ileocolic v.　215, **220**, 221
回結腸動脈　Ileocolic a.　207, **212**, 213, 220, 221, 241
— 回腸枝　Ileal branch of ileocolic a.　212, 213, 220
— 結腸枝　Colic branch of ileocolic a.　212, 213, 220
回結腸リンパ節　Ileocolic lymph node　232, 233
回旋筋　Rotatores muscles　32

回旋枝《左冠状動脈の》　Circumflex a. of left coronary a.　88
回腸　Ileum　142-145, 148, 153, **162**, 165, 182
— 終末部　Terminal of ileum　164
回腸口　Ileocecal orifice　164
回腸口小帯　Frenulum of ileal orifice　164
回腸静脈　Ileal vv.　215, 220, **221**
回腸動脈　Ileal aa.　212, 220, **221**
回盲唇（下唇）　Inferior lip　164
海馬　Hippocampus　596, 609, **621**
海馬采　Fimbria of hippocampus　596
海綿静脈洞　Cavernous sinus　496, 497, 510, 567, **607**
解剖学的嗅ぎタバコ入れ（橈骨窩）　Anatomic (anatomical) snuffbox　346, 351-353
外陰部静脈　External pudendal vv.　57, 202, **225**, 422, 434, 436
外陰部動脈　External pudendal aa.　202, **225**, 420, 436, 440
外果　Lateral malleolus　356, 357, **380**, 381, 394, 404, 405, 442, 444, 450
外果関節面　Lateral malleolar articular surface　404, 405
外果面《距骨の》　Lateral malleolar surface of talus　403, 405, 407
外顆粒層　External granular layer (Ⅱ)　595
外眼筋　Extraocular muscle　508
外頸静脈　External jugular v.　496, 499, 557, **567**, 578-580, 582, 583
外頸動脈　External carotid a.　490, **491**, 492-494, 556, 566, 580, 581, 608
— 後枝　Posterior branches of external carotid a.　491, 493
— 終枝　Terminal branches of external carotid a.　491, 494
— 前枝　Anterior branches of external carotid a.　491, 492
— 内側枝　Medial branches of external carotid a.　491, 492
外頸動脈神経叢　External carotid plexus　75
外口蓋静脈　External palatine v.　497
外肛門括約筋　External anal sphincter　136, 137, 150, 151, 166, **167**, 182-184, 194, 203
— 深部　Deep part of external anal sphincter　167
— 浅部　Superficial part of external anal sphincter　167
— 皮下部　Subcutaneous part of external anal sphincter　167
外後頭隆起　External occipital protuberance　24, 25, **456**, 458, 588
外後頭稜　External occipital crest　458
外子宮口　External os of uterus　189, **190**, 191
— 後唇　Posterior lip of uterine os　190
— 前唇　Anterior lip of uterine os　190
外耳　External ear　528
外耳孔　External acoustic opening　526
外耳道　External auditory canal (external acoustic meatus)　454, 526, **528**, 529, 530
— 骨性部　Bony part of external auditory canal　528
— 軟骨性部　Cartilaginous part of external auditory canal　528
外錐体細胞層　External pyramidal layer (Ⅲ)　595
外生殖器　External genitalia　186, 192
外精筋膜　External spermatic fascia　132, 196, 198, **199**, 202
外側横膝蓋支帯　Lateral transverse patellar retinaculum　384

外側下膝動脈　Lateral inferior genicular a.　420, 421, **443**
外側顆《脛骨の》　Lateral condyle of tibia　356, 357, 380-382, 393, 450
外側顆《大腿骨の》　Lateral condyle of femur　356, 360, 361, 382
外側顆上線《大腿骨の》　Lateral supracondylar line of femur　360
外側顆上稜《上腕骨の》　Lateral supracondylar ridge of humerus　256
外側弓状靱帯　Lateral arcuate l.　52, 53
外側嗅条　Lateral olfactory stria　472, 620
外側胸筋神経　Lateral pectoral n.　320, 321, **326**, 334-336
外側胸静脈　Lateral thoracic v.　**60**, 62
外側胸動脈　Lateral thoracic a.　56, **60**, 62, 316, 335-337
— 外側乳腺枝　Lateral mammary branches of lateral thoracic a.　62
外側頸三角部（後頸三角）　Lateral cervical region (posterior triangle)　576, 582
外側頸リンパ節の浅リンパ節　Lateral superficial cervical lymph nodes　587
外側楔状骨　Lateral cuneiform　**400**, 401-403, 410
外側広筋　Vastus lateralis　366, 367, 371, 373, **378**, 429, 440, 448, 450
外側後頭動脈, P3区　Lateral occipital a. (P3)　**608**, 609
外側溝　Lateral sulcus　593, 595
外側骨半規管　Lateral semicircular canal　**481**, 528, 530, 531
外側根《正中神経の》　Lateral root of median n.　328
外側鎖骨上神経　Lateral supraclavicular nn.　582, 583
外側臍ヒダ　Lateral umbilical fold　**135**, 144, 145, 148, 149, 152, 153, 182, 183
外側膝状体　Lateral geniculate body　**473**, 598, 616, 617
外側手根側副靱帯　Radial carpal collateral l.　302
外側縦膝蓋支帯　Lateral longitudinal patellar retinaculum　384
外側上顆《上腕骨の》　Lateral epicondyle of humerus　253, **256**, 257, 285, 350
外側上顆《大腿骨の》　Lateral epicondyle of femur　357, 360, 382, **451**
外側上膝動脈　Lateral superior genicular a.　**420**, 421, 443
外側上腕筋間中隔　Lateral intermuscular septum of arm　333
外側神経束　Lateral cord　320, 321, **326**, 327, 328, 336-338
外側髄板　External medullary lamina　597
外側仙骨静脈　Lateral sacral vv.　216, **222**, 223
外側仙骨動脈　Lateral sacral aa.　34, 208, **222**
外側仙骨稜　Lateral sacral crest　10, 11
外側前庭脊髄路　Lateral vestibulospinal tract　618
外側前頭底動脈　Lateral frontobasal a.　609
外側前腕皮神経　Lateral antebrachial cutaneous n.　327, **330**, 331, 339
外側鼠径窩　Lateral inguinal fossa　**135**, 153, 182
外側足根動脈　Lateral tarsal a.　420, 445
外側足底溝　Lateral plantar sulcus　446
外側足底静脈　Lateral plantar v.　**422**, 446, 447
外側足底神経　Lateral plantar n.　424, **433**, 443, 446, 447
— 筋枝　Muscular branches of lateral plantar n.　433

（かんせつえんばん）

― 深枝　Deep branch of lateral plantar n.　446, 447
― 浅枝　Superficial branch of lateral plantar n.　433, 446
外側足底中隔　Lateral plantar septum　412
外側足底動脈　Lateral plantar a.　**420**, 443, 446, 447
外側足背皮神経　Lateral dorsal cutaneous n.　433, **435**, 444, 445
外側足放線　Lateral rays of foot　410
外側側副靱帯《膝関節の》　Lateral collateral l. of knee joint　384-386, 388-390
外側側副靱帯《上橈尺関節の》　Radial collateral l. of proximal radio-ulnar joint　284-286, 301
外側帯《手の》　Lateral bands of hand　311
外側大静脈リンパ節　Lateral caval lymph node　228
外側大腿回旋静脈　Lateral circumflex femoral vv.　422
外側大腿回旋動脈　Lateral circumflex femoral a.　**420**, 440
― 下行枝　Descending branch of lateral circumflex femoral a.　440
― 上行枝　Ascending branch of lateral circumflex femoral a.　440
外側大腿皮神経　Lateral femoral cutaneous n.　424-426, **427**, 434-436, 440
外側大動脈リンパ節　Lateral aortic lymph node　226, 227, **228**, 229
― 右外側大動脈リンパ節　Right lateral aortic lymph node　226, 227, 229
― 左外側大動脈リンパ節　Left lateral aortic lymph node　226-229
外側中葉区　Lateral segment of lung　108
外側中葉動脈《右肺の》　Lateral segmental a. of right lung　115
外側直筋　Lateral rectus　475, **508**, 509, 513, 516
外側ツチ骨靱帯　Lateral l. of malleus　532
外側頭直筋　Rectus capitis lateralis　29, 465, **565**
外側肺底区　Lateral basal segment of lung　108
外側肺底動脈　Lateral basal segmental a. of lung　115
外側半規管　Lateral semicircular duct　536, 537
外側半規管隆起　Prominence of lateral semicircular canal　531
外側半月　Lateral meniscus　386, **387**, 388-390
外側腓腹皮神経　Lateral sural cutaneous n.　**432**, 434, 435, 442, 444
外側鼻軟骨　Lateral nasal cartilage　520
外側腹側核　Ventral lateral nucleus　615
外側膨大部神経　Lateral ampullary n.　**481**, 536, 537
外側毛帯　Lateral lemniscus　619
外側毛帯核　Nuclei of lateral lemniscus　619
外側腰リンパ節　Lateral lumbar lymph node　156
外側翼突筋　Lateral pterygoid　463-465, 467, **468**, 469, 541
― 下頭　Inferior head (part) of lateral pterygoid　469, 541
― 上頭　Superior head (part) of lateral pterygoid　469, 541
外側翼突筋神経　Lateral pterygoid n.　477, 488, 503, **546**
外側輪状披裂筋　Lateral cricoarytenoid　572
外側裂孔　Lateral lacuna　602
外側裂孔リンパ節　Lateral lacunar lymph node　229
外側肋横突靱帯　Lateral costotransverse l.　49

外腸骨静脈　External iliac v.　151, 155, 184, 216, 222, **223**, 224, 225, 436, 440
外腸骨動脈　External iliac a.　149, 151, 152, 155, 184, 208, 222, **223**, 224, 225, 420, 440
外腸骨リンパ節　External iliac lymph node　227-229, **234**, 235, 436
外椎骨静脈叢　External vertebral venous plexus　35, 497, 606
外転神経　Abducent n. (CN Ⅵ)　470, 475, **509**, 511-513, 599, 608
外転神経核　Nucleus of abducent n.　**471**, 474, 618
外尿道口　External urethral orifice　136, **185**, 190, 192, 194, 197
外腹斜筋　External oblique　22, 26, 40, 53, 61, 130, 131, 134, 138, **139**, 248, 264, 268, 269
外腹斜筋腱膜　External oblique aponeurosis　**130**, 132-134, 139, 436, 440
外閉鎖筋　Obturator externus　155, 367, 372, **377**
外包　External capsule　594
外肋間筋　External intercostal muscles　26, 27, 50, **51**, 61, 130
外肋間膜　External intercostal membrane　51
蓋膜《外側環軸関節の》　Tectorial membrane of lateral atlanto-axial joint　16-18
角切痕《胃の》　Angular notch of stomach　158
角膜　Cornea　514, 516, **518**
角膜縁　Corneoscleral limbus　516
顎下三角　Submandibular (digastric) triangle　576
顎下神経節　Submandibular ganglion　479, **547**, 549
顎下腺　Submandibular gland　501, **551**, 580
顎下腺管　Submandibular duct　549, 551
顎下リンパ節　Submandibular lymph nodes　587
顎関節　Temporomandibular joint　540, 541
― 外側靱帯　Lateral l. of temporomandibular joint　463, 468, 540
顎静脈　Maxillary vv.　**496**, 497, 567
顎舌骨筋　Mylohyoid　465, 544, 548, 554, 562, **563**
顎舌骨筋神経　Mylohyoid n.　489, 503, **547**
顎舌骨筋神経溝　Mylohyoid groove　540
顎舌骨筋線　Mylohyoid line　539, 563
顎舌骨筋縫線　Mylohyoid raphe　544, 563
顎動脈　Maxillary a.　491-494, **495**, 502-504, 524, 534
顎二腹筋　Digastric muscle　464, 465, 544, 554, 555, 562, **563**, 580
― 後腹　Posterior belly of digastric muscle　544, 554, 555, 563
― 前腹　Anterior belly of digastric muscle　464, 544, 554, **563**
― 中間腱　Intermediate tendon of digastric muscle　544
滑車　Trochlea　508
滑車下神経　Infratrochlear n.　477, 500, **511**, 512, 513
滑車上静脈　Supratrochlear v.　510
滑車上神経　Supratrochlear n.　477, 489, 498, 499, **511**, 512, 513
滑車上動脈　Supratrochlear a.　490, 492, **510**, 513
滑車上リンパ節　Supratrochlear lymph node　64
滑車神経　Trochlear n. (CN Ⅳ)　470, **474**, 475, 509, 512, 513, 599
滑車神経核　Nucleus of trochlear n.　471, **474**, 618

滑車切痕《尺骨の》　Trochlear notch of ulna　280, 281, 283
滑膜　Synovial membrane　365
肝胃間膜　Hepatogastric l.　143, 148, **159**, 163, 168
肝円索　Ligamentum teres of liver　163, 168, **170**, 171
肝鎌状間膜　Falciform l. of liver　144, 159, **171**
肝冠状間膜　Coronary l. of liver　170, 171
肝管　Hepatic duct　177
― 左肝管　Left hepatic duct　171-173
肝区域　Segments of liver　170
肝十二指腸間膜　Hepatoduodenal l.　146, 148, 149, **159**, 163, 168, 177
肝静脈　Hepatic vv.　82, 216, **218**, 219
肝食道間膜　Hepato-esophageal l.　159
肝神経叢　Hepatic plexus　238, 240, 245
肝臓　Liver　146, 156, **168**, 170
― 胃圧痕　Gastric impression of liver　170
― 右葉　Right lobe of liver　146, 156, 168, 171
― 下縁　Inferior border of liver　171
― 結腸圧痕　Colic impression of liver　170
― 左葉　Left lobe of liver　146, 168, 171
― 十二指腸圧痕　Duodenal impression of liver　170
― 腎圧痕　Renal impression of liver　170
― 線維付着　Fibrous appendix of liver　171
― 臓側面　Visceral surface of liver　170
― 尾状突起　Caudate process of liver　171
― 尾状葉　Caudate lobe of liver　146, 170, 171
― 副腎圧痕　Suprarenal impression of liver　170
― 方形葉　Quadrate lobe of liver　171
― 無漿膜野　Bare area of liver　170, 171
[肝]門脈（肝静脈）　Portal v.　82, 171, 210-212, 215, **218**, 219-221
肝葉　Lobes of liver　170
肝リンパ節　Hepatic lymph node　230, 231
冠状溝　Coronary sulcus　84, 85
冠状静脈口　Valved orifice of coronary sinus　85
冠状静脈洞　Coronary sinus　84, 86, 88
冠状静脈弁　Valve of coronary sinus　85
冠状縫合　Coronal suture　454, 457
貫通静脈　Perforator vv.　**318**, 339
貫通動脈　Perforating aa.　420, 440, 445
― 第2貫通動脈　2nd perforating a.　**421**, 441
― 第3貫通動脈　3rd perforating a.　421, 441
間脳　Diencephalon　594, **596**, 599
間膜縁　Mesovarial margin　188, 189
間膜ヒモ　Taenia mesocolica　164
寛骨　Hip bone　124, 125, 356, **358**
― 坐骨恥骨枝　Ischiopubic ramus of hip bone　197
寛骨臼　Acetabulum　124-126, 129, **358**, 361, 363
― 寛骨臼縁　Acetabular rim　124-126, 358, **359**, 362
― 寛骨臼窩　Acetabular fossa　125, **359**, 363, 364, 421
― 寛骨臼切痕　Acetabular notch　125, 359
― 寛骨臼の関節唇　Acetabular labrum　361, 363, 421
― 月状面　Lunate surface of acetabulum　125, 359, 364
寛骨臼横靱帯　Transverse l. of acetabulum　364
寛骨臼蓋　Acetabular roof　364, 421
関節円板《顎関節の》　Articular disk of temporomandibular joint　540, 541
関節円板《胸鎖関節の》　Articular disk of sternoclavicular joint　259

663

(かんせつげき)

関節隙《胸肋関節の》 Joint space of sternocostal joint 49
関節結節《顎関節の》 Articular tubercle of temporomandibular joint 526, 540, 541
関節上腕靱帯 Glenohumeral ll. 261
関節唇《肩甲骨の》 Glenoid labrum of scapula 262
関節内肋骨頭靱帯 Intra-articular l. of head of rib 49
関節包《遠位指節間(DIP)関節の》 Distal interphalangeal joint capsule 302
関節包《顎関節の》 Joint capsule of temporomandibular joint 463, 540, 541
関節包《近位指節間(PIP)関節の》 Proximal interphalangeal joint capsule 302
関節包《肩関節の》 Joint capsule of glenohumeral joint 261, 262
関節包《膝関節の》 Joint capsule of knee joint 390
関節包《中足趾節関節の》 Metatarsophalangeal joint capsules 408, 409, 419
関節包《肘関節の》 Joint capsule of elbow joint 285
関節包《椎間関節の》 Capsule of zygapophyseal joint 16, 18
環椎(第1頚椎, C1) Atlas(C1) 4, 6, 7, 47, 600
― 横突起 Transverse process of atlas 29
― 外側塊 Lateral masses of atlas 7
― 後弓 Posterior arch of atlas 6, 7
― 後結節 Posterior tubercle of atlas 7, 17, 558
― 前弓 Anterior arch of atlas 7
― 前結節 Anterior tubercle of atlas 7, 558
環椎横靱帯 Transverse l. of atlas 17, 19
環椎後頭関節 Atlanto-occipital joint 14, 16, 18
環椎後頭靱帯 Atlanto-occipital l. 17
眼窩 Orbit 455, **506**, 522
眼窩下縁 Infraorbital margin 455, 589
眼窩下管 Infraorbital canal **506**, 507
眼窩下孔 Infraorbital foramen 454, 455, 477, **506**, 515
眼窩下溝 Infraorbital groove 506
眼窩下静脈 Infraorbital v. 510
眼窩下神経 Infraorbital n. 477, 498-500, **505**, 512
― 上唇枝 Superior labial branches of infraorbital n. 546
眼窩下動脈 Infraorbital a. 492, 495, 498, 503, **504**, 512
眼窩下壁 Orbital floor 507, 514
眼窩隔膜 Orbital septum 512, 514, 515
眼窩骨膜 Periorbita 511, **514**
眼窩脂肪体 Adipose tissue of orbit 511, **514**
眼窩上縁 Supraorbital margin 455, 589
眼窩上孔 Supraorbital foramen 455, **506**
眼窩上神経 Supraorbital n. 475, 477, 489, **498**, 499, 511-513
― 外側枝 Lateral branch of supraorbital n. 498
― 内側枝 Medial branch of supraorbital n. 498
眼窩上動脈 Supraorbital a. 490, **510**, 512, 513
眼窩板《篩骨の》 Orbital plate of ethmoid bone 460, 506, 507, 523
眼角静脈 Angular v. 496-499, 502, **510**, 512, 567
眼角動脈 Angular a. 492, 498, 502, **512**
眼球 Eyeball 514, **516**
眼球結膜 Ocular conjunctiva 516, 518
眼球鞘(テノン嚢) Bulbar fascia(Tenon's capsule) 514
眼瞼 Eyelid 514
眼静脈 Ophthalmic v. 510

眼神経 Ophthalmic division(CN V₁) 476, **477**, 489, 525
― テント枝 Recurrent meningeal branch of ophthalmic division 477
眼動脈 Ophthalmic a. 490, 492, **510**, 512, 524
眼房水 Aqueous humor 518
眼輪筋 Orbicularis oculi **462**, 463, 464, 466
― 眼窩部 Orbital part of orbicularis oculi 464
― 涙嚢部 Lacrimal part of orbicularis oculi 464
顔面横動脈 Transverse facial a. 494, **498**, 499
顔面静脈 Facial v. **496**, 497-501, 512, 567
顔面神経 Facial n.(CN Ⅶ) **478**, 479, 488, 498, 500, 501, 547, 551, 599
― 運動枝 Motor branches of facial n. 478
― 下顎縁枝 Marginal mandibular branch of facial n. 478, **488**, 498, 500, 580
― 頬枝 Buccal branches of facial n. 478, 488, 498, 500
― 頬骨枝 Zygomatic branches of facial n. 478, 488, 498, 500
― 茎突舌骨筋枝 Stylohyoid branch of facial n. 547
― 頚枝 Cervical branch of facial n. 478, 488, 500, 578, 582
― 側頭枝 Temporal branches of facial n. 478, 488, 498, 500
― 二腹筋枝 Digastric branch of facial n. 547
顔面神経核 Facial nucleus 471, 478
顔面神経管 Facial canal 478
顔面神経丘 Facial colliculus 599
顔面神経膝(内膝) Internal genu of facial n. 478
顔面頭蓋 Viscerocranium 454
顔面動脈 Facial a. **298**, 491-493, 498, 500, 501, 512

き

キーゼルバッハ部位 Kiesselbach's area 524
キヌタ-アブミ関節 Incudo-stapedial joint 532
キヌタ-ツチ関節 Incudo-malleolar joint 532
キヌタ骨 Incus 528, 530, 531, **532**
― キヌタ骨体 Body of incus 532
― 短脚 Short process of incus 532
― 長脚 Long process of incus 532
― 豆状突起 Lenticular process of incus 532
ギヨン管(尺骨神経管) Ulnar tunnel 342-344
気管 Trachea 23, 108, **110**, 570
― 胸部 Thoracic part of trachea 110
― 頚部 Cervical part of trachea 110
気管気管支リンパ節 Tracheobronchial lymph node 73, 100, 101, **118**
気管支樹 Bronchial tree 108, **111**
気管支周囲リンパ管叢 Peribronchial network 118
気管支縦隔リンパ本幹 Bronchomediastinal trunk 72
気管支静脈 Bronchial vv. 117
気管支動脈 Bronchial a. 68, 116
気管支肺リンパ節 Bronchopulmonary lymph node 73, 100, 101, 118, **119**
気管軟骨 Tracheal cartilages 110
気管分岐部 Tracheal bifurcation 110
気管傍リンパ節 Paratracheal lymph node 73, 100, 101, 118, **119**
奇静脈 Azygos v. 35, 54, 55, 57, 61, **70**, 71, 78, 99, 611
基節骨《足の》 Proximal phalanx of foot 401
― 基節骨の体 Shaft of proximal phalanx 400
― 基節骨の底 Base of proximal phalanx 400
― 基節骨の頭 Head of proximal phalanx 400

― 第1基節骨 1st proximal phalanx of foot 402, 410
― 第5基節骨 5th proximal phalanx of foot 400, 401
基節骨《手の》 Proximal phalanx of hand 298, 300, 301, 304
― 第2基節骨 2nd proximal phalanx of hand 298
― 第4基節骨 4th proximal phalanx of hand 252
基靱帯(子宮頚横靱帯) Transverse cervical l. 152, 155
亀頭 Glans penis 137
亀頭冠 Corona of glans 197, 202
疑核 Nucleus ambiguus 471, 482, **484**, 486
脚間窩 Interpeduncular fossa 599
脚間核 Interpeduncular nucleus 472, 620
脚間静脈 Interpeduncular vv. 607
脚間線維 Intercrural fibers 133, 437
脚間槽 Interpeduncular cistern 604
弓下動脈 Subarcuate a. 535
弓状膝窩靱帯 Arcuate popliteal l. 385
弓状静脈《腎臓の》 Arcuate v. of kidney 179
弓状動脈《腎臓の》 Arcuate a. of kidney 179, **209**, 420, 445
求心性核 Afferent nuclei 612
求心性線維 Afferent fibers 54
球海綿体筋 Bulbospongiosus 136, 137, 155, 184, 185, 191, 193, 197
球形嚢 Saccule **481**, 536, 618
球形嚢神経 Saccular n. **481**, 536, 537
球形嚢膨大部神経 Sacculoampullary n. 481
嗅球 Olfactory bulb **472**, 524, 525, 594, 620
嗅索 Olfactory tract 472, 594, **620**
嗅三角 Olfactory trigone 472, 594, 620
嗅神経 Olfactory n. 470, **472**, 593-595
嗅神経糸 Olfactory fibers 472, 524, 525
嗅粘膜 Olfactory mucosa 472, 620
挙筋門 Levator hiatus 141
距骨 Talus 400-406, **407**
― 外果面 Lateral malleolar surface of talus 403, 405, 407
― 距骨頚 Neck of talus 400, 401, 405
― 距骨溝 Sulcus tali of talus 407
― 距骨体 Body of talus **400**, 401
― 距骨頭 Head of talus 400, 401, 405
― 内果面 Medial malleolar surface of talus 403, 405, 407
距骨下関節 Subtaler(talocalcaneal) joint 402, **404**, 406
距骨滑車 Trochlea of talus 403-405, 407
― 後径 Posterior diameter of trochlea of talus 405
― 前径 Anterior diameter of trochlea of talus 405
距骨後突起 Posterior process of talus 400, 401, 407
― 外側結節 Lateral tubercle of posterior process of talus 401, 405, 407
― 内側結節 Medial tubercle of posterior process of talus **401**, 405, 407
距舟関節 Talonavicular joint 402
距腿関節 Talocrural joint 356, 402, 404, **405**
距踵舟関節 Talocalcaneonavicular joint 405
鋸状縁 Ora serrata 519
強膜 Sclera 514, 516, **518**, 519
強膜外隙 Episcleral space 514
強膜篩板 Lamina cribrosa of sclera 516
強膜静脈洞 Scleral venous sinus 517
胸横筋 Transversus thoracis 50, **51**

胸郭横径　Transverse thoracic diameter　48
胸郭下口　Inferior thoracic aperture　44
胸郭矢状径　Sagittal thoracic diameter　48
胸郭上口　Superior thoracic aperture　44
胸管　Thoracic duct　72，79，**100**，119，226，579
胸棘筋　Spinalis thoracis　27，30，**31**
胸筋腋窩リンパ節　Pectoral axillary lymph node　64
胸筋間腋窩リンパ節　Interpectoral axillary lymph node　64
胸腔　Thoracic cavity　66
胸肩峰動脈　Thoracoacromial a.　56，**316**，334-337
— 胸筋枝　Pectoral branch of thoracoacromial a.　316
— 肩峰枝　Acromial branch of thoracoacromial a.　316
— 三角筋枝　Deltoid branch of thoracoacromial a.　316
胸骨　Sternum　44，45，**46**，49，61，130，131
— 胸骨角　Sternal angle of sternum　44，**46**，120
— 胸骨体　Body of sternum　44，**46**
— 剣状突起　Xiphoid process of sternum　44，46，120
胸骨下角　Infrasternal angle　48
胸骨関節面　Sternal articular surface　254
胸骨甲状筋　Sternothyroid　465，562，**563**，578，580
胸骨舌骨筋　Sternohyoid　465，562，**563**，578，581
胸骨端《鎖骨の》　Sternal end of clavicle　254，259
胸骨柄　Manubrium of sternum　44，**46**，47
胸骨傍リンパ節　Parasternal lymph node　**64**，73，118
胸鎖関節　Sternoclavicular joint　47，258，**259**
胸鎖乳突筋　Sternocleidomastoid　24，120，264，464，560，**561**，578，583
— 胸骨頭　Sternal head of sternocleidomastoid　561
— 鎖骨頭　Clavicular head of sternocleidomastoid　561
胸鎖乳突筋部　Sternocleidomastoid region　576
胸最長筋　Longissimus thoracis　27，30，**31**
胸神経　Thoracic n.　321
— 第1胸神経　T1 spinal n.　321，600
胸神経節　Thoracic ganglion　74，78，91
胸腺　Thymus　66，77，78，**80**
— 右葉　Right lobe of thymus　80
— 左葉　Left lobe of thymus　80
胸大動脈　Thoracic aorta　55，56，61，**68**，77，79，93，98，99，104，316，610
— 外側皮枝　Lateral cutaneous branch of thoracic aorta　34
— 後枝　Posterior(dorsal) branch(ramus) of thoracic aorta　34，610
— 脊髄枝　Spinal branch of thoracic aorta　34
— 前枝　Anterior ramus of thoracic aorta　34
— 内側皮枝　Medial cutaneous branch of thoracic aorta　34
胸大動脈神経叢　Thoracic aortic plexus　75，91
胸短回旋筋　Rotatores thoracis breves　27
胸長回旋筋　Rotatores thoracis longi　27
胸腸肋筋　Iliocostalis thoracis　27，**31**
胸椎　Thoracic vertebrae[T1-T12]　2，4，**8**
— 第6胸椎　6th thoratic vertebra　8
胸内筋膜　Endothoracic fascia　53，61，**103**
胸内臓神経　Thoracic splanchnic nn.　244，245
胸背静脈　Thoracodorsal v.　**318**，336
胸背神経　Thoracodorsal n.　320，321，**323**，337

胸背動脈　Thoracodorsal a.　316，336，**337**
胸半棘筋　Semispinalis thoracis　33
胸部　Thorax　44，77
胸部狭窄(中食道狭窄)　Thoracic(middle esophageal) constriction　96
胸腹壁静脈　Thoracoepigastric v.　57，60，**318**
胸膜下結合組織　Subpleural connective tissue　116
胸膜下リンパ管叢　Subpleural network　118
胸膜腔　Pleural cavity　**66**，77，102，176
胸腰筋膜　Thoracolumbar fascia　22，**23**，26，27，40，268，269，277
— 深葉　Deep layer of thoracolumbar fascia　23，27
— 浅葉　Superficial layer of thoracolumbar fascia　22，23，26
胸腰椎境界　Thoracolumbar junction　2
胸肋関節　Sternocostal joints　**49**，259
胸肋三角　Sternocostal triangle　53
頬筋　Buccinator　462，464，**467**，554
頬骨　Zygomatic bone　**454**，455，458，506，507，523
— 眼窩面　Orbital surface of zygomatic bone　507
— 側頭面　Temporal surface of zygomatic bone　458
頬骨眼窩孔　Zygomatico-orbital foramen　506，507
頬骨眼窩動脈　Zygomatico-orbital a.　494，499
頬骨弓　Zygomatic arch　458
頬骨神経　Zygomatic n.　505，546
頬骨神経との交通枝　Communicating branch to zygomatic n.　477
頬骨突起《側頭骨の》　Zygomatic process of temporal bone　458，526
頬神経　Buccal n.　**477**，488，489，502，503，546
頬動脈　Buccal a.　495，502，503，**504**
橋　Pons　474，478，593，**598**，599，605
橋延髄槽　Pontomedullary cistern　604
橋核(三叉神経主感覚核)　Pontine nucleus(principal sensory nucleus)　471，476
橋枝　Pontine aa.　608
橋中脳静脈　Pontomesencephalic v.　607
曲精細管　Convoluted seminiferous tubules　199
曲精巣上体管　Epididymal duct　199
棘下窩《肩甲骨の》　Infraspinous fossa of scapula　255，260，261
棘下筋　Infraspinatus　22，262，269，270，**273**，351
棘下筋膜　Infraspinous fascia　332
棘間筋　Interspinales　32，**33**
棘間靱帯　Interspinous ll.　12，18，19，**20**
棘筋　Spinalis　26，27，**30**
棘孔　Foramen spinosum　458，459，**461**
棘上窩《肩甲骨の》　Supraspinous fossa of scapula　47，255
棘上筋　Supraspinatus　22，262，265，266，269，270，**273**，332
棘上靱帯　Supraspinous l.　18，19，**20**，559
棘突起　Spinous process　2，4，**5**，6-9，12，18，44，45，49
近位横手掌線　Proximal transverse crease　353
近位指節間(PIP)関節　Proximal interphalangeal joint　300，301，**302**，304，311，352
— 関節包　Proximal interphalangeal joint capsule　302
— 側副靱帯　Collateral ll. of proximal interphalangeal joint　**302**，304，305
近位指節間関節線　PIP joint crease　353

近位趾節間(PIP)関節　Proximal interphalangeal joints　402
近位手根線　Proximal wrist crease　353
近位伸筋線　Proximal extension creases　353
筋横隔動脈　Musculophrenic a.　**54**，55，56，61
筋三角　Muscular triangle　120，576，589
筋皮神経　Musculocutaneous n.　320，321，**327**，330，331，336，338，339，341
筋裂孔　Lacuna musculorum　437

く

クーパー靱帯(乳房提靱帯)　Cooper's(suspensory) ll. of breast　63
クモ膜　Arachnoid　602
クモ膜下腔　Subarachnoid space　601，**602**，604
クモ膜顆粒　Arachnoid granulations　602，604
クモ膜顆粒小窩　Granular foveolae　457，602
クモ膜絨毛　Arachnoid villi　602
クモ膜小柱　Arachnoid trabeculae　602
グラーフ卵胞　Graafian follicle　188
グランフェルト三角(上腰三角)　Fibrous lumbar triangle of Grynfeltt　39
区域気管支　Segmental bronchus　111
区域静脈　Segmental vv.　179
区域動脈　Segmental aa.　179
空腸　Jejunum　142-145，160，161，**162**，165，173，174
空腸静脈　Jejunal vv.　215，**220**，221
空腸動脈　Jejunal aa.　**212**，220，221
隅角　→虹彩角膜角　Chamber(iridocorneal) angle
屈筋支帯《足の》　Flexor retinaculum of foot　**415**，442，443
屈筋支帯《手の》　Flexor retinaculum of hand　303，**306**，307，308，328，329，344

け

ケルクリングヒダ　Valves of Kerckring　160
茎状突起《尺骨の》　Styloid process of ulna　253，**281**，286，287，351-353
茎状突起《側頭骨の》　Styloid process of temporal bone　16，454，456，458，**526**，527，528，556
茎状突起《橈骨の》　Styloid process of radius　253，**280**，281，286，287，351，352
茎突咽頭筋　Stylopharyngeus　465，482，**554**，555，556
茎突咽頭筋腱膜　Stylopharyngeal aponeurosis　556
茎突下顎靱帯　Stylomandibular l.　540
茎突舌筋　Styloglossus　465，**548**，554，556
茎突舌骨筋　Stylohyoid　465，**544**，554，555，563
茎乳突孔　Stylomastoid foramen　458，478，479，503，**526**，547
茎乳突孔動脈　Stylomastoid a.　534，535
脛骨　Tibia　356，**380**，381，382，404，405，448，450
— 下関節面　Inferior articular surface of tibia　381，405
— 顆間隆起　Intercondylar eminence of tibia　380-382
— 外側顆　Lateral condyle of tibia　356，357，380-382，393，450
— 外側面　Lateral surface of tibia　380
— 脛骨粗面　Tibial tuberosity　356，357，373，380，381，392，450
— 脛骨体　Shaft of tibia　380，397
— 脛骨頭　Head of tibia　380

（けいこつ）

脛骨（つづき）
― 後顆間区　Posterior intercondylar area of tibia　381
― 後面　Posterior surface of tibia　380
― 上関節面　Tibial plateau　356, 380, 382
― 前縁　Anterior border of tibia　380
― 前顆間区　Anterior intercondylar area of tibia　381, 391
― 内果　Medial malleolus of tibia　380, 381
― 内果関節面　Articular surface of medial malleolus（medial malleolar articular surface）381, 404, 405
― 内果溝　Malleolar groove of tibia　380
― 内側顆　Medial condyle of tibia　356, 357, 380-382, 450
― 内側面　Medial surface of tibia　357, 380, 450
― ヒラメ筋線　Soleal line of tibia　380, 382
脛骨神経　Tibial n.　424, 425, **433**, 434, 435, 442, 443
― 内側踵骨枝　Medial calcaneal branch of tibial n.　433, 442, 443
脛腓関節　Tibiofibular joint　380, 382
脛腓靱帯結合　Tibiofibular syndesmosis　380, 404, 409
頸横静脈　Transverse cervical v.　334
頸横神経　Transverse cervical n.　**568**, 569, 578, 582, 583
頸横動脈　Transverse cervical a.　39, 317, **579**
頸横突間筋　Intertransversarii cervicis　25
頸胸椎境界　Cervicothoracic junction　2
頸棘間筋　Interspinales cervicis　25, 27
頸棘筋　Spinalis cervicis　27, 30, **31**
頸筋膜　Cervical fascia　23, 556, 574, **577**, 578
― 気管前筋膜　Pretracheal lamina of cervical fascia　577
― 気管前葉　Pretracheal layer of cervical fascia　23, 574, 577, 578
― 浅葉　Investing layer（superficial layer）of cervical fascia　23, 574, 577, 578, 580
― 椎前葉　Prevertebral layer of cervical fascia　23, 577
頸鼓神経　Caroticotympanic n.　483
頸鼓動脈　Caroticotympanic aa.　534, 535
頸後横突間筋　Cervical posterior intertransversarius　585
頸最長筋　Longissimus cervicis　30, 31
頸心臓神経　Cervical cardiac nn.　75
頸静脈　Jugular vv.　496
頸静脈窩　Jugular fossa　526
頸静脈弓　Jugular venous arch　567, 578
頸静脈孔　Jugular foramen **458**, 459, 486, 607
頸神経　Cervical nn.　584
― 後皮枝　Posterior cutaneous branches of cervical nn.　584
― 硬膜枝　Meningeal branches of cervical nn.　603
― 前根　Ventral root of cervical nn.　599
― 前枝　Anterior ramus of cervical nn.　547, 569
― 第1頸神経　C1 spinal n.　487, 547, 569
― 第2頸神経　C2 spinal n.　569, 600
― 第4頸神経　C4 spinal n.　322
― 第5頸神経　C5 spinal n.　321
― 第5頸神経の後枝　Posterior ramus of C5 spinal n.　37
― 第8頸神経　C8 spinal n.　321
― 第8頸神経の前根　Anterior root of C8　579
頸神経叢　Cervical plexus　500
頸神経ワナ　Ansa cervicalis　547, **568**, 569, 578, 580, 581

― 下根　Inferior root of ansa cervicalis　547, 568, 569
― 甲状舌骨筋枝　Thyrohyoid branch of ansa cervicalis　578, 580
― 上根　Superior root of ansa cervicalis　547, 568, 569, 580
頸髄　Cervical cord　593
頸切痕　Jugular notch　44, **46**, 120
頸長筋　Longus colli　23, **29**, 565
― 下斜部　Inferior oblique part of longus colli　29, 565
― 上斜部　Superior oblique part of longus colli　29, 565
― 垂直部　Vertical part of longus colli　29, 565
頸腸肋筋　Iliocostalis cervicis　27, **30**, 31
頸椎　Cervical vertebrae[C1-C7]　**2**, 4, 6
― 後結節　Posterior tubercle of cervical vertebrae　6
― 鉤状突起　Uncinate process of cervical vertebrae　6, 7
― 前結節　Anterior tubercle of cervical vertebrae　6
― 第1頸椎　→環椎　C1 vertebra[Atlas(C1)]
― 第2頸椎　→軸椎　C2 vertebra[Axis(C2)]
― 第4頸椎　C4 vertebra　601
頸椎後頭境界　Craniocervical junction　2
頸動脈管　Carotid canal　458, 526
頸動脈三角　Carotid triangle　**576**, 580
頸動脈小体　Carotid body　556, **580**, 581
頸動脈鞘　Carotid sheath　23, 577
頸動脈洞　Carotid sinus　482
頸動脈分岐部　Carotid bifurcation　490, 491, 581
頸半棘筋　Semispinalis cervicis　24, **32**, 33, 269
頸板状筋　Splenius cervicis　24, 26, 27, **30**, 31
頸膨大　Cervical enlargement　600
頸リンパ節　Cervical lymph node　64
頸リンパ本幹　Jugular trunk　72
鶏冠　Crista galli　460, 507, 520
血管冠　Vasocorona　610
血管裂孔　Lacuna vasorum　437
結合管　Ductus reuniens　536
結節間滑液鞘　Intertubercular synovial sheath　261
結節間溝《上腕骨の》　Intertubercular groove of humerus　**256**, 257, 259-262
結腸　Colon　164
結腸圧痕《肝臓の》　Colic impression of liver　170
結腸静脈　Colic vv.　215
結腸壁リンパ節　Epicolic lymph node　233
結腸辺縁動脈　Marginal a.　212
結腸傍溝　Paracolic gutter　149
結腸傍リンパ節　Paracolic lymph node　233
結腸膨起　Haustra of colon　164, 165
結膜　Conjunctiva　514
楔間関節　Intercuneiform joints　402
楔舟関節　Cuneonavicular joint　402
楔状結節　Cuneiform tubercle　553, **572**, 573
楔状骨群　Cuneiforms　405
楔状束核　Nucleus cuneatus　614
楔状束核小脳線維　Cuneocerebellar fibers　614
楔状束結節　Tubercle of nucleus cuneatus　599
楔立方関節　Cuneocuboid joint　402
月状骨　Lunate　**298**, 299-301
犬歯　Canine　542
肩関節　Shoulder joint　252, **258**, 263
肩甲下腋窩リンパ節　Subscapular axillary lymph node　64
肩甲下窩　Subscapular fossa　255
肩甲下筋　Subscapularis　258, 262, 265, 266, **273**

― 腱下包　Subtendinous bursa of subscapularis　262, 263
肩甲下神経　Subscapular n.　320, 321
肩甲下動脈　Subscapular a.　**316**, 317, 335, 337
肩甲回旋動脈　Circumflex scapular a.　316, **317**, 333, 336, 337
肩甲挙筋　Levator scapulae　22, 23, 269, **276**, 561
肩甲胸郭関節　Scapulothoracic joint　258
肩甲棘　Scapular spine　4, 22, 40, 252, 253, **255**, 260, 261, 268, 269, 332, 351, 561
肩甲孔　Scapular foramen　254
肩甲骨　Scapula　40, 52, 252, 253, **255**, 262, 269, 272
― 下角　Inferior angle of scapula（inferior scapular angle）4, 40, 253, **255**, 351
― 外側縁　Lateral border of scapula　**255**, 260, 262
― 外側角　Lateral angle of scapula　255
― 関節下結節　Infraglenoid tubercle　**255**, 260
― 関節窩　Glenoid cavity　**255**, 259, 260, 262
― 関節上結節　Supraglenoid tubercle　**255**, 260
― 棘下窩　Infraspinous fossa of scapula　255, 260, 261
― 棘上窩　Supraspinous fossa of scapula　47, 255
― 肩甲頸　Neck of scapula　255, 261
― 後面　Posterior surface of scapula　255
― 上縁　Superior border of scapula　255
― 上角　Superior angle of scapula　253, **255**, 259, 351
― 内側縁　Medial border of scapula　22, 40, 253, **255**, 259, 269
― 肋骨面　Costal surface of scapula　255, 259
肩甲鎖骨三角　Omoclavicular triangle　576
肩甲上静脈　Suprascapular v.　496
肩甲上神経　Suprascapular n.　320, 321, **322**, 333, 579
肩甲上動脈　Suprascapular a.　316, **317**, 332, 333, 335
― 肩峰枝　Acromial branch of suprascapular a.　317
肩甲上腕関節　Glenohumeral joint　258, 260
肩甲切痕　Scapular notch　47, 255, 259, **260**, 261
肩甲舌骨筋　Omohyoid　332, 465, **563**, 578
― 下腹　Inferior belly of omohyoid　563
― 上腹　Superior belly of omohyoid　563
― 中間腱　Intermediate tendon of omohyoid　563
肩甲背神経　Dorsal scapular n.　320, 321, **322**
肩甲背動脈　Dorsal scapular a.　317
肩鎖関節　Acromioclavicular joint　47, 252, 258, **259**
肩鎖靱帯　Acromioclavicular l.　259, 261
肩峰　Acromion　22, 40, 253, **255**, 258-262
肩峰下腔　Subacromial space　258
肩峰下包　Subacromial bursa　262, 263
肩峰角《肩甲骨の》　Acromial angle of scapula　255
肩峰関節面　Acromial articular surface　254, 262
肩峰端《鎖骨の》　Acromial end of clavicle　253, 254, 259
肩峰皮下包　Subcutaneous acromial bursa　263
肩峰部《三角筋の》　Acromial part of deltoid　265, 272
剣状突起《胸骨の》　Xiphoid process of sternum　44, 46, 120
腱画　Tendinous intersections　131, 139
腱索　Chordae tendineae　85, 87

腱鞘　Tendon sheath　415
腱中心《横隔膜の》　Central tendon of diaphragm　52，53，55，61，134
腱裂孔　→［内転筋］腱裂孔　Adductor hiatus
瞼板腺　Tarsal glands　514
原皮質　Archicortex　594

こ

コケットの静脈群　Cockett's vv.　423
コリース筋膜　→浅会陰筋膜　Colles' fascia (superficial perineal fascia)
コルチ器　Corti organ　619
古皮質　Paleocortex　594
呼吸細気管支　Respiratory bronchiole　111，116
固有蝸牛動脈　Cochlear a. proper　537
固有肝動脈　Proper hepatic a.　171，207，**210**，211，212，220，221
　—　右枝　Right branch of proper hepatic a.　171，210
　—　左枝　Left branch of proper hepatic a.　171，210
固有口腔　Oral cavity proper　550
固有掌側指神経　Proper palmar digital nn.　328-330，331，**344**
固有掌側指動脈　Proper palmar digital a.　317，344
固有底側趾神経　Proper plantar digital nn.　433，445，**446**，447
固有底側趾動脈　Proper plantar digital aa.　420，**446**，447
固有背筋　Intrinsic back muscles　23，53，61
固有卵巣索　Proper ovarian l.　151，152，183，184，**188**，189，205
孤束核　Nucleus of solitary tract　471，478，479，**482**，484
　—　下部　Inferior part of nucleus of solitary tract　482，484
　—　上部　Superior part of nucleus of solitary tract　482，484
股関節　Hip joint　356，**362**，363，364
鼓索神経　Chorda tympani　478，479，**481**，503，531，532，534，536，547
鼓室　Tympanic cavity　481，528，**530**，531
　—　鼓室蓋　Roof of tympanic cavity (tegmen tympani)　481
　—　後壁（乳突壁）　Posterior wall of tympanic cavity　481
　—　前壁（頸動脈壁）　Anterior wall of tympanic cavity　481
鼓室階　Scala tympani　536
鼓室神経　Tympanic n.　481，482，**483**，531
鼓室神経小管　Tympanic canaliculus　483
鼓室神経叢　Tympanic plexus　481，**483**，531，547
　—　耳管枝　Tubarian branch of tympanic plexus　483
鼓室乳突裂　Tympanomastoid fissure　526
鼓膜　Tympanic membrane　478，528，531，**532**，534
　—　緊張部　Pars tensa of tympanic membrane　532
　—　弛緩部　Pars flaccida of tympanic membrane　532
鼓膜臍　Umbo　532
鼓膜切痕　Tympanic incisure　532
鼓膜張筋　Tensor tympani　**528**，531，534
鼓膜張筋神経　N. of tensor tympani　503
鼓膜張筋の腱　Tendon of tensor tympani　531

鼓膜張筋半管　Semicanal of tensor tympani　481，531
口蓋咽頭弓　Palatopharyngeal arch　548，550，**552**，553
口蓋咽頭筋　Palatopharyngeus　555，556
口蓋腱膜　Palatine aponeurosis　545
口蓋骨　Palatine bone　458，521，**538**
　—　水平板　Horizontal plate of palatine bone　521
　—　垂直板　Perpendicular plate of palatine bone　521，538
　—　錐体突起　Pyramidal process of palatine bone　538
口蓋骨鞘突起管　Palatovaginal (pharyngeal) canal　458
口蓋垂　Uvula　525，**545**，550，552，553
口蓋垂筋　Musculus uvulae　**545**，555
口蓋舌弓　Palatoglossal arch　548，550，**552**
口蓋舌筋　Palatoglossus　548
口蓋突起《上顎骨の》　Palatine process of maxilla　456，458，507，521，**538**
口蓋帆（軟口蓋）　Soft palate　524，**545**，550，552，553
口蓋帆挙筋　Levator veli palatini　465，530，**545**，555
口蓋帆張筋　Tensor veli palatini　530，**545**，555
口蓋帆張筋神経　N. of tensor veli palatini　503
口蓋扁桃　Palatine tonsil　548，550，**552**，556
口角下制筋　Depressor anguli oris　462-464，**467**，561
口角挙筋　Levator anguli oris　462，464，**467**
口峡峡部　Faucial isthmus　550，553
口腔　Oral cavity　550
口腔前庭　Oral vestibule　550，556
口腔粘膜　Oral mucosa　544
光錐　Cone of light　532
広筋内転筋膜　Vastoadductor membrane　429
広頸筋　Platysma　462-464，**561**，578
広背筋　Latissimus dorsi　22，26，40，268，**277**，332，351
　—　肩甲骨部　Scapular part of latissimus dorsi　277
　—　広背筋腱膜　Latissimus dorsi aponeurosis　26
　—　腸骨部　Iliac part of latissimus dorsi　277
　—　椎骨部　Vertebral part of latissimus dorsi　277
甲状頸動脈　Thyrocervical trunk　34，56，68，316，317，335，491，566，**575**，579
甲状喉頭蓋靱帯　Thyroepiglottic l.　571
甲状舌骨筋　Thyrohyoid　554，562，**563**，578，580
甲状舌骨靱帯　Thyrohyoid l.　550，**571**，573
甲状舌骨膜　Thyrohyoid membrane　558，**571**
甲状腺　Thyroid gland　66，77，550，553，**574**，580，581
　—　右葉　Right lobe of thyroid gland　574
　—　甲状腺峡部　Isthmus of thyroid gland　574
　—　左葉　Left lobe of thyroid gland　574
　—　錐体葉　Pyramidal lobe of thyroid grand　574
甲状腺静脈叢　Thyroid venous plexus　575
甲状腺被膜（外被膜）　Capsule (external capsule) of thyroid gland　574
甲状軟骨　Thyroid cartilage　110，120，558，563，**570**，571，574，578，579
　—　右板　Right lamina of thyroid cartilage　570
　—　下角　Inferior horn of thyroid cartilage　558，570，571
　—　左板　Left lamina of thyroid cartilage　570
　—　斜線　Oblique line of thyroid cartilage　570
　—　上角　Superior horn of thyroid cartilage　558，**570**，571

甲状披裂筋　Thyroarytenoid　572
　—　甲状喉頭蓋部　Thyroepiglottic part of thyroarytenoid　572
交感神経　Sympathetic n.　622
交感神経幹　Sympathetic trunk　74，75，78，79，91，98，237，239，243，245-247，556，557，579，581，623
　—　節間枝　Interganglionic trunk　237
交感神経幹神経節　Sympathetic ganglion　36，600
交感神経系　Sympathetic nervous system　75，244
交感神経根　Sympathetic root　511
交感神経節後線維　Postsynaptic sympathetic fiber　622
交連尖　Commissural cusp　87
肛門　Anus　136，137，167，192，194，203
肛門管　Anal canal　166，167
肛門挙筋　Levator ani　136，137，**140**，141，150-153，155，167，182-184，191，193-195，203
肛門挙筋腱弓　Tendinous arch of levator ani　141
肛門三角　Anal triangle　136
肛門櫛（白帯）　Anal pecten (white zone)　167
肛門皺皮筋　Corrugator cutis ani　167
肛門柱　Anal columns　167
肛門洞　Anal sinuses　167
肛門皮膚線　Anocutaneous line　167
肛門尾骨神経　Anococcygeal nn.　203
肛門尾骨靱帯　Anococcygeal l.　136，137，140，141
肛門尾骨縫線　Anococcygeal raphe　141
肛門弁　Anal valves　167
岬角《仙骨の》　Promontory of sacrum (sacral promontory)　**2**，3，5，10，11，126，365，366，531
岬角《腸骨の》　Promontory of ilium　127
岬角リンパ節　Promontory lymph node　229，234，235
虹彩　Iris　514，516，**518**，519
虹彩角膜角（隅角）　Iridocorneal (chamber) angle　516，518
虹彩支質　Iris stroma　518
虹彩色素上皮　Pigmented iris epithelium　518
咬筋　Masseter　462-465，467，**468**，555，556，582
　—　深部　Deep part of masseter　463，467，468
　—　浅部　Superficial part of masseter　463，467，468
咬筋神経　Masseteric n.　477，488，489，503，541，**546**
咬筋動脈　Masseteric a.　495，504
後胃神経叢　Posterior gastric plexus　98，245
後胃動脈　Posterior gastric a.　211
後陰唇交連　Posterior labial commissure　136，**192**，193
後陰唇静脈　Posterior labial vv.　195
後陰唇神経　Posterior labial nn.　194
後陰嚢静脈　Posterior scrotal v.　202，**222**，223
後陰嚢神経　Posterior scrotal nn.　202，203，**243**
後下行枝（後室間枝）　Posterior descending (interventricular) a.　88
後下小脳動脈　Posteroinferior cerebellar a.　608
後下膵十二指腸動脈　Posterior branch of inferior pancreaticoduodenal a.　211，212，**219**
後海綿間静脈洞　Posterior intercavernous sinus　607
後外側溝　Posterolateral sulcus　599
後外側束　Posterolateral bundle　423
後外側裂《小脳の》　Posterolateral fissure of cerebellum　598

（こうかく）

後角《脊髄の》 Posterior horn of spinal cord　610, 612
後角《側脳室の》 Posterior (occipital) horn of lateral ventricle　594, 596, 605
後環椎後頭膜 Posterior atlanto-occipital membrane　**16**, 17-19, 25
後眼房 Posterior chamber of eyeball　516, 518
後キヌタ骨靱帯 Posterior l. of incus　532
後脚動脈 Posterior crural a.　535
後弓状静脈 Posterior arch v.　422, 423
後距骨関節面《踵骨の》 Posterior talar articular surface of calaneus　407
後距腓靱帯 Posterior talofibular l.　409
後鋸筋 Posterior serratus　30
後胸鎖靱帯 Posterior sternoclavicular l.　258
後区動脈《腎臓の》 Posterior segmental a. of kidney　209
後脛骨筋 Tibialis posterior　394, 395, **399**, 404, 410, 412, 413, 415, 442, 443
後脛骨筋の腱 Tibialis posterior tendon　399, **413**, 443
後脛骨静脈 Posterior tibial vv.　404, **422**, 423
後脛骨動脈 Posterior tibial a.　404, 420, **421**, 442
― 内果枝 Medial malleolar branches of posterior tibial a.　421, 443
後脛骨反回動脈 Posterior tibial recurrent a.　421, 443
後脛腓靱帯 Posterior tibiofibular l.　408, 409
後頸三角（外側頸三角部） Posterior triangle (lateral cervical region)　576, 582
後頸部 Posterior cervical region　576, 584
後結節間束 Posterior internodal bundles　90
後鼓室動脈 Posterior tympanic a.　532, **534**, 535
後交通動脈 Posterior communicating a.　490, 608
後骨間動脈 Posterior interosseous a.　316, 317, **340**, 341
後骨半規管 Posterior semicircular canal　481, 528, **530**, 531
後根《脊髄神経の》 Posterior (dorsal) root of spinal n.　59, 321, 601, 615
後根糸 Posterior rootlets　600
後根静脈 Posterior radicular v.　611
後根動脈 Posterior radicular a.　56
後索《脊髄の》 Posterior funiculus of spinal cord　613
後篩骨孔 Posterior ethmoidal foramen　460, **506**
後篩骨神経 Posterior ethmoidal n.　**477**, 513, 603
後篩骨洞 Posterior ethmoid sinus　521
後篩骨動脈 Posterior ethmoidal a.　490, 510, 513, **524**, 525
後耳介筋 Auricularis posterior (posterior auricular muscles)　463, 466, **529**
後耳介静脈 Posterior auricular v.　496, 567
後耳介神経 Posterior auricular n.　478, 488
後耳介動脈 Posterior auricular a.　491-493, 529, **534**
後室間溝 Posterior interventricular sulcus　84
後室間枝（後下行枝） Posterior interventricular (descending) a.　88
後室間静脈（中心静脈） Posterior interventricular v.　88
後斜角筋 Scalenus posterior (posterior scalene)　51, 317, 564, **565**
後十字靱帯 Posterior cruciate l.　387, **388**, 389
後縦隔 Posterior mediastinum　67, **76**
後縦靱帯 Posterior longitudinal l.　16, 17, **18**, 19, 21, 559
後床突起 Posterior clinoid process　459, 461

後踵骨関節面《距骨の》 Posterior calcaneal articular surface of talus　407
後上歯槽動脈 Posterior superior alveolar a.　495, 502, 503, **504**
後上膵十二指腸静脈 Posterior superior pancreaticoduodenal v.　215
後上膵十二指腸動脈 Posterior superior pancreaticoduodenal a.　207, 210, 211, 218, **219**
後上葉区《右肺の》 Posterior segment of right lung　108
後上葉静脈《右肺の》 Posterior v. of upper lobe of right lung　115
後上葉動脈《肺の》 Posterior segmental a. of lung　115
後上腕回旋動脈 Posterior circumflex humeral a.　316, 317, **333**
後上腕皮神経 Posterior brachial cutaneous n.　325, **331**, 332, 337, 338
後静脈洞交会 Posterior venous confluence　607
後神経束 Posterior cord　320, 321, 337
後深側頭動脈 Posterior deep temporal a.　504
― 翼突筋枝 Pterygoid branches of posterior deep temporal a.　495, 504
後膵動脈 Dorsal pancreatic a.　211
後髄節動脈 Posterior segmental medullary a.　610
後正中延髄静脈 Posteromedian medullary v.　606, 607
後脊髄静脈 Posterior spinal v.　611
後脊髄動脈 Posterior spinal a.　610
後仙骨孔 Posterior sacral foramen　4, **10**, 11, 126, 430
後仙腸靱帯 Posterior sacroiliac ll.　128, 129, **364**, 365
後［前腕］骨間神経 Posterior interosseous n.　325, 341
後前腕皮神経 Posterior antebrachial cutaneous n.　325, **331**, 346
後足 Hindfoot　400
後大腿神経 Posterior femoral cutaneous n.　194, 203, 424, 425, **430**, 435, 438, 441
― 会陰枝 Perineal branches of posterior femoral cutaneous n.　194, 430, 438
後大脳動脈 Posterior cerebral a.　608, 609
― 背側脳梁枝 Dorsal callosal branch of posterior cerebral a.　609
後ツチ骨ヒダ Posterior malleolar fold　532
後殿筋線 Posterior gluteal line of ilium　125, 375
後頭下筋 Suboccipital muscles　28
後頭下神経 Suboccipital n.　37, 38, **568**, 585
後頭顆 Occipital condyle　16, 456, **458**
後頭蓋窩（小脳窩） Posterior cranial (cerebellar) fossa　459
後頭極 Occipital pole　473, 595
後頭筋《後頭前頭筋の》 Occipital belly of occipitofrontalis　463, 464
後頭孔 Occipital foramen　606
後頭骨 Occipital bone　454, **456**, 457
後頭三角 Occipital triangle　576
後頭静脈 Occipital v.　496, 497, 499, 567, **584**, 606
後頭静脈洞 Occipital sinus　607
後頭前頭筋 Occipitofrontalis　462, 463
後頭頂動脈 Posterior parietal a.　609
後頭頂野 Posterior parietal cortex　613
後頭動脈 Occipital a.　38, 491-493, 499, 534, 556, 557, **584**, 585
― 下行枝 Descending branch of occipital a.　493
― 後枝 Posterior branch of occipital a.　493

― 後頭枝 Occipital branches of occipital a.　493
― 乳突枝 Mastoid branch of occipital a.　603
後頭導出静脈 Occipital emissary v.　497
後頭葉 Occipital lobe　593
後頭リンパ節 Occipital lymph node　**584**, 587
後突起《鼻軟骨の》 Posterior process of nasal cartilage　520
後内側腹側核《視床の》 Ventral posteromedial nucleus of thalamus　619
後内椎骨静脈叢 Posterior internal vertebral venous plexus　35, **57**, 601, 611
後乳頭筋 Posterior papillary muscle　85, 87
後肺底区 Posterior basal segment of lung　108
後肺底動脈 Posterior basal segmental a. of lung　115
後半規管 Posterior semicircular duct　**536**, 537
後半月大腿靱帯 Posterior meniscofemoral l.　387, 388
後半月弁《大動脈弁の》 Posterior cusp of aortic valve　86
後被蓋核 Dorsal tegmental nucleus　619, 620
後腓骨頭靱帯 Posterior l. of fibular head　386, 388
後鼻棘 Posterior nasal spine　538
後鼻孔 Choana　458, **520**, 521, 524, 538
後膨大部神経 Posterior ampullary n.　481, **536**, 537
後迷走神経幹 Posterior vagal trunk　98, 237, **238**, 239, 240, 245-247
― 肝枝 Hepatic branch of posterior vagal trunk　238
― 腹腔枝 Celiac branch of posterior vagal trunk　237, 238, 240
後盲腸動脈 Posterior cecal a.　212, 213, 220, **221**
後輪状披裂筋 Posterior cricoarytenoid　555, 557, **572**
鉤《辺縁葉の》 Uncus of limbic lobe　472
鉤状突起《頸椎の》 Uncinate process of cervical vertebrae　6, 7
鉤状突起《篩骨の》 Uncinate process of ethmoid bone　420, 521, 523
鉤状突起《尺骨の》 Coronoid process of ulna　280-283, 285, 286
鉤状突起《膵臓の》 Uncinate process of pancreas　143, 174, 175
鉤椎関節 Uncovertebral joint　15
鉤突窩《上腕骨の》 Coronoid fossa of humerus　256, 283, 285
喉頭蓋 Epiglottis　550, 552, 553, 558, **573**
喉頭蓋茎 Stalk of epiglottis　570
喉頭蓋軟骨 Epiglottic cartilage　570, 571
喉頭口 Laryngeal inlet　553
喉頭室 Ventricle　573
喉頭小嚢 Laryngeal saccule　573
喉頭腺 Laryngeal glands　573
喉頭前庭（声門上腔） Layngeal vestibule (supraglottic space)　573
喉頭隆起 Laryngeal prominence　558, **570**, 571
硬口蓋 Hard palate　**524**, 530, 538, 550
硬膜《頭蓋冠の》 Dura mater of calvaria　457, 537, 601, **602**
硬膜上腔 Epidural space　601
硬膜静脈洞 Dural sinus　457
硬膜嚢 Dural sac　601
項筋膜 Nuchal fascia　**23**, 26
― 深葉 Deep layer of nuchal fascia　23, 26
― 浅葉 Superficial layer of nuchal fascia　23
項靱帯 Nuchal l.　16, 17, 19, 276, **559**, 588
溝静脈 Sulcal v.　611

溝動脈　Sulcal a.　610
黒質　Substantia nigra　474, 615
骨間距踵靱帯　Interosseous talocalcanean l.　402, 405, 406, **409**
骨間筋《足の》　Interossei of foot　392, 402, 415
骨間筋《手の》　Interossei of hand　307-309
骨間筋腱線維　Interosseous slip　311
骨間仙腸靱帯　Interosseous sacroiliac ll.　128, 129
骨軟骨性接合部　Chondro-osseous junction　51
骨半規管　Semicircular canals　480, 536
骨盤　Pelvis　154
骨盤下口　Pelvic outlet　129
骨盤隔膜　Pelvic diaphragm　167
骨盤上口　Pelvic inlet　127
骨盤神経叢（下下腹神経叢）　Inferior hypogastric plexus　236, **239**, 244-247, 623
骨盤底　Pelvic floor　136, **141**
骨盤底の筋　Pelvic floor muscles　140
骨盤内臓神経　Pelvic splanchnic nn.　237, 239, 242, **243**, 244-247, 623
根嚢　Root sleeve　601

さ

サーファクタント（表面活性物質）　Surfactant　111
左胃静脈　Left gastric v.　99, 215, **218**, 219-221
左胃大網静脈　Left gastro-omental v.　215, **218**, 219
左胃大網動脈　Left gastro-omental a.　207, 210, 211, **218**, 219
左胃大網リンパ節　Left gastro-omental lymph node　230
左胃動脈　Left gastric a.　147, 207, 210-212, **218**, 219-221
左胃リンパ節　Left gastric lymph node　**230**, 231
左下肺静脈　Left inferior pulmonary v.　114, 115
左下葉気管支　Left inferior lobar bronchi　110
左肝静脈　Left hepatic vv.　171
左肝部　Left liver　170
— 左外側区　Left lateral division of left liver　170
— 左外側後区域（区域Ⅱ）　Left posterior lateral segment (Segment Ⅱ) of left liver　170
— 左外側前区域（区域Ⅲ）　Left anterior lateral segment (Segment Ⅲ) of left liver　170
— 左内側区　Left medial division of left liver　170
— 左内側区域（区域Ⅳ）　Left medial segment (Segment Ⅳ) of left liver　170
左冠状動脈　Left coronary a.　83, **88**
— 回旋枝　Circumflex a. of left coronary a.　88
— 外側枝　Lateral branch of left coronary a.　88
— 前室間枝（前下行枝）　Anterior interventricular (left anterior descending) branch of left coronary a.　83, 88
左冠状リンパ本幹　Left coronary trunk　100
左気管支縦隔リンパ本幹　Left broncho-mediastinal trunk　119
左頸リンパ本幹　Left jugular trunk　100
左結腸曲　Left colic flexure　144, 145, 148, 156, 161, **164**, 165, 175
左結腸静脈　Left colic v.　149, **215**
左結腸動脈　Left colic a.　149, **207**, 221
左結腸リンパ節　Left colic lymph node　233
左交感神経幹　Left sympathetic trunk　98
左鎖骨下リンパ本幹　Left subclavian trunk　119
左三角間膜　Left triangular l.　170, 171
左主気管支　Left main bronchus　68, 79, **110**
左上肺静脈　Left superior pulmonary v.　85, 114, 115
左上葉気管支　Left superior lobar bronchus　110
左上肋間静脈　Left superior intercostal v.　79

左心耳　Left auricle　83, **84**, 85, 88
左心室　Left ventricle　82-84, **85**, 93
左心室後枝　Posterior left ventricular branch　88
左心室後静脈　Posterior v. of left ventricle　88
左心房　Left atrium　82, 84, **85**, 87, 88, 93
左心房斜静脈　Oblique v. of left atrium　88
左精巣静脈　Left testicular v.　179, 180, 214, **217**, 219
左精巣動脈　Left testicular a.　179, 180, **217**, 219
左線維三角　Left fibrous trigone　86
左線維輪　Left fibrous anulus　86
左肺　Left lung　66, 93, 104, **105**
— 下葉　Inferior lobe of left lung　93, 104
— 斜裂　Oblique fissure of left lung　93, 104, 105, 109
— 上葉　Superior lobe of left lung　93, 104
左肺静脈　Left pulmonary vv.　70, 77, 79, 84, 88, **114**
左肺動脈　Left pulmonary a.　66, 68, 77, 79, 83, 84, 104, **114**, 115
左半月弁《大動脈弁の》　Left cusp of aortic valve　87
左半月弁《肺動脈弁の》　Left cusp of pulmonary valve　86
左尾状葉胆管　Left duct of caudate lobe　172
左副腎静脈　Left suprarenal v.　176, 179, 180, 214, 216, **217**, 219
左辺縁静脈　Left marginal v.　88
左辺縁動脈　Left marginal a.　88
左房室弁　Left atrioventricular valve　85, **86**, 87
— 後尖　Posterior cusp of left atrioventricular valve　86, 87
— 前尖　Anterior cusp of left atrioventricular valve　86, 87
左腰リンパ節　Left lumbar lymph node　229, 234
左腰リンパ本幹　Left lumbar trunk　72, **226**, 228
左卵巣静脈　Left ovarian v.　214, 216, 217, 219, **225**
左卵巣動脈　Left ovarian a.　179, 216, 217, 219, **225**
左腕頭静脈　Left brachiocephalic v.　35, 54
鎖骨　Clavicle　47, 120, 252, 253, **254**, 258-260, 350
— 胸骨端　Sternal end of clavicle　254, 259
— 肩峰端　Acromial end of clavicle　253, 254, 259
— 鎖骨体　Shaft of clavicle　254
— 内側頭　Medial head of clavicle　120
鎖骨下窩　Infraclavicular fossa　334
鎖骨下筋　Subclavius　265, 266, **275**
鎖骨下筋溝　Groove for subclavius muscle　254
鎖骨下筋神経　N. to subclavius　320, 321, **322**
鎖骨下静脈　Subclavian v.　35, 62, 66, 215, **318**, 334, 335, 567, 575, 579
— 右鎖骨下静脈　Right subclavian v.　70, 71, 78, 114, 583
— 左鎖骨下静脈　Left subclavian v.　54, 70, 77, 79, 114
鎖骨下静脈溝　Groove for subclavian v.　47
鎖骨下動脈　Subclavian a.　34, 56, 62, 66, 316, **317**, 335, 490, 491
— 右鎖骨下動脈　Right subclavian a.　34, 68, 78
— 左鎖骨下動脈　Left subclavian a.　54, 68, 77, 79, 84, 99, 557, 566, 575
鎖骨下動脈溝　Groove for subclavian a.　47, 565
鎖骨下動脈神経叢　Subclavian plexus　75
鎖骨下リンパ本幹　Subclavian trunk　72
鎖骨間靱帯　Interclavicular l.　259

鎖骨上神経　Supraclavicular nn.　37, 58, 62, 330-332, 334, **568**, 569, 578, 582
鎖骨上リンパ節　Supraclavicular lymph node　64
鎖骨切痕　Clavicular notch　44, **46**, 49
鎖骨中線　Midclavicular line (MCL)　120
坐骨　Ischium　**124**, 125, 126, 359
— 坐骨枝　Ischial ramus　124-126, 136, 137, 359
— 坐骨体　Body of ischium　**124**, 125, 358, 359
— 小坐骨切痕　Lesser sciatic notch　125, 126, 359, 439
— 大坐骨切痕　Greater sciatic notch　125, 126, 359, 439
坐骨海綿体筋　Ischiocavernosus　136, 137, **140**, 155, 191, 193, 194, 197, 203
坐骨棘　Ischial spine　**124**, 125-127, 129, 136, 141, 157, 356, 358, 359, 362, 364, 365
坐骨結節　Ischial tuberosity　40, **124**, 125, 126, 129, 136, 137, 141, 194, 203, 356-359, 362, 365, 450
坐骨肛門窩（坐骨直腸窩）　Ischioanal fossa　154, 155
坐骨神経　Sciatic n.　157, 424, 425, 431, **432**, 434, 435, 438, 439, 441, 448
坐骨大腿靱帯　Ischiofemoral l.　364, 365
坐骨恥骨枝《寛骨の》　Ischiopubic ramus of hip bone　197
坐骨直腸窩　→坐骨肛門窩　Ischioanal fossa
細気管支　Bronchiole　111
最小内臓神経　Least splanchnic n.　245-247
最外包　Extreme capsule　594
最上胸動脈　Superior thoracic a.　56, 316, **335**, 336, 337
最上項線　Supreme nuchal line　456, 458
最上肋間静脈　Supreme intercostal v.　70
最上肋間動脈　Supreme intercostal a.　317
最長筋　Longissimus　26, **30**, 560
最内肋間筋　Innermost intercostals　50, **51**, 61
載距突起　Sustentaculum tali　**401**, 403-407, 410
臍　Umbilicus　94, 95, 120, 121, 130, 131, 134
臍静脈　Umbilical v.　94
臍帯　Umbilical cord　95
臍動脈　Umbilical a.　**94**, 95, 208, 222, 223, 225
— 開存部　Patent part of umbilical a.　225
— 閉塞部　Occluded part of umbilical a.　225
臍ヒダ　Umbilical folds　135
臍平面　Transumbilical plane　248
臍傍静脈　Paraumbilical (periumbilical) vv.　57, 215
臍輪　Umbilical ring　139
三角窩　Triangular fossa　529
三角筋　Deltoid　22, 40, 120, 264-266, 268, 270, **272**, 332, 350, 351
— 肩甲棘部　Spinal part of deltoid　272
— 肩峰部　Acromial part of deltoid　265, 272
— 鎖骨部　Clavicular part of deltoid　272
三角筋下包　Subdeltoid bursa　262, 264
三角筋胸筋溝　Deltopectoral groove　120, 318
三角筋粗面《上腕骨の》　Deltoid tuberosity of humerus　256, 272
三角骨　Triquetrum　253, **298**, 299, 301, 351, 352
三角靱帯　Deltoid l.　**408**, 409
— 脛舟部　Tibionavicular part of deltoid l.　408
— 脛踵部　Tibiocalcanean part of deltoid l.　408

(さんかくじんたい)

三角靱帯(つづき)
　— 後脛距部　Posterior tibiotalar part of deltoid l.　408
　— 前脛距部　Anterior tibiotalar part of deltoid l.　408
三叉神経　Trigeminal n.(CN Ⅴ)　470, **476**, 483, 546, 598, 599, 607
　— 運動根　Motor root of trigeminal n.　511, 599
　— 感覚根　Sensory root of trigeminal n.　511, 599
三叉神経運動核　Motor nucleus of trigeminal n.　471, 476
三叉神経核群　Trigeminal n. nuclei　471
三叉神経主感覚核(橋核)　Principal sensory (pontine) nucleus　471, 476
三叉神経脊髄路核　Spinal nucleus of trigeminal n.　471, **476**, 482, 484, 619
三叉神経節　Trigeminal ganglion　**476**, 477, 478, 488, 489, 525, 547
三叉神経中脳路核　Mesencephalic nucleus of trigeminal n.　471, 476
三尖弁　tricuspid valve　→右房室弁
山頂　Culmen　598
産科的真結合線　True conjugate　129

【し】

シュレム管　Canal of Schlemm　516, 518
ショパール関節(横足根関節)　Transverse tarsal joint　402
子宮　Uterus　151, 152, 181, 183, 184, 186, **188**, 189-191, 205, 235
　— 後面　Posterior surface of uterus　181
　— 子宮峡部　Uterine isthmus　188
　— 子宮腔　Uterine cavity　188, 189
　— 子宮体　Uterine body(corpus)　151, 184, 188-190
　— 子宮端　Uterine pole　188
　— 子宮底　Uterine fundus　151, 152, 155, 181, 184, 188, 189, 191, 225
子宮円索　Round l. of uterus　151, 152, **181**, 183, 184, 186, 191, 205, 223, 225
子宮外膜(漿膜)　Perimetrium(serosa)　188, 190
子宮間膜　Mesometrium　**188**, 189, 235
子宮筋層　Myometrium　188, 189
子宮頸　Uterine cervix　151, 155, 157, 184, 186, **188**
　— 腟上部　Supravaginal part of uterine cervix　188, 189
　— 腟部　Vaginal part of uterine cervix　188, 189
子宮頸横靱帯(基靱帯)　Transverse cervical l.　152, 155
子宮頸管　Cervical canal　188, 189
子宮頸軸　Longitudinal cervical axis　188
子宮広間膜　Broad l. of uterus　152, **181**, 183
子宮静脈　Uterine vv.　216, 222, **223**, 225
子宮静脈叢　Uterine venous plexus　216, 222, **223**
子宮仙骨靱帯(直腸子宮靱帯)　Uterosacral l.　157, **181**, 189, 190
子宮仙骨ヒダ(直腸子宮ヒダ)　Uterosacral fold　152, **166**, 181, 183
子宮体軸　Longitudinal uterine axis　188
子宮動脈　Uterine a.　208, 222, **223**, 225
　— 腟枝　Vaginal branch of uterine a.　222
　— 卵管枝　Tubal branch of uterine a.　225
子宮腟神経叢　Uterovaginal plexus　242, 247
子宮腟静脈叢　Uterovaginal venous plexus　157, 190

子宮内膜　Endometrium　188
四角小葉《小脳の》　Quadrangular lobule of cerebellum　598
四角膜《喉頭腔の》　Quadrangular membrane of laryngeal cavity　573
四丘体板　Quadrigeminal plate　598, 599, 605
　— 上丘　Superior colliculus of quadrigeminal plate　599, 616
　— 下丘　Inferior colliculus of quadrigeminal plate　599
矢状縫合　Sagittal suture　456, 457
糸状乳頭　Filiform papillae　548
指屈筋の総腱鞘　Common flexor tendon sheath　306
指節間関節　Interphalangeal(IP) joint　253, 301, 350
指節間関節線　IP joint crease　353
指節関節靱帯　Phalangoglenoid l.　304
指(節)骨　Phalanx(phalanges)　252, 253, **298**, 300, 351, 352, 356
[指(節)]骨体　Shaft of phalanges　300
[指(節)]骨底　Base of phalanges　300
[指(節)]骨頭　Head of phalanges　300
指背腱膜　Dorsal digital expansion　297, **311**, 353
脂腺《眼瞼の》　Sebaceous glands　514
脂肪被膜　Perirenal fat capsule　156
視蓋前野　Pretectal area　616, 617
視覚野(有線野)　Visual cortex(striate area)　616
視交叉　Optic chiasm　473, 511, 598, 605, 609, 616
視交叉上核　Suprachiasmatic nucleus　616
視交叉槽　Chiasmatic cistern　604
視索　Optic tract　**473**, 616, 617
視索上陥凹　Supraoptic recess　596, 605
視索前野　Preoptic area　596
視床　Thalamus　473, 594, **596**, 598, 609, 614, 618
視床下核　Subthalamic nucleus　597
視床下溝　Hypothalamic sulcus(ventral diencephalic sulcus)　596
視床下部　Hypothalamus　593, **596**, 598, 618
視床外側腹側核群　Ventrolateral thalamic nuclei　597
視床間橋　Interthalamic adhesion　596, 605
視床室傍核群　Paraventricular nuclei of thalamus　597
視床髄条　Stria medullaris of thalamus　596, 620
視床線条体静脈　Thalamostriate v.　606
視床前核　Anterior nuclei of thalamus(anterior thalamic nuclei)　597, 621
視床帯状回路　Thalamocingular tract　621
視床内側核群　Medial nuclei of thalamus　597
視床枕　Pulvinar of thalamus　598, 616
視床網様核　Reticular nucleus of thalamus　597
視神経　Optic n.(CN Ⅱ)　470, **473**, 475, 511, 513, 616, 617
視神経円板(視神経乳頭)　Optic disk　516
視神経外鞘　Dural sheath　514
視神経管　Optic canal　459, 461, 473, **506**, 507, 538
視神経乳頭(視神経円板)　Optic disk　516
視放線　Optic radiation　473, **594**, 616
趾節間関節　Interphalangeal joints of the foot　357, 450
趾(節)骨　Phalanx(phalanges)　356
趾背腱膜　Dorsal aponeurosis　415
歯　Teeth　455, 456, **542**
歯冠　Crown of tooth　542
歯頸　Neck of tooth　542

歯根　Root of tooth　542
歯根尖　Apex of root　542
歯状回　Dentate gyrus　596
歯状靱帯　Denticulate l.　601
歯髄腔　Pulp chamber　542
歯尖靱帯　Apical l. of dens　17, 559
歯槽　Alveoli(tooth sockets)　539
歯槽骨　Alveolar bone　542
歯突起《第2頸椎の》　Dens of axis(C2)　3, 4, 7, 47, 524, 556
歯肉縁　Gingival margin　542
篩骨　Ethmoid bone　454, 455, **460**, 506, 507, 520, 523, 538
　— 眼窩板　Orbital plate of ethmoid bone　460, 506, 507, 523
　— 鉤状突起　Uncinate process of ethmoid bone　460, 521, 523
　— 垂直板　Perpendicular plate of ethmoid bone　455, 460, 507, 520, 523, 538
篩骨洞(篩骨蜂巣)　Ethmoid sinus　522, 523
篩骨胞　Ethmoid bulla　460, 521
篩骨蜂巣(篩骨洞)　Ethmoid sinus　522, 523
篩骨漏斗　Ethmoid infundibulum　460
篩板　Cribriform plate　459, **460**, 520-525, 603
示指伸筋　Extensor indicis　290, 291, **297**, 309, 310, 353
示指伸筋の腱　Extensor indicis tendon　352
耳下腺　Parotid gland　499, **551**, 556, 582, 583
　— 深部　Deep part of parotid gland　551
　— 浅部　Superficial part of parotid gland　551
耳下腺管　Parotid duct　499, 501, **551**, 556
耳下腺神経叢　Parotid plexus　478, 488, 499, 500, **551**
耳介　Auricle　529
耳介横筋　Transversus auriculae　529
耳介後リンパ節　Retroauricular lymph nodes　587
耳介斜筋　Obliquus auriculae　529
耳介側頭神経　Auriculotemporal n.　477, 488, 489, 499, 500, **502**, 503, 529, 541, 546
　— 耳下腺枝　Parotid branches of auriculotemporal n.　503
耳管　Pharyngotympanic(auditory) tube　528, **530**, 531
　— 耳管咽頭口　Pharyngeal orifice of pharyngotympanic tube　524, 530, 550, 552
　— 軟骨部　Cartilaginous part of pharyngotympanic tube　530, 555
　— 膜性板　Membranous lamina of pharyngotympanic tube　530
耳管咽頭筋　Salpingopharyngeus　530
耳管咽頭ヒダ　Salpingopharyngeal fold　525, 550, 552
耳管動脈　Tubal a.　535
耳管扁桃　Tubal tonsil　552
耳管隆起　Torus tubarius　524, 550, 552
耳甲介　Concha　529
耳甲介舟　Cymba conchae　529
耳珠　Tragus　529, 589
耳珠筋　Tragicus　529
耳小骨　Auditory ossicles　532
耳小骨連鎖　Ossicular chain　533
耳神経節　Otic ganglion　483, 503
耳垂　Earlobe　529
耳側半月　Temporal crescent　616
耳道腺　Cerumen glands　528
耳輪　Helix　529, 589
自由ヒモ　Taeniae coli　144, 145, 148, 150, 151, 162-164, 166, 182

茸状乳頭　Fungiform papilla　548
軸椎(第2頸椎)　Axis(C2)　4, 6, 7
室間孔　Interventricular foramen　604, 605
室上稜　Supraventricular crest　85
膝横靱帯　Transverse l. of knee　387, 388
膝蓋下脂肪体　Infrapatellar fat pad　390, 391
膝蓋血管網　Patellar vascular network　440
膝蓋骨　Patella　356, 357, 361, 366, 382, **383**, 390, 391, 450
　― 関節面　Articular surface of patella　383, 390
　― 膝蓋骨尖　Apex of patella　383
　― 前面　Anterior surface of patella　383
膝蓋上陥凹　Suprapatellar pouch　390, 391
膝蓋靱帯　Patellar l.　366, 367, 369, 373, **384**, 386, 390, 392, 393
膝蓋前皮下包　Prepatellar bursa　391
膝蓋大腿関節　Femoropatellar joint　386
膝関節　Knee joint　356, 382
膝関節筋　Articularis genus　367
膝静脈　Genicular vv.　422
膝神経節　Geniculate ganglion　**478**, 479, 536, 547, 619
膝窩　Popliteal fossa　370, 451
膝窩筋　Popliteus　379, 385, 394, **399**, 442
膝窩筋下陥凹　Subpopliteal recess　385, 390
膝窩静脈　Popliteal v.　422, 441, **443**
膝窩動脈　Popliteal a.　420-442, **443**
櫛状筋　Pectinate muscles　85
射精管　Ejaculatory duct　187, **200**, 201
斜角筋　Scalene　23, **50**, 565
斜角筋隙　Interscalene space　321, 565
斜径　Oblique diameter　127
斜索　Oblique cord　286
斜膝窩靱帯　Oblique popliteal l.　385
斜台　Clivus　459, 509, 524
斜披裂筋　Oblique arytenoid　555, 557, **572**
尺骨　Ulna　252, 253, **280**, 309, 352
　― 滑車切痕　Trochlear notch of ulna　280, 281, 283
　― 関節環状面　Articular circumference of ulna　280, 287
　― 茎状突起　Styloid process of ulna　253, **281**, 286, 287, 351-353
　― 後縁　Posterior border of ulna　280
　― 後面　Posterior surface of ulna　280
　― 鉤状突起　Coronoid process of ulna　280-283, 285, 286
　― 骨間縁　Interosseous border of ulna　280, **281**
　― 尺骨粗面　Ulnar tuberosity　278, 280, **281**
　― 尺骨体　Shaft of ulna　280, 351
　― 尺骨頭　Head of ulna　280, 281, 286
　― 橈骨切痕　Radial notch of ulna　280, 281, 287
　― 内側面　Medial surface of ulna　280
尺骨静脈　Ulnar vv.　318
尺骨神経　Ulnar n.　60, 321, **329**, 330, 331, 335-346
　― 掌枝　Palmar branch of ulnar n.　329, 330
　― 深枝　Deep branch of ulnar n.　329, 342, 343, 345
　― 浅枝　Superficial branch of ulnar n.　329, 342, 343, 345
　― 背側枝　Dorsal branch of ulnar n.　329, 331, 346
尺骨神経管(ギヨン管)　Ulnar tunnel　342-344
尺骨神経溝《上腕骨の》　Ulnar groove of humerus　256, 257
尺骨切痕《橈骨の》　Ulnar notch of radius　287
尺骨動脈　Ulnar a.　316, 317, 339-341, **342**, 343-345, 347

― 深枝　Deep branch of ulnar a.　342-345
― 浅枝　Superficial branches of ulnar a.　343
― 背側手根枝　Dorsal carpal branch of ulnar a.　317, 341, 347
尺側手根屈筋　Flexor carpi ulnaris　268, 270, 288, 290, **293**, 306, 309, 350, 351
尺側手根屈筋の腱　Flexor carpi ulnaris tendon　302, 307, 308, 352
尺側手根伸筋　Extensor carpi ulnaris　268, 270, **290**, 297, 309, 310, 351
尺側手根隆起　Ulnar carpal eminence　303
尺側正中皮静脈　Median basilic v.　318, 339
尺側反回動脈　Ulnar recurrent a.　316
尺側皮静脈　Basilic v.　**318**, 330, 339, 350, 351
尺側皮静脈の裂孔　Basilic hiatus　**318**, 330
尺側リンパ管群　Ulnar group of lymphatics　319
尺側リンパ管束領域　Ulnar bundle territory　319
手　Hand　252
手根　Carpal region　342
手根管　Carpal tunnel　303, 342
手根骨　Carpal bones　252, **298**
手根中央関節　Midcarpal joint　300, 301
手根中手関節　Carpometacarpal joint　300, 301
手掌　Palm　350
手掌腱膜　Palmar aponeurosis　293, 306, 330
手掌静脈網　Palmar venous network　350, 353
手背静脈網　Dorsal venous network of hand　**318**, 331, 353
珠間切痕　Intertragic incisure　529
種子骨　Sesamoids　299, **401**, 403, 404
舟状窩　Scaphoid fossa　529
舟状骨《足の》　Navicular　**400**, 401-406
舟状骨《手の》　Scaphoid　298, **300**, 301
舟状骨関節面《距骨の》　Articular surface for navicular(navicular articular surface) of talus　403, 407
舟状骨結節《手の》　Tubercle of scaphoid　253, 299, 350, 352
舟状骨粗面《足の》　Navicular tuberosity　357, 403, 450, 451
周原皮質　Periarchicortex　594
終板槽　Cistern of lamina terminalis　604
終末細気管支　Terminal bronchiole　111
皺眉筋　Corrugator supercilii　462, 464
十二指腸　Duodenum　142, 143, 146, 148, 149, 156, 159, **160**, 172-175, 210, 213
　― 下行部　Descending part of duodenum　147, 149, **160**, 161, 172, 174, 176
　― 外筋層　Muscularis externa of duodenum　160, 172
　― [十二指腸]球部　Duodenal bulb　160
　― 縦筋層　Longitudinal layer of duodenum　160, 172
　― 上行部　Ascending part of duodenum　149, **160**, 161, 174
　― 上部　Superior part of duodenum　148, 149, **160**, 161, 172, 174
　― 水平部　Horizontal part of duodenum　143, 148, 149, **160**, 161, 172, 174
　― 輪筋層　Circular layer of duodenum　**160**, 172
十二指腸圧痕《肝臓の》　Duodenal impression of liver　170
十二指腸空腸曲　Duodenojejunal flexure　148, 160, 162
十二指腸憩室　Duodenal diverticula　161
十二指腸上動脈　Supraduodenal a.　211
十二指腸提筋　Suspensory l. of duodenum　160
重心線　Line of gravity　3, 357
縦隔　Mediostinum　77

縦隔胸膜(壁側胸膜の縦隔部)　Mediastinal part of parietal pleura　54, 55, 66, 77, 80, 83, 97, **103**
縦条　Longitudinal striae　472, 620
縦束　Longitudinal fascicles　17, 19, 306, 559
女性骨盤　Female pelvis　126
女性尿道　Female urethra　185
鋤骨　Vomer　455, 507, **520**, 523, 538
小陰唇　Labium minus(minor)　136, 185, 186, 190, 191, **192**, 194
小円筋　Teres minor　40, 262, 269, 270, **273**
小角結節　Corniculate tubercle　553, 573
小角軟骨　Corniculate cartilage　570, 571
小丘《披裂軟骨の》　Colliculus of arytenoid cartilage　570, 571
小臼歯　Premolars　542
小胸筋　Pectoralis minor　265, 266, **275**
小頬骨筋　Zygomaticus minor　462-464, **467**
小結節《上腕骨の》　Lesser tubercle(tuberosity) of humerus　253, **256**, 257, 259, 260, 262, 350
小結節稜《上腕骨の》　Crest of lesser tuberosity of humerus　256, 257
小口蓋孔　Lesser palatine foramen　458, 538
小口蓋神経　Lesser palatine nn.　**505**, 525, 546
小口蓋動脈　Lesser palatine a.　495, **504**, 546
小虹彩動脈輪　Lesser arterial circle of iris　517, 518
小後頭神経　Lesser occipital n.　37, 38, 499, 568, **569**, 582-584
小後頭直筋　Rectus capitis posterior minor　24, 25, 27, 28, 464, 465, 564, **565**, 585
小鎖骨上窩　Lesser supraclavicular fossa　120, 576
小坐骨孔　Lesser sciatic foramen　129, 439
小坐骨切痕　Lesser sciatic notch　125, 126, 359, 439
小指外転筋　Abductor digiti minimi　301, 306-310, 312, **313**
小指球　Hypothenar eminence　350, 352, 353
小指伸筋　Extensor digiti minimi　290, 296, **297**, 309, 310, 353
小指対立筋　Opponens digiti minimi　307-309, 312, **313**
小趾外転筋　Abductor digiti minimi　402, 412, 413, 415, **417**, 433, 446
小趾対立筋　Opponens digiti minimi　413, 414, 418, **419**
小耳輪筋　Helicis minor　529
小十二指腸乳頭　Minor duodenal papilla　160, 172
小心臓静脈　Small cardiac v.　88
小腎杯　Minor calix　179
小錐体神経　Lesser petrosal n.　483, 503
小節　Nodule　598
小帯線維　Zonular fibers　516, **518**, 519
小腸　Small intestine　142, 160
小腸傍リンパ節　Juxtaintestinal lymph node　232
小転子　Lesser trochanter　356, **360**, 362, 364, 365
小殿筋　Gluteus minimus　367, 370-372, 374, **375**, 439, 441, 448
小頭滑車溝　Capitulotrochlear groove　285
小内臓神経　Lesser splanchnic n.　**237**, 238-240, 245-247
小内転筋　Adductor minimus　377
小脳　Cerebellum　593, **598**, 599
　― 外側部　Lateral parts of cerebellum　598
　― 水平裂　Horizontal fissure of cerebellum　598
　― 正中部　Median part of crebellum　598
小脳延髄槽(大槽)　Cerebellomedullary cistern (cisterna magna)　604

(しょうのうか)

小脳窩(後頭蓋窩) Cerebellar (posterior cranial) fossa 459
小脳脚 Cerebellar peduncles 598
小脳後葉 Posterior lobe of cerebellum 598
小脳谷 Vallecula of cerebellum 598
小脳小舌 Lingula of cerebellum 598
小脳前葉 Anterior lobe of cerebellum 598
小脳中心小葉 Central lobule of cerebellum 598
小脳虫部 Vermis of cerebellum 598
小脳虫部槽 Vermian cistern of cerebellum 604
小脳テント Tentorium cerebelli 602, **603**, 607
小脳扁桃 Tonsil of cerebellum 598
小鼻翼軟骨 Minor alar cartilages 520
小伏在静脈 Short saphenous v. **422**, 423, 435, 442, 443
小網 Lesser omentum 146, 148, **159**, 163, 168, 210
小葉間動脈 Interlobular a. 209
小腰筋 Psoas minor 52, 369, 374, **375**
小翼《蝶形骨の》 Lesser wing of sphenoid bone 455, **461**, 507, 521, 523
小菱形筋 Rhomboid minor 22, 26, 269, **276**, 561
小菱形骨 Trapezoid **298**, 299-301, 315
小弯《胃の》 Lesser curvature of stomach 158, 159
松果体 Pineal body 593, 598, 599, **605**
松果体陥凹 Pineal recess 605
松果体上陥凹 Suprapineal recess 605
笑筋 Risorius 462, 463
掌側骨間筋 Palmar interossei 314, 315
— 第1掌側骨間筋 1st palmar interosseus 308, 309, 315
— 第2掌側骨間筋 2nd palmar interosseus 308, 309, 315
— 第3掌側骨間筋 3rd palmar interosseus 308, 309, 315
掌側指静脈 Palmar digital vv. 318
掌側指神経 Palmar digital nn. 344, 345
— 背側枝 Dorsal branches of palmar digital nn. 344, 346
掌側指動脈 Palmar digital aa. 316, 317, 344, **345**
掌側尺骨手根靱帯 Palmar ulnocarpal l. 302
掌側手根間靱帯 Palmar intercarpal ll. 302
掌側手根中手靱帯 Palmar carpometacarpal ll. 302
掌側手根動脈網 Palmar carpal network 317
掌側靱帯 Palmar ll. **302**, 305, 308, 311
掌側中手静脈 Palmar metacarpal vv. 318
掌側中手靱帯 Palmar metacarpal ll. 302
掌側中手動脈 Palmar metacarpal aa. 317, 345
掌側橈骨尺骨靱帯 Palmar radioulnar l. 286, 287, 302
掌側橈骨手根靱帯 Palmar radiocarpal l. 302
硝子体 Vitreous body 516
硝子体窩 Hyaloid fossa 516
硝子軟骨性関節面 Hyaline cartilage end plate 12
睫毛腺 Ciliary 514
漿膜(子宮外膜) Serosa (perimetrium) 190
漿膜下組織 Subserosa 133
漿膜性心膜 Serous pericardium 80, 81
— 臓側板 Visceral layer of serous pericardium 80, 81
— 壁側板 Parietal layer of serous pericardium, 80, 81
鞘状突起 Processus vaginalis 196
踵骨 Calcaneus 356, **400**, 401-407, 410
— 載距突起 Sustentaculum tali **401**, 403-407, 410
— 踵骨溝 Sulcus calcanei 407

— 足根洞 Sinus tarsi of calcaneum 407
踵骨腱(アキレス腱) Achilles' tendon 393, 394, 398, 405, 411, **415**, 442, 443, 448, 451
踵骨動脈網 Calcaneal rete 442
踵骨隆起 Calcaneal tuberosity 357, **400**, 401, 404, 407, 412, 415
— 外側突起 Lateral process of calcaneal tuberosity 400, 407
— 内側突起 Medial process of calcaneal tuberosity 400, 401, 407
踵腓靱帯 Calcaneofibular l. 409
踵立方関節 Calcaneocuboid joint 402, 403
上咽頭収縮筋 Superior pharyngeal constrictor **554**, 555
— 顎咽頭部 Mylopharyngeal part of superior pharyngeal constrictor 554
— 頰咽頭部 Buccopharyngeal part of superior pharyngeal constrictor 554
— 舌咽頭部 Glossopharyngead part of superior pharyngeal constrictor 554
— 翼突咽頭部 Pterygopharyngeal part of superior pharyngeal constrictor 554
上腋窩リンパ節 Apical axillary lymph node 64
上オリーブ核 Superior olivary nucleus 619
上横隔動脈 Superior phrenic aa. 54, 55, 61
上横隔リンパ節 Superior phrenic lymph node 79, 100
上下垂体動脈 Superior hypophyseal a. 490
上下腹神経叢 Superior hypogastric plexus 236, **237**, 239, 241-243, 246, 247
上-下葉区《肺の》 Superior segment [S VI] of lung 108
上-下葉静脈《肺の》 Superior v. of lower lobe of lung 115
上-下葉動脈《肺の》 Superior segmental a. of lung 115
上外側上腕皮神経 Superior lateral brachial cutaneous n. 324, 330-332
上外側浅鼠径リンパ節 Superolateral lymph node of superficial inguinal nodes 423, 436
上顎骨 Maxilla **454**, 455, 456, 458, 507, 521, 524, 538
— 眼窩面 Orbital surface of maxilla 506, 507
上顎神経 Maxillary division (n.) (CN V₂) 476, **477**, 489, 511, 525, 546
— 外側上後鼻枝 Lateral superior posterior nasal branches (posterior superior lateral nasal branches) of maxillary n. 505, 525
— 外側鼻枝 Lateral nasal branches of maxillary n. 525
— 外鼻枝 External nasal branch of maxillary n. 525
— 眼窩枝 Orbital branches of maxillary n. 505
— 硬膜枝 Meningeal branch of maxillary n. 477, 603
— テント枝 Tentorial branches of maxillary n. 603
— 内側上後鼻枝 Medial superior posterior nasal branches (posterior superior medial nasal branches) of maxillary n. 505, **524**, 525
— 内鼻枝 Internal nasal branches of maxillary n. 525
上顎洞 Maxillary sinus 506, 507, 514, **522**, 523, 538
上顎洞裂孔 Maxillary hiatus 506, 521
上関節突起 Superior articular process **5**, 6-11, 126, 127
上関節面《脛骨の》 Tibial plateau 356, 380, 382

上眼窩裂 Superior orbital fissure 461, 477, **506**, 507, 509, 523, 538
上眼瞼 Upper eyelid 514, 515
上眼瞼挙筋 Levator palpebrae superioris 475, **508**, 509, 514
上眼静脈 Superior ophthalmic v. 496, 497, **510**, 512, 513, 567, 607
上眼動脈 Superior ophthalmic a. 512
上キヌタ骨靱帯 Superior ll. of incus 532
上気管気管支リンパ節 Superior tracheobronchial lymph node 118, 119
上丘《四丘体板の》 Superior colliculus of quadrigeminal plate 599, 616
上丘腕 Brachium of superior colliculus 599
上区動脈《腎臓の》 Superior segmental a. of kidney 209
上頸神経節 Superior cervical ganglion 75, 500, 501, **556**, 557, 580, 581, 623
— 喉頭咽頭枝 Laryngopharyngeal branch of superior cervical ganglion 117
上結膜円蓋 Superior conjunctival fornix 514
上肩甲横靱帯 Superior transverse scapular l. 259, 261, 262
上肩甲下神経 Upper subscapular n. 323, 337
上瞼板 Superior tarsus 514
上瞼板筋 Superior tarsal muscle 514
上鼓室 Epitympanum 531
上鼓室動脈 Superior tympanic a. 534
上鼓膜陥凹 Superior recess of tympanic membrane 532
上甲状結節 Superior thyroid tubercle 570
上甲状切痕 Superior thyroid notch 570
上甲状腺静脈 Superior thyroid v. **496**, 567, 575
上甲状腺動脈 Superior thyroid a. 490, 492, **493**, 500, 501, 556, 566, 574, 578-581
— 後腺枝 Posterior glandular branches of superior thyroid a. 566
— 舌骨下枝 Infrahyoid branch of superior thyroid a. 566
— 前腺枝 Anterior glandular branches of superior thyroid a. 566
— 輪状甲状枝 Cricothyroid branch of superior thyroid a. 566, 575
上行咽頭動脈 Ascending pharyngeal a. 491, 492, **493**, 534, 556, 566
上行頸動脈 Ascending cervical a. 317, 579, 610
上行結腸 Ascending colon 142, 145, 147-149, 162, **164**, 165
上行大動脈 Ascending aorta **68**, 82-84, 87, 114
上行腰静脈 Ascending lumbar v. 35, **215**, 216, 219, 611
— 右上行腰静脈 Right ascending lumbar v. 70, 71
— 左上行腰静脈 Left ascending lumbar v. 55, 70, 71
上行路《求心路》《脊髄の》 Ascending (afferent) tracts of spinal cord 613
上後鋸筋 Serratus posterior superior 26, 31
上後腸骨棘 Posterior superior iliac spine 40, 124-126, 129, **357**, 358, 359, 362, 439, 451
上喉頭静脈 Superior laryngeal v. 575
上喉頭神経 Superior laryngeal n. 117, 484, **485**, 556, 557, 575, 578-580
— 外枝 External branch of superior laryngeal n. 485, **575**, 578, 579
— 内枝 Internal branch of superior laryngeal n. 485, **575**, 578, 580

上喉頭動脈　Superior laryngeal a.　557, **566**, 575, 578, 579
上項線　Superior nuchal line　16, 24, 25, 28, 269, **456**, 458
上骨盤隔膜筋膜　Superior fascia of pelvic diaphragm　152, 153, **167**
上根《頸神経ワナの》　Superior root of ansa cervicalis　547, **568**, 569, 580
上矢状静脈洞　Superior sagittal sinus　35, 496, 497, 567, 602, 604, **606**, 607
上矢状洞溝　Groove for superior sagittal sinus　457
上肢　Upper limb　252
上肢帯　Shoulder girdle　252
上歯槽神経　Superior alveolar nn.　505, 546
　— 後上歯槽枝　Posterior superior alveolar branches of superior alveolar nn.　505, 546
　— 前上歯槽枝　Anterior superior alveolar branches of superior alveolar nn.　477, 546
　— 中上歯槽枝　Middle superior alveolar branches of superior alveolar nn.　477, 546
上耳介筋　Auricularis superior（superior auricular muscles）　463, **466**, 529
上斜筋　Superior oblique　475, 508
上尺側側副動脈　Superior ulnar collateral a.　**316**, 338-340
上十二指腸陥凹　Superior duodenal recess　161
上十二指腸曲　Superior duodenal flexure　160
上縦隔　Superior mediastinum　**66**, 76
上縦舌筋　Superior longitudinal muscle of tongue　548
上縦束　Superior longitudinal fasciculus　594
上小脳脚　Superior cerebellar peduncle　598, 599
上小脳静脈　Superior cerebellar v.　602, 606, 607
上小脳動脈　Superior cerebellar a.　608
上上皮小体（上副甲状腺）　Superior pair of parathyroid glands　574
上食道狭窄　Upper esophageal constriction　96
上伸筋支帯　Superior extensor retinaculum　415, 443, 445
上神経幹（第5・6頸神経）　Upper trunk（C5-C6）　321
上神経節　Superior ganglion　482-484
上唇　Upper lip　524
上唇（回結腸唇）　Superior lip　164
上唇挙筋　Levator labii superioris　462, 463, **467**
上唇小帯　Frenulum of upper lip　550
上唇動脈　Superior labial a.　492
上唇鼻翼挙筋　Levator labii superioris alaeque nasi　462-464, **466**
上錐体静脈　Superior petrosal v.　607
上錐体静脈洞　Superior petrosal sinus　497, 607
上膵リンパ節　Superior pancreatic lymph node　231
上髄帆　Superior medullary velum　598, 599
上前区動脈《腎臓の》　Anterior superior segmental a. of kidney　209
上前腸骨棘　Anterior superior iliac spine　40, 120, **124**, 125, 126, 129, 136, 137, 248, 356-359, 362
上前腸骨棘間径　Interspinous distance of anterior iliac spines　127
上双子筋　Gemellus superior　370-372, 374, **375**, 438, 439, 448
上唾液核　Superior salivatory nucleus　471, 478, 479
上大静脈　Superior vena cava　35, 54, 57, 66, **70**, 77, 78, 83, 88, 114, 611
上腸間膜静脈　Superior mesenteric v.　149, 156, 160, 211, 215, **220**, 221

上腸間膜動脈　Superior mesenteric a.　143, 149, 156, 160, 174, 175, 180, 206-208, 211, **212**, 219-221
上腸間膜動脈神経節　Superior mesenteric ganglion　237, 239, 240, 245, 247
上腸間膜動脈神経叢　Superior mesenteric plexus　236, 238, 240, 244, 245
上腸間膜リンパ節　Superior mesenteric lymph node　**226**, 227, 228, 231-233
上直筋　Superior rectus　475, **508**, 509, 514
上直腸横ヒダ　Superior transverse rectal fold　167
上直腸静脈　Superior rectal v.　215, **221**, 224
上直腸動脈　Superior rectal a.　**207**, 213, 221, 224
上直腸動脈神経叢　Superior rectal plexus　245
上直腸リンパ節　Superior rectal lymph node　233
上ツチ骨靱帯　Superior ll. of malleus　532
上ツチ骨ヒダ　Superior malleolar fold　532
上椎切痕　Superior vertebral notch　**5**, 8, 9, 12
上殿静脈　Superior gluteal v.　216, 222, **224**, 438, 441
　— 右上殿静脈　Right superior gluteal v.　223, 224
　— 左上殿静脈　Left superior gluteal v.　180, 216
上殿神経　Superior gluteal n.　425, **431**, 438, 439, 441
上殿動脈　Superior gluteal a.　208, 222, 223, **224**, 420, 438-441
　— 右上殿動脈　Right superior gluteal a.　223, 224
　— 左上殿動脈　Left superior gluteal a.　208
上殿皮神経　Superior cluneal nn.　37, 39, 58, 203, 430, **435**, 438, 441
上頭斜筋　Obliquus capitis superior　24, 25, 27, 28, 464, 465, 564, **565**
上橈尺関節　Proximal radioulnar joint　281, **282**, 286, 287
上内側浅鼠径リンパ節　Superomedial lymph node of superficial inguinal nodes　423
上肺底静脈　Superior basal v. of lower lobe of lung　115
上半月小葉　Superior semilunar lobule　598
上皮小体（副甲状腺）　Parathyroid glands　574
上腓骨筋支帯　Superior fibular retinaculum　415
上鼻甲介　Superior nasal concha　460, 507, **521**, 522, 525
上鼻道　Superior meatus　460, **521**, 523, 525
上副甲状腺（上皮小体）　Superior pair of parathyroid glands　574
上副腎動脈　Superior suprarenal aa.　178, 179, 208, **217**
　— 右上副腎動脈　Right superior suprarenal a.　55, 177
　— 左上副腎動脈　Left superior suprarenal a.　55, 177, 180
上腹壁静脈　Superior epigastric v.　215
上腹壁動脈　Superior epigastric a.　56
上吻合静脈　Superior anastomotic v.　606
上膀胱静脈　Superior vesical v.　223
上膀胱動脈　Superior vesical a.　222, 223, 225
上葉気管支　Superior lobar bronchi　77, 78, 104
上腰三角（グランフェルト三角）　Fibrous lumbar triangle（of Grynfeltt）　39
上涙小管　Superior lacrimal canaliculi　515
上涙点　Superior puncta　515
上肋横突靱帯　Superior costotransverse l.　49
上肋骨窩　Superior costal facet　5, 8, **49**
上腕　Arm　252
上腕腋窩リンパ節　Humeral axillary lymph node　64

上腕横靱帯　Transverse l. of humerus　261, 262
上腕筋　Brachialis　264, 267, **278**, 288, 289
上腕骨　Humerus　252, 253, **256**, 257, 259, 260
　— 解剖頸　Anatomical neck of humerus　**256**, 257, 260
　— 外側縁　Lateral border of humerus　256
　— 外側顆上稜　Lateral supracondylar ridge of humerus　256
　— 外側上顆　Lateral epicondyle of humerus　253, 256, 257
　— 外科頸　Surgical neck of humerus　256
　— 鈎突窩　Coronoid fossa of humerus　256, 283, 285
　— 結節間溝　Intertubercular groove of humerus　**256**, 257, 259-262
　— 三角筋粗面　Deltoid tuberosity of humerus　**256**, 272
　— 尺骨神経溝　Ulnar groove of humerus　256, 257
　— 小結節　Lesser tubercle（tuberosity）of humerus　253, **256**, 257, 259, 260, 262, 350
　— 小結節稜　Crest of lesser tuberosity of humerus　256, 257
　— 小頭滑車溝　Capitulotrochlear groove of humerus　257
　— 上腕骨顆　Condyle of humerus　256
　— 上腕骨小頭　Capitelum of humerus　**256**, 257, 282, 285
　— 上腕骨体　Shaft of humerus　256, 257
　— 上腕骨頭　Head of humerus　**256**, 257-260
　— 前外側面　Anterolateral surface of humerus　256
　— 前内側面　Anteromedial surface of humerus　256
　— 大結節　Greater tubercle（tuberosity）of humerus　253, 256, 257, 259, **260**, 350, 351
　— 大結節稜　Crest of greater tuberosity of humerus　256
　— 肘頭窩　Olecranon fossa of humerus　**256**, 257, 283
　— 内側縁　Medial border of humerus　257
　— 内側顆上稜　Medial supracondylar ridge of humerus　256, 257
　— 内側上顆　Medial epicondyle of humerus　253, **256**, 257, 264, 339, 350
上腕骨滑車　Trochlea of humerus　**256**, 257, 282, 283, 285
上腕三頭筋　Triceps brachii　22, 40, 268, 270, **279**, 288, 290, 333, 350, 351
　— 外側頭　Lateral head of triceps brachii　268, 270, **279**, 333, 350, 351
　— 長頭　Long head of triceps brachii　268, 270, 279, 333
　— 内側頭　Medial head of triceps brachii　270, 279
上腕静脈　Brachial v.　**318**, 336, 337, 339
上腕深動脈　Profunda brachii a.　**316**, 317, 333
上腕中間領域　Middle arm territory　319
上腕動脈　Brachial a.　**316**, 317, 336-339, 341
上腕二頭筋　Biceps brachii　262, 264, 266, **267**, 288, 289, 341, 350
　— 短頭　Short head of biceps brachii　262, 264, 266-278
　— 長頭　Long head of biceps brachii　262, 264, 266, 278
　— 停止腱　Tendon of insertion of biceps brachii　266, 288
上腕二頭筋腱膜　Bicipital aponeurosis　266, 288

（じょうわんはいがいそくりょういき）

上腕背外側領域　Dorsolateral arm territory　319
上腕背内側領域　Dorsomedial arm territory　319
上腕リンパ節　Brachial lymph node　64
静脈管索　Ligamentum venosum　95，171
静脈洞交会　Confluence of sinuses　496，497，602，604，**606**，607
静脈輪　Venous ring　611
食道　Esophagus　23，77-79，**96**，97，104，158，159
—胸部　Thoracic part of esophagus　77，96，104
—筋層　Muscular coat(Muscularis) of esophagus　97
—頸部　Cervical part of esophagus　77，96
—縦筋層　Longitudinal layer of esophagus　97
—縦走ヒダ　Longitudinal folds of esophagus　97
—粘膜　Mucosa of esophagus　97
—粘膜下組織　Submucosa of esophagus　97
—腹部　Abdominal part of esophagus　96
—輪筋層　Circular layer of esophagus　97
食道と胃粘膜との境界(Z線)　Junction of esophageal and gastric mucosae(Z line)　97
食道静脈　Esophageal vv.　**99**，215，218
食道神経叢　Esophageal plexus　74，75，**98**
食道動脈　Esophageal branches　68，99
食道入口　Esophageal inlet　96
食道傍リンパ節　Paraesophageal lymph node　73，101
食道裂孔　Esophageal hiatus(aperture) of diaphragm　52，55，70，77，**97**
心圧痕　Cardiac impression　105
心外膜　Cardiac surface　80
心室中隔　Interventricular septum　**85**，87，90，93
—筋性部　Muscular part of interventricular septum　87
—肉柱　Trabeculae carneae of interventricular septum　85
—膜性部　Membranous part of interventricular septum　87
心切痕　Cardiac notch　105
心尖　Cardiac apex　83-85，87
心臓　Heart　82，**84**
心臓刺激伝導系　Conducting system of heart　90
心臓神経叢　Cardiac plexus　75，91
—心臓枝　Cardiac branches of cardiac plexus　75
心房間束　Interatrial bundle　90
心房枝《右冠動脈の》　Atrial branch of right coronary a.　88
心房中隔　Interatrial septum　85，87
心膜　Pericardium　55，66，**80**，84
心膜横隔静脈　Pericardiacophrenic v.　**55**，66，77，80
心膜横隔動脈　Pericardiacophrenic a.　**54**，55，66，77，80
心膜横洞　Transverse pericardial sinus　81
心膜外側リンパ節　Lateral pericardial lymph node　79
心膜腔　Pericardial cavity　81
伸筋支帯《足の》　Extensor retinaculum of foot　353
伸筋支帯《手の》　Extensor retinaculum of hand　310
神経下垂体　Neurohypophysis　598
—後葉　Posterior lobe of neurohypophysis　596
神経核　Terminal nuclei　616
神経線維　Nerve fiber　471
神経点(エルブ点)　Erb's point　582
神経内腔　Endoneural space　604
唇交連　Commissure of lips　589
真肋　True ribs　45

深陰核背静脈　Deep dorsal clitoral v.　191，195
深陰茎筋膜　Deep penile fascia　197，201，202
深陰茎背静脈　Deep dorsal penile v.　181，197，**202**，203，222，223，225
深会陰横筋　Deep transverse perineal　151，**155**，184，190，191，193-195，197，200，201
深横中手靱帯　Deep transverse metacarpal l.　**302**，304-307，311
深横中足靱帯　Deep transverse metatarsal l.　410
深顔面静脈　Deep facial v.　497
深頸静脈　Deep cervical v.　567，611
深頸動脈　Deep cervical a.　317
深頸リンパ節　Deep cervical lymph node　119
深指屈筋　Flexor digitorum profundus　289-291，**293**，307，309，311
深指屈筋の腱　Flexor digitorum profundus tendons　288，289，304，305，**306**，307，308，311，315
深耳下リンパ節　Deep parotid lymph nodes　587
深耳介動脈　Deep auricular a.　495，504，**534**，535
深掌静脈弓　Deep palmar venous arch　318
深掌動脈弓　Deep palmar arch　316，317，343，**345**
—貫通枝　Perforating branches of deep palmar arch　317
深膝窩リンパ節　Deep popliteal lymph nodes　443
深膝蓋下包　Infrapatellar bursa　390，391
深錐体神経　Deep petrosal n.　479，505
深鼠径リンパ節　Deep inguinal lymph node　227-229，**234**，235，436
深鼠径輪　Deep inguinal ring　131，**133**，152，183
深足底動脈　Deep plantar a.　445
深足底動脈弓　Deep plantar arch　420，447
深側頭静脈　Deep temporal vv.　497
深側頭神経　Deep temporal nn.　477，488，502，**503**，541
深側頭動脈　Deep temporal aa.　495，502，**504**
深中大脳静脈　Deep middle cerebral v.　607
深肘正中皮静脈　Deep median cubital v.　318，339
深腸骨回旋静脈　Deep circumflex iliac v.　216，225
深腸骨回旋動脈　Deep circumflex iliac a.　**208**，216，225，420
深腓骨神経　Deep fibular n.　424，**432**，434，444，445
—皮枝　Cutaneous branch of deep fibular n.　444，445
人中　Philtrum　589
腎圧痕《肝臓の》　Renal impression of liver　170
腎盂(腎盤)　Renal pelvis　178，179
腎筋膜　Renal fascia　176
—後葉　Retrorenal layer of renal fascia　176
—前葉　Anterior layer of renal fascia　176
腎神経節　Renal ganglia　247
腎神経叢　Renal plexus　236，**237**，239，240，246
腎錐体　Renal pyramid　179
腎髄質　Renal medulla　179
腎静脈　Renal vv.　179，214，216，**217**
—右腎静脈　Right renal v.　177，178，**214**，216，217
—左腎静脈　Left renal v.　71，143，160，177-180，212，**214**，216，217
腎臓　Kidney　23，142，147，149，156，159，161，175，**176**，177-180，186，187，209，218
—下端　Inferior pole of kidney　178

—外側縁　Lateral border of kidney　178
—後面　Posterior surface of kidney　178
—脂肪被膜　Pararenal fat pad(perirenal fat capsule) of kidney　176-178
—上端　Superior pole of kidney　178
—髄放線　Medullary rays of kidney　179
—線維被膜　Fibrous capsule of kidney　23，178，179，209
—前面　Anterior surface of kidney　178
—内側縁　Medial border of kidney　178
腎柱　Renal column　179
腎動脈　Renal a.　179，206，208，**209**，217，220，221
—右腎動脈　Right renal a.　156，175，177，178，217
—後枝　Posterior branch of renal a.　209
—左腎動脈　Left renal a.　143，177，179，180，208，**209**，212，217，220，221
—前枝　Anterior branch of renal a.　209
—尿管枝　Ureteral branches of renal a.　209
—被膜枝　Capsular branches of renal a.　209
腎乳頭　Renal papilla　179
腎盤(腎盂)　Renal pelvis　178，179
腎皮質　Renal cortex　178，179
腎門　Renal hilum　176，178

す

水晶体　Lens　514，516，**518**，519
水平板《口蓋骨の》　Horizontal plate of palatine bone　521
垂直舌筋　Vertical muscle of tongue　548
垂直板《口蓋骨の》　Perpendicular plate of palatine bone　521，538
垂直板《篩骨の》　Perpendicular plate of ethmoid bone　455，**460**，507，520，523，538
膵管　Pancreatic duct(Main pancreatic duct)　160，172，173，**174**
膵管括約筋　Sphincter of pancreatic duct　172
膵十二指腸静脈　Pancreaticoduodenal v.　218，219
膵十二指腸動脈　Pancreaticoduodenal a.　220
膵十二指腸リンパ節　Pancreaticoduodenal lymph node　231
膵静脈　Pancreatic vv.　215
膵神経叢　Pancreatic plexus　238，245
膵臓　Pancreas　142，143，146-149，156，160，161，173，**174**，177，210
—胃面　Gastric surface of pancreas　174
—横隔面　Diaphragmatic surface of pancreas　174
—下縁　Inferior border of pancreas　174
—結腸面　Colic surface of pancreas　174
—後端　Posterior extremity of pancreas　174
—鉤状突起　Uncinate process of pancreas　143，174，175
—膵体　Body of pancreas　174，175
—膵頭　Head of pancreas　174，175
—膵尾　Tail of pancreas　174，175
膵尾動脈　A. of pancreatic tail　211
膵リンパ節　Pancreatic lymph node　230
錐体　Pyramid　615
錐体外路系　Extrapyramidal motor system　615
錐体筋　Pyramidalis　131，139
錐体鼓室裂　Petrotympanic fissure　458，478，526，**533**
錐体交叉　Decussation of pyramids　599，615
錐体上縁　Petrous ridge　459
錐体静脈　Petrosal v.　606
錐体神経節　Petrosal ganglion　619

錐体尖　Petrous apex　526
錐体葉《甲状腺の》　Pyramidal lobe of thyroid gland　574
錐体路（皮質脊髄路）　Pyramidal (corticospinal) tract　615
髄核　Nucleus pulposus　12
髄鞘（ミエリン鞘）　Myelin sheath　592
髄条　Medullary striae　619
髄節動脈《肋間動脈の》　Segmental medullary a. of posterior intercostal a.　610
髄膜　Meninges　602

せ

セメント質　Cementum　542
正円孔　Foramen rotundum　461, **477**, 506
正中環軸関節　Median atlantoaxial joint　16, 17
正中弓状靱帯　Median arcuate l.　52, 53
正中口蓋縫合　Median palatine suture　458, 538
正中甲状舌骨靱帯　Median thyrohyoid l.　**571**, 578, 579
正中臍ヒダ　Median umbilical fold　**135**, 144, 145, 148, 149, 152, 153, 182, 183
正中臍索　Median umbilical l.　180, **181**, 186, 187
正中神経　Median n.　60, 320, **328**, 330, 331, 335-342, 345, 346
　― 外側根　Lateral root of median n.　328
　― 関節枝　Articular branch of median n.　328
　― 掌枝　Palmar branch of median n.　328, 330
　― 内側根　Medial root of median n.　328
　― 母指球枝　Thenar branch of median n.　342
正中神経根　Median n. roots　336
正中仙骨静脈　Median sacral v.　**180**, 216, 224, 225
正中仙骨動脈　Median sacral a.　**34**, 180, 208, 216, 222-225
正中仙骨稜　Median sacral crest　5, **10**, 11, 126, 127
正中輪状甲状靱帯　Median cricothyroid l.　110, 571
正中輪状披裂靱帯　Median cricoarytenoid l.　572
生殖器《女性の》　Genital organs of female　186
生殖器《男性の》　Genital organs of male　187
声帯筋　Vocalis　572
声帯靱帯　Vocal l.　571
声帯突起《披裂軟骨の》　Vocal process of arytenoid cartilage　570, 571
声帯ヒダ　Vocal fold　550, 573
声門下腔　Subglottic space (infraglottic cavity)　573
声門間腔（喉頭室）　Intermediate laryngeal cavity (transglottic space)　573
声門上腔（喉頭前庭）　Supraglottic space (layngeal vestibule)　573
声門裂　Rima glottidis　573
性腺原基　Gonad primordium　205
星状神経節　Stellate ganglion　75, **557**, 579, 623
精管　Ductus deferens　157, 180-182, 187, **196**, 198, 199, 205, 225
精管静脈　V. of ductus deferens　196, 199
精管神経叢　Deferential plexus　243, 247
精管動脈　A. of ductus deferens　196, 199, **222**, 223
精管膨大部　Ampulla of ductus deferens　143, 150, 187, 200
精丘　Seminal colliculus　155, 185, **197**, 200
精細管　Seminiferous tubules　199
精索　Spermatic cord　130-133, **196**, 203, 205, 223, 436, 440

精巣　Testis　187, **198**, 205, 225, 234
精巣挙筋　Cremaster muscle　130, 131, **132**, 133, 196
精巣挙筋静脈　Cremasteric v.　196, 199
精巣挙筋動脈　Cremasteric a.　196, 199
精巣挙筋膜　Cremasteric (cremaster) fascia　132, 133, 196, 198
精巣縦隔　Mediastinum testis (testicular mediastinum)　198, 199
精巣鞘膜　Tunica vaginalis　196, 198
　― 臓側板　Visceral layer of tunica vaginalis　196, 198
　― 壁側板　Parietal layer of tunica vaginalis　196, 198
精巣鞘膜腔　Peritoneal cavity of scrotum　199
精巣上体　Epididymis　187, 196, **198**, 205, 225, 234
　― 精巣小葉　Lobule of epididymis　198, 199
　― 精巣上体垂　Appendix of epididymis　198
　― 精巣上体体　Body of epididymis　198
　― 精巣上体頭　Head of epididymis　198
　― 精巣上体尾　Tail of epididymis　198
精巣静脈　Testicular v.　196, 198, 199, **225**
精巣垂　Appendix of testis　198, 205
精巣中隔　Septum　198, 199
精巣動脈　Testicular a.　196, 198, 199, **225**
精巣動脈神経叢　Testicular plexus　196, 198, 236, **237**, 239, 240, 247
精巣網　Rete testis　198, 199
精巣輸出管　Efferent ductules　198, 199
精嚢　Seminal vesicle　150, 157, 182, 187, 201, 205, **223**, 243
赤核　Red nucleus　474, 615
脊髄　Spinal cord　3, 23, 36, 61, 592, **600**, 604
脊髄の白質　White matter (substance) of spinal cord　613
脊髄円錐　Conus medullaris of spinal cord　3, 600
脊髄クモ膜　Spinal arachnoid　600, 601
脊髄硬膜　Spinal dura mater　600, 601
脊髄根　Spinal root　486
脊髄静脈　Spinal v.　611
脊髄神経　Spinal n.　36, 37, 39, 58, 59, 592, **600**, 601, 604
　― 外側皮枝　Lateral cutaneous branch of spinal n.　**36**, 59
　― 関節枝　Articular branch of spinal n.　36
　― 後根　Dorsal root of spinal n.　59
　― 後枝　Posterior (dorsal) ramus of spinal n.　**36**, 39, 58, 59, 321, 332, 600
　― 硬膜枝　Meningeal branch (ramus) of spinal nerves　**36**, 600
　― 前根　Anterior (ventral) root of spinal n.　59, 430
　― 前枝　Anterior (ventral) rami of spinal n.　**36**, 59, 321
　― 前皮枝　Anterior cutaneous branch of spinal n.　**36**, 59
　― 内側枝　Medial branch of spinal n.　36
　― 内側皮枝　Medial cutaneous branches of spinal n.　37, 58
　― 白交通枝　White ramus communicans of spinal n.　59, 600, 622
脊髄神経溝　Sulcus for spinal n.　6, 7
脊髄神経節　Spinal ganglion　36, 59, **600**, 601, 622
脊柱　Vertebral column　2
脊柱管　Vertebral canal　3
脊柱起立筋　Erector spinae　**31**, 41, 53, 269
脊柱溝　Spinal furrow　41

切歯　Incisors　542
切歯窩　Incisive fossa　538, 542
切歯管　Incisive canal　520, 538
切歯孔　Incisive foramen　456, 458, 538
切歯縫合　Incisive suture　542
節状神経節　Nodose ganglion　619
舌　Tongue　548
　― 舌根　Root of tongue　548, 553
　― 舌尖　Apex of tongue　548
　― 舌体　Body of tongue　548
　― 舌背　Dorsum of tongue　548, 550
舌咽神経　Glossopharyngeal n. (CN Ⅸ)　470, **482**, 483, 547, 549, 599, 619
　― 咽頭枝　Pharyngeal branches of glossopharyngeal n.　482
　― 茎突咽頭筋枝　Stylopharyngeal branch of glossopharyngeal n.　482
　― 頸動脈枝　Carotid branch of glossopharyngeal n.　482
　― 舌枝　Lingual branch of glossopharyngeal n.　482
　― 扁桃枝　Tonsillar branch of glossopharyngeal n.　482
舌下小丘　Sublingual papilla　544, 549
舌下神経　Hypoglossal n. (CN XII)　470, **487**, 501, 547, 549, 580, 581, 599
舌下神経核　Nucleus of hypoglossal n.　471, 487
舌下神経管　Hypoglossal canal　458, 459, 487
舌下神経管静脈叢　Venous plexus of hypoglossal canal　606
舌下神経三角　Hypoglossal trigone　487
舌下神経前位核　Nucleus prepositus hypoglossi　618
舌下腺　Sublingual gland　548, **551**, 556
舌下動脈　Sublingual a.　549
舌下ヒダ　Sublingual fold　544, 549
舌筋　Lingual muscles　465, 548
舌腱膜　Lingual aponeurosis　548
舌骨　Hyoid bone　465, **539**, 544, 558
　― 小角　Lesser horn of hyoid bone　539, 558, 570
　― 舌骨体　Body of hyoid bone　539, 558
　― 大角　Greater horn of hyoid bone　539, 558, 570
舌骨下筋群　Infrahyoid muscles　544, 569
舌骨筋　Hyoid muscles　464
舌骨喉頭蓋靱帯　Hyoepiglottic l.　573
舌骨上筋群　Suprahyoid muscles.　544
舌骨舌筋　Hyoglossus　465, **544**, 545, 548, 554
舌小帯　Frenulum of tongue　549
舌静脈　Lingual v.　549, 567
舌神経　Lingual n. (CN V₃)　477-479, 488, 489, 503, 546, **547**, 549, 619
舌深静脈　Deep lingual v.　549
舌深動脈　Deep lingual a.　549
舌正中溝　Median furrow　548
舌中隔　Lingual septum　548
舌動脈　Lingual a.　491, **492**, 549, 580
舌乳頭　Lingual papilae　548
舌粘膜　Lingual mucosa　548
舌盲孔　Foramen cecum　548
舌扁桃　Lingual tonsil　**548**, 550, 552, 556, 573
仙棘靱帯　Sacrospinous l.　**128**, 129, 141, 157, 364, 365, 439
仙結節靱帯　Sacrotuberous l.　**128**, 129, 141, 364, 365, 370, 371, 375, 438, 439, 441
仙骨　Sacrum　2, 4, 5, **10**, 40, 126, 129, 136, 137, 141, 357, 358, 364, 451
　― 横線　Transverse lines　10

仙骨（つづき）
— 外側仙骨稜　Lateral sacral crest　10, 11
— 外側部　Lateral part of sacrum　5, 10, 11
— 岬角　Promontory of sacrum　5, 10, 11, 126
— 後仙骨孔　Posterior sacral foramen　4, **10**, 11, 126, 430
— 耳状面　Auricular surface of sacrum　10, 11
— 上関節面　Superior articular facet of sacrum　10
— 正中仙骨稜　Median sacral crest　5, **10**, 11, 126, 127
— 仙骨角　Sacral cornua　10
— 仙骨管　Sacral canal　5, 10, 11, 126, 129
— 仙骨尖　Apex of sacrum　10
— 仙骨粗面　Sacral tuberosity　10, 11, 129
— 仙骨底　Base of sacrum　5, 11
— 仙骨翼　Wing of sacrum　5, 10, 11
— 仙骨裂孔　Sacral hiatus　10, 126, 129, 600
— 前仙骨孔　Anterior sacral foramina　10, 11, 126, 129
— 前面　Pelvic surface of sacrum　126
— 内側仙骨稜　Medial sacral crest　10
仙骨三角　Sacral triangle　41
仙骨神経　Sacral n.　36, **430**
— 外側枝　Lateral branch of sacral n.　36
— 後枝　Dorsal (posterior) ramus of sacral n.　36, 430
— 前根　Anterior root of sacral n.　36
— 前枝　Anterior ramus of sacral n.　36
— 第1仙骨神経　1st sacral n.　237, 239, 242, 600
— 第1仙骨神経の前枝　Anterior ramus of 1st sacral n.　237, 239, 242
— 背側根（後根）　Dorsal (posterior) root of sacral n.　36, 430
仙骨神経節　Sacral ganglia　236, 237, 239
仙骨神経叢　Sacral plexus　194, 202, 237, 242, **425**, 440, 601
仙骨内臓神経　Sacral splanchnic n.　244-246
仙骨リンパ節　Sacral lymph node　227, 228, 234, 235
仙腸関節　Sacroiliac joint　124, 126, 127, 129, 358
仙尾関節　Sacrococcygeal joint　10
浅陰茎筋膜　Superficial penile fascia　197, 201, 202
浅陰茎背静脈　Superficial dorsal penile vv.　197, 201, 202
浅会陰横筋　Superficial transverse perineal　**136**, 137, 193-195, 203
浅会陰筋膜　Superficial perineal fascia　**136**, 137, 152, 155, 191
浅横中手靱帯　Superficial transverse metacarpal l.　306
浅横中足靱帯　Superficial transverse metatarsal l.　412
浅筋膜　Superficial fascia　198
浅頸静脈　Superficial cervical v.　582, 583
浅頸動脈　Superficial cervical a.　**317**, 581-583
浅頸リンパ節　Superficial cervical lymph node　582
浅骨盤隔膜筋膜　Superficial pelvic diaphragmatic fascia　154
浅指屈筋　Flexor digitorum superficialis　288, 289, 292, **293**, 306, 309, 311, 342
— 尺骨頭　Ulnar head of flexor digitorum superficialis　289, 292
— 上腕頭　Humeral head of flexor digitorum superficialis　292
— 橈骨頭　Radial head of flexor digitorum superficialis　289

浅指屈筋の腱　Flexor digitorum superficialis tendon　288, 304-308, 311
浅耳下腺リンパ節　Superficial parotid lymph nodes　587
浅膝窩リンパ節　Superficial popliteal lymph node　423
浅掌静脈弓　Superficial palmar venous arch　318
浅掌動脈弓　Superficial palmar arch　316, 317, 342, 343, **345**
浅錐体動脈　Superficial petrosal a.　535
— 下行枝　Descending branch of superficial petrosal a.　535
— 上行枝　Ascending branch of superficial petrosal a.　535
浅前頸リンパ節　Anterior superficial cervical lymph nodes　587
浅鼠径リンパ節　Superficial inguinal lymph node　227, 228, 229, 234, 235, 423, 436
浅鼠径輪　Superficial inguinal ring　130, **132**, 133, 139, 196, 202, 248, 436
— 外側脚　Lateral crus of superficial inguinal ring　132, 133, 437
— 内側脚　Medial crus of superficial inguinal ring　132, 133, 437
浅側頭静脈　Superficial temporal v.　496, **497**, 498, 502, 503, 567
浅側頭動脈　Superficial temporal a.　491-493, **494**, 499, 502, 503, 529
— 前頭枝　Frontal branch of superficial temporal a.　494, 499
— 頭頂枝　Parietal branch of superficial temporal a.　494, 499
浅中大脳静脈　Superficial middle cerebral v.　606, 607
浅腸骨回旋静脈　Superficial circumflex iliac v.　57, **422**, 434, 436
浅腸骨回旋動脈　Superficial circumflex iliac a.　420, 436, 440
浅腓骨神経　Superficial fibular n.　424, **432**, 434, 444, 445
浅腹筋膜　Superficial abdominal fascia　132, 133, **134**, 201, 436
— 膜様層　Membranous layer of superficial abdominal fascia　134
浅腹壁静脈　Superficial epigastric v.　57, 422, 434, **436**
浅腹壁動脈　Superficial epigastric a.　420, 440
腺下垂体　Adenohypophysis　598
— 前葉　Anterior lobe of adenohypophysis　596
腺房　Acinus　111
［線維鞘の］十字部　Cruciform ll.　304-306, 412, 417
［線維鞘の］輪状部　Annular l.　305, 306, 311, 412
線維性間質　Fibrous stroma　196
線維性心膜　Fibrous pericardium　77-79, **80**, 81, 83
線維膜　Fibrous membrane　365
線維輪　Anulus fibrosus　12, 20
線条体　Corpus striatum　594
前陰唇交連　Anterior labial commissure　192
前陰唇枝　Anterior labial branches　195
前陰嚢静脈　Anterior scrotal v.　202
前陰嚢動脈　Anterior scrotal a.　202
前右心室静脈　Anterior vv. of right ventricle　88
前下小脳動脈　Anteroinferior cerebellar a.　608
前下膵十二指腸動脈　Anterior branch of inferior pancreaticoduodenal a.　211, 212, 219
前下腿筋間中隔　Anterior crural intermuscular septum　444

前顆間区　Anterior intercondylar area　381, 391
前海綿間静脈洞　Anterior intercavernous sinus　607
前外果動脈　Anterior lateral malleolar a.　420, 445
前外側橋静脈　Anterolateral pontine v.　607
前外側溝　Anterolateral sulcus　599
前外側脊髄視床路　Anterolateral system（spinothalamic tract）　614
前外椎骨静脈叢　Anterior external vertebral venous plexus　**35**, 57, 611
前角《脊髄の》　Anterior horn of spinal cord　612
前角《側脳室の》　Anterior horn of lateral ventricle　594, 605
前環椎後頭膜　Anterior atlantooccipital membrane　18, 19, **559**
前眼房　Anterior chamber of eyeball　516, 518
前脚動脈　Anterior crural a.　535
前距骨関節面《踵骨の》　Anterior talar articular surface of calcaneus　407
前距腓靱帯　Anterior talofibular l.　408
前鋸筋　Serratus anterior　22, 61, 120, 130, 258, 264, 266, 269, **275**
前鋸筋結節　Tuberosity for serratus anterior　47
前胸鎖靱帯　Anterior sternoclavicular l.　258, 259
前脛骨筋　Tibialis anterior　369, 373, 392, 393, **397**, 404, 415, 443, 450
前脛骨静脈　Anterior tibial vv.　**422**, 445
前脛骨動脈　Anterior tibial a.　420, 421, 445
前脛骨反回動脈　Anterior tibial recurrent a.　420, 421
前脛腓靱帯　Anterior tibiofibular l.　408, 409
前頸三角（前頸部）　Anterior cervical triangle (region)　576, 578
前頸静脈　Anterior jugular v.　**496**, 567, 578
前結節間束　Anterior internodal bundles　90
前結膜動脈　Anterior conjunctival a.　517
前鼓室動脈　Anterior tympanic a.　495, 504, 534
前交通静脈　Anterior communicating v.　607
前交通動脈　Anterior communicating a.　608
前交連　Anterior commissure　596, 598, 605, 609
前骨間静脈　Anterior interosseous vv.　318
前骨間動脈　Anterior interosseous a.　316, **317**, 340, 345
— 後技　Posterior branch of anterior interosseous a.　317
前骨半規管　Anterior semicircular canal　528, 530, 531, **536**
前根《頸神経》　Ventral root of of cervical n.　599
前根《脊髄神経の》　Anterior (ventral) root of spinal n.　59, 321, 430, **600**, 601, 615
前根《仙骨神経の》　Anterior root of sacral n.　36
前根糸　Anterior rootlets　600
前根静脈　Anterior radicular v.　611
前根動脈　Anterior radicular a.　56
前索《脊髄》　Anterior funiculus of spinal cord　613
前篩骨孔　Anterior ethmoidal foramen　460, 506
前篩骨神経　Anterior ethmoidal n.　477, 513, **525**
— 硬膜枝　Meningeal branches of anterior ethmoidal n.　603
— 内側鼻枝　Medial nasal branches of anterior ethmoidal n.　524, 525
前篩骨動脈　Anterior ethmoidal a.　510, 513, **524**, 525
— 中隔前鼻枝　Anterior septal branches of anterior ethmoidal a.　524
前耳介筋　Auricularis anterior　463, 466, **529**
前耳介動脈　Anterior auricular aa.　529

前室間溝　Anterior interventricular sulcus　84
前室間枝（前下行枝）《左冠状動脈の》　Anterior interventicular（left anterior descending）branch of left coronary a.　83，88
前斜角筋　Scalenus anterior（anterior scalene）　51，77，317，321，564，**565**，579，581
前斜角筋結節　Scalene tubercle　565
前十字靱帯　Anterior cruciate l.　387，**388**，389，391
前縦隔　Anterior mediastinum　67，76
前縦靱帯　Anterior longitudinal l.　**18**，19，20，51，128，365，366，559
前床突起　Anterior clinoid process　459，461，538
前障　Claustrum　594，609
前踵骨関節面《距骨の》　Anterior calcaneal articular surface of talus　407
前上歯槽動脈　Anterior superior alveolar aa.　495
前上膵十二指腸動脈　Anterior superior pancreaticoduodenal a.　207，**211**，212，218，219
　─ 十二指腸枝　Duodenal branch of anterior superior pancreaticoduodenal a.　211
前上葉静脈《肺の》　Anterior v. of upper lobe of lung　115
前上葉動脈《肺の》　Anterior segmental a. of lung　115
前上腕回旋動脈　Anterior circumflex humeral a.　316，317
前深側頭動脈　Anterior deep temporal a.　504
前髄節動脈　Anterior segmental medullary a.　610
前正中裂　Anterior median fissure　599
前脊髄小脳路　Anterior spinocerebellar tract　598
前脊髄静脈　Anterior spinal v.　611
前脊髄動脈　Anterior spinal a.　608，610
前舌腺　Anterior lingual glands　549
前仙骨孔　Anterior sacral foramina　10，11，126，129
前仙腸靱帯　Anterior sacroiliac ll.　**128**，129，141，365
前仙尾靱帯　Anterior sacrococcygeal l.　129
前［前腕］骨間神経　Anterior antebrachial interosseous n.　320，328
前足　Forefoot　400
前足骨（趾骨）　Forefoot（phalanges）　400
前大腿皮静脈　Anterior femoral cutaneous v.　422，436
前大脳静脈　Anterior cerebral v.　606，607
前大脳動脈　Anterior cerebral a.　608，609
　─ 楔前部枝　Precuneal branches of anterior cerebral a.　609
　─ 中心傍小葉枝　Paracentral branches of anterior cerebral a.　609
前ツチ骨靱帯　Anterior l. of malleus　532
前ツチ骨ヒダ　Anterior malleolar fold　532
前庭　Vestibule　528，530
前庭蝸牛動脈　Vestibulocochlear a.　537
前庭階　Scala vestibuli　536
前庭器　Vestibular apparatus　536
前庭球　Vestibular bulb　155，185，186，191，**192**，193
前庭小脳線維　Vestibulocerebellar fibers　618
前庭神経　Vestibular root（CN Ⅷ）　480，**481**，528
前庭神経下核　Inferior vestibular nucleus　480，618
前庭神経外側核　Lateral vestibular nucleus　480，618
前庭神経核　Vestibular nuclei　618
前庭神経上核　Superior vestibular nucleus　480，618

前庭神経節　Vestibular ganglion　480，**481**，536，537，618
　─ 下部　Inferior part of vestibular ganglion　481，536，537
　─ 上部　Superior part of vestibular ganglion　481，536，537
前庭神経内側核　Medial vestibular nucleus　480，618
前庭神経野　Vestibular area　599
前庭靱帯　Vestibular l.　571
前庭水管　Vestibular aqueduct　537
前庭水管静脈　V. of vestibular aqueduct　537
前庭窓　Oval window　**481**，531，532，536
前庭動脈　Vestibular a.　537
前庭ヒダ　Vestibular fold　550，573
前庭裂　Rima vestibuli　573
前殿筋線《腸骨の》　Anterior gluteal line of ilium　125，359
前透明中隔静脈　Anterior v. of septum pellucidum　606
前頭蓋窩　Anterior cranial fossa　459，523
前頭極　Frontal pole　595
前頭極動脈　Polar frontal a.　609
前頭筋《後頭前頭筋の》　Frontal belly of occipitofrontalis　462，463
前頭骨　Frontal bone　454，**455**，457，459，506，507，520，523
　─ 眼窩面　Orbital surface of frontal bone　506，507
前頭神経　Frontal n.　475，477，**511**，512，513
前頭切痕　Frontal incisure　455，506
前頭前動脈　Prefrontal a.　609
前頭前野　Prefrontal cortex　613
前頭側頭束　Frontotemporal fasciculus　594
前頭直筋　Rectus capitis anterior　29，465
前頭洞　Frontal sinus　457，459，472，**507**，520-524
前頭突起《上顎骨の》　Frontal process of maxilla　506，520，521
前頭葉　Frontal lobe　593
前頭稜　Frontal crest　457，459
前内果動脈　Anterior medial malleolar a.　420
前内側橋静脈　Anteromedian pontine v.　607
前内側束《下肢リンパ管の》　Anteromedial bundle of lymphatics of lower limb　423
前内椎骨静脈叢　Anterior internal vertebral venous plexus　35，**57**，601，611
前乳頭筋　Anterior papillary muscle　85，87，90
前肺底区　Anterior basal segment of lung　108
前肺底静脈　Anterior basal v. of lung　115
前肺底動脈　Anterior basal segmental a. of lung　115
前半規管　Anterior semicircular duct　536，537
前腓骨頭靱帯　Anterior l. of fibular head　388
前鼻棘　Anterior nasal spine　454，455，538
前膨大部神経　Anterior ampullary n.　481，536，**537**
前脈絡叢動脈　Anterior choroidal a.　490，608
前迷走神経幹　Anterior vagal trunk　74，**98**，237-240，245
　─ 肝枝　Hepatic branch of anterior vagal trunk　238，240
　─ 幽門枝　Pyloric branch of anterior vagal trunk　238，240，245
前毛様体動脈　Anterior ciliary aa.　517
前盲腸動脈　Anterior cecal a.　212，213，**220**，221
前有孔質　Anterior perforate substance　472，620
前立腺　Prostate　150，153，155，182，184，185，187，197，**200**，201，205，223

　─ 右葉　Right lobe of prostate　200
　─ 左葉　Left lobe of prostate　200
　─ 前立腺峡部　Prostatic isthmus of prostate　200
　─ 前立腺尖　Apex of prostate　200
　─ 前立腺底　Base of prostate　200
前立腺管　Prostatic ductules　185，197
前立腺原基　Primordium of prostate duct　205
前立腺小室　Prostatic utricle　205
前立腺静脈叢　Prostatic venous plexus　202，222
前立腺神経叢　Prostatic plexus　239，**243**，247
前立腺被膜　Prostatic capsule　200
前涙嚢稜　Anterior lacrimal crest　506
前肋間静脈　Anterior intercostal vv.　35，57
前腕　Forearm　252
前腕筋膜　Antebrachial fascia　306
前腕屈筋　Flexors of forearm　289
前腕骨間膜　Interosseous membrane of forearm　281，**286**，292，293，295，301，317
前腕正中皮静脈　Median antebrachial v.　**318**，330，339
　─ 貫通枝　Perforating branches of median antebrachial v.　330
前腕正中皮神経　Median antebrachial cutaneous n.　321
前腕中間領域　Middle forearm territory　319

そ

咀嚼筋　Muscles of mastication　463
鼠径管　Inguinal canal　**133**，187
鼠径靱帯　Inguinal l.　**128**，130，131，133，135，139，225，248，364-366，436，437，440，450
鼠径部　Inguinal region　**132**，436
僧帽筋　Trapezius　23-26，40，264，266，268，**276**，332，464，465，560，561
　─ 横行部（水平部）　Transverse part of trapezius　22，268，276，332，561
　─ 下行部　Descending part of trapezius　22，268，276，332，561
　─ 上行部　Ascending part of trapezius　22，268，276，332
僧帽弁　mitral valve　→左房室弁
総蝸牛動脈　Common cochlear a.　537
総肝管　Common hepatic duct　172，173
総肝動脈　Common hepatic a.　55，147，173，207，**210**，211，212，218
総顔面静脈　Common facial v.　501，502，580
総頸動脈　Common carotid a.　34，68，317，335，491-494，556，557，**566**，575，578，579，581，608
　─ 左総頸動脈　Left common carotid a.　68，77，84，99
総頸動脈神経叢　Common carotid plexus　75
総腱輪　Common tendinous ring　475，**508**，509
総骨間動脈　Common interosseous a.　**316**，317，340
［総］指伸筋　Extensor digitorum　268，270，290，296，**297**，309，310，347，351，353
　─ 腱間結合　Intertendinous connections of extensor digitorum　290，310
［総］指伸筋の腱　Extensor digitorum tendon　290，305，351，353
［総］趾伸筋の腱　Extensor digitorum tendons　450
総掌側神経　Common palmar digital nn.　328-330
総掌側指動脈　Common palmar digital aa.　316，317，**344**，345
総胆管　Bile duct　171，**172**，173，175，179，210

（そうたんかんかつやくきん）

総胆管括約筋　Sphincter of bile duct　172
総腸骨静脈　Common iliac v.　57, **214**, 215, 216, 221, 224, 225, 611
　― 右総腸骨静脈　Right common iliac v.　149-151, 182, 216, 224
　― 左総腸骨静脈　Left common iliac v.　71, 143, 151, 216, 221, 223, 225
総腸骨動脈　Common iliac a.　206, **208**, 213, 221-225, 420
　― 右総腸骨動脈　Right common iliac a.　149-151, 180, 182, 208, 213, 224, 227
　― 左総腸骨動脈　Left common iliac a.　143, 151, 206, 221, 223, 225
総腸骨リンパ節　Common iliac lymph node　**226**, 227-229, 234, 235
　― 右総腸骨リンパ節　Right common iliac lymph node　226
　― 左総腸骨リンパ節　Left common iliac lymph node　226
総底側趾神経　Common plantar digital nn.　433, 446
総底側趾動脈　Common plantar digital aa.　420
総肺底静脈　Common basal v. of lower lobe of lung　115
総腓骨神経　Common fibular n.　424, 425, **432**, 434, 435, 441-444
槽間中隔　Interalveolar septum　542
象牙質　Dentin　542
臓側胸膜　Visceral pleura　66
臓側骨盤筋膜　Visceral pelvic fascia　150, 151, **154**, 182, 183, 185
臓側腹膜　Visceral peritoneum　103, **142**, 143, 167, 182-184, 201
足　Foot　356
足関節窩　Ankle mortise　356, 380, **404**, 405
足根　Tarsals　356
足根管　Tarsal tunnel　443
足根骨　Tarsus (tarsal bones)　400
足根中足関節　Tarsometatarsal joints　402, 403
足根洞《踵骨の》　Sinus tarsi of calcaneum　407
足底　Sole of foot　451
足底弓　Arches of foot　410
足底筋　Plantaris　370, 371, 394, **398**, 442, 448
足底筋の腱　Plantaris tendon　394, 398
足底腱膜　Plantar aponeurosis　406, 411, **412**, 446, 447
足底交叉　Plantar chiasm　395, 399
足底静脈弓　Plantar venous arch　422
足底靱帯　Plantar ll.　410
足底方形筋　Quadratus plantae　404, 411, 413, 418, **419**, 446, 447
足背静脈弓　Dorsal venous arch of foot　422
足背静脈網　Dorsal venous network of foot　422
足背動脈　Dorsal pedal a.　420, 445
側角《脊髄の》　Lateral horn of spinal cord　612
側索《脊髄の》　Lateral funiculus of spinal cord　613
側頭下窩　Infratemporal fossa　502, 503
側頭窩　Temporal fossa　501
側頭筋　Temporalis　463-465, **468**, 501
側頭骨　Temporal bone　16, 454, 456, 458, 459, 525, **526**, 527
　― 岩様部　Petrous part of temporal bone　456, 459, **527**
　― 頬骨突起　Zygomatic process of temporal bone　458, 526
　― 茎状突起　Styloid process of temporal bone　16, 454, 456, 458, **526**, 527, 528, 556

　― 鼓室部　Tympanic part of temporal bone　527
　― 乳突切痕　Mastoid notch of temporal bone　458, 526
　― 乳様突起　Mastoid process of temporal bone　16, 24, 454, 456, 458, **526**, 588
　― 鱗部　Squamous part of temporal bone　454, 456, **527**
側頭錐体鱗部静脈洞　Petrosquamous sinus　607
側頭頭頂筋　Temporoparietalis　463
側頭葉　Temporal lobe　593
側脳室　Lateral ventricle　473, 594, **605**, 609, 616
　― 下角　Inferior (temporal) horn of lateral ventricle　596, 605
　― 後角　Posterior (occipital) horn of lateral ventricle　594, 596, 605
　― 前角　Anterior horn of lateral ventricle　594, 605
　― 側副三角　Collateral trigone of lateral ventricle　605
　― 中心部　Central part of lateral ventricle　605
側脳室脈絡叢　Choroid plexus of lateral ventricle　604
側副三角　Collateral trigone of lateral ventricle　605
側腹筋　Lateral abdominal wall muscles　23

【た】

ダグラス窩　→直腸子宮窩　Rectouterine pouch
手綱核　Habenular nuclei　472, 620
多形細胞層　Multiform layer　595
多裂筋　Multifidus　27, 32, **33**
唾液核　Salivatory nuclei　471
対角結合線　Diagonal conjugate　129
対角帯　Diagonal stria　472, 620
対珠　Antitragus　529, 589
対珠筋　Antitragicus　529
対輪　Antihelix　529, 589
対輪脚　Crura of antihelix　529
帯状回　Cingulate gyrus　593, 595, 596, **621**
帯状回海馬線維　Cingulo-hippocampal fibers　621
帯状回枝《脳梁縁動脈の》　Cingular branch of callosomarginal a.　609
胎盤　Placenta　94
大陰唇　Labium majus　136, 185, 186, 191, **192**
大円筋　Teres major　22, 40, 264-270, **277**, 332, 351
大鉗子　Forceps major　594
大臼歯　Molars　542
大胸筋　Pectoralis major　120, 130, 264-266, **274**, 334, 350
　― 胸肋部　Sternocostal part of pectoralis major　130, 264, 274, 334
　― 鎖骨部　Clavicular part of pectoralis major　264, 274, 334
　― 腹部　Abdominal part of pectoralis major　130, 264, 274
大頬骨筋　Zygomaticus major　462-464, **467**, 498
大結節《上腕骨の》　Greater tubercle (tuberosity) of humerus　253, 256, 257, 259, **260**, 350, 351
大結節稜《上腕骨の》　Crest of greater tuberosity of humerus　256
大口蓋管　Greater palatine canal　538
大口蓋孔　Greater palatine foramen　458, 538
大口蓋神経　Greater palatine n.　**505**, 525, 546

　― 下後鼻枝　Inferior posterior nasal branches of greater palatine n.　525
大口蓋動脈　Greater palatine a.　495, **504**, 524, 525, 546
大虹彩動脈輪　Greater arterial circle of iris　517, 518
大後頭孔　Foramen magnum　**458**, 459, 486
大後頭孔周囲静脈叢　Venous plexus around foramen magnum　497, 606
大後頭神経　Greater occipital n.　37, 38, 499, **568**, 584, 585
大後頭直筋　Rectus capitis posterior major　24, 25, 27, 28, 464, 465, **565**, 585
大坐骨孔　Greater sciatic foramen　129, 439
大坐骨切痕　Greater sciatic notch　**125**, 126, 359, 439
大耳介神経　Great auricular n.　37, 38, 334, 499, **568**, 569, 578, 582-585
大耳輪筋　Helicis major　529
大十二指腸乳頭　Major duodenal papilla　160, 172
大静脈孔《横隔膜の》　Caval hiatus (aperture) of diaphragm　**52**, 53, 55, 70, 77
大静脈後リンパ節　Retrocaval lymph node　228, 229
大静脈溝　Groove for vena cava　171
大静脈靱帯　L. of vena cava　171
大心臓静脈　Great cardiac v.　88
大腎杯　Major calix　179, 209
大膵動脈　Great pancreatic a.　211
大錐体神経　Greater petrosal n.　**478**, 479, 481, 505
大錐体神経管裂孔　Hiatus of canal for greater petrosal n.　478
大前髄節動脈　Great anterior segmental medullary a.　610
大前庭腺　Greater vestibular gland　186, 205
大前庭腺開口部　Opening of greater vestibular glands　192
大槽　Cisterna magna　604
大唾液腺　Major salivary glands　551
大腿　Thigh　356
大腿筋膜　Fascia lata　133, **438**, 440, 441
大腿筋膜張筋　Tensor fasciae latae　366, 367, 370, 371, 373, 374, **375**, 439, 440, 448, 450
大腿骨　Femur　356, **360**, 361, 362, 364, 365, 448
　― 顆間窩　Intercondylar notch of femur　360, 382
　― 顆間線　Intercondylar line of femur　360
　― 外側顆　Lateral condyle of femur　356, 360, 361, 382
　― 外側顆上線　Lateral supracondylar line of femur　360
　― 外側上顆　Lateral epicondyle of femur　360, 382
　― 外側唇　Lateral lip of femur　360
　― 骨端線　Epiphyseal line　363
　― 膝窩面　Popliteal surface of femur　360, 382
　― 膝蓋面　Patellar surface of femur　360, 361, 389
　― 小転子　Lesser trochanter　356, **360**, 362, 364, 365
　― 粗線　Linea aspera　360, 362
　― 大腿骨頸　Neck of femur　356, 360-363, 365
　― 大腿骨体　Shaft of femur　360, 363

― 大腿骨頭　Head of femur　155, 157, **360**, 361-363, 421
― 大転子　Greater trochanter　40, 356, 357, **360**, 361-365, 370, 450
― 恥骨筋線　Pectineal line　360
― 転子窩　Trochanteric fossa　360
― 転子間線　Intertrochanteric line　360, 362, 365
― 転子間稜　Intertrochanteric crest　360, 362, 365
― 殿筋粗面　Gluteal tuberosity　360, 362
― 内側顆　Medial condyle of femur　356, 360, 361, 382, 389
― 内側顆上線　Medial supracondylar line of femur　360
― 内側上顆　Medial epicondyle of femur　356, 357, 360, 382, 451
― 内側唇　Medial lip of linea aspera　360
― 内転筋結節　Adductor tubercle　360
大腿骨頭窩　Fovea of femoral head　360, 361, 364
大腿骨頭靱帯　L. of head of femur　157, 363, **364**, 421
大腿四頭筋　Quadriceps femoris　248, **378**, 429, 440
大腿膝窩静脈　Femoropopliteal v.　422
大腿静脈　Femoral v.　57, 157, 196, 208, 225, **422**, 423, 434, 436, 440
大腿神経　Femoral n.　135, 157, 424-426, **429**, 434, 435, 440
― 筋枝　Muscular branches of femoral n.　425, 429
― 前皮枝　Anterior cutaneous branches of femoral n.　425, 426, 429, 434
大腿深静脈　Deep femoral v.　422
大腿深動脈　Profunda femoris a.　420, 440
大腿直筋　Rectus femoris　366, 367, 369, 373, **378**, 429, 440, 448, 450
大腿動脈　Femoral a.　157, 196, 208, 225, **420**, 434, 436, 440
大腿二頭筋　Biceps femoris　373, **379**, 394, 441, 442, 448, 451
― 短頭　Short head of biceps femoris　371, 373, 379, 394, 441, 448
― 長頭　Long head of biceps femoris　370, 371, 373, 379, 441, 448
大腿方形筋　Quadratus femoris　155, 370, 371, 374, **375**, 438, 439, 441, 448
大腿方形筋神経　Quadratus femoris n.　431
大腿輪　Femoral ring　135, 437
大大脳静脈　Great cerebral v.　606, 607
大腸　Large intestine　164
大転子　Greater trochanter　40, 356, 357, **360**, 361-365, 370, 450
大殿筋　Gluteus maximus　40, 136, 137, 157, 194, 203, 369-374, **375**, 438, 441, 451
大動脈　Aorta　77, 82
大動脈弓　Aortic arch　34, **68**, 77, 79, 83, 84, 90, 95, 99, 114
大動脈後リンパ節　Retroaortic lymph node　226, 228
大動脈腎動脈神経節　Aorticorenal ganglia　236, 237, 239
大動脈前リンパ節　Preaortic lymph node　226, 229
大動脈洞　Aortic sinus　87
大動脈分岐部　Aortic bifurcation　56, 206, 213
大動脈弁　Aortic valve　**86**, 87

― 右半月弁　Right cusp of aortic valve　87
― 左半月弁　Left cusp of aortic valve　87
大動脈裂孔《横隔膜の》　Aortic hiatus (aperture) of diaphragm　**52**, 53, 68, 70
大内臓神経　Greater splanchnic n.　55, 74, 78, 98, **237**, 238-240, 245, 623
大内転筋　Adductor magnus　194, 203, 366-372, **377**, 421, 439-441, 448
大脳　Telencephalon　594
大脳窩　Cerebral fossa　459
大脳鎌　Falx cerebri　602, 603
大脳基底核　Basal ganglia　592, 594
大脳脚　Cerebral peduncle　**594**, 598, 599, 605
大脳弓状線維　Cerebral arcuate fibers (U fibers)　594
大脳縦裂　Longitudinal cerebral fissure　593, 595
大脳動脈　Cerebral a.　602
大脳皮質　Cerebral cortex　592, **594**, 595, 602
大鼻翼軟骨　Major alar cartilage　520
― 外側脚　Lateral crus of major alar cartilage　520
― 内側脚　Medial crus of major alar cartilage　520
大伏在静脈　Long saphenous v.　57, **422**, 423, 434, 436, 442
大網　Greater omentum　143, **144**, 146-148, 156, 159, 175
大網ヒモ　Taenia omentalis　164
大腰筋　Psoas major　23, 52, 135, 139, 180, 225, 366, 367, 369, 374, **375**
大翼《蝶形骨の》　Greater wing of sphenoid bone　454, 455, 459, **461**, 507, 523
大菱形筋　Rhomboid (romboideus) major　22, 26, 269, **276**
大菱形骨　Trapezium　**298**, 300, 301
大菱形骨結節　Tubercle of trapezium　253, **299**, 350, 352, 353
大弯《胃の》　Greater curvature of stomach　158, 159
台形体核　Nucleus of trapezoid body　619
第3後頭神経　3rd occipital n.　37-39, **568**, 584, 585
第3腓骨筋　Fibularis tertius　392, 393, 396, **397**, 415, 441
第一裂　Primary fissure　598
第三脳室　3rd ventricle　596, **605**, 609
第三脳室脈絡叢　Choroid plexus of 3rd ventricle　604
第四脳室　4th ventricle　598, 599, **605**
第四脳室外側陥凹　Lateral recess of 4th ventricle　605
第四脳室外側口　Lateral aperture of 4th ventricle　599
第四脳室髄条　Striae medullaris of 4th ventricle　599
第四脳室正中口　Median aperture of 4th ventricle　604, 605
第四脳室ヒモ　Taenia cinerea of 4th ventricle　599
第四脳室脈絡叢　Choroid plexus of 4th ventricle　604
単小葉　Simple lobule　598
胆管　Bile ducts　172
胆膵管　Hepatopancreatic duct　173
胆膵管膨大部　Hepatopancreatic ampulla　172
胆膵管膨大部括約筋　Sphincter of hepatopancreatic ampulla　172

胆嚢　Gallbladder　142, 144, 146-148, 156, 159, 163, 168, 171, **172**, 173, 175, 210
― 胆嚢頸　Neck of gallbladder　172
― 胆嚢体　Body of gallbladder　172
― 胆嚢底　Fundus of gallbladder　172
胆嚢管　Cystic duct　171-173
胆嚢静脈　Cystic v.　215
胆嚢動脈　Cystic a.　171, **210**, 211
胆嚢リンパ節　Cystic lymph node　231
胆嚢漏斗　Infundibulum of gallbladder　172
淡蒼球　Globus pallidus　594, 609
― 外節　Lateral segment of globus pallidus　597
― 内節　Medial segment of globus pallidus　597
短胃静脈　Short gastric vv.　215, 218, 219
短胃動脈　Short gastric aa.　211
短回旋筋　Rotatores breves　33
短後毛様体動脈　Short posterior ciliary aa.　**510**, 513, 517
短趾屈筋　Flexor digitorum brevis　404, 411, 412, **417**, 446, 447
短趾屈筋の腱　Flexor digitorum brevis tendons　412, 413, 446, 447
短趾伸筋　Extensor digitorum brevis　392, 393, 415, **416**
短趾伸筋の腱　Extensor digitorum brevis tendons　415, 416
短小指屈筋　Flexor digiti minimi brevis　306-309, **312**, 313
短小趾屈筋　Flexor digiti minimi brevis　412-414, **418**, 419
短掌筋　Palmaris brevis　306, 353
短橈側手根伸筋　Extensor carpi radialis brevis　268, 270, 288, 290, 291, 294, **295**, 309, 310
短内転筋　Adductor brevis　367, 372, **376**, 440, 448
短腓骨筋　Fibularis brevis　392-394, **396**, 404, 413-415, 442, 445
短母指外転筋　Abductor pollicis brevis　306-309, 312, **313**, 353
短母指屈筋　Flexor pollicis brevis　306, 308, 309, 312, **313**, 353
― 深頭　Deep head of flexor pollicis brevis　308
― 浅頭　Superficial head of flexor pollicis brevis　307
短母指伸筋　Extensor pollicis brevis　290, 291, 297, 307-309, **310**, 353
短母趾屈筋　Flexor hallucis brevis　411-414, 418, **419**, 447
― 外側頭　Lateral head of flexor hallucis brevis　413, 419
― 内側頭　Medial head of flexor hallucis brevis　413, 419
短母趾伸筋　Extensor hallucis brevis　392, 415, **416**
短毛様体神経　Short ciliary nn.　477, **511**, 513, 617
短肋骨挙筋　Levatores costarum breves　27, 32, **33**
男性骨盤　Male pelvis　126
男性尿道　Male urethra　185
弾性円錐　Conus elasticus　571, 572

【ち】

チン動脈輪　Arterial circle of Zinn　517
恥丘　Mons pubis　136, 192

恥骨　Pubis　**124**, 125, 126, 157, 166, 181, 359
ー 弓状線　Arcuate line of pubis　129
ー 恥骨下角　Subpubic angle　127
ー 恥骨下枝　Inferior pubic ramus　124-126, 136, 137, 150-153, 155, 191, 358, 359
ー 恥骨櫛　Pecten pubis　124, 126, 129
ー 恥骨上枝　Superior pubic ramus　124-126, 133, 137, 150, 151, 197, 358, 359
ー 恥骨体　Body of pubis　124, 125, 359
恥骨弓状靱帯　Pubic arcuate l.　141
恥骨筋　Pectineus　133, 157, 366, 367, **376**, 436, 440, 450
恥骨筋線　Pectineal line　362
恥骨結合　Pubic symphysis　124, 126, 127, **128**, 129, 141, 150, 151, 191, 201, 248, 357, 358, 365, 366, 369, 450
恥骨結合面　Symphyseal surface　124, 129, 358
恥骨結節　Pubic tubercle　124, 126, 127, **128**, 141, 248, 356-359, 362, 364, 450
恥骨後隙　Retropubic space　150, 152, 153, 201
恥骨櫛　Pecten pubis　**127**, 358
恥骨櫛靱帯　Pectineal l.　133
恥骨大腿靱帯　Pubofemoral l.　364, 365
恥骨直腸筋　Puborectalis　141, 166
恥骨尾骨筋　Pubococcygeus　141, 166
腟　Vagina　151, 152, 155, 183, 184, 186, 189, **190**, 191, 205
ー 後部　Posterior part of vagina　190
ー 後壁　Posterior wall of vagina　190
ー 前皺柱　Anterior vaginal column　190
ー 前部　Anterior part of vagina　190
ー 前壁　Anterior wall of vagina　189, 190
ー 尿道隆起　Urethral carina of vagina　190
腟円蓋　Vaginal fornix　151, 188-190
ー 外側部　Lateral part of vaginal fornix　189
ー 後部　Posterior vaginal fornix　151, 184, 188
ー 前部　Anterior vaginal fornix　151, 184, 188
腟口　Vaginal orifice　136, 190-192, 194
腟軸　Longitudinal axis in vagina　188
腟静脈叢　Vaginal venous plexus　222, 223
腟前庭　Vestibule of vagina (vaginal vestibule)　155, 186, **190**, 191, 194
腟前庭球静脈　V. of vestibular bulb　195
腟前庭球動脈　A. of vestibular bulb　191, 195
腟動脈　Vaginal a.　**222**, 223, 225
腟粘膜ヒダ　Vaginal rugae　190, 191
腟傍組織　Paravaginal tissue　155
中位小掌線　Middle crease　353
中咽頭収縮筋　Middle pharyngeal constrictor　554, 555
ー 小角咽頭部　Chondropharyngeal part of middle pharyngeal constrictor　554
ー 大角咽頭部　Ceratopharyngeal part of middle pharyngeal constrictor　554
中隔縁柱　Septomarginal trabecula　85, 87, 90
中隔乳頭筋　Septal papillary muscle　85, 87
中間肝静脈　Intermediate hepatic vv.　171
中間楔状骨　Intermediate cuneiform　**400**, 401-403, 410
中間腱《顎二腹筋の》　Intermediate tendon of digastric muscle　544
中間腱《肩甲舌骨筋の》　Intermediate tendon of omohyoid　563
中間広筋　Vastus intermedius　366, 367, 371, **378**, 429, 440, 448
中間鎖骨上神経　Intermediate supraclavicular nn.　582, 583
中間神経　Nervus intermedius　478, **481**, 537, 557, 599

中間足背皮神経　Intermediate dorsal cutaneous n.　432, 434, 444, 445
中間帯　Central slip　311
中間腸間膜リンパ節　Intermediate mesenteric lymph node　232
中間腰リンパ節　Intermediate lumbar lymph node　156, **228**, 229, 234, 235
中間裂孔リンパ節　Intermediate lacunar lymph node　228, 229, 235
中距骨関節面《踵骨の》　Middle talar articular surface of calcaneus　407
中頚神経節　Middle cervical ganglion　74, 75, 91, 98, 557, **579**, 623
中結節間束　Middle internodal bundles　90
中結腸静脈　Middle colic v.　162, **215**, 218-221
中結腸動脈　Middle colic a.　143, 162, **207**, 212, 213, 220, 221
中結腸リンパ節　Middle colic lymph node　233
中鼓室　Mesotympanum　531
中甲状腺静脈　Middle thyroid vv.　575
中硬膜静脈　Middle meningeal v.　607
中硬膜動脈　Middle meningeal a.　**495**, 503, 504, 510, 534, 603
ー 岩様部枝　Petrous branch of middle meningeal a.　495
ー 前頭枝　Frontal branch of middle meningeal a.　495, 603
ー 頭頂枝　Parietal branch of middle meningeal a.　495, 603
ー 涙腺動脈との吻合枝　Anastomotic branch with lacrimal a.　495
中篩骨洞　Middle ethmoid sinus　523
中耳　Middle ear　528, 530
中膝動脈　Middle genicular a.　421, 443
中斜角筋　Middle scalene (scalenus medius)　51, 317, **564**, 565
中手骨　Metacarpals　252, 253, **298**, 300, 304, 351, 352
ー 体　Shaft of metacarpals　299, 300
ー 第1中手骨　1st metacarpal　252, 253, 298, 300, 301, 315
ー 第2中手骨　2nd metacarpal　253, 315
ー 第3中手骨　3rd metacarpal　304, 305, 311, 315
ー 第4中手骨　4th metacarpal　315
ー 第5中手骨　5th metacarpal　301, 315
ー 底　Base of metacarpals　299, 300
ー 頭　Head of metacarpals　299, 300, 353
中手骨頭間静脈　Intercapitular vv.　318, 331
中手指節 (MCP) 関節　Metacarpophalangeal (MCP) joint　253, 300, 301, **302**, 304, 311, 344, 350, 352
ー 側副靱帯　Collateral ll. of metacarpophalangeal joint　301, **302**, 304, 305
中手指節関節線　MCP joint crease　353
中縦隔　Middle mediastinum　67, 76
中小脳脚　Middle cerebellar peduncle　598, 599
中踵骨関節面《距骨の》　Middle calcaneal articular surface of talus　407
中食道狭窄 (胸部狭窄)　Middle esophageal (thoracic) constriction　96
中心腋窩リンパ節　Central axillary lymph node　64
中心窩　Fovea centralis　516, 616
中心灰白質　Central gray substance　474
中心管《脊髄の》　Central canal of spinal cord　604, 605
中心後回　Postcentral gyrus　593, 613-615, 619
中心後溝動脈　A. of postcentral sulcus　609
中心溝　Central sulcus　593, 595, 613
中心溝動脈　A. of central sulcus　609

中心前回　Precentral gyrus　593, 613, 615
中心前溝動脈　A. of precentral sulcus　609
中心臓静脈 (後室間静脈)　Posterior interventricular v.　88
中心被蓋路　Central tegmental tract　598
中神経幹 (第7頚神経)　Middle trunk (C7)　321
中腎管 (ウォルフ管)　Mesonephric (wolffian) duct　205
中節骨《足の》　Middle phalanx of foot　400
ー 第5中節骨　5th middle phalanx of foot　400-402
中節骨《手の》　Middle phalanx of hand　**299**, 300, 301, 305
ー 体　Shaft of middle phalanx of hand　299
ー 第2中節骨　2nd middle phalanx of hand　298
ー 第4中節骨　4th middle phalanx of hand　252
ー 底　Base of middle phalanx of hand　299
ー 頭　Head of middle phalanx of hand　299
中足　Midfoot　400
中足間関節　Intermetatarsal joints　402
中足骨　Metatarsus (metatarsal)　356, 400, 403
ー 第1中足骨　1st metatarsal　400, **401**, 402-404, 406, 410
ー 第2中足骨　2nd metatarsal　405
ー 第5中足骨　5th metatarsal　400, 401, 406
ー 第5中足骨粗面　Tuberosity of 5th metatarsal　400, **401**, 403, 404, 410, 412, 413, 415, 417, 450, 451
中足趾節関節　Metatarsophalangeal joint　357, 450
ー 関節包　Metatarsophalangeal joint capsules　408, 409, 419
ー 第1中足趾節関節　1st metatarsophalangeal joint　402
中側頭動脈　Middle temporal a.　494
中側副動脈　Middle collateral a.　316
中大脳動脈　Middle cerebral a.　**608**, 609
ー 角回枝　Angular gyral branch of middle cerebral a.　609
ー 後側頭枝　Posterior temporal branch of middle cerebral a.　609
ー 前側頭枝　Anterior temporal branch of middle cerebral a.　609
ー 中側頭枝　Middle temporal branch of middle cerebral a.　609
ー 蝶形骨部 (M1区)　Sphenoidal part (M1) of middle cerebral a.　608
ー 島部 (M2区)　Insular part (M2) of middle cerebral a.　608
ー 頭頂後頭枝　Parieto-occipital branch of middle cerebral a.　609
中直腸横ヒダ　Middle transverse rectal fold　167
中直腸静脈　Middle rectal vv.　215, 216, **222**, 223, 224
中直腸動脈　Middle rectal a.　202, 208, **222**, 223-225
中直腸動脈神経叢　Middle rectal plexus　239, **242**, 243, 245
中殿筋　Gluteus medius　40, 367, 370-374, **375**, 437, 448, 451
中殿皮神経　Middle cluneal nn.　37, 39, 203, 430, **435**, 438, 441
中頭蓋窩　Middle cranial fossa　459
中脳　Mesencephalon　595, 599
中脳蓋　Tectum of midbrain　474
中脳水道　Cerebral aqueduct　474, 599, **604**, 605, 609
中鼻甲介　Middle nasal concha　455, 460, 507, **521**, 522, 523, 525, 538, 553
中鼻道　Middle meatus　**521**, 523, 525

中副腎動脈　Middle suprarenal a.　**178**, 179, 217
— 左中副腎動脈　Left middle suprarenal a.　177, 180, 208
中葉静脈《右肺の》　Middle lobe v. of right lung　115
中葉動脈《右肺の》　Middle lobe a. of right lung　115
虫垂　Vermiform appendix　142, 153, **164**, 182
虫垂間膜　Mesoappendix　149, 164
虫垂口　Orifice of vermiform appendix　164
虫垂静脈　Appendicular v.　215, 220
虫部垂　Uvula vermis　598
虫部錐体　Pyramid of vermis　598
虫部葉　Folium vermis　598
虫様筋《足の》　Lumbricals of foot　411-413, 418, **419**, 447
虫様筋《手の》　Lumbricals of hand　307, 308, 314, **315**
— 第1虫様筋　1st lumbrical of hand　315
— 第2虫様筋　2nd lumbrical of hand　311, 315
— 第3虫様筋　3rd lumbrical of hand　315
— 第4虫様筋　4th lumbrical of hand　315
虫様筋腱線維　Lumbrical slip　311
肘窩　Cubital fossa　339
肘関節　Elbow joint　252, **282**, 284, 285
肘筋　Anconeus　268, 270, **279**, 290
肘正中皮静脈　Median cubital v.　**318**, 330, 339, 350
肘頭　Olecranon　22, 252, 253, **268**, 280, 281, 283, 290, 351
肘頭窩《上腕骨の》　Olecranon fossa of humerus　**256**, 257, 283
肘頭皮下包　Olecranoan bursa　283
肘リンパ節　Cubital lymph node　64, **319**
長回旋筋　Rotatores longi　32, 33
長胸神経　Long thoracic n.　320, 321, **322**, 335-337
長後毛様体動脈　Long posterior ciliary aa.　510, 517
長趾屈筋　Flexor digitorum longus　394, 395, **399**, 411-413, 415, 419, 442, 443
長趾屈筋の腱　Flexor digitorum longus tendon　**413**, 418, 419, 446, 447, 451
長趾伸筋　Extensor digitorum longus　392, **397**, 404, 415
長趾伸筋の腱　Extensor digitorum longus tendon　397, 415
長掌筋　Palmaris longus　288, **292**, 293
長掌筋の腱　Palmaris longus tendon　306, 350, 352, 353
長足底靱帯　Long plantar l.　406, **408**, 409, 411, 413, 414, 419
長橈側手根伸筋　Extensor carpi radialis longus　268, 270, 288, 290, 291, 294, **295**, 309, 310, 350, 351
長橈側手根伸筋の腱　Extensor carpi radialis longus tendon　290
長内転筋　Adductor longus　366, 367, 369, 372, **376**, 440, 448, 450
長腓骨筋　Fibularis longus　373, 392-394, **396**, 404, 410, 412, 413, 415, 442, 450
長腓骨筋の腱　Fibularis longus tendon　**396**, 411, 413, 414, 419, 451
長腓骨筋腱溝　Groove for fibularis longus tendon　401
長母指外転筋　Abductor pollicis longus　288, 290, 291, 296, **297**, 307, 309, 310
長母指外転筋の腱　Abductor pollicis longus tendon　307, 308

長母指屈筋　Flexor pollicis longus　288, 289, 292, **293**, 306, 307, 309
長母指屈筋の腱　Flexor pollicis longus tendon　288, **289**, 306, 308
長母指伸筋　Extensor pollicis longus　290, 291, 296, **297**, 309, 310, 352, 353
長母指伸筋の腱　Extensor pollicis longus tendon　290
長母趾屈筋　Flexor hallucis longus　394, 395, **399**, 404, 411-413, 415, 442, 443
長母趾屈筋の腱　Flexor hallucis longus tendon　399, **412**, 413, 446, 447
長母趾屈筋腱溝《距骨の》　Groove for flexor hallucis longus tendon of talus　407
長母趾屈筋腱溝《踵骨の》　Groove for flexor hallucis longus tendon of calcaneus　407
長母趾伸筋　Extensor hallucis longus　392, 393, **397**, 404, 415, 450
長母趾伸筋の腱　Extensor hallucis longus tendon　397, **415**, 443
長毛様体神経　Long ciliary nn.　477, **511**, 513
長肋骨挙筋　Levatores costarum longi　27, 32, **33**
鳥距溝　Calcarine sulcus　595
腸間膜　Mesentery　142, 143, 145, 146, **148**, 163, 165, 175
腸間膜根　Mesenteric root（root of mesentery）　149, 161
腸間膜動脈間神経叢　Intermesenteric plexus　236, **237**, 239, 241-244, 247
腸脛靱帯　Iliotibial tract　366, 367, 370, **373**, 440, 441, 448, 451
腸骨　Ilium　**124**, 125-127, 129, 181, 359
— 下後腸骨棘　Posterior inferior iliac spine　124-126, **359**, 362
— 下前腸骨棘　Anterior inferior iliac spine　124-126, 128, 136, 137, **358**, 359
— 下殿筋線　Inferior gluteal line of ilium　125, 359
— 弓状線　Arcuate line of ilium　**124**, 127, 129, 358
— 岬角　Promontory of ilium　127
— 後殿筋線　Posterior gluteal line of ilium　125, 375
— 耳状面　Auricular surface of ilium　124, 358
— 前殿筋線　Anterior gluteal line of ilium　125, 359
— 腸骨窩　Iliac fossa　124, 126, 127
— 腸骨粗面　Iliac tuberosity　**124**, 126, 127, 129, 358
— 腸骨体　Body of ilium　**124**, 125, 358, 359
— 腸骨翼　Iliac wing　125, 126, 359
— 殿筋面　Gluteal surface of ilium　125, 126, 359
腸骨下腹神経　Iliohypogastric n.　37, 58, 133, 176, 178, 179, 424-426, **427**, 434, 435, 438, 441
— 外側枝　Lateral branch of iliohypogastric n.　430, 438, 441
— 外側皮枝　Lateral cutaneous branch of iliohypogastric n.　58, 426, 427, 435
— 前皮枝　Anterior cutaneous branch of iliohypogastric n.　133, 426, 427
腸骨筋　Iliacus　134, 135, 139, 180, 225, 366, 367, 369, 374, **375**, 376
腸骨鼠径神経　Ilioinguinal n.　132, 176, 178, 179, 194, 196, 202, 203, 424-426, **427**, 434, 436
腸骨大腿靱帯　Iliofemoral l.　364, 365, 367
腸骨動脈神経叢　Iliac plexus　239, 243
腸骨尾骨筋　Iliococcygeus　140, 141

腸骨稜　Iliac crest　4, 22, 40, 120, **124**, 125-127, 268, 356-359, 362, 364, 365, 450, 451
— 外唇　Outer lip of iliac crest　127
— 中間線　Intermediate line of iliac crest　127
— 腸骨結節　Iliac tubercle　126, 127
— 内唇　Inner lip of iliac crest　127
腸恥筋膜弓　Iliopectineal arch　135, 437
腸恥包　Iliopectineal bursa　437
腸恥隆起　Iliopubic eminence　127, 437
腸腰筋　Iliopsoas　135, 138, **139**, 157, 366, 367, 429, 440
腸腰靱帯　Iliolumbar l.　**128**, 365
腸腰動脈　Iliolumbar a.　208, 222, 223
腸リンパ本幹　Intestinal trunk　226, 228
腸肋筋　Iliocostalis　26, 30, 560
蝶下顎靱帯　Sphenomandibular l.　540
蝶形骨　Sphenoid bone　454-456, 459, **461**, 507, 521, 523
— 下垂体窩　Hypophyseal fossa（sella turcica）of sphenoid bone　459, **461**, 520, 521, 524
— 外側板　Lateral plate of sphenoid bone　521
— 眼窩面　Orbital surface of sphenoid bone　**461**
— 小翼　Lesser wing of sphenoid bone　455, 459, **461**, 507, 521, 523
— 側頭面　Temporal surface of sphenoid bone　461
— 大脳面　Cerebral surface of sphenoid bone　461
— 大翼　Greater wing of sphenoid bone　454, 455, 459, **461**, 507, 523
— 蝶形骨体　Body of sphenoid bone　461
— 内側板　Medial plate of sphenoid bone　521
— 翼状突起　Pterygoid process of sphenoid bone　456, 458, **461**, 521, 538
蝶形[骨]頭頂静脈洞　Sphenoparietal sinus　607
蝶形骨洞　Sphenoid sinus　**520**, 521, 522, 524, 525
— 蝶形骨洞口　Aperture of sphenoid sinus　461
— 蝶形骨洞中隔　Septum of sphenoid sinus　538
蝶形骨隆起　Jugum sphenoidale　459, 461
蝶形骨稜　Sphenoid crest　461
蝶口蓋孔　Sphenopalatine foramen　525
蝶口蓋動脈　Sphenopalatine a.　**495**, 503, 504, 524, 546
— 外側後鼻枝　Lateral posterior nasal aa. of sphenopalatine a.　525
— 中隔後鼻枝　Posterior septal branches of sphenopalatine a.　495, 504, 524, 546
蝶篩陥凹　Sphenoethmoid recess　525
蝶前頭縫合（プテリオン）　Sphenofrontal suture（pterion）　454
蝶鱗縫合　Sphenosquamous suture　454
聴覚器　Auditory apparatus　536
聴放線　Acoustic radiation　619
直細動脈　Vasa recta　212
直精細管　Straight seminiferous tubules　199
直静脈洞　Straight sinus　604, **606**, 607
直腸　Rectum　143, 150-153, 157, **166**, 167, 180-183, 201
— 外筋層　Muscularis externa of rectum　167
— 縦筋層　Longitudinal layer of rectum　167
— 輪筋層　Circular layer of rectum　167
直腸横ヒダ　Transverse rectal fold　166
直腸子宮窩（ダグラス窩）　Rectouterine pouch　151, 152, 157, **181**, 183, 184, 188, 190
直腸子宮靱帯（子宮仙骨靱帯）　Uterosacral l.　157, **181**, 189, 190

直腸子宮ヒダ（子宮仙骨ヒダ） Uterosacral fold 152, **166**, 181, 183
直腸静脈叢 Rectal venous plexus 216
直腸前線維 Prerectal fibers 141
直腸前立腺筋膜 Rectoprostatic fascia 150, 182, 201
直腸膀胱窩 Rectovesical pouch 143, 150, 153, 182, **184**, 201
直腸膀胱中隔 Rectovesical septum 150, **153**, 157, 184
直腸膨大部 Rectal ampulla 167
直腸腟中隔 Rectovaginal septum 152, 190

つ

ツチ骨 Malleus 528, 530, 531, **532**
— 外側突起 Lateral process of malleus 532
— 前突起 Anterior process of malleus 532
— ツチ骨頸 Neck of malleus 532
— ツチ骨頭 Head of malleus 532
— ツチ骨柄 Handle of malleus 532, 534
ツチ骨条 Malleolar stria 532
ツチ骨隆起 Malleolar prominence 532
椎管 Vertebral canal 12, 20
椎間円板 Intervertebral disk 2-4, **12**, 20, 21, 44, 49, 129
— 髄核 Nucleus pulposus 12, 20
— 線維輪 Anulus fibrosus 12, 20
椎間関節 Zygapophyseal joint 6, 8, 9, **14**, 558
— 関節包 Capsule of zygapophyseal joint 16, 18
椎間孔 Intervertebral foramen 2, **8**, 9, 12, 601
椎間静脈 Intervertebral v. 35, 611
椎間面 Intervertebral surface 12
椎弓 Vertebral arch **5**, 6, 7, 9, 12
— 椎弓根 Pedicle of vertebral arch 5, 7, 8
— 椎弓板 Lamina of vertebral arch 5, 7, 8
椎孔 Vertebral foramen **5**, 7, 9, 12, 45
椎骨 Vertebra 5
— 下関節面 Inferior articular facet of vertebra 6-9
— 後関節面 Posterior articular facet of vertebra 6
— 上関節面 Superior articular facet of vertebra **5**, 6-9
— 前関節面 Anterior articular facet of vertebra 7
— 前結節 Anterior tubercle of vertebra 5, 7, 18
椎骨静脈 Vertebral v. 567, 601, 611
椎骨静脈叢 Vertebral venous plexus 35, 156, 604
椎骨動脈 Vertebral a. 34, 38, 56, 68, 316, 317, 490, 491, 556, **566**, 579, 601, 608, 610
椎骨動脈溝 Groove for vertebral a. **6**, 7, 16, 17
椎骨動脈神経叢 Vertebral plexus 75
椎前神経節 Prevertebral ganglion 622
椎前リンパ節 Prevertebral lymph node 100
椎体 Vertebral body 4-6, 8, 12, 45
椎体静脈 Basivertebral v. 611
椎傍神経節 Paravertebral ganglia 244
土踏まず Plantar vault 410
爪 Nail 305
蔓状静脈叢 Pampiniform plexus 196, 198, 199, **225**

て

テノン嚢（眼球鞘） Tenon's capsule（bulbar fascia） 514
テント切痕 Tentorial notch 603
底側骨間筋 Plantar interossei 414
— 第1底側骨間筋 1st plantar interosseus 414
— 第3底側骨間筋 3rd plantar interosseus 412-414, 419
底側趾静脈 Plantar digital vv. 422
底側踵舟靱帯 Plantar calcaneonavicular l. 406, **408**, 411, 414, 419
底側中足静脈 Plantar metatarsal vv. 422
底側中足動脈 Plantar metatarsal aa. **420**, 446, 447
転子窩 Trochanteric fossa 360
転子間線 Intertrochanteric line 360, 362, 365
転子間稜 Intertrochanteric crest 360, 362, 365
転子包 Trochanteric bursa 363, 439, 441
殿筋腱膜 Gluteal aponeurosis 22
殿筋粗面 Gluteal tuberosity 360, 362
殿筋膜 Gluteal fascia 438, 441
殿溝 Gluteal fold（sulcus） 41, 438, 451
殿部 Gluteal region 438
殿裂 Anal cleft 41, 136

と

ドッドの静脈群 Dodd's vv. 423
豆状骨 Pisiform 253, 299, 301, 350, 352, 353
島 Insula 595, 609, 619
透明中隔 Septum pellucidum 595, 605, 609
等皮質 Isocortex 595
頭蓋 Skull 454
頭蓋窩 Cranial fossa 459
頭蓋冠 Calvaria 457
— 外板 Outer table of clavaria 457, 602
— 硬膜 Dura mater of calvaria 457, 537, 601, **602**
— 内板 Inner table of clavaria 457, 602
— 板間層 Diploë of calvaria 457, 602
頭最長筋 Longissimus capitis 24, 25, 27, 30, **31**, 464, 465, 585
頭長筋 Longus capitis **29**, 465, 565
頭頂孔 Parietal foramen 457, 606
頭頂後頭溝 Parieto-occipital sulcus 595
頭頂骨 Parietal bone 454-456, **457**, 458, 523
頭頂導出静脈 Parietal emissary v. 497, 606
頭半棘筋 Semispinalis capitis 24-27, 32, **33**, 268, 269, 464, 465
頭板状筋 Splenius capitis 24-27, 30, **31**, 268, 269, 464, 465
頭皮 Scalp 457, 602
橈骨 Radius 252, 253, **280**, 309
— 外側面 Lateral surface of radius 280
— 関節窩 Articular fovea of radius 280, 281, 286
— 関節環状面 Articular circumference of radius 281, 287
— 茎状突起 Styloid process of radius 253, **280**, 281, 286, 287, 351, 352
— 後縁 Posterior border of radius 280
— 後面 Posterior surface of radius 280
— 骨間縁 Interosseous border of radius 280, **281**
— 尺骨切痕 Ulnar notch of radius 287
— 手根関節面 Carpal articular surface of radius 280, 281
— 前縁 Anterior border of radius 280, 281
— 橈骨頸 Neck of radius 280, 286
— 橈骨粗面 Radial tuberosity 278, 280, **281**
— 橈骨体 Shaft of radius 280
— 橈骨頭 Head of radius 252, 253, **281**, 282, 285, 351
— 橈骨頭の関節環状面 Aticular circumference of head of radius 280-282
— 背側結節 Dorsal tubercle of radius **280**, 281, 290, 291, 310
橈骨窩 →解剖学的嗅ぎタバコ入れ Anatomic（anatomical）snuffbox
橈骨手根関節 Radiocarpal joint 300, 301
橈骨静脈 Radial vv. 318
橈骨神経 Radial n. 320, **325**, 330, 331, 333, 337, 339-341, 346
— 運動枝 Motor branches of radial n. 337
— 筋枝 muscular branches of radial n. 333, 339, 341
— 深枝 Deep branch of radial n. 320, 339, 341
— 浅枝 Superficial branch of radial n. 320, 325, 330, 331, 339-341, 346
橈骨神経管 Radial tunnel 325, 339
橈骨切痕《尺骨の》 Radial notch of ulna 280, 281, 287
橈骨動脈 Radial a. **316**, 317, 339-342, 344, 345, 347
— 浅掌枝 Superficial palmar branch of radial a. 316, 342, 344, 345
— 背側手根枝 Dorsal carpal branch of radial a. 347
橈骨輪状靱帯 Annular l. of radius 284-287
橈尺関節 Radioulnar Joints 286
橈側手根屈筋 Flexor carpi radialis 288, **292**, 293, 306, 309, 350
橈側手根屈筋の腱 Flexor carpi radialis tendon 307, 308, 352
橈側手根隆起 Radial carpal eminence 303
橈側正中皮静脈 Median cephalic v. 318
橈側側副動脈 Radial collateral a. 316, 341
橈側反回動脈 Radial recurrent a. 316, 339
橈側皮静脈 Cephalic v. 57, 60, **318**, 330, 331, 334-336, 339, 350, 351
橈側リンパ管群 Radial group of lymphatics 319
橈側リンパ管束領域 Radial bundle territory 319
洞房結節 Sinoatrial（SA）node 90
動眼神経 Oculomotor n.（CN Ⅲ） 470, **474**, 475, 509, 511-513, 599, 608, 617
— 下枝 Inferior branch of oculomotor n. 475, 511, 512
— 上枝 Superior branch of oculomotor n. 475, 511, 512
動眼神経核 Nucleus of oculomotor n. 471, **474**, 617, 618
動眼神経副核（エディンガー-ウェストファル核） Visceral oculomotor（Edinger-Westphal）nuclei 471, **474**, 617
動脈円錐 Conus arteriosus 85
動脈円錐腱 Tendon of conus 86
動脈管索 Ligamentum arteriosum 77, 79, **83**, 84, 95, 115
動脈溝 Arterial groove 457, 459, 526
導出静脈 Emissary v. 457, 602
瞳孔 Pupil 519
瞳孔括約筋 Pupillary sphincter 518, 617
瞳孔散大筋 Pupillary dilator 518
特殊臓性遠心性線維 Special visceral efferent fiber 471

な

内陰部静脈　Internal pudendal v.　195, 202, 203, 216, 222, 223, **224**, 439
－ 右内陰部静脈　Right internal pudendal v.　216, 224
－ 左内陰部静脈　Left internal pudendal v.　223
内陰部動脈　Internal pudendal a.　195, 202, 203, 208, 222, 223, **224**, 439
－ 右内陰部動脈　Right internal pudendal a.　208
－ 左内陰部動脈　Left internal pudendal a.　223, 224
内果　Medial malleolus　380, 381
内果皮下包　Subcutaneous bursa of medial malleolus　443
内顆粒層　Internal granular layer（Ⅳ）　595
内胸静脈　Internal thoracic vv.　35, 55, **57**, 60-62, 66, 70, 77, 155, 156, 185, 215
内胸動脈　Internal thoracic a.　34, 54, 55, **56**, 60-62, 64, 68, 77, 99, 156, 316, 317
－ 貫通枝　Perforating branches of internal thoracic a.　62
－ 胸骨枝　Sternal branches of internal thoracic a.　34
－ 前肋間枝　Anterior intercostal branches of internal thoracic a.　34, 56
－ 内側乳腺枝　Medial mammary branches of internal thoracic a.　56, 62
内頸静脈　Internal jugular v.　23, 35, 57, 70, 71, 114, 335, **496**, 497, 500, 501, 556, 557, 567, 575, 578, 580, 581, 606, 611
－ 右内頸静脈　Right internal jugular v.　70, 119
－ 左内頸静脈　Left internal jugular v.　54, 70, 77, 114
内頸動脈　Internal carotid a.　34, 481, **490**, 491-493, 500, 501, 510, 524, 532, 556, 566, 580, 581, 608
－ 海綿静脈洞枝　Cavernous sinus branch of internal carotid a.　490
－ 海綿静脈洞部　Cavernous part of internal carotid a.　490
－ 頸部　Cervical part of internal carotid a.　490, **608**
－ 硬膜枝　Meningeal branch of internal carotid a.　490
－ 三叉神経枝　Neural branch of internal carotid a.　490
－ 三叉神経節枝　Trigeminal ganglion branch of internal carotid a.　490
－ 錐体部　Petrous part of internal carotid a.　490, **608**
－ 大脳部　Cerebral part of internal carotid a.　490, **608**
－ テント縁枝　Marginal tentorial branch of internal carotid a.　490
－ テント底枝　Basal tentorial branch of internal carotid a.　490
内頸動脈神経叢　Internal carotid plexus　75, 481, **483**, 505
内肛門括約筋　Internal anal sphincter　167
内後頭静脈　Internal occipital v.　606
内後頭隆起　Internal occipital protuberance　18
内子宮口　Internal os　189
内耳介動脈　Internal auditory a.　535
内耳孔　Internal acoustic opening　526
内耳神経　Vestibulocochlear n.（CN Ⅷ）　470, **480**, 481, 528, 598, 599
内耳道　Internal acoustic meatus　459

内錐体細胞層　Internal pyramidal layer（Ⅴ）　595
内生殖器　Internal genitalia　186
内精筋膜　Internal spermatic fascia　133, 196, 198, **199**, 225
内臓神経　Splanchnic nn.　600, 622
内側横膝蓋支帯　Medial transverse patellar retinaculum　384
内側下膝動脈　Medial inferior genicular a.　420, 421, **443**
内側顆《脛骨の》　Medial condyle of tibia　356, 357, 380-382, 450
内側顆《大腿骨の》　Medial condyle of femur　356, 360, 361, 382, 389
内側顆上線《大腿骨の》　Medial supracondylar line of femur　360
内側顆上稜《上腕骨の》　Medial supracondylar ridge of humerus　256, 257
内側眼瞼靱帯　Medial palpebral l.　515
内側眼瞼動脈　Medial palpebral a.　510
内側弓状靱帯　Medial arcuate l.　52, 53
内側嗅条　Medial olfactory stria　472, 620
内側胸筋神経　Medial pectoral n.　320, 321, **326**, 334-336
内側結合腕傍核　Medial parabrachial nucleus　619
内側楔状骨　Medial cuneiform　**400**, 401-403, 406, 410
内側広筋　Vastus medialis　366, 367, 369, **378**, 429, 440, 448, 450
内側後頭動脈（P4区）　Medial occipital a.（P4）　608, 609
内側鎖骨上神経　Medial supraclavicular nn.　582
内側臍索　Medial umbilical ll.　95
内側臍ヒダ　Medial umbilical（umbilicus）fold　135, 145, 148, 149, 152, 153
内側膝状体　Medial geniculate body　473, 617
内側膝状体核　Nucleus of medial geniculate body　619
内側手根側副靱帯　Ulnar carpal collateral l.　302
内側縦膝蓋支帯　Medial longitudinal patellar retinaculum　384
内側縦束　Medial longitudinal fasciculus（MLF）　618
内側上顆《上腕骨の》　Medial epicondyle of humerus　253, **256**, 257, 264, 339, 350
内側上顆《大腿骨の》　Medial epicondyle of femur　356, 357, **360**, 382, 451
内側上膝動脈　Medial superior genicular a.　420, 421, **443**
内側上腕筋間中隔　Medial intermuscular septum of arm　338
内側上腕皮神経　Medial brachial cutaneous n.　320, 321, **326**, 330, 331, 338
内側神経束　Medial cord　320, 321, **326**, 328, 329, 337, 338
内側髄板　Internal medullary lamina　597
内側仙骨稜　Medial sacral crest　10
内側前腕静脈　Medial antebrachial v.　339
内側前腕皮神経　Medial antebrachial cutaneous n.　**326**, 330, 331, 338, 339
内側鼠径窩　Medial inguinal fossa　135
内側足根動脈　Medial tarsal aa.　443
内側足底溝　Medial plantar sulcus　446
内側足底静脈　Medial plantar v.　422
内側足底神経　Medial plantar n.　424, 433, 443, **446**, 447
－ 浅枝　Superficial branch of medial plantar n.　446
内側足底中隔　Medial plantar septum　412

内側足底動脈　Medial plantar a.　420, 421, 443, 446, **447**
－ 深枝　Deep branch of medial plantar a.　420, 446, 447
－ 浅枝　Superficial branch of medial plantar a.　420, 443, 446
内側足背皮神経　Medial dorsal cutaneous n.　432, **434**, 444, 445
内側足放線　Medial rays　410
内側側副靱帯《膝関節の》　Medial collateral l. of knee joint　384-386, **388**
内側側副靱帯《肘関節の》　Ulnar collateral l. of elbow joint　**284**, 285, 286, 301
－ 横部　Transverse part of ulnar collateral l.　284
－ 後部　Posterior part of ulnar collateral l.　284
－ 前部　Anterior part of ulnar collateral l.　284
内側大腿回旋静脈　Medial circumflex femoral vv.　422
内側大腿回旋動脈　Medial circumflex femoral a.　**420**, 421, 440, 441
内側中葉区　Medial segment of lung　108
内側中葉動脈《右肺の》　Medial segmental a. of right lung　115
内側直筋　Medial rectus　475, **508**, 509, 516, 617
内側肺底区　Medial basal segment of lung　108
内側肺底動脈　Medial basal segmental a. of lung　115
内側半月　Medial meniscus　386, **387**, 388-390
内側腓腹皮神経　Medial sural cutaneous n.　**433**, 435, 442, 444
内側毛帯　Medial lemniscus　614
内側翼突筋　Medial pterygoid　463-465, **469**, 502, 553, 555, 556
－ 深頭　Deep head of medial pterygoid　468
－ 浅頭　Superficial head of medial pterygoid　468
内側翼突筋神経　Medial pterygoid n.　477, 488, 503, **546**
内側隆起《第四脳室底の》　Medial eminence of floor of 4th ventride　599
内側裂孔リンパ節　Medial lacunar lymph node　229
内大脳静脈　Internal cerebral v.　606, 607
内腸骨静脈　Internal iliac v.　**35**, 202, 216, 222-225, 611
－ 左内腸骨静脈　Left internal iliac v.　180, 225
－ 前枝　Anterior trunk of internal iliac v.　180
内腸骨動脈　Internal iliac a.　**34**, 202, 208, 222-225, 420
－ 右内腸骨動脈　Right internal iliac a.　208, 216, 223, 224
－ 左内腸骨動脈　Left internal iliac a.　180, 225
－ 前枝　Anterior trunk of internal iliac a.　180
内腸骨リンパ節　Internal iliac lymph node　**227**, 228, 229, 235
内転筋管　Adductor canal　420, 422
内転筋群　Adductor muscles　155
[内転筋]腱裂孔　Adductor hiatus　367, 377, 420-422, 441
内尿道口　Internal urethral orifice　155, 185
内皮様細胞層　Neurothelium　602
内腹斜筋　Internal oblique　22, 26, 27, 130, 131, 133, 138, **139**, 268, 269, 525
内腹斜筋腱膜　Internal oblique aponeurosis　**130**, 134, 139
内閉鎖筋　Obturator internus　136, 137, 140, 141, 152, 153, 155, 157, 369-372, 374, **375**, 438, 439, 448
内閉鎖筋筋膜　Obturator internus fascia　141

(ないへいさきんしんけい)

内閉鎖筋神経　Obturator internus n.　431
内包　Internal capsule　594, 609
　― 後脚　Posterior crus of internal capsule　594
　― 前脚　Anterior crus of internal capsule　594
内包膝　Genu of internal capsule　594
内有毛細胞　Inner hair cells　619
内リンパ管　Endolymphatic duct　536
内リンパ嚢　Endolymphatic sac　530, 536, 537
内肋間筋　Internal intercostals　50, **51**, 61, 130
内弯点　Inflection points　3
軟口蓋（口蓋帆）　Soft palate　524, 545, 550, **552**, 553
軟膜　Pia mater　602
軟膜血管叢　Pial vascular plexus　517

に

ニューロン　Neurons　592
Ⅱ型肺小葉上皮細胞　Type Ⅱ pneumocyte　111
二腹小葉前裂　Prebiventral fissure　598
二分靱帯　Bifurcate l.　406, **408**, 409
肉柱《心室中隔の》　Trabeculae carneae of interventricular septum　85
肉様膜　Tunica dartos　196, 198, **199**
乳腺　Mammary gland　63
　― 乳管　Lactiferous duct　63
　― 乳管洞　Lactiferous sinus　63
　― 乳腺小葉　Lobules of mammary gland　63
　― 乳腺葉　Mammary lobes　63
乳頭　Nipple　62, 63, 121
乳頭視床路　Mammillothalamic tract　621
乳頭体　Mammillary body　595, **596**, 598, 621
乳頭体視床束　Mammillothalamic fasciculus　597
乳突孔　Mastoid foramen　456, 458, **526**, 606
乳突切痕《側頭骨の》　Mastoid notch of temporal bone　458, 526
乳突洞　Mastoid antrum　534
乳突洞口　Aditus (inlet) to mastoid antrum　531
乳突導出静脈　Mastoid emissary v.　497, 606
乳突蜂巣　Mastoid cells (mastoid air cells)　481, 530, **531**, 547
乳突リンパ節　Mastoid lymph nodes　587
乳ビ槽　Cisterna chyli　72, **226**, 228
乳房　Breast　**62**, 63, 121
乳房提靱帯（クーパー靱帯）　Suspensory (Cooper's) ll. of breast　63
乳輪　Areola　62, 121
乳輪静脈叢　Areolar venous plexus　57
乳輪腺　Areolar glands　62
尿管　Ureter　142, 149-151, 157, 166, 177, 178, **180**, 181, 183-187, 216, 225
　― 骨盤部　Pelvic part of ureter　180
　― 腹部　Abdominal part of ureter　180
尿管間ヒダ　Interureteric fold　185
尿管口　Ureteral orifice　185-187
尿管神経叢　Ureteral plexus　**237**, 239, 242, 243, 246
尿生殖三角　Urogenital triangle　136
尿生殖洞　Urogenital sinus　205
尿道　Urethra　155, **184**, 185, 186, 190, 197, 200
　― 海綿体部　Spongy part of urethra　185, 187, 197, 200, 201
　― 隔膜部　Membranous part of urethra　155, 185, 197, 200
　― 縦走ヒダ　Longitudinal folds of urethra　185
　― 前立腺部　Prostatic (preprostatic) part of urethra　185, 197, 200
　― 膨大部　Urethral ampulla　185

尿道海綿体　Corpus spongiosum　184, 185, 187, **197**, 201, 203
尿道海綿体白膜　Tunica albuginea of corpus spongiosum　197
尿道括約筋　Sphincter urethrae　150, 152, 153
尿道球　Bulb of penis　155, **185**, 187, 197
尿道球静脈　Bulbar penile vv.　202, 222
尿道球腺　Bulbourethral gland　150, 184, 185, 187, 197, **200**, 201, 203, 205
尿道球動脈　Bulbar penile a.　202
尿道舟状窩　Navicular fossa of urethra　185, 197, 201
尿道腺　Urethral glands　185, 197
尿道動脈　Urethral a.　197, 202
尿道傍腺　Paraurethral gland　205
尿道稜　Urethral crest　197

の

脳　Brain　592
脳幹　Brainstem　599
脳弓　Fornix　595, **596**, 598, 605, 621
　― 脳弓脚　Crus of fornix　596
　― 脳弓体　Body of fornix　596
　― 脳弓柱　Column of fornix　596
脳弓ヒモ　Taenia of fornix　596
脳室　ventricle　605
脳神経　Cranial nn.　470, 592
脳神経核　Nucleus of cranial nerve　471
脳底静脈　Basilar v.　606, 607
脳底静脈叢　Basilar plexus　607
脳底槽　Basal cistern　604
脳底動脈　Basilar a.　490, **608**, 610
脳頭蓋　Neurocranium　454
脳梁　Corpus callosum　593-595, **596**, 598, 605, 609, 621
脳梁縁動脈　Callosomarginal a.　609
　― 帯状回枝　Cingular branch of callosomarginal a.　609
脳梁灰白層　Indusium griseum　596
脳梁周囲槽　Interhemispheric cistern　604
脳梁周囲動脈　Pericallosal a.　609
囊状陥凹《肘関節の》　Sacciform recess of elbow joint　284-286, 301

は

バルトリン腺　Bartholin's gland　186, 192
パイエル板　Peyer's patches　162
破裂孔　Foramen lacerum　458, 459
馬尾　Cauda equina　3, 430, 592, 600, **601**
背側距舟靱帯　Dorsal talonavicular l.　**408**, 409
背側骨間筋《足の》　Dorsal interossei of foot　411, 413
　― 第1背側骨間筋　1st dorsal interosseus of foot　414, 419
　― 第2背側骨間筋　2nd dorsal interosseus of foot　414
　― 第4背側骨間筋　4th dorsal interosseus of foot　412-414
背側骨間筋《手の》　Dorsal interossei of hand　309, 314, 315
　― 第1背側骨間筋　1st dorsal interosseous of hand　301, 307-310, 315, 352
　― 第2背側骨間筋　2nd dorsal interosseous of hand　308-311, 315
　― 第3背側骨間筋　3rd dorsal interosseus of hand　308-311, 315
　― 第4背側骨間筋　4th dorsal interosseus of hand　301, 308-310, 315

背側指静脈　Dorsal digital vv.　318, 331
背側指神経　Dorsal digital nn.　329, 331, 344, **346**
背側指動脈　Dorsal digital aa.　**317**, 344, 347
背側趾神経　Dorsal digital nn.　445
背側趾動脈　Dorsal digital aa.　445
背側手根間靱帯　Dorsal intercarpal ll.　302
背側手根腱鞘　Dorsal carpal tendon sheaths　310
背側手根中手靱帯　Dorsal carpometacarpal ll.　302
背側手根動脈　Dorsal carpal a.　317, 347
背側手根動脈網　Dorsal carpal network　317, 347
背側縦束　Dorsal longitudinal fasciculus　472
背側踵立方靱帯　Dorsal calcaneocuboid ll.　406, 409
背側足根靱帯　Dorsal tarsal ll.　408, 409
背側中手動脈　Dorsal metacarpal aa.　317, 347
背側中足靱帯　Dorsal metatarsal ll.　408
背側中足動脈　Dorsal metatarsal aa.　420, 445
背側橈骨尺骨靱帯　Dorsal radioulnar l.　286, 287, **302**
背側橈骨手根靱帯　Dorsal radiocarpal l.　302
肺　Lungs　104, **105**
　― 横隔面　Diaphragmatic surface of lung　105
　― 下縁　Inferior border of lung　105
　― 下葉　Inferior lobe of lung　105
　― 斜裂　Oblique fissure of lung　93, 104, 105, 109
　― 縦隔面　Mediastinal surface of lung　105
　― 小舌　Lingula of lung　105
　― 上葉　Superior lobe of lung　105
　― 水平裂　Horizontal fissure of lung　105
　― 前縁　Anterior border of lung　105
　― 中葉　Middle lobe of lung　105
　― 肺尖　Apex of lung　105
　― 肺底　Base of lung　105
　― 肋骨面　Costal surface of lung　105
肺間膜　Pulmonary l.　105
肺区域　Bronchopulmonary Segments　108
肺静脈　Pulmonary vv.　82, 114
肺神経叢　Pulmonary plexus　75, 91, 117
肺舌静脈　Lingular v.　115
肺舌動脈　Lingular a.　115
肺尖区　Apical segment of right lung　108
肺尖後静脈　Apicoposterior v. of upper lobe of right lung　115
肺尖静脈　Apical v. of upper lobe of right lung　115
肺尖動脈　Apical segmental a. of lung　115
肺動脈　Pulmonary aa.　114
肺動脈幹　Pulmonary trunk　68, 77, 83, 84, 87, 90, 91, 104, **114**, 115
肺動脈弁　Pulmonary valve　**86**, 87, 88
　― 右半月弁　Right cusp of pulmonary valve　86
　― 左半月弁　Left cusp of pulmonary valve　86
　― 前半月弁　Anterior cusp of pulmonary valve　86, 87
肺内リンパ節　Intrapulmonary lymph node　73, 118, **119**
肺胞　Alveolus (pulmonary alveolus)　111, 116
肺胞管　Alveolar duct　111
肺胞大食細胞　Alveolar macrophage　111
肺胞中隔　Interalveolar septum　111
肺胞嚢　Alveolar sac　111
肺門　Hilum of lung　105
排出管　Excretory duct　187
排尿筋　Detrusor vesicae　185
白質　White matter　592, 594, 613
白線　Linea alba　120, **130**, 131, 134, 139, 248, 436
白膜　Tunica albuginea　198, 199

薄筋　Gracilis　194, 203, 366, 367, 369-371, **376**, 438-442, 448
薄束核　Nucleus gracilis　614
薄束結節　Tubercle of nucleus gracilis　599
反回骨間動脈　Interosseous recurrent a.　317, 341
反回神経　Recurrent laryngeal n.　66, 74, 75, 77, 79, 91, 98, 117, **485**, 557, 575, 579
― 右反回神経　Right recurrent laryngeal n.　575
― 左反回神経　Left recurrent laryngeal n.　557, 575
― 食道枝　Esophageal branches of recurrent laryngeal n.　98, 99
反転靱帯　Reflex [inguinal] l.　436, 437
半奇静脈　Hemiazygos v.　35, 54, 55, 57, **70**, 71, 79, 99, 117, 214, 215, 611
半規管　Semicircular ducts　481, 537
― 総脚　Common crus of semicircular ducts　537
半棘筋　Semispinalis　**32**, 560
半月回　Semilunar gyrus　472, 620
半月線　Semilunar line　120, **131**, 248
半月弁結節　Nodule of semilunar cusps　87
半月弁半月《大動脈弁の》　Lunules of semilunar cusps of aortic valve　87
半月弁半月《肺動脈弁の》　Lunules of semilunar cusps of pulmonary valve　87
半月ヒダ　Semilunar folds　164
半腱様筋　Semitendinosus　369, 370, **379**, 438, 439, 441, 442, 448, 451
半側視野　Visual hemifield　616
半膜様筋　Semimembranosus　369-371, **379**, 394, 438, 441, 442, 448, 451
板間静脈　Diploic vv.　457, 602
板間層　Diploë of calvaria　457, 602
板状筋　Splenius muscles　30, 31, **560**

【ひ】

ヒス束　Bundle of His　90
ヒラメ筋　Soleus　392, 394, **398**, 442, 445, 448
ヒラメ筋［の］腱弓　Tendinous arch of soleus　398, 442
ヒラメ筋線　Soleal line of tibia　380, 382
皮下静脈叢　Subcutaneous venous plexus　167
皮質延髄線維　Corticobulbar fibers　486
皮質縁　Cortical margin　609
皮質核線維　Corticonuclear fibers　615
皮質脊髄線維　Corticospinal fibers　615
皮質脊髄路（錐体路）　Corticospinal (pyramidal) tract　615
皮静脈　Cutaneous v.　57
披裂筋　Arytenoid　557
披裂喉頭蓋ヒダ　Aryepiglottic fold　553, 572, **573**
披裂軟骨　Arytenoid cartilage　570, 571
― 関節面　Articular facet of arytenoid cartilage　570
― 筋突起　Muscular process of arytenoid cartilage　570, 571
― 後面　Posterior surface of arytenoid cartilage　570
― 小丘　Colliculus of arytenoid cartilage　570, 571
― 声帯突起　Vocal process of arytenoid cartilage　570, 571
― 前外側面　Anterolateral surface of arytenoid cartilage　570
― 内側面　Medial surface of arytenoid cartilage　570
― 披裂軟骨尖　Apex of arytenoid cartilage　570

被蓋核　Tegmental nucleus　472, 615
被殻　Putamen　594, 609
脾静脈　Splenic v.　143, **174**, 175, 179, 211, 215, 218-221
脾神経叢　Splenic plexus　238, 240, 245
脾臓　Spleen　142, 146-148, 156, 159, 161, 168, 173, **174**, 210, 218
― 胃面　Gastric surface of spleen　148, 175
― 上縁　Superior border of spleen　148, 174, 175
― 前端　Anterior extremity of spleen　174
脾動脈　Splenic a.　55, 143, 147, 173, **174**, 175, 177, 179, 207, 210-212, 218-221
― 膵枝　Pancreatic branches of splenic a.　207
脾門　Hilum of spleen　174
脾リンパ節　Splenic lymph node　230, 231
腓骨　Fibula　356, **380**, 381, 404, 405, 415, 448
― 外果　Lateral malleolus　356, 357, **380**, 381, 394, 404, 405, 442, 444, 450
― 外果窩　Lateral malleolar fossa of fibula　380, 381
― 外果関節面　Articular surface of lateral malleolus of fibula　381
― 外側面　Lateral surface of fibula　380
― 後面　Posterior surface of fibula　380
― 内側面　Medial surface of fibula　380
― 腓骨頚　Neck of fibula　380, 382
― 腓骨体　Shaft of fibula　380
― 腓骨頭　Head of fibula　356, 357, **380**, 381, 382, 393, 451
腓骨静脈　Fibular vv.　422
腓骨動脈　Fibular a.　**420**, 421, 442, 445
― 外果枝　Lateral malleolar branches of fibular a.　421
― 貫通枝　Perforating branch of fibular a.　421, 442
― 筋枝　Muscular branches of fibular a.　421
― 交通枝　Communicating branch of fibular a.　421
― 踵骨枝　Calcaneal branches of fibular a.　421
腓腹筋　Gastrocnemius　392, 394, **398**, 442, 448, 450, 451
― 外側腱下包　Lateral subtendinous bursa of gastrocnemius　385
― 外側頭　Lateral head of gastrocnemius　370, 371, 393, 394, 398, 442
― 内側腱下包　Medial subtendinous bursa of gastrocnemius　385
― 内側頭　Medial head of gastrocnemius　370, 371, 392, 394, 398, 442
腓腹神経　Sural n.　424, 433-435, **442**, 444
― 外側踵骨枝　Lateral calcaneal branches of sural n.　433, 444
腓腹動脈　Sural aa.　421
尾骨　Coccyx　2, 3, 4, **10**, 11, 126, 127, 129, 136, 137, 141, 157, 166
― 尾骨角　Coccygeal cornu　10
尾骨筋　Coccygeus　140, 141
尾骨神経　Coccygeal n.　425
― 筋枝　Muscular branches of Coccygeal n.　425
尾骨神経叢　Coccygeal plexus　425
尾状核　Caudate nucleus　594, 609
― 尾状核頭　Head of caudate nucleus　594
― 尾状核尾　Tail of caudate nucleus　594
尾状突起《肝臓の》　Caudate process of liver　171
尾状葉《肝臓の》　Caudate lobe of liver　146, 170, 171
尾側性腺靱帯（導帯）　Caudal gonadal l. (gubernaculum)　205

眉間　Glabella　454, 520
鼻筋　Nasalis　462-464, **466**
― 横部　Transverse part of nasalis　464
― 翼部　Alar part of nasalis　464
鼻腔　Nasal cavity　520, 522
鼻限　Limen nasi　525
鼻口蓋神経　Nasopalatine n.　**524**, 525, 546
鼻甲介　Nasal conchae　552
鼻骨　Nasal bone　454, 455, 506, **520**
鼻根筋　Procerus　462, 466
鼻根点　Nasion　455
鼻前庭　Nasal vestibule　525
鼻中隔　Nasal septum　522, **524**, 553
鼻中隔下制筋　Depressor septi nasi　464
鼻背静脈　Dorsal nasal v.　510, 512
鼻背動脈　Dorsal nasal a.　490, 492, 498, **510**, 512
鼻毛様体神経　Nasociliary n.　477, **511**, 513
鼻毛様体神経根　Nasociliary root　477, 511
鼻稜　Nasal crest　520, 538
鼻涙管　Nasolacrimal duct　**515**, 522
［左-］　→［さ-］の項をみよ
表情筋　Muscles of facial expression　462
表面活性物質（サーファクタント）　Surfactant　111

【ふ】

ファロービウス管　Fallopian tube　151
プチ三角（下腰三角）　Iliolumbar triangle of Petit　39
プテリオン（蝶前頭縫合）　Pterion (sphenofrontal suture)　454
プルキンエ線維　Purkinje's fibers　90
不対神経節　Ganglion impar　236, 237
付属生殖腺　Accessory sex glands　200
浮遊肋　Floating ribs　45
伏在神経　Saphenous n.　424, 425, **429**, 434, 435, 440, 442
― 膝蓋下枝　Infrapatellar branch of saphenous n.　429, 434
― 内側下腿皮枝　Medial cutaneous branches of saphenous n.　429
伏在裂孔　Saphenous hiatus　225, 436
副楔状束核　Accessory nucleus cuneatus　614
副甲状腺（上皮小体）　Parathyroid glands　574
副交感神経系　Parasympathetic nervous system　75, 244
副交感神経根　Parasympathetic root　511
副交感神経節　Parasympathetic ganglia　623
副耳下腺　Accessory parotid gland　551
副神経　Accessory n. (CN XI)　470, **486**, 501, 556, 579-584, 599
― 外枝　External branch of accessory n.　580, 581, 583
副神経脊髄核　Spinal nucleus of accessory n.　471, 486
副腎　Suprarenal gland　142, 147, 149, 156, 161, 175, **176**, 177-180
― 上縁　Superior border of suprarenal gland　176
― 腎面　Renal surface of suprarenal gland　176
― 髄質　Medulla of suprarenal gland　176
― 線維被膜　Fibrous capsule of suprarenal gland　176
― 前面　Anterior surface of suprarenal gland　176
― 中心静脈　Central v. of suprarenal gland　176
― 内側縁　Medial border of suprarenal gland　176
― 皮質　Cortex of suprarenal gland　176
副腎圧痕《肝臓の》　Suprarenal impression of liver　170

(ふくじんじょうみゃく)

副腎静脈　Suprarenal v.　178
副腎神経叢　Suprarenal plexus　236, **237**, 239
副膵管　Accessory pancreatic duct　160, 172, 174
副側副靱帯　Accessory collateral l.　304
副橈側皮静脈　Accessory cephalic v.　318, 331
副突起　Accessory process　5, 9
副半奇静脈　Accessory hemiazygos v.　35, 57, **70**, 71, 79, 99, 117, 611
副鼻腔　Paranasal air sinuses　522
副伏在静脈　Accessory saphenous v.　422, 434
腹横筋　Transversus abdominis　27, 52, 131, 133-135, **138**, 139
腹横筋腱膜　Aponeurosis of transversus abdominis (transversus abdominis aponeurosis)　131, **134**, 139
腹腔神経節　Celiac ganglia　240, 245
腹腔神経叢　Celiac plexus　236
腹腔動脈　Celiac trunk　54, 55, 143, 147, 178, 206-208, **210**, 211, 216-219
腹腔リンパ節　Celiac lymph node　100, **226**, 228, 230-232
腹大動脈　Abdominal aorta　23, 34, 55, 56, 143, 146, 149, 156, 175, 180, 206, 207, **208**, 210, 213
腹直筋　Rectus abdominis　55, 120, 130, 131, 133, 134, 138, **139**, 143, 150-153, 157, 182, 183, 248
腹直筋鞘　Rectus sheath　**134**, 139, 264
　─ 弓状線　Arcuate line of rectus sheath　131, 134, 135, 139
　─ 後葉　Posterior layer or rectus sheath　134
　─ 前葉　Anterior layer of rectus sheath　134
腹膜　Peritoneum　142, 143, 154
腹膜下隙　Subperitoneal space　154
腹膜腔　Peritoneal cavity　142, 143, **144**, 148, 154, 176
腹膜後域　Retroperitoneum　176
腹膜後隙　Retroperitoneal space　152, 153
腹膜垂　Epiploic appendices　144, **145**, 162, 164
噴門　Cardia　158, 159
噴門口　Cardiac orifice　146, 148, 149
噴門リンパ輪　Cardiac lymphatic ring　101, 230
分界溝　Sulcus terminalis　548
分界条　Stria terminalis　620
分界線　Linea terminalis　127, 129
分界稜　Crista terminalis　85
分子層　Molecular layer (I)　595

へ

ヘッセルバッハ三角　Hesselbach's triangle　133
ペルリア核　Perlia's nucleus　617
閉鎖管　Obturator canal　141, 157
閉鎖筋膜　Obturator fascia　136, 137, 141, 152
閉鎖孔　Obturator foramen　**124**, 125, 126, 141, 358, 359
閉鎖静脈　Obturator vv.　135, 157, 216, **222**, 223-225
閉鎖神経　Obturator n.　135, 157, 242, 243, 424, 425, **428**, 434, 435, 440
　─ 筋枝　Muscular branches of obturator n.　428
　─ 後枝　Posterior branch of obturator n.　425, 428
　─ 前枝　Anterior branch of obturator n.　425, 428
　─ 皮枝　Cutaneous branch of obturator n.　428, 435, 440
閉鎖動脈　Obturator a.　135, 157, 208, **222**, 223-225, 421
閉鎖膜　Obturator membrane　128, 129, 364

閉鎖リンパ節　Obturator lymph node　235
壁側胸膜　Parietal pleura　103
　─ 横隔部(横隔胸膜)　Diaphragmatic part of parietal pleura　54, 55, 66, 77, 97, **103**, 104, 134
　─ 頸部　Cervical part of parietal pleura　77
　─ 縦隔部(縦隔胸膜)　Mediastinal part of parietal pleura　54, 55, 66, 77, 80, 83, 97, **103**
　─ 肋骨部(肋骨胸膜)　Costal part of parietal pleura　55, 61, 66, 78, 79, **103**, 104
壁側骨盤筋膜　Parietal pelvic fascia　154
壁側腹膜　Parietal peritoneum　23, 103, **134**, 135, 143-145, 149-153, 159, 161, 166, 167, 176, 181-184
片葉　Flocculus　598
片葉脚　Peduncle of flocculus　598
片葉小節葉　Flocculonodular lobe　598
辺縁静脈洞　Marginal sinus　607
扁桃　Tonsils　552
扁桃窩　Tonsillar fossa　552
扁桃体　Amygdala　472, 594, **620**

ほ

ボイドの静脈群　Boyd's vv.　423
ボクダレク三角(腰肋三角)　Bochdalek's triangle (lumbocostal triangle)　52, 53
補助運動野　Supplementary motor cortex　613, 615
母指球　Thenar eminence　350, 352, 353
母指線　Thenar crease　353
母指対立筋　Opponens pollicis　301, 306-309, **312**, 313
母指内転筋　Adductor pollicis　306, 308, 309, 312, **313**
　─ 横頭　Transverse head of adductor pollicis　307, 308, 313
　─ 斜頭　Oblique head of adductor pollicis　307, 308, 313
母趾外転筋　Abductor hallucis　402, 404, 411-414, **417**, 420, 443, 446, 447
母趾内転筋　Adductor hallucis　411, 413, 418, **419**, 447
　─ 横頭　Transverse head of adductor hallucis　410, 413, 419, 447
　─ 斜頭　Oblique head of adductor hallucis　410, 413, 414, 419, 447
方形回内筋　Pronator quadratus　288, 289, 292, **293**, 306
方形葉《肝臓の》　Quadrate lobe of liver　171
包皮　Prepuce　201
放線冠　Corona radiata　594
放線状胸肋靱帯　Radiate sternocostal ll.　49, 51
放線状肋骨頭靱帯　Radiate l. of head of rib　49
胞状垂《卵巣上体の》　Vesicular appendices of epoöphoron　189
縫工筋　Sartorius　248, 366, 367, 369, 373, **378**, 440, 448
房室結節　Atrioventricular (AV) node　90
房室束　Atrioventricular bundle　90
　─ 右脚　Right bundle branch of atrioventricular bundle　90
　─ 左脚　Left bundle branch of atrioventricular bundle　90
傍正中橋網様体　Paramedian pontine reticular formation (PPRF)　618
帽状腱膜　Galea aponeurotica　462, 463, 602

膀胱　Urinary bladder　142, 143, 150-153, 155, 157, 180, 182, 183, **184**, 185-187, 190, 197, 225, 235
　─ 外膜　Adventitia of urinary bladder　185
　─ 筋層　Muscularis of urinary bladder　185
　─ 粘膜　Mucosa of urinary bladder　185
　─ 粘膜下組織　Submucosa of urinary bladder　185
　─ 膀胱頸　Neck of bladder　185, 200, 201
　─ 膀胱垂　Uvula of bladder　185
　─ 膀胱尖　Apex of bladder　181, 201
　─ 膀胱体　Body of (urinary) bladder　181, 185, 201
　─ 膀胱底　Fundus of bladder　201
膀胱三角　Bladder trigone　185
膀胱子宮窩　Vesicouterine pouch　151, 152, **181**, 183, 184, 188, 190
膀胱上窩　Supravesical fossa　135, 152, 183
膀胱静脈　Vesical vv.　222, 225
膀胱静脈叢　Vesical venous plexus　**202**, 216, 222
膀胱神経叢　Vesical plexus　239, **242**, 243, 246, 247
膀胱前立腺静脈叢　Vesicoprostatic venous plexus　157
膀胱腟中隔　Vesicovaginal septum　190
膀胱傍陥凹　Paravesical fossa　152, 155, 183
膀胱傍結合組織　Paravesicular fascia　153
膨大部稜　Ampullary crests　618

ま

マイヤーのループ　Meyer's loop　473, 616
膜性壁《気管の》　Membranous wall of trachea　573
膜迷路　Membranous labyrinth　537
末節骨《足の》　Distal phalanges of foot　397
　─ 第1末節骨　1st distal phalanx of foot　400, **401**, 402
　─ 第5末節骨　5th distal phalanx of foot　400, **401**
末節骨《手の》　Distal phalanx of hand　**298**, 300, 301, 305, 311
　─ 第1末節骨　1st distal phalanx of hand　253, 300
　─ 第2末節骨　2nd distal phalanx of hand　298
　─ 第4末節骨　4th distal phalanx of hand　252
　─ 末節骨粗面　Tuberosity of distal phalanx of hand　299, 300, 305

み む め も

ミエリン鞘(髄鞘)　Myelin sheath　592
ミハエリス菱形窩　Michaelis' rhomboid　41
ミュラー管　Müllerian (paramesonephric) duct　205
「右-」→「う-」の項をみよ
脈絡叢　Choroid plexus　596, 598
脈絡膜　Choroid　516, 519
無漿膜野《肝臓の》　Bare area of liver　170, 171
迷走神経　Vagus n. (CN X)　23, 66, 74, 75, 77-79, 91, 98, 244, 470, 482, **484**, 485, 549, 556, 579-581, 599, 619, 622
　─ 咽頭枝　Pharyngeal branch of vagus n.　482, 484, 485
　─ 頸心臓枝　Cervical cardiac branches of vagus n.　485
　─ 硬膜枝　Meningeal branches of vagus n.　603
迷走神経三角　Trigone of CN X　599
迷走神経背側核　Dorsal vagal nucleus　471, **484**, 619

迷路動脈　Labyrinthine a.　608
毛様体　Ciliary body　514, 516, 518, **519**
　— 皺襞部　Pars plicata of ciliary body　519
　— 平滑部　Pars plana of ciliary body　519
毛様体筋　Ciliary muscle　516, 518, **519**, 617
毛様体色素上皮　Pigment epithelium of ciliary body　516
毛様体神経節　Ciliary ganglion　475, 477, **511**, 513, 617
毛様体突起　Ciliary processes　519
盲腸　Cecum　142, 145, 148, 152, 153, 162, **164**, 165, 182, 183
盲腸静脈　Cecal vv.　220, 221
盲腸前リンパ節　Prececal lymph node　233
盲点　Blind spot　616
網嚢　Omental bursa (lesser sac)　**146**, 156, 175
　— 下陥凹　Inferior recess of omental bursa　146
　— 脾陥凹　Splenic recess of omental bursa　146
網嚢孔　Omental foramen　143, 148, 168
網嚢前庭　Vestibule of omental bursa　146, 147
網膜　Retina　514, 516
網膜視部　Optical part of retina　519
網膜中心静脈　Central retinal v.　517
網膜中心動脈　Central retinal a.　**510**, 516, 517
網様体　Reticular formation　472, 616
網様体脊髄路　Reticulospinal tract　618

ゆ よ

有鈎骨　Hamate　298, 301
有鈎骨鈎　Hook of hamate　299, 350, 352
有郭乳頭　Circum (vallate) papilla　548
有線野　Striate area　473, 616
有頭骨　Capitate　253, **298**, 299-301, 351, 352
幽門下リンパ節　Subpyloric lymph node　230, 231
幽門括約筋　Pyloric sphincter　160
幽門管　Pyloric canal　158, 159
幽門口　Pyloric orifice　158, 160
幽門後リンパ節　Retropyloric lymph node　231
幽門上リンパ節　Suprapyloric lymph node　230, 231
幽門洞　Pyloric antrum　158, 159
葉間静脈　Interlobar v.　179
葉間動脈　Interlobar a.　179, 209
腰外側横突間筋　Intertransversarii laterales lumborum　27, 32, **33**
腰棘間筋　Interspinales lumborum　27, 32, **33**
腰筋筋膜　Psoas fascia　23
腰三角　Lumbar triangle　22
腰静脈　Lumbar v.　35, 71, 214, 216
　— 第1腰静脈　1st lumbar v.　57
腰神経　Lumbar nn.　242, 243
　— 前枝　Anterior rami of lumbar nn.　242, 243
腰神経節　Lumbar ganglia　**237**, 239, 242, 243
腰神経叢　Lumbar plexus　425
腰仙骨神経幹　Lumbosacral trunk　**242**, 243, 425
腰仙椎境界　Lumbosacral junction　2
腰腸肋筋　Iliocostalis lumborum　27, 30, **31**
腰椎　Lumbar vertebrae [L1-L5]　2, 4, **9**
　— 第1腰椎　L1 vertebra　4
　— 第2腰椎　L2 vertebra　600, 601
　— 第4腰椎　L4 vertebra　9
　— 第5腰椎　L5 vertebra　150, 151, 364, 365, 600
　— 乳頭突起　Mammillary process of lumber vertebrae　9
腰動脈　Lumbar aa.　208, 610
　— 第2腰動脈　2nd lumbar aa.　56
　— 第3腰動脈　3rd lumbar aa.　56

腰内臓神経　Lumbar splanchnic nn.　**242**, 243-247
腰内側横突間筋　Intertransversarii mediales lumborum　27, 32, **33**
腰方形筋　Quadratus lumborum　23, 27, 52, 138, **139**
腰膨大　Lumbosacral enlargement　600
腰リンパ節　Lumbar lymph node　226
腰肋三角（ボクダレク三角）　Lumbocostal triangle (Bochdalek's triangle)　52, 53
翼棘靱帯　Pterygospinous l.　540
翼口蓋窩　Pterygopalatine fossa　504, 506
翼口蓋神経節　Pterygopalatine ganglion　477-479, 489, **505**, 525, 546
翼状靱帯　Alar ll.　17
翼状突起　Pterygoid process of sphenoid bone　456, 458, **461**, 521, 538
　— 外側板　Lateral plate of pterygoid process　458, 461, 538
　— 内側板　Medial plate of pterygoid process　458, 461, 538
翼状ヒダ　Alar folds　390
翼突窩　Pterygoid fossa　461, 538
翼突管　Pterygoid canal　538
翼突管神経　Nerve of pterygoid canal　479, 505
翼突管動脈　A. of pterygoid canal　490, 504
翼突筋窩　Pterygoid fovea　539, 540
翼突筋静脈叢　Pterygoid plexus　496, **497**, 567
翼突鈎　Pterygoid hamulus　461, 545

ら

ラセン神経節　Spiral ganglion　**480**, 481, 536, 537, 619
ラムダ縫合　Lambdoid suture　454, **456**, 457
卵円窩　Fossa ovalis　85
卵円窩縁　Limbus of fossa ovalis　85
卵円孔　Foramen ovale　**458**, 459, 461, 477, 503, 538
卵円孔静脈叢　Venous plexus of foramen ovale　607
卵円孔弁　Valve of foramen ovale　85
卵管　Uterine tube　152, 155, 181, 183, 184, 186, 188, **189**, 191, 205, 225, 235
　— 子宮部　Uterine part of uterine tube　189
　— 卵管峡部　Isthmus of uterine tube　189
　— 卵管子宮口　Uterine ostium of uterine tube　189
卵管間膜　Mesosalpinx　188, 189
卵管膨大部　Ampulla of uterine tube　189
卵管漏斗　Infundibulum of uterine tube　189
卵形核　Oval nucleus　619
卵形嚢　Utricle　536, 618
卵形嚢神経　Utricular n.　536, 537
卵形嚢膨大部神経　Utriculoampullary n.　481
卵巣　Ovary　151, 152, 155, 181, 183, 186, **188**, 189, 191, 205, 225, 235
　— 血管極　Vascular pole of ovary　188, 189
　— 自由縁　Free margin of ovary　188
　— 内側面　Medial surface of ovary　188
卵巣間膜　Mesovarium　188
卵巣上体　Epoöphoron　189, 205
　— 胞状垂　Vesicular appendices　189
卵巣静脈　Ovarian v.　179, 188, 189, **223**
卵巣提索　Suspensory l. of the ovary　155
卵巣提靱帯　Ovarian suspensory l.　151, 152, **183**, 184, 186, 205
卵巣動脈　Ovarian a.　188, 189, 208, **223**
卵巣動脈神経叢　Ovarian plexus　**236**, 237, 240, 242, 247

卵胞口　Follicular stigm　188

り

リスフラン関節線　Lisfranc's joint line　402
リンパ管　Lymphatic vessel　72
リンパ小節　Lymphatic follicles　162
リンパ節　Lymph node　73
梨状陥凹　Piriform recess　553, 573
梨状筋　Piriformis　140, **141**, 222, 366, 367, 369-371, 375, 420, 438, 439, 441, 448
梨状筋神経　Piriformis n.　431
梨状口　Piriform (anterior nasal) aperture　455, 521
梨状前野　Prepiriform area　472, 620
立方骨　Cuboid　**400**, 402, 403, 406, 410
　— 立方骨粗面　Tuberosity of cuboid　**401**, 417
立方骨関節面《踵骨の》　Cuboid articular surface of calaneus　407
隆椎（第7頸椎）　Vertebra prominens (C7)　4, 6, 40, 558, 600
菱形窩　Rhomboid fossa　599
菱形靱帯　Trapezoid l.　259
輪気管靱帯　Cricotracheal l.　571
輪状甲状関節　Cricothyroid joint　571
輪状甲状筋　Cricothyroid　485, 554, **572**, 574, 578, 579
　— 斜部　Oblique part of cricothyroid　572
　— 直部　Straight part of cricothyroid　572
輪状甲状靱帯　Cricothyroid l.　571, 574
輪状骨端　Epiphyseal ring　12
輪状靱帯　Annular l.　110
輪状軟骨　Cricoid cartilage　96, 110, 550, 558, **570**, 571
　— 甲状関節面　Articular facet for thyroid cartilage　570
　— 披裂関節面　Articular facet for arytenoid cartilage　570
　— 輪状軟骨弓　Arch of cricoid cartilage　570, 571
　— 輪状軟骨板　Lamina of cricoid cartilage　570, 571
輪状披裂関節　Cricoarytenoid joint　571
輪状披裂靱帯　Cricoarytenoid l.　571
輪状ヒダ　Circular folds　160, 162
鱗状縫合　Squamous suture　454

る れ ろ

涙器　Lacrimal apparatus　515
涙丘　Lacrimal caruncle　515
涙骨　Lacrimal bone　454, 506, 521
涙腺　Lacrimal gland　475, **515**
　— 眼窩部　Orbital part of lacrimal gland　515
　— 眼瞼部　Palpebral part of lacrimal gland　515
涙腺静脈　Lacrimal v.　510
涙腺神経　Lacrimal n.　475, 477, **511**, 512, 513
涙腺動脈　Lacrimal a.　510, 513
涙点　Lacrimal punetun　515
涙嚢　Lacrimal sac　515
涙嚢窩　Fossa of lacrimal sac　506
裂孔靱帯　Lacunar l.　132, 133, **436**, 437
ローゼンミュラーのリンパ節　Rosenmüller's lymph node　436
漏斗　Infundibulum of hypophysis　596, 598, 605
漏斗陥凹　Infundibular recess　596, 605
肋横突関節　Costotransverse joint　44, 49
肋横突靱帯　Costotransverse l.　49
肋下筋　Subcostal muscles　51
肋下静脈　Subcostal v.　35, 57, 611

(ろくかしんけい)

肋下神経　Subcostal n.　36，**58**，176，179，425
肋下動脈　Subcostal a.　34
肋間筋　Intercostal muscles　50
肋間上腕神経　Intercostobrachial nn.　**36**，58，321，326，330，331
肋間静脈　(Posterior) intercostal vv.　35，54，**57**，60，61，70，71，99，156，611
― 外側皮枝　Lateral cutaneous branches of posterior intercostal vv.　39
肋間神経　Intercostal nn.　36，37，39，55，**58**，60-62，74，78，79，98，156，330
― 外側乳腺枝　Lateral mammary branches of intercostal nn.　62
― 外側皮枝　Lateral cutaneous branch of intercostal nn.　37，58，61，330
― 胸骨枝　Sternal branches of intercostal nn.　58
― 後枝　Posterior ramus of intercostal nn.　61，326
― 前枝　Anterior (ventral) rami of intercostal nn.　61
― 前皮枝　Anterior cutaneous branch of intercostal nn.　58，61，330
― 側副枝　Collateral branch of intercostal nn.　61
― 第1肋間神経　1st intercostal nn.　58
― 第2肋間神経　2nd intercostal nn.　58
― 第2肋間神経の前皮枝　Anterior cutaneous branch of 2nd intercostal nn.　326
― 第3肋間神経　3rd intercostal nn.　58
― 第4肋間神経　4th intercostal nn.　58
― 第4肋間神経の外側皮枝　Lateral cutaneous branch of 4th intercostal nn.　326
― 内側乳腺枝　Medial mammary branches of intercostal nn.　62

肋間動脈　Posterior intercostal aa.　34，39，**56**，61，68，77，98，99，610
― 外側皮枝　Lateral cutaneous branch of posterior intercostal aa.　39，**56**，610
― 後枝　Posterior (dorsal) ramus of posterior intercostal aa.　56，61
― 脊髄枝　Spinal branch of posterior intercostal aa.　56，610
― 側副枝　Collateral branch of posterior intercostal aa.　56
― 第1肋間動脈　1st posterior intercostal a.　34
― 第2肋間動脈　2nd posterior intercostal a.　34
― 内側皮枝　Medial cutaneous branch of posterior intercostal aa.　56，610
肋間リンパ管　Intercostal lymphatics　72，100
肋間リンパ節　Intercostal lymph node　73，118
肋頸動脈　Costocervical trunk　34，317
肋剣靱帯　Costoxiphoid l.　49
肋骨　Rib　45，**47**
― 第1肋骨　1st rib　44，47，263
― 第2肋骨　2nd rib　47
― 第5肋骨　5th rib　47
― 第6肋骨　6th rib　45
― 肋骨角　Costal angle of rib　44，45，47
― 肋骨頸　Neck of rib　45，47
― 肋骨頸稜　Crest of neck of rib　47
― 肋骨結節　Costal tubercle　44，45，47，49
― 肋骨体　Body (shaft) of rib　45，47
― 肋骨頭　Head of rib　45，47
肋骨横隔洞　Costodiaphragmatic recess　103，104
肋骨下平面　Subcostal plane　120
肋骨窩　Costal facet　2，5
肋骨弓　Costal margin (arch)　44，265

肋骨挙筋　Levatores costarum　27，32
肋骨胸膜　→壁側胸膜の肋骨部　Costal part of parietal pleura
肋骨結節　Costal tubercle　44，45，47，49
肋骨溝　Costal groove　61
肋骨縦隔洞　Costomediastinal recess　93
肋骨切痕　Costal notch　46
肋骨頭関節　Joint of head of rib　49
肋骨突起　Costal process　5，9
肋鎖靱帯　Costoclavicular l.　259
肋鎖靱帯圧痕　Impression for costoclavicular l.　254
肋椎関節　Costovertebral joints　49
肋軟骨　Costal cartilage　**44**，45，49，130，259，265

わ

Y軟骨　Triradiate cartilage　125，359
腕尺関節　Humeroulnar joint　282，283
腕神経叢　Brachial plexus　23，66，77，91，320，**321**，326，335，579，581，583
腕頭静脈　Brachiocephalic v.　35，57，**70**，71，77，78，83，99，114
腕頭動脈　Brachiocephalic trunk　34，68，78，83，84，**316**，557
腕頭リンパ節　Brachiocephalic lymph node　78，100
腕橈関節　Humeroradial joint　282
腕橈骨筋　Brachioradialis　270，288，290，291，294，**295**，310，350
― 停止腱　Tendon of insertion of brachioradialis　295